# Fundamental and Advanced

# Fetal Imaging

## Ultrasound and MRI

# Fundamental and Advanced
# Fetal Imaging
## Ultrasound and MRI

EDITORS

**Beth M. Kline-Fath, MD**

Chief of Fetal and Neonatal Imaging
Associate Professor of Radiology
Department of Radiology
Cincinnati Children's Hospital Medical Center
Cincinnati, Ohio

**Dorothy I. Bulas, MD**

Program Director for Fetal Imaging
Fetal and Transitional Medicine
Vice Chief of Academic Affairs
Division of Diagnostic Imaging and Radiology
Children's National Health System
Professor of Pediatrics and Radiology
George Washington University
Washington, DC

**Ray Bahado-Singh, MD, MBA**

Professor of Obstetrics and Gynecology
Oakland University William Beaumont School
    of Medicine
Rochester Michigan
Health System Chair, Department Obstetrics
    and Gynecology
William Beaumont Health System
Royal Oak, Michigan

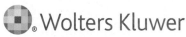
Health

Philadelphia • Baltimore • New York • London
Buenos Aires • Hong Kong • Sydney • Tokyo

*Acquisitions Editor:* Ryan Shaw
*Product Development Editor:* Amy G. Dinkel
*Production Project Manager:* David Salztberg
*Design Coordinator:* Stephen Druding
*Prepress Vendor:* S4Carlisle Publishing Services

9  8  7  6  5  4  3  2  1

Printed in China

**Library of Congress Cataloging-in-Publication Data**
Fundamental and advanced fetal imaging : ultrasound and MRI / editors, Beth M. Kline-Fath, Dorothy I. Bulas, Ray Bahado-Singh.
     p. ; cm.
   Includes bibliographical references and index.
   ISBN 978-1-4511-7583-7 (hardback) — ISBN 1-4511-7583-3 (hardback)
   I. Kline-Fath, Beth M., editor.    II. Bulas, Dorothy I., editor.    III. Bahado-Singh, Ray, editor.
   [DNLM: 1. Magnetic Resonance Imaging—methods.    2. Ultrasonography, Prenatal—methods.    3. Congenital Abnormalities—diagnosis.    4. Fetal Diseases—diagnosis.    5. Fetus—abnormalities.    WQ 209]
   RC78
   616.07'57—dc23

                                                                                            2014019723

LWW.com

*To my husband, Tom, who without his love and support, this book would not be possible. To my daughters, Kelsey and Abby, I will always love you more. To my father who is looking down on me and my mother by my side, thank you for your love and guidance and for teaching me to always reach for more. And to my family, especially my nieces Natasha and Naomi, thank you for believing in me; for it is through your lives that I understood the importance of this field.*

*BMKF*

*To my husband, Neal, who despite all the hours and weekends spent on this book, was always encouraging and supportive. To Mark and Adam for the love and joy you bring to my life. And to my parents who continue to inspire me to enjoy the gifts medicine has to offer.*

*DIB*

# CONTRIBUTORS

**Fred E. Avni, MD PhD**
Department of Pediatric Imaging
Jeanne de Flandre Hospital
Lille University
Lille, France

**Ray Bahado-Singh, MD, MBA**
Professor of Obstetrics and Gynecology
Oakland University William Beaumont School of Medicine
Rochester Michigan
Health System Chair, Department Obstetrics and Gynecology
William Beaumont Health System
Royal Oak, Michigan

**Richard A. Barth, MD**
Professor of Radiology
Stanford University
Radiologist-in-Chief
Stanford Children's Health
Palo Alto, California

**Krista L. Birkemeier**
Assistant Professor of Radiology
Texas A&M Health Science Center College of Medicine
Department of Radiology
McLane Children's Hospital, Scott and White
Temple, Texas

**Richard A. Bronsteen, MD**
Associate Professor of Obstetrics & Gynecology
Oakland University William Beaumont School of Medicine
Rochester, Michigan
Co-director of Fetal Imaging
William Beaumont Health System
Royal Oak, Michigan

**Dorothy I. Bulas, MD**
Program Director for Fetal Imaging
Fetal and Transitional Medicine
Vice Chief of Academic Affairs
Division of Diagnostic Imaging and Radiology
Children's National Health System
Professor of Pediatrics and Radiology
George Washington University
Washington, DC

**Maria A. Calvo-Garcia, MD**
Associate Professor of Radiology
Cincinnati Children's Hospital Medical Center
Cincinnati, Ohio

**Christopher Cassady MD**
Chief of Fetal and Neonatal Imaging
Department of Pediatric Radiology
Texas Children's Hospital and Fetal Center
Houston, Texas

**Tinnakorn Chaiworapongsa, MD**
Professor
Director of Biomarker Discovery Unit
Perinatology Research Branch, NICHD
National Institutes of Health
Department of Health and Human Services
Department of Obstetrics and Gynecology
Wayne State University School of Medicine
Detroit, Michigan

**Teresa Chapman, MD**
Associate Professor of Radiology
Department of Radiology
Seattle Children's Hospital
University of Washington School of Medicine
Seattle, Washington

**Sarah B. Clauss, MD**
Assistant Professor of Pediatrics
Division of Cardiology
Children's National Medical Center
George Washington University
Washington, DC

**Cedric Clouchoux, PhD**
Diagnostic Imaging and Radiology
Fetal and Transitional Medicine
Children's National Medical Center
Washington, DC

**Beverly G. Coleman, MD**
Professor and Associate Chairman Radiology
Director of Ultrasound Imaging
University of Pennsylvania Health System
Philadelphia, Pennsylvania

**Kimberly Ann Dannull, MD**
Assistant Professor of Radiology
University of Colorado School of Medicine
Staff, Pediatric Radiology
Children's Hospital Colorado
Aurora, Colorado

**Greggory R. DeVore, MD**
Clinical Professor
Department of Obstetrics and Gynecology
David Geffen School of Medicine at UCLA
Los Angeles, California
Director of Fetal Diagnostic Centers
Pasadena, Tarzana, Mission Hills, California
Director of Perinatology
Providence Tarzana Medical Center
Tarzana, California

**Mary T. Donofrio, MD**
Director of the Fetal Heart Program and Critical Care Delivery Service
Director of Advanced Cardiac Imaging Fellowship
Division of Cardiology
Children's National Medical Center
Professor of Pediatrics
George Washington University
Washington, DC

**Judy A. Estroff, MD**
Division Chief of Fetal-Neonatal Imaging
Department of Radiology
Boston Children's Hospital
Associate Professor of Radiology
Harvard Medical School
Boston, Massachusetts

**Henry L. Galan, MD**
Professor
Department of Obstetrics and Gynecology
University of Colorado School of Medicine
Codirector of the Colorado Fetal Care Center
Colorado Institute for Maternal and Fetal Health
The University of Colorado Hospital and Children's Hospital of Colorado
Aurora, Colorado

**Katherine R. Goetzinger, MD**
Department of Obstetrics and Gynecology
Washington University School of Medicine
St. Louis, Missouri

**Luís F. Gonçalves, MD**
Professor of Radiology and Obstetrics and Gynecology
Oakland University William Beaumont School of Medicine
Rochester, Michigan
Staff Physician
Departments of Radiology and Obstetrics and Gynecology
Division of Fetal Imaging
William Beaumont Hospital
Royal Oak, Michigan

**Mounira Habli, MD**
Assistant Professor
Co-Chair of Perinatal Research Institute at Good Samaritan Hospital
Maternal Fetal Medicine Division
Department of Pediatric Surgery
Fetal Care Center of Cincinnati
Good Samaritan Hospital
Cincinnati, Ohio

**Sonia S. Hassan, MD**
Associate Dean for Maternal, Perinatal, and Child Health
Professor, Division of Maternal-Fetal Medicine
Department of Obstetrics and Gynecology
Wayne State University School of Medicine
Director, Center for Advanced Obstetrical Care and Research
Perinatology Research Branch
Eunice Kennedy Shriver NICHD
National Institutes of Health
Detroit, Michigan

**Edgar Hernández-Andrade, MD**
Associate Professor
Department of Obstetrics and Gynecology
Division of Maternal Fetal Medicine
Hutzel Women Hospital
Wayne State University Director of Maternal and Fetal Imaging
Perinatology Research Branch
NICHD, National Institutes of Health
Detroit, Michigan

**Robert J. Hopkin, MD**
Associate Professor
University of Cincinnati College of Medicine
Cincinnati Children's Hospital Medical Center
Division of Human Genetics and Fetal Care Center
Cincinnati, Ohio

**John Hyett, MD**
Clinical Professor
Head of High Risk Obstetrics
RPA Women and Babies
Joint Head of Academic Department of Obstetrics, Gynaecology and Neonatology
University of Sydney
Royal Prince Alfred Hospital
Sydney, Australia

**Cristiano Jodicke, MD**
Assistant Professor
Associate Program Director
Maternal-Fetal Medicine Fellowship Program
University of Missouri–Kansas City School of Medicine
Kansas City, Missouri

**Jennifer H. Johnston, MD**
Assistant Professor
Department of Diagnostic and Interventional Imaging
The University of Texas Medical School at Houston
Houston, Texas

**Beth M. Kline-Fath, MD**
Chief of Fetal and Neonatal Imaging
Associate Professor of Radiology
Department of Radiology
Cincinnati Children's Hospital Medical Center
Cincinnati, Ohio

**Anita Krishnan, MD**
Division of Cardiology
Children's National Medical Center
Assistant Professor of Pediatrics
George Washington University
Washington, DC

**Jennifer Lam-Rachlin, MD**
Fellow, Division of Maternal-Fetal Medicine
Department of Obstetrics and Gynecology
Wayne State University School of Medicine
Perinatology Research Branch, NICHD National Institutes of Health
Detroit, Michigan

**Catherine Limperopoulos, PhD**
Director, MRI Research of the Developing Brain
Children's National Medical Center
Director, Advanced Pediatric Brain Imaging Research Laboratory
Associate Professor of Neurology, Radiology, and Pediatrics
Division of Diagnostic Imaging and Radiology/Fetal
and Transitional Medicine
George Washington University
Washington, DC

**Leanne E. Linam, MD**
Assistant Professor of Radiology
University of Arkansas for Medical Sciences
Arkansas Children's Hospital
Little Rock, Arkansas

**Dev Maulik, MD, PhD**
Professor and Chair
Department of Obstetrics and Gynecology
Senior Associate Dean of Women's Health
Professor of Basic Science
University of Missouri Kansas City School of Medicine
Chair, Department of Obstetrics and Gynecology
Truman Medical Center
Cahir, Department of Maternal-Fetal Medicine
Children's Mercy Hospital
Kansas City, Missouri

**Margaret B. Menzel, MS, CGC**
Genetics and Metabolism
Fetal Medicine Institute
Children's National Health System
Clinical Instructor, Pediatrics
George Washington University
Washington, D.C.

**Mariana Laura Meyers, MD**
Director of Fetal Imaging
Assistant Professor of Radiology
University of Colorado School of Medicine
Staff Pediatric Radiology
Children's Hospital Colorado
Aurora, Colorado

**Kypros H. Nicolaides, MD**
Professor of Fetal Imaging
Harris Birthright Research Center of Fetal Medicine
King's College Hospital
London, United Kingdom

**Marta Nucci, MD**
Research Fellow
Harris Birthright Research Center of Fetal Medicine
Department of Obstetrics and Gynecology
King's College Hospital
London, United Kingdom

**Anthony O. Odibo, MD**
Professor of Obstetrics and Gynecology
Department of Obstetrics and Gynecology
University of South Florida,
Morsani School of Medicine
Tampa, Florida

**Ashok Panigrahy, MD**
Radiologist-in-Chief
Associate Professor of Radiology
Children's Hospital of Pittsburgh of UPMC
Pittsburgh, Pennsylvania

**Jodi I. Pike, MD**
Division of Cardiology
Children's National Medical Center
Assistant Professor of Pediatrics
George Washington University
Washington, DC

**Shane Reeves, MD**
Assistant Professor
Department of Obstetrics and Gynecology
University of Colorado School of Medicine
Medical Director, Maternal-Fetal Care Unit
The University of Colorado Hospital and Children's
Hospital of Colorado
Aurora, Colorado

**Jason D. Retzke, MD**
Maternal-Fetal Medicine
Riverside Methodist Hospital
Columbus, Ohio

**Ashley James Robinson, MD**
Staff Radiologist
BC Children's Hospital
Clinical Assistant Professor
University of British Columbia
Vancouver, British Columbia, Canada

**Robert Romero, MD, D.Med.Sci.**
Chief, Perinatology Research Branch
Program Head, Program for Perinatal Research
and Obstetrics Division of Intramural Research
Eunice Kennedy Shriver National Institute of Child Health
and Human Development, NIH Bethesda, Maryland
and Detroit, Michigan
Department of Obstetrics and Gynecology, University
of Michigan
Ann Arbor, Michigan
Department of Epidemiology and Biostatics, Michigan State
University
East Lansing, Michigan

**Eva I. Rubio, MD**
Medical Unit Director
Division of Diagnostic Imaging and Radiology
Children's National Health System
Assistant Professor of Pediatrics and Radiology
George Washington School of Medicine
Washington, DC

**Stephanie L. Santoro, MD**
Resident Physician
Division of Human Genetics
University of Cincinnati College of Medicine
Cincinnati Children's Hospital Medical Center
Cincinnati, Ohio

**William T. Schnettler, MD**
Maternal-Fetal Medicine Physician
Department of Obstetrics and Gynecology
Tri-Health
Cincinnati, Ohio

**Carmen Sciorio, MD**
Medical Doctor
Resident in Obstetrics and Gynecology
Research Fellow
Harris Birthright Research Center of Fetal Medicine
King's College Hospital
London, United Kingdom

**Mike Seed, MD**
Staff Cardiologist and Radiologist Hospital for Sick Children
Division of Paediatric Cardiology
Department of Paediatrics
University of Toronto
Toronto, Ontario, Canada

**Paul Singh, MD**
Clinical Instructor
Department of Obstetrics and Gynecology
Division of Maternal-Fetal Medicine
Kansas City, Missouri

**Jiri D. Sonek, MD**
Clinical Professor, Department of Obstetrics and Gynecology
Wright State University
Director, Fetal Medicine Foundation of USA
Medical Director, Center for Maternal Fetal Medicine, Ultrasound, and Genetics
Miami Valley Hospital
Dayton, Ohio

**Eleazar Soto, MD**
Assistant Professor
University of Texas Health Science Center-Houston
Department of Obstetrics and Gynecology
Division of Maternal Fetal-Medicine
Houston, Texas

**Gayathri Sreedher, MD**
Instructor
Children's Hospital of Pittsburgh of UPMC
Pittsburgh, Pennsylvania

**Teresa Victoria MD PHD**
Assistant Professor of Radiology
Perelman School of Medicine
University of Pennsylvania
Philadelphia, PA

**Amy E. Whitten, MD**
Division of Maternal Fetal Medicine
William Beaumont Health System
Royal Oak, Michigan

The development of prenatal ultrasound ushered in an exciting new age in fetal assessment and represented the proverbial great leap forward. The systematic investigation of both fetal behavior and anatomy became a reality. Subsequent technological advances have ensued at a relentless pace. Pulse and color Doppler facilitated the near complete interrogation of the fetal vasculature while 3-dimensional ultrasound provided enhanced realism and novel perspectives of fetal structure.

The introduction of fetal MR imaging is proving equally transformational. Structural details have been dramatically enhanced with the promise of providing previously unachievable metabolic fingerprint of fetal tissues. Techniques such as bright blood imaging, diffusion spectroscopy and other functional modalities promise to transform our understanding of intrauterine life with the anticipated rewards being improved clinical management and fetal outcome.

Initial concerns that MRI development would be at the expense of ultrasound now appear unsubstantiated. Evidence suggests that these two modalities are deeply complementary and that their simultaneous deployment is critical for optimal fetal assessment for many important fetal disorders.

In this book, the specialties of radiology and obstetrics converge to provide a reference on the complex field of fetal imaging. The first part of the book is dedicated to normal prenatal US and MR imaging. In that section, US evaluation in the first and second trimesters, growth, Doppler, and basic cardiac anatomy of fetus are reviewed. Normal MR imaging discussion includes a how-to technical section and provides normal examples of the entire fetal anatomy, with emphasis on the fetal brain. Advanced fetal brain and cardiac MR techniques are also detailed. The second part of the book reviews the major fetal pathologies by organ system with a separate chapter dedicated to common genetic and chromosomal disorders. This section of the book reflects the approach in a prior edition by Nyberg. The incidence, pathogenesis, etiology, and diagnosis with US and MRI, as well as prognosis and management for fetal pathologies are examined. Color diagrams, tables, and, most importantly, images utilizing both US and MRI provide the reader with an enhanced understanding of the anomalies. The appendix offers important biometry tables for easy reference. These tables contain normal MR values, including essential measurements of the fetal brain at different gestational ages.

Another unique feature of this book is that a diverse group of fetal subspecialists graciously helped author chapters, including cardiologists, geneticists, and Doppler specialists. International experts, including Kypros Nicolaides and Fred Avni, provided a global perspective of this discipline.

Our goal for *Fundamental and Advanced Fetal Imaging* was to provide the most up-to-date and encompassing reference for fetal imaging. We hope all fetologists, including radiologists and obstetricians, as well as pediatric specialists such as surgeons, geneticists, counselors, neurologists, urologists, and neurosurgeons, will turn to this reference for basic and advanced imaging information. This book should also serve as an excellent resource for the resident and medical student.

Understanding normal development and pathologies in the fetus is essential for optimal prenatal and postnatal care. We hope you find this book illuminating and that it will contribute to fetal research, therapeutic techniques, perinatal care, and counseling. Our objective has been the integration of two critical technologies for fetal assessment. We believe that the finished product is in alignment with our original intent.

*Beth M. Kline-Fath*
*Dorothy I. Bulas*
*Ray Bahado-Singh*

# ACKNOWLEDGMENTS

First and foremost, we would like to thank all the authors from so many different specialties who have generously shared their expertise, research and images.

We cannot thank them enough for their hard work, and leadership in this growing field of fetology.

We want to acknowledge the authors of the first edition of Diagnostic Imaging of Fetal Anomalies, David A. Nyberg, John P. McGahan, Dolores H. Pretorius, and Gianluigi Pilu, whose important initial work was the basis of this new text.

We thank the sonographers, obstetricians, radiologists, and fetal specialists who have worked together to improve the care of the fetus.

We thank the fellows, residents and students in training who have asked questions pushing us to search for better answers.

We would like to thank Glenn Minano for his creative assistance with regard to the artwork presented in this book.

We thank the staff of Lippincott Williams and Wilkins/ Wolters Kluwer Health; Charley Mitchell for getting us started, Ryan Shaw, Amy Dinkel, Emilie Moyer, Jonathan Pine for their guidance, Grace Caputo for keeping us on track and Mohamed Hameed for his gracious efficiency.

*BMKF, DIB, RBS*

I would like to thank my coworkers at Cincinnati Children's, especially Juanita Hunter, for their constant support and enthusiasm about this project. To those who encouraged and directed my medical career, I would like to express gratitude to Ben Felson, Hugh Hawkins, Alan Chambers, John Egelhoff and Lane Donnelly. For those who taught me the importance of team work to improve fetal and neonatal care, I would like to thank Constance Bitters, Maria Calvo-Garcia, Bill Polzin, Foong-Yen Lim, Tim Crombleholme and all of my fetal co-workers, many of whom have gone to other institutions to continue work in this innovative field. Finally, I would like to thank all families who entrust the care of their unborn; it is their lives that inspire me to learn more to improve fetal care.

*BMKF*

I want to thank my department and coworkers for their support during this process. I could not have completed this work without them. I am grateful to all my colleagues who have shared my enthusiasm for caring for the fetus. Their collaboration has been a source of inspiration through the years. Lastly, I want to thank all the families I have had the privilege to work with. It is their stories that move me to continue to work in this field.

*DIB*

I wish to express my gratitude to the contributing authors, chosen for their expertise and leadership in the field, who so selflessly gave of their valuable time. A very special thank you to my associate editors, Drs. Dorothy Bulas (George Washington University) and Beth Kline-Fath (Cincinnati Children's). It is their vision and limitless reserves of energy and commitment that made this book a reality.

On a personal note, may I also express my profound gratitude to my mentors who have made transformative contributions in the field of prenatal imaging, and women's health: Drs. Jeremiah Mahoney, John Hobbins, Roberto Romero, Frederick Naftolin and Joshua Copel. Their example has served as a beacon over these many years. In like manner, I am indebted to Drs. Roger Freeman, Thomas Garite and Mike Nageotte for opening our eyes to both the challenges and bountiful rewards that flow from the care of the pregnant woman and her fetus. Finally, to the thousands of such women without whose permission we could not have gained this knowledge, a my most sincere- Thank you!

*RBS*

# CONTENTS

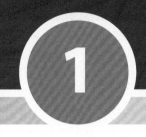

# 1 Normal Fetal Ultrasound Survey

Jiri D. Sonek • Jason D. Retzke • John Hyett

Prenatal ultrasound represents one of the most important advances in modern obstetrics. Prior to the advent of this technology, the contents of the uterus were essentially a black box. Ultrasound has evolved significantly since Ian Donald et al. first demonstrated its potential value. It provides an effective means of evaluating the fetus from both a structural and a functional perspective. As a consequence, obstetrics has evolved from a discipline that dealt almost exclusively with maternal health concerns to one that also focuses on the health and development of the fetus.[1,2]

A complete obstetric ultrasound includes evaluation of the uterus, the adnexa, and the intrauterine contents.[3–7] In this chapter, we focus on examination of the fetus. Examinations of the umbilical cord, placenta, and amniotic fluid are discussed in Chapter 7, and assessment of the uterine cervix is discussed in Chapter 10.

The obstetric ultrasound is a comprehensive exam with different components of the exam emphasized at various stages of fetal development. While examination at 8 weeks' gestation is not currently considered the optimal gestational age for fetal ultrasound assessment, it does provide an opportunity to assess viability and intrauterine location of the pregnancy, to reliably determine chorionicity in the case of a multiple gestation, and to date the pregnancy with a great degree of accuracy. The 12-week scan is a relatively recent addition, but is now accepted as a point for routine assessment and is rapidly gaining recognition as one of the most important points for fetal evaluation. Most fetal chromosomal and severe structural abnormalities can be detected even at this early stage of development. Recognition of a problem at this point in pregnancy allows the parents ample time for counseling with a wide range of options regarding termination or continuation of pregnancy.[8–12] More recently, the 12-week scan has also been shown to be valuable in the prediction of obstetric complications such as preeclampsia and growth restriction, allowing obstetricians to take preventive action at a point early in gestation, potentially reducing the risk of adverse pregnancy outcome.[13]

For many years, the 20-week scan has been the cornerstone of obstetric imaging. Systematic examination at this stage identifies a high proportion of major structural anomalies. At this gestation, the fetus is already relatively large, and the formation of major fetal structures except for the brain has been completed. Therefore, more anomalies can be detected at this point than at 12 weeks, and those that are suspected at an earlier gestational age can now be confirmed and better defined. Still, some important abnormalities such as neuronal migration defects will remain undetectable until the late third trimester or until after birth. Finally, most data regarding the value of cervical assessment also pertain to the 20-week gestational age window.

Even though a complete structural survey can be performed at ≥28 weeks' gestation, scans at this stage are limited by bone shadowing from the calvarium, ribs, spine, and limbs. However, investigation at this point in gestation provides invaluable information regarding fetal well-being and placental function. In addition to the evaluation of fetal growth and amniotic fluid volume, Doppler ultrasound can be employed to evaluate placental and fetal hemodynamics, and to look for changes indicative of placental insufficiency and fetal hypoxia. This information is helpful in determining timing and mode of delivery of growth restricted fetuses. This approach is also useful in identifying late onset growth restriction and the failing placenta at term.[14–23]

Obstetric ultrasound has its limitations, a fact that both clinicians and patients need to recognize. Anomalies may be missed for a variety of reasons. In early pregnancy, structures may be too small for examination, the embryologic development process may be incomplete, or secondary pathologic change may have not yet occurred. As noted above, development of some structures, such as the central nervous system, continues throughout the pregnancy and even into infancy; therefore, anomalies may not be evident at the time of a routine 20-week ultrasound examination. Other important abnormalities, such as autism, are functional rather than structural and therefore cannot be detected by ultrasound.[24]

The exact prognosis associated with a particular anomaly finding might be unclear. For example, with certain ultrasound findings most fetuses might have a normal outcome, yet a small proportion may be severely incapacitated. Clinicians that report ultrasound findings have to be able to define risks as clearly as possible, recognize the inherent uncertainties, and have the skill to communicate them effectively to the patient.[25]

The quality of the ultrasound image may be affected by a number of maternal and fetal factors, including maternal obesity and fetal position. Increased maternal body mass index (BMI) has become a notable impediment to the performance of obstetric ultrasound. Ultrasound does not penetrate adipose tissue well, leading to decreased image quality and prolonged examination time. The increased study length and physical stress is a major health issue for sonographers.[26,27] Nonetheless, it also needs to be kept in mind that increased maternal BMI is associated with an increased risk of a number of fetal anomalies such as neural tube defects, cardiac defects, and facial clefts.[28] It therefore becomes important to attempt to maximize the diagnostic potential of the ultrasound examination, while minimizing risks to staff. This can be accomplished by defining a maximum time limit for an exam and termination of an exam at a point where it is determined that optimal images are not obtainable. Difficulties relating to fetal position are relatively easier to deal with by alteration of the angle of insonation, manipulation of the fetus, combined transabdominal and transvaginal imaging, or simply waiting until the fetus spontaneously changes its position. Despite these difficulties, we need to remember that image interpretation is fundamentally dependent on image quality, and sonographers should be encouraged to be single-minded in their pursuit of excellence.

## Table 1.1    Summary of Recommendations for Diagnostic Ultrasound Parameters and Indices

In the low-megahertz frequency range, there have been no independently confirmed adverse biologic effects in mammalian tissues exposed in vivo under experimental ultrasound conditions, as follows:

1. Thermal mechanisms
   a. No effects have been observed for an unfocused beam having free-field spatial-peak temporal-average (SPTA) intensities[a] below 100 mW/cm², or a focused[b] beam having intensities below 1 W/cm², or thermal index values of <2.
   b. For fetal exposures, no effects have been reported for a temperature increase above the normal physiologic temperature, $\Delta T$, when $\Delta T$ < 4.5 – ($\log_{10} t$/0.6), where $t$ is exposure time ranging from 1 to 250 min, including off time for pulsed exposure.[30]
   c. For postnatal exposures producing temperature increases of 6°C or less, no effects have been reported when $\Delta T$ < 6 – ($\log_{10} t$/0.6), including off time for pulsed exposure. For example, for temperature increases of 6.0°C and 2.0°C, the corresponding limits for the exposure durations $t$ are 1 and 250 min.[31]
   d. For postnatal exposures producing temperature increases of 6°C or more, no effects have been reported when $\Delta T$ < 6 – ($\log_{10} t$/0.3), including off time for pulsed exposure. For example, for a temperature increase of 9.6°C, the corresponding limit for the exposure duration is 5 s (=0.083 min).[31]

2. Nonthermal mechanisms
   a. In tissues that contain well-defined gas bodies, e.g., lung, no effects have been observed for in situ peak rarefactional pressures below approximately 0.4 MPa or mechanical index values approximately <0.4.
   b. In tissues that do not contain well-defined gas bodies, no effects have been reported for peak rarefactional pressures below approximately 4.0 MPa or mechanical index values approximately <4.0.[29]

[a]Free-field SPTA intensity for continuous wave and pulsed exposures.
[b]Quarter-power (−6 dB) beam width smaller than 4 wavelengths or 4 mm, whichever is less at the exposure frequency.
Modified from American Institute of Ultrasound in Medicine. *AIUM Statement on Mammalian In Vivo Ultrasonic Biological Effects*. November 8, 2008. http://www.aium.org/.

Sound waves transmit energy, which has the potential to heat and disrupt tissue.[29-44] While diagnostic grayscale imaging delivers a low amount of energy, other forms of ultrasound such as pulse wave and color Doppler, focus higher levels of energy on small areas of tissue. The limited data available suggest that the application of diagnostic ultrasound to human pregnancy is safe and that the value of the information gained through examination easily outweighs any risk to the fetus. All ultrasound machines report power output as the thermal index (TI), a measure of the potential increase in temperature that ultrasound causes in tissue, and the mechanical index (MI), a measure of the potential for tissue cavitation (Table 1.1).[29-32] Ultrasound technology should always be applied according to the "as low as reasonably achievable" (ALARA) principle, which states that one should perform the shortest exam with the lowest amount of ultrasound energy required to successfully complete a diagnostic examination. The Bioeffects Committee of the American Institute of Ultrasound in Medicine, comprising 35 experts in various fields pertaining to ultrasound safety, has defined acceptable limits for diagnostic investigation. Selected safety recommendations are included in Table 1.2.[33,34]

Effective prenatal diagnosis relies on a high standard of imaging. Several national and international bodies have described standards for imaging in the first, second, and third trimester of pregnancy. These include organizations such as the American College of Obstetricians and Gynecologists (ACOG), American Institute of Ultrasound in Medicine (AIUM), Australasian Society of Ultrasound in Medicine (ASUM), National Health Service (NHS) in the United Kingdom, and the International Society of Ultrasound in Obstetrics and Gynecology (ISUOG) (Table 1.3).[3-7] Guidelines typically describe the essential components of an obstetric ultrasound examination. However, many experts in the field advocate the use of additional views to improve diagnostic performance. In addition to describing the basic components of an obstetrical ultrasound examination in this chapter, we also present extended views that improve the quality of the examination and the detection of pregnancy-related problems. This chapter deals with normal fetal anatomy; however, frequent

## Table 1.2    Selected Safety Recommendations for Diagnostic Ultrasound

- Ultrasound exposures that elevate fetal temperature by 4°C above normal for 5 min or more have the potential to induce severe developmental defects

- Apply the ALARA principle if the tissues to be exposed contain stabilized gas bodies (lung) and the MI exceeds 0.4

- There is no epidemiologic support for a causal relationship between diagnostic ultrasound during pregnancy and adverse biologic effects to the fetus observed for outputs under a spatial-peak temporal-average intensity of 94 mW/cm²

- The temperature of the fetus should not safely rise more than 0.5°C above its normal temperature

- When MI is above 0.5 or the TI is above 1.0, the NCRP recommends that the risks of ultrasound be weighed against the benefits

From Fowlkes JB; Bioeffects Committee of the American Institute of Ultrasound in Medicine. American Institute of Ultrasound in Medicine consensus report on potential bioeffects of diagnostic ultrasound. *J Ultrasound Med*. 2008;27:503–515. National Council on Radiation Protection and Measurements. *Exposure Criteria for Medical Ultrasound, II: Criteria Based on All Known Mechanisms*. Bethesda, MD: National Council on Radiation Protection and Measurements; 2002. NRCP report 140.

| Table 1.3 | Summary of Recommendations Regarding Evaluation of Fetal Anatomy on Prenatal Ultrasound | | | |
|---|---|---|---|---|
| | *ISUOG* | *AIUM and ACOG* | *ASUM* | *NHS (UK)* |
| **Head and Neck** | | | | |
| Skull bones, calvarium | X | | X | X (shape) |
| - Biparietal diameter (measure) | X | X | X | |
| - Head circumference (measure) | X | X | X | X |
| - Nuchal fold | X | X (measure if increased age) | X | X (measure if increased) |
| **Brain** | | | | |
| - Cavum septum pellucidum | X | X | X | X |
| - Cerebral ventricles, choroid plexus | X | X | X | X (measure) |
| - Cerebellum | X | X | X | X (measure) |
| - Cisterna magna | X | X | X | |
| - Midline falx | X | X | X | |
| **Face** | | | | |
| Orbits | X | | X | |
| Nose | X (if tech feas) | | X | |
| Lips | X (upper) | X (upper) | X | X (coronal) |
| Mouth | X | | | |
| Jaw | | | X | |
| Profile | X (if tech feas) | | X | |
| **Chest** | | | | |
| Heart | | | | |
| - Cardiac activity | X | X | X | |
| - Four-chamber view | X | X | X | X |
| - Outflow tracts | X (if tech feas) | X (if tech feas) | X | X |
| Lungs | X | | | X |
| Diaphragm | X | | X (right/left) | |
| **Abdomen and Pelvis** | | | | |
| Stomach | X (presence, situs) | X (presence, size, situs) | X (presence, situs) | X |
| Abdominal wall | | | X | X |
| - Abdominal circumference (measure) | X | X | X | X |
| - Umbilical cord insertion | X | X | X | |
| - Umbilical cord vessel number | X | X | X | |
| Bowel | X | | | X |
| Kidneys | X | X | X | X |
| - Renal pelvis (measure if increased) | X | | | X |
| Bladder | X | X | X | X |
| **Spine** | | | | |
| Vertebrae | X | X | X | X |
| Skin covering | | | X | X |

*(continued)*

| Table 1.3 | Summary of Recommendations Regarding Evaluation of Fetal Anatomy on Prenatal Ultrasound *(continued)* | | | |
|---|---|---|---|---|
| | *ISUOG* | *AIUM and ACOG* | *ASUM* | *NHS (UK)* |
| **Limbs** | | | | |
| Upper extremity | X | X | X | X |
| - Metacarpals (right and left) | X | | X | X |
| Lower extremity | X | X | X | X |
| - Femur length | X (measure) | X (measure) | X | X (measure) |
| - Metatarsals (right and left) | X | | X | X |
| **Uterus, Cervix, and Adnexa** | | | | |
| Cervical length | | X (if tech feas) | X | |
| Adnexa | X (if tech feas) | X (if tech feas) | X | |
| Amniotic fluid volume (subj or meas) | X | X | X | X |
| Placental position | X | X | X | X |

ISUOG, International Society of Ultrasound in Obstetrics and Gynecology; AIUM, American Institute of Ultrasound in Medicine; ACOG, American College of Obstetricians and Gynecologists; ASUM, Australasian Society of Ultrasound in Medicine; NHS, National Health Service, UK.
From Salomon LJ, Alfirevic Z, Berghella V, et al. Practice guidelines for performance of the routine mid-trimester fetal ultrasound scan (ISUOG). *Ultrasound Obstet Gynecol.* 2011;37:116–126. American Institute of Ultrasound in Medicine. AIUM practice guideline for the performance of obstetric ultrasound examinations. *J Ultrasound Med.* 2010;29:157–166. American College of Obstetricians and Gynecologists. Ultrasonography in pregnancy. *Obstet Gynecol.* 2009;113:451–461. ACOG Practice Bulletin No. 101. Australasian Society for Ultrasound in Medicine. *Policies and Statements, D2: Guidelines for the Mid Trimester Obstetric Scan.* http://www.asum.com.au/open/P&S/D2_policy.pdf. National Collaborating Centre for Women's and Children's Health. *Antenatal Care: Routine Care for the Healthy Pregnant Woman.* 2nd ed. London, England: RCOG Press; 2008.

references to anomalies are made to underscore the pertinence of a good anatomic evaluation. Each image used in this chapter was obtained using two-dimensional (2D) ultrasound. Three-dimensional (3D) ultrasound can be a useful adjunct to 2D ultrasound in select circumstances and will be discussed in Chapter 2. All stated gestational ages are according to last menstrual period dating.

## EARLY FIRST TRIMESTER SCAN (5 TO 10 WEEKS' GESTATION)

The embryonic stage, ending at 10 weeks' gestation, is a time of very rapid change in the small, developing conceptus.[45] Ultrasound before 11 weeks' gestation is not typically regarded as a routine part of pregnancy assessment. When performed, the examination is generally limited to determination of the location and number of gestations present, determination of chorionicity in cases of multiple gestations, assessment for viability, and estimation of gestational age.[46] Although the anatomy of embryo is not typically examined in detail, a variety of severe congenital anomalies (e.g., severe amniotic band syndrome, body-stalk anomalies, and conjoined twins) may be identified even at this point. A finding that is commonly seen in the early first trimester and that deserves special mention is physiologic herniation of the midgut into the root of the abdominal cord insertion (Fig. 1.1).[47] This finding is considered normal until the early portion 12th week of gestation and should not be mistaken for an omphalocele.

Most examinations at this stage are performed for a specific clinical indication such as pain or vaginal bleeding associated with a positive pregnancy test. Systematic evaluation is needed to accurately distinguish between a viable intrauterine pregnancy,

a miscarriage, or an ectopic pregnancy. Ultrasound findings are frequently best interpreted in combination with quantitative maternal serum hCG (human chorionic gonadotropin) with or without progesterone levels. Serial examinations may be needed to reach a diagnosis. The transvaginal approach should be used in all circumstances where a viable intrauterine pregnancy is not obvious on transabdominal assessment. The uterus and adjacent structures should be assessed in both longitudinal and axial sections, taking care to pass completely from side to side and from fundus to cervix to determine the number and location of gestational sacs and embryos. In the early first trimester, the transvaginal approach is ideal to detect any adnexal pathology or free fluid.

Using transvaginal ultrasound, the presence of an intrauterine gestational sac can be consistently demonstrated by the

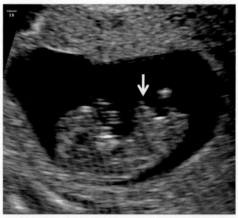

**FIGURE 1.1:** Sagittal view of a 10- to 11-week fetus demonstrating a physiologic midgut herniation *(arrow).*

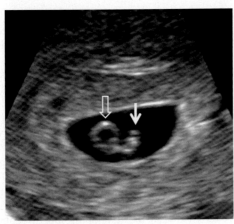

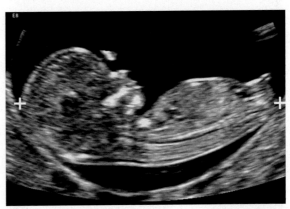

**FIGURE 1.2:** Embryo at 6.5 weeks' gestation. *Solid arrow*, embryo; *open arrow*, yolk sac.

**FIGURE 1.4:** Sagittal view of an 11- to 12-week fetus. The fetus is in a neutral position and occupies the majority of the image. *Calipers*, CRL measurement.

completion of the 5th week of gestation. At this early stage, the gestational age is being estimated by determination of the mean sac diameter (MSD): the average of the sac length, width, and depth. The yolk sac becomes visible within the gestational sac by the midportion of the 6th gestational week, corresponding to an MSD of approximately 10 mm. An embryonic pole with a heartbeat is generally detected by the middle of the 7th gestational week (MSD of approximately 18 mm). When an embryonic pole becomes identifiable, the best method of establishing the gestational age is measurement of the crown-rump length (CRL). Prior to the completion of the 7th gestational week, the anatomy of the embryonic pole is difficult to clearly delineate. At this stage, the CRL is defined as the longest dimension of the embryonic pole (Fig. 1.2). Beginning with the 8th week of gestation, the embryonic head and torso become identifiable. At this point, the CRL is defined as measurement between the top of the fetal head and the fetal rump along its longitudinal axis (Fig. 1.3).[48] Whereas some investigators advocate using the average of three CRL measurements to establish gestational age, most use the single best measurement. In the 11th week of gestation, the fetus begins to flex and extend its body to a degree that may significantly affect CRL; therefore, CRL measurements need to be carefully standardized from this point on (Fig. 1.4).[49,50]

The accuracy of CRL measurement decreases with gestational age. Between 7 and $11^{+6}$ weeks' gestation measurements should

be within 4 days of dates by LMP (last menstrual period). At 12 to $13^{+6}$ weeks, an error of $\pm7$ days is considered to be acceptable.[51,52]

## LATE FIRST TRIMESTER SCAN ($11^{+1}$ TO $13^{+6}$ WEEKS' GESTATION)

The late first trimester scan is generally considered to be the first scheduled point for routine ultrasound assessment in pregnancy. It provides the same information as the early first trimester scan with a number of additional benefits. Since it includes highly accurate estimation of gestational age, routine implementation of the late first trimester scan would lead to a significant reduction in postterm pregnancies. During this time frame, the fetus reaches a size and stage of development sufficient to allow for the performance of an informative anatomic survey.[10,11,53] A number of markers, the most important of which is the nuchal translucency measurement, can be employed to provide an accurate risk assessment for aneuploidy. It should also be stressed that an increased translucency and the presence of other markers, most notably tricuspid valve regurgitation and an abnormal ductus venosus (DV) Doppler waveform, increase the risk of structural abnormalities even in chromosomally normal fetuses.[54]

Optimal timing of the first trimester scan involves some compromise. Nuchal translucency assessment is easier to perform and more sensitive at an earlier gestation (11 to 12 weeks), whereas anatomy is best assessed at a slightly later gestation (12 to 13 weeks).[8] The examination may be performed transabdominally, and if necessary transvaginally, but a combination of the two approaches often yields the best results. Regardless of the approach used, the fetus needs to be assessed in all planes: Longitudinal, axial, and coronal.

The midsagittal section of the fetus is very important, as this allows accurate measurement of CRL and, when adequately magnified, nuchal translucency (Fig. 1.5). Nuchal translucency measurement is typically increased in fetuses affected by chromosomal abnormality. Measurement according to standardized methodology allows individualized levels of risk for trisomy 21, 18, and 13 to be calculated. Another marker for aneuploidy, the fetal nasal bone, can be examined in the same section. Absence of the nasal bone is associated with an increased risk of trisomy 21.[55] Similarly, the intracranial anatomy of the posterior

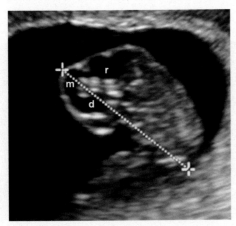

**FIGURE 1.3:** Sagittal view of an 8-week gestation. *Calipers*, CRL measurement; *d*, diencephalon; *m*, mesencephalon; *r*, rhombencephalon.

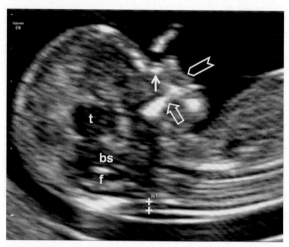

**FIGURE 1.5:** Sagittal view of a 12- to 13-week fetus. The fetal head and upper torso occupy the majority of the image, and the fetus is in a neutral position. *Calipers*, NT measurement; *solid arrow*, nasal bone; *t*, thalamus; *bs*, brain stem; *f*, fourth ventricle; *open arrow*, maxilla; *chevron*, upper lip.

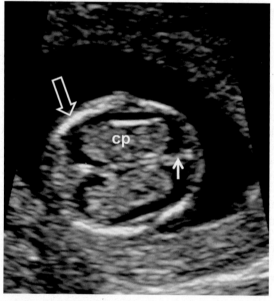

**FIGURE 1.6:** Axial view of the fetal head at 12 weeks' gestation. *cp*, choroid plexus; *solid arrow*, falx cerebri; *open arrow*, ossified portion of calvarium.

fossa can be examined and used to screen for spina bifida in this view.[12] The methodology for assessment of these features as well as the overall utility of the 11 to 13$^{+6}$ week scan is discussed in detail in Chapter 8.

Fetal anatomy is most readily assessed with a transverse sweep, running from head to toe. In this section, the intracranial anatomy essentially consists of the lateral ventricles and a very thin layer of brain parenchyma. The lateral ventricles are essentially filled by choroid plexi, which are seen as paired echogenic structures, one within each hemisphere ("butterfly view"). The midline falx is visible as an echogenic line running antero-posteriorly in the midline bisecting the "butterfly" (Fig. 1.6). The posterior fossa contains the developing cerebellum. Since the cerebellar vermis is not yet fused, a large midline communication is seen between the developing fourth ventricle and the cisterna magna (CM) (Fig. 1.7). The posterior fossa undergoes rapid change during the late first trimester, and by 13 to 14 weeks the cerebellum begins to assume a shape resembling that seen in the mid-second trimester (Fig. 1.8). Occasionally, the third ventricle can be detected in a midcoronal section of the head (Fig. 1.9).

After 11 weeks' gestation, the calvarium should be ossified and is seen as an echogenic ring around the intracranial structures (see Fig. 1.6). Absence of an ossified calvarium in association with abnormal intracranial anatomy is consistent with exencephaly/anencephaly sequence. As the transducer is moved caudally, the orbits can be identified. However, these are often better seen in a coronal section of the face (Fig. 1.10). The face, specifically lips and nose, are best examined in sagittal section (see Fig. 1.5). In this view, an upper lip seen extending beyond the tip of the nose raises the possibility of cleft lip and palate.

In an axial section at the superior aspect of the thorax, clavicles can be seen even early in gestation (Fig. 1.11). The four-chamber view and outflow tracts can be assessed using both grayscale and color Doppler imaging (Figs. 1.12 to 1.14). The stomach should be visible in the upper abdomen, and the integrity of the diaphragm can be assessed in sagittal or coronal sections (Figs. 1.15 and 1.16). Returning to an axial section, the anterior abdominal wall and cord insertion are evaluated (Fig. 1.17). The kidneys are generally difficult to see owing to their small size and echogenicity, which is similar to that of the small bowel. Both axial and coronal views are often required in order to identify them with confidence (Figs. 1.18 and 1.19). Color Doppler may be used to look for the renal arteries. However, it should be kept in mind that since the vessels are very

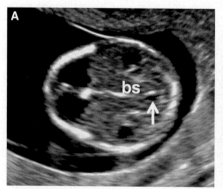
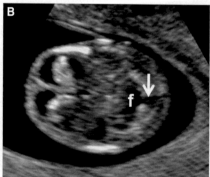
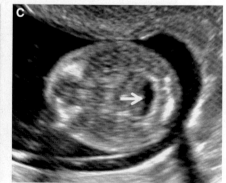

**FIGURE 1.7:** Transverse views of a fetal head at 12 weeks' gestation demonstrating hindbrain appearance at various levels in descending order. **A:** *Arrow*, developing aqueduct of Sylvius; *bs*, brain stem. **B:** *Arrow*, open communication with cisterna magna; *f*, fourth ventricle. **C:** *Arrow*, cisterna magna.

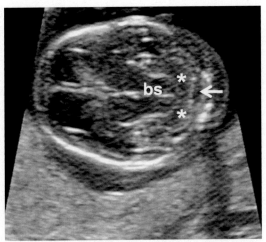

**FIGURE 1.8:** Transverse views of a fetal head at 13.5 weeks' gestation demonstrating progressive development of the cerebellum. Compare with Figure 1.7. *bs*, brainstem; *asterisks*, cerebellar hemispheres; *arrow*, cisterna magna.

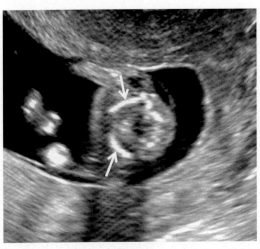

**FIGURE 1.11:** Transverse view of the lower neck at 12 to 13 weeks' gestation. *Solid arrows*, clavicles.

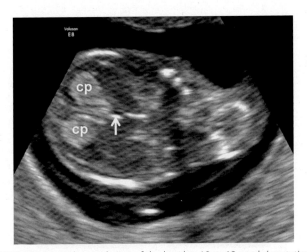

**FIGURE 1.9:** Midcoronal view of the head at 12 to 13 weeks' gestation. *cp*, choroid plexus; *arrow*, third ventricle.

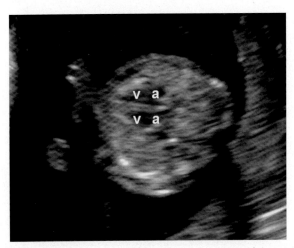

**FIGURE 1.12:** Transverse view of the chest at 12 to 13 weeks' gestation containing a four-chamber heart view. *v*, ventricles; *a*, atria.

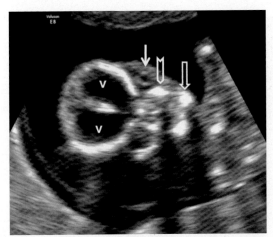

**FIGURE 1.10:** Coronal view of the fetal face. *v*, lateral ventricles; *solid arrow*, ocular orbit with a lens within it; *chevron*, maxilla; *open arrow*, body of the mandible.

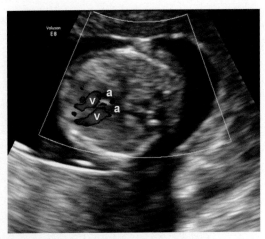

**FIGURE 1.13:** Transverse view of the chest at 12 to 13 weeks' gestation containing a four-chamber heart view in diastole with the ventricles *(v)* highlighted using color Doppler. *a*, atria.

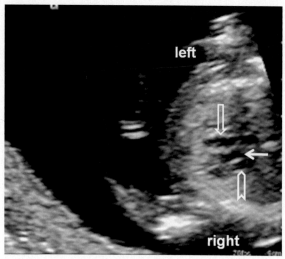

**FIGURE 1.14:** Transverse view of the chest at 12 to 13 weeks' gestation at the level of the three-vessel view. *Open arrow*, pulmonary artery; *solid arrow*, aorta; *chevron*, superior vena cava.

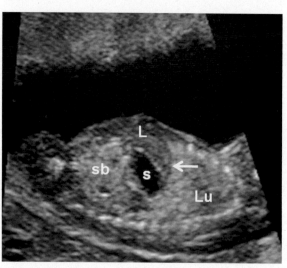

**FIGURE 1.16:** Left longitudinal view of the abdomen at 12 weeks' gestation demonstrating the left lung *(Lu)*, intact diaphragm *(arrow)*, left lobe of the liver *(L)*, stomach *(s)*, and small bowel *(sb)*. Note the difference in echogenicities between the various organs.

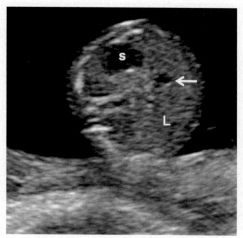

**FIGURE 1.15:** Transverse view of the abdomen at 13 weeks' gestation at the level of the abdominal circumference. *s*, stomach; *L*, liver; *arrow*, portal sinus.

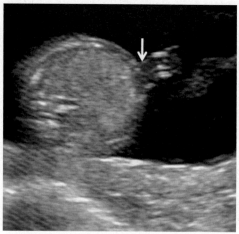

**FIGURE 1.17:** Transverse view of the abdomen at 13 weeks' gestation at the level of abdominal cord insertion *(arrow)*.

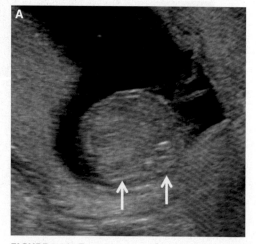
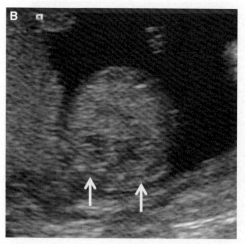

**FIGURE 1.18:** Transverse view of the abdomen at the level of the kidneys *(arrows)* at 12 weeks' gestation **(A)** and at 13 weeks' gestation **(B)**.

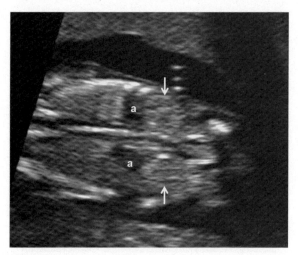

**FIGURE 1.19:** Coronal view of the abdomen at 12 weeks' gestation at the level of the kidneys *(arrows)*. Note the relatively prominent adrenal glands *(a)*, which need to be kept in mind in order not to mistake them for the kidneys.

small, only small adjustments of the transducer can affect their visualization (Fig. 1.20).[56,57]

The bladder should be visible in all cases from 12 weeks' onward. It is best assessed in the midsagittal section. A standardized longitudinal measurement of the bladder in the first trimester should be performed in this view if it appears to be enlarged.[58] The same section provides information regarding fetal gender by qualitative evaluation or measurement of the angle between the genital tubercle and the fetal longitudinal axis. A small angle, which is essentially parallel to the longitudinal axis of the fetus, indicates a female gender, whereas an angle measuring 30° or more suggests a male gender (Figs. 1.21 and 1.22). Using this method, the accuracy of sex determination is only 70% at 11 weeks' gestation but increases to nearly 100% at 13 to 14 weeks' gestation.[59]

A skeletal survey is best performed by utilizing both axial and transverse sections. Both hands are commonly held in front of the chest or fetal face, and the legs are generally flexed at the hip at this gestation. The number of fingers is relatively easy to assess in the first trimester as all fingers, including the thumb, lie in approximately the same ultrasound plane (Fig. 1.23). Fetal feet can also be identified, though evaluating the number of toes may be difficult because of their small size (Fig. 1.24). There is a tendency of the ankles to turn inward, making the diagnosis of clubfoot in the first trimester challenging. Both the femur and the humerus can be identified and measured (Figs. 1.25 and 1.26).

Color Doppler may be used to help define the cord insertion and the number of arteries in the cord (Fig. 1.27). It can also be used to localize the DV in a right parasagittal section, allowing pulse wave assessment of this vessel for aneuploidy and cardiac screening. The hepatic artery peak systolic velocity may be evaluated in the same section to aid in aneuploidy risk assessment (Fig. 1.28).[8] Doppler examination involves higher power levels and consequently should generally be avoided during the embryonic period (≤10 weeks' menstrual gestational age) unless the benefits clearly outweigh the risks. When using Doppler during the 11 to 13[+6] week scan, power indices should be reduced to a minimum, and the region of interest should be interrogated for the minimum time necessary. Often, the region of interest can be effectively identified using grayscale prior to employing Doppler, resulting in reduced energy exposure to the fetus.

## ASSESSING FETAL ANATOMY DURING THE SECOND AND THIRD TRIMESTERS

Standard assessment of the fetus is quite complex. It is best to develop a systematic approach to the examination. A complete examination of the uterine contents in pregnancy includes much more than evaluation of the fetal anatomy; the remaining issues will be discussed in later chapters. The issue of fetal biometry is discussed in this chapter only to illustrate the proper technique rather than clinical applicability.

Fetal anatomy is best assessed at 20 to 24 weeks' gestation. At this point, the pregnant uterus is out of the pelvis and is located well within the maternal abdomen. The fetus usually presents

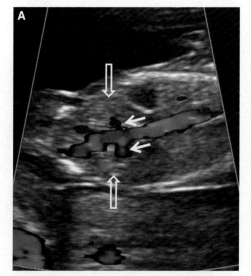
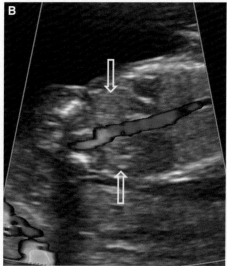

**FIGURE 1.20:** Coronal view of the abdomen at the level of the kidneys *(open arrows)* in a 12- to 13-week fetus. Color Doppler is used to demonstrate the renal arteries *(solid arrows)* in **A**, which can become nondetectable with only a slight adjustment of the transducer, as in **B**.

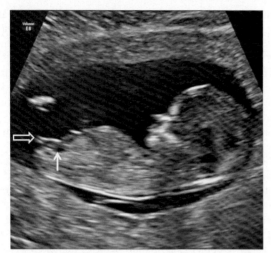

**FIGURE 1.21:** Sagittal view of a 12- to 13-week fetus demonstrating the presence of a small urinary bladder *(solid arrow)*. The genital tubercle *(open arrow)* points in a direction parallel to the longitudinal axis of the fetus, indicating a female gender.

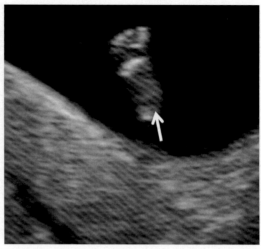

**FIGURE 1.24:** Fetal foot *(arrow)* with all five toes visible (12 to 13 weeks' gestation).

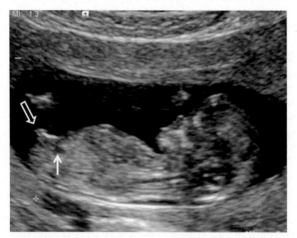

**FIGURE 1.22:** Sagittal view of a 12- to 13-week fetus demonstrating the presence of a small urinary bladder *(solid arrow)*. The genital tubercle *(open arrow)* up from the fetal longitudinal axis (>30°).

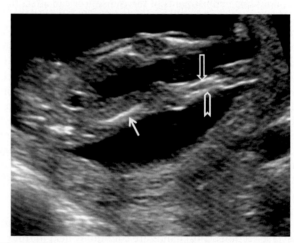

**FIGURE 1.25:** Both lower extremities visible at 13 to 14 weeks' gestation. *Solid arrow,* femur; *open arrow,* tibia; *chevron,* fibula.

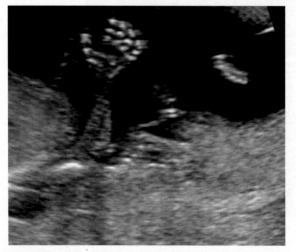

**FIGURE 1.23:** Fetal hand with all phalangeal ossification centers visible (13 to 14 weeks' gestation).

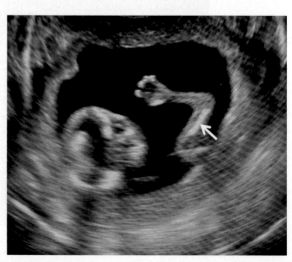

**FIGURE 1.26:** Upper extremity at 12 to 13 weeks' gestation. *Arrow,* humerus.

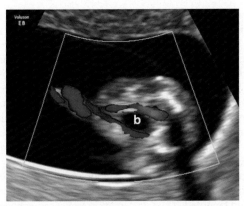

**FIGURE 1.27:** Transverse/oblique section of the lower abdomen and the pelvis showing the urinary bladder *(b)* with two umbilical arteries coursing around it in a 12- to 13-week fetus.

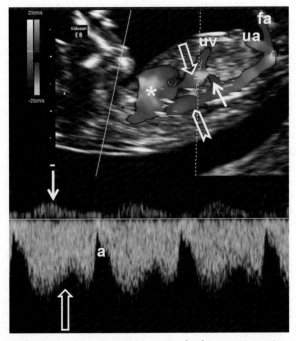

**FIGURE 1.28:** Right parasagittal section of a fetus at 12 to 13 weeks' gestation with color and pulsed Doppler. *Asterisk,* heart; *chevron,* aorta; *open arrows,* ductus venosus and its corresponding waveform; *solid arrows,* hepatic artery and its corresponding waveform; *uv,* umbilical vein; *ua,* umbilical artery; *fa,* femoral artery.

itself in a better axis for examination. The fetus is also larger and more developed, making the detection of anomalies easier.[60–73] In some jurisdictions, the anomaly scan is performed earlier (e.g., at 18 to 20 weeks' gestation) in view of the legal restrictions related to interruption of pregnancy if there are abnormal findings. However, it should be pointed out that there is a statistically significant difference in being able to complete the fetal anatomic survey if it is performed at 18 to 18+6 (in 76% of cases) versus 20 to 22+6 weeks' gestation (in 90% of cases).[74]

The approach to the anatomical survey is essentially the same in both the second and the third trimesters. However, fetal position, reduction in amniotic fluid volume, and increased bony ossification often make the third trimester examination more challenging. It is, however, good practice to briefly check fetal anatomy at the third trimester scan, even if a more comprehensive survey has previously been done at 20 to 24 weeks. Some

anomalies may be more readily detectable with the fetus in a different position and others (e.g., duodenal atresia, X-linked aqueductal stenosis, certain skeletal dysplasias, and fetal tumors) generally only become apparent after the mid-second trimester examination. The exact timing of the examination may also depend on maternal habitus. Increased BMI can significantly compromise the ultrasound examination and may require a change in the usual strategy. One reasonable approach to evaluating a fetus in an obese patient is to perform a thorough examination at 12 weeks' gestation using the transvaginal route and delay the anomaly scan until 22 to 24 weeks' gestation to increase the likelihood of successfully completing the structural examination.

Immediately after starting the scan, the fetal heart is checked, establishing viability and providing some reassurance to the mother. The uterus should then be scanned in cross section, from left to right and from top to bottom, determining the number of fetuses that are present and defining the lie of the fetus. Placental site and cervical length can then be assessed, although true cervical assessment requires a transvaginal approach, which is best performed at the end of the examination.

Standard fetal biometry includes the following measurements: biparietal diameter (BPD), head circumference (HC), abdominal circumference (AC), and femur length (FL).[75–80] Other measurements that are commonly performed as a part of a routine examination in some centers are the humerus length (HL) and the transcerebellar diameter (TCD).[81,82] The correct manner in which each of these measurements should be obtained is described in the individual sections below. Additional fetal biometry is performed if clinically appropriate. Standard measurements of essentially all fetal structures have been published.

## Calvarium

The shape, measurements, and integrity of the calvarium are best assessed utilizing axial and sagittal views. In the axial section, the contour of the fetal head is normally oval in shape. In order to assess the symmetry of the two halves of the brain, regardless of the level of the axial view, care should be taken to keep the falx cerebri truly in the midline. The BPD is assessed using an axial image of the head at a level where standard anatomic landmarks are visible: The globular and slightly hypoechoic paired structures representing the thalami in the midportion of the head with a slit-like hypoechoic structure representing the third ventricle located between them, the cavum septi pellucidi (CSP) in front of the thalami, and the lateral ventricles, with the frontal horns seen anteriorly and the atria (trigones) seen posteriorly. Care should be taken with caliper placement as the authors of some charts measure from the outer aspect of the calvarium in the near field to the inner aspect of the calvarium in the far field, while others use an outer–outer approach. The HC is measured by tracing around the outside of the calvarium in the same axial section as the BPD. In addition to measuring the BPD and HC, the occipitofrontal diameter (OFD) can be measured and expressed in ratio to the BPD (BPD/OFD) as the cephalic index (CI) (Fig. 1.29). This ratio is valuable in describing the shape of the head. The normal range for CI is 0.74 to 0.83. A CI, which is below 0.74, connotes a relatively flat head (dolichocephaly), while a CI above 0.83 describes a relatively round head (brachycephaly).[83] Dolichocephaly is not uncommon and is often seen in fetuses that are in a persistently breech presentation or in association with chronic oligohydramnios. Dolichocephaly has been reported in fetuses with sagittal synostosis. Brachycephaly

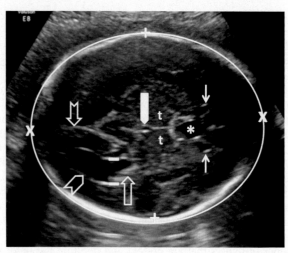

**FIGURE 1.29:** Axial view of the fetal head at the BPD level. *Calipers,* BPD measurement; *chevron,* lateral ventricle (occipital horn); *open arrow,* lateral ventricle (atrium containing echogenic choroid plexus); *thin solid arrows,* lateral ventricle (frontal horns); *notched arrow,* lateral ventricle (occipital horn); *thick solid arrow,* third ventricle; *t,* thalamus; *asterisk,* cavum septi pellucidi. Please note the difference in anatomic detail between the proximal and distal half of the brain.

may also be a normal variant but has been described in association with trisomy 21. It can also be seen in conditions where the skull is poorly ossified such as certain types of osteogenesis imperfecta and hypophosphatasia. In these conditions, the skull is also easily compressible, which can be demonstrated by applying gentle pressure with the ultrasound transducer.

The shape of the skull may be abnormal in association with a number of specific fetal anomalies. In the mid-second trimester, bifrontal scalloping occurs in >95% of open neural tube defects resulting in a "lemon"-shaped calvarium seen in the axial section.[84,85] The occipital portion of the skull is typically flattened in trisomy 18, while the frontal and parietal portions of the skull gently slope toward one another anteriorly, creating a "strawberry" shape in axial view. Premature closure of multiple cranial sutures restricts expansion of the skull, particularly with advancing gestation, resulting in a "cloverleaf" appearance. The sagittal section offers the best view of the fetal forehead. Abnormalities such as frontal bossing, which are part of a number of skeletal dysplasias or a sloping forehead present in conditions such as microcephaly, are best visualized in this fashion.

The calvarium should be systematically examined to ensure that it is intact. The most common defects are a cephalocele or an encephalocele. These are generally located in the occipital portion of the calvarium, but can be seen less frequently in the area of the nasal root anteriorly or parietally. Disruption of the skull can also occur at more unusual sites, especially when it is caused by amniotic bands. The calvarium will be completely absent in anencephaly.

## Intracranial Anatomy

Intracranial anatomy is complex and gestational age–dependent owing to rapid embryologic and later fetal development.[86] The sections most commonly employed to look at the fetal anatomy are axial ones. This is because of the fact that they are the easiest to obtain and are very familiar to operators who are involved in fetal scanning.

The half of the brain that is closest to the transducer is much more difficult to image clearly when compared with the distal half. This is due to ossification of the skull, which casts an acoustic shadow over the proximal portion of the fetal brain. With advancing gestation, increasing calcification of the calvarium limits resolution. Images can often be improved by rotating the probe so the brain is imaged through the suture lines and fontanelles, using techniques similar to those applied during neonatal examination. Employing the transvaginal route to image a fetus that is cephalic in presentation can facilitate a detailed examination of the intracranial anatomy.

The general symmetry of the fetal brain is first assessed using standard axial views. The presence and position of the falx cerebri should be noted. The falx cerebri is seen as an echogenic line running in the anteroposterior direction. It is a structure that is usually very easy to visualize, and if absent, the possibility of a severe structural defect such as alobar holoprosencephaly should be entertained. The cerebral cortex is a hypoechoic structure, which is fairly thin and difficult to visualize at early gestations. The proportion of the cranial cavity that it fills progressively increases as the gestation advances. The structures that are easiest to identify because of their well-delineated boundaries and greatest differences in echogenicity from the surrounding cortex are the lateral ventricles and the CSP. Routine examination of the intracranial anatomy should always include identification of these structures.

Each lateral ventricle is divided into five parts: The frontal horn, the body of the lateral ventricle, the occipital horn, the inferior (temporal) horn, and the atrium (trigone). The atrium is the point of confluence between the occipital horn, inferior horn, and the body of the lateral ventricle and is the largest, most easily identifiable portion of the lateral ventricle. In axial section at the level of the thalami, the atrium can be measured. This is normally done at the level of the posterior margin of the choroid plexus using a magnified image so that calipers can be accurately placed on the inner margins of the ventricular walls (Fig. 1.29). Enlargement of the lateral ventricle (ventriculomegaly) will be recognized by measurement at this point. At 20 weeks' gestation, the upper limit of normal is considered to be 10 mm, although recently some authors have suggested that even measurements up to 12 mm are very unlikely to be associated with significant pathology.[87–90] The ventricles become less prominent with advancing gestation although a threshold of measurement <10 mm is typically also used in the third trimester.

It needs to be kept in mind that the shape of the lateral ventricle is 3D complex; unless it is enlarged, it is difficult to visualize in its entirety in a single ultrasound plane. The atrium is located medially. The body and the anterior horn of the lateral ventricle radiate anteriorly, superiorly, and laterally from the atrium. The occipital horns project posteriorly. The temporal horn extends from the atrium in an inferior and anterior direction. Additionally, the bodies of the lateral ventricle and their continuation, the frontal horns, are domed in shape in the sagittal section; therefore, their appearance differs significantly when viewed in various axial planes. The inferior (temporal) horns run through the area of the temporal lobe and are difficult to identify unless they are enlarged. The shape of the ventricles is best assessed using the combination of longitudinal and coronal views (Figs. 1.30 to 1.33). The atrium contains a globular and echogenic structure, the glomus of the choroid plexus. In the majority of cases, the glomus is homogeneous in its ultrasound appearance. However, occasionally echolucent

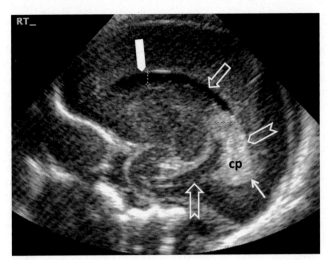

**FIGURE 1.30:** Sagittal view of the lateral ventricle at 24 weeks' gestation. Note that this is a neonatal image to show the anatomy in its entirety. *cp*, choroid plexus; *thick solid arrow*, frontal horn; *open arrow*, body of the lateral ventricle; *chevron*, trigone; *thin solid arrow*, portion of the occipital horn; *notched arrow*, inferior (temporal) horn.

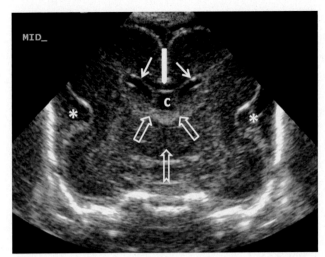

**FIGURE 1.32:** Midcoronal view of the brain at 24 weeks' gestation. Please note the increased echogenicity of the roof of the third ventricle extending into the foramina of Monro. This represents the choroid plexus. Note that this is a neonatal image to show the anatomy in its entirety. *Thin solid arrows*, bodies of the lateral ventricles; *thick solid arrow*, corpus callosum; *open arrows*, location of the foramina of Monro; *notched arrow*, third ventricle; *asterisk*, operculization of the insula; *c*, cavum septi pellucidi.

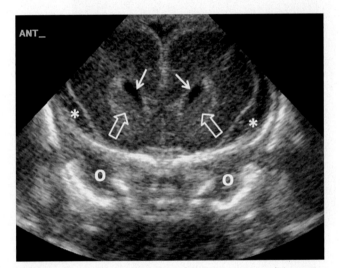

**FIGURE 1.31:** Anterior coronal view of the brain at 24 weeks' gestation. Please note the increased amount of extra-axial fluid, which is normal early in gestation. Note that this is a neonatal image to show the anatomy in its entirety. *Solid arrows*, frontal horns of the lateral ventricles; *open arrows*, caudate nuclei; *o*, orbit; *asterisk*, extra-axial fluid.

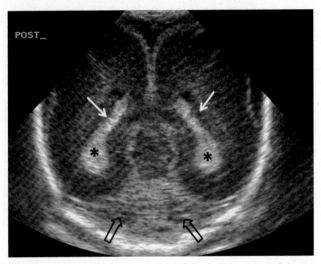

**FIGURE 1.33:** Posterior coronal view of the brain at 24 weeks' gestation. Note that this is a neonatal image to show the anatomy in its entirety. *White arrows*, trigones; *asterisks*, choroid plexi; *black arrows*, section through a portion of the cerebellum.

structures of varying complexity and size called choroid plexus cysts (CPCs) are present.[91–93] They can develop in any portion of the choroid plexus, but those that are ≥3 mm tend to be located in the glomus. Unilateral or bilateral CPCs are a common finding affecting 1% to 4% of euploid fetuses but have also been associated with aneuploidy, particularly trisomy 18. They invariably resolve spontaneously and do not represent a true pathologic entity. When found in isolation, risk for aneuploidy is not increased, but it is worth reviewing the results of first trimester screening, and in particular of first trimester biochemistry (both free β-hCG (beta human chorionic gonadotropin) and PAPP-A (pregnancy-associated plasma protein A) are low in trisomy 18), to check there are no common themes through different modalities of screening. The choroid plexus does not extend into the anterior horn of the lateral ventricle; therefore,

cystic structures seen anterior to the caudothalamic notch will have a different underlying etiology.

The CSP and its posterior extension, the cavum septi vergae (CSV), are seen as a continuous hypoechoic structure located in the midline. It represents a space between the two septi pellucidi, which is filled with cerebrospinal fluid (CSF). Not infrequently, the cavum septi pellucidi et vergae (CSPV) contains septations, especially in its posterior portion (Fig. 1.34). The CSPV begins to close in the third trimester, a process that is completed in infancy.

There is no direct communication between the ventricular system and CSPV; it is diffusion across the thin septi pellucidi that allows CSF to enter this space. This space begins to close in late gestation, a process that is completed during infancy. It is bounded by the corpus callosum anteriorly and superiorly, the fornix posteriorly, and the anterior commissure inferiorly.

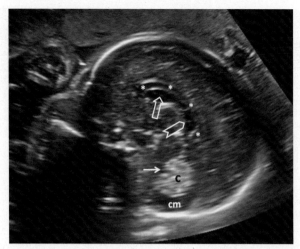

**FIGURE 1.34:** Sagittal view of the fetal head at 24 weeks' gestation. Please note the septations in the cavum septi vergae seen as echogenic lines running anteroposteriorly. *Asterisks*, corpus callosum; *open arrow*, cavum septi pellucidi; chevron, cavum septi vergae; *solid arrow*, fourth ventricle; *c*, cerebellum; *cm*, cisterna magna.

In a midsagittal section, the CSPV is arched in shape. Therefore, in the standard axial section at the level of the BPD, usually it is only the CSP that is visible. In this section, the CSP appears as a hypoechoic roughly rectangular structure located anteriorly to the thalami. As a normal variant, the CSV can be unusually large and visible in this section. Since the CSPV is arched in shape, may appear to be separate from the cavum septi pellucid, simulating a cyst (Fig. 1.35). Examination of the CSPV in the sagittal section will help to elucidate the diagnosis (see Fig. 1.34). A cystic midline structure that is occasionally seen located posteriorly and inferiorly to the CSV is the cavum veli interpositi (Fig. 1.36). This is a normal variant and is part of the leptomeningeal space between the roof of the third ventricle and the body of the fornices. The size of this structure normally does not exceed 1 cm. It can be difficult to distinguish from an arachnoid cyst located at the quadrigeminal cistern.[94,95]

The importance of positively identifying the CSPV lies in the fact that it can be absent in association with midline defects. It should be remembered that the anterior pillars of the fornices lie in the same general area as the CSP. They are hypoechoic and have a generally rectangular shape in the axial plane. This can lead to a

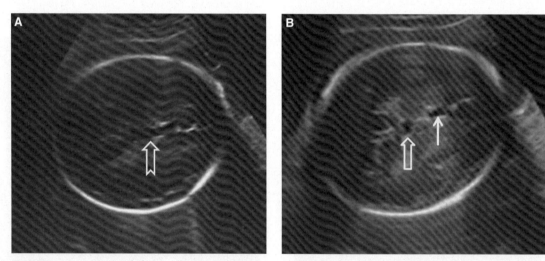

**FIGURE 1.35:** Axial view of a fetal head at 32 weeks. **A:** Section through the cavum septum pellucidi et vergae at a point when continuity between two is evident *(arrow)*. **B:** Axial view in a plane slightly caudal to **A**, where the cavum septi pellucidi *(solid arrow)* and cavum septi vergae *(open arrow)* are seen as two separate structures. The latter should not be mistaken for a cyst.

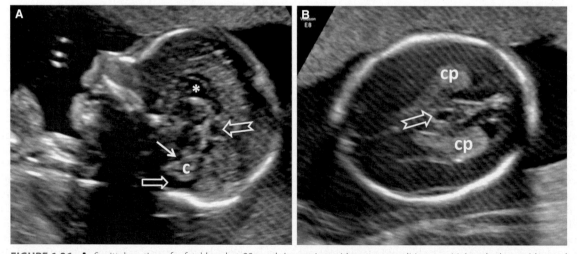

**FIGURE 1.36: A:** Sagittal section of a fetal head at 22 weeks' gestation with a cavum veli interpositi *(notched arrow)* located posteriorly and inferiorly to CSPV *(asterisk)*. *Solid arrow*, fourth ventricle; *open arrow*, cisterna magna; *c*, cerebellum. **B:** Axial view of the same fetus. *Arrow*, cavum veli interpositi; *cp*, choroid plexus.

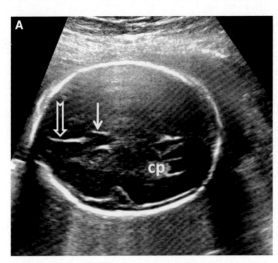
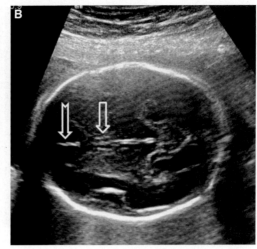

**FIGURE 1.37: A:** Axial section of a fetal head at 22 weeks' gestation at the level of the cavum septi pellucidi *(solid arrow)*. *Notched arrow,* falx cerebri; *cp,* choroid plexus. **B:** Axial view of the same fetus in slightly more caudal section. Note the two juxtaposed pillars of the fornix *(open arrow)* with a midline echogenic division. *Notched arrow,* falx cerebri.

false impression that the CSP is present, consequently missing the diagnosis of anomalies that can be associated with absent CSPV such as agenesis of corpus callosum, septo-optic dysplasia, lobar holoprosencephaly, and neuronal migration defects. However, unlike the CSP, a thin echogenic line can be seen between the two fornices, which helps to differentiate between the two entities (Fig. 1.37).[96] In the sagittal view, visualization of the pericallosal artery helps to confirm the presence of the corpus callosum (Fig. 1.38). Since the corpus callosum is a structure that completes its formation relatively late in pregnancy, the CSPV should not be expected to be visible prior to 18 to 19 weeks' gestation.

The third ventricle is located inferiorly to the CSP, between the paired thalami. This slit-like structure is filled with CSF and is hypoechoic in its ultrasound appearance (see Fig. 1.29). It is normally small (<3 mm diameter) and may be difficult to visualize. Enlargement of the third ventricle is typically only seen in association with enlargement of the lateral ventricles.

Examination of the cerebral cortex focuses on ruling out any space occupying lesions, either cystic or solid in nature. Cortical maturation continues throughout pregnancy, as the brain develops gyri and loses its smooth appearance (Fig. 1.39).

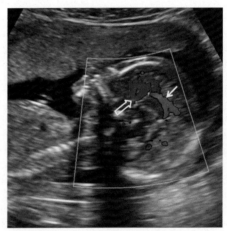

**FIGURE 1.38:** Sagittal view of the fetal head at 22 weeks. Anterior cerebral *(open arrow)* and pericallosal *(solid arrow)* arteries with some of their branches are demonstrated using color Doppler.

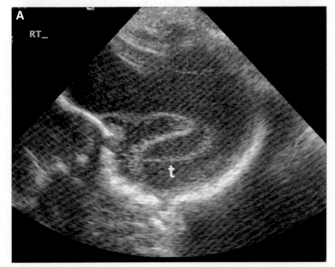
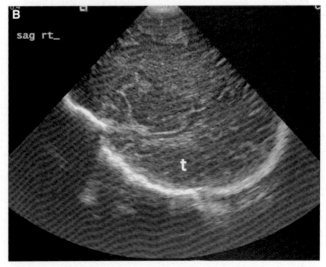

**FIGURE 1.39:** Parasagittal section of the fetal head with the temporal lobe *(t)* visible. Please note the difference in the texture of the surface of the cortex, with absent sulci and gyri at 22 weeks' gestation **(A)** and well-developed pattern of sulci and gyri at term **(B)**.

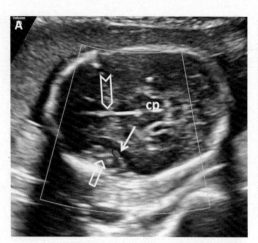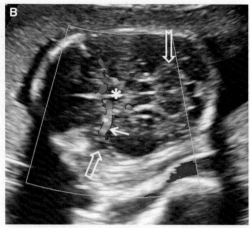

**FIGURE 1.40: A:** Axial section of a fetal head at 20 weeks' gestation demonstrating the insula at an early stage of operculization *(open arrow)* with the middle cerebral artery (color Doppler) at its base *(solid arrow). Chevron,* falx cerebri; *cp,* cerebral peduncles. **B:** Slightly more caudal section of the same fetus demonstrating the course of the middle cerebral artery *(solid arrow)* to the base of the insula *(open arrow)* with color Doppler. *Asterisk,* center of the circle of Willis; *notched arrow,* cerebellum.

The process of cortical maturation can be most easily observed in the insula. Even though operculization of the insula begins at approximately 14 weeks' gestation, on ultrasound, this process does not become evident until approximately 19 weeks' gestation. It begins as infolding of the cerebral cortex at the lateral edge of the cerebrum located initially in the anterior half of the distance between the occiput and the forehead. It first appears as a heterogeneous depression, which is increased in echogenicity. Prominent pulsations can be seen at the bottom of the depression, which represents the Sylvian segment of the middle cerebral artery (Fig. 1.40). As operculization progresses, the depression is roofed over by the temporal lobe. By the completion of the process at the beginning of the third trimester, it remains as only a slit-like structure, representing the Sylvian fissure (Fig. 1.41). Absence of normal operculization raises the possibility of a neuronal migration defect such as lissencephaly.

### Posterior Fossa

Another axial section routinely employed to evaluate the intracranial anatomy is the suboccipitobregmatic view: Starting with the BPD view, the posterior aspect of the probe is rotated caudally until the posterior fossa becomes visible. Even though this view is primarily designed to evaluate the posterior fossa and the back of the fetal head, it also offers a good view of the CSP, thalami, and the midbrain as well as their anatomic relationship (Fig. 1.42). Sagittal views of the posterior fossa are also very informative. Coronal sections add very little information to the axial ones, but depending on the position of the fetus, this approach may provide the clearest view.

Routine examination of the posterior fossa is critical to detect not only anomalies that originate in the posterior fossa but also changes that are indicative of problems in the spine. In addition to the bifrontal scalloping of the cranium described earlier, open spine defects are accompanied by the Chiari Type II

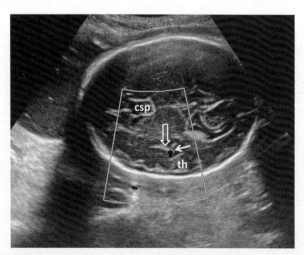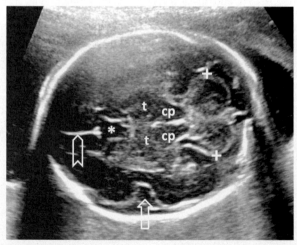

**FIGURE 1.41:** Axial view of a fetal head in the third trimester after the completion of insular operculization. *th,* temporal horn; *solid arrow,* color Doppler of the middle cerebral artery; *open arrow,* Sylvian fissure; *csp,* cavum septi pellucidi.

**FIGURE 1.42:** Suboccipitobregmatic view of the head. *Calipers,* transcerebellar diameter; *cp,* cerebral peduncles; *t,* thalami; *open arrow,* insula; *asterisk,* cavum septi pellucidi; *chevron,* falx cerebri.

malformation (herniation of the cerebellar tonsils through the foramen magnum and downward displacement of the cerebellar vermis). In the axial view, this defect translates into flattening of the cerebellar hemispheres with an anterior bend (so-called banana sign) and obliteration of the CM.[84,85,97–99] Finally, since most cephaloceles and encephaloceles are located in the occipital region of the skull, examination of the posterior fossa must also include a careful evaluation of the calvarium in that region.[100]

The formation of the cerebellar hemispheres and the connecting vermis continues throughout the first half of the pregnancy. Since the vermis is not fully developed until mid-gestation, vermian defects, especially small ones, are difficult to diagnose prior to 18 to 20 weeks' gestation. Using axial planes, the mid-second trimester cerebellum is seen as a dumbbell-shaped structure consisting of two hemispheres connected by the vermis. The shape of the cerebellar hemispheres becomes somewhat flattened on its anterior surface. As gestation advances, the vermis increases in echogenicity in relation to the hemispheres, and the caudal part of the vermis becomes notched (cerebellar tonsils). The hemispheres develop gyri through the third trimester, which are visible on ultrasound, and the cerebellar tonsils become more elongated. An axial view of the inferior aspect of the cerebellum at this point in pregnancy may reveal

a fluid-filled space between the tonsils, which may lead to the erroneous diagnosis of a defect in the vermis. The TCD is measured in an axial section using the suboccipitobregmatic view. Care must be taken so that the cerebellar hemispheres are symmetrical, and the measurement is done at a point where the distance between the lateral edges of the two hemispheres is the greatest.[101,102]

Every attempt should be made to visualize both cerebellar hemispheres to allow a comparison of their size and echotexture. There are conditions that may affect only one of the cerebellar hemispheres such as unilateral hypoplasia, hemorrhage, or infarction. If a cerebellar defect or ventriculomegaly is suspected, the fourth ventricle should be evaluated. It is seen as a hypoechoic structure between the cerebral peduncles and the cerebellum (Fig. 1.43). Isolated enlargement of the fourth ventricle is unlikely to occur and is of limited clinical significance.

The CM is a CSF-filled structure that is located behind the cerebellum. If it appears to be exceptionally large, it can be objectively assessed by measurement of its anteroposterior diameter in an axial section of the posterior fossa (Fig. 1.44). Even though normal CM diameter is below 10 mm, isolated CM enlargement (mega-cisterna magna) is considered to be a normal variant. Nonetheless, a large CM should lead to a detailed evaluation of the fetal anatomy overall and the cerebellar vermis

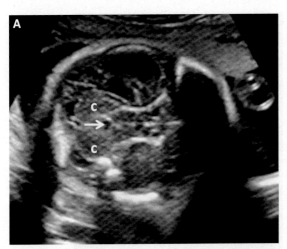
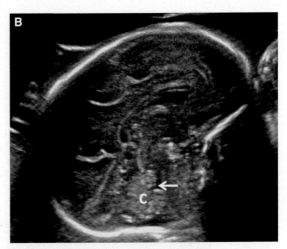

**FIGURE 1.43: A:** Axial section of a fetal head in the mid-second trimester weeks demonstrating the fourth ventricle *(arrow)*. *c,* cerebellar hemispheres. **B:** Sagittal section of a fetal head in the early third trimester. *Arrow,* fourth ventricle; *c,* cerebellum.

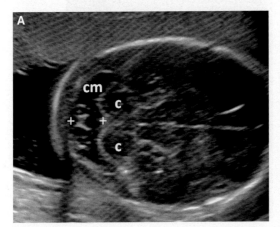
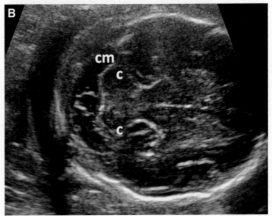

**FIGURE 1.44: A, B:** Suboccipitobregmatic views of the head demonstrating a variety of normal septations within the cisterna magna *(cm)*. Note the formation of a cyst-like structure in **B**. *Calipers,* cisterna magna measurement; *c,* cerebellar hemispheres.

specifically, as this finding has a weak association with trisomy 13 and 21 and verminan defects. Septations within the CM are a common finding and occasionally they can simulate a small cyst. These are due to subarachnoid trabeculae and represent a normal finding.[103–105]

With the exception of the above-described Chiari Type II malformation, most defects affecting the posterior fossa are cystic in nature (Dandy–Walker malformation, Blake's pouch, arachnoid cysts, and dysgenesis of the cerebellar vermis). These diagnoses can be difficult to tease out and depend on findings in axial, midsagittal, and coronal sections. The posterior fossa anomalies are one area where a fetal MRI may be especially helpful in arriving at the correct diagnosis.

Finally, the suboccipitobregmatic view is also used as a standardized view for nuchal fold measurement. Thickened (>6 mm) nuchal fold is associated with an increased risk of trisomy 21.

### Fetal Spine

Assessment of the central nervous system is not complete without detailed examination of the fetal spine. This involves evaluation of the vertebrae and the contents of the spinal canal. Open spinal defects also disrupt the skin, so careful examination of the cutaneous covering of the spine is also important. The vertebral column should be evaluated in at least two of the three planes: coronal, axial, and longitudinal (midsagittal). The vertebrae have three ossification centers visible prenatally: Vertebral body anteriorly and one in each of the vertebral arches (laminae) posteriorly. In the axial section, the three ossification centers are in a triangular arrangement. The vertebral body ossification center is round and is located in the midline. The paired laminar ossification centers are slightly offset from the midline. They are linear in shape and form a roof over the spinal canal (Fig. 1.45).[106,107] In the presence of an open spine defect, this arrangement is disrupted, and the laminar ossification centers are displaced laterally, forming the shape of the letter U or V in the axial view of the spine. Often, axial views are best for assessing the integrity of the skin. Both individual vertebrae and their skin covering should be evaluated by sliding the transducer along the entire length of the spine.

The whole length of the vertebral column can be seen in both a coronal and in a sagittal section, and the ossification centers should be spaced evenly in these views. In the coronal view, the two lateral points of ossification can be visualized cleanly, and by moving the probe anteriorly, ossification of the vertebral body can be brought into view. As the spine is curved, it is common to be able to visualize the vertebral bodies at some levels and the arches at other levels in the same view (Fig. 1.46). In longitudinal section, the line of ossification of vertebral bodies

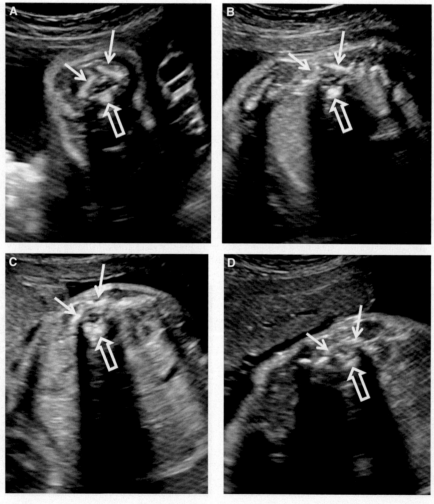

**FIGURE 1.45:** A transverse view of vertebrae at various levels of the vertebral column: cervical (**A**); thoracic (**B**); lumbar (**C**); sacral (**D**). The three ossification centers (*solid arrows*, vertebral arches; *open arrow*, vertebral body) are seen. Note the differences in their appearance depending on the level.

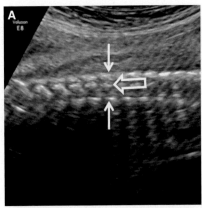
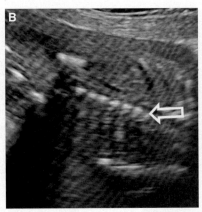
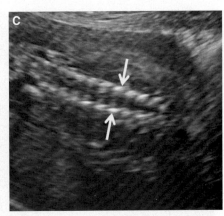

**FIGURE 1.46:** Coronal views of the vertebral column. **A:** Section demonstrating all three types of ossification centers in the same view. *Solid arrows,* vertebral arch ossifications; *open arrow,* vertebral body ossification. **B:** Section demonstrating vertebral body ossification centers *(open arrow)* only. **C:** Section demonstrating vertebral arch ossification centers *(solid arrows)* only.

is seen anteriorly and, if there is a slight oblique cut, one set of posterior ossification sites will be visualized. In the anteroposterior axis, the spine is curved, being convex in the thoracic region and concave in the lumbosacral region. The sacral portion of the spine usually has a more persistent curvature, with the tip of the spine pointing posteriorly (Fig. 1.47). This sacral upswing may be absent in the presence of an open spine defect and in the presence of caudal regression syndrome.

Overcurvature of the thoracic spine, kyphosis, or lateral curvature of the spine, scoliosis, can be detected by careful assessment of at least two of the three standard planes. Abnormal curvature may be due to the presence of a hemivertebra, which is a feature of a number of genetic syndromes such as VACTERL; therefore, other anomalies known to be associated with this syndrome should be actively sought.

The spinal cord can be delineated within the spinal canal using ultrasound on most exams (Fig. 1.48). However, the presence of multiple vertebral ossification centers does obscure it to a variable degree, especially later in gestation. The ultrasound appearance of the spinal cord is fairly uniform with slightly decreasing size moving cranial to caudal. The conus medullaris can be identified as the place where the spinal cord comes to its end point (Fig. 1.49). Measuring the distance between the tip of the conus medullaris to the tip of the spine is potentially useful in diagnosing tethered cord, and therefore spina bifida

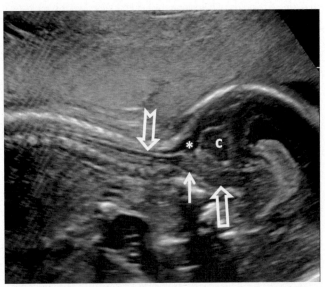

**FIGURE 1.48:** Sagittal view of the cervical spinal cord *(notched arrow)* in late second trimester. *Solid arrow,* medulla oblongata; *open arrow,* pons; *asterisk,* cisterna magna; *c,* cerebellum.

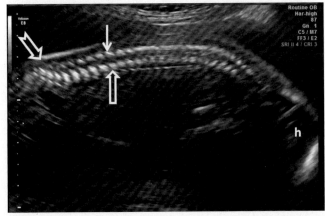

**FIGURE 1.47:** Sagittal view of the spine in mid-second trimester demonstrating its normal curvature. *Open arrow,* vertebral body ossification center; *solid arrow,* vertebral arch ossification center. Note the sacral upswing *(notched arrow)*. *h,* head.

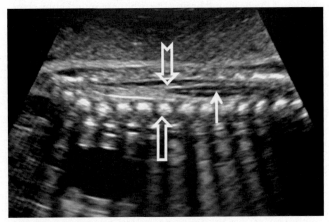

**FIGURE 1.49:** Sagittal view of the lumbar spinal cord *(solid arrow)* ending in the conus medullaris *(notched arrow)* in late second trimester. *Open arrow,* vertebral body ossification center.

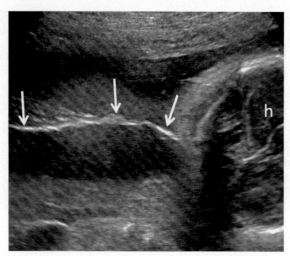

**FIGURE 1.50:** Superficial coronal view along the fetal back in the third trimester. A thin line of hair along the fetal back *(arrows)* is seen. *h*, fetal head.

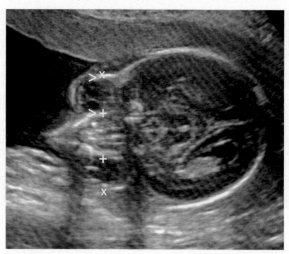

**FIGURE 1.51:** Axial view of the fetal head at the level of the orbits in mid-second trimester. The distance between two orbits is designated by + (interocular diameter), external ocular diameter by ×, and the ocular diameter by >.

occulta.[108] Fetal hair can occasionally be seen on ultrasound, especially in the third trimester.[109] It can also form a prominent echogenic line behind the fetal back generally following the outline of the spine, which may be a confusing finding for those that are not aware of this possibility (Fig. 1.50).

## Fetal Face

The face is a large and complex structure. As such, it needs to be examined at multiple levels and in multiple planes.[110] At a minimum, complete examination requires axial sections to evaluate the orbits and maxilla, a midsagittal section that identifies the nasal bone and demonstrates the profile, and a coronal section demonstrating the lips. The face should be investigated for right–left symmetry and defects of fusion. Since the formation of the face involves fusion in the midline, many of the defects are located close to the midline. Also, since the cleavage of the prosencephalon is intimately associated with formation of the facial structures, in cases where holoprosencephaly is suspected, the facial structures also need to be evaluated carefully.

The orbits should be assessed in an axial section. This is best achieved by moving the probe caudally from the standard axial section of the head and brain. The orbits are round bony structures, each containing a hypoechoic bulbus oculi. Although gestational charts for intraorbital and extraorbital diameter are available, these measurements are not routinely made. However, visually, the interorbital distance should be approximately one-third of the extraorbital distance (Fig. 1.51). A number of fetal syndromes are associated with decreased (hypotelorism) or increased (hypertelorism) interorbital distance.[111,112] Visualization of the lens of the eye will rule out anophthalmia or aphakia. This can be done in both the axial and the coronal sections. In the coronal view, the lens is a round hypoechoic structure with a thin echogenic border (Fig. 1.52). Congenital cataracts can be demonstrated as an additional thick echogenic ring within the lens oculi. In the axial view, an echogenic linear structure, the hyaloid artery, can be visualized running from the midposterior aspect of the lens to the back of the ocular orbit (Fig. 1.53). This vessel is easily visualized in the mid-second trimester but starts to become obliterated at about 28 weeks' gestation, eventually becoming the hyaloid (Cloquet) canal.

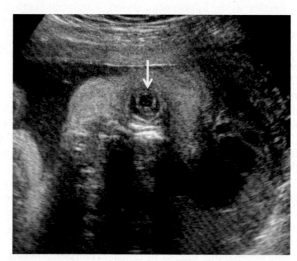

**FIGURE 1.52:** Coronal view of the eye demonstrating a normal lens *(arrow)* in the third trimester.

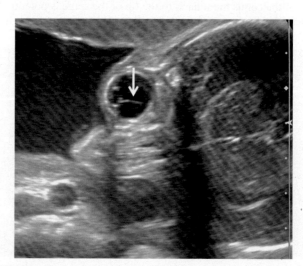

**FIGURE 1.53:** Axial view of the fetal head at the level of the orbits late second trimester. The echogenic line *(arrow)* extending from the posterior aspect of the lens to the posterior border of bulbus oculi is the hyaline artery, the future hyaline (Cloquet) canal.

Moving the probe caudally, the maxilla, alveolar ridge, and upper lip can also be examined in transverse section (Fig. 1.54). These structures should be examined to ensure continuity over the midline. The presence of a defect would be indicative of the presence of a cleft lip and/or palate, which is by far the most common facial anomaly (approximately 1:700 pregnancies). The lips should also be examined in a coronal section (Fig. 1.55), taking care not to identify the natural depression of the philtrum as an anomaly (Fig. 1.56). Any cleft in the lip or palate will effectively be filled by amniotic fluid and will therefore be hypoechoic. Fetal small parts or a loop of umbilical cord positioned in front of the lips may create a false impression of a defect (Fig. 1.57).

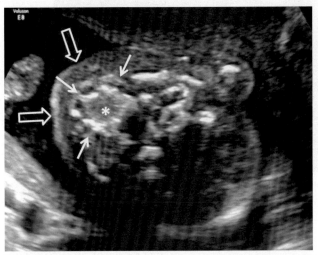

**FIGURE 1.54:** Axial view of the fetal head at the level of the maxilla *(asterisk)* and the upper lip *(open arrows)*. Multiple hypoechoic structures within the alveolar ridge are dental alveoli, with the two large ones in front being the incisors. *Solid arrows,* external border of the alveolar ridge.

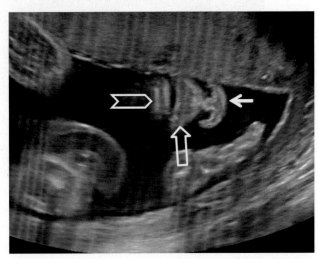

**FIGURE 1.55:** Coronal view of the upper lip *(open arrow)* with both the tip of the nose *(solid arrow)* and the lower lip *(chevron)* visible.

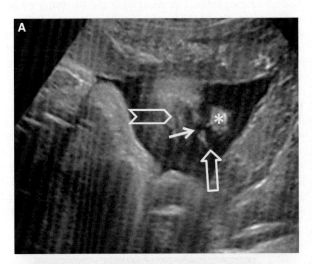

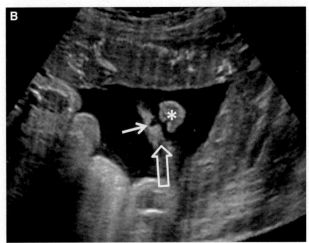

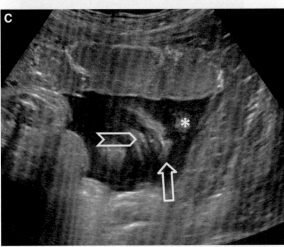

**FIGURE 1.56:** Coronal view of the upper lip in a fetus with a deep philtrum. **A, B:** Sections through the philtrum simulate a midline defect *(solid arrow)*. **C:** A deeper section through the face demonstrates an intact upper lip. *Open arrow,* upper lip; *chevron,* lower lip; *asterisk,* tip of the nose.

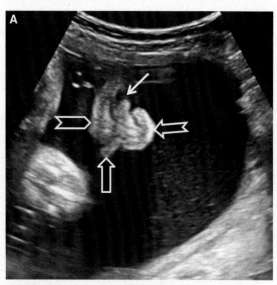 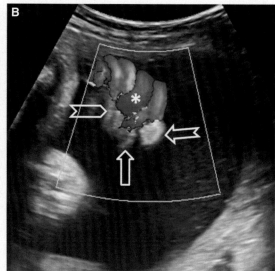

**FIGURE 1.57: A:** Coronal view of the upper lip with an apparent deep defect *(solid arrow)*. **B:** Color Doppler demonstrating that the false impression of a defect is being created by a loop of umbilical cord *(asterisk)*. *Chevron,* lower lip; *open arrow,* upper lip; *notched arrow,* tip of the nose.

Therefore, if a facial cleft is suspected, it needs to be confirmed in a number of different views.

The front of the maxilla can be evaluated in the coronal view as well. In this view, generally only the two alveolar processes, the incisors, are seen. The alveolar processes with a thin bony division between them and bones on each side create the so-called three-line view (Fig. 1.58). However, an axial examination of the maxilla allows for the entire alveolar ridge to be visualized (see Fig. 1.54).

Isolated cleft palate involves the posterior aspect of the palate. This can vary from just a bifid uvula or a defect in the soft palate to a defect that involves the palatine portion of the maxilla. The usual views to detect cleft palate in association with a cleft lip are not useful. Isolated cleft palate is extremely difficult to diagnose, especially if it just involves the soft palate. Evaluation of fluid flow through the nasal cavity and the nasopharynx using color Doppler can aid in making the diagnosis of an isolated cleft palate as fluid will be noted to flow directly between the nasal and oral cavities in the presence of a large defect (Fig. 1.59).

The fetal mandible can be seen in the axial plane (Fig. 1.60). Its contour in severe micrognathia tends to be less domed than seen in normal cases.

The fetal profile is best evaluated in a sagittal section (Fig. 1.61). The evaluation is done subjectively by visually evaluating the contour of the profile. The nasal bone can be simply evaluated for its presence or absence, or it can be measured. Delayed ossification (absence of the nasal bone) and hypoplasia of the nasal bone are strong markers for trisomy 21. Prenasal skin and the prefrontal space ratio evaluation and measurements are useful markers for Down syndrome, although they are not currently included in the routine anomaly scan in most departments.[113–115] The portion of the mandible, which is seen in the midline, is the mentum. Its position relative to the front of the maxilla provides a subjective assessment for the presence of micrognathia. A parasagittal section can be used to assess the ear (Fig. 1.62). This is not routinely done, but can be of value in defining risk for aneuploidy and may be significant in identifying a number of genetic syndromes.[116] As the ear is a small, complex and irregular structure, 3D ultrasound may be a useful adjunct to evaluation.

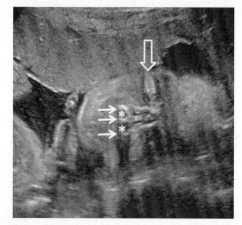

**FIGURE 1.58:** Coronal view of the front of the maxilla in the early third trimester demonstrating the two hypoechoic alveoli of the incisors *(asterisks)* with the surrounding bone creating the so-called "three-line view" *(solid arrows)*. *Open arrow,* eyelids.

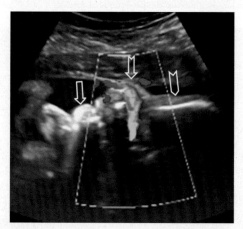

**FIGURE 1.59:** Sagittal view of the fetal face demonstrating normal flow of amniotic fluid across the upper palate with color Doppler. *Open arrow,* chin; *notched arrow,* tip of the nose; *chevron,* forehead.

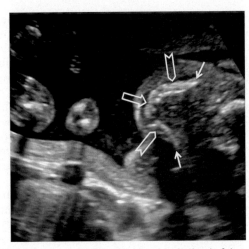

**FIGURE 1.60:** Axial view of the fetal head at the level of the mandible in the mid-second trimester. Note the small hypoechoic structures representing dental alveoli within the mandibular alveolar ridge. Note also its normal domed appearance. *Open arrow,* chin; *chevrons,* bodies of the mandible; *solid arrows,* portions of the mandibular rami.

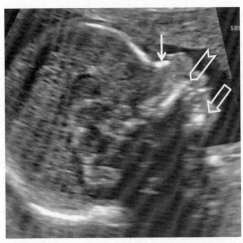

**FIGURE 1.61:** Sagittal view of the fetal profile. *Solid arrow,* nasal bone; *chevron,* front of the maxilla; *open arrow,* mandibular mentum.

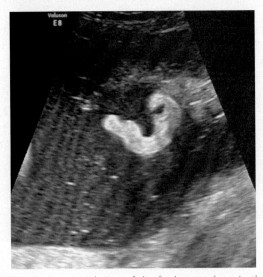

**FIGURE 1.62:** Parasagittal view of the fetal external ear in the third trimester.

## Neck

Examination typically centers on the identification of any abnormal fluid accumulation (nuchal edema or cystic hygroma) in the posterior aspect of the neck. In a transverse section, normal anatomy includes the cervical vertebrae, muscles, vessels, pharynx, upper trachea, and fetal thyroid, which can be identified as a slightly echogenic paired organ in the lower anterior aspect of the neck (Fig. 1.63). The thyroid becomes more obvious when enlarged, and a fetal goiter can be readily apparent. Any protrusion in the skin line, either anteriorly or posteriorly, should raise the suspicion of fetal abnormality. Cervical meningomyeloceles are a rare but well-recognized subgroup of neural tube defects, and cervical teratomas (epignathus; with mixed cystic and solid components), and lymphatic malformations can be found both anteriorly and posteriorly.

Nuchal fold measurement at 16 to 20 weeks is performed in the suboccipitobregmatic view (see Fig. 1.41). Increased thickness ($\geq$6 mm) is associated with trisomic aneuploidy.[117] A septated cystic lesion (cystic hygroma) is more commonly associated with monosomy X (Turner syndrome). Assessment of nuchal fold thickness at 20 weeks has value in screening for aneuploidy, but the efficacy of the test at this gestation is significantly lower than that performed at 11 to $13^{+6}$ weeks.

## Thorax

Examination of the thorax may be split into three parts: The thoracic cage and mediastinum, the lungs, and the heart. Most information about thoracic anatomy can be obtained using transverse sections. The thoracic cage is comprised of the thoracic vertebrae posteriorly, the ribs laterally, and the sternum anteriorly. The ribs can be examined in both transverse and parasagittal sections. They will normally wrap around the lateral wall of the abdomen and remain visible in the part of the chest. Ribs may be shortened, fractured, or have areas of focal echogenicity in a variety of skeletal dysplasias, and this can affect the size of the chest. The circumference of the lower portion of the thorax should be similar to the AC. If there is concern that the chest may be small, then axial sections of the thorax and abdomen can be compared directly. Gestational age–adjusted ranges for measurement of the anteroposterior and transverse

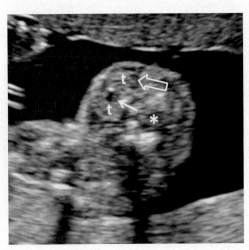

**FIGURE 1.63:** Transverse view of the neck demonstrating the trachea *(solid arrow),* thyroid *(t),* and the neck vessels *(open arrow). Asterisk,* spine.

diameters and the thoracic circumference are also available.[118] The fetus with a small chest will also look abnormal in sagittal section, with an apparent "step" between the thorax and the abdomen at the level of the diaphragm.

The fetal thymus can be identified within the thoracic inlet, located anteriorly to the great vessels within the mediastinum (Fig. 1.64). Its echogenicity is similar to or slightly less than that of the lung. Occasionally, it is seen to extend to the level of the heart and may lead to the erroneous diagnosis of an anterior intrathoracic mass. In fetuses with cardiac abnormalities that are associated with 22q11 deletion, the identification of the thymus provides some reassurance, as it may be absent in this chromosomal abnormality. Lesions of the anterior mediastinum are exceptionally rare. Generally, these are echogenic in nature, and teratomas are most common.

The trachea lies to the right and slightly anterior to the spine. It is relatively small and difficult to visualize on ultrasound. It is best seen in the upper thorax at the level used to demonstrate the cardiac three-vessel view (see below). The trachea bifurcates into right and left main stem bronchi between the lower portion of the fourth and the seventh thoracic vertebrae. A dilated and distended trachea is more easily seen as in congenital high airway obstructive sequence (CHAOS). The whole lower airway below the level of obstruction becomes visible in coronal or sagittal section, while the lungs are large and hyperechoic, the diaphragms depressed, and the heart and mediastinum compressed.

The esophagus runs posteriorly and to the left of the trachea. It is normally collapsed and free of fluid, and consequently difficult to identify on ultrasound. It is most easily seen in sagittal or coronal section as two or more parallel, echogenic lines.[119,120] Occasionally, if the esophagus is insonated during fetal swallowing, it has hypoechoic content (Fig. 1.65). In esophageal atresia, the proximal esophagus (the "esophageal pouch") may be seen as a dilated tubular structure in the upper chest.

The lungs fill the major part of each hemithorax. Abnormalities of the lung are rare, and the process of examination is relatively straightforward. The lungs are homogeneous with a moderately hyperechoic appearance on ultrasound (see Figs. 1.64 and 1.65). The periphery of the lungs should be inspected carefully to identify a pleural effusion as a hypoechoic layer surrounding the lung. Lesions of the lung can be either cystic or solid in appearance and of variable echogenicity. Furthermore, lesions within the thorax may be extrathoracic in origin such as a diaphragmatic hernia. Displacement of the heart may be the first indication of the presence of a lung abnormality. It can be displaced to one side or the other depending on the location and size of the lesion. It can also be displaced with congenital agenesis of the lung. As the pregnancy progresses beyond the mid-second trimester, the shadowing by the fetal ribs increases due to their ossification. The resultant alternating areas of echogenicity and acoustic shadows located within the thorax may give the false impression of a mass (see Fig. 1.65). Therefore, if a mass is suspected, it should be evaluated in multiple sections to rule out an artifact.

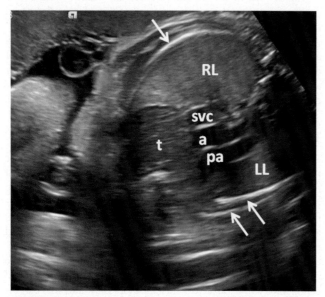

**FIGURE 1.64:** Axial view of the thoracic cavity demonstrating the presence of the thymus *(t)* at the level of the three-vessel view. *RL*, right lung; *LL*, left lung; *svc*, superior vena cava; *a*, aorta; *pa*, pulmonary artery; *solid arrows*, ribs.

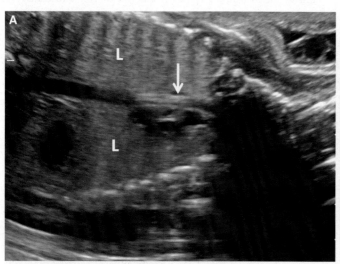
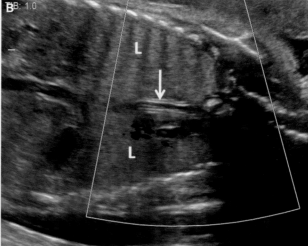

**FIGURE 1.65:** Coronal view of the esophagus *(arrow)* in late second trimester. Note the presence of echogenic dots around the periphery of the chest representing cross sections of the ribs and their acoustic shadows within the proximal lung. *L*, lungs. **A:** The esophagus is at rest consisting of three solid lines. **B:** The esophagus of the same fetus containing hypoechoic fluid during swallowing.

## Heart

Cardiac defects are very common, affecting approximately 1% of infants. However, they are also commonly missed on prenatal ultrasound.[70] The two main reasons for this are the fact that the range of cardiac abnormalities is wide and that the 3D anatomy of the heart is very complex. However, over 90% of cardiac defects are detectable, so it is important to develop an effective screening strategy that will alert clinicians to the risk of an abnormality. The basic components of this strategy include the four-chamber view, outflow tracts, and three-vessel view in the mid-second trimester. Not only do cardiac anomalies have a high association with neonatal and childhood morbidity and mortality, but they are also markers for chromosomal and genetic anomalies. Therefore, the importance of a careful cardiac cannot be overstated.[121–123]

The cardiac examination begins outside the chest by checking situs. First, fetal position is assessed to define the left and right sides of the fetus. The abdomen is then examined in axial sections to define the position of the stomach and of the great vessels. The stomach should normally be on the left side of the abdomen, and the aorta should be anterior to the spine and slightly to the left of the midline (see section on abdomen). The vena cava normally is more anterior and to the right of the aorta (see below). Once abdominal situs is established, the examination moves to the chest. In axial section, the apex of the heart should lie to the left side of the midline. The heart occupies one-third of the surface area of the chest, and the axis of the ventricular septum should be at 45° (±7°) to the anteroposterior axis of the thorax (Fig. 1.66).[124] An abnormal position of the heart may arise as a result of an abnormal space-occupying lesion in the left or right chest. The cardiac axis can also be displaced in the setting of certain cardiac malformations (e.g., tetralogy of Fallot and truncus arteriosus) and is a useful screening tool for cardiac defects.

Once situs and basic relationships are established, heart rate and rhythm are evaluated. Primary detection of rhythm anomalies is done by qualitative observation of cardiac motion. Detailed analysis of cardiac rhythm requires measurement of heart rate, the time intervals in the cardiac cycle, and, in particular, the relationship between atrial and ventricular contractions. The exact rate can be determined using either pulse wave Doppler or

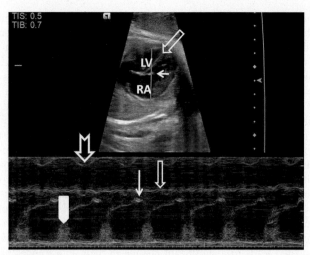

**FIGURE 1.67:** Axial view of the four-chamber heart with an M-mode through the left ventricle (*LV, notched arrow* on M-mode) and the right atrium (*RA, thick solid arrow* on M-mode). The cursor also includes the ventricular septum (*open arrow* on both grayscale and M-mode) and the medial leaflet of the tricuspid valve (*thin solid arrow* on both grayscale and M-mode).

M-mode ultrasound, both of which document movement over time (Fig. 1.67). When using M-mode ultrasound, the sampling line is placed across both ventricle and atrium to display the temporal relationship of ventricular and atrial motion on one image. The timing and frequency of atrial and ventricular contractions may be used to classify the specific form of arrhythmia present. Premature atrial or ventricular contractions are a common benign finding and, in the absence of a cardiac structural defect, are of no clinical significance.

Before discussing issues regarding the circulation, it is appropriate to briefly review some of the specialized aspects of fetal circulatory anatomy. The fetal circulation is oxygenated by the placenta and therefore has several anatomical differences compared with the postnatal circulation. The fetal cardiovascular system is designed in such a way that the most highly oxygenated blood is delivered to the myocardium and brain. This is achieved in the fetus by both the preferential streaming of oxygenated blood and the presence of intracardiac and extracardiac shunts. The fetal circulation runs in parallel and is shunt dependent. The three vascular structures most important in the fetal circulation are the DV, foramen ovale (FO), and ductus arteriosus (DA). Briefly, during fetal life, DV delivers highly oxygenated blood from the umbilical vein directly into the inferior vena cava (IVC). The IVC also contains poorly oxygenated blood from the lower abdomen and pelvis. The blood coming from the DV is preferentially streamed across the FO into the left atrium owing to anatomic adaptations in the right atrium and a differential in flow velocity between the blood coming from the DV and the rest of the blood in the IVC. The oxygenated blood then empties into the left ventricle to be expelled into the aorta. In this way, the most oxygen-rich blood is delivered to the coronary arteries and the upper portion of the body, including the brain. Most of the deoxygenated blood from the IVC joins the deoxygenated blood returning via the superior vena cava (SVC) in the right atrium and is preferentially directed into the right ventricle and subsequently the pulmonary artery. The majority of this blood reenters the systemic circulation through the DA, which enters the aorta below the isthmus and mixes with more oxygenated blood coming from the left ventricle. In this way, the organs of

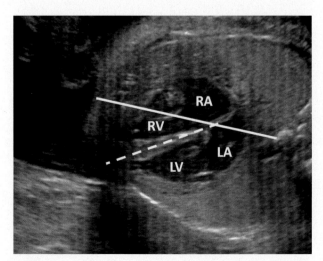

**FIGURE 1.66:** Axial view of the thoracic cavity at the level of the four-chamber view of the heart in diastole. The cardiac axis is formed by the anteroposterior axis of the thorax (*solid line*) and the longitudinal axis of the ventricular septum (*dashed line*) and is within normal limits. *LV*, left ventricle; *RV*, right ventricle; *LA*, left atrium; *RA*, right atrium.

the lower part of the body, which have a lower oxygen demand than the brain and the heart, receive blood with lower oxygen content. Also, the relatively deoxygenated blood is pumped to the placenta for re-oxygenation via the umbilical arteries, which originate from the internal iliac arteries.

Comprehensive evaluation of anatomy is best performed in a sequential fashion. Because of the 3D complexity of the anatomy of the heart and its arterial and venous connections, many views and transducer positions have been developed to assist in their examination. To complicate matters even further, optimal positions of the transducer are also greatly influenced by the position of the fetus, which changes during the examination as the fetus moves. Optimization of views requires frequent adjustment of the position of the transducer and the angle of insonation. It is important to recognize that even a slight alteration in angle or level at which the heart or great vessels are insonated leads to a significant change in their appearance. An added degree of difficulty is added by the fact that multiple cardiac structures lie in close proximity to each other. The operator should frequently return to a familiar and easily obtainable view such as the four-chamber, which acts as a point of reference. In the following section, we present the views that produce the highest yield and efficiency.

The four chambers of the heart can be seen in an axial section through the lower portion of the thorax. Normally, the heart is primarily located in the left hemithorax but does extend slightly to the right side. A line drawn along the anteroposterior axis transects the heart close to its crux. The entire left ventricle and a portion of the right ventricle will be located in the left hemithorax, whereas the entire right atrium and portion of the left atrium will be on the right (see Fig. 1.66). A careful search for a thoracic mass needs to be performed for cases in which the heart's location significantly deviates from this relationship. A small amount of pericardial fluid is usually present (Fig. 1.68). The amount of fluid is considered increased if the measurement between the wall of the heart and the pericardial sac exceeds 2 mm. In the four-chamber view, two atria and two ventricles with a septum at midcavity are present. There are two atrioventricular valves; the tricuspid valve opens in to the right ventricle

and the mitral valve opens in the left ventricle. The crux is the center of the heart where the atrial septum meets the ventricular septum and at which the atrioventricular valves also insert.[125,126]

The two ventricles are approximately equal in size. The right ventricle lies anteriorly, just behind the anterior chest wall, and the left ventricle is located behind it. The right ventricle can be identified morphologically by the fact that the tricuspid valve inserts into the interventricular septum (IVS) at a slightly lower level than the mitral valve and has a septal attachment, whereas the mitral valve has only a free wall attachment. The right ventricle is more coarsely trabeculated than the left and contains a thick band of tissue called the moderated band, which is located close to its apex (Fig. 1.69). While the right ventricle extends toward the apex, the left ventricle makes the apex of the heart (Fig. 1.70). In the short axis view, the shapes of the two ventricles also differ: The right ventricle appears to slightly wrap around the more rounded left ventricular lumen (Fig. 1.71). The two atrioventricular valves should be visualized and seen to open

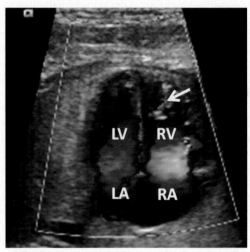

**FIGURE 1.69:** Axial and apical view of the four-chamber heart during early diastole with color Doppler demonstrating inflow of blood. Please note the moderator band *(arrow)* in the right ventricle *(RV)*. *LV*, left ventricle; *LA*, left atrium; *RA*, right atrium.

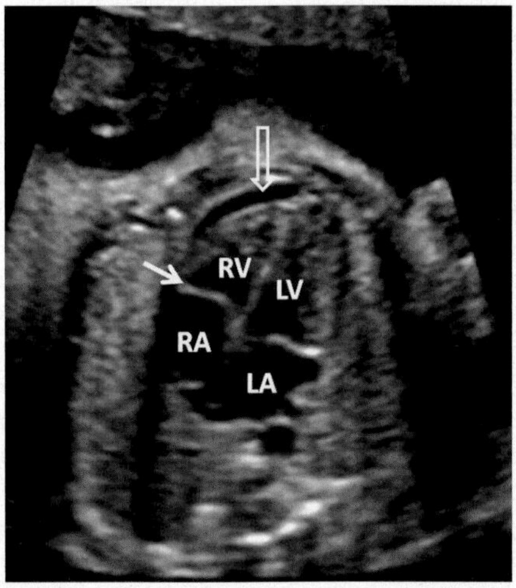

**FIGURE 1.68:** Axial view of the four-chamber heart demonstrates a prominent layer of pericardial fluid *(open arrow)* and apical displacement of the tricuspid valve *(solid arrow)*. Compare the location of this valve to that of the mitral valve. *LV*, left ventricle; *RV*, right ventricle; *LA*, left atrium; *RA*, right atrium.

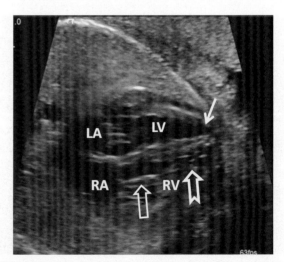

**FIGURE 1.70:** Axial view of the four-chamber heart. Please note that the tip of the left ventricle *(LV)* forms the apex of the heart *(solid arrow)* and the more "full" appearance of the right ventricular *(RV)* lumen due to chordae tendinae/papillary muscles *(open arrow)* and trabeculations *(notched arrow)*. *LA*, left atrium; *RA*, right atrium.

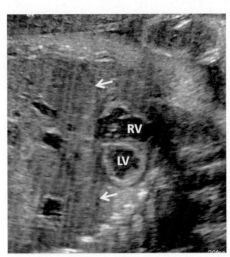

**FIGURE 1.71:** Short axis of the heart demonstrating the differences between the ventricular shapes. Note the rounded appearance of the left ventricle *(LV)* and the more flattened appearance of the right ventricle *(RV)*, which appears to "wrap" around the left one. Also note the echogenic projections into the right ventricular lumen representing trabeculations and chordae tendinae/papillary muscles. *Arrows*, domes of the diaphragm.

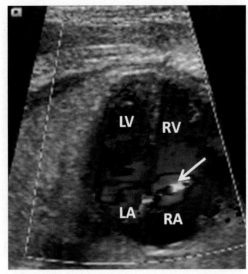

**FIGURE 1.72:** Apical view of the four-chamber heart at the time of valve closure. There is an area of turbulent flow *(arrow)* across the tricuspid valve, which is often seen at the time of valve closure and should not be mistaken for regurgitation. *LV*, left ventricle; *RV*, right ventricle; *LA*, left atrium; *RA*, right atrium.

and close through the cardiac cycle. Color flow and pulse wave Doppler can be used to demonstrate filling of the ventricular chambers and to look for valvular regurgitation (Fig. 1.72).

A common finding is an intracardiac echogenic focus, which is usually located in the left ventricle. As an isolated finding, it is of no consequence, though it is considered to be a weak marker for trisomy 21. It is thought to represent an area of calcification in a papillary muscle, though it may be caused by reflection from a papillary muscle surface during diastole (Fig. 1.73).[92,93,127,128]

The IVS separates the two ventricular cavities. It has muscular (basal) and membranous (inlet) parts. A number of different views should be employed to assure its integrity from the apex to the crux as ventricular septal defects (VSDs) are relatively common but often difficult to detect. The septum is best examined with the ultrasound beam perpendicular to the longitudinal axis. In this view, the entire septum, including both muscular and membranous portions, can be seen, and large defects can be visualized. Color Doppler is a valuable adjunct for smaller muscular VSDs, which may be identified owing to the presence of flow across the septum. However, generally, this method is limited to the detection of muscular septal defects. Color Doppler evaluation of the subaortic portion of the septum is compromised by its proximity to the outflows and valves, rendering it less helpful due to "color bleed." Demonstration of bidirectional flow on Doppler helps to identify a VSD as outflow tracts will contain unidirectional flow only. The septum can also be insonated apically, that is, with the direction of the ultrasound beam parallel to the longitudinal axis of the septum. In this view, the membranous portion of the septum, which is close to the crux cordis, is not well imaged. This portion of the IVS is particularly thin, creating a "drop out," giving the erroneous impression of a VSD (Fig. 1.74).

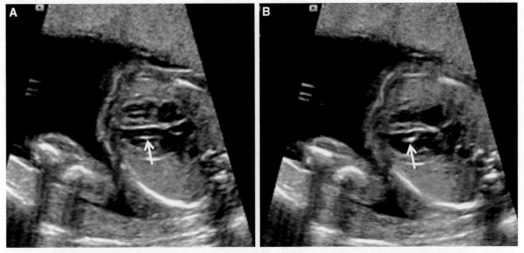

**FIGURE 1.73:** Axial view of the four-chamber heart. **A:** Appearance of the papillary muscle *(arrow)* when it is stretched during ventricular systole. **B:** Papillary muscle in the same patient presenting as an intracardiac echogenic focus *(arrow)* when it is relaxed during ventricular diastole.

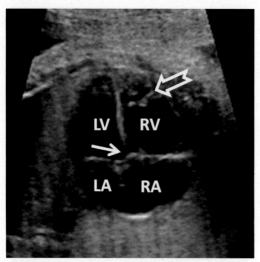

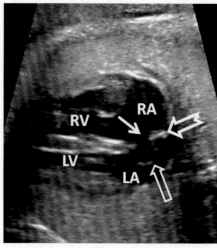

**FIGURE 1.74:** Apical view of the four-chamber heart. Note the "fall-out" in the membranous portion of the ventricular septum *(solid arrow)*. *Notched arrow*, moderator band; *LV*, left ventricle; *RV*, right ventricle; *LA*, left atrium; *RA*, right atrium.

**FIGURE 1.75:** Axial view of the four-chamber heart showing the foramen ovale *(solid arrow)* with a foramen flap forming a small aneurysm *(open arrow)*. Most of the time, foramen ovale flap aneurysm is of limited clinical significance. *LV*, left ventricle; *RV*, right ventricle; *LA*, left atrium; *RA*, right atrium; *notched arrow*, atrial septum.

However, an echogenic dot (so-called "flashlight" sign) is often seen at the margin of a true VSD. This may in fact be the initial indication of its presence.

The two atria are also approximately the same in size and are of similar appearance. The atria are separated by the interatrial septum (IAS), which is significantly thinner than the IVS. The IAS contains a prominent conduit (FO) that lets oxygenated blood to stream into the left atrium from the right. A flap valve, which is associated with FO, is seen fluttering in the left atrium, reflecting the right to left direction of blood flow. Occasionally, it assumes the shape of an aneurysm, which is considered a benign variant (Fig. 1.75). Atrial septal defects are very difficult to detect prenatally as the majority are ostium secundum defects involving the FO. Ostium primum atrial septal defects are located close to the atrioventricular valves and are considered to be part of an atrioventricular septal (AV canal) defect spectrum.

The objective of imaging the left and right ventricular outflow tracts is to determine their size and relationship to each other, and to their respective ventricles (Fig. 1.76).[129,130] These

views are necessary for identification of a number of cardiac anomalies not detectable using the four-chamber view alone. Evaluation of the left then right outflow tract involves moving the probe progressively cranially in an axial section from the four-chamber view. The left ventricular outflow tract appears first, and this view can be improved by tilting the probe slightly toward the left shoulder of the fetus. As one continues to move cranially in axial section, the right ventricular outflow tract becomes apparent. The left ventricular outflow tract courses from left to right as it exits the left ventricle. The continuity of the IVS with the anterior wall of the aorta is more clearly seen in this view. An interruption in the IVS in this region is indicative of a perimembranous or outlet VSD. An overriding aorta is frequently found in association with an outlet VSD. The pulmonary trunk normally runs posteriorly, directly toward the spine, so the two vessels effectively cross one another at the level of their origin. Absence of this crossing suggests the presence of transposition of the great vessels. The pulmonary trunk divides into the right and left pulmonary arteries, a finding which is useful to differentiate between the two great

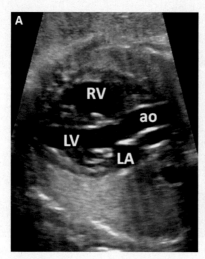

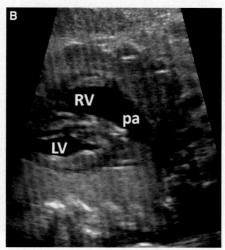

**FIGURE 1.76:** Axial views of the outflow tracts. **A:** Aortic outflow *(ao)* tract exiting from the left ventricle *(LV)*. *LA*, left atrium. **B:** Pulmonary artery outflow *(pa)* exiting from the right ventricle *(RV)*.

arteries. An additional major vessel, which originates from the point of bifurcation of the pulmonary trunk or from the left pulmonary artery, is the DA. It is a fetal vessel, which connects the pulmonary circulation with the descending thoracic aorta. Color Doppler is useful to define the direction of flow through the great arteries as they leave the heart.

Moving the probe further cranially into the upper mediastinum allows the outflow tracts to be imaged in the three-vessel view. This view includes from left to right: The main pulmonary trunk, a transverse section of the aorta, and of the SVC. The lumen of the aorta and pulmonary trunk are similar in size, though the pulmonary artery tends to be slightly larger, and the SVC is the smallest. The DA is usually but not always seen in this view coursing posteriorly toward the descending aorta (Figs. 1.77 and 1.78). The DA is usually a fairly straight vessel,

but occasionally a highly tortuous DA is found (Fig. 1.79). This is of no apparent clinical significance.

The tracheal view is obtained by moving the probe further cranially. This view also includes the aorta, the pulmonary artery, and the DA (Fig. 1.80). However, they are seen more along their long axis running anteroposteriorly from right to left. The cross section of the trachea is also seen in this section located anteriorly to the vertebral body and to the right of both the pulmonary artery and the aorta.

In addition to the axial views described above, the course of the great arteries can also be defined using longitudinal views of the chest (aortic and ductal arch views). Since the two lie close to each other, it is important to be able to differentiate them on the basis of their morphology. The ductal arch is formed by the DA as it travels from its origin at the pulmonary artery to

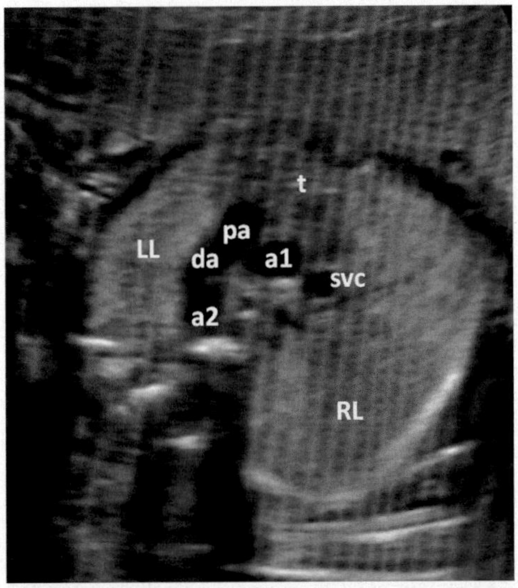

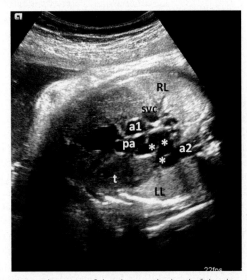

**FIGURE 1.77:** Axial section of the chest at the level of the three-vessel view with the ductus arteriosus *(da)* visible. *a1*, ascending thoracic aorta; *a2*, descending thoracic aorta; *LL*, left lung; *RL*, right lung; *pa*, pulmonary artery; *svc*, superior vena cava; *t*, thymus.

**FIGURE 1.79:** Axial section of the chest at the level of the three-vessel view. The convoluted vessel *(asterisks)* is an unusually tortuous ductus arteriosus. *a1*, ascending thoracic aorta; *a2*, descending thoracic aorta; *LL*, left lung; *RL*, right lung; *pa*, pulmonary artery; *svc*, superior vena cava; *t*, thymus.

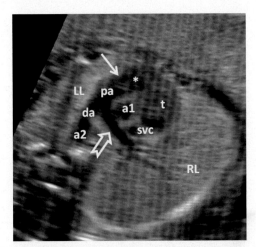

**FIGURE 1.78:** Modified (oblique) axial section of the chest at a similar level to Figure 1.16, demonstrating the right branch *(notched arrow)* of the pulmonary artery *(pa)* and ductus arteriosus *(da)*. *Solid arrow*, pulmonary valve; *asterisk*, upper portion of the right ventricle; *a1*, ascending thoracic aorta; *a2*, descending thoracic aorta; *LL*, left lung; *RL*, right lung; *t*, thymus; *da*, ductus arteriosus; *svc*, superior vena cava.

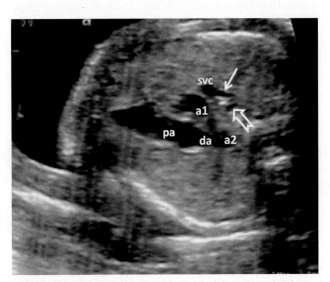

**FIGURE 1.80:** Tracheal view with the entry of the azygos *(solid arrow)* vein visible. *Notched arrow*, trachea; *a1*, ascending thoracic aorta; *a2*, descending thoracic aorta; *da*, ductus arteriosus; *pa*, pulmonary artery; *svc*, superior vena cava.

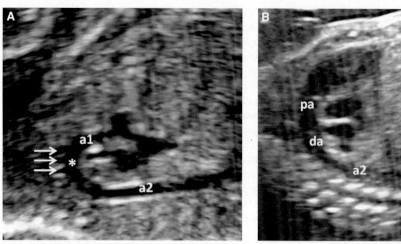

**FIGURE 1.81:** Axial views of the aortic **(A)** and ductal **(B)** arches demonstrating the difference in shape between the two. *Asterisk*, aortic arch; *solid arrows*, three branches of the aortic arch; *a1*, ascending thoracic aorta; *a2*, descending thoracic aorta; *da*, ductus arteriosus; *pa*, pulmonary artery.

the point of entry into the descending aorta. Its distinguishing features include a relatively flat shape ("hockey stick") and the fact that it does not give off any branches. The aortic arch, on the other hand, is more rounded (like a candy cane) and gives off branch vessels from its superior aspect (brachiocephalic, left common carotid, and left subclavian arteries) (Fig. 1.81).

Short axis views are defined as the views at right angles to the longitudinal axis of the IVS. The two views that are most helpful are a cross section of the ventricles and a cross section at the level of the aortic valve. The easiest method for obtaining short axis views is to first obtain the four-chamber view and then rotate the transducer at right angles to the longitudinal axis of the heart.

As mentioned above, the short axis view of the ventricles is useful for defining right and left ventricular morphology (see Fig. 1.71). Also, sweeping the entire ventricular septum in this view while employing color Doppler is helpful for the detection of VSDs.

A short axis view at the level of the aortic valve is very informative. However, it needs to be kept in mind that the components of this view change depending on even slight adjustments in angulation of the transducer. Nonetheless, the aortic valve ring should always be seen in a transverse section and should be located in the center of the image. The structures of the right heart are organized radially around the aortic valve: The upper portion of the right ventricle and the longitudinal view of the right outflow tract are located anteriorly, the right pulmonary artery wraps around the aortic root, the superior portion of the right atrium is located to the right of the aortic root and posteriorly to the right ventricle (Fig. 1.82). Since both the aortic and the pulmonary valves are seen in the same view, comparison of their relative size can be readily performed.

The venous connections of the heart also should be examined. The SVC and IVC are relatively large and are readily identifiable using grayscale ultrasound. The SVC can be seen on axial views of the chest (see Figs. 1.1, 1.77 to 1.80). Of note is that the azygos vein can be identified at its point of entry into the posterior aspect SVC in this view (see Fig. 1.80). Significant enlargement of this vessel indicates an interruption of IVC. In the longitudinal view, both the SVC and the IVC can be identified as they enter the right atrium. The DV can frequently be seen entering the IVC anteriorly just before its entry into the right atrium (Fig. 1.83).

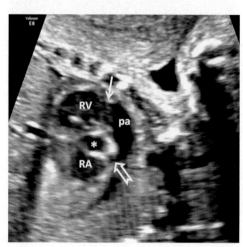

**FIGURE 1.82:** Short axis view at the level of the aortic valve. *Asterisk*, aortic valve annulus; *RV*, right ventricle; *pa*, pulmonary artery; *RA*, right atrium; *notched arrow*, right pulmonary artery; *solid arrow*, pulmonary valve annulus.

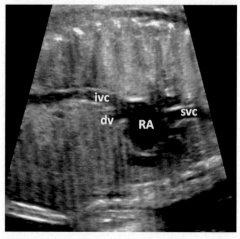

**FIGURE 1.83:** Longitudinal view of the superior and inferior venae cavae (*svc* and *ivc*, respectively) entering the right atrium (*RA*). Note the entry of the ductus venosus (*dv*) into the anterior aspect of the IVC.

The pulmonary veins are much smaller than the IVC and SVC; therefore, they are much more difficult to visualize with grayscale imaging. Color Doppler (with a low PRF setting) is very helpful. Normally, there are four pulmonary veins that enter the left atrium. Usually, it is the left and right lower veins that are seen on the four-chamber view, and it is reasonable to expect to be able to identify connection of only these two. The pulmonary veins may become confluent behind the left atrium without being connected, and it is important to demonstrate flow into the atria, not merely flow behind the atria (Fig. 1.84). In a total anomalous pulmonary venous drainage, the pulmonary veins cannot be seen connecting to the left atrium.

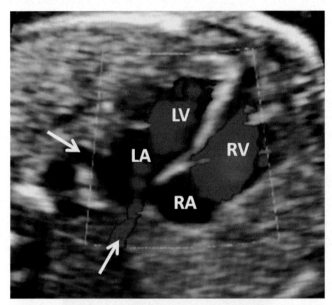

**FIGURE 1.84:** Axial view of the four-chamber heart with right and left pulmonary veins *(arrows)* visible entering the left atrium *(LA)* during diastole. Color Doppler is used to improve the ease of visualization. *LV*, left ventricle; *RV*, right ventricle; *RA*, right atrium.

## Diaphragm

The diaphragm forms the division between the abdomen and the chest. It is identified and examined most easily utilizing sweeping longitudinal and coronal views (Figs. 1.85 and 1.86). The diaphragm is a thin, hypoechoic, membrane-like structure that may be difficult to clearly visualize on ultrasound. If not directly visualized, the presence of the diaphragm may be implied by a clearly defined interface between the lungs and the intra-abdominal contents. If this border appears blurred, detailed examination of the diaphragm is indicated, and the relative levels of the intra-abdominal organs with respect to the heart should be determined. There should be no abdominal structures visible in a transverse view of the chest at the level of the four-chamber heart.

The coronal view offers the additional advantage of viewing both domes of the diaphragm at the same time. This is an important view for establishing that they are at approximately the same level. In some fetal disorders, such as eventration, both domes are present, but one is significantly higher than the other. Flattening or even inversion of the diaphragm may be seen in association with congenital upper airway obstruction.

## Abdomen and Pelvis

During the morphology scan, the abdomen and pelvis are traditionally examined in four main axial planes. The landmarks used to assess the upper abdomen and to obtain the proper level for an AC measurement are the stomach, a portion of the umbilical vein, the portal sinus, and a portion of the right portal vein (RPV) (the so-called J sign). A true axial section is verified by ensuring that a single rib is visible through its length rather than a number of ribs cut in cross section. The adrenal glands are often seen in this section (Fig. 1.87). However, visualization of any portion of the kidneys indicates an improper plane for AC measurement. Moving caudally, the next axial section is taken at the level of the renal pelves. The kidneys are best visualized with the fetal back being closest to the transducer, and

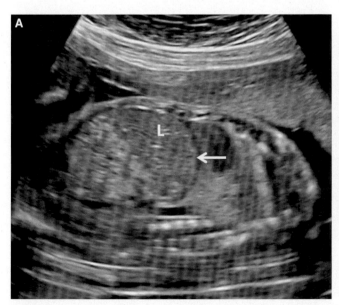
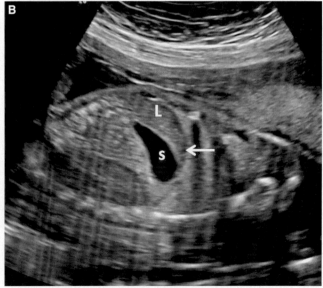

**FIGURE 1.85:** Longitudinal views of the domes of the diaphragm *(arrows)* on the right *(A)* and left *(B)*. *L*, liver; *s*, stomach.

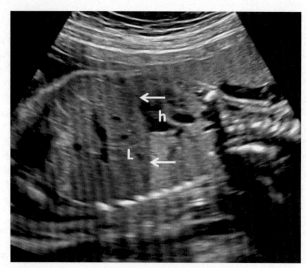

**FIGURE 1.86:** Coronal view of the dome of the diaphragm *(arrows). H,* heart; *L,* liver.

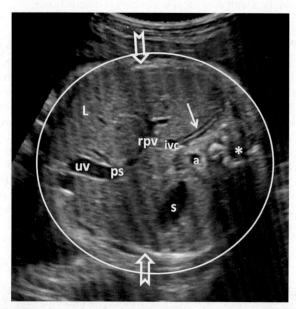

**FIGURE 1.87:** Axial view of the upper abdomen in the late second trimester at the level of the abdominal circumference *(circle). Notched arrows,* ribs along their longitudinal axis; *solid arrow,* adrenal; *asterisk,* vertebra; *uv,* hepatic portion of the umbilical vein; *ps,* portal sinus; *rpv,* right portal vein; *s,* stomach; *L,* liver; *ivc,* inferior vena cava; *a,* aorta.

the probe should be manipulated to achieve this whenever possible. The next axial section is at the level of the umbilical cord, and is used to document the integrity of the anterior abdominal wall. Defects at the umbilicus can be subtle, so care needs to be taken to visualize this clearly. Finally, an axial section of the pelvis, showing the bladder and, with color Doppler, the umbilical arteries around its lateral margins, should be recorded. In real time, these views can be linked by sweeping the probe through the abdomen and pelvis. This allows the sonographer to identify any cystic or solid masses within the abdomen and to determine whether the bowel is abnormally echogenic. Some intra-abdominal anomalies, such as duodenal atresia or obstruction of the bowel, are not readily visualized at the time of the 20-week scan. Assessment of intra-abdominal anatomy during any third trimester scan is therefore worthwhile.

In an axial section of the upper abdomen, the liver fills the right upper abdominal quadrant, and the stomach is seen on the left. The liver is homogeneous and slightly less echogenic than the lung. There are three interconnected vessels coursing through the liver, which are large enough to be easily visualized using gray-scale ultrasound only: The intrahepatic portion of the umbilical vein, the RPV, and the portal sinus located between the two. The umbilical vein enters the abdomen at the abdominal cord insertion and courses a short distance through the falciform ligament to the anterior and inferior edge of the liver. It then courses obliquely in a posterior and caudal direction along the inferior aspect of the liver (Fig. 1.88). It changes into the portal sinus after the junction with the inferior left portal vein (LPV). The portal sinus ends at the point of origin of the RPV. The portal sinus and the RPV form a J-like shape in the axial section. There are additional branches originating from the portal sinus (superior

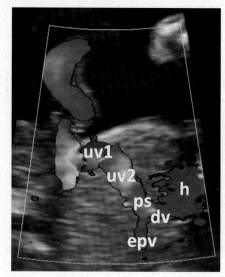

**FIGURE 1.88:** Anatomy of the hepatic portion of the umbilical vein and portal circulation in a longitudinal view. *uv1,* intra-abdominal portion of the umbilical vein; *uv2,* intrahepatic portion of the umbilical vein; *ps,* portal sinus; *dv,* ductus venosus; *epv,* extrahepatic portal vein; *h,* heart.

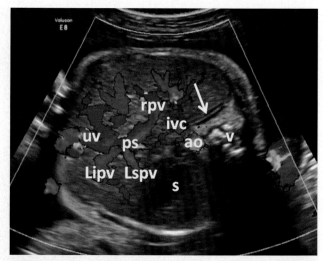

**FIGURE 1.89:** Anatomy of the hepatic portion of the umbilical vein and portal circulation in an axial section. Additional portions of the hepatic circulation are also seen. *Solid arrow,* adrenal; *uv,* umbilical vein; *Lipv,* left inferior portal vein; *Lspv,* left superior portal vein; *ps,* portal sinus; *rpv,* right portal vein; *s,* stomach; *ao,* aorta; *ivc,* inferior vena cava; *v,* vertebra.

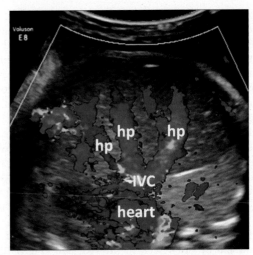

**FIGURE 1.90:** Color Doppler demonstrating the three hepatic veins *(hp)* in an axial oblique view of the liver. *IVC,* inferior vena cava.

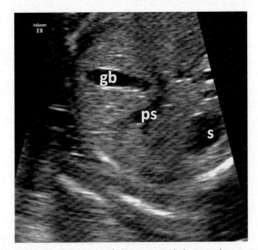

**FIGURE 1.91:** Axial section of the upper abdomen demonstrating a gallbladder *(gb)* in its normal location to the right of the portal sinus *(ps)*. *s,* stomach.

LPV, extrahepatic portal vein, and the DV), all of which are difficult to see without the aid of color Doppler (Fig. 1.89). The DV originates at the point where the portal sinus takes a sharp bend toward the right. It travels in a posterior and cephalad direction without giving off any branches until it joins the IVC. The course that it takes is more directly cephalad than is the direction of the hepatic portion of the umbilical vein.[131]

Detailed analysis of hepatic vasculature is not part of the routine 20-week scan. Despite this, it is important to have a good understanding of hepatic vasculature (Figs. 1.88 to 1.90), as identification and assessment of the DV is necessary for assessment of cardiovascular compensation then decompensation in the severely growth restricted fetus. Pulse wave Doppler evaluation of the DV normally shows forward flow throughout the cardiac cycle. In the later stage of intrauterine growth restriction, as the myocardium becomes hypoxic and dysfunctional, resistance to atrial filling increases and reversal of the DV a-wave is seen. Additionally, this investigation can lead to the rare diagnosis of congenitally absence of the DV, a condition that has an increased risk of poor perinatal outcome.

Moving the probe a fraction caudally from the axial section of the upper abdomen brings another elongated cystic structure that runs along the inferior surface of the liver into view. The gallbladder is pear-like in shape, with the stem pointing toward the hepatic hilum (porta hepatis).[132] It is usually located between the right and the left hepatic lobes, and is located to the right of the intrahepatic portion of the umbilical vein and portal sinus (Fig. 1.91). On grayscale, the appearance of the vascular structures and the gallbladder can be fairly similar. However, color Doppler can be used to distinguish between them by identifying flow in the vessels.

Congenital persistence of the right umbilical vein will lead to the intrahepatic portion of the umbilical vein being located to the right of the gallbladder (Fig. 1.92). This is not an uncommon finding (1:500 to 1:1,000) and is of no clinical significance when isolated. However, it does increase the risk of extrahepatic abnormalities such as cardiac and renal defects being present.

As a normal variant, the gallbladder may also contain septations or have an unusual shape such as the "Phrygian cap"

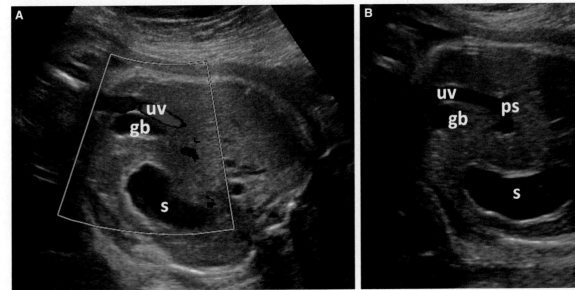

**FIGURE 1.92:** Axial section of the upper abdomen demonstrating the location of the gallbladder *(gb),* which is here to the left of the hepatic portion of the umbilical vein *(uv).* The direction of the curvature of the portal sinus *(ps)* is to the left rather than in its usual direction. These findings are indicative of persistent right umbilical vein. *s,* stomach.

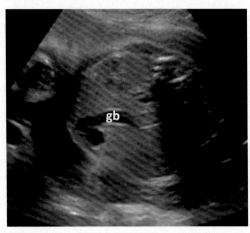

**FIGURE 1.93:** Axial section of the upper abdomen demonstrating a Phrygian cap gallbladder (gb).

gallbladder (Fig. 1.93). The gallbladder is congenitally absent in 1:1,000 infants. Nonvisualization on prenatal ultrasound is usually a transient finding due to variable and intermittent emptying of biliary contents. However, a persistently absent gallbladder may be indicative of congenital hepatic problems, such as biliary atresia. Occasionally, in the third trimester, the gallbladder contains echogenic structures, which are consistent with sludge or gallstones (Fig. 1.94). These generally resolve in the neonatal period and are of limited clinical significance. Occasionally, a calcification can be seen at the periphery of the liver (Fig. 1.95). As an isolated finding, these are usually of no clinical significance.

The fetal stomach is normally located in the left upper quadrant of the abdomen. Its normal ultrasound appearance is that of an elongated cystic structure with uniformly hypoechoic contents (see Figs. 1.85, 1.87, 1.91, 1.92, 1.94). However, the contents occasionally include structures with increased echogenicity, which usually represent swallowed intra-amniotic debris such as blood (Fig. 1.96). Small echogenic foci may be seen associated with the gastric wall (Fig. 1.97). These are of unclear etiology and have been shown not to be associated with an increase in adverse fetal outcome.

The stomach varies in size depending on fetal swallowing and gastric emptying. Nonvisualization or enlargement of the stomach is typically transient, and serial examination may help in elucidating any abnormality. If obstruction is suspected, then assessment of the amniotic fluid index (AFI) may also be helpful to determine whether there is concurrent polyhydramnios. Obstruction may not become apparent until the fetus is swallowing more actively in the late second or third trimester.[133,134]

The spleen is located in the left upper quadrant of the abdomen along the periphery of the stomach. In the axial section, it is roughly oval in shape (Fig. 1.98). The spleen has similar echogenicity to the liver and, as such, is often difficult to clearly delineate (Fig. 1.99). It is not routinely evaluated at 20 weeks' gestation, but an attempt to image it should be made in circumstances where polysplenia or asplenia are suspected.[135]

The fetal adrenals are also imaged within the upper abdomen, and can be often seen in the AC view (Fig. 1.100; see Figs. 1.87 and 1.89).[136] As such, it is often visualized during the 20-week anomaly scan, though a formal assessment is normally done only if a mass is discovered in this area. The adrenal gland is draped as a pyramidal structure over the upper pole of the kidney. Therefore, an axial view of the cephalic tip of the kidney can result in an image of the adrenal with a highly echogenic center. This is an artifact resulting from the anatomic relationship of the two organs and not an adrenal hemorrhage. A longitudinal view of the kidney and adrenal resolves this question: The interface between the two organs can be visualized in this section, and the appearance of the adrenal can be evaluated independently of the kidney (Fig. 1.101).

Moving caudally, the kidneys are also imaged in axial section. They are in a posterior, retroperitoneal location next to the spine. Their visualization may be compromised by several factors, including the decreased penetration of ultrasound if scanning from the anterior aspect of the fetus, and one or the other kidney being obscured by the spine if scanning from the lateral aspect of the fetus. Similar to the first trimester, kidneys in the mid-second trimester are homogeneous and only slightly more echogenic than neighboring structures, making them difficult to delineate (Fig. 1.102). In addition to scanning the kidneys with the ultrasound probe being pointed toward the fetal

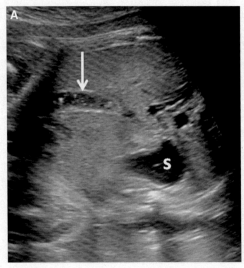
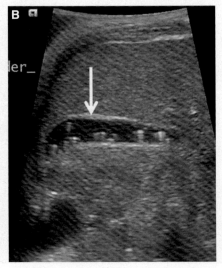

**FIGURE 1.94:** Axial sections of the upper abdomen demonstrating a gallbladder (arrows) with multiple small luminal echogenicities, which are suggestive of either gallstones or sludge. s, stomach.

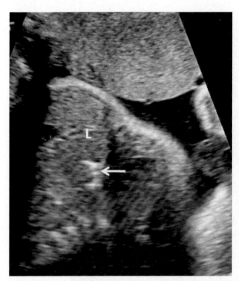

**FIGURE 1.95:** Sagittal view of the liver *(L)* of a fetus in the late second trimester. An isolated calcification of the liver capsule *(arrow)* is seen.

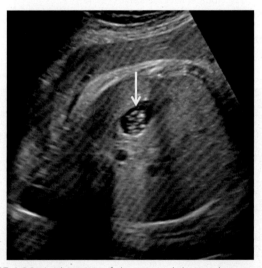

**FIGURE 1.96:** Axial section of the upper abdomen demonstrating a stomach *(arrow)* filled with echogenic debris.

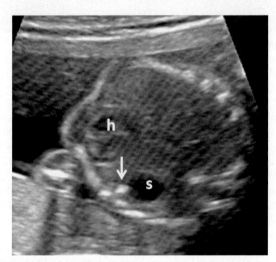

**FIGURE 1.97:** Axial/oblique section of the upper abdomen and the lower chest demonstrating a perigastric echogenic focus *(arrow). s,* stomach; *h,* heart.

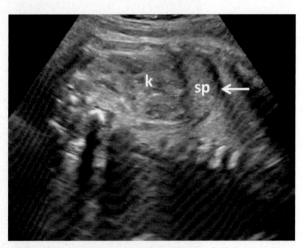

**FIGURE 1.98:** Longitudinal view of the left side of a fetus in the late second trimester. *k,* kidney; *sp,* spleen; *arrow,* diaphragm.

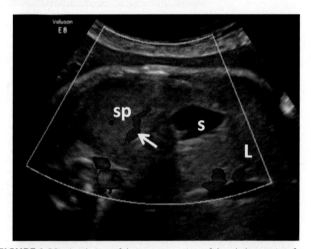

**FIGURE 1.99:** Axial view of the upper portion of the abdomen in a fetus in the late second trimester. Please note the similarity in echogenicity of the spleen *(sp)* and the liver *(L). Arrow,* splenic artery; *s,* stomach.

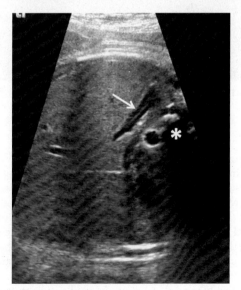

**FIGURE 1.100:** Axial view of the upper portion of the abdomen in a fetus in the early third trimester demonstrating the normal adrenal gland *(arrow)* appearance. The thin echogenic line located in the middle of the adrenal is a normal finding. *Asterisk,* vertebra.

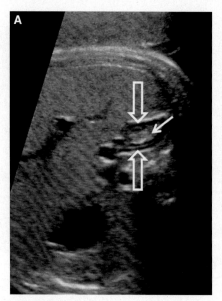
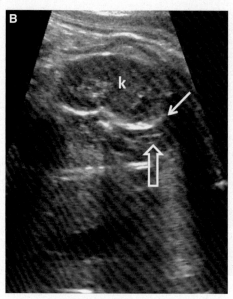

**FIGURE 1.101: A:** Axial view of the upper portion of the abdomen of the same fetus as in Figure 1.100. However, the section is slightly more caudal in location and includes the renal capsule over the superior pole of the kidney *(solid arrow)*, which is surrounded by normal adrenal parenchyma *(open arrows)*. This should not be mistaken for an adrenal hemorrhage. **B:** Longitudinal view of the same region depicting the anatomic relationship of the renal capsule *(solid arrow)* and the adrenal *(open arrow)* that produces the artifact presented in **A**. Note that the adrenal gland is partially obscured by rib shadowing. *k,* kidney.

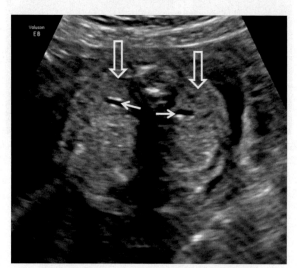

**FIGURE 1.102:** Axial view of the abdomen at the level of the renal pelves *(solid arrows)* in a midtrimester fetus. Please note that the echogenicity of the kidneys *(open arrows)* is very similar to that of the surrounding structures.

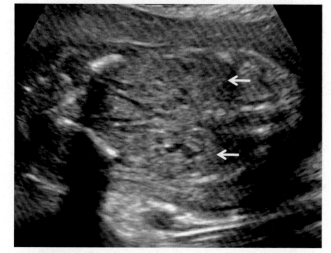

**FIGURE 1.103:** Coronal view of both kidneys in a midtrimester fetus *(arrows,* upper renal poles). The echogenicity of the kidneys is very similar to that of the surrounding structures.

back, employing coronal and longitudinal views may be very helpful in establishing the presence of the kidneys (Fig. 1.103). Similarly, color Doppler can be used to help define the renal vessels, which also helps in distinguishing renal presence versus absence (Fig. 1.104). The renal cortex becomes less echogenic in the third trimester, and the capsule is more sharply delineated, making them easier to see (Fig. 1.105). The surface of the kidney is often undulating in contour, consistent with fetal lobulations (Fig. 1.106).[137,138]

The renal hilum is located on the medial side of the kidney. The renal pelvis is located at the hilum and can be identified on ultrasound as a small, slit-like structure with anechoic content (see Figs. 1.102 and 1.105). Although the kidneys are not normally measured during the course of the 20-week anomaly scan, charts of measurements of the kidney throughout the gestation are available. The renal pelvis is typically assessed in AP diameter and is commonly measured, as mild pyelectasis (measurement ≥4 mm) is recognized as a potential marker for trisomy 21 (see Fig. 1.105). This is, however, a weak marker of limited value within the context of modern screening strategies. However, pyelectasis, especially if associated with caliectasis, requires follow-up later in pregnancy and after delivery, as in some cases these can become clinically significant. A wide variety of renal abnormalities may be seen during the 20-week scan, or become apparent at later gestations. It is important to ensure that both kidneys are properly assessed and to remember that

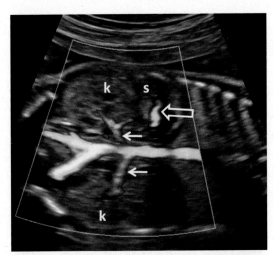

**FIGURE 1.104:** Coronal view of both kidneys *(k)* in a midtrimester fetus demonstrating the presence of renal vessels *(solid arrows)* bilaterally with color Doppler. *Open arrow,* splenic artery; *s,* spleen.

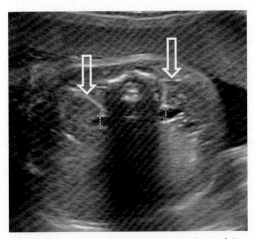

**FIGURE 1.105:** Axial view of the abdomen at the level of the renal pelves *(calipers)* in a third trimester fetus. The renal parenchyma is now more hypoechoic as compared with Figure 1.102, and the renal capsule *(arrows)* is better defined and increased in echogenicity.

it is not uncommon for a fetus with one renal anomaly to have another problem affecting the contralateral kidney.[139–141]

Each kidney should be evaluated along its entire length in either a longitudinal or coronal section. Occasionally, isolated renal cysts may be present. These are generally not clinically significant but rarely may be an early sign of autosomal dominant polycystic kidney disease. It is important to include a sweep through the entire length of the kidney, as the cysts may be isolated. Large cysts are readily defined and are hypoechoic. Highly echogenic kidneys should undergo careful evaluation and follow-up. This finding may be due to perinatal type of polycystic kidney disease, which is a serious problem with a grave prognosis. In these circumstances, the kidneys are enlarged and diffusely echogenic, and the normal internal anatomy is absent. However, occasionally the renal parenchyma will be noted as highly echogenic, but the anatomy is otherwise normal as is the renal size (Fig. 1.107). The prognosis in these cases is generally good, but the risk of poor renal function later in childhood is increased.

The renal pyramids become better delineated as the pregnancy progresses. They are seen as hypoechoic structures surrounded by echogenic cortical projections, containing the straight tubules of the nephrons (see Fig. 1.106). Understanding that this represents normal architecture, especially in the third trimester, helps to prevent the incorrect diagnosis of renal cysts from being made.

Renal agenesis may be unilateral or bilateral. Unilateral agenesis does not normally complicate the postnatal period, and the amniotic fluid volume around the fetus is typically normal. The contralateral kidney is often enlarged, which appears to be a compensatory change. It is important to remember that an empty renal fossa does not necessarily mean that the kidney is absent; it may be present in an ectopic location, most commonly in the pelvis. Therefore, the finding of an empty renal fossa should always first lead to a careful search for a kidney in an unusual location. Fetuses with bilateral renal agenesis develop anhydramnios by mid-gestation. The absence of fluid around the fetus reduces the quality of imaging and makes the decision whether or not kidneys are absent that much more difficult. In the presence of anhydramnios, it is especially important to employ all views of the fetal abdomen (axial, longitudinal, and

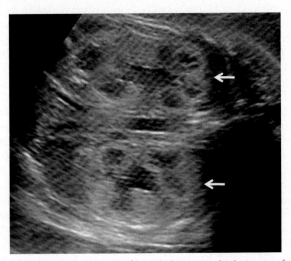

**FIGURE 1.106:** Coronal view of both kidneys in a third trimester fetus. The hypoechoic structures within the renal parenchyma are renal pyramids with the surrounding cortical projections that are more echogenic. Also note the slightly undulating contour of the surface of the kidneys, consistent with fetal lobulations. *Arrows,* upper renal poles.

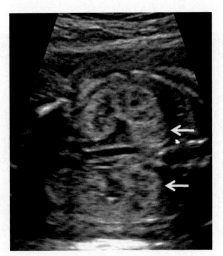

**FIGURE 1.107:** Coronal view of both kidneys in late second trimester fetus. The echogenicity of the renal parenchyma is increased. However, the normal renal architecture, including the hypoechoic pyramids, is preserved, and the kidneys are not enlarged. *Arrows,* upper renal poles.

coronal) as well as undertake a detailed search for the kidneys in ectopic locations. This should also include an attempt to identify renal arteries using color Doppler. This is best accomplished by scanning through the aorta and IVC in a coronal section.

Ureters are not normally visible during a prenatal scan. An obstructed, dilated ureter appears as a convoluted hypoechoic tubular structure; therefore, a cross section of a significantly dilated ureter will often have the appearance of multiple anechoic cysts. Common causes of pelvic and ureteral dilatation include vesicoureteral reflux and ureteral obstruction. Both of these problems can also be associated with renal duplication. Therefore, abnormal ureteral findings should always lead to a careful examination of the renal hilum (looking for a duplicated collecting system) and the urinary bladder (looking for a ureterocele), both of which can be seen in renal duplication.[142,143] A hypoechoic structure extending from the lower portion of the kidney to the pelvis is frequently noted in longitudinal views. This represents the psoas muscle and should not be mistaken for a prominent ureter (Fig. 1.108).

Defects of the anterior abdominal wall can occur anywhere along the midline but are most common at the level of the umbilicus. Therefore, the abdominal cord insertion should be clearly imaged. Although this is typically done in a transverse section, it may also be achieved with a midsagittal view (Fig. 1.109). Herniation of abdominal contents into the root of the umbilical cord beyond 12 weeks' gestation is never normal and constitutes an omphalocele. While an omphalocele has a membranous covering, and the umbilical cord is noted to insert directly into this membranous sac, gastroschisis is an open abdominal wall defect located immediately to the right of an otherwise normal abdominal cord insertion. This diagnosis is also made in a transverse section, but in contrast to an omphalocele, the protruding bowel in a gastroschisis does not have a covering membrane and is free-floating in the amniotic fluid.

The umbilical cord normally contains a single vein, which carries oxygenated blood to the fetus and two arteries, which return deoxygenated blood to the placenta. These vessels are encased in Wharton's jelly up to the point where the cord meets the anterior abdominal wall. A detailed discussion regarding the umbilical cord is included in Chapter 7. The umbilical vessels separate within the fetal abdomen. The umbilical vein first

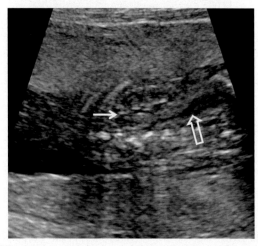

**FIGURE 1.108:** Longitudinal and slightly oblique view of the right kidney. The psoas muscle (*open arrow*) is clearly visible and should not be mistaken for a dilated ureter. *Solid arrow*, upper renal pole.

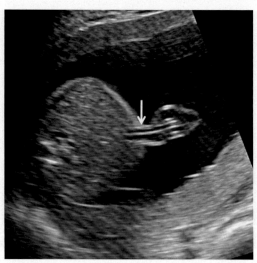

**FIGURE 1.109:** An axial view of the fetal abdomen at the level of the abdominal cord insertion (*arrow*).

courses along the anterior abdominal wall in a cephalad direction and then enters the liver, following a course as described above. Between the umbilical cord insertion and the liver, the size of the umbilical vein is variable. If it is excessively large, it is termed a varix. This finding has been associated with other fetal anomalies and poor perinatal outcome. From the umbilical cord insertion, the direction of umbilical arteries is in the posterior and inferior direction around the bladder (Fig. 1.110). They originate from the internal iliac arteries (Fig. 1.111). Following delivery, the segments of the umbilical arteries that bridge the distance between the dome of the bladder and the cord insertion become obliterated and become the medial umbilical ligaments. The remaining portions of the umbilical arteries stay patent and become the superior vesical arteries.

The bowel can be examined as the transducer is swept in transverse section from the upper abdomen, through the level of the umbilicus to the pelvis. The appearance of fetal bowel changes with gestation. In the first and early second trimester, the bowel is fairly uniform in appearance, and individual bowel loops are difficult to identify. The overall echogenicity is normally slightly greater and more heterogeneous than that of the liver parenchyma (Fig. 1.112). In the latter half of the second trimester and the third trimester, a variable amount of fluid may be visualized within some of the small bowel loops, and the differentiation between the small and large bowels becomes possible (Figs. 1.113 and 1.114). Under normal circumstances, the amount of fluid within the small bowel is relatively small. However, small bowel dilatation, defined as a diameter >6 mm,[144] may be indicative of bowel pathology such as jejunal or ileal atresia. The bowel may be abnormally echogenic, appearing as bright as bone, during the 20-week scan. This is most commonly due to a benign cause such as intra-amniotic bleeding, where the fetus has swallowed bloodstained amniotic fluid. However, it can also be associated with fetal aneuploidy, fetal hypoxia, intrauterine growth restriction, cystic fibrosis, meconium ileus, and fetal infection. The colon is identifiable on prenatal ultrasound consistently from 24 weeks onward. Its diameter is variable but tends to be significantly greater than small bowel. The contents have greater echogenicity than those of the small bowel. Dilated large bowel may be associated with obstruction or neurologic diseases affecting the bowel wall. Significantly increased echogenicity of the large

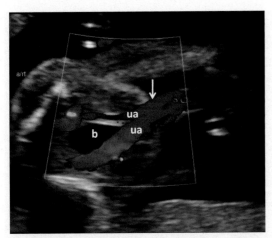

**FIGURE 1.110:** An axial/oblique view of the fetal lower abdomen and pelvis demonstrating the two umbilical arteries *(ua)* coursing from the abdominal cord insertion *(arrow)* around the bladder *(b)*.

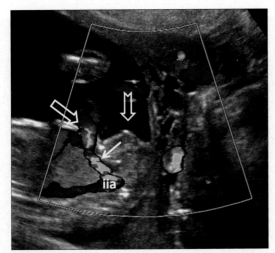

**FIGURE 1.111:** A longitudinal view of the umbilical cord insertion *(open arrow)* and the course of the intra-abdominal portion of the umbilical artery *(solid arrow)* to the point of its origin from the internal iliac artery *(iia)*. This is a female fetus *(notched arrow)*.

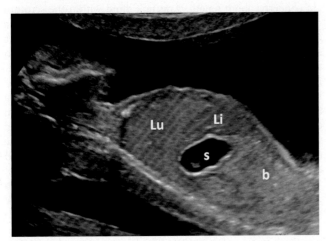

**FIGURE 1.112:** A longitudinal view of the torso and abdomen in the mid-second trimester demonstrating the differences in echogenicity of the lung *(Lu)*, liver *(Li)*, and the bowel *(b)*. Note the homogeneous appearance of the bowel. *s,* stomach.

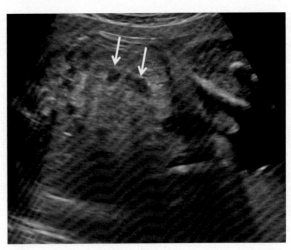

**FIGURE 1.113:** Transverse/oblique view of the fetal abdomen in the third trimester. Note the multiple hypoechoic spaces *(arrows)* representing fluid-filled small bowel loops. This is a normal finding in the third trimester.

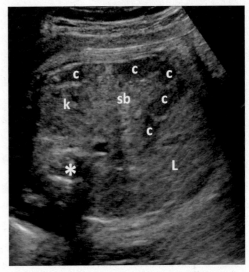

**FIGURE 1.114:** Transverse/oblique view of the fetal abdomen in the third trimester with the colon *(c)* clearly visible separately from the rest of the abdominal structures. *Asterisk,* vertebra; *L,* liver; *sb,* small bowel; *k,* kidney.

colon contents may be associated with disease processes such as cystic fibrosis. Occasionally, the rectum is seen to have anechoic contents, which is a normal finding. The anus and the anal sphincter can be identified readily as a hypoechoic ring with an echogenic center on careful examination of the posterior fetal pelvis (Fig. 1.115).[144–147]

The urinary bladder is visualized as an anechoic cystic structure within the fetal pelvis (Fig. 1.116; see Fig. 1.110). The size of the bladder is highly variable and dependent on the amount of fetal urine production and output at any point in time. After emptying, the bladder may be difficult to visualize, but this is normally a transient issue. Sustained absence of the urinary bladder throughout the examination is never a normal finding. If the bladder proves difficult to visualize, color Doppler can be used to locate the intra-abdominal portions of the umbilical arteries, and therefore the location where the bladder should be seen (see Fig. 1.110). Persistent absence of a urinary bladder in

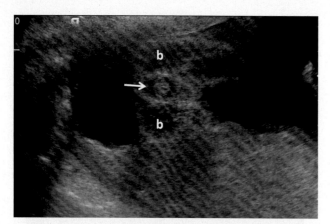

**FIGURE 1.115:** Transverse view of the anus *(arrow)*. The anal sphincter is hypoechoic, forming a ring around the anus, known as the "target sign." *b*, buttocks.

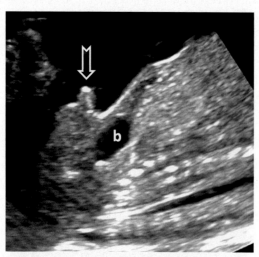

**FIGURE 1.116:** A longitudinal view of the abdomen demonstrating a normal size bladder *(b)*. This is a male fetus *(arrow)*.

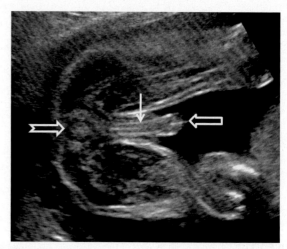

**FIGURE 1.117:** A transverse view of external male genitalia in mid-second trimester. *Open arrow*, penis; *solid arrow*, corpus cavernosum; *notched arrow*, anus.

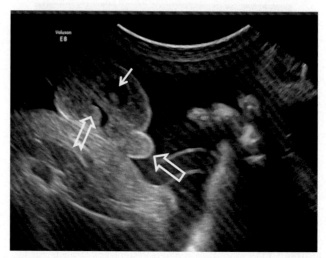

**FIGURE 1.118:** A coronal/oblique view of external male genitalia in mid-third trimester. *Open arrow*, penis; *notched arrow*, testis; *solid arrow*, small hydrocele.

association with a normal amniotic fluid volume is indicative of rare but serious fetal anomalies such as bladder or cloacal exstrophy. At the other extreme, a large bladder may be observed when there is outflow obstruction. There are a number of potential causes, but in male fetuses a "key hole" appearance with dilatation of the proximal portion of the urethra is indicative of the presence of posterior urethral valves. When an anomaly of the urinary tract is suspected, assessment of the amniotic fluid volume provides valuable information about its functional effect.

## External Genitalia

The gender of the fetus can be determined with a high degree of accuracy by using transverse and midsagittal planes. Accurate definition of fetal gender is important in a number of genetic conditions. It may help define the need for invasive testing in pregnancies at risk of X-linked dominant conditions. Alternatively, it may direct need for therapeutic intervention, e.g., steroid therapy to prevent virilization in female fetuses at risk of congenital adrenal hyperplasia.

At the 20-week anomaly scan, the diagnosis of a male depends on demonstration of the penis and scrotum. The penis appears to be short compared with infancy, but this is normal (Fig. 1.117). Charts of penile length have been published if there

are concerns about length. Anechoic fluid within the scrotum representing hydroceles is fairly common, and in the absence of hydrops fetalis or ascites, it is not associated with any specific fetal and neonatal problems. One or both testes appear within the scrotum at variable times during (Fig. 1.118) the third trimester. Both the penis and the scrotum may also be visualized in the same view in a sagittal section of the genital area (Fig. 1.119). The fetal urethra is not identifiable under normal circumstances. However, in the presence of posterior urethral valves, the proximal urethra can be very dilated. Also, in the rare instance of a megalourethra, the urethra may be dilated and contain anechoic fluid along its entire length.

The diagnosis of female gender should not be reliant on merely being unable to demonstrate the presence of the penis/scrotum. In transverse section, the swelling of the labial folds can be visualized (Fig. 1.120). The clitoris is best identified in a sagittal section (Fig. 1.121). The labia minora, and later in pregnancy the labia majora, are seen as two elongated somewhat hypoechoic structures with an echogenic line dividing the two (Figs. 1.122 and 1.123). The latter represents the interface

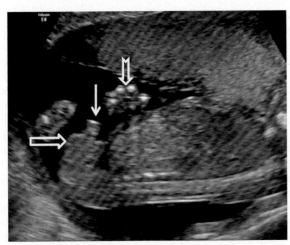

**FIGURE 1.119:** A sagittal view of external male genitalia in mid-second trimester. *Solid arrow,* penis; *open arrow,* scrotum; *notched arrow,* transverse view of fingers.

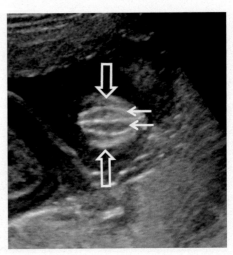

**FIGURE 1.122:** A transverse view of external female genitalia in early third trimester with prominent labia minora. *Solid arrows,* labia minora; *open arrows,* labia majora.

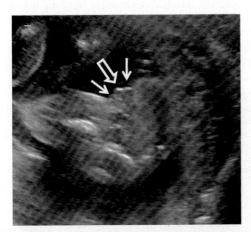

**FIGURE 1.120:** A transverse view of external female genitalia in mid-second trimester. *Solid arrows,* labia majora; *open arrow,* confluence of labia minora.

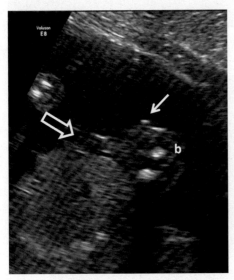

**FIGURE 1.121:** A sagittal view of external female genitalia in mid-second trimester. *Solid arrow,* clitoris; *open arrow,* abdominal cord insertion; *b,* buttock.

between the two labia. The echogenicity of the labia majora is the same as of the fetal skin and, therefore, greater than of the labia minora.

Identification of fetal gender is made more difficult by several factors such as early gestational age (see section on first trimester ultrasound evaluation), positioning of the fetal legs close together, umbilical cord coursing between the legs, maternal habitus, and fetal position. In both sagittal and transverse views, care should be taken to ensure the structures visualized represent male anatomy and not the rare case of ambiguous genitalia. If the labia majora are especially prominent in the third trimester, they may be erroneously identified as the scrotum. If the labia minora are particularly prominent, especially in the presence of clitoromegaly, the appearance of the external genitalia may be ambiguous. Erroneous assignment of female gender may occur in the presence of severe hypospadias.

## Extremities

Careful, systematic sequential examination of the extremities is important as anomalies may affect one or more limbs and be seen at any level. These anomalies are frequently isolated. However, a wide range of fetal problems, including aneuploidy and genetic syndromes, are associated with limb defects. Therefore, a limb anomaly should lead to a careful examination of the rest of the fetal anatomy.[148]

Starting proximally, both humeri and femora should be examined to make sure they are an appropriate length, are straight with normal mineralization, and have no evidence of fractures (Fig. 1.124). Both the femur and the humerus are measured in exactly the same fashion: The bone is insonated along its longitudinal axis with the ends of the bone being as sharply delineated as possible, and it is measured from one end to the other. In the second trimester, shortening of the humerus has a slightly better predictive value than shortening of the femur when screening for trisomy 21. Moving distally, the forearm or lower leg should contain two long bones, which are also assessed for mineralization and fractures. They are not routinely measured unless an anomaly is suspected. Identification of both bones in the forearm is important, as radial hypoplasia or aplasia is part of the phenotype of a number of syndromes. At the elbow, the ulna is located medially

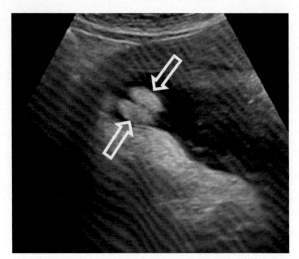

**FIGURE 1.123:** A transverse view of external female genitalia in late third trimester with only labia majora *(arrows)* visible.

to the radius. Their relative position at the level of the wrist depends on the degree of rotation of the forearm (Fig. 1.125). Many skeletal dysplasias will be defined on the basis of shortening or fracture of long bones, and the pattern of shortening is often important in reaching a firm diagnosis. Unilateral limb deficiencies

are rare but can be detected at 20 weeks' gestation. These can involve any portion of the limb; therefore, it is important to always attempt to evaluate each limb in its entirety (Fig. 1.126).

In the presence of normal amniotic fluid volume, the limbs should move freely at each of the joints. Freedom of movement is implied by documentation that the hip, knee, elbow, ankle, and wrist joints are held in normal anatomical positions. Abnormal angulation of the ankle joint (ankle clubbing, talipes equinovarus) is common, with a prevalence of 1 in 100 live births. The most useful view for ruling out this diagnosis is a coronal section of the ankle. The ankle normally extends straight along the same axis as the lower leg (Fig. 1.127). However, in the presence of ankle clubbing, the ankle deviates medially. The longitudinal view is also useful to evaluate the relationship between the lower leg and the ankle. Slight angulation of the ankle is common, especially in the third trimester due to intrauterine crowding (Fig. 1.128). Two findings help to differentiate positional angulation of the ankles from true clubbing. Firstly, the angulation of the ankle due to positional changes is not as severe as with true clubbing. Secondly, a clubbed ankle stays in a fixed position and never straightens out. Unilateral ankle clubbing is generally an isolated defect. However, bilateral clubbing can be seen in association with chromosomal or genetic conditions.

The wrist is very flexible and may be seen in a variety of positions. The position of the fingers is also variable. In a resting

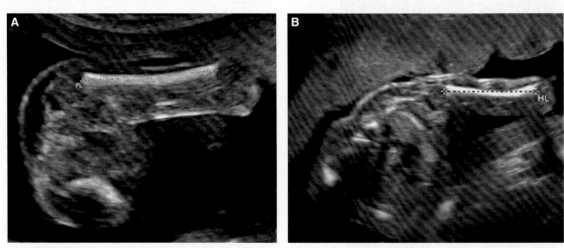

**FIGURE 1.124:** Longitudinal views of femur (*FL* in **A**) and humerus (*HL* in **B**). *Calipers* denote their measurements.

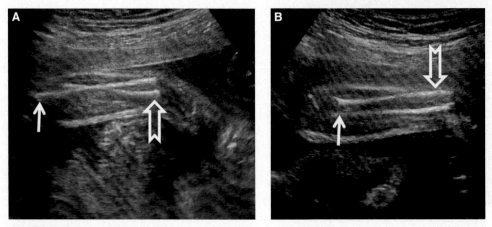

**FIGURE 1.125:** Views of ulna *(solid arrow)* and radius *(open arrow)*. **A:** The bones are crossed during pronation. **B:** The bones are parallel in a supine position.

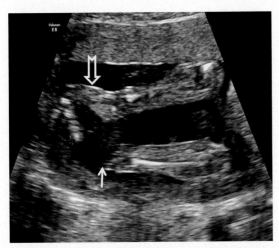

**FIGURE 1.126:** Longitudinal view of both forearms with a normal left hand *(open arrow)* and a completely absent right hand *(solid arrow).*

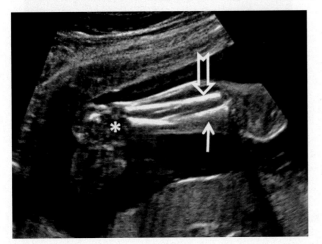

**FIGURE 1.127:** Coronal view of the lower leg and the ankle *(asterisk).* The edges of the ankle are a fairly straight continuation of the lower leg, ruling out ankle clubbing. *Solid arrow,* tibia; *open arrow,* fibula.

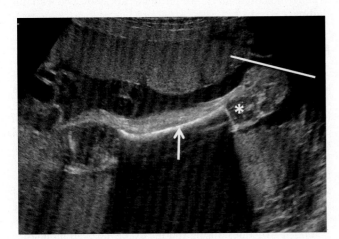

**FIGURE 1.128:** Coronal view of the lower leg and the ankle *(asterisk).* Please note that the ankle is straight but the foot is turned in *(solid line* is parallel to the sole of the foot). This is related to fetal position rather than clubbing. *Arrow,* tibia.

position, the fingers often form a fist, but the hand can be stimulated to open, showing all four fingers and thumb (Fig. 1.129). Unlike in the first trimester, in the second and third trimesters the thumb is visible in a different plane from the rest of the fingers (Fig. 1.130). The most consistently reliable method for counting the fingers is in a transverse section that lines up the proximal phalanges or their respective metacarpals in a row (Fig. 1.131). Polydactyly is more common in some ethnic groups, such as African Americans. It may be seen in isolation and may affect both hands and feet. Both abnormal number of fingers or abnormal position of fingers (campylodactyly or clinodactyly) is associated with an increased risk of an underlying fetal syndrome. Fingers also can be missing, often due to the amniotic band syndrome. However, certain rare syndromes such as Ectrodactyly–ectodermal dysplasia–cleft syndrome are associated with missing fingers as well.

The foot is best imaged with a superficial transverse section showing the heel, sole, and toes (Fig. 1.132). The position of the big toe with respect to the other toes can be evaluated for a "sandal gap" anomaly, which has a weak association with trisomy 21. The length of the foot can also be assessed in the same view. This is especially useful in assessment of skeletal dysplasias, where the femur is short but the foot length is typically preserved; therefore, the femur to foot length ratio will be significantly decreased (0.9). A normal ratio will be preserved in a fetus with a constitutionally short femur.

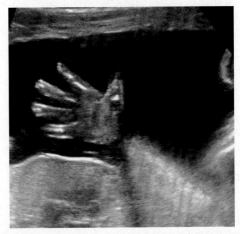

**FIGURE 1.129:** Image of an open hand demonstrating portions of all five fingers.

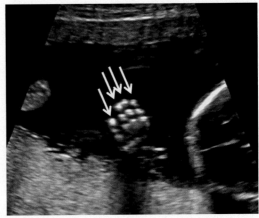

**FIGURE 1.130:** Image of four fingers *(arrows)* with all three phalangeal ossification centers visible in each digit.

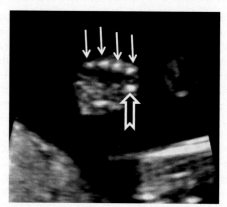

**FIGURE 1.131:** Transverse section of the hand allowing visualization of the phalanges of all four fingers *(solid arrows)* and the thumb *(open arrow)* in the same view.

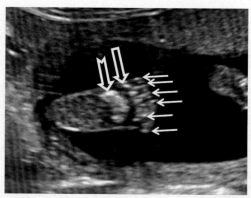

**FIGURE 1.134:** Transverse section of the foot with a row of metatarsals *(notched arrow)* and a row of digits *(open arrow)* visible. Note the echogenic skin *(solid arrows)* on the surface of the toes, which can often be even more prominent than presented here.

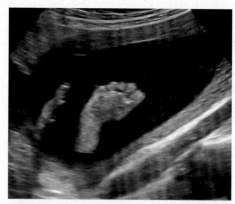

**FIGURE 1.132:** Superficial transverse section of the foot with all five toes evident.

The phalangeal and/or metatarsal ossification centers can occasionally be counted in a transverse section (Fig. 1.133). However, the interfaces between the toes can often be seen as thin echogenic lines and can be mistaken for phalanges (Fig. 1.134). Therefore, toes should also be counted in coronal section (Fig. 1.135). This view has the advantage of presenting the phalanges and/or metatarsals as discrete echogenic points that are easier to define individually. Essentially the same differential diagnosis applies to lower extremity polydactyly or missing toes as to their upper extremity counterparts.

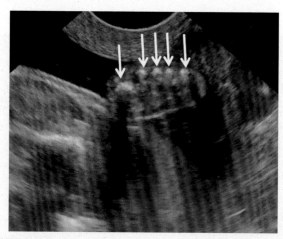

**FIGURE 1.135:** Coronal section of the foot with all five metatarsals or digits easily identified as separate echogenic dots *(arrows)*.

The lower extremities should be visually evaluated for the presence of fluid accumulation since certain syndromes, such as congenital (hereditary) lymphedema, are associated with this finding.

## Miscellaneous Bony Structures

There are a number of other bony structures that can be evaluated and/or measured, although this is not normally done as a routine. Extended, specialized examinations are generally performed as needed, based on recognized family history or on other abnormalities that are identified. For example, the fetal clavicles can be readily examined and measured as early as the first trimester (Fig. 1.136; see Fig. 1.11). This evaluation is helpful in those individuals who are at risk for cleidocranial dysplasia. Fetal scapulae are also readily identifiable, and may be of value in defining skeletal dysplasia, where the scapulae may be dysplastic (Fig. 1.137). Defining the anatomy of less commonly examined structures during routine exams helps to familiarize the operator with their typical appearance, experience that is very valuable in the event that they need to be assessed to clarify a diagnosis.

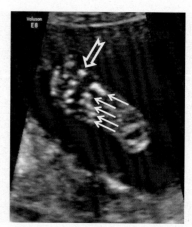

**FIGURE 1.133:** Transverse section of the foot with five metatarsals *(solid arrows)* and the row of their corresponding digits *(open arrow)*.

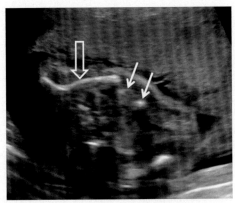

**FIGURE 1.136:** Axial view of the clavicle *(open arrow)* in the late second trimester. *Solid arrows,* upper portion of the manubrium.

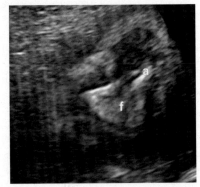

**FIGURE 1.137:** Coronal/oblique section of the fetal back in late second trimester demonstrating the scapula. *a,* acromion and spina scapulae; *f,* fossa infraspinata.

## CONCLUSION

The list of complications that can affect pregnancy outcome is long and varied. Many of these issues can be assessed by a high-quality ultrasound performed by qualified personnel. The effectiveness of ultrasound is improved by taking a systematic approach to the examination. It cannot be overstated that thorough understanding of normal fetal anatomy is the first step toward fetal anomaly detection.[149] It is critical for individual ultrasound centers to perform ongoing audit, which includes a periodic review of image quality for each sonographer and to collect data related to pregnancy outcome. A detailed image review needs to be performed in each case where a fetal anomaly went unrecognized on prenatal ultrasound. If deficiencies are noted on the review, appropriate and prompt changes need to be made to improve techniques and methods of assessment.

## REFERENCES

1. Donald I, MacVicar J, Brown TG. Investigation of abdominal masses by pulsed ultrasound. *Lancet.* 1958;1:1188–1195.
2. Donald I, Abdulla U. Ultrasonics in obstetrics and gynaecology. *Br J Radiol.* 1967;40:604–611.
3. Salomon LJ, Alfirevic Z, Berghella V, et al. Practice guidelines for performance of the routine mid-trimester fetal ultrasound scan (ISUOG). *Ultrasound Obstet Gynecol.* 2011;37:116–126.
4. American Institute of Ultrasound in Medicine. AIUM practice guideline for the performance of obstetric ultrasound examinations. *J Ultrasound Med.* 2010;29:157–166.
5. American College of Obstetricians and Gynecologists. Ultrasonography in pregnancy. *Obstet Gynecol.* 2009;113:451–461 ACOG Practice Bulletin No. 101.
6. Australasian Society for Ultrasound in Medicine. *Policies and Statements, D2: Guidelines for the Mid Trimester Obstetric Scan.* http://www.asum.com.au/open/P&S/D2_policy.pdf.
7. National Collaborating Centre for Women's and Children's Health. *Antenatal Care: Routine Care for the Healthy Pregnant Woman.* 2nd ed. London, England: RCOG Press; 2008.
8. Nicolaides KH. Screening for fetal aneuploidy at 11 to 13 weeks. *Prenat Diagn.* 2011;31:7–15.
9. Sonek JD. First trimester ultrasonography in screening and detection of fetal anomalies. *Am J Med Genet C Semin Med Genet.* 2007;145:45–61.
10. Souka AP, Pilalis A, Kavalakis Y, et al. Assessment of fetal anatomy at the 11–14-week ultrasound examination. *Ultrasound Obstet Gynecol.* 2004;24:730–734.
11. Becker R, Wegner RD. Detailed screening for fetal anomalies and cardiac defects at the 11–13 week scan. *Ultrasound Obstet Gynecol.* 2006;27:613–618.
12. Lanchmann R, Chaoui R, Moratalla J, et al. Posterior brain in fetuses with open spina bifida at 11–13 weeks. *Prenat Diagn.* 2011;31:103–106.
13. Poon LCY, Kametas NA, Chelemen T, et al. Maternal risk factors for hypertensive disorders in pregnancy: a multivariate approach. *J Hum Hypertens.* 2010;24:104–110.
14. Brenner WE, Edelman DA, Hendricks CH. A standard of fetal growth for the United States of America. *Am J Obstet Gynecol.* 1976;126:555–564.
15. Campbell S, Thoms A. Ultrasound measurement of fetal head to abdomen circumference ratio in the assessment of growth retardation. *Br J Obstet Gynaecol.* 1977;84:165–174.
16. Hadlock FP, Harrist RB, Martinez-Poyer J. In utero analysis of fetal growth: a sonographic weight standard. *Radiology.* 1991;181:129–133.
17. Robson SC, Gallivan S, Walkinshaw SA, et al. Ultrasonic estimation of fetal weight: use of targeted formulas in small for gestational age fetuses. *Obstet Gynecol.* 1993;82:359–364.
18. David C, Gabrielli S, Pilu G, et al. The head-to-abdomen circumference ratio: a reappraisal. *Ultrasound Obstet Gynecol.* 1995;5:256–259.
19. Gardosi J, Chang A, Kalyan B, et al. Customised antenatal growth charts. *Lancet.* 1992;339:283–287.
20. Clausson B, Gardosi J, Francis A, et al. Perinatal outcome in SGA births defined by customised versus population-based birthweight standards. *Br J Obstet Gynecol.* 2001;108:830–834.
21. Smith-Bindman R, Chu PW, Ecker JL, et al. US evaluation of fetal growth: prediction of neonatal outcomes. *Radiology.* 2002;223:153–161.
22. Nyberg DA, Abuhamad A, Ville Y. Ultrasound assessment of abnormal fetal growth. *Semin Perinatol.* 2004;28:3–22.
23. Bricker L, Neilson JP, Dowswell T. Routine ultrasound in late pregnancy (after 24 weeks' gestation). *Cochrane Database Syst Rev.* 2008;8:CD001451.
24. Prayer D, Kasparian F, Krampl E, et al. MRI of normal brain development. *Eur J Radiol.* 2006;57:199–216.
25. Eurenius K, Axelsson O, Gallstedt-Fransson I, et al. Perception of information, expectations and experiences among women and their partners attending a second-trimester routine ultrasound scan. *Ultrasound Obstet Gynecol.* 1997;9:86–90.
26. Pike I, Russo A, Berkowitz J, et al. The prevalence of musculoskeletal disorders among diagnostic medical sonographers. *JDMS.* 1997;13:219–227.
27. Magnavita N, Bevilacqua L, Mirk P, et al. Work-related musculoskeletal complaints in sonologists. *J Occup Environ Med.* 1999;41:981–988.
28. Stothard KJ, Tennant PW, Bell R, et al. Maternal overweight and obesity and the risk of congenital anomalies: a systematic review and meta-analysis. *JAMA.* 2009;301:636–650.
29. Church CC, Carstensen EL, Nyborg WL, et al. The risk of exposure to diagnostic ultrasound in postnatal subjects: nonthermal mechanisms. *J Ultrasound Med.* 2008;27:565–592.
30. Miller MW, Nyborg WL, Dewey WC, et al. Hyperthermic teratogenicity, thermal dose and diagnostic ultrasound during pregnancy: implications of new standards on tissue heating. *Int J Hyperthermia.* 2002;18:361–384.
31. O'Brien WD Jr, Deng CX, Harris GR, et al. The risk of exposure to diagnostic ultrasound in postnatal subjects: thermal effects. *J Ultrasound Med.* 2008;27:517–535.
32. American Institute of Ultrasound in Medicine. *AIUM Statement on Mammalian In Vivo Ultrasonic Biological Effects.* November 8, 2008. http://www.aium.org/.
33. Fowlkes JB; Bioeffects Committee of the American Institute of Ultrasound in Medicine. American Institute of Ultrasound in Medicine consensus report on potential bioeffects of diagnostic ultrasound. *J Ultrasound Med.* 2008;27:503–515.
34. National Council on Radiation Protection and Measurements. *Exposure Criteria for Medical Ultrasound, II: Criteria Based on All Known Mechanisms.* Bethesda, MD: National Council on Radiation Protection and Measurements; 2002 NRCP report 140.
35. Cavicchi TJ, O'Brien WD. Heat generated by ultrasound in an absorbing medium. *J Acoust Soc Am.* 1984;76:1244–1245.
36. Barnett SB, Rott HD, ter Haar GR, et al. The sensitivity of biological tissue to ultrasound. *Ultrasound Med Biol.* 1997;23:805–812.
37. Hershkovitz R, Sheiner E, Mazor M. Ultrasound in obstetrics: a review of safety. *Eur J Obstet Gynecol Reprod Biol.* 2002;101:15–18.
38. Stark CR, Orleans M, Haverkamp AD, et al. Short- and long-term risks after exposure to diagnostic ultrasound in utero. *Obstet Gynecol.* 1984;63:194–200.

39. Lyons EA, Dyke C, Toms M, et al. In utero exposure to diagnostic ultrasound: a 6-year follow-up. *Radiology.* 1988;166:687–690.

40. Tarantal AF, Hendrickx AG. Evaluation of the bioeffects of prenatal ultrasound exposure in the cynomolgus macaque (*Macaca fascicularis*), II: growth and behavior during the first year. *Teratology.* 1989;39:149–162.

41. Kossoff G. Contentious issues in safety of diagnostic ultrasound. *Ultrasound Obstet Gynecol.* 1997;10:151–155.

42. Rott HD. Clinical safety statement for diagnostic ultrasound: European Committee for Medical Ultrasound Safety, Tours, France, March 1998. *Eur J Ultrasound.* 1998;8:67–68.

43. Zhu J, Lin J, Zhu Z, et al. Effects of diagnostic levels of color Doppler ultrasound energy on the cell cycle of newborn rats. *J Ultrasound Med.* 1999;18:257–260.

44. Ang ES, Gluncic V, Duque A, et al. Prenatal exposure to ultrasound waves impacts neuronal migration in mice. *Proc Natl Acad Sci U S A.* 2006;103:12903–12910.

45. Warren WB, Timor-Tritsch I, Peisner DB, et al. Dating the early pregnancy by sequential appearance of embryonic structures. *Am J Obstet Gynecol.* 1989;161:747–753.

46. Sepulveda W, Sebire NJ, Hughes K, et al. The lambda sign at 10–14 weeks of gestation as a predictor of chorionicity in twin pregnancies. *Ultrasound Obstet Gynecol.* 1996;7:421–423.

47. Bowerman RA. Sonography of fetal midgut herniation: normal size criteria and correlation with crown-rump length. *J Ultrasound Med.* 1993;5:251–254.

48. Robinson HP, Fleming JEE. A critical evaluation of sonar "crownrump length" measurements. *Br J Obstet Gynecol.* 1975;82:702–710.

49. Chalouhi GE, Bernard JP, Ville Y, et al. A comparison of first trimester measurements for prediction of delivery date. *J Matern Fetal Neonatal Med.* 2011;24:51–57.

50. Salomon LJ, Bernard M, Amarsy R, et al. The impact of crown-rump length measurement error on combined Down syndrome screening: a simulation study. *Ultrasound Obstet Gynecol.* 2009;33:506–511.

51. Hadlock FP, Shah YP, Kanon DJ, et al. Fetal crown-rump length: reevaluation of relation to menstrual age (5–18 weeks) with highresolution real-time US. *Radiology.* 1992;182:501–505.

52. Robinson HP. Gestational age determination: first trimester. In: Chervenak FA, Isaacson GC, Campbell S, eds. *Ultrasound in Obstetrics and Gynecology.* Boston, MA: Little, Brown and Company; 1993:295–304.

53. Blaas HG, Eik-Nes SH, Kiserud T, et al. Early development of the abdominal wall, stomach and heart from 7 to 12 weeks of gestation: a longitudinal ultrasound study. *Ultrasound Obstet Gynecol.* 1995;6:240–249.

54. Souka AP, Von Kaisenberg CS, Hyett JA, et al. Increased nuchal translucency with normal karyotype. *Am J Obstet Gynecol.* 2005;192:1005–1021.

55. Sonek J, Nicolaides KH. Additional first trimester ultrasound markers. *Clin Lab Med.* 2010;30:573–592.

56. Rosati P, Guariglia L. Transvaginal sonographic assessment of the fetal urinary tract in early pregnancy. *Ultrasound Obstet Gynecol.* 1996;7:95–100.

57. Haak MC, Twisk JW, Van Vugt JM. How successful is fetal echocardiographic examination in the first trimester of pregnancy? *Ultrasound Obstet Gynecol.* 2002;20:9–13.

58. Liao AW, Sebire NJ, Geerts L, et al. Megacystis at 10–14 weeks of gestation: chromosomal defects and outcome according to bladder length. *Ultrasound Obstet Gynecol.* 2003;21:338–341.

59. Efrat Z, Akinfenwa O, Nicolaides KH. First-trimester determination of fetal gender by ultrasound. *Ultrasound Obstet Gynecol.* 1999;13:305–307.

60. Saari-Kemppainen A, Karjalainen O, Ylostalo P, et al. Ultrasound screening and perinatal mortality: controlled trial of systematic onestage screening in pregnancy: the Helsinki Ultrasound Trial. *Lancet.* 1990;336:387–391.

61. Chitty LS, Hunt GH, Moore J, et al. Effectiveness of routine ultrasonography in detecting fetal structural abnormalities in a low risk population. *BMJ.* 1991;303:1165–1169.

62. Brocks V, Bang J. Routine examination by ultrasound for the detection of fetal malformations in a low risk population. *Fetal Diagn Ther.* 1991;6:37–45.

63. Levi S, Hyjazi Y, Schaapst JP, et al. Sensitivity and specificity of routine antenatal screening for congenital anomalies by ultrasound: the Belgian Multicentric Study. *Ultrasound Obstet Gynecol.* 1991;1:102–110.

64. Shirley IM, Bottomley F, Robinson VP. Routine radiographer screening for fetal abnormalities by ultrasound in an unselected low risk population. *Br J Radiol.* 1992;65:564–569.

65. Luck CA. Value of routine ultrasound scanning at 19 weeks: a four year study of 8849 deliveries. *BMJ.* 1992;304:1474–1478.

66. Roberts AB, Hampton E, Wilson N. Ultrasound detection of fetal structural abnormalities in Auckland 1988–1989. *N Z Med J.* 1993;106:441–443.

67. Romero R. Routine obstetric ultrasound. *Ultrasound Obstet Gynecol.* 1993;3:303–307.

68. Vintzileos AM, Campbell WA, Rodis JF, et al. The use of secondtrimester genetic sonogram in guiding clinical management of patients at increased risk for fetal trisomy 21. *Obstet Gynecol.* 1996;87:948–952.

69. VanDorsten JP, Hulsey TC, Newman RB, et al. Fetal anomaly detection by second-trimester ultrasonography in a tertiary center. *Am J Obstet Gynecol.* 1998;178:742–749.

70. Grandjean H, Larroque D, Levi S. The performance of routine ultrasonographic screening of pregnancies in the Eurofetus Study. *Am J Obstet Gynecol.* 1999;181:446–454.

71. Vintzileos AM, Ananth CV, Smulian JC, et al. Routine second-trimester ultrasonography in the United States: a cost-benefit analysis. *Am J Obstet Gynecol.* 2000;182:655–660.

72. Filly RA. Obstetrical sonography: the best way to terrify a pregnant woman. *J Ultrasound Med.* 2000;19:1–5.

73. Timor-Tritsch IE. As technology evolves, so should its application: shortcomings of the "18-week anatomy scan." *J Ultrasound Med.* 2006;25:423–428.

74. Schwarzler P, Senat MV, Holden D, et al. Feasibility of the second-trimester fetal ultrasound examination in an unselected population at 18, 20 or 22 weeks of pregnancy: a randomized trial. *Ultrasound Obstet Gynecol.* 1999;14:92–97.

75. Hadlock FP, Deter RL, Harrist RB, et al. Fetal biparietal diameter: rational choice of plane of section for sonographic measurement. *AJR Am J Roentgenol.* 1982;138:871–874.

76. Shepard M, Filly RA. A standardized plane for biparietal diameter measurement. *J Ultrasound Med.* 1982;1:145–150.

77. Hadlock FP, Harrist RB, Deter RJ, et al. Fetal head circumference: relation to menstrual age. *AJR Am J Roentgenol* 1982;138:649–653.

78. Hadlock FP, Deter RL, Harrist RB, et al. Fetal abdominal circumference as a predictor of gestational age. *AJR Am J Roentgenol.* 1982;139:367–370.

79. Queenan JT, O'Brien GD, Campbell S. Ultrasound measurement of fetal limb bones. *Am J Obstet Gynecol.* 1980;138:297–302.

80. Hadlock FP, Harrist RB, Deter RJ, et al. Fetal femur length as a predictor of menstrual age: sonographically measured. *AJR Am J Roentgenol.* 1982;138:875–878.

81. Jeanty P, Rodesch F, Delbeke D, et al. Estimation of gestational age form measurements of fetal long bones. *J Ultrasound Med.* 1984;3:75–79.

82. Smith PA, Johansson D, Tzannatos C, et al. Prenatal measurement of the fetal cerebellum and cisterna cerebellomedullaris by ultrasound. *Prenat Diagn.* 1986;6:133–141.

83. Hadlock FP, Deter RL, Carpenter RLL, et al. The effect of head shape on the accuracy of BPD on estimating fetal gestational age. *AJR Am J Roentgenol.* 1981;137:83–85.

84. Nicolaides KH, Campbell S, Gabbe SG, et al. Ultrasound screening for spina bifida: cranial and cerebellar signs. *Lancet.* 1986;2:72–74.

85. Van den Hof MC, Nicolaides KH, Campbell S, et al. Evaluation of the lemon and banana signs in one hundred thirty fetuses with open spina bifida. *Am J Obstet Gynecol.* 1990;162:322–327.

86. Nyberg DA. Recommendations for obstetric sonography in the evaluation of the fetal cranium. *Radiology.* 1989;172:309–311.

87. Cardoza JD, Goldstein RB, Filly RA. Exclusion of fetal ventriculomegaly with a single measurement: the width of the lateral ventricular atrium. *Radiology.* 1988;169:711–714.

88. Alagappan R, Browning PD, Laorr A, et al. Distal lateral ventricular atrium: reevaluation of normal range. *Radiology.* 1994;193:405–408.

89. Farell TA, Hertzberg BS, Kliewer MA, et al. Fetal lateral ventricles: reassessment of normal values for atrial diameter at US. *Radiology.* 1994;193:409–411.

90. Pilu G, Falco P, Gabrielli S, et al. The clinical significance of fetal isolated cerebral borderline ventriculomegaly: report of 31 cases and review of the literature. *Ultrasound Obstet Gynecol.* 1999;14:320–326.

91. Ghidini A, Strobelt N, Locatelli A, et al. Isolated fetal choroid plexus cysts: role of ultrasonography in establishment of the risk of trisomy 18. *Am J Obstet Gynecol.* 2000;182:972–977.

92. Filly RA, Benacerraf BR, Nyberg DA, et al. Choroid plexus cyst and echogenic intracardiac focus in women at low risk for chromosomal anomalies. *J Ultrasound Med.* 2004;23:447–449.

93. Doubilet PM, Copel JA, Benson CB, et al. Choroid plexus cyst and echogenic intracardiac focus in women at low risk for chromosomal anomalies: the obligation to inform the mother. *J Ultrasound Med.* 2004;23:883–885.

94. D'Addario V, Pinto A, Rossi AC, et al. Cavum veli interpositi cyst: prenatal diagnosis and postnatal outcome. *Ultrasound Obstet Gynecol.* 2009;34:52–54.

95. Bannister CM, Russell SA, Rimmer S, et al. Fetal arachnoid cysts: their site, progress, prognosis and differential diagnosis. *Eur J Pediatr Surg.* 1999;9(suppl 1):27–28.

96. Callen PW, Callen AL, Glenn OA, et al. Columns of the fornix, not be mistaken for the cavum septi pellucidi on prenatal sonography. *J Ultrasound Med.* 2008;27:25–31.

97. Ulm B, Ulm MR, Deutinger J, et al. Dandy-Walker malformation diagnosed before 21 weeks of gestation: associated malformations and chromosomal abnormalities. *Ultrasound Obstet Gynecol.* 1997;10:167–170.

98. Bernard JP, Moscoso G, Renier D, et al. Cystic malformations of the posterior fossa. *Prenat Diagn.* 2001;21:1064–1069.

99. Boddaert N, Klein O, Ferguson N, et al. Intellectual prognosis of the Dandy-Walker malformation in children: the importance of vermian lobulation. *Neuroradiology.* 2003;45:320–324.

100. Bannister CM, Russell SA, Rimmer S, et al. Can prognostic indicators be identified in a fetus with an encephalocele? *Eur J Pediatr Surg.* 2000;10(suppl 1):20–23.

101. McLeary RD, Kuhns LR, Barr M Jr. Ultrasonography of the fetal cerebellum. *Radiology.* 1984;151:439–442.

102. Serthatlioglu S, Kocakoc E, Kiris A, et al. Sonographic measurement of the fetal cerebellum, cisterna magna, and cavum septum pellucidum in normal fetuses in the second and third trimesters of pregnancy. *J Clin Ultrasound.* 2003;31:194–200.

103. Mahony BS, Callen PW, Filly RA, et al. The fetal cisterna magna. *Radiology.* 1984;153:773–776.

104. Knutzon R, McGahan JP, Salamat MS, et al. Fetal cisterna magna septa: a normal anatomic finding. *Radiology*. 1991;180:799–801.

105. Laing FC, Frates MC, Brown DL, et al. Sonography of the fetal posterior fossa: false appearance of mega-cisterna magna and Dandy-Walker variant. *Radiology*. 1994;192:247–251.

106. Filly RA, Simpson GF, Linkowski G. Fetal spine morphology and maturation during the second trimester. *J Ultrasound Med*. 1987;6:631–636.

107. Gray DL, Crane JP, Rudolff MA. Prenatal diagnosis of neural tube defects: origin of midtrimester vertebral ossification centers as determined by sonographic water-bath studies. *J Ultrasound Med*. 1988;7:421–427.

108. Hoopman M, Able H, Yazdi B, et al. Prenatal evaluation of the position of the fetal conus medullaris. *Ultrasound Obstet Gynecol*. 2011;38:548–552.

109. Petrikovsky BM, Vintzileos AM, Rodis JF. Sonographic appearance of occipital fetal hair. *J Clin Ultrasound*. 1989;17:425–427.

110. Bowerman RA. Ultrasound of the fetal face. *Ultrasound Q*. 1993;11:211–258.

111. Mayden KL, Tortora M, Berkowitz RL, et al. Orbital diameters: a new parameter for prenatal diagnosis and dating. *Am J Obstet Gynecol*. 1982;144:289–297.

112. Jeanty P, Cantraine F, Cousaert E, et al. The binocular distance: a new way to estimate gestational age. *J Ultrasound Med*. 1984;3:241–243.

113. Sonek JD, Cicero S, Neiger R, et al. Nasal bone assessment in prenatal screening for trisomy 21. *Am J Obstet Gynecol*. 2006;195:1219–1230.

114. Persico N, Borenstein M, Molina F, et al. Prenasal thickness in trisomy 21 fetuses at 16–24 weeks of gestation. *Ultrasound Obstet Gynecol*. 2008;32(6):751–754.

115. Sonek J, Molina F, Hiett AK, et al. Prefrontal space ratio: comparison between trisomy 21 aneuploid fetuses in the second trimester. *Ultrasound Obstet Gynecol*. 2012;40:293–296.

116. Bimholz JC, The fetal external ear. *Radiology*. 1983;147:819–821.

117. Benacerraf BR, Frigoletto FD Jr. Soft tissue nuchal fold in the second trimester fetus: standards for normal measurements compared with those in Down syndrome. *Am J Obstet Gynecol*. 1987;157:1146–1149.

118. Fong K, Ohlsson A, Zaley A. Fetal thoracic circumference: a prospective cross-sectional study with real-time ultrasound. *Am J Obstet Gynecol*. 1988;158:1154–1160.

119. Cooper C, Mahony BS, Bowie JD, et al. Ultrasound evaluation of the normal fetal upper airway and esophagus. *J Ultrasound Med*. 1985;4:343–346.

120. Avni EF, Rypens F, Milaire J. Fetal esophagus: normal sonographic appearance. *J Ultrasound Med*. 1994;13:175–180.

121. Hess LW, Hess DB, McCaul JF, et al. Fetal echocardiography. *Obstet Gynecol Clin North Am*. 1990;17:41–79.

122. Bromley B, Estroff A, Sandets SP. Fetal echocardiography: accuracy and limitations in a population at high and low risk for heart defects. *Am J Obstet Gynecol*. 1992;166:1473–1481.

123. Abuhamad A. *A Practical Guide to Fetal Echocardiography*. Philadelphia, PA: Lippincott-Raven; 1997.

124. Comstock CH. Normal fetal heart axis and position. *Obstet Gynecol*. 1987;70:255–259.

125. McGahan JP. Sonography of the fetal heart: findings on the four-chamber view. *AJR Am J Roentgenol*. 1991;156:547–553.

126. Brown DL, Cartier MS, Emerson DS, et al. The peripheral hypoechoic rim of the fetal heart. *J Ultrasound Med*. 1989;8:603–608.

127. Levy DW, Mintz MC. The left ventricular echogenic focus: a normal finding. *AJR Am J Roentgenol*. 1988;150:85–86.

128. Petrikovsky BM, Challenger M, Wyse LJ. Natural history of echogenic foci within the ventricle of the fetal heart. *Ultrasound Obstet Gynecol*. 1995;5:92–94.

129. DeVore GR. The aortic and pulmonary outflow tract screening examination in the human fetus. *J Ultrasound Med*. 1992;11:345–348.

130. DeVore GR. Color Doppler examination of the outflow tracts of the fetal heart: a technique for identification of cardiovascular malformation. *Ultrasound Obstet Gynecol*. 1994;4:463–471.

131. Mavrides E, Moscoso G, Carvalho JS, et al. The anatomy of the umbilical, portal and hepatic venous systems in the human fetus at 14–19 weeks of gestation. *Ultrasound Obstet Gynecol*. 2001;18:598–604.

132. Hata K, Aoki S, Hata T, et al. Ultrasound identification of the human fetal gall bladder in utero. *Gynecol Obstet Invest*. 1987;23:79–83.

133. Pretorius DH, Gosink BB, Clautice-Engle T, et al. Sonographic evaluation of the fetal stomach: significance of non-visualization. *AJR Am J Roentgenol*. 1988;151:987–989.

134. Millener PB, Anderson NG, Chisholm RJ. Prognostic significance of non-visualization of the fetal stomach by sonography. *AJR Am J Roentgenol*. 1993;160:827–830.

135. Schmidt W, Yarkoni S, Jeanty P, et al. Sonographic measurements of the fetal spleen: clinical implications. *J Ultrasound Med*. 1985;4:667–672.

136. Rosenberg R, Bowie JD, Andreotti RF, et al. Sonographic evaluation of the fetal adrenal glands. *AJR Am J Roentgenol*. 1982;139:1145–1147.

137. Lawson TL, Foley WD, Berland LL, et al. Ultrasonic evaluation of fetal kidneys: analysis of normal size and frequency of visualization as related to stage of pregnancy. *Radiology*. 1981;138:153–156.

138. Bowie JD, Rosenberg R, Andreotti RF, et al. The changing sonographic appearance of the fetal kidneys during pregnancy. *J Ultrasound Med*. 1983;2:505–507.

139. Grannum P, Bracken M, Silverman R, et al. Assessment of fetal kidney size in normal gestation by comparison of ratio of kidney circumference to abdominal circumference. *Am J Obstet Gynecol*. 1980;136:249–254.

140. Cohen HL, Cooper J, Eisenberg P, et al. Normal length of fetal kidneys: sonographic study in 397 obstetric patients. *AJR Am J Roentgenol*. 1991;157:545–548.

141. Anderson N, Clautice-Engle T, Allan R, et al. Detection of obstructive uropathy in the fetus: predictive value of sonographic measurements of renal pelvic diameter at various gestational ages. *AJR Am J Roentgenol*. 1995;164:719–723.

142. Corteville JE, Gray DL, Crane JP. Congenital hydronephrosis: correlation of fetal ultrasonographic findings with infant outcome. *Am J Obstet Gynecol*. 1991;165:384–388.

143. Mandell J, Blyth BR, Peters CA, et al. Structural genitourinary defects detected in utero. *Radiology*. 1991;178:193–196.

144. Parulekar SG. Sonography of normal fetal bowel. *J Ultrasound Med*. 1991;10:211–220.

145. Nyberg DA, Mack LA, Pattern RM, et al. Fetal bowel: normal sonographic findings. *J Ultrasound Med*. 1987;6:3–6.

146. Vincoff S, Callen PW, Smith-Bindman R, et al. Effect of ultrasound transducer frequency on the appearance of the fetal bowel. *J Ultrasound Med*. 1999;18:799–803.

147. Fakhry J, Reiser M, Shapiro LR, et al. Increased echogenicity in the lower fetal abdomen: a common normal variant in the second trimester. *J Ultrasound Med*. 1986;5:489–492.

148. Mahony BS, Filly RA. High-resolution sonographic assessment of the fetal extremities. *J Ultrasound Med*. 1984;3:489–498.

149. Bowerman RA. *Atlas of Normal Fetal Ultrasonographic Anatomy*. 2nd ed. Chicago, IL: Year Book Medical Publishers; 1992.

# 2 Three-Dimensional Ultrasonography

Luís F. Gonçalves • Richard A. Bronsteen

The first attempts at three-dimensional ultrasonography (3DUS) began in the early 1980s. Tanaka et al.[1] developed a computerized ultrasound system capable of reconstructing and displaying sagittal and coronal planes from images acquired in the transverse plane. Subsequently, Baba et al.[2] reported the first 3DUS examination of a fetus using a system with linear and convex array probes mounted on the position-sensing arm of a manual compound ultrasound machine. Once the technology became commercially available in the 1990s several investigators began experimenting with it and reporting the first clinical applications of 3DUS in obstetrical imaging.[3–5] 3DUS eventually evolved to incorporate a temporal component to the three spatial components that define volumetric imaging in order to capture and depict motion.[6,7] The term four-dimensional ultrasound (4DUS) was coined to describe this capability,[8] and commercial ultrasound systems have evolved to the point that the dynamic volumetric images of the beating heart can be acquired, making volumetric assessment of cardiac function a reality.[6,7,9–18]

In this chapter, we introduce the reader to the basic principles of 3DUS, provide tips for successful volume acquisition, and describe the most commonly used techniques to explore 3DUS volume datasets, including 4DUS datasets of the fetal heart. Examples of clinical applications are provided with a brief discussion of the complementary roles of 2DUS and 3DUS in clinical fetal imaging.

## PRINCIPLES OF 3DUS IMAGING

Volumetric imaging is used to enhance an examiner's ability to look at an anatomical structure or disease process simultaneously in multiple planes or as a rendered realistic 3D depiction of the structure that is otherwise not possible by cross-sectional planar imaging alone. The expectation is to improve the understanding of the spatial relationships between anatomical structures and enhance diagnostic capabilities to elucidate complex pathology, including congenital malformations of the cranium and spine, facial trauma, fractures, vascular disorders leading to stroke, and cancer, to name a few.

The primary volumetric imaging modality in prenatal diagnosis is 3DUS. Three-dimensional ultrasonography can be performed in several ways, the most common of which is to generate a 3DUS volume dataset departing from a sequence of 2DUS planar images acquired with a dedicated mechanical volumetric probe or by real-time volumetric acquisition using an electronic matrix array transducer. Other techniques that are seldom used nowadays rely on the acquisition of a series of 2DUS with regular ultrasound transducers that may or not be attached to a position-sensing device, with 3D reconstruction performed on external computer workstations.

### Mechanical 3DUS Transducers

The mechanical volumetric probe consists of a 2DUS ultrasound array mounted on a mechanical wobble, both of which located within a compartment in the transducer head.[3,5] Once the sonographer identifies the structure to be examined, he or she activates the transducer by pressing a button on the ultrasound machine, and volume acquisition starts. While the transducer remains stationary in the patient's abdomen, the mechanical wobble drives the array to sweep the region of interest (ROI) at a predetermined spatial interval and speed. The series of 2DUS images acquired by this process are combined into a volume dataset that can then be resliced into any desired plane or segmented using 3D rendering techniques (Fig. 2.1).

### Matrix Array Transducers

Matrix array transducers are full electronic transducers that consist of multiple (usually thousands) transducer elements arranged in a 2D matrix array configuration (Fig. 2.2). The face of the transducer has either a rectangular or a square shape.

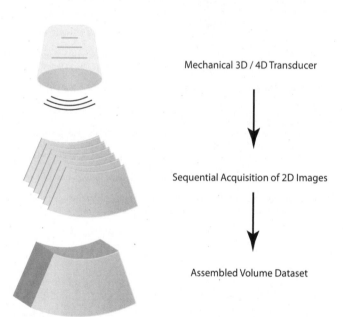

Mechanical 3D / 4D Transducer

Sequential Acquisition of 2D Images

Assembled Volume Dataset

**FIGURE 2.1:** Scanners equipped with mechanical 3D transducers generate 3D volume datasets by automatically acquiring a sequence of 2D images through a ROI selected by the examiner. The images are reassembled into a final volume dataset that can be explored using postprocessing tools. The examiner can reslice the volume in virtually any plane, either to obtain rendered 3D images or to perform volumetric measurements. Most mechanical 3D transducers are also capable of 4DUS imaging, whereby multiple volume datasets are continuously acquired and quickly updated on the screen. With this technology, motion (temporal dimension) is added to the three spatial dimensions, allowing real-time visualization of 3D images. The primary limitation of 4DUS is that spatial resolution is often sacrificed at the expense of temporal resolution. (Reproduced with permission from Gonçalves LF, Joshi A, Mody S, et al. Volume US of the urinary tract in pediatric patients—a pilot study. *Pediatr Radiol.* 2011;41:1047–1056.)

Matrix transducers can scan one line at a time (similar to mechanical probes described above), two planes simultaneously (orthogonal to each other or not), or an entire volume dataset by using multiple transducer elements simultaneously. Matrix array transducers are capable of real-time volumetric imaging, were originally designed for cardiac applications, but are now used in general and obstetrical imaging as well.[15,19-23]

## Tips for Successful Volume Acquisition

Regardless of the choice of ultrasound equipment and type of volumetric probe, the reader is reminded that 3DUS is just an extension of 2DUS technology. Therefore, the same physics-related limitations apply. One cannot expect to compensate for poor 2DUS image quality caused by common problems such as patient obesity, oligohydramnios, and excessive bone shadowing by using 3DUS technology. Therefore, high-quality 2DUS imaging is a prerequisite for diagnostic 3DUS volume datasets.

Another issue that requires attention during volume acquisition is fetal movement. 3DUS technology has evolved over time to minimize movement-related artifacts by increasing acquisition speed while still maintaining acceptable image resolution, by the development of 4DUS technology for mechanical probes, and real-time volumetric imaging using matrix array probes. Still, excessive fetal movement can be a significant problem, not only because it can degrade image quality but also because it tends to generate artifacts that can affect image interpretation.[24] Therefore, the sonographer has to scan smarter to compensate for fetal movement. Our anecdotal experience is that fetuses tend to move less during the early part of the exam, before the maternal abdomen is manipulated by the act of scanning. Our suggestion is that, if the purpose of the exam is the acquisition of volumetric data, the sonographer should begin the exam with a volumetric probe and attempt volume acquisition early. We also recommend careful attention to gentle scanning, avoiding excessive transducer movement and pressure, in an effort to prevent the initiation of movements by the fetus. In addition, once the 2DUS image is optimized and a good acoustic window to the structure of interest is present, volume acquisition should start without delay. The sonographer should avoid the trap of thinking that perfect 2D views (for example, a perfect facial profile or a perfect four-chamber view) are a prerequisite for high-quality 3DUS imaging. Although ideal, this is not necessary, since once a high-quality volume is acquired, these views can be obtained offline by image postprocessing. In fact, we propose that all that is needed for a good volume acquisition is a good acoustic window to the structure of interest in the absence of fetal movement. Therefore, if the target is the fetal face, all that is needed is that the face is oriented toward the transducer and that fluid is present between the face and the transducer. If the target is the fetal heart, similarly, all that is required is that the fetal chest faces the examiner and that no limbs are interposed between the fetal chest and the transducer. Again, the objective is an excellent acoustic window to the structure of interest, and not to pursue a perfect conventional 2DUS view prior to volume acquisition.

## Postprocessing

Once the volume dataset is acquired, image postprocessing can take place at the scanner or at dedicated computer workstations. In the next few sections, we will review common approaches to explore 3DUS volume datasets.

### Multiplanar Display

The multiplanar display is a simple but practical method to examine 3DUS volume datasets.[5,25] This type of display typically shows three images, one representing the original plane of acquisition and another two orthogonal planes. A reference

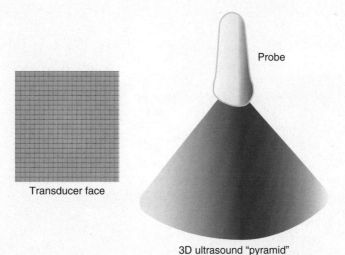

**FIGURE 2.2:** The "transducer face" diagram illustrates the typical configuration of a matrix array transducer, with thousands of elements arranged as a 2D matrix array, with each tiny square representing a single element. All elements, a portion of them, or two simultaneous lines can be activated simultaneously to produce real-time 3D images. The diagram "3D ultrasound pyramid" illustrates the pyramid of ultrasound that is emitted when all elements are fired simultaneously. The elements can also be fired in sequence, one line at a time, to produce volumetric data in a manner similar to the mechanical probe illustrated in Figure 2.1, just much faster.

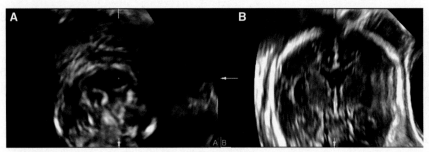
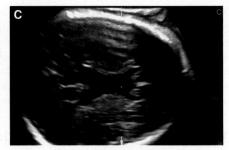

**FIGURE 2.3:** Multiplanar display of a volume dataset of the fetal brain acquired transabdominally using axial sections through the fetal head. The volume was manipulated so that the sagittal plane is shown in **A**, the coronal plane in **B**, and the original plane of acquisition, the axial plane, in **C**. The original plane of acquisition has the best resolution. The reference *dot* represents the intersection of the three orthogonal planes and, in this example, shows the typical imaging features of absence of the cavum septi pellucidi in the coronal **(A)**, sagittal **(B)**, and axial **(C)** planes.

"dot" or "cross," depending on the manufacturer, marks the intersection of the three orthogonal planes. As the user moves the reference "dot" or "cross" with a mouse or another electronic pointing device, any structure present in the volume dataset can be simultaneously displayed in three different planes. Figure 2.3 illustrates the basic principles of the multiplanar display method.

### Multiple Slice Imaging

An alternative display method presents multiple slices of the volume dataset as a series of images in a single screen.[26,27] This method, variously known as tomographic ultrasound imaging (TUI), multislice, or iSlice, depending on the manufacturer, permits simultaneous display of several consecutive planes of an organ or abnormality and may facilitate interpretation and/or teaching. Figure 2.4 shows features of

tricuspid atresia with ventricular septal defect (VSD) using the TUI method.

### 3D Rendering

The term 3D rendering refers to the display method whereby a 3D object is displayed on a 2D screen using 3D photorealistic effects. The capability of presenting an image of the fetal face with surface rendering technology captured the attention of fetal imaging specialists and parents alike, and helped foster the initial interest in 3D obstetrical imaging.[3,5,25,28]

**Surface Rendering:** As the name implies, the surface rendering method is used when the intention is to display a 3D image of the surface of an object. This method works by displaying the first hyperechogenic voxel along the projection path of a volume dataset whose brightness is higher than a threshold determined

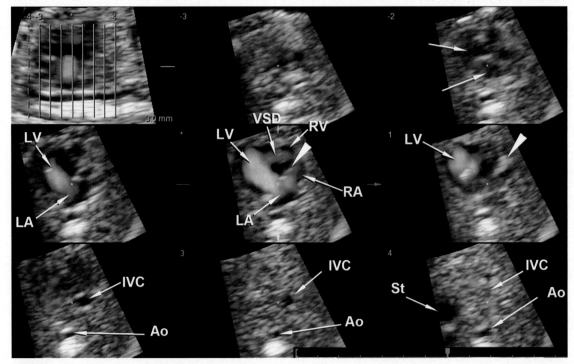

**FIGURE 2.4:** Multiple slice display of a volume dataset of the fetal heart acquired with color Doppler and spatiotemporal correlation (STIC). The left upper panel represents the scout sagittal view, with eight consecutive lines representing eight axial planes from the superior mediastinum to the upper abdomen shown in the next eight panels. The *arrowhead* points to the atretic tricuspid valve. Ao, abdominal aorta; IVC, inferior vena cava; VSD, ventricular septal defect; LV, left ventricle; RV, right ventricle; LA, left atrium; RA, right atrium.

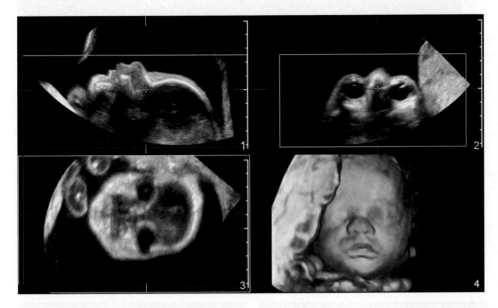

**FIGURE 2.5:** Multiplanar and volume rendered images of a normal fetal face acquired from a 2DUS facial profile view. **Panels 1–3** show the sagittal, axial, and coronal orthogonal planes, respectively. A generous amount of amniotic fluid is interposed between the transducer and the skin surface of the fetal face. The *boxes* in **panels 1–3**, defined the ROI. The direction of view (or projection path) is determined by the user and, in this example, is given by the *yellow line*. Therefore, the first echo brighter than amniotic fluid (the threshold level) along the projection path is displayed as a pixel in **panel 4** in order to form the rendered view of the fetal face.

by the user. The typical example is a rendered image of the fetal face (Fig. 2.5).

**Maximum Intensity Projection:** In this rendering method, the voxel with the highest brightness signal along the projection path is displayed on the screen.[4,25,29–32] In fetal imaging, this is typically used to display osseous structures, as illustrated in Figure 2.6.

**Minimum Intensity Projection:** The minimum intensity projection method, as the name implies, displays the voxel with the lowest brightness signal along the projection path.[25,33] This method is useful to display rendered images of fluid-filled

structures. Figure 2.7 shows a rendered view of jejunal atresia displayed in the coronal plane.

**Average Intensity Projection:** With average intensity projection, as the name implies, the average brightness of the voxels along the projection path are displayed as a pixel on a 2D screen. We use this method when we want to show rendered views of fetal limbs that simultaneously show the bones and soft tissues. Figure 2.8 shows the same fetal arm, forearm, and hand displayed using just the multiplanar display or volume contrast imaging (VCI, see detailed description below) with a slice thickness of 20 mm using the average intensity projection method.

**Inversion Mode:** Inversion mode is a rendering method that inverts the grayscale of the voxels with the lowest brightness signal along the projection path. It is used for demonstration of fluid-filled structures.[34–37] Figure 2.9 shows the same case of jejunal atresia previously seen using the minimum intensity project, now displayed using inversion mode. Although analogous, the inversion mode display allows further segmentation of the volume dataset and provides a better depiction of the anatomical relationships of the structures of interest.

**Volume Contrast Imaging:** VCI is a rendering method that combines multiple consecutive frames together into a thick slab that can be displayed using any of the other rendering methods described above. Besides the example already provided in Figure 2.8, Figure 2.10 illustrates the improved tissue contrast resolution that can be obtained with this technology.

**Postprocessing in the Ultrasound Equipment versus External PACS Systems and 3D Workstations:** Image postprocessing is an integral part of volumetric imaging, and excellent results can only be expected once the examiner becomes comfortable with both volume acquisition and volume postprocessing. All ultrasound manufacturers provide volume manipulation and rendering capabilities directly in the ultrasound system. However, particularly when an examiner is learning 3DUS, volume manipulation and segmentation can be time consuming, and it may not be practical to tie the ultrasound equipment for this purpose (since it could otherwise be used to scan other patients).

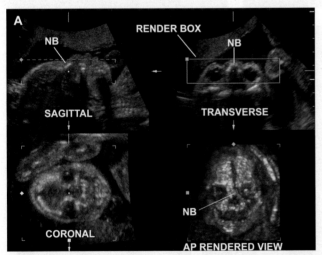

**FIGURE 2.6:** Normally developed nasal bones in a fetus with no abnormalities at 23 weeks of gestation. Multiplanar and anteroposterior rendered views of the fetal skull using the maximum intensity projection mode. The *render box* delimits the ROI, and the *green line* determines the direction of view for reconstruction of the 3D image. The paired nasal bones (*NB*) are visualized as a single structure fused in the midline. (Reproduced with permission from Gonçalves LF, Espinoza J, Lee W, et al. Phenotypic characteristics of absent and hypoplastic nasal bones in fetuses with Down syndrome: description by 3-dimensional ultrasonography and clinical significance. *J Ultrasound Med.* 2004;23(12):1619–1627.)

**FIGURE 2.7:** Multiplanar display of a volume dataset of a fetus with jejunal atresia. *A–C* show axial, sagittal, and coronal views of the fetal abdomen, respectively. The dilated loops of bowel are seen in the coronal plane. **Panel 3D** shows a rendered view of the abdomen using the minimum intensity projection mode. In this mode, the voxels with the lowest brightness signal along the projection path are preferentially displayed. In this case, a portion of the heart, the stomach (*St*), and the dilated bowel loops are the structures with the lowest brightness signal. They are simultaneously displayed in a single coronal view allowing the examiner to compare the relative positions of the bowel loops to the stomach, to determine that there are only a few dilated loops, and to note that the dilated bowel ends as a blind pouch in the left lower quadrant.

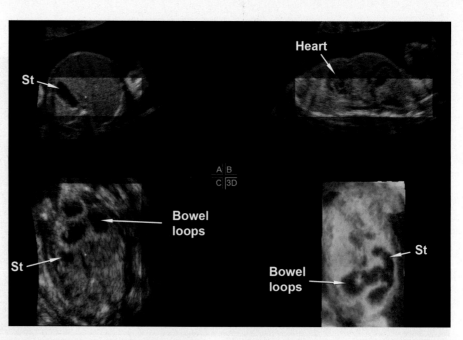

**FIGURE 2.8: A:** Single view of a fetal arm, forearm, and hand displayed using the multiplanar method. **B:** Volume contrast imaging (VCI) rendered view of the same arm using a 20-mm thick slab rendered using the average intensity projection method. Note that all fingers and the humerus are better seen on **B** when compared with **A**, with better demonstration of the soft tissues as well.

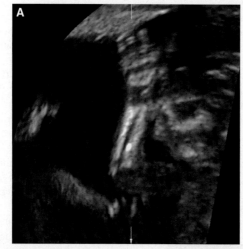
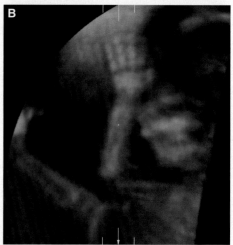

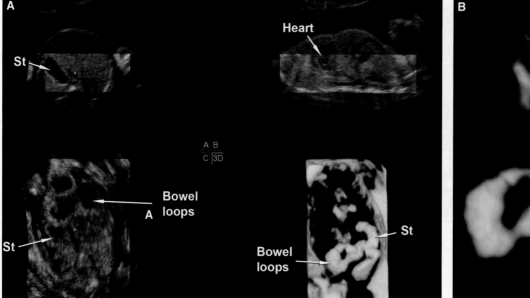
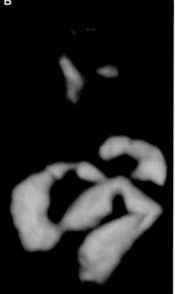

**FIGURE 2.9: A:** Multiplanar display of a volume dataset of a fetus with jejunal atresia. *A–C* show axial, sagittal, and coronal views, respectively, of the fetal abdomen. The dilated loops of bowel are seen in the coronal plane. **Panel 3D** shows a rendered view of the abdomen using the inversion mode method. The method is analogous to the minimum intensity projection mode, only that the voxels with the lowest brightness along the projection path are displayed with the grayscale inverted. **B:** In this image, further segmentation of the volume dataset was performed to display only the stomach (*St*), the duodenum, and the proximal jejunum. Part of the fetal heart is included only as a point of reference.

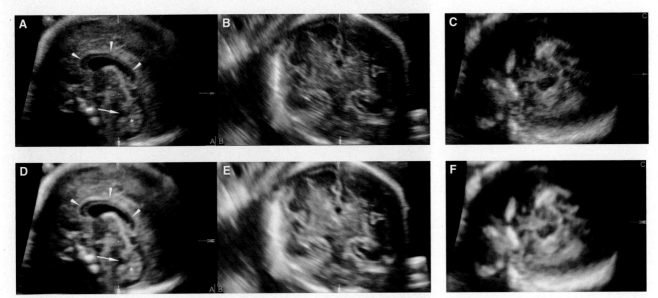

**FIGURE 2.10:** Multiplanar display of a volume dataset of the fetal brain obtained using a sagittal acquisition through the anterior fontanelle without **(A–C)** and with VCI **(D–F)**. The corpus callosum (*arrowheads*), cisterna magna, fourth ventricle (*arrow*), and cerebellar vermis (*star*) are well depicted in both images; however, contrast resolution is better with VCI.

The good news is that volume datasets can be manipulated in dedicated 3D workstations. Once exported, all capabilities available in the equipment are also available in 3D workstations. The problem that users face today is that ultrasound manufacturers use proprietary data formats that can only be opened using vendor-specific programs. Therefore, if the lab uses equipment from multiple manufacturers, the program interface to manipulate and segment volumes will be different, and programs from one manufacturer will not open volume datasets from the other, and vice versa. The hope of the ultrasound community is that full implementation of the 3DUS DICOM (Digital Imaging and Communications in Medicine) protocol will make 3DUS volumetric data available to all PACS systems with 3D manipulation and segmentation capabilities, regardless of the ultrasound system that generated the images, improving the learning process and workflow of 3DUS in clinical practice.[38]

## FOUR-DIMENSIONAL ULTRASONOGRAPHY (4DUS)

4DUS is a term that describes the incorporation of a temporal component to the three spatial dimensions of a 3DUS volume dataset.[8] Therefore, 4DUS allows the sequential display of multiple volumes as they are acquired and hence the capability of appreciating motion in volumetric imaging. This technology allows examiners to look not only at gross fetal movements (e.g., limbs) but also at more subtle fetal behavioral characteristics such as facial expressions (Fig. 2.11). Several investigators have applied this technology to study fetal behavioral states in utero, including the effect of adverse maternal and fetal disorders on expected behavioral patterns.[39–46]

### 4DUS of the Fetal Heart

Four-dimensional ultrasound of the fetal heart is possible by using spatiotemporal correlation (STIC) or real-time volumetric matrix array technology.[7,11,13–15,47] STIC is a rendering algorithm that was developed specifically for fetal echocardiography

applications. The algorithm essentially performs retrospective gating of the fetal heart rate to the acquired volume. The heart rate is calculated retrospectively from the raw volume dataset.[7] The end result is that the multiple volumes of the fetal heart obtained in sequence through a single automated sweep of the fetal chest are reshuffled according to the phase of the cardiac cycle at which they were acquired. Provided that there is not excessive fetal motion during acquisition, excellent volume datasets of the fetal heart can be acquired, manipulated, and segmented using any of the display and rendering methods described in the "postprocessing" section above. Figure 2.12 shows the multiplanar display and rendered views of the atrioventricular valve orifices of a normal fetal heart acquired through a transverse sweep of the fetal chest.

## FETAL ANATOMY BY VOLUMETRIC IMAGING WITH ABNORMAL EXAMPLES

In this section, we present a series of images that illustrate examples of both normal structures and pathology depicted by 3DUS and 4DUS, including the fetal heart.

### Fetal Head

Figure 2.13 shows the sagittal corpus callosum reconstructed from a volume dataset originally acquired using a coronal sweep through the anterior fontanelle. This method is also suited for examination of the neonatal head using volumetric probes.[48–50] Contrast the findings of this normal image with that of a fetus with absent cavum septi pellucidi shown in Figure 2.3. The same volume dataset is shown in Figure 2.14, now displayed using the multiplanar method with VCI set to a slice thickness of 3 mm to show the optic nerves and optic tracts at the level of the suprasellar cistern. Preliminary data show that the optic tracts and nerves can be successfully imaged using 3DUS rendering methods, and that optic tract measurements in the case of absent cavum septi pellucidi may help to identify those fetuses at high risk for septo-optic dysplasia.[51]

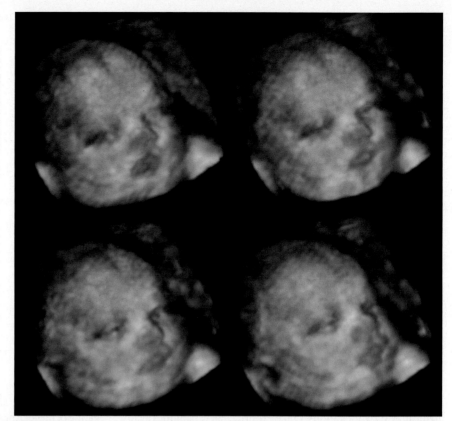

**FIGURE 2.11:** Series of rendered images of the face from a term fetus obtained with a real-time matrix array transducer. The images illustrate the capability of 4DUS to depict subtle changes of facial expression, such as eye opening.

**FIGURE 2.12:** Volume dataset of the fetal heart acquired with STIC. **A** shows a four-chamber view of the fetal heart, **B** shows an orthogonal sagittal section through the ventricular septum (VS) displayed "en face," and **C** shows a coronal section at the level of the atrioventricular (AV) valves. The rendered view of the AV valves is seen in **panel 3D**. Please note that the green line that determines the projection path is positioned within the atrial chambers **(panels A and B)** and, therefore, the rendered view is seen as if the examiner is looking at the AV valve orifices from the atrial chambers toward the ventricles. LV, left ventricle; LA, left atrium; RV, right ventricle; RA, right atrium; Ao, descending aorta; VS, ventricular septum; Ao root, Aortic root; PA, pulmonary artery; M, mitral valve orifice; T, tricuspid valve orifice.

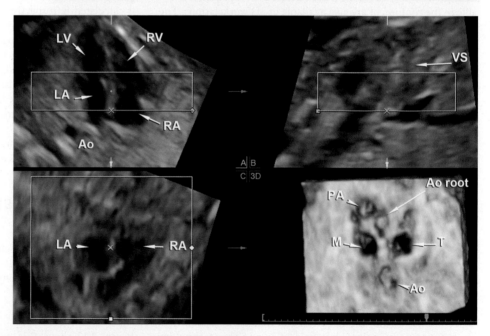

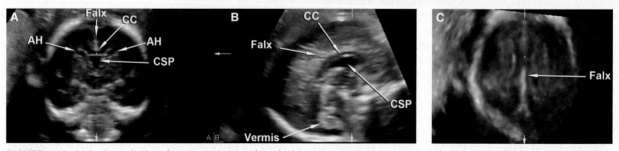

**FIGURE 2.13:** Multiplanar display of a volume dataset of the fetal head acquired using an automated coronal sweep through the anterior fontanelle. **A** shows the original coronal plane of acquisition, **B** shows the sagittal plane, and **C** shows the coronal plane. The reference dot is positioned at the anterior body of the corpus callosum, which is seen in its full length on the reconstructed sagittal plane. AH, anterior horns of the lateral ventricles; CC, corpus callosum; CSP, cavum septi pellucidi.

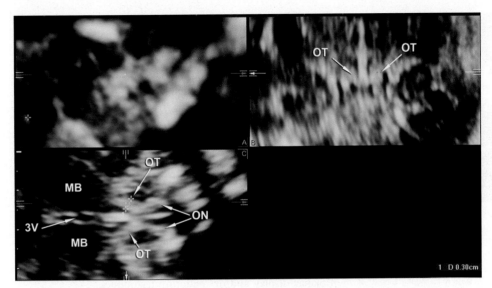

**FIGURE 2.14:** This image was produced from exactly the same volume dataset of the fetus with absent cavum septi pellucidi shown in Figure 2.3. The view is now magnified and displayed using VCI with a slice thickness of 3 mm. The sagittal, coronal, and axial orthogonal planes at the level of the suprasellar cistern are shown in **panels A–C**. The optic tracts and optic nerves can be clearly seen. OT, optic tracts; ON, optic nerves; MB, mid brain; 3V, third ventricle.

## Fetal Face and Calvarium

3DUS is well suited for the evaluation of facial anomalies, with several studies documenting additional diagnostic information or better diagnostic accuracy when compared with 2DUS. 3DUS is useful for the evaluation of cranial sutures,[4,52,53] facial bones,[54–61] as well as cleft lip and palate.[52,62–74]

Figures 2.5, 2.6, and 2.11 illustrate the capabilities of 3DUS to depict normal facial structures and demonstrate subtle movements such as eye opening. The next few images illustrate the capabilities of 3DUS in the evaluation of selected craniofacial abnormalities. Figure 2.15 shows examples of hypoplastic and absent nasal bones in fetuses with trisomy 21.[56,58] Figure 2.16 shows widened cranial sutures in a fetus with cleidocranial dysostosis. The same fetus had pseudoarthrosis of the right clavicle shown in Figure 2.17.

### Evaluation of Orofacial Clefts

Volumetric imaging plays an important role in the evaluation of orofacial clefts and, therefore, deserves a separate discussion.

Orofacial clefts are common birth defects, being second in prevalence only to trisomy 21 according to a recent publication from the Centers of Disease Control of the United States.[75] The most common types of orofacial clefts are isolated cleft lip, cleft lip with cleft palate, and isolated cleft palates. Median clefts are much less common and usually associated with chromosomal and structural brain anomalies. The adjusted United States prevalence of cleft lip with or without cleft palate was estimated as 1 in 1,574 live births, and that of isolated cleft palate as 1 in 940 live births. The prevalence in Asian and Native American populations is higher (as high as 1 in 500), whereas African-derived populations have a lower prevalence, estimated as 1 in

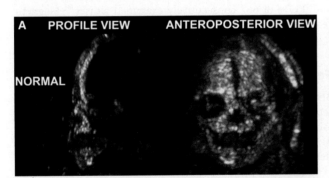

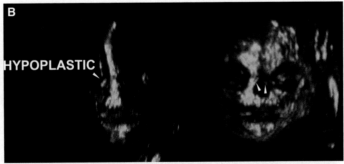

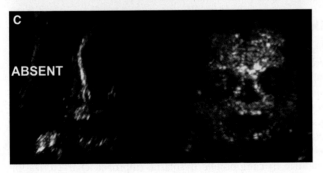

**FIGURE 2.15:** **A:** Normally developed nasal bones in a fetus with no abnormalities at 23 weeks of gestation. **B:** Delayed ossification or hypoplastic: Two small ossification centers can be seen away from the midline in the frontal projection and can be seen as a single hyperechogenic linear structure (owing to superimposition) in the sagittal projection. **C:** Absent nasal bones: No ossified nasal bones are present either in the frontal or in the sagittal projection. (Reproduced with permission from Gonçalves LF, Espinoza J, Lee W, et al. Phenotypic characteristics of absent and hypoplastic nasal bones in fetuses with Down syndrome: description by 3-dimensional ultrasonography and clinical significance. *J Ultrasound Med.* 2004;23[12]:1619–1627.)

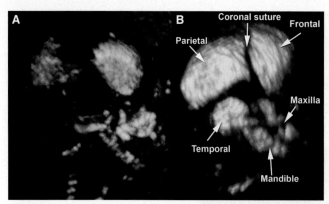

**FIGURE 2.16: A:** Three-dimensional (3D) rendering of the fetal skull at 18 + 3 weeks of gestation using the maximum intensity projection mode demonstrates widening of the coronal suture, absence of the squamous portion of the temporal bone, and absence of the nasal bones. **B:** Labeled 3D image of a normal fetal skull at 18 + 3 weeks (control). (Reproduced with permission from Soto E, Richani K, Gonçalves LF, et al. Three-dimensional ultrasound in the prenatal diagnosis of cleidocranial dysplasia associated with B-cell immunodeficiency. *Ultrasound Obstet Gynecol.* 2006;27[5]:574–579.)

2,500. Approximately 70% of cases of cleft lip and palate, and 50% of cases of isolated cleft palate are nonsyndromic. The rest are associated with a wide range of malformation syndromes, chromosomal abnormalities and teratogen exposure. For a detailed review of the genetics and environmental factors associated with cleft lip and palate, the reader is referred to the excellent review article of Dixon et al.[76]

A diagram illustrating the anatomy of the palate is presented in Figure 2.18. Facial clefts can be unilateral or bilateral midline. When clefts involve only the lip, they are called isolated cleft lip or labioalveolar cleft. Clefts can extend to involve the primary palate (alveolus and premaxillary part of the maxilla, anterior to the incisive foramen) and/or the secondary palate (palatine process of the maxillary bones and palatine bone) (Fig. 2.19). In a large prospective ultrasound screening study from the Netherlands that included 35,000 low-risk and 2,800 high-risk patients,

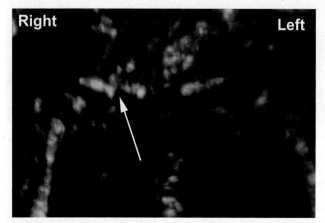

**FIGURE 2.17:** Three-dimensional rendering of the fetal shoulders using maximum intensity projection. The *arrow* points to the pseudoarthrosis of the right clavicle. (Reproduced with permission from Soto E, Richani K, Gonçalves LF, et al. Three-dimensional ultrasound in the prenatal diagnosis of cleidocranial dysplasia associated with B-cell immunodeficiency. *Ultrasound Obstet Gynecol.* 2006;27[5]:574–579.)

40% of the clefts were clefts of the lip and palate, 29% were isolated cleft lip, and 27% were isolated cleft palate. Median and atypical clefts were rare and observed in only two fetuses. Sixty one per cent of the clefts were unilateral.

Figure 2.20 shows the technique to properly acquire a volume dataset of the hard palate.[74] Figure 2.21 shows how poor volume acquisition leads to shadowing artifact posterior to the tooth buds and, therefore, limited diagnostic value for the evaluation of the secondary palate.

Figure 2.22 shows an example of a rendered view of a unilateral cleft lip and palate with the 3D surface mode. Figures 2.23 and 2.24 show extension through the primary and secondary palates.

Several investigators have compared the diagnostic performance of 2DUS versus 3DUS for correct classification of the type and extent of orofacial clefts. Collectively, the evidence supports 3DUS as a more accurate method, largely because of better characterization of the extent of hard palate involvement using multiplanar display and/or rendering techniques.[64–67,69–71,73,74,77–85] In one of the comparative studies, Johnson et al.[67] showed that 2DUS overestimated the severity of the defect in 41.9% (13/31) of the cases. Of interest, a recent study performed with 3DUS in the first trimester reported sensitivities of 100% and 86% for the diagnosis of clefts of the primary and secondary palate, with a 0.9% false-positive rate.[86]

### Pitfalls

3DUS rendered images of the fetal face provide a visual realistic view of the defect that may help explain the abnormality to the parents and perhaps the surgeon who is involved in counseling. However, one must be careful in interpreting 3D rendered images alone and take into consideration the possibility of rendering artifacts or shadows that may create artificial clefts.[87–89]

In addition, ultrasound has traditionally not performed well for the evaluation of the soft palate, except for a recent series from Germany that reported on a new sign ("equal sign") for evaluation of the soft palate and uvula. In that study, adequate visualization of the soft palate and uvula was possible in 85.3% and 90.7% of 667 consecutively examined fetuses.[90] Magnetic resonance imaging (MRI) is a good adjunctive imaging modality for visualization of the soft palate.[91–93]

### Fetal Spine

3DUS is a useful adjunct to 2DUS for the examination of the fetal spine. Besides its role in the characterization of segmentation abnormalities and abnormal curvature of the spine, 3DUS has proven accurate with one vertebral segment to determine the level of the defect in cases of spinal dysraphism (Fig. 2.25).[30–32,94–99]

### Skeletal Dysplasias

The ability of 3DUS to obtain rendered images of the fetal skeleton makes it a useful adjunctive modality in the diagnostic workup of skeletal dysplasias (see Figs. 2.16 and 2.17) and musculoskeletal disorders (Fig. 2.26). Several case reports have been published highlighting potential benefits of 3DUS for the visualization of specific features of skeletal abnormalities, for example, enhanced visualization of femoral and tibial bowing in a case of platyspondylic lethal chondrodysplasia, hypoplastic scapulae in campomelic dysplasia, improved characterization

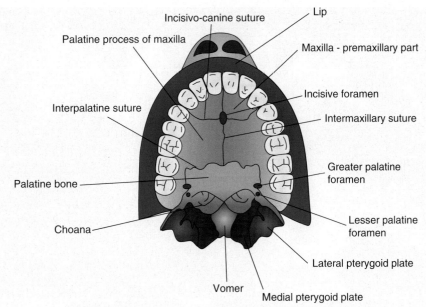

**FIGURE 2.18:** Normal palate anatomy.

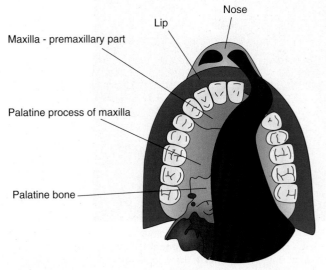

**FIGURE 2.19:** Diagram illustrating a unilateral cleft lip and palate involving the nose, lip, primary palate (anterior to the incisive foramen), and secondary palate.

of frontal bossing in thanatophoric dysplasia, demonstration of caudal narrowing of the interpedicular distance of the lumbar spine in achondroplasia, improved visualization of epiphyseal stippling in chondrodysplasia punctata, better characterization of the abnormal spine and ribs in Jarcho-Levin syndrome, visualization of genu recurvatum in Larsen syndrome, and pseudoarthrosis of the clavicle in cleidocranial dysostosis.[100–108] Few studies, however, have directly compared 3DUS versus 2DUS for the prenatal diagnosis of skeletal dysplasias, with the exception of the study of Ruano et al.,[109] who showed higher visualization rates for skeletal structures by 3DUS (77.1%) when compared with 2DUS (51.4%), but lower than helical CT reconstructions (94.1%).

## Congenital Heart Disease

Accurate prenatal diagnosis of congenital heart disease (CHD) is an important goal of prenatal care. Besides affording the parents appropriate and timely counseling, advanced knowledge of ductal-dependent anomalies allows planned delivery at institutions equipped to handle such cases, both from the medical and from the surgical standpoints. Indeed, prenatal diagnosis of CHD, including hypoplastic left heart syndrome, transposition of the great arteries, and coarctation of the aorta, is associated with improved perinatal morbidity and mortality.[110–113] Recent evidence indicates the prenatal diagnosis of transposition of the great arteries is also associated with improved long-term neurocognitive outcomes when compared with children diagnosed only in the neonatal period.[114]

### Volumetric Imaging of the Fetal Heart

As briefly described earlier in this chapter, volumetric imaging of the fetal heart can be performed using STIC or real-time matrix array technology.[7,11,13–15,47] Once volume datasets are acquired, the same postprocessing methods that are used to evaluate other fetal organs can be applied to the examination of the fetal heart. Because of the complexity of cardiac anatomy and the fact that standardized planes of section are recommended for the examination of the fetal heart, it was natural that several techniques have emerged to describe how these planes of section can be extracted from volume datasets.[13,14,26,27,34,36,115–120] The techniques that we most commonly use in our clinical practice are illustrated in the following sections, along with examples of their application to cases of CHD.

**Scrolling through the Volume Dataset:** Evaluation of the volume dataset in its original plane of acquisition is an intuitive and easy way to examine the heart. We usually begin our examination with volume datasets acquired through transverse automated sweeps through the fetal chest, since these include a four-chamber view. The volume is displayed using a single large frame, and the examiner scrolls up and down to identify

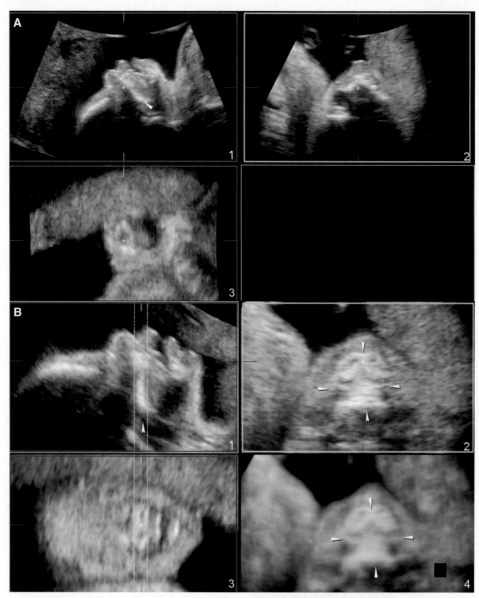

**FIGURE 2.20:  A:** The ideal position of the fetal face for volume acquisition of the secondary palate. Note that the angle between the palate *(arrowhead)* and the transducer is approximately 45° **(panel 1)**. **B:** Manipulation of the volume dataset to show the hard palate in its entirety. In **panel 1**, the volume is rotated around the z-axis so that the hard palate *(arrowhead)* is oriented at a 0° angle. In **panel 2**, the full extent of the hard palate can be seen in the axial plane *(four arrowheads)*. **Panel 3** shows the anterior maxillary tooth buds. **Panel 4** shows a rendered view of the hard palate *(four arrowheads)* using the maximum intensity projection method.

the following planes: Transverse view of the fetal abdomen, four-chamber view, five-chamber view, three-vessel view, and three-vessel and trachea view, as originally proposed by Yagel et al.[121] (Fig. 2.27).

**Multiple Slice Method:** An alternative way to simultaneously display multiple equally spaced planes of section in the same screen is to use the multiple slice method.[26,27] This method automatically slices the volume dataset, and with minimal adjustment, one is usually able to demonstrate the five axial planes of section shown in Figure 2.27 in the majority of cases. Figure 2.28 illustrates the use of this method in a volume dataset of a normal fetal heart, and Figure 2.29 shows all planes of section needed to

make the diagnosis of hypoplastic right heart due to pulmonary atresia in a single image. A case of tricuspid atresia with VSD is illustrated in Figure 2.4.

**Three-Step Technique for Evaluation of the Outflow Tracts:** This technique was designed specifically to demonstrate, in the same image, the long axis view of the left ventricular outflow tract and the short axis view of the right ventricular outflow tract (Fig. 2.30).[14] This technique has been validated both from the standpoint of reproducibility as well as clinical applicability.[117,122] It is particularly useful to diagnose conotruncal anomalies, including transposition of the great arteries and conotruncal defects with overriding of the aorta (e.g., tetralogy

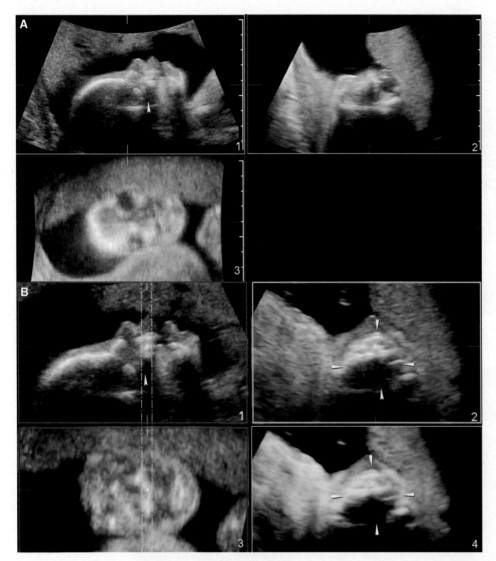

**FIGURE 2.21:** Contrast the volume acquisition in this figure with that in Figure 2.20. **A:** The facial profile is oriented in such a way that the hard palate is 0° with the transducer and therefore, a strong acoustic shadow is present posterior to the tooth buds (**panel 1**, *arrowhead*). **B:** The shadowing artifact is related exclusively to poor acquisition, and it cannot be corrected by postprocessing techniques. The same shadow seen in **panel 1** *(arrowhead)* is seen posterior to the tooth buds in **panel 2** and also in the maximum intensity projection rendered image displayed in **panel 4**. The anterior maxillary tooth buds can be well seen in **panel 3**.

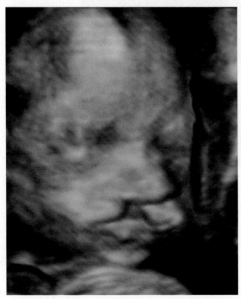

**FIGURE 2.22:** Three-dimensional surface rendered view of the fetal face. Unilateral cleft lip is seen on the left side.

of Fallot, pulmonary atresia with VSD, truncus arteriosus, and double outlet right ventricle).[122,123] Figure 2.31 shows a case of transposition of the great arteries demonstrated with this technique.

### Rendered Images

***Cardiac Valves:*** Rendered images of the cardiac valves can be easily obtained, as illustrated in Figure 2.12. Figure 2.32 shows the technique to obtain an "en face" rendered view of the atrioventricular valves in a case of complete atrioventricular canal. Figure 2.33 shows a comparative example of a rendered "en face" view of a normal atrioventricular valve, a closed single atrioventricular valve, and an open single atrioventricular valve in a case of complete atrioventricular canal.

***Great Vessels:*** Rendered views of the great vessels, and, for that matter, also of the venous return to the fetal heart can be obtained using several techniques, including inversion mode, color or power Doppler imaging, or B-flow imaging. For volume datasets acquired using color Doppler imaging, the reader is reminded that the color Doppler settings must be adjusted prior to acquisition to maintain the highest frame

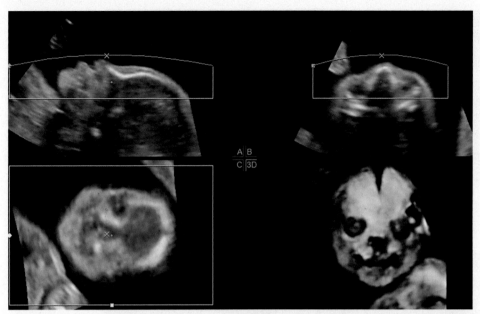

**FIGURE 2.23:** Multiplanar display and rendered views of the fetal face using the maximum intensity projection method to highlight the skull. A unilateral cleft lip can be seen going through the left alveolar ridge.

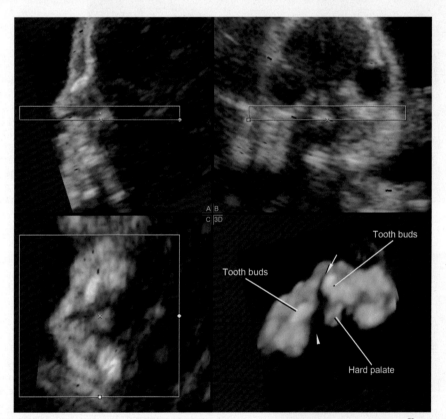

**FIGURE 2.24:** Reconstruction of the hard palate using the technique proposed by Platt et al.[73] The rendered view using a combination of surface and maximum intensity projection modes shows that the unilateral cleft extends through the primary and secondary palates. Arrow, cleft of the primary palate; arrowhead, extension to the secondary palate.

rate possible. Failure to do so will result in poor temporal resolution of the volume dataset. Color Doppler optimization steps include narrowing the field of view on the grayscale image, using a single focal zone adjusted to the depth of the structure of interest, and narrowing the color Doppler ROI. Figures 2.34 to 2.36 illustrate normal outflow tracts displayed using color Doppler, inversion mode, and B-flow imaging.[27,123] Figure 2.37 shows the application of 3D rendered reformats to the prenatal diagnosis of transposition of the great arteries.[123]

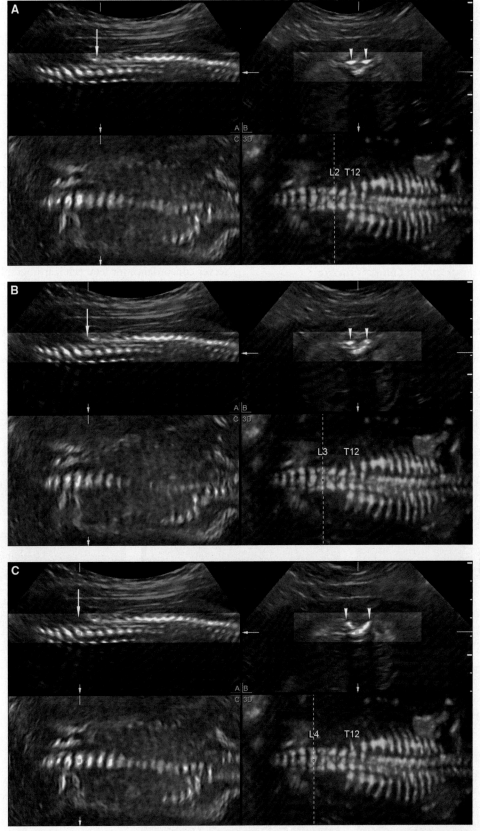

**FIGURE 2.25:** Multiplanar display (*A* is sagittal; *B*, transverse; and *C*, coronal) and rendered views **(panel 3D)** of the fetal spine in a fetus with open spinal dysraphism and a mild scoliosis. **A:** A vertical *dashed line* corresponds to the level at which the three planes intersect at *L2*. The posterior laminae of the spine are closed at this level (*arrowheads* in *B*). **B:.** The vertical *dashed line* is at the level of *L3*; the posterior elements begin to splay at this level (*arrowheads* in *B*). **C:** The posterior elements are clearly splayed at the level of *L4* (*arrowheads* in *B*).

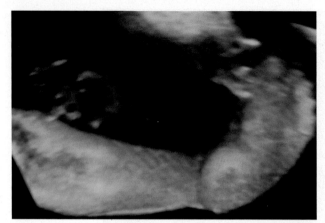

**FIGURE 2.26:** Three-dimensional rendered view of the fetal leg and feet showing clubfoot.

## 4D Fetal Echocardiography in Clinical Practice

A few studies have addressed the feasibility of 4D fetal echocardiography in clinical practice. The first study included 148 high-risk fetuses examined by two experienced sonographers with no more than four acquisition attempts allowed during the exam. Successful volume dataset acquisition was possible in 76% of the cases, with 65% of these volumes deemed to have enough quality for diagnostic purposes. Only 25% of the volume datasets were considered high quality.[124] The second study allowed 40 minutes for volume dataset acquisition per exam, and showed that the four-chamber view and outflow tracts could be adequately visualized in 70% and 83% of the cases, respectively.[125] The main factors associated with poor volume dataset quality were maternal obesity, anterior placenta, and unfavorable fetal position (spine up).[124,125]

The next question is whether a diagnostic quality volume dataset can be used in clinical practice. The evidence available to date indicates that examiners can rely on volume datasets of the fetal heart for diagnostic purposes. Viñals et al.[17,126] conducted studies in Chile, where volume datasets of the fetal heart were obtained by examiners with little experience in fetal echocardiography and then transmitted to a remote server via an internet link. The volumes were evaluated by an expert in fetal echocardiography, with a complete exam possible in 96.2% of the cases obtained in the second trimester[17] and a high degree of interobserver concordance for fetal echocardiography views extracted from volume datasets obtained between 11 and 14 weeks of gestation.[126] Bennasar et al. compared 4DUS against 2DUS for diagnostic accuracy in detecting CHD. Volume datasets were analyzed blindly one year after acquisition. The study included 342 fetuses with suspected CHD and showed similar diagnostic accuracy for both methods (91% for 4DUS vs. 94.2% for 2DUS,

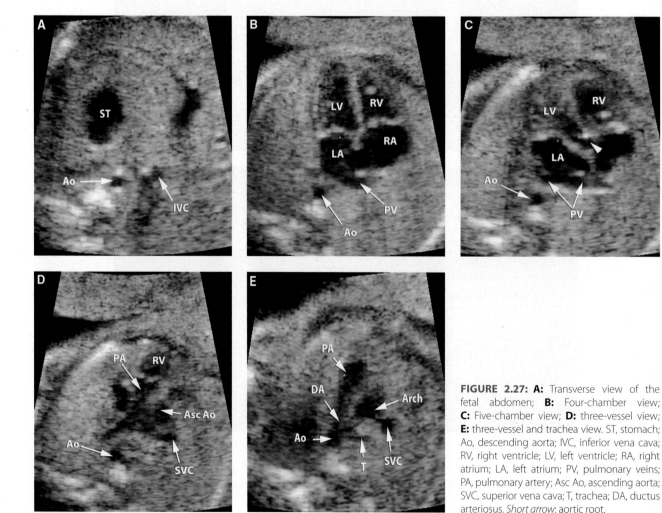

**FIGURE 2.27: A:** Transverse view of the fetal abdomen; **B:** Four-chamber view; **C:** Five-chamber view; **D:** three-vessel view; **E:** three-vessel and trachea view. ST, stomach; Ao, descending aorta; IVC, inferior vena cava; RV, right ventricle; LV, left ventricle; RA, right atrium; LA, left atrium; PV, pulmonary veins; PA, pulmonary artery; Asc Ao, ascending aorta; SVC, superior vena cava; T, trachea; DA, ductus arteriosus. *Short arrow*: aortic root.

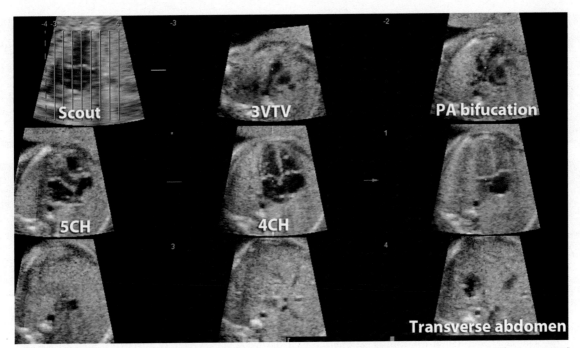

**FIGURE 2.28:** Multiple slice images of a normal fetal heart applied to the same volume dataset as in Figure 2.27. The "scout view" is sagittal and located in the left upper corner of the image. The vertical lines represent the planes displayed in the other eight images, from the superior mediastinum to the upper abdomen. Note that most of the planes seen in Figure 2.27 are automatically and simultaneously displayed, except the three-vessel view. 3VTV, three-vessel and trachea view; 5CH, five-chamber view; 4CH, four-chamber view; PA, pulmonary artery.

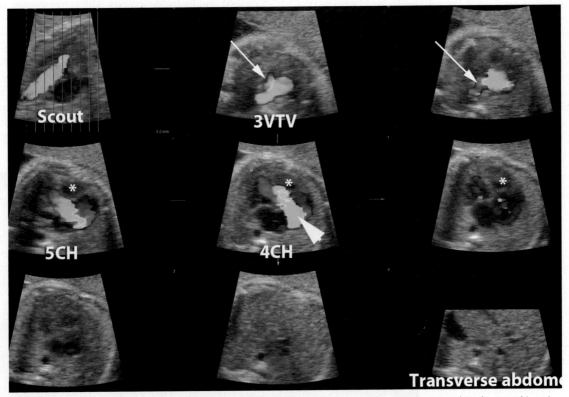

**FIGURE 2.29:** Volume dataset of an abnormal heart acquired with color Doppler imaging. Tomographic ultrasound imaging sliced from the superior mediastinum to the upper abdomen as in Figure 2.28. Note the hypoplastic right ventricle *(asterisk)*, the severe tricuspid regurgitation *(arrowhead)*, and the retrograde perfusion of the pulmonary artery through the ductus arteriosus *(arrow)* in this case of pulmonary atresia with intact ventricular septum 3VTV, three-vessel and trachea view; 5CH, five-chamber view; 4CH, four-chamber view.

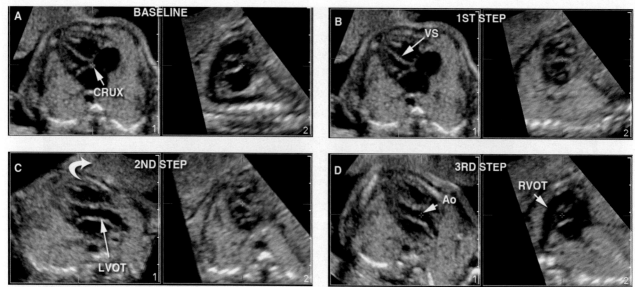

**FIGURE 2.30:** Simultaneous visualization of the left ventricular outflow tract and right ventricular outflow tract, obtained with the "3-step" technique.[14] Only the original transverse plane of acquisition *(1)* and the reconstructed sagittal plane *(2)* for each step are shown. **Baseline: A** shows the four-chamber view with the fetal spine down and oriented horizontally on *2* (as if the fetus was lying on a flat surface). The reference crosshair is at the crux of the heart. **Step 1:** In **A**, the crosshair has been moved to the middle of the ventricular septum *(VS)*. **Step 2:** Once the crosshair in "anchored" in the middle of the septum, rotating the volume dataset around the y-axis *(curved arrow)* will "open up" the septum, showing its normal continuity with the anterior wall of the aorta *(Ao)*. In the same image, the posterior wall of the aorta continues with the anterior leaflet of the mitral valve. Thus, this second step displays the long-axis view of the left ventricular outflow tract *(LVOT)*. **Step 3:** The crosshair is moved to the region of the *Ao*, and the short-axis view of the right ventricular outflow tract *(RVOT)* can be seen on the reconstructed sagittal plane. (Reproduced from Gonçalves LF, et al. 3D-4D fetal echocardiography. *Appl Radiol.* 2012;3:31–43, Copyright 2012, with permission from Anderson Publishing Ltd.)

$P > 0.05$), with 10 false-negative diagnoses by 4DUS (VSD [$n = 9$], interrupted aortic arch [$n = 1$]) and 3 by 2DUS (VSD [$n = 2$], persistent left superior vena cava [$n = 1$]). 4DUS had 19 false-positive diagnoses (VSD [$n = 10$], coarctation of the aorta [$n = 4$], persistent left superior vena cava [$n = 2$], pulmonary stenosis [$n = 1$], tricuspid dysplasia [$n = 1$], rhabdomyoma [$n = 1$]), while 2DUS have 17 false-positive diagnoses (VSD [$n = 11$], coarctation of the aorta [$n = 4$], tricuspid dysplasia [$n = 1$], ostium primum atrial septal defect [$n = 1$]).[127] Espinoza et al.[127a] conducted a multicenter study that included experts at seven international institutions. Ninety volume datasets of fetuses with and without CHD were uploaded to a server and examined blindly by the experts. The study showed very good sensitivity and specificity for the diagnosis of CHD (93% and 96%, respectively) with excellent intercenter agreement (kappa = 0.97). The study conducted by Yagel et al. demonstrated additional value of 4DUS when compared with 2DUS in 193 cases of CHD analyzed blindly. The study showed that 12 cardiac anomalies were correctly diagnosed only by 4DUS, including a right aortic arch with anomalous branching, transposition of the great arteries with pulmonary atresia, interrupted aortic arch, right ventricular aneurysm, and total anomalous

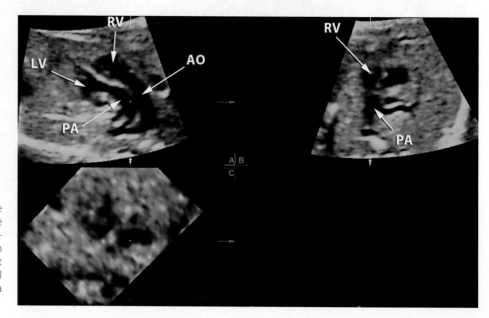

**FIGURE 2.31:** D-Transposition of the great arteries demonstrated using the three-step technique. Note that the bifurcating pulmonary artery *(PA)* arises from the left ventricle *(LV)*. The vessel that leaves the right ventricle *(RV)* in parallel with the pulmonary artery is the aorta arising transposed. Ao, Aorta.

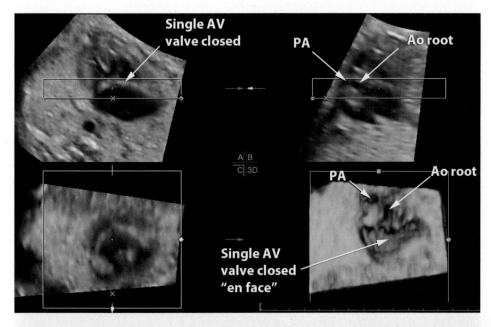

**FIGURE 2.32:** Multiplanar **(A–C)** and rendered **(D)** views of the atrioventricular valve seen "en face" in a case of complete atrioventricular canal. Note the size of the ROI box as well as the direction of the projection path, which is determined by the *green line*. In this case the closed single atrioventricular valve in a case of complete atrioventricular canal is seen as if the examiner is looking from the atrial chambers toward the ventricles. PA, pulmonary artery; Ao root, aortic root; AV, atrioventricular.

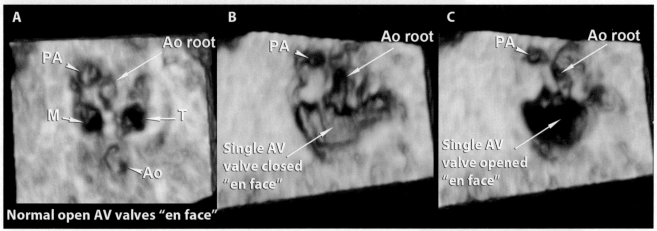

**FIGURE 2.33:** Rendered "en face" views of normal atrioventricular valves **(A)**, single closed atrioventricular canal valve **(B)**, and single opened atrioventricular valve **(C)**. *PA*, pulmonary artery; *Ao root*, aortic root; *AV*, atrioventricular; *T*, Trachea.

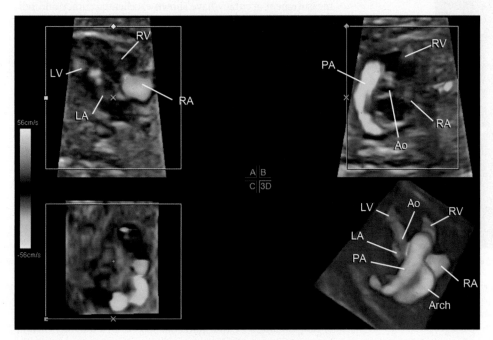

**FIGURE 2.34:** Multiplanar **(A–C)** and rendered **(D)** views of a normal fetal heart acquired using a transverse sweep through the fetal chest and color Doppler imaging. Note the ROI box adjusted in **panels A–C** to include the entire heart. Also note the projection direction given in **panels B** and **C** by the position of the *green line*. In this case, the projection direction is from the superior mediastinum down toward the abdomen. Therefore, the resulting rendered image **(D)** displays, in sequence, the pulmonary artery crossing over the aortic root, the ascending aorta and part of the arch, and then the atrial and ventricular chambers seen in the background in red. PA, pulmonary artery; Ao, aorta; RA, right atrium; RV, right ventricle; LA, left atrium; LV, left ventricle.

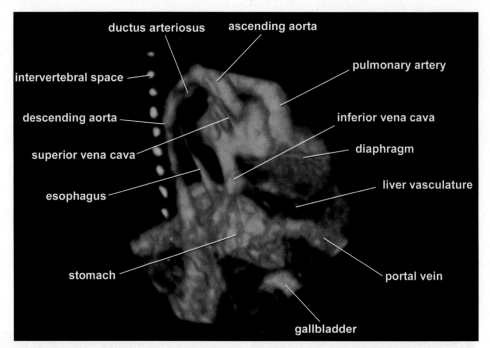

**FIGURE 2.35:** Three-dimensional rendered image of the aortic and ductal arches in a normal fetus at 22 + 2 weeks using the inversion mode technique. (Reproduced with permission from Gonçalves LF, Espinoza J, Lee W, et al. Three- and four-dimensional reconstruction of the aortic and ductal arches using inversion mode: a new rendering algorithm for visualization of fluid-filled anatomical structures. *Ultrasound Obstet Gynecol.* 2004;24[6]:696–698.)

pulmonary venous return. In that study, the sensitivity of 2DUS was 87.6% (95% confidence interval [CI], 81.8% to 91.7%), and the sensitivity of 4DUS was 93.8% (95% CI, 89.1% to 96.6%). Both imaging modalities had a specificity of 100% (95% CI, 99.9% to 100%).[128]

## VOLUMETRIC MEASUREMENTS

Before widespread availability of 3DUS equipment, fetal volumetric measurements could be obtained only with the use of formulas based on 2D measurements of the structure of interest.

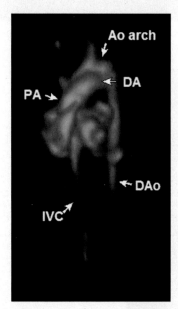

**FIGURE 2.36:** Rendered image of the aortic and ductal arches obtained from a volume dataset acquired with B-flow imaging. Ao arch, aortic arch; DA, ductus arteriosus; Dao, descending aorta; IVC, inferior vena cava; PA, pulmonary artery. (Reproduced with permission from Gonçalves LF, Lee W, Espinoza J, et al. Examination of the fetal heart by four-dimensional [4D] ultrasound with spatio-temporal image correlation [STIC]. *Ultrasound Obstet Gynecol.* 2006;27[3]:336–348.)

The ellipsoid formula (transverse × anteroposterior × longitudinal dimensions × $\pi/6$), still widely used in clinical practice to estimate the volumes of various organs, assumes an approximate ellipsoid shape and regular contour. This is not true for complex anatomical structures such as the left and right ventricles of the heart, for which the mean measurement error can be as high as 25%.[129,130] Direct volumetric measurements can now be performed from 3D and 4D volume datasets obtained with most commercially available equipment. Two methods are generally used: (1) multiplanar or multiple parallel plane method and (2) rotational virtual organ computer-aided analysis (VOCAL, GE Healthcare, Milwaukee, WI). Several investigators have reported on the accuracy of volumetric measurements for a variety of organs and clinical scenarios.[37,131–158]

Even though in vitro studies evaluating 3DUS volumetric measurement accuracy have shown excellent accuracy and reliability,[159–161] a recent review of published nomograms for volumetric measurements of various fetal organs showed remarkable variability.[151] To illustrate the point, suppose one wants to know the normal fetal lung volume for a 28-week fetus. After a literature search is conducted, one finds out that the reported mean fetal lung volume at 28 weeks of gestation ranges between 17.2 and 43.3 mL among 15 peer-reviewed papers.[131,140,141,151,162–172] The implications of this observation are clinically important: a fetal lung volume of 36.12 mL at 28 weeks may lie anywhere between −2.94 standard deviations and +1.11 standard deviations of the mean for gestational age, depending on the chosen nomogram. Such a wide discrepancy makes it difficult to diagnose true pathology with confidence. Consequently, volumetric measurements must be approached with caution. Methodological sources of error, rather than true biological differences, are likely the explanation for the wide variation of reported normal values. One such source of variation is inherent to the physical principles underlying ultrasonography, which is a reflective technique and, therefore, plagued with artifacts related to shadowing from bones that limit the ability to precisely define the borders of soft tissue structures (e.g., rib shadows impairing precise tracing of lung contours). Other potential sources of variability include heterogeneity of 3DUS system platforms, inconsistency in the

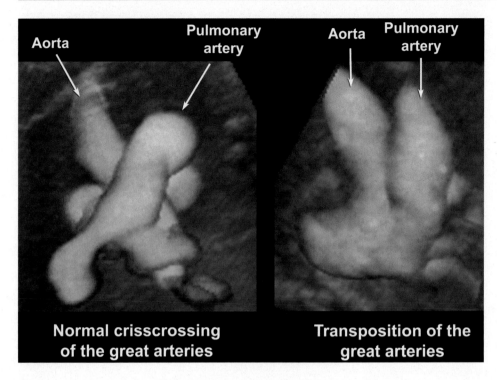

Normal crisscrossing of the great arteries

Transposition of the great arteries

**FIGURE 2.37:** Rendered images from volume datasets of the fetal heart in a normal case **(A)** and TGA **(B)**. The volumes were acquired through a transverse sweep of the fetal chest using power Doppler 4DUS with STIC. In the normal case, normal crisscrossing of the great arteries is observed, whereas in TGA, the vessels leave the ventricles in parallel. The technique used to render the volume datasets is explained in Figure 2.34. (Reproduced with permission from Gonçalves LF, Espinoza J, Romero R, et al. A systematic approach to prenatal diagnosis of transposition of the great arteries using 4-dimensional ultrasonography with spatiotemporal image correlation. *J Ultrasound Med.* 2004;23:1225–1231.)

interpretation of ultrasonographic images, problems with data analysis and reporting of measurement errors, and issues related to method validation.[151] To complicate matters further, there are a multitude of mutually incompatible 3DUS imaging formats and software measuring tools, an issue that is unlikely to improve until manufacturers adopt a 3DUS DICOM standard.

In the following sections, we review the clinical applications of 3DUS volumetry to three clinically relevant scenarios: fetal weight estimation using limb volumes, volumetric measurements of the fetal lungs to predict pulmonary hypoplasia, and volumetric measurements of the fetal heart chambers to evaluate cardiac function.

## Fetal Weight Estimation Using Volumetric Imaging

Estimated fetal weight (EFW) is routinely obtained in the second and third trimesters to assess fetal size and nutritional status. Most methods estimate fetal weight based on 2D measurements of the fetal biparietal diameter (BPD), head circumference (HC), abdominal circumference (AC), and femur length (FL). When compared with actual fetal weight, ultrasonographic EFW is associated with random errors ranging from 8.1% to 11.8%.[173]

To improve the accuracy of ultrasonographic EFW, recent efforts have focused on volumetric measurements of the fetal limbs using 3DUS.[132,145,155–158,174–181] Initial studies used total limb volumetry to predict fetal weight.[156–158] However, total limb volumetry is technically cumbersome, largely due to poor visualization of soft tissue borders at the distal ends of the limbs, and the large number of manual tracings to obtain a volume measurement. To overcome these obstacles, fractional limb volumetry (FLV) was introduced in 2001.[132] In FLV, only the midportion of the limb is measured as a fixed percentage (50%) of the diaphysis length. Either fractional thigh ($T_{vol}$) or fractional arm volume ($A_{vol}$) can be measured, as illustrated in Figures 2.38 and 2.39. Initial investigations found that a combination of either $T_{vol}$ or

$A_{vol}$ and AC could predict actual birth weight much more reliably than conventional 2DUS measurements.[132] Furthermore, $T_{vol}$ correlates strongly with the percentage of neonatal body fat measured within 48 hours of delivery by air displacement plethysmography.[179]

Subsequent studies found that $A_{vol}$ and $T_{vol}$ measurements could be performed with good intraobserver and interobserver bias and agreement (intraobserver bias and agreement: $A_{vol}$ 2.2% ± 4.2% (95% limits of agreement, −6.0% to 10.5%), $T_{vol}$ 2.0% ± 4.2% (95% limits of agreement, −6.3% to 10.3%); interobserver bias and agreement: $A_{vol}$ −1.9% ± 4.9% (95% limits of

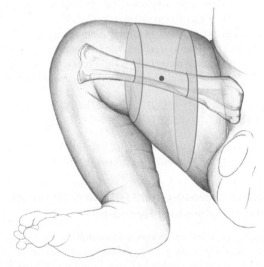

**FIGURE 2.38:** Illustration of fractional thigh volume ($T_{vol}$). $T_{vol}$ is a subvolume that includes 50% of the femoral diaphysis length. The volume is centered on the midfemoral shaft *(small circle)*. The principle is the same for fractional arm volume ($A_{vol}$). (Reproduced with permission from Lee W, Deter RL, McNie B, et al. Individualized growth assessment of fetal soft tissue using fractional thigh volume. *Ultrasound Obstet Gynecol.* 2004;24[7]:767–774.)

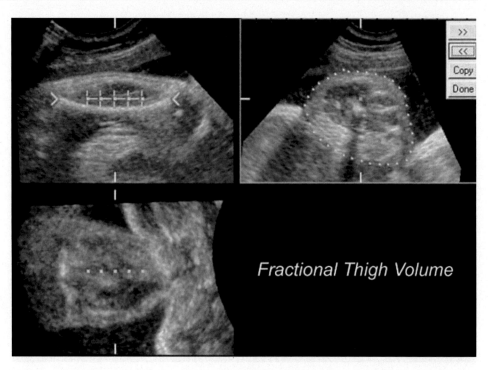

**FIGURE 2.39:** Fractional thigh volume by 3DUS. Orthogonal viewing planes (sagittal, upper left window; axial, upper right window; coronal, lower left window) are used to examine the fetal thigh by multiplanar imaging. The *arrowheads* are electronically positioned at both ends of the femoral diaphysis in the sagittal plane. A midthigh subvolume is based on 50% of the diaphysis length and is split into five sections that are manually traced from axial views. The principle is the same for fractional arm volume ($A_{vol}$). (Reproduced with permission Lee W, Deter RL, McNie B, et al. Individualized growth assessment of fetal soft tissue using fractional thigh volume. *Ultrasound Obstet Gynecol.* 2004;24[7]:767–774.)

agreement, −11.6% to 7.8%), $T_{vol}$ −2.0% ± 5.4% (95% limits of agreement, −12.5% to 8.6%). Normal reference ranges for $A_{vol}$ and $T_{vol}$ during pregnancy have been established in 2009 and are reproduced in Appendix 15 and 16.[146]

More recently, new fetal weight estimation models based on FLV and conventional 2DUS were developed[145] and subsequently validated[155] in a different population. The validation study included 164 pregnant women who delivered between 21 and 42 weeks of menstrual age and who had $T_{vol}$, $A_{vol}$, BPD, AC, and FL measured within 4 days of delivery. The best model to predict actual birth weight was a combination of the BPD, AC, and $T_{vol}$.[155] The model correctly classified a greater proportion of EFW within 5% (55.1% vs. 43.7%, $P = .03$) and 10% (86.5% vs. 75.9%, $P < .05$) of actual birth weight when compared with EFW calculated using formulas derived from 2DUS measurements (modified Hadlock formula using BPD, AC, and FL with coefficients derived from the same population[145]).

The formulas to estimate birth weight based on a combination of 2DUS parameters and $T_{vol}$ and $A_{vol}$ are provided below[145]:

$$T_{vol}: \text{Ln BW} = -0.8297 + 4.0344 \, (\ln \text{BPD}) - 0.7820 \, (\ln \text{BPD})^2 + 0.7853 \, (\ln \text{AC}) + 0.0528 \, (\ln T_{vol})^2$$

$$A_{vol}: \text{Ln BW} = 0.5046 + 1.9665 \, (\ln \text{BPD}) - 0.3040 \, (\ln \text{BPD})^2 + 0.9675 \, (\ln \text{AC}) + 0.3557 \, (\ln A_{vol})$$

## Volumetric Measurements of the Fetal Lungs to Predict Pulmonary Hypoplasia

Identification of fetuses at risk for pulmonary hypoplasia, particularly lethal pulmonary hypoplasia is important in several conditions, including congenital diaphragmatic hernia (CDH), congenital lung malformations (e.g., congenital pulmonary airway malformation), skeletal dysplasias, and prolonged premature rupture of the membranes.

The pathological criteria to diagnose pulmonary hypoplasia are a lung weight to body weight ratio of 0.015 or less before 28 weeks

of gestation, and 0.012 or less at 28 weeks of gestation or more, and/or an abnormal mean radial alveolar count.[182] The diagnosis of pulmonary hypoplasia in vivo relies on chest and/or lung measurements. The most extensively studied condition that requires in utero lung measurements is CDH, and the most widely used biometric parameter to predict pulmonary hypoplasia is the lung-to-head ratio (LHR).[183–185] The LHR indirectly assesses the risk of pulmonary hypoplasia of the contralateral lung, and is defined as the product of the longest orthogonal lung diameters measured on a 2D axial view of the fetal chest at the level of the four-chamber view divided by the fetal HC (with all measurements performed in mm). Metkus et al.[183] reported 0% survival for fetuses with a LHR < 0.6, whereas Lipshutz et al.[184] reported 0% survival for those with a LHR < 1.0. Fetuses with a LHR > 1.4 have a better prognosis. Intermediate values are associated with survival rates ranging from 38% to 61%. Because of concerns regarding LHR variability with gestational age, Jani et al.[186] have proposed the use of observed to expected LHR (O/E-LHR).

The use of 3DUS to assess lung volume was born out of the interest in improving measurement accuracy by directly measuring volume instead of relying on estimations. Several studies have been performed using either the multiplanar (Fig. 2.40) or VOCAL methods (Fig. 2.41). Kalache et al.[134] showed that both methods could be used interchangeably with excellent intermethod variability and good agreement. Several other studies have shown that volumetric measurements of the fetal lungs are accurate when compared with in vitro models and that there is also good intraobserver and interobserver reproducibility and reliability. When compared with MRI using in vitro lung models and also in vivo among fetuses with CDH in vivo, both technologies were shown to be highly correlated, reliable, and accurate.[187,188]

The current problems with both 3DUS and fetal MRI to be used as the gold standard methods for evaluation of lung hypoplasia are related mainly to the high variability in the reported normal values among the various published nomograms. Ioannou et al.[151] reviewed 15 published nomograms for fetal lung volumes using 3DUS,[131,140,141,151,162–172] and documented such a wide

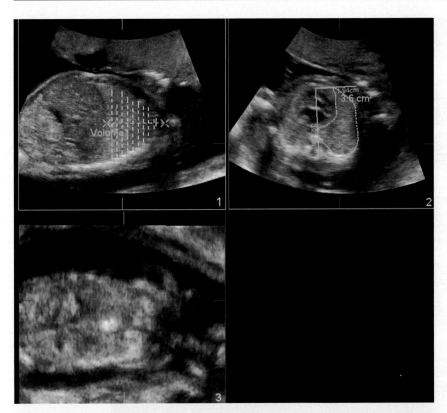

**FIGURE 2.40:** 3D fetal lung volume measurement using the multiplanar technique. **Panel 1** is sagittal, **panel 2** is axial, and **panel 3** is coronal. After the user defines the distance from the lung apex to the base (**panel 1**, *green crosses* and *dashed line*), the equipment automatically divides the distance into a number of slices that is defined by the examiner. The examiner then traces each slice in sequence (**panel 2**). After all slices are traced, the system provides the volume calculation.

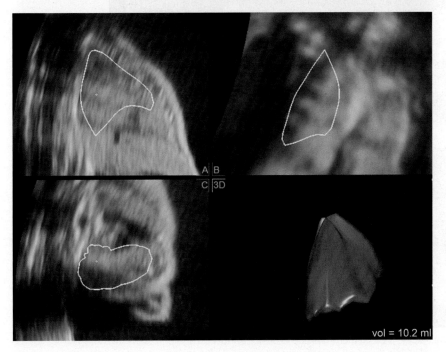

**FIGURE 2.41:** 3D fetal lung measurement using the VOCAL™ (Virtual Organ Computed Aided Analysis, 4DView, GE Healthcare, Milwaukee, WI, USA). The lung is rotated around the vertical axis. The number of rotation steps is determined by the examiner and ranges between 6 (30° increments) and 15 (6° increments). The examiner traces the lung contour multiple times during until the volume is rotated a total of 180°. The system then computes the volume.

variability for reported normal values that may hamper the applicability of the lung volumetry by 3DUS to clinical practice (see discussion on the section "Volumetric Measurements" above). Similar concerns have been reported by Deshmukh et al.[189] for fetal MRI data based on a review of 10 published studies.[190–199]

Our personal experience with 3DUS lung volumetry in skeletal dysplasias has also been disappointing, largely on account of technical difficulties in tracing the contour of the lungs when the thorax is very small, with more rib shadowing artifact than expected in normal fetal lungs. In a study of 41 fetuses with confirmed skeletal dysplasias, the sensitivity of total lung volume to detect lethal pulmonary hypoplasia was high (92.9%), but the specificity was too low (51.9%) to be useful in clinical practice.[200]

## Functional Evaluation of the Fetal Heart by 4DUS

Stroke volume (SV), cardiac output (CO), and ejection fraction (EF) are important parameters to evaluate fetal cardiac function. Until recently, these could only be estimated from 2DUS measurements that rely on imperfect geometric assumptions

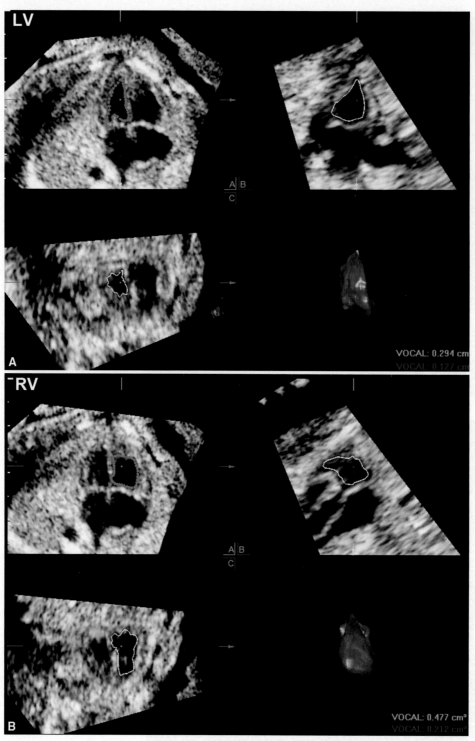

**FIGURE 2.42:** Left (LV; **A**) and right (RV; **B**) ventricular volume measurements obtained VOCAL™ (Virtual Organ Computed Aided Analysis, 4DView, GE Healthcare, Milwaukee, WI, USA) during systole and diastole. Once the measurements are obtained, several hemodynamic parameters can be calculated. For example: (1) Ejection fraction (EF) for the right ventricle *(RV)* is calculated as follows: RV end-diastolic volume (0.477 mL) − RV end-systolic volume (0.212 mL)/RV end-diastolic volume (0.477 mL) = 55.5%; (2) EF for the left ventricle *(LV)* is: LV end-diastolic volume (0.294 mL) − LV end-systolic volume (0.127 mL)/LV end-diastolic volume (0.294 mL) = 56.8%; (3) Stroke volume for the RV is RV end-diastolic volume (0.477 mL) − RV end-systolic volume (0.212 mL) = 0.265 mL, and RV cardiac output for a fetal heart rate of 140 bpm is 37.1 mL; (4) Stroke volume for the LV is LV end-diastolic volume (0.294 mL) − LV end-systolic volume (0.127 mL) = 0.167 mL, and LV cardiac output for a fetal heart rate of 140 bpm is 23.4 mL.

about ventricular shape (orthogonal measurements, multiple disc method—Simpson's rule),[201,202] or by using a combination of 2DUS and Doppler.[203] Simpson and Cook[204] showed that the repeatability of volumetric measurements using the multiple disc method is poor (the coefficient of variation exceeded 10% for the estimation for both the left ventricular end-diastolic volume [13%] and the SV [14%]), with intraobserver errors consistently higher than intraobserver errors. Furthermore, formulas that rely on geometric assumptions about ventricular morphology apply only to the left ventricle, since the right ventricle has a complex morphology.

| Table 2.1 | | Volumetric Measurements of the Fetal Heart Using Spatiotemporal Image Correlation (STIC) | | | |
|---|---|---|---|---|---|

| *Author* | *Year* | *n* | *GA Range (wk)* | *Method* | *Main Findings* |
|---|---|---|---|---|---|
| Messing et al.[209] | 2007 | 100 | 20–40 | Inversion Mode | ▪ ESV, EDV, and SV for both ventricles correlated strongly with GA<br>▪ No significant change in EF with GA, with left EF slightly larger than the right<br>▪ Good intraobserver and interobserver reproducibility |
| Rizzo et al.[214] | 2007 | 56 | 20–32 | VOCAL Manual Trace | ▪ Good intraobserver and interobserver agreement for SV measured with either Doppler or STIC<br>▪ STIC significantly faster than Doppler (3.1 ± 0.84 min vs. 7.9 ± 2.3 min, $P < .0001$) |
| Molina et al.[210] | 2008 | 140 | 12–34 | VOCAL Manual Trace | ▪ SV and CO increased with GA<br>▪ Ratio of right to left SV increased with GA from 0.97 at 12 weeks to 1.13 at 34 weeks |
| Uittenbogaard et al.[148] | 2009 | 63 | 12–30 | 3D Slice Method | ▪ Longitudinal study involving 202 STIC volumes<br>▪ Ratio of right to left SV of about 1.2 |
| Hamill et al.[144] | 2009 | 25 | | VOCAL Contour Trace VOCAL Manual Trace Inversion | ▪ Better intraobserver and interobserver agreement for the Contour Trace method<br>▪ Better agreement between measurements with 15° rotation increments<br>▪ Ventricular volume measurements were repeatable and reproducible |
| Rizzo et al.[211] | 2010 | 45 | 19–32 | VOCAL Manual Trace VOCAL SonoAVC | ▪ Good reliability between Manual Trace and SonoAVC<br>▪ SonoAVC significantly faster (2.8 ± 1.9 min vs. 11.7 ± 4.8 min $P < 0.0001$) |
| Hamill et al.[154] | 2011 | 184 | 19–42 | Vocal Contour Trace | ▪ In this study, normal fetal cardiovascular physiology was characterized by a larger right ventricular volume and a greater left ventricular ejection fraction, resulting in similar left ventricular and right ventricular stroke volume and cardiac output |

VOCAL, Virtual Organ Computer-Aided Analysis; ESV, end systolic volume; EDV, end diastolic volume; SV, stroke volume; EF, ejection fraction; GA, gestational age; CO, cardiac output.

Doppler calculations of SV and CO are accomplished by multiplying the Doppler velocity time integral (VTI) by the 2D cross-sectional valve area of either the atrioventricular or the semilunar valves. The formulas are:

$$SV = VTI \times \pi d^2/4, \text{ where } d \text{ is the diameter of the valve}$$

$$CO = SV \times Heart\ rate$$

Several sources of error are possible with the combination of 2DUS and Doppler measurements. These include: (1) poor angle of insonation ($<20°$), which may result in underestimation of the Doppler VTI; and (2) the derivation of valve area from its radius squared, which tends to amplify measurement errors, even if minimal. Poor reproducibility of Doppler measurements to evaluate SV and CO has been previously reported, with interobserver errors consistently higher than intraobserver errors.[204]

With the advent of 4DUS fetal echocardiography, left and right ventricular volumes can now be directly measured during systole and diastole, allowing direct calculation of SV, CO, and EF. The first attempt to measure ventricular volumes using 4DUS was reported by Meyer-Wittkopf et al.[205] in 2001. In that study, the investigators used a free-hand volume acquisition system composed of standard 2DUS equipment interfaced with a magnetic tracking system.

Volumetric measurements were obtained in 57 normal fetuses and in 22 fetuses with CHD. The authors found that end-systolic and end-diastolic volumes increased exponentially with gestational age for both groups. Fetuses with CHD and inequality of ventricular sizes tended to have smaller combined end-diastolic and SVs than normal fetuses. Free-hand volumetric measurements of the fetal hearts was also attempted by Esh-Broder et al.,[206] who found mean right and left ventricular EF of 54% ± 11.2% and 57.5% ± 14.6% between 20 and 24 weeks of gestation.

After the introduction of STIC technology in 2003,[13,17] several groups have reported on the ability to obtain volumetric measurements of the fetal heart using this technology. Experiments in vitro using pulsatile balloon models have validated the accuracy of STIC for measurements of small volumes such as those found in second and third trimester fetal hearts.[161,207] Several subsequent studies performed in human fetuses collectively showed that: (1) the intraobserver and interobserver repeatability and reproducibility for volumetric measurements of the fetal heart using STIC are high[144,148,208–211]; (2) that EF tends to remain stable through gestation[148,208,209]; (3) and that SV and CO for both the right and the left ventricles increase exponentially with gestation,[148,154,208–210] except when corrected for EFW (Table 2.1).[154]

Of interest is the large study of Hamill et al., who applied one of the 4D segmentation methods with best repeatability and reproducibility, namely VOCAL with contour finder, to measure end-diastolic and end-systolic volumes of the right and left ventricles in 184 fetuses examined between 19 and 42 weeks (Fig. 2.42). SV, CO, and EF were calculated. The study confirmed prior observations that ventricular volumes, SV and CO increase with advancing gestational age. However, it also showed no difference between left and right ventricles for SV and CO, as well as a drop in EF with advancing gestation, with the left EF significantly greater than the right, findings that have not been previously reported.

Regarding the feasibility of 4DUS with STIC to measure cardiac volumes in clinical practice, a few reports comment on pitfalls related to volume acquisition. Hamill et al.,[154] for example, rejected 33/217 (15%) volumes based on poor image quality, whereas Shoonderwaldt et al.[212] reported poor success rate for STIC acquisitions in a study 84 pregnancies scanned between 20 and 34 weeks of gestation. In that study, only 30/84 volumes (36%) had sufficient quality to allow volumetric measurements. The other volumes had to be excluded due to unfavorable fetal position with the spine projecting anterior or lateral, and/or fetal movements that resulted in acoustic shadows and movement artifacts. Uittenbogaard et al.[148] also noted low-image resolution at early gestational age, and a high failure rate after 30 weeks' gestation.

Volumetric imaging of the fetal heart with 4DUS is only in its infancy. Future directions in this area include determining the role of calculations of SV, CO, and EF on various fetal disease processes such as intrauterine growth restriction, preterm labor, preterm premature rupture of the membranes, preeclampsia, fetal hydrops, and fetal monitoring in the context of CHD. It will be important, in the process, to directly compare the performance of these parameters against the many others currently used for fetal hemodynamic evaluation based mainly on Doppler, such as the myocardial performance index (also known as the Tei index) that is currently used to evaluate global (systolic and diastolic) cardiac function.[213]

## CONCLUSION

3DUS provides the obstetrical imager with a tool that can improve diagnosis by enhancing the display of anatomical structures imaged by 2DUS. The workhorse of 3DUS is the multiplanar format, where a structure or lesion can be simultaneously visualized in three planes at the same time. Rendered images, that is, the ones that produce realistic 3D models of the structure of interest, also enhance the capabilities of the examiner in specific conditions, as detailed in the text above. 3DUS and 4DUS have been found particularly useful in the evaluation of facial defects, CNS and skeletal abnormalities, and CHD. The reader is reminded, however, that 3D imaging only enhances 2DUS, and, therefore, artifacts and limitations inherent to ultrasonography are unlikely to be overcome by 3D/4D technology. For additional training in 3D/4D ultrasonography, a good starting point is to explore the resources offered by the American Institute of Ultrasound in Medicine (www.aium.org).

## REFERENCES

1. Tanaka Y, Okamura S, Doi S, et al. A preliminary report of computerized ultrasonography in obstetrics and gynecology: a new technique of C-mode (author's transl) [in Japanese]. *Nihon Sanka Fujinka Gakkai Zasshi*. 1982;34:101–108.
2. Baba K, Satoh K, Sakamoto S, et al. Development of an ultrasonic system for three-dimensional reconstruction of the fetus. *J Perinat Med*. 1989;17:19–24.
3. Kratochwil A. Attempt at three-dimensional imaging in obstetrics [in German]. *Ultraschall Med*. 1992;13:183–186.
4. Pretorius DH, Nelson TR. Prenatal visualization of cranial sutures and fontanelles with three-dimensional ultrasonography. *J Ultrasound Med*. 1994;13:871–876.
5. Merz E, Bahlmann F, Weber G, et al. Three-dimensional ultrasonography in prenatal diagnosis. *J Perinat Med*. 1995;23:213–222.
6. Deng J, Gardener JE, Rodeck CH, et al. Fetal echocardiography in three and four dimensions. *Ultrasound Med Biol*. 1996;22:979–986.
7. Nelson TR, Pretorius DH, Sklansky M, et al. Three-dimensional echocardiographic evaluation of fetal heart anatomy and function: acquisition, analysis, and display. *J Ultrasound Med*. 1996;15:1–9; quiz 11–12.
8. Deng J. Terminology of three-dimensional and four-dimensional ultrasound imaging of the fetal heart and other moving body parts. *Ultrasound Obstet Gynecol*. 2003;22:336–344.
9. Sklansky MS, Nelson TR, Pretorius DH. Usefulness of gated three-dimensional fetal echocardiography to reconstruct and display structures not visualized with two-dimensional imaging. *Am J Cardiol*. 1997;80:665–668.
10. Nelson TR. Three-dimensional fetal echocardiography. *Prog Biophys Mol Biol*. 1998;69:257–272.
11. Sklansky MS, Nelson TR, Pretorius DH. Three-dimensional fetal echocardiography: gated versus nongated techniques. *J Ultrasound Med*. 1998;17:451–457.
12. Deng J, Ruff CF, Linney AD, et al. Simultaneous use of two ultrasound scanners for motion-gated three-dimensional fetal echocardiography. *Ultrasound Med Biol*. 2000;26:1021–1032.
13. DeVore GR, Falkensammer P, Sklansky MS, et al. Spatio-temporal image correlation (STIC): new technology for evaluation of the fetal heart. *Ultrasound Obstet Gynecol*. 2003;22:380–387.
14. Gonçalves LF, Lee W, Chaiworapongsa T, et al. Four-dimensional ultrasonography of the fetal heart with spatiotemporal image correlation. *Am J Obstet Gynecol*. 2003;189:1792–1802.
15. Maulik D, Nanda NC, Singh V, et al. Live three-dimensional echocardiography of the human fetus. *Echocardiography*. 2003;20:715–721.
16. Sklansky M. New dimensions and directions in fetal cardiology. *Curr Opin Pediatr*. 2003;15:463–471.
17. Viñals F, Poblete P, Giuliano A. Spatio-temporal image correlation (STIC): a new tool for the prenatal screening of congenital heart defects. *Ultrasound Obstet Gynecol*. 2003;22:388–394.
18. Chaoui R, Hoffmann J, Heling KS. Three-dimensional (3D) and 4D color Doppler fetal echocardiography using spatio-temporal image correlation (STIC). *Ultrasound Obstet Gynecol*. 2004;23:535–545.
19. Gonçalves LF, Espinoza J, Kusanovic JP, et al. Applications of 2-dimensional matrix array for 3- and 4-dimensional examination of the fetus: a pictorial essay. *J Ultrasound Med*. 2006;25:745–755.
20. Shiota T, Jones M, Chikada M, et al. Real-time three-dimensional echocardiography for determining right ventricular stroke volume in an animal model of chronic right ventricular volume overload. *Circulation*. 1998;97:1897–1900.
21. Goldberg RL, Smith SW. Multilayer piezoelectric ceramics for two-dimensional array transducers. *IEEE Trans Ultrason Ferroelectr Freq Control*. 1994;41:761–771.
22. Light ED, Davidsen RE, Fiering JO, et al. Progress in two-dimensional arrays for real-time volumetric imaging. *Ultrason Imaging* 1998;20:1–15.
23. von Ramm OT, Smith SW. Real time volumetric ultrasound imaging system. *J Digit Imaging*. 1990;3:261–266.
24. Nelson TR, Pretorius DH, Hull A, et al. Sources and impact of artifacts on clinical three-dimensional ultrasound imaging. *Ultrasound Obstet Gynecol*. 2000;16:374–383.
25. Riccabona M, Pretorius DH, Nelson TR, et al. Three-dimensional ultrasound: display modalities in obstetrics. *J Clin Ultrasound*. 1997;25:157–167.
26. Devore GR, Polanko B. Tomographic ultrasound imaging of the fetal heart: a new technique for identifying normal and abnormal cardiac anatomy. *J Ultrasound Med*. 2005;24:1685–1696.
27. Gonçalves LF, Espinoza J, Romero R, et al. Four-dimensional ultrasonography of the fetal heart using a novel Tomographic Ultrasound Imaging display. *J Perinat Med*. 2006;34:39–55.
28. Pretorius DH, Gattu S, Ji EK, et al. Preexamination and postexamination assessment of parental-fetal bonding in patients undergoing 3-/4-dimensional obstetric ultrasonography. *J Ultrasound Med*. 2006;25:1411–1421.
29. Lee A, Kratochwil A, Deutinger J, et al. Three-dimensional ultrasound in diagnosing phocomelia. *Ultrasound Obstet Gynecol*. 1995;5:238–240.
30. Nelson TR, Pretorius DH. Visualization of the fetal thoracic skeleton with three-dimensional sonography: a preliminary report. *AJR Am J Roentgenol*. 1995;164:1485–1488.
31. Riccabona M, Johnson D, Pretorius DH, et al. Three dimensional ultrasound: display modalities in the fetal spine and thorax. *Eur J Radiol*. 1996;22:141–145.
32. Johnson DD, Pretorius DH, Riccabona M, et al. Three-dimensional ultrasound of the fetal spine. *Obstet Gynecol* 1997;89:434–438.
33. Espinoza J, Gonçalves LF, Lee W, et al. The use of the minimum projection mode in 4-dimensional examination of the fetal heart with spatiotemporal image correlation. *J Ultrasound Med*. 2004;23:1337–1348.
34. Gonçalves LF, Espinoza J, Lee W, et al. Three- and four-dimensional reconstruction of the aortic and ductal arches using inversion mode: a new rendering algorithm for visualization of fluid-filled anatomical structures. *Ultrasound Obstet Gynecol*. 2004;24:696–698.
35. Espinoza J, Gonçalves LF, Lee W, et al. A novel method to improve prenatal diagnosis of abnormal systemic venous connections using three- and four-dimensional ultrasonography and "inversion mode". *Ultrasound Obstet Gynecol*. 2005;25:428–434.
36. Gonçalves LF, Espinoza J, Lee W, et al. A new approach to fetal echocardiography: digital casts of the fetal cardiac chambers and great vessels for detection of congenital heart disease. *J Ultrasound Med*. 2005;24:415–424.

37. Lee W, Gonçalves LF, Espinoza J, et al. Inversion mode: a new volume analysis tool for 3-dimensional ultrasonography. *J Ultrasound Med.* 2005;24:201–207.
38. Association N-NEM. Digital imaging and communications in medicine (DICOM). In: *Supplement 43: Storage of 3D Ultrasound Images.* Rosslyn, VA: National Electrical Manufacturers Association; 2009:102.
39. Kurjak A, Stanojevic M, Andonotopo W, et al. Fetal behavior assessed in all three trimesters of normal pregnancy by four-dimensional ultrasonography. *Croat Med J.* 2005;46:772–780.
40. Kurjak A, Stanojevic M, Azumendi G, et al. The potential of four-dimensional (4D) ultrasonography in the assessment of fetal awareness. *J Perinat Med.* 2005;33:46–53.
41. Rustico MA, Mastromatteo C, Grigio M, et al. Two-dimensional vs. two- plus four-dimensional ultrasound in pregnancy and the effect on maternal emotional status: a randomized study. *Ultrasound Obstet Gynecol.* 2005;25:468–472.
42. Andonotopo W, Kurjak A. The assessment of fetal behavior of growth restricted fetuses by 4D sonography. *J Perinat Med.* 2006;34:471–478.
43. Yigiter AB, Kavak ZN. Normal standards of fetal behavior assessed by four-dimensional sonography. *J Matern Fetal Neonatal Med.* 2006;19:707–721.
44. Kurjak A, Tikvica A, Stanojevic M, et al. The assessment of fetal neurobehavior by three-dimensional and four-dimensional ultrasound. *J Matern Fetal Neonatal Med.* 2008;21:675–684.
45. Kim TH, Lee JJ, Chung SH, et al. Efficacy of assessment in fetal behaviour by four dimensional ultrasonography. *J Obstet Gynaecol.* 2010;30:439–443.
46. Lebit DF, Vladareanu PD. The role of 4D ultrasound in the assessment of fetal behaviour. *Maedica (Buchar).* 2011;6:120–127.
47. Sklansky M, Miller D, Devore G, et al. Prenatal screening for congenital heart disease using real-time three-dimensional echocardiography and a novel "sweep volume" acquisition technique. *Ultrasound Obstet Gynecol.* 2005;25:435–443.
48. Salerno CC, Pretorius DH, Hilton SW, et al. Three-dimensional ultrasonographic imaging of the neonatal brain in high-risk neonates: preliminary study. *J Ultrasound Med.* 2000;19:549–555.
49. Riccabona M, Fritz G, Ring E. Potential applications of three-dimensional ultrasound in the pediatric urinary tract: pictorial demonstration based on preliminary results. *Eur Radiol.* 2003;13:2680–2687.
50. Riccabona M, Nelson TR, Weitzer C, et al. Potential of three-dimensional ultrasound in neonatal and paediatric neurosonography. *Eur Radiol.* 2003;13:2082–2093.
51. Bault JP, Salomon LJ, Guibaud L, et al. Role of three-dimensional ultrasound measurement of the optic tract in fetuses with agenesis of the septum pellucidum. *Ultrasound Obstet Gynecol.* 2011;37:570–575.
52. Devonald KJ, Ellwood DA, Griffiths KA, et al. Volume imaging: three-dimensional appreciation of the fetal head and face. *J Ultrasound Med.* 1995;14:919–925.
53. Faro C, Wegrzyn P, Benoit B, et al. Metopic suture in fetuses with holoprosencephaly at 11 + 0 to 13 + 6 weeks of gestation. *Ultrasound Obstet Gynecol.* 2006;27:162–166.
54. Lee W, DeVore GR, Comstock CH, et al. Nasal bone evaluation in fetuses with Down syndrome during the second and third trimesters of pregnancy. *J Ultrasound Med.* 2003;22:55–60.
55. Radlanski RJ. Prenatal craniofacial morphogenesis: four-dimensional visualization of morphogenetic processes. *Orthod Craniofac Res.* 2003;6(suppl 1):89–94.
56. Gonçalves LF, Espinoza J, Lee W, et al. Phenotypic characteristics of absent and hypoplastic nasal bones in fetuses with Down syndrome: description by 3-dimensional ultrasonography and clinical significance. *J Ultrasound Med.* 2004;23:1619–1627.
57. Rembouskos G, Cicero S, Longo D, et al. Assessment of the fetal nasal bone at 11–14 weeks of gestation by three-dimensional ultrasound. *Ultrasound Obstet Gynecol.* 2004;23:232–236.
58. Benoit B, Chaoui R. Three-dimensional ultrasound with maximal mode rendering: a novel technique for the diagnosis of bilateral or unilateral absence or hypoplasia of nasal bones in second-trimester screening for Down syndrome. *Ultrasound Obstet Gynecol.* 2005;25:19–24.
59. Pilu G, Visentin A, Ambrosini G, et al. Three-dimensional sonography of unilateral Tessier number 7 cleft in a mid-trimester fetus. *Ultrasound Obstet Gynecol.* 2005;26:98–99.
60. Sleurs E, Gonçalves LF, Johnson A, et al. First-trimester three-dimensional ultrasonographic findings in a fetus with frontonasal malformation. *J Matern Fetal Neonatal Med.* 2004;16:187–197.
61. Ramos GA, Ylagan MV, Romine LE, et al. Diagnostic evaluation of the fetal face using 3-dimensional ultrasound. *Ultrasound Q.* 2008;24:215–223.
62. Kuo HC, Chang FM, Wu CH, et al. The primary application of three-dimensional ultrasonography in obstetrics. *Am J Obstet Gynecol.* 1992;166:880–886.
63. Lee A, Deutinger J, Bernaschek G. Three dimensional ultrasound: abnormalities of the fetal face in surface and volume rendering mode. *Br J Obstet Gynaecol.* 1995;102:302–306.
64. Pretorius DH, House M, Nelson TR, et al. Evaluation of normal and abnormal lips in fetuses: comparison between three- and two-dimensional sonography. *AJR Am J Roentgenol.* 1995;165:1233–1237.
65. Merz E, Weber G, Bahlmann F, et al. Application of transvaginal and abdominal three-dimensional ultrasound for the detection or exclusion of malformations of the fetal face. *Ultrasound Obstet Gynecol.* 1997;9:237–243.
66. Ulm MR, Kratochwil A, Ulm B, et al. Three-dimensional ultrasonographic imaging of fetal tooth buds for characterization of facial clefts. *Early Hum Dev.* 1999;55:67–75.
67. Johnson DD, Pretorius DH, Budorick NE, et al. Fetal lip and primary palate: three-dimensional versus two-dimensional US. *Radiology.* 2000;217:236–239.
68. Lee W, Kirk JS, Shaheen KW, et al. Fetal cleft lip and palate detection by three-dimensional ultrasonography. *Ultrasound Obstet Gynecol.* 2000;16:314–320.
69. Chmait R, Pretorius D, Jones M, et al. Prenatal evaluation of facial clefts with two-dimensional and adjunctive three-dimensional ultrasonography: a prospective trial. *Am J Obstet Gynecol.* 2002;187:946–949.
70. Campbell S, Lees C, Moscoso G, et al. Ultrasound antenatal diagnosis of cleft palate by a new technique: the 3D "reverse face" view. *Ultrasound Obstet Gynecol.* 2005;25:12–18.
71. Benacerraf BR, Sadow PM, Barnewolt CE, et al. Cleft of the secondary palate without cleft lip diagnosed with three-dimensional ultrasound and magnetic resonance imaging in a fetus with Fryns' syndrome. *Ultrasound Obstet Gynecol.* 2006;27:566–570.
72. Chmait R, Pretorius D, Moore T, et al. Prenatal detection of associated anomalies in fetuses diagnosed with cleft lip with or without cleft palate in utero. *Ultrasound Obstet Gynecol.* 2006;27:173–176.
73. Platt LD, Devore GR, Pretorius DH. Improving cleft palate/cleft lip antenatal diagnosis by 3-dimensional sonography: the "flipped face" view. *J Ultrasound Med.* 2006;25:1423–1430.
74. Pilu G, Segata M. A novel technique for visualization of the normal and cleft fetal secondary palate: angled insonation and three-dimensional ultrasound. *Ultrasound Obstet Gynecol.* 2007;29:166–169.
75. Parker SE, Mai CT, Canfield MA, et al. Updated National Birth Prevalence estimates for selected birth defects in the United States, 2004–2006. *Birth Defects Res A Clin Mol Teratol.* 2010;88:1008–1016.
76. Dixon MJ, Marazita ML, Beaty TH, et al. Cleft lip and palate: understanding genetic and environmental influences. *Nat Rev Genet.* 2011;12:167–178.
77. Mueller GM, Weiner CP, Yankowitz J. Three-dimensional ultrasound in the evaluation of fetal head and spine anomalies. *Obstet Gynecol.* 1996;88:372–378.
78. Hata T, Aoki S, Hata K, et al. Three-dimensional ultrasonographic assessments of fetal development. *Obstet Gynecol.* 1998;91:218–223.
79. Chen ML, Chang CH, Yu CH, et al. Prenatal diagnosis of cleft palate by three-dimensional ultrasound. *Ultrasound Med Biol.* 2001;27:1017–1023.
80. Ghi T, Perolo A, Banzi C, et al. Two-dimensional ultrasound is accurate in the diagnosis of fetal craniofacial malformation. *Ultrasound Obstet Gynecol.* 2002;19:543–551.
81. Mangione R, Lacombe D, Carles D, et al. Craniofacial dysmorphology and three-dimensional ultrasound: a prospective study on practicability for prenatal diagnosis. *Prenat Diagn.* 2003;23:810–818.
82. Mittermayer C, Blaicher W, Brugger PC, et al. Foetal facial clefts: prenatal evaluation of lip and primary palate by 2D and 3D ultrasound. *Ultraschall Med.* 2004;25:120–125.
83. Sommerlad M, Patel N, Vijayalakshmi B, et al. Detection of lip, alveolar ridge and hard palate abnormalities using two-dimensional ultrasound enhanced with the three-dimensional reverse-face view. *Ultrasound Obstet Gynecol.* 2010;36:596–600.
84. Faure JM, Captier G, Baumler M, et al. Sonographic assessment of normal fetal palate using three-dimensional imaging: a new technique. *Ultrasound Obstet Gynecol.* 2007;29:159–165.
85. Baumler MA, Faure JM, Bigorre M, et al. Accuracy of prenatal three-dimensional ultrasound in the diagnosis of cleft hard palate when cleft lip is present. *Ultrasound Obstet Gynecol.* 2011;38(4):440–444.
86. Martinez-Ten P, Adiego B, Illescas T, et al. First-trimester diagnosis of cleft lip and palate using three-dimensional ultrasound. *Ultrasound Obstet Gynecol.* 2012;40:40–46.
87. Leung KY, Ngai CS, Tang MH. Facial cleft or shadowing artifact? *Ultrasound Obstet Gynecol.* 2006;27:231–232.
88. Timor-Tritsch IE, Platt LD. Three-dimensional ultrasound experience in obstetrics. *Curr Opin Obstet Gynecol.* 2002;14:569–575.
89. Ramos GA, Romine LE, Gindes L, et al. Evaluation of the fetal secondary palate by 3-dimensional ultrasonography. *J Ultrasound Med.* 2010;29:357–364.
90. Wilhelm L, Borgers H. The "equals sign": a novel marker in the diagnosis of fetal isolated cleft palate. *Ultrasound Obstet Gynecol.* 2010;36:439–444.
91. Manganaro L, Savelli S, Di Maurizio M, et al. Potential role of fetal cardiac evaluation with magnetic resonance imaging: preliminary experience. *Prenat Diagn.* 2008;28:148–156.
92. Mailath-Pokorny M, Worda C, Krampl-Bettelheim E, et al. What does magnetic resonance imaging add to the prenatal ultrasound diagnosis of facial clefts? *Ultrasound Obstet Gynecol.* 2010;36:445–451.
93. Descamps MJ, Golding SJ, Sibley J, et al. MRI for definitive in utero diagnosis of cleft palate: a useful adjunct to antenatal care? *Cleft Palate Craniofac J.* 2010;47:578–585.
94. Schild RL, Wallny T, Fimmers R, et al. Fetal lumbar spine volumetry by three-dimensional ultrasound. *Ultrasound Obstet Gynecol.* 1999;13:335–339.
95. Lee W, Chaiworapongsa T, Romero R, et al. A diagnostic approach for the evaluation of spina bifida by three-dimensional ultrasonography. *J Ultrasound Med.* 2002;21:619–626.
96. Yang XH, Chen M, Leung TY, et al. Use of three-dimensional (3D) sonography to assess the true midsagittal plane of fetal spine. *J Matern Fetal Neonatal Med.* 2011;24:297–300.
97. Huissoud C, Bisch C, Charrin K, et al. Prenatal diagnosis of partial lumbar asoma by two- and three-dimensional ultrasound and computed tomography: embryological aspects and perinatal management. *Ultrasound Obstet Gynecol.* 2008;32:579–581.
98. Alvarez de la Rosa M, Padilla Perez AI, de la Torre Fernandez de Vega FJ, et al. Genetic counseling in a case of congenital hemivertebrae. *Arch Gynecol Obstet.* 2009;280:653–658.
99. Haratz K, Vinkler C, Lev D, et al. Hemifacial microsomia with spinal and rib anomalies: prenatal diagnosis and postmortem confirmation using 3-D computed tomography reconstruction. *Fetal Diagn Ther.* 2011;30:309–313.

100. Steiner H, Spitzer D, Weiss-Wichert PH, et al. Three-dimensional ultrasound in prenatal diagnosis of skeletal dysplasia. *Prenat Diagn*. 1995;15:373–377.

101. Garjian KV, Pretorius DH, Budorick NE, et al. Fetal skeletal dysplasia: three-dimensional US—initial experience. *Radiology*. 2000;214:717–723.

102. Chen CP, Chern SR, Shih JC, et al. Prenatal diagnosis and genetic analysis of type I and type II thanatophoric dysplasia. *Prenat Diagn*. 2001;21:89–95.

103. Machado LE, Bonilla-Musoles F, Osborne NG. Thanatophoric dysplasia. *Ultrasound Obstet Gynecol*. 2001;18:85–86.

104. Moeglin D, Benoit B. Three-dimensional sonographic aspects in the antenatal diagnosis of achondroplasia. *Ultrasound Obstet Gynecol*. 2001;18:81–83.

105. Viora E, Sciarrone A, Bastonero S, et al. Three-dimensional ultrasound evaluation of short-rib polydactyly syndrome type II in the second trimester: a case report. *Ultrasound Obstet Gynecol*. 2002;19:88–91.

106. Krakow D, Williams J III, Poehl M, et al. Use of three-dimensional ultrasound imaging in the diagnosis of prenatal-onset skeletal dysplasias. *Ultrasound Obstet Gynecol*. 2003;21:467–472.

107. Seow KM, Huang LW, Lin YH, et al. Prenatal three-dimensional ultrasound diagnosis of a camptomelic dysplasia. *Arch Gynecol Obstet*. 2004;269:142–144.

108. Shih JC, Peng SS, Hsiao SM, et al. Three-dimensional ultrasound diagnosis of Larsen syndrome with further characterization of neurological sequelae. *Ultrasound Obstet Gynecol*. 2004;24:89–93.

109. Ruano R, Molho M, Roume J, et al. Prenatal diagnosis of fetal skeletal dysplasias by combining two-dimensional and three-dimensional ultrasound and intrauterine three-dimensional helical computer tomography. *Ultrasound Obstet Gynecol*. 2004;24:134–140.

110. Bonnet D, Coltri A, Butera G, et al. Detection of transposition of the great arteries in fetuses reduces neonatal morbidity and mortality. *Circulation*. 1999;99:916–918.

111. Bartlett JM, Wypij D, Bellinger DC, et al. Effect of prenatal diagnosis on outcomes in D-transposition of the great arteries. *Pediatrics*. 2004;113:e335–e340.

112. Franklin O, Burch M, Manning N, et al. Prenatal diagnosis of coarctation of the aorta improves survival and reduces morbidity. *Heart*. 2002;87:67–69.

113. Tworetzky W, McElhinney DB, Reddy VM, et al. Improved surgical outcome after fetal diagnosis of hypoplastic left heart syndrome. *Circulation*. 2001;103:1269–1273.

114. Calderon J, Angeard N, Moutier S, et al. Impact of prenatal diagnosis on neurocognitive outcomes in children with transposition of the great arteries. *J Pediatr*. 2012;161:94–98.e1.

115. DeVore GR, Polanco B, Sklansky MS, et al. The "spin" technique: a new method for examination of the fetal outflow tracts using three-dimensional ultrasound. *Ultrasound Obstet Gynecol*. 2004;24:72–82.

116. Gonçalves LF, Romero R, Espinoza J, et al. Four-dimensional ultrasonography of the fetal heart using color Doppler spatiotemporal image correlation. *J Ultrasound Med*. 2004;23:473–481.

117. Gonçalves LF, Espinoza J, Romero R, et al. Four-dimensional fetal echocardiography with spatiotemporal image correlation (STIC): a systematic study of standard cardiac views assessed by different observers. *J Matern Fetal Neonatal Med*. 2005;17:323–331.

118. Espinoza J, Kusanovic JP, Gonçalves LF, et al. A novel algorithm for comprehensive fetal echocardiography using four-dimensional ultrasonography and tomographic imaging. *J Ultrasound Med*. 2006;25:947–956.

119. Yeo L, Romero R, Jodicke C, et al. Simple targeted arterial rendering (STAR) technique: a novel and simple method to visualize the fetal cardiac outflow tracts. *Ultrasound Obstet Gynecol*. 2011;37:549–556.

120. Yeo L, Romero R, Jodicke C, et al. Four-chamber view and "swing technique" (FAST) echo: a novel and simple algorithm to visualize standard fetal echocardiographic planes. *Ultrasound Obstet Gynecol*. 2011;37:423–431.

121. Yagel S, Cohen SM, Achiron R. Examination of the fetal heart by five short-axis views: a proposed screening method for comprehensive cardiac evaluation. *Ultrasound Obstet Gynecol*. 2001;17:367–369.

122. Rizzo G, Capponi A, Muscatello A, et al. Examination of the fetal heart by four-dimensional ultrasound with spatiotemporal image correlation during routine second-trimester examination: the "three-steps technique". *Fetal Diagn Ther*. 2008;24:126–131.

123. Gonçalves LF, Espinoza J, Romero R, et al. A systematic approach to prenatal diagnosis of transposition of the great arteries using 4-dimensional ultrasonography with spatiotemporal image correlation. *J Ultrasound Med*. 2004;23:1225–1231.

124. Uittenbogaard LB, Haak MC, Spreeuwenberg MD, et al. A systematic analysis of the feasibility of four-dimensional ultrasound imaging using spatiotemporal image correlation in routine fetal echocardiography. *Ultrasound Obstet Gynecol*. 2008;31:625–632.

125. Cohen L, Mangers K, Grobman WA, et al. Satisfactory visualization rates of standard cardiac views at 18 to 22 weeks' gestation using spatiotemporal image correlation. *J Ultrasound Med*. 2009;28:1645–1650.

126. Viñals F, Ascenzo R, Naveas R, et al. Fetal echocardiography at 11 + 0 to 13 + 6 weeks using four-dimensional spatiotemporal image correlation telemedicine via an Internet link: a pilot study. *Ultrasound Obstet Gynecol*. 2008;31:633–638.

127. Bennasar M, Martinez JM, Gomez O, et al. Accuracy of four-dimensional spatiotemporal image correlation echocardiography in the prenatal diagnosis of congenital heart defects. *Ultrasound Obstet Gynecol*. 2010;36:458–464.

127a. Espinoza J, Lee W, Comstock C, et al. Collaborative study on 4-dimensional echocardiography for the diagnosis of fetal heart defects-the COFEHD study. *J Ultrasound Med* 2010;29(11):1573–1580.

128. Yagel S, Cohen SM, Rosenak D, et al. Added value of three-/four-dimensional ultrasound in offline analysis and diagnosis of congenital heart disease. *Ultrasound Obstet Gynecol*. 2011;37:432–437.

129. Riccabona M, Nelson TR, Pretorius DH, et al. Distance and volume measurement using three-dimensional ultrasonography. *J Ultrasound Med*. 1995;14:881–886.

130. Riccabona M, Nelson TR, Pretorius DH, et al. In vivo three-dimensional sonographic measurement of organ volume: validation in the urinary bladder. *J Ultrasound Med*. 1996;15:627–632.

131. Laudy JA, Janssen MM, Struyk PC, et al. Three-dimensional ultrasonography of normal fetal lung volume: a preliminary study. *Ultrasound Obstet Gynecol*. 1998;11:13–16.

132. Lee W, Deter RL, Ebersole JD, et al. Birth weight prediction by three-dimensional ultrasonography: fractional limb volume. *J Ultrasound Med*. 2001;20:1283–1292.

133. Pooh RK, Pooh KH. The assessment of fetal brain morphology and circulation by transvaginal 3D sonography and power Doppler. *J Perinat Med*. 2002;30:48–56.

134. Kalache KD, Espinoza J, Chaiworapongsa T, et al. Three-dimensional ultrasound fetal lung volume measurement: a systematic study comparing the multiplanar method with the rotational (VOCAL) technique. *Ultrasound Obstet Gynecol*. 2003;21:111–118.

135. Ruano R, Joubin L, Sonigo P, et al. Fetal lung volume estimated by 3-dimensional ultrasonography and magnetic resonance imaging in cases with isolated congenital diaphragmatic hernia. *J Ultrasound Med*. 2004;23:353–358.

136. Bhat AH, Corbett V, Carpenter N, et al. Fetal ventricular mass determination on three-dimensional echocardiography: studies in normal fetuses and validation experiments. *Circulation*. 2004;110:1054–1060.

137. Lee W, Deter RL, McNie B, et al. Individualized growth assessment of fetal soft tissue using fractional thigh volume. *Ultrasound Obstet Gynecol*. 2004;24(7):766–774.

138. Lee W, Deter RL, McNie B, et al. The fetal arm: individualized growth assessment in normal pregnancies. *J Ultrasound Med*. 2005;24(6):817–828.

139. Gadelha PS, Da Costa AG, Filho FM, et al. Amniotic fluid volumetry by three-dimensional ultrasonography during the first trimester of pregnancy. *Ultrasound Med Biol*. 2006;32(8):1135–1139.

140. Gerards FA, Engels MA, Twisk JW, et al. Normal fetal lung volume measured with three-dimensional ultrasound. *Ultrasound Obstet Gynecol*. 2006;27(2):134–144.

141. Peralta CF, Cavoretto P, Csapo B, et al. Lung and heart volumes by three-dimensional ultrasound in normal fetuses at 12–32 weeks' gestation. *Ultrasound Obstet Gynecol*. 2006;27(2):128–133.

142. Gerards FA, Twisk JW, Bakker M, et al. Fetal lung volume: three-dimensional ultrasonography compared with magnetic resonance imaging. *Ultrasound Obstet Gynecol*. 2007;29(5):533–536.

143. Lee W, Deter RL, Sameera S, et al. Individualized growth assessment of fetal thigh circumference using three-dimensional ultrasonography. *Ultrasound Obstet Gynecol*. 2008;31(5):520–528.

144. Hamill N, Romero R, Hassan SS, et al. Repeatability and reproducibility of fetal cardiac ventricular volume calculations using spatiotemporal image correlation and virtual organ computer-aided analysis. *J Ultrasound Med*. 2009;28(10):1301–1311.

145. Lee W, Balasubramaniam M, Deter RL, et al. New fetal weight estimation models using fractional limb volume. *Ultrasound Obstet Gynecol*. 2009;34(5):556–565.

146. Lee W, Balasubramaniam M, Deter RL, et al. Fractional limb volume—a soft tissue parameter of fetal body composition: validation, technical considerations, and normal ranges during pregnancy. *Ultrasound Obstet Gynecol*. 2009;33(4):427–440.

147. Ruano R, Aubry MC, Barthe B, et al. Three-dimensional ultrasonographic measurements of the fetal lungs for prediction of perinatal outcome in isolated congenital diaphragmatic hernia. *J Obstet Gynaecol Res*. 2009;35(6):1031–1041.

148. Uittenbogaard LB, Haak MC, Spreeuwenberg MD, et al. Fetal cardiac function assessed with four-dimensional ultrasound imaging using spatiotemporal image correlation. *Ultrasound Obstet Gynecol*. 2009;33(3):272–281.

149. Barreto EQ, Milani HF, Araujo Júnior E, et al. Reproducibility of fetal heart volume by 3D-sonography using the XI VOCAL method. *Cardiovasc Ultrasound*. 2010;8:17.

150. Rolo LC, Nardozza LM, Araujo Júnior E, et al. Nomogram of amniotic fluid volume at 7 to 10 + 6 weeks of pregnancy by three-dimensional ultrasonography using the rotational method (VOCAL). *Arch Gynecol Obstet*. 2010;281(2):235–241.

151. Ioannou C, Sarris I, Salomon LJ, et al. A review of fetal volumetry: the need for standardization and definitions in measurement methodology. *Ultrasound Obstet Gynecol*. 2011;38(6):613–619.

152. Gindes L, Matsui H, Achiron R, et al. Comparison of ex-vivo high-resolution episcopic microscopy with in-vivo four-dimensional high-resolution transvaginal sonography of the first-trimester fetal heart. *Ultrasound Obstet Gynecol*. 2012;39:196–202.

153. Nardozza LM, Cavalcante RO, Araujo Júnior E,et al. Fetal thigh and upper arm volumes by 3D-sonography: comparison between multiplanar and XI VOCAL methods. *J Matern Fetal Neonatal Med*. 2012;25:353–357.

154. Hamill N, Yeo L, Romero R, et al. Fetal cardiac ventricular volume, cardiac output, and ejection fraction determined with 4-dimensional ultrasound using Spatio-Temporal Image Correlation (STIC) and Virtual Organ Computer-aided Analysis (VOCALTM). *Am J Obstet Gynecol*. 2011;205(1):76.e1–76.e10.

155. Lee W, Deter R, Sangi-Haghpeykar H, et al. Prospective validation of fetal weight estimation using fractional limb volume. *Ultrasound Obstet Gynecol*. 2013;41(2):198–203.

156. Chang FM, Liang RI, Ko HC, et al. Three-dimensional ultrasound-assessed fetal thigh volumetry in predicting birth weight. *Obstet Gynecol*. 1997;90:331–339.

157. Lee W, Comstock CH, Kirk JS, et al. Birthweight prediction by three-dimensional ultrasonographic volumes of the fetal thigh and abdomen. *J Ultrasound Med.* 1997;16:799–805.

158. Liang RI, Chang FM, Yao BL, et al. Predicting birth weight by fetal upper-arm volume with use of three-dimensional ultrasonography. *Am J Obstet Gynecol.* 1997;177:632–638.

159. Ioannou C, Sarris I, Yaqub MK, et al. Surface area measurement using rendered three-dimensional ultrasound imaging: an in-vitro phantom study. *Ultrasound Obstet Gynecol.* 2011;38:445–449.

160. Raine-Fenning NJ, Clewes JS, Kendall NR, et al. The interobserver reliability and validity of volume calculation from three-dimensional ultrasound datasets in the in vitro setting. *Ultrasound Obstet Gynecol.* 2003;21:283–291.

161. Bhat AH, Corbett VN, Liu R, et al. Validation of volume and mass assessments for human fetal heart imaging by 4-dimensional spatiotemporal image correlation echocardiography: in vitro balloon model experiments. *J Ultrasound Med.* 2004;23:1151–1159.

162. Bahmaie A, Hughes SW, Clark T, et al. Serial fetal lung volume measurement using three-dimensional ultrasound. *Ultrasound Obstet Gynecol.* 2000;16:154–158.

163. Chang CH, Yu CH, Chang FM, et al. Volumetric assessment of normal fetal lungs using three-dimensional ultrasound. *Ultrasound Med Biol.* 2003;29:935–942.

164. D'Arcy TJ, Hughes SW, Chiu WS, et al. Estimation of fetal lung volume using enhanced 3-dimensional ultrasound: a new method and first result. *BJOG.* 1996;103:1015–1020.

165. Hata T, Kuno A, Dai SY, et al. Three-dimensional sonographic volume measurement of the fetal lung. *J Obstet Gynaecol Res.* 2007;33:793–798.

166. Moeglin D, Talmant C, Duyme M, et al. Fetal lung volumetry using two- and three-dimensional ultrasound. *Ultrasound Obstet Gynecol.* 2005;25:119–127.

167. Osada H, Iitsuka Y, Masuda K, et al. Application of lung volume measurement by three-dimensional ultrasonography for clinical assessment of fetal lung development. *J Ultrasound Med.* 2002;21:841–847.

168. Pohls UG, Rempen A. Fetal lung volumetry by three-dimensional ultrasound. *Ultrasound Obstet Gynecol.* 1998;11:6–12.

169. Ruano R, Benachi A, Joubin L, et al. Three-dimensional ultrasonographic assessment of fetal lung volume as prognostic factor in isolated congenital diaphragmatic hernia. *BJOG.* 2004;111:423–429.

170. Sabogal JC, Becker E, Bega G, et al. Reproducibility of fetal lung volume measurements with 3-dimensional ultrasonography. *J Ultrasound Med.* 2004;23:347–352.

171. Araujo Júnior E, Nardozza LM, Pires CR, et al. Comparison of the two-dimensional and multiplanar methods and establishment of a new constant for the measurement of fetal lung volume. *J Matern Fetal Neonatal Med.* 2008;21:81–88.

172. Britto IS, de Silva Bussamra LC, Araujo Júnior E, et al. Fetal lung volume: comparison by 2D- and 3D-sonography in normal fetuses. *Arch Gynecol Obstet.* 2009;280:363–368.

173. Melamed N, Yogev Y, Meizner I, et al. Sonographic fetal weight estimation: which model should be used? *J Ultrasound Med.* 2009;28:617–629.

174. Matsumoto M, Yanagihara T, Hata T. Three-dimensional qualitative sonographic evaluation of fetal soft tissue. *Hum Reprod.* 2000;15(11):2438–2442.

175. Chang CH, Yu CH, Chang FM, et al. Three-dimensional ultrasound in the assessment of normal fetal thigh volume. *Ultrasound Med Biol.* 2003;29:361–366.

176. Patipanawat S, Komwilaisak R, Ratanasiri T. Correlation of weight estimation in large and small fetuses with three-dimensional ultrasonographic volume measurements of the fetal upper-arm and thigh: a preliminary report. *J Med Assoc Thai.* 2006;89:13–19.

177. Schild RL, Maringa M, Siemer J, et al. Weight estimation by three-dimensional ultrasound imaging in the small fetus. *Ultrasound Obstet Gynecol.* 2008;32:168–175.

178. Siemer J, Peter W, Zollver H, et al. How good is fetal weight estimation using volumetric methods? *Ultraschall Med.* 2008;29:377–382.

179. Lee W, Balasubramaniam M, Deter RL, et al. Fetal growth parameters and birth weight: their relationship to neonatal body composition. *Ultrasound Obstet Gynecol.* 2009;33:441–446.

180. Nardozza LM, Vieira MF, Araujo Júnior E, et al. Prediction of birth weight using fetal thigh and upper-arm volumes by three-dimensional ultrasonography in a Brazilian population. *J Matern Fetal Neonatal Med.* 2010;23:393–398.

181. Song TB, Moore TR, Lee JI, et al. Fetal weight prediction by thigh volume measurement with three-dimensional ultrasonography. *Obstet Gynecol.* 2000;96:157–161.

182. Askenazi SS, Perlman M. Pulmonary hypoplasia: lung weight and radial alveolar count as criteria of diagnosis. *Arch Dis Child.* 1979;54:614–618.

183. Metkus AP, Filly RA, Stringer MD, et al. Sonographic predictors of survival in fetal diaphragmatic hernia. *J Pediatr Surg.* 1996;31:148–151; discussion 51–52.

184. Lipshutz GS, Albanese CT, Feldstein VA, et al. Prospective analysis of lung-to-head ratio predicts survival for patients with prenatally diagnosed congenital diaphragmatic hernia. *J Pediatr Surg.* 1997;32:1634–1636.

185. Laudy JA, Van Gucht M, Van Dooren MF, et al. Congenital diaphragmatic hernia: an evaluation of the prognostic value of the lung-to-head ratio and other prenatal parameters. *Prenat Diagn.* 2003;23:634–639.

186. Jani J, Nicolaides KH, Keller RL, et al. Observed to expected lung area to head circumference ratio in the prediction of survival in fetuses with isolated diaphragmatic hernia. *Ultrasound Obstet Gynecol.* 2007;30:67–71.

187. Kehl S, Zirulnik A, Debus A, et al. In vitro models of the fetal lung: comparison of lung volume measurements with 3-dimensional sonography and magnetic resonance imaging. *J Ultrasound Med.* 2011;30:1085–1091.

188. Kehl S, Kalk AL, Eckert S, et al. Assessment of lung volume by 3-dimensional sonography and magnetic resonance imaging in fetuses with congenital diaphragmatic hernias. *J Ultrasound Med.* 2011;30:1539–1545.

189. Deshmukh S, Rubesova E, Barth R. MR assessment of normal fetal lung volumes: a literature review. *AJR Am J Roentgenol.* 2010;194:W212–W217.

190. Duncan KR, Gowland PA, Freeman A, et al. The changes in magnetic resonance properties of the fetal lungs: a first result and a potential tool for the non-invasive in utero demonstration of fetal lung maturation. *BJOG.* 1999;106:122–125.

191. Duncan KR, Gowland PA, Moore RJ, et al. Assessment of fetal lung growth in utero with echo-planar MR imaging. *Radiology.* 1999;210:197–200.

192. Coakley FV, Lopoo JB, Lu Y, et al. Normal and hypoplastic fetal lungs: volumetric assessment with prenatal single-shot rapid acquisition with relaxation enhancement MR imaging. *Radiology.* 2000;216:107–111.

193. Mahieu-Caputo D, Sonigo P, Dommergues M, et al. Fetal lung volume measurement by magnetic resonance imaging in congenital diaphragmatic hernia. *BJOG.* 2001;108:863–868.

194. Rypens F, Metens T, Rocourt N, et al. Fetal lung volume: estimation at MR imaging-initial results. *Radiology.* 2001;219:236–241.

195. Keller TM, Rake A, Michel SC, et al. MR assessment of fetal lung development using lung volumes and signal intensities. *Eur Radiol.* 2004;14:984–989.

196. Osada H, Kaku K, Masuda K, et al. Quantitative and qualitative evaluations of fetal lung with MR imaging. *Radiology.* 2004;231:887–892.

197. Tanigaki S, Miyakoshi K, Tanaka M, et al. Pulmonary hypoplasia: prediction with use of ratio of MR imaging-measured fetal lung volume to US-estimated fetal body weight. *Radiology.* 2004;232:767–772.

198. Kasprian G, Balassy C, Brugger PC, et al. MRI of normal and pathological fetal lung development. *Eur J Radiol.* 2006;57:261–270.

199. Ward VL, Nishino M, Hatabu H, et al. Fetal lung volume measurements: determination with MR imaging—effect of various factors. *Radiology.* 2006;240(1):187–193.

200. Gonçalves LF, Kusanovic JP, Espinoza J, et al. OC34: lung volume measurements by 3D ultrasound are not superior to biometry by 2D ultrasound to predict pulmonary hypoplasia in fetuses with musculoskeletal disorders. *Ultrasound Obstet Gynecol.* 2006;28(4):368–369.

201. Schmidt KG, Silverman NH, Hoffman JI. Determination of ventricular volumes in human fetal hearts by two-dimensional echocardiography. *Am J Cardiol.* 1995;76:1313–1316.

202. Wladimiroff JW, McGhie J. Ultrasonic assessment of cardiovascular geometry and function in the human fetus. *BJOG.* 1981;88:870–875.

203. De Smedt MC, Visser GH, Meijboom EJ. Fetal cardiac output estimated by Doppler echocardiography during mid- and late gestation. *Am J Cardiol.* 1987;60:338–342.

204. Simpson JM, Cook A. Repeatability of echocardiographic measurements in the human fetus. *Ultrasound Obstet Gynecol.* 2002;20:332–339.

205. Meyer-Wittkopf M, Cole A, Cooper SG, et al. Three-dimensional quantitative echocardiographic assessment of ventricular volume in healthy human fetuses and in fetuses with congenital heart disease. *J Ultrasound Med.* 2001;20:317–327.

206. Esh-Broder E, Ushakov FB, Imbar T, et al. Application of free-hand three-dimensional echocardiography in the evaluation of fetal cardiac ejection fraction: a preliminary study. *Ultrasound Obstet Gynecol.* 2004;23:546–551.

207. Uittenbogaard LB, Haak MC, Peters RJ, et al. Validation of volume measurements for fetal echocardiography using four-dimensional ultrasound imaging and spatiotemporal image correlation. *Ultrasound Obstet Gynecol.* 2010;35:324–331.

208. Simioni C, Nardozza LM, Araujo Júnior E, et al. Heart stroke volume, cardiac output, and ejection fraction in 265 normal fetus in the second half of gestation assessed by 4D ultrasound using spatio-temporal image correlation. *J Matern Fetal Neonatal Med.* 2011;24:1159–1167.

209. Messing B, Cohen SM, Valsky DV, et al. Fetal cardiac ventricle volumetry in the second half of gestation assessed by 4D ultrasound using STIC combined with inversion mode. *Ultrasound Obstet Gynecol.* 2007;30:142–151.

210. Molina FS, Faro C, Sotiriadis A, et al. Heart stroke volume and cardiac output by four-dimensional ultrasound in normal fetuses. *Ultrasound Obstet Gynecol.* 2008;32:181–187.

211. Rizzo G, Capponi A, Pietrolucci ME, et al. Role of sonographic automatic volume calculation in measuring fetal cardiac ventricular volumes using 4-dimensional sonography: comparison with virtual organ computer-aided analysis. *J Ultrasound Med.* 2010;29:261–270.

212. Schoonderwaldt EM, Groenenberg IA, Hop WC, et al. Reproducibility of echocardiographic measurements of human fetal left ventricular volumes and ejection fractions using four-dimensional ultrasound with the spatio-temporal image correlation modality. *Eur J Obstet Gynecol Reprod Biol.* 2012;160:22–29.

213. Godfrey ME, Messing B, Cohen SM, et al. Functional assessment of the fetal heart: a review. *Ultrasound Obstet Gynecol.* 2012;39:131–144.

214. Rizzo G, Capponi A, Cavicchioni O, et al. Fetal cardiac stroke volume determination by four-dimensional ultrasound with spatio-temporal image correlation compared with two-dimensional and Doppler ultrasonography. *Prenat Diagn.* 2007;27:1147–1150.

# Growth, Doppler, and Fetal Assessment

Henry L. Galan • Shane Reeves

Intrauterine growth restriction (IUGR), also known as fetal growth restriction (FGR), is a common complication of pregnancy. There is a lack of consensus regarding optimal terminology, diagnostic criteria, and management options. Elucidating these factors is important as IUGR has been associated with a variety of adverse perinatal outcomes including increased risk of intrauterine demise, neonatal morbidity and mortality, as well as the long-term sequelae of neurodevelopmental delay, cardiovascular disease, and diabetes.[1-3] The purpose of this chapter is to review the topic of FGR with a focus on methods for determining gestational age, definitions of fetal undergrowth, and diagnostic biometric and surveillance tools. An algorithm for management and for timing the delivery of the IUGR fetus is provided.

## ESTABLISHMENT OF GESTATIONAL AGE

The *menstrual age* is defined as the age of a pregnancy when compared with the first day of the last menstrual period (LMP). This is the most commonly used method to determine the due date in clinical practice. The *conceptional age* is the true fetal age of the pregnancy, as it estimates the gestational age when compared with the day of conception. The difficulty with using the conceptional age is that it is truly known only in cases of assisted reproduction such as in vitro fertilization. Even in these cases, it is common in clinical practice to refer to the menstrual age by calculating backward 14 days from the day of conception and using this as a guide to determine the menstrual age. In this chapter, the gestational age of the pregnancy will be synonymous with the menstrual age.

Knowledge of the menstrual age is important, as risk assessment, diagnosis, and interventions in pregnancy depend upon knowing the exact duration of the pregnancy. In the first trimester, for example, screening for aneuploidy through ultrasound assessment of the nuchal translucency is performed in a narrow window between 10 weeks 4 days and 13 weeks 6 days.[4] Chorionic villus sampling can be performed after 10 weeks, and performing this procedure earlier than this will increase the risk of limb reduction defects.[5] Amniocentesis can be performed after 15 weeks, but prior to this gestational age, there is a significant increase in the number of newborns with talipes equinovarus.[6] Therefore, if the precise gestational age is not known, there could be an increased risk of pregnancy complications from the diagnostic procedures. Additionally, once a due date is established, the fetus will be compared with other fetuses at the same gestational age to determine whether the fetus is measuring too large or too small. This is particularly important in identifying pregnancies at risk for poor perinatal outcome because of IUGR. If the gestational age is incorrect, then accurate classification of fetal growth is impossible. Similarly, therapeutic response to preterm labor also depends upon accurate determination of gestational age, as administration of tocolytics would be inappropriate after a certain gestational age. Finally, planning induction of labor or timed cesarean delivery is critically dependent upon accurate knowledge of the gestational age so as not to incur iatrogenic prematurity or stillbirth from a post-dates pregnancy. Virtually all clinical decisions depend upon accurate determination of gestational age.

The due date is commonly calculated by adding 280 days to the first day of the LMP. This assumes a normal menstrual cycle of 28 days with ovulation occurring on the 14th day. Many women may not remember the first day of their LMP. Even in women with reliable recall, the LMP could be misleading as it is common for women to have cycle lengths that vary between 21 and 35 days. One study showed that up to 20% of women will have early or late ovulation,[7] increasing the probability of an inaccurate gestational age determination. For all of these reasons, determination of the due date by using the LMP alone is fraught with inaccuracy.

## FIRST TRIMESTER ULTRASOUND

In the first trimester, the first ultrasonographic sign of pregnancy is the identification of the gestational sac. This is a fluid-filled structure containing mostly chorionic fluid. In the early days of ultrasonography, this could not reliably be seen until approximately 6 weeks' gestational age. However, with high-resolution, real-time sonography and transvaginal imaging, the sac can be seen as early as during the 4th or 5th week of gestation. Menstrual age can be estimated by measuring the size of the gestational sac. The mean sac diameter (MSD) is the average of the measurement of the gestational sac in three orthogonal planes. This measurement is obtained from the interface of the chorionic fluid, and the sac wall. The sac wall is not included in the measurement (Fig. 3.1). The gestational sac can be seen with measurements as small as 2 to 3 mm, and the MSD increases approximately 1 mm per day in early gestation.[8] Table 1A and 1B in Appendix A1 shows the relationship between MSD, menstrual age, and human chorionic gonadotropin level.

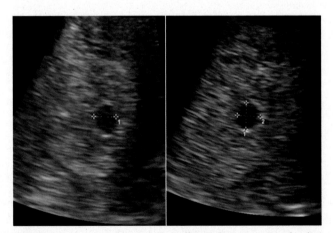

**FIGURE 3.1:** Mean sac diameter. The gestational sac is measured in three planes with the *calipers* placed at the interface between the wall of the sac and the embryonic fluid. Notice that the sac wall is not incorporated in the measurement. The MSD is the average of the three measurements.

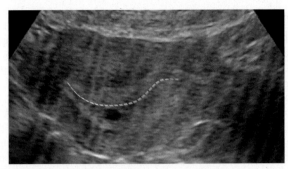

**FIGURE 3.2:** Characteristics of a gestational sac. In this image, the gestational sac is seen eccentrically located in the endometrial cavity. It is displaced inferiorly such that it is located in the decidua rather than the endometrial canal *(line)*. The sac also has a hypoechoic rim around a hyperechoic sac wall.

The gestational sac can often be confused with a pseudo-sac seen in ectopic pregnancy. To distinguish a true gestational sac, one must identify a double sac sign. This is a finding that is created by visualization of the two layers of the decidua parietalis. The deep layer of the decidua parietalis and early villi is more echogenic, and this can be seen as separated from the less echogenic layer of the superficial layer. Also, the intradecidual sign can be seen, where the sac is imbedded in the decidua rather than between two layers of the endometrium (Fig. 3.2).

As the first trimester advances, the reliability of the MSD in predicting menstrual age decreases. Between 2 and 14 mm, the MSD is quite precise in determination of age, but after a MSD of 14 mm, an embryo can be seen. Once an embryo is seen, the measurement of the crown rump length (CRL) can be obtained, and this is now more accurate in obtaining the true estimation of gestational age. The CRL is not the true measurement of the length of the fetus, as fetuses in early gestation have flexion. In truth, the CRL is the measurement of the longest straight line from the head of the fetus to the caudal end. Figure 3.3 depicts measurements of the CRL at different gestational ages. When obtaining the CRL, the sonologist should obtain at least three measurements and average the values to obtain the gestational age (see Table 1 in Appendix A1).

The accuracy of gestational age determination based on CRL is best in the middle of the first trimester. As the pregnancy advances, the CRL loses precision in gestational age determination.[9] When examining pregnancies conceived through IVF, where the precise gestational age is known, from 7 to 11 weeks,

the 95% confidence interval shows that the CRL is within 3 days of true gestational age. From 11 to 13 weeks, the 95% confidence interval is within 5 days.[10] Hadlock et al.[11] showed that the variability in the CRL remained fairly constant from 2 mm to 12 cm, where the 95% confidence interval for gestational age was 8%. Therefore, if a pregnancy measured 8 weeks 0 days, the true gestational age was 8 weeks 0 days $\pm$ 0.64 weeks. If the pregnancy measured 12 weeks, the true gestational age was 12 $\pm$ 0.96 weeks. Variation in fetal growth in the late second and third trimesters is an expectation in any given population reflecting individual genetic determinants of growth, but deviation in fetal CRL size may be a predictor of growth pathology. Using pregnancies resulting from assisted reproductive technology, the FASTER trial showed that fetuses who measured small in the first trimester had a higher risk of being small for gestational age (SGA) later at birth.[12] Alternatively, fetuses measuring larger than expected by CRL in the first trimester also may be at risk for macrosomia at birth.[13] Therefore, CRL is a useful tool not only for gestational dating, but it may also predict patients at risk for developing abnormalities in fetal growth as pregnancy advances.

Other measurements can be obtained in the first trimester that can help in the determination of gestational age. First trimester biparietal diameter (BPD) and abdominal circumference (AC) have been investigated by multiple authors. Two independent authors evaluated first trimester measurement of BPD and compared this with CRL between 7 and 13 weeks. Both showed that the CRL was superior to BPD in determining menstrual age.[14,15] This has come into question in a more recent analysis evaluating BPD and CRL in pregnancies conceived through IVF. In this study, the two measurements were similar in ability to predict gestational age, but the BPD had the advantage of having lower random measurement error.[16] Another recent analysis showed similar findings when evaluating first trimester BPD, CRL, and AC. This analysis showed that both CRL and BPD were accurate in determining when a pregnancy will actually deliver, and both were superior to the fetal AC.[17] Given the precision and ease of obtaining a first trimester CRL with high-resolution abdominal and vaginal ultrasonography, most practitioners utilize this measurement as the primary means of determining gestational age. However, in the event that CRL cannot be obtained because of fetal position, uterine anomalies, or maternal body habitus, first trimester use of the BPD could be an alternative measurement in determining gestational age.

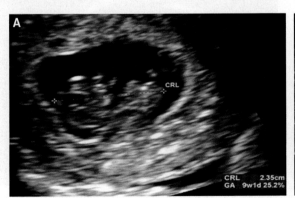
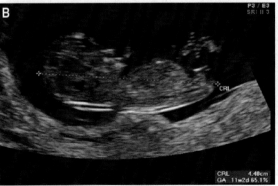

**FIGURE 3.3:** Crown rump length *(CRL)*. **A:** The CRL is measured in a sagittal plane through the fetus. The image contains the head and body. *Calipers* are placed from the tip of the head to the edge of the caudal end. **B:** The CRL at later gestational ages *(GA)* allows for a clearer distinction of the fetal edges.

First trimester ultrasound is the most accurate method of determining gestational age. The measurement of the gestational MSD between 2 and 14 mm, followed by CRL determination once a fetal pole is seen, will appropriately assign an estimated due date. Biological variability in the first trimester is present, but it is much smaller than later in gestation. Once a due date is determined from a precise first trimester ultrasound, this due date should not be changed later in gestation. If a future ultrasound shows significant deviation from the due date established by first trimester ultrasound, this identifies a fetus with abnormal growth. As detailed later in this chapter, these fetuses may be at risk for poor perinatal outcome and should have further evaluation.

## SECOND AND THIRD TRIMESTER BIOMETRY

In order to calculate a second or third trimester gestational age, multiple structures should be evaluated with rigorous criteria, and those criteria will be discussed below.

### Biparietal Diameter

The BPD was originally defined as the widest distance between the parietal eminences. However, this measurement is often more cephalad in location when compared with the thalami.[18] Since standardization is the goal, the BPD is measured when certain landmarks are identified. The BPD can be measured in any plane that traverses the third ventricle and the thalami. By convention, the BPD is measured in a similar plane as the head circumference (HC), but since it is a single line that crosses through the thalamus, it can be measured in any plane. For the BPD to be accurate, the third ventricle and thalamus need to be identified and located centrally in the image. The calvarial walls should be symmetric, and the midline of the fetal brain should be equidistant from the parietal bones to ensure that an oblique measurement is not obtained as this will falsely increase the distance. The calipers are then placed on the outer edge of the proximal calvaria and measured to the inner edge of the distal calvaria (Fig. 3.4). With this measurement, the BPD is compared with a dataset to determine the percentile of the value, which can help to identify normal and abnormal growth (see Table 9 in Appendix A1).

### Head Circumference

Unlike the BPD, the HC requires a specific plane for proper acquisition. To appropriately obtain the measurement, the proper plane needs to parallel the base of the skull, the transducer must be perpendicular to the parietal bones, and the image must transect the third ventricle and thalami. To ensure the correct plane of measurement, the cavum septum pallucidum (CSP) must be visualized as a box-like structure in the anterior portion of the fetal brain. The thalamus needs to be visualized around the third ventricle, and the cerebellum should not be in the image. If the cerebellum is seen, the image was obtained in an oblique plane, and this will increase the overall circumference measurement. Once the appropriate plane is obtained with identification of the appropriate structures, the HC is measured as an ellipse around the perimeter of the fetal skull. The HC does not include the skin edge; rather, an accurate HC traces around the calvarial margins. Ideally, the entire calvarium is visualized (Fig. 3.5). Often, images of the head shape appear abnormal, as in cases of breech presentation or fetal head molding. The fetal head is called dolichocephalic when transverse diameter appears flattened with the A-P diameter elongated. Conversely, the head is called brachycephalic when it appears more rounded than long. In both of these instances, the BPD may appear abnormal, but the overall size of the fetal head is within a normal range. The HC will not be altered by the relative shape of the head, and this provides an advantage over the BPD in determining whether a fetus has abnormal growth. Table 7 & 9 in Appendix A1 shows normal values for HC.

### Abdominal Circumference

The AC is similar to the HC in that it requires a precise plane of obtainment in order to be accurate. Inclusive in the AC is the fetal liver, an organ that can be affected by pathological growth in that it will be small in instances of growth restriction because of glycogenolysis and large in instances of fetal macrosomia secondary to excessive glycogen storage. The appropriate AC incorporates the stomach, ribs, spine, and portal vein. The location of the confluence of the left portal vein and the right portal vein will create a "C-shape" in the fetal liver on ultrasound imaging, indicating an appropriate plane of obtainment. If the "C" is not seen in the fetal liver, either the transducer is too cephalad in the fetal abdomen or oblique to the correct plane. There should be one or two ribs seen

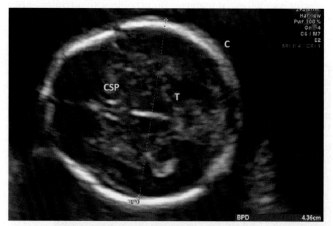

**FIGURE 3.4:** Biparietal diameter *(BPD)*. The BPD is taken in an axial plane with the midline perpendicular to the transducer. The thalamus *(T)* is seen in the center, and the cavum septum pellucidum *(CSP)* is noted in the front of the image. The calipers are placed from the outer edge of the proximal calvarium *(C)* to the inside edge of the distal calvarium.

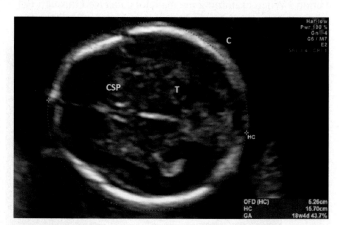

**FIGURE 3.5:** Head circumference *(HC)*. The HC is taken in an axial plane. In the image, the landmarks of the thalamus *(T)* and cavum septum pellucidum *(CSP)* are visible. The midline is noted to be equidistant from both calvarial *(C)* edges. The HC is measured as the perimeter around the bone.

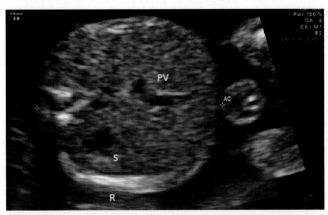

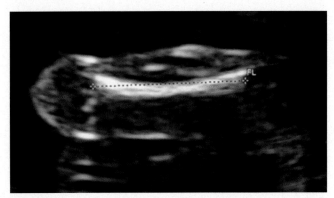

**FIGURE 3.7:** Femur length *(FL)*. The femur length is measured with the longest portion of the bone perpendicular to the transducer. If the femur is not horizontal, shadowing from the ossified bone may shorten the length. The calipers are placed in the center of the femur and measured to the end of the bright edges, ensuring not to include the femoral tip.

**FIGURE 3.6:** Abdominal circumference *(AC)*. The AC is taken in an axial plain through the section of the abdomen containing the fetal liver. In this image, the liver is the proximal structure in the fetal abdomen. The portal vein *(PV)* can be seen curving away from the stomach *(S)*. The PV makes a "C" shape, indicating that the image is taken appropriately. Additionally, the three bright spots on the left side of the image mark the spine. The rib *(R)* is seen at the bottom of the image of the abdomen. There is only one rib seen, indicating that the plane is not oblique to the fetal lie.

in the image, but if the ribs are seen in cross-section with multiple segments visualized, the measurement will be falsely elevated. Figure 3.6 shows an appropriate image of the AC, including the stomach, portal vein, spine, and ribs. Tables 6 and 9 in Appendix A1 show measurements of the AC as gestational age progresses.

## Femur Length

The femur is measured by aligning the transducer to the long axis of the femoral diaphysis. To measure the femur length (FL) correctly, the shaft should be aligned horizontally on the image. If the femur is not horizontal, shadowing from the edges of the bone will shorten the true length. Of note, ultrasound will detect only the ossified region of the femur, including the diaphysis and metaphysis. The cartilaginous regions are not well seen by ultrasound imaging. Once the entire length of the ossified bone is horizontal on the image, the calipers are placed on the central part of the femoral head and extended to the distal condyle. The calipers should be at the edge of the ossified site, between the bright bone and the dark cartilage. The correct measurement also does not incorporate the distal femoral point, as this is nonstandard and will incorrectly lengthen the measurement. Figure 3.7 depicts the proper measurement of the FL, and Tables 8 and 9 in Appendix A1 show the predicted gestational age for measured FL.

## ACCURACY IN MEASUREMENTS

### Biparietal Diameter Accuracy

The BPD has been well studied in its accuracy in determining gestational age. Between 14 and 21 weeks, Hadlock et al.[19] investigated 1,770 chromosomally normal fetuses, and they showed that the 95% confidence interval for measuring the BPD was within 1 week of the known gestational age. Other authors showed similar findings in accuracy between 14 and 20 weeks when looking at pregnancies dated either by known dates of conception or first trimester CRL.[20–22] In all of these studies, two standard deviations (SDs) for the accuracy of BPD in determining gestational age ranged between 0.92 and 1.02 weeks

for gestational ages between 14 and 20 weeks. As gestational age advances, the variability of BPD measurement increases, diminishing the accuracy of gestational age determination. Benson and Doubilet[23] looked at pregnancies dated by early CRL, and they showed that the variability ($\pm 2$ SD) in determining gestational age increased from 2.1 weeks at 20 to 26 weeks to 4.1 weeks from 32 to 42 weeks (Table 3.1). Similar to early CRL, BPD measurements are most accurate the earlier the study is performed, and as pregnancy progresses, deviation from normal will be more of a measure of abnormal growth rather than assigning gestational age.

As mentioned previously, the BPD can be significantly affected by the fetal head shape. In cases of breech presentation, uterine anomalies, fibroids, and multiple gestations, the fetal calvarium can be compressed so that the BPD is shortened or elongated relative to the true gestational age. The cephalic index (CI) is a ratio that assesses dolichocephaly and brachycephaly, and it is calculated from the BPD and the fronto-occipital diameter (FOD). This measurement is from the outside of the anterior portion of the fetal skull to the outside of the posterior calvarium. The CI is calculated as follows:

$$CI = (BPD/FOD) \times 100$$

Hadlock et al. demonstrated that the CI remained relatively stable from 14 to 40 weeks, with a mean value of 78.3 and a SD of 4.4. In this study, CI measurements that were greater than 1 SD from the mean had BPD measurements that were inaccurate in

| Table 3.1 | Variability in Predicting Gestational Age in the Second Half of Pregnancy | | |
|---|---|---|---|
| *Parameter* | *20–26 wk* | *26–32 wk* | *32–42 wk* |
| BPD | 2.1 | 3.8 | 4.1 |
| HC | 1.9 | 3.4 | 3.8 |
| AC | 3.7 | 3.0 | 4.5 |
| FL | 2.5 | 3.1 | 3.5 |

The variability is expressed as $\pm 2$ SD. BPD, biparietal diameter; HC, head circumference; AC, abdominal circumference; FL, femur length.
Adapted from Benson CB, Doubilet PM. Sonographic prediction of gestational age: accuracy of second and third trimester fetal measurements. *AJR Am J Roentgenol.* 1991;157:1275.

determining gestational age. In such instances, the HC is a better measure as it is not as dependent upon head shape.[24]

## Head Circumference Accuracy

The HC is not dependent upon fetal head shape, and its measurement has also been shown to be an accurate predictor of gestational age. In fact, at less than 20 weeks, the HC may be more predictive of gestational age than BPD, as shown by Law and MacRae[25] Like the BPD, this measurement is accurate to within 1 week ($\pm$2 SD) of the gestational age when the precise due date is known. Like other measures in pregnancy, the best prediction of gestational age occurs with earlier measurement with error in accuracy increasing as gestational age advances.[19,21] In the third trimester, the inaccuracies of HC parallel that of BPD in gestational age determination with a margin of error of $\pm$3.8 weeks (2 SD) after 32 weeks.[23]

## Abdominal Circumference Accuracy

The AC is the most difficult measure to obtain of all of the biometric assessments. Also, the AC contains the liver, which is subject to acute and subacute changes in metabolism by the fetus. In pathological states, it has been theorized that the liver size may shrink because of metabolic demands from nutrient deficiency. In instances of glucose excess, such as diabetes, the fetal liver should increase in size as glucose is stored in this organ. For these reasons, the AC would be expected to have the highest level of variability when predicting gestational age. This was observed by Benson and Doubilet[23] in their analysis, where they saw that the AC had the highest variability in predicting gestational age when compared with the other measures.

## Femur Length Accuracy

With the ease of measuring the FL, this biometric parameter has been well studied in determining gestational age. Similar to other measures, the earlier the measurement is obtained, the more accurate the FL is in determining gestational age. As shown by Benson and Doubilet,[23] the FL has similar variability to other bony measures (e.g., BPD, HC) in the late second and third trimesters.

## OTHER BIOMETRIC PARAMETERS

Multiple other structures have been investigated for determining gestational age. These include measurements of the binocular distance, clavicular length, ulna, tibia, radius, and foot. Similar to the other measurements, earlier assessment is most accurate. One structure that shows promise in accuracy is the transcerebellar diameter (TCD). This measurement can be obtained during evaluation of the posterior fossa. The best image is obtained by having the transducer perpendicular to the parietal bones, in a plane slightly diagonal to that used for the BPD. The optimal image has the CSP seen anteriorly and the cerebellum seen posteriorly. The calipers are placed on the outer edge of the cerebellum and measured to the opposite side (Fig. 3.8). Table 22 in Appendix A1 shows the measurements of the cerebellar length as gestational age advances.

The accuracy in gestational age determination for the TCD is quite high. Chavez et al. studied the TCD in the second and third trimesters in singleton, nonanomalous, well-dated pregnancies. Between 17 and 21 weeks, the TCD predicted gestational age accurately within 4 days. In fact, as pregnancy advanced, the TCD maintained a higher accuracy than any other biometric parameter.

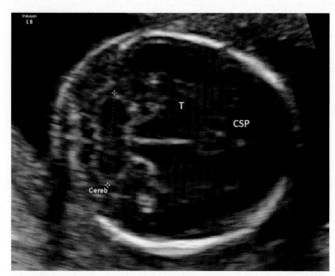

**FIGURE 3.8:** Cerebellar measurement. The cerebellum *(Cereb)* is measured from an axial plane in the fetal head. The plane is in the correct location when the cavum septum pellucidum *(CSP)* is located anteriorly with the thalamus *(T)* seen in the midline. The midline is equidistant from both calvarial edges.

Between 29 and 36 weeks, the predicted age was within 5 days of the actual age, and at greater than 37 weeks, it was within 9 days.[26] However, measurement of the TCD may be challenging late in pregnancy. Fetal positioning and calcification of the skull can make visualization of cerebellar landmarks difficult. Unlike the BPD, HC, AC, and FL, the TCD is particularly important in determining gestational age at extremes of fetal growth. When evaluating pregnancies with good dating criteria, even in fetuses with growth restriction (estimated weight <10th percentile) and macrosomia (estimated weight >90th percentile), the TCD maintained accuracy in predicting gestational age.[27] Of note, like other measurements, chromosomally abnormal fetuses can have a TCD smaller than predicted,[28] which could further complicate assessment of gestational age. Despite this finding, clinicians are often challenged with patients presenting late in pregnancy with an uncertain gestational age. The TCD can be a measurement that will help in determining whether a fetus is measuring small or large for gestational age, as it seems to be less subject to variability when compared with other biometric parameters.

Although other long bone measurements do not provide any clear additional benefit for dating a pregnancy or for EFW calculation, in certain circumstances, they may be beneficial relative to bony abnormalities. Measurements for the humerus, radius, ulna, tibia, and fibula are captured in Table 17 in Appendix A1. The fetal foot length can be measured throughout gestation beginning as early as the end of the first trimester. The literature on newborn and fetal foot length has been summarized elsewhere,[29] and the foot length percentiles across gestation are shown in Table 18 in Appendix A1. In IUGR, Meirowitz and colleagues showed that 60% of fetuses have foot length measurements that are less than the 10th percentile. Thus, the foot length may not be sufficiently spared to provide clinical utility.[30]

## ESTIMATION OF FETAL WEIGHT

Up until this point, this chapter has focused on gestational age determination using ultrasound biometric parameters. This is crucial in determining the true due date and assigning an appropriate age to the pregnancy. Once the due date from early measurement has been established, it should not be altered later in pregnancy. In cases of deviation from the predicted gestational age, the fetus is demonstrating growth abnormalities—either in the case of excess fetal growth called macrosomia, or inhibited growth called FGR. Gestational age is not the only issue in assessing normal progression of a pregnancy; fetal weight is another key element in determining the status of growth.

## Formulae

Shortly after the application of ultrasound to modern obstetrics, measurements of the fetus were evaluated in predicting birth weight (BW). One of the first publications showed that the AC alone was predictive of newborn weight with a moderate degree of accuracy if the AC was measured within 48 hours of delivery.[31] With this observation, multiple other investigators started adding additional biometric parameters in an attempt to improve accuracy. Several authors added the BPD as the first measurement, and regression analysis was used to create standardized formulae for estimating fetal weight. Warsof et al.[32] found that the addition of the BPD could improve accuracy with a SD of 106 g per kg if performed within 48 hours of delivery. Other investigators followed and generated other equations using the BPD and AC to estimate fetal weight.[33–36] Over time, FL was added to the equations in an attempt to improve prediction as the prior measurements did not take long bone growth into consideration. Additionally, BPD was recognized as being influenced by head shape, so HC was added to the equation in some instances, and replaced the BPD in others.[37–41] Table 3.2 shows some of the most commonly used equations in calculating an estimated fetal weight (EFW).

## Accuracy of Specific Formulae

Numerous formulae exist for the estimation of fetal weight. Since none of the formulae has perfect accuracy, institutions may choose a particular formula as a standard or in specific scenarios. When looking at accuracy, investigators will assess bias (the systematic overprediction or underprediction of weight) and precision (random error). Systematic bias is often defined as the mean percentage error (MPE), where percentage error = $100 \times (BW - EFW) / BW$, and the MPE is the mean of per cent errors in a given population. Random error is the SD of the MPE. This method has been used to compare the accuracies of different formulae, and it is one tool that can help to determine which formula may be best. Of note, if an estimate of weight is calculated and the fetus progresses beyond one week from the measures, the EFW would be expected to be incorrect because of ongoing fetal growth. Additionally, maternal body habitus has a significant effect on accuracy, where the MPE in women with a body mass index (BMI) > 30 is almost double that in women with a BMI < 25.[42] Therefore, appropriate comparisons can be made only if the EFW is made close to the time of delivery in a population where visualization of the fetus is possible.

Multiple factors can play a part in EFW accuracy, but how important is the specific formula used? When looking at each formula, using the same measurements from an individual fetus can provide considerable differences in values. Anderson et al. evaluated 12 different formulae for accuracy in population data from 1991 and 2000. They compared intraobserver and interobserver variability, and also looked at different formulae in the accuracy of predicting BW. They found that observer error (that obtained from multiple measures or from multiple sonologists on the same fetus) provided far less error than the

---

| Table 3.2 | Common Formulae for Fetal Growth | |
|---|---|---|
| **Parameters** | **References** | **Formula** |
| AC, BPD | Thurnau et al.[33] | BW = (BPD × AC × 9.337) − 229 |
| | Shepard et al.[36] | Log₁₀ BW = 0.166(BPD) + 0.046(AC) − 0.002546(AC)(BPD) − 1.7492 |
| | Hadlock et al.[35] | Log₁₀ BW = 1.1134 + 0.05845(AC) − 0.000604(AC)2 − 0.007365(BPD)2 + 0.000595(BPD)(AC) + 0.1694(BPD) |
| | Vintzileos et al.[34] | Log₁₀ BW = 1.879 + 0.084(BPD) + 0.026(AC) |
| | Warsof et al.[32] | Log₁₀ BW = 0.144(BPD) + 0.032(AC) − 0.000111(BPD)2(AC) − 1.599 |
| AC, HC | Weiner et al.[37] | Log₁₀ BW = 1.6575 + 0.04035(HC) + 0.01285(AC) |
| AC, FL, BPD | Hadlock et al.[35] | Log₁₀ BW = 1.182 + 0.0273(HC) + 0.07057(AC) − 0.00063(AC)2 − 0.0002184(HC)(AC) |
| | Combs et al.[40] | BW = 0.23718(AC)2(FL) + 0.03312(HC)3 |
| | Hadlock et al.[38] | Log₁₀ BW = 1.326 − 0.00326(AC)(FL) + 0.0107(HC) + 0.0438(AC) + 0.158(FL) |
| | Weiner et al.[37] | Log₁₀ BW = 1.6961 + 0.02253(HC) + 0.01645(AC) + 0.06439(FL) |
| | Ott et al.[39] | Log₁₀ BW = −2.0661 + 0.04355(HC) + 0.05394(AC) − 0.0008582(HC)(AC) + 1.2594(FL/AC) |
| AC, FL, BPD, HC | Hadlock et al.[38] | Log₁₀ BW = 1.3596 + 0.0064(HC) + 0.0424(AC) + 0.174(FL) + 0.00061(BPD)(AC) − 0.00386(AC)(FL) |
| AD, FL, BPD | Rose and McCallum[41] | Ln BW = 0.143(BPD + AD + FL) + 4.198 |

AC, abdominal circumference; BPD, biparietal diameter; HC, head circumference; FL, femur length; BW, birth weight.
Reproduced with permission from Burd I, Srinivas S, Pare E, et al. Is sonographic assessment of fetal weight influenced by formula selection? *J Ultrasound Med.* 2009;28:1019–1024.

use of different formulae. In fact, only six formulae were able to provide an MPE within 7%.[43] Edwards et al.[44] found that Hadlock[35] and Shepard[18] provided more accurate results than other formulae. A systematic review of articles comparing EFW formulae was performed in an attempt to determine accuracy. In this analysis, the formulae by Hadlock et al. using BPD, HC, AC, and FL[35,38] seemed to provide the most consistent MPEs when used on various populations with the same amount of precision as other formulae. However, all formulae presented a fairly wide MPE and SD, and the authors conclude that no particular formula is ideal.[45] Other authors found that between 2,500 and 3,999 g, the Schild et al.[46] formula is the most accurate in determining weight (EFW = − 4,035.275 + 1.143 $BPD^3$ + 1,159.878 $AC^{1/2}$ + 10.079 $FL^3$ − 81.277 × $FL^2$). However, in this study most formulae performed similarly, and the MPE was still around 7% for the best ones.[47] Another group looked at multiple formulae and determined that for a general population, the formula by Hadlock [$Log_{10}$ EFW = 1.335 − 0.0034(AC) (FL) + 0.0316(BPD) + 0.0457(AC) + 0.1623(FL)][38] had the lowest MPE with a sensitivity of 72% to 100% and specificity of 41% to 88% for detecting FGR.[48] The above studies have consistent findings, and Hadlock's formula may be more accurate than others in determining fetal weight, but most formulae are similar and even the best do not have an MPE <5%. Further studies may help to identify the optimal formula given a specific population.

## Accuracy at Extremes of Measurement

EFW accuracy can be affected by multiple factors, and one of the most significant factors influencing inaccuracies is the fetus demonstrating abnormal growth. In the EFW formulae, FL, BPD, and HC are all measures of bony structures. The AC is the only measurement incorporating soft tissue, as it encompasses the outer perimeter of the abdomen, which includes the liver and subcutaneous tissue. Investigators have argued that formulae based on bone structures may be less accurate with abnormal growth. In growth restriction, nutrient deficiency may lead to a more pronounced decline in muscle and fat cell growth compared with bone growth. In macrosomia, subcutaneous tissues would be expected to be increased, and the current formulae could be particularly inaccurate owing to the lack of accounting for this tissue development.

Multiple studies have been published addressing the issue of accuracy in EFW determination at extremes of newborn weight. Dudley showed that regardless of EFW formula, all methods showed wide variation in accuracy when the BW was less than 1,500 g. Additionally, for macrosomic newborns, the formulae were also more inaccurate with a tendency to underestimate weight.[45] Ben-Haroush et al. studied 840 pregnancies that were induced for various reasons and had an ultrasound EFW from 1 to 3 days prior to delivery. In this cohort, ultrasound EFW underestimated suspected macrosomic fetuses by a mean of 110 g and overestimated suspected growth-restricted fetuses by 113 g.[49] The same group also looked at 26 different formulae and found that models that incorporated 3 or 4 biometric indices were more accurate than those that only used 1 to 2. All models confirmed previous findings that the accuracy decreased at the extremes of newborn weight, where they overestimated low BW and underestimated large BW.[50] Regardless of the formula used, inaccuracy in EFW calculation exists when fetuses are small or large.

EFW is crucial in pregnancy management, where pregnancies identified as growth restricted will have increased surveillance and earlier delivery. Pregnancies identified as macrosomic will have changes in delivery planning in regard to route and timing. Clearly, improving accuracy at extremes of fetal weight will better guide the clinician in management of a specific pregnancy. As mentioned above, certain EFW models may be superior to others given a small or large fetus. In one study, when evaluating pregnancies with BW <2,500 g, Hadlock's formulae ($Log_{10}$ EFW = 1.3596 − 0.00386 AC × FL + 0.0064 HC + 0.00061 BPD × AC + 0.0424 AC + 0.174 FL) and ($Log_{10}$ EFW = 1.335 − 0.0034 AC × FL + 0.0316 BPD + 0.0457 AC + 0.1623 FL)[38] were the most accurate when compared with 11 other formulae in predicting EFW.[47] In a different study, for fetuses expected to be <10th percentile, investigators found that symmetric (all measures small) versus asymmetric (AC and FL smaller than head measurements) growth restriction also affected accuracy in EFW. For symmetrically grown fetuses, Hadlock formulae incorporating three or more measures were the most accurate in determining weight. However, in asymmetric fetuses, the Hadlock formula with only two measures that excluded FL was more accurate.[51] Studies investigating small fetuses show that Hadlock's formulae have the highest degree of accuracy, but in the macrosomic fetus, other formulae could provide more appropriate EFWs. When comparing 36 commonly used formulae for EFW on 350 singleton fetuses with BW >4,000 g, Hoopmann et al. showed that Hart's formula ($e^{\land}7.6377445039$ + 0.0002951035 × Maternal Weight + 0.0003949464 × HC + 0.0005241529 × AC + 0.0048698624 × FL [g, mm])[52] had the lowest MPE and the highest detection rate for macrosomic fetuses. This method also showed that 96% of fetuses fell within 10% of the EFW.[53]

Certain formulae may be more accurate than others at the extremes of fetal weight, but it may be that customizing a calculation provides the most accuracy. In a Chinese study of 1,034 patients, comparing 25 existing models failed to demonstrate a superior formula for EFW calculation. In this group, they created a regional-specific EFW model that could be used on the whole population. When the model predicted fetuses >90th percentile or <10th percentile, two different formulae were used: one for small fetuses and one for large fetuses. Using this method, they were able to more accurately predict fetal weight in growth-restricted and macrosomic fetuses.[54] Estimates of fetal soft tissue mass have been attempted to be measured through three-dimensional (3D) fractional thigh volume, which is an attractive addition to EFW formulae for the accurate prediction of weight in fetuses at the extremes of gestational age.[55] In one study, it showed superiority over conventional formulae for predicting actual BW in diabetic pregnancies.[56]

## Accuracy Conclusions

The literature has yet to declare a clear superior formula in the prediction of fetal and newborn weight. Factors affecting EFW include maternal body habitus, formula used, individual variability of the measures taken, and extremes of fetal weight. Although new models incorporating 3D technology have promise because they can evaluate fetal soft tissue mass, their clinical utility has not yet been adequately studied, and they have not yet entered into common practice. It seems that formulae involving three to four measures are more accurate than those involving one to two except in asymmetrically growth-restricted fetuses.

It is recommended that each institution use a consistent formula for assigning an EFW rather than altering the formula for each patient. Universal application would lead to less confusion and more uniform care.

## GROWTH CURVES

A growth curve is a graphic model of data that identifies the normal range of growth given a specific gestational age. Outliers are classified as too large or too small. Usually, a fetus measuring greater than the 90th percentile is defined as large for gestational age (LGA), while a fetus measuring less than the 10th percentile is defined as SGA. SGA was originally defined in 1967 by neonatologists to categorize a newborn with a birth weight of <10th percentile.[57] Over time, SGA was adopted by obstetricians to broadly classify the undergrown fetus regardless of etiology. The correct classification of fetuses as large or small is needed to accurately identify those fetuses that are at risk for poor perinatal outcome. An ideal standard would therefore allow a clinician to appropriately identify a pregnancy as high risk, and a good growth curve is the screening tool that would inform a clinician that increased surveillance is necessary.

### Population-Specific Growth Curves

Normal neonatal birth weight differs depending upon the population studied. Race and ethnicity are key factors in determining normal weight, where black infants have lower mean birth weights than white infants.[58,59] Chinese neonates are lighter than newborns in the United States,[60] and Asian newborns are smaller than European newborns.[61] It is not surprising that newborns of different races and different locations across the globe have different birth weights, but even when looking at birth weight ranges in Europe, regional differences exist. Knowing that differences exist is one thing, but does a birth weight in one region portend a different prognosis than the same birth weight in another region? One study by Graafmans and coworkers tried to answer this question. They compared the modal birth weights in specific countries, and they investigated their relationship to country-specific mortality curves. They found that shifts in the modal birth weight values paralleled the shift in the perinatal mortality curve. For example, Scotland has a modal birth weight of 3,446 g, with the lowest perinatal mortality found at 3,888 g. Norway has a heavier modal birth weight of 3,622 g, and the perinatal mortality nadirs at 4,305 g.[62] This shows that perinatal outcome related to birth weight is regionally specific, and each population has an "ideal birth weight." Many countries and institutions have created locally derived birth weight standards, and the curves generated from the data sources identify newborns at risk for poor outcome based on the individualized regional population. This seems to be a good strategy to identify those pregnancies that should be truly classified as high risk.

### Fetal versus Neonatal Growth Curves

Neonatal birth weight standards vary by population, and European standards have been created identifying different normal weights depending upon the country of birth.[63] In the United States, many birth weight curves have been created, with one of the first standards defined by Lula Lubchenco in Denver.[64] The use of this birth weight curve to the general population came into question as this standard reported the birth weights of newborns born at moderately high altitude, a known factor leading to smaller newborn size. This again emphasizes the importance of regional standards.

Questions began to arise about the validity of using a birth weight growth standard for in utero fetal weight standards as investigators realized that preterm birth was a pathological condition. In fact, at preterm gestational ages, the normal population is one in which the mother is still pregnant. As ultrasound technology improved, it was possible to estimate fetal weight using mathematical modeling by measuring certain fetal characteristics as described previously in this chapter. In 1991, Ott and coworkers compared birth weight percentile at various gestational ages as determined by an ultrasound-derived EFW curve versus a standard BW curve. When using the ultrasound fetal weight curve as the standard, they showed that the number of fetuses classified as IUGR (<10th percentile) decreased as gestational age advanced. If the birth weight curve was used to classify a newborn's weight, the number of babies identified as IUGR remained static. This caused the authors to draw the conclusion that growth restriction and preterm birth are related.[65] Hadlock et al.[66] created the most commonly used fetal growth curve, which was based on cross-sectional analysis of ultrasound data. By comparing EFW curves and newborn BW curves, the questions to be answered are: (a) how do these curves differ, and (b) which growth standard better identifies fetuses at risk for adverse perinatal outcome?

To address the first question, Bernstein and colleagues created a regional ultrasound-derived EFW curve based on 1,331 normal pregnancies. They compared this curve with the same region's BW data from 9,553 births at various gestational ages. The estimates for the 10th percentile at each gestational age were different for all ages except 37 and 38 weeks. In preterm gestations, less than 2% of EFWs fall below the 10th percentile on the birth weight standard. Conversely, more than 26% of ultrasound EFWs were greater than the 90th percentile on the birth weight standard.[67] In a French population, Salomon et al. compared an EFW standard with a birth weight standard created from 18,989 singleton, nonanomalous fetuses and neonates. The growth curves were significantly different, showing that the 50th percentile on the birth weight standard matched the 10th percentile on the estimated weight standard from 28 to 32 weeks' gestation.[68] These two studies showed that a birth weight standard will underestimate the number of IUGR fetuses and overestimate the number of LGA fetuses when compared with a growth curve created by EFW.

If a growth curve derived from EFW differs from that derived from birth weight, which curve is better at predicting adverse pregnancy and neonatal outcome? A Canadian study compared the outcomes of 37,377 nonanomalous pregnancies between 25 and 40 weeks classified as IUGR on either a birth weight curve or Hadlock's curve.[66] This study showed that infants classified as IUGR from a fetal weight standard were more likely to have preterm birth than those that were appropriately grown; however, if a fetus was classified as IUGR on the birth weight standard, there was no association with preterm birth. The fetal standard identified 90 fetuses that eventually experienced a perinatal death compared with 57 fetuses identified employing the birth weight standard.[69] By classifying a fetus as IUGR on a fetal weight standard, the ability to predict adverse pregnancy outcome is improved over that of using a birth weight standard. Like pregnancy outcomes, neonatal outcomes have also been investigated. Zaw et al. compared the outcomes of 1,267 newborns at less than 34 weeks and classified them as IUGR using either a Canadian birth weight curve or Hadlock's curve. In this study, babies classified as IUGR on the fetal weight standard were more likely to have the neonatal outcomes of respiratory distress syndrome (RDS), bronchopulmonary dysplasia, intraventricular hemorrhage, and retinopathy of prematurity. If the birth weight curve was used, newborns classified as IUGR were more likely to have neonatal mortality, retinopathy of prematurity, and necrotizing enterocolitis.[70] The differences in predictive ability likely hinge on the fact that newborns identified as IUGR on the birth weight curve are the smallest infants using either schema.

Using a fetal standard on ongoing pregnancies will better identify fetuses at risk for pregnancy and perinatal morbidity, whereas using a birth weight standard will better identify those fetuses destined for neonatal mortality. It is the obligation of the obstetrician to identify a diseased state, where fetuses classified as high risk are at an increased probability of developing poor outcome. Mortality is only one factor when considering poor outcome; therefore, the authors suggest using a fetal weight standard, such as that created by Hadlock et al.,[66] when determining the percentile of a given EFW.

## Individualized Growth Chart

Population growth curves can be generated using databases on either birth weight or EFW, but many have advocated that designing a regionally specific population curve is still not sensitive enough to appropriately identify those fetuses truly at risk for poor outcome. A baby born at 39 weeks weighing 3,000 g to parents both under 65 inches tall may not be at the same risk as a baby born at the same weight to parents who are above 70 inches tall. This has led some investigators to generate an individualized growth chart to more accurately identify the fetus at high risk.

Gardosi and coworkers have proposed a novel method for an individualized growth curve. This group observed that multiple factors influence a neonatal birth weight, including maternal height, weight in early pregnancy, parity, and ethnic group.[71] Paternal height was also a minor variable that contributes to the infant's weight.[72] This group developed a software program to calculate a fetus' "term optimal weight" using coefficients of adjustment for each of the aforementioned variables. These coefficients were generated from multivariate analysis of large, well-dated birth weight databases of term infants. The confidence interval for the optimal birth weight was determined by the coefficient of variation for the mean term birth weight of the population database. A growth curve for each gestational age is then created using a log polynomial equation described by Hadlock.[73] This novel approach allows for the generation of a growth curve that takes into consideration normal term birth weight and normal preterm EFW, while adjusting for factors specific to the parents of a fetus.

Using this methodology, Clausson and coworkers compared perinatal outcomes of infants identified as IUGR on a Swedish birth weight standard versus the individualized growth curve. Infants identified as appropriately grown for their individualized standard but <10th percentile on the birth weight standard were not at risk for poor outcome. Conversely, infants identified as appropriately grown by birth weight standards but <10th percentile on the customized curve had an increased odds ratio of having poor outcome.[74] The individualized growth curve had a better ability to predict perinatal outcomes such as stillbirth, neonatal death, and APGAR scores <4 at 5 minutes.[73] The findings from this study were confirmed in French, Spanish, and US

populations.[75–77] Additionally, the methodology has been used to generate customized growth standards for multiple gestations. When comparing a growth curve customized for twins to a customized curve for singletons, the curve for twins was more accurate in predicting fetal demise.[78] From multiple studies, the individualized growth curve is superior to birth weight standards at identifying fetuses at risk for poor perinatal outcome.

The concept of an individualized growth chart that takes into consideration maternal characteristics, paternal factors, and fetal number and sex is an attractive one. However, few data are available comparing this model directly to a fetal growth curve. A large study by Hutcheon and collegues compared the individualized curve to a birth weight curve and Hadlock's curve. When looking at 782,303 infants, compared with the birth weight standard, both the individualized standard and the fetal standard identified more fetuses as <10th percentile at preterm gestations. However, they identified a statistically similar number of patients as IUGR when compared with each other. Additionally, the study confirmed that the birth weight standard was inferior in predicting which fetuses will have stillbirth or neonatal death; however, the individualized curve was similar to the fetal standard in predicting these outcomes.[79] This study suggests that the true benefit of an individualized curve rests on establishing an in utero standard, and the effect of maternal and paternal characteristics is minimal. Further study is needed to confirm these findings; and until data are available, the use of a fetal growth curve, such as that provided by Hadlock et al.,[66] seems to provide as much accuracy as the individualized curve in identifying fetuses that are at high risk of poor perinatal outcome.

## MAGNETIC RESONANCE IMAGING

Ultrasound is the gold standard method for assessing fetal growth, but some authors have started using magnetic resonance imagining (MRI) as an adjunctive imaging modality in the assessment of at-risk fetuses. MRI has the advantage of a larger field of view, it is not affected by maternal body habitus or fetal position, and it has multiplanar and modal capabilities. One attractive feature of MRI is the ability to measure volume in 3D planes. In one of the first studies, Baker et al. measured fetal liver, placental, and brain volumes in 32 fetuses to see whether there was any association with newborn weight below the 10th percentile. Interestingly, the liver volume was <2.5th percentile in 10 of 11 fetuses who ultimately weighed less than the 10th percentile at birth. The placenta and brain did not show any reduction in measured volume compared with normally grown newborns.[80] Duncan et al. compared MRI with ultrasound in 74 fetuses, roughly half of which were growth restricted at birth. In this analysis, ultrasound fetal weight was superior to MRI in identifying fetuses that were measuring SGA. In contrast to the prior study, asymmetric IUGR fetuses (head size preserved) had reduced brain volume on MRI, suggesting that cerebral growth is still affected by growth restriction.[81] This was not confirmed by another group in 2012. In this study, MRI was performed on 20 growth-restricted fetuses and 19 normal fetuses. There was a significant reduction in whole body volume and of all internal organs in growth-restricted fetuses except the fetal brain. In fact, with a brain: liver volume ratio above 3.0, there was a 3.3-fold increased risk of perinatal mortality.[82] All three of these studies were small, and their assessments should be confirmed with larger analysis. However, the results parallel those seen by ultrasound in that fetuses that demonstrate growth abnormalities will have reduction in size of the fetal liver, which is incorporated in the ultrasonographic measurement of the AC. MRI is a relatively new technology in pregnancy assessment, and future studies could be performed to assess whether there is any benefit with assessment of fetal body composition, the macrosomic fetus, fetal brain perfusion, and the obese mother, all of which have limitations by current ultrasound technology.

## USE OF DOPPLER VELOCIMETRY IN IUGR

### Doppler Physics

The Doppler effect, described by Johann Christian Doppler in 1842, shows that when energy is reflected from a moving boundary, the frequency of the reflected energy varies in relation to the velocity and direction of the moving boundary. In ultrasound terms, Doppler depends upon the ability of an ultrasound beam to be changed in frequency when encountering a moving object (e.g., red blood cells; RBCs). The change in frequency, or frequency shift, is directly proportional to the speed with which the RBCs are moving within a particular vessel, and it is also dependent on the cosine of the angle that the ultrasound beam makes with the direction of blood flow, also referred to as the angle of insonation (Fig. 3.9). After some cosmetic manipulation by ultrasound programming, a flow velocity waveform is generated with the velocity in centimeter per second (reflecting the Doppler frequency shift) on the $y$-axis and time on the $x$-axis. For arterial waveforms, there is a clear systolic and diastolic component, while venous waveforms are typically steady and without pulsations (exceptions are centrally located veins such as the hepatic veins (HV), ductus venosus (DV), inferior vena cava (IVC), and pulmonary veins). Two general characteristics of vascular flow can be determined from the flow velocity waveforms. One of these is resistance or impedance to blood flow, and the second is the velocity of the blood moving through the vessel. To get the true velocity of the RBCs within a blood vessel, one needs to reduce the angle of insonation to 0°, as shown in Figure 3.10. Ultrasound machines that have pulsed wave Doppler capabilities generally have the ability to have the operator angle correct the Doppler signal. Several indices of resistance have been described, and the more commonly used indices are shown in Figure 3.11. The systolic/diastolic ratio (S/D ratio) is the most

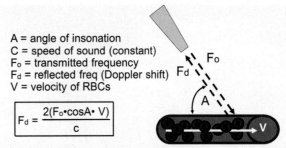

A = angle of insonation
C = speed of sound (constant)
$F_o$ = transmitted frequency
$F_d$ = reflected freq (Doppler shift)
V = velocity of RBCs

$$F_d = \frac{2(F_o \cdot \cos A \cdot V)}{c}$$

**FIGURE 3.9:** Relationship between the pulsed wave. Doppler signals transmitted *(Fo)* and received *(Fd)* by the transducer and the velocity of the red blood cells *(RBCs)*. This relationship is defined in the above formula. The Doppler (frequency) shift is directly proportional to the speed with which the RBCs are moving within a particular vessel, and it is also dependent on the cosine of the angle the Doppler beam makes with the blood vessel (as shown in the equation).

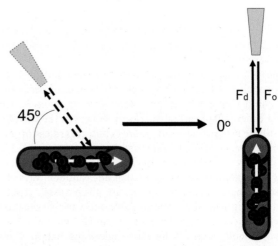

**FIGURE 3.10:** Example of angle correction with elimination of the angle between the Doppler beam and the interrogated vessel. This brings the angle of insonation to 0°, whereby the reflected Doppler signal *(Fd)* represents the actual speed of the blood. Fo, transmitted frequency; Fd, reflected frequency or Doppler shift.

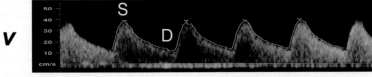

| Index | Calculation |
|---|---|
| Systolic to Diastolic (S/D) ratio | $\dfrac{\text{systolic peak velocity}}{\text{diastolic peak velocity}}$ |
| Resistance Index (RI) | $\dfrac{\text{systolic - end-diastolic peak velocity}}{\text{systolic peak velocity}}$ |
| Pulsatility Index (PI) | $\dfrac{\text{systolic - end-diastolic peak velocity}}{\text{time averaged maximum velocity}}$ |

**FIGURE 3.11:** Commonly used indices of resistance to assess blood flow velocity.

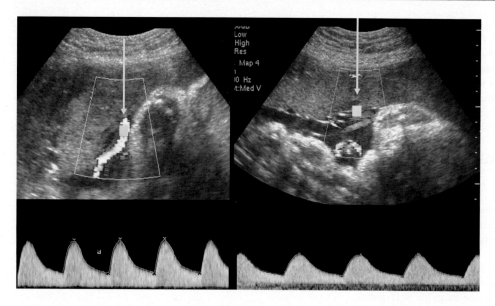

**FIGURE 3.12:** Two ultrasound images with color Doppler depicting different angles of insonation with flow velocity waveforms that are different in appearance, but proportionate in nature.

commonly used clinically in the United States, although all three are used throughout the literature. All three of these indices correlate very highly.

One of the characteristics of these resistance indices is angle independence. Changing the angle of insonation between the ultrasound Doppler beam and blood flow direction will produce a different appearing waveform. However, the waveforms will still be proportionate in nature. Thus, regardless of the index of resistance used, the same value will be obtained (e.g., the S/D ratios will be the same; Fig. 3.12). This is an advantage in the interrogation of vessels given that one cannot always obtain the same angle of insonation for any given vessel, especially when dealing with the uncontrollable and variable position of the fetus. A technical pearl to keep in mind is that the best waveform attainable is one in which the angle of insonation is closest to 0°. Obtaining the best possible waveform can be particularly useful when trying to determine whether there is low or absent end-diastolic flow in the umbilical artery. In clinical practice, an angle <30° is generally acceptable for Doppler measurement.

## Umbilical Artery Doppler

The fetal vessel most commonly interrogated with color and pulsed wave Doppler is the umbilical artery, which was first reported in 1977 by Fitzgerald and Drumm.[83] There is a gestational age-related increase in diastolic flow velocity in the umbilical artery both in human and in sheep pregnancies. This corresponds to the decreasing resistance to blood flow resulting from growth of placental vessels that branch from the umbilical arteries. Figure 3.13 depicts the progressive increase in diastolic flow velocity across gestation in normal pregnancy. Assessment of the flow velocity waveform in the umbilical artery has been described numerous times in the clinical setting of IUGR. The abnormal flow velocity waveform in the umbilical artery of IUGR fetuses was first described by Trudinger et al.[84] in 1985. In this study, 85% of 43 infants less than the 10th percentile birth weight had S/D ratios >95th percentile for gestational age, and this was secondary to a decrease in diastolic velocity in turn due to high resistance to blood flow downstream in the placenta. The degree of resistance in the umbilical artery, and thus the smaller downstream placental arterial vasculature to

which it is connected can be determined by analysis of the flow velocity waveform. The three common resistance indices used for arterial flow are shown in Figure 3.11. Figure 3.14 shows an initially normal flow velocity waveform that becomes progressively abnormal in an IUGR fetus. In IUGR pregnancies where there is an increase in the umbilical artery resistance indices, approximately 30% of the placental villous vessels are abnormal.[85] As the IUGR placental disease worsens, the velocity waveforms show absent flow and then reversed end-diastolic flow (AEDF; REDF). At this stage, 60% to 70% of the villous vessels will be abnormal.[86,87] In addition, there is a rate of 50% to 80% of intrauterine hypoxia by the time AEDF is apparent.[88–90] From a clinical standpoint, AEDF in the umbilical artery is associated with an 80-fold increase in perinatal mortality.[91]

## Middle Cerebral Artery Doppler

The middle cerebral artery (MCA) is another commonly interrogated fetal vessel in the setting of IUGR. The MCA is easy to visualize by obtaining a suboccipitobregmatic axial plane through the fetus and applying color Doppler. This will allow the circle of Willis to be visualized with six cerebral vessels extending from the circle of Willis. These vessels are paired and named the anterior, middle, and posterior cerebral arteries. The MCA tends to be the easiest to visualize given the lateral orientation of the vessel and the fact that the vessel carries approximately 80% of the cerebral blood flow. In normal circumstances, the flow velocity waveform in the MCA reflects the normally high impedance of the cerebral circulation in comparison with the normal umbilical artery waveform. Several studies in humans and in animal models have shown that an increase in diastolic flow velocity in the MCA is consistent with a chronic hypoxemic state in the fetus (Fig. 3.15). In addition, there is a redistribution of blood flow from nonvital organ systems and the torso of the fetus toward the fetal heart, brain, and adrenal glands.[92–95]

Clinically, the MCA Doppler in IUGR management is useful primarily in two ways. The first is a combination of the MCA PI and the umbilical artery PI in the form of a ratio and reported as the cerebroplacental ratio (CPR = MCA PI / Umb art PI) by Arbeille et al.[96] and subsequently by others.[95,97] CPR values < 1.0 or 1.08 have been reported as abnormal. Bahado-Singh et

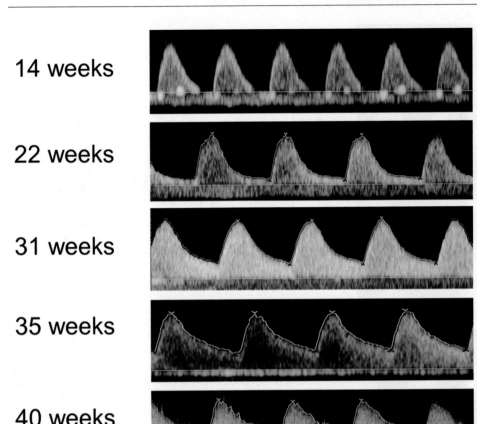

14 weeks

22 weeks

31 weeks

35 weeks

40 weeks

**FIGURE 3.13:** Umbilical artery flow velocity waveforms showing an increase in diastolic flow with advancing gestational age. This increase in diastolic flow is a result of the processes of placental branching angiogenesis at the end of the first trimester and beginning of the second, and nonbranching angiogenesis that starts at the end of the second and into the third trimesters.

al. reported that the CPR correlates well with birth weights <5th percentile with and without neonatal complications compared with the umbilical artery alone. They also showed that among 123 IUGR fetuses, those with an abnormal CPR were born 5 weeks earlier, weigh 850 g less, and had a significantly greater number of neonatal complications. Importantly, this chapter identifies that the CPR beyond 34 weeks loses its predictive ability and thus clinical utility. This was because the umbilical artery waveform often did not become abnormal in IUGR pregnancies beyond 34 weeks. Their observation supports prior studies that report that the umbilical artery Doppler may not become abnormal in the late (>34 week) IUGR fetuses (Fig. 3.16).[97] A second area where the MCA Doppler alone has begun to show some potential clinical utility is in the late IUGR fetus. IUGR fetuses with a normal umbilical artery, but a reduced MCA PI, show higher rates of neurological behavioral problems and a higher rate of nonreassuring fetal heart rate (FHR) pattern in labor, often leading to an emergency cesarean section.[98–100] Thus, although the late onset IUGR (>34 weeks) fetus may not develop abnormal umbilical artery Doppler velocimetry, the fetus may still develop an abnormal MCA Doppler waveform and still identify a pregnancy at risk for adverse outcome. In clinical practice, use of the CPR to identify pregnancies at greater risk for adverse outcomes can be used for counseling purposes. However, insufficient data are available to use CPR as a trigger for delivery. A reduction in the MCA peak systolic velocity, an index used clinically to assess for fetal anemia, has been associated with fetal polycythemia in IUGR; however, the clinical utility of this measurement has yet to be determined.

## Venous Vessel Doppler

The precardiac venous vessels have been studied extensively in IUGR. These "venous structures" are a general reference to the DV, HV, and the IVC. The anatomic relationship of these venous structures to one another and the liver are elegantly described and illustrated in the 16-week human fetus microdissections by Mavrides et al.[101] Figure 3.17 depicts the vasculature of the hepatic and portal circulations. The umbilical vein is a conduit vessel that delivers nutrient and oxygen-rich blood from the placenta to the fetus. After entering the abdominal wall, the umbilical vein courses anteriorly through the falciform ligament entering the liver becoming the portal sinus. On ultrasound, this portal sinus is depicted as the characteristic hypoechoic vascular structure with an L or hockey stick appearance (Fig. 3.18) and has a typical steady venous flow velocity waveform Doppler pattern. The portal sinus delivers blood to the left lobe of the liver via the inferior and superior portal veins and venules, and terminates in the right lobe of the liver, where this fresh blood coalesces with flows from the portal circulation. Ultrasound resolution is now sufficiently high that even the echolucent lines representing the left portal veins can be seen (see Fig. 3.18). At the approximate bend of the L-shaped portal sinus, about 50% of the blood delivered by the umbilical veins is shunted through the cone-shaped DV vessel, allowing this fresh blood to bypass the highly metabolic liver and stream toward the fetal heart. These vessels coalesce into an area just beneath the diaphragm that has been described as the subdiaphragmatic vestibulum, where the process of differential streaming is initiated. Preferential streaming

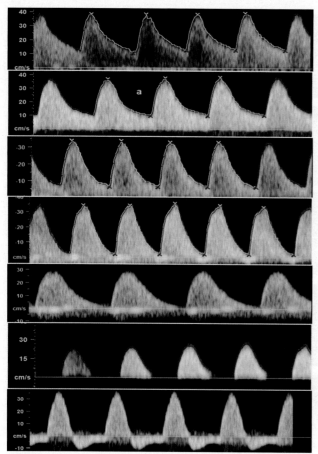

**FIGURE 3.14:** Multiple sequential umbilical artery flow velocity waveforms depicting a progressive increase in resistance over time in an IUGR fetus with advancing placental disease. Note that the end-diastolic flow progresses from normal in the first waveform to abnormal with absent end-diastolic flow and then to reversed end-diastolic flow.

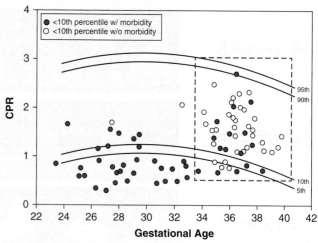

**FIGURE 3.16:** The cerebroplacental ratio (CPR) is shown across gestation in 123 IUGR fetuses. Note that the CPR loses its ability to identify morbidity in fetuses <10th percentile after 34 weeks (box). (From Bahado-Singh RO, Kovanci E, Jeffres A, et al. The Doppler cerebroplacental ratio and perinatal outcome in intrauterine growth restriction. *Am J Obstet Gynecol.* 1999;180:750–756, copyright © 1999 with permission from Elsevier.)

directs the more nutrient and oxygen-rich blood across the foramen ovale into the left atrium and left ventricle. This results in the fetal heart (via coronary vessels) and the fetal brain through the aorta to receive this oxygen-rich blood.

The central venous vessels (DV, HV, and IVC) have characteristic triphasic pulsed-wave Doppler waveforms that reflect the central venous pressures, while the peripheral venous vessels (umbilical vein and portal sinus) have steady-flow velocity waveforms. The normal triphasic flow velocity waveforms of the central venous vessels have three components, which are shown in Figure 3.19. The highest pressure gradient between the venous vessels and the right atrium occurs during ventricular systole, resulting in the highest blood flow velocity. This is the first peak of forward flow. The second phase of forward flow occurs during early diastole when the AV valves open with passive early filling of the ventricles. The nadir of flow velocities occurs with atrial contraction during late diastole, at which time the foramen ovale flap and crista dividens meet. One advantage of venous Doppler interrogation is that it provides assessment of cardiac forward function. The forward function is complex and

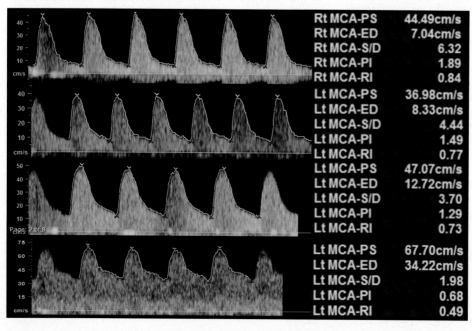

| | |
|---|---|
| Rt MCA-PS | 44.49cm/s |
| Rt MCA-ED | 7.04cm/s |
| Rt MCA-S/D | 6.32 |
| Rt MCA-PI | 1.89 |
| Rt MCA-RI | 0.84 |
| Lt MCA-PS | 36.98cm/s |
| Lt MCA-ED | 8.33cm/s |
| Lt MCA-S/D | 4.44 |
| Lt MCA-PI | 1.49 |
| Lt MCA-RI | 0.77 |
| Lt MCA-PS | 47.07cm/s |
| Lt MCA-ED | 12.72cm/s |
| Lt MCA-S/D | 3.70 |
| Lt MCA-PI | 1.29 |
| Lt MCA-RI | 0.73 |
| Lt MCA-PS | 67.70cm/s |
| Lt MCA-ED | 34.22cm/s |
| Lt MCA-S/D | 1.98 |
| Lt MCA-PI | 0.68 |
| Lt MCA-RI | 0.49 |

**FIGURE 3.15:** Normal and abnormal middle cerebral artery (MCA) flow velocity waveforms in an IUGR fetus. There is a progressive increase in the diastolic flow velocity resulting in a progression from a normal waveform with a high resistance to flow to an abnormal waveform with very low resistance. The abnormal waveforms with increase in diastolic flow velocity are consistent with chronic hypoxemia of IUGR.

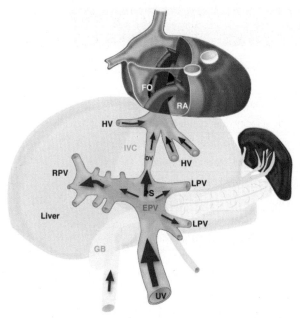

**FIGURE 3.17:** Schematic representation of the fetal umbilical, portal, and hepatic venous circulations. The *arrows* indicate the direction of blood flow. The *red color* reflects the more oxygenated blood and the *blue color* the lesser oxygenated blood. FO, foramen ovale; RA, right atrium; DV, ductus venosus; UV, umbilical vein; HV, hepatic veins; IVC, inferior vena cava; PS, portal sinus; LPV, left portal vein; RPV, right portal vein; EPV, extrahepatic portal vein; GB, gall bladder. (From Mavrides E, Moscoso G, Carvalho JS, et al. The anatomy of the umbilical, portal and hepatic venous systems in the human fetus at 14–19 weeks of gestation. *Ultrasound Obstet Gynecol.* 2001;18:598–604, with permission.)

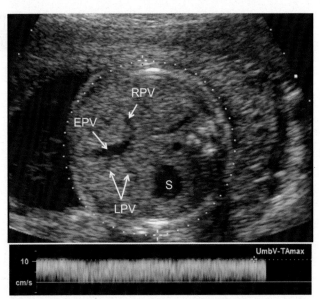

**FIGURE 3.18:** Axial ultrasound image of the fetal abdomen showing the portal sinus vasculature with the characteristic "hockey-stick" appearance. Also shown is a steady, non-pulsatile Doppler flow velocity waveform characteristic of the portal and umbilical venous vessels. LPV = left portal vein; RPV = right portal vein; EPV = extrahepatic portal vein; S = stomach.

is determined by afterload, compliance, and contractility. The DV waveform normally has forward flow throughout the cardiac cycles, whereas the IVC and HV waveforms have reverse or absent flow at the atrial kick. The complex triphasic waveform has been described by multiple venous Doppler indices, none of which has been shown to have a clear advantage (Table 3.3). Hecher et al.[102] and Rizzo et al.[103] performed fetal blood sampling in fetuses who had reversal of flow in the DV or greatly reversed flow in the IVC and showed that this is consistent with an acidemic state in the fetus. The utility of umbilical artery and venous Dopplers in IUGR management is discussed further below.

## Uterine Artery Dopplers

The uterine arteries that emanate from the maternal hypogastric arteries bilaterally have a variable and at times tortuous course along the lateral aspects of the uterus before terminating in the much smaller caliber spiral arteries embedded in the myometrium. In the nonpregnant state and early pregnancy period, the spiral arteries are characterized by a high vascular impedance state. Under normal circumstances, in the first trimester of pregnancy, placental cytotrophoblast differentiate into invasive and noninvasive cytotrophoblast.[104] These specialized trophoblast cells penetrate and cross the decidualized endometrium, invading the maternal and spiral radial arteries. This results in physiologic remodeling of arterial musculature, transforming these normally high-resistance vessels into low-resistance vessels. If the trophoblast invasion remains confined to the decidualized endometrial portion of the myometrium, maternal spiral and radial arteries fail to undergo the physiologic transformation into low-resistance vessels. Blood flow impedance in these small caliber vessels can be detected upstream in the larger caliber uterine artery vessels through the use of color and pulsed-wave Doppler velocimetry. The normal

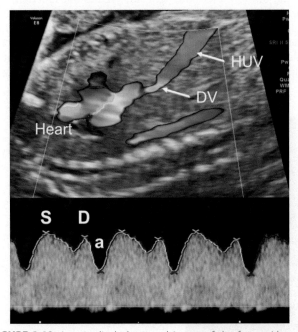

**FIGURE 3.19:** Longitudinal ultrasound image of the fetus with color Doppler showing the hepatic portion of the umbilical vein (*HUV*; also termed extrahepatic portal vein), the ductus venosus *(DV)*, and fetal heart. Note the aliasing of the DV that allows for easy identification of the DV. Also shown triphasic flow velocity waveform of the ductus venosus obtained by PW Doppler. S, systole; D, early diastole; a, atrial contraction. (Courtesy of Simona Ivanov, RDMS, and Henry L. Galan, MD.)

| Table 3.3 | Formulae for the Doppler Indices Commonly Used for the Central Venous Vessels |
|---|---|
| **Index** | **Calculation** |
| Ductus venosus (DV) preload index | $\dfrac{\text{systolic} - \text{diastolic peak velocity}}{\text{systolic peak velocity}}$ |
| Inferior vena cava (IVC) preload index | $\dfrac{\text{peak velocity during atrial contraction}}{\text{systolic peak velocity}}$ |
| IVC and DV pulsatility index for veins (PIV) | $\dfrac{\text{systolic} - \text{diastolic peak velocity}}{\text{time} - \text{averaged maximum velocity}}$ |
| IVC and DV peak velocity index for veins (PVIV) | $\dfrac{\text{systolic} - \text{atrial contraction peak velocity}}{\text{diastolic peak velocity}}$ |
| Percentage reverse flow | $\dfrac{\text{systolic time averaged velocity}}{\text{diastolic time averaged velocity}} \times 100$ |

flow velocity waveform in the uterine artery after vascular remodeling is characterized by a smooth gentle peak systolic component, absence of an early or protodiastolic notch, and high end-diastolic flow velocity that results in low-resistance indices. Normal and abnormal flow velocity waveforms in the uterine artery are shown in Figure 3.20. The low-resistance transformation in the small caliber vessels is generally expected by 22 to 24 weeks. Many studies and reviews have illustrated that failure to achieve low resistance in these vessels is associated with an increased risk for adverse pregnancy outcomes, including the development of preeclampsia, IUGR, placental abruption, and other adverse pregnancy outcomes.[105] While the evidence is strong that uterine artery Doppler abnormalities are associated with and predictive of adverse pregnancy outcomes, the benefit and application of uterine artery Doppler in pregnancy as a screening tool, either for routine use in low- or high-risk pregnancies, remain controversial and is currently not recommended.[106]

## Cardiac Dopplers

The fetal heart is probably the most challenging organ to interrogate in the fetus as blood flows into, through, and out of the heart are affected by several factors including preload, afterload, heart rate, and compliance. Several investigators have reported on cardiac Doppler changes and function in IUGR, and some of these have been conducted in longitudinal fashion. In addition to functional cardiac status, numerous sites in the fetal heart have been interrogated by real-time, color and Doppler ultrasound. These include, but are not limited to, E/A ratios, DV, aortic isthmus, myocardial performance indices, cardiac outflow tracts, the right and left diastolic function, and coronary arteries.[102,107–114] The more commonly interrogated sites in the fetal heart are the aortic and pulmonary outflow tracts, DV, and atrioventricular (AV) valves. Because flow indices at the level of the heart are quantitative in nature, it is important to be cognizant of the angle of insonation and try to

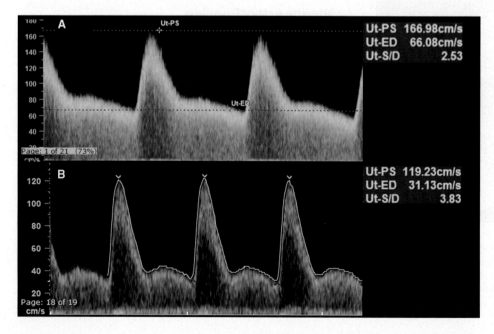

**FIGURE 3.20:** Normal **(A)** and abnormal **(B)** flow velocity waveforms in the uterine artery. Note the softer peak, absence of early diastolic notching, higher end-diastolic flow, and lower S/D ratio in the normal uterine artery waveform in **A** compared with that of the abnormal waveform in **B**.

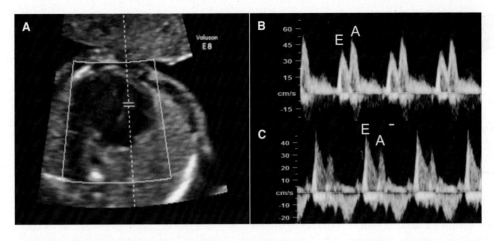

**FIGURE 3.21: A:** Four-chamber view of the heart showing the location of the Doppler sample volume at the distal point of the opening of the A-V valve. **B:** The characteristic M shape of the flow velocity waveform with the E and A components through the valve. Reversal of the E/A waveform is seen in extrauterine life and can be seen in IUGR **(C)**. (Courtesy of Lisa Howley, MD.)

maintain it <20° since at greater angles than this, the measurements are less reliable.

The AV valve Doppler investigation is best obtained in a four- or five-chamber view with the sample volumes placed just distal to the opening of the AV valves within the ventricular chamber. The Doppler beam should be nearly parallel to the flow of blood in order to obtain the best and most consistent waveforms possible. The waveform should have a characteristic "M" configuration from which the E/A ratio, which expresses the diastolic ventricular function, can be calculated. This M configuration is similar in the tricuspid and mitral valves, which suggests similar diastolic function in the two ventricles.[115] The E component of the ratio (initial peak velocity) represents early and fast ventricular filling, while the A component (second peak velocity) represents peak velocity with atrial contraction (Fig. 3.21). Under normal circumstances in utero, the E peak velocity is less than the A peak velocity. Because the ratio is related to preload and cardiac compliance, the ratio increases with advancing gestational age.[116] Postnatally, the E/A ratio reverses and assumes the adult pattern of the E peak velocity being greater than the A peak velocity. In IUGR, diastolic function can be damaged by insufficient ventricular filling and can appear either as a lower E/A ratio or as a significant reduction of the atrial peak in the flow velocity waveform.[102,112,117,118]

Normally, the contributions of the right and left ventricles to the combined fetal cardiac output (CCO) are 60% and 40%, respectively. Approximately, 40% of the CCO is delivered to the low-resistance vascular bed of the placenta. In IUGR, there are several mechanisms involved in affecting the flows through the fetal heart. These include (a) increase in afterload secondary to increases in placental blood flow resistance, (b) reduced blood flow volume, (c) reduction in diastolic function due to inadequate ventricular filling via the AV valves, and (d) progressive enlargement of the cardiac structures such as the AV valves and the outflow tract vessels. The net result is a decrease in CCO with an approximate 10% shift from the right ventricle to the left, resulting in a decrease in the right to left cardiac output ratio.[119] There is also a decrease in the peak velocities in both the aortic and the pulmonary outflow tracts.[110] In addition, the reduction of peak velocity in the pulmonary outflow tract is seen with more frequency (95% of IUGR cases) than in the aortic tract (57% of IUGR cases), which is understandable given that it is the right side of the heart (via the ductus arteriosus) that is most affected by the increase in afterload. The reduction in ventricular peak velocities is considered to be a relatively late cardiovascular finding in the decompensating IUGR fetus.[111] The

ventricle damage that is seen in IUGR because of inadequate filling of the ventricles is reflected in the AV valves where either a decrease in the E/A ratio or an isolated atrial peak systolic waveform may be seen.[102,112,117,118]

A less commonly discussed cardiac vascular structure in the setting of IUGR is the coronary artery. In 1998, Baschat et al.[113] reported that fetal coronary artery blood flow could be visualized in normal fetuses at 32 weeks and beyond. Coronary artery blood flow identification requires close attention to color Doppler ultrasound setting, as described by these authors, including: (1) adjustment of color Doppler velocity scale between 27 and 48 cm per second, depending on the depth of insonation and the transducer used, (2) reduction in size of the color Doppler box and gate as much as possible to optimize both temporal and spatial resolution, (3) setting the color filter to a high degree of motion discrimination, (4) setting the color amplification gain to eliminate color background noise on the screen, and (5) selection of a persistence setting from a range of 0 (no averaging of frames) to 3. They also verify the identification of coronary vessels by color Doppler, with pulsed wave Doppler showing the typical flow velocity waveform.[113] In a follow-up study, these authors also showed that coronary artery blood flow could be visualized at an earlier gestational age in IUGR fetuses (e.g., <32 weeks) with abnormal arterial and venous Doppler findings, and that these fetuses with AREDV and centralization of blood flow are at high risk for hypoxemia, acidemia, and adverse outcome.[120] The authors speculated that the visualization of coronary blood flow <32 weeks represents another example of the "sparing" effects seen in IUGR. While interrogation of coronary vessels was seen in conjunction with venous Doppler abnormalities, further investigation is needed to show whether there is additional benefit to interrogating the coronary vessels.

## SURVEILLANCE OF THE IUGR FETUS

The IUGR fetus is at increased risk for progressive placental dysfunction, deterioration of acid-base balance, and stillbirth. As such, fetal surveillance in this condition is warranted. Several tools are available to assess the status of the IUGR fetus, and these are listed in Table 3.4.

### Fetal Movement

Several methods have been described for maternal assessment of fetal movement. A simple technique involves having the patient

| Table 3.4 | Surveillance Tools in IUGR |
|-----------|---------------------------|

Maternal monitoring of fetal activity
Amniotic fluid volume (AFV)
Nonstress testing
Biophysical profile
Modified biophysical profile (NST + AFV assessment)
Doppler velocimetry
Interval growth

lie on her side and record any fetal movement one or two times per day. The fetus should move 10 times within a 2-hour period, although most pregnant patients will feel their fetuses achieve the target movements in the first 5 to 10 minutes of maternal monitoring. Failure to achieve 10 movements in a 2-hour period warrants further fetal evaluation with nonstress testing (NST). In a 1975 study, Matthews[121] showed the predictive value of fetal activity counts in 50 IUGR fetuses who subsequently demonstrated distress in labor.

## Amniotic Fluid Volume

Assessment of amniotic fluid volume is important as the amniotic fluid is a reflection of fetal renal perfusion and an indirect measure of fetal vascular status.

Amniotic fluid assessment by ultrasound can be determined by one of the three general methods: amniotic fluid index (AFI) absolute value of <5 cm, AFI of <5th percentile for gestational age, or deepest or maximal vertical pocket (DVP or MVP). A nomogram for amniotic fluid across gestation is shown in Table 4 in Appendix A1. There are limitations to the use of ultrasound to assess the amniotic fluid volume. Ultrasound sources of error when estimating the amniotic fluid volume include excess abdominal pressure by the sonographer, multiple loops of cord, umbilical or placental cysts, and particulate variation in the amniotic fluid (e.g., meconium). Controversy exists regarding the best cut-offs to use to define oligohydramnios and polyhydramnios. Assessment by ultrasound is only an indirect measurement of amniotic fluid volume, and previous studies of amniotic fluid volume determination comparing ultrasound with intraamniotic dye tests have shown the limited accuracy of ultrasound at both extremes of amniotic fluid volumes.[122] Although there is no consensus regarding the best ultrasound method to predict adverse neonatal outcome, the single MVP has higher specificity than AFI and reduces the likelihood of intervention without a demonstrable benefit.[123–125]

While low amniotic fluid (anhydramnios or oligohydramnios) itself is a poor screening tool for IUGR, it may be the first sign of a growth-restricted fetus. Up to 96% of fetuses with fluid pockets less than 1 cm in depth may be IUGR.[126] A gradual reduction in amniotic fluid volume is due to redistribution of blood flow favoring the fetal heart, brain, and adrenal glands, and away from the lungs, digestive tract, kidneys, and torso, has been well described with hypoxia in lambs.[127] This "brain-sparing" effect has been described in human IUGR pregnancies, and the reduction in renal blood flow is felt to account for the oligohydramnios.[128,129] The relationship of oligohydramnios and progressive worsening of both arterial and venous Doppler velocimetry findings has been previously

described.[130] The large PORTO trial on IUGR demonstrated that low AFI is most valuable clinically when the IUGR fetus is <3rd percentile.[131]

## Antepartum Testing

The nonstress test (NST) and the biophysical profile (BPP) are the two most commonly used standard surveillance tools in high-risk pregnancies. The NST is a method of fetal heart rate (FHR) analysis that uses Doppler technology to record and trace the FHR concomitantly with contraction monitoring. NST reactivity is defined as two accelerations (15 bpm above baseline for 15 seconds' duration) within a 20-minute window, and this must occur within 40 minutes of monitoring. In fetuses less than 32 weeks, reactivity has been defined as accelerations greater than 10 bpm above baseline for greater than 10 seconds. Antepartum testing with the NST is combined with amniotic fluid assessment, and when the testing is normal, it identifies a fetus with a normal fetal acid–base status and low risk of stillbirth.[132,133] While 80% of fetuses beyond 32 weeks have a reactive NST, the rate of reactivity is lower in IUGR fetuses. Studies have shown that there is delay of CNS maturation, including a delay in the normal decline of FHR with advancing gestation, decreased short- and long-term variability, and delay in reactivity, especially in early IUGR.[134,135] Thus, additional testing with the BPP or prolonged monitoring is commonly required for IUGR fetuses.

While CNS maturation is delayed, centrally regulated responses to hypoxia remain preserved.[136] Because of delay in reactivity in IUGR fetuses and because IUGR is seen early in pregnancy before reactivity is expected, the four-point BPP is commonly used. A BPP score of 4 or less is strongly associated with a pH less than 7.20. Further, a BPP score of 2 or less has 100% sensitivity for prediction of acidemia. With progressive fetal hypoxemia and acidemia, the IUGR fetus will show a progressive loss of fetal breathing motions, body movements, and tone, and eventually cessation of all activity.[137–139] If the decrease in activity is acute, amniotic fluid volume may not be decreased. In contrast, if it is more gradual, the amniotic fluid volume may decrease. Given that reactivity is not expected in early IUGR (<30 weeks), the four-component BPP that excludes FHR assessment makes clinical sense. However, although reactivity is not necessarily anticipated, monitoring the fetus with the FHR tracing will allow for assessment of FHR decelerations. A BPP score of 4 or less, recurrent decelerations, or nonreactive FHR tracing by computerized cardiac monitoring is associated with an increased rate of fetal hypoxemia, acidemia, cord compression from oligohydramnios, and increased perinatal mortality.[90,132,133,140] The frequency of fetal monitoring using these techniques is dependent on the gestational age of the fetus and the severity of the IUGR condition. This is further elucidated in an algorithm for IUGR management in Figure 3.22. Monitoring of the IUGR fetus with pulsed-wave Doppler velocimetry has been used effectively for three decades to assess the status of the IUGR fetus. Use of Doppler as a trigger for delivery is discussed further below. Interval growth of the fetus reflects the ongoing ability of the placenta to provide adequate nutrition to the fetus over time. Interval growth assessment is discussed earlier in the chapter, but in general, the timing of these ultrasounds should not occur any more frequently than every 2 to 3 weeks. In practical terms, the frequency of interval growth prior to 34 weeks impacts pregnancy management less than other parameters of fetal assessment.

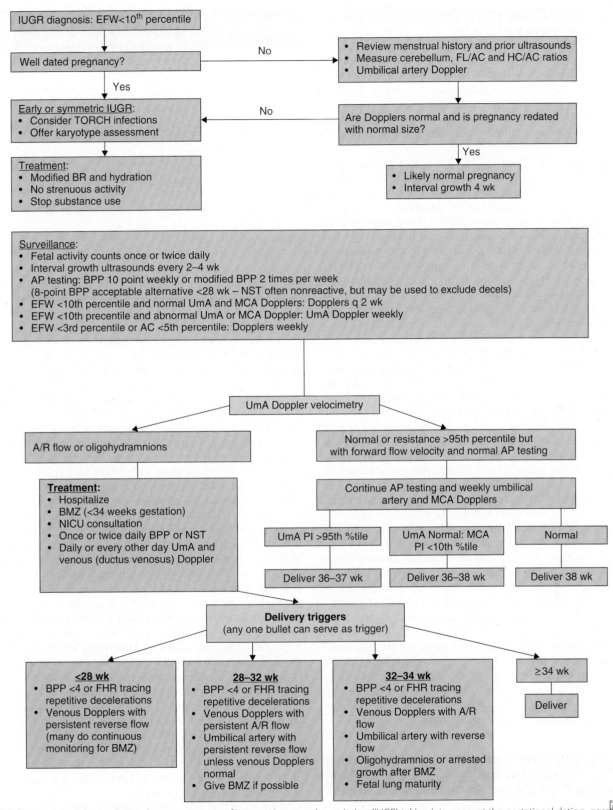

**FIGURE 3.22:** Algorithm outlining the management of intrauterine growth restriction (IUGR) taking into account the gestational dating, possible etiologies, and potential treatments, as well as providing a guideline for fetal surveillance (antepartum testing and Doppler studies) and timing of delivery. AP, antepartum; AR, absent/reverse; BPP, biophysical profile; BR, bedrest; BMZ, betamethasone; EFW, estimated fetal weight; NST, nonstress test; MCA, middle cerebral artery; UmA, umbilical artery; NICU, neonatal intensive care unit; PI, pulsatility index; FHR, fetal heart rate.

# MANAGEMENT AND DELIVERY OF PRETERM AND TERM IUGR FETUSES

Timing delivery of the IUGR fetus requires close consideration of a variety of key factors listed in Table 3.5, which are discussed further in this section. These determinants represent different aspects of the IUGR pregnancy. While any one determinant might serve as a trigger for delivery, in general, they are used in combination to assess the overall health and developmental status of the pregnancy.

The etiology of IUGR for a given fetus is important to establish when the diagnosis of IUGR is first assigned. While this is not always possible, efforts should be made as this not only allows for appropriate counseling of the patient, but may have a significant impact on the timing of delivery. For example, a fetus affected by aneuploidy or a congenital viral infection may not have its outcome affected by delaying delivery until term gestation. Furthermore, if a lethal condition is present, maternal preference and her safety take precedence in regard to the timing of delivery. In counseling patients with a new diagnosis of IUGR, it is important to share that 70% of fetuses <10th percentile will be small for normal reasons and not at risk for IUGR complications; this is referred to as "constitutional" smallness.[141] This will help alleviate some of the patient's anxiety and give her hope that the pregnancy may still be normal. Often the obstetrical provider will note that there are individuals of short stature in the family, which may account for the small constitutional size of the fetus. In contrast, 30% of fetuses <10th percentile will be at risk for adverse perinatal outcomes and require surveillance. The risk of adverse outcomes has been shown to be highest in newborns with birth weights <3rd percentile.[142] Once poor pregnancy dating, aneuploidy (either with fetal karyotype or cell-free fDNA testing), structural abnormalities (e.g., gastroschisis), and congenital infection (CMV, toxoplasmosis, herpes simplex virus, rubella, etc.) have been determined to be unlikely or excluded, the majority of the remaining cases will be due to constitutional smallness or placental insufficiency. Placental insufficiency may be due to a primary placental problem (circumvallate placenta), substance abuse, or chronic maternal disease, which may impact placentation, uterine blood flow, and placental perfusion. Table 3.6 depicts the typical phenotype of the IUGR fetus due to placental insufficiency. Even with the use of this phenotype, distinguishing between placental insufficiency and small constitutional size can be challenging, and at times, the two may overlap. As such, fetuses that are constitutionally small should still be considered at risk and will require additional surveillance. Testing for the above-mentioned congenital infections is generally not performed unless there is ultrasound evidence for infections (e.g., periventricular or hepatic calcifications).

| Table 3.5 | Determinants of Delivery in the IUGR Fetus |
|---|---|

Etiology
Gestational age
Biophysical assessment (NST/BPP)
Umbilical artery Doppler velocimetry
Maternal comorbidity
Low amniotic fluid volume (anhydramnios/oligohydramnios)
Interval growth

| Table 3.6 | Phenotype of the Fetus with Uteroplacental Insufficiency |
|---|---|

Biometry: symmetric
Anatomic abnormalities: absent
Evidence of brain-sparing effect:
    Head circumference size maintained
    Cerebellum size maintained
    MCA Doppler Index reduced
Amniotic fluid: reduced
Fetal Doppler velocimetry:
    Umbilical artery with elevated indices, absent or reversed end-diastolic flow
    Precordial venous Dopplers showing elevated indices or absent/reversed flow in the a-wave
Biophysical assessment:
    Nonstress test: nonreactive or with late decelerations
    Biophysical profile score: ≤4
Maternal comorbidity: Preeclampsia or chronic medical disease

The use of these delivery determinants, either alone or in combination, as an indication for delivery is largely dependent on the gestational age of the fetus. While fetuses weighing <500 g may survive, achieving an EFW of at least 500 g is generally considered to be a threshold for intervening on fetal behalf. While fetal weight is important, work by several groups has demonstrated that gestational age is a more important determinant of survival and intact survival. Beyond 27 weeks, survival and intact survival first exceed 50%; however, a birth weight less than 550 g is associated with a very high risk of neonatal death.[143,144] In 604 IUGR fetuses between 24 and 32 weeks, Baschat et al. assessed the relationship between a variety of perinatal variables (Doppler studies, GA, BW, acid–base status, and Apgar scores) and major neonatal complications, survival, and intact survival. They found that gestational age was the most significant determinant of survival until 26 6/7 weeks and intact survival until 29 2/7 weeks. Beyond these cut-offs, DV Doppler and cord artery pH predicted survival, and only DV Doppler predicted intact survival.[143] Mari et al. similarly showed in 41 IUGR fetuses delivered <32 weeks that gestational age is a critical factor in survival. Perinatal mortality decreased by 48% for each additional week gained, and 94% of deaths occurred when the delivery was less than 29 weeks.[145] The importance of both fetal size and gestational age further emphasized their inverse relationship with neonatal morbidities underscored by the work of McIntire and colleagues. These investigators demonstrated a decrease in respiratory distress syndrome (RDS) in more than 12,000 preterm infants with increasing gestational age and birthweight when stratified by these variables.[142] For example, the incidence of RDS at 35 to 36 weeks at <10th percentile birth weight was approximately 5%, and the incidence decreased with increasing birth weight percentiles.

There is little argument that over the past 25 years, the use of color and spectral Doppler velocimetry has increased our understanding of the pathophysiology of IUGR. Resultant studies have led to the use of Doppler as a primary tool for assessing the vascular status and managing the IUGR fetus. Initial Doppler studies were focused on the umbilical and cerebral circulations, and subsequently the venous circulations. As discussed above, absent or reverse flow in the umbilical artery is associated with

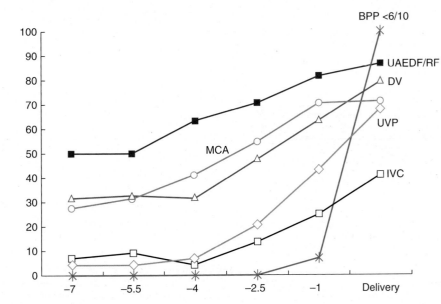

**FIGURE 3.23:** The percentage of abnormal Doppler findings in individual vessels and the incidence of a biophysical profile score below 6 in the week prior to delivery. UAEDF/RF, umbilical artery absent or reversed end-diastolic flow; MCA, abnormal middle cerebral artery flow; IVC, abnormal inferior vena cava flow; DV, abnormal ductus venosus flow; UVP, umbilical vein pulsations. Deterioration of Doppler findings precedes the decline in biophysical profile score. (Modified with permission from Baschat AA, Gembruch U, Harman CR. The sequence of changes in Doppler and biophysical parameters as severe fetal growth restriction worsens. *Ultrasound Obstet Gynecol.* 2001;18:571–577.)

high rates of intrauterine hypoxemia (50% to 80%) and increased risk of perinatal mortality (80-fold). A 2010 Cochrane database systematic review of 18 studies and over 10,000 women demonstrated that the use of umbilical artery Doppler reduces the rate of perinatal deaths (RR = 0.71; 95% CI, 0.52 to 0.98). It also reduced the rate of inductions of labor (RR = 0.89; 95% CI 0.80 to 0.99) and cesarean sections (RR = 0.90; 95% CI 0.87 to 0.94).[146] In 1997, the American College of Obstetricians and Gynecologists reported that use of umbilical artery Doppler in conjunction with standard antepartum testing (e.g., NST) reduced mortality.[147] In the 1990s, interrogation of the fetal venous structures gained significant attention. Fetal Doppler studies by investigators, such as those by Hecher et al.[102] and Rizzo et al.[103] demonstrated that venous back flow during the atrial contraction in precordial venous structures is reflective of fetal metabolic acidemia. Subsequent studies were published to address longitudinal Doppler changes and biophysical testing in IUGR fetuses in order to better understand the progressive nature of the IUGR pathologic process. Several of these studies depicted how venous Doppler changes (especially the DV) precede BPP and FHR tracing abnormalities. Baschat and colleagues[139] showed that 70% of fetuses demonstrate Doppler abnormalities in the DV and other vessels prior to an abnormal BPP defined as <6/10 (Fig. 3.23). Ferrazzi et al.[111] similarly showed that as IUGR fetuses decompensate, there is a fairly consistent pattern to which vessels show abnormal Dopplers. These are depicted as early and late Doppler changes in Figure 3.24. Work by Hecher and colleagues in the IUGR fetus with deteriorating condition very nicely demonstrated the close relationship between the DV and short-term variability.[130] This may be the first clear link between an abnormal Doppler vessel and the FHR parameter of short-term variability that reflects the balance between the parasympathetic and sympathetic nervous system in the fetus. More specifically, they showed a clear inverse relationship, namely, as the DV Doppler index became abnormal, so did the short-term variability (Fig. 3.25). This could suggest that as the DV becomes abnormal, so does the autonomic nervous system.

These last three studies collectively suggest that before a fetus becomes acidotic as indicated by an abnormal biophysical test, the majority of fetuses (50% to 70%) will demonstrate Doppler

abnormalities, particularly the DV. These types of data have led several groups to propose that abnormal venous Dopplers, and the DV in particular, be considered as triggers for delivery of the IUGR fetus. A randomized clinical trial comparing outcomes between fetuses delivered by DV Doppler and standard delivery indicators is near completion (TRUFFLE study). Another publication from the previously mentioned PORTO trial of 1,100 IUGR fetuses demonstrated that the DV abnormality was seen in only 11% of the 1,100 IUGR cases and that there was no specific or dominant sequence of abnormal Doppler changes seen in these 1,100 cases. However, this study also did not categorize the severity of umbilical artery Doppler findings. More specifically, they did not report on the rate of occurrence of absent or reversed end-diastolic flow (A/REDF) in the umbilical artery. A/REDF changes are far more

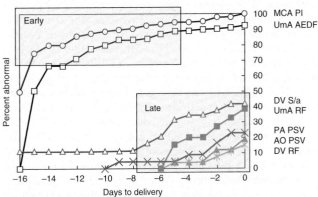

**FIGURE 3.24:** Temporal sequence of Doppler changes prior to delivery in decompensating IUGR fetuses. Fourteen days prior to delivery, the umbilical artery pulsatility index *(PI)* was abnormal in 100% of cases (not shown graphically). Early and late Doppler changes are depicted. MCA PI, middle cerebral artery PI; UmA AEDF, umbilical artery absent end-diastolic flow; DV S/a, ductus vensosus S/a ratio; UmA RF, umbilical artery reverse end-diastolic flow; PA PSV, pulmonary artery peak systolic velocity; AO PSV, aortic peak systolic velocity; DV RF, ductus venosus reverse flow. (Modified with permission from Ferrazzi E, Bozzo M, Rigano S, et al. Temporal sequence of abnormal Doppler changes in the peripheral and central circulatory systems of the severely growth-restricted fetus. *Ultrasound Obstet Gynecol.* 2002;19:140–149.)

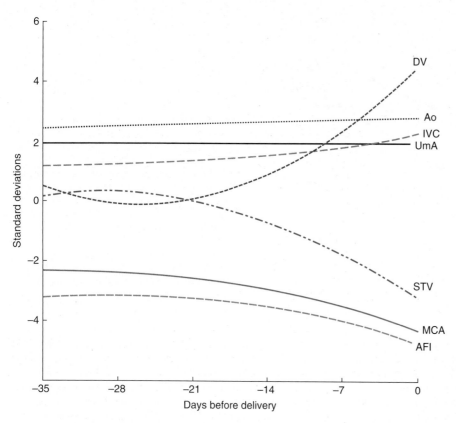

**FIGURE 3.25:** Trends over time of variables in relation to time before delivery and reference ranges (±2 SD; for fetuses delivered before or at 32 weeks of gestation). UmA, umbilical artery; DV, ductus venosus; Ao, aorta; IVC, inferior vena cava; STV, short-term variation; MCA, middle cerebral artery; AFI, amniotic fluid index. (Modified with permission from Hecher K, Bilardo CM, Stigter RH, et al. Monitoring of fetuses with intrauterine growth restriction: a longitudinal study. *Ultrasound Obstet Gynecol.* 2001;18:564–570.)

severe Doppler findings, and it is likely in this subgroup of fetuses where DV Doppler changes are likely to occur.

Like other determinants of delivery listed in Table 3.5, Doppler triggers and timing of delivery need to be reconciled with the gestational age of the fetus, given that gestational age, at least until 29 weeks, is the strongest predictor of intact survival.[139,145] The timing of delivery of the IUGR fetus is best answered in randomized clinical trials (RCT). There is one reported RCT addressing IUGR fetuses <36 weeks and one RCT for delivery beyond 36 weeks, and each of these have some long-term follow-up studies on the original study cohort. The Growth Restriction Intervention Trial (GRIT) had 548 study subjects, of which 196 were between 24 and 30 weeks, and 352 between 30 and 36 weeks. In this trial, patients were enrolled when physicians were unsure about delivery timing, and they were then randomized to a delivery-now or delayed-delivery group. The interval of time between randomization and delivery was 0.9 and 4.9 days, respectively. The cesarean delivery rates were 91% and 79%, respectively. There was no difference in mortality.[148] In a two-year follow-up study, the GRIT study group reported similar neurological outcomes between groups for gestational age at delivery >31 weeks. In contrast, they found a slightly higher rate of disability <31 weeks in the delivery-now group (14% vs. 5%). Clinically significant differences between immediate and deferred delivery were not found.[149] A 6- to 13-year follow-up report on one-half of the original cohort did not show the higher disability rate findings of the two-year follow-up study. This long-term report showed similar cognitive, language, behavior, and motor ability between groups.[150] Although there were some limitations to the GRIT trial, such as the small difference in the interval of delivery between groups (0.9 to 4.9 days) and the possibility that the delivery-now group may not have had sufficient benefit from steroids (range of delivery from time

of randomization 0.4 to 1.3 days), this study may suggest that the timing of delivery may not make a difference in early-onset IUGR fetuses. The neurologic injury in IUGR may already be set by the time the usual triggers for delivery are used.

Available literature on fetal Doppler interrogation and its application to fetuses beyond 34 weeks is limited for two primary reasons: the overwhelming majority of fetal vascular Doppler studies have been performed on fetuses less than 34 weeks of gestation, and umbilical artery Doppler interrogation has been found to be less reliable after 34 weeks. The uteroplacental insufficiency seen in IUGR fetuses diagnosed late in gestation (>34 weeks' gestation) is depicted by more mild placental dysfunction in which the elevated umbilical artery Doppler indices are often not seen. Other studies further show that the cerebroplacental Doppler ratio loses its predictive accuracy after 34 weeks' gestation.[95,97] Curiously, more recent data suggest that the only sign of placental dysfunction and nutrient and oxygen transfer insufficiency may be MCA Doppler changes characterized by an elevated diastolic flow velocity (e.g., brain-sparing effect), and these fetuses may still be at risk.[98–100]

As mentioned above, amniotic fluid is an important component of evaluation of the IUGR fetus and is an integral part of the standard antepartum testing modalities (e.g., modified BPP and BPP). In addition, anhydramnios and oligohydramnios may also serve as triggers for delivery. There are no randomized trials of delivery on the basis of low amniotic fluid volume in IUGR pregnancies. However, data have shown that the combination of IUGR and oligohydramnios is associated with fetal hypoxia, abnormal Doppler studies and biophysical testing, and increased rates of fetal distress in labor and perinatal mortality.[151,152] This has led to expert opinion and committee consensus that delivery should occur as early as 34 weeks and probably not later than 37 weeks gestation when IUGR is complicated by oligohydramnios.[124]

| Table 3.7 | Risk of Stillbirth beyond 37 Weeks' Gestation | | |
|---|---|---|---|
| **Gestational Age (wk)** | **Ongoing SGA Pregnancies** | **SGA Stillbirths (n = 20)** | **Stillbirth risk/10,000 ongoing SGA pregnancies (95% CI)** |
| 37–37 6/7 | 3,333 | 7 | 21 (13.0–32.1) |
| 38–38 6/7 | 2,776 | 3 | 11 (5.5–19.7) |
| 39–39 6/7 | 1,953 | 5 | 26 (17.0–38.1) |
| >40 | 832 | 5 | 60 (45.9 – 77.2) |

Adapted with permission from Trudell AS, Cahill AG, Methodius G, et al. Risk of stillbirth after 37 weeks in pregnancies complicated by small-for-gestational-age fetuses. *Am J Obstet Gynecol*. 2013;208:376.e1–376.e7.

Timing delivery of the IUGR fetus beyond 34 to 36 weeks has generally been based on the concern for stillbirth risk at a time when prematurity complications wane. In a study of 76 fetal demises with postmortem validated exams and 582 controls, Froen et al.[153] found that 52% of the fetal death cases were growth restricted. Vergani et al.[154] assessed independent predictors of adverse neonatal outcomes in 481 IUGR fetuses and, using a scoring model, determined that beyond 37.5 weeks, gestational age no longer had an independent impact on outcome. A more recent report demonstrates a progressive increase in the risk of stillbirth beyond 37 weeks (Table 3.7).[155] The only randomized clinical trial for timing the delivery of the late IUGR fetus (beyond 36 weeks) is the Disproportionate Intrauterine Growth Intervention Trial at Term (DIGITAT). Boers et al. reported the initial results of this trial that included 650 study subjects who were randomized after 36 weeks of gestation to induction of labor (n = 321) or expectant management (n = 329). Compared with the expectant management group, the induction of labor group delivered on average 10 days earlier, weighed 130 g less, and had similar composite adverse neonatal outcomes. Maternal outcomes showed no differences for spontaneous or operative vaginal delivery or for cesarean section rate. Preeclampsia was significantly more common in the expectant management group (7.9% vs. 3.7%).[156] A follow-up subanalysis of this study using a more sensitive analytic technique for neonatal morbidities (MAIN: Morbidity Index for Newborns) showed that while NICU admissions were higher in the induction of labor group, the percentage of adverse outcomes was similar between the two groups.[157] In a two-year neurodevelopmental follow-up study, induction of labor and expectant management had similar developmental and behavioral outcomes.[158] Drawing clinical strategies about timing delivery of the late preterm/early term IUGR fetus from the DIGITAT trial is limited by an absence of Doppler interrogation of these fetuses. Umbilical artery Doppler was performed in the trial, and only 10% of cases were affected, which has been a previously described finding in late IUGR. However, the MCA Doppler may be the only abnormal Doppler finding in late IUGR, and it is suggestive of fetal hypoxemia, and these were not reported. This type of information may help distinguish between the constitutionally small fetus at or near term that may benefit from delivery at 39 weeks versus the pathologically small fetus that may benefit from earlier delivery. As such, the guidelines provided by the American College of Obstetricians and Gynecologists that recommends delivery of the otherwise uncomplicated (absence of maternal comorbidity, normal umbilical artery Dopplers, and amniotic fluid) late IUGR fetus between 38 0/7 and 39 6/7 weeks is reasonable, at least until other studies show benefit of earlier delivery.[159]

Figure 3.22 depicts an algorithm for the management of IUGR that is intended to serve as a guideline. The guideline begins with the most common definition used clinically for diagnosis of IUGR: an EFW of <10th percentile for gestation. Ascertainment of pregnancy dating remains a cornerstone for the correct diagnosis, something that at times is not possible when patients present late in gestation for prenatal care. A surveillance approach is outlined using BPPs, NST, and Doppler velocimetry tools. As previously discussed in this chapter, the BPP may be used prior to 28 weeks as a primary tool for fetal surveillance since the FHR tracing may not show reactivity; however, a FHR tracing may still be used to see whether variable or late decelerations are present. As mentioned above, the umbilical artery Doppler may not become abnormal in late-onset IUGR, whereas the MCA Doppler may become abnormal. Thus, the algorithm incorporates the use of Dopplers in both types of vessels to evaluate near-term or term IUGR. Once absent or reversed umbilical artery diastolic flow or oligohydramnios are present, hospitalization is suggested for further evaluation and surveillance. In some cases, IUGR may precede the development of preeclampsia in the mother. The triggers for delivery are divided into gestational age epochs based on the knowledge that IUGR fetuses have less morbidity and mortality at certain gestational ages. The recent publication on multivessel fetal Dopplers from the PORTO trial showed that the interval of a Doppler abnormality to the time of delivery can be roughly predicted by the specific abnormality seen. For example, reverse flow in the umbilical artery has a very short interval to delivery (mean of 5 days), while an abnormal umbilical artery PI is nearly 40 days.[160] An abnormal MCA carried a mean interval to delivery of 30 days, while the DV interval was about 37 days. While this is useful for counseling, in reality, there are many variables that need to be taken into account that can shorten or lengthen the interval to delivery. Beyond 34 weeks, delivery is recommended for persistent oligohydramnios or anhydramnios, absence of interval growth, or for absent end-diastolic velocity in the umbilical artery. For IUGR fetus with isolated oligohydramnios beyond 34 weeks, timing the delivery can be individualized, and the American College of Obstetricians and Gynecologists has recommended delivery anytime between 34 0/7 and 37 6/7 weeks.[159] Finally, when delivery is anticipated prior to 34 weeks, the following should be considered: (1) betamethasone administration to reduce complications of prematurity and improve outcomes,[161–164] (2) magnesium sulfate administration for neuroprotection based on published protocols,[165–167] and (3) delivery at a facility that has neonatal intensive care unit capabilities.[168]

## Doppler Abnormalities and Long-Term Neurologic Outcome

There are few studies relating neurodevelopment to antenatal surveillance parameters including Doppler studies. A 2004 study consisting primarily of preterm growth-restricted pregnancies and that evaluated developmental outcomes for two years reported that gestational age at delivery, birthweight, and reversal of umbilical artery end-diastolic velocity were the main determinants of motor and neurosensory morbidity. Fetal deterioration of venous Doppler or biophysical parameters did not have an impact on neurodevelopment.[149] Furthermore, a recent study assessed the long-term (age 6 to 13 years of age) impact on neurologic outcomes that were reported for the GRIT study. This was a randomized clinical trial of immediate versus delayed delivery of IUGR fetuses with the majority born <34 weeks. Cognitive development was identical in both groups. In short, these findings are concerning in that they suggest that the intrauterine environment has a significant impact on neurodevelopment before delivery criteria arise and, accordingly, it suggests that any neurologic injury may already be set by the time delivery is required and that it may not be mitigated by any specific delivery criteria.[150] There are few data on long-term neurologic outcomes and delivery timing in late IUGR fetuses. A two-year follow-up study from patients enrolled in the DIGITAT trial concluded that in term IUGR fetuses, neither a policy of labor induction nor one of expectant management has an effect on developmental or behavioral outcomes.[158] This study did not report on Doppler findings. As previously mentioned, changes in the MCA Doppler may be the only Doppler changes noted in late IUGR fetuses, and these may be associated with neurologic sequelae.[98,99] Currently, there is insufficient evidence to warrant early delivery of the IUGR fetus <36 weeks for the sole purpose of reducing neurologic injury.

## Doppler Velocimetry Reference Ranges

Longitudinal reference ranges for Doppler velocimetry flow velocities and indices for the uterine arteries, umbilical arteries, MCA, and DV are shown in Appendix A1 in Tables 48-57.

## REFERENCES

1. Resnik R. Intrauterine growth restriction. *Obstet Gynecol.* 2002;99:490–496.
2. Pallotto EK, Kilbride HW. Perinatal outcome and later implications of intrauterine growth restriction. *Clin Obstet Gynecol.* 2006;49:257–269.
3. Barker DJ. Adult consequences of fetal growth restriction. *Clin Obstet Gynecol.* 2006;49:270–283.
4. ACOG Committee on Practice Bulletins. ACOG practice bulletin number 77: screening for fetal chromosomal abnormalities. *Obstet Gynecol.* 2007;109:217–227.
5. Firth HV, Boyd PA, Chamberlain P, et al. Severe limb abnormalities after chorion villus sampling at 56–66 days of gestation. *Lancet.* 1991;337:762–763.
6. Sundberg K, Bang J, Smidt-Jensen S, et al. Randomized study of the risk of fetal loss related to early amniocentesis versus chorionic villus sampling. *Lancet.* 1997;350:697–703.
7. Matsumoto S, Nogami Y, Ohkuri S. Statistical studies on menstruation: a criticism on the definition of normal menstruation. *J Med Sci.* 1962;11:294.
8. Batzer IR, Weiner S, Corson SL, et al. Landmarks during the first forty-two days of gestation demonstrated by the beta-subunit of human chorionic gonadotropin and ultrasound. *Am J Obstet Gynecol.* 1983;146:973–979.
9. MacGregor SN, Tamura RK, Sabbagha RE, et al. Underestimation of gestational age by conventional crown-rump length dating curves. *Obstet Gynecol.* 1987;70:344–348.
10. Daya S. Accuracy of gestational age estimation by means of fetal crown-rump length measurement. *Am J Obstet Gynecol.* 1993;168:903–908.
11. Hadlock RP, Shah YP, Kanon DJ, et al. Fetal crown-rump length: reevaluation of relation to menstrual age (5–18 weeks) with high resolution real-time US. *Radiology.* 1992;182:501–505.
12. Bukowski R, Smith GC, Malone FD, et al. Fetal growth in early pregnancy and risk of delivering low birth weight infant: prospective cohort study. *BMJ.* 2007;334:836.
13. Hackmon R, LeScale KB, Horani J, et al. Is severe macrosomia manifested at 11–14 weeks of gestation? *Ultrasound Obstet Gynecol.* 2008;32:740–743.
14. Selbing A. Gestational age and ultrasonic measurement of gestational sac, crown-rump length and biparietal diameter during first 15 weeks of pregnancy. *Acta Obstet Gynecol Scand.* 1982;61:233–235.
15. Silva PD, Mahairas G, Schaper AM, et al. Early crown-rump length: a good predictor of gestational age. *J Reprod Med.* 1990;35:641–644.
16. Wu FS, Hwu YM, Lee RK, et al. First trimester ultrasound estimation of gestational age in pregnancies conceived after in vitro fertilization. *Eur J Obstet Gynecol Reprod Biol.* 2012;160:151–155.
17. Chalouhi GE, Bernard JP, Benoist G, et al. A comparison of first trimester measurements for prediction of delivery date. *J Matern Fetal Neonatal Med.* 2011;24:51–57.
18. Shepard M, Filly RA. A standarized plane for biparietal diameter measurement. *J Ultrasound Med.* 1982;1:145–150.
19. Hadlock FP, Harrist RB, Martinez-Poyer J. How accurate is second trimester fetal dating? *J Ultrasound Med.* 1991;10:557–561.
20. Persson PH, Weldner BM. Reliability of ultrasound fetometry estimating gestational age in the second trimester. *Acta Obstet Gynecol Scand.* 1986;65:481–483.
21. Rossavik IK, Fishburne JI. Conceptual age, menstrual age, and ultrasound age: a second-trimester compariso of pregnancies of know conception datewith pregnancies dated from the last menstrual period. *Obstet Gynecol.* 1989;73:243–249.
22. De Crespigny LC, Speirs AL. A new look at biparietal diameter. *Aust N Z J Obstet Gynaecol.* 1989;29(1):26–29.
23. Benson CB, Doubilet PM. Sonographic prediction of gestational age: accuracy of second- and third-trimester fetal measurements. *AJR Am J Roentgenol.* 1991;157:1275–1277.
24. Hadlock FP, Deter RL, Harrist RB, et al. The effect of head shape on the accuracy of BPD in estimating fetal gestational age. *AJR Am J Roentgenol.* 1981;137:83–85.
25. Law RG, MacRae KD. Head circumference as an index of fetal age. *J Ultrasound Med.* 1982;1:281–288.
26. Chavez MF, Ananath CV, Smulian JC, et al. Fetal transcerebellar diameter measurement with particular emphasis in the third trimester: a reliable predictor of gestational age. *Am J Obstet Gynecol.* 2004;191:979–984.
27. Chavez MR, Ananth CV, Smulian JC, et al. Fetal transcerebellar diameter measurement for prediction of gestational age at the extremes of fetal growth. *J Ultrasound Med.* 2007;26:1167–1171.
28. Vinkesteijn AS, Jansen CL, Los FJ, et al. Fetal transcerebellar diameter and chromosomal abnormalities. *Ultrasound Obstet Gynecol.* 2001;17:502–505.
29. Gottlieb AG, Galan HL. Nontraditional sonographic pearls in estimating gestational age. *Semin Perinatol.* 2006;32(3):154–160.
30. Meirowitz NB, Ananth CV, Smulian JC, et al. Foot length in fetuses with abnormal growth. *J Ultrasound Med.* 2000;19:201–205.
31. Campbell S, Wilkins D. Ultrasonic measurement of fetal abdomen circumference in the estimation of fetal weight. *Br J Obstet Gynaecol.* 1975;82:689–697.
32. Warsof SL, Gohari P, Berkowitz RL, et al. The estimation of fetal weight by computer-assisted analysis. *Am J Obstet Gynecol.* 1977;128:881–892.
33. Thurnau GR, Tamura RK, Sabbagha R, et al. A simple estimated fetal weight equation based on real-time ultrasound measurements of fetuses less than thirty-four weeks' gestation. *Am J Obstet Gynecol.* 1983;145:557–561.
34. Vintzileos AM, Campbell WA, Rodis JF, et al. Fetal weight estimation formulas with head, abdominal, femur, and thigh circumference measurements. *Am J Obstet Gynecol.* 1987;157:410–414.
35. Hadlock FP, Harrist RB, Carpenter RJ, et al. Sonographic estimation of fetal weight: the value of femurlength in addition to head and abdomen measurements. *Radiology.* 1984;150:535–540.
36. Shepard MJ, Richards VA, Berkowitz RL, et al. An evaluation of two equations for predicting fetal weight by ultrasound. *Am J Obstet Gynecol.* 1982;142:47–54.
37. Weiner CP, Sabbagha RE, Vaisrub N, et al. Ultrasonic fetal weight prediction: role of head circumference and femur length. *Obstet Gynecol.* 1985;65:812–817.
38. Hadlock FP, Harrist RB, Sharman RS, et al. Estimation of fetal weight with the use of head, body, and femur measurements: a prospective study. *Am J Obstet Gynecol.* 1985;151:333–337.
39. Ott WJ, Doyle S, Flamm S, et al. Accurate ultrasonic estimation of fetal weight: prospective analysis of new ultrasonic formulas. *Am J Perinatol.* 1986;3:307–310.
40. Combs CA, Jaekle RK, Rosenn B, et al. Sonographic estimation of fetal weight based on a model of fetal volume. *Obstet Gynecol.* 1993;82:365–370.
41. Rose BI, McCallum WD. A simplified method for estimating fetal weight using ultrasound measurements. *Obstet Gynecol.* 1987;69:671–675.
42. Gandhi M, Ferrara L, Belogolovkin V, et al. Effect of increased body mass index on the accuracy of estimated fetal weight by sonography in twins. *J Ultrasound Med.* 2009;28:301–308.
43. Anderson NG, Jolley IJ, Wells JE. Sonographic estimation of fetal weight: comparison of bias, precision and consistency using 12 different formulae. *Ultrasound Obstet Gynecol.* 2007;30:173–179.
44. Edwards A, Goff J, Baker L. Accuracy and modifying factors of the sonographic estimation of fetal weight in a high-risk population. *Aust N Z J Obstet Gynaecol.* 2001;41:187–190.
45. Dudley N. A systematic review of the ultrasound estimation of fetal weight. *Ultrasound Obstet Gynecol.* 2005;25:80–90.

46. Schild RL, Sachs C, Fimmers R, et al. Sex-specific fetal weight prediction by ultrasound. *Ultrasound Obstet Gynecol.* 2004;23:30–35.

47. Siemer J, Egger N, Hart N, et al. Fetal weight estimation by ultrasound: comparison of 11 different formulae and examiners with differing skill levels. *Ultraschall Med.* 2008;29:159–164.

48. Burd I, Srinivas S, Paré E, et al. Is sonographic assessment of fetal weight influenced by formula selection? *J Ultrasound Med.* 2009;28:1019–1024.

49. Ben-Haroush A, Yogev Y, Bar J. Accuracy of sonographically estimated fetal weight in 840 women with different pregnancy complications prior to induction of labor. *Ultrasound Obstet Gynecol.* 2004;23:172–176.

50. Melamed N, Yogev Y, Meizner I, et al. Sonographic fetal weight estimation: which model should be used? *J Ultrasound Med.* 2009;28:617–629.

51. Proctor LK, Rushworth V, Shah PS, et al. Incorporation of femur length leads to underestimation of fetal weight in asymmetric preterm growth restriction. *Ultrasound Obstet Gynecol.* 2010;35:442–448.

52. Hart N, Hilbert A, Meurer B. Macrosomia: a new formula for optimized fetal weight estimation. *Ultrasound Obstet Gynecol.* 2010;35:42–47.

53. Hoopmann M, Abele H, Wagner N, et al. Performance of 36 different weight estimation formulae in fetuses with macrosomia. *Fetal Diagn Ther.* 2010;27:204–213.

54. Chen P, Yu J, Li X, et al. Weight estimation for low birth weight fetuses and macrosomic fetuses in Chinese population. *Arch Gynecol Obstet.* 2011;284:599–606.

55. Lee W, Balasubramaniam M, Deter RL, et al. New fetal weight estimation models using fractional limb volume. *Ultrasound Obstet Gynecol.* 2009;34:556–565.

56. Pagani G, Palai N, Zatti S, et al. Fetal weight estimation in gestational diabetic pregnancies: comparison between conventional and three-dimensional fractional thigh volume methods using gestation-adjusted projection. *Ultrasound Obstet Gynecol.* 2014;43(1):72–76 doi:10.1002/uog.12458.

57. Battaglia FC, Lubchenco LO. A practical classification of newborn infants by weight and gestational age. *J Pediatr.* 1967;71:159–163.

58. Hulsey TC, Levkoff AH, Alexander GR, et al. Differences in black and white infant birth weights: the role of maternal demographic factors and medical complications of pregnancy. *South Med J.* 1991;84:443–446.

59. Goldenberg RL, Cliver SP, Cutter GR. Black-white differences in new born anthropometric measurements. *Obstet Gynecol.* 1991;78:782–788.

60. Yip R, Li Z, Chong WH. Race and birth weight: the Chinese example. *Pediatrics.* 1991;87:688–693.

61. Alver J, Brooke OG. Fetal growth in different racial groups. *Arch Dis Child.* 1978;53:27–32.

62. Graafmans WC, Richardus JH, Borsboom GJ, et al. Birth weight and perinatal mortality: a comparison of "optimal" birth weight in seven Western European countries. *Epidemiology.* 2002;13:569–574.

63. Hemming K, Hutton JL, Glinianaia SV, et al. Differences between European birthweight standards: impact on classification of "small for gestational age". *Dev Med Child Neurol.* 2006;48:906–912.

64. Lubhcneco L. Classification of high risk infants by birth weight and gestational age: an overview. *Major Probl Clin Pediatr.* 1976;14:1–279.

65. Ott WJ. Intrauterine growth retardation and preterm delivery. *Am J Obstet Gynecol.* 1993;168:1710–1715.

66. Hadlock FP, Harrist RB, Martinez-Poyer J. In utero analysis of fetal growth: a sonograpic weight standard. *Radiology.* 1991;181:129–133.

67. Bernstein IM, Mohs G, Rocquoi M, et al. Case for hybrid "fetal growth curves": a population-based estimation of normal fetal size across gestational age. *J Matern Fetal Med.* 1996;5:124–127.

68. Salomon LJ, Bernard JP, Ville Y. Estimation of fetal weight: reference range at 20–36 weeks' gestation and comparison with actual birth weight reference range. *Ultrasound Obstet Gynecol.* 2007;29:550–555.

69. Lackman F, Capewell V, Richardson B, et al. The risks of spontaneous preterm delivery and perinatal mortality in relation to size at birth according to fetal versus neonatal growth standards. *Am J Obstet Gynecol.* 2001;184:946–953.

70. Zaw W, Gagnon R, da Silva O. The risks of adverse neonatal outcome among preterm small for gestational age infants according to neonatal versus fetal growth standards. *Pediatrics.* 2003;111:1273–1277.

71. Gardosi J, Mongelli M, Wilcox M, et al. An adjustable fetal weight standard. *Ultrasound Obstet Gynecol.* 1995;6:168–174.

72. Wilcox MA, Newton CS, Johnson IR. Paternal influences on birthweight. *Acta Obstet Gynecol Scand.* 1995;74(1):15–18.

73. Gardosi J. Customized fetal growth standards: rationale and clinical application. *Semin Perinatol.* 2004;28:33–40.

74. Clausson B, Gardosi J, Francis A, et al. Perinatal outcome in SGA births defined by customized versus population-based birth weight standards. *Br J Obstet Gynecol.* 2001;108:830–834.

75. Ego A, Subtil D, Gilles G, et al. Customized versus population based birth weight standards for identifying growth restricted infants: a French multicenter study. *Am J Obstet Gynecol.* 2006;194:1042–1049.

76. Figueras F, Figueras J, Meler E, et al. Customised birth weight standards accurately predict perinatal morbidity. *Arch Dis Child Fetel Neonatal Ed.* 2007;92:F277–F280.

77. Odibo AO, Francis A, Cahill AG, et al. Association between pregnancy complications and small-for-gestational-age birth weight defined by customized fetal growth standard versus a population-based standard. *J Matern Fetal Neonatal Med.* 2011;24:411–417.

78. Obido AO, Cahill AG, Goetzinger KR, et al. Customized growth charts for twin gestations to optimize identification of small-for-gestational age fetuses at risk of intrauterine fetal death. *Ultrasound Obstet Gynecol.* 2013;41:637–642.

79. Hutcheon JA, Zhang X, Cnattingius S, et al. Customised birthweight percentiles: does adjusting for maternal characteristics matter? *Br J Obstet Gynecol.* 2008;115:1397–1404.

80. Baker PN, Johnson IR, Gowland PA. Measurement of fetal liver, brain and placental volumes with echo-planar magnetic resonance imaging. *Br J Obset Gynaecol.* 1995;102(1):35–39.

81. Duncan KR, Issa B, Moore R. A comparison of fetal organ measurements by echo-planar magnetic resonance imaging and ultrasound. *BJOG.* 2005;112(1):43–49.

82. Damodaram MS, Story L, Eixarch E. Foetal volumetry using magnetic resonance imaging in intrauterine growth restriction. *Hum Dev.* 2012;88(suppl 1):S35–S40.

83. Fitzgerald DE, Drumm JE. Non-invasive measurement of human fetal circulation using ultrasound: a new method. *Br Med J.* 1977;2(6100):1450–1451.

84. Trudinger BJ, Giles WB, Cook CM. Uterioplacental blood flow velocity-time waveforms in normal and complicated pregnancy. *Br J Obstet Gynaecol.* 1985;92:39–45.

85. Giles WB, Trudinger BJ, Baird PJ. Fetal umbilical artery flow velocity waveforms and placental resistance: pathologic correlation. *Br J Obstet Gynaecol.* 1985;92:31–38.

86. Kingdom JC, Burrell SJ, Kaufmann P. Pathology and clinical implications of abnormal umbilical artery Doppler waveforms. *Ultrasound Obstet Gynecol.* 1997;9:271–286.

87. Morrow RJ, Adamson SL, Bull SB, et al. Effect of placental embolization on the umbilical arterial velocity waveform in fetal sheep. *Am J Obstet Gynecol.* 1989;161:1055–1060.

88. Nicolaides KH, Bilardo CM, Soothill PW, et al. Absence of end diastolic frequencies in umbilical artery: a sign of fetal hypoxia and acidosis. *BMJ.* 1988;297:1026–1027.

89. Bilardo CM, Nicolaides KH, Campbell S. Doppler measurements of fetal and uteroplacental circulations: relationship with umbilical venous blood gases measured at cordocentesis. *Am J Obstet Gynecol.* 1990;162:115–120.

90. Pardi G, Cetin I, Marconi AM, et al. Diagnostic value of blood sampling in fetuses with growth retardation. *N Engl J Med.* 1993;328:692–696.

91. Thornton JG, Lilford RJ. Do we need randomized trials of antenatal tests of fetal wellbeing? *Br J Obstet Gynaecol.* 1993;100(3):197–200.

92. Gudmundsson S, Tulzer G, Huhta JC, et al. Venous Doppler in the fetus with absent end-diastolic flow in the umbilical artery. *Ultrasound Obstet Gynecol.* 1996;7(4):262–267.

93. Wladimiroff JW, Tonge HM, Steward PA. Doppler ultrasound assessment of cerebral blood flow in the human fetus. *Br J Obstet Gynaecol.* 1986;93(5):471–475.

94. Mari G, Deter RL. Middle cerebral artery flow velocity in waveforms in normal and small-for-gestational-age fetuses. *Am J Obstet Gynecol.* 1992;166(4):1262–1270.

95. Gramellini D, Folli MC, Raboni S, et al. Cerebral-umbilical Doppler ratio as a predictor of adverse perinatal outcome. *Obstet Gynecol.* 1992;79(3):416–420.

96. Arbeille P, Roncin A, Berson M, et al. Exploration of the fetal cerebral flow by duplex Doppler linear array system in normal and pathological pregnancies. *Ultrasound Med Biol.* 1987;13:329–337.

97. Bahado-Singh RO, Kovanci E, Jeffres A et al. The Doppler cerebroplacental ratio and perinatal outcome in intrauterine growth restriction. *Am J Obstet Gynecol.* 1999;180:750–756.

98. Oros D, Figueras F, Cruz-Martinez R, et al. Middle versus anterior cerebral artery Doppler for the prediction of perinatal outcome and neonatal neurobehavior in term small-for-gestational age fetuses with normal umbilical artery Doppler. *Ultrasound Obstet Gynecol.* 2010;35:456–461.

99. Eixarch E, Meler E, Iraola A, et al. Neurodevelopmental outcome in 2-year-old infants who were small-for-gestational age term fetuses with cerebral blood flow redistribution. *Ultrasound Obstet Gynecol.* 2008;32:894–899.

100. Cruz-Martinez R, Figueras F, Hernandez-Andrade E, et al. Fetal brain Doppler to predict cesarean delivery for nonreassuring fetal status in term small-for-gestational age fetuses. *Obstet Gynecol.* 2011;117:618–626.

101. Mavrides E, Moscoso G, Carvalho JS, et al. The anatomy of the umbilical, portal and hepatic venous systems in the human fetus at 14–19 weeks of gestation. *Ultrasound Obstet Gynecol.* 2001;18:598–604.

102. Hecher K, Snijders R, Campbell S, et al. Fetal venous, intracardiac, and arterial blood flow measurements in intrauterine growth retardation: relationship with fetal blood gases. *Am J Obstet Gynecol.* 1995;173:10–15.

103. Rizzo G, Capponi A, Arduini D, et al. The value of fetal arterial, cardiac and venous flows in predicting pH and blood gases measured in umbilical blood at cordocentesis in growth retarded fetuses. *Br J Obstet Gynaecol.* 1995;102:963–969.

104. Zhou Y, Fisher SJ, Janatpour M, et al. Human cytotrophoblasts adopt a vascular phenotype as they differentiate: a strategy for successful endovascular invasion? *J Clin Invest.* 1997;99:2139–2151.

105. Lovgren TR, Dugoff L, Galan HL. Uterine artery Doppler and prediction of preeclampsia. *Clin Obstet Gynecol.* 2010;53(4):888–898.

106. Berkley E, Chauhan SP, Abuhamad A. Doppler assessment of the fetus with intrauterine growth restriction. Society for Maternal-Fetal Medicine Publications Committee. *Am J Obstet Gynecol.* 2012;206(4):300–308.

107. Figueras F, Puerto B, Martinez JM, et al. Cardiac function monitoring of fetuses with growth restriction. *Eur J Obstet Gynecol Reprod Biol.* 2003;110:159–163.

108. Benavides-Serralde A, Scheier M, Cruz-Martinez R, et al. Changes in central and peripheral circulation in intrauterine growth-restricted fetuses at different stages of umbilical artery flow deterioration: new fetal cardiac and brain parameters. *Gynecol Obstet Invest.* 2011;71(4):274–280.

109. Mari G, Hanif F, Kruger M. Sequence of cardiovascular changes in IUGR in pregnancies with and without preeclampsia. *Prenat Diagn.* 2008;28:377–383.

110. Groenenberg IAL, Wladimiroff JW, Hop WCJ. Fetal cardiac and peripheral flow velocity waveforms in intrauterine growth retardation. *Circulation.* 1989;80:1711–1717.

111. Ferrazzi E, Bozzo M, Rigano S, et al. Temporal sequence of abnormal Doppler changes in the peripheral and central circulatory systems of the severely growth-restricted fetus. *Ultrasound Obstet Gynecol.* 2002;19:140–149.

112. Reed KI, Anderson CF, Shenker L. Changes in intracardiac Doppler blood flow velocities in fetuses with absent umbilical artery diastolic flow. *Am J Obstet Gynecol.* 1987;157:774–779.

113. Baschat AA, Gembruch U, Harman CR. Coronary blood flow in fetuses with intrauterine growth restriction. *J Perinat Med.* 1998;26:143–156.

114. Baschat AA, Muench MV, Gembruch U. Coronary artery blood flow velocities in various fetal conditions. *Ultrasound Obstet Gynecol.* 2003;21:426–429.

115. Kenny JF, Plappert T, Doubilet P, et al. Changes in intracardiac blood flow velocities and right and left ventricular stroke volumes with gestational age in the normal human fetus: a prospective Doppler echocardiographic study. *Circulation.* 1986;74:1208–1216.

116. Stottard MF, Pearson AC, Kern MJ, et al. Influence of alteration in preload of left ventricular diastolic filling as assessed by Doppler echocardiography in humans. *Circulation.* 1989;79:1226–1236.

117. Rizzo G, Arduini D, Romanini C. Doppler echocardiographic assessment of fetal cardiac function. *Ultrasound Obstet Gynecol.* 1992;2:434–445.

118. Forouzan I, Graham E, Morgan MA. Reduction of right atrial peak systolic velocity in growth-restricted discordant twins. *Am J Obstet Gynecol.* 1996;175:1033–1035.

119. Al-Ghazali W, Chita SK, Chapman MG, et al. Evidence of redistribution of cardiac output in asymmetrical growth retardation. *Br J Obstet Gynaecol.* 1989;96:697–704.

120. Baschat AA, Gembruch U, Gortner L, et al. Coronary blood flow visualization signifies hemodynamic deterioration in growth-restricted fetuses. *Ultrasound Obstet Gynecol.* 2000;16:425–431.

121. Matthews DD. Maternal assessment of fetal activity in small-for-dates infants. *Obstet Gynecol.* 1975;45:488–493.

122. Chauhan SP, Magann EF, Morrison JC, et al. Ultrasonographic assessment of amniotic fluid does not reflect actual amniotic fluid volume. *Am J Obstet Gynecol.* 1997;177:291–296.

123. Spong CY, Mercer BM, D'Alton M, et al. Timing of indicated late-preterm and early-term birth. *Obstet Gynecol.* 2011;118:323–333.

124. Chauhan SP, Doherty DD, Magann EF, et al. Amniotic fluid index vs. single deepest pocket technique during modified biophysical profile: a randomized clinical trial. *Am J Obstet Gynecol.* 2004;191:661–668.

125. Nabhan AF, Abdelmoula YA. Amniotic fluid index versus single deepest vertical pocket as a screening test for preventing adverse pregnancy outcome. *Cochrane Database Syst Rev.* 2008;16(3):CD006593.

126. Manning FA, Hill LM, Platt LD. Qualitative amniotic fluid volume determination by ultrasound: antepartum detection of intrauterine growth retardation. *Am J Obstet Gynecol.* 1981;139:254–258.

127. Peeters JH, Sheldon RE, Jones MD, et al. Blood flow to fetal organs as a function of arterial oxygen content. *Am J Obstet Gynecol.* 1979;135:637–646.

128. Arabin B, Bergman PL, Saling E. Simultaneous assessment of blood flow velocity in uteroplacental vessels, the umbilical artery, the fetal aorta and the fetal common carotid artery. *Fetal Ther.* 1987;2:17–26.

129. Veille JC, Kanaan C. Duplex Doppler ultrasonography evaluation of the fetal renal artery in normal and abnormal fetuses. *Am J Obstet Gynecol.* 1989;161:1502–1507.

130. Hecher K, Bilardo CM, Stigter RH, et al. Monitoring of fetuses with intrauterine growth restriction: a longitudinal study. *Ultrasound Obstet Gynecol.* 2001;18:564–570.

131. Unterscheider J, Daly S, Geary MP, et al. Optimizing the definition of intrauterine growth restriction: the multicenter prospective PORTO study. *Am J Obstet Gynecol.* 2013;208:290.e1–290.e6.

132. Nageotte MP, Towers CV, Asrat T, et al. Perinatal outcome with the modified biophysical profile. *Am J Obstet Gynecol.* 1994;170(6):1672–1676.

133. Baschat AA, Galan HL, Bhide A, et al. Doppler and biophysical assessment in growth restricted fetuses: distribution of test results. *Ultrasound Obstet Gynecol.* 2006;27:41–47.

134. Arduini D, Rizzo G, Caforio L, et al. Behavioural state transitions in healthy and growth retarded fetuses. *Early Hum Dev.* 1989;19:155.

135. Henson G, Dawes GS, Redman CW. Characterization of the reduced heart rate variation in growth-retarded fetuses. *Br J Obstet Gynaecol.* 1984;91:751.

136. Pillai M, James D. Continuation of normal neurobehavioural development in fetuses with absent umbilical arterial end diastolic velocities. *Br J Obstet Gynaecol.* 1991;98:277–281.

137. Visser GH, Dawes GA, Redman CW. Numerical analysis of the normal human antenatal fetal heart rate. *Br J Obstet Gynaecol.* 1981;88:792–802.

138. Ribben LS, Nicolaides KH, Visser GH. Prediction of fetal acidaemia in intrauterine growth retardation: comparison of quantified fetal activity with biophysical profile score. *Br J Obstet Gynaecol.* 1993;100:653–656.

139. Baschat AA, Gembruch U, Harman CR. The sequence of changes in Doppler and biophysical parameters as severe fetal growth restriction worsens. *Ultrasound Obstet Gynecol.* 2001;18:571–577.

140. Vintzileos AM, Fleming AD, Scorza WE, et al. Relationship between fetal biophysical activities and umbilical cord blood gas values. *Am J Obstet Gynecol.* 1991;165:707–713.

141. Ott WJ. The diagnosis of altered fetal growth. *Obstet Cynecol Clin North Am.* 1988;15:237–263.

142. McIntire DD, Bloom SL, Casey BM, et al. Birth weight in relation to morbidity and mortality among newborn infants. *N Engl J Med.* 1999;340:1234–1238.

143. Baschat AA, Cosmi E, Bilardo CM, et al. Predictors of neonatal outcome in early-onset placental dysfunction. *Obstet Gynecol.* 2007;109:253–261.

144. Garite TJ, Clark R, Thorp JA. Intrauterine growth restriction increases morbidity and mortality among premature neonates. *Am J Obstet Gynecol.* 2004;191:481–487.

145. Mari G, Hanif F, Treadwell MC, et al. Gestational age at delivery and Doppler waveforms in very preterm intrauterine growth-restricted fetuses as predictors of perinatal mortality. *J Ultrasound Med.* 2007;26(5):555–559.

146. Alfirevic Z, Stampalija T, Gyte GM. Fetal and umbilical Doppler ultrasound in high-risk pregnancies. *Cochrane Database Syst Rev.* 2010;20(1):CD007529.

147. American College of Obstetricians and Gynecologists. Committee on Obstetric Practice. Utility of antepartum umbilical artery Doppler velocimetry in intrauterine growth restriction. Committee Opinion No 188. October 1997.

148. The Grit Study Group. A randomized trial of timed delivery for the compromised preterm fetus: short term outcomes and Bayesian interpretation. *Br J Obstet Gynaecol* 2003;110(1):27–32.

149. The Grit Study Group. Infant wellbeing at 2 years of age in the Growth Restriction Intervention Trial (GRIT): multicentred randomized controlled trial. *Lancet.* 2004;364:513–520.

150. Walker DM, Marlow N, Upstone L, et al. The growth restriction intervention trial: long-term outcomes in a randomized trial of timing of delivery in fetal growth restriction. *Am J Obstet Gynecol.* 2011;204:34.e1–34.e9.

151. Groome LJ, Owen J, Neely CL, et al. Oligohydramnios: antepartum fetal urine production and intrapartum fetal distress. *Am J Obstet Gynecol.* 1991;165:1077–1080.

152. Peipert JF, Donnenfeld AE. Oligohydramnios: a review. *Obstet Gynecol Surv.* 1991;46(6):325–339.

153. Froen JF, Gardosi JO, Thurmann A, et al. Restricted fetal growth in sudden intrauterine unexplained death. *Acta Obstet Gynecol Scand.* 2004;83:801–807.

154. Vergani P, Roncaglia N, Ghidini A, et al. Can adverse neonatal outcome be predicted in late preterm or term fetal growth restriction? *Ultrasound Obstet Gynecol.* 2010;36:166–170.

155. Trudell AS, Cahill AG, Methodius G, et al. Risk of stillbirth after 37 weeks in pregnancies complicated by small-for-gestational-age fetuses. *Am J Obstet Gynecol.* 2013;208:376.e1–376.e7.

156. Boers KE, Vijgen SMC, Bijlenga D, et al. Induction versus expectant monitoring for intrauterine growth restriction at term: randomised equivalence trial (DIGITAT). *BMJ.* 2010;341:c7087.

157. Boers KE, van Wyk L, van der Post JAM. Neonatal morbidity after induction vs expectant monitoring in intrauterine growth restriction at term: a subanalysis of the DIGITAT RCT. *Am J Obstet Gynecol.* 2012;206:344.e1–344.e7.

158. Van Wyk L, Boers KE, van der Post JAM, et al. Effects on (neuro)developmental and behavioral outcome at 2 years of age of induced labor compared with expectant management in intrauterine growth-restricted infants: long-term outcomes of the DIGITAT trial. *Am J Obstet Gynecol.* 2012;206:406.e1–406.e7.

159. American College of Obstetricians and Gynecologists. Medically indicated late-preterm and early-term deliveries. Committee Opinion No 560. *Obstet Gynecol.* 2013;121:908–910.

160. Unterscheider J, Daly S, Geary MP, et al. Predictable progressive Doppler deterioration in IUGR: does it really exist? *Am J Obstet Gynecol.* 2013;209:539.e1–539.e7.

161. Effect of corticosteroids for fetal maturation on perinatal outcomes. *NIH Consens Statement.* 1994;12(2):1–24.

162. Antenatal corticosteroids revisited: repeat courses. *NIH Consens Statement.* 2000;17:1–18.

163. Roberts D, Dalziel SR. Antenatal corticosteroids for accelerating fetal lung maturation for women at risk of preterm birth. *Cochrane Database Syst Rev.* 2006;(3):CD00445.

164. Bernstein IM, Horbar JD, Badger GJ, et al. Morbidity and mortality among very-low-birth-weight neonates with intrauterine growth restriction. The Vermont Oxford Network. *Am J Obstet Gynecol.* 2000;182:198–206.

165. American College of Obstetricians and Gynecologists. Magnesium sulfate before anticipated preterm birth for neuroprotection. Committee Opinion No 455. *Obstet Gynecol.* 2010;115:669–671.

166. Marret S, Marpeau L, Zupan-Simunetk V, et al. Magnesium sulphate given before very-preterm birth to protect infant brain: the randomized controlled PREMAG trial. PREMAG Trial Group. *BJOG.* 2007;114:310–318.

167. Rouse DJ, Hirtz DG, Thorn E, et al. A randomized controlled trial of magnesium sulfate for the prevention of cerebral palsy. Eunice Kennedy Shriver NICHD Maternal-Fetal Medicine Units network. *N Engl J Med.* 2008;359:895–905.

168. American College of Obstetricians and Gynecologists. ACOG practice bulletin no. 134: fetal growth restriction. *Obstet Gynecol.* 2013;121(5):1122–1133.

# 4 Normal Fetal Heart Survey

Jodi I. Pike • Anita Krishnan • Mary T. Donofrio

Structural cardiac disease is the most commonly diagnosed congenital malformation. The incidence of congenital heart disease (CHD) has been estimated to be between 6 and 12 per 1,000 live births,[1–4] or approximately 1% of the general population. It is likely that the incidence prenatally is much higher, given that some pregnancies affected by CHD are terminated and other fetuses may die in utero. One study from Belgium[5] reported a CHD incidence of 8.3% in chromosomally normal infants born at 26 weeks gestation.

## INDICATIONS FOR REFERRAL

There are many fetal, maternal, and familial factors that can increase the risk of CHD in the fetus above that of the general population (Table 4.1). It is often these fetuses who are referred for additional cardiac evaluation beyond the routine mid-gestation obstetric ultrasound. All of these indications for referral increase the risk of identifying CHD somewhat above that of the general population, but with varying effects on relative risk.

### Maternal Factors

#### Diabetes Mellitus

Pregestational diabetes mellitus (DM) is found in approximately 1% of all pregnant women and, in the fetuses of these women, approximately 3% to 5% show CHD, which is significantly higher than the general population.[6] There are conflicting data regarding whether or not strict glycemic control prior to pregnancy affects the incidence of CHD.[7,8] As the fetal heart is fully formed within the first trimester of pregnancy, and gestational DM usually does not develop until the third trimester, it is not considered to be a reason for routine fetal cardiac evaluation. However, some fetuses may develop ventricular hypertrophy in the setting of poor glycemic control. Gestational diabetes, acquired late in pregnancy, is not thought to carry a risk of CHD[9]; however, there may be women with pregestational diabetes not uncovered until pregnancy whose fetuses are at risk for CHD.

#### Autoimmune Disease

Maternal autoimmune disease such as systemic lupus erythematosus (SLE) and Sjogren syndrome have been shown to be associated with congenital complete heart block (CHB) in the fetus, especially in those women demonstrating the autoantibodies anti-Ro/SSA and/or anti-La/SSB, and even in the setting of a mother who demonstrates no clinical symptoms of autoimmune disease. The incidence of CHB can be as low as 1% in those with no previously affected fetuses, but rise to nearly 20% in those with a previously affected child. Although there is no consensus regarding initiation and frequency of monitoring, antibody-positive women are usually referred for serial fetal heart evaluation between 16 and 28 weeks gestation. This includes structural and functional assessment, as well as measurement of the mechanical PR interval to evaluate for first- or second-degree heart block.[10] The mechanical PR interval (Fig. 4.1) measures the time for the electrical signal to travel from the atria to the ventricle. It has been hypothesized that prolongation of this measurement may represent an early marker of inflammation of the conduction system, though multiple studies have shown reversal to normal sinus rhythm with no intervention. The types of structural disease and arrhythmias associated with anti-SSA antibodies include ventricular arrhythmias,[11] sinus bradycardia,[12,13] junctional ectopic tachycardia,[14] structural cardiac disease,[15,16] valve regurgitation,[17–19] and aortic root dilation.[20,21] Multicenter collaborations in this area may lead to a consensus regarding standardized management of anti-SSA antibody exposed fetuses, but it is clear that evaluation of more than heart rate and PR interval is needed.

#### Medication Exposure

Fetal exposure to many different maternal medications has been shown to increase the risk of CHD in the fetus. This is dependent on the potential teratogenicity of the substance, when during gestation the fetus is exposed, and how likely it is to cross the placenta in significant quantities. Maternal medications that have been shown to lead to an increased risk of CHD in the fetus include anticonvulsants such as carbamazepine,[22] lithium (though more recent literature has suggested that the relative risk is not as high as initially thought),[23,24] retinoic acid,[25] antihypertensives such as ACE inhibitors,[26] selective

| Table 4.1 | Indications for Fetal Echocardiography |
| --- | --- |

Maternal or Familial Factors
Hereditary disorders of connective tissue disease, i.e., Marfan syndrome
In vitro fertilization
Maternal CHD or heart disease in a first-degree relative
Maternal systemic disease (DM, phenylketonuria, carriage of anti-SSA or anti-SSB antibodies)
Maternal teratogenic exposure
Assisted reproductive technologies
Fetal Factors
Suspected cardiac disease on prior imaging
Suspected cardiac arrhythmia
Fetal chromosomal abnormality
Fetal genetic syndrome
Fetal extracardiac anomaly
Increased nuchal translucency
Nonimmune hydrops fetalis
Single umbilical artery
Monochorionic twin gestation (concern for twin–twin transfusion syndrome)
Unexplained polyhydramnios

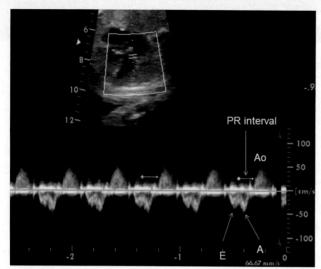

**FIGURE 4.1:** The mechanical PR or AV interval corresponds to the ECG measurement of the *PR interval*, the time for the electrical impulse to travel from atrium to ventricle. A pulse waved Doppler is placed to simultaneously sample mitral inflow and aortic outflow in the four-chamber view. The mitral inflow during diastole consists of two phases, *E* or passive filling and *A* or active atrial contraction. *Ao* indicates aortic outflow during ventricular systole. The PR interval is measured from the beginning of the mitral A wave to the beginning of the aortic ejection phase. Normative data for 2 and 3 standard deviations exist in the literature.

serotonin reuptake inhibitors,[27] and nonsteroidal anti-inflammatory drugs.[28]

### Metabolic Diseases

Uncontrolled phenylketonuria may lead to an increased risk of CHD in the fetus.[29,30] Phenylketonuria, with elevated phenylalanine level >10 mg per dL may carry up to 12% to 14% risk of CHD for the fetus.

### Viral Infections

Maternal rubella,[31] parvovirus, or other infections, including coxsackievirus,[32] adenovirus, and cytomegalovirus, can have adverse effects on fetal myocardial function. HIV is not associated with structural CHD[23]; however, fetuses of HIV-infected women may have alterations of left ventricular function.[33] Parvovirus infection is a common cause of nonimmune hydrops fetalis in the fetus. It can cause direct myocardial damage, with reports of conduction system disease,[34] or fetal anemia with secondary congestive heart failure. Cardiovascular changes can include chamber dilation, ventricular thickening, and valvular regurgitation.

### Assisted Reproductive Technology

An increasingly common indication for fetal echocardiography is the use of assisted reproductive technologies such as in vitro fertilization (IVF), which may or may not be combined with intracytoplasmic sperm injection (ICSI). It is difficult to accurately assess the increase in risk imposed by IVF and/or ICSI on the development of CHD in the fetus, as its use is often more common in mothers of advanced parental age and also leads to an increased risk of monozygous twins, both of which can slightly increase the incidence of CHD. Regardless, the risk of CHD in infants conceived through such assisted reproductive

technologies is considered increased and is an indication for fetal echocardiography.[35–37]

### Family History

Another common indication for fetal cardiac evaluation is a family history of CHD. The incidence of recurrence in subsequent family members can vary depending on what the relationship of the fetus to the proband is, and what the nature of the CHD is. The highest risk of recurrence occurs when CHD is present in the mother of the fetus, and fetal echocardiography is indicated in all such cases.[38,39] The increase in risk overall is 3% to 7%, but is lesion-dependent, with the most pronounced increase for lesions of atrioventricular septal defect (10% to 14%) and aortic stenosis (13% to 18%). There is also an increased risk of CHD in the fetuses of affected fathers; though the risk of 2% to 3% is not as significant, fetal echocardiography remains reasonable. The recurrence risk for siblings is approximately 3%, though higher for hypoplastic left heart syndrome. The risk to the fetus increases as the number of previously affected siblings increases, and it is not unusual for multiple fetuses of the same parents to be affected with heterotaxy syndrome or aortic valve stenosis.[39] Although fewer data are available for the incidence of recurrence in second-degree relatives of affected patients, the risk is thought to be somewhat above that of the general population, but not significant enough to require routine screening in these fetuses.[38]

### Fetal Factors

Multiple factors relating to the fetus itself can be indications for fetal echocardiography.

### Suspected Fetal Cardiac Disease

The indication for fetal echocardiography yielding the greatest likelihood of CHD is an abnormal four-chamber view on obstetrical ultrasound. The detection rate of the four-chamber view for significant CHD in the fetus is over 40%.[40,41] When outflow tract views are included in the obstetrical screening examination, this number increases to over 50%.[40]

### Suspected Fetal Arrhythmia

All fetuses thought to have an abnormal cardiac rhythm, whether it be tachycardia, bradycardia, or an irregular rhythm, should have a fetal echocardiogram to better assess the specific rhythm abnormality and to diagnose any associated structural heart disease. This can help both in guiding therapy and in evaluating for the underlying cause of the arrhythmia.

### Chromosomal Abnormalities

Previously diagnosed or suspected chromosomal abnormalities that are associated with CHD are a common indication for referral for fetal echocardiography. The incidence of detecting CHD varies with the specific chromosomal abnormality in the fetus.[42] Commonly referred chromosomal abnormalities include Trisomy 21, 18, or 13, DiGeorge syndrome, and Turner syndrome.

### Extracardiac Abnormalities

Even in a genetically normal fetus, extracardiac abnormalities may warrant an echocardiogram. Some abnormalities that are highly associated with CHD in the affected fetus include omphalocele, congenital diaphragmatic hernia, genitourinary abnormalities, and central nervous system abnormalities.[43–46]

### Increased Nuchal Translucency

An increased nuchal translucency found in fetuses between 11 and 14 weeks gestational age has been shown to increase the risk of aneuploidy and other congenital anomalies, including CHD.[47,48] The risk of CHD in the fetus rises with increasing NT, even in the absence of known aneuploidy or other genetic abnormality.[49]

### Vascular Malformations

Vascular abnormalities in the fetus that are indications for fetal cardiac evaluation include a single umbilical artery or absence of the ductus venosus. Single umbilical artery is associated with CHD of various types, and in association with renal and vertebral anomalies in the VACTERL syndrome.

### Twin Pregnancy

Monochorionic twin gestation carries an overall risk of 2% for CHD. A second indication for fetal echocardiography is to evaluate the heart in fetuses with twin–twin transfusion syndrome. If twin–twin transfusion syndrome is present, structural cardiac anomalies including pulmonary valve stenosis have been described.

### Fetal Hydrops

Fetal echocardiography is indicated to rule out structural cardiac disease, arrhythmia, tumor, or vascular anomalies in fetuses with hydrops fetalis. Additionally, scoring systems based on heart size, function, and umbilical Doppler parameters have been created and shown to correlate with outcome.[50]

## FETAL ECHOCARDIOGRAPHY

### Timing and Technical Considerations

Timing of fetal echocardiography can vary depending on the indication for referral. The major cardiac structures are present by 9 weeks, and the developmental sequence has been delineated in anatomic specimens using advanced imaging techniques.[51] During pregnancy, Doppler assessment of cardiac function can be performed in the early first trimester, even before fetal cardiac development is complete.[52] A complete fetal echocardiogram, with the exception of pulmonary vein assessment, is possible at 12 to 16 weeks, with a high level of sensitivity for major CHD.[53] However, in general, screening echocardiography for maternal risk factors such as family history or pregestational DM occurs between 18 and 22 weeks gestational age. Follow-up examinations should be performed whenever the initial cardiac evaluation occurs earlier in gestation and/or if any abnormalities are suspected. Once CHD is diagnosed, interval follow-up occurs throughout pregnancy.

Imaging of the fetal heart is limited by the small size of the fetal heart, the rapid heart rate, and the depth of imaging in all cases, and can be additionally compromised by factors such as maternal body habitus and fetal positioning. To optimize imaging, the highest frequency transducer (usually between 4 and 12 MHz) that sufficiently penetrates the maternal abdomen should be used. This may become more difficult later in gestation as the need for increased depth penetration necessitates using a lower frequency transducer. The ultrasound system used should be able to perform two-dimensional (2D) imaging, M-mode, color Doppler, and pulsed-wave Doppler.

## Evaluation of the Normal Fetal Heart

### Fetal Visceral Situs

The initial step in evaluating the fetal heart is to determine the visceral situs of the fetus, or the laterality of the organs. The normal arrangement of the visceral organs is described as situs solitus, with morphologic right atrium, major hepatic lobe, inferior vena cava, trilobed lung, and short eparterial bronchus on the right side. Situs inversus refers to a reversal in laterality, when these anatomic findings occur on the left side of the fetus. In situs ambiguous, the laterality cannot be determined, and does not fit easily into the solitus or inversus description. Visceral/atrial situs ambiguous is commonly associated with significant CHD, most notably heterotaxy.[54] (See Chapter 16)

The first step in determining fetal visceral situs is to determine the exact position of the fetus within the maternal abdomen. By sweeping from maternal foot to head, and from maternal right to left, the exact position of the fetus can be determined. A transverse view of the fetal abdomen and thorax should be obtained, and it can confirm that the fetal heart is pointing to the left side of the chest, as well as the stomach and descending aorta. Typically, the inferior vena cava can be seen on the right side, and the atria into which the inferior vena cava enters is the morphologic right atrium. The inferior vena cava can be interrupted, with azygous continuation to the superior vena cava.

### Fetal Cardiac Axis

A transverse view of the chest at the level of the four-chamber view of the heart is found to determine the cardiac axis. A normal cardiac axis lies at approximately 45° from the midline, with the apex of the heart pointing leftward[55] (Fig. 4.2). Abnormal cardiac axis, either significantly more or less, can indicate either

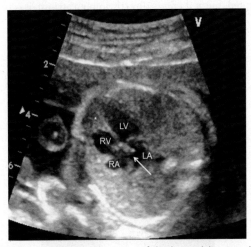

**FIGURE 4.2:** The four-chamber view of the heart delineates the right atrium *(RA)*, left atrium *(LA)*, right ventricle *(RV)* and left ventricle *(LV)*. The *asterisk* indicates the moderator band characteristic of a morphologic right ventricle. The foramen ovale, indicated with an *arrow*, bows into the left atrium. Note a line drawn through the apex of the left ventricle is at a 45° angle with the midline, which is a normal cardiac axis. The heart lies in the left chest, with apex pointing leftward, and occupies less than one-third of the area of the thorax.

structural heart disease or other abnormality within the thorax of the fetus such as congenital cystic malformation of the lung or congenital diaphragmatic hernia.

### Fetal Cardiac Size

The fetal heart occupies approximately one-third of the area in the thorax. This can be evaluated by tracing the circumference of both the heart and the thorax, and comparing either the area or the circumference. The cardiothoracic area ratio remains fairly consistent throughout gestation and should range between 0.25 and 0.35. Greater ratios may indicate cardiomegaly in the fetus[56] and are associated with hydrops fetalis, volume overload lesions such as arteriovenous malformations or sacrococcygeal teratoma, fetal anemia, or myocardial injury from structural heart disease, valvular regurgitation, or arrhythmia.

### Fetal Cardiac Position

The position of the heart within the fetal chest is referred to as cardiac position. The normal position is described as levocardia, with the heart located in the left chest (see Fig. 4.2). In dextrocardia, the heart is located in the right chest, and in mesocardia, the heart is located in the midline. The determination of cardiac position is independent of the cardiac axis. For example, with a left-sided congenital diaphragmatic hernia, the heart is positioned in the right chest, but the apex is still pointing leftward. This is known as dextroposition of the heart.

## Evaluation of the Fetal Cardiac Chambers

As ultrasound uses 2D images to evaluate the three-dimensional anatomy of the heart, multiple views of all of the fetal cardiac chambers should be obtained.

### The Right Atrium

The normal right atrium is located anterior and to the right of the left atrium. Typically, the right atrium receives desaturated blood from the inferior vena cava, superior vena cava, and coronary sinus (Fig. 4.3). At times, the inferior vena cava can be interrupted, but if it enters directly into an atrium, it is typically

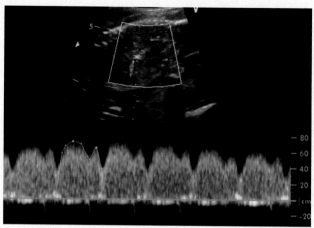

**FIGURE 4.4:** The ductus venosus should be identified and a pulse wave Doppler performed in a fetal echocardiogram. Here, a normal Doppler flow pattern is seen, with continuous flow entering the fetal heart. Ductus venosus tissue restricts the volume of highly oxygenated maternal blood returning to the fetal heart. Absence of the ductus venosus can cause right heart volume overload. Reversed flow in the ductus venosus is abnormal and can indicate right ventricular diastolic dysfunction or early atrial contraction/arrhythmia, where the atrium contracts against a closed valve.

the morphologic right atrium. The right atrial body is smooth posteriorly and trabeculated anteriorly, with a broad-based right atrial appendage.[57] The Eustachian valve, which is located over the opening of the inferior vena cava, directs the highly oxygenated blood from the maternal circulation and, subsequently, the ductus venosus (Fig. 4.4), across the foramen ovale to the left side of the heart, so that the most oxygenated blood supplies the head vessels of the aorta.[58]

The atrial septum separates the right and left atria, which is formed by the septum primum and septum secundum. The fossa ovalis is on the right atrial side, flow across the fossa ovalis is typically right to left (Fig. 4.5). Septum primum forms the valve of the foramen ovale, and is located within the left atrium. Atrial septal defects are classified by where they lie within the atrial septum.

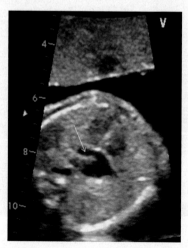

**FIGURE 4.3:** The coronary sinus is a normal structure located in the posterior–inferior aspect of the heart. Care should be taken not to mistake this normal structure for a primum atrial septal defect. An enlarged coronary sinus, highlighted by the *arrow*, can be associated with a left superior vena cava, anomalous pulmonary venous connection to the coronary sinus, or with elevated right-sided pressure.

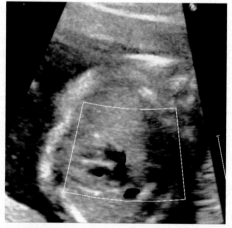

**FIGURE 4.5:** Unrestricted foramen ovale flow is seen crossing from right to left (normal) in this fetus. Restriction of the atrial septum can be seen in CHD as well as as an isolated finding, and careful attention should be paid to the size and direction of the foramen flow. The foramen ovale typically constitutes less than one-third of the atrial septum.

### The Left Atrium

The normal left atrium is located posteriorly within the chest cavity and is smooth-walled. It should receive all four pulmonary veins in the normal heart and is smooth-walled throughout. The left atrial appendage is narrow and fingerlike.[57] It contains the septum primum or the flap valve of the foramen ovale (see Fig. 4.2).

### The Right Ventricle

Located behind the sternum, the right ventricle is the most anterior chamber in the normal heart. It is coarsely trabeculated in contrast to the smooth trabeculations of the left ventricle. It is crescent shaped as opposed to elliptical like the left ventricle. Although the left ventricle is designed to handle the demands of the systemic circulation after birth, in utero it is the right ventricle that pumps against high resistance of the pulmonary circulation. It contains a moderator band (see Fig. 4.2).

### Tricuspid Valve

The atrioventricular valve is defined by its ventricle, with the tricuspid valve directing blood into the right ventricle. The tricuspid valve should be slightly more apically displaced within the heart than the mitral valve. The tricuspid valve is comprised of three leaflets—the anterior, posterior, and septal leaflets—which are anchored by the chordae tendineae to the three papillary muscles within the body of the right ventricle. Chordae tendineae from the tricuspid valve attach directly to the septal wall in the right ventricle, a feature that is not found in the left ventricle.

### The Left Ventricle

The left ventricle is smooth-walled, and located posterior and leftward of the right ventricle. It is elliptical or bullet shaped and should form the apex of the heart. It does not have a moderator band and has two distinct papillary muscles that should be clearly separated (the anterolateral and posteromedial papillary muscles).

### Mitral Valve

The mitral valve is the atrioventricular valve associated with the morphologic left ventricle. The mitral valve has two leaflets—the anterior and posterior leaflets—that attach to the anterolateral and posteromedial papillary muscles, which then insert into the free wall of the left ventricle, without the septal attachments apparent in the morphologic right ventricle.

### The Pulmonary Valve, Conus, and Pulmonary Arteries

The subpulmonic conus separates the pulmonary valve anteriorly from the tricuspid valve and the body of the right ventricle.[57] The main pulmonary artery arises from the right ventricle and crosses the aorta, with the pulmonary valve located anterior and leftward of the aortic valve. The pulmonary valve has three leaflets. The main pulmonary artery then divides into the right and left branch pulmonary arteries (Fig. 4.6) and the ductus arteriosus, which subsequently joins the descending aorta.

### The Aortic Valve and Aorta

The aortic semilunar valve has three leaflets, the right and left coronary cusps, and the posterior or noncoronary cusp. The ascending aorta arises from the left ventricle and is crossed by the pulmonary artery so that the aortic valve is posterior and rightward of the pulmonary valve. The valve is in fibrous

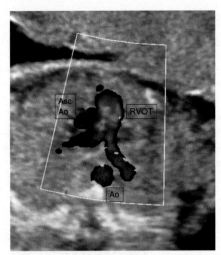

**FIGURE 4.6:** The branch pulmonary arteries are seen in the right ventricular outflow tract *(RVOT)* view in the transverse imaging plane. Asc Ao, Ascending aorta; Ao, aorta.

continuity with the mitral valve. The ascending aorta curves posteriorly into the aortic arch and gives rise to the three main head vessels—the innominate artery, which divides into the right subclavian and right common carotid artery, the left common carotid artery, and the left subclavian artery. The descending thoracic aorta lies posterior to the left atrium and becomes the abdominal aorta at the level of the diaphragm.[59] Arch sidedness is typically leftward, which means that the arch crosses to the left of the trachea. A right aortic arch is common in conotruncal abnormalities, but can occur as an isolated finding or in association with a vascular ring (Fig. 4.7). Arch sidedness is delineated in the trachea view, described later. A right aortic arch carries an increased risk of 22q microdeletion syndrome.[60]

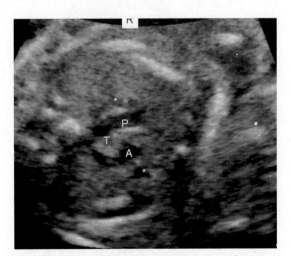

**FIGURE 4.7:** Three-vessel view with trachea is seen in a fetus diagnosed with right aortic arch and a left-sided superior vena cava (*). In this fetus, the pulmonary artery (P) is seen to the left of the trachea. The ascending aorta (A) is seen crossing right of the trachea, and a left-sided ductus is seen posterior to the trachea. This provides the substrate for a vascular ring at birth that can cause compression of the trachea and esophagus. If symptoms of emesis or respiratory difficulties are noted, this type of lesion would need surgical repair. A right aortic arch can also be associated with 22q microdeletion syndrome.

## Standard Imaging Planes

Depending on the source, the standard imaging views may carry different names. For the purposes of this discussion, the imaging planes described by the American Institute of Ultrasound in Medicine will be used.[61]

### Transverse Views

The transverse scanning planes consist of the four-chamber view, the left and right arterial outflow tract views, and the three-vessel and trachea view.

**Four-Chamber View:** A four-chamber view of the heart can be obtained by imaging transversely through the fetal chest (Fig. 4.8). In the normal four-chamber view, the apex of the heart should be pointing leftward at approximately 45° (see Fig. 4.2). The descending aorta should be visualized to the left and anterior to the fetal spine. The atria should be approximately equal in size, and the ventricles should be approximately equal in size and contractility (though this can vary by gestational age). The ventricular septum should appear intact, and the foramen ovale (see Fig. 4.5) should be visible within the atrial septum. In addition, the anatomic right atrium and ventricle should be

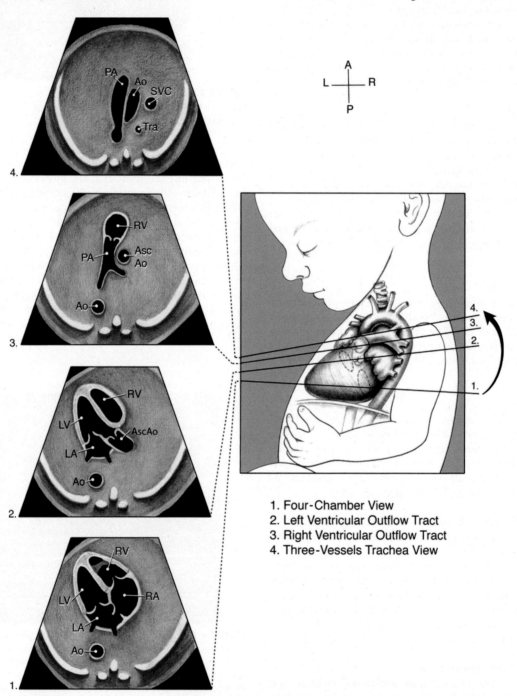

1. Four-Chamber View
2. Left Ventricular Outflow Tract
3. Right Ventricular Outflow Tract
4. Three-Vessels Trachea View

**FIGURE 4.8:** The transverse scanning planes. Desc Ao, descending aorta; Asc Ao, ascending aorta; LA, left atrium; LV, left ventricle; PA, pulmonary artery; RA, right atrium; RV, right ventricle; Tra, trachea; SVC, superior vena cava. (Reproduced with permission from American Institute of Ultrasound in Medicine. AIUM practice guideline for the performance of fetal echocardiography. *J Ultrasound Med.* 2013;32:1067–1082.)

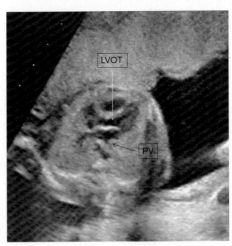

**FIGURE 4.9:** The left ventricular outflow tract view in the transverse imaging plane. The *PV* indicates a left pulmonary vein entering the left atrium. Note the normal unobstructed left ventricular outflow tract *(LVOT)*.

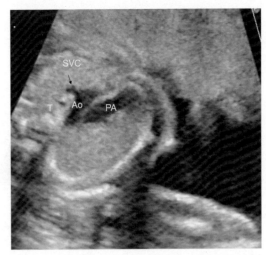

**FIGURE 4.10:** The three-vessel view shows the relative size of the main pulmonary artery and aorta, and their position relative to the trachea. This figure highlights a typical left arch in which both the aorta and pulmonary artery cross to the left of the trachea. SVC, superior vena cava; Ao, aorta; PA, pulmonary artery; T, trachea.

rightward, and the anatomic left atrium and ventricle should be leftward, as described below. It can be challenging to assess the pulmonary venous return to the left atrium as only a small amount of blood is directed to the lungs during fetal life. Often, the transverse, four-chamber view of the fetal heart yields the most helpful images of the pulmonary veins entering the left atrium (Fig. 4.9). Ideally, at least one left and one right pulmonary vein is visualized draining normally.

**Outflow Tract Views:** Following initial determination of situs and evaluation of the four-chamber fetal heart from the transverse view, the transducer can be tipped anteriorly within the fetus (toward the fetal head) to obtain the "five-chamber view" of the fetal heart, which includes the left ventricular outflow tract (see Fig. 4.9). The membranous ventricular septum and much of the muscular portion of the ventricular septum can also be assessed in this view. Moving the transducer cranially will bring in the right ventricular outflow tract view (see Fig. 4.6), and then moving it again cranially will define the three-vessel view with trachea.

**Three-Vessel and Trachea View:** In the three-vessel and trachea view (Fig. 4.10), the aorta, main pulmonary artery, and superior vena cava are visualized. This angulation of the three-vessel view shows the relationship of the arch to the trachea. Relative size can be evaluated as can arch sidedness. A right aortic arch, suggested by an aorta positioned rightward of the trachea, warrants further evaluation for associated structural heart disease. From the three-vessel view, tilting the transducer cranially can yield a transverse view of the ductus arteriosus with the ductus joining the descending aorta leftward of the spine.

### Sagittal Views
The sagittal views consist of the bicaval view, the aortic arch view, and the ductal arch views.

**Bicaval Sagittal View:** From a sagittal view of the fetus (parallel to the fetal spine), the systemic venous anatomy can be assessed (Fig. 4.11). The bicaval view (Fig. 4.12) can be obtained by tilting the probe rightward in the fetus from the midline sagittal

plane. The superior and inferior vena cava can be seen entering the right atrium posteriorly. A portion of the atrial septum and left atrium can be visualized. The superior vena cava is seen anterior to the right pulmonary artery. At the junction of the inferior vena cava and right atrium, the Eustachian valve can sometimes be appreciated.[55]

**Aortic Arch View:** From a sagittal view of the fetus (parallel to the fetal spine), the aortic and ductal arches can be assessed. In the left sagittal plane, a view of the aortic arch can be obtained (Fig. 4.13). The aortic arch arises from the middle of the chest and curves in a "candy-cane" appearance posteriorly. The three head vessels can be seen arising from the aortic arch and heading superiorly toward the neck and head of the fetus. The right pulmonary artery is seen in cross section posterior to the ascending aorta. The aortic isthmus can be visualized distal to the left subclavian artery, before the insertion of the ductus arteriosus. This is the most narrow aspect of the aortic arch, and most aortic coarctations are located just distal to this part of the arch.

**Ductal Arch View:** By sweeping further leftward with a slight change of angulation, the ductal arch can be imaged (Figs. 4.14 and 4.15). The ductal arch arises more anteriorly within the chest and has a more acute curvature, previously described as having a "hockey stick" appearance. The ductal arch connects to the descending aorta distal to the aortic isthmus.

### Short Axis Views
Oblique, or short axis, views of the fetal heart can be obtained (Fig. 4.16). The short-axis view of the fetal heart can assist in evaluation of the right ventricular outflow tract (Fig. 4.17) and can be obtained by orienting the transducer from right fetal hip to left fetal shoulder. The right ventricle is visualized anteriorly, as is the main pulmonary artery as it crosses over the aorta, which is viewed in cross section. The main pulmonary artery then divides into the right pulmonary artery and the ductus arteriosus. Both the atrium and the foramen ovale can also be visualized from this plane.

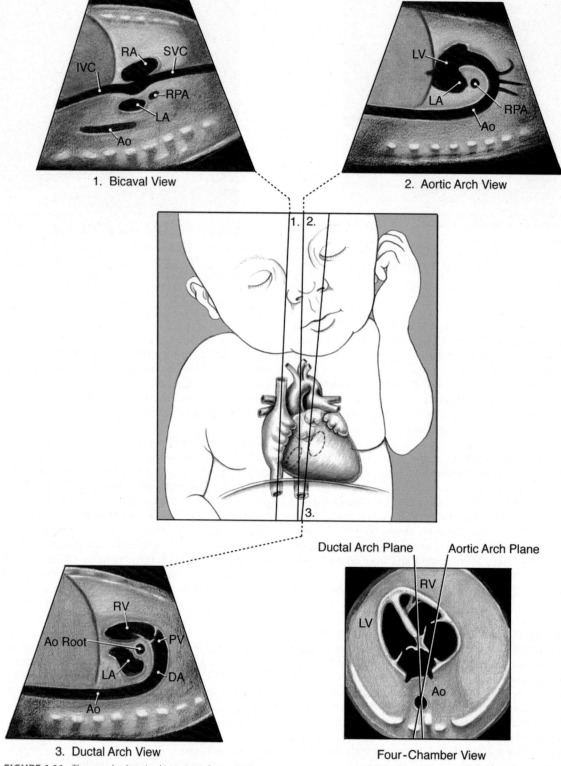

1. Bicaval View

2. Aortic Arch View

3. Ductal Arch View

Four-Chamber View

**FIGURE 4.11:** The standard sagittal imaging planes. Ao, aorta; Ao Root, aortic root; DA, ductus arteriosus; IVC, inferior vena cava; LA, left atrium; LV, left ventricle; PV, pulmonary valve; RA, right atrium; RPA, right pulmonary artery; RV, right ventricle; SVC, superior vena cava. (Reproduced with permission from American Institute of Ultrasound in Medicine. AIUM practice guideline for the performance of fetal echocardiography. *J Ultrasound Med.* 2013;32:1067–1082.)

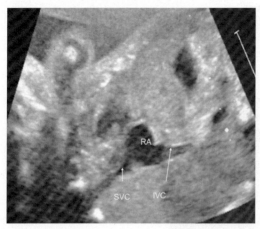

**FIGURE 4.12:** The bicaval sagittal view illustrates the inferior and superior vena cava *(SVC)* entering the right atrium *(RA)*. A portion of the atrial septum is seen. The inferior vena cava *(IVC)* can be interrupted in certain types of CHD, specifically the heterotaxy syndromes. Anomalous pulmonary venous drainage to the superior or inferior vena cava can cause dilation of these vessels.

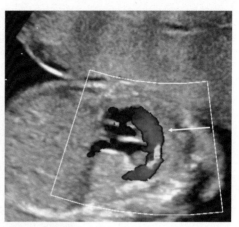

**FIGURE 4.15:** Color imaging of the ductal arch is helpful in evaluating for critical CHD. Reversed color flow in the ductus arteriosus is abnormal and can indicate ductal-dependent pulmonary blood flow.

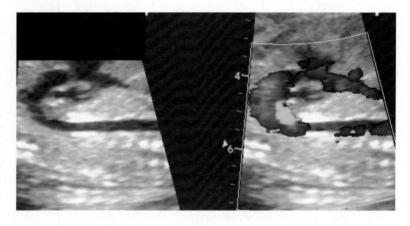

**FIGURE 4.13:** The aortic arch is seen in black and white, and color imaging. It typically has a candy cane appearance, although this is altered in diseases like transposition of the great arteries. The head vessels are usually equally spaced. Color imaging of the arches is helpful in ruling out critical CHD, in which there will be reversed flow in one of the arches, but can obfuscate finer details about the size of the distal ductus and aortic isthmus. Relying on only color imaging may cause the clinician to miss milder disease.

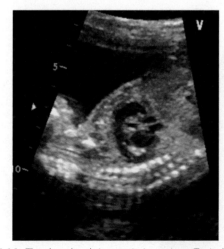

**FIGURE 4.14:** The ductal arch is seen in its entirety. Typically, the peak systolic velocity in the ductus arteriosus is less than 2 m/s, and diastolic velocity is 0.35 m/s. Restriction of the ductus can be caused by maternal ingestion of nonsteroidal anti-inflammatory medications. It is imperative to image the entire ductus, particularly where it enters the aortic isthmus, as restriction may occur primarily in this area.

By adjusting the transducer from apical to basal within the fetal heart, multiple short-axis views can be obtained. With these views, the ventricular chamber size, ventricular wall thickness, ventricular septum, and systolic function can be assessed (Fig. 4.18). The left ventricle should appear posterior, circular, and smooth-walled, while the right ventricle is more trabeculated, crescent-shaped, and anterior.

## CARDIAC BIOMETRY

Quantitative assessment of cardiac structure and function is valuable in both structurally normal and abnormal hearts. Normative values and Z-score equations are available for all valves and chambers of the heart, at all periods during gestation.[62–65] Measurement of atrioventricular and semilunar valves, ventricular length, and subsequent comparison of left- and right-sided structures can give significant insight into underlying structural cardiac disease. For example, a small pulmonary valve annulus may be the first indication of tetralogy of Fallot in a fetal heart with a relatively normal four-chamber view with a questionable ventricular septal defect, while a small aortic valve may be the first indication of coarctation of the aorta. Both by

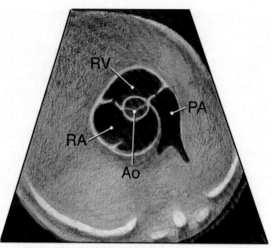

1. High Short Axis View - Great Arteries

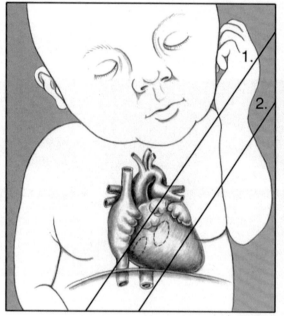

Fetal Heart - Coronal View

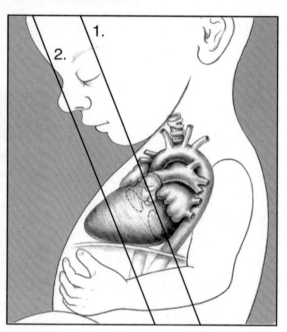

Fetal Heart - Sagittal View

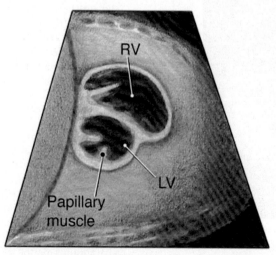

2. Low Short Axis View - Ventricles

**FIGURE 4.16:** The standard short axis views of the heart. Ao, aortic valve; LV, left ventricle; PA, pulmonary artery; RA, right atrium; RV, right ventricle. (Reproduced with permission from American Institute of Ultrasound in Medicine. AIUM practice guideline for the performance of fetal echocardiography. *J Ultrasound Med.* 2013;32:1067–1082.)

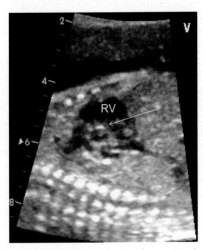

**FIGURE 4.17:** In the "high" short axis view, the aortic valve in cross section is indicated with an *arrow*. The right ventricular outflow tract crosses anteriorly. This view is helpful in evaluating for diseases like tetralogy of Fallot, in which there is small and anteriorly deviated right ventricular outflow tract. RV, right ventricle.

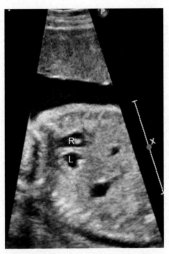

**FIGURE 4.18:** In the "low" short axis view, the two ventricles are seen in cross section. This view can be used to obtain the shortening fraction, a measure of function.

qualitative assessment and by established normative values, the right-sided atrioventricular and semilunar valves should be slightly larger than their left-sided counterparts, while the right and left ventricles should be approximately equal in length and width.[62–65] However, in late gestation, the right ventricular width can be noticeably larger than the left.

## COLOR DOPPLER EVALUATION

The fetal heart is a moving, beating organ, and full assessment of it should include evaluation of blood flow. Color Doppler can be useful in the assessment of atrioventricular and semilunar valve stenosis or regurgitation, anatomy and flow through the ductal and aortic arches, drainage of the systemic and pulmonary veins, as well as evaluation of septal defects,[66,67] and is now recommended as part of a comprehensive fetal echocardiographic examination.[68]

## Technical Considerations

A high frame rate improves the quality of 2D imaging of the fetal heart. Once color Doppler imaging commences, the frame rate decreases, and a balance must be reached between optimizing frame rate and allowing for adequate color Doppler assessment. The narrower the width of the color box, the higher the frame rate, yielding improved quality of images. The quality of color Doppler imaging can also be affected by the velocity scale. For the majority of the fetal cardiac evaluation, a relatively high velocity scale can be used (>40 cm per second). This allows for adequate imaging across the atrioventricular and semilunar valves as well as the great vessels, without color aliasing that would be apparent at a lower scale. Lower velocity scales are more appropriate for low-velocity vessels such as the pulmonary and systemic veins. Doppler interrogation of the heart with the probe angled parallel to blood flow will optimize color imaging. All standard views, including the four-chamber view, outflow tracts, three-vessel view with trachea, and arch, should be acquired with 2D and color. Two-dimensional images allow assessment of anatomic features, and color adds physiologic information.

## OTHER CARDIAC EVALUATIONS

### Pulsed-Wave Doppler Evaluation

Less commonly used in routine obstetrical ultrasound screening, but important to the full fetal cardiac assessment, is pulsed-wave Doppler, which will be discussed in more detail in the subsequent chapter (see Chapter 5). Normative data for peak velocities and typical blood flow patterns are available for all of the cardiac valves and great vessels, and should be applied in the comprehensive evaluation of the fetal heart. An example of a pulse wave Doppler tracing in the aortic isthmus is seen in Figure 4.19.

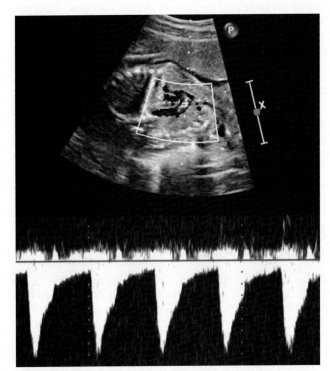

**FIGURE 4.19:** A pulse wave Doppler tracing in the aortic isthmus.

## Fetal Rhythm Assessment

Suspected fetal arrhythmias are a common indication for referral for fetal echocardiography. In addition to a comprehensive assessment of the structure of the fetal heart, an assessment of fetal rhythm should be performed. M-mode or pulsed-wave Doppler imaging allows assessment of the mechanical measure of fetal cardiac rhythm.

### M-Mode Echocardiography

M-mode imaging allows for the visual representation of the movement of a structure over time. To evaluate the rhythm of the heart, the sample line is placed through the right atrium and either ventricle. The M-mode images show the change in wall motion over time, so that the relationship between atrial and ventricular contractions can be assessed, and the fetal heart rate and rhythm can be measured.[69]

### Pulsed-Wave Doppler

Another method of assessing mechanical atrial and ventricular systole as a means of fetal rhythm assessment is through pulsed-wave Doppler. This can be evaluated by simultaneous Doppler of the left ventricular inflow and outflow and/or the superior vena cava and ascending aorta so that the fetal rhythm can be more accurately assessed.[70,71] In this way, the relationship between atrial and ventricular contractions can be more clearly visualized than using 2D ultrasound alone. In women with anti-SSA antibodies, the mechanical PR interval can be measured and followed over the duration of pregnancy using simultaneous left ventricular inflow and outflow Dopplers.

## Fetal Cardiac Functional Assessment

In addition to an assessment of fetal cardiac structure and rhythm, an assessment of function of the fetal heart is also an integral part of a comprehensive fetal cardiac evaluation. Persistent arrhythmias, cardiomyopathies, maternal infections, and structural heart disease are some of the factors that can affect fetal cardiac function. A qualitative assessment of fetal cardiac function is part of the basic cardiac evaluation. Cardiomegaly can indicate impaired fetal cardiac function or altered loading conditions.[72] Quantitatively, the shortening fraction of the left ventricle can be evaluated from 2D or M-mode imaging (Shortening fraction [%] = [End diastolic diameter-end systolic diameter]/End diastolic diameter).[73] The Tei index is a global additional assessment of cardiac function, calculated from the inflow–outflow Doppler of the mitral and aortic valve. Additional measures for evaluating fetal cardiac function use pulsed-wave Doppler, and will be discussed in more detail in the subsequent chapter (see Chapter 5).

## LIMITATIONS OF FETAL ECHOCARDIOGRAPHY

There are limitations to fetal echocardiography due to the small size of the fetal heart, the rapid fetal heart rate, and the fact that imaging occurs through the maternal abdomen and uterus. In addition, factors such as maternal body habitus and fetal position may worsen already suboptimal imaging. Fortunately, major structural heart disease can usually be identified with a complete fetal echo, and most of the lesions less consistently diagnosed prenatally often have little impact on neonatal

well-being or hemodynamic stability. These include small ventricular or atrial septal defects, minor valve abnormalities, and partial pulmonary venous drainage abnormalities.[74] Imaging with the four-chamber view alone cannot detect major malformations such as tetralogy of Fallot or transposition of the great arteries, making the outflow views essential in accurately diagnosing cardiac defects. Because of the nature of fetal cardiac circulation, a patent foramen ovale and patent ductus arteriosus cannot be predicted. Additionally, some cardiac anomalies develop later in gestation or progress throughout gestation, and may not be apparent at the routine mid-gestation evaluation. These include fetal arrhythmias, cardiomyopathies, rhabdomyomas, and some obstructive lesions.[75-77] Certain conditions, such as coarctation and anomalous pulmonary venous return, are challenging but possible to detect prenatally by experienced clinicians. Coarctation often becomes more severe when ductal tissue in the aortic isthmus constricts after birth. Prenatally, a small aorta relative to the pulmonary outflow may be seen in the three-vessel view with trachea,[78] and bidirectional or low velocity flow may be seen in the aortic isthmus. In total anomalous pulmonary venous connection, an additional venous structure entering either the superior vena cava or crossing below the diaphragm may be noted.

## REFERENCES

1. Ferencz C, Rubin JD, McCarter RJ, et al. Congenital heart disease: prevalence at livebirth. The Baltimore-Washington Infant Study. *Am J Epidemiol.* 1985;121(1):31–36.
2. Hoffman JI. Congenital heart disease: incidence and inheritance. *Pediatr Clin North Am.* 1990;37(1):25–43.
3. Tegnander E, Williams W, Johansen OJ, et al. Prenatal detection of heart defects in a non-selected population of 30,149 fetuses—detection rates and outcome. *Ultrasound Obstet Gynecol.* 2006;27(3):252–265.
4. Wren C, Richmond S, Donaldson L. Temporal variability in birth prevalence of cardiovascular malformations. *Heart.* 2000;83(4):414–419.
5. Moons P, Sluysmans T, De Wolf D, et al. Congenital heart disease in 111 225 births in Belgium: birth prevalence, treatment and survival in the 21st century. *Acta Paediatr.* 2009;98(3):472–477.
6. Moore T. *Maternal-Fetal Medicine: Principles and Practice.* Philadelphia, PA: WB Saunders; 1999.
7. Miller E, Hare JW, Cloherty JP, et al. Elevated maternal hemoglobin A1c in early pregnancy and major congenital anomalies in infants of diabetic mothers. *N Engl J Med.* 1981;304(22):1331–1334.
8. Lisowski LA, Verheijen PM, Copel JA, et al. Congenital heart disease in pregnancies complicated by maternal diabetes mellitus: an international clinical collaboration, literature review, and meta-analysis. *Herz.* 2010;35(1):19–26.
9. Hagay Z, Reece A. *Reece and Hobbins: Medicine of the Fetus and Mother.* Philadelphia, PA: Lippincott Williams & Wilkins; 1999.
10. Friedman DM, Kim MY, Copel JA, et al. Utility of cardiac monitoring in fetuses at risk for congenital heart block: the PR Interval and Dexamethasone Evaluation (PRIDE) prospective study. *Circulation.* 2008;117(4):485–493.
11. Hornberger LK, Al Rajaa N. Spectrum of cardiac involvement in neonatal lupus. *Scand J Immunol.* 2010;72(3):189–197.
12. Chockalingam P, Jaeggi ET, Rammeloo LA, et al. Persistent fetal sinus bradycardia associated with maternal anti-SSA/Ro and anti-SSB/La antibodies. *J Rheumatol.* 2011;38(12):2682–2685.
13. Askanase AD, Friedman DM, Copel J, et al. Spectrum and progression of conduction abnormalities in infants born to mothers with anti-SSA/Ro-SSB/La antibodies. *Lupus.* 2002;11(3):145–151.
14. Zhao H, Cuneo BF, Strasburger JF, et al. Electrophysiological characteristics of fetal atrioventricular block. *J Am Coll Cardiol.* 2008;51(1):77–84.
15. Costedoat-Chalumeau N, Amoura Z, Villain E, et al. Anti-SSA/Ro antibodies and the heart: more than complete congenital heart block? A review of electrocardiographic and myocardial abnormalities and of treatment options. *Arthritis Res Ther.* 2005;7(2):69–73.
16. Eronen M. Long-term outcome of children with complete heart block diagnosed after the newborn period. *Pediatr Cardiol.* 2001;22(2):133–137.
17. Krishnan AN, Sable CA, Donofrio MT. Spectrum of fetal echocardiographic findings in fetuses of women with clinical or serologic evidence of systemic lupus erythematosus. *J Matern Fetal Neonatal Med.* 2008;21(11):776–782.
18. Cuneo BF, Fruitman D, Benson DW, et al. Spontaneous rupture of atrioventricular valve tensor apparatus as late manifestation of anti-Ro/SSA antibody-mediated cardiac disease. *Am J Cardiol.* 2011;107(5):761–766.

19. Cuneo BF, Strasburger JF, Niksch A, et al. An expanded phenotype of maternal SSA/SSB antibody-associated fetal cardiac disease. *J Matern Fetal Neonatal Med.* 2009;22(3):233–238.

20. Davey DL, Bratton SL, Bradley DJ, et al. Relation of maternal anti-Ro/La antibodies to aortic dilation in patients with congenital complete heart block. *Am J Cardiol.* 2011;108(4):561–564.

21. Radbill AE, Brown DW, Lacro RV, et al. Ascending aortic dilation in patients with congenital complete heart block. *Heart Rhythm.* 2008;5(12):1704–1708.

22. Matalon S, Schechtman S, Goldzweig G, et al. The teratogenic effect of carbamazepine: a meta-analysis of 1255 exposures. *Reprod Toxicol.* 2002;16(1):9–17.

23. Jenkins KJ, Correa A, Feinstein JA, et al. Noninherited risk factors and congenital cardiovascular defects: current knowledge: a scientific statement from the American Heart Association Council on Cardiovascular Disease in the Young: endorsed by the American Academy of Pediatrics. *Circulation.* 2007;115(23): 2995–3014.

24. Warner JP. Evidence-based psychopharmacology 3—assessing evidence of harm: what are the teratogenic effects of lithium carbonate? *J Psychopharmacol.* 2000;14(1):77–80.

25. Lammer EJ, Chen DT, Hoar RM, et al. Retinoic acid embryopathy. *N Engl J Med.* 1985;313(14):837–841.

26. Cooper WO, Hernandez-Diaz S, Arbogast PG, et al. Major congenital malformations after first-trimester exposure to ACE inhibitors. *N Engl J Med.* 2006;354(23):2443–2451.

27. Louik C, Lin AE, Werler MM, et al. First-trimester use of selective serotonin-reuptake inhibitors and the risk of birth defects. *N Engl J Med.* 2007;356(26):2675–2683.

28. Moise KJ Jr, Huhta JC, Sharif DS, et al. Indomethacin in the treatment of premature labor: effects on the fetal ductus arteriosus. *N Engl J Med.* 1988;319(6):327–331.

29. Levy HL, Waisbren SE. Effects of untreated maternal phenylketonuria and hyperphenylalaninemia on the fetus. *N Engl J Med.* 1983;309(21):1269–1274.

30. Platt LD, Koch R, Hanley WB, et al. The international study of pregnancy outcome in women with maternal phenylketonuria: report of a 12-year study. *Am J Obstet Gynecol.* 2000;182(2):326–333.

31. Botto LD, Lynberg MC, Erickson JD. Congenital heart defects, maternal febrile illness, and multivitamin use: a population-based study. *Epidemiology.* 2001;12(5):485–490.

32. Ornoy A, Tenenbaum A. Pregnancy outcome following infections by coxsackie, echo, measles, mumps, hepatitis, polio and encephalitis viruses. *Reprod Toxicol.* 2006;21(4):446–457.

33. Hornberger LK, Lipshultz SE, Easley KA, et al. Cardiac structure and function in fetuses of mothers infected with HIV: the prospective PCHIV multicenter study. *Am Heart J.* 2000;140(4):575–584.

34. Fishman SG, Pelaez LM, Baergen RN, et al. Parvovirus-mediated fetal cardiomyopathy with atrioventricular nodal disease. *Pediatr Cardiol.* 2011;32(1):84–86.

35. Reefhuis J, Honein MA, Schieve LA, et al. Assisted reproductive technology and major structural birth defects in the United States. *Hum Reprod.* 2009;24(2):360–366.

36. Bahtiyar MO, Campbell K, Dulay AT, et al. Is the rate of congenital heart defects detected by fetal echocardiography among pregnancies conceived by in vitro fertilization really increased?: a case-historical control study. *J Ultrasound Med.* 2010;29(6):917–922.

37. Tararbit K, Houyel L, Bonnet D, et al. Risk of congenital heart defects associated with assisted reproductive technologies: a population-based evaluation. *Eur Heart J.* 2010;32(4):500–508.

38. Oyen N, Poulsen G, Boyd HA, et al. Recurrence of congenital heart defects in families. *Circulation.* 2009;120(4):295–301.

39. Burn J, Brennan P, Little J, et al. Recurrence risks in offspring of adults with major heart defects: results from first cohort of British collaborative study. *Lancet.* 1998;351(9099):311–316.

40. Carvalho JS, Mavrides E, Shinebourne EA, et al. Improving the effectiveness of routine prenatal screening for major congenital heart defects. *Heart.* 2002;88(4):387–391.

41. Simpson LL. Indications for fetal echocardiography from a tertiary-care obstetric sonography practice. *J Clin Ultrasound.* 2004;32(3):123–128.

42. Pierpont ME, Basson CT, Benson DW Jr, et al. Genetic basis for congenital heart defects: current knowledge: a scientific statement from the American Heart Association Congenital Cardiac Defects Committee, Council on Cardiovascular Disease in the Young: endorsed by the American Academy of Pediatrics. *Circulation.* 2007;115(23):3015–3038.

43. Copel JA, Pilu G, Kleinman CS. Congenital heart disease and extracardiac anomalies: associations and indications for fetal echocardiography. *Am J Obstet Gynecol.* 1986;154(5):1121–1132.

44. Greenwood RD, Rosenthal A, Nadas AS. Cardiovascular malformations associated with omphalocele. *J Pediatr.* 1974;85(6):818–821.

45. Greenwood RD, Rosenthal A, Nadas AS. Cardiovascular abnormalities associated with congenital diaphragmatic hernia. *Pediatrics.* 1976;57(1):92–97.

46. Greenwood RD, Rosenthal A, Nadas AS. Cardiovascular malformations associated with congenital anomalies of the urinary system: observations in a series of 453 infants and children with urinary system malformations. *Clin Pediatr.* 1976;15(12):1101–1104.

47. Nicolaides KH, Heath V, Cicero S. Increased fetal nuchal translucency at 11–14 weeks. *Prenat Diagn.* 2002;22(4):308–315.

48. Snijders RJ, Noble P, Sebire N, et al. UK multicentre project on assessment of risk of trisomy 21 by maternal age and fetal nuchal-translucency thickness at 10–14 weeks of gestation. Fetal Medicine Foundation First Trimester Screening Group. *Lancet.* 1998;352(9125):343–346.

49. Atzei A, Gajewska K, Huggon IC, et al. Relationship between nuchal translucency thickness and prevalence of major cardiac defects in fetuses with normal karyotype. *Ultrasound Obstet Gynecol.* 2005;26(2):154–157.

50. Huhta JC, Paul JJ. Doppler in fetal heart failure. *Clin Obstet Gynecol.* 2010;53(4):915–929.

51. Dhanantwari P, Lee E, Krishnan A, et al. Human cardiac development in the first trimester: a high-resolution magnetic resonance imaging and episcopic fluorescence image capture atlas. *Circulation.* 2009;120(4):343–351.

52. Wloch A, Rozmus-Warcholinska W, Czuba B, et al. Doppler study of the embryonic heart in normal pregnant women. *J Matern Fetal Neonatal Med.* 2007;20(7):533–539.

53. Moon-Grady A, Shahanavaz S, Brook M, et al. Can a complete fetal echocardiogram be performed at 12 to 16 weeks' gestation? *J Am Soc Echocardiogr.* 2012;25(12):1342–1352.

54. Salomon LJ, Baumann C, Delezoide AL, et al. Abnormal abdominal situs: what and how should we look for? *Prenat Diagn.* 2006;26(3):282–285.

55. Tacy TA, Silverman NH. Systemic venous abnormalities: embryologic and echocardiographic considerations. *Echocardiography.* 2001;18(5):401–413.

56. Chaoui R, Bollmann R, Goldner B, et al. Fetal cardiomegaly: echocardiographic findings and outcome in 19 cases. *Fetal Diagn Ther.* 1994;9(2):92–104.

57. Van Praagh R. Morphologic anatomy. In: Keane JF, Lock JE, Fyler DC, eds. *Nadas Pediatric Cardiology.* Philadelphia, PA: Saunders; 1992:17–26.

58. Rudolph AM, Heymann MA. The circulation of the fetus in utero: methods for studying distribution of blood flow, cardiac output and organ blood flow. *Circ Res.* 1967;21:163–184.

59. Van Praagh R. Segmental approach to diagnosis. In: Keane JF, Lock JE, Fyler DC, eds. *Nadas Pediatric Cardiology.* Philadelphia, PA: Saunders; 1992:27–35.

60. Berg C, Bender F, Soukup M, et al. Right aortic arch detected in fetal life. *Ultrasound Obstet Gynecol.* 2006;28(7):882–889.

61. Fetal Echocardiography Task Force, American Institute of Ultrasound in Medicine Clinical Standards Committee, American College of Obstetricians and Gynecologists, Society for Maternal-Fetal Medicine. AIUM practice guideline for the performance of fetal echocardiography. *J Ultrasound Med.* 2011;30(1):127–136.

62. Schneider C, McCrindle BW, Carvalho JS, et al. Development of Z-scores for fetal cardiac dimensions from echocardiography. *Ultrasound Obstet Gynecol.* 2005;26(6):599–605.

63. Sharland GK, Allan LD. Normal fetal cardiac measurements derived by cross-sectional echocardiography. *Ultrasound Obstet Gynecol.* 1992;2(3):175–181.

64. St John Sutton MG, Gewitz MH, Shah B, et al. Quantitative assessment of growth and function of the cardiac chambers in the normal human fetus: a prospective longitudinal echocardiographic study. *Circulation.* 1984;69(4):645–654.

65. Tan J, Silverman NH, Hoffman JI, et al. Cardiac dimensions determined by cross-sectional echocardiography in the normal human fetus from 18 weeks to term. *Am J Cardiol.* 1992;70(18):1459–1467.

66. Copel JA, Morotti R, Hobbins JC, et al. The antenatal diagnosis of congenital heart disease using fetal echocardiography: is color flow mapping necessary? *Obstet Gynecol.* 1991;78(1):1–8.

67. Stewart PA, Wladimiroff JW. Fetal echocardiography and color Doppler flow imaging: the Rotterdam experience. *Ultrasound Obstet Gynecol.* 1993;3(3):168–175.

68. Lee W, Allan L, Carvalho JS, et al. ISUOG consensus statement: what constitutes a fetal echocardiogram? *Ultrasound Obstet Gynecol* 2008;32(2):239–242.

69. Allan LD, Anderson RH, Sullivan ID, et al. Evaluation of fetal arrhythmias by echocardiography. *Br Heart J.* 1983;50(3):240–245.

70. Strasburger JF, Huhta JC, Carpenter RJ Jr, et al. Doppler echocardiography in the diagnosis and management of persistent fetal arrhythmias. *J Am Coll Cardiol.* 1986;7(6):1386–1391.

71. Fouron JC, Fournier A, Proulx F, et al. Management of fetal tachyarrhythmia based on superior vena cava/aorta Doppler flow recordings. *Heart.* 2003;89(10):1211–1216.

72. Pedra SR, Smallhorn JF, Ryan G, et al. Fetal cardiomyopathies: pathogenic mechanisms, hemodynamic findings, and clinical outcome. *Circulation.* 2002;106(5):585–591.

73. Wladimiroff JW, McGhie J. Ultrasonic assessment of cardiovascular geometry and function in the human fetus. *Br J Obstet Gynaecol.* 1981;88(9):870–875.

74. Gottliebson WM, Border WL, Franklin CM, et al. Accuracy of fetal echocardiography: a cardiac segment-specific analysis. *Ultrasound Obstet Gynecol.* 2006;28(1):15–21.

75. Hornberger LK, Barrea C. Diagnosis, natural history, and outcome of fetal heart disease. *Semin Thorac Cardiovasc Surg Pediatr Card Surg Annu.* 2001;4:229–243.

76. Sivasankaran S, Sharland GK, Simpson JM. Dilated cardiomyopathy presenting during fetal life. *Cardiol Young.* 2005;15(4):409–416.

77. Tworetzky W, McElhinney DB, Margossian R, et al. Association between cardiac tumors and tuberous sclerosis in the fetus and neonate. *Am J Cardiol.* 2003;92(4):487–489.

78. Slodki M, Rychik J, Moszura T, et al. Measurement of the great vessels in the mediastinum could help distinguish true from false-positive coarctation of the aorta in the third trimester. *J Ultrasound Med.* 2009;28(10):1313–1317.

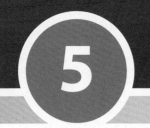

# Advanced Assessment of Fetal Cardiac Function

Greggory R. DeVore

Abnormal cardiac function cannot be assessed by a single measurable entity. Dysfunction of the fetal heart may alter the size and shape of the heart and great vessels, the direction of blood flow within the atrial and ventricular chambers and outflow tracts, as well as the contractility of the right and left ventricular walls and interventricular septum. Because of the changes in size and function, multiple ultrasound modalities are used to evaluate each of these parameters. This chapter will discuss the use of M-Mode, B-Mode and pulsed Doppler ultrasound to evaluate cardiac function.

## UNDERSTANDING THE INTERRELATIONSHIPS BETWEEN Z-SCORES, PERCENTILES, AND STANDARD DEVIATIONS

Postnatally, scientists have used anthropometric techniques to study the interrelationships between body measurements. Investigators have reported measurements of cardiac structures and their distribution as percentiles and Z-scores as a function of age and biometric measurements such as the biparietal diameter, head circumference, abdominal circumference, and femur length.[1-9] Before discussing the various anthropometric fetal studies of cardiac measurements, it is important to understand the terminology and relationships between standard deviations, Z-scores, and percentiles.

### Standard Deviation

The standard deviation represents the variation or the dispersion that exists from the mean. A small standard deviation indicates that the data points tend to cluster very close to the mean, while a large standard deviation indicates that the data points are spread out over a larger range of values. The *Standard Error of the Estimate* is the standard deviation of the differences between the observed values of the dependent variables (results) and the predicted values. This statistic is derived from regression analysis.

### Z-Score

A Z-score is a dimensionless quantity obtained by subtracting the population *mean* from an *individual measurement* obtained from that population, and then dividing the difference by the population *standard deviation*. A positive Z-score represents a datum above the mean, while a negative Z-score represents a datum below the mean. For example, a standard deviation that is 2.35 above the mean has an equivalent Z-score of +2.35. A standard deviation that is 2.35 below the mean has a corresponding Z-score of −2.35. It is important to realize that the Z-score and computed standard deviation are equivalent except that the Z-score assigns a + or − to the value.

### Percentile

A percentile is the value below which a given percentage of observations in a group of observations fall. The mean of a group of measurements is the 50th percentile. The 10th percentile is the value below which 10% of the observations may be found, while the 90th percentile is a value below which 90% of the values fall. The distribution of percentiles is >0 and <100. There is a direct relationship between the percentile and the Z-score, the latter being a computed value for the corresponding percentile in a normally distributed sample population.

### Computing Percentiles from Z-scores

Statisticians have created Z-score tables that allow the user to compute the corresponding percentile from the Z-score (Tables 5.1 and 5.2). For example, if a Z-score is 1.65, the clinician would use Table 5.1 and find 1.6 along the left column, and 0.05 along the top column. Where these two intersect is the 95th percentile. The following is an example of the computation of the 5th and 95th percentiles:

If the measurement for the mean aortic diameter is 4 mm for a given gestational age, and the standard deviation is 0.6, what would be the 5th and 95th percentiles?

The computations are as follows:

1. The Z-score for the 95th percentile is +1.65
2. The Z-score for the 5th percentile is −1.65
3. The Z-score is multiplied by the standard deviation.
   a. 95th Percentile = mean + (1.65 × SD) = 4 + (1.65 × 0.6) = 4.99
   b. 5th Percentile = mean − (1.65 × SD) = 4 − (1.65 × 0.6) = 3.01

Table 5.3 lists the Z-scores for commonly used percentiles.

Another use of this table would be computation of the standard deviation from the percentiles. The first step would be to find the percentile of interest from Tables 5.1 or 5.2 and then identify the corresponding Z-score that is equal to the standard deviation. For example, if one wanted to find the standard deviation for the 10th percentile, the user would refer to Table 5.2 and find the value closest to the 10th percentile. Once identified, the examiner would find the value on the left side of the table, which is 1.2 and the value at the top of the table, which is 0.08. Therefore, the corresponding Z-score (standard deviation) is −1.28.

### Creating Percentile Graphs

Authors from the studies cited in this chapter have reported various types of data analysis in the form of regression equations, percentiles, standard deviations, and standard error of the estimate. Even though data may be reported in different

| Table 5.1 | Computing Percentiles from Positive Z-scores | | | | | | | | |
|---|---|---|---|---|---|---|---|---|---|
| | **Positive Z-score (%)** | | | | | | | | |
| **Z** | **0** | **0.01** | **0.02** | **0.03** | **0.04** | **0.05** | **0.06** | **0.07** | **0.08** | **0.09** |
| 0 | 50.00 | 50.40 | 50.80 | 51.20 | 51.60 | 51.99 | 52.39 | 52.79 | 53.19 | 53.59 |
| 0.1 | 53.98 | 54.38 | 54.78 | 55.17 | 55.57 | 55.96 | 56.36 | 56.75 | 57.14 | 57.53 |
| 0.2 | 57.93 | 58.32 | 58.71 | 59.10 | 59.48 | 59.87 | 60.26 | 60.64 | 61.03 | 61.41 |
| 0.3 | 61.79 | 62.17 | 62.55 | 62.93 | 63.31 | 63.68 | 64.06 | 64.43 | 64.80 | 65.17 |
| 0.4 | 65.54 | 65.91 | 66.28 | 66.64 | 67.00 | 67.36 | 67.72 | 68.08 | 68.44 | 68.79 |
| 0.5 | 69.15 | 69.50 | 69.85 | 70.19 | 70.54 | 70.88 | 71.23 | 71.57 | 71.90 | 72.24 |
| 0.6 | 72.57 | 72.91 | 73.24 | 73.57 | 73.89 | 74.22 | 74.54 | 74.86 | 75.17 | 75.49 |
| 0.7 | 75.80 | 76.11 | 76.42 | 76.73 | 77.04 | 77.34 | 77.64 | 77.94 | 78.23 | 78.52 |
| 0.8 | 78.81 | 79.10 | 79.39 | 79.67 | 79.95 | 80.23 | 80.51 | 80.78 | 81.06 | 81.33 |
| 0.9 | 81.59 | 81.86 | 82.12 | 82.38 | 82.64 | 82.89 | 83.15 | 83.40 | 83.65 | 83.89 |
| 1 | 84.13 | 84.38 | 84.61 | 84.85 | 85.08 | 85.31 | 85.54 | 85.77 | 85.99 | 86.21 |
| 1.1 | 86.43 | 86.65 | 86.86 | 87.08 | 87.29 | 87.49 | 87.70 | 87.90 | 88.10 | 88.30 |
| 1.2 | 88.49 | 88.69 | 88.88 | 89.07 | 89.25 | 89.44 | 89.62 | 89.80 | 89.97 | 90.15 |
| 1.3 | 90.32 | 90.49 | 90.66 | 90.82 | 90.99 | 91.15 | 91.31 | 91.47 | 91.62 | 91.77 |
| 1.4 | 91.92 | 92.07 | 92.22 | 92.36 | 92.51 | 92.65 | 92.79 | 92.92 | 93.06 | 93.19 |
| 1.5 | 93.32 | 93.45 | 93.57 | 93.70 | 93.82 | 93.94 | 94.06 | 94.18 | 94.29 | 94.41 |
| 1.6 | 94.52 | 94.63 | 94.74 | 94.84 | 94.95 | 95.05 | 95.15 | 95.25 | 95.35 | 95.45 |
| 1.7 | 95.54 | 95.64 | 95.73 | 95.82 | 95.91 | 95.99 | 96.08 | 96.16 | 96.25 | 96.33 |
| 1.8 | 96.41 | 96.49 | 96.56 | 96.64 | 96.71 | 96.78 | 96.86 | 96.93 | 96.99 | 97.06 |
| 1.9 | 97.13 | 97.19 | 97.26 | 97.32 | 97.38 | 97.44 | 97.50 | 97.56 | 97.61 | 97.67 |
| 2 | 97.72 | 97.78 | 97.83 | 97.88 | 97.93 | 97.98 | 98.03 | 98.08 | 98.12 | 98.17 |
| 2.1 | 98.21 | 98.26 | 98.30 | 98.34 | 98.38 | 98.42 | 98.46 | 98.50 | 98.54 | 98.57 |
| 2.2 | 98.61 | 98.64 | 98.68 | 98.71 | 98.75 | 98.78 | 98.81 | 98.84 | 98.87 | 98.90 |
| 2.3 | 98.93 | 98.96 | 98.98 | 99.01 | 99.04 | 99.06 | 99.09 | 99.11 | 99.13 | 99.16 |
| 2.4 | 99.18 | 99.20 | 99.22 | 99.25 | 99.27 | 99.29 | 99.31 | 99.32 | 99.34 | 99.36 |
| 2.5 | 99.38 | 99.40 | 99.41 | 99.43 | 99.45 | 99.46 | 99.48 | 99.49 | 99.51 | 99.52 |
| 2.6 | 99.53 | 99.55 | 99.56 | 99.57 | 99.59 | 99.60 | 99.61 | 99.62 | 99.63 | 99.64 |
| 2.7 | 99.65 | 99.66 | 99.67 | 99.68 | 99.69 | 99.70 | 99.71 | 99.72 | 99.73 | 99.74 |
| 2.8 | 99.74 | 99.75 | 99.76 | 99.77 | 99.77 | 99.78 | 99.79 | 99.79 | 99.80 | 99.81 |
| 2.9 | 99.81 | 99.82 | 99.82 | 99.83 | 99.84 | 99.84 | 99.85 | 99.85 | 99.86 | 99.86 |
| 3 | 99.87 | 99.87 | 99.87 | 99.88 | 99.88 | 99.89 | 99.89 | 99.89 | 99.90 | 99.90 |
| 3.1 | 99.90 | 99.91 | 99.91 | 99.91 | 99.92 | 99.92 | 99.92 | 99.92 | 99.93 | 99.93 |
| 3.2 | 99.93 | 99.93 | 99.94 | 99.94 | 99.94 | 99.94 | 99.94 | 99.95 | 99.95 | 99.95 |
| 3.3 | 99.95 | 99.95 | 99.95 | 99.96 | 99.96 | 99.96 | 99.96 | 99.96 | 99.96 | 99.97 |
| 3.4 | 99.97 | 99.97 | 99.97 | 99.97 | 99.97 | 99.97 | 99.97 | 99.97 | 99.97 | 99.98 |

| Table 5.2 | Computing Probabilities from Negative Z-scores |

| | Negative Z-score (%) | | | | | | | | | |
| --- | --- | --- | --- | --- | --- | --- | --- | --- | --- | --- |
| Z | 0.09 | 0.08 | 0.07 | 0.06 | 0.05 | 0.04 | 0.03 | 0.02 | 0.01 | 0 |
| −3.4 | 0.02 | 0.03 | 0.03 | 0.03 | 0.03 | 0.03 | 0.03 | 0.03 | 0.03 | 0.03 |
| −3.3 | 0.03 | 0.04 | 0.04 | 0.04 | 0.04 | 0.04 | 0.04 | 0.05 | 0.05 | 0.05 |
| −3.2 | 0.05 | 0.05 | 0.05 | 0.06 | 0.06 | 0.06 | 0.06 | 0.06 | 0.07 | 0.07 |
| −3.1 | 0.07 | 0.07 | 0.08 | 0.08 | 0.08 | 0.08 | 0.09 | 0.09 | 0.09 | 0.10 |
| −3 | 0.10 | 0.10 | 0.11 | 0.11 | 0.11 | 0.12 | 0.12 | 0.13 | 0.13 | 0.13 |
| −2.9 | 0.14 | 0.14 | 0.15 | 0.15 | 0.16 | 0.16 | 0.17 | 0.18 | 0.18 | 0.19 |
| −2.8 | 0.19 | 0.20 | 0.21 | 0.21 | 0.22 | 0.23 | 0.23 | 0.24 | 0.25 | 0.26 |
| −2.7 | 0.26 | 0.27 | 0.28 | 0.29 | 0.30 | 0.31 | 0.32 | 0.33 | 0.34 | 0.35 |
| −2.6 | 0.36 | 0.37 | 0.38 | 0.39 | 0.40 | 0.41 | 0.43 | 0.44 | 0.45 | 0.47 |
| −2.5 | 0.48 | 0.49 | 0.51 | 0.52 | 0.54 | 0.55 | 0.57 | 0.59 | 0.60 | 0.62 |
| −2.4 | 0.64 | 0.66 | 0.68 | 0.69 | 0.71 | 0.73 | 0.75 | 0.78 | 0.80 | 0.82 |
| −2.3 | 0.84 | 0.87 | 0.89 | 0.91 | 0.94 | 0.96 | 0.99 | 1.02 | 1.04 | 1.07 |
| −2.2 | 1.10 | 1.13 | 1.16 | 1.19 | 1.22 | 1.25 | 1.29 | 1.32 | 1.36 | 1.39 |
| −2.1 | 1.43 | 1.46 | 1.50 | 1.54 | 1.58 | 1.62 | 1.66 | 1.70 | 1.74 | 1.79 |
| −2 | 1.83 | 1.88 | 1.92 | 1.97 | 2.02 | 2.07 | 2.12 | 2.17 | 2.22 | 2.28 |
| −1.9 | 2.33 | 2.39 | 2.44 | 2.50 | 2.56 | 2.62 | 2.68 | 2.74 | 2.81 | 2.87 |
| −1.8 | 2.94 | 3.01 | 3.07 | 3.14 | 3.22 | 3.29 | 3.36 | 3.44 | 3.51 | 3.59 |
| −1.7 | 3.67 | 3.75 | 3.84 | 3.92 | 4.01 | 4.09 | 4.18 | 4.27 | 4.36 | 4.46 |
| −1.6 | 4.55 | 4.65 | 4.75 | 4.85 | 4.95 | 5.05 | 5.16 | 5.26 | 5.37 | 5.48 |
| −1.5 | 5.59 | 5.71 | 5.82 | 5.94 | 6.06 | 6.18 | 6.30 | 6.43 | 6.55 | 6.68 |
| −1.4 | 6.81 | 6.94 | 7.08 | 7.21 | 7.35 | 7.49 | 7.64 | 7.78 | 7.93 | 8.08 |
| −1.3 | 8.23 | 8.38 | 8.53 | 8.69 | 8.85 | 9.01 | 9.18 | 9.34 | 9.51 | 9.68 |
| −1.2 | 9.85 | 10.03 | 10.20 | 10.38 | 10.56 | 10.75 | 10.93 | 11.12 | 11.31 | 11.51 |
| −1.1 | 11.70 | 11.90 | 12.10 | 12.30 | 12.51 | 12.71 | 12.92 | 13.14 | 13.35 | 13.57 |
| −1 | 13.79 | 14.01 | 14.23 | 14.46 | 14.69 | 14.92 | 15.15 | 15.39 | 15.62 | 15.87 |
| −0.9 | 16.11 | 16.35 | 16.60 | 16.85 | 17.11 | 17.36 | 17.62 | 17.88 | 18.14 | 18.41 |
| −0.8 | 18.67 | 18.94 | 19.22 | 19.49 | 19.77 | 20.05 | 20.33 | 20.61 | 20.90 | 21.19 |
| −0.7 | 21.48 | 21.77 | 22.06 | 22.36 | 22.66 | 22.96 | 23.27 | 23.58 | 23.89 | 24.20 |
| −0.6 | 24.51 | 24.83 | 25.14 | 25.46 | 25.78 | 26.11 | 26.43 | 26.76 | 27.09 | 27.43 |
| −0.5 | 27.76 | 28.10 | 28.43 | 28.77 | 29.12 | 29.46 | 29.81 | 30.15 | 30.50 | 30.85 |
| −0.4 | 31.21 | 31.56 | 31.92 | 32.28 | 32.64 | 33.00 | 33.36 | 33.72 | 34.09 | 34.46 |
| −0.3 | 34.83 | 35.20 | 35.57 | 35.94 | 36.32 | 36.69 | 37.07 | 37.45 | 37.83 | 38.21 |
| −0.2 | 38.29 | 38.97 | 39.36 | 39.74 | 40.13 | 40.52 | 40.90 | 41.29 | 41.68 | 42.07 |
| −0.1 | 42.47 | 42.86 | 43.25 | 43.64 | 44.04 | 44.43 | 44.83 | 45.22 | 45.62 | 46.02 |
| 0 | 46.41 | 46.81 | 47.21 | 47.61 | 48.01 | 48.40 | 48.80 | 49.20 | 49.60 | 50.00 |

| Table 5.3 | Commonly Used Percentiles and Their Corresponding Z-scores |
|---|---|

| Percentile | Z-score |
|---|---|
| 1 | −2.33 |
| 2.5 | −1.96 |
| 5 | −1.65 |
| 10 | −1.28 |
| 20 | −0.84 |
| 25 | −0.67 |
| 50 | 0 |
| 75 | 0.67 |
| 80 | 0.84 |
| 90 | 1.28 |
| 95 | 1.65 |
| 97.5 | 1.96 |
| 99 | 2.33 |

formats, using the concepts described above, the 1st, 5th, 50th, 95th, and 99th percentiles for various cardiac measurements can be computed using an Excel spreadsheet. Tables 5.4 and 5.5 are examples of the linear and quadratic equations used to create percentile curves used in this chapter.

## M-MODE QUANTITATION OF FETAL CARDIAC STRUCTURES

### Techniques for Obtaining M-Mode Measurements of the Ventricular Chambers

The use of M-mode ultrasound to detect cardiac motion was first reported in 1971 followed by its use to detect fetal death in 1976.[10,11] In 1980, Kleinman et al.[12] published the first paper using M-Mode to diagnose abnormal cardiac rhythm and function. In 1981, DeVore et al.[13] reported using M-Mode to measure the pre-ejection and ventricular ejection time of the right and left ventricles. Between 1982 and 2011, several investigators reported the use of real-time-directed M-mode echocardiography and cardio-STIC-M-mode to obtain M-mode recordings from which they made cardiac and outflow tract measurements.[1–5,14–17] Table 5.6 contains a summary of each of

| Table 5.4 | Biventricular Outer Dimensions (BVOD) DeVore (1984)<br>Upper table contains equations to compute the BVOD 50th,1st, 5th, 95th, 99th %.<br>The Z-score of 1% = −1.65, 95% = +1.65, 99% = +2.33. SD is a fixed value.<br>The bottom table contains the results from the computations. |
|---|---|

| | A | B | C | D | E | F | G |
|---|---|---|---|---|---|---|---|
| 1 | | | | Computed Percentiles | | | |
| 2 | Standard Deviation | Biparietal Diameter (cm) | BVOD 50th Percentile | BVOD 1st Percentile | BVOD 5th Percentile | BVOD 95th Percentile | BVOD 99th Percentile |
| 3 | 0.2387 | 4 | =+(−0.5038) + (0.5091 * B3) | =+C3 − (2.33 * 0.2387) | =+C3 − (1.65 * 0.2387) | =+C3 + (1.65 * 0.2387) | =+C3 + (2.33 * 0.2387) |
| 4 | 0.2387 | 9.5 | =+(−0.5038) + (0.5091 * B4) | =+C4 − (2.33 * 0.2387) | =+C4 − (1.65 * 0.2387) | =+C4 + (1.65 * 0.2387) | =+C4 + (2.33 * 0.2387) |

5  DeVore (1985):
   Mean: Linear Equation: $(Y) = +a + bX$
   $a = -0.5038$, $b = 0.5091$
   BVOD (cm) Mean = (−0.5038) + (0.5091 × BPD)
   Standard error of the estimate = standard deviation = constant = 0.2387

| | A | B | C | D | E | F | G |
|---|---|---|---|---|---|---|---|
| 1 | | | | Computed Percentiles | | | |
| 2 | Standard Deviation | Biparietal Diameter (cm) | BVOD 50th Percentile | BVOD 1st Percentile | BVOD 5th Percentile | BVOD 95th Percentile | BVOD 99th Percentile |
| 3 | 0.2387 | 4 | 1.5326 | 0.976429 | 1.138745 | 1.926455 | 2.088771 |
| 4 | 0.2387 | 9.5 | 4.33265 | 3.776479 | 3.938795 | 4.726505 | 4.888821 |

| Table 5.5 | Biventricular Outer Dimensions (BVOD) Luewan(2011)<br>Upper table contains equations to compute the BVOD 50th, 1st, 5th, 95th, 99th %.<br>The Z-score of 1% = −2.33, 5% = −1.65%, 95% = +1.65, 99% = +2.33. SD is a function of BPD.<br>The bottom table contains the results from the computations. |
|---|---|

| | A | B | C | D | E | F | G |
|---|---|---|---|---|---|---|---|
| 1 | | | **Computed Percentiles** | | | | |
| 2 | *Standard Deviation* | *Biparietal Diameter (cm)* | *BVOD 50th Percentile* | *BVOD 1st Percentile* | *BVOD 5th Percentile* | *BVOD 95th Percentile* | *BVOD 99th Percentile* |
| 3 | =+(0.0274) + (0.0364 * B3) | **4** | =+(−0.8278) + (0.7088 * B3) + (−0.0213 * B3 * B3) | =+C3 − (2.33 * A3) | =+C3 − (1.65 * A3) | =+C3 + (1.65 * A3) | =+C3 + (2.33 * A3) |
| 4 | =+(0.0274) + (0.0364 * B4) | 5 | =+(−0.8278) + (0.7088 * B4) + (−0.0213 * B4 * B4) | =+C4 − (2.33 * A4) | =+C4 − (1.65 * A4) | =+C4 + (1.65 * A4) | =+C4 + (2.33 * A4) |
| 5 | =+ (0.0274) + (0.0364 * B5) | 6 | =+(−0.8278) + (0.7088 * B5) + (−0.0213 * B5 * B5) | =+C5 − (2.33 * A5) | =+C5 − (1.65 * A5) | =+C5 + (1.65 * A5) | =+C5 + (2.33 * A5) |
| 6 | =+(0.0274) + (0.0364 * B6) | 7 | =+(−0.8278) + (0.7088 * B6) + (−0.0213 * B6 * B6) | =+C6 − (2.33 * A6) | =+C6 − (1.65 * A6) | =+C6 + (1.65 * A6) | =+C6 + (2.33 * A6) |
| 7 | =+(0.0274) + (0.0364 * B7) | 8 | =+ (−0.8278) + (0.7088 * B7) + (−0.0213 * B7 * B7) | =+C7 − (2.33 * A7) | =+C7 − (1.65 * A7) | =+C7 + (1.65 * A7) | =+C7 + (2.33 * A7) |
| 8 | =+(0.0274) + (0.0364 * B8) | 9.5 | =+(−0.8278) + (0.7088 * B8) + (−0.0213 * B8 * B8) | =+C8 − (2.33 * A8) | =+C8 − (1.65 * A8) | =+C8 + (1.65 * A8) | =+C8 + (2.33 * A8) |

9 Luewan, 2011

Mean: Second-Order Quadratic Equation: $(Y) = + a + bX + cX^2$

$a = -0.8278, b = 0.7088, c = -0.0213$

BVOD (cm) Mean = (−0.8278) + (0.7088 × BPD) + (−0.0213 × BPD2)

Standard Deviation: Linear equation

$a = 0.0274$

$b = 0.0364$

BVOD Standard Deviation = (0.0274) + (0.0364 × BPD)

| | A | B | C | D | E | F | G |
|---|---|---|---|---|---|---|---|
| 1 | | | **Computed Percentiles** | | | | |
| 2 | *Standard Deviation* | *Biparietal Diameter (cm)* | *BVOD 50th Percentile* | *BVOD 1st Percentile* | *BVOD 5th Percentile* | *BVOD 95th Percentile* | *BVOD 99th Percentile* |
| 3 | 0.173 | **4** | 1.6666 | 1.2635 | 1.3812 | 1.9521 | 2.0697 |
| 4 | 0.2094 | 5 | 2.1837 | 1.6958 | 1.8382 | 2.5292 | 2.6716 |
| 5 | 0.2458 | 6 | 2.6582 | 2.0855 | 2.2526 | 3.0638 | 3.2309 |
| 6 | 0.2822 | 7 | 3.0901 | 2.4326 | 2.6245 | 3.5557 | 3.7476 |
| 7 | 0.3186 | 8 | 3.4794 | 2.7371 | 2.9537 | 4.0051 | 4.2217 |
| 8 | 0.3732 | 9.5 | 3.9835 | 3.1139 | 3.3677 | 4.5993 | 4.8530 |

the above studies. Allan, DeVore, Cartier, and Luewan provided regression equations, while St. John Sutton only performed correlation analysis.[1–5,14–17] Investigators compared cardiac measurements with gestational age and/or biometric measurements from the fetus (biparietal diameter, head circumference, abdominal circumference, and femur length).[1–5,14–17] Figure 5.1 compares the two methods by which the M-mode was recorded from the above studies to measure the ventricular diameters and the corresponding measurements as defined in Table 5.6. The first method obtains the M-mode from a location just below the movement of the mitral and tricuspid valve leaflets (Fig. 5.1). When the M-mode is obtained at this level, often the left

| Table 5.6 | Comparing M-Mode Studies |
| --- | --- |

| | Allan et al.[1] | DeVore et al.[2,3,15] | DeVore et al.[14] | St John Sutton et al.[17] | Cartier et al.[4] | Luewan et al.[5] |
| --- | --- | --- | --- | --- | --- | --- |
| **Study Parameters** | | | | | | |
| Gestational age range | 14–40 | 18–41 | 18–41 | 20–40 | 14–42 | 14–42 |
| Number of fetuses studied | 200 | 82 | 43 | 16 | 403 | 657 |
| Type of study | Cross-sectional | Cross-sectional | Cross-sectional | Sequential | Cross-sectional | Cross-sectional |
| **Data Analysis** | | | | | | |
| Statistical analysis | Linear regression | Linear regression | Linear regression | Correlation | Linear regression | Linear and polynomial regression |
| Display of data | Mean, standard error of the estimate | Mean, standard error of the estimate | Mean, standard error of the estimate | Correlation analysis, standard error of the estimate | | |
| Regression equations provided | Yes | Yes | Yes | No | Yes | Yes |
| Weeks of gestation | X | | | X | X | X |
| Biparietal diameter | | X | X | | | X |
| Head circumference | | | X | | X | X |
| Abdominal circumference | | X | X | | | |
| Femur length | | X | X | | | |
| **Ventricular Measurements** | | | | | | |
| Biventricular outer dimension | | X | | | | X |
| Biventricular inner dimension | | X | | | | |
| Left ventricular dimension | X | X | | X | | X |
| Mitral valve excursion | | X | | | | |
| Left ventricular mass | | X | | X | | |
| Right ventricular dimension | X | X | | X | | X |
| Tricuspid valve excursion | | X | | | | |
| Right/left ventricular ratio | | X | | X | | |
| Left/right ventricular ratio | | | | | | X |
| Change in septal and wall thickness | | | | X | | |
| Left ventricular wall thickness | X | X | | X | | X |
| Interventricular wall thickness | X | X | | X | | X |
| Right ventricular wall thickness | | X | | X | | X |
| Right/left ventricular wall thickness ratio | | | | X | | |
| Ventricular systolic function | | X | | X | | |
| **Atrial Measurements** | | | | | | |
| Right atrial dimension | | | | | | |
| Left atrial dimension | | | | X | | |

| Outflow Tracts | Allan et al.[1] | DeVore et al.[2,3,15] | DeVore et al.[14] | St John Sutton et al.[17] | Cartier et al.[4] | Luewan et al.[5] |
|---|---|---|---|---|---|---|
| Aortic valve dimension | | | X | | | |
| Aortic dimension | X | | X | X | X | |
| Pulmonary valve dimension | | | | | | |
| Pulmonary artery dimension | | | | | X | |
| Aorta/left atrial ratio | | | | X | | |
| Aortic valve/mitral valve | | | X | | | |
| Aortic valve/biventricular dimension | | | X | | | |
| Aortic valve/left ventricular dimension | | | X | | | |
| Aortic diameter/mitral valve | | | X | | | |
| Aortic root/biventricular dimension | | | X | | | |
| Aortic root/left ventricular dimension | | | X | | | |

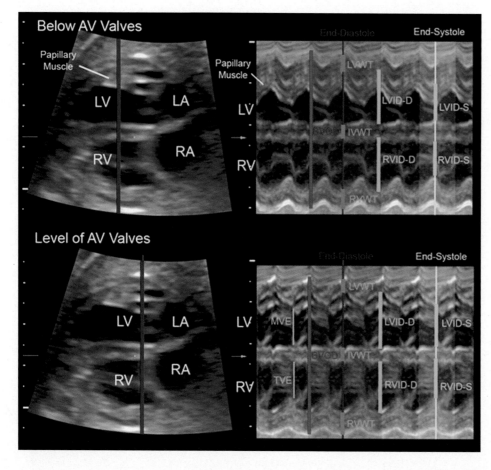

**FIGURE 5.1:** This illustrates the M-mode recording obtained when the cursor is placed below the level of the atrioventricular (AV) valve leaflets **(upper panel)** and at the level of the leaflets **(lower panel)**. When the cursor is placed at the level of the valves, the papillary muscle of the left ventricle does not obscure the boundary of the left ventricular wall. In addition, the mitral valve opening excursion (MVE) and tricuspid opening excursion (TVE) can be identified for the measurement of valve size. LV, left ventricle; RV, right ventricle; LA, left atrium; RA, right atrium; BVOD, biventricular outer dimension; RVID-D, right ventricular inner dimension at end-diastole; RVID-S, right ventricular inner dimension at end-systole; LVID-D, left ventricular inner dimension at end-diastole; LVID-S, left ventricular inner dimension at end-systole; LVWT, left ventricular wall thickness at end-diastole; RVWT, right ventricular wall thickness at end-diastole; IVWT, interventricular septal wall thickness at end-diastole; Fractional shortening is computed as follows: Right ventricle: [(RVID-D − RVID-S)/RVID-D]; Left ventricle: [(LVID-D − LVID-S)/LVID-D].

ventricular wall is obscured because of the adjacent papillary muscle. The second method obtains the recording at the level of the atrioventricular valves, which is the largest diameter of the chambers (Fig. 5.1). As a result, I prefer measuring all chamber dimensions using this approach.

## Comparison of 5% and 95% Percentile Graphs for Right and Left Ventricular Inner Dimensions

### Gestational Age

Figure 5.2 compares the end-diastolic right and left ventricular inner dimensions between Allan et al.[1] and Luewan et al.[5] The difference between the 5% and 95% percentiles is narrower during the second trimester but wider in the third trimester when polynomial regression is used (Luewan et al.[5]) compared with linear regression (Allan et al.[1]). Allan et al.[1] obtained the M-mode measurements at the level just below the mitral and tricuspid valves, while Luewan et al.[5] obtained the measurements at the level of the valves.

### Biparietal Diameter

Figure 5.3 compares the end-diastolic right and left inner dimensions between DeVore et al.[2] and Luewan et al.[5] The 5% and 95% confidence intervals are wider in the third trimester when polynomial regression is used (Luewan et al.[5]) compared with linear regression (DeVore et al.[2]). Both DeVore et al.[2] and

Luewan et al.[5] obtained the measurements of the ventricles at the level of the opening and closing of the mitral and tricuspid valve leaflets (Fig. 5.1).

## Comparison of 5% and 95% Percentile Graphs for the Biventricular Outer Dimension

### Biparietal Diameter

Figure 5.4 compares the end-diastolic biventricular outer dimension between DeVore et al.[2] and Luewan et al.[5] The 5% and 95% percentile graphs are wider in the third trimester when polynomial regression is used (Luewan et al.[5]) compared with linear regression (DeVore et al.[2]). Both DeVore et al.[2] and Luewan et al.[5] obtained the measurements of the ventricles at the level of the opening and closing of the mitral and tricuspid valve leaflets (Fig. 5.1).

## Comparison of 5% and 95% Percentile Graphs for the Right and Left Ventricular and Interventricular Wall Thickness

### Biparietal Diameter

Figure 5.5 compares the end-diastolic wall and interventricular wall thickness between DeVore et al.[2] and Luewan et al.[5] The 5% and 95% percentile graphs are narrower in the second and third trimesters when polynomial regression is used (Luewan[5]) compared with linear regression (DeVore et al.[2]).

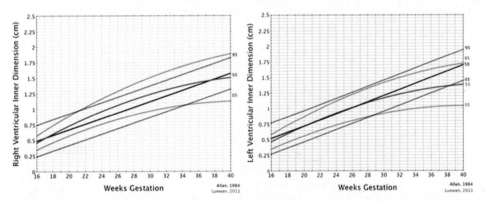

**FIGURE 5.2:** Comparison of the mean, 95% and 5% for the left and right inner dimensions between studies by Allan et al.[1] and Luewan et al.[5] Allan et al. found that the best fit for the regression analysis was linear, while Luewan et al. found that it was a second-order polynomial. Luewan's data demonstrated a narrower band for the 5% and 95% during the second trimester and a larger band in the third trimester.

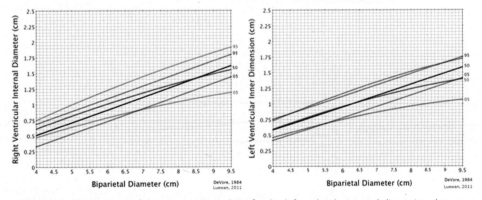

**FIGURE 5.3:** Comparison of the mean, 95% and 5% for the left and right internal dimensions between studies by DeVore et al.[2] and Luewan et al.[5] DeVore et al. found that the best fit for the regression analysis was linear, while Luewan et al. found that it was a second-order polynomial. Comparing the two graphs, Luewan's data showed a wider band for the 5% and 95% during the third trimester for both ventricles.

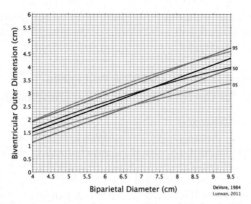

**FIGURE 5.4:** Comparison of the mean, 95% and 5% for the biventricular outer dimension between studies by DeVore[14] and Luewan.[5] DeVore found that the best fit for the regression analysis was linear, while Luewan found that it was a second-order polynomial. Comparing the two graphs, Luewan's data showed a wider band for the 5% and 95% during the third trimester.

Both DeVore et al.[2] and Luewan et al.[5] obtained the measurements of the ventricles at the level of the opening and closing of the mitral and tricuspid valve leaflets (Fig. 5.1).

## Comparison of 5% and 95% Percentile Graphs for Ventricular Ejection Fraction

### Biparietal Diameter

Figure 5.6 compares the ventricular fractional shortening ([diastolic dimension-systolic dimension]/diastolic dimension) between DeVore et al.[2] and Luewan et al.[5] Both studies found the best fit was using linear regression. Comparing the two graphs, Luewan's et al.[5] data showed a narrower band for the 5% and 95% for the right ventricle, but similar percentiles for the left ventricle. Both DeVore et al.[2] and Luewan et al.[5] obtained the measurements of the ventricles at the level of the opening and closing of the mitral and tricuspid valve leaflets.

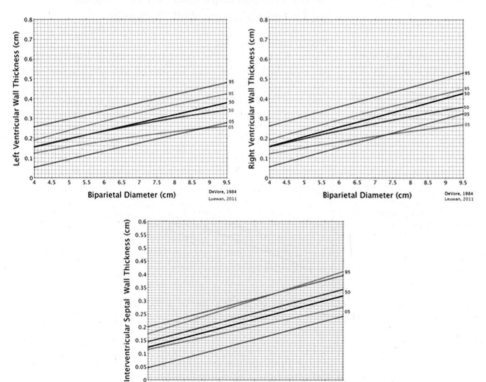

**FIGURE 5.5:** Comparison of the mean, 95% and 5% for the ventricular walls and interventricular septum between studies by DeVore[6] and Luewan.[13] DeVore found that the best fit for the regression analysis was linear, while Luewan found that it was a second-order polynomial. Comparing the two graphs, Luewan's data showed a narrower band for the 5% and 95% throughout pregnancy.

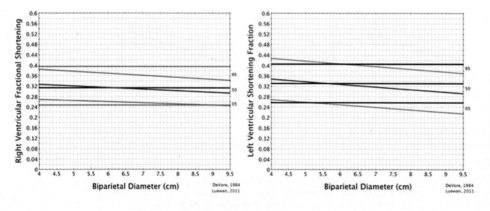

**FIGURE 5.6:** Comparison of the mean, 95% and 5% for the shortening fraction between studies by DeVore[6] and Luewan.[13] Both studies found the best fit was using linear regression. Comparing the two graphs, Luewan's data showed a narrower band for the 5% and 95% for the right ventricle, but similar confidence intervals for the left ventricle.

## Comparison of 5% and 95% Percentile Graphs for a Fetus with a Dilated Right Ventricle

Figure 5.7 is an M-mode from a fetus with a dilated ventricle. In the normal fetus, the excursion of the tricuspid valve leaflet touches the right ventricular wall as the leaflets open at the beginning of diastole. When the right ventricle is dilated, the tricuspid valve leaflet opens but does not touch the lateral right ventricular wall, revealing a space between the full extension of the valve leaflet and the right ventricular wall. From this tracing, the right and left ventricular inner dimension was plotted against gestational age and biparietal diameter[1,2,5] (Fig. 5.8). The right ventricular inner dimension was at the 95% using the data

from DeVore et al.,[2] but normal for Luewan et al.[5] The fractional shortening of the right ventricle was 0.238, below the 5% for both DeVore et al.[2] and Luewan et al.[5] The left ventricular inner dimension was normal for both DeVore et al.[2] and Luewan et al.,[5] as was the fractional shortening (0.394).

## M-Mode Graphs For Evaluating Ventricular Size and Function

From a practical perspective, the reader often desires to use graphs or tables that have been published for clinical purposes. For this chapter, I have created graphs that display the 1st, 5th,

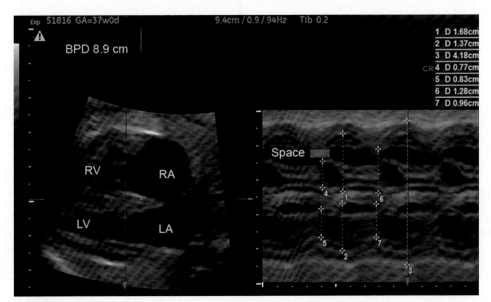

**FIGURE 5.7:** This is an M-mode recording from a fetus with a dilated right ventricle as manifest by the space between the tricuspid valve excursion and the right lateral wall. The white bar on the M-mode tracing demonstrates this space. The M-mode measurements are listed from numbers 1 to 7 and correspond as follows: 1, right ventricular inner dimension-diastole; 2, left ventricular inner dimension-diastole; 3, biventricular outer dimension-diastole; 4, tricuspid valve excursion; 5, mitral valve excursion; 6, right ventricular inner dimension-systole; 7, left ventricular inner dimension-systole. Fractional shortening = (RVID Diastole – RVID Systole)/RVID Diastole = (Measurement 1 – Measurement 6)/Measurement 1 = (1.68 − 1.28)/1.68 = 0.238.

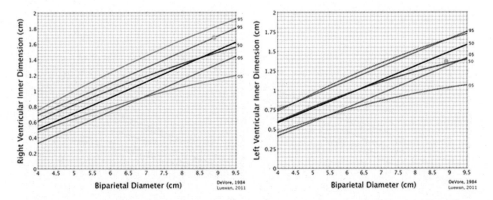

**FIGURE 5.8:** The case illustrated in Figure 5.7 demonstrates measurement of the right ventricular inner dimension to be at the 95% for DeVore, but in the normal range for Luewan. Comparing weeks of gestation, Allan demonstrated the right ventricular inner dimension to be at the 95%, while Luewan showed that it was in the upper range of normal. The left ventricular inner dimension is normal for DeVore, Allan, and Luewan. The fractional shortening of the right ventricle is decreased for both DeVore and Luewan. It is increased for the left ventricle for Luewan but not for DeVore.

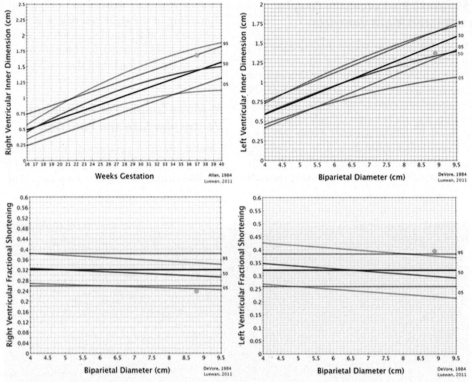

**FIGURE 5.8:** (continued)

50th, 95th, and 99th percentiles for each of the measurements reported in the literature.[1-5] The raw data used to create the graphs were derived from regression equations published by the authors.[1-5] From the standard deviations, the percentiles were computed for each measurement using the concepts described in Tables 5.4 and 5.5. The x and y axes for each measurement have been normalized between the various authors for consistency.

### End-Diastolic Biventricular
### Outer Dimension (BVOD)

When cardiomegaly is suspected, the BVOD can be useful to quantitate the overall size of the heart. Depending upon the underlying pathology, the user can select the biparietal diameter, head circumference, femur length, or gestational age

(Fig. 5.9). For example, if a fetus is brachycephalic and has a short femur, the examiner may select the head circumference or weeks' gestation as a reference standard to evaluate the size of the heart other than say the femur length

### End-Diastolic Left Ventricular
### Inner Dimension (LVID)

An enlarged left ventricle is observed in early critical aortic stenosis in which the left ventricle is poorly contractile. The LVID is decreased in size in fetuses with coarctation of the aorta, as well as those with varying degrees of the hypoplastic left heart syndrome. Figure 5.10 lists the LVID graphs reference to the biparietal diameter, head circumference, femur length, and gestational age.

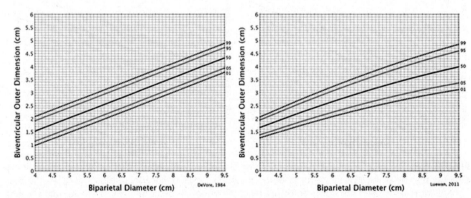

**FIGURE 5.9:** These graphs demonstrate the 1st, 5th, 50th, 95th, and 99th percentiles for the end-diastolic biventricular outer dimension for the biparietal diameter, head circumference, femur length, and weeks of gestation.

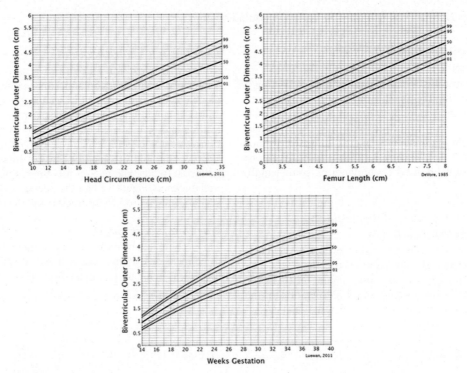

**FIGURE 5.9:** (*Continued*)

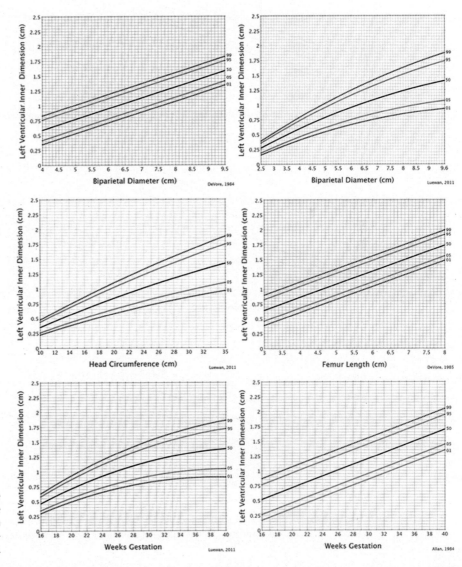

**FIGURE 5.10:** These graphs demonstrate the 1st, 5th, 50th, 95th, and 99th percentiles for the end-diastolic left ventricular inner dimension refer to the biparietal diameter, head circumference, femur length, and weeks of gestation.

### End-Diastolic Right Ventricular Inner Dimension (RVID)

An enlarged right ventricle is the most common finding I observe when evaluating the fetal heart. It can be present with intrauterine growth restriction, postterm pregnancies, coarctation of the aorta, and other fetal conditions that result in either volume loading of the right ventricle and/or increased pulmonary vascular resistance.[18–20] Figure 5.11 lists the RVID graphs for the biparietal diameter, head circumference, femur length, and gestational age.

### End-Diastolic Right Ventricle/Left Ventricle and Left Ventricle/Right Ventricle Ratios

When disproportion between the right and left ventricular chambers is suspected, the ratio between the chambers may be useful in evaluating cardiac function.[21] Figure 5.12 lists the graphs for the RVID/LVID as well as LVID/RVID ratios for the biparietal diameter, head circumference, and gestational age.

### End-Diastolic Ventricular and Interventricular Wall Thickness

Ventricular wall hypertrophy occurs as a result of primary cardiomyopathy, cardiomyopathy secondary to maternal diabetes, and fetal conditions that are associated with increased volume loading and/or increased outflow tract resistance. For the experienced examiner, a thickened wall or septum is easily visualized. However, the ability to quantify the wall thickness is important for following trends. Figure 5.13 lists the graphs for left ventricular wall thickness, Figure 5.14 for the thickness of the interventricular septum, and Figure 5.15 the thickness of the right ventricular wall.

### Fractional Shortening

This is computed by measuring the right or left ventricular chamber dimensions at end-diastole and end-systole (Fig. 5.1). From these measurements, fractional shortening is computed as follows:

$$(\text{Diastolic measurement} - \text{Systolic measurement}) / \text{Diastolic measurement}$$

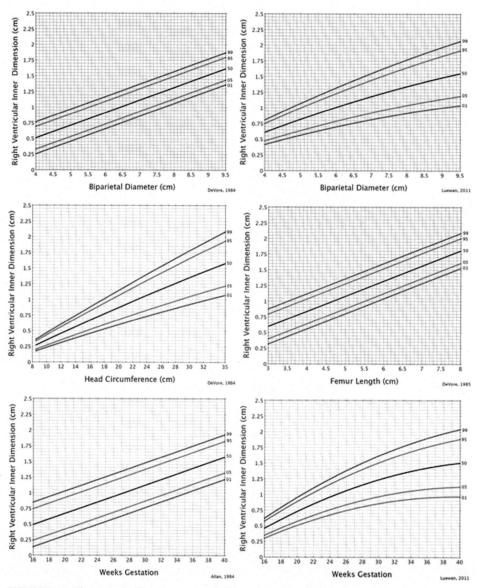

**FIGURE 5.11:** These graphs demonstrate the 1st, 5th, 50th, 95th, and 99th percentiles for the end-diastolic right ventricular inner dimension for the biparietal diameter, head circumference, femur length, and weeks of gestation.

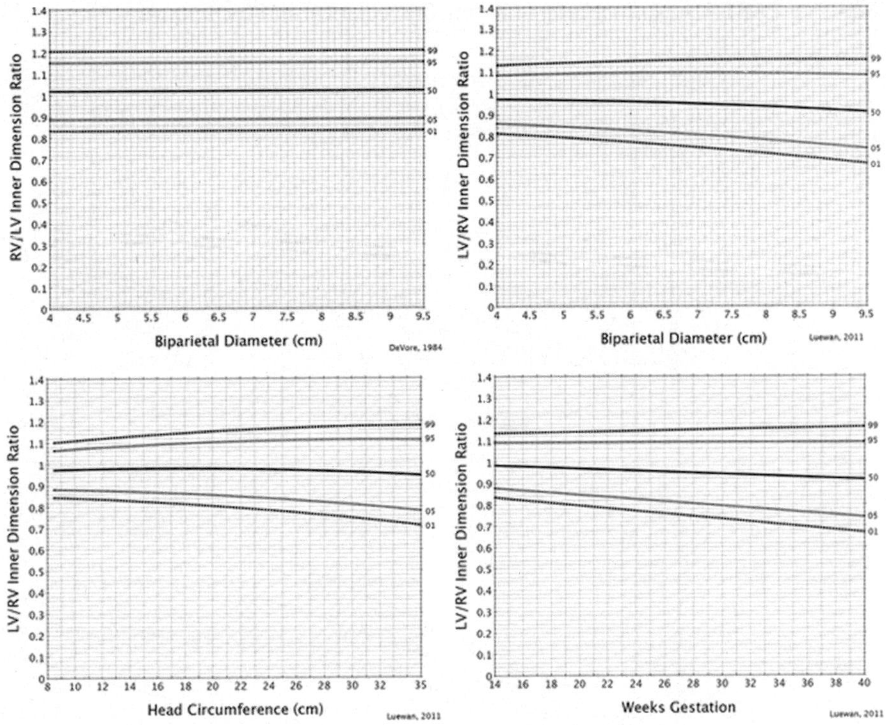

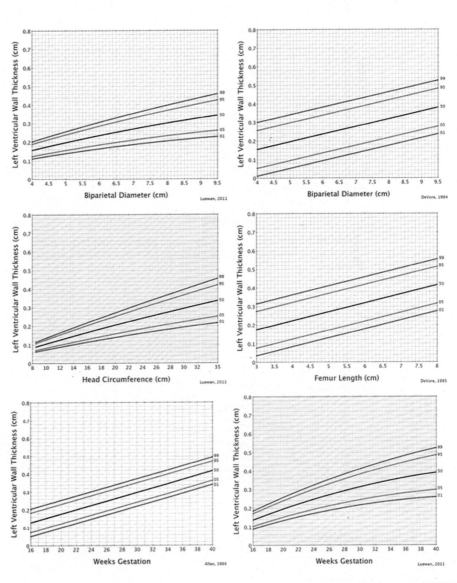

**FIGURE 5.12:** These graphs demonstrate the 1st, 5th, 50th, 95th, and 99th percentiles for the LVID/RVID ratios for the biparietal diameter, head circumference, femur length, and weeks of gestation.

**FIGURE 5.13:** These graphs demonstrate the 1st, 5th, 50th, 95th, and 99th percentiles for the end-diastolic left ventricular wall thickness for the biparietal diameter, head circumference, femur length, and weeks of gestation.

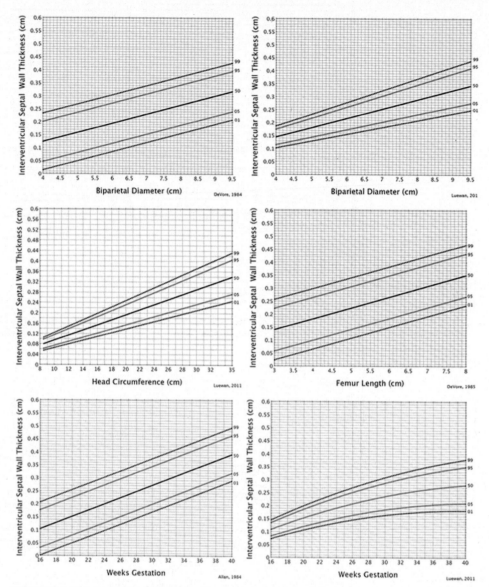

**FIGURE 5.14:** These graphs demonstrate the 1st, 5th, 50th, 95th, and 99th percentiles for the end-diastolic interventricular wall thickness for the biparietal diameter, head circumference, femur length, and weeks of gestation.

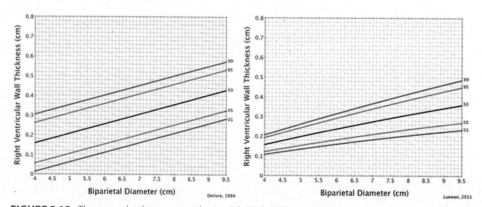

**FIGURE 5.15:** These graphs demonstrate the 1st, 5th, 50th, 95th, and 99th percentiles for the end-diastolic right ventricular wall thickness for the biparietal diameter, head circumference, femur length, and weeks of gestation.

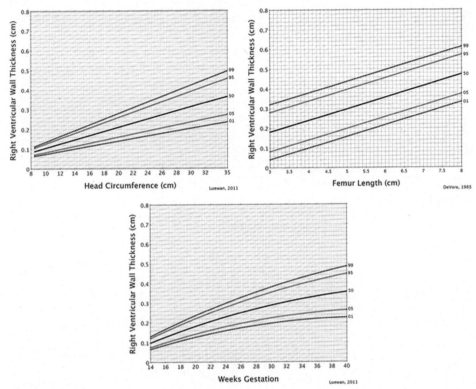

**FIGURE 5.15:** (*Continued*)

Figure 5.16 lists the graphs for right ventricular fractional shortening, and Figure 5.17 for left ventricular fractional shortening.

### *Opening Excursion of the Mitral and Tricuspid Valve Leaflets*

The opening of these valve leaflets is useful when detecting a small left or right ventricular valve orifice. In addition, investigators have measured the Doppler inflow waveform to compute the cardiac output for the right and left ventricles. Measurement of the valve opening excursion represents the diameter of the valves from which the area can be computed. Figure 5.18 lists the graphs for the mitral and tricuspid valve opening excursion.

## M-Mode Graphs for Evaluating the Aorta and Pulmonary Artery

Measurements of the aorta and main pulmonary artery diameter are important when computing Doppler blood flow through these vessels. Investigators reported using measurements from these vessels to detect fetuses with tetralogy of Fallot, as well as hypoplastic outflow tracts.[1,4,13,14,16] Figure 5.19 illustrates the M-mode recording from the aorta and the main pulmonary artery. Figures 5.20 and 5.21 list the percentile graphs for the aorta and the main pulmonary artery.

## B-Mode Quantitation of Fetal Cardiac Structures

B-mode ultrasound has an advantage over M-mode in that measurements of cardiac structures do not have to be aligned perpendicular to the specific structure to be measured. Therefore, B-mode measurements of chamber and outflow tracts can be more easily obtained. The limitation is that the timing at end-diastole or end-systole may be more difficult because the examiner has to scroll through the cine loop to find the exact phase of the cardiac cycle from which to make the measurement.

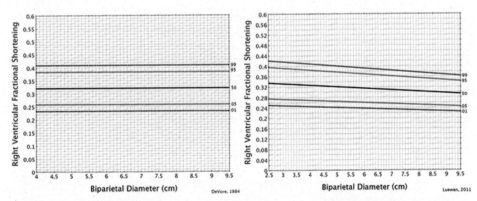

**FIGURE 5.16:** These graphs demonstrate the 1st, 5th, 50th, 95th, and 99th percentiles for the right ventricular fractional shortening for the biparietal diameter, head circumference, femur length, and weeks of gestation.

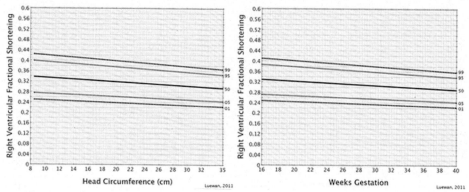

**FIGURE 5.16:** (*Continued*)

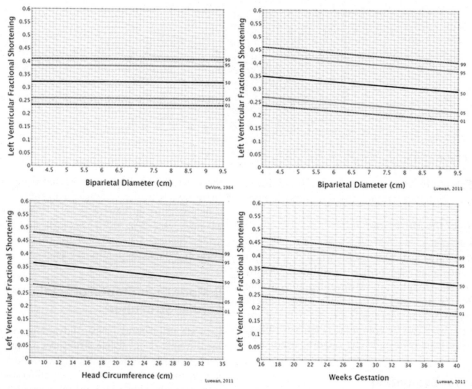

**FIGURE 5.17:** These graphs demonstrate the 1st, 5th, 50th, 95th, and 99th percentiles for the left ventricular fractional shortening for the biparietal diameter, head circumference, femur length, and weeks of gestation.

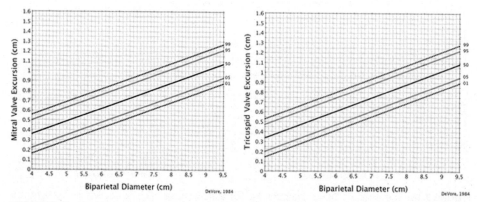

**FIGURE 5.18:** These graphs demonstrate the 1st, 5th, 50th, 95th, and 99th percentiles for the mitral and tricuspid valve opening excursion for the biparietal diameter and femur length.

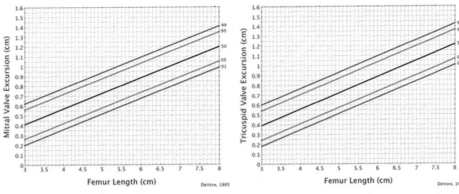

**FIGURE 5.18:** (Continued)

Figure 5.22 illustrates examples of B-mode images and where specific measurements are made.

## B-Mode Percentile Graphs for Evaluating the Size of the Ventricular and Outflow Tracts Using Gestational Age

In 1992, Sharland and Allan[8] reported measuring ventricular chamber dimensions and the diameters of the outflow tracts from still frames of B-mode images of the heart (Table 5.7).

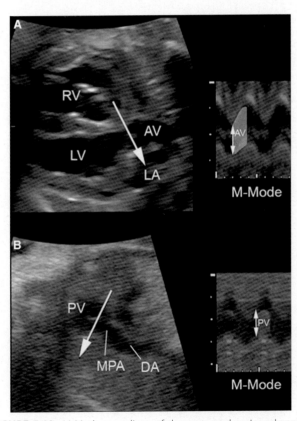

**FIGURE 5.19:** M-Mode recordings of the aorta and main pulmonary artery. Using traditional M-mode, the cursor is placed perpendicular to the aorta and main pulmonary artery at the level of the aortic valve (AV) and the pulmonary valve (PV). When the M-mode is obtained from a STIC volume, the M-mode line can be drawn through the aorta and main pulmonary artery (MPA) at the level of the valves. RV, right ventricle; LV, left ventricle; LA, left atrium.

They reported that quadratic polynomial regression equations best described the distribution of cardiac measurements and provided a graphical display of the mean and 95th percentile for each measurement as a function of gestational age.[8] When I compared the graphical display of the percentiles with the published equations and computed the intervals, they were not the same. Therefore, I have not used their data in this chapter.

In the same year, Tan et al.[9] reported results from their study that included more measurements than Sharland and Allan, and found that linear and quadratic regression equations best fit their data (Table 5.7). They computed the mean and standard error of the estimate, using gestational age as the independent variable.[9]

In 1998, Shapiro et al. studied a larger number of patients than those from the two previous studies but measured fewer cardiac structures (Table 5.7).[8,9,22] Shapiro et al.[22] also reported that linear and quadratic polynomial equations best described their dataset and provided regression equations for the 95% confidence intervals. This resulted in narrower distribution bands for the confidence intervals earlier in pregnancy when compared with later in pregnancy and used gestational age as the independent variable.[22] In 2001, Firpo et al.[23] expanded on the dataset of Tan et al.[9] However, when I compared the graphical analysis and the corresponding regression equations provided in this study, I found several errors that were confirmed by the authors (personal communication). Therefore, this dataset should not be used until the errors have been corrected.

While the previous studies by Tan et al.[9] and Shapiro et al.[22] are important contributions to our understanding of the growth of fetal cardiac structures from B-mode measurements, their use has the limitation that their data were described for only gestational age. This is important because gestational age does not take into account variations in fetal size for a given gestational age. For example, a fetus at 34 weeks could be normal, macrocosmic, or have intrauterine growth restriction. Therefore, using gestational age to compare cardiac dimensions could erroneously suggest pathology when none is present. For this reason, one should use these data only if the fetus is of normal growth for gestational age. Figures 5.23 to 5.26 lists the graphs for gestational age for the right ventricular inner dimension, left ventricular inner dimension, aortic root diameter, and the pulmonary root diameter.

## Z-Scores

Recent papers have focused on converting cardiac measurements to Z-scores, which are simply a measurement of the

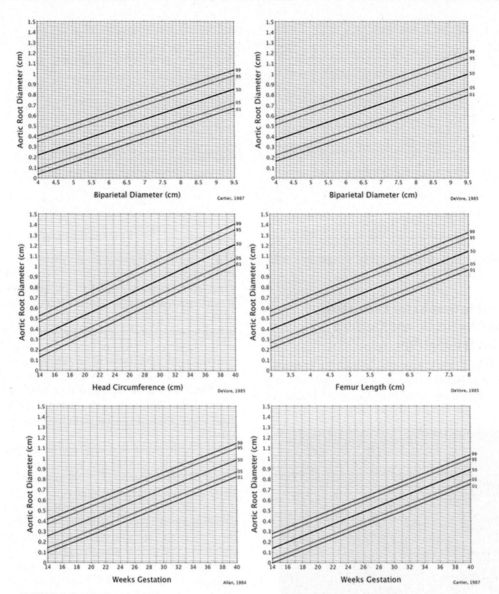

**FIGURE 5.20:** These graphs demonstrate the 1st, 5th, 50th, 95th, and 99th percentiles for aortic root diameter obtained at the level of the opening of the aortic valve for the biparietal diameter, head circumference, femur length, and weeks of gestation.

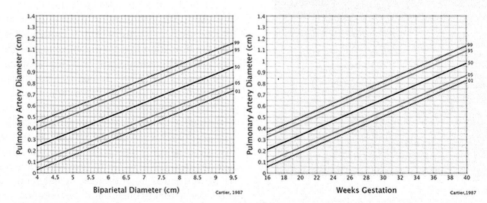

**FIGURE 5.21:** These graphs demonstrate the 1st, 5th, 50th, 95th, and 99th percentiles for the main pulmonary artery diameter obtained at the level of the opening of the pulmonary valve for the biparietal diameter, and weeks of gestation.

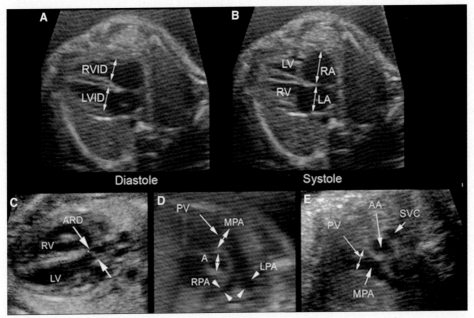

**FIGURE 5.22:** B-Mode Images of Measurements. **A:** The right and left ventricular inner dimensions *(RVID, LVID)* are measured at end-ventricular systole. **B:** The right and left atrial dimensions *(RA, LA)* are measured at end-ventricular systole. The aorta and main pulmonary artery *(MPA)* dimensions are measured at the level of the aortic valve *(A)*. **C:** Measurement of the aortic diameter *(ARD)* from the left ventricular outflow tract view. **D:** The measurement of the aorta and main pulmonary artery from the short-axis view. **E:** Measurement of the main pulmonary artery at the level of the PV from the three-vessel view. LV, left ventricle; RV, right ventricle; RPA, right pulmonary aretery; LPA, left pulmonary artery; AA, ascending aorta; SVC, superior vena cava.

| Table 5.7 | **B-Mode Measurements of the Fetal Heart** |
| --- | --- |

| | Percentiles | | | Z-scores | | |
| --- | --- | --- | --- | --- | --- | --- |
| | **Sharland et al.**[8] | **Tan et al.**[9] | **Shapiro et al.**[22] | **Schneider et al.**[6] | **Pasquini et al.**[27] | **Lee et al.**[7] |
| **Study Parameters** | | | | | | |
| Gestational age range | 16–40 | 18–40 | 14–40 | 15–39 | 18–37 | 17–41 |
| Number of fetuses studied | 337 | 100 | 637 | 130 | 204 | 2735 |
| **Data Analysis** | | | | | | |
| Statistical analysis | Quadratic polynomial regression | Linear and quadratic regression | Linear and quadratic regression | | | |
| Display of data | Percentiles | Percentiles | Percentiles | Z-scores | Z-scores | Z-scores |
| Regression equations provided | | | | | | |
| Weeks of gestation | X | X | X | X | X | X |
| Femur length | | | | X | X | X |
| Biparietal diameter | | | | X | | X |
| **Ventricular Measurements** | | | | | | |
| Right ventricle end-diastolic dimension | X | X | X | X | | X |
| Left ventricle end-diastolic dimension | X | X | X | X | | X |
| Right ventricle length | X | X | | X | | |
| Left ventricle length | X | X | | X | | |

|  | Percentiles | | | Z-scores | | |
|---|---|---|---|---|---|---|
|  | *Sharland et al.*[8] | *Tan et al.*[9] | *Shapiro et al.*[22] | *Schneider et al.*[6] | *Pasquini et al.*[27] | *Lee et al.*[7] |
| Right ventricle area |  |  |  | X |  |  |
| Left ventricle area |  |  |  | X |  |  |
| Chest circumference |  |  |  |  |  | X |
| Tricuspid valve | X |  |  | X |  |  |
| Mitral valve | X |  |  | X |  |  |
| Right ventricle wall thickness |  | X |  |  |  |  |
| Left ventricle wall thickness |  | X |  |  |  |  |
| Interventricular septum thickness |  | X |  |  |  |  |
| **Atrial Measurements** | | | | | | |
| Right atrial width |  | X | X |  |  |  |
| Right atrial length |  | X |  |  |  |  |
| Left atrial width |  | X | X |  |  |  |
| Left atrial length |  | X |  |  |  |  |
| **Outflow Tracts** | | | | | | |
| Aortic valve |  |  |  |  |  | X |
| Pulmonary valve |  |  |  | X |  | X |
| Ascending aorta | X | X | X | X |  |  |
| Main pulmonary artery | X | X | X | X |  |  |
| Descending aorta |  | X |  | X | X |  |
| Right pulmonary artery |  | X |  | X |  |  |
| Left pulmonary artery |  | X |  | X |  |  |
| Ductus arteriosus |  | X |  | X | X |  |
| Three-vessel view |  |  |  |  | X |  |
| Tracheal view |  |  |  |  | X |  |
| **Venous System** | | | | | | |
| Inferior vena cava |  | X |  | X |  |  |
| Superior vena cava |  | X |  |  |  |  |

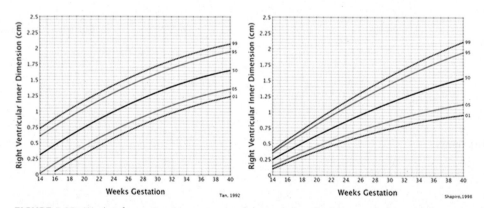

**FIGURE 5.23:** Weeks of gestation. Measurement of the end-diastolic right ventricular inner dimension. These graphs demonstrate the 1st, 5th, 50th, 95th, and 99th percentiles obtained at the level of the four-chamber view. The bottom graph illustrates the 5th, 50th, and 95th percentiles for the curves from Tan,[9] Shapiro,[22] Schneider,[6] and Lee.[7]

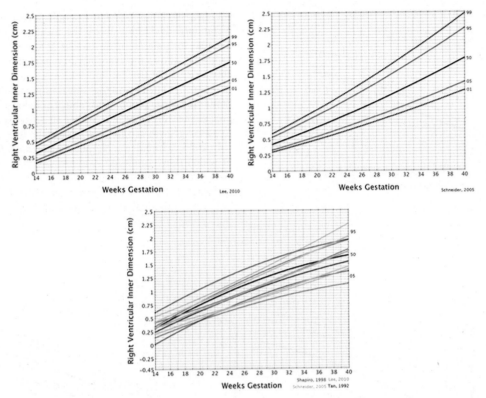

**FIGURE 5.23:** (Continued)

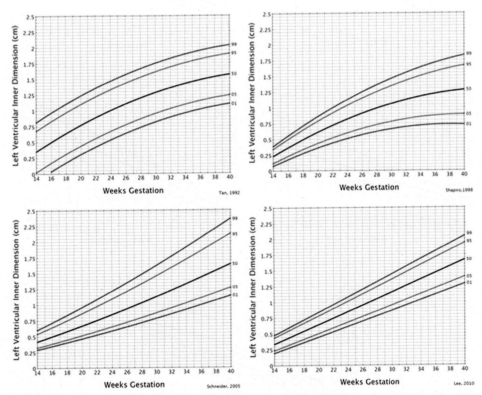

**FIGURE 5.24:** Weeks of gestation. Measurement of the end-diastolic left ventricular inner dimension. The upper four graphs demonstrate the 1st, 5th, 50th, 95th, and 99th percentiles obtained at the level of the four-chamber view. The bottom graph illustrates the 5th, 50th, and 95th percentiles for the curves from Tan, Shapiro, Schneider, and Lee.

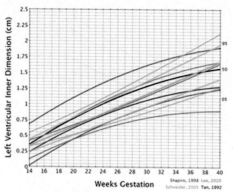

**FIGURE 5.24:** (*Continued*)

standard deviation.[6,7,24] For example, a Z-score of 3 is equal to 3 standard deviations above the mean, while a Z-score of −3 is equal to 3 standard deviations below the mean. Using this technique allows the examiner to report measurements that are above or below the 1st and 99th percentiles in a quantitative manner.[8,9,22] The reason that this is important is that once a particular measurement extends above or below these percentiles, a precise measurement of a cardiac structure is preferable so that trends in growth can more accurately be followed.

In 2005, Schneider et al.[6] published results from a large study in which they computed Z-scores as a function of the biparietal diameter, femur length, and gestational age (Table 5.7). Although Schneider et al. provided the raw data for computation of individual Z-scores as well as a graphical display of

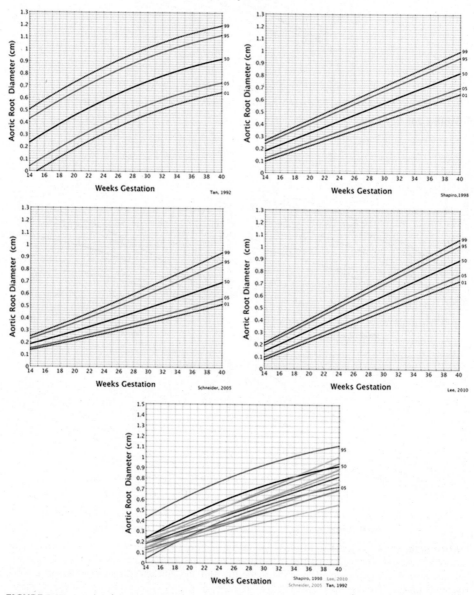

**FIGURE 5.25:** Weeks of gestation. Measurement of the aortic root diameter at the level of the valve. These graphs demonstrate the 1st, 5th, 50th, 95th, and 99th percentiles. The bottom graph illustrates the 5th, 50th, and 95th percentiles for the curves from Tan, Shapiro, Schneider, and Lee.

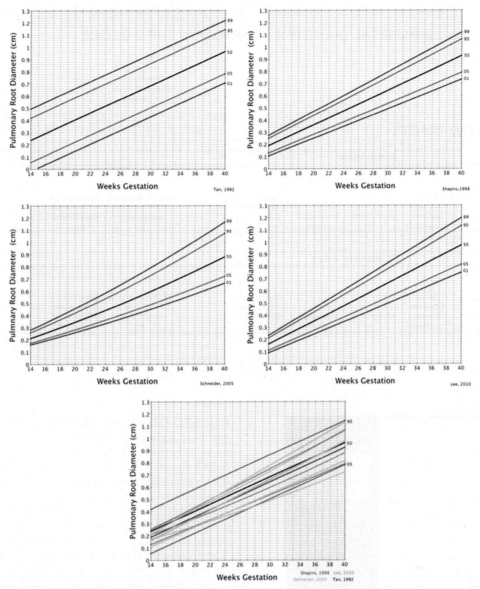

**FIGURE 5.26:** Weeks of gestation. Measurement of the pulmonary root diameter at the level of the valve. These graphs demonstrate the 1st, 5th, 50th, 95th, and 99th percentiles. The bottom graph illustrates the 5th, 50th, and 95th percentiles for the curves from Tan, Shapiro, Schneider, and Lee.

Z-scores in their paper and supplementary material on the journal's website, this was inconvenient for some to compute, especially if a computer reporting system is used. At the time of the publication, a companion opinion paper was also published.[25] Because of the difficulty for the average clinician to compute Z-scores, I provided an Excel spreadsheet based upon their data that made the computations easier to obtain (Fig. 5.27).[25] Since the publication of these papers, a number of investigators have reported using these data in the cardiac evaluation of fetuses with different pathologies.[7,26–51]

In 2010, Lee et al.[7] published a Z-score paper based on a larger database, but fewer cardiac measurements (Table 5.7). Several authors have referred to this study in recent publications.[36,44,52,53]

Of interest, there is no single paper that provides data for all of the measurements listed in Table 5.7.

Figure 5.28 illustrates a graphical display representing 2 standard deviations and the computed Z-score from an interactive multimedia program created for the iPad, Mac, and Windows platforms using data from Schneider et al.,[6] Pasquini et al.,[27] and Lee et al.[7]

## B-Mode Percentile Graphs for Evaluating the Size of the Ventricular and Outflow Tracts Using Biparietal Diameter and Femur Length

Unlike Tan et al.[9] and Shapiro et al.,[22] the studies by Schneider et al.[6] and Lee et al.[7] also provided equations from which to compute percentile graphs based on the biparietal diameter and femur length. Figures 5.29 to 5.33 lists the graphs for gestational age for the right ventricular inner dimension, tricuspid valve opening excursion of the valve leaflets, mitral valve opening excursion of the valve leaflets, left ventricular inner dimension, aortic root diameter, and the pulmonary root diameter.

## BIPARIETAL DIAMETER - COMPUTING THE Z SCORE

**Step 1:** Enter the Measured Biparietal Diameter in centimeters

**Step 2:** Enter the Measured STRUCTURE in centimeters

**Step 3:** Read the Z Score

### OUTFLOW TRACTS

#### Aortic Valve

| ENTER Measured Biparietal Diameter in centimeters | LN of Biparietal Diameter | Multiplier M | Intercept C | Computed Ln of predicted STRUCTURE | ENTER Measured STRUCTURE in centimeters | Computed Ln of Measured STRUCTURE | Root Mean Square | Z Score |
|---|---|---|---|---|---|---|---|---|
| 4 | 1.386294361 | 1.039 | -2.848 | -1.4076 | 0.3 | -1.2039728 | 0.1307 | 1.558281 |

#### Pulmonary Valve

| ENTER Measured Biparietal Diameter in centimeters | LN of Biparietal Diameter | Multiplier M | Intercept C | Computed Ln of predicted STRUCTURE | ENTER Measured STRUCTURE in centimeters | Computed Ln of Measured STRUCTURE | Root Mean Square | Z Score |
|---|---|---|---|---|---|---|---|---|
| 4 | 1.386294361 | 1.126 | -2.813 | -1.2520 | 0.3 | -1.2039728 | 0.1171 | 0.410416 |

**FIGURE 5.27:** This is from the Microsoft Excel spreadsheet that can be downloaded from http://onlinelibrary.wiley.com/doi/10.1002/uog.2605/suppinfo. To view the computed Z-score, the user enters the biometric measurement (Step 1) and the measured cardiac structure (Step 2) and then reads the Z-score (Step 3).[25]

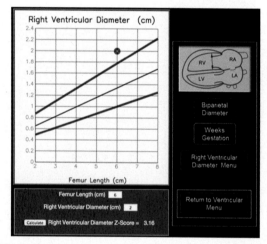

**FIGURE 5.28:** This is from the multimedia program entitled "Z-scores of the Fetal Heart." The user can compute the Z-score and display the findings on a graph that shows the mean, ±2 SD. (http://www.fetalecho.com/z_score.html.)

## PULSED DOPPLER EXAMINATION OF THE FETAL HEART

Pulsed Doppler examination provides information regarding the direction and the characteristics of blood flow within the heart. Pulsed Doppler devices use one crystal that transmits and receives the ultrasound signal. This is performed by placing a small box that is a sample volume on the cursor that can be steered through any sector line or depth of the image (Fig. 5.34). Doppler signals that are received from moving red blood cells are then displayed either above or below the baseline. They are displayed above the baseline if the red blood cells are traveling toward the transducer, and displayed below the baseline if the red blood cells are flowing away from the transducer. It is ideal to obtain the Doppler signal parallel or at a zero degree angle to the main direction of blood flow, as the more perpendicular the Doppler sample volume recording is to the flowing blood, the less is the frequency shift (change in frequency between the incident and reflected ultrasound beams) of the displayed Doppler

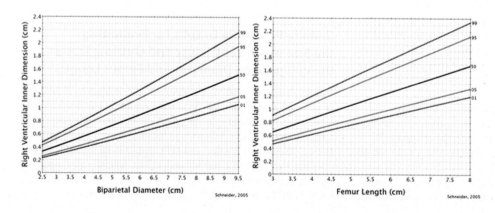

**FIGURE 5.29:** Biparietal diameter and femur length. Measurement of the end-diastolic right ventricular inner dimension. These graphs demonstrate the 1st, 5th, 50th, 95th, and 99th percentiles obtained at the level of the four-chamber view.

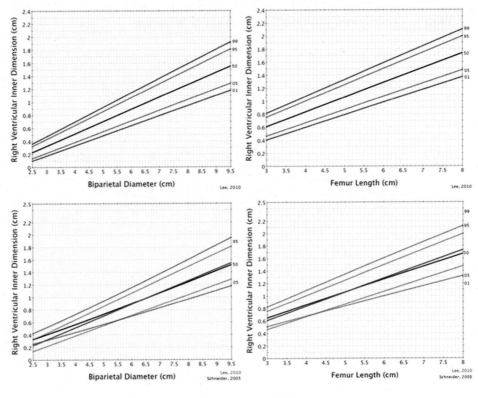

**FIGURE 5.29:** *(Continued)*

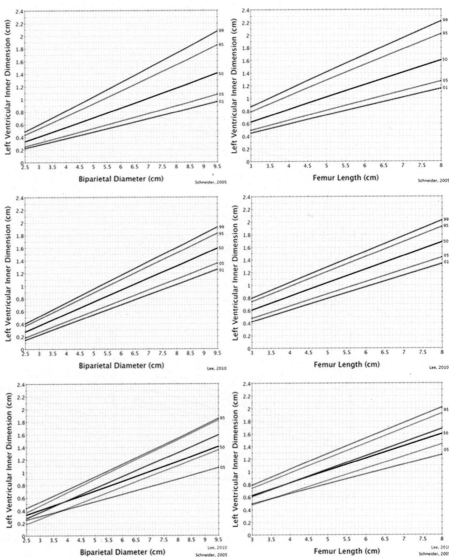

**FIGURE 5.30:** Biparietal diameter and femur length. Measurement of the end-diastolic left ventricular inner dimension. These graphs demonstrate the 1st, 5th, 50th, 95th, and 99th percentiles obtained at the level of the four-chamber view.

**139**

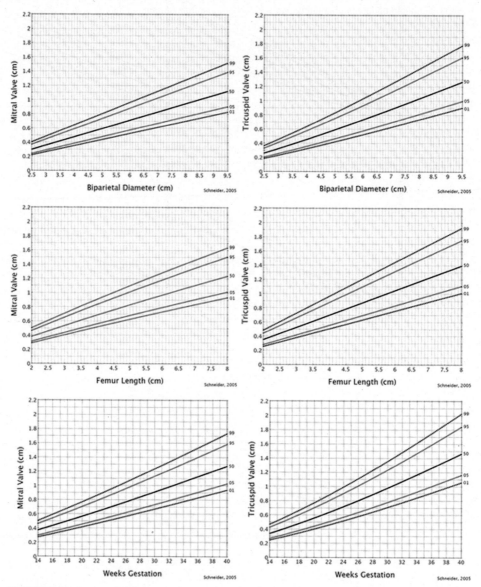

**FIGURE 5.31:** Biparietal diameter, femur length, and weeks of gestation. Measurement of the mitral and tricuspid valve dimension. These graphs demonstrate the 1st, 5th, 50th, 95th, and 99th percentiles obtained at the level of the four-chamber view.

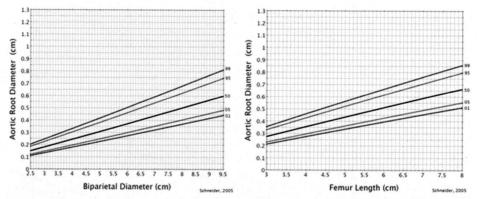

**FIGURE 5.32:** Biparietal diameter and femur length. Measurement of the aortic root diameter. These graphs demonstrate the 1st, 5th, 50th, 95th, and 99th percentiles obtained at the level of the four-chamber view.

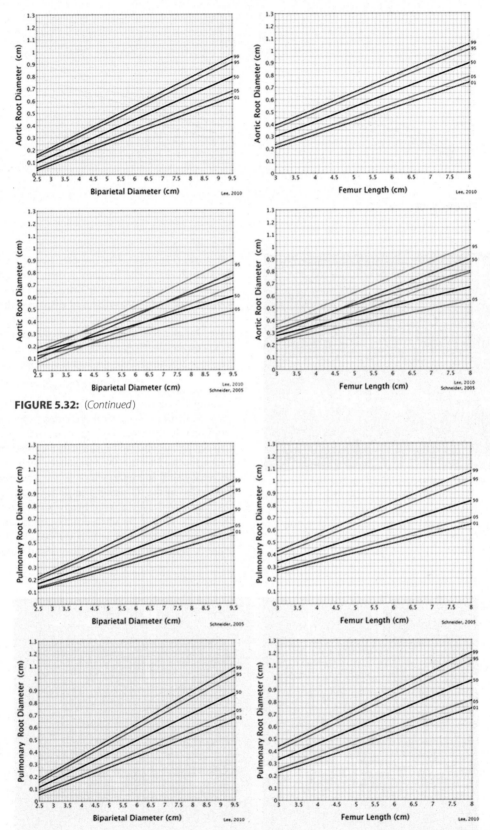

**FIGURE 5.32:** (Continued)

**FIGURE 5.33:** Biparietal diameter and femur length. Measurement of the pulmonary root diameter. These graphs demonstrate the 1st, 5th, 50th, 95th, and 99th percentiles obtained at the level of the four-chamber view.

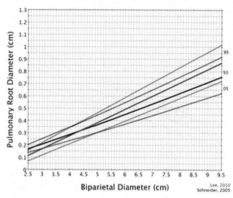

**FIGURE 5.33:** (Continued)

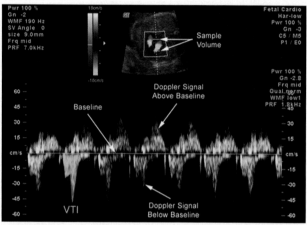

**FIGURE 5.34:** Doppler waveform and sample volume. The sample volume is placed over the left ventricle and the pulsed Doppler waveform recorded. The pulsed Doppler waveform is recorded demonstrating a waveform above the baseline and below the baseline. The velocity time integral *(VTI)* is the area under the curve of the Doppler waveform, which represents one cardiac cycle.

waveform (Fig. 5.35). The Doppler frequency, which returns to the transducer, is the frequency shift that can be displayed as a signal on the output of the ultrasound monitor. Older ultrasound equipment measured and displayed the frequency shift, whereas most current equipment using state-of-the-art pulse wave Doppler technology automatically use fast Fourier analysis to convert the frequency shift into a velocity display. Velocity display is obtained from the formula in which

$$V = (f_d \times c) / (2f_0 \times \cos \emptyset)$$

Using this formula, the velocity ($V$) is recorded in meters per second and recorded on the video output of the ultrasound monitor. $C$ is the velocity of sound in water, which is a constant at 1,560 m per second, and $f_0$ is the transmitted frequency (i.e., the frequency used within the transducer such as 3 MHz). $f_d$ is the frequency shift in Hertz, which is the returning frequency that is recorded by the ultrasound equipment, and ($\emptyset$) is the angle of insonation of the ultrasound beam ($f_0$) as it interrogates the red blood cells. Thus, if the ultrasound beam is parallel to the flow of red blood cells, the angle is zero and cos Ø is 1. If the ultrasound beam is perpendicular to the flow of red blood cells, the angle

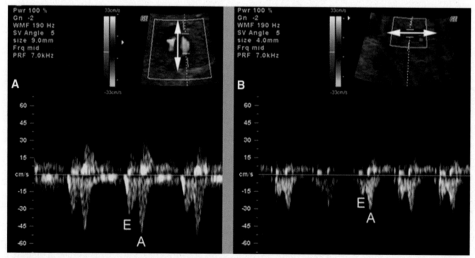

**FIGURE 5.35:** Comparing the Doppler waveforms obtained parallel and perpendicular to flow. **A:** This illustrates the pulsed Doppler waveform obtained when the sample volume was placed parallel *(white double arrow)* to blood flow identified with the color Doppler. **B:** The four-chamber view is perpendicular *(white double arrow)* and the Doppler waveform recorded. Because the angle is 90°, the pulsed Doppler waveform is decreased in size for the same Doppler scale used in **A.**

| Table 5.8 | Doppler Measurements | |
|---|---|---|
| **Measurement[a]** | **Method** | **Units** |
| Peak or maximal velocity | Zero line to peak of the waveform | Centimeters/second or meters/second |
| Mean velocity | Time velocity integral/time of cardiac cycle | Centimeters/second or meters/second |
| Volume flow | Mean velocity × area[b] × 60 | Milliliters/minute or liters/minute |
| Time-to-peak velocity or acceleration time | Time from onset to the peak of the waveform | Milliseconds |
| Deceleration time | Time from peak to zero line along slope of descent | Milliseconds |
| Velocity time integral | Area under the curve of the Doppler waveform | |

[a]Velocities should be measured within 30° of the estimated direction of flow or be angle-corrected.
[b]Area obtained from diameters measured with two-dimensional ultrasound.

is 90°, and the cos Ø is 0. The angle Ø should always be less than 60° and ideally less than 30° for most accurate measurements. Thus, using this formula, velocity is recorded in meters per second.

Velocities can be measured using continuous wave instrumentation. With continuous wave instrumentation, two transducers are used—one to transmit and the other to receive the Doppler signal. Use of continuous wave Doppler is nonselective in that all signals along the ultrasound beam are recorded. Therefore, most individuals use pulsed wave Doppler for examining the fetal heart.

Doppler ultrasound also exposes the fetus to higher levels of ultrasound energy than real-time imaging or M-mode ultrasound. As such, the amount of time one uses in performing pulsed Doppler ultrasound of the fetus should be limited. For this reason, most clinicians will use color Doppler to identify the structure of interest and then place the sample volume for pulsed Doppler recording.[54] This shortens the time required to obtain the pulsed Doppler waveform. It is known that the Doppler ultrasound energy should be kept below 100 mW per cm$^2$ spatial peak-temporal average.

Measurement of blood volume ($Q$) requires measurement of the cross-sectional area of the vessel ($A$) through which blood is flowing, which is then multiplied by an average velocity.

$$Q = V \times A$$

Let us examine how the above equation can be used to compute blood volume. The average velocity ($V$) can be computed by multiplying the velocity time integral (VTI) by the heart rate. The VTI is the area under the curve of the Doppler waveform for one cardiac cycle (Fig. 5.34). Multiplying the VTI by the heart rate (beats per minute) provides an estimate of the average velocity of blood flow during one minute. The second component of the equation to compute blood volume is to measure the area of the orifice through which blood is flowing. Since all structures in the fetal heart (mitral valve, tricuspid valve, aortic valve, and the pulmonary valve) approximate a circle, measurements of their diameter can be obtained and the area computed ((diameter/2)$^2$ × 3.14). Once these values are measured, the volume of blood flow can be determined as follows:

$$Q = 3.14 \times (D / 2)^2 \times \text{VTI} \times \text{HR}$$

Table 5.8 lists common measurements that are made from the Doppler waveform that include the peak or maximal velocity, volume flow, time-to-peak velocity (acceleration time), deceleration time, and the velocity time integral.

## INTRACARDIAC DOPPLER

Intracardiac Doppler examination can be performed for either the tricuspid or the mitral valve. In most instances, it is best to have the pulsed Doppler cursor placed as parallel to the moving red blood cells as possible. As such, it is best to image the four-chamber view of the heart so that the interventricular septum is parallel to the ultrasound beam (Fig. 5.35A). Velocities can be angle corrected, but small errors in estimation of the angle may result in an unacceptably large error of velocity measurements (Fig. 5.35). Ideally, angle measurement between the ultrasound beam and the direction of the flowing blood should be less than 30° and must always be less than 60°.

When examining either the tricuspid or the mitral valve, the Doppler sample volume is placed immediately distal to the valve leaflets in the right or the left ventricle, respectively (Fig. 5.36). When velocity flow is detected across the tricuspid or the mitral valve with the cursor placed within either of their respective ventricles, there is usually a biphasic Doppler signal (Fig. 5.37). The flow velocity waveform across the valve is characterized by an E component, followed by a higher A component. The E component is a result of the rapid filling phase of diastole and is entirely passive. The A component is the result of atrial contraction. Several studies have examined the velocities of the E and A wave as a function of gestational age, and reported an increase in the E wave, with little or no change in the A wave (Table 5.9).[55-60] The E/A wave ratio increases with gestational age as a function of reversal of flow of the E-wave as it increases in velocity (Table 5.9, Fig. 5.38).[55,56] Increased velocities through the valve may indicate valvular stenosis.[61] If valvular insufficiency is suspected, the Doppler sample may be placed through the mitral or tricuspid valve into their respective atrium for

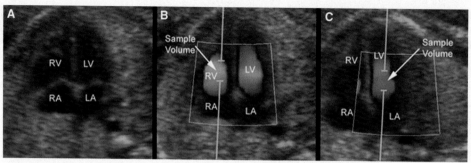

**FIGURE 5.36:** Placement of the Doppler sample volume. **A:** This is the four-chamber view when the mitral and tricuspid valves are closed during ventricular systole. **B:** The four-chamber view when the mitral and tricuspid valves are open as identified by color Doppler ultrasound. The sample volume is placed within the right ventricular chamber and increased in size to record as much of the blood flow entering the chamber as possible. **C:** The sample volume is placed within the left ventricular chamber and increased in size to record as much of the blood flow entering the chamber as possible. RV, right ventricle; LV, left ventricle; RA, right atrium; LA, left atrium.

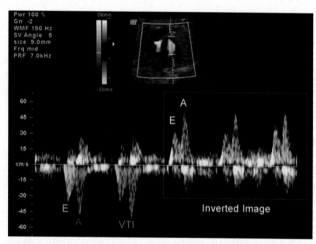

**FIGURE 5.37:** The sample volume is placed within the left ventricular chamber. Since the spine is a 1 o'clock, the flow into the ventricular chambers is away from the baseline. The colored portions of the waveform represent the *E* and *A* waves, and the velocity time integral *(VTI)*. The inverted image illustrates the waveforms if the blood flow were above the baseline.

detection of valvular insufficiency. Studies have shown changes in the E/A ratio as the result of intrauterine growth restriction (no change, increased, or decreased), fetal inflammatory response syndrome, and maternal diabetes (Fig. 5.39).[62–71]

Investigators have also attempted to measure cardiac output from the mitral and tricuspid valve Doppler waveforms by measuring the VTI (Fig. 5.37) and using the following equation to compute flow (Table 5.10, Figs. 5.40 and 5.41)[72–76]:

$$Q = 3.14 \times (D/2)^2 \times \text{VTI} \times \text{HR}$$

The difficulty, however, is the determination of the area of the mitral and tricuspid valves.

## AORTIC AND PULMONARY OUTFLOW TRACT DOPPLER EXAMINATION

Aortic or pulmonary arterial Doppler waveforms may be obtained from either the aorta or the pulmonary artery as they exit their respective ventricles. The aortic blood flow velocities

| Table 5.9 | Diastolic Function of the Right and Left Ventricles in Normal Fetuses | | | |
|---|---|---|---|---|
| | *All Subjects* | *17–24 (w)* | *25–31 (wk)* | *32–39 (wk)* |
| Gestational age (wk) | 27 ± 7 | 21 ± 2 | 27 ± 2 | 35 ± 2 |
| Heart rate (beats/min) | 142 ± 10 | 146 ± 9 | 140 ± 10 | 138 ± 11 |
| **Left Ventricle** | | | | |
| Mitral valve studies | 307 | 130 | 91 | 86 |
| E wave peak velocity (cm/s) | 31 ± 7 | 26 ± 4 | 31 ± 5 | 38 ± 6 |
| A wave peak velocity (cm/s) | 44 ± 11 | 41 ± 6 | 45 ± 7 | 47 ± 6 |
| E/A ratio | 0.7 ± 0.11 | 0.63 ± 0.07 | 0.70 ± 0.09 | 0.80 ± 0.10 |
| **Right Ventricle** | | | | |
| Tricuspid valve studies | 258 | 118 | 71 | 69 |
| E wave peak velocity (cm/s) | 33 ± 7 | 29 ± 5 | 35 ± 6 | 39 ± 6 |
| A wave peak velocity (cm/s) | 48 ± 7 | 45 ± 6 | 49 ± 8 | 51 ± 8 |
| E/A ratio | 0.70 ± 0.09 | 0.64 ± 0.07 | 0.70 ± 0.08 | 0.77 ± 0.09 |

Values are mean ± 1 SD.

From Harada K, Rice MJ, Shiota T, et al. Gestational age- and growth-related alterations in fetal right and left ventricular diastolic filling patterns. *Am J Cardiol.* 1997;79:173–177.

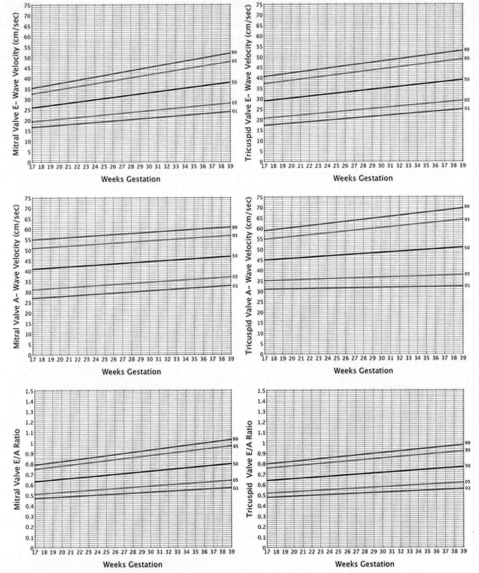

**FIGURE 5.38:** Mitral and Tricuspid *E* and *A* wave velocities and *E/A* ratios as a function of gestational age.

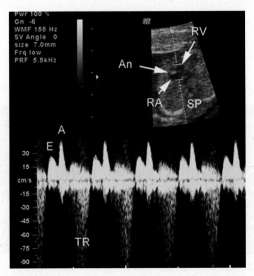

**FIGURE 5.39:** The sample volume has been placed in the right ventricle and atrium. The pulsed Doppler waveform records the inflow of blood into the right ventricle during diastole, as manifest by the *E* and *A* waveforms. During ventricular systole, there is holosystolic regurgitation of blood back into the right atrium *(TR)*. RV, right ventricle; RA, right atrium; SP, spine; An, annulus.

can be obtained using the long axis of the five-chamber view of the heart (Fig. 5.42), whereas pulmonary Doppler flow velocities are best obtained from a short axis view of the heart or through a transverse plane above the five-chamber view in the chest (Fig. 5.43). Using these approaches, the pulmonary artery and the aorta are parallel to the ultrasound beam and the pulsed Doppler sample volume placed distal to the valves so that accurate Doppler recordings of their respective waveforms can occur. For the pulmonary artery and the aorta, there is usually only one peak noted on the Doppler waveform, rather than the two peaks as noted for either the tricuspid or the mitral valve (Figs. 5.44 and 5.45). The peak or maximum velocity is obtained by measuring the highest velocity of the time velocity Doppler signal that is angle corrected. Maximum velocities for the aorta and the pulmonary artery increase as a function of gestational age (Fig. 5.46).[73] The time-to-peak velocity can be measured for each vessel and is measured from the beginning of the waveform to the point of the peak velocity (Fig. 5.47). As gestational age increases, the resistance in the aorta decreases as manifest by an increasing time-to-peak velocity. Conversely, the resistance in the main pulmonary artery increases as manifest by a

| Table 5.10 | **Reported Values of Volume Flow Estimations from the Atrioventricular (AV) Valves for Left Cardiac Output (LCO), Right Cardiac Output (RCO), and Combined Cardiac Output (CCO) Corrected for Fetal Weight** | | | | | | | |
|---|---|---|---|---|---|---|---|---|

| Author | Site of Recording | LCO (mL/min) | | | RCO (mL/min) | | | CCO (mL/min/kg) |
|---|---|---|---|---|---|---|---|---|
| | | 19–21 | 29–31 | 36–40 | 19–21 | 29–31 | 36–40 | |
| De Smedt et al.[75] | AV valves | 84 | 333 | 820 | 105 | 372 | 915 | 553 |
| Allan et al.[76] | AV valves | 109 | 333 | 686 | 140 | 428 | 883 | - |
| Rizzo et al.[65] | AV valves | 91 | 320 | 693 | 134 | 435 | 890 | 546 |

From DeVore GR, Donnerstein RL, Kleinman CS, et al. Real-time—directed M-mode echocardiography: a new technique for accurate and rapid quantitation of the fetal preejection period and ventricular ejection time of the right and left ventricles. *Am J Obstet Gynecol.* 1981;141:470–471.

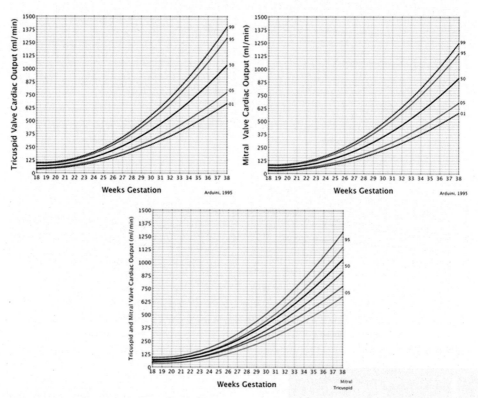

**FIGURE 5.40:** Normal values for gestation of left and right cardiac outputs obtained from the atrioventricular valves in 284 normal fetuses studied cross-sectionally.

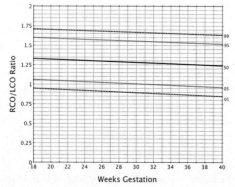

**FIGURE 5.41:** Normal values for gestation of left cardiac output *(RCO)* divided by right cardiac output *(LCO)* obtained from the atrioventricular valves in 284 normal fetuses studied cross-sectionally.

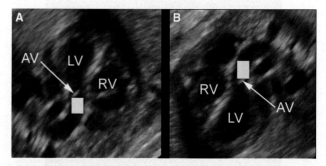

**FIGURE 5.42:** Five-chamber view of the heart demonstrating the aorta parallel to the Doppler sample volume. The sample volume is placed distal to the aortic valve and the pulsed Doppler waveform recorded. Apex of the heart at 12 o'clock **(A)**, apex at 6 o'clock **(B)**. AV, aortic valve; LV, left ventricle; RV, right ventricle; yellow box, location of pulsed Doppler sample volume.

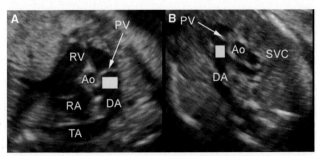

**FIGURE 5.43: A:** Short-axis view of the heart imaged in a sagittal plane demonstrating the placement of the Doppler sample volume distal to the pulmonary valve *(PV)*. **B:** Main pulmonary artery imaged in a transverse plane of the chest, cephalad to the five-chamber view. RV, right ventricle; RA, right atrium; Ao, aorta; DA, ductus arteriosus; TA, thoracic aorta; SVC, superior vena cava.

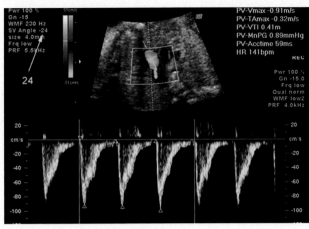

**FIGURE 5.45:** Pulsed Doppler waveform recorded distal to the pulmonary valve. The sample volume was at a 24° angle.

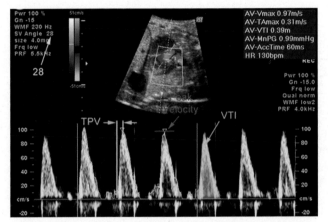

**FIGURE 5.44:** Pulsed Doppler recording from the ascending aorta with the apex of the ventricles at 6 o'clock. TPV, time-to-peak velocity or acceleration time; VTI, velocity time integral. The angle of insonation is 28°. Note the computed measurements in the upper right portion of the image.

shorter time-to-peak velocity. In addition to measuring cardiac output from the atrioventricular valves, investigators have measured cardiac output from the aorta and main pulmonary artery by using the following equation:

$$Q = 3.14 \times (D/2)^2 \times \text{VTI} \times \text{HR}$$

They found that the cardiac output increased as a function of gestational age (Table 5.11) (Figs. 5.48 and 5.49).[73,77] Figure 5.50 compares cardiac output between that obtained from the atrioventricular valves and the outflow tracts. Another indirect method to measure cardiac output is to simply measure the velocity time integral (VTI) and multiply this by the heart rate (Figs. 5.51 and 5.52). The benefit of this approach is that the examiner does not have to measure the dimension of the outflow tracts, which, if an error is made, can markedly alter

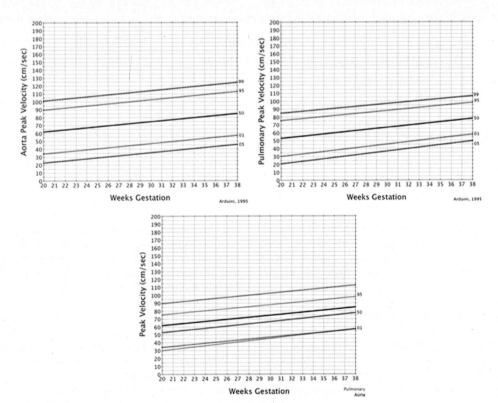

**FIGURE 5.46:** Peak velocity for the aorta and main pulmonary artery.

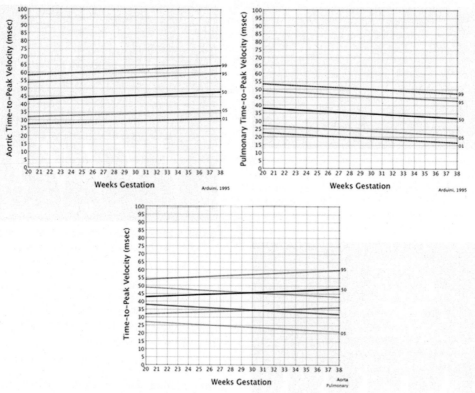

**FIGURE 5.47:** Time-to-peak velocity of the aorta and main pulmonary artery. As gestational age increases, the resistance decreases in the aorta and increases in the main pulmonary artery.

| | | LCO (mL/min) | | | RCO (mL/min) | | | |
|---|---|---|---|---|---|---|---|---|
| **Author** | **Site of Recording** | **19–21** | **29–31** | **36–40** | **19–21** | **29–31** | **36–40** | **CCO (mL/min/kg)** |
| Kenny | Outflow tracts | 118 | 282 | 676 | 132 | 302 | 692 | — |
| Allan | Outflow tracts | 70 | 269 | 647 | 93 | 361 | 886 | 450 |
| Rizzo | Outflow tracts | 78 | 284 | 670 | 100 | 390 | 866 | 525 |

**Table 5.11** — Reported Values of Volume Flow Estimations from the Aorta and Main Pulmonary Artery Outflow Tracts for Left Cardiac Output (LCO), Right Cardiac Output (RCO), and Combined Cardiac Output (CCO) Corrected for Fetal Weight

From Arduini D, Rizzo G, Romanini C, et al. (1995) *Fetal cardiac output measurement in normal and pathologic states.* In: Copel JA and Reed KL, Doppler Ultra-sound in Obstetrics and Gynecology, Springer Publishing Company, New York, Chap 27.

the computation of the cardiac output. Investigators have found that there is a decrease in cardiac output in fetuses with growth restriction and fetal anemia, while others have reported no difference between control and IUGR fetuses when the cardiac output is corrected for fetal weight.[69,73,74,77–81]

## DOPPLER MECHANICAL PR INTERVAL

Several investigators have examined the use of pulsed Doppler to identify the mechanical PR interval in utero.[82–86] Although the PR interval can be obtained following delivery using an electrocardiogram, this is not feasible in utero. Prolongation of the fetal mechanical PR interval has been observed with first- and second-degree heart block in fetuses at risk for complete heart block as the result of abnormal maternal Sjogren antibodies as well as other fetal conditions.[86,87] To obtain this waveform, the sample volume is placed at the junction of the anterior mitral valve leaflet and the ascending aorta (Fig. 5.53). The Doppler mechanical PR interval is measured from the onset of the A wave of the mitral waveform to the onset of the aortic waveform. The fetal Doppler mechanical PR interval has been found to be fairly constant and is not altered by gestational age or fetal heart rate. The normal value is 120 milliseconds (95% confidence interval 10 to 140 milliseconds).

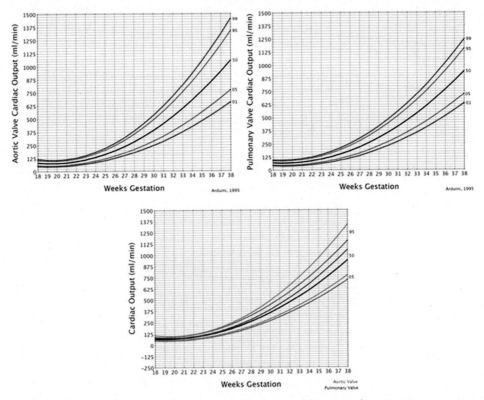

**FIGURE 5.48:** Measurement of cardiac output from the aorta and the main pulmonary artery.

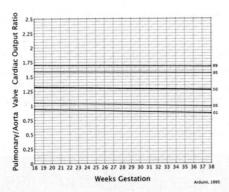

**FIGURE 5.49:** Normal values for gestation of left cardiac output divided by right cardiac output obtained from the pulmonary artery and aorta.

## MYOCARDIAL PERFORMANCE INDEX (MPI) OR TEI INDEX USING PULSED DOPPLER VELOCITY WAVEFORMS

### Historical Background

In 1995, Tei et al. reported a new technique for evaluating myocardial function called the myocardial performance index.[88–90] Since systolic and diastolic dysfunction frequently coexist, it was hypothesized that a combined measure of left ventricular chamber performance could be more reflective of overall cardiac dysfunction than systolic or diastolic measures alone. They

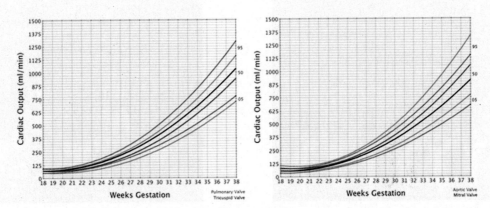

**FIGURE 5.50:** This compares the cardiac outputs determined by measuring either the ventricular inflow (mitral and tricuspid valves) or the outflow tracts (aorta and pulmonary artery). For the left ventricle, the range is higher for the aorta than the mitral valve. For the right ventricle, the range is higher for the tricuspid valve than the pulmonary artery.

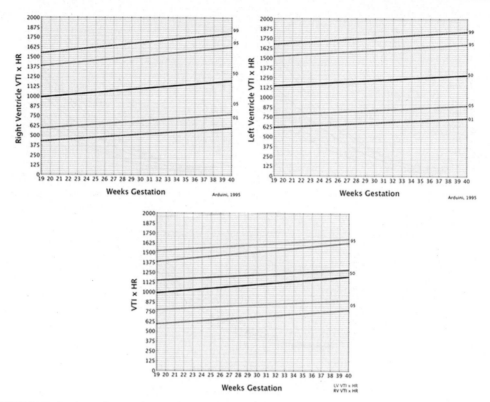

**FIGURE 5.51:** Products of time velocity integral multiplied by heart rate (TVI × HR) in aortic and pulmonary valves.

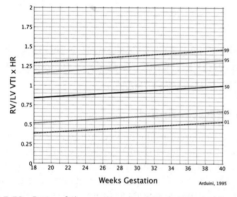

**FIGURE 5.52:** Ratio of the aortic valve (VTI × HR) to the pulmonary valve (VTI × HR).

measured three parameters from the Doppler velocity waveform (Fig. 5.54):

1. Isovolumetric Contraction Time (ICT). This is the period of time between closure of the atrioventricular valves and the opening of the semilunar valves. During this time, the increased pressure resulting from myocardial contraction opens the aortic and pulmonary valves.

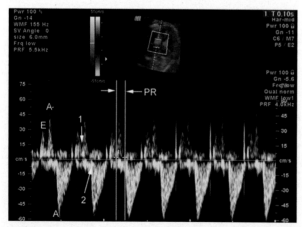

**FIGURE 5.53:** Measurement of the mechanical PR interval. This is obtained by measuring the time between the beginning of the *A* wave *(1)* and the beginning of the aortic waveform *(2)*. In this example, the time is 10 milliseconds.

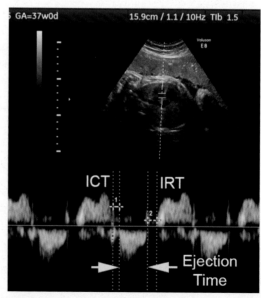

**FIGURE 5.54:** Simultaneous recording of the pulsed Doppler blood flow waveforms from the mitral inflow and aortic outflow tracts. ICT, isovolumetric contraction time; IRT, isovolumetric relaxation time. The myocardial performance index is computed as follows: (ICT + IRT)/Ejection Time.

2. Ejection time (ET). This is the time that the aortic and pulmonary valves are open. The ET may be decreased when cardiac dysfunction is present.

3. Isovolumetric Relaxation Time (IRT). This is the time after all the blood has been ejected from the ventricles following closure of the semilunar valves until the atrioventricular valves open. During this time, the pressure is reduced and the reuptake of calcium occurs.[91] Reduction in calcium uptake is a manifestation of deterioration of cardiac function. The IRT is the main component that alters the MPI in fetal pathological states. When the IRT is increased, the ET is often decreased.

From these time intervals, the MPI is computed as follows:

$$(ICT + IRT) / ET$$

Since the ICT + IRT is the difference between the intervals from the closure of the A wave to the beginning of the E wave minus the ejection time, the MPI equation becomes the following (Fig. 5.55):

$$(\text{Time from closure of the A wave to the beginning of the E wave} - \text{Ejection Time}) / \text{Ejection Time}.$$

In adults, the normal values were 0.39 ± 0.05 (SD), while individuals with abnormal cardiac function had increased values of 0.59 (±0.10 and 1.06 ± 0.24. Tei found that the MPI was not related to heart rate or ventricular size/shape.[88–90]

## Measuring the Myocardial Performance Index for the Left Ventricle

Three approaches have been reported in the literature to compute MPI for the left ventricle.

1. Nonsimultaneous recording of the mitral and aortic Doppler flow velocity waveforms[92]: The pulsed Doppler is placed within the left ventricular inflow tract, and the mitral waveform is recorded. The time between the closure of the A wave and the beginning of the E wave is measured. The pulsed

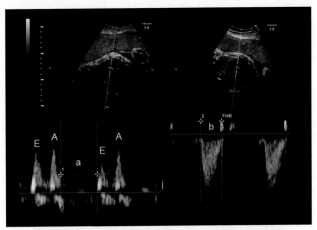

**FIGURE 5.56:** Nonsimultaneous recording of the mitral and aortic pulsed Doppler waveforms from the left ventricle. A, time from the closure of the mitral *A* wave to the opening of the *E* wave. B, the ejection time. The myocardial performance index is computed as follows: (*a* − *b*)/*b*.

Doppler waveform of the aorta is recorded, and the ET is measured. All recordings are not simultaneously recorded (Fig. 5.56). The problem with this approach is that it is impossible to compute the individual isovolumetric times. In addition, small differences in heart rate can affect the MPI calculation because of the change in ET.

2. Simultaneous recording of the Mitral Doppler flow velocity waveform[93]: To avoid the problems listed in the above approach, the pulsed Doppler is placed in a location in which the mitral and aortic waveforms are simultaneously recorded. The time between the closure of the A wave and the beginning of the E wave is measured. The pulsed Doppler waveform of the aorta is recorded, and the ejection time is measured. The landmarks for the measurements are a "best visual estimate" of the beginning and end of the waveforms (Fig. 5.54).

3. Simultaneous recording of the "clicks" of the opening and closing of the mitral and aortic valve leaflets[94]: In 2005, Hernandez-Andrade et al.[94] reported that using the valve "clicks" improved the reproducibility of the MPI. This approach has been termed the Modified-MPI, or Mod-MPI.[94] To accomplish this, the pulsed Doppler is placed at a location in which the mitral and aortic valves are simultaneously recorded. The time between the closure of the A wave and the beginning of the E wave is measured from valve "click" to valve "click." The pulsed Doppler waveform of the aorta is recorded and the ET is measured from "click" to "click" (Fig. 5.57). The landmarks for the measurements are more accurate than the method listed above under option 2. This technique can be applied to the left ventricle throughout gestation, but can only be used for the right ventricle up to 20 weeks of gestation because the distance between the tricuspid and the pulmonary valves increases such that both valves cannot simultaneously be recorded.[95] Criteria for obtaining the proper waveform are listed in Table 5.12.

## Measuring the Myocardial Performance Index for the Right Ventricle

Because the tricuspid inflow and the pulmonary outflow tracts are separated, simultaneous recording of the Doppler

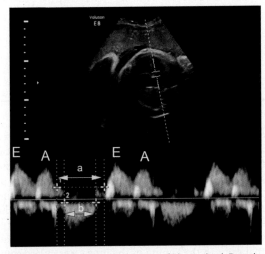

**FIGURE 5.55:** Simultaneous recording of the pulsed Doppler blood flow waveforms from the mitral inflow and aortic outflow tracts. A, time from the closure of the mitral *A* wave to the opening of the *E* wave. B, the ejection time. The myocardial performance index is computed as follows: (*a* − *b*)/*b*.

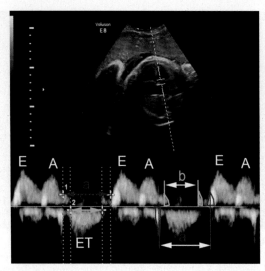

**FIGURE 5.57:** Simultaneous recording of the pulsed Doppler blood flow waveforms from the mitral inflow and aortic outflow tracts using the valve clicks to compute the a and b times. The valve clicks for *a* are in *red* and the clicks for *b* in *green*. A, time from the closure of the mitral *A* wave to the opening of the *E* wave. B, the ejection time. The myocardial performance index is computed as follows: $(a − b)/b$.

waveforms is not possible with conventional ultrasound equipment. Therefore, the pulsed Doppler is placed within the right ventricular inflow tract and the waveform recorded. The time between the closure of the A wave and the beginning of the E wave is measured. The pulsed Doppler waveform of the pulmonary artery is recorded, and the ejection time is measured (Table 5.12, Fig. 5.58).

## Studies of MPI in Fetuses

### Normal Fetuses

Table 5.13 lists studies from normal fetuses that have evaluated the MPI for the left ventricle or both ventricles. The 95th percentile has been computed for the MPI. As the result of refining the technique for obtaining the MPI and measuring the peaks of the waveforms, as described above, the studies reported after 2005 may have better reproducibility than those prior to 2005.[94] Figure 5.59 is the MPI reported by Hernandez-Andrade et al.,[96] in which 557 fetuses were examined. This nomogram has been tested in several subsequent studies of fetuses with pathology.[69,95,97]

### Abnormal Fetuses

The MPI of the left ventricle has been studied in fetuses who are the recipient and donor in the twin-to-twin transfusion syndrome, fetuses of pre-diabetic and diabetic mothers, and fetuses with intrauterine growth restriction.

**Twin-to-twin Transfusion:** The MPI has been reported to be significantly increased in the recipient twin in the twin-to-twin syndrome, in both the right and the left ventricles.[98–101] Michelfelder et al.[102] found that abnormal (increased values) changes in the MPI occurred in the recipient twin early in the disease process. Habli et al.[103] reported that following laser therapy, improvement in left ventricular MPI was associated with an improved outcome.

| Table 5.12 | Criteria That Must Be Followed to Optimally Record the Modified MPI Using the "Click" Method[95,146,147,148] |
|---|---|

**Left Ventricle**

| | |
|---|---|
| Step 1 | Recording obtained from the apical four-chamber view |
| Step 2 | The angle of insonation should be less than 15° |
| Step 3 | The transducer beam is angled cephalad to simultaneously visualize the mitral and aortic valves |
| Step 4 | The sample gait should be 3–4 mm |
| Step 5 | The sample gait is placed over the leaflets of the mitral and aortic valves |
| Step 6 | Reduce the gain to exclude noise and artifacts |
| Step 7 | Increase the speed of the Doppler waveform display to the maximum value (5 cm/s) |
| Step 8 | Set the wall motion filter to 300 Hz |
| Step 9 | Clear valve "clicks" must be observed |
| Step 10 | Three waveforms should be analyzed |
| Step 11 | Measure the ICT from the peak of the mitral valve closure click to the beginning of the aortic valve opening click |
| Step 12 | Measure the IRT from the peak of the aortic valve closure click to the beginning of the mitral valve opening click |
| Step 13 | Measure the ejection time from the beginning of the aortic valve opening click to the aortic valve closure click |
| Step 14 | Compute the Mod-MPI as (ICT + IRT) / ET |

**Right Ventricle**

| | |
|---|---|
| Step 1 | Two individual recordings must be obtained: One from the tricuspid valve leaflets, and one from the pulmonary valve leaflets |
| Step 2 | Isovolumetric time (*a*-interval): measured from the peak of the tricuspid valve closure click to the beginning of the tricuspid valve opening click. |
| Step 3 | Ejection time (*b*-interval): Measured from the beginning of the pulmonary valve opening click to the peak of the pulmonary valve closing click. |
| Step 4 | Compute the Mod-MPI: $(a − b)/b$ |
| Step 5 | The heart rate should be measured |
| Step 6 | If the heart rate differs by more than 10 beats, the recordings should be repeated |

**Maternal Diabetes:** During the 2nd and 3rd trimesters of pregnancy, hyperglycemia puts the fetus at risk for myocardial hypertrophy and dysfunction, which, when abnormal, increases the risk for stillbirth five times higher than the normal population.[104] Studies have demonstrated that changes in the left MPI in fetuses of mothers with diabetes increase during the last trimester of pregnancy and was associated with large for gestational age fetuses.[92,99] The MPI has also been found to become abnormal prior to thickening of the interventricular septum in fetuses of mothers with pregestational diabetes that occurred as early as the first trimester.[105] However, one of the studies of fetuses whose mothers had mild gestational diabetes found

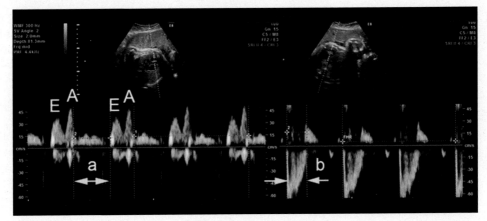

**FIGURE 5.58:** Nonsimultaneous recording of the tricuspid and pulmonary pulsed Doppler waveforms from the right ventricle. A, time from the closure of the mitral *A* wave to the opening of the *E* wave. B, the ejection time. The myocardial performance index is computed as follows: $(a - b)/b$.

**Table 5.13    Normal Myocardial Performance Index Values for the Left and Right Ventricles**

| Reference | Number of Fetuses | MPI | Gestational Age (weeks) | Left MPI Mean (SD) | Left MPI 95% | Right MPI Mean (SD) | Right MPI 95% |
|---|---|---|---|---|---|---|---|
| Tsutsumi et al.[92] | 50 | Left ventricle[72] | 20 | 0.65 (0.03) | 0.70 | | |
| | | | 40 | 0.43 (0.03) | 0.48 | | |
| Eidem et al.[149] | 125 | Both ventricles | 20–40 | 0.36 (0.06) | 0.46 | 0.32 (0.03) | 0.37 |
| Falkensammer et al.[150] | 23 | Both ventricles | 24–34 | 0.41 (0.05) | 0.49 | 0.38 (0.04) | 0.45 |
| Friedman et al.[93] | 74 | Left ventricle | 18–31 | 0.53 (0.13) | 0.74 | | |
| Chen et al.[151] | 225 | Both ventricles | 18–27 + M6 | 0.37 (0.08) | 0.50 | 0.39 (0.04) | 0.46 |
| | | | 28–36 + 6 | 0.27 (0.05) | 0.35 | 0.30 (0.05) | 0.38 |
| | | | 37–42 | 0.22 (0.05) | 0.30 | 0.24 (0.04) | 0.31 |
| Figueroa-Diesel et al.[152] | 209 | Left ventricle | 30–40 | 0.37 (0.06) | 0.47 | | |
| Wong et al.[106] | 41 | Both ventricles | 34–37 | 0.54 (0.16) | 0.80 | 0.58 (0.17) | 0.86 |
| Hernandez-Andrade et al.[96] | 557 | Left ventricle | 19 | 0.35 (0.27) | 0.39 | | |
| | | | 39 | 0.37 (0.29) | 0.42 | | |
| Russell et al.[105] | 30 | Both ventricles | 20 | 0.53 (0.09) | 0.68 | 0.54 (0.12) | 0.74 |
| | | | 36 | 0.57 (0.09) | 0.72 | 0.60 (0.11) | 0.78 |
| Acharya et al.[153] | 87 | Left ventricle | 28 + 3 | 0.38 (0.1) | 0.55 | | |
| Van Mieghem et al.[154] | 117 | Left ventricle | 20–36 | 0.34 (0.05) | 0.42 | | |
| Api et al.[155] | 40 | Left ventricle | 26–40 | 0.43 (0.045) | 0.50 | | |
| Wood et al.[156] | 3,200 | Left ventricle | 11 | 0.4 (0.05) | 0.48 | | |
| | | | 40 | 0.58 (0.05) | 0.66 | | |
| Romiti et al.[157] | 49 | Both ventricles | 14–26 | 0.42 (0.14) | 0.65 | 0.49 (0.14) | 0.72 |
| | 61 | | 27–34 | 0.40 (0.17) | 0.68 | 0.49 (0.16) | 0.75 |
| | 17 | | 35–40 | 0.41 (0.14) | 0.64 | 0.52 (0.18) | 0.82 |
| Clur et al.[158] | 120 | Both ventricles | 11–15 | 0.36 (0.12) | 0.56 | 0.35 (0.14) | 0.58 |
| | 98 | | 18–22 | 0.31 (0.12) | 0.51 | 0.32 (0.16) | 0.58 |
| | 35 | | 28–32 | 0.31 (0.25) | 0.51 | 0.35 (0.22) | 0.71 |
| Hamela-Olkowska and Szymkiewicz-Danger[159] | 117 | Both ventricles | 18–40 | 0.47 (0.07) | 0.59 | 0.48 (0.1) | 0.65 |
| Ghawi et al.[160] | 250 | Both ventricles | Second and third trimesters (averaged) | 0.464 (0.08) | 0.60 | 0.466 (0.09) | 0.615 |

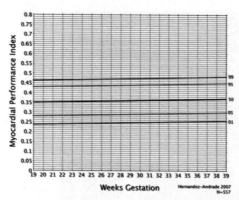

**FIGURE 5.59:** This is the graph for the myocardial performance index for the left ventricle.

that the MPI for both ventricles decreased in the third trimester instead of increasing.[106] Abnormal MPI of both ventricles examined in the first trimester has been reported to be associated with increasing levels of HbA1c.[107]

**Intrauterine Growth Restriction:** Similar to diabetic pregnancies, the MPI in fetuses with IUGR was abnormal in the third trimester, which is shown in Figure 5.60.[92,108–113] Fetuses with IUGR who have a normal umbilical artery pulsatility index have been shown to have an abnormal MPI of both ventricles.[114] Preeclampsia did not change the incidence of an abnormal MPI in fetuses with IUGR.[115] The MPI has also been evaluated as an independent predictor of perinatal death in preterm IUGR fetuses and found to have an accuracy similar to an abnormal ductus venosus waveform.[97]

**Spontaneous Rupture of the Membranes:** In 2010, Letti et al.[116] reported evaluating fetuses with premature rupture of the membranes prior to 34 weeks of gestation (24 to 33 weeks). They found the left ventricular MPI was significantly greater in fetuses with preterm PROM compared with controls (0.63 ± 0.13 vs. 0.51 ± 0.10, $P = .007$). While there was no difference in isovolumetric times, the left ventricular ejection time was significantly shorter in the preterm PROM group (164 ± 17 ms vs.

184 ± 16 ms, $P = .003$). In the preterm PROM group, neonatal sepsis was diagnosed in 73.3%, and funisitis and chorionic vasculitis confirmed fetal inflammatory response syndrome in 53.3%, compared with 6.7% for these three diagnoses in controls ($P = .001$).[116]

**Cardiovascular Malformations:** The MPI has been reported to be abnormal in fetuses with pulmonary insufficiency or atresia, compared with those with forward flow, fetuses with Ebstein anomaly, as well as fetuses with tetralogy of Fallot with an absent pulmonary valve.[117–119] In fetuses with a hypoplastic left ventricle, the MPI of the right ventricle has been reported to be increased.[120–122]

**Constriction of the Ductus Arteriosus:** In 2001, Mori et al.[123] reported that in fetuses with indomethacin-induced ductal constriction (pulsatility index <1.9) the right ventricular MPI was elevated, but decreased when the drug was withdrawn. Ductal constriction did not alter the MPI of the left ventricle. They postulated that the MPI was a sensitive indicator of cardiac function in fetuses with constriction of the ductus arteriosus.

## MYOCARDIAL PERFORMANCE INDEX USING PULSED TISSUE DOPPLER IMAGING (TDI)

Unlike conventional Doppler imaging of flow velocity in which flow through the atrioventricular and semilunar valves is obtained, TDI is a measure of the velocity and timing of myocardial wall motion of the right and left ventricles and the interventricular septum (Fig. 5.61). TDI is a sensitive marker of mildly impaired systolic and diastolic function, and is useful in the identification of subtle cardiac dysfunction in preclinical stages in postnatal life.[124,125] The TDI measured in adults and children has been shown to predict future cardiovascular disease.[118,126] The recording of TDI is obtained by placing the pulsed Doppler sample volume at the base of the right and left ventricular walls or septum and recording the wall motion (Fig. 5.62). Unlike the flow velocity waveform, the TDI demonstrates specific movement of the walls during the ICT and IRT times (Fig. 5.63). Previous studies have measured the parameters listed in Table 5.14 (Fig. 5.64).[125,127] Investigators have reported TDI in normal fetuses as well as those with IUGR and pregestational diabetes,

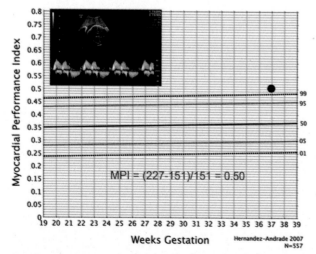

**FIGURE 5.60:** This is the myocardial performance index from the left ventricle in a fetus with intrauterine growth restriction. The MPI is increased above the 99th percentile, suggesting myocardial dysfunction.

MPI = (227−151)/151 = 0.50

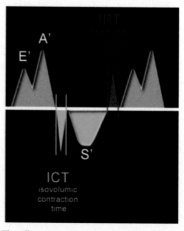

**FIGURE 5.61:** This illustrates the tissue Doppler image (TDI) waveform recorded from the right and left ventricular walls. The ICT and the IRT are distinct waveforms.

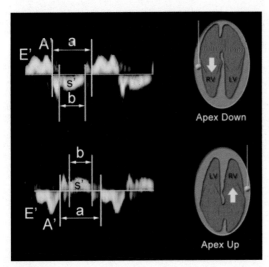

**FIGURE 5.62:** This illustrates TDI recordings from the right ventricular wall illustrating the direction of the waveforms, depending upon the position of the heart.

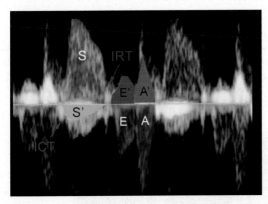

**FIGURE 5.63:** Simultaneous recording from the left ventricle that includes the pulsed Doppler flow velocity waveforms and the movement of the interventricular wall TDI. This demonstrates the timing relationships and the movement of the waveforms in opposite directions. For example, as the flow velocity waveform moves downward in diastole (E, A), the movement of the ventricular wall is upward (E', A'). The same relationship is observed for ventricular systole (S, S').

and found that it is more sensitive for detection of cardiovascular dysfunction than pulsed Doppler velocity of the mitral, tricuspid, aortic, and pulmonary valve waveforms.[69,111,126–135]

## Normal Values

Several studies have published normal fetal values for the measured TDI parameters listed in Table 5.14.[69,127–131,134] However, the most comprehensive study performed in normal fetuses was published by Comas et al.[127] in 2011. They examined 213 singleton pregnancies and published the mean, 5th, and 95th percentile ranges for all measurements listed in Table 5.14 for gestational age and estimated fetal weight. In addition, they provided regression equations for computing percentiles, as well as a calculator for computing Z-scores for each measurement. At the time of this writing, it is my opinion that these data should be the standard that clinicians should use for comparison between normal fetuses and those with suspected pathology. Figures 5.65 to 5.67 are the graphs for the E', A', and S' waves, E'/A', E/E' ratios, and the MPI' for the right and left ventricles. Table 5.15 contains the equations used for calculating the Z-score for each of the above measurements using an Excel spreadsheet.

## Small-for-Gestational Age (SGA) Fetuses

In the past, SGA fetuses were thought to be constitutionally small versus having intrauterine growth restriction of whether the Doppler of the umbilical artery was normal. Recent studies, however, have suggested that the SGA fetus may indeed have components of IUGR without abnormal umbilical artery Doppler waveforms and have adverse perinatal events and postnatal cardiovascular complications when compared with normal-weight newborns of the same gestational age.[70,132,133,136–141] Recent studies have suggested that echocardiographic and biochemical abnormalities are present in subclinical cardiac dysfunction that further deteriorates as the IUGR process becomes more severe.[69,70,81,142] In 2011, Comas et al. studied 58 SGA fetuses and 58 controls and compared pulsed Doppler flow velocity variables with tissue Doppler (Table 5.16). They found that the only flow velocity variable that was abnormal was a smaller A wave velocity in both ventricles, while tissue Doppler showed significantly lower peak velocities for the right E', A', and S' waves. In addition, the MPI' for both ventricles was significantly increased in the SGA fetuses. The authors postulated that because the TDI annular peak velocities reflect the motion of the longitudinal

| Table 5.14 | Definitions of Pulsed Tissue Doppler Waveforms | | | |
|---|---|---|---|---|
| *Location* | *Abbreviation* | *Weeks* | *Fetal Weight* | *Definition* |
| LV wall | PVE' | X | X | Peak left ventricular wall velocity of the diastolic E' wave from the tissue Doppler waveform |
| | PVA' | X | X | Peak left ventricular wall velocity of the diastolic A' wave from the tissue Doppler waveform |
| | PVS' | X | X | Peak left ventricular wall velocity of the systolic (S') wave from the tissue Doppler waveform |
| | E'/A' ratio | X | | Left ventricular wall velocity E'/A' ratio |
| | E/E' ratio | X | | Left ventricular flow velocity peak velocity (E) divided by the left ventricular peak wall velocity (E') ratio |

| Location | Abbreviation | Weeks | Fetal Weight | Definition |
|---|---|---|---|---|
| | MPI' | X | | Left ventricular myocardial performance index [(IVC' + IVR') / EF' |
| RV wall | PVE' | X | X | Peak right ventricular wall velocity of the diastolic E' wave from the tissue Doppler waveform |
| | PVA' | X | X | Peak right ventricular wall velocity of the diastolic A' wave from the tissue Doppler waveform |
| | PVS' | X | X | Peak right ventricular wall velocity of the systolic (S') wave from the tissue Doppler waveform |
| | E'/A' ratio | X | | Right ventricular velocity E'/A' ratio |
| | E/E' ratio | X | | Right ventricular flow velocity peak velocity (E) divided by the left ventricular peak wall velocity (E') ratio |
| | MPI' | X | | Right ventricular myocardial performance index [(IVC' + IVR')/EF' |
| Interventricular septal wall | PVE' | X | X | Peak interventricular septal wall velocity of the diastolic E' wave from the tissue Doppler waveform |
| | PVA' | X | X | Peak interventricular septal wall velocity of the diastolic A' wave from the tissue Doppler waveform |
| | PVS' | X | X | Peak interventricular septal wall velocity of the systolic (S') wave from the tissue Doppler waveform |
| | MPI' | X | | Left ventricular myocardial performance index [(IVC' + IVR')/EF' |

The ' next to the abbreviations refers to the pulsed Doppler recordings from the walls of the right and left ventricles and interventricular septum.

From Comas M, Crispi F, Gomez O, et al. Gestational age- and estimated fetal weight-adjusted reference ranges for myocardial tissue Doppler indices at 24–41 weeks' gestation. *Ultrasound Obstet Gynecol.* 2011;37:57–64.

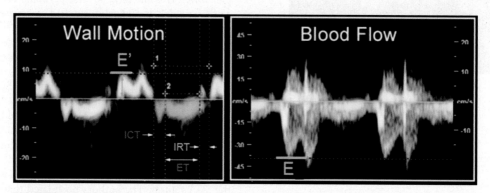

**FIGURE 5.64:** This illustrates the TDI recordings of the ICT, IRT, ET, *E'*, and the *E* velocity form the blood velocity waveform.

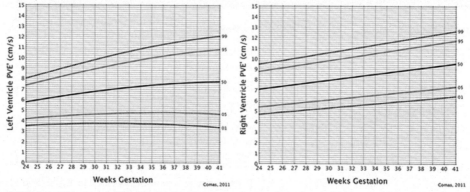

**FIGURE 5.65:** Left and right peak *E'*, *A'*, and *S'* peak velocities in centimeter per second for gestational age.[127]

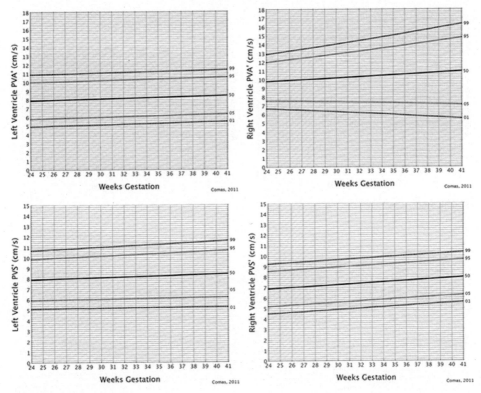

**FIGURE 5.65:** (continued)

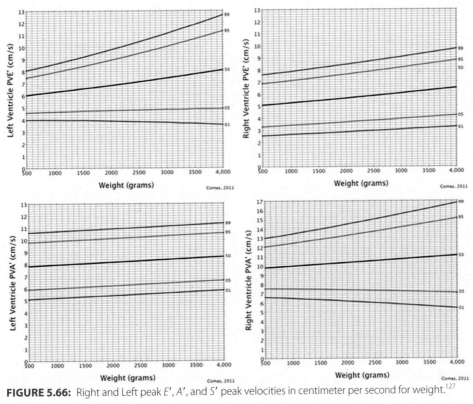

**FIGURE 5.66:** Right and Left peak *E'*, *A'*, and *S'* peak velocities in centimeter per second for weight.[127]

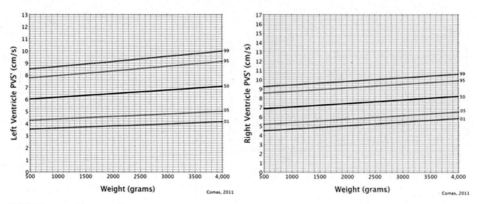

**FIGURE 5.66:** (*continued*)

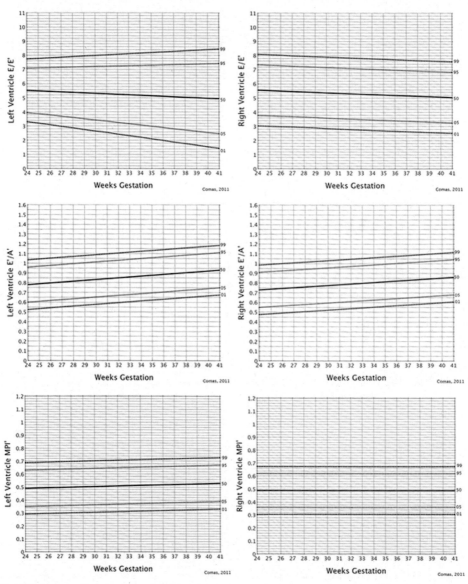

**FIGURE 5.67:** Left and right peak *E'/A'* peak velocities in centimeter per second and the corresponding MPI for gestational age.[127]

## Table 5.15  Equations for Computing the Z-score for Mitral, Tricuspid, and Septal Tissue Doppler Measurements.

| A | B | C GA (wks) | D GA (d) | E Value | F Log | G Median | H SD | I Z-score |
|---|---|---|---|---|---|---|---|---|
| LV wall | PVE' | | =D2 * 7 | | =LN(F2) | =0.475 + E2 * 0.0105901 − E2 * E2 * 0.0000178 | =0.071 + (E2 * 0.0004596) | =(G2 − H2)/I2 |
| | PVA' | | =D3 * 7 | | =LN(F3) | =7.1352 + 0.00456 * E3 | 1.2733 | =(F3 − H3)/I3 |
| | PVS' | | =D4 * 7 | | =LN(F4) | =(1.618801 + 0.00108 * E4) | 0.1711 | =(G4 − H4)/I4 |
| | E'/A' ratio | | =D5 * 7 | | =LN(F5) | =(0.56586) + (0.00127 * E5) | 0.11137 | =(F5 − H5)/I5 |
| | E/E' ratio | | =D6 * 7 | | =LN(F6) | =(6.33933 − 0.00485 * E6) | =(0.17383 + 0.004647 * E6) | =(F6 − H6)/I6 |
| | MPI' | | =D7 * 7 | | =LN(F7) | =(0.43462 + 0.00033 * E7) | 0.08577 | =(F7 − H7)/I7 |
| RV Wall | PVE' | | =D9 * 7 | | =LN(F9) | =(3.64026 + 0.02054 * E9) | =(0.58457 + 0.00262 * E9) | =(F9 − H9)/I9 |
| | PVA' | | =D10 * 7 | | =LN(F10) | =(2.12331078 + 0.000937 * E10) | =EXP(0.03985 + 0.000498 * E10) | =(G10 − H10)/I10 |
| | PVS' | | =D11 * 7 | | =LN(F11) | =(5.3016404 + 0.009366 * E11) | 1.02489 | =(F11 − H11)/I11 |
| | E'/A' ratio | | =D12 * 7 | | =LN(F12) | =(0.5501) + (0.00108 * E12) | 0.1106 | =(F12 − H12)/I12 |
| | E/E' ratio | | =D13 * 7 | | =LN(F13) | =(6.28218 − 0.00432 * E13) | 1.0877 | =(F13 − H13)/I13 |
| | MPI' | | =D14 * 7 | | =LN(F14) | =0.49432 | 0.07929 | =(F14 − H14)/I14 |
| Interventricular septal wall | PVE' | | =D16 * 7 | | =LN(F16) | =(1.33919 + 0.00176 * E16) | =EXP(0.18285) | =(G16 − H16)/I16 |
| | PVA' | | =D17 * 7 | | =LN(F17) | =(1.647171 + 0.001197 * E17) | 0.17911 | =(G17 − H17)/I17 |
| | PVS' | | =D18 * 7 | | =LN(F18) | =(1.36718 + 0.001517 * E18) | 0.15752 | =(G18 − H18)/I18 |
| | E'/A' ratio | | =D19 * 7 | | =LN(F19) | 0.8377 | 0.08888 | =(F19 − H19)/I19 |
| | MPI' | | =D20 * 7 | | =LN(F20) | 0.5098 | 0.06826 | =(F20 − H20)/I20 |

The Excel spreadsheet for these computations can be downloaded from the following website: http://onlinelibrary.wiley.com/doi/10.1002/uog.8870/suppinfo

From Comas M, Crispi F, Gomez O, et al. Gestational age- and estimated fetal weight-adjusted reference ranges for myocardial tissue Doppler indices at 24–41 weeks' gestation. *Ultrasound Obstet Gynecol.* 2011;37:57–64.

| Table 5.16 | Comparison of Doppler Velocity and Ventricular Wall Motion Measurements in Fetus with Intrauterine Growth Restriction Who Did Not Have Absent Flow in the Umbilical Artery | | |
|---|---|---|---|
| **Measurements** | **Control** | **IUGR** | **P Value Adjusted for Fetal Weight** |
| **Pulsed Doppler Flow Velocity** | | | |
| *Variable* | | | |
| Left E wave velocity | 38 (8) | 36 (6) | NS |
| **Left A wave velocity** | **49 (8)** | **44 (6)** | **<.001** |
| Left E/A ratio | 0.78 (0.12) | 0.83 (0.13) | NS |
| Right E wave velocity | 47 (9) | 43 (7) | NS |
| **Right A wave velocity** | **59 (10)** | **53 (9)** | **.007** |
| Right E/A ratio | 0.80 (0.8) | 0.82 (0.11) | NS |
| Left MPI | 0.49 (0.08) | 0.53 (0.11) | NS |
| **Pulsed Tissue Doppler** | | | |
| *Annular Peak Velocities (cm/s)* | | | |
| Left PVE′ | 7.89 (1.56) | 7.60 (1.39) | NS |
| Left PVA′ | 8.56 (1.37) | 8.17 (1.86) | NS |
| Left PVS′ | 6.94 (1.19) | 6.64 (1.35) | NS |
| **Right PVE′** | **9.25 (1.42)** | **8.48 (1.47)** | **.039** |
| **Right PVA′** | **11.23 (2.15)** | **10.13 (1.64)** | **.033** |
| **Right PVS′** | **8.09 (1.29)** | **7.39 (1.29)** | **.049** |
| Septal PVE′ | 6.24 (1.13) | 6.11 (1.07) | NS |
| Septal PVA′ | 7.41 (1.37) | 6.97 (1.34) | NS |
| Septal PVS′ | 6.03 (1.02) | 5.99 (1.14) | NS |
| *Myocardial Performance Index* | | | |
| **Left MPI′** | **0.52 (0.09)** | **0.55 (0.09)** | **.001** |
| **Right MPI′** | **0.49 (0.09)** | **0.56 (0.10)** | **<.001** |
| *Septal MPI′* | 0.52 (0.09) | 0.59 (0.11) | NS |

From Comas M, Crispi F, Cruz-Martinez R, et al. Tissue Doppler echocardiographic markers of cardiac dysfunction in small-for-gestational age fetuses. *Am J Obstet Gynecol.* 2011;205:57.e1–57.e6.

myocardial fibers, which are located in the subendocardial layer, they are the earliest to be altered in the presence of decreased oxygen.[143] They suggested that pulsed tissue Doppler measurements are more sensitive than velocity measurements.[114] The SGA fetuses had an increased trend for higher rates of intervention for fetal distress, cesarean section, and preeclampsia, and longer days in the newborn intensive care unit.

## Early-Onset Intrauterine Growth Restriction (IUGR)

Fetuses with IUGR have been shown to have cardiac dysfunction, while maintaining appropriate cardiac output for their specific weight.[69,70,81] Prior studies reported abnormal cardiac dysfunction at more advanced stages of IUGR.[66,67,71] However, recent studies have suggested that subclinical cardiac dysfunction occurs at earlier stages of fetal deterioration.[69,111] In 2010, Comas et al. studied 25 IUGR fetuses whose estimated fetal weight was below the 10th percentile and umbilical artery pulsatility index above the 95th percentile. Fetuses who were delivered between 26 and 34 weeks of gestation were evaluated. Fetuses with structural and/or chromosomal anomalies and those with infection were excluded. Fifty normally growth fetuses, matched for gestational age, were used as controls. Table 5.17 lists their findings for velocity flow measurements and TDI measurements for diastolic function, systolic function, and combined diastolic and systolic dysfunction. The pulsed Doppler flow measurements demonstrated decreased right and left ventricular E and A wave velocities, but the E/A ratios were normal. While the peak velocities for the aorta and pulmonary artery were decreased in the

| Table 5.17 | Comparison of Doppler Velocity and Ventricular Wall Motion Measurements in Fetuses with Early-Onset Intrauterine Growth Restriction Who Had Abnormal Doppler of the Umbilical Artery | | |
|---|---|---|---|

| Measurements (cm/s) | Control | IUGR | P Value Adjusted for Fetal Weight |
|---|---|---|---|
| **Pulsed Doppler Flow Velocity** | | | |
| *Diastolic Parameters* | | | |
| **Left E wave velocity** | **37 (5.4)** | **31 (7.4)** | **<.002** |
| **Left A wave velocity** | **50 (8.5)** | **41 (10.1)** | **<.001** |
| Left E/A ratio | 0.74 (0.1) | 0.78 ((0.2) | NS |
| **Right E wave velocity** | **43 (7.9)** | **32 (7.5)** | **<.001** |
| **Right A wave velocity** | **57 (9.2)** | **39 (7.2)** | **<.001** |
| Right E/A ratio | 0.76 (0.1) | 0.81 (0.1) | NS |
| *Systolic Parameters* | | | |
| Aortic peak velocity | 94 (20.2) | 81 (16.5) | NS |
| Pulmonary artery peak velocity | 91 (20.9) | 84 (24.5) | NS |
| *Myocardial Performance Index (diastolic and systolic dysfunction)* | | | |
| **Left MPI** | **0.45 (0.06)** | **0.52 (0.09)** | **.006** |
| Right MPI | 0.47 (0.19) | 045 (0.13) | NS |
| **Pulsed Tissue Doppler** | | | |
| *Diastolic Parameters* | | | |
| Left PVE′ | 7.3 (1.3) | 6.7 (0.8) | NS |
| **Left PVA′** | **8.5 (1.4)** | **6.2 (0.7)** | **<.001** |
| **Left E′/A′** | **0.85 (0.13)** | **1.09 (0.17)** | **<.001** |
| **Right PVE′** | **8.5 (1.13)** | **7.2 (1.3)** | **.007** |
| **Right PVA′** | **10.8 (1.5)** | **9.1 (1.2)** | **.01** |
| Right E′/A′ | 0.79 (0.1) | 0.82 (0.1) | NS |
| Septal PVE′ | 6.3 (1.1) | 5.4 (1) | NS |
| **Septal PVA′** | **7.4 (1.3)** | **6.2 (0.6)** | **.049** |
| Septal E′/A′ | 0.86 (0.1) | 0.88 (0.1) | NS |
| *Systolic Parameters* | | | |
| **Left PVS′** | **6.9 (1.2)** | **5.6 (0.6)** | **.002** |
| **Right PVS′** | **7.6 (1.2)** | **6.6 (1.4)** | **.049** |
| Septal PVS′ | 5.8 (0.88) | 5.3 (1.1) | NS |
| *Myocardial Performance Index (diastolic and systolic dysfunction)* | | | |
| **Left MPI′** | **0.49 (0.08)** | **0.56 (0.09)** | **.007** |
| **Right MPI′** | **0.47 (0.09)** | **0.61 (0.11)** | **.006** |
| **Septal MPI′** | **0.49 (0.06)** | **0.58 (0.05)** | **<.001** |

From Comas M, Crispi F, Cruz-Martinez R, et al. Usefulness of myocardial tissue Doppler vs conventional echocardiography in the evaluation of cardiac dysfunction in early-onset intrauterine growth restriction. *Am J Obstet Gynecol.* 2010;203:45.e1–45.e7.

IUGR fetuses, the decrease was not statistically significant. Only the left ventricle demonstrated an increased MPI. While the TDI measurements demonstrated similar significant decreases for E' and A' for both ventricles and an increased MPI' for the left ventricle, the approach also showed a significant increase in the left E'/A' ratio, decreased left and right ventricular S', and abnormal MPI' for the right ventricle and septum. The authors concluded that TDI is a more sensitive tool for evaluating systolic and diastolic dysfunction than conventional pulsed Doppler evaluation of the flow velocity waveforms.[111] They also concluded that the aortic and pulmonary artery flow velocities were similar, when corrected for fetal weight.[111]

## Diabetes

In 2008, Hatem et al. examined fetuses of mothers with pregestational diabetes from 25 weeks to term and reported the following:

1. The right and left myocardial velocities of E' and A' were significantly higher in fetuses of diabetic mothers.
2. The E'/A' ratios were higher than in normal fetuses
3. In fetuses of mothers with pregestational diabetes, the ratio of early diastolic peak inflow velocity (E) to peak annular velocity (E') was lower in fetuses of mothers with diabetes.

They concluded that the changes in diastolic dysfunction were independent of fetal myocardial hypertrophy, and thus an earlier indication of cardiovascular dysfunction.[144]

In 2013, Bui et al.[145] reported a study performed between 17 and 23 weeks in which they evaluated the MPI for right ventricle in 69 normal fetuses and 51 fetuses of diabetic mothers. They found that there were no significant differences between the two groups for the E', A', E'/A' ratio, peak E and Peak A wave velocities. However, the E/E'ratio had a P value of <.05. The right ventricular pulsed wave MPI was not statistically significant between the two groups, but the TDI MPI was significantly higher in the diabetic population (0.563 [SD 0.104]) than in controls (0.512 [SD 0.098]) ($P < .01$). They concluded that the MPI of the TDI was more sensitive than spectral Doppler MPI for detecting cardiac dysfunction in the mid-trimester fetus of the diabetic mother.

## ACKNOWLEDGMENTS

The librarians and volunteers of the Health Sciences Library, Huntington Memorial Hospital, Pasadena, CA, provided full text articles through the Document Delivery service.

## REFERENCES

1. Allan LD, Joseph MC, Boyd EG, et al. M-mode echocardiography in the developing human fetus. *Br Heart J.* 1982;47:573–583.
2. DeVore GR, Siassi B, Platt LD. Fetal echocardiography, IV: M-mode assessment of ventricular size and contractility during the second and third trimesters of pregnancy in the normal fetus. *Am J Obstet Gynecol.* 1984;150:981–988.
3. De Vore GR, Siassi B, Platt LD. Use of femur length as a mans of assessing M-mode ventricular dimensions during second and third trimesters of pregnancy in normal fetus. *J Clin Ultrasound.* 1985;13:619–620.
4. Cartier MS, Davidoff A, Warneke LA, et al. The normal diameter of the fetal aorta and pulmonary artery: echocardiographic evaluation in utero. *AJR Am J Roentgenol.* 1987;149:1003–1007.
5. Luewan S, Yanase Y, Tongprasert F, et al. Fetal cardiac dimensions at 14–40 weeks' gestation obtained using cardio-STIC-M. *Ultrasound Obstet Gynecol.* 2011;37:416–422.
6. Schneider C, McCrindle BW, Carvalho JS, et al. Development of Z-scores for fetal cardiac dimensions from echocardiography. *Ultrasound Obstet Gynecol.* 2005;26:599–605.
7. Lee W, Riggs T, Amula V, et al. Fetal echocardiography: z-score reference ranges for a large patient population. *Ultrasound Obstet Gynecol.* 2010;35:28–34.
8. Sharland GK, Allan LD. Normal fetal cardiac measurements derived by cross-sectional echocardiography. *Ultrasound Obstet Gynecol.* 1992;2:175–181.
9. Tan J, Silverman NH, Hoffman JI, et al. Cardiac dimensions determined by cross-sectional echocardiography in the normal human fetus from 18 weeks to term. *Am J Cardiol.* 1992;70:1459–1467.
10. Murata Y, Takemura H, Kurachi K. Observation of fetal cardiac motion by M-mode ultrasonic cardiography. *Am J Obstet Gynecol.* 1971;111:287–294.
11. O'Malley BP, Salem S. Ultrasonic diagnosis of intrauterine fetal death. *J Can Assoc Radiol.* 1976;27:273–277.
12. Kleinman CS, Hobbins JC, Jaffe CC, et al. Echocardiographic studies of the human fetus: prenatal diagnosis of congenital heart disease and cardiac dysrhythmias. *Pediatrics.* 1980;65(6):1059–1067.
13. DeVore GR, Donnerstein RL, Kleinman CS, et al. Real-time—directed M-mode echocardiography: a new technique for accurate and rapid quantitation of the fetal preejection period and ventricular ejection time of the right and left ventricles. *Am J Obstet Gynecol.* 1981;141:470–471.
14. DeVore GR, Siassi B, Platt LD. Fetal echocardiography, V: M-mode measurements of the aortic root and aortic valve in second- and third-trimester normal human fetuses. *Am J Obstet Gynecol.* 1985;152:543–550.
15. DeVore GR, Siassi B, Platt LD. The use of the abdominal circumference as a means of assessing M-mode ventricular dimensions during the second and third trimesters of pregnancy in the normal human fetus. *J Ultrasound Med.* 1985;4:175–182.
16. DeVore GR, Siassi B, Platt LD. Fetal echocardiography, VIII: aortic root dilatation—a marker for tetralogy of Fallot. *Am J Obstet Gynecol.* 1988;159:129–136.
17. St John Sutton MG, Gewitz MH, Shah B, et al. Quantitative assessment of growth and function of the cardiac chambers in the normal human fetus: a prospective longitudinal echocardiographic study. *Circulation.* 1984;69:645–654.
18. DeVore GR. Examination of the fetal heart in the fetus with intrauterine growth retardation using M-mode echocardiography. *Semin Perinatol.* 1988;12(1):66–79.
19. DeVore GR. Assessing fetal cardiac ventricular function. *Semin Fetal Neonatal Med.* 2005;10:515–541.
20. Horenstein J, DeVore GR, Platt LD, et al. The use of fetal echocardiography for predicting intrapartum fetal heart rate patterns in the post-term pregnancy. *Ultrasound Obstet Gynecol.* 1991;1:395–400.
21. DeVore GR, Siassi B, Platt LD. Ventricular disproportion—the prenatal manifestation of coarctation of the aorta. *J Perinatol.* 1986;6:265–273.
22. Shapiro I, Degani S, Leibovitz Z, et al. Fetal cardiac measurements derived by transvaginal and transabdominal cross-sectional echocardiography from 14 weeks of gestation to term. *Ultrasound Obstet Gynecol.* 1998;12:404–418.
23. Firpo C, Hoffman JI, Silverman NH. Evaluation of fetal heart dimensions from 12 weeks to term. *Am J Cardiol.* 2001;87:594–600.
24. Rimoldi HJA, Lev M. A note on the concept of normality and abnormality in quantitation of pathologic findings in congenital heart disease. *Pediatr Clin North Am.* 1963;10:589–591.
25. Devore GR. The use of Z-scores in the analysis of fetal cardiac dimensions. *Ultrasound Obstet Gynecol.* 2005;26:596–598.
26. Galindo A, Gutierrez-Larraya F, Martinez JM, et al. Prenatal diagnosis and outcome for fetuses with congenital absence of the pulmonary valve. *Ultrasound Obstet Gynecol.* 2006;28:32–39.
27. Pasquini L, Mellander M, Seale A, et al. Z-scores of the fetal aortic isthmus and duct: an aid to assessing arch hypoplasia. *Ultrasound Obstet Gynecol.* 2007;29:628–633.
28. Wald RM, Tham EB, McCrindle BW, et al. Outcome after prenatal diagnosis of tricuspid atresia: a multicenter experience. *Am Heart J.* 2007;153:772–778.
29. Gardiner HM, Belmar C, Tulzer G, et al. Morphologic and functional predictors of eventual circulation in the fetus with pulmonary atresia or critical pulmonary stenosis with intact septum. *J Am Coll Cardiol.* 2008;51:1299–1308.
30. Lee W, Allan L, Carvalho JS, et al. ISUOG consensus statement: what constitutes a fetal echocardiogram? *Ultrasound Obstet Gynecol.* 2008;32:239–242..
31. Kaski JP, Daubeney PE. Normalization of echocardiographically derived paediatric cardiac dimensions to body surface area: time for a standardized approach. *Eur J Echocardiogr.* 2009;10:44–45.
32. Seale AN, Ho SY, Shinebourne EA, et al. Prenatal identification of the pulmonary arterial supply in tetralogy of Fallot with pulmonary atresia. *Cardiol Young.* 2009;19:185–191.
33. Wan AW, Jevremovic A, Selamet Tierney ES, et al. Comparison of impact of prenatal versus postnatal diagnosis of congenitally corrected transposition of the great arteries. *Am J Cardiol.* 2009;104:1276–1279.
34. Hamdan MA, El-Zoabi BA, Begam MA, et al. Antenatal diagnosis of pompe disease by fetal echocardiography: impact on outcome after early initiation of enzyme replacement therapy. *J Inherit Metab Dis.* 2010;33(suppl 3):S333–S339.
35. Hirji A, Bernasconi A, McCrindle BW, et al. Outcomes of prenatally diagnosed tetralogy of Fallot: implications for valve-sparing repair versus transannular patch. *Can J Cardiol.* 2010;26:e1–e6
36. Hornberger LK. Role of quantitative assessment in fetal echocardiography. *Ultrasound Obstet Gynecol.* 2010;35:4–6.
37. Kohl T. Chronic intermittent materno-fetal hyperoxygenation in late gestation may improve on hypoplastic cardiovascular structures associated with cardiac malformations in human fetuses. *Pediatr Cardiol.* 2010;31:250–263.

38. Arzt W, Wertaschnigg D, Veit I, et al. Intrauterine aortic valvuloplasty in fetuses with critical aortic stenosis: experience and results of 24 procedures. *Ultrasound Obstet Gynecol.* 2011;37:689–695.

39. Byrne FA, Lee H, Kipps AK, et al. Echocardiographic risk stratification of fetuses with sacrococcygeal teratoma and twin-reversed arterial perfusion. *Fetal Diagn Ther.* 2011;30:280–288.

40. Escribano D, Herraiz I, Granados M, et al. Tetralogy of Fallot: prediction of outcome in the mid-second trimester of pregnancy. *Prenat Diagn.* 2011;31:1126–1133.

41. Hirai M, Vernon L. The role of disgust propensity in blood-injection-injury phobia: comparisons between Asian Americans and Caucasian Americans. *Cogn Emot.* 2011;25:1500–1509.

42. Jowett V, Miller O. Prenatal diagnosis of left ventricular aneurysm in association with interruption of the aortic arch. *Cardiol Young.* 2011;21:113–115.

43. Stressig R, Fimmers R, Eising K, et al. Intrathoracic herniation of the liver ('liver-up') is associated with predominant left heart hypoplasia in human fetuses with left diaphragmatic hernia. *Ultrasound Obstet Gynecol.* 2011;37:272–276.

44. Tutschek B, Schmidt KG. Techniques for assessing cardiac output and fetal cardiac function. *Semin Fetal Neonatal Med.* 2011;16:13–21.

45. Seale AN, Carvalho JS, Gardiner HM, et al. Total anomalous pulmonary venous connection: impact of prenatal diagnosis. *Ultrasound Obstet Gynecol.* 2012;40:310–318.

46. Kwon EN, Parness IA, Srivastava S, et al. Subpulmonary stenosis assessed in midtrimester fetuses with tetralogy of fallot: a novel method for predicting postnatal clinical outcome. *Pediatr Cardiol.* 2013;34(6):1314–1320.

47. Marantz P, Aiello H, Grinenco S, et al. Foetal aortic valvuloplasty: experience of five cases. *Cardiol Young.* 2013;23(5):675–681.

48. Quartermain MD, Glatz AC, Goldberg DJ, et al. Pulmonary outflow tract obstruction in fetuses with complex congenital heart disease: predicting the need for neonatal intervention. *Ultrasound Obstet Gynecol.* 2013;41:47–53.

49. Thakur V, Fouron JC, Mertens L, et al. Diagnosis and management of fetal heart failure. *Can J Cardiol.* 2013;29(7):759–767.

50. Weber RW, Ayala-Arnez R, Atiyah M, et al. Foetal echocardiographic assessment of borderline small left ventricles can predict the need for postnatal intervention. *Cardiol Young.* 2013;23:99–107..

51. Wertaschnigg D, Jaeggi M, Chitayat D, et al. Prenatal diagnosis and outcome of absent pulmonary valve syndrome: contemporary single-center experience and review of the literature. *Ultrasound Obstet Gynecol.* 2013;41:162–167.

52. Riggs T, Saini AP, Comstock CH, et al. Comparison of cardiac Z-score with cardiac asymmetry for prenatal screening of congenital heart disease. *Ultrasound Obstet Gynecol.* 2011;38:332–336.

53. Tongprasert F, Srisupundit K, Luewan S, et al. Reference ranges of fetal aortic and pulmonary valve diameter derived by STIC from 14 to 40 weeks of gestation. *Prenat Diagn.* 2011;31:439–445.

54. DeVore GR, Horenstein J, Siassi B, et al. Fetal echocardiography, VII: Doppler color flow mapping: a new technique for the diagnosis of congenital heart disease. *Am J Obstet Gynecol.* 1987;156:1054–1064.

55. Harada K, Rice MJ, Shiota T, et al. Gestational age- and growth-related alterations in fetal right and left ventricular diastolic filling patterns. *Am J Cardiol.* 1997;79:173–177.

56. Carceller-Blanchard AM, Fouron JC. Determinants of the doppler flow velocity profile through the mitral valve of the human fetus. *Br Heart J.* 1993;70:457–460.

57. Pacileo G, Paladini D, Pisacane C, et al. Role of changing loading conditions on atrioventricular flow velocity patterns in normal human fetuses. *Am J Cardiol.* 1994;73:991–993.

58. Reed KL, Sahn DJ, Scagnelli S, et al. Doppler echocardiographic studies of diastolic function in the human fetal heart: changes during gestation. *J Am Coll Cardiol.* 1986;8:391–395.

59. Tulzer G, Khowsathit P, Gudmundsson S, et al. Diastolic function of the fetal heart during second and third trimester: a prospective longitudinal Doppler-echocardiographic study. *Eur J Pediatr.* 1994;153:151–154.

60. Weiner Z, Efrat Z, Zimmer EZ, et al. Fetal atrioventricular blood flow throughout gestation. *Am J Cardiol.* 1997;80:658–662.

61. Reed KL. Fetal Doppler echocardiography. *Clin Obstet Gynecol.* 1989;32:728–737.

62. Romero R, Espinoza J, Goncalves LF, et al. Fetal cardiac dysfunction in preterm premature rupture of membranes. *J Matern Fetal Neonatal Med.* 2004;16:146–157.

63. Weiner Z, Zloczower M, Lerner A, et al. Cardiac compliance in fetuses of diabetic women. *Obstet Gynecol.* 1999;93:948–951.

64. Tsyvian P, Malkin K, Artemieva O, et al. Assessment of left ventricular filling in normally grown fetuses, growth-restricted fetuses and fetuses of diabetic mothers. *Ultrasound Obstet Gynecol.* 1998;12:33–38.

65. Rizzo G, Arduini D, Romanini C. Doppler echocardiographic assessment of fetal cardiac function. *Ultrasound Obstet Gynecol.* 1992;2:434–445.

66. Hecher K, Campbell S, Doyle P, et al. Assessment of fetal compromise by Doppler ultrasound investigation of the fetal circulation: arterial, intracardiac, and venous blood flow velocity studies. *Circulation.* 1995;91:129–138.

67. Figueras F, Puerto B, Martinez JM, et al. Cardiac function monitoring of fetuses with growth restriction. *Eur J Obstet Gynecol Reprod Biol.* 2003;110:159–163.

68. Rizzo G, Arduini D, Romanini C, et al. Doppler echocardiographic assessment of atrioventricular velocity waveforms in normal and small-for-gestational-age fetuses. *Br J Obstet Gynaecol.* 1988;95:65–69.

69. Crispi F, Hernandez-Andrade E, Pelsers MM, et al. Cardiac dysfunction and cell damage across clinical stages of severity in growth-restricted fetuses. *Am J Obstet Gynecol.* 2008;199:254.e1–254.e8.

70. Girsen A, Ala-Kopsala M, Makikallio K, et al. Cardiovascular hemodynamics and umbilical artery N-terminal peptide of proB-type natriuretic peptide in human fetuses with growth restriction. *Ultrasound Obstet Gynecol.* 2007;29:296–303.

71. Makikallio K, Vuolteenaho O, Jouppila P, et al. Ultrasonographic and biochemical markers of human fetal cardiac dysfunction in placental insufficiency. *Circulation.* 2002;105:2058–2063.

72. Arduini D, Rizzo G, Romanini C, et al. (1995) *Fetal cardiac output measurement in normal and pathologic states.* In: Copel JA and Reed KL, Doppler Ultra-sound in Obstetrics and Gynecology, Springer Publishing Company, New York, Chap 27.

73. Rizzo G, Arduini D. Fetal cardiac function in intrauterine growth retardation. *Am J Obstet Gynecol.* 1991;165:876–882.

74. Copel JA, Grannum PA, Green JJ, et al. Fetal cardiac output in the isoimmunized pregnancy: a pulsed Doppler-echocardiographic study of patients undergoing intravascular intrauterine transfusion. *Am J Obstet Gynecol.* 1989;161:361–365.

75. De Smedt MC, Visser GH, Meijboom EJ. Fetal cardiac output estimated by Doppler echocardiography during mid- and late gestation. *Am J Cardiol.* 1987;60:338–342.

76. Allan LD, Chita SK, Al-Ghazali W, et al. Doppler echocardiographic evaluation of the normal human fetal heart. *Br Heart J.* 1987;57:528–533.

77. Mielke G, Benda N. Cardiac output and central distribution of blood flow in the human fetus. *Circulation.* 2001;103:1662–1668.

78. Copel JA, Grannum PA, Green JJ, et al. Pulsed Doppler flow-velocity waveforms in the prediction of fetal hematocrit of the severely isoimmunized pregnancy. *Am J Obstet Gynecol.* 1989;161:341–344.

79. Severi FM, Rizzo G, Bocchi C, et al. Intrauterine growth retardation and fetal cardiac function. *Fetal Diagn Ther.* 2000;15:8–19.

80. Di Renzo GC, Luzi G, Cucchia GC, et al. The role of Doppler technology in the evaluation of fetal hypoxia. *Early Hum Dev.* 1992;29:259–267.

81. Kiserud T, Ebbing C, Kessler J, et al. Fetal cardiac output, distribution to the placenta and impact of placental compromise. *Ultrasound Obstet Gynecol.* 2006;28:126–136.

82. Bolnick AD, Borgida AF, Egan JF, et al. Influence of gestational age and fetal heart rate on the fetal mechanical PR interval. *J Matern Fetal Neonatal Med.* 2004;15:303–305.

83. Glickstein J, Buyon J, Kim M, et al. The fetal Doppler mechanical PR interval: a validation study. *Fetal Diagn Ther.* 2004;19:31–34.

84. Glickstein JS, Buyon J, Friedman D. Pulsed Doppler echocardiographic assessment of the fetal PR interval. *Am J Cardiol.* 2000;86:236–239.

85. Rosenthal D, Friedman DM, Buyon J, et al. Validation of the Doppler PR interval in the fetus. *J Am Soc Echocardiogr.* 2002;15:1029–1030.

86. Van Bergen AH, Cuneo BF, Davis N. Prospective echocardiographic evaluation of atrioventricular conduction in fetuses with maternal Sjogren's antibodies. *Am J Obstet Gynecol.* 2004;191:1014–1018.

87. Friedman DM, Rupel A, Glickstein J, et al. Congenital heart block in neonatal lupus: the pediatric cardiologist's perspective. *Indian J Pediatr.* 2002;69:517–522.

88. Tei C, Dujardin KS, Hodge DO, et al. Doppler index combining systolic and diastolic myocardial performance: clinical value in cardiac amyloidosis. *J Am Coll Cardiol.* 1996;28:658–664.

89. Tei C, Ling LH, Hodge DO, et al. New index of combined systolic and diastolic myocardial performance: a simple and reproducible measure of cardiac function—a study in normals and dilated cardiomyopathy. *J Cardiol.* 1995;26:357–366.

90. Tei C, Nishimura RA, Seward JB, et al. Noninvasive Doppler-derived myocardial performance index: correlation with simultaneous measurements of cardiac catheterization measurements. *J Am Soc Echocardiogr.* 1997;10:169–178.

91. Browne VA, Stiffel VM, Pearce WJ, et al. Activator calcium and myocardial contractility in fetal sheep exposed to long-term high-altitude hypoxia. *Am J Physiol.* 1997;272:H1196–H1204

92. Tsutsumi T, Ishii M, Eto G, et al. Serial evaluation for myocardial performance in fetuses and neonates using a new Doppler index. *Pediatr Int.* 1999;41:722–727.

93. Friedman D, Buyon J, Kim M, et al. Fetal cardiac function assessed by Doppler myocardial performance index (Tei Index). *Ultrasound Obstet Gynecol.* 2003;21:33–36.

94. Hernandez-Andrade E, Lopez-Tenorio J, Figueroa-Diesel H, et al. A modified myocardial performance (Tei) index based on the use of valve clicks improves reproducibility of fetal left cardiac function assessment. *Ultrasound Obstet Gynecol.* 2005;26:227–232.

95. Hernandez-Andrade E, Benavides-Serralde JA, Cruz-Martinez R, et al. Evaluation of conventional Doppler fetal cardiac function parameters: E/A ratios, outflow tracts, and myocardial performance index. *Fetal Diagn Ther.* 2012;32:22–29.

96. Hernandez-Andrade E, Figueroa-Diesel H, Kottman C, et al. Gestational-age-adjusted reference values for the modified myocardial performance index for evaluation of fetal left cardiac function. *Ultrasound Obstet Gynecol.* 2004;29:321–325.

97. Hernandez-Andrade E, Crispi F, Benavides-Serralde JA, et al. Contribution of the myocardial performance index and aortic isthmus blood flow index to predicting mortality in preterm growth-restricted fetuses. *Ultrasound Obstet Gynecol.* 2009;34:430–436.

98. Szwast A, Tian Z, McCann M, et al. Impact of altered loading conditions on ventricular performance in fetuses with congenital cystic adenomatoid malformation and twin-twin transfusion syndrome. *Ultrasound Obstet Gynecol.* 2007;30:40–46.

99. Ichizuka K, Matsuoka R, Hasegawa J, et al. The Tei index for evaluation of fetal myocardial performance in sick fetuses. *Early Hum Dev.* 2005;81:273–279.

100. Stirnemann JJ, Mougeot M, Proulx F, et al. Profiling fetal cardiac function in twin-twin transfusion syndrome. *Ultrasound Obstet Gynecol.* 2010;35:19–27.

101. Van Mieghem T, Klaritsch P, Done E, et al. Assessment of fetal cardiac function before and after therapy for twin-to-twin transfusion syndrome. *Am J Obstet Gynecol.* 2009;200:400.e1–400.e7.

102. Michelfelder E, Gottliebson W, Border W, et al. Early manifestations and spectrum of recipient twin cardiomyopathy in twin-twin transfusion syndrome: relation to Quintero stage. *Ultrasound Obstet Gynecol.* 2007;30:965–971.

103. Habli M, Michelfelder E, Livingston J, et al. Acute effects of selective fetoscopic laser photocoagulation on recipient cardiac function in twin-twin transfusion syndrome. *Am J Obstet Gynecol.* 2008;199(4):412.e1–412.e6.

104. Casson IF, Clarke CA, Howard CV, et al. Outcomes of pregnancy in insulin dependent diabetic women: results of a five year population cohort study. *BMJ.* 1997;315:275–278.

105. Russell NE, Foley M, Kinsley BT, et al. Effect of pregestational diabetes mellitus on fetal cardiac function and structure. *Am J Obstet Gynecol.* 2008;199(3):312.e1–312.e7.

106. Wong ML, Wong WH, Cheung YF. Fetal myocardial performance in pregnancies complicated by gestational impaired glucose tolerance. *Ultrasound Obstet Gynecol.* 2007;29:395–400.

107. Turan S, Turan OM, Miller J, et al. Decreased fetal cardiac performance in the first trimester correlates with hyperglycemia in pregestational maternal diabetes. *Ultrasound Obstet Gynecol.* 2011;38:325–331.

108. Niewiadomska-Jarosik K, Lipecka-Kidawska E, Kowalska-Koprek U, et al. Assessment of cardiac function in fetuses with intrauterine growth retardation using the Tei Index [in Polish]. *Med Wieku Rozwoj.* 2005;9:153–160.

109. Cruz-Martinez R, Figueras F, Benavides-Serralde A, et al. Sequence of changes in myocardial performance index in relation to aortic isthmus and ductus venosus Doppler in fetuses with early-onset intrauterine growth restriction. *Ultrasound Obstet Gynecol.* 2011;38:179–184.

110. Cruz-Martinez R, Figueras F, Hernandez-Andrade E, et al. Changes in myocardial performance index and aortic isthmus and ductus venosus Doppler in term, small-for-gestational age fetuses with normal umbilical artery pulsatility index. *Ultrasound Obstet Gynecol.* 2011;38:400–405.

111. Comas M, Crispi F, Cruz-Martinez R, et al. Usefulness of myocardial tissue Doppler vs conventional echocardiography in the evaluation of cardiac dysfunction in early-onset intrauterine growth restriction. *Am J Obstet Gynecol.* 2010;203:45.e1–45.e7.

112. Benavides-Serralde A, Scheier M, Cruz-Martinez R, et al. Changes in central and peripheral circulation in intrauterine growth-restricted fetuses at different stages of umbilical artery flow deterioration: new fetal cardiac and brain parameters. *Gynecol Obstet Invest.* 2011;71:274–280.

113. Bahtiyar MO, Copel JA. Cardiac changes in the intrauterine growth-restricted fetus. *Semin Perinatol.* 2008;32:190–193.

114. Comas M, Crispi F, Cruz-Martinez R, et al. Tissue Doppler echocardiographic markers of cardiac dysfunction in small-for-gestational age fetuses. *Am J Obstet Gynecol.* 2011;205:57.e1–57.e6.

115. Crispi F, Comas M, Hernandez-Andrade E, et al. Does pre-eclampsia influence fetal cardiovascular function in early-onset intrauterine growth restriction? *Ultrasound Obstet Gynecol.* 2009;34:660–665.

116. Letti Muller AL, Barrios Pde M, Kliemann LM, et al. Tei index to assess fetal cardiac performance in fetuses at risk for fetal inflammatory response syndrome. *Ultrasound Obstet Gynecol.* 2010;36:26–31.

117. Inamura N, Taketazu M, Smallhorn JF, et al. Left ventricular myocardial performance in the fetus with severe tricuspid valve disease and tricuspid insufficiency. *Am J Perinatol.* 2005;22:91–97.

118. Inamura N, Kado Y, Nakajima T, et al. Left and right ventricular function in fetal tetralogy of Fallot with absent pulmonary valve. *Am J Perinatol.* 2005;22:199–204.

119. Lasa JJ, Tian ZY, Guo R, et al. Perinatal course of Ebstein's anomaly and tricuspid valve dysplasia in the fetus. *Prenat Diagn.* 2012;32:245–251.

120. Brooks PA, Khoo NS, Mackie AS, et al. Right ventricular function in fetal hypoplastic left heart syndrome. *J Am Soc Echocardiogr.* 2012;25:1068–1074.

121. Natarajan S, Szwast A, Tian Z, et al. Right ventricular mechanics in the fetus with hypoplastic left heart syndrome. *J Am Soc Echocardiogr.* 2013;26:515–520.

122. Szwast A, Tian Z, McCann M, et al. Right ventricular performance in the fetus with hypoplastic left heart syndrome. *Ann Thorac Surg.* 2009;87:1214–1219.

123. Mori Y, Rice MJ, McDonald RW, et al. Evaluation of systolic and diastolic ventricular performance of the right ventricle in fetuses with ductal constriction using the Doppler Tei index. *Am J Cardiol.* 2001;88:1173–1178.

124. Waggoner AD, Bierig SM. Tissue Doppler imaging: a useful echocardiographic method for the cardiac sonographer to assess systolic and diastolic ventricular function. *J Am Echocardiogr.* 2001;14:1143–1152.

125. Price DJ, Wallbridge DR, Stewart MJ. Tissue Doppler imaging: current and potential clinical applications. *Heart.* 2000;84(suppl 2):II11–II18.

126. Ganame J, Claus P, Uyttebroeck A, et al. Myocardial dysfunction late after low-dose anthracycline treatment in asymptomatic pediatric patients. *J Am Soc Echocardiogr.* 2007;20:1351–1358.

127. Comas M, Crispi F, Gomez O, et al. Gestational age- and estimated fetal weight-adjusted reference ranges for myocardial tissue Doppler indices at 24–41 weeks' gestation. *Ultrasound Obstet Gynecol.* 2011;37:57–64.

128. Aoki M, Harada K, Ogawa M, et al. Quantitative assessment of right ventricular function using doppler tissue imaging in fetuses with and without heart failure. *J Am Soc Echocardiogr.* 2004;17:28–35.

129. Chan LY, Fok WY, Wong JT, et al. Reference charts of gestation-specific tissue Doppler imaging indices of systolic and diastolic functions in the normal fetal heart. *Am Heart J.* 2005;150:750–755.

130. Harada K, Tsuda A, Orino T, et al. Tissue Doppler imaging in the normal fetus. *Int J Cardiol.* 1999;71:227–234.

131. Huhta JC, Kales E, Casbohm A. Fetal tissue Doppler—a new technique for perinatal cardiology. *Curr Opin Pediatr.* 2003;15:472–474.

132. Larsen LU, Sloth E, Petersen OB, et al. Systolic myocardial velocity alterations in the growth-restricted fetus with cerebroplacental redistribution. *Ultrasound Obstet Gynecol.* 2009;34:62–67.

133. Naujorks AA, Zielinsky P, Beltrame PA, et al. Myocardial tissue Doppler assessment of diastolic function in the growth-restricted fetus. *Ultrasound Obstet Gynecol.* 2009;34:68–73.

134. Paladini D, Lamberti A, Teodoro A, et al. Tissue Doppler imaging of the fetal heart. *Ultrasound Obstet Gynecol.* 2000;16:530–535.

135. Watanabe S, Hashimoto I, Saito K, et al. Characterization of ventricular myocardial performance in the fetus by tissue Doppler imaging. *Circ J.* 2009;73:943–947.

136. Barker DJ, Osmond C, Simmonds SJ, et al. The relation of small head circumference and thinness at birth to death from cardiovascular disease in adult life. *BMJ.* 1993;306:422–426.

137. Crispi F, Bijnens B, Figueras F, et al. Fetal growth restriction results in remodeled and less efficient hearts in children. *Circulation.* 2010;121:2427–2436.

138. Doctor BA, O'Riordan MA, Kirchner HL, et al. Perinatal correlates and neonatal outcomes of small for gestational age infants born at term gestation. *Am J Obstet Gynecol.* 2001;185:652–659.

139. Eixarch E, Meler E, Iraola A, et al. Neurodevelopmental outcome in 2-year-old infants who were small-for-gestational age term fetuses with cerebral blood flow redistribution. *Ultrasound Obstet Gynecol.* 2008;32:894–899.

140. Figueras F, Oros D, Cruz-Martinez R, et al. Neurobehavior in term, small-for-gestational age infants with normal placental function. *Pediatrics.* 2009;124:e934–e941

141. Illa M, Coloma JL, Eixarch E, et al. Growth deficit in term small-for-gestational fetuses with normal umbilical artery Doppler is associated with adverse outcome. *J Perinat Med.* 2009;37:48–52.

142. Tsyvian P, Malkin K, Artemieva O, et al. Cardiac ventricular performance in the appropriate-for-gestational age and small-for-gestational age fetus: relation to regional cardiac non-uniformity and peripheral resistance. *Ultrasound Obstet Gynecol.* 2002;20:35–41.

143. Bijnens B, Claus P, Weidemann F, et al. Investigating cardiac function using motion and deformation analysis in the setting of coronary artery disease. *Circulation.* 2007;116:2453–2464.

144. Hatem MA, Zielinsky P, Hatem DM, et al. Assessment of diastolic ventricular function in fetuses of diabetic mothers using tissue doppler. *Cardiol Young.* 2008;18:297–302.

145. Bui YK, Kipps AK, Brook MM, et al. Tissue Doppler is more sensitive and reproducible than spectral pulsed-wave Doppler for fetal right ventricle myocardial performance index determination in normal and diabetic pregnancies. *J Am Soc Echocardiogr.* 2013;26:507–514.

146. Meriki N, Izurieta A, Welsh AW. Fetal left modified myocardial performance index: technical refinements in obtaining pulsed-Doppler waveforms. *Ultrasound Obstet Gynecol.* 2012;39:421–429.

147. Meriki N, Welsh AW. Development of Australian reference ranges for the left fetal modified myocardial performance index and the influence of caliper location on time interval measurement. *Fetal Diagn Ther.* 2012;32:87–95.

148. Meriki N, Izurieta A, Welsh A. Reproducibility of constituent time intervals of right and left fetal modified myocardial performance indices on pulsed Doppler echocardiography: a short report. *Ultrasound Obstet Gynecol.* 2012;39:654–658.

149. Eidem BW, Edwards JM, Cetta F. Quantitative assessment of fetal ventricular function: establishing normal values of the myocardial performance index in the fetus. *Echocardiography.* 2001;18:9–13.

150. Falkensammer CB, Paul J, Huhta JC. Fetal congestive heart failure: correlation of Tei-index and cardiovascular-score. *J Perinat Med.* 2001;29:390–398.

151. Chen Q, Sun XF, Liu HJ. Assessment of myocardial performance in fetuses by using Tei index [in Chinese]. *Zhonghua Fu Chan Ke Za Zhi.* 2006;41:387–390.

152. Figueroa-Diesel H, Silva MC, Illanes S, et al. Evaluation of the modified myocardial performance index in pregnancies complicated with gestational and pregestational diabetes. *Ultrasound Obstet Gynecol.* 2007;30:524.

153. Acharya G, Pavlovic M, Ewing L, et al. Comparison between pulsed-wave Doppler- and tissue Doppler-derived Tei indices in fetuses with and without congenital heart disease. *Ultrasound Obstet Gynecol.* 2008;31:406–411.

154. Van Mieghem T, Gucciardo L, Lewi P, et al. Validation of the fetal myocardial performance index in the second and third trimesters of gestation. *Ultrasound Obstet Gynecol.* 2009;33:58–63.

155. Api O, Emeksiz MB, Api M, et al. Modified myocardial performance index for evaluation of fetal cardiac function in pre-eclampsia. *Ultrasound Obstet Gynecol.* 2009;33:51–57.

156. Wood DC, Bisulli M, Ashraf S, et al. Fetal myocardial performance (Tei) index and left ventricular shortening fraction (LVSF). *Ultrasound Obstet Gynecol.* 2009;34:11.

157. Romiti A, Caforio L, Mappa I, et al. Fetal cardiac function assessed by myocardial performance index in normal pregnancy. *Ultrasound Obstet Gynecol.* 2010;36:214.

158. Clur SA, Oude Rengerink K, Mol BW, et al. Fetal cardiac function between 11 and 35 weeks' gestation and nuchal translucency thickness. *Ultrasound Obstet Gynecol.* 2011;37:48–56.

159. Hamela-Olkowska A, Szymkiewicz-Dangel J. Quantitative assessment of the right and the left ventricular function using pulsed Doppler myocardial performance index in normal fetuses at 18 to 40 weeks of gestation [in Polish]. *Ginekol Pol.* 2011;82:108–113.

160. Ghawi H, Gendi S, Mallula K, et al. Fetal left and right ventricle myocardial performance index: defining normal values for the second and third trimesters—single tertiary center experience. *Pediatr Cardiol.* 2013;34(8):1805–1815.

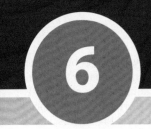

## Basic Technique

### 6.1

Dorothy I. Bulas and Ashley James Robinson

## BACKGROUND

Magnetic resonance imaging (MRI) is an alternative modality to evaluate the fetus. It uses no ionizing radiation, has excellent tissue contrast, large field of view, is not limited by obesity or overlying bone, and can image the fetus in multiple planes no matter the fetal lie. Fetal MRI was initially attempted in the 1980s but was limited because of slow sequences requiring fetal and/or maternal sedation. Since then, the development of faster sequences has been fundamental in the success of imaging the moving fetus without the use of sedation.[1-3] Faster scanning techniques now allow studies to be performed without sedation in the second and third trimesters with excellent tissue contrast, good signal-to-noise ratio (SNR), and minimal motion artifact.

### Utility

With advances in fetal management, there is an increasing need for precise depiction of abnormalities. Ultrasound (US) remains the screening modality of choice in the assessment of the fetus. When additional information is needed, MRI is a useful adjunct in the assessment of complex fetal anomalies. The use of fetal MRI can help confirm or exclude the presence of lesions noted by US. MRI can demonstrate additional subtle anomalies not visualized by US that may alter outcome. These additional findings can aid in the planning of fetal intervention, delivery, and postnatal therapeutic planning as well as in counseling parents regarding long-term prognosis.

MRI has numerous advantages that make it a complementary study in the evaluation of the fetus. MRI, in comparison with US, is not limited by fetal lie, overlying maternal or fetal bone, obesity, or oligohydramnios. MRI offers excellent soft tissue contrast and multiplanar visualization of all organs. Evidence-based data for the performance of fetal MRI is strongest for CNS anomalies and for cases being considered for fetal intervention such as neural tube defects.[4] Advanced techniques are being developed that may provide physiologic information, including fetal spectroscopy and functional MRI[5,6] (see Chapter 6.3). Much research is currently being performed on the use of MRI to estimate lung volumes, particularly in cases of congenital diaphragmatic hernia as well as lung masses and lung hypoplasia.[7,8] With the airway filled with fluid in fetal life, MRI can directly visualize the larynx, pharynx, and trachea, assessing the need for ex utero intrapartum treatment (EXIT) procedure when an oral or neck mass is present compressing the airway.[2,3] Various T1w, T2w, and echo planar sequences can distinguish blood, fat, meconium, and cartilage, increasing the accuracy of diagnosis. Large field of view with multiplanar capability enables other specialists as well as family members to

better visualize and understand the abnormalities. The ability to view images as a team is a powerful tool in counseling families and planning potential interventions.[4] Indeed, the ability to view images has pulled many specialists into fetology, including neonatologists, pediatric surgeons, neurosurgeons, neurologists, and urologists who may feel more comfortable reviewing MRI images.[9-11] This team approach is particularly useful in planning fetal surgery or complex deliveries in cases of neck masses, sacrococcygeal teratomas, and conjoined twins. In addition, fetal studies can be used for postnatal surgical planning, decreasing the need for emergent studies in the unstable newborn.

### Timing

MRI can be a useful adjunct when a targeted sonogram performed by an experienced sonographer raises questions that could benefit from further assessment. MRI may provide additional information when an abnormality is identified by US or when findings are equivocal and require clarification.[4,11] The optimal timing of a fetal MRI depends on what questions need to be answered.

As the theoretical risk of MRI is potentially greatest during organogenesis, and the size of the developing fetus is so small early gestation, fetal MRI in the first trimester is not recommended.[12-14] At times, owing to maternal indications, MRI has been performed with limited visualization of the embryo. Anomalies are better visualized by US during this gestation.

From 12 to 16 weeks, fetal MRI remains limited because of the small size of the fetus, increased fetal motion, and the fact that some anomalies may have not yet evolved (such as cortical dysplasias).

MRI between 17 and 24 weeks' gestation is useful to further evaluate or confirm findings noted on target sonograms that can impact pregnancy planning and intervention.

MRI in the third trimester is optimal for the assessment of anomalies, particularly of the cerebral cortex, owing to improved spatial resolution. Decreased motion, head engagement in the lower pelvis, and larger targets allow for advanced imaging such as spectroscopy, DTI, and fMRI. Later studies, however, risk identifying anomalies too late for optimal intervention. MRI studies performed in the second trimester may, at times, benefit from a follow-up exam in the third trimester, particularly those requiring complex delivery planning such as neck masses.

### Limitations

Technical challenges include motion artifact, limited fast sequences, optimizing SNR, and lack of technical expertise. Motion comes mainly from the fetus, but also from the mother, who can be uncomfortable and anxious, making it difficult to obtain adequate images. The moving fetus makes obtaining appropriate planes challenging for the technologist, and repeat sequences are often required to obtain a quality image. If the MRI technologist is inexperienced, the physician will need to help as anatomy can be confusing in a moving fetus, particularly when complex anomalies are distorting normal landmarks.

Fast scanning sequences are limited. T1- and T2-weighted sequences must be optimized to decrease the scanning time and motion artifact. Some sequences require the breath to be held to improve image quality (T1w). This can be difficult for a mother lying uncomfortably with diaphragms elevated by the gravid uterus. Fetal gating is currently not commercially available, limiting evaluation of the fetal heart. When fetal motion is problematic, particularly when polyhydramnios is present, dynamic steady-state free process (SSFP) can be useful.

Interpreting fetal MRIs can be challenging as structures are small and change with fetal maturation. Great care must be made when interpreting as well as performing these studies. Prognosis of abnormalities can be highly varied with limited long-term data available. This can make counseling difficult at times, even when anomalies are well delineated. Additional long-term follow-up studies are necessary to provide more accurate data for improved counseling.[4]

## SAFETY

While there is currently no evidence that fetal MRI produces harmful effects to the fetus, long-term safety has not been firmly established. There is a lack of consensus as to whether there are true risks to the fetus.[12-16] Saunders[16] noted in a review of the literature that while no adverse effects have been consistently demonstrated, the evidence is inconclusive, numbers are small, data variable with potential confounders, and few studies include data obtained at fields greater than 1 T.

Several potential safety issues have been raised. These include acoustic damage and teratogenic effects due to torque, acceleration by the static field, nerve stimulation by the gradient fields, and/or tissue heating by radio frequency (RF) fields.[12-18]

In terms of acoustic damage, MRI produces a loud tapping noise when coils are exposed to rapidly oscillating electromagnetic currents. Initially, concern was raised regarding potential acoustic damage to the developing ear. A study by Baker et al.[19] suggested that hearing was preserved but sample size was small. A study in 1995 simulated the acoustic environment of the gravid uterus by passing a microphone through the esophagus of a volunteer. This demonstrated a sufficient attenuation of sound to an acceptable level not harmful to the developing fetal ear.[20]

Some studies have raised the concern for teratogenic effects of MRI when performed early in pregnancy, secondary to the heating effect of MRI gradient changes and a direct nonthermal interaction of the electromagnetic field.[16,21,22] Static magnetic fields produce short-term high-field exposure to the patient from 0.2 to 3 T and long-term low-field exposure to MRI staff (0.5 mT to 200 mT). Animal studies have demonstrated effects such as a decrease in crown rump length when mice were exposed to MRI in mid-gestation[21]; eye malformations in genetically predisposed mice[22]; and demise of chick embryos when exposed to strong magnetic fields.[12] These studies are not applicable to humans and cannot be extrapolated, but they do raise concerns.

RF fields generate heat and are measured by specific absorption rate (SAR). Mathematical models on simulations have identified RF levels that are tolerable to humans; however, fetal dosimetry is only now being developed.[23-25] Fast sequences use high-specification magnetic field gradients. Db/dt exposure

needs to be further researched not only in adults but in the fetus as well. Murbach et al.[17] investigated whether children and fetuses were at higher risk than adults when current RF regulations were applied. In their limited series, they noted local exposure was smaller for children and fetuses than adults. Local thermal load, however, could be increased to the fetus because of high exposure average of the nonperfused amniotic fluid.[17]

Effective exposure time during a fetal MRI has not been well studied, making estimation of RF deposition and noise exposure difficult. Brugger and Prayer noted that actual imaging time accounts for only about 33% of total study time. Exposure time is not continuous with the remaining time taken up by repositioning of the coil/mother and planning sequences.[26]

Kanal et al.[27] produced a worker survey on female MRI technologists concerning low-field exposure. There were over 1,900 responses with no statistically significant associations revealed.

While several series have described no adverse long-term effects of fetal MRI in children imaged as fetus, the samples have been small, and no long-term studies are currently available regarding higher strength magnets greater than 3 T.[19,20,28-32]

It is unknown whether higher magnet strengths and prolonged imaging times may have biological effects if applied at sensitive stages of development. The United States' Food and Drug Administration (US FDA) and the International Commission on Non-Ionizing Radiation Protection (ICNIRP) recommend performing studies with caution, including a close control of SAR values.[12-14] In the United Kingdom, the Medical Device Agency (MDA) guidelines require SAR to be a maximum of 10 W per kg.[31,32]

With no conclusive documentation of deleterious effects of MRI at 1.5 T, no specific recommendations may be required for any trimester in pregnancy.[33] Pregnant patients should undergo an MRI, if the attending radiologist determines a need, and benefits outweigh any potential risks. However, with the advent of 3 T and higher Tesla magnets, radiologists should be aware of increased power deposition with high-field studies and make sure established guidelines are not exceeded.[34-37]

### Gadolinium

MRI contrast agents should not be routinely administered to the pregnant patient. While there are no specific fetal indications for the use of MRI contrast, rarely, contrast may be needed for assessing maternal pathology.

The use of intravenous gadolinium and its toxic effects to the fetus has been tested in animals, but not adequately in humans. Gadolinium crosses the placenta and is excreted in urine by the fetus and later reabsorbed/swallowed, prolonging the elimination time.[38-44] When excreted into the amniotic fluid, the gadolinium chelate molecules may remain for an indeterminate amount of time before being eliminated. The longer the chelate molecule remains in the amniotic fluid, the greater the potential of dissociation of the gadolinium ion from its chelate molecule. The impact of free gadolinium ion on the human fetus remains unclear.[45]

In a study with rabbits, a high concentration of gadolinium was noted 5 minutes after its administration, with a subsequent decrease of 50% after 60 minutes.[41,43] At high (two to seven times the dose used in humans) and repeated doses, teratogenic effects (including growth retardation, visual problems, and bone and visceral anomalies) have been described in animals.[38,41-43] No carcinogenic or mutagenic effects have been noted.[38] Other preclinical studies using contrast have not shown negative effects on the fetus, including detectable chromosomal damage, abortions, stillbirth, and grossly detectable anomalies, even at 11 to 16 times the clinical dose.[38]

In the human fetus, the concentration of gadolinium in different organs is low, except for the kidneys, which show an increase in concentration over the first 60 minutes.[38,44] A few human clinical studies using contrast have been performed with no adverse effects to the fetus or neonate reported, even when given during the first trimester.[38] When clinical doses have been administered, side effects have not been observed.[46,47] However, as contrast may remain within the amniotic fluid for long periods of time, unless absolutely needed, its use is not recommended during pregnancy, particularly during the early period of organogenesis. Use of gadolinium late in gestation may be appropriate for specific maternal or obstetric indications. The decision to administer MRI contrast to the pregnant patient should be well documented with thoughtful risk to benefit analysis. Benefits should outweigh theoretical risks of fetal exposure to free gadolinium ions.[38,45]

## TECHNIQUE

### Patient Positioning (Table 6.1-1)

The patient should go through appropriate metal screening. Heavy clothing should be removed and light gowns offered to increase comfort during the study. The bladder should be emptied just prior to getting on the scanner.

The patient can lie either supine with a pillow under her knees, or in a decubitus position. The left lateral position has been thought to reduce the risk of vena cava compression syndrome. However, a study by Kienzl et al. has suggested that vena cava compression syndrome is actually rare during MRI scanning in the supine position. Despite narrowing of the IVC, there appear to be physiologic compensatory mechanisms.[48] Nonetheless, the lateral decubitus position can have additional

---

| Table 6.1-1 | Fetal MR Technique Tips |
| --- | --- |

- USE the largest bore magnet available.
- POSITION the patient so she is comfortable, feet first.
- USE distracting techniques. Have a family member accompany the patient in the scanner.
- PLACE a surface coil when possible. Multichannel better, more elements better. Two surface coils work well in series, especially with larger patients.
- LOCALIZE to the uterus with a large field of view. Check cervical length and placental location.
- REDUCE field of view.
- 3-Point PLAN a standard plane in the fetus.
- HAVE a protocol planned, but remain flexible with order of sequences. Acquire the sequences most likely to answer the question first. Consider leaving the loudest sequences and breath-hold sequences until last. If there is significant fetal motion, consider repeating a key sequence until the fetus rests, or use dynamic SSPE.
- OBTAIN images of the entire fetus.
- REVIEW images with the technologist before ending the exam.

---

advantages. It can help in patients with back pain or sciatica, or in the third trimester when the mother may have shortness of breath lying supine because of elevation of the diaphragm.

Because of claustrophobia, patients prefer to go into the bore of the magnet feet first. This allows the uterus to be in the center of the bore with their head at the level of the flanged opening so they can see out into the room. Having a family member accompany the mother into the scanning room can be helpful. If the mother is anxious, holding her hand may be calming. An alarm ball or other method of direct communication to the technologist should be offered to the mother. Listening to music or watching a movie is a useful distraction technique. If a patient is extremely claustrophobic or anxious, oral sedation and/or oxygen supplementation may be required.

### Coils

Depending on the size of the mother and fetal gestation, either a torso or cardiac-phased array surface coil is placed over the gravid uterus. One or two flexible phased array surface coils can be wrapped over the patient sandwiching the uterus between the table-top coils and surface coils.[49] Elements closest to the uterus can then be selected, which can increase the SNR ratio. If the patient is too large to fit into the magnet with a surface coil, the coil intrinsic to the magnet may be used. Large bore magnets are particularly advantageous when the BMI is high or there are multiple gestations.

### Imaging Protocol (Table 6.1-2)

The development of single-shot rapid acquisition with relaxation enhancement sequences has been key to decreasing fetal and maternal movement artifact. A series of images can be performed in as little as 15 to 20 seconds. Slices are acquired one at a time, each slice produced in less than 400 milliseconds by a single excitation pulse. Examination times overall average 20 to 40 minutes, depending on how many sequences have to be repeated owing to fetal movement and protocol.

An initial three-plane localizer sequence should be performed. This will demonstrate the cranial and caudal extent of the uterus, and can be followed with T2-weighted Half Fourier Single-Shot Echo (SSFSE/Haste/ssTSE/Fast FE) (Table 6.1-2), large FOV,[36–48] thick (5 to 10 mm) sections through the entire uterus, coronal to the mother. This can be followed by T2w SSFSE or SSFP sagittal and/or axial planes of the maternal pelvis. These sequences will allow assessment of fetal lie, placental position and signal, cervix, and fetal situs. These sequences also help determine whether the surface coils need to be repositioned to get the best signal from the fetal anatomy in question.

At this point, there are several ways to get into a fetal orthogonal plane. Advanced technology allows user selection of three points within the images that will appear on the same plane in the next sequence. For example, two points can be selected in the lumbar spinal canal, and one at the umbilicus, which would result in a perfect sagittal stack. If this technology is not available, it is possible to pick two points that are symmetric on either side of the body, for example, the orbits and place the center "eye" of the stack on the one point, then page through the images until the second point is visible and rotate the stack so that the center line passes through the second point. This will result in images between axial and coronal, from which a perfect sagittal can then be obtained.[50]

| Table 6.1-2 | Vendor Sequences Used in Fetal MRI |
|---|---|

| Sequence Type | GE (Milwaukee, WI) | Siemens (Erlangen, Germany) | Philips (Eindhoven, The Netherlands) | Hitachi (Twinsburg, OH) | Toshiba (Otawara, Japan) |
|---|---|---|---|---|---|
| Half Fourier single-shot echo (T2w) | SSFSE | HASTE | SSTSE | SSFSE | FASE |
| Steady-state free precess (SSFP) (T2w) | FIESTA | TruFISP | Balanced FFE | Balanced SARGE | True SSFP |
| Spoiled gradient echo (T1w) | SPGR | FLASH | T1-FFE | RF spoiled SARGE, RSSG | FastFE |
| 3D ultrafast (T1w) | 3D FGRE, 3D Fast SPGR | MPRAGE | 3D TFE | MPRAGE | 3D Fast FE |
| Ultrafast gradient echo | Fast GRE, Fast SPGR | Turbo FLASH | | RGE | FastFE |
| Rapid acquisition relaxation enhancement | FSE | TSE | TSE | FSE | FSE |
| Diffusion-weighted imaging | DWI | DWI | DWI | DWI | DWI |
| Diffusion tensor imaging | Diffusion tensor imaging | DTI | Diffusion tensor imaging | | DTI |
| Echo-planar imaging | EPI | EPI | EPI | EPI | EPI |
| Susceptibility-weighted imaging | SWAN | SWI | | | |
| Parallel imaging | ASSET | iPAT, mSENSE | SENSE | RAPID | SPEEDER |

Because the fetus continues to move throughout the study, each sequence is typically planned using a plane perpendicular to the prior sequence. Images of the head then body or vice versa should be protocoled depending on which anomaly needs to be evaluated first. In the sagittal and coronal planes, the entire head, chest, and abdomen can often be included particularly in earlier gestation. Dedicated axial sequences of the fetal brain and abdomen, however, are typically needed for optimal image interpretation. At times, the fetus will move but then quickly return to its initial position. Therefore, it can be helpful to simply repeat the sequence without changing parameters. If the fetus truly has moved into another position, the above techniques can be used to rapidly get another appropriate orthogonal plane.

Quiet maternal breathing is typically adequate; however, breath-hold techniques are needed for certain series, particularly T1w gradient-echo (GRE) sequences. Breath-holding can be useful if the fetus is breech, when the maternal diaphragmatic motion is more readily transmitted to the fetus. Breath-holding is successful only if the length of the sequence is relatively short, less than 20 seconds. Allowing the mother to gently release the breath-hold toward the end of the series can help if the sequence is longer than this.

Phase oversampling is often used in fetal MRI. It has the advantages of reducing the field of view to include just the fetus and exclude maternal anatomy by eliminating phase-wrap, and it also increases the SNR, which can be particularly important early in gestation when the fetus is small. The disadvantage is that it increases the scan time according to the number of phase-encoding steps. If this is problematic, the phase oversampling ratio can be reduced or turned off completely. This will result in phase-wrap, but with careful positioning and sizing of the field of view, often the maternal structures will only phase-wrap into the maternal structures on the opposite side of the body, and not overlie onto the fetal anatomy.

When scanning the fetus, a smaller 24- to 30-cm FOV should be used. Slices as thin as 2 to 3 mm can be obtained; however, the smaller the slice thickness, the lower the SNR. In larger fetuses, slice thicknesses of 4 to 6 mm work well, decreasing time per series and improving signal.

A typical matrix size is 256 px. Counterintuitively, increasing the matrix size in the attempt to increase in-plane resolution will typically have the opposite effect because of loss of signal from smaller voxels. This can be partly countered by increasing the slice thickness but results in more volume-averaging.

**T2-weighted half Fourier single-shot echo sequences** (SSFSE/HASTE/ssTSE/SsFSE/FASE) (Table 6.1-2) provide the highest SNR and resolution, and are fast.[50] Slices as thin as 2 to 3 mm with no skip can be obtained. These T2-weighted images are most useful for anatomic detail, particularly of the fetal surface structures at the interface with amniotic fluid and the various body cavities that are fluid-filled such as the brain, ventricles, eyes, nasal cavities, oral cavity, airway, GI tract, and GU tract. Typically, axial, sagittal, and coronal images angled to the brain and then body should be obtained.

**Heavy T2-weighted hydrography** takes longer to acquire, but produces excellent SNR contrast. Slice thickness choices are dependent on gestational age; 3 mm works well at <24 weeks, and 4 mm at >24 weeks decreases the length of this longer sequence.[51-53]

**Steady-state free precess** (SSFP/FIESTA/TruFISP/Balanced FFE/Balanced SARGE/True SSFP) images demonstrate bright blood imaging. The cardiac chambers and great vessels may be discreetly identified. Images can be obtained in all three planes at 3- to 4-mm increments. This sequence is also quite useful for the assessment of fluid-filled structures such as dilated renal collecting systems or cystic masses. Because of its high contrast, inner ear anatomy, clefts of the palate, and fluid surrounding the spinal cord are particularly well demonstrated. Extremities are outlined by the amniotic fluid with fingers and toes often visualized. There is less contrast between gray and white matter in the brain and meconium in the abdomen due to lower flip angles and banding artifacts.

**Thick slab T2w** are useful for assessing fetal surface contours. Thick slab acquisitions of 40 to 60 mm give an overall three-dimensional (3D) effect. Transparency is increased using shorter echo times or by using SSFP sequences that can similarly be acquired with thick slices. To maximize SNR, overlapping slices of 5- to 6-mm thickness can be used; however, this approach typically makes this sequence less useful for volumetry. These images can be useful for parents and health care workers not used to evaluation of two-dimensional (2D) anatomy.[54]

**T1-weighted sequences** are fast multiplanar spoiled gradient recall acquisitions in the steady state (SPGR/FLASH/T1-FFE/Fast FE) sequences (Table 6.1-2) require breath-hold with thicker slices (5-7 skip 0) for sufficient SNR. It can be useful to perform a T1 sequence immediately after a T2 sequence with the same slice parameters so they can be directly compared. T1-weighted images are particularly useful for detecting hemorrhage, calcification, meconium, thyroid tissue, and fat.

**Dynamic SSFP sequences** (Cine, real time) can be used to assess fetal movements. Multiple frames per second can be obtained at each slice with slice thicknesses ranging from 7 to 50 mm. Assessment of fetal breathing, swallowing, cardiac motion, and gastrointestinal activity is possible. When there is a burst of fetal activity that precludes use of other imaging sequences, it can be a useful backup sequence. When the fetus settles down, other sequences can then be acquired.

**Echoplanar imaging** (EPI) is useful in assessment of the musculoskeletal system with high-signal cartilage and low-signal bone. The fetal liver has significant hypointense signal, while other organs are intermediate in signal. Flow voids make vessels and heart hypointense. Susceptibility-weighted imaging can be used to detect hemorrhage and calcification.

**Long-Tau inversion recovery sequences** can be useful to further characterize fluid that appears high-intensity on T2-weighted imaging, but that may contain proteinaceous fluid such as hemorrhage.

**Diffusion-weighted sequences** (DWI) can be acquired with three phase-encoding directions. The area of interest should be as centered as possible. DWI can demonstrate ischemic lesions in white matter. It can be used in the identification of renal tissue, particularly if kidneys are not visible sonographically or by routine MRI.

Advanced imaging with **spectroscopy and diffusion tensor imaging** is becoming available and is discussed in Chapter 6.3.

Whatever the indication for the fetal MRI, the entire fetus from head to toe should be examined. Fetal pathologies and malformations frequently involve multiple organs. Thus, identification of other anomalies can further elucidate an underlying genetic or chromosomal syndrome.

Because of the risk of maternal fatigue, anxiety, or discomfort, it is important to complete the study as quickly and efficiently as possible. Protocols should be well thought out prior to placing the mother on the scanner. If a brain anomaly is present, planes angled to the brain should first be obtained, then sequences angled to the chest and abdomen. Most protocols benefit from a combination of T2-weighted sequences (SSFSE and /or SSFP) in all three planes and T1-weighted imaging in at least one plane.

### Postprocessing

Volumetry of fetal organs by MRI has become a useful tool, particularly in the determination of fetal lung volumes (see Chapter 17). A region of interest can be manually segmented and its total area multiplied by the slice thickness to calculate volumes. Continuous motion-free images are needed for accurate volumetry. Sequences may need to be repeated to ensure continuity of images if volumes are to be obtained. Spatial resolution of reformatted images can be limited owing to large slice thickness. Advanced methods to develop 3D volume images are being developed so that even when motion occurs, accurate data can be generated (see Chapter 6.3).[6]

Three-dimensional virtual model reconstruction using techniques such as stereolithography or fused deposition modeling can create life-size physical models using T2w MRI data.[55,56]

## 3 Tesla MRI

As the push for improved resolution and increased signal continues, and more 3 T scanners become available for use, centers have begun to address the use of 3 T scanners for fetal imaging. The use of 3 T magnets, however, represents another technical challenge with its increased susceptibility to motion artifact and the need to closely follow SAR limits.[35,37]

The US FDA approved the use of 3 T for human use in 2002. Advantages include improved SNR at higher strengths as more protons are available to increase magnetization. The gain of SNR may be up to 1.7 to 1.8 times that of 1.5 T.[37,57] Image quality, temporal and/or special resolution can thus be improved. With greater SNR, parallel imaging can be implemented to speed SSFSE protocols, reduce echo time, and potentially decrease RF heating by decreasing the number of pulses required.[37]

With 3 T, unfortunately, more artifacts are encountered. RF field inhomogeneity is a major challenge, with the larger the field of view, the worse the artifact. RF shielding artifact "conductivity effect" from amniotic fluid results in blackout areas often where the fetus is lying. Dielectic pads, RF cushions, or saline pads can help decrease these dielectric resonance artifacts.[37,58] Multichannel transmission coils, RF shimming with parallel imaging may also help decrease RF field inhomogeneity.

Magnetic susceptibility artifacts and chemical shift artifacts are also accentuated with 3 T requiring additional modifications. Changing the field of view, scan orientation, frequency, or bandwidth may move the artifact away from the fetal area of interest.

The US FDA limits of exposure to changing magnetic fields are independent of magnetic field strength. FDA safety limits prevent exposure to changing magnetic fields (dB/dt) of more than 60 T per second with failsafe software limiting scanners from exposures above these limits. With the fetus near the center of the FOV exposure, dB/dt changes are usually low with slew rates similar at both 1.5 and 3 T.[37]

RF pulses deposit energy into the imaged subject. The energy deposition is measured by the SAR reported in Watts per kilogram. The amplitude of applied RF fields increases with increasing magnetic field strength and quadruples from 1.5 to 3 T. Decreasing number of slices, lowering flip angles, increasing repetition time, and shorter echo train length can decrease SAR. The FDA safety limits are set at 4 W per kg independent of magnetic field strength with failsafe controls prohibiting additional exposure. Studies by Victoria et al.[37] have demonstrated SAR well below whole body exposure limits for both 1.5 and 3 T.

Focal SAR hotspots are of concern because of RF field inhomogeneity, dielectric, and standing wave effects. Modeling of fetal environment by Hand et al.[25,59] suggests that maximum energy deposited to the fetus is a fraction of that received by the mother. The fetus may be exposed to a peak of 50% to 70% of maternal SAR at 3 T. In their study, average temperature of the fetus remained below 38°C. However, they noted that continuous exposures over 7.5 minutes can exceed the 38°C limit, so long continuous exposures should be avoided.[59]

While 3 T has inherent artifact issues and potential increased safety risks, limiting SAR levels to those associated with 1.5 T and developing methods to decrease inhomogeneity appear to be feasible and will likely continue to progress.

## Indications (Table 6.1-3)

Fetal MRI is a valuable complement to prenatal US. Because of higher contrast resolution, large field of view, and ability to image both sides of the fetus at once, fetal MRI can be more precise than US for anatomic evaluation. There are multiple indications for performing a fetal MRI, some of which are listed in Table 6.1-3. As MRI technology advances, additional indications will continue to develop, many described in the chapters in this book.

| Table 6.1-3 | Fetal MRI Indications |
|---|---|
| Brain | Congenital anomalies such as ventriculomegaly, agenesis of the corpus callosum, holoprosencephaly, posterior fossa anomalies, cortical dysplasias, tuberous sclerosis, lissencephaly, microcephaly, family history |
| | Vascular abnormalities such as malformations, infarctions, hydranencephaly, twin-to-twin complications |
| | Craniosynostosis |
| | Tumors |
| | Infection |
| Spine | Neural tube defects/vertebral anomalies |
| | Sacrococcygeal teratoma |
| | Caudal regression/sirenomelia |
| Face and neck | Facial and palate clefts, micrognathia, dacrocystocele, anophthalmia |
| | Masses—lymphatic malformations, hemangioma, teratoma, goiter |
| | Airway obstruction |
| Thorax | Masses—congenital pulmonary airway malformations, congenital diaphragmatic hernia, effusions |
| | Lung hypoplasia—oligohydramnios, skeletal dysplasia |
| | Cardiac—heterotaxy |
| Abdomen | Masses/cysts |
| | Complex ventral wall defects |
| | Genitourinary anomalies/cloaca |
| | Bowel anomalies |
| Musculoskeletal | Limb anomalies |
| | Muscle abnormalities |
| | Soft tissue masses—lymphangiomas, hemangiomas |
| | Skeletal dysplasia |
| Twins | Monochorionic, twin-to-twin complications |
| | Conjoined |
| Fetal intervention/surgery Delivery planning Postnatal surgical planning | EXIT procedures for airway obstruction Congenital diaphragmatic hernia repair Myelomeningocele repair Complex lesions requiring immediate neonatal surgery |
| Maternal | Placenta implantation abnormalities Poor evaluation due to obesity/oligohydramnios |

### Maternal

Initial large FOV images are an opportunity to identify maternal abnormalities such as fibroids and ovarian pathology (Figs. 6.1-1 and 6.1-2). At times, maternal renal or skeletal anomalies are identified that should be described if noted. Pelvic inlet measures can be obtained as needed, but require large field of view pelvic images in all three planes for complete assessment of sagittal inlet and outlet, transverse inlet diameter, and interspinous distance.[60-63]

### Placenta/Umbilical Cord

Placental location and thickness are well delineated by MRI (Fig. 6.1-3). When a placental anomaly is present, all three planes of the uterus should be obtained for adequate assessment.[64,65] The placenta appears as an intermediate signal soft tissue structure along the margin of the uterus. The myometrial decidual interface is visible as a low-signal intensity line deep to the placenta.

MRI has been used to evaluate placenta accreta with an overall sensitivity of 80% to 88% and a specificity of 65% to 100%.[66-68]

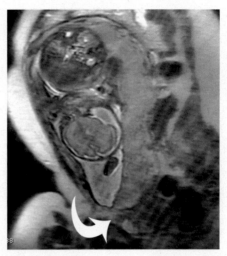

**FIGURE 6.1-3:** Placenta previa. Sagittal SSFSE image of a gravid uterus demonstrates the placenta completely covering the cervix *(curved arrow).*

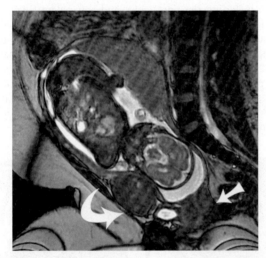

**FIGURE 6.1-1:** Fibroid. Sagittal SSFSE image of a gravid uterus demonstrates an anterior fibroid compressing the fetal head *(curved arrow). Straight arrow* points to the closed cervix.

MRI features include uterine bulging, heterogeneous placental signal, and dark intraplacental bands.[67,68] Some studies have used intravenous gadolinium contrast to assess for accreta, though the use remains controversial due to safety concerns. If contrast is being considered, the study should be timed as close to delivery as possible.[64]

Cervical length can be measured in the sagittal plane with location of placenta in relation to the cervix best noted on this view.

While MRI volumetry of amniotic fluid can be calculated, simple estimation of amniotic fluid is usually adequate.[69] Uterine synechia and amniotic sheets may be well visualized in all three planes[70] (Figs. 6.1-4 and 6.1-5).

The number of umbilical vessels is best determined in a transverse plane either by SSFSP or SSFP. The two umbilical arteries can be followed as they course along the fetal bladder. Placental cord insertion as well as fetal cord insertion should be identified with note made of length and configuration of the umbilical cord (Fig. 6.1-6).

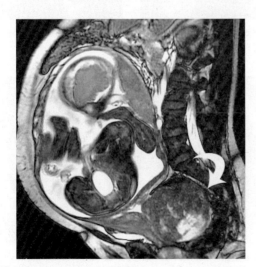

**FIGURE 6.1-2:** Fibroid. Sagittal SSFP image of a gravid uterus demonstrates a large cervical fibroid *(curved arrow)* deep in the pelvis.

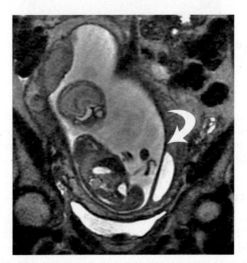

**FIGURE 6.1-4:** Uterine synechia. Coronal SSFSE image of a gravid uterus at 21 weeks' gestation demonstrates a thick band *(curved arrow)* along the lateral inferior uterus. No fetal entrapment was noted.

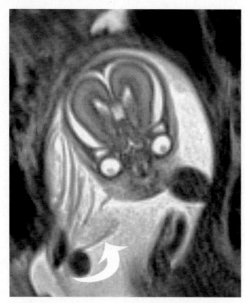

**FIGURE 6.1-5:** Amniotic bands. Numerous thin sheets *(curved arrow)* are adjacent to the fetal face. There were limb deformities, but no facial cleft was noted.

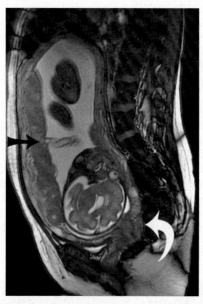

**FIGURE 6.1-6:** Placental cord insertion. Sagittal SSFP image of a gravid uterus demonstrates an anterior placenta with central cord insertion *(black arrow)*. Note the closed cervix *(curved white arrow)*.

*Situs*

Fetal orientation should be evaluated on the basis of fetal and maternal anatomy using the initial large FOV sequences. Identifying the location of the fetal heart and stomach may not automatically identify the left side of the fetus in cases of heterotaxy.

## Brain (see Chapters 6.2 and 6.3)

Coronal, axial, and sagittal orthogonal planes should be acquired with T2-weighted sequences. T1-weighted and diffusion-weighted sequences may provide additional information. Long-Tau inversion recovery, spectroscopy, volumetric data, and DTI are advanced techniques that may be useful in cranial assessment and are described further in Chapter 6.3.

| Table 6.1-4 | Fetal Face |
|---|---|

| Anatomy | Sequences |
|---|---|
| Craniofacial ratio, profile | Sagittal T2w SSFSE, SSFP |
| Nose | Sagittal, coronal T2w SSFSE, SSFP |
| Lips, palate, teeth | Coronal, axial T2w SSFSE, SSFP |
| Pharynx | Sagittal T2w SSFSE, SSFP |
| Swallow, breathing | Sagittal dynamic SSFP |

SSFSE, single-shot fast spin-echo sequences; SSFP, steady-state free precession sequences.
Reproduced with permission from Prayer D, Brugger P. Investigation of normal organ development with fetal MRI. *Eur Radiol.* 2007;17:2458–2471.

### Face (Table 6.1-4)

The sagittal midline plane is important for assessing the facial profile, including the nose, chin, and soft palate (Fig. 6.1-7). Fluid motion may be seen because of fetal exhalation. Coronal planes of the face are useful in assessing symmetry of the face, lips (for clefts), orbits, and nose (Fig. 6.1-8). External ears should be evaluated for their presence, location, and shape. Axial plane of the maxilla demonstrates tooth buds as a continuous arc (Fig. 6.1-9). The primary palate is triangular and includes the alveolar ridge. The secondary palate includes the remaining hard and soft palates.

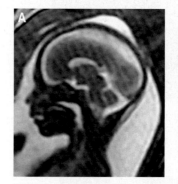
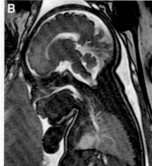

**FIGURE 6.1-7:** Fetal profile. Sagittal SSFP midline image demonstrates fetal lips, chin, soft palate, and pharynx: 21 weeks GA **(A)**, 32 weeks GA **(B)**.

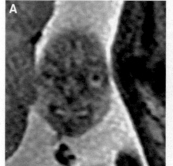
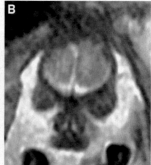

**FIGURE 6.1-8:** Fetal face coronal SSFSE. **A:** 21-Week gestation demonstrates orbits, nose, and mouth. **B:** Slightly more superficial coronal section at 29 weeks' gestation demonstrates intact lip and nares.

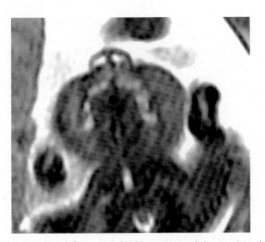

**FIGURE 6.1-9:** Fetal face axial SSFSE at 29 weeks' gestation demonstrates the maxilla with tooth buds in a continuous arc.

## Neck (Table 6.1-5)

Axial and sagittal T2w best detect the fluid-filled larynx and trachea. Epiglottis and laryngeal folds are typically noted only in the late second and third trimester (Fig. 6.1-10). The cervical

| Table 6.1-5 | Fetal Neck |
|---|---|

| Anatomy | Sequences |
|---|---|
| Larynx, trachea | Sagittal, coronal, axial T2w SSFSE, SSFP |
| Thyroid | Axial, coronal T1w GRE |
| Vessels | Axial, coronal, sagittal SSFP, GRE |

SSFSE, single-shot fast spin-echo sequences; SSFP, steady-state free precession sequences; GRE, gradient echo sequences.
Reproduced with permission from Prayer D, Brugger P. Investigation of normal organ development with fetal MRI. *Eur Radiol.* 2007;17:2458–2471.

esophagus is usually not seen unless caught during a swallow. The thyroid gland is poorly seen on T2w, but is high signal on T1w imaging from 18 weeks GA onward (Fig. 6.1-11). Cervical vessels can be identified on all three planes using SSPE sequences (Fig. 6.1-12).

## Thorax (Table 6.1-6)

Fetal lungs increase in volume throughout gestation and can be measured with MRI volumetry. Normal lung volumes have been documented by MRI as demonstrating growth proportionate to fetal body size.

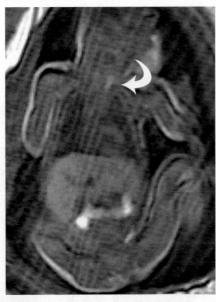

**FIGURE 6.1-11:** Coronal T1w at 29 weeks' gestation demonstrates high-signal thyroid glands *(curved arrow)*, high-signal meconium in the transverse colon, and intermediate signal liver.

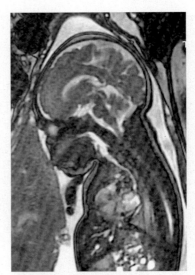

**FIGURE 6.1-10:** Sagittal SSFP at 32 weeks' gestation demonstrates the larynx, epiglottis, and trachea.

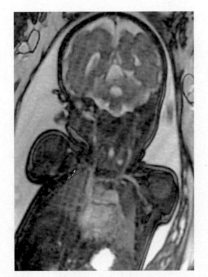

**FIGURE 6.1-12:** Coronal SSFP at 32 weeks' gestation demonstrates bilateral subclavian and jugular veins as well as superior vena cava.

| Table 6.1-6 | **Fetal Thorax** |
|---|---|

| Anatomy | Sequences |
|---|---|
| Lung parenchyma | Coronal, axial, sagittal SSFSE; volumetry |
| Diaphragmatic hernia | Coronal, axial, sagittal SSFSE; volumetry; coronal, sagittal T1w GRE |
| Heart | Axial, long and short axis SSFP, dynamic SSFP |
| Thymus | Axial, coronal T2w SSFSE |
| Diaphragm | Coronal, sagittal SSFSE, dynamic SSFP |
| Esophagus | Thick-slab sagittal SSFSE, SSFP; Axial SSFSE, SSFP; dynamic SSFP |

SSFSE, single-shot fast spin-echo sequences; SSFP, steady-state free-precession sequences; GRE, gradient echo sequences.

Reproduced with permission from Prayer D, Brugger P. Investigation of normal organ development with fetal MRI. *Eur. Radiol.* 2007;17:2458–2471.

The trachea, carina, and bronchi are often seen filled with fluid on T2w. Repeating sequences with thinner slices may be required for adequate evaluation as needed (Fig. 6.1-13).

Lung parenchyma is homogeneously brighter than muscle on T2w and increases in signal after 24 weeks' gestation, while T1w signal decreases with gestational age (Fig. 6.1-14). Apparent diffusion coefficient has been used in addition to T2w signal to assess lung maturation.[71]

The diaphragms are dome-shaped bands between the lungs and the abdomen. They have low signal on T2w, slightly lower than adjacent liver. Breathing may be noted on dynamic SSFP sequences. The esophagus is rarely seen unless caught during a swallow (Fig. 6.1-15). If an atresia is present, fluid may be identified proximal to the obstruction, but is not a constant finding. Thick dynamic SSFP sequences in the sagittal midline plane may best demonstrate transient dilatation of a proximal esophageal pouch.

The thymus is homogeneous, intermediate signal in the anterior mediastinum. It is best seen in the third trimester and should not have any mass effect on adjacent vessels or the trachea (Fig. 6.1-16).

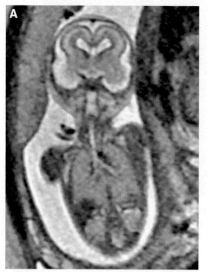
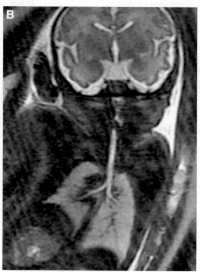
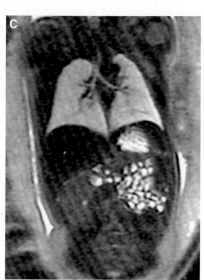

**FIGURE 6.1-13:** Trachea and bronchi. Coronal SSFSE images: 21 weeks **(A)**, 31 weeks **(B)**, 37 weeks **(C)**.

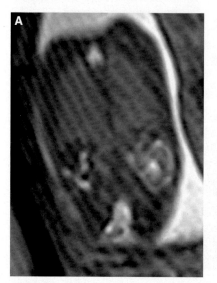
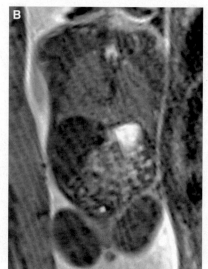
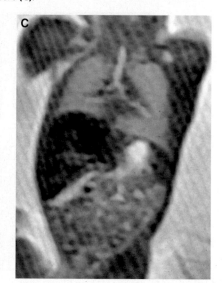

**FIGURE 6.1-14:** Lungs. Coronal SSFSE at various gestational ages demonstrating progressive increase in T2w signal: 17 weeks **(A)**, 21 weeks **(B)**, 23 weeks **(C)**, 27 weeks **(D)**, 30 weeks **(E)**, 34 weeks **(F)**, 37 weeks **(G)**.

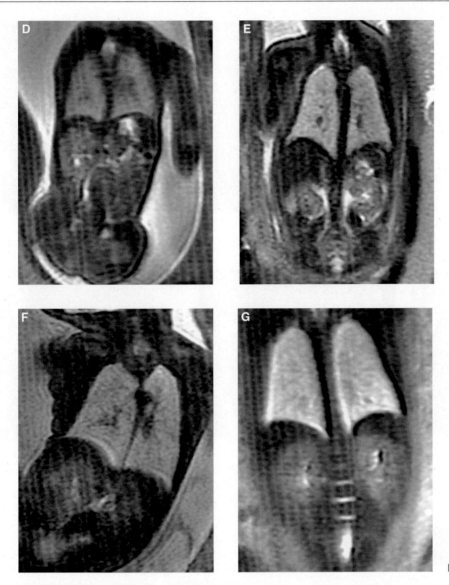

**FIGURE 6.1-14:** (*continued*)

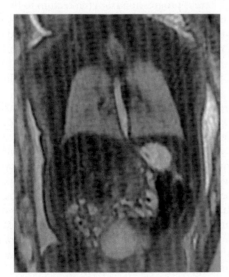

**FIGURE 6.1-15:** Fluid-filled esophagus. Coronal SSFSE image at 33 weeks' gestation.

The heart is low signal on T2w SSFSE due to flowing blood. This sequence is limited to identification of the position and size of the heart. SSFP sequences are more useful in delineating the myocardium, septum, and valves (Fig. 6.1-17). Dynamic SSFP sequences can demonstrate cardiac motion. These sequences may be particularly useful in cases of oligohydramnios and maternal obesity when fetal echocardiography may be limited. While ultrasound remains the primary method of assessing fetal heart dynamics, Chapter 6.4 describes advances in cardiac MRI that may provide additional information.

## Abdomen (Tables 6.1-7 and 6.1-8)

The fetal abdomen is well visualized by MRI with progressive changes as gestation advances. The dominant fluid-filled abdominal structures throughout the second and third trimesters include the stomach, gallbladder, and bladder (Fig. 6.1-18). The stomach is a fluid-filled structure in the left upper quadrant, high signal on T2w, and low signal on T1w. While the stomach may be transiently small, it should always be seen during a 30-minute scan.

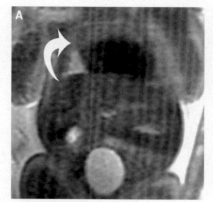
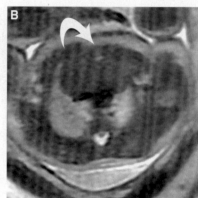

**FIGURE 6.1-16:** Thymus. Coronal **(A)** and axial **(B)** SSFSE images at 32 weeks' gestation demonstrates an intermediate signal soft tissue mass *(curved arrow)* in the anterior mediastinum consistent with thymus.

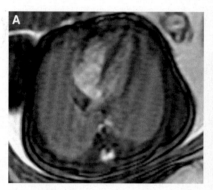
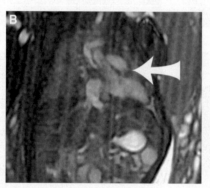
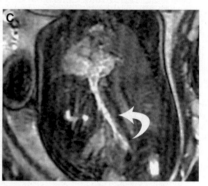

**FIGURE 6.1-17:** Fetal heart. **A:** SSFPaxial image of the four chambers. **B:** Oblique SSFP demonstrates the left ventricular outflow track *(straight arrow)*. **C:** Oblique coronal SSFP demonstrates the inferior vena cava *(curved arrow)* draining into the right atrium.

| Table 6.1-7 | Fetal Abdomen |
|---|---|
| **Anatomy** | **Sequences** |
| Liver, spleen | Coronal, axial, sagittal T2w SSFSE; coronal T1w GRE, EPI |
| Gallbladder | Axial, sagittal T2w SSFSE, SSFP |
| Bowel/meconium | Axial, coronal, sagittal T2w SSFSE; coronal, sagittal T1w GRE |
| Kidneys, adrenals | Coronal, sagittal, axial T2w SSFSE; coronal thick-slab SSFP; axial DWI |
| Bladder | Axial, sagittal, coronal T2w SSFSPR, SSFP |
| Vessels—aorta, IVC, umbilical, azygous | Coronal, sagittal, axial SSFP |
| Internal genitalia | Not well visualized; axial, sagittal T2w SSFSE |
| External genitalia | Sagittal, axial T2w SSFSE, SSFP |

SSFSE, single-shot fast spin-echo sequences; SSFP, steady-state free-precession sequences; GRE, gradient echo sequences; DWI, diffusion-weighted imaging; EPI, echoplanar.
Reproduced with permission from Prayer D, Brugger P. Investigation of normal organ development with fetal MRI. *Eur Radiol.* 2007;17:2458–2471.

Before 25 weeks' gestation, small bowel is typically collapsed containing minimal fluid. In the third trimester, small bowel becomes fluid-filled, high signal on T2w and low signal on T1w (Fig. 6.1-19). Meconium, which is typically low signal on T2w and high signal on T1w likely because of protein and/or paramagnetic minerals, initially fills the rectum at 19 to 20 weeks' gestation. There is progression from the rectum to the descending colon by 22 to 23 weeks.[72] Meconium will variably extend to the transverse and ascending colon during the third trimester with continuous colonic filling closer to term (Fig. 6.1-20) (see Chapter 18.1). MRI can provide information regarding level of bowel obstruction if present and assess size of colon in later gestation.

The liver is homogeneous low to intermediate signal on T2w, slightly high signal on T1w (Fig. 6.1-21) (Table 6.1-8). Iron causes low signal on T2w. Thus, early in gestation when there is a large amount of iron bound to fetal hemoglobin in the liver, parenchyma is relatively low in signal best assessed by echoplanar sequences. By the third trimester, there is less iron, a change that can help assess fetal physiology.[72,73] Splenic signal changes may also be noted on echoplanar sequences, possibly due to red pulp volume in the third trimester.[72] The spleen is noted posterior to the stomach, best seen on sagittal and axial images. The two hepatic lobes are equal in size with the ductus venosus and portal vein noted best on SSFP sequences.

MRI appearance of the fetal gallbladder is variable. Signal intensity changes over time, likely due to accumulation

| Table 6.1-8 | T1 and T2 Appearance of Organs | |
|---|---|---|
| | *T2w* | *T1w* |
| Orbits (vitreous) | High signal | Low signal |
| Nasopharynx, oropharynx, trachea | High-signal lumen, low-signal wall | Low signal |
| Thyroid gland | Intermediate signal | High signal |
| Thymus | Intermediate signal | Intermediate signal |
| Lungs | Intermediate signal, increasing with GA | Low signal, decreasing with GA |
| Aorta, heart, vessels | Low signal (flow void) | |
| Stomach | High signal | Low signal |
| Fluid-filled bowel | High signal | Low signal |
| Meconium | Low signal | High signal |
| Liver, spleen, gallbladder | Low or high signal second trimester, intermediate or high signal third trimester | Slightly high signal or low signal |
| Kidneys | Cortex = intermediate signal | |
| | Medulla = slightly high signal | |
| Bladder | High signal | Low signal |
| Bone, cartilage | Low signal/high signal—EPI | Low signal |

of paramagnetic substances/sludge in bile. Brugger et al.[74] described T2w high signal exclusively in fetuses younger than 27 weeks' gestation. Lower signal gallbladders were noted only after 30 weeks' gestation and may cause nonvisualization of

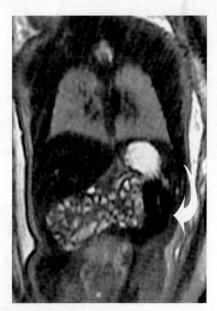

**FIGURE 6.1-19:** T2w bowel. Coronal SSFSE at 32 weeks' gestation demonstrates fluid-filled high-signal small bowel and low-signal meconium-filled descending colon *(curved arrow).*

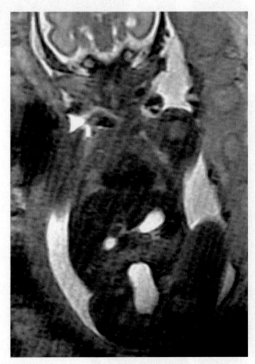

**FIGURE 6.1-18:** Fluid-filled stomach, gallbladder, and bladder. Coronal SSFSE image at 30 weeks' gestation.

an otherwise normal gallbladder. When the gallbladder is not visualized in the second trimester, diagnosis of biliary atresia, particularly in cases of heterotaxy, should be considered. Cystic fibrosis should also be included in the differential.

The cord insertion is best visualized by axial or sagittal SSFSE or SSFP sequences (Fig. 6.1-22). In the third trimester, the cord insertion may be difficult to identify owing to overlying limbs.

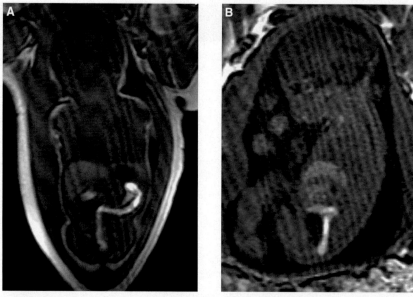

**FIGURE 6.1-20:** T1w bowel. Coronal **(A)** and sagittal **(B)** images at 30 weeks' gestation demonstrate high-signal meconium in the rectum, sigmoid, and descending colon.

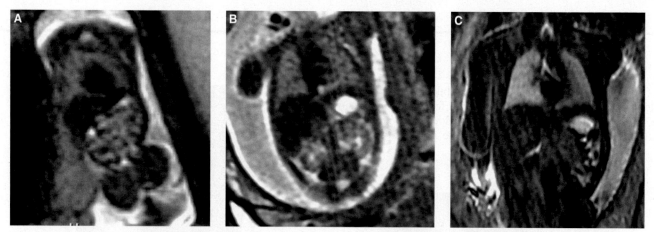

**FIGURE 6.1-21:** Liver. Coronal SSFSE images of the liver and spleen at 17 weeks' **(A)**, 21 weeks' **(B)**, and 29 weeks' **(C)** gestation.

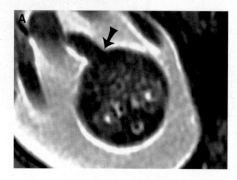

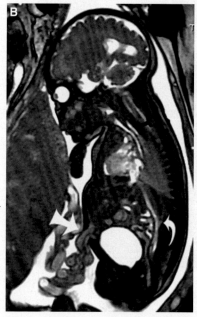

**FIGURE 6.1-22:** Cord insertion. **A:** Axial SSFSE at 20 weeks demonstrates cord insertion *(black arrow)* at the ventral abdomen. **B:** Sagittal SSFP image at 32 weeks demonstrates cord insertion *(straight arrow)*, inferior vena cava draining into the right atrium *(white curved arrow)* as well as the fluid-filled trachea and partially filled proximal esophagus *(black arrow)*.

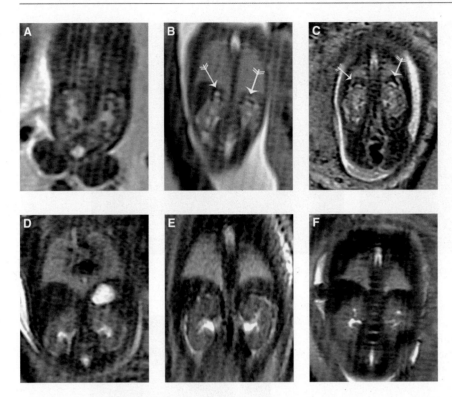

**FIGURE 6.1-23:** Kidneys. Coronal SSFSE at various gestational ages: 17 weeks **(A)**, 20 weeks **(B)**, 23 weeks **(C)**, 28 weeks **(D)**, 32 weeks **(E)**, 37 weeks **(F)**. Note low-signal adrenals surrounding by high signal fat at 20 and 23 weeks gestation *(arrows)*.

The genitourinary track requires assessment of the kidneys, adrenal glands, ureters, bladder, and genitalia. The fetal kidneys are relatively well seen early in the second trimester, intermediate in signal on T2w. Perinephric fat is high signal on T2w and can be mistaken for perirenal fluid. Fluid in the renal pelvis is well depicted separate from the renal tissue. With maturation, the renal cortex and the medulla become more differentiated (Fig. 6.1-23). Diffusion-weighted imaging is useful in identifying renal parenchyma, particularly if not in the expected location (Fig. 6.1-24). Apparent diffusion coefficient of the kidneys increases with advancing gestation.[75] The adrenal glands are noted above the kidneys. In the early second trimester, the adrenal are hypointense on T2w and relatively well seen because of surrounding hyperintense perirenal fat (Fig. 6.1-23). They can be triradiate or lambda-shaped. As they grow becoming pyramidal in shape, they become higher in signal, becoming more difficult to visualize in the third trimester.

The ureters are typically not visualized. When dilated, sagittal and coronal SSFSE T2w and SSPE sequences help document level of ureteral insertion. Thick slab coronal imaging can simulate MRI urography[54] (Fig. 6.1-25).

The bladder should always contain high-signal fluid on T2w sequences and should be identified some time during a 30-minute exam.

The uterus, vagina, ovaries, and prostate are not well separated from surrounding tissues. If ascites or an anomaly such as an ovarian cyst or hydrometrocolpos is present, they can be

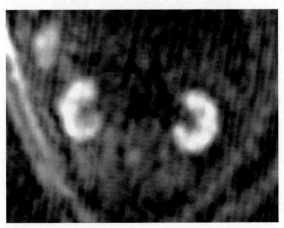

**FIGURE 6.1-24:** Oblique diffusion-weighted image (DWI) of both kidneys at 32 weeks gestation.

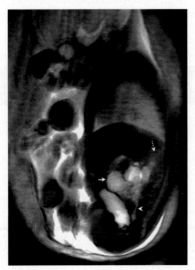

**FIGURE 6.1-25:** Sagittal thick slab SSFSE of a kidney with hydroureteronephrosis *(dotted arrow)* and a contralateral multicystic dysplastic kidney *(solid arrow)*. *Arrowhead* points to the distal hydroureter.

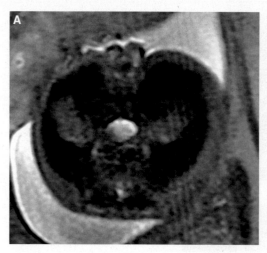
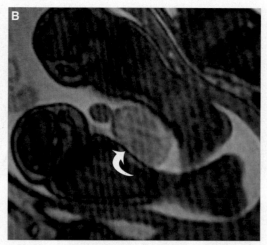

**FIGURE 6.1-26:** Genitalia. **A:** Axial SSFSE demonstrates labia at 33 weeks gestation. **B:** Oblique SSFP image of testes within the scrotal sacs *(curved arrow)* in this 32-week male fetus.

depicted. Identifying labia or penis and scrotum is best noted on axial or sagittal T2w sequences with amniotic fluid outlining the surface (Fig. 6.1-26) (see Chapter 19.3).Testicles within the scrotum may be seen after 28 weeks' gestation.[76,77]

## Musculoskeletal (Table 6.1-9)

While US remains the cornerstone of fetal skeletal assessment, MRI has become an important adjunct. Large FOV can help assess configuration of limbs, with thick slab delineating fetal surface contours[54,78,79] (Figs. 6.1-27 and 6.1-28). Dynamic SSFP images may characterize extremity movement.

T2w sequences demonstrate skin and muscle. Muscle is relatively homogeneous hypointense on T2w so discreet muscles cannot be delineated. High signal or thin musculature may suggest an abnormality[47,80] (Fig. 6.1-29). The subcutaneous tissue layer becomes more prominent as subcutaneous fat develops in the third trimester, high signal on T1w (Fig. 6.1-30).[81]

EPI sequences provide a way of evaluating bone (low signal) and cartilage (high signal) maturation[80] (Fig. 6.1-31). With US only moderately accurate in the diagnosis of specific skeletal

| Table 6.1-9 | Fetal Musculoskeletal |
|---|---|
| *Anatomy* | *Sequences* |
| Hands, feet | Coronal, sagittal SSFP; dynamic SSFP; thick slab SSFP; EPI |
| Arms, legs | Sagittal, coronal EPI, SSFP; dynamic SSFP |
| Spine | Axial, sagittal T2w SSFSE; EPI; T1w GRE to look for fat |

Single-shot fast spin-echo sequences (SSFSE), steady-state free precession sequences (SSFP), gradient echo sequences (GRE). Reproduced with permission from Prayer D, Brugger P. Investigation of normal organ development with fetal MRI. *Eur Radiol.* 2007;17:2458–2471.

**FIGURE 6.1-27:** SSFSE coronal image of the arm at 26 weeks gestation demonstrates amniotic fluid outlining the fingers of the hand.

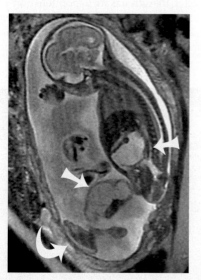

**FIGURE 6.1-28:** Lymphangioma. Large field of view SSFSE sagittal image at 24 weeks gestation demonstrates large subcutaneous cysts along the femur, loculated septated cysts within the abdomen *(straight arrows)* as well as swelling of the foot *(curved arrow)* in this fetus with extensive lymphangioma.

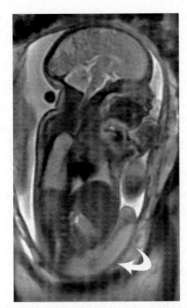

**FIGURE 6.1-29:** Amyoplasia. SSFSE sagittal image at 34 weeks gestation demonstrates abnormal high signal of the muscles of the thigh *(curved arrow)*. Amyoplasia is characterized by absence of limb muscles that are replaced by fibrous and fatty tissue. Fetal activity was decreased.

dysplasias, fetal MRI may become a useful adjunct in arriving at a more definitive diagnosis (see Chapter 21).[82]

## Normal Measurements

Reference values of fetal organs are available from numerous US studies. Various studies evaluating measurements by either fetal MRI alone or by comparison with US have been performed. MRI measurements have shown good correlation with US.[83–87] Volumetric data for lung, fetal weight may be more accurate by MRI than US.[88–90] MRI measures continue to be established, including brain, lungs, liver, and kidney.

## CONCLUSION

MRI has been increasingly used as a problem-solving tool in the assessment of the fetus. It is important when using this modality to be aware of potential safety risks, know how to optimize protocols, and understand how fetal anatomy develops over gestation. With appropriate use, this exciting modality will continue to evolve, further advancing the care of the fetus.

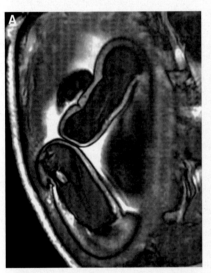
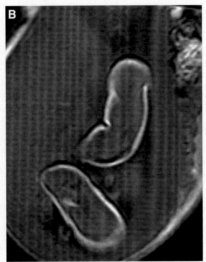

**FIGURE 6.1-30:** Subcutaneous fat at 37-week gestation. **A:** Sagittal SSPE image demonstrates low-signal muscle bone and cartilage. **B:** T1w image in the same plane delineates high-signal subcutaneous fat which develops in the third trimester.

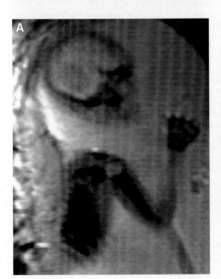
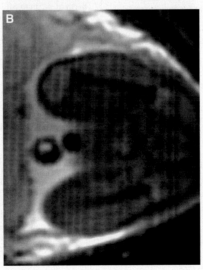

**FIGURE 6.1-31:** Skeleton. A: Sagittal EPI of a 21-week fetus demonstrates hyperintense cartilage and hypointense bone that is well delineated against the adjacent high-signal muscle. B: Axial EPI of both femurs at 33-week GA demonstrates less contrast between muscle and bone.

# REFERENCES

1. Coakley FV, Glenn OA, Qayyum A, et al. Fetal MRI: a developing technique for the developing patient. *AJR Am J Roentgenol.* 2004;182(1):243–252.
2. Reddy UM, Filly RA, Copel JA. Prenatal imaging: ultrasonography and magnetic resonance imaging. *Clin Obstet Gynecol.* 2008;112(1):145–157.
3. Levine D. Obstetric MRI. *J Magn Reson Imaging.* 2006;24:1–15.
4. Bulas D. Imaging of fetal anomalies. In: Medina LS, et al, eds. *Evidence Based Imaging.* New York, NY: Springer; 2009:615–632.
5. Garel C. Fetal MRI: what is the future? *Ultrasound Obstet Gynecol.* 2008;31(2):123–128.
6. Clouchoux C, Limperopoulos C. Novel applications of quantitative MRI for the fetal brain. *Pediatr Radiol.* 2012;42(suppl 1):S24–S32.
7. Kline-Fath BM. Current advances in prenatal imaging of congenital diaphragmatic hernia. *Pediatr Radiol.* 2012;42(suppl 1):S74–S90.
8. Victoria T, Bebbington MW, Danzer E, et al. Use of magnetic resonance imaging in prenatal prognosis of the fetus with isolated left congenital diaphragmatic hernia. *Prenat Diagn.* 2012;32(8):715–723.
9. Wieseler KM, Bhargava P, Kanal KM, et al. Imaging in pregnant patients: examination appropriateness. *Radiographics.* 2010;30:1215–1233.
10. Benacerraf BR, Shipp TD, Bromley B, et al. What does magnetic resonance imaging add to the prenatal sonographic diagnosis of ventriculomegaly? *J Ultrasound Med.* 2007;26(11):1513–1522.
11. Garel C, Brisse H, Sebag G, et al. Magnetic resonance imaging of the fetus. *Pediatr Radiol.* 1998;28:201–211.
12. Yip YP, Capriotti C, Talagala SL, et al. Effects of MR exposure at 1.5 T on early embryonic development of the chick. *J Magn Reson Imaging.* 1994;4:742–748.
13. Yip YP, Capriotti C, Yip JW. Effects of MR exposure on axonal outgrowth in the sympathetic nervous system of the chick. *J Magn Reson Imaging.* 1995;5:457–462.
14. Mevissen M, Buntenkotter S, Loscher W. Effects of static and time varying (50-Hz) magnetic fields on reproduction and fetal development in rats. *Teratology.* 1994;50:229–237.
15. Magin RL, Lee JK, Klintsova A, et al. Biological effects of long-duration, high-field (4 T) MRI on growth and development of the mouse. *J Magn Reson Imaging.* 2000;12:140–149.
16. Saunders R. Static magnetic fields: animal studies. *Prog Biophys Mol Biol.* 2005;87(2–3):225–239.
17. Murbach M, Cabot E, Neufeld E, et al. Local SAR enhancements in anatomically correct children and adult models as a function of position within 1.5 T MR body coil. *Prog Biophys Mol Biol.* 2011;107(3):428–433.
18. Neufeld E, Gosselin MC, Murbach M, et al. Analysis of the local worst case SAR exposure caused by an MRI multi transmit body coil in anatomical models of the human body. *Phys Med Biol.* 2011;56(15):4649–4659.
19. Baker P, Johnson I, Harvey R, et al. A three-year follow-up of children imaged in utero with echo-planar magnetic resonance. *Am J Obstet Gynecol.* 1994;170:32–33.
20. Glover P, Hykin J, Gowl P, et al. An assessment of the intrauterine sound intensity level during obstetric echo-planar magnetic resonance imaging. *Br J Radiol.* 1995;68(814):1090–1094.
21. Heinrichs WL, Fong P, Flannery M, et al. Midgestational exposure of pregnant BALB/c mice to magnetic resonance imaging conditions. *Magn Reson Imaging.* 1988;6(3):305–313.
22. Tyndall DA, Sulik KK. Effects of magnetic resonance imaging on eye development in the C57BL/6J mouse. *Teratology.* 1991;43:263–275.
23. Levine D, Zuo C, Faro CB, et al. Potential heating effect in the gravid uterus during MR HASTE imaging. *J Magn Reson Imaging.* 2001;13(6):856–861.
24. Dimbylow P. Development of pregnant female, hybrid voxel-mathematical models and their application to the dosimetry of applied magnetic and electric fields at 50 Hz. *Phys Med Biol.* 2006;51(10):2383–2394.
25. Hand JW, Li Y, Hajnal JV. Numerical study of RF exposure and the resulting temperature rise in the foetus during a magnetic resonance procedure. *Phys Med Biol.* 2010;55(4):913–930.
26. Brugger PC, Prayer D. Actual imaging time in fetal MRI. *Eur J Radiol.* 2012;81(3):e194–e196.
27. Kanal E, Gillen J, Evans JA, et al. Survey of reproductive health among female MR workers. *Radiology.* 1993;187(2):395–399.
28. Myers C, Duncan KR, Gowland PA, et al. Failure to detect intrauterine growth restriction following in utero exposure to MRI. *Br J Radiol.* 1998;71:549–551.
29. Clements H, Duncan KR, Fielding K, et al. Infants exposed to MRI in utero have a normal paediatric assessment at 9 months of age. *Br J Radiol.* 2000;73:190–194.
30. Kok RD, de Vries MM, Heerschap A, et al. Absence of harmful effects of magnetic resonance exposure at 1.5 T in utero during the third trimester of pregnancy: a follow-up study. *Magn Reson Imaging.* 2004;22:851–854.
31. International Commission on Non-Ionizing Radiation Protection. Medical magnetic resonance (MR) procedures: protection of patients. *Health Phys.* 2004;87(2):197–216.
32. De Wilde JP, Rivers AW, Price DL. A review of the current use of magnetic resonance imaging in pregnancy and safety implications for the fetus. *Prog Biophys Mol Biol.* 2005;87(2–3):335–353.
33. Kanal E, Borgstede JP, Barkovich AJ, et al. American College of Radiology white paper on MR safety. *AJR Am J Roentgenol.* 2002;178(6):1335–1347.
34. Bulas D, Egloff A. Benefits and risks of MRI in pregnancy. *Semin Perinatol.* 2013;37(5):301–304.
35. Welsh R, Nemec U, Thomason M. Fetal magnetic resonance imaging at 3.0 T. *Top Magn Reson Imaging.* 2011;1:1–13.
36. Merkle EM, Dale BM, Paulson EK. Abdominal MR imaging at 3 T. *Magn Reson Imaging Clin N Am.* 2006;14(1):17–26.
37. Victoria T, Jaramillo D, Roberto T, et al. Fetal MRI: jumping from 1.5 to 3 T MRI-preliminary experience. *Pediatr Radiol.* 2014, in press.
38. Sundgren PC, Leander P. Is administration of gadolinium-based contrast media to pregnant women and small children justified? *J Magn Reson Imaging.* 2011;34(4):750–757.
39. Runge VM. Safety of approved MR contrast media for intravenous injection. *J Magn Reson Imaging.* 2000;12:205–213.
40. Webb JAW, Thomsen HS, Morcos SK. The use of iodinated and gadolinium contrast media during pregnancy and lactation. *Eur Radiol.* 2005;15(6):1234–1240.
41. Okuda Y, Sagami F, Tirone P, et al. Reproductive and developmental toxicity study of gadobenate dimeglumine formulation (E7155) (3): study of embryo-fetal toxicity in rabbits by intravenous administration [in Japanese]. *J Toxicol Sci.* 1999;24(suppl 1):79–87.
42. Rofsky NM, Pizzarello DJ, Weinreb JC, et al. Effect on fetal mouse development of exposure to MR imaging and gadopentate dimeglumine. *J Magn Reson Imaging.* 1994;4:805–807.
43. Novak Z, Thurmond AS, Ross PL, et al. Gadolinium DTPA transplacental transfer and distribution in fetal tissue in rabbits. *Invest Radiol.* 1993;28:828–830.
44. Vanhaesebrouck P, Verstratet AG, De Prater C, et al. Transplacental passage of a nonionic contrast agent. *Eur J Pediatr.* 2005;164:408–410.
45. Coletti PM, Sylvestre PB. MRI in pregnancy. *Magn Reson Imaging Clin N Am.* 1994;2:291–307.
46. Marcos HB, Semelka RC, Worawattanakkul S. Normal placenta: gadolinium enhanced dynamic MR imaging. *Radiology.* 1997;205:493–496.
47. Prayer C, Brugger P. Investigation of normal organ development with fetal MRI. *Eur Radiol.* 2007;17:2458–2471.
48. Kienzl D, Berger-Kulemann V, Kasprian G, et al. Risk of inferior vena cava compression syndrome during fetal MRI in the supine position: a retrospective analysis. *J Perinat Med.* 2013;16:1–6.
49. Serai SD, Merrow AC, Kline-Fath BM. Fetal MRI on a multi-element digital coil platform. *Pediatr Radiol.* 2013;43(9):1213–1217.
50. Hosseinzadeh K, Owens E. Optimization of acquisition time for MRI of fetal head: the eyes have it. *AJR Am J Roentgenol.* 2005;185(4):1060–1062.
51. Chaumoitre K, Wikberg E, Shojai R, et al. Fetal magnetic resonance hydrography: evaluation of a single-shot thick-slab RARE (rapid acquisition with relaxation enhancement) sequence in fetal thoracoabdominal pathology. *Ultrasound Obstet Gynecol.* 2006;27(5):537–544.
52. Huisman TAGM, Solopova A. MR fetography using heavily T2-weighted sequences: comparison of thin- and thick-slab acquisitions. *Eur J Radiol.* 2009;71(3):557–563.
53. Kline-Fath BM, Calvo-Garcia MA, O'Hara SM, et al. Water imaging (hydrography) in the fetus: the value of a heavily T2-weighted sequence. *Pediatr Radiol.* 2007;37(2):133–140.
54. Brugger PC, Mittermayer C, Prayer D. A new look at the fetus thick slab T2w sequence on fetal MRI. *Eur J Radiol.* 2006;57:182–186.
55. Werner H, Lopes dos Santos JR, Fontes R, et al. Virtual bronchoscopy for evaluating cervical tumors of the fetus. *Ultrasound Obstet Gynecol.* 2013;41(1):90–94.
56. Werner H, dos Santos JR, Fontes R, et al. Additive manufacturing models of fetuses built from three-dimensional ultrasound, MRI and CT scan data. *Ultrasound Obstet Gynecol.* 2010;36(3):355.
57. Barth MM, Smith MP, Pedrosa I, et al. Body MR imaging at 3.0 T: understanding the opportunities and challenges. *Radiographics.* 2007;27:1445–1462.
58. Kataoka M, Isoda H, Maetani Y, et al. MR imaging of the female pelvis at 3 Tesla: evaluation of image homogeneity using different dielectric pads. *J Magn Reson Imaging.* 2007;26:1572–1577.
59. Hand JW, Li Y, Thomas EL, et al. Predication of SAR in mother and fetus associated with MRI examination during pregnancy. *Magn Reson Med.* 2006;55:883–893.
60. Zaretsky MV, Alexander JM, McIntire DD, et al. MRI pelvimetry and the prediction of labor dystocia. *Obstet Gynecol.* 2005;106:919–926.
61. Korhonen U, Solja R, Laitinen J, et al. MR pelvimetry measurements, analysis of inter and intraobserver variation. *Eur J Radiol.* 2010;75:56–61.
62. Keller T, Rake A, Michel S, et al. Obstetric MR pelvimetry: reference values and evaluation of inter and intraobserver error and intraindividual variability. *Radiology.* 2003;227:37–43.
63. Tukeva TA, Aronen HJ, Karjalainen PT, et al. Low field MRI pelvimetry. *Eur Radiol.* 1997;7:230–234.
64. Gowlan P. Placental MRI. *Semin Fetal Neonatal Med.* 2005;10:485–490.
65. Nguyen D, Nguyen C, Yavobozzi M, et al. Imaging of the placenta with pathologic correlation. *Semin Ultrasound CT MR.* 2012;33:65–77.
66. Elsayes KM, Trout A, Friedkin A, et al. Imaging of the placenta: a multimodality pictorial review. *Radiographics.* 2009;29:1371–1391.
67. Baughman WC, Corteville JE, Shah RR. Placenta accreta: spectrum of US and MR findings. *Radiographics.* 2008;28:1905–1916.

68. Warshak CR, Eskander R, Hull AD, et al. Accuracy of US and MRI in the diagnosis of placenta accrete. *Obstet Gynecol.* 2006;108:573–581.

69. Zaretsky MV, McIntire DD, Reichel TF, et al. Correlation of measured amniotic fluid volume to sonographic and MR predictions. *Am J Obstet Gynecol.* 2004;191:2148–2153.

70. Kato K, Shiozawa T, Ashida T, et al. Prenatal diagnosis of amniotic sheets by MRI. *Am J Obstet Gynecol.* 2005;193:881–884.

71. Moore RJ, Stradchan B, Tyler DJ, et al. In vivo diffusion measurements as an indication of fetal lung maturation using echo planar imaging at 0.5 T. *Magn Reson Med.* 2001;45:247–253.

72. Brugger P, Prayer D. Fetal abdominal MRI. *Eur J Radiol.* 2006;57:278–293.

73. Goitein O, Eshet Y, Hoffmann C, et al. Fetal liver T2* values: defining a standardized scale. *J Magn Reson Imaging.* 2013;38(6):1342–1345.

74. Brugger PC, Weber M, Prayer D. MRI of the fetal gallbladder and bile. *Eur Radiol.* 2010;20:2862–2869.

75. Witzani L, Brugger P, Horman M, et al. Normal renal development investigated with fetal MRI. *Eur J Radiol.* 2006;57:294–302.

76. Nemec SF, Nemec U, Weber M, et al. Female external genitalia on fetal MRI. *Ultrasound Obstet Gynecol.* 2011;38:695–700.

77. Nemec SF, Nemec U, Weber M, et al. Penile biometry on prenatal MRI. *Ultrasound Obstet Gynecol.* 2012;39:330–335.

78. Nemec SF, Nemec U, Grugger PC, et al. Skeletal development on fetal MRI. *Top Magn Reson Imaging.* 2011;22:101–106.

79. Nemec SF, Nemec U, Brugger PC, et al. MR imaging of the fetal musculoskeletal system. *Prenat Diagn.* 2012;32:205–213.

80. Witters I, Moerman P, Fryns FP. Fetal akinesia deformation sequence: a study of 30 consecutive in utero diagnoses. *Am J Med Genet.* 2002;113:23–28.

81. Anblagan D, Deshpande R, Jones NW, et al. Measurement of fetal fat in utero in normal and diabetic pregnancies using magnetic resonance imaging. *Ultrasound Obstet Gynecol.* 2013;42(3):335–340.

82. Applegate KE. Can MR imaging be used to characterize fetal musculoskeletal development? *Radiology.* 2004;233:305–306.

83. Garel C. Fetal cerebral biometry: normal parenchymal findings and ventricular size. *Eur Radiol.* 2005;15:809–813.

84. Parazzini C, Righini A, Rustico M, et al. Prenatal MRI: brain normal linear biometric values below 24 gestation weeks. *Neuroradiology.* 2008;50:877–883.

85. Duncan KR, Issa B, Moore R, et al. A comparison of feral organ measurement by echoplanar magnetic resonance imaging and ultrasound. *BJOG.* 2005;112:43–49.

86. Cannie M, Neirrynck V, DeKeyzer F, et al. Prenatal MRI demonstrates linear growth of the human fetal kidneys during gestation. *J Urol.* 2007;178:1570–1574.

87. Kacem Y, Cannie MM, Kadji C, et al. Fetal weight estimation: comparison of 2 dimensional US and MRI assessment. *Radiology.* 2013;267:902–910.

88. Lo Zito L, Kadfi C, Cannie M, et al. Determination of fetal body volume measurement at term with MRI effect of various factors. *J Matern Fetal Neonatal Med.* 2013;26:1254–1258.

89. Willimas G, Coakley FV, Qayyum A, et al. Fetal relative lung volume: quantification by using prenatal MRI lung volumetry. *Radiology.* 2004;233:456–462.

90. Cannie MM, Jani JC, Van Kerhove F, et al. Fetal body volume at MRI to quantify total fetal lung volume: normal ranges. *Radiology.* 2008;247:197–203.

# Normal Brain Imaging

Beth M. Kline-Fath

## BACKGROUND

Fetal magnetic resonance imaging (MRI) is often performed when the fetus is at increased risk for neurologic abnormalities or a central nervous system abnormality has been detected on a prenatal ultrasound (US). It has been repeatedly demonstrated that fetal MRI can detect abnormalities that are not apparent on prenatal sonography. These abnormalities may influence decisions regarding pregnancy management and site of delivery. However, because the fetal brain changes dramatically through different gestational ages, it is imperative to understand the normal anatomy so that correct interpretation of the imaging occurs. The supplement at the end of this chapter, Normal Brain Imaging by Gestational Age, contains figures of the brain in 2-week increments.

## Imaging

The fetal brain has lower protein content and higher water content than the normal adult brain, with extracellular space 40% in the fetus and 20% in the adult. Therefore, subtle differences in the brain parenchyma are best depicted by utilizing heavily T2-weighted imaging. MRI of the fetal brain should be performed in axial, sagittal, and coronal planes. Superior interpretation is obtained if anatomic imaging is performed as then symmetry of the fetal brain can be utilized. The interhemispheric fissure is an excellent midline landmark that can be used to set up the anatomic sequences. The best depiction of fetal brain morphology is achieved by utilizing single-shot rapid acquisition with refocused echoes (SS-RARE or SSFSE). This the sequence provides the highest signal to noise and resolution. Imaging of the fetal brain should include at least two sets of axial, coronal, and sagittal images at a 3-mm slice and no gap and field of view (FOV) 24 to 30. If the fetal gestational age is >28 weeks and more signal to noise is desired, then a 4-mm slice with no gap can be considered. Sometimes, a 2-mm slice thickness may be utilized, especially in evaluation of the fetal posterior fossa. True fast imaging with steady precession (SSFP) is often helpful as it provides good resolution, bright blood imaging, and high definition between fluid and soft tissue interfaces. It is very helpful in evaluating the face, especially the palate, and skull base, including temporal bones, and to diagnose old hemorrhage or lipoma in the brain.[1] The disadvantages include less signal and contrast between gray and white matter than SSFSE because of lower flip angle and banding artifacts.[2] SSFP imaging is typically obtained at a slice thickness of 3 to 4 mm in axial, coronal, and sagittal plane. Three-dimensional SSFP imaging may be helpful as with 1.6-mm thick sections, midline anatomy as well as cortical sulcation can be well defined.[1] Additional imaging should include axial or coronal gradient echo planar T2-weighted images (3 mm skip 0) to detect hemorrhage and fast multiplanar spoiled gradient recall acquisition in the steady-state (FMPSPGR) T1-weighted images (5 mm skip 0) for detection of hemorrhage, fat, or calcification (Table 6.2-1).

Advanced imaging of the fetal brain includes diffusion-weighted imaging (DWI). Diffusion exploits the properties of randomly moving water molecules in a magnetic field. Within tissue, diffusion of water can be restricted by cell membranes, axons, small vessels, etc. The components that do not allow water to move in all directions move anisotropically. A high fractional anisotropy (FA) value reflects water motion limited in direction. The apparent diffusion coefficient (ADC) serves as a measure of freedom of diffusion of protons. Low ADC values reflect a restriction in diffusion of water, while high ADC values reflect little restriction in water diffusion. The T2 trace or diffusion-weighted (DW) image reflects similar changes but with opposite signal, respectively. Diffusion allows depiction of fetal brain development, including early areas of myelination, and cytotoxic edema related to injury. Imaging is typically obtained at a slice thickness of 5 mm with no gap and field of view of 32 to 40.

When imaging the fetal brain, the entire fetus from head to toe should be examined. Fetal pathologies and malformations frequently involve multiple organs. Identification of other anomalies may give the imager a clue to underlying genetic or chromosomal syndrome. When imaging the body, typical sequences should include anatomic planes utilizing SSFSE, SSFP, and T1-weighted imaging. Anatomy of the bowel is important, so do not skip the T1 sequence.

## Indications

MRI is a valuable complement to prenatal US in evaluation of the fetal brain. Because of higher soft tissue contrast, resolution, large field of view, and ability to image both sides of the fetus at once, fetal MRI is more precise than US in evaluating parenchymal architecture, cortical development, sulcation, brainstem anatomy, and cerebellar lesions. Most cases of fetal MRI are performed to investigate the cause of ventriculomegaly or to evaluate a cerebral malformation. In the presence of maternal infection, trauma, coagulation disorder or a twin gestation at risk for twin twin transfusion syndrome, fetal MRI is often utilized to screen for intracranial hemorrhage or injury. If there are extracerebral malformations such as cardiac or lymphatic, fetal brain imaging is helpful to exclude intracranial findings. In the presence of a family history of genetic disorder, fetal MRI may be appropriate.

| Table 6.2-1 | Fetal Brain Imaging |
| --- | --- |

| Anatomy | Sequences |
| --- | --- |
| Cerebrum | Sagittal, axial, and coronal T2w SSFSE (run twice) and SSFP |
| Midline structures | Sagittal T2w SSFSE, SSFP |
| Temporal bones | Axial and coronal T2w SSFP |
| Blood or fat | T1 and GRE |
| Ischemia | Diffusion |
| Calvarium | EPI |

SSFSE, single-shot fast spin-echo sequences; SSFP, steady-state free-precession sequences; GRE, gradient echo sequences; and EPI, ecoplanar imaging.

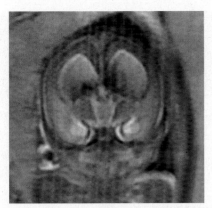

**FIGURE 6.2-1:** Coronal T2 image of a fetus with severe ventriculomegaly. Dark signal is related to CSF pulsation artifact in large ventricles.

## Limitations

Pitfalls in interpretation are possible if the imager is not familiar with the normal patterns of development. The fetal brain changes dramatically, and lack of knowledge of normal for each gestational age may lead to incorrect pathologic diagnosis. Two of the most common misdiagnoses include lissencephaly prior to 24 weeks and misinterpreting the germinal matrix as hemorrhage early in gestation.[3] Accurate interpretation can be more difficult if the gestational age of the fetus is not defined. Knowing the correct imaging sequences is important, such as gradient echo for hemorrhage and diffusion for ischemia. Artifacts related to maternal and fetal motion can make interpretation difficult. Therefore, imaging in the same plane at least two to three times can prevent over reading or missing findings. Flow artifact related to amniotic fluid and cerebral spinal fluid (CSF) in the ventricles should not be interpreted as hemorrhage (Fig. 6.2-1). The small size of the fetus also creates difficulties in imaging and interpretation. The smallest field of view without wraparound, anatomic imaging planes, and thinnest slices are necessary for diagnostic fetal imaging. Typically, it is helpful if pathology is confirmed on two different imaging planes and/or sequences.

## BASIC EMBRYOLOGY

A short review of embryology is necessary for understanding the different developmental appearances of the fetal brain. Important time lines described below include the embryonic period, which is the first 8 weeks after conception, and the fetal period, which represents the time from the end of the embryonic period to birth. Embryology time lines tend to reflect postconception or postovulatory dating, whereas in fetal imaging we refer to age via last menstrual period which can allow for a 2 week difference. Therefore, please note that embryology in this chapter will be dated by postconception/postovulatory age, and fetal MRI age reflects fetal age by last menstrual period.

The stages of embryonic development are primary neurulation, also known as dorsal induction, ventral induction, neuronal cell lineage, proliferation, differentiation, neuronal migration, organization, and finally brain myelination (Table 6.2-2). Primary neurulation (dorsal induction) and ventral induction will be described here. The following stages will be emphasized as it relates to fetal imaging.

### Table 6.2-2   Stages of Embryonic Development

| Major Developmental Event | Time of Occurrence |
| --- | --- |
| Primary neurulation | 3–5 wk |
|    Anterior neuropore closure | 24 d |
|    Posterior neuropore closure | 26 d |
|    Development of prosencephalon/ rhombencephalon | 4–5 wk |
| Ventral induction[a] | 5–6 wk |
| Midline/commissure | 8–20 wk |
|    Anterior commissure | 8–9 wk |
|    Hippocampal | 9–11 wk |
|    Septum pellucidum | 10–17 wk |
|    Corpus callosum | 10–17 wk |
| Neuronal lineage, proliferation, and migration | |
|    Cerebral | 5–24 wk |
|      Ventricular zone | 5–14 wk |
|      Subventricular zone | 14–24 wk |
|    Cerebellar: ventricular and rhombic lips | 8 wk to postnatal |
| Neuronal organization | 24 wk to postnatal |
| Myelination | 20 wk to postnatal |

[a]Formation of cerebral hemispheres, cerebellum, brainstem, optic vesicles, olfactory bulbs and tracts, pituitary gland and stalk, and face.

Initially, ectodermal cells at day 23, through dorsal induction, differentiate into a neural plate. The plate will thicken and fold to the midline, giving rise to a neural tube with central embryonic vesicle (Fig. 6.2-2). The neural tube closes at the anterior neuropore (lamina terminalis) at day 24 and the posterior neuropore (lumbosacral) on day 26. During this time, early development of the ear and eye is noted by visualization of the otic disc and optic sulcus, respectively. The final phase of primary neurulation is separation of the neural tissue and surface ectoderm.[4]

At the end of the 4th week, the cranial aspect of the neural tube forms three primary vesicles: prosencephalon (forebrain), mesencephalon (midbrain), and rhombencephalon (hindbrain). At the same time, two flexures develop: the cervical flexure at the junction of the hindbrain and spinal cord and the cephalic flexure at the level of the midbrain. During the 5th week, the prosencephalon divides into the telencephalon and the diencephalon defined by further visualization of the optic vesicles. The mesencephalon remains unchanged, but an area is defined between the hindbrain and the midbrain known as the mesencephalic isthmus. The rhombencephalon will further differentiate into the metencephalon and myelencephalon. Flexure in the hindbrain (pontine) will occur with this division (Fig. 6.2-3). Persistence of the central embryonic canal in each of these areas will give rise to the ventricular system: telencephalon—lateral ventricles, diencephalon—third ventricle, mesencephalon—cerebral aqueduct, and rhombencephalon—fourth ventricle (Fig. 6.2-4). As the

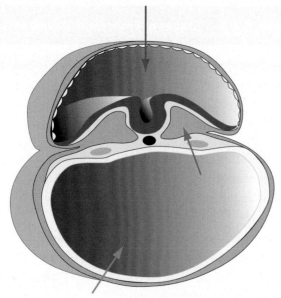

**FIGURE 6.2-2:** Section through the trilaminar germ disc. The neural tissue, blue tissue marked by *green arrow*, arises from ectoderm along the dorsal aspect of the embryo and contains amniotic fluid due to continuity with the amniotic sac. The mesodermal layer is delineated by *blue arrow*, and yolk sac by *brown arrow*.

vesicles form, the choroid plexus will develop from blood vessels that invade the ventricular walls.

A sulcus hemispheric divides the developing telencephalon and diencephalon. The dorsal medial corresponds to the velum interpositum, and the basal medial corresponds to the lamina terminalis. The walls of the telencephalic cerebral vesicle are extremely thin but are connected in the midline by the lamina terminalis, the site of the anterior neuropore closure. Ventral induction is the formation of the brain into two cerebral hemispheres. The telencephalon does not cleave, but instead at the beginning of the 5th week, bilateral evaginations around the foramen of Monro develop as outgrowths of the dorsolateral walls of the prosencephalon, forming caudal wards and bending in ventral and rostral directions, eventually completely covering

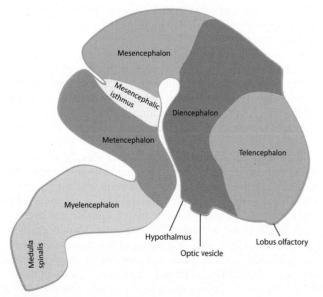

**FIGURE 6.2-3:** The primitive brain and its embryologic origins.

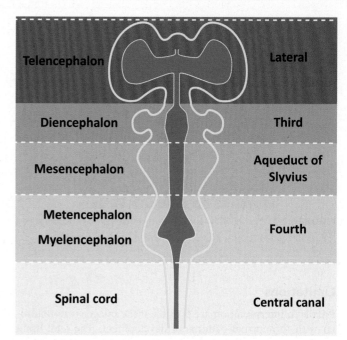

**FIGURE 6.2-4:** The primitive vesicles with embryologic origins.

the diencephalon. This C-shaped growth results in the formation of the temporal lobes. The interhemispheric fissure will be present at approximately 10 weeks, forming anterior to posterior.[5] A loose mesenchyme will form the primary meninges at 5 weeks. The dural layer is present at 6 weeks, and as the dura develops, the attachment between the tentorium cerebelli and falx move more caudal, causing a reduction in size of the posterior fossa relative to the supratentorial brain.[4] Concurrently, during ventral induction, the cerebellum, brainstem, optic vesicles, olfactory bulbs and tract, pituitary gland and stalk, and face are developing.

There is emerging evidence that the development of the brain is influenced by innumerable genes and that normal development cannot occur without their direction. However, the discussion of genetic embryology is beyond the space allotment and will not be discussed further here.

## VENTRICLES

The ventricles develop from cavities of the primitive cerebral vesicles and should be smooth throughout fetal life. Life for the developing brain arises from the surface of the ventricles, as it is in the ventricular wall that the germinal matrix proliferates and gives rise to the developing neurons and glial cells of the fetal brain.

### Lateral Ventricles

#### Embryology

The lateral ventricles begin as a primitive cerebral cavity that becomes paired with development of the telencephalon. The cavities communicate with each other and the third ventricle through the intraventricular foramina (Fig. 6.2-5). Along the medial wall of the primitive ventricles, the choroid plexus develops as a fold covered by pseudostratified epithelium with proliferation of underlying blood vessels. The choroid is anchored at the foramen Monro and present in the body, atrium, and temporal horns of the lateral ventricles. Early in the pregnancy,

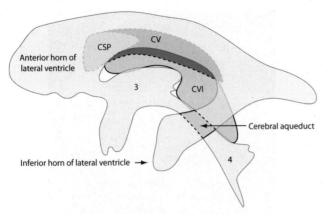

**FIGURE 6.2-5:** Lateral view of the ventricles, cavum septum pellucidum *(CSP)*, cavum vergae *(CV)*, cavum velum interpositum *(CVI)*, 3 third ventricle, and 4 fourth ventricle.

the choroid has a high glycogen content, which is believed to be a major energy supply for the growing cerebrum, but after 19 weeks, the choroid will also be responsible for CSF production.

### Imaging

The lateral ventricles are visible at 13 to 14 weeks and change dramatically with the development of the cerebrum. Before 16 weeks, the primitive lateral ventricles appear large and are composed primarily of globular frontal horns, body, and atrium (Fig. 6.2-6A). With growth of the occipital and temporal lobes, periventricular structures, and corpus callosum, the ventricles narrow gradually, achieving an adult configuration. Growth of the thalamus and corpus striatum results in the development of the foramen of Monro. The caudate nuclei reshape the frontal horn, so that they appear biconcave rather than lobular. The occipital horns may appear prominent until 24 weeks (Fig. 6.2-6B) but demonstrate typical internal and medial deviation early third trimester owing to evolution of the calcar avis.[6] Between 24 and 28 weeks, the lateral ventricles appear less prominent (Fig. 6.2-7). At 34 to 36 weeks, the ventricles appear small.[7] Despite the apparent change in the lateral ventricles, the atrial diameter is relatively constant from 14 to 40 weeks' gestation, with normal values being <10 mm on prenatal US.[8,9] Measurements performed with fetal MRI have confirmed that atrial width is not dependent on gestational age with average normal values of 6 to 7 mm with threshold for

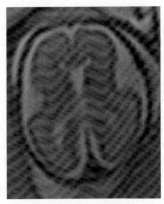

**FIGURE 6.2-7:** Axial SSFSE T2 of fetus at 28 weeks with mature ventricular configuration.

ventriculomegaly being >10 mm.[6,10,11] Axial measurements on fetal MRI at the level of the thalamic nuclei can be obtained but may be 1 to 2 mm inconsistent with US measurements.[10] Coronal measurements inside the lateral ventricular wall at the level of the choroid plexus are highly concordant between both US and MRI and probably provide the best technique for lateral ventricular measurement (Fig. 6.2-8).[11] The atriocerebral ratio (ratio of the diameter of the atrium and the brain biparietal diameter) progressively decreases during gestation (13.6% and 8% at 22 and 38 weeks, respectively), reflecting fetal brain growth combined with constant ventricular size.[12]

## Cavum Septum Pellucidum

### Embryology

The cavum septum pellucidum (CSP) is an important space defined by two thin translucent membranes that extend from the anterior part of the body, genu, and rostrum of the corpus callosum, inferior to the superior surface of the fornix and lateral along the inner walls of the lateral ventricles. The cavum vergae is a cavity within the septum pellucidum, located posterior to the foramina of Monro or, anatomically, the vertical plane formed by the columns of the fornix (see Fig. 6.2-5). The embryologic development of the CSP is closely associated with formation of the corpus callous, thought to represent a space caused by thinning of the commissural plate and disappearance of the glial sling and may be understood as the bridge scaffolding that remains after the corpus callosum has formed (see corpus callosum).[13,14] The structure begins to develop at 10 to 12 weeks

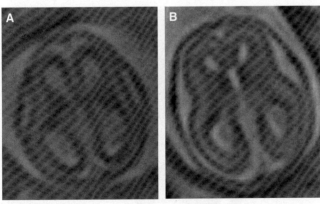

**FIGURE 6.2-6: A:** Axial SSFSE T2 of fetus at 16 weeks with large rudimentary ventricles. **B:** Axial imaging of fetus at 21 weeks with prominent occipital horns.

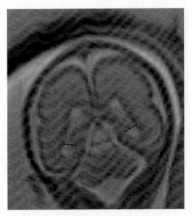

**FIGURE 6.2-8:** Measurement of the lateral ventricle on coronal imaging.

and reaches adult form by 17 weeks.[13] Although visually the cavum is a CSF space, the septal leaflets, which contain neurons, are important, serving as a relay station for the hippocampus and hypothalamus.

### Imaging

The CSP is not typically apparent before 18 weeks and increases in size from 19 to 27 weeks, plateauing at 28 weeks (Fig. 6.2-9).[15] Diameter usually varies between 2 and 10 mm in size. Closure of cavum begins at approximately 24 weeks from posterior to anterior. The cavum vergae fuses by 40 weeks, the CSP as early as 37 weeks but often persists postnatal from 3 to 6 months of age.[14,16] Sometimes, the cavum can become prominent in the late fetal period and resemble an interhemispheric cyst.

## Third Ventricle and Aqueduct

The third ventricle becomes visible in the late first trimester and demonstrates an unchanging adult appearance as a slit-like CSF structure located between the thalamic nuclei. It is easiest to visualize and measure the third ventricle on the coronal plane (Fig. 6.2-10).[12] A normal 3rd ventricle should measure less than 4 mm in transverse dimension (also see Table 24 in Appendix A1).[12] The aqueduct of Slyvius is closely related to the development of the mesencephalon, representing a thin linear CSF space

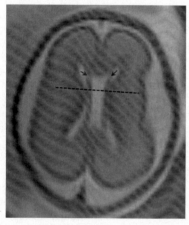

**FIGURE 6.2-9:** Axial T2 image of fetus at 25 weeks with cavum septum pellucidum and vergae. The septal leaflets of the septum pellucidum are defined by *arrows*. The cavum pellucidum is anterior to the foramen of Monro (*anterior to dotted line*) and the cavum vergae is posterior (*posterior to dotted line*).

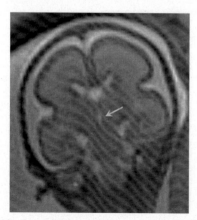

**FIGURE 6.2-10:** Coronal T2 image at 25 weeks with slit-like normal third ventricle (*arrow*).

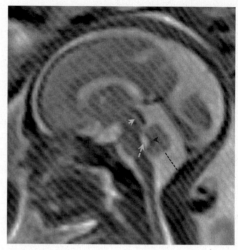

**FIGURE 6.2-11:** Sagittal T2 image at 27 weeks with fluid in the aqueduct of Sylvius (*white arrowhead*). The fourth ventricle (*dotted arrow*) is normal in size and configuration. Fastigial point denoted with *black arrowhead*. Cisterna magna is labeled with *dotted black line*.

(Fig. 6.2-11). Anatomic midline sagittal imaging of 3 mm or less is important to document CSF signal in the aqueduct of Slyvius.

## Fourth Ventricle

### Embryology

The fourth ventricle undergoes unusual development. Early between 5 and 7 weeks, a large ellipsoid CSF cavity develops owing to focal dilatation of the central canal of the neural tube in the hindbrain.[17,18] This rhombencephalic vesicle will eventually become the fourth ventricle. Choroid plexus will develop within the primitive vesicle. The inferior roof of this vesicle will evaginate caudal and dorsal to the developing cerebellar vermis as an ependyma-lined diverticulum to form Blake pouch (Fig. 6.2-12).[17,18] The pouch contains an inner layer of ependymal, middle layer of attenuated neuroglial tissue, and outer layer of pia-arachnoid. Blake pouch will fenestrate down to the obex, leaving a hole that is termed Blake metaphore. This hole will go on to create the foramen of Magendie at 7 to 8 postovulatory weeks.[19] The foramen of Luschka will open later, resulting in equilibrium of the CSF between ventricles and subarachnoid space. Before fenestration, there is enlargement of the fourth

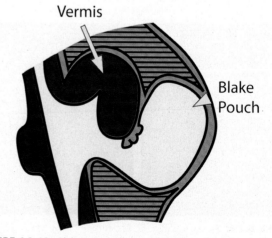

**FIGURE 6.2-12:** Blake pouch. There is dilatation of the fourth ventricle forming a diverticulum called Blake pouch. The subarachnoid space (*striped purple*) does not communicate with Blake pouch.

ventricle with a likely transient increase in intraaxial CSF pressure. The fourth ventricle enlarges between 14 and 16 weeks and decreases to normal size around 22 to 23 weeks.[18] The septae in the cisterna magna are remnants of Blake pouch walls.[18]

### Imaging

The fourth ventricle development is therefore closely tied to the development of the vermis and cisterna magna (see also Chapter 12.3. The fourth ventricle is best evaluated on a sagittal midline image of the fetal brain. Table 24 in appendix A1 provides biometry for normal values via gestational age, but in general, the normal fourth ventricle anterior to posterior dimensions on midline sagittal imaging should be below 7 mm (see Fig. 6.2-11).[12,20–23]

## SUBARACHNOID SPACES

### Supratentorial Space

#### Embryology

Early in gestation, the subarachnoid spaces appear enlarged because of immaturity and small size of the fetal brain (Fig. 6.2-13). As the brain develops and increases in weight, the spaces appear less prominent. The extraaxial spaces remain constant until 30 weeks from which they decrease in size, although prominent spaces can persist in some fetuses in the parieto-occipital area.[24]

#### Imaging

Subarachnoid spaces can be measured from the cortex of the brain to the inner table of the cranium. The frontal subarachnoid space measured on the axial plane at the level of the anterior horn of the lateral ventricle from 18 to 30 weeks should measure <6 mm with a mean of 3 to 4 mm.[25] After 32 weeks, the frontal subarachnoid space decreases in size and measures a mean of 1 to 2 mm. The parieto-occipital space measured on a sagittal image at the level of the parieto-occipital sulcus reaches a maximum of 11 mm between 26 and 28 weeks and decreases in size after 34 weeks to 5 to 7 mm.[25] Interhemispheric and opercular space dimensions by gestational age are shown in Table 24 Appendix A1. Comparing brain BPD to bone BPD may also provide clues to enlarged spaces.

### Infratentorial Space

#### Embryology

The cisterna magna has two compartments. The mesial compartment between the cisterna magna septa is derived from the rhombencephalic vesicle or Blake pouch. These septae can typically be seen on fetal and neonatal US as linear echos or bridging septations in the cisterna magna. The remnant septal leaflets of Blake pouch can also often be detected on a heavily weighted SSFSE or SSFP sequence (Fig. 6.2-14). The lateral compartment is derived from cavitation of the meninx primitiva to form subarachnoid space.

#### Imaging

The cisterna magna can be measured on an axial or sagittal image from midline posterior cerebellar vermis to the inner margin of the occiput (see Fig. 6.2-11). The cisterna magna increases with gestational age (see Table 24 Appendix A1), but normal range should be >2 and <10 mm.[10,25]

## SUPRATENTORIAL BRAIN

### Cerebral Parenchyma

#### Embryology

The supratentorial brain (forebrain) is derived from the telencephalon and diencephalon. The dorsal telencephalon (pallium) gives rise to the cerebral cortex and hippocampus, the ventral telencephalon (subpallium) to the striatum and globus pallidus, and the diencephalon to the thalamus and hypothalamus (Fig. 6.2-15). Initially, cell lineage (glial, neuronal, or ependymal cell) will be decided, and proliferation will then ensue in the germinal matrix. Refined differentiation of the cell then occurs. Important cortical neurons include motor or pyramidal neurons of excitatory type that are glutamate mediated. Interneurons or sensory granule cells are inhibitory or γ-aminobutyric acid (GABA) mediated. Astrocytes are present for neuronal support, and oligodendrocytes are important for myelination. Two types of neuronal migration are described by pathology: radial and tangential (cells migrate perpendicular to radial). In the fetal period from the 8th week to the 24th week, the time is dominated by cortical neuronal migration.[26] From 24 weeks to term, the period is characterized by structural neuronal organization and maturation.[26] Beginning in the fetal period and continuing postnatal is a time of myelination (see Table 6.2-1).

Initially, the embryonic cerebral vesicle is composed of a single layer of neuroepithelial cells, the primitive germinal matrix (ventricular zone). However, at 5 weeks postconception, the forebrain is composed of two layers because of cellular proliferation and migration. At this time, there is a deep neuroepithelial layer and more superficial layer, known as the preplate.

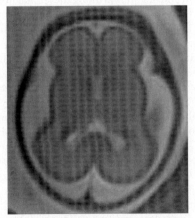

**FIGURE 6.2-13:** Axial T2 image at 25 weeks with prominent but normal extraaxial fluid spaces.

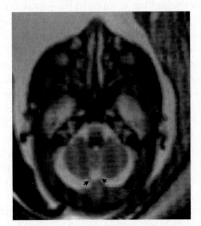

**FIGURE 6.2-14:** Axial T2 image at 24 weeks, there are thin septations paramidline (*arrows*) that are septal leaflets remnant of Blake pouch.

Pallium ⟶ Cerebral cortex

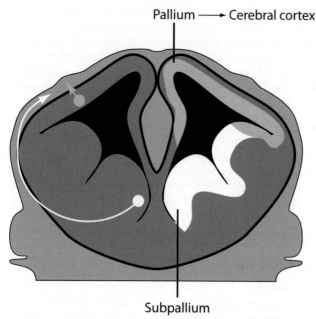

Subpallium

**FIGURE 6.2-15:** Cortical development and neuronal migration.

Subventricular zone    Ventricular zone

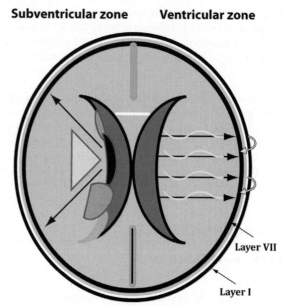

Layer VII

Layer I

**FIGURE 6.2-16:** Cerebral cortical development ventricular zone and subventricular zone. **Ventricular zone (right side):** Migration from the ventricular zone demonstrate neurons traveling radial from the ependymal surface of the lateral ventricles (*purple lining ventricles*) with guidance of radial glial cells (*yellow curvy lines*) to the cortex. The neurons then migrate in an inside-out configuration (*yellow curved arrows*) after splitting the preplate into layers I and VII. **Subventricular zone (left side):** The cells avoid the striatum (*light tan*) and thalamus (*brown*) and migrate tangentially from the medial ganglionic eminence (*red*). The lateral ganglionic eminence is light blue and caudal orange. The SVZ cells also line the entire ventricular surface (*dark purple*).

The development of the preplate is considered the beginning of neurogenesis. These cells rather than arising from the ventricular zone (VZ) migrate from the basal telencephalon and travel tangentially to arrive below the pia before neural tube closure is complete.[27] After the formation of the preplate, the deep neuroepthelial area, also known as the VZ, gives rise to cortical projection neurons with long axons that migrate along radial glial cells.[28] These neurons extend to the preplate, separating it into a thin superficial (future layer I of the cortex or marginal layer) and large deeper subplate zone, also known as layer VII (Fig. 6.2-16). This splitting occurs at the end of the first 8 weeks and marks the transition from the embryonic to the fetal period.[26] With migration of these cells, the white matter, known as the intermediate zone, becomes evident. Also with continued proliferation and intense mitotic activity, the VZ gives rise to a secondary germinal matrix termed the subventricular zone (SVZ) at 7th week gestation.[29]

The VZ cells are direct descendant neurons for the cerebral cortex.[28] Continuing to 14 weeks, waves of glutaminergic projection (pyramidal) neurons arising from the VZ migrate mainly along specialized radial glial cells to form layers of the cortex in an inside out manner, with the first neurons residing in the deep layers and later migrating neurons in the superficial layer of the cortex.[29] The marginal zone, composed largely of Cajal–Retzius neurons, secretes a protein, Reelin, which is required for normal inside to outside positioning of the cells.[4] The subplate contains pioneer projection neurons. With migration of VZ neurons, further differentiation of the cortical plate and subplate will occur.

Initially, the VZ is the source of neurons in the embryonic and early fetal period, but at approximately 15 weeks, the task is transferred to the SVZ, which will lie superficial to the VZ and deep in developing white matter, known as the intermediate zone. The SVZ is a highly proliferative and heterogeneous zone that contributes to both neurogenesis and gliogenesis.[30] The SVZ becomes the remaining source of neurons for the cortex, deep gray nuclei and supplies subplate and interneurons to other areas of the brain, which result in the formation of the transient subplate layer (see Fig. 6.2-16).[30] The SVZ is also a site of proliferation of astrocytes and oligodendrocytes.

The SVZ is complex and can be histologically difficult to separate from the deep VZ. The SVZ can be separated into medial and lateral compartments. The medial compartment includes the ganglionic eminences (GEs) and subependymal ventricular area cells (Fig. 6.2-16). The lateral compartment is made up of a less cellular fiber-rich area medial and a more superficial cellular zone of cells.[30] The less cellular area of the lateral compartment will become part of the periventricular fiber-rich zone, whereas the lateral cellular area will merge into the intermediate white matter layer (Fig. 6.2-18).

The cells in thickened GE are small and compact, and lie along the lateral walls of the frontal and to a lesser extent temporal/occipital horns of the lateral ventricles. Two eminences lie along the subpallium and are present along the frontal horns. The medial, derived from the diencephalon, lies closer to midline at the level of the globus pallidus near the developing third ventricle, and the lateral, derived from the telencephalon, is adjacent but continues along the frontal horn more superior. The caudal GE lies along the temporal/occipital horns. Thin layers of dense SVZ cells are also present diffusely along the ventricles superficial to the VZ in the subependymal layer (see Fig. 6.2-16).[31,32]

The medial and, to a lesser extent, lateral GE contribute cells for the developing neocortex.[32] Cells from primarily the medial GE of the SVZ migrate tangential, providing interneurons to the neocortex up till 20 weeks' gestation.[32,33] Twenty percent of the cells of the human cortex are supplied by SVZ interneurons and during migration astrocytes provide the primary support.[1] Cortical interneurons arising primarily from the medial GE avoid areas of the developing striatum.[28] The complex migration of these cells to the cerebral cortex is complete by 24 weeks.[26]

Caudal and, in a lesser amount, medial GE cells are also a source of neurons for the hippocampus and amygdala.[32]

The lateral and medial GE provides neurons for the striatum until 25 weeks.[32] The medial GE gives rise to neurons of the globus pallidus. The lateral gives rise to the caudate and putamen. But the caudal GE also provides neurons for the posterior striatum and globus pallidus.[32] The medial, lateral, and caudal GE contribute to the development of the thalamus.[32] The dorsal thalamus develops from 15 to 34 weeks' gestation via a transient fetal structure beneath the thalamic surface called the gangliothalamic body.[31,34] The gangliothalamic body extends from the GE to the thalamus and to form GABA-producing cells that migrate tangentially to form association nuclei, such as the pulvinar and mediodorsal as well as anterior (limbic) and other relay nuclei. GEs and originating structures are listed in Table 6.2-3.

The cells lining the ventricular wall are incompletely understood but likely give rise to neurons in the olfactory bulb.[30] Superficial to the ventricular cells is a zone of cell scarcity followed by a more lateral region of increased cellularity, with cells in this region being a major source of glial cells for the developing cortex, striatum, and white matter.[32] The VZ, after depletion at about 27 weeks, transforms into ependymal cells, while the involution of the GE at approximately 34 to 36 weeks results in a subependymal layer.[30,31] Small quantities of pluripotent SVZ cells persist along the ventricular walls into adulthood, including a population along the rostral lateral ventricle that generates olfactory neurons after birth.[35]

Following proliferation and migration, cortical organization and differentiation occur. The subplate is a transient layer formed by the preplate split and important for cortical organization (see Fig. 6.2-17). The subplate, representing layer VII of the

| Table 6.2-3 | Ganglionic Eminences and Originating Structures |
|---|---|
| **Eminence** | **Originating Structures** |
| Lateral | Caudate, putamen, olfactory, late neocortical interneurons, glial cells |
| Medial | Globus pallidus, basal nucleus of Meynert, most striatal interneurons, neocortical, hippocampal interneurons, GABA thalamic nuclei, glial |
| Caudal | Amygdaloid and thalamic nuclei Hippocampal and interneuron cortex |

developing cortex, is comprised of one of the oldest populations of neurons in the developing forebrain as well as neurotransmitters, abundant hydrophilic extracellular matrix and transient synapses.[29] This layer is thickest between 27 and 29 weeks and disappears at 32 to 34 weeks after conception.[36] The function of the subplate is not fully understood but presumed to be a waiting compartment for afferent fibers, especially from the thalamus but also brainstem nuclei and the contra and ipsilateral hemisphere, that are destined to synapse with the developing cortex, thus building a framework for cortical columnar organization.[36] The subplate is also a reservoir for maturing neurons. Remnants of this layer remain postnatal as interstitial neurons in the destined subcortical white matter.[36]

During organization and maturation from 28 to 40 weeks, differentiating neurons will emit axons that will guide cellular progression to a specific target, with which neurons will establish a specialized junction termed a synapse. Many connections occur to areas such as the thalamus, brainstem, cerebellum, and spinal cord, resulting in a complex axonal network. The cortex will organize in six final vertical layers, with each containing a specific neuron and network. For example, layers II and III will connect with the ipsilateral or contralateral cortex, layer IV is afferent from the thalamus and VI efferent to the thalamus, and V provides connection with structures other than the thalamus. These changes result in further development of the cortex with the appearance of sulci and increase in brain weight and volume.[1]

The prospective central white matter, referred to as the intermediate layer, is generated by the VZ at 8 weeks, but increases dramatically in size from 13 to 20 weeks GA.[37] Immature glial cells and migrating neurons pass through this area to reach their final cortical destinations.[38,39] Since neurons need several weeks to reach their final destination, radial neurons and tangential migrating neurons can be simultaneously present in the intermediate zone. This zone also contains growing axonal pathways. Growing thalamocortical fibers form an extensive system that interacts with the subplate and SVZ periventricular-rich zone. Glial progenitors from the SVZ migrate into the WM and give rise to oligodendrocytes and astrocytes. The astrocyte cells are needed to guide neuronal migration and support the oligodendrocytes before the onset of myelination. The oligodendrocyte progenitor differentiates into the preoligodendrocytes, which makes up 90% of the population until 28 weeks.[40] The astrocyte in contact with the oligodendrocyte cell plays a major role in initiation of the myelination process (also known as myelination gliosis). The preoligodendrocytes will begin proliferation and ensheathment of the neuronal axons. In a term infant,

**5 layer (20–28 wk)**        **3 layer (<20 wk)**

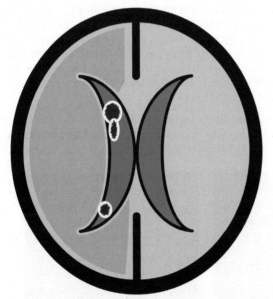

**FIGURE 6.2-17:** The layers of the fetal brain less than 20 weeks, and between 20 and 28 weeks. **Less than 20 weeks or three layer:** germinal matrix (*purple along ventricles*), intermediate layer (*gray*), and cortex (*dark peripheral purple*). **20 to 28 weeks or 5 layer pattern:** subependymal germinal matrix of SVZ (*purple along ventricles*), ganglionic eminences (*starry structures*), periventricular-rich zone or cell sparse layer of the SVZ (*light gray by ventricles*), intermediate zone containing cell dense SVZ (*light purple*), subplate (*outer light gray*), and cortex (*dark peripheral purple*).

50% of preoligodendrocytes have differentiated into immature oligodendrocytes. These cells are important in the continued encasement of the axons, resulting in directionality of water diffusion.[40]

Two important white matter tracts to discuss include the internal capsule and pyramidal (corticospinal tracts), both of which are phylogenetically older than the corpus callosum.[29] The internal capsule is visible in the late embryonic period, being mainly derived from the subplate and shaped by the developing thalamus.[41] The pyramidal tracts also are derived from the subplate and decussation of these fibers occurs early by 17 GW.[42] From 17 to 24 weeks, the internal and external capsules continue to grow. From 20 to 30 weeks, periventricular crossroads become evident, representing areas of crossing efferent, afferent, associative, and callosal fibers.[43] From 24 to 34 weeks, the corona radiata develops because of enlargement of the thalamocortical, commissural, and associative fibers. As the afferent fibers relocate from the subplate to the cortex, the white matter architecture changes from predominately tangential to radial, and sulcation becomes active.[43]

### Imaging

The fetal brain changes and grows considerably from 16 weeks to term. Fronto-occipital, brain biparietal, and bone biparietal measurements increase and can be compared with normative values (see Table 24 Appendix A1) to assure normal growth. The brain parenchymal signal changes with gestational age, as discussed below.

**16 to 20 Weeks:** The appearance of the fetal brain reflects the embryology in its development. Imaging prior to 20 weeks tends to demonstrate a three-layer pattern likely because of the limited spatial resolution in the presence of a small fetal brain.[39,44] The three layers include, from deep to superficial, the germinal matrix, fetal white matter, and cortex (Fig. 6.2-17). The three-layer pattern on T2 imaging is comparable to an oreo cookie, dark on the ends and white in the middle (Fig. 6.2-18A,B):

- Germinal matrix, composed of ventricular and SVZ GEs, is high in cellularity, and demonstrates T1 hyperintensity and T2 hypointensity. Because of high cellularity, the germinal matrix demonstrates a high T2 trace and low ADC (Fig. 6.2-19).
- Intermediate zone (premature white matter) shows higher water content owing to lack of myelination and appears low on T1 and high on T2. Because of low cellularity, the

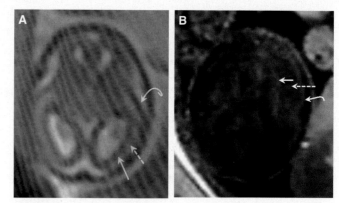

**FIGURE 6.2-18: A:** Axial T2 image of a 17-week fetus with three-layered pattern. *Solid arrow* is germinal matrix, *dotted arrow* intermediate zone or white matter, and *curved arrow* cortex. **B:** T1 axial image of fetus showing hyperintense germinal matrix *(solid arrow)* and cortex *(curved arrow)* and dark white matter *(dotted arrow)*.

intermediate zone demonstrates a low T2 trace and high ADC (see Fig. 6.2-19).
- Cortex is similar to the germinal matrix owing to high cellularity and demonstrates high T1 and low T2 signal. Because of high cellularity, the germinal matrix demonstrates a high T2 trace and low ADC (see Fig. 6.2-19).

At this early gestation, the germinal matrix is thick due to high neuronal proliferation and incomplete migration. The VZ and SVZ cannot be separated, but prominent thickening is noted at the GEs at the caudothalamic groove and along the temporal/occipital horn, creating a "C" configuration (Fig. 6.2-20A,B). These areas should not be mistaken for hemorrhage. The germinal matrix should be smooth without nodularity. The cortex of the brain is thin owing to incomplete development.

**20 to 30 Weeks:** From approximately 20 to 28 weeks, there is a five-layered pattern observed (see Fig. 6.2-17).[39,44–49] The five-layer pattern on T2 imaging appears similar to a double oreo cookie, being dark, white, dark, white, and dark from germinal matrix to cortex (Fig. 6.2-21A,B). During this time, the subplate is clearly evident. On fetal MRI, from central to peripheral the pattern shows:

- *Germinal matrix* includes both the VZ and the GEs of the SVZ. The GEs appear as pronounced areas of thickening primarily along the frontal but also, to a lesser extent, along

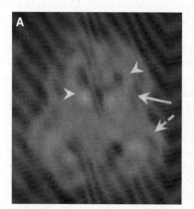
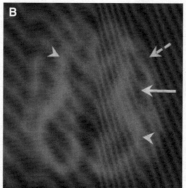
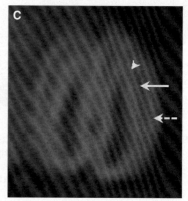

**FIGURE 6.2-19:** Diffusion of the fetal brain at 19 weeks. **A, B,** and **C** show high T2 trace in germinal matrix *(arrowheads)* and cortex *(dotted arrows)* and low in the intermediate zone *(solid arrows)*.

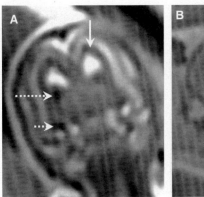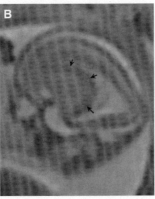

**FIGURE 6.2-20: A:** Coronal image of fetus at 17 weeks GA. The germinal matrix *(solid arrow and dotted arrows)* is very thick and prominent. The ganglionic eminences medial/lateral *(dotted long arrow)* and caudal *(dotted short arrow)* are large and can simulate hemorrhage. **B:** On sagittal oblique T2 imaging, the germinal matrix *(arrows)* has a "C" configuration in this 20 week fetus.

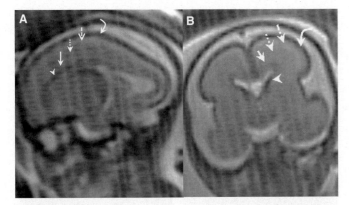

**FIGURE 6.2-21:** Fetus at 25 weeks' gestation sagittal **(A)** and coronal **(B)** T2 imaging. The brain is five layered with dark thin germinal matrix *(arrowheads)*, thin high-signal periventricular-rich zone *(solid arrows)*, dark intermediate zone *(dotted arrow)*, thick high T2 signal subplate *(dot dash arrows)*, and thick cortex *(curved arrows)*.

the temporal/occipital horns. Because of the high density of cellular nuclei, this area appears hyperintense on T1 and hypointense on T2-weighted imaging. On diffusion sequences, the DW images show high signal and ADC low signal due to high cell density, radial organization, and microvascularity.[50] Fractional anistropy (FA) shows inverse correlation with gestational age owing to loss of proliferating radially oriented cells leaving the germinal matrix and migrating to the cortex.[51]

■ *Subventricular-periventricular fiber-rich zone* (most medial lateral compartment of the SVZ) is cell sparse and demonstrates a low signal on T1 imaging and a high signal on the T2-weighted images. The fibers in this area are primarily derived from the corpus callosum with a small contribution from those which merge with the fountainhead of the internal capsule.[43] Diffusion signal changes in this area are difficult to separate from the adjacent intermediate zone, but visually on imaging appear low signal on DW and high on ADC.[52]

■ *Subventricular cellular/intermediate zone* represents the fetal white matter that medially contains cellular areas of the SVZ and is marginated laterally by the external capsule. Thalamocortical fibers are tangentially oriented in the intermediate

zone. Because of the migrating glia, astrocyte, and neuronal cells, this layer appears slightly hypointense T2 and hyperintense T1 signal.[49] At this time, the DW image is slightly bright and ADC lower.[52] After 22 weeks, the neuronal and glial cell population diminishes, and there is an increase in projecting fibers and acid mucopolysaccharide resulting in higher T2 and lower T1 signals. The ADC values show a slow decline with increase in FA with gestation, which may reflect organization of the white matter and axons.[53,54]

■ *Subplate* contains abundant hydrophilic extracellular matrix. Because of the high water content, the area appears hyperintense on T2 images and hypointense on T1. The DW is low signal with a corresponding medium signal on ADC.[50] After 25-week gestation, the hydrophilic extracellular matrix diminishes in conjunction with the thalamocortical neuron accumulation in the upper part of the subplate before relocating to the cortex. Because of this, the FA values are low but increase from 18 to 25 weeks.[55]

■ *Cortical plate*, similar to the germinal matrix, is dark T2 and bright T1 signal owing to high cellularity. The cortex thickens with increasing gestational age owing to an increase in cell number and organization of the six cellular layers. The DW is high in signal and ADC has low intensity. The FA values increase from 15 to 26 weeks consistent with migration and radial organization of the cells. After 27 weeks, the FA in the cortex is noted to decline, likely reflecting alteration in radial organization due to elaboration of dendrites, formation of synapses, and proliferation and transition of glia to astrocytes.[51]

In the developing fetal WM, encompassing the subventricular periventricular fiber-rich, intermediate and subplate zone, there are identified six periventricular crossroads that represent areas of major intersecting developing fibers. These crossroads can be identified by 22-week GA and contain axonal guidance material and abundant hydrophilic extracellular matrix like the subplate, and are thus decreased signal on T1 and hyperintense on T2 imaging. Six locations are described: lateral margin of the frontal horn and body of lateral ventricle, frontal along the dorsal aspect of the lateral ventricle, frontal inferolateral to the frontal horn and ventral to the putamen, occipital crossroad lateral to the atrium/occipital horn, the parietal crossroad anterolateral to the atrium and centered over the retrolenticular internal capsule and the temporal anterolateral to the temporal horn (Fig. 6.2-22A).[43] The two main

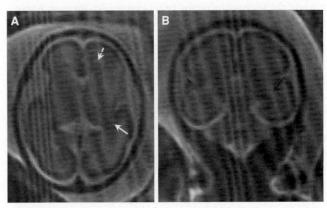

**FIGURE 6.2-22:** Periventricular crossroads. **A:** Axial T2 image in fetus at 26 weeks showing periventricular crossroad lateral to the atrium *(solid arrow)* and adjacent to the frontal horns *(dotted arrow)*. **B:** Coronal T2 image demonstrates focal hyperintense areas adjacent to the atrial horns.

crossroads that are most evident on fetal imaging are the frontal, lateral to frontal horn, and posterior at the fountainhead of the anterior and posterior limb of internal capsule, also known as Wetterwinkel (Fig. 6.2-22B).[44]

At 28 weeks, the SVZ/VZ decreases in size as the neurons migrate to their respective sites. As the germinal matrix decreases in size, the hydrophilic extracellular matrix in the subplate and periventricular crossroads decreases. At the same time, there is a decline in migrating neurons in the intermediate zone, which results in blurring and loss of the multilayer pattern.[49,55] However, the multilayer pattern often persists longer in the frontal and anterior temporal lobes because of persistence of the subplate, following known developmental patterns of myelination and sulcation such that more primitive functions develop earlier and higher cortical functions later.[36] As a result, the subplate in the anterior temporal lobes can persist to 30 to 32 weeks.[3]

**30 to 40 Weeks:** After 30 weeks, there is continued blurring and loss of the multilayer pattern. The germinal matrix completely surrounds the ventricular walls until 30 weeks' gestation.[46] At approximately 33 weeks, small rests of the GE persist caudothalamic and in the roof of the temporal horn and lateral wall of the occipital horn (Fig. 6.2-23A). Germinal matrix becomes increasing less evident with small persistent areas of cells at the caudate heads in the GEs till approximately 36 weeks to 2 months postnatal (Fig. 6.2-23B). Thus, the layered pattern is only three in areas of residual GE and appears as two layered, white and cortical gray, in most areas of the fetal brain.[39] From 28 to 40 weeks, the white matter, including corona radiata, increases in size. The development of the white matter is associated with high ADC values that decline with increasing gestational age, except, to a lesser extent, frontal WM.[56,57] These changes reflect WM maturation related to reduced water content and increase in lipid and macromolecules important for myelination. The cortex of the brain reaches maximum thickness and gyration/sulcation is increasingly evident.

### Deep Gray Nuclei

#### Embryology
As described above, the striatum (caudate and putamen) and globus pallidus arise through tangential migration of neurons from the GEs. The thalamus originates as part of the diencephalon and the telencephalon via cells from the GE through a transient structure known as the gangliothalamic body.

#### Imaging
The basal ganglia are variable in signal depending on gestational age. The thalamus and pallidum are isointense on T1- and T2-weighted imaging when compared with the internal capsule and WM before 27 weeks (Fig. 6.2-24A). Though not well described, the superior thalamus may demonstrate accentuated T2 hyperintensity early before 22 and 24 weeks (Fig. 6.2-24B). After 28 weeks, the pallidum and thalamus appear hyperintense on T1 and hypointense on T2 imaging (Fig. 6.2-24C). The putamen and caudate are T1 hypointense and T2 hyperintense with regard to the internal capsule until 34 weeks. After that time, similar to the thalamus and pallidum, the two structures appear high on T1 and dark on T2 imaging (Fig. 6.2-24D).[39] With change in signal of the basal ganglia and thalamus, the internal capsule becomes defined as an unmyelinated

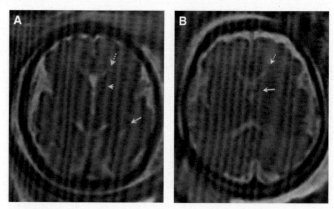

**FIGURE 6.2-23:** 30 to 40 weeks. **A:** Axial T2 image at 33 weeks demonstrating small germinal matrix at the caudothalamic groove *(arrowhead)* and by the temporal horns *(long arrow)*. Note small germinal matrix by frontal horns, which is olfactory in origin and will persist postnatal *(dotted arrow)*. **B:** Axial T2 in 35-week fetus with germinal matrix at caudothalamic groove *(solid arrow)* and by frontal horns *(dotted arrow)*.

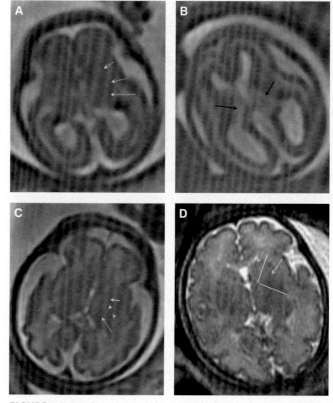

**FIGURE 6.2-24:** Deep gray nuclei. **A:** Axial T2 image at 21 weeks demonstrates homogeneous signal in the basal ganglia and internal capsule *(arrows)*. **B:** Axial T2 in 20-week fetus, with accentuated high T2 signal in the area of the superior thalami *(arrows)*. **C:** Axial T2 image in a fetus at 30 weeks shows the thalamus *(dotted arrow)* and pallidum *(solid arrow)* being hypointense with regard to the internal capsule *(arrowheads)*. **D:** Axial T2 at 36 weeks shows caudate *(dotted arrow)* and putamen *(solid arrow)* hypointense on T2-weighted imaging, and there is clear definition of the T2 hyperintense internal capsule *(straight lines)*.

T1 hypointense and T2 hyperintense structure. Diffusion ADC values decrease in the basal ganglia and thalamus with advancing gestational age related to the increase in neuronal cell density.[53,56,57]

## COMMISSURES/CORPUS CALLOSUM

### Embryology

Commissures are bundles of white matter that connect structures on both sides of the central nervous system (Fig. 6.2-25). The commissures develop in the area of the supratentorial brain in closest apposition to the anterior wall of the third ventricle or lamina terminalis. At 5 weeks, in the upper/dorsal area of the lamina terminalis, active cellular proliferation results in a joining plate, also known as the lamina reunions of His. There are three main commissures: the anterior (olfactory and inferior temporo-occipital cortex), hippocampal (hippocampal and posterior neocortex), and corpus callosum (hemispheric neocortex). The anterior commissure forms from the ventral lamina reuniens during weeks 8 and 9. The hippocampal commissure arises in the dorsal lamina reuniens at 9 to 11 weeks.[13]

The development of the largest commissure, the corpus callosum, is initiated at 10 weeks in the interhemisphere midline, which is filled with primitive meninges. Deeping in the interhemispheric fissure results in a cleft, known as the sulcus medianus telencephali medii, which is in continuity with the upper lamina reunions of His. The banks of this groove approximate and form the massa commissuralis. Glial and neuronal cells migrate medially from the SVZ to midline to form a glial sling/zipper at the corticoseptal boundary.[14] These cells express surface molecules and secrete chemicals that will guide axons across the midline. Two specialized glial structures also direct axons to the midline and glial sling. These include the indusium griseum glia anterior at the corticoseptal boundary and the other below is the glial wedge along the dorsomedial aspect of the lateral ventricle. The glial cell foundations will support the first pioneer axons at 12 to 13 weeks and guide axons across midline by chemoattractive and chemoreplusive factors. During the 13th week, the first axons begin to cross initially arising from the area of the cingulate cortex followed by neocortical areas.[58] At week 14, the corpus callosum is short and stretches from the anterior to the hippocampal commissures, anatomically representing the anterior body of the corpus callosum.[59] From that moment, growth of the structure occurs by addition of fibers. Rather than growing from front to back, as previously described, the corpus callosum grows in as two independent portions with the anterior crossing by the glial sling and the posterior via the hippocampal commissure. The two then meet in the midline posterior body area. However, due to disproportionate growth of the frontal lobes, the hippocampus and splenium are shifted posterior above the posterior third ventricle and the anterior aspect of the corpus callosum appears prominent.[59] Because of this, the anterior sections of the corpus callosum are identified by 14 to 15 weeks and the posterior at 18 to 19 weeks. At the 20th week, the shape of the corpus callosum is final, but only 5% of its mature sagittal section.[14] Continued growth is noted throughout fetal and into postnatal life.

### Imaging

The corpus callosum is present on a sagittal T2-weighted imaging as a uniform thickness hypointense structure superior to the fornix.[44,45] Below 20 weeks, the callosum is short in the midline and rather horizontal in shape (Fig. 6.2-26A). At 20 weeks, the structure shows a crescent shape and can be identified above the septum pellucidum (Fig. 6.2-26B). Its length grows through fetal gestation and normal values are shown in Table 24 of Appendix A1. The rostrum, genu, body, and splenium should be apparent after 20 weeks (Fig. 6.2-26C). The structure is verified on coronal imaging as a crescent of tissue crossing above the walls of the lateral ventricles and the lower margin of the interhemispheric fissure (Fig. 6.2-26D). It is important to separate the corpus callosum from the fornix. The anterior commissure is not well delineated until the third trimester. Crossing fibers of the corpus callosum demonstrate low ADC.[52]

## TEMPORAL LOBE

### Embryology

The hippocampus develops similar to the neocortex with neurons arising from the VZ migrating radial along glial cells and SVZ tangential. The neurons in the developing hippocampus form similar to the cerebral cortex in an inside-out manner.[60] The only significant difference in development of the hippocampus when compared with the neocortex is that the marginal layer (layer I of the cortex) is increased in size containing prominent hydrophilic extracellular matrix, as it is the primary site of afferent synapse formation.[16,60] The subplate layer in the hippocampus is thus significantly thinner.[49,60] White matter tracts of the hippocampus merge and extend to the hippocampal commissure/fornix.

Development of the hippocampal anatomy occurs in fetal life. The hippocampal sulcus is one of the oldest sulci, forming as a shallow structure in embryology around 10 weeks.[61] The sulcus is initially wide and vertical but with growth of the cortex, becomes progressively smaller and more horizontal. By 18 to 24 weeks, the hippocampus has become the typical C-shaped configuration with near complete obliteration of the hippocampal sulcus.[61]

The amygdala is nuclei that develop primarily from the GE of the SVZ. This structure lies anterior to the developing

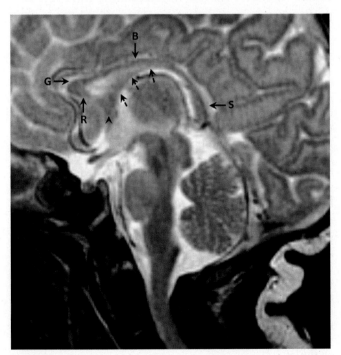

**FIGURE 6.2-25:** Midline commissures in a neonate at 6 days of life. The parts of the corpus callosum are clearly delineated (*R*, rostrum; *G*, genu; *B*, body; and *S*, splenium). The *dotted arrows* represent the fornix/hippocampal commissure and the *arrowhead*, anterior commissure.

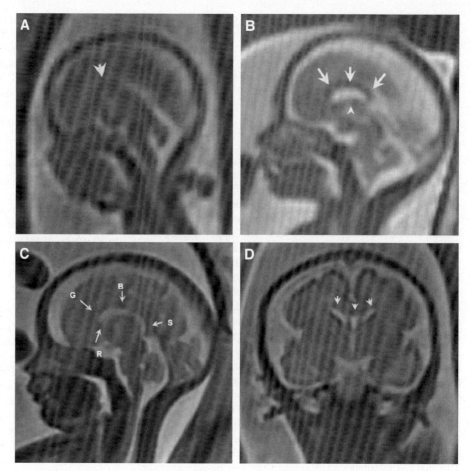

**FIGURE 6.2-26: A:** Sagittal T2 of 16-week fetus. The corpus collosum is seen but short, horizontal, and incompletely formed *(arrow)*. **B:** Sagittal T2 of 21-week fetus. The corpus callosum is crescentic, fully formed but short *(arrows)*. Note the fornix below *(arrowhead)*. **C:** Sagittal T2 of 30-week fetus. The corpus callosum is elongated and C-shaped. All parts are clearly delineated (*R*, rostrum; *G*, genu; *B*, body; and *S*; splenium). **D:** Coronal T2 image of 30-week fetus showing the crossing fibers of the corpus callosum *(arrows)*.

hippocampus. The ventrolateral portion of the amygdala is covered by VZ and SVZ, and the dorsolateral by complex crossroad fibers.

## Imaging

The cortex of the hippocampus demonstrates T1 hyperintensity and T2 hypointensity, as expected. However, the marginal layer (layer I of the cortex) owing to the highly hydrophilic extracellular matrix, can be visualized as a band of T1 hypointensity and T2 hyperintensity.[49] The subplate is small and thus not as well delineated.

The hippocampus is best depicted on coronal T2-weighted imaging (Fig. 6.2-27A). As early as 18 weeks, the hippocampus appears as a slim "C"-shaped T2 hypointense structure along the medial temporal lobe (Fig. 6.2-27B).[44] By 22 to 24 weeks, owing to growth of the cortex, there is progressive infolding, which results in a horizontal orientation of the hippocampal sulcus.[45] After 24 weeks, the hippocampal sulcus is horizontal and nearly completely obliterated, appearing similar to the adult (Fig. 6.2-27C). If measurement is obtained of the infolding angle of the hippocampal sulcus, it is noted that the infolding angle increases with gestational age.[62] Subsequently, the hippocampus increases in thickness and volume.[63] The amygdala is a cellular but inhomogeneous nucleus showing primarily T1 hyperintensity and T2 hypointensity anterior to the temporal horn on coronal T2 imaging and anterior to the hippocampus on axial imaging (Fig. 6.2-27D).[44] The amygdala signal is stable throughout gestation.

## SULCATION

### Embryology

The exact mechanism by which sulcation occurs is still poorly understood. Hypotheses include cortical infolding initiated by cortical differentiation into inner and outer layers,[64] physical tension exerted by axons in the white matter pulling on the developing cortex,[65] or genetic and/or growth factors that shape the cortical surface.[66] It is interesting that the appearance of the primary sulci coincides with the migration of the thalamocortical axons to the cortical plate. The secondary gyri are established with development of corticocortical connections.[47]

### Imaging

Cortical sulcation is one of the most accurate ways to date pregnancy on fetal MRI as it follows a predictable pattern, delayed by an average of 1 to 2 weeks behind the neuropathologic correlative.[5,67,68] A larger lag of 2 to 3 weeks has been described in twin gestations.[5,67] When imaging a fetus, it is important to note that there can be a delay of 2 weeks from the time the sulcus is identified on MRI to when it is present in 75% of fetuses.[69] Cortical sulcation has also proven to be asymmetric, with the right superior temporal gyrus appearing prior to that on the left.[5,70]

On imaging, primary sulci develop first as a shallow depression. With time, the sulcus becomes deeper, and the adjacent surface more angular. Eventually, the sulcus deepens

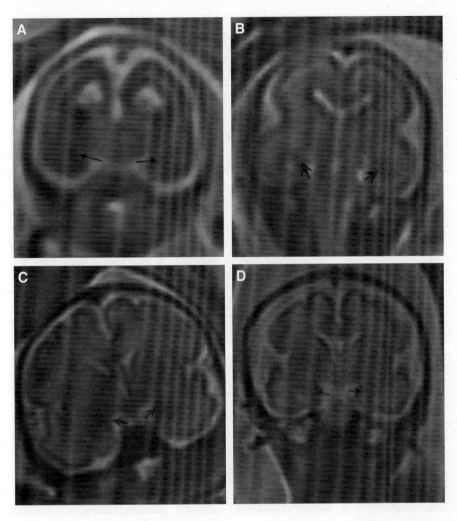

**FIGURE 6.2-27: A:** Coronal T2 of 16-week fetus with open hippocampal fissures and dark oblique hippocampi *(arrows)*. **B:** Coronal T2 21-week fetus with dark C-shaped hippocampus *(arrows)* along the medial temporal lobes. **C:** Coronal T2 of 33 weeks with horizontal hippocampus *(arrows)*. **D:** Coronal T2 of 30-week fetus demonstrating dark T2 amygdala *(arrows)*.

and narrows as the gyrus transforms from a round to square configuration.[71] The primary sulcus with maturation develops branches that become secondary sulci. The secondary sulci will also branch, creating tertiary sulci.[70]

Cortical gyration occurs late in fetal life. In the first half, less than 20 weeks, the brain is smooth and lissencephalic in appearance. In the second half of pregnancy, the brain develops sulci and becomes complex in appearance. The appearance of the fetal brain therefore provides important information with regard to gestational age and can be utilized as a time line for normal fetal development, with sulci identified in 75% of fetuses at ages described below and listed in Table 6.2-4.[67,69] The SSFSE T2 images are very sensitive to detection of the fissures. SSFP sequences can be helpful as there is sharp separation of the CSF from the adjacent cortical indentation.

**14 to 15 Weeks:** Pathologically, the first fissure to develop is the interhemispheric fissure, which appears at 8 weeks, forming anteriorly and extending posterior by 10 weeks. The interhemispheric fissure can be identified as early as 14 to 15 weeks' gestation. The fetal brain is absent of other sulci, smooth in configuration (Fig. 6.2-28A).

**16 Weeks:** The first sulcus to become evident is the sylvian fissure, visualized as a shallow infolding along the surface of the brain (Fig. 6.2-28A).

| Table 6.2-4 | Fetal Sulcation |
|---|---|
| **Gestational Age (wk)** | **New Sulci (Detected in 75% of Fetuses)** |
| 14–15 | Interhemispheric |
| 16 | Sylvian |
| 22–23 | Callosal Parieto-occipital Hippocampal |
| 24–25 | Calcarine Cingular |
| 26 | Central Collateral |
| 27 | Precentral Superior temporal Marginal |
| 28 | Postcentral Intraparietal |
| 29 | Superior frontal Inferior frontal |
| 33–34 | Inferior temporal Occipitotemporal |

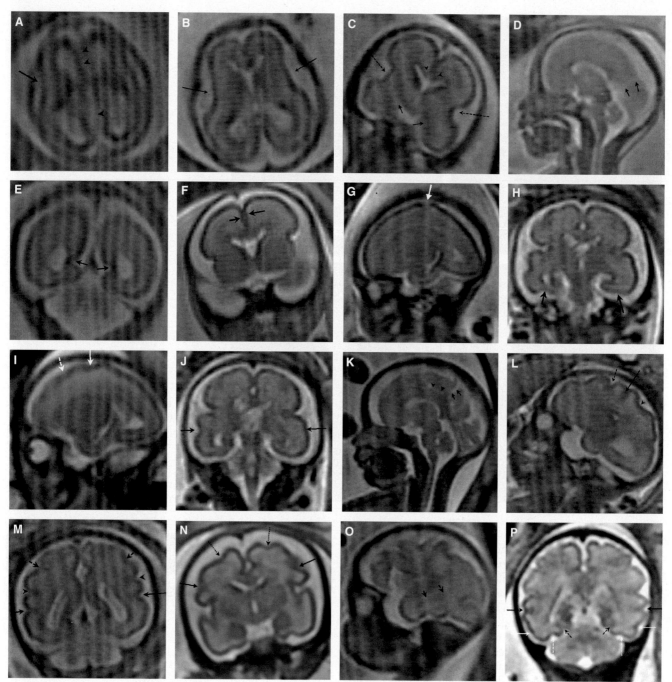

**FIGURE 6.2-28:** SSFSE T2 images of fetal sulcation. **A:** Axial: 16-week fetus with interhemispheric *(arrowheads)* and sylvian fissures *(arrow)*. **B:** Axial: fetus at 20 weeks with deeper sylvian *(arrows)*. Note the brain is still smooth. **C:** Coronal: 23-week fetus with subtle visualization of the callosal *(arrowheads)* and hippocampal fissure *(arrows)*. The sylvian fissure is angular *(dotted arrows)*. **D:** Sagittal: parietal-occipital fissure *(arrows)* in 22-week fetus. **E:** Coronal: calcarine *(arrows)* in 24-week fetus. **F:** Coronal: cingular fissure *(arrows)* in 25-week fetus. **G:** Sagittal: central sulcus *(arrow)* in 26-week fetus. **H:** Coronal: collateral sulcus *(arrows)* in 27-week fetus. **I:** Sagittal: precentral *(dotted arrow)* sulcus at 27 weeks. Note deeper central sulcus *(solid arrow)*. **J:** Coronal: superior sulcus *(arrows)*. Right is more developed than left, which is typical. **K:** Sagittal: the marginal *(solid arrows)* is now noted extending from the cingulate sulcus *(arrowheads)*. **L:** Sagittal: postcentral *(arrowhead)* is shallow in 28-week fetus. Note deep central *(solid long arrow)* and moderately undulated precentral sulcus *(dotted short arrow)*. **M:** Coronal: intraparietal sulcus *(dotted arrows)* is present at 28 weeks. Also note deep posterior sylvian *(arrowheads)* and superior temporal *(solid arrows)*. **N:** Coronal: superior *(dotted arrows)* and inferior frontal sulcus *(solid long arrow)* at 29 weeks. **O:** Sagittal: deep cortical indentation of the superior temporal sulcus *(arrows)* in 30-week fetus. **P:** Coronal: occipitotemporal sulcus *(dotted white arrows)* and subtle inferior temporal *(solid white arrows)* are noted in this 34-week fetus. Note deep superior temporal *(black solid arrows)* and posterior collateral sulcus *(short black dotted arrows)*.

**17 to 21 Weeks:** Only the interhemispheric and sylvian fissures are identified. The sylvian fissure increases in depth with increase in gestational age (Fig. 6.2-28B).

**22 to 23 Weeks:** The callosal, parieto-occipital, and hippocampal fissures can be identified. The callosal and hippocampal fissures are best depicted on coronal imaging (Fig. 6.2-28C). In general, the callosal fissure is more difficult to visualize. The parieto-occipital fissure is defined on the sagittal plane (Fig. 6.2-28D). The sylvian fissure has become angular in configuration with increased formation of the posterior operculum (see Fig. 6.2-28C).

**24 to 25 Weeks:** The calcarine (Fig. 6.2-28E) and cingular fissures (Fig. 6.2-28F) are evident, both best depicted on the coronal plane.

**26 Weeks:** The central sulcus (Fig. 6.2-28G) is identified as a shallow indentation along the lateral aspect of the brain. This sulcus is best depicted on sagittal and axial imaging. The collateral sulcus (Fig. 6.2-28H) is noted, on a coronal sequence, along the inferior temporal lobe.

**27 Weeks:** The precentral sulcus (Fig. 6.2-28I) is seen as a shallow indentation on the lateral aspect of the cerebral hemisphere ventral to the central sulcus. The posterior portion of the superior temporal sulcus (Fig. 6.2-28J) is noted, best depicted on a sagittal or coronal imaging. The marginal sulcus (Fig. 6.2-28K) is also best identified on sagittal imaging, representing a posterior extension of the cingulate sulcus.

**28 Weeks:** The postcentral sulcus (Fig. 6.2-28L) is now identified dorsal to the central sulcus as a lateral indentation along the lateral cerebral hemisphere, best appreciated on axial and sagittal imaging. The intraparietal sulcus, located on the lateral surface of the brain, runs perpendicular and dorsal to the postcentral sulcus, and is best depicted on a coronal or sagittal imaging (Fig. 6.2-28M).

**29 Weeks:** The superior and inferior frontal sulci (Fig. 6.2-28N) are identified best on a coronal imaging.

**30 to 32 Weeks:** By 30 weeks, the central sulcus has extended medially such that it abuts the interhemispheric fissure. The anterior portion of the superior temporal sulcus is now present (Fig. 6.2-28O). There is continued evolution of primary sulcation with development of multiple secondary gyri.

**33 to 34 Weeks:** The inferior temporal sulcus, inferior to the superior temporal, and the occipitotemporal sulcus, medial to the inferior temporal and lateral to the collateral sulcus, are now identified (Fig. 6.2-28P). At 34 weeks, all primary and most of the secondary gyri are present.

**35 to 40 Weeks:** Fetal brain demonstrates an appearance similar to that of a term infant. The sulci continue to deepen, and gyri become square in configuration. Tertiary sulci are evident.

If sulcation is abnormal, follow-up imaging in 4 to 6 weeks should be considered to reassess development. As gyration progresses later in gestation, performing MR imaging in the fetus beyond 25 to 28 weeks typically provides the most information with regard to cortical development. In the United States, this is usually not possible, given legalities with regard to termination.

## PITUITARY AND OLFACTORY BULBS

### Embryology

During ventral induction from 5 to 6 weeks postconception, there is also development of the optic vesicles, pituitary gland and stalk, and olfactory bulbs. The optic chiasm develops from the rostral wall of the diencephalon.[4] The pituitary is derived from two areas: an ectodermal outpouching of the oral cavity, known as Rathke's pouch, and downward extension of the diencephalon through the infundibulum. At 3 weeks, Rathke's pouch appears as an evagination of the stomodeum and grows

toward the infundibulum. By the end of the second month, the tissue loses connection with the oral cavity, and cells proliferate to form the adenohypophysis. The infundibulum gives rise to the stalk and the posterior lobe of the pituitary.[4]

Olfactory bulb development is primarily through stimulation of olfactory sensory afferents that arise in the epithelium of the nasal cavity. These axons project to the rostral forebrain and induce neurogenesis, followed by interneurons that will result in the development of the olfactory bulb.[72] As the bulbs form, cells from the lateral GE SVZ migrate into each bulb along a rostral migratory stream (RMS). The olfactory sulci are horizontal structures separating the medial rectus gyrus and lateral orbital gyrus and are present at 8 weeks. The olfactory sulci are seen at 16 weeks' gestation as initially shallow open indentations.[5] The sulci will increase in depth from a posterior to anterior direction.[5]

The areas of residual GE tissue from the SVZ adjacent to the frontal horns represent RMS. This specialized migratory route along with neuronal precursors continue to travel to reach the olfactory cortex, tract and bulb after birth and may be a source of neurogenesis postnatal.

## Imaging

The normal expansion of the subarachnoid space in the frontal and suprasellar area allows reliable visualization of the optic chiasm, pituitary and olfactory bulbs. As the frontal space decreases later in gestation, olfactory visualization may be more difficult.

### Optic Chiasm/Nerves

The optic chiasm can be seen normally in 89% of fetal cases, increasing significantly in detection with increase in gestational age.[73] Early in gestation, it is often difficult to separate the chiasm from the floor of the third ventricle/hypothalamic tissue (Fig. 6.2-29A). All three planes of imaging are suitable for identification as gestation progresses (Fig. 6.2-29B, C). SSFP imaging can be helpful in evaluation of the optic nerves as the structures are highlighted against the high signal of the adjacent CSF (Fig. 6.2-29D).

### Pituitary Gland and Stalk

The pituitary stalk, a thin T2 and T1 isointense structure, is well delineated on fetal MRI, best detected on sagittal and coronal planes (Fig. 6.2-29B, C).[73] An increase in detection is noted on the basis of gestational age, with sensitivity at 72% below 25 weeks and 100% beyond 26 weeks.[74] The pituitary gland on T2-weighted imaging demonstrates homogeneous hypointensity (Fig. 6.2-29B,C). On T1-weighted images, the gland can be detected in 60% of fetuses and is noted to increase in diameter (2 to 6 mm) with increasing gestational age.[73] Separation of the anterior and posterior lobe is not possible as the gland diffusely demonstrates increased T1 signal, which is similar to the appearance of the normal gland in a neonate (Fig. 6.2-29E).[75] The posterior lobe is felt to be high T1 signal due to neurosecretory granules and phospholipids.[75] At this early age, the anterior lobe is believed to demonstrate high T1 signal due to higher hormonal synthetic activity and less free water molecules.[75]

### Olfactory System

Coronal T2-weighted imaging (SSFP or SSFSE) is the best sequence to detect the olfactory bulbs.[73,76] The bulbs are identified under the ventral frontal lobes as punctate structure with lower T2 signal intensity (Fig. 6.2-29F). The sensitivity in detection of the olfactory bulbs increases with gestation age to approximately 35 weeks, being approximately 85% to 90% between 30 and 34 weeks. After 35 weeks, the detection falls to 66%, likely on account of a decrease in frontal subarachnoid space.[76]

The olfactory sulci are also best delineated on coronal T2 imaging and can be detected in 47% of fetuses prior to 30 weeks. After 30 weeks, the sulci can be identified in 90% to 100% of fetuses (Fig. 6.2-29G).[76] Prior to 31 weeks, the sulci appear open and shallow. From 32 weeks to term, the sulci become progressively deeper, closed and visualized on more anterior slices.[76]

The RMS can be defined from 24 weeks to postnatal as caps of medial low T2 and high T1 signal adjacent to the frontal horns of the lateral ventricles (Fig. 6.2-23A,B).[77]

## INFRATENTORIAL BRAIN

The infratentorial brain is derived from the mesencephalon and the rhombencephalon. The rhombencephalon is further divided into the metencephalon, future pons and cerebellum, and myelencephalon, which will become the medulla oblongata. Although

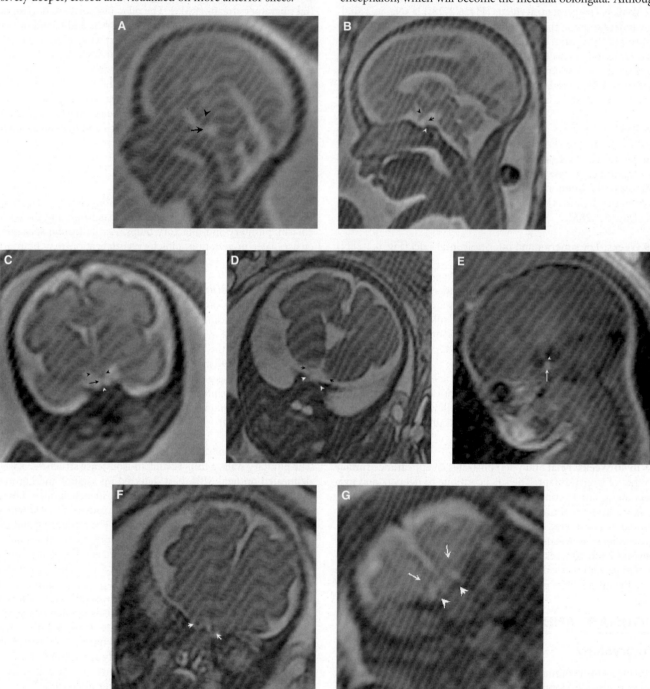

**FIGURE 6.2-29:** Optic chiasm, nerve, pituitary, and olfactory **A:** Sagittal T2 SSFSE in 16 weeks. It is difficult to separate the optic chiasm *(arrowhead)* from hypothalamic tissue. The infundibulum is well delineated *(solid arrow)*. **B:** Sagittal T2 in fetus at 28 weeks showing optic chiasm *(arrowhead)*, infundibulum *(short arrow)*, and dark pituitary *(white arrowhead)*. **C:** Coronal T2 in same fetus with same structures as noted in **B. D:** SSFP coronal image highlights the prechiasmatic optic nerves *(white arrows)*. Also noted are the olfactory bulbs *(black arrows)*. **E:** Sagittal T1 image shows homogeneous hyperintense pituitary gland *(arrow)* and pituitary stalk *(arrowhead)*. **F:** Coronal SSFP in 28-week fetus nicely highlights the olfactory bulbs *(arrows)*. The sulci are not well delineated. **G:** Coronal SSFSE in 34 weeks shows olfactory sulci *(short arrows)* and olfactory bulbs *(arrowheads)*.

each segment has been designated to result in direct growth of these organs, it has recently been discovered that in the mesencephalon at the midbrain–hindbrain boundary, there is an area known as the isthmic organizer, which influences the development of the cerebellar hemispheres, vermis, and pons.[78,79] Recent data have also proved that the cerebellar hemispheres are derived primarily from the metencephalon, while the vermis is derived at least partly from the mesencephalon.[80] As with other regions of the brain, normal development of the brainstem and cerebellum are also dependent on temporal and spatial expression of multiple genes and hormones that are beyond discussion in this book.

## Cerebellum Parenchyma

### Embryology

The cerebellum plays a central role in the coordination of motion and control of balance. The cerebellum is also important in learning and higher cognitive functions. The flocculonodular or vestibulocerebellum participates primarily in balance and spatial orientation via vestibular nuclei. The vermis or spinocerebellum (paleocerebellum) functions mainly to fine-tune body and limb movements via input from the dorsal column of the spinal cord and trigeminal nerve. The cerebellar hemiphers or cerebrocerebellum (neocerebellum) receive input from the cerebral cortex via pontine nuclei and send output to the red nucleus and premotor and primary motor area via the ventral lateral thalamus.

The cerebellar system includes the deep cerebellar nuclei (DCN) that represent efferent pathways for the cerebellum. The cerebellar cortex has five different cellular populations in a 3-layered laminar pattern encompassing from deep to superficial, the granule cell layer (GCL), Purkinje cell layer (PCL), and molecular layer (ML). The dominant neurons are the Purkinje cells and granule cells. The Purkinje cell is the heart of the cerebellar circuit and represents the efferent neurons with projections to the DCN. Although the cell body is primarily present in the PCL, the dendrite arborization spreads out into the ML. The stellate and basket cells in this layer modulate the activity of the Purkinje cell. The granule cells are small, numerous, and spherical but have axons that extend to the ML and bifurcate in a T shape to communicate via parallel fibers with Purkinje dendrites. The precerebellar nuclei are present in the brainstem and represent afferent cerebellar pathways. Two axons that enter from these nuclei outside the cerebellum include the mossy and climbing fibers. The mossy

fibers project directly to the DCN but also connect to granule cells, which then connect via parallel fibers to the Purkinje cell and then finally DCN. The climbing fibers arise from the inferior olivary nucleus and project directly to Purkinje cells and DCN.

The cerebellum is one of the first structures in the brain to develop but one of the last to mature, with cellular organization continuing for many months after birth. The cerebellum develops from two germinal matrix locations: a VZ in the roof of the fourth ventricle and the rhombic lips (Fig. 6.2-30). The VZ provides inhibitory neurons or GABAergic neurons. The cells from the VZ migrate radial with the help of glial cells and give rise to DCN, Purkinje neurons, and interneurons. Additionally, glial cells, specialized ones termed Bergmann glia and oligodendrocytes also arise from the VZ. The rhombic lips are dorsolaterally located in the metencephalon between the roof plate and the neuroepithelium at the caudal aspect of the fourth ventricle and give rise to glutamatergic or excitatory neurons. The cells from the RL travel via tangential migration.[81] Cells arising from the RL include DCN, unipolar brush cells, granule cells, and precerebellar nuclei.[82]

The DCN relay all output from the cerebellar cortex to the cortical and subcortical targets. There are three DCN, the fastigial which receive from the vermis, the interposed (emboliform and globose) from the paravermis and large dentate from lateral cerebellar hemispheres. The first neurons born are the DCN at approximately 5 weeks. Initially, DCN were thought to arise only in the VZ, migrating outward first to form a nuclear transitory zone where they differentiate and then migrate inward to their ultimate location. However, recently it has been determined that RL also give rise to DCN at the same time or slightly earlier than VZ.[83]

The VZ will give rise to the Purkinje cells beginning at 9 to 10 weeks' postconception.[81] The Purkinje cells migrate radial along radial glial cells to their future location.[84] The full number of Purkinje cells is present early, but development of extensive dendritic arbors and synapses will occur up to 24 weeks in the vermis and 30 weeks in the hemispheres.[81] Till after birth, the Purkinje neurons will mature projecting their axons to the DCN. In addition, from late embryonic to postnatal, interneurons will migrate from the VZ to the cerebellar parenchyma in an inside out sequence to give rise to neurons in the DCN, granular layer (Golgi and Lugaro cells), and finally ML (stellate and basket cells). These progenitors continue to divide while migrating through the white matter to their final destination in the nuclei or cortex.[85]

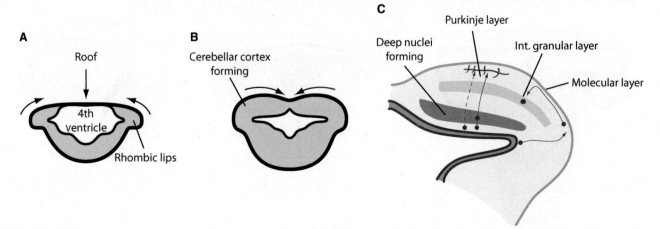

**FIGURE 6.2-30: A:** The germinal matrix of the cerebellum includes the roof of the fourth ventricle and rhombic lips. **B:** With continued growth, the hemispheres form first. **C:** Demonstrates the migration of cells with development of final cell layers, including deep nuclei, internal granular, Purkinje, and molecular.

At the end of the embryonic period, the RL will give rise to unipolar brush cells which, similar to VZ neurons, will colonize the cerebellar white matter before making it to their final home in the internal granular layer.[85] At approximately 11 to 13 weeks, the upper portion of the RL will give rise to granule cell precursors, which will migrate tangentially to the superficial aspect of the cerebellum and form the external granular layer (EGL). The outer EGL will become a germinative zone with proliferative activity, continuing after birth. Granule neuron precursors migrate from the outer to the inner ECL where they become postmitotic.[81] The EGL cells will migrate along Bergmann glia cells to the definitive internal granular layer beginning at 16 weeks. A transient layer known as the lamina dessicans is visible superficial to the IGL and deep to the Purkinje cells from 20 to 32 weeks.[86] This layer acts as a transient zone for proliferating and migrating cells, and disappears first from the archicerebellum and last neocerebellum. The ECL will disappear months to 1 to 2 years after birth, leaving a three-layered cerebellar cortex.[87] The lower RL gives rise to the precerebellar nuclei, including the pontine and inferior olivary nucleus, which will migrate primarily tangential but over complex pathways.[84] These nuclei give rise to major afferent systems, mossy and climbing fibers, which will eventually converge on the Purkinje cells in the cerebellar cortex.

While the rate of differentiation of neuronal groups in the vermis precedes the hemipheres, the overall bulk growth of the vermis lags behind that of the hemispheres.[88] Cortical organization occurs in all areas resulting in the development of dendrites and synapsis to form a functioning neuron.[86]

With the appearance of the pontine flexure at approximately the 5th gestational week, the cerebellum arises due to bending of the fourth ventricle (see Fig. 6.2-4). As this occurs between the 28th and the 32nd postconception day, tissue develops in the form of an inverted V, resulting in a thin roof and dorsal alar plate, which represents the cerebellar primordium, (tuberculum cerebelli) (Fig. 6.2-31).[80,84] At 6 weeks postconception, the tuberculum cerebelli first grows laterally and caudally, giving rise to an inner cerebellar bulge which will represent the hemispheres.

An external bulge will develop in the 7th week, which will represent the flocculi delineated by the posterolateral fissures. This fissure is the first fissure to appear and separates the cerebellum from the flocculonodular lobe.[84] The midline component then accelerates, resulting in the formation of the vermis at 9 weeks.[89] Fissures then begin to form transversely across the cerebellum, first on the vermis and then laterally into the hemispheres. The second fissure to develop, the primary fissure, divides the cerebellar vermis and hemipheres into anterior and posterior lobes and is present by 11 to 12 weeks.[81,84,90] The primary fissure is first identified midline, penetrating deeply into the vermis and extending laterally onto the medial cerebellar hemispheres, where it will remain as a shallow fissure. However, the horizontal fissure is more prominent within the cerebellar hemispheres than the vermis. The vermis and cerebellar hemispheres share the same fissures. Main fissures and nine vermian subdivisions are present at approximately 14 weeks (Fig. 6.2-32).[81] The foliated appearance of the hemispheres is detected by 30 weeks' gestation.[90]

### Imaging

The parenchymal signal of the cerebellum changes as described below.

**16 to 20 Weeks:** The cerebellar hemispheres and the vermis are small but can be identified along the rostral aspect of the fourth ventricle. The hemispheres first enlarge dorsolaterally and later caudolaterally. The cerebellum demonstrates homogeneous intermediate signal from 16 to 19 weeks (Fig. 6.2-33A). The early fastigial point of the fourth ventricle should be visible as a crease along the ventral surface of the developing vermis (Fig. 6.2-33B).[91] The fourth ventricle appears large and is in continuity with the cisterna magna. However, as the vermis grows exophytically from the roof of the rhombencephalic vesicle, the ventricle will decrease in size. The vermis should cover the developing fourth ventricle as early as 18 to 20 weeks.[18,81] At this time, the craniocaudal length of the vermis should be nearly equal to the cerebellar hemispheres.[91] The primary fissure can be recognized by 18 weeks but is better

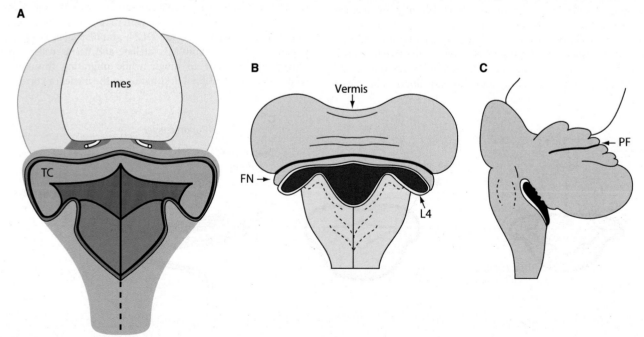

**FIGURE 6.2-31: A:** Below the mesencephalon *(mes)* is the tuberculum cerebelli *(TC)*, which is an inverted V-shaped tissue that will develop into the cerebellum. **B:** The hemispheres and flocculonodular lobe *(FN)* develop first, followed by the vermis. *L4* is lateral recess of fourth ventricle. **C:** First fissure on the vermis is the primary fissure *(PF)*.

appreciated by 20 weeks (Fig. 6.2-33C).[24,81,91] At 20 weeks, the tentorium has a definitive orientation perpendicular to the occipital bone with insertion at the level of the torcula.[81]

**20 to 30 Weeks:** A three-layered pattern in the cerebellum is identified corresponding to the development of the cerebellar cortex, white matter, and DCN (Fig. 6.2-33D).[81,89] From deep to superficial, the layers are as follows:

- *DCN* are highly cellular and appear T1 hyperintense and T2 hypointense.
- *Central cerebellar white matter* is devoid of myelination and mainly water, reflected by low T1 and high T2 signal. The middle cerebellar peduncles appear as low T2 signal between 23 and 26 weeks owing to high cellularity.[44,90]
- *Cerebellar cortex* is highly cellular with neuronal development, demonstrating increased T1 and decreased T2 signal. In the cerebellar cortex, there is lack of anistrophy owing to the many directions of migrating neurons.[44] Progressive decline in mean diffusivity is noted with increasing gestational age, reflecting neuron proliferation and organization.[56,57]

During this time, the fissures of the cerebellum become increasingly evident (Table 6.2-5). The posterolateral fissure that separates the flocculonodular lobe and primary, separating the vermis into anterior and posterior lobes, are present before or by 20 weeks. By 27 weeks, all vermian foliation will be detected (Fig. 6.2-33E, F). The cerebellar hemisphere foliation will follow a few weeks later, appearing between 24 and 29 weeks (Fig. 6.2-33G).[24,81,91]

**30 to 40 Weeks:** The three layered pattern persists but gyration of the DCN results in signal changes such that the central core is T2 hyperintense and peripheral gyri hypointense (Fig. 6.2-33H).[44,90] By 30 to 33 weeks, prominent folia can be identified throughout the cerebellum, although the surface remains smooth.[24,90] By 31 to 32, the flocculi and nodulus are detectable (Fig. 6.2-33I). After 34 weeks, the lateral cerebellum becomes convoluted.

Growth and development of the cerebellum should be assessed by measurements, as between 19 and 37 weeks the cerebellum grossly doubles in diameter.[89] The greatest transverse cerebellar diameter should be obtained via either the axial or the coronal plane (see Table 24 in Appendix A1). The vermis should be measured craniocaudal and anterior to posterior on midsagittal section as greatest height and distance from the fastigium to the posterior surface of the vermis.[89] The tegmento-vermian angle is an excellent way to follow vermian growth. The angle is obtained by drawing a line along the dorsal surface of the brain stem parallel to the tegmentum and should transect at the obex. A second line is drawn along the ventral surface of the vermis. The normal fetal tegmento-vermian angle is close to 0 degrees[91] (Fig. 6.2-34). A significantly elevated angle (>40 degrees) is associated with pathology. Another helpful line is one drawn through the fastigial point and declive (lobule below primary fissure) (Fig. 6.2-35). The anterior and posterior lobes are defined, and normal ratios should be 47% for anterior lobe and 53% posterior lobe or subjectively 1:2.[81,91] After 20 weeks, the vermis lags in growth compared with the hemispheres, so a normal height ratio of the vermis to the hemisphere is on average 0.8 but should definitely be >0.7.[92]

## BRAIN SYSTEM

### Embryology

The brainstem is formed between 6 and 7 weeks postconception and matures caudally to rostrally, thus forming first the medulla, then the pons and finally the midbrain.[44] The brainstem does not mature before the 7th postnatal month. Formation results from direct and indirect migration of cells from the periventricular germinal zones. For the most part, direct migration results in cells destined to become motor and sensory brainstem nuclei.[88] Although the cranial nerves originate very early in the 4th week, their eventual positions change as a result of ingrowth of fiber tracts and migration of neurons from the rhombic lips.[88] The olfactory bulbs arises from the telencephalon and the optic nerves from diencephalon. The oculomotor nerve arises from the mesencephalon. The rest of the cranial nerves are derived from rhombencephalic neuronal precursors.[93]

### Imaging

It is important to evaluate the configuration of the brainstem, which should be straight, and the contour of the pons, which should be rounded at every gestational age (Fig. 6.2-36). The

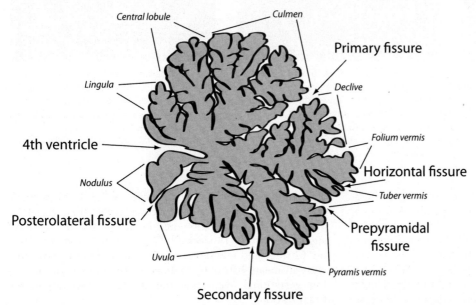

**FIGURE 6.2-32:** Fissures and lobules of the cerebellum with attention to vermis.

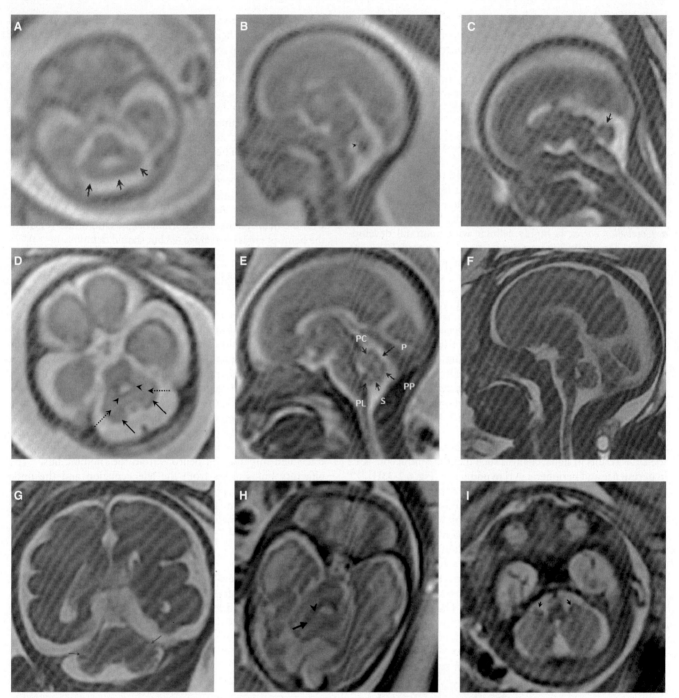

**FIGURE 6.2-33:** SSFSE T2 and SSFP images of cerebellum. **A:** Axial: fetus at 16 weeks with homogeneous cerebellum *(arrows)*. **B:** Sagittal: Fetus at 17 weeks with fastigial point *(arrowhead)* and incomplete coverage of the fourth ventricle by vermis. **C:** Sagittal SSFP: fetus at 19 weeks. Vermis covers the fourth ventricle, and primary fissure is seen *(arrow)*. **D:** Axial: fetus at 24 weeks with three-layered pattern. DCN *(arrowheads)*, white matter *(dotted arrows)*, and cortex *(solid arrows)*. **E:** Sagittal: fetus at 26 weeks with almost all fissures identified. P, primary; PP, prepyramidal; S, secondary; PL, posterolateral; PC, preculminate. **F:** Sagittal SSFP: fetus is 28 weeks. All foliation is present. **G:** Coronal SSFP: fetus at 29 weeks shows prominent foliation of cerebellar hemispheres with deepest being horizontal *(arrows)*. **H:** Axial: fetus at 33 weeks with central high T2 *(arrowhead)* and peripheral dark signal *(arrow)* in the DCN. **I:** Axial image of 34-week fetus. The flocculus lobes are noted *(arrows)*. DCN represents deep cerebellar nuclei.

pons can be measured in the anterior to posterior and craniocaudal dimension (see Table 24 in Appendix A1) to ensure normalcy. The brainstem prior to myelination is overall T2 hyperintense with the exception of hypointense signal in the tectum, especially the inferior colliculus, and the solitary nucleus due to high neuronal cellularity (Fig. 6.2-36).[81,94] The inferior colliculus is the relay station for auditory input and is T2 hypointense as early as 16 weeks but reliably by 20 weeks.

The solitary nucleus/tract is located in the dorsal medulla and receives cardiovascular, visceral, respiratory, gustatory, and orotactile information, and demonstrates decreased T2 signal as early as 18 weeks.[81] The brainstem appears bright on T2 trace and low signal on ADC maps.[52] Progressive decline in mean diffusivity is noted in the pons with increasing gestational age, reflecting neuron proliferation and organization.[56,57]

| Table 6.2-5 | Visualization of Fissures for the Cerebellar Vermis | |
|---|---|---|
| Timing (wk) | Fissure | Landmarks/Adjacent Lobules |
| 20 | Posterolateral | Uvula and nodulus |
| | Primary | Culmen and declive |
| 21 | Prepyramidal | Tuber and pyramis |
| 21–22 | Preculminate | Central and culmen |
| 24 | Secondary/ postpyramidal | Pyramis and uvula |
| 27 | Horizontal | Folium and tuber |

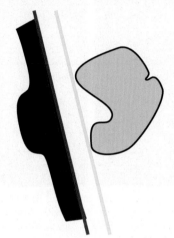

**FIGURE 6.2-34:** Temento-vermian angle should be close to 0 degrees. The tegmentum *(red line)* should be parallel to line drawn along the ventral vermis *(yellow line).*

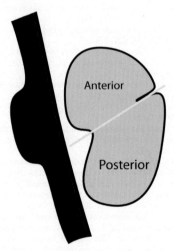

**FIGURE 6.2-35:** Fastigial and declive line *(yellow line)* to separate anterior and posterior lobes.

## MYELINATION

### Embryology

Myelin is an organized multilamellar structure formed by the plasma membrane of the oligodendrocyte. The membrane surrounds neuronal axons and facilitates electric impulse conduction. The process of myelination includes proliferation and

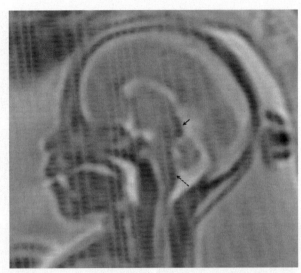

**FIGURE 6.2-36:** Sagittal SSFSE T2 in fetus 21 weeks with homogeneous mainly hyperintense brainstem except dark signal in tectum/inferior colliculus *(short solid arrow)* and medulla/solitary nucleus *(long dotted arrow).* Note that the brainstem is straight and the pons is rounded in contour.

differentiation of oligodendryocytes, proliferation of astrocytes for neuronal support and connection, and increased lipid synthesis via olidgodendrocytes. Myelin is rich in lipids and, to a lesser extent, proteins, and with its development water content decreases. Myelination follows an organized pattern, progressing from caudal to cranial, central to peripheral, and occipital to frontal and then temporal. Areas important to sensory show myelination prior to motor, and projection fibers demonstrate myelination prior to associative fibers.

### Imaging

On fetal MRI, myelination appears high signal on T1 and low signal on T2, likely related to an increase in cholesterol and glycolipid content but also owing to an increase in cellular density. Myelination begins at 12 to 13 weeks in the spinal cord, followed by the brainstem, and progresses cranially.[73] Prior to 18 weeks, the brainstem is homogeneous in signal with the exception of low signal in the tectum.[81,94]

**18 Weeks:** Myelination is noted in the medulla in the ventral ascending sensory tracts and dorsal solitary nucleus tract.[81]

**20 Weeks:** Beginning posterior medial medulla and pons, myelination is noted in the area of the medial longitudinal fasciculus (MLF), medial and lateral lemniscus.[52,94] The medial lemniscus is important for sensory, lateral lemniscus for sound, and the MLF for eye movement and control of the muscles of the neck (Fig. 6.2-37A).

**28 to 29 Weeks:** The inferior and superior cerebellar peduncles are myelinated (Fig. 6.2-37B).[90]

**32 Weeks:** Myelination has reached the dorsal midbrain (Fig. 6.2-37C).[94]

**32 to 33 Weeks:** The inferior colliculus, lateral putamen, and ventrolateral thalami are myelinated (Fig. 6.2-37D).[90] Hyperintense T1 signal may be present as a dot in the posterior limb of the internal capsule.[1,52]

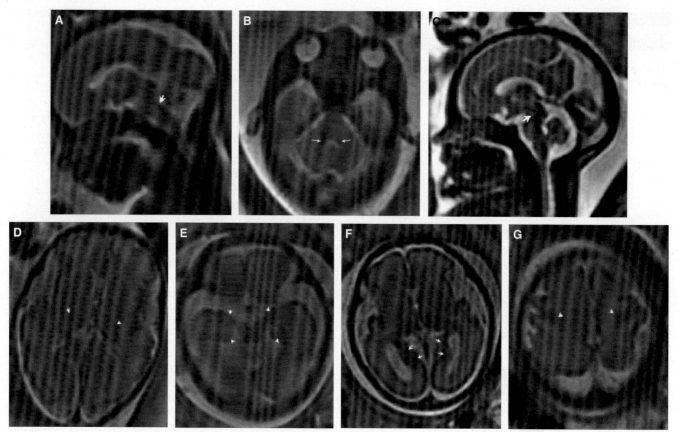

**FIGURE 6.2-37:** T2 imaging in myelination. **A:** Sagittal: fetus at 23 weeks with dark myelination in dorsal brainstem *(arrow)*. **B:** Axial: fetus at 29 weeks with dark myelinated superior cerebellar peduncles *(arrows)*. **C:** Sagittal: fetus at 32 weeks with myelination now dorsal midbrain *(arrow)*. Note myelination along the entire brainstem. **D:** Axial: fetus at 33 weeks with dark signal in posterior lateral thalami *(arrows)*. **E:** Axial: early myelination medial temporal *(arrowheads)*. **F:** Axial: early myelination medial occipital *(arrows)*. **G:** Early myelination perirolandic *(arrows)*.

**35 Weeks:** Hyperintense T1 signal may be present in the posterior limb of the internal capsule.[1,52] The optic tracts show evidence of myelination, and there are similar changes within the perirolandic subcortical white matter.[24] Other areas of high metabolic activity will begin to show myelination in the subcortical white matter of the calacarine, perirolandic and medial temporal lobes during the late fetal period to 2 months postnatal (Fig. 6.2-37E–G).[1]

**38 to 40 Weeks:** The posterior limb of the internal capsule will show focal T2 myelination. The superior vermis is myelinated at term.[90]

## REFERENCES

1. Fogliarini C, Chaumoitre K, Chapon F, et al. Assessment of cortical maturation with prenatal MRI, part I: normal and cortical maturation. *Eur Radiol.* 2005;15:1671–1685.
2. Chung HW, Chen CY, Zimmerman RA, et al. T2-weighted fast MR imaging with true FISP versus HASTE: comparative efficacy in the evaluation of normal fetal brain maturation. *AJR Am J Roentgenol.* 2000;175:1375–1380.
3. Al-Mukhtar A, Kasprian G, Schmook MT, et al. Diagnostic pitfalls in fetal brain MRI. *Semin Perinatol.* 2009;33:251–258.
4. Ten Donkelaar H, Lammens M, Hori A. *Clinical Neuroembryology.* Berlin, Germany: Springer; 2006.
5. Chi JG, Dooling EC, Gilles FH. Gyral development of the human brain. *Ann Neurol.* 1977;1:86–93.
6. Levine D, Trop I, Mehta TS, et al. MR imaging appearance of fetal cerebral ventricular morphology. *Radiology.* 2002;223:652–660.
7. Huisman TA, Martin E, Kubik-Huch R, et al. Fetal magnetic resonance imaging of the brain: technical considerations and normal brain development. *Eur Radiol.* 2002;12:1941–1951.
8. Filly RA, Goldstein RB. The fetal ventricular atrium: fourth down and 10 mm to go. *Radiology.* 1994;193:315–317.
9. Farrell TA, Hertzberg BS, Kliewer MA, et al. Fetal lateral ventricles: reassessment of normal values for atrial diameter at US. *Radiology.* 1994;193:409–411.
10. Twickler DM, Riechel T, Mcintire DD, et al. Fetal central nervous system ventricle and cisterna magna measurements by magnetic resonance imaging. *Am J Obstet Gynecol.* 2002;187:927–931.
11. Garel C, Alberti C. Coronal measurement of the fetal lateral ventricles: comparison between ultrasonography and magnetic resonance imaging. *Ultrasound Obstet Gynecol.* 2006;27:23–27.
12. Garel C. *MRI of the Fetal Brain: Normal Development and Cerebral Pathologies.* Stuttgart, Germany: Springer; 2004.
13. Sarwar M. The septum pellucidum: normal and abnormal. *AJNR Am J Neuroradiol.* 1989;10:989–1005.
14. Raybaud C. The corpus callosum, the other great forebrain commissures, and the septum pellucidum: anatomy, development, and malformation. *Neuroradiology.* 2010;52:447–477.
15. Jou HJ, Shyu MK, Wu SC, et al. Ultrasound measurement of the fetal cavum septi pellucidi. *Ultrasound Obstet Gynecol.* 1998;12:419–421.
16. Falco P, Gabriella S, Visentin A, et al. Transabdominal sonography of the cavum septum pellucidum in normal fetuses in the second and third trimesters of pregnancy. *Ultrasound Obstet Gynecol.* 2000;16:549–553.
17. Blake JA. The roof and lateral recesses of the fourth ventricle, considered morphologically and embryologically. *J Comp Neurol.* 1900;10:78–108.
18. Robinson AJ, Goldstein R. The cisterna magna septa: vestigial remnants of Blake's pouch and a potential new marker for normal development of the rhombencephalon. *J Ultrasound Med.* 2007;26:83–95.
19. Nelson MD, Maher K, Gilles FH. A different approach to cysts of the posterior fossa. *Pediatr Radiol.* 2004;34:720–732.
20. Reichel TF, Ramus RM, Caire JT, et al. Fetal central nervous system biometry on MR imaging. *AJR Am J Roentgenol.* 2003;180:1155–1158.
21. Tilea B, Albert C, Adamsbaum C, et al. Cerebral biometry in fetal magnetic resonance imaging: new reference data. *Ultrasound Obstet Gynecol.* 2009;33:173–181.
22. Parazzini C, Righini A, Rustico M, et al. Prenatal magnetic resonance imaging: brain normal linear biometric values below 24 gestational weeks. *Neuroradiology.* 2008;50:877–883.
23. Garel C. Fetal cerebral biometry: normal parenchymal findings and ventricular size. *Eur Radiol.* 2005;15:809–813.
24. Girard NJ, Chaumoitre K. The brain in the belly: what and how of fetal neuroimaging. *J Magn Reson Imaging.* 2012;36:788–804.

25. Watanabe Y, Abe S, Takagi K, et al. Evolution of subarachnoid space in normal fetuses using magnetic resonance imaging. *Prenat Diagn.* 2005;25:1217–1222.

26. Marin-Padilla M. Origin, formation, and prenatal maturation of the human cerebral cortex: an overview. *J Craniofac Genet Dev Biol.* 1990;10:137–146.

27. Bystron I, Rakic P, Molnar Z, et al. The first neurons of the human cerebral cortex. *Nat Neurosci.* 2006;9:880–886.

28. Marin O, Rubenstein JL. Cell migration in the forebrain. *Annu Rev Neurosci.* 2003;26:441–483.

29. Bystron I, Blakemore C, Rakic P. Development of the human cerebral cortex: Boulder Committee revisited. *Nat Rev Neurosci.* 2008;9:110–122.

30. Zecevic N, Chen Y, Filipovic R. Contributions of cortical subventricular zone to the development of the human cerebral cortex. *J Comp Neurol.* 2005;491:109–122.

31. Del Bigio MR. Cell proliferation in human ganglionic eminence and suppression after prematurity-associated haemorrhage. *Brain.* 2011;134:1344–1361.

32. Brazel CY, Romanko MJ, Rothstein RP, et al. Roles of mammalian subventricular zone in brain development. *Prog Neurobiol.* 2003;69:49–69.

33. Petanjek Z, Dujmovic A, Kostovic I, et al. Distinct origin of GABA-ergic neurons in forebrain of man, nonhuman primates and lower mammals. *Coll Antropol.* 2008;32(suppl 1):9–17.

34. Letinic K, Kostovic I. Transient fetal structure, the gangliothalamic body, connects telencephalic germinal zone with all thalamic regions in the developing human brain. *J Comp Neurol.* 1997;384:373–395.

35. Kam M, Curtis MA, McGlashan SR, et al. The cellular composition and morphological organization of the rostral migratory stream in the adult human brain. *J Chem Neuroanat.* 2009;37:196–205.

36. Kostovic I, Jovanov-Milosevic N. Subplate zone of the human brain: historical perspective and new concepts. *Coll Antropol.* 2008;32(suppl 1):3–8.

37. Samuelsen GB, Larsen KB, Bogdanovic N, et al. The changing number of cells in the human fetal forebrain and its subdivisions: a stereological analysis. *Cereb Cortex.* 2003;13:115–122.

38. Menezes JRL, Luskin MB. Expression of neuron-specific tubulin defines a novel population in the proliferative layers of the developing telencephalon. *J Neurosci.* 1994;14:5399–5416.

39. Brisse H, Fallet C, Sebag G, et al. Supratentorial parenchyma in the developing fetal brain: in vitro MR study with histologic comparison. *AJNR Am J Neuroradiol.* 1997;18:1491–1497.

40. Back SA, Han BH, Luo NL, et al. Selective vulnerability of late oligodendrocyte progenitors to hypoxia-ischemia. *J Neurosci.* 2002;22:455–463.

41. Molnar Z, Blakemore C. How do thalamic axons find their way to the cortex. *Trends Neurosci.* 1995;18:389–397.

42. Eyre JA, Miller S, Clowry GJ, et al. Functional corticospinal projections are established prenatally in the human foetus permitting involvement in the development of the spinal motor centres. *Brain.* 2000;123:51–64.

43. Judas M, Rados M, Jovanov-Milosevic N, et al. Structural, immunocyto-chemical and MR imaging properties of periventricular crossroads of growing cortical pathways in preterm infants. *AJNR Am J Neuroradiol.* 2005;26:2671–2784.

44. Prayer D, Kasprian G, Krampl E, et al. MRI of normal fetal brain development. *Eur J Radiol.* 2006;57:199–216.

45. Glenn OA. Normal development of the fetal brain by MRI. *Semin Perinatol.* 2009;33:208–219.

46. Girard N, Raybaud C, Poncet M. In vivo MR study of brain maturation in normal fetuses. *AJNR Am J Neuroradiol.* 1995;16:407–413.

47. Kostovic I, Judas M, Rados M, et al. Laminar organization of the human fetal cerebrum revealed by histochemical markers and magnetic resonance imaging. *Cereb Cortex.* 2002;12:536–544.

48. Kostovic I, Vasung L. Insights from in vitro fetal magnetic resonance imaging of the cerebral development. *Semin Perinatol.* 2009;33:220–233.

49. Rados M, Judas M, Kostovic I. In vitro MRI of brain development. *Eur J Radiol.* 2006;57:187–198.

50. Maas LC, Mukherjee P, Carballido-Gamio J, et al. Early laminar organization of the human cerebrum demonstrated with diffusion tensor imaging in extremely premature infants. *Neuroimage.* 2004;22:1134–1140.

51. Gupta RK, Hasan KM, Trivedi R, et al. Diffusion tensor imaging of the developing human cerebrum. *J Neurosci Res.* 2005;81:172–178.

52. Girard N, Confort-Gouny S, Schneider J, et al. MR imaging of brain maturation. *J Neuroradiol.* 2007;34:290–310.

53. Righini A, Bianchini E, Parazzini C, et al. Apparent diffusion coefficient determination in normal fetal brain: a prenatal MR imaging study. *AJNR Am J Neuroradiol.* 2003;24:799–804.

54. Glenn O. Contributions of diffusion-weighted imaging to fetal and neonatal imaging. *Top Magn Reson Imaging.* 2011;22:3–9.

55. Widjaja E, Geiprasert S, Mahmoodabadi SZ, et al. Alteration of human fetal subplate layer and intermediate zone during normal development on MR and diffusion tensor imaging. *AJNR Am J Neuroradiol.* 2010;31:1091–1099.

56. Schneider JF, Confort-Gouny S, Le Fur Y, et al. Diffusion-weighted imaging in normal fetal brain maturation. *Eur Radiol.* 2007;17:2422–2429.

57. Schneider MM, Berman JI, Baumer FM, et al. Normative apparent diffusion coefficient values in the developing fetal brain. *AJNR Am J Neuroradiol.* 2009;30:1799–1803.

58. Koester SE, O'Leary DDM. Axons of early generated neurons in cingulate cortex pioneer the corpus callosum. *J Neurosci.* 1994;14:6608–6620.

59. Kier EL, Truwit CL. The normal and abnormal genu of the corpus callosum: an evolutionary, embryologic, anatomic and MR analysis. *AJNR Am J Neuroradiol.* 1996;17:1631–1641.

60. Supèr H, Soriano E, Uylings HBM. The functions of the preplate in development and evolution of the neocortex and hippocampus. *Brain Res Brain Res Rev.* 1998;27:40–64.

61. Kier EL, King JH, Fulbright RK, et al. Embryology of the human fetal hippocampus: MR imaging, anatomy and histology. *AJNR Am J Neuroradiol.* 1997;18:525–532.

62. Righini A, Zirpoli S, Parazzini C, et al. Hippocampal infolding angle changes during brain development assessed by prenatal MR imaging. *AJNR Am J Neuroradiol.* 2006;27:2093–2097.

63. Jacob FD, Habas P, Kim K, et al. Fetal hippocampal development: analysis by magnetic resonance imaging volumetry. *Pediatr Res.* 2011;65:425–429.

64. Richman DP, Stewart RM, Hutchinson JW, et al. Mechanical model of brain: convolutional development. *Science.* 1975;189:18–21.

65. Van Essen DC. A tension-based theory of morphogenesis and compact wiring in the central nervous system. *Nature.* 1997;385:313–318.

66. Lefèvre J, Mangin JF. A reaction-diffusion model of human brain development. *PLoS Comput Biol.* 2010;6:1–10.

67. Levine D, Barnes PD. Cortical maturation in normal and abnormal fetuses as assessed with prenatal MR imaging. *Radiology.* 1999;210:751–758.

68. Garel C, Chantrel E, Brisse H, et al. Fetal cerebral cortex: normal gestational landmarks identified using prenatal MR imaging. *AJNR Am J Neuroradiol.* 2001;22:184–189.

69. Garel C, Chantrel E, Elmaleh M, et al. Fetal MRI: normal gestational landmarks for cerebral biometry, gyration and myelination. *Childs Nerv Syst.* 2003;19:422–425.

70. Kasprian G, Langs G, Brugger PC, et al. The prenatal origin of hemispheric asymmetry: an in utero neuroimaging study. *Cereb Cortex.* 2011;21:1076–1083.

71. Van der Knaap MS, van Wezel-Meijler G, Barth PC, et al. Normal gyration and sulcation in preterm and term neonates: appearance on MR images. *Radiology.* 1996;200:389–396.

72. Fritz A, Gorlick DL, Burd GD. Neurogenesis in the olfactory bulb of the frog xenopus laevis shows unique patterns during embryonic development and metamorphosis. *Int J Dev Neurosci.* 1996;14:931–943.

73. Schmook MT, Brugger PC, Weber M, et al. Forebrain development in fetal MRI: evaluation of anatomical landmarks before gestational week 27. *Neuroradiology.* 2010;52:495–504.

74. Righini A, Parazzini C, Doneda C, et al. Prenatal MR imaging of the normal pituitary stalk. *AJNR Am J Neuroradiol.* 2009;30:1014–1016.

75. Dietrich RB, Lis LE, Greensite FS, et al. Normal MR appearance of the pituitary gland in the first 2 years of life. *AJNR Am J Neuroradiol.* 1995;16:1413–1419.

76. Azoulay R, Fallet-Bianco C, Garel C, et al. MRI of the olfactory bulbs and sulci in human fetuses. *Pediatr Radiol.* 2006;36:97–107.

77. Battin M, Rutherford MA. Magnetic resonance imaging of the brain in preterm infants: 24 weeks' gestation to term. In: Rutherford MA, ed. *MRI of the Neonatal Brain.* pp 1–28. Available at: http://www.mrineonatalbrain.com.

78. Nakamura H, Katahira T, Matsunaga E, et al. Isthmus organizer for midbrain and hindbrain development. *Brain Res Brain Res Rev.* 2005;49:120–126.

79. Basson MA, Echevarria D, Ahn CP, et al. Specific regions within the embryonic midbrain and cerebellum require different levels of FGF signaling during development. *Development.* 2008;135:889–898.

80. Hashimoto M, Hibi M. Development and evolution of cerebellar neural circuits. *Dev Growth Differ.* 2012;54:373–389.

81. Adamsbaum C, Moutard ML, André C, et al. MRI of the fetal posterior fossa. *Pediatr Radiol.* 2005;35:124–140.

82. Fink AJ, Englund C, Daza RA, et al. Development of the deep cerebellar nuclei: transcription factors and cell migration from the rhombic lip. *J Neurosci.* 2006;26:3066–3076.

83. Leto K, Carletti B, Williams IM, et al. Different types of cerebellar GABAergic interneurons originate from a common pool of multipotent progenitor cells. *J Neurosci.* 2006;26:11682–11694.

84. Ten Donkelaar HJ, Lammens M. Development of the human cerebellum and its disorders. *Clin Perinatol.* 2009;36:513–530.

85. Carletti B, Rossi F. Neurogenesis in the cerebellum. *Neuroscientist.* 2008;14:91–100.

86. Ten Donkelaar HJ, Lammens M, Wesseling P, et al. Development and developmental disorders of the human cerebellum. *J Neurol.* 2003;250:1025–1036.

87. Larroche JC. Morphological criteria of the central nervous system development in the human foetus. *J Neuroradiol.* 1981;8:93–108.

88. Yachnis AT, Rorke LB. Cerebellar and brainstem development: an overview in relation to Joubert syndrome. *J Child Neurol.* 1999;14:570–573.

89. Triulzi F, Parazzini C, Righini A. Magnetic resonance imaging of fetal cerebellar development. *Cerebellum.* 2006;5:199–205.

90. Triulzi F, Parazzini C, Righini A. MRI of fetal and neonatal cerebellar development. *Semin Fetal Neonatal Med.* 2005;10:411–420.

91. Robinson AJ, Blaser S, Toi A, et al. The fetal cerebellar vermis: assessment for abnormal development by ultrasonography and magnetic resonance imaging. *Ultrasound Q.* 2007;23:211–223.

92. Kapur RP, Mahony BS, Finch L, et al. Normal and abnormal anatomy of the cerebellar vermis in midgestational human fetuses. *Birth Defects Res A Clin Mol Teratol.* 2009;85:700–709.

93. Barkovich AJ, Millen KJ, Dobyns WB. A developmental and genetic classification for midbrain-hindbrain malformations. *Brain.* 2009;132:3199–3230.

94. Stazzone MM, Hubbard AM, Bilaniuk LT, et al. Ultrafast MR imaging of the normal posterior fossa in fetuses. *AJR Am J Roentgenol.* 2000;175:835–839.

## 16 TO 17 WEEKS

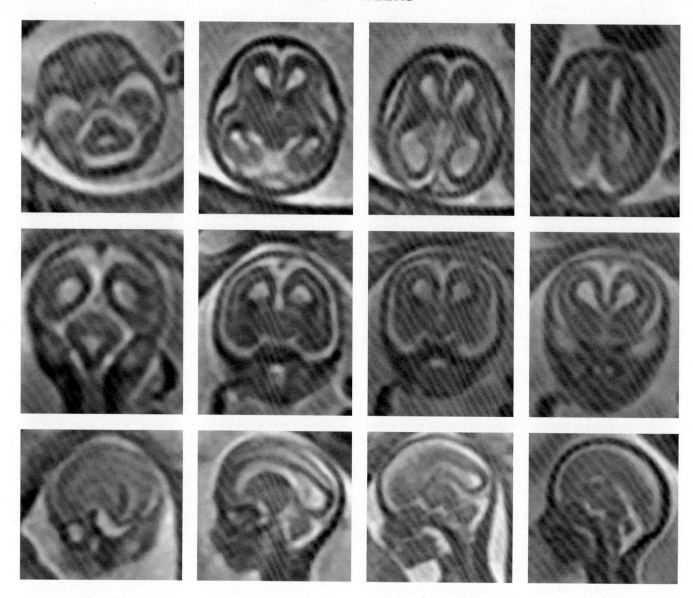

## SUPRATENTORIAL

**SULCATION:** Interhemispheric, slyvian

**PARENCHYMA:** 3 layer

**BASAL GANGLIA:** Difficult to separate from germinal matrix

**GERMINAL MATRIX:** Thick, prominent GE

**CORPUS CALLOSUM:** Short and horizontal

**LATERAL VENTRICLES:** Primitive lateral

## INFRATENTORIAL

**PARENCHYMA:** Homogeneous

**VERMIS:** Incomplete coverage of 4th

  **SULCATION:** Smooth

**CEREBELLAR HEMISPHERES:**

  **SULCATION:** Smooth

**MYELINATION:** Possible medulla

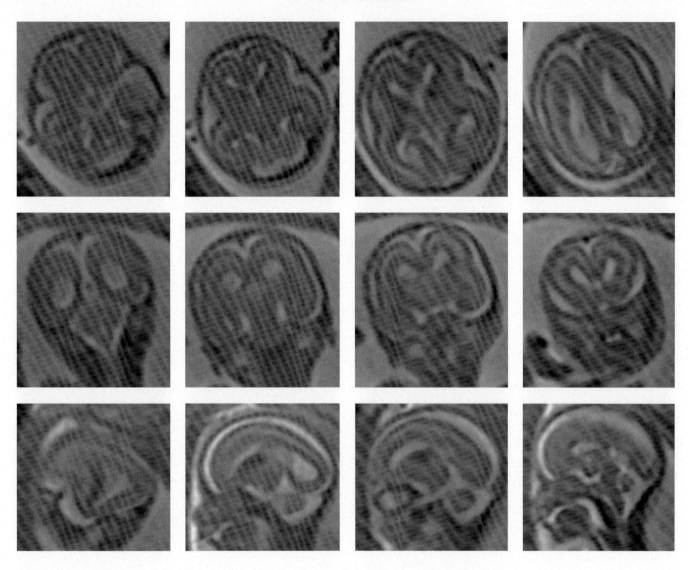

## SUPRATENTORIAL

**SULCATION:** Interhemispheric, sylvian

**PARENCHYMA:** 3 layer

**BASAL GANGLIA:** Homogeneous to white matter

**GERMINAL MATRIX:** Thick, prominent GE

**CORPUS CALLOSUM:** Short

**LATERAL VENTRICLES:** Biconcave frontal, but occipital horns prominent

## INFRATENTORIAL

**PARENCHYMA:** Homogeneous

**VERMIS:** Near coverage of 4th

  **SULCATION: Primary**

**CEREBELLAR HEMISPHERES:**

  **SULCATION:** Smooth

**MYELINATION: Medulla**

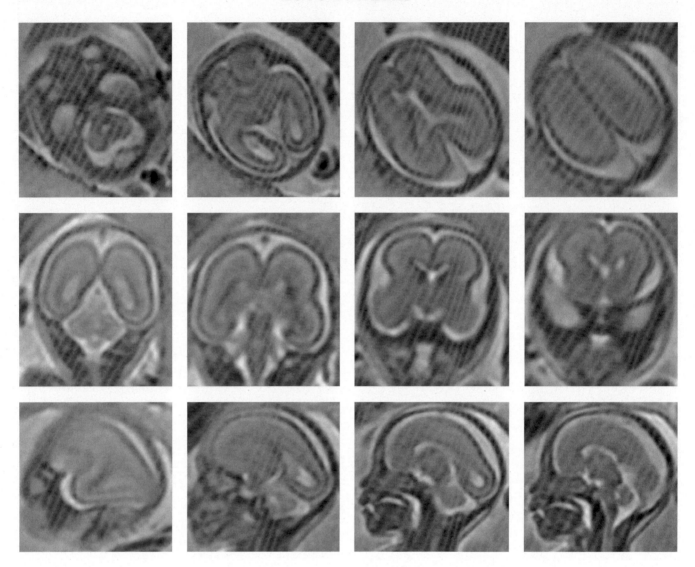

## SUPRATENTORIAL

**SULCATION:** Interhemispheric, **sylvian deepens**

**PARENCHYMA:** 5 layer

**BASAL GANGLIA:** Homogeneous to white matter with thalamus mildly T2 hyperintense

**GERMINAL MATRIX:** Thick, prominent GE

**CORPUS CALLOSUM:** Crescent, short but fully formed

**LATERAL VENTRICLES:** Mature configuration but prominent occipital horns

## INFRATENTORIAL

**PARENCHYMA:** 3 layer

**VERMIS:** Coverage of 4th

   **SULCATION:** Primary, **prepyramidal**

**CEREBELLAR HEMISPHERES:**

   **SULCATION:** **Flocculonodular,** hemispheres smooth

**MYELINATION:** Medulla, **pons**

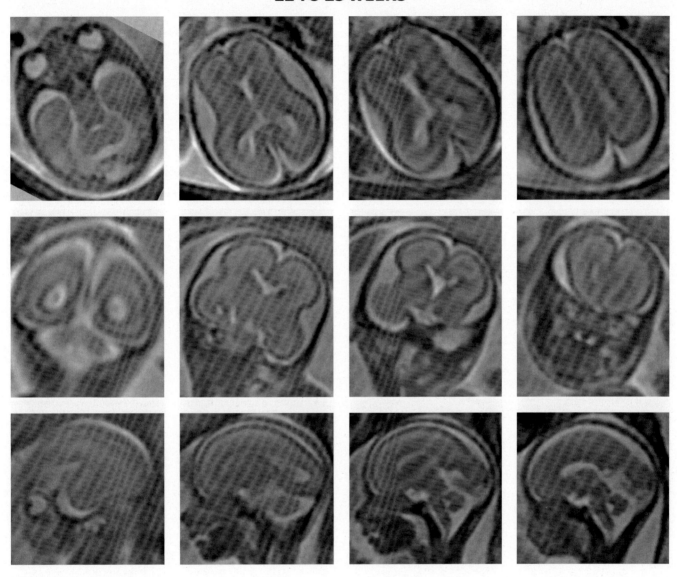

## SUPRATENTORIAL

**SULCATION:** Interhemispheric, **sylvian angular**, **callosal**, **parieto-occipital**, **hippocampal**

**PARENCHYMA:** 5 layer

**BASAL GANGLIA:** Homogeneous to white matter with thalamus mildly hyperintense

**GERMINAL MATRIX:** Thinning, less prominent GE

**CORPUS CALLOSUM:** Crescentic

**LATERAL VENTRICLES:** Mature configuration but prominent occipital horns

## INFRATENTORIAL

**PARENCHYMA:** 3 layer

**VERMIS:** Coverage of 4th

   **SULCATION:** Primary, prepyramidal, **preculminate**

**CEREBELLAR HEMISPHERES:**

   **SULCATION:** Flocculonodular, hemispheres smooth

**MYELINATION:** Medulla, pons

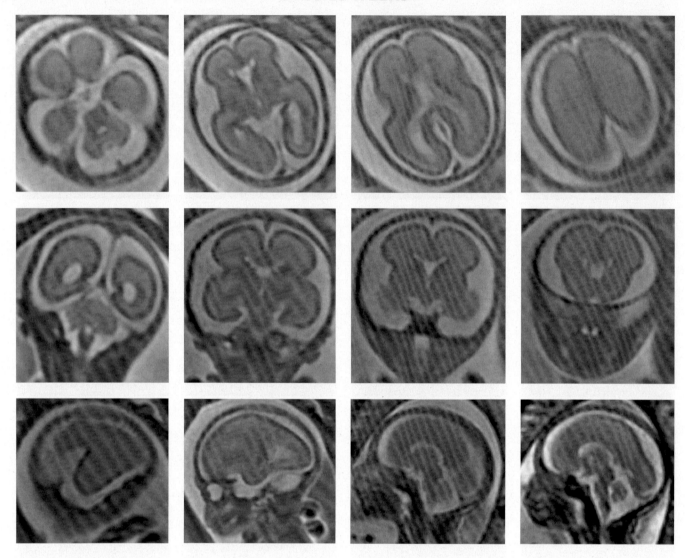

## SUPRATENTORIAL

**Sulcation:** Interhemispheric, sylvian, callosal, parieto-occipital, hippocampal, **calcarine, cingular**

**Parenchyma:** 5 layer

**Basal ganglia:** Homogeneous to white matter with thalamus mildly hyperintense

**Germinal matrix:** Moderate prominent

**Corpus callosum:** Crescentic

**Lateral ventricles:** Normal configuration and less prominent

## INFRATENTORIAL

**Parenchyma:** 3 layer

**Vermis:** Coverage of 4th

    **Sulcation:** Primary, prepyramidal, preculminate, **postpyramidal (secondary)**

**Cerebellar hemispheres:**

    **Sulcation:** Early foliation

**Myelination:** Medulla, pons

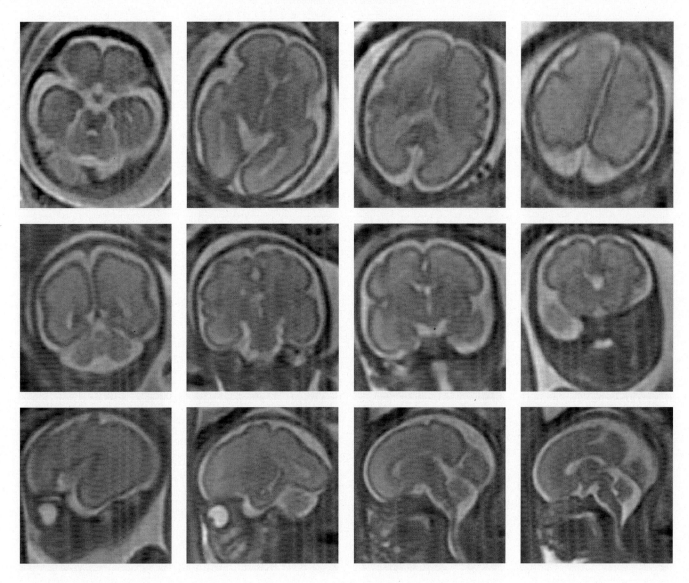

## SUPRATENTORIAL

**SULCATION:** Interhemispheric, sylvian, callosal, parieto-occipital, hippocampal, calcarine, cingular, **central, collateral, precentral, superior temporal, marginal**

**PARENCHYMA:** 5 layer

**BASAL GANGLIA:** Homogeneous to white matter

**GERMINAL MATRIX:** Less prominent

**CORPUS CALLOSUM:** Crescentic

**LATERAL VENTRICLES:** Normal configuration and less prominent

## INFRATENTORIAL

**PARENCHYMA:** 3 layer

**VERMIS:** Coverage of 4th

    **SULCATION:** Primary, prepyramidal, preculminate, postpyramidal (secondary), **horizontal**

**CEREBELLAR HEMISPHERES:**

    **SULCATION:** Partial foliation

**MYELINATION:** Medulla, pons

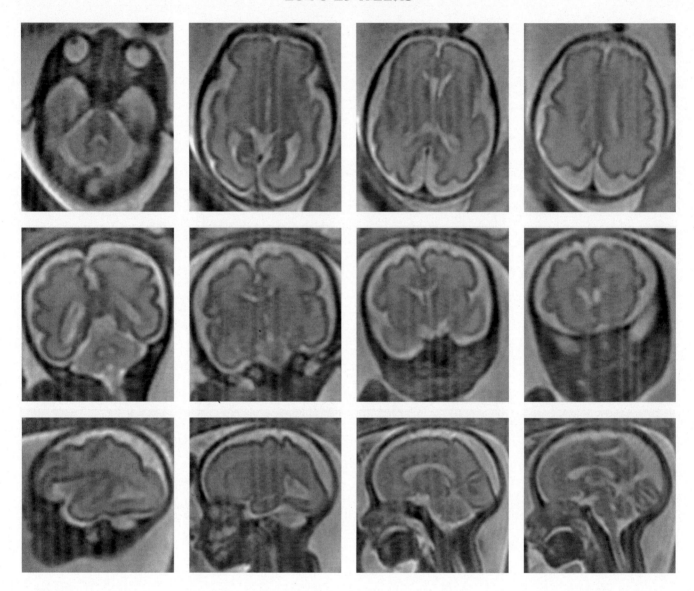

## SUPRATENTORIAL

**SULCATION:** Interhemispheric, sylvian, callosal, parieto-occipital, hippocampal, calcarine, cingular, central, collateral, precentral, superior temporal, marginal, **postcentral, intraparietal, superior frontal, and inferior frontal**

**PARENCHYMA:** Blurring of multilayer with residual 5-layer frontal and temporal

**BASAL GANGLIA:** Thalamus and pallidum T2 hypointense

**GERMINAL MATRIX:** Less prominent but still along lateral ventricles

**CORPUS CALLOSUM:** Crescentic

**LATERAL VENTRICLES:** Normal

## INFRATENTORIAL

**PARENCHYMA:** 3 layer

**VERMIS:** Coverage of 4th

    **SULCATION:** All fissures

**CEREBELLAR HEMISPHERES:**

    **SULCATION:** Completely foliated

**MYELINATION:** Medulla, pons, **inferior and superior cerebellar peduncles**

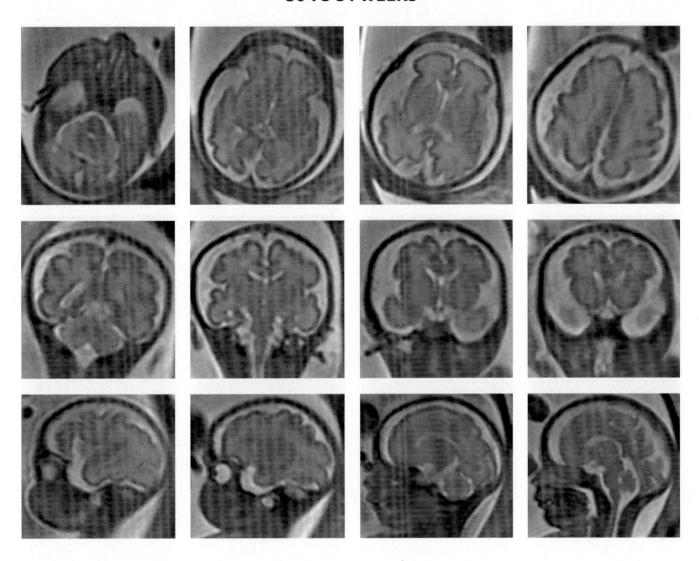

## SUPRATENTORIAL

**SULCATION:** Interhemispheric, sylvian, callosal, parieto-occipital, hippocampal, calcarine, cingular, central, collateral, precentral, superior temporal, marginal, postcentral, intraparietal, superior frontal, and inferior frontal. **Central sulcus now extends medially and superior temporal anteriorly**

**PARENCHYMA:** Blurring of layers with residual 5-layer anterior temporal lobes

**BASAL GANGLIA:** Thalamus and pallidum T2 hypointense

**GERMINAL MATRIX:** Inconsistent along lateral ventricles

**CORPUS CALLOSUM:** Crescentic

**LATERAL VENTRICLES:** Normal

## INFRATENTORIAL

**PARENCHYMA:** 3 layer with T2 hyperintense central and peripheral hypointense DCN

**VERMIS:** Coverage of 4th

    **SULCATION:** All fissures

**CEREBELLAR HEMISPHERES:**

    **SULCATION:** Folia diffusely, with flocculi noted

**MYELINATION:** Medulla, pons, inferior and superior cerebellar peduncles

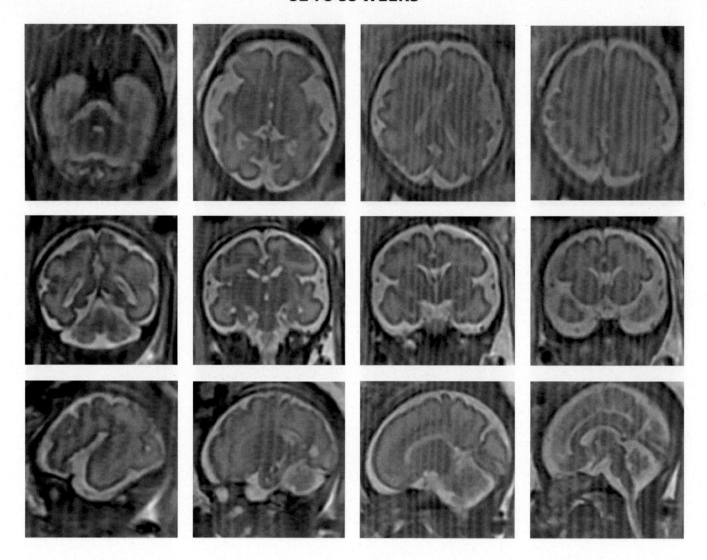

## SUPRATENTORIAL

**SULCATION:** Interhemispheric, sylvian, callosal, parieto-occipital, hippocampal, calcarine, cingular, central, collateral, precentral, superior temporal, marginal, postcentral, intraparietal, superior frontal, and inferior frontal. Central sulcus now extends medially and superior temporal anteriorly. **Inferior temporal and occipitotemporal**

**PARENCHYMA:** 2 layer in absence of germinal matrix

**BASAL GANGLIA:** Thalamus and pallidum T2 hypointense

**GERMINAL MATRIX:** Small rests at caudate head and temporal/occipital horn in the ganglionic eminences

**CORPUS CALLOSUM:** Crescentic

**LATERAL VENTRICLES:** Normal

## INFRATENTORIAL

**PARENCHYMA:** 3 layer with T2 hyperintense central and peripheral hypointense DCN

**VERMIS:** Coverage of 4th

   **SULCATION:** All fissures

**CEREBELLAR HEMISPHERES:**

   **SULCATION:** Folia diffusely, with flocculi noted

**MYELINATION:** Medulla, pons, inferior and superior cerebellar peduncles, **dorsal midbrain, inferior colliculus, lateral putamen, ventrolateral thalami, possible T1 high signal dot posterior limb of internal capsule**

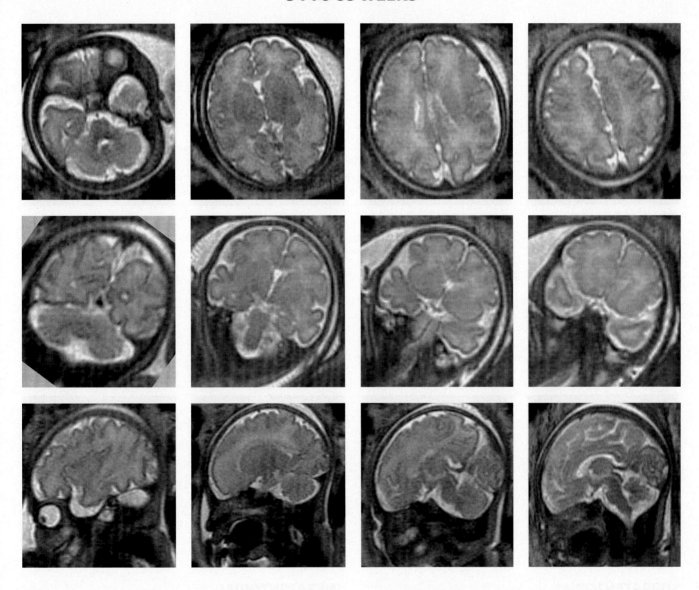

## SUPRATENTORIAL

**SULCATION: All primary with most secondary**

**PARENCHYMA:** 2 layer in absence of germinal matrix

**BASAL GANGLIA:** Thalamus, pallidum, caudate, and putamen T2 hypointense

**GERMINAL MATRIX:** Small rest at caudate heads

**CORPUS CALLOSUM:** Crescentic

**LATERAL VENTRICLES:** Normal

## INFRATENTORIAL

**PARENCHYMA:** 3 layer with T2 hyperintense central and peripheral hypointense DCN

**VERMIS:** Coverage of 4th

**SULCATION:** All fissures

**CEREBELLAR HEMISPHERES:**

**SULCATION:** Folia diffusely, with flocculi noted

**MYELINATION:** Medulla, pons, inferior and superior cerebellar peduncles, dorsal midbrain, inferior colliculus, lateral putamen, ventrolateral thalami, T1 high signal posterior limb of internal capsule, **optic tracts and subcortical white matter perirolandic, calcarine, medial temporal lobe**

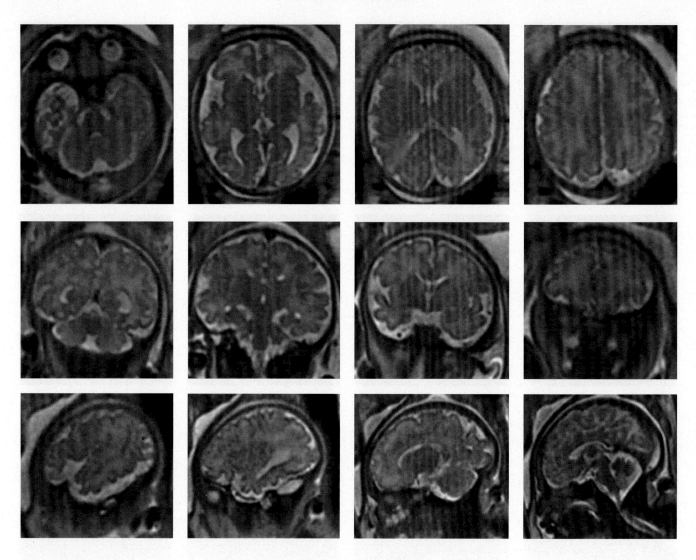

## SUPRATENTORIAL

**SULCATION:** **All primary, secondary, and tertiary sulci**

**PARENCHYMA:** 2 layer

**BASAL GANGLIA:** Thalamus, pallidum, caudate, and putamen T2 hypointense

**GERMINAL MATRIX:** Thick, less prominent GE

**CORPUS CALLOSUM:** Crescentic

**LATERAL VENTRICLES:** Normal

## INFRATENTORIAL

**PARENCHYMA:** 3 layer with T2 hyperintense central and peripheral hypointense DCN

**VERMIS:** Coverage of 4th

**SULCATION:** All fissures

**CEREBELLAR HEMISPHERES:**

**SULCATION:** Folia diffusely, with flocculi noted

**MYELINATION:** Medulla, pons, inferior and superior cerebellar peduncles, dorsal midbrain, inferior colliculus, lateral putamen, ventrolateral thalami, T1 high signal posterior limb of internal capsule, optic tracts and subcortical white matter perirolandic, calcarine, medial temporal lobes

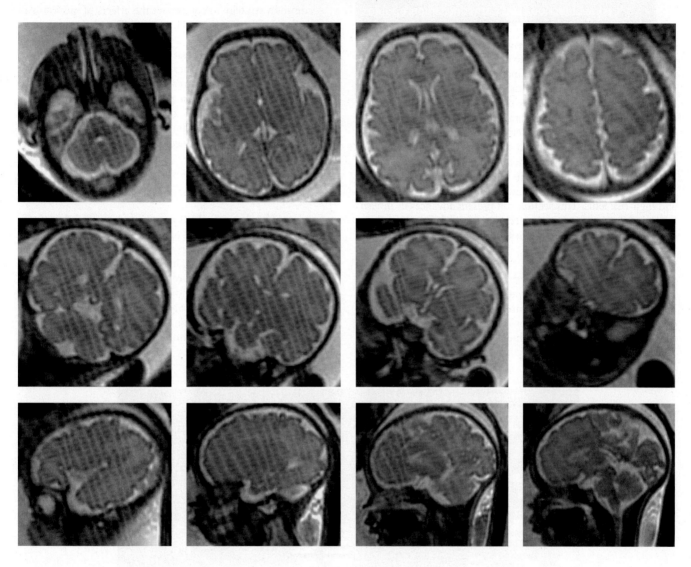

## SUPRATENTORIAL

**SULCATION:** All primary, secondary, and tertiary sulci

**PARENCHYMA:** 2 layer

**BASAL GANGLIA:** Thalamus, pallidum, caudate, and putamen T2 hypointense

**GERMINAL MATRIX:** Absent

**CORPUS CALLOSUM:** Crescentic

**LATERAL VENTRICLES:** Normal

## INFRATENTORIAL

**PARENCHYMA:** 3 layer with T2 hyperintense central and peripheral hypointense DCN

**VERMIS:** Coverage of 4th

**SULCATION:** All fissures

**CEREBELLAR HEMISPHERES:**

**SULCATION:** Folia diffusely, with flocculi noted

**MYELINATION:** Medulla, pons, inferior and superior cerebellar peduncles, dorsal midbrain, inferior colliculus, lateral putamen, ventrolateral thalami, T1 high signal posterior limb of internal capsule, optic tracts and subcortical white matter perirolandic, calcarine, medial temporal lobes. **T2 focal dark signal in the posterior limb of the internal capsule and superior vermis**

The successful application of *in vivo* magnetic resonance imaging (MRI) in the living fetus has led to unprecedented advances in our understanding of the elaborate maturational processes that take place in the healthy fetal brain, and in how these critical maturational events can be derailed by developmental aberrations and acquired injury. The availability of a growing set of MRI sequences, together with the advent of dedicated image-processing pipelines is providing us with unparalleled access to fetal brain micro- and macrostructure, metabolism, function, and behavior. These quantitative methods are affording us with increasingly reliable and reproducible quantitative neuroimaging biomarkers of the healthy and high-risk fetus. This section will present advances in *in vivo* fetal quantitative neuroimaging techniques and demonstrate their clinical application in the high-risk fetus.

## TECHNIQUE

Image degradation frequently accompanies nonsedated fetal MRI studies.[1,2] Although the most common culprit for image degradation is fetal and maternal motion occurring during the acquisition, the inherent high water content of the fetal brain and surrounding intrauterine tissue also negatively impacts the signal. Consequently, fetal MR images are often corrupted by motion artifact and resulting low tissue contrast (Fig. 6.3-1).[3–5]

A common strategy to counteract the effects of motion is to reduce the acquisition time.[3] However, MR imaging in nonsedated patients often involves a trade-off between high-image quality and resolution, and fast scanning. A reduced acquisition time leads to the use of increased slice thickness and lower resolution images. Current research efforts are focused on implementing new acquisition protocols in order to decrease scanning time, increase tissue contrast, and to develop specific image postprocessing algorithms that are dedicated to collectively enhance image quality, signal-to-noise (SNR) ratio, contrast, and spatial resolution.

## Fetal MRI Acquisitions

A number of fetal-specific MRI acquisition protocols have been developed, providing a large set of modalities with which to study fetal brain *in vivo*,[3,6–8] particularly SSFSE T2-weighted sequences. Standard T1-weighted imaging in the *in utero* fetus is not always feasible as T1 sequences require a longer acquisition time, are prone to image degradation, and offer a low gray and white matter contrast.[7] As an alternative, SNAPIR imaging has been shown to effectively overcome motion artifact, and offers improved anatomical detail in comparison with standard T1-weighted

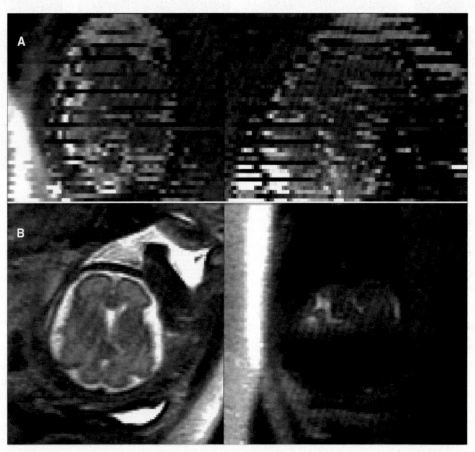

**FIGURE 6.3-1:** Image degradation during fetal MRI acquisition. **A:** Interslice motion, observed from out-of-plane directions. **B:** Intraslice motion, resulting in a loss of image contrast and intensity.

acquisitions. Other imaging modalities, including diffusion-weighted imaging (DWI) and diffusion tensor imaging (DTI), functional MRI, and spectroscopy, are actively being developed and refined, and will be described further in this section.

## Fetal MR Image Processing

Once the raw MR images have been acquired, the quality is often suboptimal for subsequent quantitative analysis, particularly as it relates to decreased spatial resolution and tissue contrast. A recent body of work has emerged that focuses on developing fetal-specific imaging processing pipelines that address the unique complexities encountered with fetal imaging, including specific image artifacts, noise, poor SNR, low voxel resolution, low tissue contrast, and intensity field nonuniformity.[4,5,9,10]

A common artifact encountered in fetal MRI is the inhomogeneity of the voxel intensities. This degradation is due to several factors, including coil design, poor radio frequency field uniformity, loss of signal (due to the position of the coil, the distance between the fetus and the coil), and/or patient anatomy. Consequently, this leads to variation of the signal intensity across the image. Intensity nonuniformity can be particularly strong in fetal imaging, in situations where the coil is not often properly positioned, or if the fetus is too far from the coil. Another common artifact encountered in fetal MRI is "noise," which gives the images a grainy appearance, frequently making brain tissues boundary (e.g., white matter/gray matter) delineation difficult to achieve. Several algorithms have been proposed to compensate for these artifacts,[9-14] and are summarized below.

Novel methods have been developed that increase fetal MR image contrast and resolution.[5,15-17] These methods typically rely on multiple low-resolution acquisitions of the same fetal brain (typically 2- to 4-mm slice thickness), in all three directions (coronal, axial, and sagittal). The in-plane resolution of these images usually ranges from 0.8 to 1.6 mm. Several approaches have been proposed to overcome this issue, either by compensating interslice motion[15] or by reconstructing a single high-resolution isotropic volume, using the available multiple low-resolution MR images of a single fetal brain.[5,12,17] These super-resolution methods result in the creation of a single high-resolution volume as well as an increase in tissue contrast (Fig. 6.3-2), and are now readily incorporated in advanced fetal brain imaging pipelines,[17,18] to allow for an accurate representation of the fetal brain anatomy, which is mandatory in order to delineate brain tissues and extract quantitative features such as brain volumes.

## QUANTIFYING FETAL BRAIN STRUCTURE

### Brain Volumetry

The availability of high-resolution image reconstruction is enabling us to accurately quantify *in utero* brain development, by extracting anatomical features such as brain tissue (e.g., cortical white matter, white matter) volumes, and regional brain structures (e.g., cerebellum, brainstem). Although previous studies have reported three-dimensional (3D) fetal brain growth measurements using manual delineation of brain volumes,[19-21] manual segmentations remain problematic, mainly for two reasons: the resulting labeling can be operator-biased; and manual editing of a high-resolution segmentation is a very tedious and time-consuming process. For example, segmenting a single fetal brain can take several hours, even for a well-trained operator.[22] Consequently, this cannot be applied to large-scale databases.

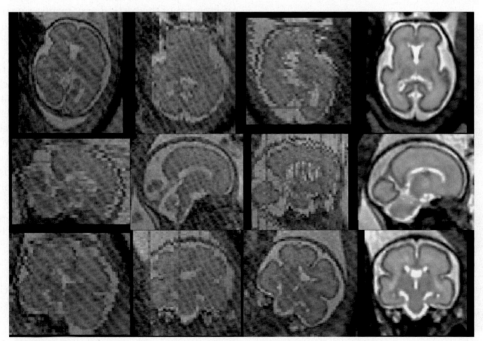

**FIGURE 6.3-2:** High-resolution reconstruction of a fetal brain MR image **(right column)**, using initial low-resolution images, acquired in three different (axial, sagittal, and coronal) directions **(three left columns, left to right)**.

A growing number of methods are becoming available to automatically delineate and quantify global and regional brain volumes in the fetus, including intracranial cavity volume, total brain volume, cerebellar volume, cerebrum volume, lateral ventricular volume, and brainstem volume (Fig. 6.3-3).[5,23,24] The quantification of brain tissue volumes, including cortical gray matter, unmyelinated white matter, and basal ganglia, has also been investigated.[25,26] These methods may be single-[18,23–25] or multiatlas based.[27] However, caution must be used when applying these methods to fetuses with advanced gestational age given the increasing complexity of the fetal brain, lamination, and gyrification. Although most of these automated methods provide satisfactory segmentations before 30 weeks of gestation, manual editing is often required to correct brain tissue delineation beyond this gestational age.[18] To date, fully automated methods have been mostly described in second trimester fetuses (20 to 28 weeks of gestation).[28,29] However, ongoing validation studies are needed for automated brain tissue quantification in fetuses greater than 28 weeks of gestation.

Quantification of fetal brain growth is relevant in the clinical setting in order to reliably ascertain the timing and progression of aberrant brain trajectories. Recent studies have employed sophisticated segmentation tools to characterize normal *in utero* brain maturation, and to compare cerebral tissue development in healthy and high-risk fetal populations. In fact, normative fetal brain growth trajectories are now readily available (Fig. 6.3-4).[23,24,30] It has been shown that cerebral volume increases 250% between 25 and 36 weeks of gestation, and that cerebellar volume shows an exponential growth rate of 366% over the same period.[24] These segmentation methods have also been shown to be very informative when studying high-risk fetuses.[21,26,27,31] For example, Limperopoulos and colleagues[21] showed a progressive third trimester impairment in brain growth in fetuses with complex congenital heart disease (CHD) compared with healthy control fetuses. Noteworthy is the fact that the conventional brain MRI studies of these fetuses were considered

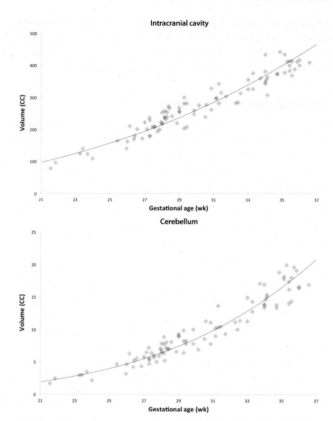

**FIGURE 6.3-4:** Example of normative volumetric fetal brain growth trajectories for intracranial cavity and cerebellum. (From Clouchoux C, Guizard N, Evans AC, et al. Normative fetal brain growth by quantitative *in vivo* magnetic resonance imaging. *Am J Obstet Gynecol.* 2012;206[2]:173. e1–173.e8.)

normal. These findings were extended in a subgroup of fetuses with hypoplastic left heart syndrome (HLHS),[26] and delayed development of the cortical gray matter, subcortical gray matter, and white matter volumes was also reported in the third trimester. Two other studies used automated fetal brain segmentation methods to characterize lateral ventricular volume and shape in fetuses with ventriculomegaly.[27,31] The first study used a multiatlas, multishape segmentation approach to delineate and quantify volume and shape of the lateral ventricles.[27] Scott and colleagues[31] used automatically segmented fetal brain tissues to characterize the surface of the lateral ventricles in fetuses with ventriculomegaly, and reported significant differences in ventricular surface curvature between cases and controls.

Taken together, MRI volumetric methods are increasingly demonstrating valuable clinical utility. Ongoing clinical implementation will largely depend on the ability to decrease computational burden associated with quantitative MRI in order to provide expedited diagnostic information to the clinical team.

## Cortical Development

Cerebral cortical anatomy has been directly related to cytoarchitecture and brain function.[32–34] From a developmental perspective, cortical gyrification is closely linked to the maturation of underlying brain structures.[35] The formation of gyri and sulci follows a highly orchestrated developmental process, which was first described in *postmortem* fetuses.[36] Initial studies relied on

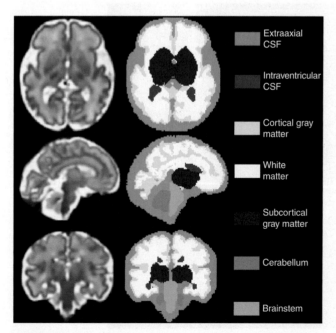

**FIGURE 6.3-3:** Segmentation of a high-resolution reconstructed fetal brain **(left)** in seven tissue classes **(right)**. CSF, cerebrospinal fluid.

conventional MRI to describe the timetable of cortical folding using visual/clinical description[37] or geometric measurements in *ex vivo*[38] and *in vivo* fetuses.[39] More recently, advances in brain imaging have permitted the development of quantitative methods to delineate the emergence of the sulcal pattern *in vivo*.

Several studies have characterized cortical folding processes using 3D reconstruction of the fetal cortical surface.[18,25] These techniques offer global measurements of the cortical surface, including surface area and gyrification index, but also very specific measurements of the sulci and gyri, including shape, location, curvature, depth, or length, and offer probabilistic maps of the sulcal patterns.[18] It has been demonstrated that during the second and third trimesters of pregnancy, the complexity of the cortical surface is dramatically increasing in several regions, including the frontal, temporal, and occipital lobes.[18,25]

In addition, cortical surface-based morphometry has been used to investigate the prenatal origin of sulcal asymmetries.[18,25,40] These studies reported a developing asymmetry in the temporal lobe as early as 18 weeks, where the left temporal lobe appears to be larger and more folded when compared with the right hemisphere. These observations confirm what has been reported in ex-utero premature babies.[34]

Clinically, surface-based methods have demonstrated their potential to provide unique insights into developmental brain disturbances. Clouchoux et al.[26] investigated differences in cortical maturation between healthy fetuses and fetuses with HLHS. The study demonstrated delayed cortical folding in fetuses with HLHS compared with the controls in several cortical areas, including the frontal, parietal, calcarine, temporal, and collateral regions (Fig. 6.3-5). Interestingly, this cortical folding delay appears to precede volumetric growth impairments, and may represent an important, early marker for subsequent disturbances in growth. Similarly, Scott and colleagues[31] showed reduced

cortical folding in the parieto-occipital region in fetuses with ventriculomegaly compared with healthy controls.

In summary, available studies suggest that cortical folding quantification provides a promising and powerful tool for investigating the timing and extent of cerebral cortical aberrations in high-risk fetuses.

## Fetal Brain Microstructure

During fetal brain maturation, the cerebral white matter undergoes a rapid set of changes in its microstructural organization.[41-47] These changes can be observed and quantified using DWI and DTI. DWI allows us to characterize the diffusion of water molecules in the brain, reflecting the degree of organization of the white matter fibers, and can be measured by calculating the apparent diffusion coefficient (ADC). Several studies have described normal and abnormal microstructure using DWI. These studies have reported a decrease in ADC from 30 weeks of gestation onward.[43,48-50] DWI has been shown to provide valuable information in cases of fetal brain hemorrhage and acute ischemia.[42,43,47] In CHD fetuses, ADC values have been shown to be higher when compared with the controls.[51] DWI has also been used to investigate brain maturation between fetuses and infants born prematurely infants.[52] Differences in ADC were reported between the two groups in the pons and the parietal white matter, where higher ADC values were reported in fetuses, suggesting increased regional brain maturation in *in utero* fetuses compared with ex-utero preterm infants.

DTI allows us to quantify the direction and magnitude of water molecules diffusion, and is measured using fractional anisotropy (FA)[52a]. Complementary to DWI, DTI provides an indirect assessment of axonal/fiber connectivity in the developing brain.[45,51,53-57] Although DTI can provide important insights

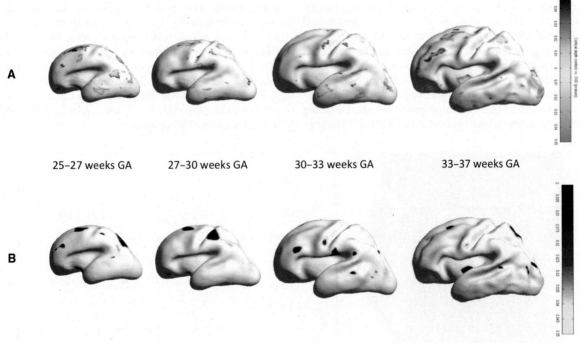

25–27 weeks GA      27–30 weeks GA      30–33 weeks GA      33–37 weeks GA

**FIGURE 6.3-5:** Local cortical development delays in fetuses with hypoplastic left heart syndrome, compared with healthy controls. **A:** Delays in cortical depth. **B:** Delays in sulcation. (From Clouchoux C, du Plessis AJ, Bouyssi-Kobar M, et al. Delayed cortical development in fetuses with complex congenital heart disease. *Cereb Cortex.* 2013;23:2932–2943.)

into fetal brain microstructural development, its successful application to the living fetus remains technically challenging secondary to fetal and maternal motion, and low voxel resolution. Consequently, very few studies have investigated this modality *in vivo.*[58–60] Hierarchical regional distribution of FA values has been described in the *in utero* fetal brain, with gradually decreasing FA in the splenium, the genu of the corpus callosum, and lastly the internal capsule with increasing gestational age.[58] Zanin and colleagues[60] also reported a gradual maturation of the cerebral white matter, which they divided into three different phases, potentially reflecting axonal organization, myelination gliosis, and myelination.

Fetal DWI and DTI will undoubtedly continue to benefit from ongoing technical advances in both MRI pulse sequence development and postprocessing methods to circumvent motion-related artifact and increase image resolution and clinical applicability.

## QUANTIFYING FETAL BRAIN METABOLISM AND FUNCTION

### Spectroscopy

Metabolite mapping of the fetal brain can provide crucial insights into brain maturation, in both healthy and high-risk pregnancies. The recent successful application of proton MR spectroscopy (¹HMRS) has enabled the quantification of metabolic profiles in the living fetus.[21,61–64] Despite the length of the acquisition (approximately 3 to 4 minutes), recent studies showed that unsedated single voxel spectroscopy can be successfully performed in about two-thirds of fetuses.[21,65]

The most commonly reported metabolites in the fetal brain include creatine (Cr), reflecting cellular mitochondrial metabolism, choline (Cho), a marker of myelination, and *N*-acetylaspartate (NAA), a neuroaxonal marker reflecting dendrites and synapse development (Fig. 6.3-6).[6–69] Creatine can be detected as early as at 22 weeks' gestation and increases with gestational age. Similarly, NAA has been shown to significantly increase with advancing gestational age, while choline steadily decreases with increasing maturation. This evolution in metabolic concentrations is associated with myelination and the development of synapses and dendrites. Lactate, the product of anaerobic metabolism has been reported in compromised fetuses, including those with intrauterine growth restriction (IUGR) and complex

CHD.[61–64,70] Moreover, decreased NAA:Cr and NAA:Cho ratios have also been found to be lower in these high-risk fetuses.[21,63] These emerging studies suggest that fetal brain ¹HMRS may serve as an important early marker of fetal compromise.

### Fetal Resting-State Functional MRI

Functional MRI (fMRI) is a noninvasive MR imaging modality that enables the quantification of local blood oxygenation, using the blood oxygen-level–dependent (BOLD) response. Functional MRI provides an indirect measure of regional activation of the brain. To date, functional assessment of the living fetus has been largely limited to Doppler ultrasound, changes in fetal activity or heart rate, or magnetoencephalography (MEG).[71–74] Understandably, task-related fMRI is not possible in the fetus. A very small number of stimulus-driven fetal fMRI experiments have been performed to date, where fetal brain oxygenation level was measured during auditory,[75–77] vibroacoustic,[78] or visual stimuli.[79] For example, Jardri and colleagues[77] reported fetal activation in the left temporal cortex in six fetuses (33 weeks of gestation), when an auditory stimulus was applied. Noteworthy is the fact that mothers were sedated during the study, and the authors reported that signal variance was not corrupted by fetal motion during the acquisition.

More recently, resting-state fMRI has been explored in the living fetus.[80,81] Resting-state fMRI is designed to quantify regional brain activity and interactions when the subject is not performing any given task.[82] The goal is then to extract the "default mode" functional network, representing regions with a functional activity, even when the subject is not performing an explicit task.[83] Schopf and colleagues[80] used resting-state fMRI in a cohort of 16 healthy fetuses from 16 to 36 weeks of gestation, to analyze fetal brain networks. This study reported a bilateral occipital network, as well as medial and lateral prefrontal networks. A more recent study from Thomason and colleagues[81] using resting-state fMRI in healthy fetuses reported bilateral connectivity in 20 cortical regions including visual, somatosensory, ventral, dorsal, and cingulate cortex. Functional connectivity was shown to increase with gestation age. Although fMRI remains technically challenging, available studies are demonstrating the feasibility of measuring functional brain connectivity *in utero*, and will likely provide a critical foundation for understanding the role of early life insults on later disturbances in neural functional connectivity.

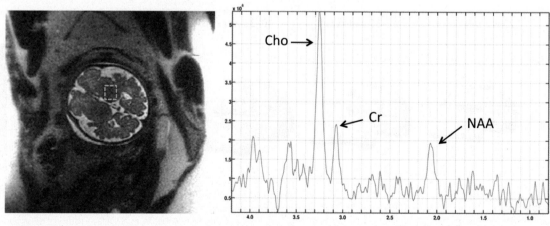

**FIGURE 6.3-6:** MR spectroscopy in a 32-week gestation age fetus. Metabolite peaks measured from the resulting spectra **(right)**, including Choline *(Cho)*, Creatine *(Cr)*, and *N*-acetylaspartate *(NAA)*.

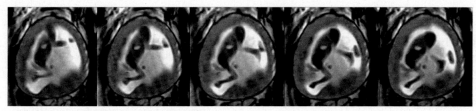

**FIGURE 6.3-7:** Sample frames of a cine-MRI acquisition in a 32-week gestational age fetus.

## Fetal Behavior

Fetal movements, reflexive and voluntary, are closely related to fetal brain function.[2,84] With advancing gestational age, these movements become increasingly complex,[84] and specific patterns of movements have been described at each developmental stage.[2,85] Given that fetal movements rely on an intact central nervous system,[86] their quantification can potentially provide important biomarkers of fetal health and well-being (Fig. 6.3-7).

Dynamic MRI cine sequences have been used to investigate fetal movements.[87,88] Hayat and colleagues[87] reported a multislice balanced steady-state free precision cine sequence, originally developed for adult cardiac dynamic MRI, to image fetal movements in 37 healthy fetuses (10 to 37 weeks of gestation). The study demonstrated three levels of fetal activity at 22, 28, and 36 weeks of gestation. These stages were described as (a) whole body movements, (b) low-intensity movements (single limb), and (c) complete inactivity. Moreover, a gradual decrease in activity was associated with decreasing free space available in the uterus. Guo and colleagues[88] also investigated fetal movements using cine MRI in 25 fetuses, from 18 to 33 weeks of gestation, with and without central nervous system abnormalities. The study demonstrated significantly diminished and/or abnormal fetal movements among fetuses with major central nervous system abnormalities. Although ongoing development of MR imaging sequences is needed, alongside the quantification of fetal movements, cine MRI may provide clinically important, adjunct four-dimensional information for high-risk fetuses.

## QUANTIFYING PLACENTAL STRUCTURE AND FUNCTION

The placenta is an essential organ that provides nutrients to the fetus and plays an endocrine function.[89] Abnormal placental anatomy has been associated with neonatal death and small for gestational age (SGA) neonates.[90,91] Moreover, vascular placental pathologies detected through T1 MRI have also been shown to be strongly predictive of adverse neonatal outcome, including fetal demise.[91] In vivo placental anatomy and perfusion is conventionally assessed using Doppler ultrasound. Recently, different MRI modalities have emerged that are beginning to quantify placental anatomy, microstructure, perfusion, and metabolism. These are summarized below.

## Placental Volume/Microstructure

The relationship between placental volume and outcome has been recently interrogated in a small number of high-risk pregnancies.[90,92,93] Decreased placental volume has been reported in association with maternal smoking during pregnancy,[93] IUGR,[94] and SGA neonates.[90] Interestingly, Anblagan and colleagues[93] also demonstrated a concomitant reduction in volumetric growth of the fetal brain, lung, and kidneys in fetuses exposed to maternal smoking.

To date, placental microstructure has also been explored using diffusion MRI in two studies. Morita and colleagues[94] showed that DWI could be used to investigate placental invasion, and to determine the microarchitecture of the myometrium. Placental DWI has also been studied in fetuses with placental insufficiency.[95] Restricted diffusion and reduced ADC were found in IUGR pregnancies when compared with healthy fetuses controls.[95] These preliminary findings suggest that diffusion MRI may have an important role for early detection of placental-based disorders.

## Placental Function

The placenta represents the primary source of nutrients for the developing fetus, and therefore the ability to noninvasively quantify placental function, including blood flow, oxygenation, and metabolism, is critical. In vivo placental perfusion has been explored using the intravoxel incoherent motion (IVIM) technique.[96,97] Indirectly, the volume of blood moving in the placental capillary networks can be measured using IVIM, as a signal attenuation caused by phase dispersion of randomly moving water protons under a magnetic field gradient.[96] Using the same technique, decreased placental perfusion was described in a small cohort of pregnancies complicated by IUGR.[97] In a very recent study, placental perfusion measurements were compared between IVIM and arterial spin labeling (ASL) using a flow-sensitive alternating inversion recovery (FAIR) sequence. The results were then related to impedance to flow in the uterine artery, measured by Doppler ultrasound. This preliminary study demonstrated that MR-based placental perfusion was associated with pregnancy outcome.[98] Specifically, pregnancies resulting in SGA newborns were found to show reduced placental perfusion when compared with healthy control pregnancies using both ASL and IVIM techniques. These observations were correlated with uterine artery pulsatility index measured by Doppler observations,[98] suggesting that placental perfusion MRI measurements in high-risk pregnancies may reliably predict pregnancy outcomes.

Oxygenation measurements of the placental tissue have also been the focus of recent studies.[99,100] Intact placental oxygenation is critical for normal fetal growth and development; however, the relationship between placental oxygenation and supply of oxygen to the fetal organs is not yet fully understood. Huen and colleagues[100] investigated the feasibility of placental oxygenation quantification using oxygen-enhanced MRI ($R^1$ contrast) and BOLD MRI (R2* contrast) in vivo. The study showed an increase in R1 and a concomitant decrease in R2* signals in the placenta when oxygen was administered to pregnant women compared with breathing in room air.[100] Placental oxygenation using BOLD MRI in a second study was found to increase by 6.5% when oxygen was delivered to the mother over 10 minutes (12 L $O^2$ per minute).[99] Interestingly, other fetal organs showed an increase in oxygen levels, including liver, spleen, and kidney; however, no change in oxygenation was detected in the fetal brain. The authors speculate that reduced fetal brain perfusion may reflect a "reverse" brain-sparing mechanism.[99] Future studies are needed to answer this intriguing question.

## Placental Metabolism

One study has reported [1]HMRS as a potential noninvasive method to assess placental metabolism.[101] In this preliminary study, [1]HMRS was used to quantify metabolic profiles of the placenta in three women with IUGR and three matched controls. When compared with the controls, the IUGR placenta showed a lower Cho/lipid ratio compared with healthy control pregnancies, suggesting that [1]HMRS could be used to detect early signs of critical placental insufficiency.

Collectively, these preliminary studies suggest that the application of advanced placental MRI techniques has the potential to provide important, currently unavailable diagnostic information of placental functional integrity. However, these exciting placental-based MR techniques need ongoing validation before they can be translated into the clinical milieu.

## CONCLUSION

Advanced fetal MRI is becoming a powerful obstetrical tool that is transforming our ability to noninvasively assess health and wellness in the living fetus. Faster, more robust MRI pulse sequences are now adept at freezing fetal motion, while advanced postprocessing pipelines are capable of reconstructing 3D representations of the fetal brain, allowing for the precise delineation of critical maturational processes that occur throughout pregnancy. The increasing availability of normative values for fetal brain structure, microstructure, and metabolic function is revolutionizing our ability to accurately identify and monitor the compromised fetus. The successful streamlining and adoption of these emerging fetal imaging biomarkers in the clinical setting will require ongoing validation and necessitate a significant reduction in the current computational encumbrance that is inherent to these techniques. This in turn will offer advanced fetal diagnostic capabilities to guide clinical management of the high-risk fetus and the development of prenatal interventions.

## REFERENCES

1. Garel C. Fetal MRI: what is the future? *Ultrasound Obstet Gynecol.* 2008;31:123–128.
2. Prayer D. Investigation of the normal organ development with fetal MRI. *Eur Radiol.* 2006;17:2458–2471.
3. Jiang S, Xue H, Counsell S, et al. In-utero three dimension high resolution fetal brain diffusion tensor imaging. *Med Image Comput Comput Assist Interv.* 2007;10(pt 1):18–26.
4. Rousseau F, Glenn OA, Iordanova B, et al. Registration-based approach for reconstruction of high-resolution in utero fetal MR brain images. *Acad Radiol.* 2006;13:1072–1081.
5. Gholipour A, Estroff JA, Warfield SK. Robust super-resolution volume reconstruction from slice acquisitions: application to fetal brain MRI. *IEEE Trans Med Imaging.* 2010;29:1739–1758.
6. Malamateniou C, McGuinness AK, Allsop JM, et al. Snapshot inversion recovery: an optimized single-shot T1-weighted inversion-recovery sequence for improved fetal brain anatomic delineation. *Radiology.* 2011;258:229–235.
7. Sandrasegaran K, Laal C, Aisen AA, et al. Fast fetal magnetic resonance imaging. *J Comput Assist Tomogr.* 2005;29:487–498.
8. Li Y, Pang Y, Vigneron D, et al. Investigation of multichannel phased array performance for fetal MR imaging on 1.5 T clinical MR system. *Quant Imaging Med Surg.* 2011;1:24–30.
9. Coupé P, Yger P, Prima S, et al. An optimized blockwise nonlocal means denoising filter for 3D magnetic resonance images. *IEEE Trans Med Imaging.* 2008;27(4):425–441.
10. Tustison NJ, Avants BB, Cook PA, et al. N4ITK: improved N3 bias correction. *IEEE Trans Med Imaging.* 2010;29(6):1310–1320.
11. Sled JG, Zijdenbos AP, Evans AC. A nonparametric method for automatic correction of intensity nonuniformity in MRI data. *IEEE Trans Med Imaging.* 1998;17(1):87–97.
12. Kim K, Habas P, Rajagopalan V, et al. Non-iterative relative bias correction for 3D reconstruction of in utero fetal brain MR imaging. *Conf Proc IEEE Eng Med Biol Soc.* 2010;2010:879–882.
13. Rasmussen PM, Abrahamsen TJ, Madsen KH, et al. Nonlinear denoising and analysis of neuroimages with kernel principal component analysis and pre-image estimation. *Neuroimage.* 2012;60(3):1807–1818.
14. Erturk M, Bottomley P, El-Sharkawy A. De-noising MRI using spectral subtraction. *IEEE Trans Biomed Eng.* 2013;60(6):1556–1562.
15. Guizard N, Evans AC, Lepage C, et al. Automatic model-based fetal brain parcellation to quantify in vivo fetal brain development. In: OHBM Conference; 2009; San Francisco, CA. Abstract.
16. Kim K, Habas PA, Rousseau F, et al. Intersection based motion correction of multislice MRI for 3D in utero fetal brain image formation. *IEEE Trans Med Imaging.* 2010;29(1):146–158.
17. Rousseau F, Oubel E, Pontabry J, et al. BTK: an open-source toolkit for fetal brain MR image processing. *Comput Methods Programs Biomed.* 2013;109(1):65–73.
18. Clouchoux C, Kudelski D, Gholipour A, et al. Quantitative in-vivo MRI measurement of cortical development in the fetus. *Brain Struct Funct.* 2012;217(1):127–139.
19. Grossman R, Hoffman C, Mardor Y, et al. Quantitative MRI measurements of human fetal brain development in utero. *Neuroimage.* 2006;33:463–470.
20. Kazan-Tannus JF, Dialani V, Kataoka ML, et al. MR volumetry of brain and CSF in fetuses referred for ventriculomegaly. *AJR Am J Roentgenol.* 2007;189:145–151.
21. Limperopoulos C, Tworetzky W, McElhinney DB, et al. Brain volume and metabolism in fetuses with congenital heart disease: evaluation with quantitative magnetic resonance imaging and spectroscopy. *Circulation.* 2010;5:26–33.
22. Fischl B, Dale A. Measuring the thickness of the human cerebral cortex from magnetic resonance images. *Proc Natl Acad Sci U S A.* 2000;97:11050.
23. Jacob FD, Habas PA, Kim K, et al. Fetal hippocampal development: analysis by magnetic resonance imaging volumetry. *Pediatr Res.* 2011;69(5, pt 1):425–429.
24. Clouchoux C, Guizard N, Evans AC, et al. Normative fetal brain growth by quantitative in vivo magnetic resonance imaging. *Am J Obstet Gynecol.* 2012;206(2):173.e1–173.e8.
25. Habas PA, Scott JA, Roosta A, et al. Early folding patterns and asymmetries of the normal human brain detected from in utero MRI. *Cereb Cortex.* 2012;22(1):13–25.
26. Clouchoux C, du Plessis AJ, Bouyssi-Kobar M, et al. Delayed cortical development in fetuses with complex congenital heart disease. *Cereb Cortex.* 2013;23(12):2932–2943.
27. Gholipour A, Akhondi-Asl A, Estroff JA, et al. Multi-atlas multi-shape segmentation of fetal brain MRI for volumetric and morphometric analysis of ventriculomegaly. *Neuroimage.* 2012;60(3):1819–1831.
28. Corbett-Detig J, Habas PA, Scott JA, et al. 3D global and regional patterns of human fetal subplate growth determined in utero. *Brain Struct Funct.* 2010;215:255–263.
29. Rajagopalan V, Scott JA, Habas PA, et al. Local tissue growth patterns underlying normal fetal human brain gyrification quantified in utero. *J Neurosci.* 2011;31:2878–2887.
30. Scott JA, Habas PA, Kim K, et al. Growth trajectories of the human fetal brain tissues estimated from 3D reconstructed in utero MRI. *Int J Dev Neurosci.* 2012;29(5):529–536.
31. Scott JA, Habas PA, Rajagopalan V, et al. Volumetric and surface-based 3D MRI analyses of fetal isolated mild ventriculomegaly: brain morphometry in ventriculomegaly. *Brain Struct Funct.* 2013;218(3):645–655.
32. Kostović I, Judas M. Correlation between the sequential ingrowth of afferents and transient patterns of cortical lamination in preterm infants. *Anat Rec.* 2002;267:1–6.
33. Fischl B, Rajendran N, Busa E, et al. Cortical folding patterns and predicting cytoarchitecture. *Cereb Cortex.* 2008;18(8):1973–1980.
34. Dubois J, Benders M, Borradori-Tolsa C, et al. Primary cortical folding in the human newborn: an early marker of later functional development. *Brain.* 2008;131(pt 8):2028–2041.
35. Van Essen D. A tension-based theory of morphogenesis and compact wiring in the central nervous system. *Nature.* 1997;385(23):313–318.
36. Chi JG, Dooling EC, Gilles FH. Gyral development of the human brain. *Ann Neurol.* 1977;1:86–93.
37. Garel C, Chantrel E, Brisse H, et al. Fetal cerebral cortex: normal gestational landmarks identified using prenatal MR imaging. *AJNR Am J Neuroradiol.* 2001;22(1):184–189.

38. Batchelor PG, Castellano Smith AD, Hill DL, et al. Measures of folding applied to the development of the human fetal brain. *IEEE Trans Med Imaging.* 2002;21:953–965.

39. Hu H-H, Guo W-Y, Chen H-Y, et al. Morphological regionalization using fetal magnetic resonance images of normal developing brains. *Eur J Neurosci.* 2009;29:1560–1567.

40. Kasprian G, Langs G, Brugger PC, et al. The prenatal origin of hemispheric asymmetry: an in utero neuroimaging study. *Cereb Cortex.* 2010;21:1076–1083.

41. Garel C, Delezoide AL, Delezoide L, et al. *MRI of the Fetal Brain: Normal Development and Cerebral Pathologies.* New York, NY: Springer-Verlag, 2004.

42. Baldoli C, Righini A, Parazzini C, et al. Demonstration of acute ischemic lesions in the fetal brain by diffusion magnetic resonance imaging. *Ann Neurol.* 2002;52:243–246.

43. Righini A, Bianchini E, Parazzini C, et al. Apparent diffusion coefficient determination in normal fetal brain: a prenatal MR imaging study. *AJNR Am J Neuroradiol.* 2003;24:799–804.

44. Agid R, Lieberman S, Nadjari M, et al. Prenatal MR diffusion-weighted imaging in a fetus with hemimegalencephaly. *Pediatr Radiol.* 2006;36:138–140.

45. Bui T, Daire JL, Chalard F, et al. Microstructural development of human brain assessed in utero by diffusion tensor imaging. *Pediatr Radiol.* 2006;36:1133–1140.

46. Kim DH, Chung S, Vigneron DB, et al. Diffusion-weighted imaging of the fetal brain in vivo. *Magn Reson Med.* 2008;59:216–220.

47. Brunel H, Girard N, Confort-Gouny S, et al. Fetal brain injury. *J Neuroradiol.* 2004;31:123–137.

48. Schneider JF, Confort-Gouny S, Le Fur Y, et al. Diffusion-weighted imaging in normal fetal maturation. *Eur Radiol.* 2007;17:2422–2429.

49. Schneider MM, Berman JI, Baumer FM, et al. Normative apparent diffusion coefficient values in the developing fetal brain. *AJNR Am J Neuroradiol.* 2009;30:1799–1803.

50. Manganaro L, Perrone A, Savelli S, et al. Evaluation of normal brain development by prenatal MR imaging. *Radiol Med.* 2007;112:444–445.

51. Berman JI, Hamrick SE, McQuillen PS, et al. Diffusion-weighted imaging in fetuses with severe congenital heart defects. *AJNR Am J Neuroradiol.* 2011;32:E21–E22.

52. Ozcan UA, Isik U, Dincer A, et al. Identification of fetal precentral gyrus on diffusion weighted MRI. *Brain Dev.* 2013;35(1):4–9.

52a. Basser PJ, Mattiello J, LeBihan D. http://www.ncbi.nlm.nih.gov/pubmed/8130344 MR diffusion tensor spectroscopy and imaging. *Biophys J.* 1994 Jan;66(1):259–67.

53. Hüppi PS, Warfield S, Kikinis R. Quantitative magnetic resonance imaging of brain development in premature and mature newborns. *Ann Neurol.* 1998;43:224–235.

54. Partridge SC, Mukherjee P, Henry RG, et al. Diffusion tensor imaging: serial quantitation of white matter tract maturity in premature newborns. *Neuroimage.* 2004;22:1302–1314.

55. Huang H, Xue R, Zhang J, et al. Anatomical characterization of human fetal brain development with diffusion tensor magnetic resonance imaging. *J Neurosci.* 2009;29:4263–4273.

56. Anjari M, Srinivasan L, Allsop JM, et al. Diffusion tensor imaging with tract-based spatial statistics reveals local white matter abnormalities in preterm infants. *Neuroimage.* 2007;35:1021–1027.

57. Dubois J, Dehaene-Lambertz G, Soarès C, et al. Microstructural correlates of infant functional development: example of the visual pathways. *J Neurosci.* 2008;28:1943–1948.

58. Kasprian G, Brugger PC, Weber M, et al. In utero tractography of fetal white matter development. *Neuroimage.* 2008;43:213–224.

59. Mitter C, Kasprian G, Brugger PC, et al. Three-dimensional visualization of fetal white-matter pathways in utero. *Ultrasound Obstet Gynecol.* 2011;37:252–253.

60. Zanin E, Ranjeva JP, Confort-Gouny S, et al. White matter maturation of normal human fetal brain: an in vivo diffusion tensor tractography study. *Brain Behav.* 2011;1(2):95–108.

61. Borowska-Matwiejczuk K, Lemancewicz A, Tarasow E, et al. Assessment of fetal distress based on magnetic resonance examinations: preliminary report. *Acad Radiol.* 2003;10:1274–1282.

62. Wolfberg AJ, Robinson JN, Mulkern R, et al. Identification of fetal cerebral lactate using magnetic resonance spectroscopy. *Am J Obstet Gynecol.* 2007;196:e9–e11.

63. Azpurua H, Alvarado A, Mayobre F, et al. Metabolic assessment of the brain using proton magnetic resonance spectroscopy in a growth-restricted human fetus: case report. *Am J Perinatol.* 2008;25:305–309.

64. Story L, Damodaram MS, Allsop JM, et al. Brain metabolism in fetal intrauterine growth restriction: a proton magnetic resonance spectroscopy study. *Am J Obstet Gynecol.* 2011;205(5):483.

65. Berger-Kulemann V, Brugger PC, Pugash D, et al. MR spectroscopy of the fetal brain: is it possible without sedation? *AJNR Am J Neuroradiol.* 2013;34(2):424–431.

66. Fenton BW, Lin CS, Macedonia C, et al. The fetus at term: in utero volume-selected proton MR spectroscopy with breath-hold technique—a feasibility study. *Radiology.* 2001;219:563–566.

67. Kok RD, van der Bergh AJ, Heerschap A, et al. Metabolic information from the human fetal brain obtained with proton magnetic resonance spectroscopy. *Am J Obstet Gynecol.* 2001;185:1011–1015.

68. Kok RD, van der Berg PP, van der Bergh AJ, et al. Maturation of the human fetal brain as observed by 1H MR spectroscopy. *Magn Reson Med.* 2002;48:611–616.

69. Kreis R. Brain metabolite composition during early human brain development as measured by quantitative in vivo $^1$H magnetic resonance spectroscopy. *Magn Reson Med.* 2002;48:949–958.

70. Limperopoulos C, Tworetzky W, Robertson RL, et al. Impaired brain metabolism in fetuses with congenital heart disease. *Circulation.* 2008;118:S651–S652.

71. Preissl H, Lowery CL, Eswaran H. Fetal magnetoencephalography: current progress and trends. *Exp Neurol.* 2004;190(suppl 1):S28–S36.

72. Blum T, Saling E, Bauer R. First magnetoencephalography recordings of the brain activity of a human fetus. *BJOG.* 1985;92:1224–1229.

73. Lengel JM, Chen M, Wakai RT. Improved neuromagnetic detection of fetal and neonatal auditory evoked responses. *Clin Neurophysiol.* 2001;112:785–792.

74. Eswaran H, Wilson JD, Preissl H, et al. Magnetoencephalographic recordings of visual evoked brain activity in the human fetus. *Lancet.* 2002;360:779–780.

75. Moore RJ, Vadeyar S, Tyler DJ, et al. Antenatal determination of fetal brain activity in response to an acoustic stimulus using functional magnetic resonance imaging. *Proc Intl Soc Magn Reson Med.* 2000;8:875.

76. Hykin J, Moore R, Duncan K, et al. Fetal brain activity demonstrated by functional magnetic resonance imaging. *Lancet.* 1999;35:645–646.

77. Jardri R, Pins D, Houfflin-Debarge V, et al. Fetal cortical activation to sound at 33 weeks of gestation: a functional MRI study. *Neuroimage.* 2008;42:10–18.

78. Fulford J, Vadeyar SH, Dodampahala SH, et al. Fetal brain activity and hemodynamic response to a vibroacoustic stimulus. *Hum Brain Mapp.* 2004;22:116–121.

79. Fulford J, Vadeyar SH, Dodampahala SH, et al. Fetal brain activity in response to a visual stimulus. *Hum Brain Mapp.* 2003;20:239–245.

80. Schopf V, Kasprian G, Brugger PC, et al. Watching the fetal brain at "rest." *Int J Dev Neurosci.* 2011;30(1):11–17.

81. Thomason ME, Dassanayake MT, Shen S, et al. Cross-hemispheric functional connectivity in the human fetal brain. *Sci Transl Med.* 2013 February 20; 5(173): 173ra24. doi:10.1126/scitranslmed.3004978.

82. Biswal BB, VanKylen J, Hyde, JS. Simultaneous assessment of flow and BOLD signals in resting-state functional connectivity maps. *NMR Biomed.* 1997;10(4–5):165–170.

83. Raichle ME, MacLeod AM, Snyder AZ, et al. A default mode of brain function. *Proc Natl Acad Sci U S A.* 2001;98(2):676–682.

84. Sparling JW. *Concepts in Fetal Movements Research.* New York, NY: Haworth Press; 1993.

85. Prechtl HF, Einspieler C. Is neurological assessment of the fetus possible? *Eur J Obstet Gynecol Reprod Biol.* 1997;75(1):81–84.

86. Olesen AG, Svare JA. Decreased fetal movements: background, assessment, and clinical management. *Acta Obstet Gynecol Scand.* 2004;83(9):818–826.

87. Hayat TT, Nihat A, Martinez-Biarge M, et al. Optimization and initial experience of a multislice balanced steady-state free precession cine sequence for the assessment of fetal behavior in utero. *AJNR Am J Neuroradiol.* 2011;32:331–338.

88. Guo WY, Ono S, Oi S, et al. Dynamic motion analysis of fetuses with central nervous system disorders by cine magnetic resonance imaging using fast imaging employing steady-state acquisition and parallel imaging: a preliminary result. *J Neurosurg.* 2006;105(suppl 2):94–100.

89. Pasca AM, Penn AA. The placenta: the lost neuroendocrine organ. *Neoreviews.* 2010;11:e64–e77.

90. Derwig IE, Akolekar R, Zelata FO, et al. Association of placental volume measured by MRI and birth weight percentile. *J Magn Reson Imaging.* 2011;34:1125–1130.

91. Messerschmidt A, Baschat A, Linduska N, et al. Magnetic resonance imaging of the placenta identifies placental vascular abnormalities independently of Doppler ultrasound. *Ultrasound Obstet Gynecol.* 2011;37(6):717–722.

92. Javor D, Nasel C, Schweim T, et al. In vivo assessment of putative functional placental tissue volume in placental intrauterine growth restriction (IUGR) in human fetuses using diffusion tensor magnetic resonance imaging. *Placenta.* 2013;34(8):676–680.

93. Anblagan D, Jones NW, Costigan C, et al. Maternal smoking during pregnancy and fetal organ growth: a magnetic resonance imaging study. *PLoS One.* 2013;8(7):e67223.

94. Morita S, Ueno E, Fujimura M, Muraoka M, Takagi K, Fujibayashi M. http://www.ncbi.nlm.nih.gov/pubmed/19711415 Feasibility of diffusion-weighted MRI for defining placental invasion. *J Magn Reson Imaging.* 2009 Sep;30(3):666–71.

95. Bonel HM, Stolz B, Diedrichsen L, et al. Diffusion-weighted MR imaging of the placenta in fetuses with placental insufficiency. *Radiology.* 2010;255(3):810–819.

96. Moore RJ, Issa B, Tokarczuk P, et al. In vivo intravoxel incoherent motion measurement in the human plancenta using echo-planar imaging at 0.5 T. *Magn Reson Med.* 2000;43:295–302.

97. Moore RJ, Strachan BK, Tyler DJ, et al. In utero perfusing fraction maps in normal and growth restricted pregnancy measured using IVIM echo-planar MRI. *Placenta.* 2000;21(7):726–732.

98. Derwig I, Barker GJ, Poon L, et al. Association of placental T2 relaxation times and uterine artery Doppler ultrasound measures of placental blood flow. *Placenta.* 2013;34(6):474–479.

99. Sørensen A, Peters D, Simonsen C, et al. Changes in human fetal oxygenation during maternal hyperoxia as estimated by BOLD MRI. *Prenat Diagn.* 2013;33(2):141–145.

100. Huen I, Morris DM, Wright C, et al. R(1) and R(2) * changes in the human placenta in response to maternal oxygen challenge. *Magn Reson Med.* 2013;70(5):1427–1433.

101. Denison FC, Semple SI, Stock SJ, et al. Novel use of proton magnetic resonance spectroscopy (1HMRS) to non-invasive assess placental metabolism. *PLoS One.* 2012;7(8):e42926.

Fetal cardiovascular physiology is routinely examined using Doppler in a range of conditions, including congenital heart disease (CHD), intrauterine growth restriction (IUGR), multiple pregnancies, and fetal anemia. However, it is worth noting that ultrasound is not commonly used to measure one key hemodynamic parameter, namely blood flow, because of inherent inaccuracies in the technique.[1] Furthermore, although an important aim of Doppler assessment is the identification of fetal hypoxia, ultrasound provides no information about the oxygen content of arterial and venous blood. By contrast, MRI offers the potential to measure both, allowing quantification of such fundamental elements of fetal cardiovascular physiology as oxygen delivery ($Do_2$), oxygen consumption ($Vo_2$), fetal cardiac output, the distribution of blood flow across the fetal circulation, and oxygen transport from the placenta to the fetal brain.

IUGR affects up to 10% of pregnancies and is associated with changes in fetal cerebral, peripheral, and placental vascular resistance resulting in circulatory redistribution commonly referred to as "brain-sparing physiology."[2] This is routinely identified through detection of velocity waveform changes in the cerebral and umbilical arteries using Doppler ultrasound.[3] However, late onset IUGR is currently difficult to detect because ultrasound measurements of fetal growth become less accurate toward the end of the pregnancy, and the typical Doppler changes seen in early onset IUGR are frequently absent.[4] Furthermore, animal studies suggest that chronic fetal hypoxia results in a reduction in fetal $Vo_2$ that tends to normalize blood flow distribution, but which is nevertheless associated with delayed fetal growth and development.[5,6]

The detection of chronic IUGR might therefore be improved by the identification of reduced fetal $Vo_2$ in the setting of normal Doppler findings. This could be particularly useful toward the end of the pregnancy, when the potential benefits of delivery from in utero hypoxia and starvation outweigh the risks of premature birth.[7] Uncertainty about the presence of fetal hypoxia currently leads to a high incidence of avoidable iatrogenic morbidity following induction of labor or cesarean section in late gestation small for gestational age fetuses. As an example, 33.4% of 650 women recruited to the recently published DIGITAT (Disproportionate Intrauterine Growth Intervention Trial at Term) trial had no postnatal evidence of IUGR (birthweight <10th centile).[8]

Fetal $Vo_2$ can be calculated when the oxygen content of blood in the umbilical artery and vein, and placental blood flow are known.[9] This has been achieved in human fetuses using invasive cordocentesis and ultrasound.[10] However, the risks associated with direct cordocentesis make it unsuitable for routine clinical use. However, by providing a non-invasive technique to measure blood flow and oxygen content, fetal cardiovascular MRI could become a useful adjunct to the usual ultrasound assessment of conditions like IUGR and CHD.

## THEORY

Techniques for measuring blood flow using phase contrast (PC) MRI[11] and oxygen content using quantitative T2 MRI[12,13] are well established, but imaging fetal vessels requires modification of the existing techniques. Specific challenges include the small size of the vessels, the virtually constant movement of the fetus, and difficulty detecting the fetal electrocardiogram (ECG) for cardiac triggering.

The latter can be overcome with alternatives to ECG gating such as self-gating[14] and cardiotocographic gating,[15] which have both been shown to be feasible in fetal animal models. Alternatively, a retrospective technique can be used that acquires temporally oversampled data and then iteratively sorts the data using hypothetical ECG trigger times until artifact in the associated images is minimized.[16] This approach (Fig. 6.4-1) is termed metric-optimized gating (MOG) and has been used successfully for PC MRI and steady-state free precession (SSFP) cine imaging.[17,18]

Regarding fetal oximetry, a novel approach to myocardial T2 mapping with nonrigid motion correction has been developed, which holds promise for improving fetal MR oximetry in the presence of small fetal movements.[19,20] This approach may improve T2 accuracy by aligning target vessels across images used to construct a T2 map.

For fetal MRI, short scan times are essential to reduce artifact from gross fetal motion. As a result, there is a practical limit to the spatial resolution and signal-to-noise ratio that can be achieved. PC MR and T2 mapping techniques, however, perform well in the majority of late gestation fetuses, whose vessel sizes are similar to neonates and whose body motion is partly restricted by the uterine walls.

Assuming a normal hematocrit, the PC MRI and T2 data may be used to calculate fetal $Do_2$ and $Vo_2$.[9] This requires calculation of the oxygen content, $C$, of umbilical venous (UV) blood, which is given by the equation:

$$C_{UV} = [Hb] \times 1.36 \times Y_{UV}$$

where $Y_{UV}$ is the oxygen saturation of blood in the UV, and 1.36 is the amount of oxygen (mL at 1 atm) bound per gram of hemoglobin.

Fetal $Do_2$ can then be calculated from the product of UV flow ($Q_{UV}$) and $C_{UV}$. To calculate fetal $Vo_2$, the arteriovenous difference in oxygen content ($\Delta C$) between the UV and the umbilical artery (UA) must be calculated, as follows:

$$\text{Fetal } Vo_2 = Q_{UV} \times \Delta C_{UV-UA}$$

Because of the small size of the UA, the T2 in the descending aorta (DAo) is used for this calculation.

If it is assumed that the majority of the flow in the superior vena cava (SVC) is venous return from the brain, then fetal cerebral $Vo_2$ can also be approximated:

$$\text{Fetal cerebral } Vo_2 = Q_{SVC} \times \Delta C_{AAo-SVC}$$

## FETAL CMR METHODOLOGY AND PROTOCOL

### Field Strength

Fetal cardiovascular MRI can be performed on 1.5 and 3 T systems. Specific absorbed rate (SAR) is limited to 2 W per kg

## Oversampled Data Acquisition

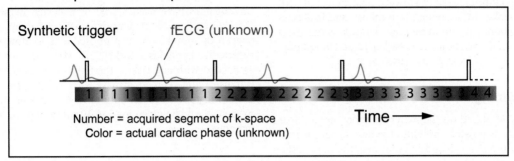

## Iterative Reconstruction

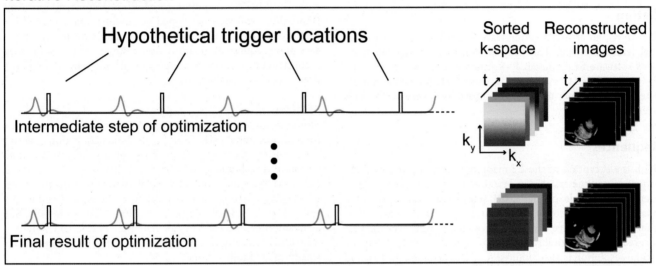

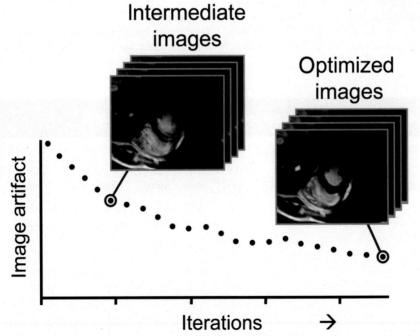

**FIGURE 6.4-1:** Metric-optimized gating. A synthetic trigger with longer R–R interval is used to acquire the k-space data. Hypothetic trigger locations are then retrospectively applied to the data and iteratively reconstructed with the correct average R–R interval identified as the reconstruction with the least image artifact.

("normal mode"). 1.5 T systems are less prone to SSFP banding artifacts from field inhomogeneity. However, the increased SNR available at 3 T makes PC imaging more robust, and facilitates MOG reconstruction. An important consideration is the effect of field strength on the relationship between T2 and blood oxygenation, with shorter T2 values encountered at 3 T.[21]

## Patient Positioning and Coil Selection

A body-matrix coil placed on the maternal abdomen, as close to the fetal thorax as possible, provides the best signal for fetal imaging. The addition of a second coil may help to improve signal across the whole field of view, particularly if the mother is in a lateral decubitus position, which many women find most comfortable later on in pregnancy.

## Gating

For MOG, an artificial gating trace is used in place of the actual fetal waveform. This may be controlled using the scanner's software to define an R–R interval. For most fetuses, an R–R interval of 545 milliseconds, which corresponds to a heart rate of 110 beats per minute, will ensure that every heartbeat is oversampled.

## Sequences

With the exception of the T2 mapping "work in progress," the sequence parameters shown in Table 6.4-1 are based on commercially available cardiac MRI sequences, and represent a possible approach to fetal CMR at 1.5 T. For PC vessel flow quantification, we use a minimum of eight voxels over the vessel area and a temporal resolution of 50 milliseconds. Adequate spatial resolution is also required for T2 measurements to avoid partial volume artifacts.[22] We use an interval of 4 seconds (8 cardiac cycles) between T2 preparation pulses for T2 mapping to ensure adequate recovery of magnetization. Figure 6.4-2 shows how we orient the PC and T2 acquisitions for the target vessels.

## Maternal Hyperoxygenation

Investigators have used a trial of maternal hyperoxygenation (MH) to enhance fetal hemodynamic assessment, and maternal oxygen therapy has been proposed as a treatment for cardiac ventricular hypoplasia and IUGR. MH does not appear to be associated with any risk to the fetus or mother. One approach is to use a non-rebreather mask with 12 L per minute of oxygen to administer an $F_{IO_2}$ of 60% to 70%. Previous studies suggest oxygen should be given for 5 to 10 minutes prior to and during imaging.[23]

## Postprocessing

### Flow

The MOG technique currently requires transfer of the raw data from the MRI to a computer for offline reconstruction using stand-alone software developed at our institution (MATLAB, Mathworks, USA). This software is available from our laboratory upon request. To quantify flow from the resulting PC MRI reconstructions, commercially available software is used (Q-flow, Medis, the Netherlands).

### Fetal Weight

Flows are indexed to fetal weight based on a high-resolution three-dimensional (3D) SSFP breath-hold acquisition covering the whole fetus to calculate the fetal volume. We use a combination of thresholding and other tools in Mimics (Materialise, Belgium) to segment the fetus. Fetal volume is converted to fetal weight using the conversion proposed by Baker (fetal weight [g] = 120 + fetal volume [mL] × 1.03).[24] The same 3D SSFP acquisition can be used to calculate the volume and weight of individual fetal organs, including the fetal brain, where brain weight (g) = brain volume × 1.04.[25]

### T2 Mapping

Regions of interest covering the central 50% of the vessel area are used for measuring T2. We currently convert the

| Table 6.4-1 | **Proposed Imaging Parameters for Fetal Cardiovascular MRI** |

| Sequence | Type | Gating | Resp. Comp. | Parallel Imaging Factor | NSA | TE (ms) | TR (ms) | Slice Thick (mm) | Matrix Size | FOV (mm) | Temp. Resol. (ms) | Scan Time (s) |
|---|---|---|---|---|---|---|---|---|---|---|---|---|
| 3D-SSFP | 3D | — | Breath hold | 2 | 1 | 1.74 | 3.99 | 2 | 256 × 205 × 80 | 400 | — | 13 |
| Static SSFP | 2D | — | — | — | 1 | 1.3 | 6.33 | 4 | 320 × 211 | 350 | 1,336 | 24 (15 slices) |
| Cine SSFP | 2D | MOG | — | 2 | 1 | 1.26 | 3.04 | 5 | 340 × 310 | 340 | 46 | 55 (10 slices) |
| Phase contrast[a] | 2D | MOG | — | — | 1 | 3.15 | 6.78 | 3 | 240 × 240 | 240 | 54 | 36 |
| T2 mapping[b] | 2D | PG | — | 2 | 1 | 1.15[c] | 3.97[c] | 6 | 224 × 181 | 350 | 4,000 | 12 |

[a]Velocity encoding sensitivity tailored according to vessel: 150 cm per second for arteries, 100 cm per second for veins, and 50 cm per second for umbilical vein. Number of segments per cardiac cycle = 4.
[b]T2 mapping used four T2 preparation times, tailored to span the expected T2 of a given vessel (0 ms, 0.33 × T2, 0.66 × T2, and 1.00 × T2), with 4,000 ms of magnetization recovery between successive T2 preparations.
[c]Rapid imaging of the T2-prepared magnetization was performed using a SSFP sequence with the indicated TE/TR values. NSA, number of signal averages; TE, echo time; TR, repetition time; FOV, field of view; MOG, metric-optimized gating (R–R interval 545 ms); PG, pseudo-gating (based on estimated R–R interval).

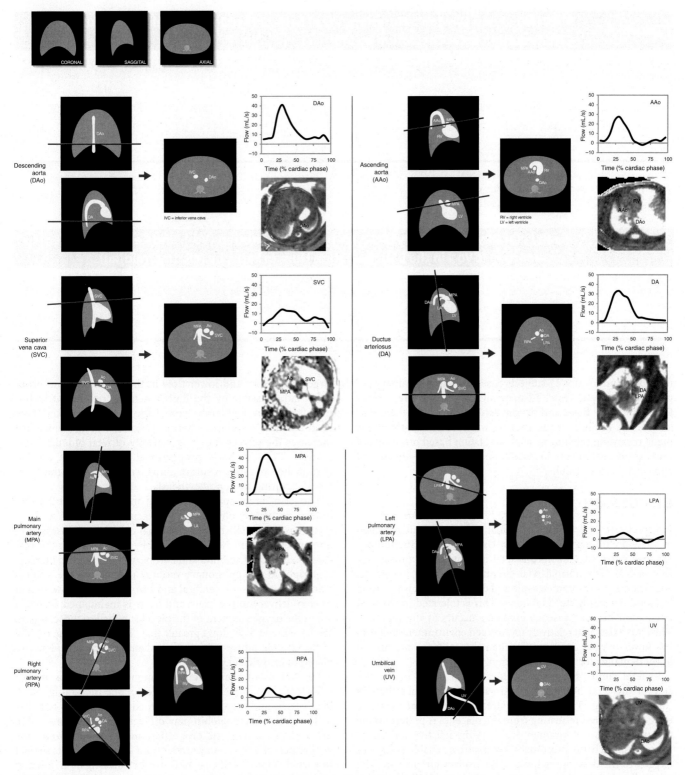

**FIGURE 6.4-2:** Slice prescriptions for fetal cardiovascular MRI. Orientation of slices for phase contrast and T2 mapping of the major fetal vessels is based on three-plane static SSFP survey of the fetal thorax showing representative flow curves and T2 maps.

T2 values to saturations using the relationship described by Wright et al.[12] for adult blood. The accurate conversion of the T2 of blood to oxygen saturation is dependent on hemoglobin [Hb] concentration. We assume a fetal [Hb] of 15 g per dL at 36 to 37 weeks.[26]

## REFERENCE VALUES

Tables 6.4-2 and 6.4-3 show the mean vessel flows and ranges of flows in 30 subjects (mean gestational age, 37 weeks; SD 1.2) by PC MRI. We also present preliminary mean oxygen saturations,

| Table 6.4-2 | Mean Flows and Oxygen Saturations (Y) in Each of the Major Vessels in the Human Late Gestation Fetal Circulation by MRI | | | | | | | | |
|---|---|---|---|---|---|---|---|---|---|
| | **CVO** | **MPA** | **AAo** | **SVC** | **DA** | **PBF** | **DAo** | **UV** | **FO** |
| Mean flow (mL/min/kg) | 473 | 250 | 210 | 135 | 189 | 78 | 254 | 129 | 145 |
| 95% CI | (376, 595) | (174, 376) | (120, 261) | (82, 200) | (97, 205) | (18, 182) | (181, 338) | (97, 205) | (9, 255) |
| Modeled mean flow (% CVO) | | 53 | 45 | 29 | 41 | 17 | 54 | 28 | 31 |
| Y (%) | | 52 | 60 | 46 | | | 53 | 79 | |

CVO, combined ventricular output; MPA, main pulmonary artery; AAo, ascending aorta; SVC, superior vena cava; DA, ductus arteriosus; PBF, pulmonary blood flow; DAo, descending aorta; UV, umbilical vein; FO, foramen ovale.

| Table 6.4-3 | Mean Fetal Oxygen Delivery ($Do_2$), Oxygen Consumption ($Vo_2$), and Cerebral Oxygen Consumption ($CVo_2$) in the Late Gestation Human Fetus by MRI (mL/min/kg) | | |
|---|---|---|---|
| | **$Do_2$** | **$Vo_2$** | **$CVo_2$** |
| Mean | 20.4 | 6.4 | 3.6 |
| SD | 3.5 | 1.7 | 0.8 |

fetal $Do_2$, and $Vo_2$ for 15 subjects based on our preliminary experience with fetal vessel T2 mapping. Figure 6.4-3 represents the mean vessel flows and oxygen saturations across the circulation. The findings are in keeping with previous estimations made regarding the human fetal circulation based on results of invasive measurements in fetal lambs and human ultrasound and cordocentesis results.[9,10]

## DISCUSSION

Interpretation of fetal cardiovascular MRI is currently limited to a few preliminary observations. Understanding the findings requires knowledge of normal fetal cardiovascular physiology (Fig. 6.4-3). The normal fetal circulation operates in parallel with shunts at the foramen ovale and ductus arteriosus resulting in blood bypassing the fetal lungs. This is tolerated in the fetal circulation because gaseous exchange occurs at the placenta. The fetus exists in a relatively low oxygen environment, but also has lower oxygen consumption than the newborn because of lower demands for thermoregulation.[9]

In fetal lambs, the oxygen saturation of blood in the left side of the fetal heart is approximately 10% higher than in the right owing to a remarkable streaming mechanism where oxygenated blood returning from the placenta is preferentially directed across the foramen ovale via the left liver and ductus venosus. This is presumably to ensure a reliable source of oxygen to the developing brain and coronary circulation. The less well-oxygenated blood returning from the SVC and lower body is preferentially routed toward the tricuspid valve and then on to the ductus arteriosus and pulmonary circulation. As pulmonary vascular resistance in the third trimester is inversely proportional to the oxygen content of the blood in the pulmonary arteries, a high pulmonary vascular resistance is maintained in the fetal lamb. Pulmonary vascular resistance is also high in the human fetus, although there is higher pulmonary blood flow compared with that in lambs.[9] There is also higher flow in the SVC in the human, likely reflecting the larger brain size, and lower flow in the umbilical vein, probably made possible by the higher hematocrit present in human fetuses. In fetal lambs exposed to chronic hypoxia, there is an adaptive response, where a 20% increase in hematocrit increases the oxygen carrying capacity of fetal blood.[6] Interestingly, T2 is inversely proportional to hematocrit, so that chronic hypoxia may result in a further reduction in the T2 of blood resulting from polycythemia.[27]

The term "brain-sparing" refers to an important mechanism in fetal circulatory physiology. This acute response to fetal hypoxia has been well studied in animal models and observed in human fetuses, and is characterized by a reduction in the vascular resistance of cerebral and coronary vessels and an increase in peripheral and pulmonary vascular resistance.[2] The result is a dramatic increase in cerebral and coronary blood flow, so that oxygen delivery to the brain and heart is maintained despite a fall in the oxygen content of the blood supplied to those organs. We have noted SVC flows greater than 250 mL/min/kg, or 50% of the CVO in fetuses with antenatal and postnatal evidence of placental insufficiency.[28]

Limitations of the current technique include gaps in our knowledge about the T2 mapping technique for fetal blood in fetal vessels and the dependence on an estimation of fetal hematocrit. Fetal hemoglobin may differ from adult hemoglobin in terms of its magnetic properties, and the small size of the fetal vessels of interest may render the T2 measurements subject to partial volume artifacts. With further investigation, a better understanding of these factors should emerge and allow MR oximetry to be reliably combined with the more established PC MRI flow quantification.

## ASSOCIATED IMAGING FINDINGS

In addition to providing information about cardiovascular anatomy and physiology, fetal MRI can provide helpful information about the respiratory system and other organs in the setting of CHD. Cardiac situs can be reliably determined in

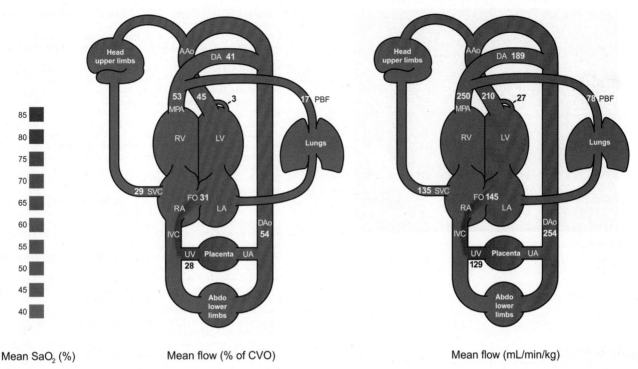

**FIGURE 6.4-3:** Mean flows and oxygen saturations in the late gestation human fetus by MRI. Mean flows as percentage of the combined ventricular output **(left)** and in mL/min/kg **(right)**. AAo, ascending aorta; DA, ductus arteriosus; MPA, main pulmonary artery; RV, right ventricle; LV, left ventricle; SVC, superior vena cava; FO, foramen ovale; LA, left atrium; PBF, pulmonary blood flow; RA, right atrium; IVC, inferior vena cava; UV, umbilical vein; UA, umbilical vein; DAo, descending aorta.

cases of isomerism using analysis of the bronchial branching pattern. Fetal hydrops due to elevated systemic venous pressures resulting from a variety of cardiovascular abnormalities is readily identified with T2W fast spin-echo sequences showing ascites, pleural effusions, pericardial effusions, and skin edema. In patients with obstructed pulmonary venous drainage because of hypoplastic left heart syndrome or totally anomalous pulmonary venous drainage, pulmonary lymphangiectasia is frequently present in the lungs, and can be identified as high-signal branching structures extending through the lung interstitium (Fig. 6.4-4).[29] In tetralogy of Fallot with absent pulmonary valve, asymmetric fluid trapping may be identified by fetal MR

because of bronchial compression by the dilated pulmonary arteries (Fig. 6.4-5). These early MR findings may help identify cases with severe pulmonary vascular disease that could benefit from early intervention.[30]

## CONCLUSION

The clinical significance regarding the distribution of flow in fetuses with CHD and IUGR is not yet known.[25,28,31] The hope is that with more experience and development, fetal CMR will gain acceptance among clinicians as an additional tool to help guide obstetric management.

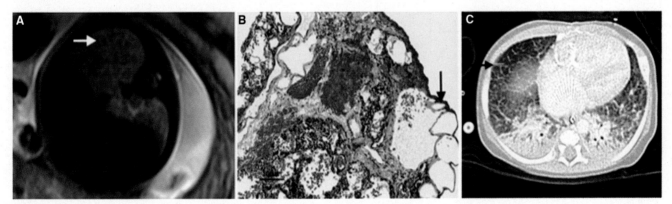

**FIGURE 6.4-4:** **A**: Axial single-shot fast spin-echo (HASTE) image of the fetal chest demonstrates high-signal branching linear structures extending to the surface of the lung (arrow) suggestive of pulmonary lymphangiectasia. **B**: The diagnosis was confirmed by lung biopsy showing dilated lymphatics (arrow). **C**: Postnatal high-resolution CT in this patient, showing thickening of the interlobular septae (arrow).

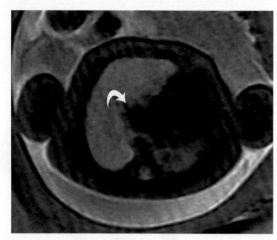

**FIGURE 6.4-5:** *Tetralogy of Fallot with absent pulmonary valve.* Axial T2W image through the thorax demonstrates hyperinflation of the right lung, which is high in signal with deviation of the heart to the left. The left lung is small and darker in signal. The pulmonary artery is prominent (*arrow*).

# REFERENCES

1. Gill RW. Measurement of blood flow by ultrasound: accuracy and sources of error. *Ultrasound Med Biol.* 1985;7:625–642.
2. Cohn HE, Sacks EJ, Heymann MA, et al. Cardiovascular responses to hypoxemia and acidemia in fetal lambs. *Am J Obstet Gynecol.* 1974;120:817–824.
3. Wladimiroff JW, Tonge HM, Stewart PA. Doppler ultrasound assessment of cerebral blood flow in the human fetus. *BJOG.* 1986;93:471–475.
4. Oros D, Figueras F, Cruz-Martinez R, et al. Longitudinal changes in uterine, umbilical and fetal cerebral Doppler indices in late-onset small-for-gestational age fetuses. *Ultrasound Obstet Gynecol.* 2011;37(2):191–195.
5. Pearce W. Hypoxic regulation of the fetal cerebral circulation. *J Appl Physiol.* 2006;100:731–738.
6. Richardson BS, Bocking AD. Metabolic and circulatory adaptations to chronic hypoxia in the fetus. *Comp Biochem Physiol A Mol Integr Physiol.* 1998;119:717–723.
7. Baschat AA. Neurodevelopment following fetal growth restriction and its relationship with antepartum parameters of placental dysfunction. *Ultrasound Obstet Gynecol.* 2011;37:501–514.
8. Boers KE, Vijgen SM, Bijlenga D, et al. Induction versus expectant monitoring for intrauterine growth restriction at term: a randomised equivalence trial (DIGITAT). *BMJ.* 2010;341:c7087.
9. Rudolph AM. *Congenital Diseases of the Heart: Clinical-Physiological Considerations.* 3rd ed. Chichester, UK: Wiley Blackwell; 2001.
10. Acharya G, Sitras V. Oxygen uptake of the human fetus at term. *Acta Obstet Gynecol Scand.* 2009;88:104–109.
11. Lotz J, Meier C, Leppert A, et al. Cardiovascular flow measurement with phase-contrast MR imaging: basic facts and implementation. *Radiographics.* 2002;22:651–671.
12. Wright GA, Hu BS, Macovski A. Estimating oxygen saturation of blood in vivo with MR imaging at 1.5 T. *J Magn Reson Imaging.* 1991;1(3):275–283.
13. Nield LE, Xiu-Ling LQ, Valsangiacomo ER. In vivo MRI measurement of blood oxygen saturation in children with congenital heart disease. *Pediatr Radiol.* 2005;35:179–185.
14. Yamamura J, Frisch M, Ecker H, et al. Self-gating MR imaging of the fetal heart: comparison with real cardiac triggering. *Eur Radiol.* 2011;21:142–149.
15. Yamamura J, Kopp I, Frisch M, et al. Cardiac MRI of the fetal heart using a novel triggering method: initial results in an animal model. *J Magn Reson Imaging.* 2012;35:1071–1076.
16. Jansz MS, Seed M, van Amerom JFP. Metric optimized gating for fetal cardiac MRI. *Magn Reson Med.* 2010;64:1304–1314.
17. Seed M, van Amerom JFP, Yoo S-J, et al. Feasibility of quantification of the distribution of blood flow in the normal human fetal circulation using CMR: a cross-sectional study. *J Cardiovasc Magn Reson.* 2012;14:14–79.
18. Roy CW, Seed M, van Amerom JF, et al. Dynamic imaging of the fetal heart using metric optimized gating. *Magn Reson Med.* 2013;70:1598–1607.
19. Giri S, Chung YC, Merchant A, et al. T2 quantification for improved detection of myocardial edema. *J Cardiovasc Magn Reson.* 2009;11:56.
20. Giri S, Shah S, Xue H, et al. Myocardial T2 mapping with respiratory navigator and automatic nonrigid motion correction. *Magn Reson Med.* 2012;68(5):1570–1578.
21. Lee T, Stainsby JA, Hong J, et al. Blood relaxation properties at 3T—effects of blood oxygen saturation. *Proc Intl Soc Mag Reson Med.* 2003;11:131.
22. Stainsby JA, Wright GA. Partial volume effects on vascular T2 measurements. *Magn Reson Med.* 2005;40:494–499.
23. Sorensen A, Peters D, Simonsen C, et al. Changes in human fetal oxygenation during maternal hyperoxia as estimated by BOLD MRI. *Prenat Diagn.* 2013;33:141–145.
24. Baker P, Johnson I, Gowland P. Fetal weight estimation by echo-planar magnetic resonance imaging. *Lancet.* 1994;343:644–645.
25. Al Nafisi B, van Amerom JF, Forsey J, et al. Fetal circulation in left-sided congenital heart disease measured by cardiovascular magnetic resonance: a case-control study. *J Cardiovasc Magn Reson.* 2013;15:65.
26. Nicolaides KH, Soothill PW, Clewell WH, et al. Fetal haemoglobin measurement in the assessment of red cell isoimmunisation. *Lancet.* 1998;331:1073–1075.
27. Bryant RG, Marill K, Blackmore C, et al. Magnetic relaxation in blood and blood clots. *Magn Reson Med.* 1990;13:133–144.
28. van Amerom JF, Roy CW, Prsa M, et al. Assessment of late-onset fetal growth restriction by phase contrast MR. In: 21st Annual Meeting of the International Society for Magnetic Resonance in Medicine; April 2013; Salt Lake City, UT. Abstract 5928.
29. Seed M, Bradley T, Bourgeois J, et al. Antenatal MR imaging of pulmonary lymphangectasia secondary to hypoplastic left heart syndrome. *Pediatr Radiol.* 2009;39:747–749.
30. Chelliah A, Berger JT, Blask A, et al. Clinical utility of fetal magnetic resonance imaging in tetralogy of Fallot with absent pulmonary valve. *Circulation.* 2013;127:757–759.
31. Porayette P, et al. MRI shows limited mixing between systemic and pulmonary circulations in fetal transposition of the great arteries: a potential cause of in utero pulmonary vascular disease. *Pediatr Radiol.* 2014.

# Placenta, Amniotic Fluid, Umbilical Cord, and Membranes

Eleazar Soto • Edgar Hernández-Andrade

The obstetric scan including ultrasound (US) and fetal magnetic resonance imaging (MRI) is traditionally dedicated to anatomical and hemodynamic fetal evaluation with less time spent on the evaluation of the placenta, umbilical cord, and membranes. While obvious abnormalities such as large placental abruption, umbilical cord cysts, or detachment of the amniotic membranes tend to be recognized immediately, other abnormalities of the placenta, amniotic fluid (AF), umbilical cord, and membranes tend to be overlooked. Given the association with adverse perinatal outcomes, knowledge of these abnormalities is of paramount importance.

## PLACENTA

### Trophoblastic Invasion

After implantation, the throphoectoderm generates a layer of cells around the blastocyst called trophoblast cells. These cells differentiate into villus and extravillous trophoblast. Villus trophoblasts form the chorionic villi that alter metabolite exchange between the fetus and the mother. The extravillous trophoblast migrates into the decidua and the myometrium, and invades the maternal spiral arteries, transforming them into low–vascular resistance vessels. The spiral arteries undergo a sequence of anatomical changes, including: lumen dilatation and transformation of the media and endothelial layers, with replacement of the muscular and elastic walls by a thick layer of fibrinoid material.[1]

Two different periods of trophoblast invasion have been described: (1) transformation of the decidual segment of the spiral arteries occurring during the first trimester of pregnancy, and (2) transformation of the myometrial segments of the spiral arteries in the second trimester of pregnancy. Abnormal transformation of the spiral arteries has been related to the development of perinatal complications. Robertson et al.[2] and Pijnenborg et al.[3] reported a lack of invasion of the myometrial segment of the spiral arteries in pregnancies complicated by preeclampsia (PE). Kim et al.[4] reported abnormal myometrial and decidual transformation of the spiral arteries in pregnancies with preterm delivery and intact membranes. Similarly, Romero et al.[5] reported that failure of physiologic transformation of the spiral arteries is associated with spontaneous second trimester abortion, preterm labor with intact membranes, preterm premature rupture of the membranes (PPROM), and placental abruption.

### Placental Anatomy

By spending a few additional minutes evaluating the placenta, the following parameters can be estimated: size, volume, echogenicity, and tissue characteristics.

#### Placental Shape

Postnatal evaluation shows that almost 90% of placentas have a circular shape and a central insertion of the cord; 10% have a different morphology.[6] Succenturiate placenta has one or more accessory lobes; the most frequent variant is the bilobed placenta.[7] Suzuki et al.[8] reported that succenturiate placentas were more frequently found in cases of assisted reproduction technologies and maternal age greater than 35 years old. The presence of succenturiate placentation is significantly correlated with retained placenta, postpartum hemorrhage, cesarean section for nonreassuring fetal status, and vasa previa.[9,10] Therefore, when there is a succenturiate placenta or accessory lobe in the lower part of the uterus careful evaluation with ultrasound for vasa previa and velamentous cord insertion should be performed.

Circumvallate placenta is characterized by a small chorionic plate with extension of placental tissue beyond the margins of the membrane insertion. A double layer of amnion and chorion with necrotic villi and fibrin forms a raised, rolled edge.[11,12] In other words, the placental membranes are attached to the fetal surface of the placenta instead of the underlying villous placental margin (Fig. 7.1). This type of placenta is reported in about 1.8% of pregnancies, and it is difficult to detect prenatally.[13] Nevertheless, prenatal diagnosis is important since the incidence of premature delivery, oligohydramnios, nonreassuring fetal heart tones, placental abruption, and fetal death increases in patients with a circumvallate placenta.[13] Some of the US findings reported in the literature are irregular and/or uplifted edge of the placenta (where the placental margin is rounded), a marginal shelf, rim, or band (where the placental edge is thin or sheet-like), and a bright border at the periphery of the placenta because of a thickened membranous rim.[11]

Placenta membranacea or placenta *diffusa* is a rare placental abnormality where part or the complete amniotic membranes are covered by chorionic villi. The reported incidence is about 1 in 21,500 deliveries; however, in cases of placenta previa, the incidence increases to 1 in 184 cases.[14] The literature about this topic is based on case reports, or small case series in which antepartum bleeding, spontaneous abortion in the second trimester, preterm delivery, fetal death, fetal growth restriction, postpartum hemorrhage, and placental retention have been reported. Placenta membranacea should be suspected when placental tissue appears to extend over most of the uterine cavity on US examination.[15]

#### Measuring the Placenta

Biometric measurements of the placenta such as thickness, area, and volume have been proposed as potentially useful methods for estimating the risk of perinatal complications.[12,16] However, to obtain reliable measurements, some factors should be considered. By using fundamental two-dimensional (2D) US, only two planes can be obtained, height and width. While theoretically a simple height measurement can be used to define the thickest part of the placenta, in practice this may be difficult as there is significant potential for variability. Identification of the thickest portion of the placenta can be technically complicated as there are only consecutive 2D US images with no depth perspective. The standard method is to locate the site of the umbilical cord insertion. In most cases, this assumption is accurate, and the umbilical cord is truly inserted at the thickest point, thus becoming the reference point for measuring thickness or obtaining placental radial measurements. However, two situations should be considered: First, in marginal umbilical cord insertion, the thickest placental region is not at the site of

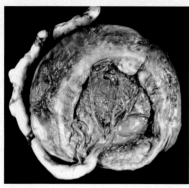

**FIGURE 7.1:** Placenta circumvallate. The main placental body is surrounded by a thick nodular ring that is formed by a double fold of the amniotic and chorionic membranes. (Courtesy of Dr. Faisal Qureshi.)

umbilical cord insertion (approximately 80% of all placentas have the umbilical cord inserted at or near to the geographic center); second, placental location and an irregular fetal surface can also affect the measurement of placental thickness.[17] Lee et al.[17] measured placental thickness in pregnancies at 18 to 22 weeks of gestation and reported a mean value of 24.6 mm. The authors also reported that posterior placentas were on average 6 mm thicker than anterior placentas. Hoddick et al.[18] proposed that an anterior placenta thickness of more than 33 mm, or a posterior placenta thickness greater than 40 mm in the midtrimester should be considered abnormal. Increased placental thickness has been associated with uncontrolled diabetes, fetal anemia, fetal hydrops, and placental floor infarction. In contrast, reduced placental thickness has been associated with intrauterine growth restriction and PE.[19] Wen et al.[20] reported that a reduced placental thickness and/or a reduced placental size were associated with high blood pressure in children. Leung et al.[21] reported that fetuses affected with alpha-thalassemia had a thickened placenta.

For volume and area calculations, it is generally assumed that the placenta has a circular shape and an equidistant distance from the center to all peripheral points. Yampolsky et al.[6] evaluated a series of 100 placentas after delivery, describing shapes and distances from the center to multiple distal points of the placenta. They found that 90% of all placentas had a circular or nearly circular shape, 5% were star-like with an average of five prominent spikes, with a distance from the center of the placenta that varied between 20% and 30%, and finally, 5%

were multilobulated placentas having on average two to three extra placental lobes. The authors commented that one of the main factors affecting the shape of the placenta is the vascular branching and ramification of the umbilical vessels.

Salafia et al.[22] further explored the characteristics of circular placentas and showed that the variation of radial measurements from different peripheral points to the center of the placenta was on average 3.4%. The same authors also evaluated the relationship between umbilical cord insertion and placental shape, and concluded that the site of umbilical cord insertion is not associated with differences in the shape of the placenta, and that central insertion is not always associated with circular placentas.[22] Placentas with a noncentral insertion of the umbilical cord (Fig. 7.2) were larger than those having a central cord insertion, and had an increased prevalence of velamentous and marginal cord insertion (Fig. 7.3). Nevertheless, no differences in birth weight were observed between circular and noncircular placentas.

The relationship between the weight of the placenta and birth weight has also been evaluated and correlated with maternal characteristics and neonatal outcome. Perry et al.[23] showed that the ratio between placental weight and birth weight did not vary with hypertensive disorders, intrauterine growth restriction, or maternal anemia during pregnancy. They documented a slight positive increment in the ratio associated with maternal obesity. Shehata et al.[24] showed a high association of placental weight/birth weight ratio with increased maternal body mass index (BMI), and uncontrolled diabetes, but no association with hypertensive disorders. In contrast, Hutcheon et al.[25] showed that lower placental weight is strongly associated with intrauterine fetal death and adverse perinatal outcomes.

### Key Points
- Nine out of ten placentas have a circular shape and a central cord insertion.
- Placenta thickness can be measured at the site of umbilical cord insertion. The normal thickness ranges from 2 to 4 cm.
- Increased placental thickness is associated with fetal hydrops, uncontrolled diabetes, and placental floor infarction.
- Reduced placenta thickness can be related to PE and intrauterine growth restriction.

## Placenta Location

Placental location can be defined by combining the following anatomical landmarks: anterior/posterior/fundal, left/right, and superior/inferior according to the main placental body position

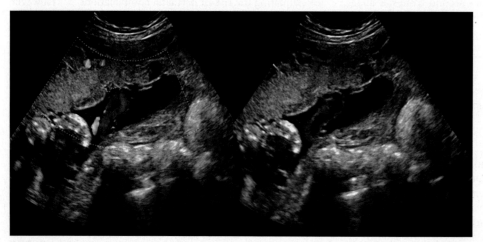

**FIGURE 7.2:** Marginal insertion of the umbilical cord.

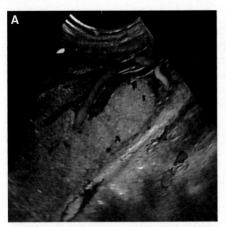
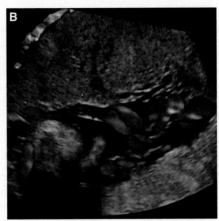
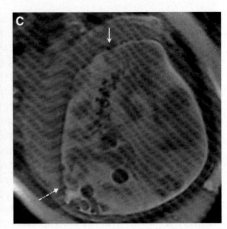

**FIGURE 7.3:** Velamentous **(A)** and marginal **(B)** insertion of the umbilical cord via US. **C:** On fetal MRI, in monochorionic twins, there is a paracentral *(solid arrow)* and marginal *(dotted arrow)* cord insertion..

from the uterus equator. A low-lying placenta is defined when the placenta edge is located in the lower uterine segment but does not reach the internal cervical os (ICO) (<2 cm away) (Fig. 7.4).

Placental location is the most frequent characteristic evaluated during US and MRI. In fact, it is so important that it can be related with life-threatening complications; the risk of placenta accreta highly increases with a low-lying placenta (OR 54, 95% CI, 18 to 166).[26] Fundally located placentas have a much lower risk of placenta accreta; however, the risk is not zero. Superior- and inferior-located placentas have the same risk of abruption and retroplacental hematomas. Low-lying placentas are also related to fetal breech presentation.[27] The lateral position of the placenta, either right or left, affects the hemodynamic parameters of the uterine arteries. The uterine artery close to the placental location shows a significantly reduced resistance compared with vessels on the opposite side of the uterus.[28] In a low-lying placenta, the most important information is the distance from the placental edge to the ICO. Either anterior or posterior low-lying placentas can partially or completely occlude the ICO. Oppenheimer et al.[29,30] measured the distance from the ICO to the placental edge and found that a distance ≥2 cm was not associated with vaginal bleeding before and during labor; therefore, a distance of 2 cm or more should be considered safe for normal vaginal delivery. Bronsteen et al.[31] found that when the placenta is within 1 cm of the ICO, 73% of cases required cesarean section due to vaginal bleeding, whereas among pregnant women with a placenta lying between 1 and 2 cm, only 23% required cesarean section due to maternal bleeding. The authors concluded that vaginal delivery in women with a placental edge

within 1 cm from the ICO carries considerable risk of maternal bleeding; but when the placenta is between 1 and 2 cm of the ICO, vaginal delivery might be considered.[31]

Measuring the distance between the edge of the placenta and the ICO should be done by transvaginal US. Farine et al.[32] compared the accuracy of transabdominal and transvaginal assessment with placenta previa, and reported that transvaginal US allowed a better visualization of the ICO and of the lower margin of the placenta than transabdominal US. They showed that transvaginal US increased by two-fold the positive predictive value for placenta previa as compared with transabdominal US. Therefore, every time that a low-lying placenta is suspected on transabdominal US, a transvaginal US should be performed.[32]

### *Imaging Recommendations*

Evaluate the lower segment of the uterus, even if the placenta has a fundal insertion. If any image is suggestive of placental tissue being present in the lower uterine segment, a transvaginal US should be performed.

## Placenta Migration

Small changes in placenta location are referred to as "placental migration." This slight displacement of the placenta can be related to the progressive increase in uterine volume moving the placental edge away from the ICO. Perhaps, the most important mechanism is the development of the lower uterine segment in the third trimester. Another hypothesized

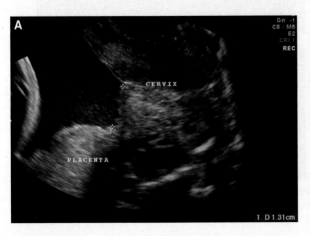
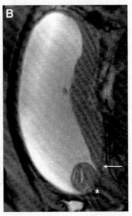

**FIGURE 7.4:** Low-lying placenta. **A:** Transvaginal ultrasound demonstrates a low lying placenta with distance from the placental edge to the ICO is less than 2 cm *(calliper)*. **B:** Fetal MRI demonstrates a low lying placenta *(solid arrow)* approximately 1.5 cm from the ICO *(asterick)*.

explanation is that the continuous renovation and reformation of placental tissue changes the relationship between the placental edge and the ICO; and finally, that the necrosis of placental tissue mainly affects the marginal parts of the placenta, resulting in a relative decrease in peripheral tissue and a change in its relationship with the ICO. Oppenheimer et al.[29] reported differences in migration related to placental position; posterior placentas tended to migrate slower than anterior placentas. These small changes in placental location can have important consequences for the clinical management of low-lying placentas. Cho et al.[33] studied 98 pregnant women, 69 with posterior and 29 with anterior placentas, and found significant differences in the weekly rate of placental migration. Posterior placentas migrate a mean distance of 1.6 mm (SD, 0.9 mm) per week, whereas anterior placentas migrate a mean of 2.6 mm (SD 1.5 mm) per week.[33] Oppenheimer et al.[29] also evaluated the placental migration in low-lying placentas and found that a migration below 1 mm per week was highly predictive of cesarean delivery because of vaginal bleeding. Similarly, Ohira et al.[34] reported that a migration rate lower than 2 mm per week is significantly associated with an increased risk of cesarean section for maternal bleeding.

Blouin and Rioux[35] investigated US scans performed in the second trimester of pregnancy and found that 8.4% of pregnancies were considered to have low-lying placentas (within 2 cm of the ICO); however, when evaluated during the third trimester, 95% of them were no longer considered low lying. Among cases identified as complete placenta previa in the second trimester, 67% had a normal delivery, and among those considered to be marginal previa, 73% had a vaginal delivery. In the overall group of low-lying placentas identified in the second trimester, only two pregnant women had a cesarean section due to antepartum hemorrhage. Contrary, Lodhi et al.[36] reported that pregnant women with complete placenta previa diagnosed between 28 and 32 weeks of gestation had no migration afterwards; in patients with partial placenta previa, migration occurred, but at a lower rate after 36 weeks of gestation. Ohira et al.[34] also reported that placental migration was reduced after 37 weeks of gestation in women with low-lying placenta.

### Measurement of Distance from Cervical Os

Transvaginal US is the gold standard to estimate the distance from the ICO to the placental edge. Transvaginal US does not increase the risk of bleeding in women with placenta previa.[37,38]

**Technique:** The bladder should be empty, avoid pressing the cervix with the transducer, visualize the entire endocervical canal (the anterior and posterior cervical lips should be of similar size), make a detailed sweep from side to side to document the location of the placental edge, measure the shortest distance between the placental edge and the ICO, do not measure during contractions or dynamic cervical changes, repeat the measurement, and select the shortest. Sonographers should report the distance in millimeters between the cervix and the placental edge. The risk of bleeding increases according to the distance.[39] A placental edge reaching the border of the ICO should be considered to be at 0 mm. If the placenta is within 20 mm from the cervical os, the US should be repeated at regular intervals; in these patients, the risk of cesarean section for vaginal bleeding is increased. When the placenta reaches or is located over the internal os at 18 to 24 weeks of pregnancy, a follow-up examination in the third trimester is recommended.[40]

### Key Points

- Low-lying placenta is diagnosed when the placental edge is within 2 cm distance of the ICO.
- Low-lying placenta is associated with placenta previa, placenta accreta, vasa previa, and breech presentation.
- The distance between the ICO and the lower placental edge should be confirmed by transvaginal US and reported in millimeters.

## Placenta Previa

The diagnosis and management of placenta previa is important as it is strongly associated with maternal hemorrhage.[41] Maternal bleeding represents a major cause of death worldwide, and may be associated with major long-term complications. The risk of maternal bleeding is related to the distance from the placental edge to the ICO.

Different terminology and definitions have been used in regard to placental location in relation to the ICO. Oppenheimer et al.[30] proposed the following classification: (a) low-lying placenta when the lowest placental edge is located at >2 cm from the ICO; (b) marginal previa when the placenta is within 2 cm of the internal os but does not cover the internal os; (c) partial previa, when only a part of the ICO is covered by the placenta (Fig. 7.5); and (d) complete previa when the entire ICO is covered by placental tissue (Fig. 7.6). Several factors increase the risk of placenta previa, including multiparity, previous abortion, smoking, advanced maternal age, and previous uterine surgical procedures. Gurol-Urganci et al.[42] reported an increase in the risk of placenta previa after one cesarean section (OR 1.60, 95% CI, 1.44 to 1.76). They concluded that from every 359 women with a prior cesarean section, one will have placenta previa.[42] Additionally, they found that having a prior history of placenta previa increases the prevalence of placenta previa in a future pregnancy to 43.3/1,000 births (OR 4.77, 95% CI, 3.55 to 6.42). Furthermore, placenta previa is associated with an increased risk of placenta accreta (1/50 after one cesarean, 1/6 after two cesareans, and 1/4 after three cesarean sections).[43] The risk of vaginal bleeding in placenta previa also increases in relation to cervical length. Ghi et al.[44] reported that pregnant women with placenta previa and a cervical length ≤30 mm have an increased risk of severe vaginal bleeding and delivery before 34 weeks of gestation. Therefore, measurement of cervical length in cases of placenta previa may have clinical value.

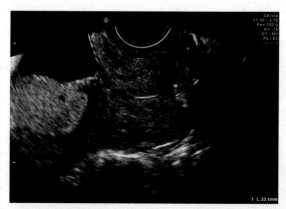

**FIGURE 7.5:** Partial placenta previa. Transvaginal ultrasound demonstrating placenta tissue covering part of the ICO.

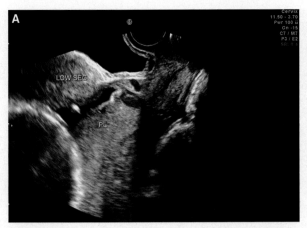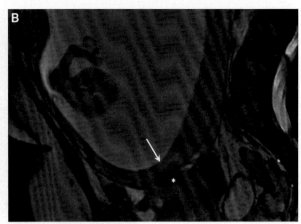

**FIGURE 7.6:** Complete placenta previa. **A:** Transvaginal ultrasound demonstrating placenta tissue completely covering the ICO. LOW SEG: lower uterine segment, PL: placenta. **B:** Sagittal SSFP T2 MR image in monochorionic twin gestation demonstrates placenta (*arrow*) covering the ICO (*asterick*).

While most diagnoses of placenta previa are made during the second trimester, the majority will no longer be considered previa during the third trimester of pregnancy. In a subset of cases, the diagnosis of complete placenta previa can be done since early pregnancy[45]; however, in all cases confirmation should be performed in the late third trimester of pregnancy.

### Imaging Recommendations
Be cautious when performing the transvaginal US; do not apply excessive pressure with the US probe. Make a detailed sweep from side to side to observe the placental edge in relation to the ICO. Apply color and/or power Doppler ultrasound (PDU) for visualization of the placental vessels close to the cervical os.

### Key Points
- Most cases of placental previa diagnosed during the second trimester will have resolved in the third trimester.
- The diagnosis of placenta previa should be confirmed during the third trimester of pregnancy.
- The risk of placenta previa increases in accordance with the number of previous cesarean sections.
- The risk of bleeding during labor increases in relation to the distance between the ICO and the placenta edge when the measurement ≤2 cm.
- A distance >2 cm between the ICO and the placenta border should be considered safe for vaginal delivery.

## Placenta Accreta

Placenta accreta is characterized by an excessive uterine invasion by the extravillous trophoblast. It complicates approximately 0.9% of all pregnancies and occurs in 9.3% of pregnant women with placenta previa.[46] Among all cases of placenta accreta, 80% to 90% are associated with placenta previa.[43] Abnormal placental invasion can be further subdivided into three types based on pathologic confirmation: (1) accreta (frequency of 81.6%) in which chorionic villi attaches to the myometrium, (2) percreta (11.8%), where the chorionic villi invades the myometrium, and (3) increta (6.6%) in which chorion villi invades through the myometrium into the serosa.[47]

Placenta accreta accounts for 33% to 50% of all emergent peripartum hysterectomies[48] and has been associated with a high maternal mortality rate. The risk for placenta accreta increases in cases with previous surgery of the uterus.[49] More important is the association of placenta previa and cesarean delivery, a circumstance that increases the risk of placenta accreta exponentially. For example, after one cesarean delivery, the risk of accreta increases from 11% to 14%; after two cesareans, it increases from 23% to 40%, after three cesareans, it increases from 35% to 61%, and after four cesareans, it increases 50% to 67%.[49] Therefore, all patients with prior history of cesarean delivery deserve a detailed placental US evaluation. Jauniaux and Jurkovic[50] reported three factors associated with placenta accreta: (1) excessive invasion of the extravillous trophoblast, (2) abnormal decidualization in the uterus, and (3) reduced perfusion in the uterine scar, which leads to local hypoxia and proliferation of the extravillous trophoblast.

### Imaging Recommendations
Findings during a first trimester US suggestive of placenta accreta include: location of the gestational sac in the lower uterine segment instead of the fundus, and a thin myometrium layer in the area of the uterine scar in the lower segment.[51] In the second and third trimesters, US findings associated with placenta accreta are the presence of multiple placenta lacunae consisting of irregular hypoechoic areas within the placenta, and loss of the placenta/myometrial interface with dilated vessels entering the myometrium creating an irregular wall between the placenta and the uterus[46,50–52] (Fig. 7.7). The placental lacunae are defined as parallel linear vascular channels extending from the placental parenchyma into the myometrium. This is the most characteristic sign of placenta accreta with a sensitivity of 78% to 93%, and the higher the number of lacunae, the higher the risk of accreta; whereas loss of the retroplacental space gives a sensitivity of 7%. Reduced myometrial thickness should be considered when the myometrium is less than 1 mm. Bulging vessels of the placenta and abnormal bladder wall have also been associated with placenta accreta. Approximately 50% to 80% of cases of placenta accreta can be detected on US. Transabdominal and transvaginal US done before emptying the bladder may help in the visualization of the interface between the uterus and the bladder.

When the diagnosis is uncertain, MRI can be used as a complementary tool to evaluate the placental/myometrial

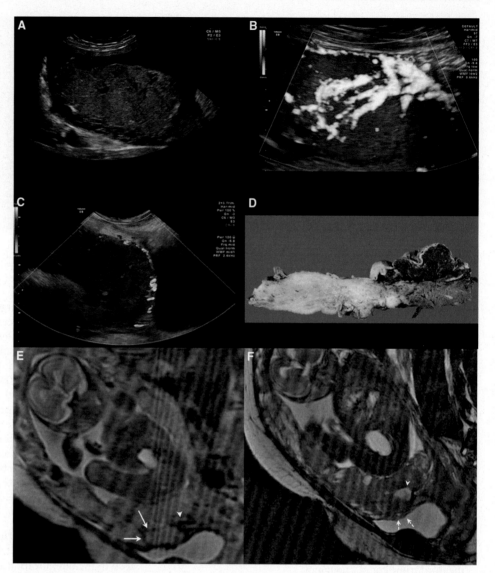

**FIGURE 7.7:** Placenta accreta. **A:** Multiple placenta lacunae (irregular hypoechoic areas distributed along the placenta) given a moth-eaten appearance. **B:** Abnormal vascularization all across the placenta. **C:** Reduced myometrial thickness and increased vascularization in the interface between the uterus and the bladder. **D:** Placenta percreta, the placenta invade the myometrium and serosa of the uterus. (Courtesy of Dr. Faisal Qureshi.) **E:** Sagittal SSFSE T2 image in a pregancy with maternal history of 2 prior C-sections. The placenta is low lying and inhomogeneous with linear bands of dark T2 signal *(arrows)* and focal round areas of disorganized vessels which are dark in signal *(arrowheads)*. **F:** Sagittal SSFP image in same pregnancy. The large vessel demonstrates bright blood flow (arrowhead). In addition, there is an abnormal lobular contour along the superior margin of the bladder *(dotted arrows)* proven to represent placental invasion of the bladder.

interface.[53] Imaging findings supportive of placenta accreta on MRI include heterogeneous signal in the placenta with large distorted vascular channels, dark intraplacental bands extending from the uterine-myometrial interface which are thought to represent fibrin deposition, outer uterine bulge or disruption of the normal uterine shape, focal interruptions in the myometrial wall with placenta invading adjacent structures particularly the bladder (Fig 7.7-E and F).[53a, 53b] Derman et al suggested that highest sensitivity for invasive placentation via MRI is by demonstrating increased placental vascularity and dark T2 intraplacental bands.[53b]

### Key Points

- The risk for placenta accreta increases according to the number of cesarean sections.
- Placenta accreta is generally (but not always) associated with placenta previa.
- Placenta lacunae is the most sensitive US finding for placenta accreta.
- Placenta lacunae, loss of interface between the placenta and the myometrium, and bulging vessels into the myometrium can detect 80% of women with placenta accreta.

- MRI may aid in diagnosis by demonstrating increased intraplacental vascularity, fibrin bands of dark T2 signal and direct placental invasion of adjacent structures.

### Vasa Previa

Vasa previa is diagnosed when fetal chorionic blood vessels are located in close proximity to the ICO without the support of the umbilical cord or placental tissue; in other words, the vessels are exposed coursing through the membranes, and are interposed between the fetal presenting part and the internal os.[54] Vasa previa is a life-threatening fetal condition, as the rupture of the membranes might lead to rupture of the fetal vessel and exsanguination.

The prevalence of vasa previa is approximately 1.5 to 4 in 10,000 pregnancies.[55] Most cases are found in association with low-lying placenta, velamentous insertion of the cord, bilobed placenta, and multiple gestations.[56] Al-Khaduri et al.[57] reported that the prevalence of vasa previa increases to 1/200 in pregnancies from assisted reproductive techniques. The reported coexistence of velamentous cord insertion and vasa praevia has been reported between at 2–6%.

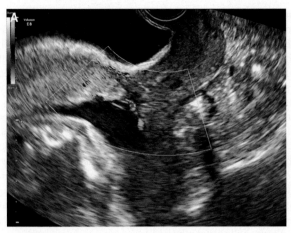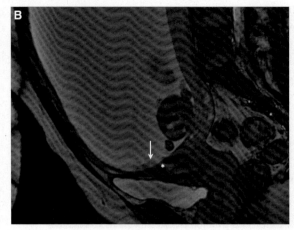

**FIGURE 7.8:** Vasa previa. **A:** On US, the fetal vessels are attached to the cervix by the amniotic membranes. **B:** On SSFP fetal MRI image there is umbilical cord *(arrow)* identified overlying the ICO *(asterick)*.

## Imaging Recommendations

The presence of an echolucent area at the placental edge suggestive of blood vessels on 2D US and confirmed using color and spectral Doppler should suggest vasa previa (Fig. 7.8A). On MRI, umbilical cord vessels crossing the placenta will demonstrate dark flow void on SSFSE T2 imaging and/or bright blood vessels on SSFP (Fig. 7.8B). Detailed examination of the lower uterine segment will assist in identifying an associated marginal placentation, velamentous insertion of the umbilical cord, or an extra placental lobe.[58,59]

Confirmation should be made by transvaginal US with clear visualization of the fetal vessel outside of the umbilical cord, in proximity to the ICO[60]. Spectral Doppler shows a venous or arterial waveform. Lack of movement of the vascular structure in relation to fetal movements also helps to define the diagnosis.[61] Serial US scans can be helpful to show a fixed location of the vascular structure. When the placenta is not in the lower part of the uterus, or in the absence of extra placenta lobes, the fetal vessels seen between the presenting part and the cervix are most probably a normal umbilical cord in a funic presentation. In this situation, serial US examinations can show changes in the position of the vascular structure in relation to the fetal part and the cervix. Other differential diagnoses include: chorioamniotic separation, fold of the amniotic membranes, amniotic band, and varicosities of the uterine veins.[62,63]

Owing to the high risk of fetal/neonatal mortality associated with vasa previa, it has been suggested that patients with this condition should be kept in the hospital after 32 weeks of gestation, with frequent monitoring of the fetal heart rate and uterine contractions, steroids therapy for lung maturation at 28 to 32 weeks of gestation, and delivery by cesarean section at 35 weeks of gestation.[37,59,60]

## Key Points

- Vasa previa is suspected when a vascular structure between the fetal presenting part and the ICO is observed.
- Vasa previa should be confirmed by transvaginal US and may be associated with low-lying placenta, velamentous insertion of the cord, multiple pregnancies, and bilobed placenta.
- Absence of movement of the vessels with fetal movements is highly suspicious of vasa previa.
- Vasa previa increases the risk of fetal bleeding and death.

## Placental Echogenicity

Grannum et al.[64] provided the first description and grading of placental echogenicity. Placental echogenicity was characterized by four different grades: grade 0, smooth chorionic plate; grade 1, subtle indentation of echogenic lines in the chorionic plate; grade 2, marked incomplete indentation from the chorionic plate to the basal layer and basal echogenic densities; grade 3, continuous and marked echogenic densities from the chorionic plate to the basal layer (Fig. 7.9). In earlier studies, grade 3 placentas were found to be significantly correlated with lung maturity, postterm pregnancies, and intrauterine growth restriction.[64,65] Subsequently, this classification lost popularity owing to its weak correlation with adverse perinatal outcome and poor agreement between operators. Moran et al.[66] reported an interobserver κ value of 0.34 for grading the placenta. Similarly, Sau et al.[67] reported only fair agreement between operators for placental grading. Nevertheless, recent studies suggest that the appearance of the placenta might provide useful information on the risk of developing perinatal complications. Kuo et al.[68] found that placentas with increased echogenicity, and increased levels of maternal serum alpha fetoprotein were associated with fetal–placental hemorrhage, as determined by the Kleihauer–Betke test. Kusanovic et al.[69] described differences in the echogenicity between the donor and the recipient placenta territories in a monchorionic twin pregnancy affected with twin-to-twin transfusion syndrome (TTTS). The authors reported and demonstrated that a hyperechoic and thicker placental in the donor twin is associated with reduced vascular Doppler signals, histologic lesions suggestive of ischemic changes, and overexpression of anti-angiogenic factors.[69]

Alternatively, reduced echogenicity and jelly-like consistency has also been associated with perinatal complications. Raio et al.[70] studied 16 pregnancies with a thick jelly-like placenta (defined as a thick placenta with patchy decrease of echogenicity and quivering like jelly to abdominal pressure) and reduced echogenicity, and found an increased risk of pregnancy-induced hypertension and fetal demise (Fig. 7.10). Jauniaux et al.[16] reported that US identification of a jelly-like placenta at 18 to 26 weeks of gestation was more prevalent in women who later developed PE. The same authors also reported a high correlation of jelly-like placentas with subchorial thrombosis and massive fibrin deposition when the pregnant woman had abnormally elevated serum hCG.[16] Therefore, the evaluation of the

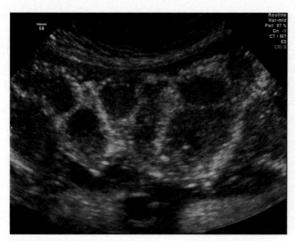

**FIGURE 7.9:** Placenta grade Grannum III showing continuous linear echogenic densities from the chorionic plate to the basal layer.

echogenicity of the placenta, whether increased or decreased, may help identify patients at risk for later pregnancy complications. Further studies in this area may add additional relevant clinical information.

### Imaging Recommendations

When increased echogenicity in the placenta is suspected, reduce the time gain compensation of the US equipment to confirm the echogenicity. In the presence of an enlarged placenta, reduce the gain to locate the jelly-like areas, create a gentle movement of the maternal abdomen to record the consistency and movements of the placenta. Measure the thickness of the placenta at the site of cord insertion.

## Placental Lesions

### Massive Perivillous Fibrin Deposition (Placental Floor Infarction)

About 10% to 15% of women with complicated pregnancies have cystic lesions surrounded by peripheral echogenicity in the placenta. Maternal floor infarction and massive perivillous fibrin deposition are linked to accumulation of serum-derived fibrin and throphoblast-derived extracellular matrix around the distal villi.[71] The reported incidence is 0.09% in all pregnant women and has been associated with adverse pregnancy

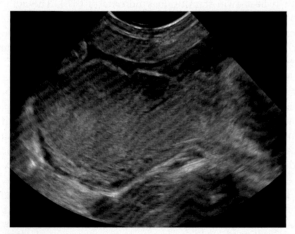

**FIGURE 7.10:** Thick jelly-like placenta with patchy decreased echogenicity and quivering in the presence of abdominal pressure.

outcomes such as fetal death, IUGR, preterm delivery, PE, and recurrent spontaneous abortion.[72–74] It is also more frequently seen in pregnant women with polymyositis[2] and antiphospholipid antibodies syndrome.[74] Some of the reported US features of massive perivillous fibrin deposition are: cystic hypoechoic areas larger than 1 cm, surrounded by an echogenic rim without blood flow inside the cyst. The hyperechogenic rim represents villi compressed by laminated fibrin and erythrocytes (Fig. 7.11). The majority of echogenic cystic lesions (72%) are 1 to 2 cm in length with a mean thickness of the echogenic rim measuring about 0.25 mm. In complicated pregnancies with echogenic lesions, Proctor et al.[75] reported a 79% prevalence of abnormal perinatal outcome, 61% risk of preterm delivery, 18% of severe IUGR, and 4% of perinatal death. During histopathology studies, between 60% and 75% cystic lesions are associated with intervillus thrombosis.

### Placental Infarcts

Placental infarcts can be documented in approximately 20% of uncomplicated pregnancies and in 70% and 40% of patients with severe and mild PE, respectively.[76,77] Vinnars et al.[78] reported that infarcts involving more than 5% of the placenta can be observed in 39% of patients with severe PE. Placental infarcts are mainly because of: (a) occlusion of spiral arteries by thrombus; (b) strangulation of the placental villi due to increased perivillous or intervillous fibrin/fibrinoid deposition; and (c) impairment of the fetal circulation due to fetal thrombotic vasculopathy.[79–81] Placental infracts can be observed as echodense or echolucid avascular areas. Fitzgerald et al.[82] reported that well-defined rounded cystic areas in the placenta were associated with a higher risk of PE and intrauterine growth restriction. The authors reported that more than 50% of these cystic lesions were associated with placental infarcts, reflecting maternal vascular underperfusion. Viero et al.[83] studied the sonographic placental features of 59 fetuses with absent end-diastolic flow in the umbilical artery (UA), and reported cystic images highly suspicious of placental lesions in 43 of 59 pregnancies. Echogenic cystic lesions had a 37% sensitivity for confirmed villous infarcts, and when combined with abnormal uterine artery Doppler velocimetry, a 53% positive predictive value for fetal death.

### Placental Lakes

Placental lakes are hypoechoic areas without villus structures that are usually larger than 2 cm and contain turbulent low-velocity flow. They are mainly seen during the third trimester of pregnancy and are not related to an adverse outcome. The shape of the lake changes dynamically and can be seen surrounded by a rich network of vessels (Fig. 7.12).

### Placental Hematomas

The ultrasonographic appearances of placental hematomas are hypoechoic or anechoic areas behind the placenta or the membranes. On MRI, hemorrhage can have different signal intensities but are often identified in the presence of bright T1 and dark T2 signal. The hematomas are classified by their location: retroplacental, subchorionic, and preplacental; however, a standard ultrasonographic definition of placental hematomas does not exist (Fig. 7.13). The identification of placental hematomas by US has been associated with an increased risk of spontaneous abortion, stillbirth, placental abruption, premature rupture of membranes, and preterm delivery.[84]

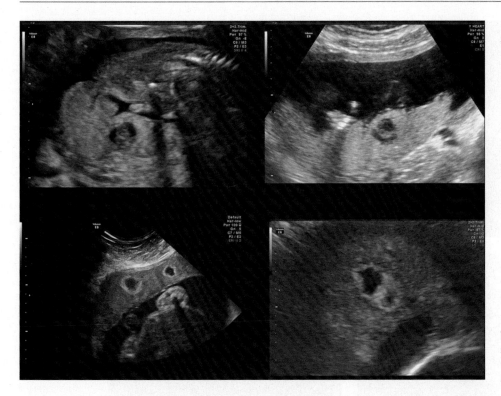

**FIGURE 7.11:** Intraplacental cystic areas surrounded by increased echogenicity (hyperechogenic rim) associated with massive perivillous fibrin deposition.

The lack of a standard definition for placental hematomas creates conflicting estimates of the incidence and risk of abnormal perinatal outcomes. Nagy et al.[85] documented a significant risk for placental abruption (RR 5.0; 95% CI, 2.8 to 11.1), PE (RR 4.0; 95% CI, 2.4 to 6.7), cotyledon retention or fragmented placenta (RR 3.2; 95% CI, 2.2 to 4.7), manual placental extraction (RR 3.4; 95% CI, 2.1 to 5.8), and NICU admission (RR 5.6; 95% CI, 4.1 to 7.6) when a large placental hematoma was observed. Fung et al.[86] reported 10 cases with massive subchorionic hematoma in which 40% of pregnancies resulted in fetal or neonatal death.

### Imaging Recommendations

A complete sweep of the placenta from side to side should be performed to exclude the presence of cystic lesions. When present, apply color directional Doppler, power Doppler, or

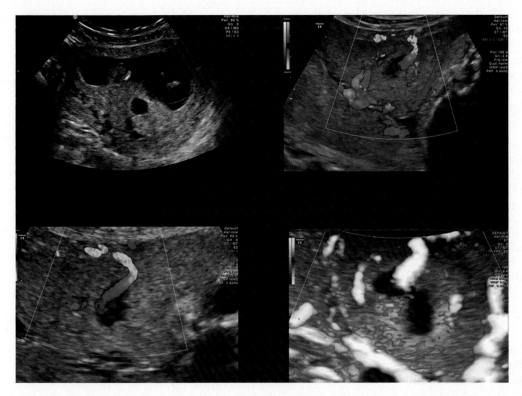

**FIGURE 7.12:** Functional cystic areas in the placenta. Hypoechoic areas of irregular shape, with no echogenic rim, and vascular supply around the cystic areas.

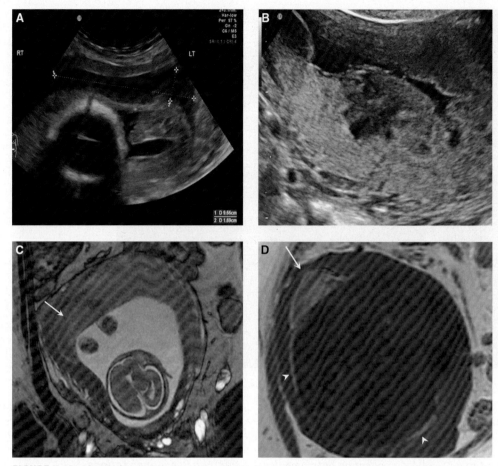

**FIGURE 7.13:** Placental Hematomas on US and MRI. Retroplacental **(A)**, and preplacental **(B)** hematomas diagnosed by US **C:** On Fetal MRI on a SSFP image, these is a crescentic area of heterogeneous dark signal *(arrow)* in a retroplacental location. **D:** Same pregancy as image **C.** The T1 weighted image depicts the hemorrhage more clearly due to bright signal *(arrow).* There is also subchorionic hemorrhages *(arrowheads)* that were not well delineated on the T2 sequence.

high-definition flow; if blood flow is documented around and/ or within the cyst, it is more likely to be a placenta lake. Careful visualization without color also allows the documentation of swirling movement inside the lake. The lake usually changes in shape and size. If the shape of the cyst is regular, does not change, has an echogenic rim and does not have flow, it is suggestive of perivillous fibrin deposition.

*Key Points*
- Increased placental echogenicity can be associated with hypoxic insult and placental hemorrhage.
- Reduced echogenicity and jelly-like appearance of the placenta can be associated with PE.
- Intraplacental cysts with echogenic rim and no blood flow are associated with massive perivillus fibrin deposition and increased risk of perinatal complications.
- Placental hematomas increase the risk of spontaneous abortion, stillbirth, abruption, PPROM, and preterm delivery.
- Large hematomas strongly correlate with fetal and neonatal demise.

## Placental Abruption

Placental abruption is defined as a premature separation of a normally implanted placenta (Fig. 7.14). The clinical manifestation is the presence of bleeding, and pain with uterine tetanic

contraction; or pain and uterine contractions without bleeding. There is not a direct association between transvaginal bleeding and the degree of abruption, as a large amount of blood can be kept in the uterus[87]; pain and contractions are the most reliable clinical signs. The risk of fetal demise increases when the abruption involves more than 50% of the placental surface. The fetal heart rate shows different pathologic patterns: from variable

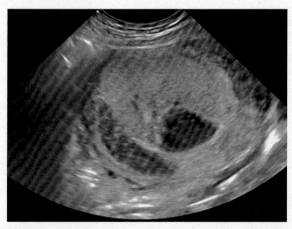

**FIGURE 7.14:** Posterior marginal placental abruption forming a retroplacental hematoma.

decelerations, bradycardia, to sinusoidal pattern.[87] Placental abruption can also be classified depending on the location of hemorrhage as: subchorionic (between the myometrium and the placental membranes), retroplacental (between the placenta and the myometrium), and preplacental (between the placenta and the AF).[88] Acute abruption can result in fetal death, activation of the coagulation cascade, and disseminated intravascular coagulation (DIC). Glantz and Purnell[89] reported that US has a sensitivity of 24% and a positive predictive value of 88% for detecting placental abruption.

The overall prevalence of placental abruption is about 1%, but increases 10-fold in preterm deliveries. In addition, a significant percentage of stillbirths are associated with placental abruption.[90] Neonates surviving from severe and acute placental abruption have a high risk of periventricular leukomalacia (PVL), and intraventricular hemorrhage (IVH).[87] Oyelese and Ananth[87] studied a series of more than 7,000 placentas after delivery and found the prevalence of abruption was about 3.8% with a majority of patients presenting without clinical symptoms; therefore, they recommended that placental abruption should only be diagnosed when clinical symptoms are present. The same authors reported that the risk of placental abruption increases from 20 weeks onward, reaching its highest prevalence between 24 and 26 weeks followed by a reduction until the end of the pregnancy. They also reported that after 24 weeks of gestation, fetal death is significantly correlated with placental abruption. The prevalence is higher in African American women than in Caucasians, perhaps related to the higher incidence of PE. Other risk factors of placental abruption include: cocaine and drug abuse, chronic hypertension, PE, chronic hypertension with superimposed PE, multiple gestation, oligohydramnios, polyhydramnios, myometrial tumors, thrombophilia disorders, PPROM, and chorioamnioitis.[87] In addition, a history of abruption in the previous pregnancy is an important risk factor of abruption in future pregnancies.

In a study by Nyberg et al.,[88] 57 cases of placental abruption that were detected by US were reviewed retrospectively. In 81% (*n* = 46) of the cases, the location of the abruption was subchorionic, in 16% (*n* = 9) was retroplacental, and in 4% (*n* = 2) preplacental; a subchorionic location of the hemorrhage was more frequent seen before 20 weeks. They described the appearance of hematomas as hyperechoic (*n* = 17), hypoechoic (*n* = 21),

and sonolucent (*n* = 19). In addition, the authors described that the echogenicity of the US appearance was related to the acuteness of the hemorrhage. For example, when there was acute hemorrhage, the area was hyperechoic compared with the rest of placenta tissue. Resolving hematomas became hypoechoic within 1 week, and sonolucent within 2 weeks.[88]

### Key Points

- The US diagnosis of placental abruption is limited, diagnosis should rely on clinical findings.
- Placental abruption should be considered in the presence of vaginal bleeding or continuous abdominal pain and uterine contractions.

## Placental Tumors

Trophoblastic disease refers to a group of clinical entities characterized by an abnormal development of trophoblastic tissue. It can be classified as: complete hydatiform mole, partial hydatidiform mole, and choriocarcinoma (Fig. 7.15).

Complete hydatidiform mole is characterized by swelling of villus tissue and trophoblastic hyperplasia with no embryonic or fetal tissue. The hydropic throphoblast tissue fills the uterus with the US appearance of multiple sonolucencies that gives the classical "snow storm" or "cluster of grapes" appearance.[91] The coexistence of complete mole and a normal fetus can be seen in dichorionic twin pregnancies with molar degeneration of one of the twins. Complete molar pregnancy is associated with severe vaginal bleeding and persistent gestational trophoblastic disease.

Partial mole is the degeneration of one or several regions of the placenta coexisting with normal placental tissue and a live fetus. The degenerated trophoblastic tissue gives an image of multiple vesicles surrounded by normal placental tissue, or the so-called "Swiss cheese" appearance. These pregnancies have an increased risk of intrauterine growth restriction, fetal anatomical defects, pregnancy-induced hypertension, and persistent gestational trophoblastic disease.[91]

Choriocarcinoma is a highly malignant tumor originating from trophoblastic epithelial cells. Approximately 50% of choriocarcinomas occur in the setting of a molar pregnancy, 30% after a miscarriage, and 20% after an apparent normal pregnancy. Clinical presentation includes vaginal bleeding, respiratory symptoms/dyspnea, and abdominal pain. The tumor is frequently metastatic to the lung, liver, and brain. Detailed placental evaluation with US might identify the primary tumor in the placenta that usually measures between 2.5 and 8 mm.[91] Placental choriocarcinoma occasionally metastasizes to the fetus resulting in infantile choriocarcinoma of the liver.[92] The sonographic appearance of this tumor is heterogeneous, echogenic, with myometrial invasion, with low-impedance circulation, and areas of marked vascularization within the mass documented with color and power Doppler imaging.

*Chorioangiomas* are the most common and benign vascular placental tumors; small chorioangiomas are identified in about 1% of placentas.[93] They are usually asymptomatic, but if the tumor is "large" (larger than 4 to 5 cm in diameter), chorioangiomas can be associated with increased fetal and neonatal morbidity, including anemia, polyhydramnios, hydrops, growth restriction, and perinatal death.[94,95] The likely reason for this increased morbidity is that chorioangiomas are supplied by the fetal circulation. The resulting fetal arteriovenous fistulas may lead to high-output cardiac failure in the fetus. The estimated

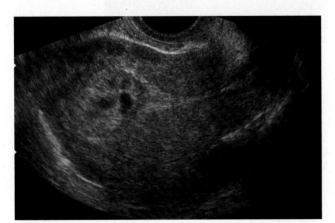

**FIGURE 7.15:** Mixed echogenic, multicystic, vascular structure in the fundus of the uterus without a gestational sac. Based on these findings, a complete molar pregnancy was suspected and subsequently confirmed on the pathology specimen after a suction/curettage procedure.

prevalence of giant chorioangiomas is about 1 in 8,000 to 1 in 50,000 pregnancies.[96] Chorioangiomas are generally diagnosed incidentally on US and have been associated with increased alpha-feto-protein concentrations in maternal serum and AF. The tumors appear solid and well circumscribed, and can be

either hyperechoic or hypoechoic protruding from the fetal surface of the placenta or near the umbilical cord insertion site (Fig. 7.16). Areas of hemorrhage, infarction, or calcification can be visualized within the mass. In addition, abundant blood flow determined by color and power Doppler is a common

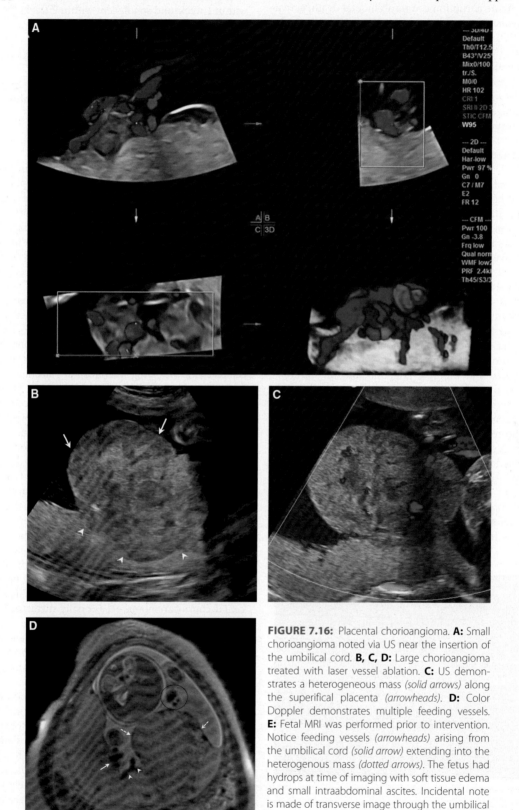

**FIGURE 7.16:** Placental chorioangioma. **A:** Small chorioangioma noted via US near the insertion of the umbilical cord. **B, C, D:** Large chorioangioma treated with laser vessel ablation. **C:** US demonstrates a heterogeneous mass *(solid arrows)* along the superifical placenta *(arrowheads)*. **D:** Color Doppler demonstrates multiple feeding vessels. **E:** Fetal MRI was performed prior to intervention. Notice feeding vessels *(arrowheads)* arising from the umbilical cord *(solid arrow)* extending into the heterogenous mass *(dotted arrows)*. The fetus had hydrops at time of imaging with soft tissue edema and small intraabdominal ascites. Incidental note is made of transverse image through the umbilical cord demonstrating dilatation of 2 arteries and vein *(black circle)*.

characteristic.[97,98] Differential diagnosis when evaluating a solid mass of the placenta include: placental teratoma, placental hematoma, partial hydatidiform mole, and metastasis to the placenta.[99] Several reports of prenatal surgery attempting to obliterate the feeding vessel of the tumor have been reported with mixed results.[100,101] MRI may be performed to confirm diagnosis and provide anatomy of the pregnancy prior to intervention. On MRI, the lesion is typically heterogeneous in signal and is supplied by large vessels, usually arising from the umbilical cord (Fig. 7-16). MRI may also be helpful to exclude brain injury in a fetus with cardiac failure. In view of the potential for adverse outcome associated with chorioangiomas, serial evaluation of fetal growth and fetal cardiac function is recommended.

## Placental Delivery

Limited studies on placental delivery are available. Krapp et al.[102] described the different phases of placental delivery as: latent, detachment, and expulsion. Herman[103] expanded this description as phase 1 or latent, characterized by thick placenta-free uterine wall and thin uterine placenta-site wall; phase 2 or contraction/detachment in which the placenta completes its separation; and phase 3 or expulsion, accompanied by sliding movement of the placenta. Krapp et al.[102] studied the vascular changes in the interphase between the placenta and the uterus during the third stage of labor, and found that absent flow in the myometrial interphase was related to successful placental delivery; whereas persistent flow in the same interphase was associated with placenta accreta. Placental delivery is related to an acute reduction in vascular supply and by the constant myometrial contraction. Detachment starts in one of the cotyledons and continues up toward the uterine fundus[104] (Fig. 7.17).

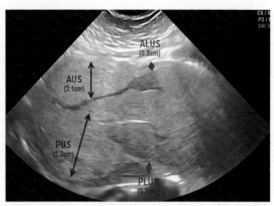

**FIGURE 7.17:** Placental delivery. Uterus in the third stage of labor where the anterior (AUS) and posterior (PUS) uterine segments are contracting, whereas the anterior and posterior low uterine segments (ALUS, PLUS) are separated allowing the expulsion of the placenta observed in the center of the image.

## Additional Placental Evaluation

### Placenta Volume

Ultrasound and MRI are imaging modalities used to estimate the placental volume.[105] Volume calculation by US can be estimated either using multiplanar measurements or Virtual Organ Computer-Aided Analysis (VOCAL). Multiplanar calculation is based on area delineation of each image included in the volume.[106] VOCAL is an algorithm applied to calculate volumes, assuming that evaluated structures have a circular shape; as the placenta is circular in 90% of cases, VOCAL can thus be used (Fig. 7.18). The main limitation is that placental size increases with gestational age. After 23 to 24 weeks of gestation, it is technically difficult to

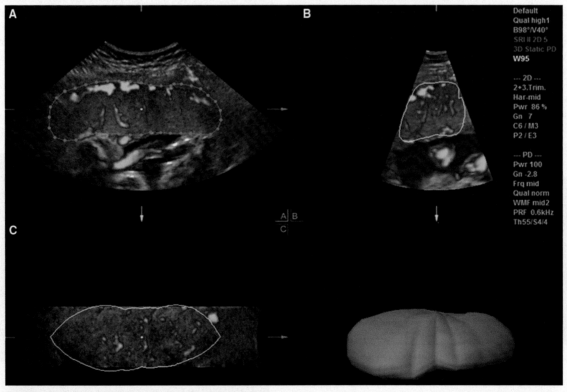

**FIGURE 7.18:** Placental volume obtained using Virtual Organ Computer-Aided Analysis (VOCAL). The **A, B,** and **C** images show the multiplanar visualization of the placenta with the selected region of interest where VOCAL was calculated. The rendered image of the placenta is created by delineating the placenta in 12 images separated by 30° in a rotational process.

include the complete placenta in the US volume. Therefore, several authors suggested that placental volume should be measured before 24 weeks of gestation. Placental volume has been associated with perinatal complications.[107] Rijken et al.[108] reported a significantly reduced placental volume before 24 weeks of gestation in women infected with *Plasmodium falciparum*. Pomorski et al.[109] showed differences in placental volume between growth restricted and normally grown fetuses. Hafner et al.[110] evaluated the placental quotient defined as placental volume/CRL during the first trimester of pregnancy and found a significant association with later development of PE. In contrast, other authors have reported that placental volume evaluation in the first trimester of pregnancy does not consistently predict perinatal complications. For example, Odeh et al.[111] reported no association between placental volume and development of PE. Rizzo et al.[112] did not detect any association between placental volume and diabetes in pregnancy. Similarly, Odibo et al.[113] did not report differences in placental volume during the first trimester of pregnancy between patients who later developed PE, gestational hypertension, or small for gestational age fetuses in comparison with those having uncomplicated pregnancies. Wegrzyn et al.[114] evaluated the association between placental volume and chromosomal abnormalities, and found that fetuses with trisomy 21 (T21) and Turner syndrome had larger placentas than fetuses with trisomy 18 (T18) and trisomy 13 (T13). On the contrary, Metzenbauer et al.[115] reported that placental volumes from chromosomal affected fetuses, including fetuses with T21, were significantly reduced when compared with normal fetuses at 10 to 13 weeks of gestation.

**Placental Blood Flow:** Evaluation of the placental blood flow with three-dimensional (3D) PDU has been proposed as a useful clinical tool for identifying cases at risk of perinatal complications[116] (Fig. 7.19). Power Doppler ultrasound expresses the changes in amplitude of the backscattered signals from the red cells. Three indices are calculated: (1) vascular index, representing the number of voxels containing power Doppler information, (2) flow index, indicating the averaged intensity of the voxels containing PDU information, and (3) the vascular/flow index, which is the ratio between the two indices.[111] These indices are calculated using the same VOCAL technique used for placental volume estimation. Vascular evaluation of the placental flow indices at the end of the first trimester of pregnancy seems to be related to the risk of developing perinatal

complications. Odeh et al.[111] reported that among the 3D PDU indices, the vascular index was significantly reduced in those patients who later developed PE. Rizzo et al.[112] reported a significant increase in 3D PDU blood flow indices in uncontrolled diabetic patents. Odibo et al.[113] found reduced 3D power Doppler indices in the group that later developed PE.

One of the main concerns of this technique is the low reproducibility between operators. Cheong et al.[117] reported a correlation coefficient of 0.33 among operators in the calculation of the blood flow indices. In contrast, Bujold et al.[118] reported a very good correlation ($R^2 > 0.8$) for all vascular indices during the first trimester of pregnancy. Standardization of US settings and clear definition of the region of interest are necessary for reproducible blood flow assessment using 3D PDU.

### Placental Circulation

The uteroplacental circulation has been mainly evaluated in the uterine and umbilical arteries, representing the maternal and fetal circulations, respectively. An abnormal process of placentation and/or placental interchange can be expressed as an increased resistance in the uterine or/and umbilical arteries.[119] Abnormal blood flow in the uterine arteries has been correlated with an abnormal trophoblastic invasion.[120] Doppler ultrasound has been applied to evaluate the uterine arteries velocimetry. By using color and spectral Doppler techniques, a histogram of vascular velocities during the cardiac cycle can be obtained, and the relationship between systolic and diastolic velocities can be expressed as resistance and pulsatility indices. Similarly, the shape of the Doppler waveform can provide important information as the presence of notch at the end of the systole is a sign of impaired placentation[121] (Fig. 7.20). An abnormal uterine arteries Doppler measurement is frequently defined as a mean pulsatility index (left and right) above the 95th percentile for gestational age and/or persistent bilateral notch.[122] Doppler evaluation of the uterine arteries between 11 and 14 weeks of gestation and between 20 and 24 weeks of gestation has been proposed as a useful screening test for the identification of cases at risk of PE and intrauterine growth restriction.[123]

### Placenta in Multiple Pregnancies

Dichorionic twins have two separate placentas with no vascular communications among them. A disproportion in placental size

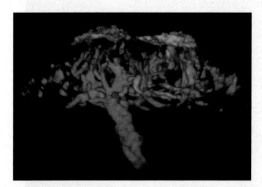

**FIGURE 7.19:** Placental blood perfusion using three-dimensional (3D) power Doppler. The placenta is delineated similarly as the previous image. When finished, only the power Doppler information is maintained showing the vascularization pattern of the placenta. The system can calculate the vascular (VI), flow (FI), and vascular/flow (VFI) 3D power Doppler vascular indices.

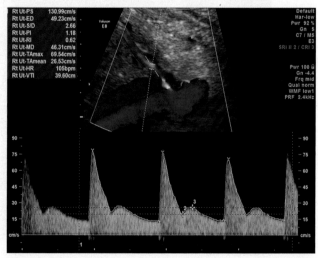

**FIGURE 7.20:** Uterine artery Doppler waveform showing the presence of early diastolic "notch."

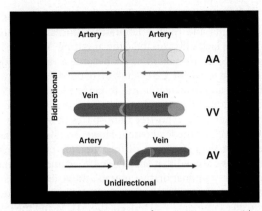

**FIGURE 7.21:** Vascular anastomoses of a twin pregnancy with a monochorionic placenta. Arterial–arterial (AA), and venous–venous (VV) are bidirectional communications occurring in the surface of the placenta. Arterial–venous (AV) are unidirectional communications, the vessels run in the surface of the placenta, but the interchange of blood occurs deep in the placental tissue (deep anastomoses).

may lead to selective intrauterine growth restriction.[124] Most monochorionic twins, on the other hand, have placental vascular anastomosis.[125] Two types of placental vascular anastomoses can be observed: unidirectional (arterial/venous), also called deep communications, and bidirectional (arterial–arterial, venous–venous), also called superficial communications (Fig. 7.21). Unidirectional communications are mainly related to twin to twin transfusion syndrome (TTTS), while bidirectional communications are associated with selective intrauterine growth restriction.[125] Differences in the placental territory for each twin have been associated with a significant impact in the fetal growth. Whereas in TTTS, twins might have similar placental territory, in selective growth restriction, there is usually a large disproportion in placental area for each twin.[125]

Clinical management of twin pregnancies is mainly based on the accurate determination of the chorionicity (number of placentas). This can be better performed during the first trimester of gestation by the identification of the lambda and T signs.[126,127] The lambda sign is produced by proliferating chorionic villi growing into the potential space between the two layers of chorion at the site of placental insertion.[128] A lambda sign

is characteristic of dichorionic twins with a sensitivity and specificity close to 100%. A clear T sign, which is an appearance due to the apposed amnion of the gestational sacs, has also a 100% sensitivity and specificity for monochorionic twins (Fig. 7.22). When either the T or lambda signs cannot be clearly defined, the pregnancy should be considered monochorionic and followed closely. The risk of selective IUGR is much lower in dichorionic than monochorionic placentas, but still higher than in singleton pregnancies. There is no risk of TTTS in dichorionic twins.[129]

### Key Points

- There are no consistent data regarding the predictive value of placental volume estimation and the risk of perinatal complications.
- The most used method for assessing placental volume is VOCAL.
- Reduced placental blood flow estimated using 3D power Doppler indices may be associated with an increased risk of perinatal complications.
- Increased pulsatility index and the presence of notch in the uterine arteries are associated with a higher risk of developing hypertensive disorders during pregnancy.
- The lambda and T signs have almost 100% sensitivity and specificity for defining dichorionic and monochorionic twins, respectively.

## AMNIOTIC FLUID

### Amniotic Fluid and Ultrasound

Amniotic fluid (AF) provides a supportive environment for fetal development. AF is fundamental for the development of the fetal respiratory, gastrointestinal, and musculoskeletal systems. AF protects the fetus from trauma and infection through its bacteriostatic properties and prevents compression of the umbilical cord. It is also believed that AF formation and maintenance reflect the integrity of the fetal cardiopulmonary and urogenital systems.

The American Institute of Ultrasound in Medicine (AIUM) and The International Society of Ultrasound in Obstetrics and Gynecology (ISUOG) recommend the assessment of the AF as part of the second and third trimester US examination.[130,131]

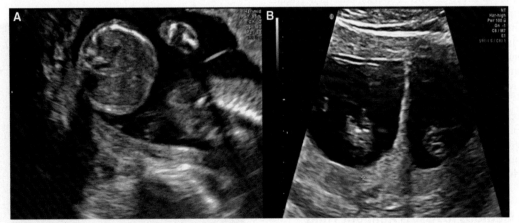

**FIGURE 7.22:** Membranes in chorionicity **A:** The T sign characteristic of monochorionic–diamniotic pregnancies. The T sign represents the amnion layers from both twins with one layer of chorion. **B:** The lambda sign characteristic of dichorionic–diamniotic twin pregnancies produced by proliferating chorionic villi growing into the space between the two layers of chorion.

## The Origin of Amniotic Fluid

In view of the difficulties of objective determination of the AF dynamics during pregnancy, most of the information regarding the physiology of the AF during pregnancy is based on animal models and, to some extent, human pregnancies. At the beginning of pregnancy, there is free transport of water, electrolytes, and other components through the chorioamniotic membranes. In addition, there is passage of water across the embryonic skin until fetal keratinization is established around 24 to 26 weeks.[132,133] This represents the origin of the AF which is considered to be a transudate.[134] AF volume measured during the first half of pregnancy increases logarithmically with advancing gestation.[135] It is estimated that at 8 weeks, there is about 23 mL of fluid, and at 14 weeks, AF has increased to approximately 100 mL.[135]

The kidneys and the lungs are two primary sources of AF later in pregnancy. Urine is first produced by the kidneys by the 9th week of gestation and is hyposmolar. After 14 weeks of gestation, approximately two-thirds of the AF is produced by fetal urination and one-third from pulmonary fluid. Urine output at term is estimated to vary from 400 to 1,200 mL per day.[136,137] The fetal lungs secrete fluid at a rate of 300 to 400 mL per day near term.[138] The AF volume increases steadily during the first half of pregnancy.

In the second half of pregnancy, the AF becomes hypotonic in comparison with maternal plasma. Between 22 and 39 weeks of gestation the AF volume is on average 800 mL (95% confidence interval (CI), 302 to 1997 mL); with its peak at 33 weeks of gestation and the greatest variation of AF volume in the third trimester.[139] These observations originated from the work of Brace et al.,[139] who reviewed information from 12 studies that included more than 700 pregnancies in which AF volume determination by dye-dilution technique or direct measurement at the time of hysterotomy were analyzed.[139] In another study, based on direct measurement of the AF at the time of cesarean section between 38 and 41 weeks, the mean AF was estimated to be 532 mL[140]; and after 42 weeks, the AF decreased approximately 150 to 170 mL per week.[141] When using US to semiquantitatively determine the AF volume, the amniotic fluid index (AFI) increases from 14 to 31 weeks and then declines thereafter. Using a different US approach (maximal vertical pocket or two-diameter pocket), the AF increases from 14 to 20 weeks' gestation, plateaus between 20 and 37 weeks, and then gradually declines through the 41st week of gestation.[142]

Amniotic fluid volume is maintained through a balance between fetal fluid production (lung liquid and urine) and fluid resorption (fetal swallowing and outflow across the amniotic and/or chorionic membranes). It is estimated that near term, the fetus removes between 200 and 500 mL of AF per day by swallowing.[143,144] Several fetal endocrine factors such as fetal arginine, vasopressin and catecholamines affect fetal renal blood flow, glomerular filtration rate, and urine flow rate.[145,146] In addition, reduction of blood flow to the fetus may elicit an endocrine response that leads to flow redistribution with reduction in fetal urine output and AF volume.

## Ultrasound Methods to Assess Amniotic Fluid

In the past, accurate estimation of actual AF volume was performed with the dye-dilution technique,[147–151] while others directly measured the amount of AF at the time of cesarean section.[139,140] The latter is not clinically useful, whereas the

dye-dilution technique requires an amniocentesis. Both are time-consuming and require laboratory processing; therefore, both methods lack utility in the clinical setting. With the introduction of US, measurement of AF became a valuable adjunct for antenatal assessment. US evaluation of the AF is noninvasive, reproducible, and relatively simple to perform. In 1980, a qualitative estimation of the AF volume was described.[152] It consisted of evaluating areas of echo-free fluid spaces between the limbs and uterine wall or the fetal trunk. However, this assessment is dependent on the experience of the operator performing US. Still, some have argued that subjective US estimation can be as reliable as the semiquantitative measurement techniques (e.g., deepest pocket and amniotic fluid index) when performed by experienced examiners.[153,154] Indeed, the AIUM and the ISUOG agreed that it might be acceptable for experienced examiners to qualitatively estimate AF volume.[130,131]

Several semiquantitative US techniques have been described to determine the amount of AF during pregnancy. These techniques are not intended to determine the exact amount of AF, but rather to provide a numerical reference that can be used for diagnosis and prognostication.

The **largest vertical pocket** was described by Manning et al.[155] in 1980 as part of the biophysical profile (BPP). A normal vertical pocket was defined as a pocket of fluid greater than 1 cm in vertical diameter visualized in any region of the uterine cavity. Subsequently, in 1984, Chamberlain et al.[156] described the largest maximal vertical pocket also referred to as the **maximal vertical pocket (MVP)** (Fig. 7.23), which included the transverse and vertical diameters of the largest pocket of AF. The authors described that the depth of the pocket should be measured at a right angle to the uterine contour (to exclude errors related to the umbilical cord). The depth of the pocket (<1.0 cm, 1.0 cm, and >2 to <8.0 cm) was used for the classification of cases into "decreased," "marginal," or "normal" groups, respectively. The authors acknowledged that the choice of less than 8 cm as the upper margin for normal AF estimate was arbitrary.[156] Based on this study, the original measurement described by Manning et al.[155] used in the BPP to define oligohydramnios was changed to a pocket of <2 cm.

The **amniotic fluid index** or **AFI** (Fig. 7.24) was then described by Phelan et al.[157] For this technique, the measurements are performed with the patient in supine position and the transducer perpendicular to the floor.[157] Real-time B-scanning is used to divide the uterus into four quadrants (defined by the linea nigra into

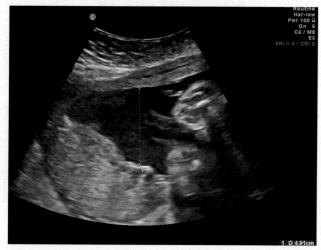

**FIGURE 7.23:** Amniotic fluid measurement using the MVP or single deepest pocket (SDP) approach.

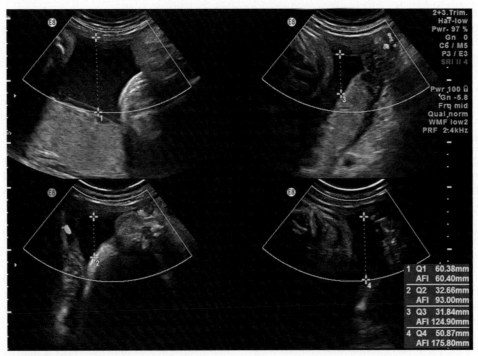

**FIGURE 7.24:** Amniotic fluid measurement using the AFI.

right and left halves, and by the umbilicus into upper and lower halves) (Fig. 7.25). The largest vertical pocket free of umbilical cord or fetal parts is measured in each quadrant, and the sum of the four measurements expressed in centimeters equals the AFI. A limitation of this technique in the second trimester is that only two quadrants may be available because of the size of the uterus. Phelan et al.[158] suggested that for pregnancies before 20 weeks, the abdomen can be divided into two halves using the linea nigra and adding each half to determine the AFI.[158] Another option at this gestational age is to use the largest or MVP. Others have suggested dividing the uterus into four quadrants along the midline and midway up the fundus, transversely, regardless of the gestational age.[159] Variability in MVP and AFI measurements have also been reported in the presence of pressure applied to the transducer by the operator on the maternal abdomen. When low pressure was applied, a 13% increase in AFI was noted along with an 11% increase in the MVP, whereas if high pressure was applied, a 21% fall in AFI and a 16% fall in the MVP were noted.[160]

Magann et al.[149] described the two-diameter pocket technique, which was calculated by multiplying the depth (vertical) and the width (horizontal) of the largest single AF pocket. Based on this technique, oligohydramnios was defined as a two-diameter pocket of 0 to 15 cm, normal fluid between 15.1 and 50 cm, and polyhydramnios as more than 50.1 cm.[149]

However, in clinical practice, both AFI and MVP are widely used, as they are the most reliable US techniques available for assessing the AF. The two-diameter pocket technique is no longer used, as it was shown to be a less reliable predictor of abnormal AF volume when compared with the AFI and the MVP.[142] The methods selected have been dependent on the experience from operator or guidelines provided by each institution (Tables 4A and 4B in Appendix A1.). One limitation of these techniques is that the values are not normally distributed during pregnancy across gestational age.[142,158,159]

The American College of Obstetricians and Gynecologists[161] recommended that either the MVP or the AFI can be used for semiquantitative assessment of the amount of AF. The Cochrane collaboration evaluated five trials, including 3,226 patients comparing the MVP and the AFI for identification of women at risk of: admission to the neonatal intensive unit care, UA pH <7.1 at birth, presence of meconium, and Apgar score <7 at 5 minutes. There was no difference in the performance of both methods; however, the AFI increased the diagnosis of oligohydramnios, the rate of induction of labor and cesarean sections, without improving the neonatal outcome; therefore, the MVP seemed to be a better option.[162]

### Recommendations for Semiquantitatively Assessing the AF Volume during Pregnancy

Technical considerations

1. The transducer should be placed sagittal to the uterine position.
2. The sonographer should look for the largest unobstructed AF pocket and measure the deepest distance.
3. The sonographer should avoid measuring gray areas on the screen, because AF is usually black on the grayscale.

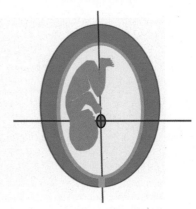

**FIGURE 7.25:** For amniotic fluid index measurement, the uterus is divided into four quadrants defined by the linea nigra in right and left halves, and by the umbilicus in upper and lower halves. The patient should be in supine position and the transducer perpendicular to the floor.

4. The sonographer should not measure between fetal anatomical structures (i.e., arm, legs, umbilical cord) and narrow spaces between fetal structures and the uterus.

5. Color Doppler should be used in areas where the umbilical cord is not clearly visualized.

6. The MVP has a reduced false positive rate for oligohydramnios as compared with the AFI.

## Oligohydramnios

Several investigators have tried to correlate US estimates of AF with dye-dilution techniques or with direct measurements (which are considered gold standards) and have shown that US techniques are poor predictors of decreased or lesser AF during pregnancy.[140,147–150,163–165] The objective of US assessment is not therefore to determine the exact volume of AF but to identify the fetus at risk for adverse perinatal outcomes.

Oligohydramnios is important to diagnose in obstetrics due to its association with adverse perinatal outcomes.[156,166–168] Indeed, in a meta-analysis published in 1999, which included antepartum AF assessment,[167] those with an AFI ≤5 cm had an increased risk of cesarean delivery for "fetal distress" (pooled RR 2.2; 95% CI, 1.5 to 3.4), and an Apgar score <7 at 5 minutes (pooled RR, 5.2; 95% CI, 2.4 to 11.3). Similar observations were noted with an intrapartum AFI ≤5 cm; however, a poor correlation was noted between oligohydramnios and neonatal acidosis (pH < 7.00).[167] One case-control study found an increased rate of stillbirth (1.4% vs. 0.3% P < .03), nonreassuring fetal heart rate (48% vs. 39%; P < .03), admission to the neonatal intensive care unit (7% vs. 2%; P < .001), meconium aspiration syndrome (1% vs. 0.1%; P < .001), and neonatal death (5% vs. 0.3%; P < .001) among women diagnosed with oligohydramnios (AFI ≤ 5 cm) in comparison with those with an AFI >5 cm.[168] The collective idea is that adverse outcomes originate from umbilical cord compression, potential "uteroplacental insufficiency," and increased incidence of meconium-stained AF (along with potential meconium aspiration). In addition, the proportion of neonates with a low birth weight (<2,500 g) was reported to be higher with oligohydramnios.[168] Similarly, oligohydramnios (AFI ≤ 5 cm) has been reported to be an independent predictor of a birth weight below the 10th percentile in uncomplicated pregnancies between 40 and 41.6 weeks.[169] In one study population, the prevalence of oligohydramnios (AFI ≤ 5 cm) in patients with preterm labor and intact membranes was 2.6% (7/272); in addition, patients with oligohydramnios had a higher rate of

intraamniotic infection/inflammation (85.7% [6/7] vs. 32.8% [87/265]; P < .01) and a shorter interval-to-delivery (median 18 hours [range 0 to 74 hours] versus median 311 hours [range 0 to 3,228 hours]; P < .01) than those with an AFI >5 cm.[170]

### Ultrasound Techniques to Determine Oligohydramnios

Two criteria have been used to define oligohydramnios based on the AFI: either using a fixed value of less than 5 cm[157] or a value below the 5th percentile according to gestational age charts[159,165] (Table 4A in Appendix A1). For the MVP, a similar approach can be used with either a fixed value of less than 2 cm[142,156] (Fig. 7.26) or less than the 5th percentile for gestational age[165] (Table 4B in Appendix A1).

Magann et al.[142] provided normal values of AFI, MVP, and two-diameter pocket by US in a group of 1,400 women with uncomplicated pregnancies. Fifty US (50) measurements for each week interval were performed between 16 and 41 weeks of gestation. The authors concluded that the MVP technique was less likely to classify patients as having inadequate (1%) fluid than either the AFI (8%) or the two-diameter pocket (30%).[142] Similar findings were reported by Alfirevic et al.[171] in a study in which 490 women at or after 290 days of gestation were randomly assigned to undergo either a MVP examination, or an AFI US evaluation. There were more women diagnosed with oligohydramnios when the AFI was used (25/250, 10%) than with the MVP (6/250, 2%).[171] In a randomized clinical trial, Moses et al.[172] compared the AFI versus the use of MVP during the intrapartum period in an attempt to identify women at risk for adverse outcomes, and concluded that oligohydramnios was diagnosed more frequently in patients in which the AFI was used (25%), versus those in whom the MVP was used (8%). However, in that study, neither technique was predictive of adverse maternal or neonatal outcomes.[172]

In 2009, a systematic review and meta-analysis was published that included four randomized trials[171–174] with 3,125 women (low risk and high risk) undergoing US measurement of AF volume as part of antepartum assessment comparing the AFI and the single deepest vertical pocket measurement. The following results were reported: (1) when the AFI was used, more cases of oligohydramnios were diagnosed (risk ratio [RR] 2.33, 95% confidence interval [CI], 1.67 to 3.24), more women had induction of labor (RR 2.10; 95% CI, 1.60 to 2.76), and more cesarean deliveries for fetal distress were performed (RR 1.45; 95% CI, 1.07 to 1.97) in comparison with the MVP and (2) there was

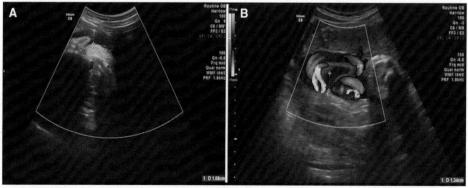

**FIGURE 7.26:** Patients with oligohydramnios after preterm premature rupture of membranes. **A:** Maximal vertical pocket—less than 2 cm without umbilical cord. **B:** Maximal vertical pocket (<2 cm) wrongly measured between the umbilical cord.

no evidence that one method was superior in the prevention of poor peripartum outcomes, such as admission to neonatal intensive care unit; UA pH of less than 7.1; presence of meconium fluid; or Apgar score <7 at 5 minutes.[175] The authors concluded that the single deepest vertical pocket measurement in the assessment of AF volume during fetal surveillance seemed a better choice, since the use of the AFI increased the rates of diagnosis of oligohydramnios and induction of labor without improvement in peripartum outcomes.[175] Other authors have stated that the higher rate of cesarean delivery and labor induction associated with oligohydramnios may be due to additional pregnancy complications such as fetal growth restriction and PE and not necessarily due to decreased AF.[176] However, many authors have reported that the outcome of pregnancies complicated with "isolated oligohydramnios" is comparable to that of low-risk pregnancies with normal AF levels.[169,177–180] Nonetheless, a limitation of those studies is the small sample size and the lack of power to study some of the adverse neonatal outcomes such as neonatal acidosis and fetal death. Based on the current available information derived from randomized studies and recent Cochrane review, the use of MVP ≤2 cm is superior over the use of AFI ≤5 cm for the assessment of AF, as it reduces the rate of false positive diagnosis of oligohydramnios.[175]

### Workup of Patients with Oligohydramnios

The reported incidence of oligohydramnios varies widely (3% to 40%), depending on the study population, whether it was determined intrapartum or antepartum, and on the US technique utilized.[167] When the AF is found to be decreased or absent, several considerations should be taken into account (Table 7.1). Most importantly, a thorough maternal history to determine rupture of amniotic membranes should be obtained. A history consistent or suspicious of rupture of membranes requires a complete examination that includes a sterile speculum examination to determine the presence of vaginal pooling, along with nitrazine and ferning testing. If rupture of membranes is ruled out, maternal medication intake should be investigated; as several drugs have been associated with decreased AF, such as angiotensin-converting-enzyme inhibitor (ACE inhibitor)[181] and chronic use of indomethacin.[182] A significant group of patients may also have oligohydramnios associated with PE,[183] diabetes,[184] and growth restriction.[142,143] For the evaluation of PE, blood pressure, urine protein measurement, as well as fetal growth assessment by US should be performed.[185,186] Placental dysfunction and fetal hypoxemia should be ruled out as these may result in decreased perfusion of the fetal kidneys with subsequent oliguria and decreasing AF volume.[187–189] In addition, US Doppler evaluation and growth assessment should be performed to determine fetal status and growth restriction. If the workup is negative, the fetal renal anatomy should be assessed by US. For example, decreased or absent AF may be a consequence of bilateral renal agenesis,[190] bilateral multi/polycystic kidneys,[191] or urinary tract obstruction.[192] Therefore, it is of utmost importance to evaluate the presence of the fetal bladder

| Table 7.1 | Factors Associated with Oligohydramnios |
|---|---|

**Maternal**

Maternal dehydration
Hypertensive disorders
Antiphospholipid syndrome
Dialysis
Myotonic dystrophy
Medications
    Angiotensin-converting enzyme (ACE) inhibitors
    Long-term use of nonsteroidal anti-inflammatory drugs (i.e., Indomethacin, Sulindac)
    Thiazide diuretics

**Fetal**

Premature rupture of membranes
Growth restriction
Postterm pregnancy
Twin-to-twin transfusion syndrome (donor)
Meckel–Gruber syndrome
Triploidy
Inborn errors of metabolism
Chorioamniotic separation
Abdominal pregnancy
Chronic abruption-oligohydramnios sequence (CHAOS)
Fetal infections
    Rubeola infection
Renal malformations
    Polycystic horseshoe-shaped kidney
    Urethral obstruction
    Polycystic kidneys
    Multicystic dysplastic kidneys
    Bilateral renal agenesis

and kidneys including Doppler confirmation of both renal arteries. When performing the anatomy survey, it is important not to mistake the adrenal glands for the kidneys as the adrenal glands can be enlarged and displaced downward ("lying down") in cases of renal agenesis, giving the false impression of a kidney when the kidneys are not present. In addition, an ectopic location of a nonfunctional kidney should be considered. Of note, the outcomes of pregnancies complicated by chronic oligohydramnios or anhydramnios of renal origin are extremely poor with a small number of survivors owing to the development of pulmonary hypoplasia.[191] In cases of urinary tract obstruction, typical US findings are dilatation of the renal pelvis and calyces, increased renal echogenicity, dilatation of the ureters, thickening of the bladder wall, and bladder enlargement. A keyhole sign is classically associated with posterior urethral valves. Another stated cause of decreased AF is maternal dehydration.[193] In these cases, the maternal hydration status should be assessed (physical exam and urinalysis), and a fluid challenge may be considered. If any of the above findings are not present, oligohydramnios can be referred to as unexplained or idiopathic oligohydramnios.

### Management of Oligohydramnios in the Third Trimester

Several randomized studies have reported that the use of oral or intravenous (IV) hydration can improve or increase the AFI in pregnancies that appear to be complicated by oligohydramnios or decreased AF if in the third trimester and with intact membranes.[194–197] Some have suggested that IV hydration increases the mean velocity of the uterine artery, leading to improvement in the uteroplacental perfusion.[198]

Doppler velocimetry has been used in the management of pregnancies complicated by oligohydramnios. In a retrospective study that consisted of 76 pregnancies complicated by oligohydramnios (defined as an AFI less than the 5th percentile for gestational age), Doppler velocimetry of the UA was assessed.[199] The women were divided into two groups based on whether they had a normal or abnormal UA systolic/diastolic (S/D) ratio. Forty-six patients had normal S/D ratios, and 17 (37%) were associated with perinatal morbidity; whereas in the group of women with abnormal Doppler ($n = 30$), 25 (80%) had associated perinatal morbidity ($P = .001$). Patients with normal UA Doppler were diagnosed at a mean of 35 weeks of gestation and delivered at 37 weeks of gestation. In contrast, the mean gestational age at diagnosis and delivery in the group with abnormal umbilical Doppler velocimetry was 31.4 and 33.8 weeks, respectively ($P < .005$ for both comparisons to patients with normal UA S/D ratio). Of note, no fetal deaths were reported in either group, but 73% of patients had IUGR in the abnormal Doppler group versus 13% in the normal Doppler group. When prematurity associated with delivery for the sole indication of oligohydramnios was excluded, morbidity occurred in 5 (11%) pregnancies instead of 17 (37%) in normal versus abnormal Doppler cases, respectively. The authors concluded that pregnancies with oligohydramnios and normal UA Doppler can be managed more conservatively, with intervention only for indications other than oligohydramnios.[199] Furthermore, this study suggests that avoiding intervention in pregnancies with oligohydramnios and normal UA Doppler velocimetry may decrease iatrogenic morbidity related to prematurity, especially in cases where no growth restriction is evident.[199] Once idiopathic oligohydramnios is diagnosed, serial AF measurements, fetal growth evaluation, fetal Doppler evaluation, and antenatal testing (including nonstress test and BPP) should be initiated.

### Key Points

- Oligohydramnios is defined as MVP <2 cm.
- MVP (<2 cm) has been found to be superior to AFI (<5 cm) as it reduces the rate of false positive diagnosis of oligohydramnios.
- Oligohydramnios is associated with increased rate of induction of labor and cesarean section for fetal distress.
- In the presence of oligohydramnios, evaluate for rupture of membranes, maternal medication intake, evidence of growth restriction or PE, and the fetal genitourinary system.
- In idiopathic oligohydramnios, maternal hydration may be of benefit.
- Use of AFI instead of MVP at term may lead to a higher rate of induction of labor and cesarean section without improving neonatal outcomes.
- Umbilical Doppler examination appears to be of value in the antenatal care of women with idiopathic oligohydramnios.

## Polyhydramnios

The reported incidence of polyhydramnios is approximately 1% to 2% in large population-based studies.[200,201] Polyhydramnios is also referred to as hydramnios by several authors. Several approaches have been suggested to define polyhydramnios using US. One method is to use a fixed value of ≥8 cm with the MVP measurement[202] (Fig. 7.27), an AFI greater than 20 cm (between 36 and 40 weeks of gestation),[157] or an AFI ≥24 cm or ≥25 cm, or to use the 95th or 97.5th according to each gestational age.[159] The second approach is to use gestational age-specific percentiles above or equal to the 95th percentile for polyhydramnios for either the AFI or MVP (see Tables 4A and 4B in Appendix A1).[142] A subjective assessment can also be considered, but this approach will depend on the operator's experience and knowledge.[154,203]

The definition of polyhydramnios based on direct measurement of the AF is >2,100 ml.[139] Regarding US method used to diagnose polyhydramnios during pregnancy, Magann et al.[142] concluded that both the MVP technique and the AFI classified patients similarly (both less than 1%) but better than the two-diameter pocket (3%).[142] Other authors have arbitrarily categorized pregnancies with polyhydramnios into three groups according to the value of the AFI: mild (AFI, 25.1 to 30.0 cm); moderate (AFI, 30.1 to 35.0 cm); or severe (AFI ≥ 35.1 cm).[204] Using the latter subcategories, the relative risk of congenital malformations increased with the severity of polyhydramnios

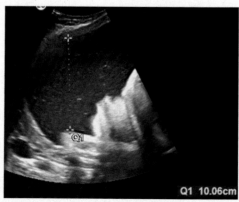

**FIGURE 7.27:** Polyhydramnios at 32 weeks of gestation with a maximal vertical pocket of 10.06 cm.

from 3.2 (95% CI, 1.5 to 6.8), to 5.7 (95% CI, 2.4 to 13.3) and 13.1 (95% CI, 5.8 to 29.5) for mild, moderate, and severe polyhydramnios, respectively.[204] However, the rate of preterm delivery did not differ significantly according to the severity of polyhydramnios unless the pregnancy was complicated with congenital anomalies and/or diabetes.[204] In a retrospective cohort study, some investigators reported that severe polyhydramnios was associated with a higher prevalence of fetal anomalies; however, the sonographic detection of the anomalies (79%) did not differ according to the degree of polyhydramnios.[205]

Using the MVP, the degree of polyhydramnios can be classified as mild (8 to 11 cm), moderate (12 to 14 cm), and severe (≥15 cm).[201] On the basis of this classification, more than 60% of patients with mild polyhydramnios will not have an identifiable cause (idiopathic), and more than 70% will have a normal healthy infant at term.[201]

Similar to the diagnosis of oligohydramnios, the method selected to define polyhydramnios should depend on the experience and data from each sonographer and institution. Polyhydramnios has been associated with an increased risk of adverse perinatal outcomes and mortality. However, the incidence of major congenital anomalies and fetal macrosomia may influence the reported adverse outcomes associated with polyhydramnios. Nonetheless, in studies that have corrected for congenital anomalies, the association of adverse outcomes such as macrosomia,[206] birth weight >4,000 g,[206–208] preterm delivery,[209] neonatal intensive care unit admission,[209] meconium-stained AF,[209] small for gestational age,[210] low and very low birth weight[209] still remains statistically significant. More importantly, a two- to five-fold increase in perinatal and neonatal mortality in pregnancies complicated with polyhydramnios has been reported in most of the studies with large datasets.[200–202,209–211] The severity of the polyhydramnios in pregnancies with fetal anomalies and diabetes correlates with the risk of preterm delivery.[212] Moreover, the rate of cesarean section has been reported to be increased in pregnancies complicated with polyhydramnios[200,206,211] primarily owing to abnormal fetal heart rate,[200] suspected macrosomia,[200] and failure to progress or cephalopelvic disproportion.[206] Of note, the combination of small for gestational age and polyhydramnios has been considered to be ominous for the fetus as it represents an independent risk factor for neonatal mortality (59%) and chromosomal abnormalities (38%).[210,213]

In a cohort study, Chen et al.[209] showed that the rate of placental abruption and placenta accreta was higher in pregnancies complicated with polyhydramnios. However, in a large case-control cohort study, pregnancies complicated with polyhydramnios did not have a higher rate of abruption, placenta previa, umbilical cord prolapse, or fetal malpresentation in comparison with those with a normal AFI.[200] It has been reported that the rate of fetal aneuploidy in cases of isolated polyhydramnios is around 1%,[200,205] but in cases when structural anomalies are detected prenatally, the rate of aneuploidy can be as high as 10%.[205] In addition, in retrospective studies that included cases of isolated polyhydramnios (no anomaly detected prenatally), 9.3% to 28.4% had an anomaly or a syndrome detected after birth (see Table 7.2).[214,215] In these cases, gastrointestinal atresia and hypospadias were more common. Other conditions such as Noonan syndrome or intrahepatic arteriovenous shunt were also detected postnatally.[214] In a cohort of 174 pregnant women with polyhydramnios that included 24 cases labeled as idiopathic polyhydramnios, 5 cases had abnormal neonatal examination and 2 experienced fetal deaths, while the rest at

| Table 7.2 | Fetal Anomalies and Syndromes Diagnosed After Birth in Idiopathic Polyhydramnios |
|---|---|

Beckwith–Wiedemann syndrome
Pulmonary valve stenosis
Bartter syndrome
Hypospadias
X-linked myotubular myopathy
Developmental and motor disorder
Hemiplegia (cerebral bleeding in utero)
Noonan syndrome
Trisomy 21
Cheiloschisis
Pierre Robin sequence
Palatoschisis
Gastrointestinal atresia (esophageal atresia)
Intrahepatic atrioventricular shunt
Pierre Robin sequence with cleft palate
Hydrocephalus

a median of 12 month of life had a normal outcome.[216] Therefore, the study suggests that idiopathic polyhydramnios can be associated with an excellent prognosis but each case should be individualized after all causes have been properly evaluated. In a series of 113 cases with polyhydramnios, 42.8% of the cases showed a reduction to mild polyhydramnios or normal AF volume with advancing gestation. In those cases, the morbidity (i.e., preterm delivery, PE, and cesarean delivery) and neonatal mortality were less in comparison with pregnancies in which marked polyhydramnios persisted.[217]

The association of polyhydramnios, increased AF pressure, and fetal acidemia and hypoxia (determined by cordocentesis) may be the reason for some adverse outcomes in fetuses with polyhydramnios and no structural anomalies.[218] It is suspected that the increased amniotic pressure may lead to abnormal uteroplacental perfusion, umbilical venous compression, or distortion of the villous trees in the placenta.[218]

In conclusion, based on the current literature, an acceptable definition of polyhydramnios in the late second and third trimesters in both singleton and multiple gestations is an MVP >8 cm.[219]

### Workup of Patients with Polyhydramnios

When evaluating a pregnant woman with polyhydramnios, several maternal and fetal conditions should be suspected (see Table 7.3). In general, polyhydramnios may be caused either by excess fetal urine or lung fluid production, or by a defect in AF resorption. One of the typical clinical findings associated with polyhydramnios is that the fundal height is greater than the current gestational age. This should prompt the clinician to perform an US examination to evaluate for polyhydramnios, a large for gestational age fetus, unrecognized multiple pregnancies, or any potential anomaly. The prevalence of either pregestational[200,220] or gestational diabetes[221–223] and polyhydramnios has been reported to be 5% to 64%[200,205,220] and 2% to 12%,[205,221] respectively. However, some authors have noted that the rate of polyhydramnios is not increased in gestational diabetes.[224] The association between polyhydramnios and central nervous system (CNS) abnormalities is common[225]; for example, cases of anencephaly, encephalocele, and hydranencephaly will develop polyhydramnios (usually in the third trimester). If the

| Table 7.3 | Factors Associated with Polyhydramnios |
|---|---|

**Maternal**

Diabetes mellitus (preexisting and gestational)
Lithium intake

**Fetal**

Erythroblastosis fetalis
Fetal arrhythmias
Macrosomia
Placental abnormalities—chorioangioma
Cystic hygromas
Beckwith–Wiedemann syndrome, Perlman syndrome
Achondrogenesis type 1-B
Fetal infections
    Cytomegalovirus infection
    Varicella zoster
    Parvovirus B19
    Toxoplasmosis
Noonan syndrome
Bartter syndrome
Multiple pregnancies
    Twin-to-twin transfusion syndrome (recipient)
    Twin-reversed arterial perfusion sequence

**Fetal malformations**

Central nervous system
    Anencephaly
    Hydrocephaly
    Iniencephaly
    Intracerebral arteriovenous malformations
    Hydranencephaly

    Encephalocele
    Microcephaly
    Sacrococcygeal teratoma
Gastrointestinal tract
    Astomia
    Congenital diaphragmatic hernia
    Annular pancreas
    Omphalocele
    Small bowel atresia
    Tracheoesophageal fistula
    Esophageal atresia
    Duodenal stenosis or atresia
    Gastroschisis
    Cleft palate
    Fetal goiter occluding the GI tract
Respiratory tract
    Congenital pulmonary airway malformation
    Bronchopulmonary sequestration
    Chylothorax
Cardiovascular system
    Valvular incompetence
    Ebstein anomaly
    Valvular stenosis
Musculoskeletal system
    Skeletal dysplasia
    Pena–Shokeir syndrome
    Myotonic dystrophy
    Fetal akinesia/hypokinesia syndrome

**Idiopathic**

---

CNS appears to be normal, gastrointestinal anomalies usually due to bowel atresia or obstruction (i.e., esophagus, small, or large bowel) should be suspected.[225] Fetuses with gastrointestinal obstructions or atresia usually develop polyhydramnios after the second trimester. The absence of the stomach bubble is noted in 30% of cases with polyhydramnios with the cause being esophageal atresia with or without tracheoesophageal fistula.[226] Of note, filling of the stomach may occur between 30 and 60 min, so it is recommended to observe the fetal stomach over this period of time when it is not properly visualized. An enlarged fetal goiter may cause esophageal obstruction and polyhydramnios.[227,228] Space-occupying thoracic lesions, such as bronchopulmonary sequestration (BPS) or congenital pumonary airway malformation (CPAM), can cause compression of the gastrointestinal tract and lead to polyhydramnios.[229,230] These lesions can also cause compression and/or obstruction of the fetal circulation or lymphatics, resulting in hydrops and polyhydramnios.[229]

Conditions that can affect the musculoskeletal system (specifically decreased or absent fetal tone or fetal movements) can be associated with polyhydramnios. In addition, if polyhydramnios and abnormal fetal posture is noted, Pena–Shokeir, Freeman–Sheldon syndrome, arthrogryposis, or an inherited neuromuscular disorder should be part of the differential diagnoses.[231–234] In cases of Prader–Willi syndrome, polyhydramnios, decreased fetal movements, and abnormal posture have been reported.[235,236] In the case of fetal growth restriction and polyhydramnios, chromosomal aneuploidy, especially T18,

should be suspected.[213] If the fetus is affected with Bartter syndrome (fetal polyuria due to an abnormal loop of Henle), the nephrons' ability to control urinary sodium, potassium, and chloride will be affected and lead to fetal polyuria and subsequent polyhydramnios.[237] Overgrowth syndromes such as Perlman syndrome and Beckwith–Wiedemann syndrome (BWS) are inherited disorders that can present with polyhydramnios.[238,239] Additional US findings of Perlman syndrome are macrosomia and nephromegaly; in BWS, there is macrosomia, renal anomalies, abdominal wall defects, and macroglossia. For these rare cases of polyhydramnios, prenatal diagnosis through AF chromosomal microarray may be available.

Polyhydramnios can be observed in cases of viral infection such as cytomegalovirus (CMV), parvovirus B19, and varicella zoster; however, this is not a characteristic feature of these antenatal infections.[240] Serology, PCR testing, and additional US findings (such as nonimmune hydrops, intracranial calcifications, ascites, and parenchymal calcifications [liver, bowel]) are more useful for diagnosis.[240]

Persistent abnormal heart rate (tachyarrhythmia) that leads to increased cardiac output and subsequent hydrops can be associated with polyhydramnios.[241] In addition, large placental chorioangiomas can cause increased cardiac output that can lead to hydrops and polyhydramnios.[242]

The literature is limited regarding the association of medications with polyhydramnios, but lithium has been reported to cause polyhydramnios probably secondary to a form of fetal nephrogenic diabetes.[243]

### Management of Polyhydramnios

The management of polyhydramnios should focus on the specific diagnosis (diabetic control, obstructive lesion), and the goal should primarily aim at improving the maternal symptoms (such as preterm contraction, difficulty ambulating, and respiratory symptoms), or to reverse/treat the fetal condition associated with polyhydramnios. Usually, mild and moderate polyhydramnios do not require intervention, as the symptoms are usually not significant. In contrast, severe polyhydramnios (leading to significant symptomology) may require some form of therapy.

Polyhydramnios can be treated by removing the AF via amniocentesis (amnioreduction). Two protocols have been described: standard or aggressive.[244] The standard protocol consists of removing the AF at a rate of 45 to 90 mL per minute for 60 to 120 minutes using a 20 g needle until an MVP below 7 to 8 cm is obtained. The aggressive protocol consists of using an 18 g needle, removing the AF at a rate of 140 mL per minute until oligohydramnios is obtained.[244] Potential complications such as contractions, rupture of membranes, and placental abruption have been noted in approximately 1.5% of procedures.[245]

Once a complete US survey of the fetus has been performed, if no anomalies have been detected, and other potential etiologies have been excluded, the pregnancy can be monitored every 10 to 14 days with AF measurements, nonstress test, and/or fetal BPP.[246] In addition, a transvaginal cervical length may be useful owing to the increased risk in preterm delivery.[247] Unfortunately, a high percentage (between 5% and 28%) of fetuses with idiopathic polyhydramnios may have a significant anomaly, syndrome, or morbidity detected postnatally.[214–216]

### Key Points

- Definition of polyhydramnios: MVP >8 cm, AFI >24 cm; or a value greater than the 95th centile for gestational age.
- Polyhydramnios is associated with increased risk of perinatal morbidity, but in most cases the outcome tends to be favorable.
- In the presence of polyhydramnios, evaluate for maternal diabetes and fetal anomalies (gastrointestinal, pulmonary, renal, or CNS).
- The greater the polyhydramnios, the higher the rate of fetal anomalies.
- Rate of aneuploidy in idiopathic polyhydramnios is 1% and 10% when structural anomalies are detected.

- Idiopathic polyhydramnios may be associated with increased postnatal morbidity because of anomalies or syndromes not detected prenatally.
- Amnioreduction is reserved for severe cases of polyhydramnios when patients are symptomatic.

## Other Ultrasound Findings in the Amniotic Fluid

On certain occasions, AF may appear to have a homogeneous echogenic material, particulate matter, or free-floating particles. Particulate matter in the first two trimesters of pregnancy has been associated with intraamniotic bleeding.[248,249] Moreover, free-floating particulate matter has also been described in uncommon cases such as excessive desquamation of the skin in congenital ichthyosis,[250] epidermolysis bullosa letalis,[251] or the acrania–anencephaly sequence.[252]

Some authors have suggested that echogenic AF material could represent meconium in the AF (especially in the third trimester).[253] However, other authors do not support this hypothesis,[254] or have reported that the echogenic material visualized in the AF during the third trimester is vernix.[255] The reason for these differences is that meconium and vernix can have a similar appearance on US.[256]

The presence of free-floating hyperechogenic material within the AF in close proximity to the uterine cervix has been described in women with an episode of preterm labor,[257] in women with a history of preterm delivery or threatened preterm labor,[258] and in asymptomatic women at risk for spontaneous preterm delivery in the midtrimester of pregnancy.[259] This particulate matter is known as AF "sludge" (Fig. 7.28) and is an independent risk factor for impending preterm delivery, histologic chorioamnionitis, and microbial invasion of the amniotic cavity in patients with spontaneous preterm labor or a short cervix and intact membranes.[257,259] Subsequent studies have confirmed that AF sludge represents a microbial biofilm in the amniotic cavity.[260,261]

## Amniotic Fluid in the Evaluation of Patients with Preterm Prelabor Rupture of Membranes (PPROM)

The sonographic examination of fetuses with PPROM may be challenging owing to the reduced AF volume. However, contrary to what is generally believed, rupture of membranes is not

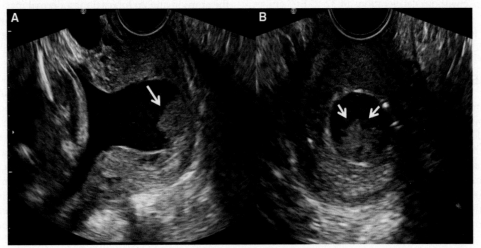

**FIGURE 7.28:** Transvaginal image of a nonmeasurable cervix with "amniotic fluid sludge" (**A**, sagittal; **B**, transverse) at 27 weeks and 2 days of gestation. The patient had spontaneous preterm delivery at 28 weeks and 4 days of gestation. Placenta pathology report: Acute chorioamnionitis and funisitis. Arrows pointing at amniotic fluid sludge.

necessarily always associated with severe oligohydramnios. For example, Harding et al.[262] noted that the AFI in patients with preterm PPROM remains stable after the rupture of membranes, with the mean AFI on admission being 5.9 ± 2.5 cm, and on the day of delivery 5.4 ± 2.0 cm. Moreover, Vintzileos et al.[263] reported that 65.5% of patients with PPROM had a MVP >2 cm, while 15.5% had a MVP between 1 and 2 cm. Only 19% had a MVP <1 cm. Patients with an AF pocket <1 cm had a shorter latency period to delivery and higher incidence of chorioamnionitis and neonatal sepsis than patients with PPROM and a vertical pocket >2 cm.[263] Similar findings were reported in another study that found that women with an MVP of <1 × 1 cm had a higher incidence of chorioamnionitis and endometritis than those with an AF pocket of >1 × 1 cm.[264] Notably, no difference in the duration of the latency period between the two groups was found, but a higher proportion of patients with reduced fluid were in labor at the time of admission.[264]

Storness-Bliss et al.[265] evaluated women with periviable PPROM (<24 weeks), those who had a MVP ≥1 cm had a longer latency period than those with a MVP <1 cm (57 vs. 13 days; P = .014). In addition, there were more surviving fetuses in the group with a MVP ≥1 cm than in the group with MVP <1 cm (6/10 [60%] vs. 1/12 [8.3%]; P = .02). The gestational age at rupture of membranes was similar in both groups (19 weeks); however, the gestational age at delivery was different (27.5 vs. 22.9 weeks) but did not reach statistical significance (P = .07).[265] Hadi et al.[266] also reported that patients with PPROM between 20 and 25 weeks of gestation with higher AFI had a longer latency to delivery and higher neonatal survival. However, others have reported that US assessment of AF is a poor predictor of survival in cases of previable PPROM after logistic regression analysis.[267]

In patients with PPROM, usually one or two pockets of AF will be found on US examination upon presentation; in these cases, an amniocentesis (if feasible) can be performed to rule out intraamniotic infection/inflammation. The rate of intraamniotic infection (positive AF culture) in patients with PPROM is approximately 30%.[268] However, if molecular techniques are used (Bacterial 16S rRNA detected by polymerase chain reaction), about 50% of cases have microbial footprints in the amniotic cavity at the time of admission.[269]

Patients with PPROM and fetal heart decelerations have a lower AFI than those without decelerations (4.32 ± 1.67 cm vs. 6.47 ± 3.59 cm, P < .01).[270] This observation suggests that cord compression due to oligohydramnios may be the mechanism behind variable decelerations observed in patients with PPROM.

## AMNIOTIC MEMBRANES

The fetal membranes are formed primarily by the chorion and amnion, and are physiologically separated during the first 12 to 13 weeks of fetal life delineating part of the extraembryonic celomic cavity. After 13 weeks of gestation, the amnion and chorion start attaching to each other to form the amniotic membrane that surrounds the amniotic cavity, and by 16 weeks, they are usually fused. Limited information regarding the membranes and US is available because the amniotic membranes are often overlooked and are difficult to visualize in the third trimester. Determination of chorionicity and number of gestational sacs is of importance because the morbidity associated with monochorionic monoamniotic and monochorionic diamniotic pregnancies is significantly higher than dichorionic diamniotic pregnancies.

When the chorioamniotic membranes remain unfused after 16 weeks of gestation, there is an association with chromosomal abnormalities, including T21, T18, Turner syndrome, and fetal structural abnormalities such as lymphatic malformations (cystic hygroma), increased nuchal translucency, and exomphalos.[271,272] Therefore, it is important to visualize the membranes if an anomaly or an abnormal aneuploidy screening is present, since an amniocentesis may be offered to the patient (Fig. 7.29).

Another incidental finding while performing an US is the observation of amniotic sheets, also referred to as synechiae. Amniotic sheets are fibrous scar bands covered with two layers of chorion and amnion during pregnancy. These are different than amniotic bands, as they cause no restriction of fetal motion or subsequent fetal deformity. The length of the sheets is between 3 and 10 cm (average 7 cm), and the thickness ranges from 3 to 8 mm (average 6 mm).[273] The reported incidence on US is approximately 0.14% to 0.6%.[273–275] Many patients who have synechiae have a clinical history of uterine instrumentation (i.e. abortion, dilatation and curettage) or uterine infections which explain scar formation.[274] Amniotic sheets have the appearance of a thick amniotic band with a broad base (Fig. 7.30). They can either be seen with a free edge or appear to traverse the entire length of the sac.[275] Although the amniotic sheet appears to be within the AF, it is anatomically external to the amniotic sac.[276] Color Doppler in the thick, less likely thin, portions of the amniotic sheets will show vascularization; the pulse rates obtained from the arterial flows are of maternal origin.[277] The overall consensus is that the presence of amniotic sheets is a benign finding; however, a higher rate of malpresentation (especially when the amniotic sheet is perpendicular to the placenta) has been reported.[274]

Amniotic band syndrome occurs when the amnion ruptures, leading to formation of fibrous bands that can cross fetal parts and cause significant anomalies in the fetus. The anomalies range from limb amputation to body wall and craniofacial defects. A characteristic US feature is the presence of an amniotic band attached to the fetus causing restriction of movement or deformity.

## UMBILICAL CORD

The umbilical cord consists of an outer layer of epithelium from the amnion and an internal mesodermal mass of gelatinous substance composed of mucopolysaccharides known as the Wharton jelly.[278] Within this jelly structure, there are two endodermal ducts, the allantois and the viteline duct, and the umbilical vessels. The umbilical cord is formed at 4 to 6 weeks of postconception by the connection between the body stalk and the yolk stalk (ductus omphaloentericus).[278] The helical course of the umbilical vessels can be observed as early as 28 days of postconception, and is clearly visible from 7 weeks in 95% of fetuses. The origin of the coiling is unknown but has been related to active or passive torsion of the embryo, differential umbilical vascular growth rates, fetal movements, and fetal hemodynamic forces and the muscular fibers in the arterial wall. There are two umbilical arteries and one vein; the left, as the right vena umbilicalis becomes obliterated. After birth, the intra-abdominal portions of the umbilical vessels degenerate. The umbilical arteries become the lateral ligaments of the bladder, and the umbilical vein becomes the round ligament of the liver. In the majority of umbilical cords, there is an anastomosis, and in few cases a fusion, within 1.5 cm of the placental insertion site, which is called Hyrtl anastomosis.[278,279]

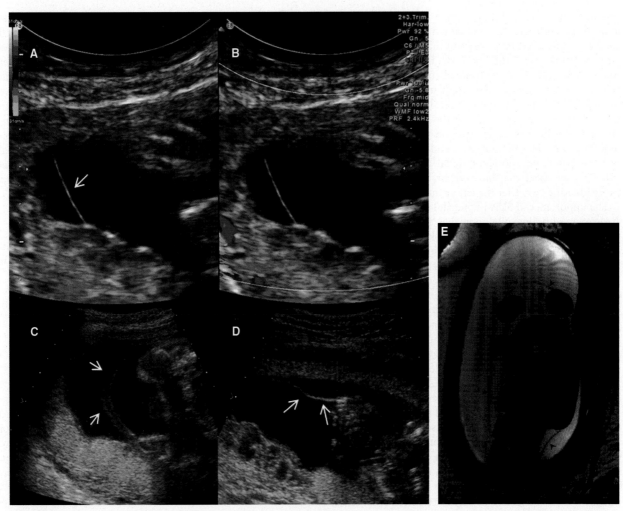

**FIGURE 7.29:** Amniotic membrane separation. (see *arrows in A-D*) **A, B:** The amniotic membrane appears thin and attached to the uterine cavity; there is no color Doppler flow within the membrane. Fetal movement may cause the membrane to undulate. This is an abnormal finding after 16 weeks of gestation. **C:** Amniotic membrane separation after fetal surgery. **D:** Small amniotic membrane separation in the anterior wall of the uterus at 15 weeks of gestation. **E:** Coronal SSFP image in a pregancy with twin reversed arterial perfusion syndrome. There is complete chorioamniotic separation *(arrowheads)*.

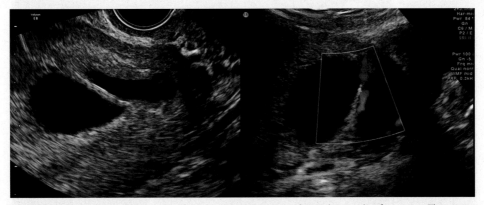

**FIGURE 7.30:** Amniotic sheets, also referred to as amniotic synechiae, at 22 weeks of gestation. There is no restriction of fetal motion or fetal deformity. The amniotic sheet crosses the entire length of the gestational sac. A maternal vessel is noted within the synechiae.

## Single Umbilical Artery

The absence of one UA, a condition known as single umbilical artery (SUA), is reported to have an incidence between 0.1% and 0.6% in singleton pregnancies.[280–282] The reported incidence in twin pregnancies is 9.2%[283] and in high-risk women (>37 years old and increased nuchal translucency) is 5.9%.[284] A SUA cord is the result of obliteration or atrophy of one of the arteries. With US and MRI, to evaluate the vessels present within the umbilical cord, a transverse view of a free loop of the cord should be obtained. Three round structures should be observed in a normal umbilical cord (two arteries and one vein) (Fig. 7.16E and 7.31). In cases of SUA, only two round structures will be observed (one vein and one artery) (Fig. 7.31). The use of color Doppler facilitates the diagnosis in longitudinal views of the umbilical cord. Another approach is to obtain a transverse view of the fetal bladder at the level of the umbilical cord insertion and use color. Normally, the umbilical arteries will course around the fetal bladder. When one UA is missing, no color signal will be observed on one side. This approach may have certain benefits because it objectively identifies whether the left or the right UA is absent.

The importance of SUA in prenatal diagnosis is related to the association with congenital anomalies (primarily cardiac and genitourinary, but also gastrointestinal, skeletal, and CNS).[280,285,286] In a review of the literature that included 1,038 cases of SUA, the prevalence of prenatally diagnosed fetal abnormalities was 33.6%.[286] This risk appears to be exaggerated in contrast to clinical experience, thus suggesting a publication bias. However, if there is a major structural abnormality detected on US in conjunction with SUA, the risk of aneuploidy increases from 2.5% (if isolated) to 41.6%.[287] Others have reported an increased risk in perinatal mortality.[281] In a recent review of the literature, including 742 fetuses with SUA, an absent left UA was detected more frequently than the right side (61.7% vs. 38.3%); however, the rate of anomalies was higher when the right UA was absent.[285]

In a retrospective cohort study that included 392 fetuses with SUA (incidence 0.62%), a SUA was associated with an increased risk of intrauterine growth restriction (adjusted OR 2.1, 95% CI, 1.6 to 2.7, $P < .01$) and preterm delivery before 34 weeks (adjusted OR 3.1, 95% CI, 2.1 to 4.8, $P < .01$).[280] Similar findings have been noted with regard to SUA and increased incidence of small for gestational age birth weight and pregnancy complications.[281,282]

### Management of Fetuses with Single Umbilical Artery

Once a SUA is detected, a detailed US evaluation of the fetus should be performed. If a fetal anomaly is detected, fetal karyotype should be offered. As part of the workup for a fetus with SUA, a fetal echocardiogram is typically recommended given the to the increased incidence in cardiac anomalies; however, a recent study suggested that evaluation of the fetal heart with the standard views (four-chamber view, outflow tracts, and transverse arches) is enough to detect the cardiac defects present in fetuses with SUA.[286] If no anomalies are detected, serial US for growth evaluation and antenatal testing are recommended in view of the association with growth restriction and perinatal complications.

### Key Points

- The incidence of SUA is between 0.1% and 0.6%.
- Color Doppler is useful for diagnosis of SUA. A transverse view of the umbilical cord or evaluation of the cord insertion at the level of the fetal bladder is helpful.
- SUA is associated with a mild increase in the risk of fetal anomalies (cardiac and genitourinary primarily) and growth restriction.
- Left absent UA is detected more frequently, but more anomalies have been associated with absent right UA.

## Umbilical Cord Coiling Index (CI)

The CI is the ratio between the number of complete coils per centimeter of umbilical cord measured after delivery. Coiling is a characteristic of the umbilical cord that is established by 9 menstrual weeks. Strong et al.[288] were the first to describe the CI in normal pregnancies and reported an estimated mean of 0.21 (SD 0.07) (Fig. 7.32). The authors reported that a CI <10th or >90th centile was associated with a high prevalence of perinatal complications such as chromosomal abnormalities, operative

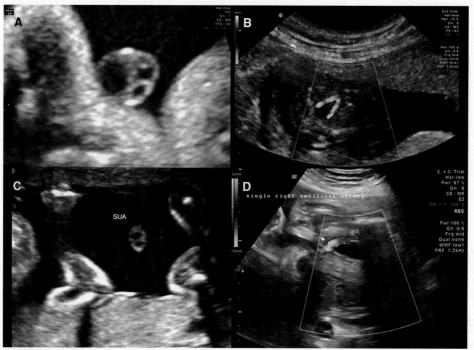

**FIGURE 7.31:** Three vessel and Two vessel cord. **A:** Cross-sectional view of the umbilical cord, two arteries, and one vein. **B:** Two umbilical arteries around the bladder. **C:** Two vessels cord in a cross-sectional view of the umbilical cord, one artery, and one vein. **D:** Single umbilical artery around the fetal bladder.

delivery for fetal stress, and severe heart rate decelerations during labor. The physiologic explanation for the coiling and the direction of coiling in the umbilical cord is still not known. Some authors considered that the fetal movements may influence coiling, as fetuses with polyhydramnios have an increased CI.[289] Others suggested that the amount of Wharton jelly, the presence of the Roach Muscle (a small muscle bundle lying just beside the UA),[290] and the thickness of the umbilical cord[291] might influence the coiling of the umbilical cord.[292] Increased CI (hypercoiling) or reduced CI (hypocoiling) is considered when the CI is >90th or <10th centiles, respectively.[293] There is not a clear difference in the association between increased or reduced CI and specific perinatal complications; however, both have been correlated with an increased risk of perinatal death, intrauterine growth restriction, and polyhydramnios.

Degani et al.[294] estimated the CI just before delivery using US. As it is not possible to measure the total length of the umbilical cord, the authors proposed the estimation of the CI in a clearly visualized segment of the umbilical cord. The calculation was done similarly to that for the CI after delivery, with an estimated CI mean of 0.44 (SD 0.11). The authors reported a significant correlation between the prenatal and the postnatal CI.[294] However, other authors attempted to correlate the prenatal CI in early pregnancy with the CI obtained after delivery without success.[295,296]

In summary, there is no consistent data on the clinical significance of an abnormal CI evaluated prenatally.[297] In addition, there are no studies on the reproducibility of the CI calculation, and there are no validation studies. The conclusion is that the CI measured before and the CI measured after delivery are likely physiologically different. Moreover, the CI can vary in the same fetus according to the anatomical location and gestational age. More data on the reliability of the CI and on the clinical implications are necessary in order to establish its clinical value.

## Umbilical Cord Cysts and Tumors

Visualization of an umbilical cord cyst in early pregnancy is relatively frequent with an estimated prevalence of 3% to 5% before 12 weeks of gestation. Most cysts disappear after the first trimester of pregnancy associated with the appearance of the coiling of the umbilical cord. Histologic examination of umbilical cord cysts demonstrate two types. Pseudocysts lack an epithelial lining, may be eccentric and are formed either by a localized

increase in Wharton jelly or by fluid collection in the presence of a urachal malformation True cysts have an epithelial lining, are typcially central within the cord and arise from remnants of the omphalomesenteric duct or allantois. There are no clear US differences between pseudocysts and true cysts as both may show similar size and imaging characteristics. On US, umbilical cord cysts are echolucent with a mean diameter of 2 cm, and no internal flow. Some imaging characteristics might provide information with regard to clinical impact and their association with adverse perinatal outcome (Fig. 7.33).

### Number of Cysts
Single and multiple cysts have a different prognostic value. Ghezzi et al.[298] studied 1,159 pregnant women between 6 and 14 weeks of gestation, and found a prevalence of umbilical cord cysts of 2.1% (21/1,159). Of the 21 cases, 6 had more than one cyst. The size and US appearance of the cysts showed no differences. All pregnancies with a single cyst resulted in a healthy newborn with no structural anomalies. However, among those with more than one cord cyst (n = 6), four miscarriaged before 14 weeks of gestation, one developed an obstructive uropathy, and one resulted in a normal uncomplicated newborn. Authors concluded that fetuses with isolated cord cysts and no structural abnormalities have a good perinatal outcome, and fetuses having more than one cord cyst, despite a normal fetal anatomy, showed a higher prevalence of adverse perinatal outcomes.

### Locations of the Cyst
Ross et al.[299] reported a prevalence of umbilical cord cysts in 29/859 (3.4%) pregnancies evaluated between 7 and 13 weeks of gestation. In most cases, the cyst resolved after 12 weeks. Among cases with persistent cyst followed until the end of the pregnancy (n = 27), 7 (26%) had structural or chromosomal anomalies, including obstructive urinary malformations, exomphalos, T18, and arthrogryposis. The authors commented that the risk of perinatal complications increased in relation to the anatomical location of the cyst, being higher when the cyst was close to the placental or fetal umbilical cord insertion.

### Isolated or Anomalies with Umbilical Cord Cyst
The presence of an umbilical cord cyst should lead to a detailed fetal structural examination. The most frequently reported associated anomalies are urinary,[300,301] gastrointestinal system (omphalomesenteric duct),[302] abdominal wall,[303] bladder exstrophy,[304] and cardiac anomalies.[305]

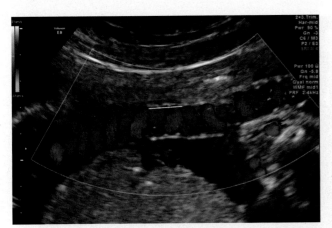

**FIGURE 7.32:** Coiling index. The antenatal umbilical coiling index (UCI) was calculated as the reciprocal of the distance between a pair of coils (antenatal UCI = 1/distance in cm). The distance between the coils is measured from the inner edge of an arterial or venous wall to the outer edge of the next coil along the ipsilateral side of the umbilical cord.

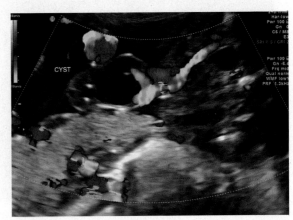

**FIGURE 7.33:** Umbilical cord cyst. Note a regular rounded, echolucent lesion within the cord without internal blood flow.

Gilboa et al.[306] showed that the presence of an isolated cyst with a normal nuchal translucency had a good prognosis. In the absence of associated structural anomalies, the prognosis is very good. Nevertheless, some authors suggested that despite good outcome, if a cyst is persistent into the second and/or third trimester, an amniocentesis for fetal karyotype might be indicated[307,308]; however, this recommendation is not universally accepted.

### Umbilical Cord Masses

Although rare, a hemangioma is one of the most common tumors of the umbilical cord.[309] They are benign tumors that may be associated with increased alpha-fetoprotein (AFP), polyhydramnios, congenital anomalies, and increased perinatal mortality.[309] Noniatrogenic umbilical cord hematoma is very rare.[310] When a hematoma is observed, it is usually secondary to invasive procedures, such as cordocentesis with a poor prognosis for the fetus.[311]

Umbilical artery aneurysm is an extremely rare vascular anomaly.[308,312] It is a cystic structure with nonpulsatile turbulent blood flow. There is a risk of fetal death due to acute umbilical venous compression.[313] Other tumors of the cord include umbilical vein varix,[314] teratoma,[315] and angiomyxomas.[316]

## Nuchal Cord

Nuchal cord is a common finding typically noted at the time of US assessment or at the time of delivery. Single and double nuchal cords are reported to be present in 33.7% and 5.8% of deliveries respectively.[317] On US or MRI, on a transverse or sagittal view of the neck, a nuchal cord is diagnosed by demonstrating the umbilical cord lying around at least three of the four sides of the neck. For accurate diagnosis, both sagittal and transverse sections (linear and circular sections, respectively of the cord) are required to avoid overdiagnosis of this condition[318] (Fig. 7.34). The diagnosis should rely on color Doppler.[319] Nuchal cord diagnosed by US remote from delivery will spontaneously reduce later in gestation[320] and is not usually associated with adverse neonatal outcomes such as five-minute Apgar score <7, NICU admission, intrapartum fetal heart rate abnormalities, and meconium-stained AF.[321] The differential

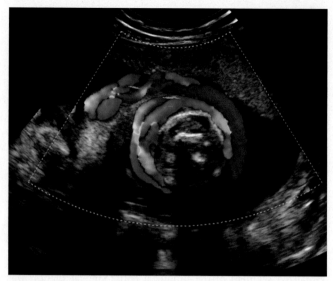

**FIGURE 7.34:** Nuchal cord. Transverse color Doppler of the fetal neck demonstrating a nuchal cord.

diagnoses of a nuchal cord includes posterior cystic neck mass, nuchal folds of the fetal skin, or AF pockets.[318]

## Funic (Cord) Presentation

A funic or cord presentation is when the umbilical cord floats or is visualized in front of the presenting fetal part in the lower uterine segment by the ICO (Fig. 7.35). It is usually associated with fetal malpresentation (breech or transverse) and low-lying placenta or marginal cord insertion. If the amniotic sac ruptures, a cord prolapse can occur with subsequent cord compression and hypoxia to the fetus. In a retrospective study, the reported incidence of funic presentation in the third trimester was 0.16% (13/8,122).[322]

The diagnosis of funic presentation by US is often incidental; however, in cases of malpresentation, it should be thoroughly investigated. Color flow Doppler is essential in diagnosing this condition and minimizing diagnostic errors.[323] Moreover, a funic presentation should always be confirmed with transvaginal US.

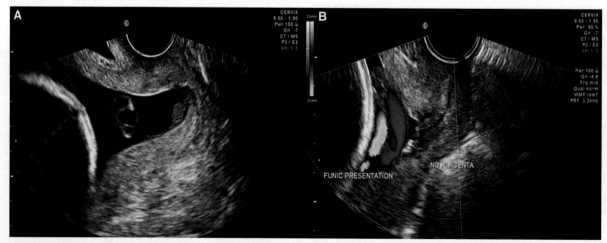

**FIGURE 7.35:** Funic presentation **A:** Transvaginal ultrasound of a patient with a short cervix and a transverse view of the umbilical cord floating between the fetal presentation and the cervix. **B:** Visualization of the umbilical cord with color Doppler ultrasound.

# REFERENCES

1. Espinoza J, Romero R, Mee Kim Y, et al. Normal and abnormal transformation of the spiral arteries during pregnancy. *J Perinat Med*. 2006;34(6):447–458.
2. Robertson WB, Brosens I, Dixon G. Uteroplacental vascular pathology. *Eur J Obstet Gynecol Reprod Biol*. 1975;5(1–2):47–65.
3. Pijnenborg R, Bland JM, Robertson WB, et al. Uteroplacental arterial changes related to interstitial trophoblast migration in early human pregnancy. *Placenta*. 1983;4(4):397–413.
4. Kim YM, Bujold E, Chaiworapongsa T, et al. Failure of physiologic transformation of the spiral arteries in patients with preterm labor and intact membranes. *Am J Obstet Gynecol*. 2003;189(4):1063–1069.
5. Romero R, Kusanovic JP, Chaiworapongsa T, et al. Placental bed disorders in preterm labor, preterm PROM, spontaneous abortion and abruptio placentae. *Best Pract Res Clin Obstet Gynaecol*. 2011;25(3):313–327.
6. Yampolsky M, Salafia CM, Shlakhter O, et al. Modeling the variability of shapes of a human placenta. *Placenta*. 2008;29(9):790–797.
7. Meizner I, Mashiach R, Shalev Y, et al. Blood flow velocimetry in the diagnosis of succenturiate placenta. *J Clin Ultrasound*. 1998;26(1):55.
8. Suzuki S, Igarashi M. Clinical significance of pregnancies with succenturiate lobes of placenta. *Arch Gynecol Obstet*. 2008;277(4):299–301.
9. Shukunami K, Tsunezawa W, Hosokawa K, et al. Placenta previa of a succenturiate lobe: a report of two cases. *Eur J Obstet Gynecol Reprod Biol*. 2001;99(2):276–277.
10. Hata K, Hata T, Aoki S, et al. Succenturiate placenta diagnosed by ultrasound. *Gynecol Obstet Invest*. 1988;25(4):273–276.
11. Harris RD, Wells WA, Black WC, et al. Accuracy of prenatal sonography for detecting circumvallate placenta. *AJR Am J Roentgenol*. 1997;168(6):1603–1608.
12. Elsayes KM, Trout AT, Friedkin AM, et al. Imaging of the placenta: a multimodality pictorial review. *Radiographics*. 2009;29(5):1371–1391.
13. Suzuki S. Clinical significance of pregnancies with circumvallate placenta. *J Obstet Gynecol Res*. 2008;34(1):51–54.
14. Hurley VA, Beischer NA. Placenta membranacea: case reports. *BJOG*. 1987;94(8):798–802.
15. Molloy CE, McDowell W, Armour T, et al. Ultrasonic diagnosis of placenta membranacea in utero. *J Ultrasound Med*. 1983;2(8):377–379.
16. Jauniaux E, Moscoso G, Campbell S, et al. Correlation of ultrasound and pathologic findings of placental anomalies in pregnancies with elevated maternal serum alpha-fetoprotein. *Eur J Obstet Gynecol Reprod Biol*. 1990;37(3):219–230.
17. Lee AJ, Bethune M, Hiscock RJ. Placental thickness in the second trimester: a pilot study to determine the normal range. *J Ultrasound Med*. 2012;31(2):213–218.
18. Hoddick WK, Mahony BS, Callen PW, et al. Placental thickness. *J Ultrasound Med*. 1985;4(9):479–482.
19. Jauniaux E, Ramsay B, Campbell S. Ultrasonographic investigation of placental morphologic characteristics and size during the second trimester of pregnancy. *Am J Obstet Gynecol*. 1994;170(1, pt 1):130–137.
20. Wen X, Triche EW, Hogan JW, et al. Association between placental morphology and childhood systolic blood pressure. *Hypertension*. 2011;57(1):48–55.
21. Leung KY, Cheong KB, Lee CP, et al. Ultrasonographic prediction of homozygous α⁰-thalassemia using placental thickness, fetal cardiothoracic ratio and middle cerebral artery Doppler: alone or in combination? *Ultrasound Obstet Gynecol*. 2010;35(2):149–154.
22. Salafia CM, Yampolsky M, Misra DP, et al. Placental surface shape, function, and effects of maternal and fetal vascular pathology. *Placenta*. 2010;31(11):958–962.
23. Perry IJ, Beevers DG, Whincup PH, et al. Predictors of ratio of placental weight to fetal weight in multiethnic community. *BMJ*. 1995;310(6977):436–439.
24. Shehata F, Levin I, Shrim A, et al. Placenta/birthweight ratio and perinatal outcome: a retrospective cohort analysis. *BJOG*. 2011;118(6):741–747.
25. Hutcheon JA, McNamara H, Platt RW, et al. Placental weight for gestational age and adverse perinatal outcomes. *Obstet Gynecol*. 2012;119(6):1251–1258.
26. Hung TH, Shau WY, Hsieh CC, et al. Risk factors for placenta accreta. *Obstet Gynecol*. 1999;93(4):545–550.
27. Filipov E, Borisov I, Kolarov G. Placental location and its influence on the position of the fetus in the uterus [in Bulgarian]. *Akush Ginekol*. 2000;40(4):11–12.
28. Ito Y, Shouno H, Yamasaki M, et al. Relationship between the placental location and the flow velocity waveforms of bilateral uterine arteries. *Asia Oceania J Obstet Gynaecol*. 1990;16(1):73–78.
29. Oppenheimer L, Holmes P, Simpson N, et al. Diagnosis of low-lying placenta: can migration in the third trimester predict outcome? *Ultrasound Obstet Gynecol*. 2001;18(2):100–102.
30. Oppenheimer LW, Farine D, Ritchie JW, et al. What is a low-lying placenta? *Am J Obstet Gynecol*. 1991;165(4, pt 1):1036–1038.
31. Bronsteen R, Valice R, Lee W, et al. Effect of a low-lying placenta on delivery outcome. *Ultrasound Obstet Gynecol*. 2009;33(2):204–208.
32. Farine D, Peisner DB, Timor-Tritsch IE. Placenta previa—is the traditional diagnostic approach satisfactory? *J Clin Ultrasound*. 1990;18(4):328–330.
33. Cho JY, Lee YH, Moon MH, et al. Difference in migration of placenta according to the location and type of placenta previa. *J Clin Ultrasound*. 2008;36(2):79–84.
34. Ohira S, Kikuchi N, Kobara H, et al. Predicting the route of delivery in women with low-lying placenta using transvaginal ultrasonography: significance of placental migration and marginal sinus. *Gynecol Obstet Invest*. 2012;73(3):217–222.
35. Blouin D, Rioux C. Routine third trimester control ultrasound examination for low-lying or marginal placentas diagnosed at mid-pregnancy: is this indicated? *J Obstet Gynaecol Can*. 2012;34(5):425–428.
36. Lodhi SK, Khanum Z, Watoo TH. Placenta previa: the role of ultrasound in assessment during third trimester. *J Pak Med Assoc*. 2004;54(2):81–83.
37. RoyalCollege of Obstetricians and Gynaecologists. *Placenta Praevia, Placenta Praevia Accreta and Vasa Praevia: Diagnosis and Management*. London, UK: Royal College of Obstetricians and Gynaecologists; 2011:2–26. Green-Top Guideline No 27.
38. Oyelese Y, Smulian JC. Placenta previa, placenta accreta, and vasa previa. *Obstet Gynecol*. 2006;107(4):927–941.
39. Dashe JS. Toward consistent terminology of placental location. *Semin Perinatol*. 2013;37(5):375–379.
40. Oppenheimer L. Diagnosis and management of placenta previa. *J Obstet Gynaecol Can*. 2007;29(3):261–273.
41. Olive EC, Roberts CL, Algert CS, et al. Placenta praevia: maternal morbidity and place of birth. *Aust N Z J Obstet Gynaecol*. 2005;45(6):499–504.
42. Gurol-Urganci I, Cromwell DA, Edozien LC, et al. Risk of placenta previa in second birth after first birth cesarean section: a population-based study and meta-analysis. *BMC Pregnancy Childbirth*. 2011;11:95.
43. Usta IM, Hobeika EM, Musa AA, et al. Placenta previa-accreta: risk factors and complications. *Am J Obstet Gynecol*. 2005;193(3, pt 2):1045–1049.
44. Ghi T, Contro E, Martina T, et al. Cervical length and risk of antepartum bleeding in women with complete placenta previa. *Ultrasound Obstet Gynecol*. 2009;33(2):209–212.
45. Ben Nagi J, Ofili-Yebovi D, Marsh M, et al. First-trimester cesarean scar pregnancy evolving into placenta previa/accreta at term. *J Ultrasound Med*. 2005;24(11):1569–1573.
46. Garmi G, Salim R. Epidemiology, etiology, diagnosis, and management of placenta accreta. *Obstet Gynecol Int*. 2012;2012:873929.
47. Belfort MA. Placenta accreta. *Am J Obstet Gynecol*. 2010;203(5):430–439.
48. Imudia AN, Awonuga AO, Dbouk T, et al. Incidence, trends, risk factors, indications for, and complications associated with cesarean hysterectomy: a 17-year experience from a single institution. *Arch Gynecol Obstet*. 2009;280(4):619–623.
49. Marshall NE, Fu R, Guise JM. Impact of multiple cesarean deliveries on maternal morbidity: a systematic review. *Am J Obstet Gynecol*. 2011;205(3):262.e1–262.e8.
50. Jauniaux E, Jurkovic D. Placenta accreta: pathogenesis of a 20th century iatrogenic uterine disease. *Placenta*. 2012;33(4):244–251.
51. Comstock CH, Lee W, Vettraino IM, et al. The early sonographic appearance of placenta accreta. *J Ultrasound Med*. 2003;22(1):19–23; quiz 24–26.
52. Comstock CH, Love JJ Jr, Bronsteen RA, et al. Sonographic detection of placenta accreta in the second and third trimesters of pregnancy. *Am J Obstet Gynecol*. 2004;190(4):1135–1140.
53. Warshak CR, Eskander R, Hull AD, et al. Accuracy of ultrasonography and magnetic resonance imaging in the diagnosis of placenta accreta. *Obstet Gynecol*. 2006;108(3, pt 1):573–581.
53a. Baughman WC, Corteville JE, Shah RR. Placenta Accreta: Spectrum of US and MR Imaging Findings. *Radiographics*. 2008; 28:1905–1916.
53b. Derman AY, Nikac V, Haberman S, et al. MRI of Placenta Accreta: A New Imaging Perspective. *AJR*. 2011;197:1514–1521.
54. Lijoi AF, Brady J. Vasa previa diagnosis and management. *J Am Board Fam Pract*. 2003;16(6):543–548.
55. Lee W, Lee VL, Kirk JS, et al. Vasa previa: prenatal diagnosis, natural evolution, and clinical outcome. *Obstet Gynecol*. 2000;95(4):572–576.
56. Baulies S, Maiz N, Munoz A, et al. Prenatal ultrasound diagnosis of vasa praevia and analysis of risk factors. *Prenat Diagn*. 2007;27(7):595–599.
57. Al-Khaduri M, Kadoch IJ, Couturier B, et al. Vasa praevia after IVF: should there be guidelines? Report of two cases and literature review. *Reprod Biomed Online*. 2007;14(3):372–374.
58. Catanzarite V, Maida C, Thomas W, et al. Prenatal sonographic diagnosis of vasa previa: ultrasound findings and obstetric outcome in ten cases. *Ultrasound Obstet Gynecol*. 2001;18(2):109–115.
59. Oyelese Y, Catanzarite V, Prefumo F, et al. Vasa previa: the impact of prenatal diagnosis on outcomes. *Obstet Gynecol*. 2004;103(5, pt 1):937–942.
60. Gagnon R, Morin L, Bly S, et al. Guidelines for the management of vasa previa. *J Obstet Gynaecol Can*. 2009;31(8):748–760.
61. Baschat AA, Gembruch U. Ante- and intrapartum diagnosis of vasa praevia in singleton pregnancies by colour coded Doppler sonography. *Eur J Obstet Gynecol Reprod Biol*. 1998;79(1):19–25.
62. Daly-Jones E, Hollingsworth J, Sepulveda W. Vasa praevia: second trimester diagnosis using colour flow imaging. *Br J Obstet Gynaecol*. 1996;103(3):284–286.
63. Clerici G, Burnelli L, Lauro V, et al. Prenatal diagnosis of vasa previa presenting as amniotic band. "A not so innocent amniotic band". *Ultrasound Obstet Gynecol*. 1996;7(1):61–63.
64. Grannum PA, Berkowitz RL, Hobbins JC. The ultrasonic changes in the maturing placenta and their relation to fetal pulmonic maturity. *Am J Obstet Gynecol*. 1979;133(8):915–922.
65. Grannum PA. The placenta. *Clin Diagn Ultrasound*. 1989;25:203–219
66. Moran M, Ryan J, Higgins M, et al. Poor agreement between operators on grading of the placenta. *J Obstet Gynaecol*. 2011;31(1):24–28.
67. Sau A, Seed P, Langford K. Intraobserver and interobserver variation in the sonographic grading of placental maturity. *Ultrasound Obstet Gynecol*. 2004;23(4):374–377.

68. Kuo PL, Lin CC, Lin YH, et al. Placental sonolucency and pregnancy outcome in women with elevated second trimester serum alpha-fetoprotein levels. *J Formos Med Assoc.* 2003;102(5):319–325.

69. Kusanovic JP, Romero R, Gotsch F, et al. Discordant placental echogenicity: a novel sign of impaired placental perfusion in twin-twin transfusion syndrome? *J Matern Fetal Neonatal Med.* 2010;23(1):103–106.

70. Raio L, Ghezzi F, Cromi A, et al. The thick heterogeneous (jellylike) placenta: a strong predictor of adverse pregnancy outcome. *Prenatal Diagn.* 2004;24(3):182–188.

71. Hung NA, Jackson C, Nicholson M, et al. Pregnancy-related polymyositis and massive perivillous fibrin deposition in the placenta: are they pathogenetically related? *Arthritis Rheum.* 2006;55(1):154–156.

72. Andres RL, Kuyper W, Resnik R, et al. The association of maternal floor infarction of the placenta with adverse perinatal outcome. *Am J Obstet Gynecol.* 1990;163(3):935–938.

73. Jindal P, Regan L, Fourkala EO, et al. Placental pathology of recurrent spontaneous abortion: the role of histopathological examination of products of conception in routine clinical practice: a mini review. *Hum Reprod.* 2007;22(2):313–316.

74. Sebire NJ, Backos M, Goldin RD, et al. Placental massive perivillous fibrin deposition associated with antiphospholipid antibody syndrome. *BJOG.* 2002;109(5):570–573.

75. Proctor LK, Whittle WL, Keating S, et al. Pathologic basis of echogenic cystic lesions in the human placenta: role of ultrasound-guided wire localization. *Placenta.* 2010;31(12):1111–1115.

76. Moldenhauer JS, Stanek J, Warshak C, et al. The frequency and severity of placental findings in women with preeclampsia are gestational age dependent. *Am J Obstet Gynecol.* 2003;189(4):1173–1177.

77. Krielessi V, Papantoniou N, Papageorgiou I, et al. Placental pathology and blood pressure's level in women with hypertensive disorders in pregnancy. *Obstet Gynecol Intern.* 2012;2012:684083.

78. Vinnars MT, Nasiell J, Ghazi S, et al. The severity of clinical manifestations in preeclampsia correlates with the amount of placental infarction. *Acta Obstet Gynecol Scand.* 2011;90(1):19–25.

79. Brosens I, Renaer M. On the pathogenesis of placental infarcts in pre-eclampsia. *J Obstet Gynaecol Br Commonw.* 1972;79(9):794–799.

80. Ogge G, Chaiworapongsa T, Romero R, et al. Placental lesions associated with maternal underperfusion are more frequent in early-onset than in late-onset preeclampsia. *J Perinat Med.* 2011;39(6):641–652.

81. SebireN. Macroscopic abnormalities of the placenta. In: Fox H, Sebire N, eds. *Pathology of the Placenta.* 3rd ed. Philadelphia, PA: Saunders Elsevier; 2007:95–146.

82. Fitzgerald B, Shannon P, Kingdom J, et al. Rounded intraplacental haematomas due to decidual vasculopathy have a distinctive morphology. *J Clin Pathol.* 2011;64(8):729–732.

83. Viero S, Chaddha V, Alkazaleh F, et al. Prognostic value of placental ultrasound in pregnancies complicated by absent end-diastolic flow velocity in the umbilical arteries. *Placenta.* 2004;25(8–9):735–741.

84. Tuuli MG, Norman SM, Odibo AO, et al. Perinatal outcomes in women with subchorionic hematoma: a systematic review and meta-analysis. *Obstet Gynecol.* 2011;117(5):1205–1212.

85. Nagy S, Bush M, Stone J, et al. Clinical significance of subchorionic and retroplacental hematomas detected in the first trimester of pregnancy. *Obstet Gynecol.* 2003;102(1):94–100.

86. Fung TY, To KF, Sahota DS, et al. Massive subchorionic thrombohematoma: a series of 10 cases. *Acta Obstet Gynecol Scand.* 2010;89(10):1357–1361.

87. Oyelese Y, Ananth CV. Placental abruption. *Obstet Gynecol.* 2006;108(4):1005–1016.

88. Nyberg DA, Cyr DR, Mack LA, et al. Sonographic spectrum of placental abruption. *AJR Am J Roentgenol.* 1987;148(1):161–164.

89. Glantz C, Purnell L. Clinical utility of sonography in the diagnosis and treatment of placental abruption. *J Ultrasound Med.* 2002;21(8):837–840.

90. Stillbirth Collaborative Research Network Writing Group. Causes of death among stillbirths. *JAMA.* 2011;306(22):2459–2468.

91. Jauniaux E. Ultrasound diagnosis and follow-up of gestational trophoblastic disease. *Ultrasound Obstet Gynecol.* 1998;11(5):367–377.

92. Sebire NJ, Jauniaux E. Fetal and placental malignancies: prenatal diagnosis and management. *Ultrasound Obstet Gynecol.* 2009;33(2):235–244.

93. Wallenburg HC. Chorioangioma of the placenta: thirteen new cases and a review of the literature from 1939 to 1970 with special reference to the clinical complications. *Obstet Gynecol Surv.* 1971;26(6):411–425.

94. Zanardini C, Papageorghiou A, Bhide A, et al. Giant placental chorioangioma: natural history and pregnancy outcome. *Ultrasound Obstet Gynecol.* 2010;35(3):332–336.

95. Sepulveda W, Alcalde JL, Schnapp C, et al. Perinatal outcome after prenatal diagnosis of placental chorioangioma. *Obstet Gynecol.* 2003;102(5, pt 1):1028–1033.

96. Benirschke K, Kaufmann P, Baergen RN. *Pathology of Human Placenta.* 5th ed. New York, NY: Springer; 2006.

97. Jauniaux E, Ogle R. Color Doppler imaging in the diagnosis and management of chorioangiomas. *Ultrasound Obstet Gynecol.* 2000;15(6):463–467.

98. Zalel Y, Weisz B, Gamzu R, et al. Chorioangiomas of the placenta: sonographic and Doppler flow characteristics. *J Ultrasound Med.* 2002;21(8):909–913.

99. Wolfe BK, Wallace JH. Pitfall to avoid: chorioangioma of the placenta simulating fetal tumor. *J Clin Ultrasound.* 1987;15(6):405–408.

100. Quintero RA, Reich H, Romero R, et al. In utero endoscopic devascularization of a large chorioangioma. *Ultrasound Obstet Gynecol.* 1996;8(1):48–52.

101. Sepulveda W, Wong AE, Herrera L, et al. Endoscopic laser coagulation of feeding vessels in large placental chorioangiomas: report of three cases and review of invasive treatment options. *Prenat Diagn.* 2009;29(3):201–206.

102. Krapp M, Baschat AA, Hankeln M, et al. Gray scale and color Doppler sonography in the third stage of labor for early detection of failed placental separation. *Ultrasound Obstet Gynecol.* 2000;15(2):138–142.

103. Herman A. Complicated third stage of labor: time to switch on the scanner. *Ultrasound Obstet Gynecol.* 2000;15(2):89–95.

104. Patwardhan M, Ahn H, Hernandez-Andrade E, et al. Dynamic myometrial changes in the upper and lower uterine segments during the third stage of labor. *Ultrasound Obstet Gynecol.* 2012;40(S1):110.

105. Hata T, Tanaka H, Noguchi J, et al. Three-dimensional ultrasound evaluation of the placenta. *Placenta.* 2011;32(2):105–115.

106. Kalache KD, Espinoza J, Chaiworapongsa T, et al. Three-dimensional ultrasound fetal lung volume measurement: a systematic study comparing the multiplanar method with the rotational (VOCAL) technique. *Ultrasound Obstet Gynecol.* 2003;21(2):111–118.

107. Hafner E, Metzenbauer M, Dillinger-Paller B, et al. Correlation of first trimester placental volume and second trimester uterine artery Doppler flow. *Placenta.* 2001;22(8–9):729–734.

108. Rijken MJ, Moroski WE, Kiricharoen S, et al. Effect of malaria on placental volume measured using three-dimensional ultrasound: a pilot study. *Malar J.* 2012;11:5.

109. Pomorski M, Zimmer M, Florjanski J, et al. Comparative analysis of placental vasculature and placental volume in normal and IUGR pregnancies with the use of three-dimensional power Doppler. *Arch Gynecol Obstet.* 2012;285(2):331–337.

110. Hafner E, Metzenbauer M, Hofinger D, et al. Comparison between three-dimensional placental volume at 12 weeks and uterine artery impedance/notching at 22 weeks in screening for pregnancy-induced hypertension, preeclampsia and fetal growth restriction in a low-risk population. *Ultrasound Obstet Gynecol.* 2006;27(6):652–657.

111. Odeh M, Ophir E, Maximovsky O, et al. Placental volume and three-dimensional power Doppler analysis in prediction of pre-eclampsia and small for gestational age between Week 11 and 13 weeks and 6 days of gestation. *Prenat Diagn.* 2011;31(4):367–371.

112. Rizzo G, Capponi A, Pietrolucci ME, et al. First trimester placental volume and three dimensional power doppler ultrasonography in type I diabetic pregnancies. *Prenat Diagn.* 2012;32(5):480–484.

113. Odibo AO, Goetzinger KR, Huster KM, et al. Placental volume and vascular flow assessed by 3D power Doppler and adverse pregnancy outcomes. *Placenta.* 2011;32(3):230–234.

114. Wegrzyn P, Faro C, Falcon O, et al. Placental volume measured by three-dimensional ultrasound at 11 to 13 + 6 weeks of gestation: relation to chromosomal defects. *Ultrasound Obstet Gynecol.* 2005;26(1):28–32.

115. Metzenbauer M, Hafner E, Schuchter K, et al. First-trimester placental volume as a marker for chromosomal anomalies: preliminary results from an unselected population. *Ultrasound Obstet Gynecol.* 2002;19(3):240–242.

116. Yu CH, Chang CH, Ko HC, et al. Assessment of placental fractional moving blood volume using quantitative three-dimensional power doppler ultrasound. *Ultrasound Med Biol.* 2003;29(1):19–23.

117. Cheong KB, Leung KY, Li TK, et al. Comparison of inter- and intraobserver agreement and reliability between three different types of placental volume measurement technique (XI VOCAL, VOCAL and multiplanar) and validity in the in-vitro setting. *Ultrasound Obstet Gynecol.* 2010;36(2):210–217.

118. Bujold E, Effendi M, Girard M, et al. Reproducibility of first trimester three-dimensional placental measurements in the evaluation of early placental insufficiency. *J Obstet Gynaecol Can.* 2009;31(12):1144–1148.

119. Aardema MW, Oosterhof H, Timmer A, et al. Uterine artery Doppler flow and uteroplacental vascular pathology in normal pregnancies and pregnancies complicated by pre-eclampsia and small for gestational age fetuses. *Placenta.* 2001;22(5):405–411.

120. Lin S, Shimizu I, Suehara N, et al. Uterine artery Doppler velocimetry in relation to trophoblast migration into the myometrium of the placental bed. *Obstet Gynecol.* 1995;85(5, pt 1):760–765.

121. Harrington KF, Campbell S, Bewley S, et al. Doppler velocimetry studies of the uterine artery in the early prediction of pre-eclampsia and intra-uterine growth retardation. *Eur J Obstet Gynecol Reprod Biol.* 1991;42(suppl):S14–S20.

122. Hernandez-Andrade E, Brodszki J, Lingman G, et al. Uterine artery score and perinatal outcome. *Ultrasound Obstet Gynecol.* 2002;19(5):438–442.

123. Gomez O, Figueras F, Martinez JM, et al. Sequential changes in uterine artery blood flow pattern between the first and second trimesters of gestation in relation to pregnancy outcome. *Ultrasound Obstet Gynecol.* 2006;28(6):802–808.

124. Acosta-Rojas R, Becker J, Munoz-Abellana B, et al. Twin chorionicity and the risk of adverse perinatal outcome. *Int J Gynaecol Obstet.* 2007;96(2):98–102.

125. Lewi L, Deprest J, Hecher K. The vascular anastomoses in monochorionic twin pregnancies and their clinical consequences. *Am J Obstet Gynecol.* 2013;208(1):19–30.

126. Carroll SG, Soothill PW, Abdel-Fattah SA, et al. Prediction of chorionicity in twin pregnancies at 10–14 weeks of gestation. *BJOG.* 2002;109(2):182–186.

127. Sepulveda W, Sebire NJ, Hughes K, et al. The lambda sign at 10–14 weeks of gestation as a predictor of chorionicity in twin pregnancies. *Ultrasound Obstet Gynecol.* 1996;7(6):421–423.

128. Finberg HJ. The "twin peak" sign: reliable evidence of dichorionic twinning. *J Ultrasound Med.* 1992;11(11):571–577.

129. Gratacos E, Deprest J. Current experience with fetoscopy and the Euro-foetus registry for fetoscopic procedures. *Eur J Obstet Gynecol Reprod Biol.* 2000;92(1):151–159.

130. American Institute of Ultrasound in Medicine. AIUM practice guideline for the performance of obstetric ultrasound examinations. *J Ultrasound Med.* 2010;29(1):157–166.

131. Salomon LJ, Alfirevic Z, Berghella V, et al. Practice guidelines for performance of the routine mid-trimester fetal ultrasound scan. *Ultrasound Obstet Gynecol.* 2011;37(1):116–126.

132. Lind T, Kendall A, Hytten FE. The role of the fetus in the formation of amniotic fluid. *J Obstet Gynaecol Br Commonw.* 1972;79(4):289–298.

133. Parmley TH, Seeds AE. Fetal skin permeability to isotopic water (THO) in early pregnancy. *Am J Obstet Gynecol.* 1970;108(1):128–131.

134. Anderson DF, Faber JJ, Parks CM. Extraplacental transfer of water in the sheep. *J Physiol.* 1988;406:75–84

135. Smith DL. Amniotic fluid volume: a measurement of the amniotic fluid present in 72 pregnancies during the first half of pregnancy. *Am J Obstet Gynecol.* 1971;110(2):166–172.

136. Gresham EL, Rankin JH, Makowski EL, et al. An evaluation of fetal renal function in a chronic sheep preparation. *J Clin Invest.* 1972;51(1):149–156.

137. Rabinowitz R, Peters MT, Vyas S, et al. Measurement of fetal urine production in normal pregnancy by real-time ultrasonography. *Am J Obstet Gynecol.* 1989;161(5):1264–1266.

138. Mescher EJ, Platzker AC, Ballard PL, et al. Ontogeny of tracheal fluid, pulmonary surfactant, and plasma corticoids in the fetal lamb. *J Appl Physiol.* 1975;39(6):1017–1021.

139. Brace RA, Wolf EJ. Normal amniotic fluid volume changes throughout pregnancy. *Am J Obstet Gynecol.* 1989;161(2):382–388.

140. Horsager R, Nathan L, Leveno KJ. Correlation of measured amniotic fluid volume and sonographic predictions of oligohydramnios. *Obstet Gynecol.* 1994;83(6):955–958.

141. Beischer NA, Brown JB, Townsend L. Studies in prolonged pregnancy, 3: amniocentesis in prolonged pregnancy. *Am J Obstet Gynecol.* 1969;103(4):496–503.

142. Magann EF, Sanderson M, Martin JN, et al. The amniotic fluid index, single deepest pocket, and two-diameter pocket in normal human pregnancy. *Am J Obstet Gynecol.* 2000;182(6):1581–1588.

143. Abramovich DR, Garden A, Jandial L, et al. Fetal swallowing and voiding in relation to hydramnios. *Obstet Gynecol.* 1979;54(1):15–20.

144. Pritchard JA. Deglutition by normal and anencephalic fetuses. *Obstet Gynecol.* 1965;25:289–297

145. Robillard JE, Weitzman RE. Developmental aspects of the fetal renal response to exogenous arginine vasopressin. *Am J Physiol.* 1980;238(5):F407–F414.

146. Lingwood B, Hardy KJ, Coghlan JP, et al. Effect of aldosterone on urine composition in the chronically cannulated ovine foetus. *J Endocrinol.* 1978;76(3):553–554.

147. Dildy GA III, Lira N, Moise KJ Jr, et al. Amniotic fluid volume assessment: comparison of ultrasonographic estimates versus direct measurements with a dye-dilution technique in human pregnancy. *Am J Obstet Gynecol.* 1992;167(4, pt 1):986–994.

148. Croom CS, Banias BB, Ramos-Santos E, et al. Do semiquantitative amniotic fluid indexes reflect actual volume? *Am J Obstet Gynecol.* 1992;167(4, pt 1):995–999.

149. Magann EF, Nolan TE, Hess LW, et al. Measurement of amniotic fluid volume: accuracy of ultrasonography techniques. *Am J Obstet Gynecol.* 1992;167(6):1533–1537.

150. Magann EF, Chauhan SP, Barrilleaux PS, et al. Amniotic fluid index and single deepest pocket: weak indicators of abnormal amniotic volumes. *Obstet Gynecol.* 2000;96(5, pt 1):737–740.

151. Queenan JT, Thompson W, Whitfield CR, et al. Amniotic fluid volumes in normal pregnancies. *Am J Obstet Gynecol.* 1972;114(1):34–38.

152. Crowley P. Non quantitative estimation of amniotic fluid volume in suspected prolonged pregnancy. *J Perinat Med.* 1980;8(5):249–251.

153. Magann EF, Chauhan SP, Whitworth NS, et al. Subjective versus objective evaluation of amniotic fluid volume of pregnancies of less than 24 weeks' gestation: how can we be accurate? *J Ultrasound Med.* 2001;20(3):191–195.

154. Magann EF, Perry KG Jr, Chauhan SP, et al. The accuracy of ultrasound evaluation of amniotic fluid volume in singleton pregnancies: the effect of operator experience and ultrasound interpretative technique. *J Clin Ultrasound.* 1997;25(5):249–253.

155. Manning FA, Platt LD, Sipos L. Antepartum fetal evaluation: development of a fetal biophysical profile. *Am J Obstet Gynecol.* 1980;136(6):787–795.

156. Chamberlain PF, Manning FA, Morrison I, et al. Ultrasound evaluation of amniotic fluid volume, I: the relationship of marginal and decreased amniotic fluid volumes to perinatal outcome. *Am J Obstet Gynecol.* 1984;150(3):245–249.

157. Phelan JP, Smith CV, Broussard P, et al. Amniotic fluid volume assessment with the four-quadrant technique at 36–42 weeks' gestation. *J Reprod Med.* 1987;32(7):540–542.

158. Phelan JP, Ahn MO, Smith CV, et al. Amniotic fluid index measurements during pregnancy. *J Reprod Med.* 1987;32(8):601–604.

159. Moore TR, Cayle JE. The amniotic fluid index in normal human pregnancy. *Am J Obstet Gynecol.* 1990;162(5):1168–1173.

160. Flack NJ, Dore C, Southwell D, et al. The influence of operator transducer pressure on ultrasonographic measurements of amniotic fluid volume. *Am J Obstet Gynecol.* 1994;171(1):218–222.

161. American College of Obstetricians and Gynecologists. ACOG Practice Bulletin No 101: ultrasonography in pregnancy. *Obstet Gynecol.* 2009;113(2, pt 1):451–461.

162. Nabhan AF, Abdelmoula YA. Amniotic fluid index versus single deepest vertical pocket as a screening test for preventing adverse pregnancy outcome. *Cochrane Database Syst Rev.* 2008;(3):CD006593.

163. Magann EF, Morton ML, Nolan TE, et al. Comparative efficacy of two sonographic measurements for the detection of aberrations in the amniotic fluid volume and the effect of amniotic fluid volume on pregnancy outcome. *Obstet Gynecol.* 1994;83(6):959–962.

164. Chauhan SP, Magann EF, Morrison JC, et al. Ultrasonographic assessment of amniotic fluid does not reflect actual amniotic fluid volume. *Am J Obstet Gynecol.* 1997;177(2):291–296; discussion 296–297.

165. Magann EF, Doherty DA, Chauhan SP, et al. How well do the amniotic fluid index and single deepest pocket indices (below the 3rd and 5th and above the 95th and 97th percentiles) predict oligohydramnios and hydramnios? *Am J Obstet Gynecol.* 2004;190(1):164–169.

166. Manning FA, Hill LM, Platt LD. Qualitative amniotic fluid volume determination by ultrasound: antepartum detection of intrauterine growth retardation. *Am J Obstet Gynecol.* 1981;139(3):254–258.

167. Chauhan SP, Sanderson M, Hendrix NW, et al. Perinatal outcome and amniotic fluid index in the antepartum and intrapartum periods: a meta-analysis. *Am J Obstet Gynecol.* 1999;181(6):1473–1478.

168. Casey BM, McIntire DD, Bloom SL, et al. Pregnancy outcomes after antepartum diagnosis of oligohydramnios at or beyond 34 weeks' gestation. *Am J Obstet Gynecol.* 2000;182(4):909–912.

169. Locatelli A, Vergani P, Toso L, et al. Perinatal outcome associated with oligohydramnios in uncomplicated term pregnancies. *Arch Gynecol Obstet.* 2004;269(2):130–133.

170. Kim BJ, Romero R, Mi Lee S, et al. Clinical significance of oligohydramnios in patients with preterm labor and intact membranes. *J Perinat Med.* 2011;39(2):131–136.

171. Alfirevic Z, Luckas M, Walkinshaw SA, et al. A randomised comparison between amniotic fluid index and maximum pool depth in the monitoring of post-term pregnancy. *BJOG.* 1997;104(2):207–211.

172. Moses J, Doherty DA, Magann EF, et al. A randomized clinical trial of the intrapartum assessment of amniotic fluid volume: amniotic fluid index versus the single deepest pocket technique. *Am J Obstet Gynecol.* 2004;190(6):1564–1569; discussion 1569–1570.

173. Chauhan SP, Doherty DD, Magann EF, et al. Amniotic fluid index vs single deepest pocket technique during modified biophysical profile: a randomized clinical trial. *Am J Obstet Gynecol.* 2004;191(2):661–667; discussion 667–668.

174. Magann EF, Doherty DA, Field K, et al. Biophysical profile with amniotic fluid volume assessments. *Obstet Gynecol.* 2004;104(1):5–10.

175. Nabhan AF, Abdelmoula YA. Amniotic fluid index versus single deepest vertical pocket: a meta-analysis of randomized controlled trials. *Int J Gynaecol Obstet.* 2009;104(3):184–188.

176. Melamed N, Pardo J, Milstein R, et al. Perinatal outcome in pregnancies complicated by isolated oligohydramnios diagnosed before 37 weeks of gestation. *Am J Obstet Gynecol.* 2011;205(3):241.e1–241.e6.

177. Conway DL, Adkins WB, Schroeder B, et al. Isolated oligohydramnios in the term pregnancy: is it a clinical entity? *J Matern Fetal Neonatal Med.* 1998;7(4):197–200.

178. Ek S, Andersson A, Johansson A, et al. Oligohydramnios in uncomplicated pregnancies beyond 40 completed weeks: a prospective, randomised, pilot study on maternal and neonatal outcomes. *Fetal Diagn Ther.* 2005;20(3):182–185.

179. Rainford M, Adair R, Scialli AR, et al. Amniotic fluid index in the uncomplicated term pregnancy: prediction of outcome. *J Reprod Med.* 2001;46(6):589–592.

180. Zhang J, Troendle J, Meikle S, et al. Isolated oligohydramnios is not associated with adverse perinatal outcomes. *BJOG.* 2004;111(3):220–225.

181. Bullo M, Tschumi S, Bucher BS, et al. Pregnancy outcome following exposure to angiotensin-converting enzyme inhibitors or angiotensin receptor antagonists: a systematic review. *Hypertension.* 2012;60(2):444–450.

182. Kirshon B, Moise KJ Jr, Mari G, et al. Long-term indomethacin therapy decreases fetal urine output and results in oligohydramnios. *Am J Perinatol.* 1991;8(2):86–88.

183. Schucker JL, Mercer BM, Audibert F, et al. Serial amniotic fluid index in severe preeclampsia: a poor predictor of adverse outcome. *Am J Obstet Gynecol.* 1996;175(4, pt 1):1018–1023.

184. Kjos SL, Leung A, Henry OA, et al. Antepartum surveillance in diabetic pregnancies: predictors of fetal distress in labor. *Am J Obstet Gynecol.* 1995;173(5):1532–1539.

185. Jang DG, Jo YS, Lee SJ, et al. Perinatal outcomes and maternal clinical characteristics in IUGR with absent or reversed end-diastolic flow velocity in the umbilical artery. *Arch Gynecol Obstet.* 2011;284(1):73–78.

186. Vink J, Hickey K, Ghidini A, et al. Earlier gestational age at ultrasound evaluation predicts adverse neonatal outcomes in the preterm appropriate-for-gestational-age fetus with idiopathic oligohydramnios. *Am J Perinatol.* 2009;26(1):21–25.

187. Veille JC, Penry M, Mueller-Heubach E. Fetal renal pulsed Doppler waveform in prolonged pregnancies. *Am J Obstet Gynecol.* 1993;169(4):882–884.

188. Selam B, Koksal R, Ozcan T. Fetal arterial and venous Doppler parameters in the interpretation of oligohydramnios in postterm pregnancies. *Ultrasound Obstet Gynecol.* 2000;15(5):403–406.

189. Veille JC, Kanaan C. Duplex Doppler ultrasonographic evaluation of the fetal renal artery in normal and abnormal fetuses. *Am J Obstet Gynecol.* 1989;161(6, pt 1):1502–1507.

190. Sepulveda W, Stagiannis KD, Flack NJ, et al. Accuracy of prenatal diagnosis of renal agenesis with color flow imaging in severe second-trimester oligohydramnios. *Am J Obstet Gynecol.* 1995;173(6):1788–1792.

191. Grijseels EW, van-Hornstra PT, Govaerts LC, et al. Outcome of pregnancies complicated by oligohydramnios or anhydramnios of renal origin. *Prenat Diagn.* 2011;31(11):1039–1045.

192. Oliveira EA, Diniz JS, Cabral AC, et al. Predictive factors of fetal urethral obstruction: a multivariate analysis. *Fetal Diagn Ther.* 2000;15(3):180–186.

193. Goodlin RC, Anderson JC, Gallagher TF. Relationship between amniotic fluid volume and maternal plasma volume expansion. *Am J Obstet Gynecol.* 1983;146(5):505–511.

194. Yan-Rosenberg L, Burt B, Bombard AT, et al. A randomized clinical trial comparing the effect of maternal intravenous hydration and placebo on the amniotic fluid index in oligohydramnios. *J Matern Fetal Neonatal Med.* 2007;20(10):715–718.

195. Kilpatrick SJ, Safford KL, Pomeroy T, et al. Maternal hydration increases amniotic fluid index. *Obstet Gynecol.* 1991;78(6):1098–1102.

196. Patrelli TS, Gizzo S, Cosmi E, et al. Maternal hydration therapy improves the quantity of amniotic fluid and the pregnancy outcome in third-trimester isolated oligohydramnios: a controlled randomized institutional trial. *J Ultrasound Med.* 2012;31(2):239–244.

197. Doi S, Osada H, Seki K, et al. Effect of maternal hydration on oligohydramnios: a comparison of three volume expansion methods. *Obstet Gynecol.* 1998; 92(4, pt 1):525–529.

198. Flack NJ, Sepulveda W, Bower S, et al. Acute maternal hydration in third-trimester oligohydramnios: effects on amniotic fluid volume, uteroplacental perfusion, and fetal blood flow and urine output. *Am J Obstet Gynecol.* 1995;173(4):1186–1191.

199. Carroll BC, Bruner JP. Umbilical artery Doppler velocimetry in pregnancies complicated by oligohydramnios. *J Reprod Med.* 2000;45(7):562–566.

200. Biggio JR Jr, Wenstrom KD, Dubard MB, et al. Hydramnios prediction of adverse perinatal outcome. *Obstet Gynecol.* 1999;94(5, pt 1):773–777.

201. Hill LM, Breckle R, Thomas ML, et al. Polyhydramnios: ultrasonically detected prevalence and neonatal outcome. *Obstet Gynecol.* 1987;69(1):21–25.

202. Chamberlain PF, Manning FA, Morrison I, et al. Ultrasound evaluation of amniotic fluid volume, II: the relationship of increased amniotic fluid volume to perinatal outcome. *Am J Obstet Gynecol.* 1984;150(3):250–254.

203. Hallak M, Kirshon B, O'Brian Smith E, et al. Subjective ultrasonographic assessment of amniotic fluid depth: comparison with the amniotic fluid index. *Fetal Diagn Ther.* 1993;8(4):256–260.

204. Lazebnik N, Many A. The severity of polyhydramnios, estimated fetal weight and preterm delivery are independent risk factors for the presence of congenital malformations. *Gynecol Obstet Invest.* 1999;48(1):28–32.

205. Dashe JS, McIntire DD, Ramus RM, et al. Hydramnios: anomaly prevalence and sonographic detection. *Obstet Gynecol.* 2002;100(1):134–139.

206. Panting-Kemp A, Nguyen T, Chang E, et al. Idiopathic polyhydramnios and perinatal outcome. *Am J Obstet Gynecol.* 1999;181(5, pt 1):1079–1082.

207. Smith CV, Plambeck RD, Rayburn WF, et al. Relation of mild idiopathic polyhydramnios to perinatal outcome. *Obstet Gynecol.* 1992;79(3):387–389.

208. Sohaey R, Nyberg DA, Sickler GK, et al. Idiopathic polyhydramnios: association with fetal macrosomia. *Radiology.* 1994;190(2):393–396.

209. Chen KC, Liou JD, Hung TH, et al. Perinatal outcomes of polyhydramnios without associated congenital fetal anomalies after the gestational age of 20 weeks. *Chang Gung Med J.* 2005;28(4):222–228.

210. Erez O, Shoham-Vardi I, Sheiner E, et al. Hydramnios and small for gestational age are independent risk factors for neonatal mortality and maternal morbidity. *Arch Gynecol Obstet.* 2005;271(4):296–301.

211. Maymon E, Ghezzi F, Shoham-Vardi I, et al. Isolated hydramnios at term gestation and the occurrence of peripartum complications. *Eur J Obstet Gynecol Reprod Biol.* 1998;77(2):157–161.

212. Many A, Hill LM, Lazebnik N, et al. The association between polyhydramnios and preterm delivery. *Obstet Gynecol.* 1995;86(3):389–391.

213. Sickler GK, Nyberg DA, Sohaey R, et al. Polyhydramnios and fetal intrauterine growth restriction: ominous combination. *J Ultrasound Med.* 1997;16(9):609–614.

214. Abele H, Starz S, Hoopmann M, et al. Idiopathic polyhydramnios and postnatal abnormalities. *Fetal Diagn Ther.* 2012;32(4):251–255.

215. Dorleijn DM, Cohen-Overbeek TE, Groenendaal F, et al. Idiopathic polyhydramnios and postnatal findings. *J Matern Fetal Neonatal Med.* 2009;22(4):315–320.

216. Touboul C, Boileau P, Picone O, et al. Outcome of children born out of pregnancies complicated by unexplained polyhydramnios. *BJOG.* 2007;114(4):489–492.

217. Golan A, Wolman I, Sagi J, et al. Persistence of polyhydramnios during pregnancy—its significance and correlation with maternal and fetal complications. *Gynecol Obstet Invest.* 1994;37(1):18–20.

218. Fisk NM, Vaughan J, Talbert D. Impaired fetal blood gas status in polyhydramnios and its relation to raised amniotic pressure. *Fetal Diagn Ther.* 1994;9(1):7–13.

219. Moise KJ Jr. Toward consistent terminology: assessment and reporting of amniotic fluid volume. *Semin Perinatol.* 2013;37(5):370–374.

220. Idris N, Wong SF, Thomae M, et al. Influence of polyhydramnios on perinatal outcome in pregestational diabetic pregnancies. *Ultrasound Obstet Gynecol.* 2010;36(3):338–343.

221. Bartha JL, Martinez-Del-Fresno P, Comino-Delgado R. Early diagnosis of gestational diabetes mellitus and prevention of diabetes-related complications. *Eur J Obstet Gynecol Reprod Biol.* 2003;109(1):41–44.

222. Jacobson JD, Cousins L. A population-based study of maternal and perinatal outcome in patients with gestational diabetes. *Am J Obstet Gynecol.* 1989;161(4):981–986.

223. Bar-Hava I, Scarpelli SA, Barnhard Y, et al. Amniotic fluid volume reflects recent glycemic status in gestational diabetes mellitus. *Am J Obstet Gynecol.* 1994;171(4):952–955.

224. Goldman M, Kitzmiller JL, Abrams B, et al. Obstetric complications with GDM: effects of maternal weight. *Diabetes.* 1991;40(suppl 2):79–82.

225. Barkin SZ, Pretorius DH, Beckett MK, et al. Severe polyhydramnios: incidence of anomalies. *AJR Am J Roentgenol.* 1987;148(1):155–159.

226. McKelvey A, Stanwell J, Smeulders N, et al. Persistent non-visualisation of the fetal stomach: diagnostic and prognostic implications. *Arch Dis Child Fetal Neonatal Ed.* 2010;95(6):F439–F442.

227. Agrawal P, Ogilvy-Stuart A, Lees C. Intrauterine diagnosis and management of congenital goitrous hypothyroidism. *Ultrasound Obstet Gynecol.* 2002;19(5):501–505.

228. Koyuncu FM, Tamay AG, Bugday S. Intrauterine diagnosis and management of fetal goiter: a case report. *J Clin Ultrasound.* 2010;38(9):503–505.

229. Pumberger W, Hormann M, Deutinger J, et al. Longitudinal observation of antenatally detected congenital lung malformations (CLM): natural history, clinical outcome and long-term follow-up. *Eur J Cardiothorac Surg.* 2003;24(5):703–711.

230. Chen WS, Yeh GP, Tsai HD, et al. Prenatal diagnosis of congenital cystic adenomatoid malformations: evolution and outcome. *Taiwan J Obstet Gynecol.* 2009;48(3):278–281.

231. MacMillan RH, Harbert GM, Davis WD, et al. Prenatal diagnosis of Pena-Shokeir syndrome type 1. *Am J Med Genet.* 1985;21(2):279–284.

232. Zelop C, Benacerraf B. Sonographic diagnosis of fetal upper extremity dysmorphology: significance and outcome. *Ultrasound Obstet Gynecol.* 1996;8(6):391–396.

233. Jungbluth H, Wallgren-Pettersson C, Laporte J. Centronuclear (myotubular) myopathy. *Orphanet J Rare Dis.* 2008;3:26.

234. Rudnik-Schoneborn S, Nicholson GA, Morgan G, et al. Different patterns of obstetric complications in myotonic dystrophy in relation to the disease status of the fetus. *Am J Med Genet.* 1998;80(4):314–321.

235. Dudley O, Muscatelli F. Clinical evidence of intrauterine disturbance in Prader-Willi syndrome, a genetically imprinted neurodevelopmental disorder. *Early Hum Dev.* 2007;83(7):471–478.

236. Geysenbergh B, De Catte L, Vogels A. Can fetal ultrasound result in prenatal diagnosis of Prader-Willi syndrome? *Genet Couns.* 2011;22(2):207–216.

237. Bhat YR, Vinayaka G, Sreelakshmi K. Antenatal bartter syndrome: a review. *Int J Pediatr.* 2012;2012:857136.

238. Alessandri JL, Cuillier F, Ramful D, et al. Perlman syndrome: report, prenatal findings and review. *Am J Med Genet A.* 2008;146A(19):2532–2537.

239. Williams DH, Gauthier DW, Maizels M. Prenatal diagnosis of Beckwith-Wiedemann syndrome. *Prenat Diagn.* 2005;25(10):879–884.

240. Degani S. Sonographic findings in fetal viral infections: a systematic review. *Obstet Gynecol Surv.* 2006;61(5):329–336.

241. Maxwell DJ, Crawford DC, Curry PV, et al. Obstetric importance, diagnosis, and management of fetal tachycardias. *BMJ.* 1988;297(6641):107–110.

242. Zalel Y, Gamzu R, Weiss Y, et al. Role of color Doppler imaging in diagnosing and managing pregnancies complicated by placental chorioangioma. *J Clin Ultrasound.* 2002;30(5):264–269.

243. Ang MS, Thorp JA, Parisi VM. Maternal lithium therapy and polyhydramnios. *Obstet Gynecol.* 1990;76(3, pt 2):517–519.

244. Coviello D, Bonati F, Montefusco SM, et al. Amnioreduction. *Acta Biomed.* 2004;75(suppl 1):31–33.

245. Elliott JP, Sawyer AT, Radin TG, et al. Large-volume therapeutic amniocentesis in the treatment of hydramnios. *Obstet Gynecol.* 1994;84(6):1025–1027.

246. ACOG practice bulletin. Antepartum fetal surveillance. Number 9, October 1999 (replaces Technical Bulletin Number 188, January 1994). Clinical management guidelines for obstetrician-gynecologists. *Int J Gynaecol Obstet.* 2000;68(2):175–185.

247. Hershkovitz R, Sheiner E, Maymon E, et al. Cervical length assessment in women with idiopathic polyhydramnios. *Ultrasound Obstet Gynecol.* 2006;28(6):775–778.

248. Vengalil S, Santolaya-Forgas J, Meyer W, et al. Ultrasonically dense amniotic fluid in early pregnancy in asymptomatic women without vaginal bleeding: a report of two cases. *J Reprod Med.* 1998;43(5):462–464.

249. Sepulveda W, Reid R, Nicolaidis P, et al. Second-trimester echogenic bowel and intraamniotic bleeding: association between fetal bowel echogenicity and amniotic fluid spectrophotometry at 410 nm. *Am J Obstet Gynecol.* 1996;174(3):839–842.

250. Vohra N, Rochelson B, Smith-Levitin M. Three-dimensional sonographic findings in congenital (harlequin) ichthyosis. *J Ultrasound Med.* 2003;22(7):737–739.

251. Dolan CR, Smith LT, Sybert VP. Prenatal detection of epidermolysis bullosa letalis with pyloric atresia in a fetus by abnormal ultrasound and elevated alpha-fetoprotein. *Am J Med Genet.* 1993;47(3):395–400.

252. Timor-Tritsch IE, Greenebaum E, Monteagudo A, et al. Exencephaly-anencephaly sequence: proof by ultrasound imaging and amniotic fluid cytology. *J Matern Fetal Med.* 1996;5(4):182–185.

253. Benacerraf BR, Gatter MA, Ginsburgh F. Ultrasound diagnosis of meconium-stained amniotic fluid. *Am J Obstet Gynecol.* 1984;149(5):570–572.

254. Sherer DM, Abramowicz JS, Smith SA, et al. Sonographically homogeneous echogenic amniotic fluid in detecting meconium-stained amniotic fluid. *Obstet Gynecol.* 1991;78(5, pt 1):819–822.

255. Brown DL, Polger M, Clark PK, et al. Very echogenic amniotic fluid: ultrasonography-amniocentesis correlation. *J Ultrasound Med.* 1994;13(2):95–97.

256. DeVore GR, Platt LD. Ultrasound appearance of particulate matter in amniotic cavity: vernix or meconium? *J Clin Ultrasound.* 1986;14(3):229–230.

257. Espinoza J, Goncalves LF, Romero R, et al. The prevalence and clinical significance of amniotic fluid "sludge" in patients with preterm labor and intact membranes. *Ultrasound Obstet Gynecol.* 2005;25(4):346–352.

258. Bujold E, Pasquier JC, Simoneau J, et al. Intra-amniotic sludge, short cervix, and risk of preterm delivery. *J Obstet Gynaecol Can.* 2006;28(3):198–202.

259. Kusanovic JP, Espinoza J, Romero R, et al. Clinical significance of the presence of amniotic fluid "sludge" in asymptomatic patients at high risk for spontaneous preterm delivery. *Ultrasound Obstet Gynecol.* 2007;30(5):706–714.

260. Romero R, Schaudinn C, Kusanovic JP, et al. Detection of a microbial biofilm in intra-amniotic infection. *Am J Obstet Gynecol.* 2008;198(1):135.e1–135.e5.

261. Romero R, Kusanovic JP, Espinoza J, et al. What is amniotic fluid "sludge"? *Ultrasound Obstet Gynecol.* 2007;30(5):793–798.

262. Harding JA, Jackson DM, Lewis DF, et al. Correlation of amniotic fluid index and nonstress test in patients with preterm premature rupture of membranes. *Am J Obstet Gynecol.* 1991;165(4, pt 1):1088–1094.

263. Vintzileos AM, Campbell WA, Nochimson DJ, et al. Degree of oligohydramnios and pregnancy outcome in patients with premature rupture of the membranes. *Obstet Gynecol.* 1985;66(2):162–167.

264. Gonik B, Bottoms SF, Cotton DB. Amniotic fluid volume as a risk factor in preterm premature rupture of the membranes. *Obstet Gynecol.* 1985;65(4):456–459.

265. Storness-Bliss C, Metcalfe A, Simrose R, et al. Correlation of residual amniotic fluid and perinatal outcomes in periviable preterm premature rupture of membranes. *J Obstet Gynaecol Can.* 2012;34(2):154–158.

266. Hadi HA, Hodson CA, Strickland D. Premature rupture of the membranes between 20 and 25 weeks' gestation: role of amniotic fluid volume in perinatal outcome. *Am J Obstet Gynecol.* 1994;170(4):1139–1144.

267. Hunter TJ, Byrnes MJ, Nathan E, et al. Factors influencing survival in previable preterm premature rupture of membranes. *J Matern Fetal Neonatal Med.* 2012;25(9):1755–1761.

268. Goncalves LF, Chaiworapongsa T, Romero R. Intrauterine infection and prematurity. *Ment Retard Dev Disabil Res Rev.* 2002;8(1):3–13.

269. DiGiulio DB, Romero R, Kusanovic JP, et al. Prevalence and diversity of microbes in the amniotic fluid, the fetal inflammatory response, and pregnancy outcome in women with preterm pre-labor rupture of membranes. *Am J Reprod Immunol.* 2010;64(1):38–57.

270. Smith CV, Greenspoon J, Phelan JP, et al. Clinical utility of the nonstress test in the conservative management of women with preterm spontaneous premature rupture of the membranes. *J Reprod Med.* 1987;32(1):1–4.

271. Lewi L, Hanssens M, Spitz B, et al. Complete chorioamniotic membrane separation: case report and review of the literature. *Fetal Diagn Ther.* 2004;19(1):78–82.

272. Ulm B, Ulm MR, Bernaschek G. Unfused amnion and chorion after 14 weeks of gestation: associated fetal structural and chromosomal abnormalities. *Ultrasound Obstet Gynecol.* 1999;13(6):392–395.

273. Sistrom CL, Ferguson JE. Abnormal membranes in obstetrical ultrasound: incidence and significance of amniotic sheets and circumvallate placenta. *Ultrasound Obstet Gynecol.* 1993;3(4):249–255.

274. Lazebnik N, Hill LM, Many A, et al. The effect of amniotic sheet orientation on subsequent maternal and fetal complications. *Ultrasound Obstet Gynecol.* 1996;8(4):267–271.

275. Tan KB, Tan TY, Tan JV, et al. The amniotic sheet: a truly benign condition? *Ultrasound Obstet Gynecol.* 2005;26(6):639–643.

276. Mahony BS, Filly RA, Callen PW, et al. The amniotic band syndrome: antenatal sonographic diagnosis and potential pitfalls. *Am J Obstet Gynecol.* 1985;152(1):63–68.

277. Ozkavukcu E, Haliloglu N. Gray-scale and color Doppler US findings of amniotic sheets. *Diagn Interv Radiol.* 2012;18(3):298–302.

278. De Laat MW, Franx A, van Alderen ED, et al. The umbilical coiling index, a review of the literature. *J Matern Fetal Neonatal Med.* 2005;17(2):93–100.

279. Fujikura T. Fused umbilical arteries near placental cord insertion. *Am J Obstet Gynecol.* 2003;188(3):765–767.

280. Hua M, Odibo AO, Macones GA, et al. Single umbilical artery and its associated findings. *Obstet Gynecol.* 2010;115(5):930–934.

281. Burshtein S, Levy A, Holcberg G, et al. Is single umbilical artery an independent risk factor for perinatal mortality? *Arch Gynecol Obstet.* 2011;283(2):191–194.

282. Gornall AS, Kurinczuk JJ, Konje JC. Antenatal detection of a single umbilical artery: does it matter? *Prenat Diagn.* 2003;23(2):117–123.

283. Klatt J, Kuhn A, Baumann M, et al. Single umbilical artery in twin pregnancies. *Ultrasound Obstet Gynecol.* 2012;39(5):505–509.

284. Rembouskos G, Cicero S, Longo D, et al. Single umbilical artery at 11–14 weeks' gestation: relation to chromosomal defects. *Ultrasound Obstet Gynecol.* 2003;22(6):567–570.

285. Santillan M, Santillan D, Fleener D, et al. Single umbilical artery: does side matter? *Fetal Diagn Ther.* 2012;32(3):201–208.

286. DeFigueiredo D, Dagklis T, Zidere V, et al. Isolated single umbilical artery: need for specialist fetal echocardiography? *Ultrasound Obstet Gynecol.* 2010;36(5):553–555.

287. Granese R, Coco C, Jeanty P. The value of single umbilical artery in the prediction of fetal aneuploidy: findings in 12,672 pregnant women. *Ultrasound Q.* 2007;23(2):117–121.

288. Strong TH Jr, Elliott JP, Radin TG. Non-coiled umbilical blood vessels: a new marker for the fetus at risk. *Obstet Gynecol.* 1993;81(3):409–411.

289. Cromi A, Ghezzi F, Durig P, et al. Sonographic umbilical cord morphometry and coiling patterns in twin-twin transfusion syndrome. *Prenat Diagn.* 2005;25(9):851–855.

290. De Laat MW, Nikkels PG, Franx A, et al. The Roach muscle bundle and umbilical cord coiling. *Early Hum Dev.* 2007;83(9):571–574.

291. Predanic M, Perni SC. Absence of a relationship between umbilical cord thickness and coiling patterns. *J Ultrasound Med.* 2005;24(11):1491–1496.

292. Di Naro E, Ghezzi F, Raio L, et al. Umbilical vein blood flow in fetuses with normal and lean umbilical cord. *Ultrasound Obstet Gynecol.* 2001;17(3):224–228.

293. Strong TH Jr, Jarles DL, Vega JS, et al. The umbilical coiling index. *Am J Obstet Gynecol.* 1994;170(1, pt 1):29–32.

294. Degani S, Lewinsky RM, Berger H, et al. Sonographic estimation of umbilical coiling index and correlation with Doppler flow characteristics. *Obstet Gynecol.* 1995;86(6):990–993.

295. Qin Y, Lau TK, Rogers MS. Second-trimester ultrasonographic assessment of the umbilical coiling index. *Ultrasound Obstet Gynecol.* 2002;20(5):458–463.

296. De Laat MW, Franx A, Nikkels PG, et al. Prenatal ultrasonographic prediction of the umbilical coiling index at birth and adverse pregnancy outcome. *Ultrasound Obstet Gynecol.* 2006;28(5):704–709.

297. Sebire NJ. Pathophysiological significance of abnormal umbilical cord coiling index. *Ultrasound Obstet Gynecol.* 2007;30(6):804–806.

298. Ghezzi F, Raio L, Di Naro E, et al. Single and multiple umbilical cord cysts in early gestation: two different entities. *Ultrasound Obstet Gynecol.* 2003;21(3):215–219.

299. Ross JA, Jurkovic D, Zosmer N, et al. Umbilical cord cysts in early pregnancy. *Obstet Gynecol.* 1997;89(3):442–445.

300. Schaefer IM, Manner J, Faber R, et al. Giant umbilical cord edema caused by retrograde micturition through an open patent urachus. *Pediatr Dev Pathol.* 2010;13(5):404–407.

301. Schiesser M, Lapaire O, Holzgreve W, et al. Umbilical cord edema associated with patent urachus. *Ultrasound Obstet Gynecol.* 2003;22(6):646–647.

302. Kita M, Kikuchi A, Miyashita S, et al. Umbilical cord cysts of allantoic and omphalomesenteric remnants with progressive umbilical cord edema: a case report. *Fetal Diagn Ther.* 2009;25(2):250–254.

303. Emura T, Kanamori Y, Ito M, et al. Omphalocele associated with a large multilobular umbilical cord pseudocyst. *Pediatr Surg Int.* 2004;20(8):636–639.

304. Tong SY, Lee JE, Kim SR, et al. Umbilical cord cyst: a prenatal clue to bladder exstrophy. *Prenat Diagn.* 2007;27(12):1177–1179.

305. Zangen R, Boldes R, Yaffe H, et al. Umbilical cord cysts in the second and third trimesters: significance and prenatal approach. *Ultrasound Obstet Gynecol.* 2010;36(3):296–301.

306. Gilboa Y, Kivilevitch Z, Katorza E, et al. Outcomes of fetuses with umbilical cord cysts diagnosed during nuchal translucency examination. *J Ultrasound Med.* 2011;30(11):1547–1551.

307. Sepulveda W, Pryde PG, Greb AE, et al. Prenatal diagnosis of umbilical cord pseudocyst. *Ultrasound Obstet Gynecol.* 1994;4(2):147–150.

308. Sepulveda W, Leible S, Ulloa A, et al. Clinical significance of first trimester umbilical cord cysts. *J Ultrasound Med.* 1999;18(2):95–99.

309. Papadopoulos VG, Kourea HP, Adonakis GL, et al. A case of umbilical cord hemangioma: Doppler studies and review of the literature. *Eur J Obstet Gynecol Reprod Biol.* 2009;144(1):8–14.

310. Seoud M, Aboul-Hosn L, Nassar A, et al. Spontaneous umbilical cord hematoma: a rare cause of acute fetal distress. *Am J Perinatol.* 2001;18(2):99–102.

311. Jauniaux E, Nicolaides KH, Campbell S, et al. Hematoma of the umbilical cord secondary to cordocentesis for intrauterine fetal transfusion. *Prenat Diagn.* 1990;10(7):477–478.

312. Sepulveda W, Corral E, Kottmann C, et al. Umbilical artery aneurysm: prenatal identification in three fetuses with trisomy 18. *Ultrasound Obstet Gynecol.* 2003;21(3):292–296.

313. Berg C, Geipel A, Germer U, et al. Prenatal diagnosis of umbilical cord aneurysm in a fetus with trisomy 18. *Ultrasound Obstet Gynecol.* 2001;17(1):79–81.

314. Mankuta D, Nadjari M, Pomp G. Isolated fetal intra-abdominal umbilical vein varix: clinical importance and recommendations. *J Ultrasound Med.* 2011;30(2):273–276.

315. Keene DJ, Shawkat E, Gillham J, et al. Rare combination of exomphalos with umbilical cord teratoma. *Ultrasound Obstet Gynecol.* 2012;40(4):481.

316. Cheng HP, Hsu CY, Chen CP, et al. Angiomyxoma of the umbilical cord. *Taiwan J Obstet Gynecol.* 2006;45(4):360–362.

317. Schaffer L, Burkhardt T, Zimmermann R, et al. Nuchal cords in term and postterm deliveries—do we need to know? *Obstet Gynecol.* 2005;106(1):23–28.

318. Sherer DM, Manning FA. Prenatal ultrasonographic diagnosis of nuchal cord(s): disregard, inform, monitor or intervene? *Ultrasound Obstet Gynecol.* 1999;14(1):1–8.

319. Jauniaux E, Mawissa C, Peellaerts C, et al. Nuchal cord in normal third-trimester pregnancy: a color Doppler imaging study. *Ultrasound Obstet Gynecol.* 1992;2(6):417–419.

320. Schaefer M, Laurichesse-Delmas H, Ville Y. The effect of nuchal cord on nuchal translucency measurement at 10–14 weeks. *Ultrasound Obstet Gynecol.* 1998;11(4):271–273.

321. Gonzalez-Quintero VH, Tolaymat L, Muller AC, et al. Outcomes of pregnancies with sonographically detected nuchal cords remote from delivery. *J Ultrasound Med.* 2004;23(1):43–47.

322. Ezra Y, Strasberg SR, Farine D. Does cord presentation on ultrasound predict cord prolapse? *Gynecol Obstet Invest.* 2003;56(1):6–9.

323. Raga F, Osborne N, Ballester MJ, et al. Color flow Doppler: a useful instrument in the diagnosis of funic presentation. *J Natl Med Assoc.* 1996;88(2):94–96.

# 8 First Trimester Evaluation

Marta Nucci • Carmen Sciorio • Kypros H. Nicolaides

In the last 30 years, the first trimester scan has evolved from an examination for the assessment of fetal viability and gestational age to become the central component of an integrated clinic for the diagnosis of fetal abnormalities and assessment of risk for a wide range of pregnancy complications. This chapter reviews the accumulated data on the role of the first trimester scan in pregnancy care.

## SCREENING FOR FETAL ANEUPLOIDIES

Aneuploidies are major causes of perinatal death and childhood handicap. Consequently, the detection of chromosomal disorders constitutes the most frequent indication for invasive prenatal diagnosis. However, invasive testing, by amniocentesis or chorionic villous sampling, is associated with a risk of miscarriage, and therefore these tests are carried out only in pregnancies considered to be at high risk for aneuploidies.[1]

In the last 40 years, prenatal screening for aneuploidies has focused on trisomy 21. The method of screening has evolved from maternal age in the 1970s with a detection rate (DR) for trisomy 21 of 30% and a false positive rate (FPR) of 5%, to a combination of maternal age and second trimester serum biochemistry in the 1980s and 1990s, with a DR of 60% to 70% and a FPR of 5%. In the last 20 years, a combination of maternal age, fetal nuchal translucency (NT) thickness, and serum-free β-hCG and PAPP-A in the first trimester has been advocated, with a DR of 90% and a FPR of 5%.[2] Studies in the last 10 years have shown that improvement in the performance of first trimester screening can be achieved by inclusion in the ultrasound assessment of the nasal bone, flow in the ductus venosus, hepatic artery, and across the tricuspid valve.

A beneficial consequence of screening for trisomy 21 is the early diagnosis of trisomies 18 and 13, which are the second and third most common chromosomal abnormalities, with a relative prevalence to trisomy 21 at 11 to 13 weeks' gestation of 1:3 and 1:7, respectively.[3,4] Since all three trisomies are similar in being associated with increased maternal age, increased fetal NT, and decreased serum PAPP-A, screening using the algorithm for trisomy 21 can detect about 90% of cases of trisomy 21 and 70% to 75% of cases of trisomies 18 and 13, at FPR of 4% to 5%.[5,6] However, with the use of specific algorithms for each trisomy, which incorporate not only their similarities but also their differences in biomarker pattern, including high serum-free β-hCG in trisomy 21 and low levels in trisomies 18 and 13 and high fetal heart rate in trisomy 13, it is possible to increase the DR of trisomies 18 and 13 to about 95% at the same overall FPR of about 4% to 5%.[5,6]

In addition to trisomies 21, 18, and 13, invasive testing in the screen positive group from the combined test detects many other clinically significant aneuploidies.[7] However, the biomarker profile for many of the rare aneuploidies and chromosomal imbalance syndromes is not clearly defined, and it is uncertain whether their incidence in the screen positive group for trisomy 21 is higher than in the screen negative group. The only exceptions are monosomy X, presenting with large fetal NT, and triploidy presenting with either very high serum-free β-hCG and large NT or very low serum-free β-hCG and PAPP-A.[2,8–10]

Several studies in the last 3 years have reported the clinical validation and implementation of screening for aneuploides by analysis of cell-free (cf) DNA in maternal blood.[11] Most studies have reported on screening for trisomies 21, 18, and 13, and a few have also reported diagnostic accuracy in sex chromosome aneuploidies. Some proof of principle studies have examined the potential value of cfDNA testing in the detection of triploidy, trisomies other than those affecting chromosomes 21, 18, and 13, and chromosomal deletions and duplications.[12–14] The combined data from studies involving a large number of affected and unaffected pregnancies indicate that with cfDNA analysis the DR for trisomies 21, 18, and 13 and monosomy X is 99.0%, 96.8%, 92.1%, and 88.6%, respectively, at FPR of 0.08%, 0.15%, 0.20%, and 0.12%.[11]

## Nuchal Translucency Thickness

NT is the sonographic appearance of a collection of fluid under the skin behind the fetal neck in the first trimester of pregnancy.[15] The term translucency is used, irrespective of whether it is separated or not and whether it is confined to the neck or envelopes the whole fetus. The incidence of chromosomal and other abnormalities is related to the size, rather than the appearance of NT.[16] During the second trimester, the translucency usually resolves and, in a few cases, it evolves into either nuchal edema alternatively referred to as increased nuchal thickness in the mid-trimester or cystic hygromas with or without generalized hydrops.

### Measurement of Nuchal Translucency Thickness

The optimal gestational age for measurement of fetal NT is $11^{+0}$ to $13^{+6}$ weeks. The minimum fetal crown rump length (CRL) should be 45 mm and the maximum 84 mm. The lower limit is selected to allow the sonographic diagnosis of many major fetal abnormalities, which would have otherwise been missed, and the upper limit is such as to provide women with affected fetuses the option of an earlier and safer form of termination. Fetal NT can be measured by either transabdominal or transvaginal sonography, and the results are similar. When measuring the NT, the magnification of the image should be such that the fetal head and upper thorax occupy the whole screen, and a midsagittal section of the fetus in a neutral position must be obtained (Fig. 8.1). The widest part of translucency must always be measured, and care must be taken to distinguish between fetal skin and amnion. Measurements should be taken with the inner border of the horizontal line of the calipers placed on the line that defines the NT thickness—the crossbar of the calipers should be such that it is hardly visible as it merges with the white line of the border, not in the nuchal fluid. During the scan, more than one measurement must be taken, and the maximum one that meets all the above criteria should be recorded.

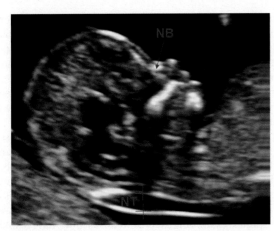

**FIGURE 8.1:** Ultrasound picture of a fetus at 12 weeks' gestation illustrating the measurement of nuchal translucency *(NT)* thickness and assessment of the nasal bone *(NB)*.

## Implications of Increased Nuchal Translucency Thickness

The measurement of fetal NT thickness provides effective and early screening for trisomy 21 and other major aneuploidies.[17-19] Furthermore, high NT is associated with fetal death, cardiac defects, and a wide range of other fetal malformations and genetic syndromes.[20-24] The heterogeneity of conditions associated with increased NT suggests that there may not be a single underlying mechanism for the collection of fluid under the skin of the fetal neck. Possible mechanisms include cardiac dysfunction in association with abnormalities of the heart and great arteries, venous congestion in the head and neck, altered composition of the extracellular matrix, failure of lymphatic drainage due to abnormal or delayed development of the lymphatic system or impaired fetal movements, fetal anemia or hypoproteinemia, and congenital infection.

In normal fetuses NT thickness increases with fetal CRL. The median and 95th percentile of NT at a CRL of 45 mm are 1.2 and 2.1 mm, and the respective values at CRL of 84 mm are 1.9 and 2.7 mm. The 99th percentile does not change significantly with CRL, and it is about 3.5 mm. Increased NT refers to a measurement above the 95th percentile.

The prevalence of fetal abnormalities and adverse pregnancy outcome increases exponentially with NT thickness (Table 8.1).

However, the parents can be reassured that the chances of delivering a baby with no major abnormalities are more than 90% if the fetal NT is between the 95th and 99th centiles, about 70% for NT of 3.5 to 4.4 mm, 50% for NT 4.5 to 5.4 mm, 30% for NT of 5.5 to 6.4 mm, and 15% for NT of 6.5 mm or more.

### Management of Pregnancies with Increased Nuchal Translucency Thickness

In pregnancies with fetal NT below the 99th percentile (3.5 mm), the decision by the parents in favor of or against fetal karyotyping will depend on the patient-specific risk for chromosomal defects, which is derived from the combination of maternal age, sonographic findings, and serum-free β-hCG and PAPP-A. In terms of the subsequent management of the pregnancy, it would be best to carry out a detailed fetal scan at 20 weeks to determine fetal growth and diagnose or exclude major abnormalities that could not be identified at the 11 to 13$^{+6}$ weeks scan.

A fetal NT above 3.5 mm is found in about 1% of pregnancies. The risk of major chromosomal abnormalities is very high and increases from about 20% for NT of 4.0 mm to 33% for NT of 5.0 mm, 50% for NT of 6.0 mm, and 65% for NT of 6.5 mm or more. Consequently, the first line of management of such pregnancies should be the offer of fetal karyotyping by CVS. In the chromosomally normal group, a detailed scan, including fetal echocardiography, should be attempted between 14 and 16 weeks to determine the evolution of the NT and to diagnose or exclude many fetal defects. If this scan demonstrates resolution of the NT with normal nuchal thickness measurement in the mid-trimester and absence of any major abnormalities, the parents can be reassured that the prognosis is likely to be good and the chances of delivering a baby with no major abnormalities is more than 95%. The only necessary additional investigation is a detailed scan at 20 to 22 weeks for the exclusion or diagnosis of both major abnormalities and the more subtle defects that are associated with certain associated genetic syndromes. If none of these is found, the parents can be counseled that the risk of delivering a baby with a serious abnormality or neurodevelopmental delay may not be higher than in the general population.

Persistence of unexplained increased NT at 14 to 16 weeks scan or evolution to nuchal edema or hydrops fetalis at 20 to 22 weeks raises the possibility of congenital infection or a genetic syndrome. Maternal blood should be tested for toxoplasmosis,

| Table 8.1 | Relation between Nuchal Translucency Thickness and Prevalence of Chromosomal Defects, Miscarriage or Fetal Death, and Major Fetal Abnormalities | | | |
|---|---|---|---|---|
| **Nuchal Translucency** | **Chromosomal Defects (%)** | **Fetal Death (%)** | **Major Fetal Abnormalities (%)** | **Alive and Well$^a$ (%)** |
| <95th centile | 0.2 | 1.3 | 1.6 | 97 |
| 95th–99th centiles | 3.7 | 1.3 | 2.5 | 93 |
| 3.5–4.4 mm | 21.1 | 2.7 | 10.0 | 70 |
| 4.5–5.4 mm | 33.3 | 3.4 | 18.5 | 50 |
| 5.5–6.4 mm | 50.5 | 10.1 | 24.2 | 30 |
| ≥6.5 mm | 64.5 | 19.0 | 46.2 | 15 |

$^a$Estimated prevalence of delivery of a healthy baby with no major abnormalities.

cytomegalovirus, and parvovirus B19. Follow-up scans to define the evolution of the edema should be carried out every 4 weeks. Additionally, consideration should be given to DNA testing for certain genetic conditions, such as spinal muscular atrophy, even if there is no family history for these conditions. In pregnancies with unexplained nuchal edema at 20 to 22 weeks scan, the parents should be counseled that there is up to a 10% risk of evolution to hydrops and perinatal death or a live birth with a genetic syndrome, such as Noonan syndrome. The risk of neurodevelopmental delay is estimated at 3% to 5%.

## Additional Ultrasound Markers

At 11 to 13 weeks absence of the fetal nasal bone, reversed a-wave in the ductus venosus, tricuspid regurgitation, and increased peak systolic velocity (PSV) in the hepatic artery are observed in about 60%, 66%, 55%, and 80% of fetuses with trisomy 21 and in 2.5%, 3.0%, 1.0%, and 5%, respectively, of euploid fetuses.[25–34]

### Absent or Hypoplastic Nasal Bone

In the assessment of the nasal bone at 11 to 13 weeks scan, a midsagittal view of the fetal profile should be obtained, and the magnification of the image should be such that the head and upper thorax occupy the whole screen. The ultrasound transducer should be parallel to the direction of the nose, and the probe must be gently tilted from one side to the other of the fetal nose. The exact midsagittal plane of the fetal face is defined by the echogenic tip of the nose and rectangular shape of the palate anteriorly, the translucent diencephalon in the center, and the nuchal membrane posteriorly.

When these criteria are satisfied, it will be possible to visualize at the level of the fetal nose three distinct lines. Two of them, proximal to the forehead, will be horizontal and parallel to each other, resembling an "equal sign." The top line represents the skin and the bottom one, usually thicker and more echogenic than the overlying skin, represents the nasal bone (see Fig. 8.1). The nasal bone is considered to be present if it is more echogenic than the overlying skin and absent if it is either not visible or its echogenicity is the same or less than that of the skin.

### Abnormal Flow Across the Ductus Venosus

The ductus venosus is a short vessel connecting the umbilical vein to the inferior vena cava that plays a critical role in preferentially shunting oxygenated blood to the fetal brain. About 20% of oxygenated blood from the placenta bypasses the liver and is directed to the heart. It enters the right atrium and then is shunted across the foramen ovale into the left atrium. From the left atrium, the blood passes into the left ventricle and then the aorta. The ductus venosus usually closes within a few minutes after birth but this may take longer in preterm neonates.

Increased impedance to flow in the fetal ductus venosus at 11 to 13 weeks' gestation is associated fetal aneuploidies, cardiac defects, and other adverse pregnancy outcomes.[29,35–39] Blood flow in the ductus venosus has a characteristic waveform with high velocity during ventricular systole (S-wave) and diastole (D-wave) and forward flow during atrial contraction (a-wave). Most studies examining ductus venosus flow have classified the waveforms as normal, when the a-wave observed during atrial contraction is positive, or abnormal, when the a-wave is absent or reversed. The preferred alternative in the estimation of patient-specific risks for pregnancy complications is measurement of the pulsatility index for veins (PIV) as a continuous variable.[40]

In the assessment of ductus venosus flow, a right ventral midsagittal view of the fetal trunk should be obtained and the magnification of the image should be such that the fetal thorax and abdomen occupy the whole screen (Fig. 8.2). The examinations should be undertaken during fetal quiescence and color flow mapping must be used to demonstrate the umbilical vein, ductus venosus, and fetal heart. The pulsed Doppler sample should be small (0.5 to 1.0 mm) to avoid contamination from the adjacent veins and it must be placed in the yellowish aliasing area, the insonation angle should be less than 30°, the filter should be set at a low frequency (50 to 70 Hz) to allow visualization of the whole waveform and the sweep speed should be high (2 to 3 cm per second) so that the waveforms were widely spread. The ductus venosus PIV is measured by the machine after manual tracing of the outline of the waveform.

### Tricuspid Regurgitation

Tricuspid regurgitation at 11 to 13 weeks' gestation is a common finding in fetal aneuploidies and major cardiac defects.[30–32,41]

In the assessment of tricuspid flow, an apical four-chamber view of the fetal heart should be obtained and the magnification of the image should be such that the fetal thorax occupies the whole screen. The pulsed Doppler sample should be large (2.0 to 3.0 mm) and positioned across the tricuspid valve, the

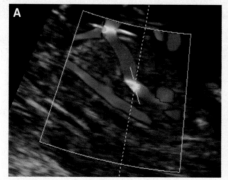
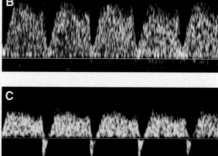

**FIGURE 8.2:** Midsagittal view of the fetal trunk demonstrating insonation of the ductus venosus **(A)** of a fetus at 12 weeks with normal waveform **(B)** and reversed a-wave **(C)**.

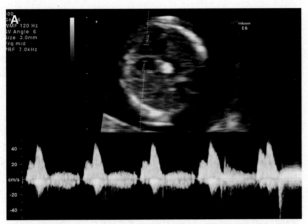 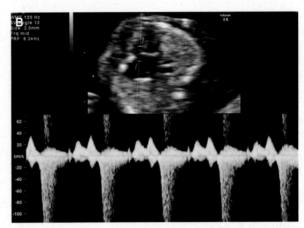

**FIGURE 8.3:** Transverse view of the fetal heart demonstrating Doppler assessment of flow across the tricuspid valve of a fetus at 12 weeks with normal waveform **(A)** and tricuspid regurgitation **(B)**.

insonation angle to the direction of flow should be less than 30° from the direction of the interventricular septum, and the sweep speed should be high (2 to 3 cm per second) so that the waveforms are widely spread (Fig. 8.3). The tricuspid valve could be insufficient in one or more of its three cusps, and therefore the sample volume should be placed across the valve at least three times, in an attempt to interrogate the complete valve. Tricuspid regurgitation is diagnosed, if it is found during at least half of the systole and with a velocity of over 60 cm per second, since aortic or pulmonary arterial blood flow at this gestation can produce a maximum velocity of 50 cm per second.

### Increased Blood Velocity in the Hepatic Artery

In fetal life, the liver is a vital organ with both metabolic and hemopoietic activities. Normally, more than 90% of the blood supply to the liver is from the umbilical and portal veins and less than 10% comes directly from the hepatic artery that is a branch of the celiac trunk from the descending aorta. In trisomy 21 fetuses at 11 to 13 weeks' gestation, the fetal hepatic artery PSV is increased and the PI is decreased.[33,34]

In the assessment of hepatic artery flow, a right ventral midsagittal view of the fetal trunk should be obtained and the magnification of the image should be such that the fetal thorax and abdomen occupy the whole screen. The examinations should be undertaken during fetal quiescence and color flow mapping should be used to demonstrate the umbilical vein, ductus venosus, descending aorta, and hepatic artery (Fig. 8.4). The pulsed Doppler sample must be set at 2.0 mm and placed so that it includes both the ductus venosus and the adjacent upper part of the hepatic artery (to ensure that this vessel rather than the celiac trunk is sampled) and it should then be reduced to 1.0 mm to include only the hepatic artery. The insonation angle to the hepatic artery must be less than 30°, the filter should be set at a high frequency (120 Hz) to avoid contamination from adjacent veins, the sweep speed should be high (2 to 3 cm per second) so that the waveforms are widely spread, and the pulsed wave pulse repetition frequency should be adjusted allowing better assessment of the PSV. When three similar consecutive waveforms are obtained, the PSV and PI are measured by the software of the machine after manual tracing.

### Clinical Implementation

In first trimester combined screening, each of the additional ultrasound markers can be assessed in all patients resulting in an increase in DR from 93% to 96% and a decrease in FPR

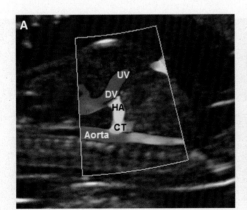 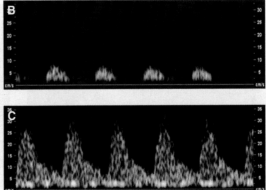

**FIGURE 8.4: A:** Right ventral midsagittal view of a fetus at 12 weeks demonstrating the umbilical vein (UV), ductus venosus (DV), descending aorta, hepatic artery (HA), and celiac trunk (CT). The peak systolic velocity in the waveform from the fetus with trisomy 21 **(C)** is much higher than in a euploid fetus **(B)**.

to less than 3%. A similar performance of screening can be achieved by a contingent policy in which first-stage screening by maternal age, fetal NT, and serum-free β-hCG and PAPP-A is offered to all cases (Fig. 8.5).[42] Patients with a risk of 1 in 50 or more are considered to be screen positive and those with a risk of less than 1 in 1,000 are screen negative. Patients with the intermediate risk of 1 in 51 to 1 in 1,000, which constitutes 15% to 20% of the total population, have second-stage screening with nasal bone, ductus venosus, or tricuspid blood flow that modifies their first-stage risk. If the adjusted risk is 1 in 100 or more, the patients are considered to be screen positive and those with a risk of less than 1 in 100 is screen negative.

## Screening in Twins

The first step in screening for trisomies in twins is to determine chorionicity by ultrasound at 11 to 13 weeks (Fig. 8.6).[43] In monochorionic twins, the average of the two NT measurements

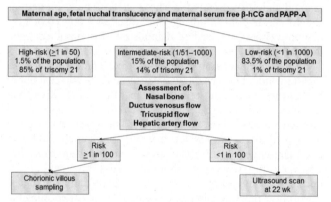

**FIGURE 8.5:** Two-stage screening for fetal aneuploidies. In the first stage, all patients have screening by a combination of maternal age, fetal nuchal translucency thickness, and maternal serum-free β-hCH and PAPP-A, and according to the results they are classified into high-risk, intermediate-risk, and low-risk groups. In the intermediate-risk group, second-stage screening is carried out by one or more sonographic markers, including nasal bone, blood flow in the ductus venosus, hepatic artery, or across the tricuspid valve, and on the basis of the results they are then classified as high-risk or low-risk groups.

can be used to calculate the pregnancy risk and in dichorionic twins, the individual NT measurements can be used to calculate the fetus-specific risk.[44,45] Measurement of serum-free β-hCG and PAPP-A is also useful in screening for trisomies in twins, but it is important to make the necessary adjustments because the levels change with gestation and they are lower in monochorionic than in dichorionic pregnancies.[46–48]

In twins, the DR of trisomy 21 by the combined test is about 90% but at a higher FPR than in singletons (6% vs. 5%).[44] In monochorionic twins, the FPR is even higher, at about 9%, because increased NT in one of the fetuses may be an early sign of twin-to-twin transfusion syndrome, rather than trisomy.[44]

## Clinical Implementation of Cell-Free DNA Testing in Maternal Blood

The performance of screening for trisomies 21, 18, and 13 by cfDNA analysis of maternal blood is superior to that of the combined test.[11] However, the test is expensive, and it is therefore unlikely that it would be used for routine screening of the whole population. We have suggested that the best model of screening is to offer cfDNA testing contingent on the results of first-line screening by the combined test.[7,49] On the basis of the combined test, the population is divided into a very high-risk group, an intermediate-risk group, and a low-risk group. In this model, it is proposed that firstly, invasive testing is carried out in all cases in the very high-risk group, and secondly, cfDNA testing is carried out in the intermediate-risk group followed by invasive testing for those with a screen positive result (Fig. 8.7).

Such strategy would retain the advantages of the first trimester scan in the diagnosis of major defects and assessment of risk for pregnancy complications and would detect about 98% of fetuses with trisomies 21, 18, and 13, at an overall invasive testing rate of less than 1%. The intermediate-risk group requiring cfDNA testing constitutes about 25% of the population. However, this proportion can be reduced to about 10%, without affecting the overall performance of screening, by a first-line method of screening that includes measurement of ductus venosus PIV, in addition to fetal NT, FHR, and serum-free β-hCG, PAPP-A, PLGF, and AFP.[49]

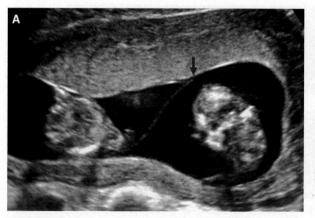

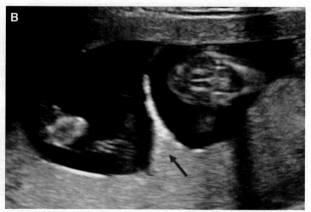

**FIGURE 8.6:** Ultrasound picture illustrating the difference in the junction of the intertwin membrane (shown by the *red arrow*) with the placenta in monochorionic **(A)** and dichorionic twins **(B)** at 12 weeks' gestation.

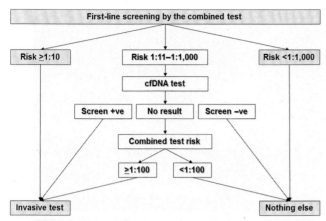

**FIGURE 8.7:** First-line screening by the combined test is carried out in all pregnancies. In those with a risk for trisomies 21, 18, or 13 ≥1:10, invasive testing is performed, and in those with a risk <1:1,000, there is no further testing. In women with risk between 1:11 and 1:1,000 cell-free (cf) DNA testing is carried out. In those with a positive cfDNA result, invasive testing is performed, and in those with a negative result, there is no further testing. In the group of women with no result from cfDNA testing, the results of the combined test are considered, and invasive testing is carried out for those with a risk for trisomy 21, 18, or 13 ≥1:100.

## DIAGNOSIS OF MAJOR FETAL DEFECTS

The 11 to 13 weeks scan evolved over the last 20 years from essentially a scan for the measurement of fetal NT and CRL to one that includes a basic checklist for examination of the fetal anatomy with the intention of diagnosing major abnormalities, which are either lethal or associated with severe handicap, so that the parents can have the option of earlier and safer pregnancy termination.

Major fetal abnormalities fall into essentially three groups in relation to whether they can be detected at the 11 to 13 weeks scan.[50] Firstly, relatively easily detectable abnormalities, including body stalk anomaly, anencephaly, alobar holoprosencephaly, omphalocele, gastroschisis, and megacystis. The second category is anomalies not detectable in the first trimester, because they manifest only during the second or third trimester of pregnancy, including microcephaly, agenesis of the corpus callosum, semilobar holoprosencephaly, hypoplasia of the cerebellum or vermis, congenital pulmonary airway malformation, and bowel obstruction. A third group includes abnormalities that are potentially detectable in the first trimester, but whose diagnosis is significantly dependent on the objectives set for such a scan and consequently the time allocated for the fetal examination, the expertise of the sonographer, the quality of the equipment used and maternal body habitus, and secondly, the presence of an easily detectable marker for an underlying abnormality. A good example of such a marker in the first trimester is high NT that is found in some fetuses with lethal skeletal dysplasias, diaphragmatic hernia, and major cardiac defects.

Several studies reported the diagnosis of a wide range of fetal abnormalities during the first trimester scan. A randomized study of 35,792 pregnancies where a routine anomaly scan was carried out at 12 or 18 weeks using a checklist (skull, neck and brain, face, chest, heart, diaphragm, abdominal wall, stomach, kidneys, bladder, spine, and limbs), reported that the rate of

prenatal detection of major abnormalities was not significantly different between the two groups (38% vs. 47%).[51] In our center, we conducted a prospective study on first trimester screening for aneuploidies that included a basic examination of the fetal anatomy in 45,191 pregnancies; the findings were compared with those at 20 to 23 weeks and with the postnatal examination.[50] Chromosomally abnormal cases were excluded from the analysis. Fetal abnormalities were observed in 488 (1.1%) cases and 213 (43.6%) of these were detected at 11 to 13 weeks. The early scan detected all cases of acrania, alobar holoprosencephaly, exomphalos, gastroschisis, megacystis, and body stalk anomaly, 77% of absent hand or foot, 50% of diaphragmatic hernia, 50% of lethal skeletal dysplasias, 60% of polydactyly, 34% of major cardiac defects, 5% of facial clefts, and 14% of open neural tube defects.

## Suggested Protocol for First Trimester Anomaly Scan

The ultrasound examination can be performed transabdominally, using 3 to 7.5 MHz curvilinear transducers, but in about 1% of cases when there are technical difficulties to obtain adequate views, a transvaginal scan (3 to 9 MHz) should also be carried out. The time allocated for the ultrasound examination of the fetus should be about 20 minutes. It should be aimed to obtain a transverse section of the head to demonstrate the skull, midline echo, and the choroid plexuses, a midsagittal view of the face to demonstrate the nasal bone, sagittal section of the spine to demonstrate kyphoscoliosis, a transverse section of the thorax to demonstrate the four-chamber view of the heart and record blood flow across the tricuspid valve, transverse and sagittal sections of the trunk, and extremities to demonstrate the stomach, bladder, and abdominal insertion of the umbilical cord, all the long bones, hands, and feet.

### Acrania and Anencephaly

The ossification of the skull and the development of the two cerebral hemispheres are usually evident at 11 weeks. In the absence of the cranial vault (acrania), the hemispheres of the brain are still recognizable. Subsequently, there is degeneration of the brain leading to exencephaly and later anencephaly. The diagnosis of anencephaly during the second trimester of pregnancy is based on the demonstration of absent cranial vault and cerebral hemispheres. In 11 to 13 weeks scan, the pathognomonic feature of anencephaly is acrania with the brain appearing either normal or at varying degrees of distortion and disruption (Fig. 8.8).[52]

### Holoprosencephaly

Holoprosencephaly, with a birth prevalence of about 1 in 10,000, is characterized by a spectrum of cerebral abnormalities resulting from incomplete cleavage of the forebrain. At 11 weeks, it is already possible to clearly visualize falx cerebri and the butterfly appearance of the cerebral hemispheres, mainly represented by the two bulky choroid plexus of the lateral ventricles (Fig. 8.9). In the standard transverse view of the fetal head, alobar and semilobar holoprosencephaly are characterized by a single

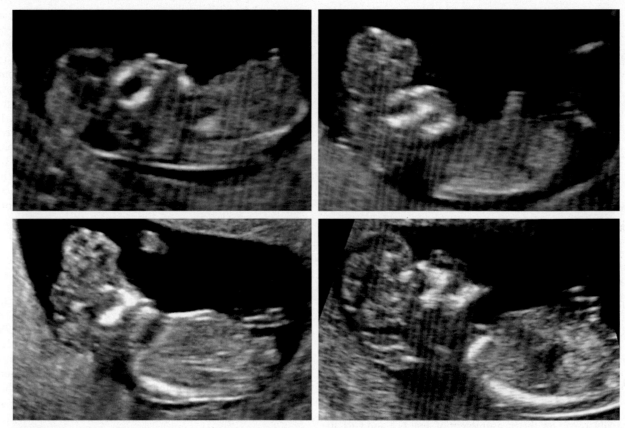

**FIGURE 8.8:** Acrania with varying degrees of distortion and disruption of the brain at 11 to 13 weeks' gestation.

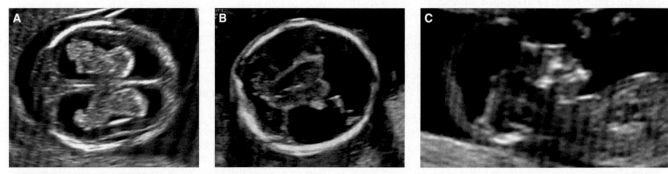

**FIGURE 8.9:** Cross-sectional view of the fetal brain at 12 weeks demonstrating the normal butterfly appearance of the lateral ventricles with the choroid plexuses **(A)** and alobar holoprosencephaly with fusion of the anterior horns of the lateral ventricles **(B)**. **C:** Sagittal view of the fetal brain demonstrating alobar holoprosencephaly.

dilated midline ventricle replacing the two lateral ventricles (fusion of the anterior horns of the lateral ventricles) or partial segmentation of the ventricles and the absence of the butterfly sign.[53] The alobar and semilobar types are often associated with facial defects, such as hypotelorism or cyclopia, facial cleft, and nasal hypoplasia or proboscis. In about 65% of cases diagnosed in the first trimester, there is an underlying aneuploidy, mainly trisomy 13.[54]

## Open Neural Tube Defects

In almost all cases of open neural tube defects, there is an associated Arnold–Chiari malformation. In the second trimester of pregnancy, the manifestations of the Arnold–Chiari malformation are the lemon and banana signs by ultrasound.[55]

It has recently been realized that in open neural tube defects caudal displacement of the brain can be apparent at 11 to 13 weeks in the same midsagittal view of the fetal face as for measurement of fetal NT and assessment of the nasal bone.[56,57] In this view, the lower part of the fetal brain between the sphenoid bone anteriorly and the occipital bone posteriorly can be divided into the brain stem in the front and a combination of the fourth ventricle and cistern magna in the back (Fig. 8.10). In fetuses with open neural tube defects, the brain stem diameter is increased and the diameter of the fourth ventricle–cisterna magna complex is decreased.

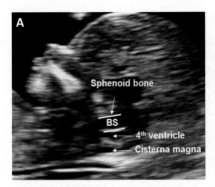
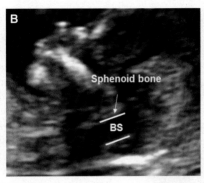

**FIGURE 8.10:** Midsagittal view of the fetal brain in a normal **(A)** and a spina bifida **(B)** fetus at 12 weeks demonstrating the measurement of brain stem *(BS)* diameter. In open spina bifida, the brain stem diameter is increased.

## Major Cardiac Defects

Abnormalities of the heart and great arteries are the most common congenital defects and they account for about 20% of all stillbirths and 30% of neonatal deaths because of congenital defects.[58] Although most major cardiac defects are amenable to prenatal diagnosis by specialist fetal echocardiography, routine ultrasound screening in pregnancy fails to identify the majority of affected fetuses.[59–61] Consequently, effective population-based prenatal diagnosis necessitates improved methods of identifying the high-risk group for referral to specialists.

The traditional method of screening for cardiac defects, which relies on family history of cardiac defects, maternal history of diabetes mellitus, and maternal exposure to teratogens, identifies only about 10% of affected fetuses.[62]

A major improvement in screening for cardiac defects came with the realization that the risk for cardiac defects increases with fetal NT thickness and is also increased in those with abnormal flow in the ductus venosus and across the tricuspid valve.[22,24,36,63–66] Reversed a-wave in the ductus venosus or tricuspid regurgitation, observed in about 2% and 1%, respectively of normal fetuses, is found in 30% of affected fetuses. Specialist fetal echocardiography for cases with NT above the 99th centile and those with reversed a-wave in the ductus venosus or tricuspid regurgitation, irrespective of NT, would require cardiac scanning in about 4% of the population and would detect about 50% of major cardiac defects.

Patients identified by first trimester screening as being at high risk for cardiac defects need not wait until 20 weeks for specialist echocardiography. First trimester fetal echocardiography is technically more difficult than at 20 weeks, because the heart is much smaller and the fetus is usually more mobile. However, it is still possible to demonstrate the four-chamber view, outflow tracts, arterial duct, and aortic arch (Fig. 8.11). The overall success rate in the assessment of the fetal heart is about 45% at 11 weeks and 90% at 13 weeks.[67] In many cases, a scan as early as at 13 weeks' gestation can effectively reassure the parents that there is no suggestion of a major cardiac defect. Similarly, in many cases with a major cardiac defect, the early scan can raise a suspicion that a defect is present, and often leads to the correct diagnosis even at this gestational age. However, an echocardiogram done later in gestation is still important, especially in those cases where the fetal heart appears to be normal during the early evaluation.

## Diaphragmatic Hernia

This is a sporadic defect with a birth prevalence of about 1 in 4,000. In up to 30% of affected fetuses, there are associated chromosomal abnormalities, mainly trisomy 18, or other anomalies. Increased NT thickness is present in about 40% of fetuses with diaphragmatic hernia, including more than 80% of those that result in neonatal death owing to pulmonary hypoplasia and in about 20% of the survivors (Fig. 8.12).[68] It is possible that in fetuses with diaphragmatic hernia and increased NT, the intrathoracic herniation of the abdominal viscera occurs in the first trimester and prolonged compression of the lungs causes pulmonary hypoplasia. In the cases where diaphragmatic hernia is associated with a good prognosis, the intrathoracic herniation of viscera may be delayed until the second or third trimesters of pregnancy.

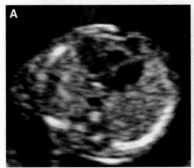
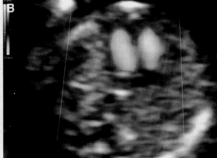
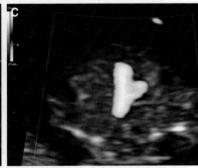

**FIGURE 8.11:** Four-chamber view of the fetal heart at 12 weeks' gestation **(A)**, color flow imaging of an apical four-chamber view demonstrating equal diastolic flows from right and left atrium into right and left ventricle **(B)**, and color flow imaging showing the V-sign formed by the ductal arch and aortic arch **(C)**.

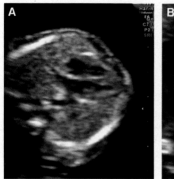
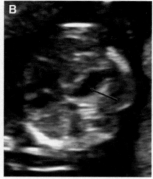

**FIGURE 8.12:** Cross-sectional view of the fetal thorax illustrating the normal position of the heart and lungs **(A)**, and intrathoracic herniation of the stomach (*arrow* in **B**) in a case of diaphragmatic hernia.

## Ventral Wall Defects

Prenatal diagnosis of omphalocele by ultrasound is based on the demonstration of the midline anterior abdominal wall defect, the herniated sac with its visceral contents, and the umbilical cord insertion at the apex of the sac (Fig. 8.13). At 8 to 10 weeks of gestation, all fetuses demonstrate herniation of the midgut that is visualized as a hyperechogenic mass in the base of the umbilical cord. Retraction into the abdominal cavity is normally completed by 12 weeks. At 11 to 13 weeks, exomphalos is observed in about 1:1,000 fetuses, and in 55% of cases there is an associated chromosomal abnormality, usually trisomy 18.[54] Omphalocele containing liver is an irreversible anatomical defect, whereas exomphalos containing only bowel can be a transient abnormality. If the fetal karyotype is found to be normal, the condition is likely to resolve spontaneously.

## Gastroschisis

This is a sporadic defect with a birth prevalence of about 1 in 4,000. It is rarely associated with chromosomal abnormalities. Evisceration of the intestine occurs through a small abdominal wall defect located just to the right of an intact umbilical cord, and the loops of intestine lie uncovered in the amniotic fluid (Fig. 8.14). The condition persists throughout pregnancy. Prenatal diagnosis by ultrasound is based on the demonstration of the normally situated umbilicus and the herniated loops of intestine, which are free floating.

## Megacystis

The fetal bladder can be visualized by sonography in about 95% of fetuses at 11 weeks of gestation and in all cases by 13 weeks. At this gestation, the fetal bladder length is normally less than 7 mm. Fetal megacystis in the first trimester, defined by a longitudinal bladder diameter 7 mm or more, is found in about 1 in 1,500 pregnancies. The condition is associated with chromosomal defects, mainly trisomies 13 and 18, which are found in about 30% of fetuses (Fig. 8.15).[54,69,70] In chromosomally normal fetuses, mild megacystis usually resolves spontaneously, but in those with bladder diameter greater than 15 mm, there is progression to severe obstructive uropathy. The presence of smooth muscle in the bladder and autonomic innervation occur only after 13 weeks, and before this gestation the bladder wall consists of epithelium and connective tissue with no contractile elements. It is therefore likely that in the majority of fetuses with mild megacystis, there is no underlying urethral obstruction but a temporary malfunction of the bladder.

## Skeletal Dysplasias

In the first trimester, it is possible to evaluate the presence of the three segments of the limbs (rhizomelic, mesomelic, and acromelic) and their movements and, therefore, to raise the suspicion of polydactyly, clenched hands, clubfoot, and some of the most severe dysplasias such as thanatophoric dysplasia, osteogenesis imperfecta, achondroplasia, achondrogenesis, and asphyxiating thoracic dystrophy. Many severe skeletal defects that can be diagnosed in the first trimester of pregnancy are usually associated with increased NT thickness. The cause of increased NT in some of the skeletal dysplasias may be venous congestion in the head and neck due to superior mediastinal compression by the narrow chest. An additional or alternative mechanism for the increased NT may be the altered composition of the extracellular matrix found in association with some of the skeletal dysplasias, such as osteogenesis imperfecta.

## Body Stalk Anomaly

This lethal sporadic anomaly has a birth prevalence of 1 in 15,000. The ultrasound features include major abdominal wall defect, severe kyphoscoliosis, and short umbilical cord with a single artery.[71] Half of the fetal body is seen in the amniotic

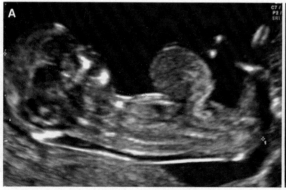
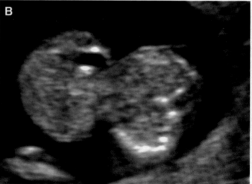

**FIGURE 8.13:** Sagittal **(A)** and transverse **(B)** views of the fetal abdomen at the level of the umbilicus illustrating cases of exomphalos containing liver at 12 weeks' gestation.

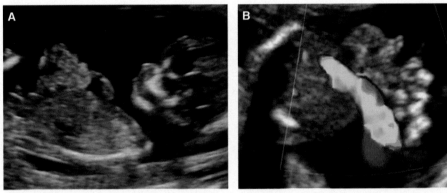

**FIGURE 8.14:** Sagittal **(A)** and transverse **(B)** views of the fetal abdomen at the level of the umbilicus illustrating cases of gastroschisis at 12 weeks' gestation.

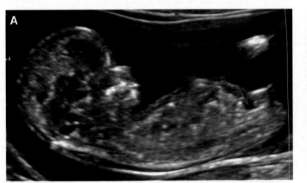
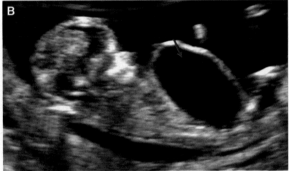

**FIGURE 8.15:** Midsagittal illustrating a normal bladder (*arrow*) in a fetus at 12 weeks gestation **(A)** and one with megacystis (*arrow*) **(B)**.

cavity and the other half in the celomic cavity, suggesting that early amnion rupture before obliteration of the celomic cavity is a possible cause of the syndrome (Fig. 8.16). A defect of somatic clefting is also a plausible contributing factor.[72] The fetal NT is increased in about 85% of the cases, but the karyotype is usually normal.

## ASSESSMENT OF RISK FOR PREGNANCY COMPLICATIONS

The current approach to prenatal care, which involves office visits at 16, 24, 28, 30, 32, 34, and 36 weeks and then weekly until delivery, was established 80 years ago.[73,74] The high concentration of visits in the third trimester implies that, firstly, most complications occur at this late stage of pregnancy and, secondly, that most major adverse outcomes are unpredictable during the first or even the second trimester.

In the last 20 years, it has become apparent that an integrated first hospital visit at 11 to 13 weeks combining data from maternal characteristics and history with findings of biophysical and biochemical tests can define the patient-specific risk for a wide spectrum of pregnancy complications, including miscarriage and stillbirth, preeclampsia, preterm birth, gestational diabetes, fetal growth restriction, and macrosomia.[75] Early estimation of patient-specific risks for these pregnancy complications would improve pregnancy outcome by shifting prenatal care from a

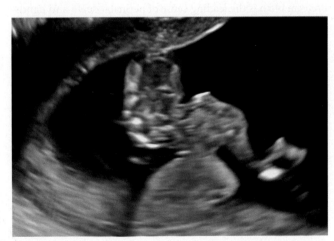

**FIGURE 8.16:** Fetus with body stalk anomaly at 12 weeks' gestation.

series of routine visits to a more individualized patient- and disease-specific approach in terms of both the schedule and the content of such visits. Each visit would have a predefined objective, and the findings will generate likelihood ratios that can be used to estimate the individual patient- and disease-specific estimated risk from the initial assessment at 11 to 13 weeks.

At 11 to 13 weeks, the great majority of women would be classified as being at low risk for pregnancy complications, and a small proportion of women would be selected as being at high risk (see Fig. 8.2). In the low-risk group, the number of routine indicated medical visits could potentially be reduced to as low as three. A subsequent visit at 20 to 22 weeks would reevaluate fetal anatomy and growth and reassess risk for such complications as preeclampsia and preterm delivery. Another visit during the third trimester will assess maternal and fetal well-being and determine the best time and method of delivery. The high-risk group can have close surveillance in specialist clinics in terms of both the investigations to be performed and the personnel involved in the provision of care. In each of these visits, their risk will be reassessed and they will either remain high-risk status or they will revert to low-risk status, in which case the intensity of their care can be reduced.

Future research will inevitably expand the number of conditions that can be identified in early pregnancy and define genetic markers of disease that will improve the accuracy of the a priori risk based on maternal characteristics and medical history. Similarly, new biophysical and biochemical markers will be described that may replace some of the current ones and modify the value of others. With the passage of time, it will become necessary to reevaluate and improve the timing and content of each visit and the likelihood ratios for each test. Early identification of high-risk groups will also stimulate further research that will define the best protocol for their follow-up and development of strategies for the prevention of disorders of pregnancy or mitigation of their adverse consequences. It is likely that the new challenge for improvement of pregnancy outcome will be met by inverting the pyramid of antenatal care (Fig. 8.17) to introduce on a large scale and in a systematic fashion a new model of antenatal care that will be based on the results of a comprehensive assessment at 11 to 13 weeks.[75]

## Preterm Birth

Preterm birth is the leading cause of perinatal death and handicap in children, and the vast majority of mortality and morbidity relates to early delivery before 34 weeks, which occurs in about 2% of singleton pregnancies. In two-thirds of the cases, this is due to spontaneous onset of labor or preterm prelabor rupture of membranes, and in the other one-third, it is iatrogenic, mainly because of preeclampsia.[76]

The patient-specific risk for spontaneous delivery before 34 weeks can be determined at 11 to 13 weeks by an algorithm combining maternal characteristics and obstetric history with the sonographic measurement of cervical length.[77,78] In the

measurement of cervical length, it is important to distinguish between the true cervix, characterized by the presence of the endocervical canal, which is bordered by the endocervical mucosa, which is usually of decreased echogenicity compared with the surrounding tissues, and the isthmus (Fig. 8.18).

Effective early identification of the high-risk group for subsequent spontaneous early delivery could potentially improve outcome by directing such patients to specialist clinics for regular monitoring of cervical length, and stimulating research for identification of potentially useful biomarkers and the investigation of the potential role of earlier intervention with such measures as prophylactic use of progesterone or cervical cerclage.

## Preeclampsia

Preeclampsia is a major cause of maternal and perinatal morbidity and mortality. Both the degree of impaired placentation and the incidence of adverse fetal and maternal short-term and long-term consequences are inversely related to the gestational age at onset of the disease. Consequently, in screening for preeclampsia, the condition should be subdivided according to gestational age at delivery.

Algorithms that combine maternal characteristics, mean arterial pressure, uterine artery PI, and maternal serum biochemical tests at 11 to 13 weeks could potentially identify about 90%, 80%, and 60% of pregnancies that subsequently develop early (before 34 weeks), intermediate (34 to 37 weeks), and late (after 37 weeks) preeclampsia, for a FPR of 5%.[79,80] Further investigations will determine whether in the high-risk group pharmacological interventions, such as low-dose aspirin, starting from the first trimester could improve placentation and reduce the prevalence of the disease.[81,82]

In the measurement of the uterine artery pulsatility index (PI) at 11 to 13 weeks' gestation, a sagittal section of the uterus should be obtained, and the cervical canal and internal cervical os identified. The transducer should be gently tilted from side to side, and color flow mapping should be used to identify each uterine artery along the side of the cervix and uterus at the level of the internal os (Fig. 8.19). Pulsed wave Doppler should be used with the sampling gate set at 2 mm to cover the whole vessel, and care should be taken to ensure that the angle of insonation is less than 30° When three similar consecutive waveforms are obtained, the uterine artery PI should be measured and the mean PI of the left and right arteries calculated.

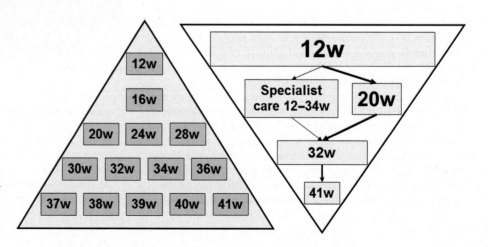

**FIGURE 8.17:** Pyramid of gestational ages according to the traditional model of prenatal care established in the 1920s **(left)** and according to the proposed new model of inverted pyramid **(right)**.

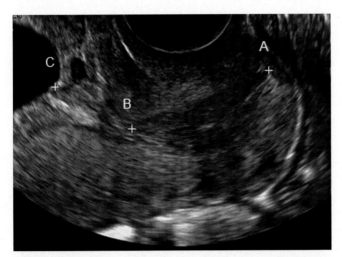

**FIGURE 8.18:** Ultrasound picture illustrating the measurement of the length of the endocervix (*A* to *B*) and the isthmus (*B* to *C*).

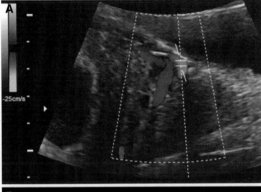

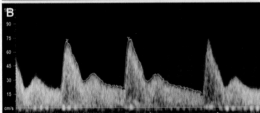

**FIGURE 8.19:** Parasagittal view of the cervix with color flow imaging to illustrate the uterine arteries **(A)** and characteristic waveform at 12 weeks' gestation **(B)**.

In conclusion, the first trimester scan has evolved recently into one of the milestones of prenatal care. As shown in this chapter, the aims of the 11 to 13 + 6 weeks scan include not only the confirmation of the viability of the pregnancy and the accurate dating of the gestation based on the CRL measurement but, especially screening for aneuploidies and various pregnancy's complications, early diagnosis of major fetal abnormalities, and the detection of multiple pregnancies with reliable identification of chorionicity.

## REFERENCES

1. Tabor A, Alfirevic Z. Update on procedure-related risks for prenatal diagnosis techniques. *Fetal Diagn Ther.* 2010;27:1–7.
2. Nicolaides KH. Screening for fetal aneuploidies at 11 to 13 weeks. *Prenat Diagn.* 2011;31:7–15.
3. Snijders RJM, Holzgreve W, Cuckle H, et al. Maternal age-specific risks for trisomies at 9–14 weeks' gestation. *Prenat Diagn.* 1994;14:543–552.
4. Snijders RJM, Sebire NJ, Nicolaides KH. Maternal age and gestational age-specific risks for chromosomal defects. *Fetal Diagn Ther.* 1995;10:356–367.
5. Kagan KO, Wright D, Valencia C, et al. Screening for trisomies 21, 18 and 13 by maternal age, fetal nuchal translucency, fetal heart rate, free beta-hCG and pregnancy-associated plasma protein-A. *Hum Reprod.* 2008;23:1968–1975.
6. Wright D, Syngelaki A, Bradbury I, et al. First trimester screening for trisomies 21, 18 and 13 by ultrasound and biochemical testing. *Fetal Diagn Ther.* 2014;35(2):118–126.
7. Syngelaki A, Pergament E, Homfray T, et al. Replacing the combined test by cell-free DNA testing in screening for trisomies 21, 18 and 13: impact on the diagnosis of other aneuploidies. *Fetal Diagn Ther.* 2014;Feb 8. [Epub ahead of print]
8. Kagan KO, Anderson JM, Anwandter G, et al. Screening for triploidy by the risk algorithms for trisomies 21, 18 and 13 at 11 weeks to 13 weeks and 6 days of gestation. *Prenat Diagn.* 2008;28:1209–1213.
9. Sebire NJ, Snijders RJ, Brown R, et al. Detection of sex chromosome abnormalities by nuchal translucency screening at 10–14 weeks. *Prenat Diagn.* 1998;18:581–584.
10. Spencer K, Tul N, Nicolaides KH. Maternal serum free beta-hCG and PAPP-A in fetal sex chromosome defects in the first trimester. *Prenat Diagn.* 2000;20:390–394.
11. Gil MM, Akolekar R, Quezada MS, et al. Analysis of cell-free DNA in maternal blood in screening for aneuploidies: meta analysis. *Fetal Diagn Ther.* 2014;Feb 8. [Epub ahead of print]
12. Nicolaides KH, Syngelaki A, Gil MM, et al. Prenatal diagnosis of triploidy from cell-free DNA testing in maternal blood. *Fetal Diagn Ther.* 2013;Oct 10. [Epub ahead of print]
13. Guex N, Iseli C, Syngelaki A, et al. A robust 2nd generation genome-wide test for fetal aneuploidy based on shotgun sequencing cell-free DNA in maternal blood. *Prenat Diagn.* 2013;33:707–710.
14. Srinivasan A, Bianchi DW, Huang H, et al. Noninvasive detection of fetal sub-chromosome abnormalities via deep sequencing of maternal plasma. *Am J Hum Genet.* 2013;92:167–176.
15. Nicolaides KH, Azar G, Byrne D, et al. Fetal nuchal translucency: ultrasound screening for chromosomal defects in first trimester of pregnancy. *BMJ.* 1992;304:867–889.
16. Molina FS, Avgidou K, Kagan KO, et al. Cystic hygromas, nuchal edema, and nuchal translucency at 11–14 weeks of gestation. *Obstet Gynecol.* 2006; 107:678–683.
17. Snijders RJ, Noble P, Sebire N, et al; Fetal Medicine Foundation First Trimester Screening Group. UK multicentre project on assessment of risk of trisomy 21 by maternal age and fetal nuchal-translucency thickness at 10–14 weeks of gestation. *Lancet.* 1998;352:343–346.
18. Wald NJ, Rodeck C, Hackshaw AK, et al; SURUSS Research Group. First and second trimester antenatal screening for Down's syndrome: the results of the Serum, Urine and Ultrasound Screening Study (SURUSS). *Health Technol Assess.* 2003;7:1–88.
19. Malone FD, Canick JA, Ball RH, et al; for the First- and Second-Trimester Evaluation of Risk (FASTER) Research Consortium. First-trimester or second-trimester screening, or both, for Down's syndrome. *N Engl J Med.* 2005;353: 2001–2011.
20. Souka AP, Snidjers RJM, Novakov A, et al. Defects and syndromes in chromosomally normal fetuses with increased nuchal translucency thickness at 10–14 weeks of gestation. *Ultrasound Obstet Gynecol.* 1998;11:391–400.
21. Souka AP, Von Kaisenberg CS, Hyett JA, et al. Increased nuchal translucency with normal karyotype. *Am J Obstet Gynecol.* 2005;192:1005–1021.
22. Hyett J, Perdu M, Sharland G, et al. Using fetal nuchal translucency to screen for major congenital cardiac defects at 10–14 weeks of gestation: population based cohort study. *BMJ.* 1999;318:81–85.
23. Hyett J, Moscoso G, Papapanagiotou G, et al. Abnormalities of the heart and great arteries in chromosomally normal fetuses with increased nuchal translucency thickness at 11–13 weeks of gestation. *Ultrasound Obstet Gynecol.* 1996;7:245–250.
24. Atzei A, Gajewska K, Huggon IC, et al. Relationship between nuchal translucency thickness and prevalence of major cardiac defects in fetuses with normal karyotype. *Ultrasound Obstet Gynecol.* 2005;26:154–157.
25. Cicero S, Curcio P, Papageorghiou A, et al. Absence of nasal bone in fetuses with trisomy 21 at 11–14 weeks of gestation: an observational study. *Lancet.* 2001; 358:1665–1667.
26. Cicero S, Avgidou K, Rembouskos G, et al. Nasal bone in first-trimester screening for trisomy 21. *Am J Obstet Gynecol.* 2006;195:109–114.
27. Kagan KO, Cicero S, Staboulidou I, et al. Fetal nasal bone in screening for trisomies 21, 18 and 13 and Turner syndrome at 11–13 weeks of gestation. *Ultrasound Obstet Gynecol.* 2009;33:259–264.
28. Matias A, Gomes C, Flack N, et al. Screening for chromosomal abnormalities at 10–14 weeks: the role of ductus venosus blood flow. *Ultrasound Obstet Gynecol.* 1998;12:380–384.
29. Maiz N, Valencia C, Kagan KO, et al. Ductus venosus Doppler in screening for trisomies 21, 18 and 13 and Turner syndrome at 11–13 weeks of gestation. *Ultrasound Obstet Gynecol.* 2009;33:512–517.
30. Huggon IC, DeFigueiredo DB, Allan LD. Tricuspid regurgitation in the diagnosis of chromosomal anomalies in the fetus at 11–14 weeks of gestation. *Heart.* 2003;89:1071–1073.

31. Faiola S, Tsoi E, Huggon IC, et al. Likelihood ratio for trisomy 21 in fetuses with tricuspid regurgitation at the 11 to 13 + 6-week scan. *Ultrasound Obstet Gynecol.* 2005;26:22–27.

32. Kagan KO, Valencia C, Livanos P, et al. Tricuspid regurgitation in screening for trisomies 21, 18 and 13 and Turner syndrome at 11+0 to 13+6 weeks of gestation. *Ultrasound Obstet Gynecol.* 2009;33:18–22.

33. Bilardo CM, Timmerman E, Robles de Medina PG, et al. Low-resistance hepatic artery flow in first trimester fetuses: an ominous sign. *Ultrasound Obstet Gynecol.* 2011;37(4):438–43. doi:10.1002/uog.7766.

34. Zvanca M, Gielchinsky Y, Abdeljawad F, et al. Hepatic artery Doppler in trisomy 21 and euploid fetuses at 11–13 weeks. *Prenat Diagn.* 2011;31:22–27.

35. Maiz N, Nicolaides KH. Ductus venosus in the first trimester: contribution to screening of chromosomal, cardiac defects and monochorionic twin complications. *Fetal Diagn Ther.* 2010;28:65–71.

36. Matias A, Huggon I, Areias JC, et al. Cardiac defects in chromosomally normal fetuses with abnormal ductus venosus blood flow at 10–14 weeks. *Ultrasound Obstet Gynecol.* 1999;14:307–310.

37. Maiz N, Kagan KO, Milovanovic Z, et al. Learning curve for Doppler assessment of ductus venosus flow at 11 + 0 to 13 + 6 weeks. *Ultrasound Obstet Gynecol.* 2008;31:503–506.

38. Maiz N, Valencia C, Emmanuel EE, et al. Screening for adverse pregnancy outcome by ductus venosus Doppler at 11–13 + 6 weeks of gestation. *Obstet Gynecol.* 2008;112:598–605.

39. Borrell A, Borobio V, Bestwick JP, et al. Ductus venosus pulsatility index as an antenatal screening marker for Down's syndrome: use with the Combined and Integrated tests. *J Med Screen.* 2009;16:112–118.

40. Maiz N, Wright D, Ferreira AF, et al. A mixture model of ductus venosus pulsatility index in screening for aneuploidies at 11–13 weeks' gestation. *Fetal Diagn Ther.* 2012;31:221–229.

41. Falcon O, Faiola S, Huggon I, et al. Fetal tricuspid regurgitation at the 11 + 0 to 13 + 6-week scan: association with chromosomal defects and reproducibility of the method. *Ultrasound Obstet Gynecol.* 2006;27:609–612.

42. Nicolaides KH, Spencer K, Avgidou K, et al. Multicenter study of first-trimester screening for trisomy 21 in 75 821 pregnancies: results and estimation of the potential impact of individual risk-orientated two-stage first-trimester screening. *Ultrasound Obstet Gynecol.* 2005;25:221–226.

43. Sepulveda W, Sebire NJ, Hughes K, et al. The lambda sign at 10–14 weeks of gestation as a predictor of chorionicity in twin pregnancies. *Ultrasound Obstet Gynecol.* 1996;7:421–423.

44. Sebire NJ, Snijders RJ, Hughes K, et al. Screening for trisomy 21 in twin pregnancies by maternal age and fetal nuchal translucency thickness at 10–14 weeks of gestation. *Br J Obstet Gynaecol.* 1996;103:999–1003.

45. Vandecruys H, Faiola S, Auer M, et al. Screening for trisomy 21 in monochorionic twins by measurement of fetal nuchal translucency thickness. *Ultrasound Obstet Gynecol.* 2005;25:551–553.

46. Spencer K, Nicolaides KH. First trimester prenatal diagnosis of trisomy 21 in discordant twins using fetal nuchal translucency thickness and maternal serum free beta-hCG and PAPP-A. *Prenat Diagn.* 2000;20:683–684.

47. Spencer K, Nicolaides KH. Screening for trisomy 21 in twins using first trimester ultrasound and maternal serum biochemistry in a one-stop clinic: a review of three years experience. *BJOG.* 2003;110:276–280.

48. Madsen H, Ball S, Wright D, et al. A re-assessment of biochemical marker distributions in T21 affected and unaffected twin pregnancies in the first trimester. *Ultrasound Obstet Gynecol.* 2011;37:38–47.

49. Nicolaides KH, Syngelaki A, Poon LC, et al. First-trimester contingent screening for trisomies 21, 18 and 13 by biomarkers and maternal blood cell-free DNA testing. *Fetal Diagn Ther.* 2013;Oct 26. [Epub ahead of print]

50. Syngelaki A, Chelemen T, Dagklis T, et al. Challenges in the diagnosis of fetal non-chromosomal abnormalities at 11–13 weeks. *Prenat Diagn.* 2011;31:90–102.

51. Saltvedt S, Almström H, Kublickas M, et al. Detection of malformations in chromosomally normal fetuses by routine ultrasound at 12 or 18 weeks of gestation—a randomised controlled trial in 39,572 pregnancies. *BJOG.* 2006;113:664–674.

52. Johnson SP, Sebire NJ, Snijders RJM, et al. Ultrasound screening for anencephaly at 10–14 weeks of gestation. *Ultrasound Obstet Gynecol.* 1997;9:14–16.

53. Sepulveda W, Dezerega V, Be C. First-trimester sonographic diagnosis of holoprosencephaly: value of the "butterfly" sign. *J Ultrasound Med.* 2004;23:761–765.

54. Kagan KO, Staboulidou I, Syngelaki A, et al. The 11–13-week scan: diagnosis and outcome of holoprosencephaly, exomphalos and megacystis. *Ultrasound Obstet Gynecol.* 2010;36:10–14.

55. Nicolaides KH, Campbell S, Gabbe SG, et al. Ultrasound screening for spina bifida: cranial and cerebellar signs. *Lancet.* 1986;2:72–74.

56. Chaoui R, Benoit B, Mitkowska-Wozniak H, et al. Assessment of intracranial translucency (IT) in the detection of spina bifida at the 11–13-week scan. *Ultrasound Obstet Gynecol.* 2009;34:249–252.

57. Lachmann R, Chaoui R, Moratalla J, et al. Posterior brain in fetuses with spina bifida at 11–13 weeks. *Prenat Diagn.* 2011;31:103–106.

58. Office for National Statistics. *Mortality Statistics, Childhood, Infancy and Perinatal.* Newport, England: Office for National Statistics; 2007. Series DH3, 40.

59. Bull C. Current and potential impact of fetal diagnosis on prevalence and spectrum of serious congenital heart disease at term in the UK. *Lancet.* 1999;35:1242–1247.

60. Bricker L, Garcia J, Henderson J, et al. Ultrasound screening in pregnancy: a systematic review of the clinical effectiveness, cost-effectiveness and women's views. *Health Technol Assess.* 2000;4:1–193.

61. Tegnander E, Williams W, Johansen OJ, et al. Prenatal detection of heart defects in a non-selected population of 30,149 fetuses-detection rates and outcome. *Ultrasound Obstet Gynecol.* 2006;27:252–265.

62. Allan LD. Echocardiographic detection of congenital heart disease in the fetus: present and future. *Br Heart J.* 1995;74:103–106.

63. Maiz N, Plasencia W, Dagklis T, et al. Ductus venosus Doppler in fetuses with cardiac defects and increased nuchal translucency thickness. *Ultrasound Obstet Gynecol.* 2008;31:256–260.

64. Martinez JM, Comas M, Borrell A, et al. Abnormal first-trimester ductus venosus blood flow: a marker of cardiac defects in foetuses with normal karyotype and nuchal translucency. *Ultrasound Obstet Gynecol.* 2010;35:267–272.

65. Chelemen T, Syngelaki A, Maiz M, et al. Contribution of ductus venosus Doppler in first trimester screening for major cardiac defects. *Fetal Diagn Ther.* 2011;31:127–134.

66. Pereira S, Ganapathy R, Syngelaki A, et al. Contribution of fetal tricuspid regurgitation in first trimester screening for major cardiac defects. *Obstet Gynecol.* 2011;117:1384–1391.

67. Persico N, Moratalla J, Lombardi CM, et al. Fetal echocardiography at 11–13 weeks by transabdominal high frequency ultrasound. *Ultrasound Obstet Gynecol.* 2011;37:296–301.

68. Sebire NJ, Snijders RJM, Davenport M, et al. Fetal nuchal translucency thickness at 10–14 weeks of gestation and congenital diaphragmatic hernia. *Obstet Gynecol.* 1997;90:943–947.

69. Sebire NJ, von Kaisenberg C, Rubio C, et al. Fetal megacystis at 10–14 weeks of gestation. *Ultrasound Obstet Gynecol.* 1996;8:387–390.

70. Liao AW, Sebire NJ, Geerts L, et al. Megacystis at 10–14 weeks of gestation: chromosomal defects and outcome according to bladder length. *Ultrasound Obstet Gynecol.* 2003;21:338–341.

71. Daskalakis G, Sebire NJ, Jurkovic D, et al. Body stalk anomaly at 10–14 weeks of gestation. *Ultrasound Obstet Gynecol.* 1997;10:416–418.

72. Paul C, Zosmer N, Jurkovic D, et al. A case of body stalk anomaly at 10 weeks of gestation. *Ultrasound Obstet Gynecol.* 2001;17:157–159.

73. Ballantyne JW. A plea for a pro-maternity hospital. *BMJ.* 1901;2101:813–814.

74. Ministry of Health Report. *1929 Memorandum on Antenatal Clinics: Their Conduct and Scope.* London, England: His Majesty's Stationery Office; 1930.

75. Nicolaides KH. Turning the pyramid of prenatal care. *Fetal Diagn Ther.* 2011;29:183–196.

76. Celik E, To M, Gajewska K, et al; for the Fetal Medicine Foundation Second Trimester Screening Group. Cervical length and obstetric history predict spontaneous preterm birth: development and validation of a model to provide individualized risk assessment. *Ultrasound Obstet Gynecol.* 2008;31:549–554.

77. Beta J, Ventura W, Akolekar R, et al. Prediction of spontaneous preterm delivery from maternal factors and placental perfusion and function at 11–13 weeks. *Prenat Diagn.* 2011;31:75–83.

78. Greco E, Lange A, Ushakov F, et al. Prediction of spontaneous preterm delivery from endocervical length at 11–13 weeks. *Prenat Diagn.* 2011;31:84–89.

79. Akolekar R, Syngelaki A, Sarquis R, et al. Prediction of preeclampsia from biophysical and biochemical markers at 11–13 weeks. *Prenat Diagn.* 2011;31:66–74.

80. Akolekar R, Syngelaki A, Poon L, et al. Competing risks model in early screening for preeclampsia by biophysical and biochemical markers. *Fetal Diagn Ther.* 2013;33:8–15.

81. Bujold E, Roberge S, Lacasse Y, et al. Prevention of preeclampsia and intrauterine growth restriction with aspirin started in early pregnancy: a meta-analysis. *Obstet Gynecol.* 2010;116:402–414.

82. Roberge S, Villa P, Nicolaides K, et al. Early administration of low dose aspirin for the prevention of preterm and term pre-eclampsia: a systematic review and meta-analysis. *Fetal Diagn Ther.* 2012;31:141–146.

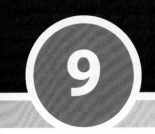

# 9

# Biochemical Screening for Neural Tube Defect and Aneuploidy Detection

Katherine R. Goetzinger • Margaret B. Menzel • Anthony O. Odibo

The use of biochemical screening in the field of obstetrics began in the 1970s with the identification of elevated levels of alpha-fetoprotein (AFP) in the amniotic fluid and maternal serum of pregnancies with fetal open neural tube defects (NTDs). Since that time, the role of biochemical screening has expanded to include multiple other maternal serum markers in both the first and the second trimesters of pregnancy, in screening not only for structural defects, but also for fetal aneuploidy, metabolic, and genetic disorders and even adverse pregnancy outcomes. This chapter will review the history of maternal biochemical serum screening, the factors that affect interpretation of these serum markers, the proposed evaluation and management of abnormal screening results, and the limitations of biochemical screening strategies. In addition, the role of ultrasound in the evaluation of abnormal serum screening results will be highlighted.

## PHYSIOLOGY OF ALPHA-FETOPROTEIN

AFP is a 70,000-Da glycoprotein with its locus on the long arm of chromosome 4. Acting as an oncofetal protein, AFP is the major serum protein produced during fetal life. Early in gestation, AFP is synthesized by the yolk sac and then later by the fetal liver. AFP enters the amniotic fluid by diffusion across fetal skin as well as by excretion into urine by the fetal kidneys.[1] The concentration of both fetal serum AFP and amniotic fluid AFP peaks toward the end of the first trimester, with fetal serum AFP peaking between 10 and 13 weeks and amniotic fluid AFP reaching peak concentration between 12 and 14 weeks. Small amounts of AFP enter maternal circulation during early gestation, likely through diffusion across the amnion and transport across the placenta. In contrast to fetal serum and amniotic fluid levels, maternal serum AFP levels continue to rise throughout gestation, reaching a peak concentration between 28 and 32 weeks and then becoming nearly undetectable at term. The concentration gradient between fetal serum and amniotic fluid is approximately 150:1 to 200:1, whereas the concentration gradient between fetal serum and maternal serum is much greater at 50,000:1.[2,3] This difference in gradient forms the basis for the use of maternal serum AFP in screening for fetal anomalies, such as open neural tube and abdominal wall defects, as only a small amount of fetal blood leakage into the amniotic fluid can lead to an exponential rise in maternal serum AFP levels.

## BIOCHEMICAL SCREENING FOR OPEN NEURAL TUBE DEFECTS

The use of AFP screening in obstetrics began in the 1970s, when Brock and Sutcliffe[4] observed that amniotic fluid AFP levels were elevated in pregnancies complicated by fetal open NTDs. They hypothesized that this elevation was due to transcapillary transudation of both cerebrospinal fluid as well as small amounts of fetal blood across the open spinal lesion and into the amniotic fluid. In the landmark United Kingdom Collaborative Study, it was demonstrated that an amniotic fluid AFP threshold of 2.5 times the multiple of the median (MoM) between 13 and 15 weeks would detect 98% of cases of anencephaly and open NTDs.[5] These findings were confirmed by other authors, yielding sensitivities ranging between 96% and 100% and specificities of greater than 99% for amniotic fluid AFP in the detection of open NTDs.[6,7] By the mid-1980s, amniotic fluid AFP as a screening test for open NTDs had been adopted into practice in the United States.

Shortly after this discovery, maternal serum AFP measurement was introduced as a screening tool for open NTDs. In 1977, Wald and colleagues[8] demonstrated that maternal serum AFP was greater than 2.5 MoMs between 16 and 18 weeks' gestation in 88% of fetuses with anencephaly and 79% with spina bifida. In 2003, the American Congress of Obstetricians & Gynecologists (ACOG) recommended that all women be offered screening for open NTDs with serum AFP in the second trimester of pregnancy.[9]

AFP levels are measured using enzyme immunoassays, and each laboratory performing this test is required to have established normal AFP reference ranges as well as undergo proficiency testing to ensure quality control. AFP levels are typically reported as MoMs of an unaffected population in order to normalize the distribution of results, accounting for interlaboratory variability and adjusting for other influential maternal factors. Today, most laboratories use thresholds of either 2.0 or 2.5 MoMs for reporting high AFP levels. Using a threshold of 2.0 MoMs, the detection rate is 95% for anencephaly and 75% to 90% for spina bifida. This results in a false positive rate (FPR) of 2% to 5%. Alternatively, when using the more stringent threshold of 2.5 MoMs, the detection rate decreases to approximately 90% for anencephaly and approximately 65% to 80% for spina bifida. However, the FPR also decreases to 1% to 3%.[6,9–11] These findings exemplify the necessary trade-off between higher detection rates at the expense of higher FPRs when defining a threshold for a screening test. Despite these promising detection rates, it is important to note that the positive predictive value (PPV) of maternal serum AFP screening is only 2% to 6%. While this PPV will increase in populations with a higher *a priori* risk of having an affected fetus, approximately 90% to 95% of NTDs occur in patients with no identifiable risk factors or family history.[9] This low PPV highlights the rather significant overlap in elevated maternal serum AFP levels in affected and unaffected pregnancies; therefore, maternal serum AFP should be used only as a screening test. All patients with positive results should undergo further diagnostic testing or imaging.

Traditionally, the gold standard for diagnosis of an open NTD following a positive screen for maternal serum AFP was amniocentesis. If amniotic fluid AFP levels were confirmed to be high, then an assay to detect the presence or absence of acetylcholinesterase (AChE) was performed. AChE is neuronally derived and, therefore, its presence in amniotic fluid is more specific to nervous system lesions. In a study of 10,000 pregnancies, the combination of amniotic fluid AFP and AChE detected 100%

of anencephaly cases and 100% of open spina bifida cases with a FPR of 0.2%.[12] Again, despite these findings, it must be noted that the presence of AChE in amniotic fluid is not 100% specific to nervous system lesions and has been reported in cases of other fetal anomalies.[13] Additionally, contamination of the amniotic fluid with fetal blood can also cause false positive results in both AFP and AChE levels. Finally, 10% to 15% of dorsal NTDs are skin-covered or "closed" and, therefore, will not be detectable using this technology.

## ULTRASOUND SCREENING FOR OPEN NEURAL TUBE DEFECTS

During the 1980s, the detection rate for fetal open NTDs was only 50% to 80% using ultrasonography.[14,15] Such detection rates led many to believe that amniocentesis for AFP and AChE was still warranted even in the setting of a normal ultrasound.[14,16] However, with improvements in ultrasound technology and in the hands of experienced operators, targeted ultrasound for NTDs in the setting of an elevated maternal serum AFP level yields a sensitivity of 97% to 100% and a specificity of 100%.[17,18] In fact, Nadel and colleagues[18] demonstrated that a maternal serum AFP-based risk for an open NTD could actually be reduced by 95% after a normal targeted ultrasound exam. Given these advances, many providers feel comfortable using ultrasound as a diagnostic tool for the detection of NTDs, thereby eliminating the risks associated with invasive testing such as amniocentesis. However, in areas with limited ultrasound expertise and lack of resources, amniocentesis for AFP and AChE can still play a role in the diagnosis of NTDs.

Typical ultrasound findings in the setting of an open NTD include a thin-walled cystic mass anterior to the lesion, splaying of the spinous processes in coronal views, and a wide separation of the lateral spinous processes in transverse views. Abnormal angulation of the spine may also be present. Depending on the size and location of the lesion, these findings may be subtle. In 1986, Nicolaides and colleagues revolutionized the concept of ultrasound screening for NTDs with the description of intracranial abnormalities that are invariably seen in a group of cases of open NTDs. He described frontal bone scalloping ("lemon sign") and obliteration of the cisterna magna with abnormal anterior curvature of the cerebellum ("banana sign") as the cerebellar vermis, fourth ventricle, and medulla are displaced through the foramen magnum[19] (Fig. 9.1). In addition, ventriculomegaly and microcephaly are frequently observed in cases of open NTDs. Of note, the "lemon" and "banana" signs are often

not observed after the midtrimester; whereas, ventriculomegaly may develop as gestation progresses. Regardless, the presence of any of these intracranial findings increases the sensitivity of ultrasound for the detection of open NTDs to greater than 99%.[20]

The majority of studies evaluating the accuracy of ultrasound have been performed in high-risk populations (i.e., patients with an elevated maternal serum AFP). More recent studies have suggested that routine second trimester ultrasonography actually may be more likely to identify an open NTD compared with routine maternal serum AFP screening in the general population.[21] Finally, *first-trimester* screening for open NTDs is currently under active investigation. It has been proposed that in fetuses with open spina bifida, the downward displacement of the fetal brain will lead to nonvisualization of the fourth ventricle in early gestation. The fourth ventricle, described as the "intracranial translucency," is typically visualized in the midsagittal view of the fetal face used to obtain first-trimester nuchal translucency measurement in normal fetuses. While larger prospective studies are warranted, preliminary results demonstrate promise.[22,23] In addition, recent studies also have demonstrated that a small biparietal diameter in the first trimester of pregnancy may be a subtle marker for open spina bifida.[24,25] In a retrospective review, Bernard and colleagues[24] observed a 10-fold increased risk of open spina bifida when the biparietal diameter measured less than the 5th percentile between 11 and 14 weeks. Combining this potential for a first-trimester screening modality with the high detection rates observed in second-trimester ultrasonography, the future role of maternal serum AFP screening for open NTDs is uncertain.

## FACTORS AFFECTING MATERNAL SERUM AFP INTERPRETATION

Accurate pregnancy dating is one of the key components to successful maternal AFP serum screening. Maternal serum AFP concentrations increase by 15% to 20% per week between 16 and 22 weeks; therefore, inaccurate dating may lead to erroneous results. The optimal timing to perform maternal serum AFP screening is between 16 and 18 weeks. Prior to this gestational age, there is considerable overlap between affected and unaffected pregnancies.[3] First-trimester crown-rump length measurement is the preferred method for accurate pregnancy dating; however, fetal biometry may be used after 14 weeks' gestation. Given that biparietal diameter measurements may lag in fetuses with open NTDs, attention to other biometric parameters is necessary.

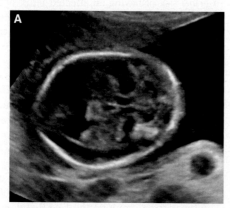 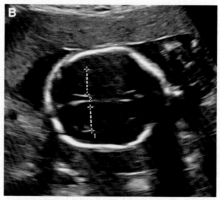

**FIGURE 9.1:** Intracranial ultrasound findings in fetuses with open NTDs: banana sign **(A)**, lemon sign **(B)**.

Other factors that must be accounted for when calculating maternal serum AFP concentration include maternal ethnicity, weight, and the diagnosis of diabetes mellitus. African Americans have a 10% to 15% higher serum AFP level compared with other races, despite the fact that African Americans have a lower incidence of NTDs overall.[26,27] While there may be small differences in serum AFP levels between other racial groups, these differences are not large enough to necessitate adjustment. Given that increasing maternal weight reflects an increased volume of distribution, higher body weights will result in a relative dilution of maternal serum AFP levels. Prior studies have shown that adjustment for maternal weight actually increases the detection rate of open NTDs and decreases the FPR.[28] The relationship between maternal serum AFP levels and diabetes mellitus remains controversial. It has been shown that serum AFP levels are approximately 20% lower in diabetic patients compared with nondiabetic patients; however, it remains uncertain whether the cause for this is the disease state itself or the state of glycemic control.[29] Notably, Baumgarten and Robinson[30] demonstrated a significant inverse relationship between maternal serum AFP and glycosylated hemoglobin, supporting the theory that uncontrolled glucose levels are the driving force behind this observed decrease. Additionally, it has been proposed that adjustment for maternal weight alone may be adequate. Although most laboratories continue to correct for diabetes in their AFP MoM calculation, the most recent literature suggests that this is likely unnecessary, regardless of insulin requirement.[31,32] Finally, maternal serum and amniotic fluid AFP levels are ineffective following multifetal or selective reduction procedures.[33] Ultrasound remains the optimal choice for open NTD screening in these patients.

## ULTRASOUND EVALUATION FOR ELEVATED AFP LEVELS

### False Positive Results

The first step in evaluating an elevated maternal serum AFP level is to perform an ultrasound to assess gestational age, if this has not previously been done. In approximately 50% of cases, underestimation of gestational age is identified, resulting in a false positive value.[3] In such cases, the initial serum AFP value can be adjusted, and often no further testing is needed. Fetal viability also should be assessed, as fetal demise can lead to an elevated maternal serum AFP level secondary to disruption in the maternal–fetal interface. Finally, it is imperative to evaluate for the presence of a multifetal gestation. Increased placental mass in multifetal gestations leads to increased AFP, approximately twofold higher in twin gestations compared with singletons. Typically, ultrasound evaluation for open NTDs is thought to be the gold standard evaluation for multifetal pregnancies; however, some laboratories do report an adjusted serum AFP value for twin gestations. Using this approach, either the maternal serum AFP MoM is divided by the median AFP level in unaffected twin pregnancies or a higher singleton threshold is used to define a positive screen. The issue with this approach is that a single serum value is being used to provide information on multiple fetuses. Cuckle and colleagues[34] demonstrated that by using a 2.5-MoM threshold, such as in a singleton pregnancy, the detection rate for open spina bifida in twin gestations was 89%; however, the FPR was as high as 30%. In order to maintain a FPR similar to that of singleton gestations, a 5.0-MoM

threshold would need to be used, resulting in an open NTD detection rate of only 39% in twin pregnancies.

Maternal–fetal hemorrhage can also result in a falsely positive elevated maternal serum AFP level. While this can often be elicited through a maternal history of vaginal bleeding, not all cases of maternal–fetal hemorrhage will lead to recognizable clinical signs. Ultrasound evaluation may demonstrate subchorionic hematoma, retroplacental hematoma, or placental sonolucencies in such cases.[35,36] Placental implantation site abnormalities such as placenta accreta have also been reported to be associated with elevated maternal serum AFP levels; therefore, ultrasound of the placental site is warranted, especially in cases of placenta previa and a prior uterine scar.[37,38] Other placental findings associated with elevated maternal serum AFP levels include chorioangiomas, angiomyxomas, and placental hypertrophy.[39,40] Rarely diagnosed during pregnancy, ovarian germ cell tumors and hepatic tumors also can cause elevated serum AFP levels; however, the magnitude of AFP increase is typically much higher than is typically observed in obstetric screening programs.

### Other Fetal Anomalies

Apart from open NTDs, elevated maternal serum AFP levels also have been associated with other fetal malformations. The second most common group of anomalies associated with elevated AFP levels are fetal abdominal wall defects, including omphalocele, gastroschisis, and bladder extrophy. As in the case of NTDs, these open defects allow for leakage of fetal serum into the amniotic fluid, resulting in high amniotic fluid and maternal serum AFP concentrations. Saller and colleagues[41] observed that pregnancies with gastroschisis and omphalocele had elevated AFP levels compared with the unaffected population, 9.42 and 4.18 MoMs, respectively. Other studies have demonstrated a greater screening sensitivity for gastroschisis compared with omphalocele at any given AFP threshold.[42]

Congenital skin disorders such as epidermolysis bullosa and aplasia cutis have also been associated with elevated AFP levels. This is hypothesized to be caused by increased diffusion of fetal AFP through the weeping skin lesions and into the amniotic fluid. Reflux of intestinal contents in cases of duodenal atresia, annular pancreas, and intestinal atresia as well as reflux of lung fluid in cases of congenital lung lesions can also cause AFP elevations. A full listing of fetal anomalies reported to be associated with elevated AFP levels is shown in Table 9.1.[1,3]

Although extremely rare in the general population, congenital nephrosis should be considered to be a potential diagnosis in cases of an extremely elevated AFP level and normal ultrasound findings.[43] This autosomal recessive disorder is most common in Finland, where the incidence ranges from 1 in 2,600 to 1 in 8,000 pregnancies.[44] This lethal disorder causes early renal failure, and death typically occurs in infancy or early childhood. Abnormal filtering capacity of the fetal glomeruli is thought to cause extreme fetal proteinuria. Consequently, elevated amniotic fluid AFP levels are present. Maternal serum levels are usually elevated on the order of 5 to 6 MoMs, whereas amniotic fluid AFP levels are typically elevated to >10.0 MoMs.[45] While the fetal kidneys may appear slightly enlarged and echogenic, ultrasound is typically normal in these fetuses. Placentomegaly may occur; however, this finding usually is not observed until the third trimester. Definitive diagnosis is made by electron microscopy of a renal biopsy. In utero kidney biopsy has been

| Table 9.1 | Fetal Anomalies Associated with Maternal Serum AFP Elevations |
|---|---|

Open NTDs
Gastroschisis
Omphalocele
Bladder extrophy
Esophageal atresia
Duodenal atresia
Annular pancreas
Pilonidal cysts
Autosomal recessive polycystic kidney disease
Epidermolysis bullosa
Aplasia cutis
Bilateral renal agenesis
Sacrococcygeal hematoma
Congenital cystic adenomatoid malformation
Cystic hygroma
Acardiac twin
Obstructive uropathy
Osteogenesis imperfecta
Triploidy

AFP, alpha-fetoprotein.

suggested and successfully performed in order to make an antenatal diagnosis in cases with high suspicion for this disorder.[46]

## Unexplained Elevated AFP

In approximately 1% of patients with an elevated AFP level, no apparent structural cause can be identified. However, these patients still remain at increased risk for adverse pregnancy outcomes, including fetal loss, preterm delivery, fetal growth restriction, oligohydramnios, placental abruption, and intrauterine fetal death.[47–49] Milunsky and colleagues[47] demonstrated that patients with an elevated maternal serum AFP level were at a twofold increased risk for preeclampsia, a threefold increased risk for placental abruption, a fourfold increased risk for low birth weight, and an eightfold increased risk for fetal death. Subsequently, Waller and colleagues conducted a case-control study and again demonstrated that elevated maternal serum AFP levels were associated with intrauterine fetal demise. The odds ratio for fetal death in that study was 10.4 (95% CI, 4.9 to 22.0) in the setting of AFP levels exceeding 3.0 MoMs.[50] Most interestingly, that study also showed that the risk of intrauterine fetal death persisted through the third trimester, suggesting that there is potential for these high-risk patients to be identified and offered increased antenatal surveillance. Most recently, elevated maternal serum AFP levels have been linked to an increased risk of sudden infant death syndrome (SIDS); however, this association may be biased by an increased incidence of fetal growth restriction and preterm delivery in those patients.[51] Despite these associations, the majority of women with an unexplained elevated AFP level do have a normal pregnancy outcome.

The optimal management strategy for patients with an unexplained elevated AFP level remains unclear. A suggested algorithm for the evaluation and management of these patients is shown in Figure 9.2. It is hypothesized that these unexplained elevations may be due to abnormal placentation; therefore, it might be possible to predict which patients are at highest risk for adverse outcome by indirectly evaluating the placental circulation through uterine artery Doppler studies. Initial studies evaluating the utility of uterine artery Doppler studies in predicting preeclampsia and fetal growth restriction produced a wide range of sensitivities and predictive values, with significant variation depending on the parameter studied (i.e., pulsatility index [PI], resistance index [RI], or diastolic notching).[52–54] A recent systematic review and meta-analysis demonstrated that an increased uterine artery PI with notching was the best predictor of preeclampsia with a positive likelihood ratio (LR) of 21.0 in high-risk populations and 7.5 in low-risk populations.[55]

Relatively few studies specifically have addressed the role of uterine artery Doppler studies in populations with unexplained elevated maternal serum AFP levels. Aristidou and colleagues[56] reported that the presence of diastolic notching was a good

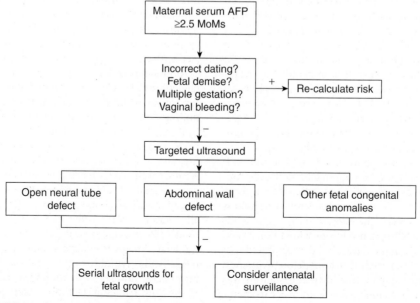

**FIGURE 9.2:** Suggested algorithm for the evaluation and management of elevated maternal serum AFP.

predictor of poor perinatal outcome in patients with an elevated maternal serum AFP level. Bromley and colleagues[57] demonstrated similar results; however, they observed that only severe grade II notching was associated with a significant increase in adverse outcomes (RR 3.4, 95% CI, 1.9 to 6.0). Finally, Konchak and colleagues demonstrated that both uterine artery notching and a RI > 95th percentile were predictive of adverse outcomes in this population. The best test characteristics were observed for the prediction of preeclampsia. Uterine artery notching demonstrated an 83.3% sensitivity and 95.6% specificity for preeclampsia, whereas an elevated RI demonstrated an 83.3% sensitivity and a 93.8% specificity for preeclampsia. Lower sensitivities were noted for the outcomes of fetal growth restriction and preterm delivery. Despite these results, PPVs ranged only between 44% and 55%.[58] While second-trimester uterine artery Doppler studies can be used in the evaluation of patients with an unexplained elevated maternal serum AFP level, there remain no specific guidelines for management and surveillance in these patients.

Umbilical artery Doppler studies as well as ultrasound evaluation of placental morphology have also been proposed as tools to evaluate patients with an unexplained elevated AFP level. Abnormal umbilical artery Doppler studies alone have not shown to be predictive of adverse outcomes in this population; however, in fetuses with identified fetal growth restriction, umbilical artery Doppler interrogation is useful in evaluating for worsening placental dysfunction.[57] Abnormal placental thickness, texture, and shape on ultrasound, especially in the setting of abnormal uterine artery Doppler studies may also be a predictor of adverse perinatal outcome in patients with elevated AFP levels.[59]

Given the increased risk for fetal growth restriction in these patients, serial ultrasound assessments for fetal growth are warranted in the third trimester of pregnancy. If abnormal growth is detected, then umbilical artery studies and antenatal testing with biophysical profiles or nonstress tests should follow. It is unclear whether the risk for intrauterine fetal demise in these patients is independent of fetal growth restriction; therefore, many institutions propose antenatal testing even in the absence of fetal growth abnormalities. In a 2001 retrospective cohort study of 136 patients with unexplained elevated maternal serum AFP levels, Huerta-Enochian and colleagues[49] demonstrated that intensive antenatal monitoring consisting of twice weekly nonstress tests and amniotic fluid volume assessment did not achieve earlier or improved detection of adverse outcome compared with routine prenatal care. The decision to perform antenatal testing in these patients remains an individualized decision between provider and patient.

## USE OF BIOCHEMICAL MARKERS IN THE FIRST TRIMESTER

### Aneuploidy Screening

In the mid-1990s, it was discovered that first-trimester alterations in pregnancy-associated plasma protein-A (PAPP-A) and free β-human chorionic gonadotropin (β-hCG) were associated with an increased risk for fetal aneuploidy.[60-62] These biochemical markers are placentally-derived, pregnancy-specific glycoproteins which are detectable in maternal serum. In pregnancies affected by trisomy 21, PAPP-A is reduced to 0.4 MoMs, and free β-hCG is increased to 1.98 MoMs between 9 and 11 weeks' gestation, on average. When combined with maternal age, low PAPP-A alone will identify approximately 50% of pregnancies

affected by trisomy 21, whereas elevated free β-hCG alone will detect only 40% of pregnancies affected by trisomy 21.[63] When combining both PAPP-A and free β-hCG with maternal age, that detection rate increases from 60% to 65% at an FPR of 5%.[62]

Prior studies have evaluated the impact of measuring the intact hCG molecule rather than the free β-hCG subunit, as discussed above. Although both serum analytes are increased in fetuses affected by Down syndrome, levels of intact hCG do not begin to increase in affected fetuses until approximately 11 weeks compared with levels of free β-hCG, which begin to increase at 9 weeks. In a meta-analysis by Evans and colleagues,[64] the use of the free β-hCG subunit achieved a higher detection rate of trisomy 21 with a lower FPR compared with the intact hCG molecule. Today, most first-trimester aneuploidy screening protocols use the free β-hCG subunit; however, its impact on screening efficiency is likely greater during the earlier gestational age window of first-trimester serum screening.

In addition to these serum analytes, the discovery that an increased size of the fluid collection on the back of the neck (i.e., the "nuchal translucency") was also associated with an increased risk for trisomy 21 further revolutionized first-trimester aneuploidy screening.[65] First-trimester nuchal translucency measurement alone has a detection rate of 64% to 70% for trisomy 21; however, combining nuchal translucency measurement with PAPP-A and free β-hCG measurement increases that detection rate from 82% to 87% at a 5% fixed FPR.[66] This combined approach to first-trimester screening is now routinely offered to all patients, regardless of maternal age, between 10 and 13 6/7 weeks' gestation.

Combined first-trimester screening can also be used in the detection of patients at high risk for other aneuploidies, including trisomy 18 and trisomy 13. In contrast to trisomy 21, both PAPP-A and free β-hCG levels are *decreased* in these particular chromosomal abnormalities, while nuchal translucency is increased.[67,68] Tul and colleagues[67] demonstrated that free β-hCG MoM levels were decreased to <5th percentile of normal in 64% of trisomy 18 cases. Similarly, PAPP-A MoM levels were decreased to <5th percentile of normal in 78% of trisomy 18 cases. Results from the BUN study by Wapner and colleagues[69] showed a 90.9% detection rate for trisomy 18 at 2% FPR. Additional studies have demonstrated similar results for combined first-trimester screening with detection rates of 92.3% for trisomy 18 and 88.9% for trisomy 13.[70]

### Adverse Pregnancy Outcomes

In the setting of a normal karyotype, low PAPP-A levels have been found to be associated with multiple adverse pregnancy outcomes. In a secondary analysis of the FASTER trial, Dugoff and colleagues demonstrated that low PAPP-A levels <5th percentile were significantly associated with fetal loss, preterm birth, gestational hypertension, preeclampsia, and low birth weight. Additionally, there was a pattern of an increased magnitude of risk as the PAPP-A level became more extreme. For example, the adjusted odds ratio (aOR) for spontaneous fetal loss <24 weeks was 1.95 (95% CI, 1.44 to 2.62) for PAPP-A levels <10th percentile; however, this risk increased to an aOR of 5.22 (95% CI, 3.09 to 8.80) for PAPP-A levels <1st percentile.[71] PAPP-A is derived from the placenta and serves as a protease for insulin-like growth factor (IGF) binding protein-4.[72] Decreased levels of PAPP-A are associated with high levels of bound IGF and, subsequently, lower levels of free IGF in the circulation.

IGF plays an important role in both fetal growth and trophoblast invasion into the maternal decidua.[73,74] Given that low PAPP-A levels are a reflection of low free circulating IGF levels, these observed associations with placenta-mediated adverse pregnancy outcomes appear to be biologically plausible.

Despite these associations, the test performance characteristics of low PAPP-A limit its use as a primary screening tool for adverse pregnancy outcomes. In a population-based cohort study, Krantz and colleagues[75] demonstrated that PAPP-A <1st percentile had a sensitivity of 3.3%, specificity of 99.3%, and PPV of 24.1% for fetal growth restriction. Pihl and colleagues[76] observed similar test characteristics for PAPP-A <5th percentile for fetal growth restriction, citing a detection rate of only 13% and a PPV of 14%. For preeclampsia, the PPV for PAPP-A <5th percentile is much lower, ranging from 3.5% to 7.6% in prior studies.[71,77,78] Incorporating a maternal risk factor-based scoring system to improve the screening efficiency of low PAPP-A for preeclampsia resulted in a sensitivity of 36.4%, specificity of 86.8%, and a positive LR of 2.8. Combining low PAPP-A, African American race, overweight maternal BMI, and maternal history of chronic hypertension and pregestational diabetes resulted in an area under the curve of 0.70, indicating only a modest predictive capability, at best, for the outcome of preeclampsia.[79]

Consideration of combining low first-trimester PAPP-A levels with elevated second-trimester maternal serum AFP levels has also been given, considering the association between elevated AFP levels and adverse outcomes, as discussed earlier in this chapter. Smith and colleagues[80] demonstrated a synergistic effect between low PAPP-A and high AFP in the identification of women at risk to develop fetal growth restriction and preterm birth. Subsequently, Dugoff and colleagues[81] demonstrated that the detection rate of patients at risk for early fetal loss <24 weeks was as high as 46% when combining low PAPP-A, high AFP, and low unconjugated estriol, another serum analyte used in second-trimester aneuploidy screening. Unfortunately, the exceedingly small number of patients who undergo sequential screening and actually have this combination of abnormal serum analytes precludes their use as clinical screening tools.

Alternatively, high levels of PAPP-A have not been consistently linked to adverse outcomes. While several studies have suggested a trend toward an increasing risk of macrosomia with high PAPP-A levels, this finding has not been confirmed in subsequent reports.[71,82]

The association between abnormal levels of first-trimester free β-hCG and adverse pregnancy outcomes has been less consistent. The most commonly cited adverse outcome associated with low free β-hCG in the first trimester has been early pregnancy loss.[71,83] Dugoff and colleagues[71] demonstrated that free β-hCG levels <1st percentile had a sensitivity of 3.7% at a 1% FPR and a PPV of 2.8% for spontaneous pregnancy loss <24 weeks. Similar to high levels of PAPP-A, high levels of free β-hCG in the first trimester have not been reliably linked to an increased risk for adverse pregnancy outcomes.

On the basis of their overall poor screening efficiency, first-trimester PAPP-A and free β-hCG cannot be recommended as primary screening tools for adverse pregnancy outcome. Additionally, subjecting a population to universal screening for outcomes for which there are currently no proven prevention strategies may lead to increases in fetal surveillance that are neither cost-effective nor clinically indicated. Nevertheless, serial ultrasounds to evaluate fetal growth may be considered in the small number of patients at the highest risk for adverse outcome such as those with PAPP-A levels <1st percentile. Conversely, patients with *normal* first-trimester PAPP-A and free β-hCG levels can be counseled so that their risk of adverse pregnancy outcome may be reduced.

## Ultrasound Evaluation

Patients with an abnormal first-trimester aneuploidy screen who decline invasive prenatal diagnostic testing should undergo a detailed genetic ultrasound during the second trimester to evaluate for major fetal anomalies as well as minor markers of aneuploidy. In patients with an abnormal first-trimester serum screen and a normal karyotype, the protocol for subsequent evaluation is less clear. As opposed to abnormal maternal serum AFP levels, abnormal first-trimester PAPP-A and free β-hCG levels have not been linked to many structural fetal defects. In a 2008 report from a secondary analysis of the FASTER trial, free β-hCG levels >2.0 MoMs were significantly associated with both unilateral and bilateral multicystic dysplastic kidney disease and hydrocele. PAPP-A levels >2.0 MoMs were also associated with hydrocele.[84] Targeted fetal renal ultrasound may be considered in this subset of patients.

In an attempt to improve the screening performance of low PAPP-A levels for the prediction of preeclampsia and fetal growth restriction, many authors have proposed the addition of uterine artery Doppler studies.[85,86] Poon and colleagues[85] demonstrated that the detection rate of early preeclampsia (requiring delivery <34 weeks) was increased when combining a model of maternal risk factors, low PAPP-A, maternal mean arterial pressure, and uterine artery Doppler PI between 11 and 13 weeks. Other authors have demonstrated that the addition of second-trimester uterine artery Doppler studies in patients with low first-trimester PAPP-A levels improves the screening efficiency for preeclampsia and fetal growth restriction; however, the optimal timing to perform this study during the second trimester remains unclear.[87,88] Currently, uterine artery Doppler studies are not routinely performed during first-trimester aneuploidy screening at all centers; however, the addition of second-trimester uterine artery Doppler studies may be considered in patients with extremely low PAPP-A levels to provide further risk stratification. The addition of novel maternal serum analytes such as A-Disintegrin and Metalloprotease 12 (ADAM12), placental protein 13 (PP13), and placental growth factor (PlGF) to uterine artery Doppler studies is actively being investigated to improve the prediction of adverse pregnancy outcomes in the first trimester.

# USE OF BIOCHEMICAL MARKERS IN THE SECOND TRIMESTER

## Aneuploidy Screening

Prior to the 1980s, aneuploidy risk assessment was based solely on maternal age. During that time, only women aged 35 or older were offered diagnostic testing with chorionic villus sampling (CVS) or amniocentesis. The risk of having a child affected by trisomy 21 is 1 in 270 at age 35; therefore, these women were considered to be of the highest risk. This threshold was chosen for two reasons: (1) The risk of having an affected child rapidly increases after age 35 and (2) the risk of pregnancy loss following amniocentesis was thought to be equivocal or less than the risk of having an affected child after this age. In 1984, Merkatz and colleagues[89] made the discovery that low levels of maternal serum AFP between 15 and 20 weeks' gestation were associated with trisomy 21. On average, maternal serum levels of AFP are 0.7 MoMs below the unaffected mean in pregnancies affected by trisomy 21.[90] This finding revolutionized the concept of aneuploidy screening, which could then be made available to all pregnant women, including those under the age of 35. Soon after this discovery, it was also noted that hCG levels were increased and unconjugated estriol levels were decreased in pregnancies with a trisomy 21 fetus. HCG levels are typically increased from 2.3 to 2.5 MoMs above the unaffected mean in trisomy 21 pregnancies, whereas unconjugated estriol levels are typically decreased below 0.7 MoMs.[91,92] Both hCG and unconjugated estriol are secreted from the syncytiotrophoblast, suggesting that aneuploid fetuses demonstrate placental immaturity, which results in both unregulated hypersecretion and undersecretion of placental products.[3]

Since AFP, hCG, and unconjugated estriol are only weakly correlated and independent of maternal age, these analytes can be combined with maternal age to assess aneuploidy risk. In 1992, Haddow and colleagues[93] demonstrated that the combination of these three serum analytes was more effective in screening for fetal trisomy 21 than screening with AFP alone. This formed the basis for the first multiple marker aneuploidy screening tool, the "triple screen." For patients under the age of 35, the detection rate for trisomy 21 is approximately 60% at a 5% screen positive rate. However, given that the *a priori* age-related risk of trisomy 21 increases with maternal age, both the detection rate and the screen positive rate of the triple screen also increase with maternal age. For women aged 35 and older, the trisomy 21 detection rate increases to >85%, at the expense of a 25% screen positive rate.[93,94] The triple screen can also be used to assess trisomy 18 risk; however, in cases of trisomy 18, levels of all three serum markers are decreased.[95]

Since the adoption of the triple screen, it has been found that pregnancies affected by trisomy 21 also have increased levels of dimeric inhibin-A in maternal serum. Levels of this protein, produced by the placenta, are elevated approximately 1.8 MoMs above the unaffected mean in trisomy 21 pregnancies.[96,97] The addition of inhibin-A to AFP, hCG, and unconjugated estriol creates what is now known as the "quadruple screen." This screening protocol results in a trisomy 21 detection rate of 81% at a 5% screen positive rate and has become the standard of care for second-trimester aneuploidy screening.[66] Using this multimarker test, a composite LR is determined on the basis of the level of the above-mentioned four serum analytes. The *a priori* maternal age-related risk is then multiplied by this LR to calculate an adjusted *posttest* aneuploidy risk. Of note, inhibin-A is not used in the risk calculation for trisomy 18. The pattern of serum analyte changes associated with trisomy 21 and 18 in both first- and second-trimester serum screening is shown in Table 9.2. The threshold at which a test is considered "screen positive" varies by individual laboratories. Given that a "screen positive" test is often a trigger for further invasive diagnostic testing, the chosen threshold must represent a balance between detection rate, FPR, and pregnancy loss risk from amniocentesis. Traditionally, a cutoff of 1 in 270 has been used, consistent with the age-related aneuploidy risk at age 35.[98]

The "quad screen" can be performed between 15 and 20 weeks' gestation; however, the screen is most accurate if performed between 16 and 18 weeks. As discussed earlier in the chapter, levels

| Table 9.2 | Pattern of Serum Analyte Alterations in Fetal Chromosomal Abnormalities |
|---|---|

First-Trimester Biochemical Screening

|  | PAPP-A | Free β-hCG |
|---|---|---|
| Trisomy 21 | ↓ | ↑ |
| Trisomy 13/18 | ↓ | ↓ |

Second Trimester Biochemical Screening

|  | AFP | hCG | Estriol | Inhibin-A |
|---|---|---|---|---|
| Trisomy 21 | ↓ | ↑ | ↓ | ↑ |
| Trisomy 18 | ↓ | ↓ | ↓ | N/A |

PAPP-A, pregnancy-associated plasma protein-A; hCG, human chorionic gonadotropin; AFP, alpha-fetoprotein.

of maternal serum AFP increase with gestational age. Unconjugated estriol levels also increase with gestational age, while hCG levels decrease; therefore, accurate pregnancy dating is essential in interpreting serum screening results. In contrast, inhibin-A levels remain relatively constant throughout gestation. Maternal weight also must be accounted for when interpreting second-trimester serum screening. The increase in maternal plasma volume observed with increasing maternal weight causes a relative dilution effect on the serum analyte concentrations. The impact of race and ethnicity on serum analyte levels has been extensively studied. While significant differences in serum analyte levels have been identified, the majority of these differences are too small to have a significant effect on screening efficiency.[26,27] The largest differences are observed when comparing African Americans to Caucasians. Watt and colleagues[99] demonstrated that African American women had serum AFP levels that were 22% higher than those of Caucasian women and hCG levels that were 19% higher. Although the overall effect of adjusting for African American race only increased the aneuploidy detection rate by approximately 0.5%, this practice is still recommended on account of its proven influence on AFP detection of open NTDs. Finally, both AFP and unconjugated estriol levels have been found to be significantly lower in pregnant women with insulin-dependent diabetes.[100,101] Controversy still exists as to whether these findings are secondary to the disease state itself or to poor glucose control.

As with open NTD screening with AFP, serum screening tests for aneuploidy are less sensitive in multiple gestations. It is possible to calculate a "pseudo-risk" for aneuploidy using maternal serum analytes in twin pregnancies; however, this approach incorporates assumptions regarding zygosity and chorionicity.[102] First-trimester screening using individual nuchal translucency measurements for each fetus is the preferred approach for aneuploidy screening at most centers.

Other serum analytes that could improve the screening efficiency for trisomy 21 have been investigated. Hyperglycosylated hCG (h-hCG), also known as invasive trophoblast antigen, initially demonstrated promise, given that both maternal serum and urinary concentrations of h-hCG were demonstrated to be elevated in pregnancies affected by trisomy 21.[103,104] Many laboratories began to incorporate h-hCG into aneuploidy screening as a fifth serum analyte, thus creating the "penta screen."

Subsequent studies demonstrated that the improvement in the trisomy 21 detection rate with the penta screen over the quadruple screen was only modest, increasing from 79% to 83% at a 5% fixed FPR, a nonsignificant increase.[105] This is likely due to the strong correlation observed between h-hCG and both intact hCG and free β-hCG. While the "penta screen" is still offered by some laboratories, it has not been adopted as routine standard of care for second-trimester serum aneuploidy screening.

ACOG currently recommends that all patients, regardless of age, be offered options for aneuploidy screening.[98] Combinations of both first- and second-trimester screening are also available that can increase the detection rate of trisomy 21 to approximately 95%.[66] While first-trimester serum screening can provide risk estimates for trisomy 13, second-trimester serum screening does not provide risk estimates for trisomy 13 or other lethal chromosomal abnormalities. This should be taken into consideration in conjunction with any potential ultrasound findings in determining whether to pursue serum screening for aneuploidy.

## Abnormal Serum Analytes in Pregnancies with Normal Karyotype

Similar to first-trimester serum screening, extreme abnormal values of the second-trimester serum analytes have also been associated with other structural defects and adverse pregnancy outcomes in the presence of a normal fetal karyotype. The association between unexplained elevations in maternal serum AFP and adverse pregnancy outcome has been discussed earlier in this chapter. Low AFP levels <0.25 MoMs also have been linked to both pregnancy loss and low birth weight; however, these associations are less robust compared with those observed with high AFP levels.[48,106-108]

Extremely elevated levels of hCG in the second trimester have also been linked to adverse pregnancy outcomes such as preeclampsia, preterm delivery, intrauterine growth restriction, pregnancy loss, and intrauterine fetal demise.[109-111] The strongest association appears to be with intrauterine fetal demise, with an increased risk as high as four fold quoted for patients with hCG levels ≥2.0 MoMs.[111] The proposed mechanism for these associations stems from the hypothesis that the placenta produces an increased amount of hCG in response to the decreased oxygen supply that occurs in the setting of early placental vascular damage.[112] This supports the theory that placental dysfunction is reflected in abnormal levels of maternal serum analytes. As with other serum analytes, the magnitude of risk appears to increase as serum hCG levels become more extreme. In a case-control study by Lepage and colleagues,[110] only 2 of 15 women with extremely high hCG levels (≥10 MoMs) gave birth to a live-born neonate without complication. The risk of these adverse pregnancy outcomes is significantly greater in patients with the rare combination of both elevated AFP and elevated hCG levels.[111]

Low estriol levels below the range of 0.5 to 0.75 MoMs have also been linked to adverse pregnancy outcome; however, this finding in a fetus with a normal karyotype should also prompt investigation into other potential genetic and metabolic disorders of the fetal–placental unit.[109,113,114] The two most common disorders associated with extremely low (<0.15 MoMs) or absent maternal serum unconjugated estriol levels are Smith–Lemli–Opitz (SLO) syndrome and placental sulfatase deficiency. To understand these associations, it is first necessary to understand the biosynthesis pathway of unconjugated estriol. Dehydroepiandrosterone sulfate (DHEAS) is produced in the fetal adrenal gland and then converted to 16α-OH-DHEAS in the fetal liver. In the placenta, 16α-OH-DHEAS is then deconjugated by placental sulfatase, yielding molecules that will later be aromatized into unconjugated estriol.[3] Any disorder that impacts any step of this biosynthesis pathway will result in low- to absent-unconjugated estriol levels in maternal serum that may be detected at the time of second-trimester serum aneuploidy screening.

First described in 1964, SLO is an autosomal recessive disorder characterized by multiple fetal anomalies, moderate to severe mental retardation, growth failure, and characteristic-appearing facies.[115] The primary defect for this disorder involves cholesterol biosynthesis, leading to an increased amount of the cholesterol precursor 7-dehydrocholesterol and, subsequently, a decreased or absent amount of unconjugated estriol in maternal serum. In a case series of 33 women with SLO, 24 of 26 women who had second trimester unconjugated estriol levels measured had values <0.5 MoMs.[116] While universal risk assessment for SLO is possible using second-trimester screening, the yield of positive cases is low.[117,118] Consideration of the diagnosis of SLO is typically entertained in fetuses with a normal karyotype and an extremely low unconjugated estriol level, typically <0.3 MoMs. Prenatal diagnosis is currently based on the detection of increased levels of the cholesterol precursor 7-dehydrocholesterol in amniotic fluid.[119]

Placental sulfatase deficiency is another disorder associated with extremely low unconjugated estriol levels.[120] Lack of the placental sulfatase enzyme leads to decreased estrogen biosynthesis in the placenta. Placental sulfatase deficiency is X-linked and manifested clinically as icthyosis. Although usually mild and treatable, a small proportion of patients can have a more severe phenotype, including mental retardation. Prenatal diagnosis is available through molecular cytogenetic testing. Other disorders that have been associated with low unconjugated estriol levels include congenital adrenal hyperplasia, adrenocorticotropin deficiency, Kallman syndrome, hypothalamic corticotropin deficiency, and anencephaly.

Elevated levels of inhibin-A have been most extensively studied for their association with preeclampsia.[121,122] Aquilina and colleagues[123] demonstrated that inhibin-A levels ≥2.0 MoMs had a sensitivity of 48.6% and a specificity of 90% for preeclampsia, a predictive efficiency that was significantly greater than that of elevated hCG. A subsequent study demonstrated elevated inhibin-A levels to have a sensitivity of 71.4%, a specificity of 96.3%, and a PPV of 62.5% for preeclampsia.[124] In summary, abnormal levels of second-trimester serum analytes have a significant association with many adverse pregnancy outcomes in the absence of fetal aneuploidy; however, their relatively low predictive capability limits their use as primary screening tools for this purpose. Although it has been demonstrated that having two or more abnormal serum markers does increase sensitivity and PPVs, even when used in combination with each other and with first-trimester markers, serum analytes display only a modest accuracy for predicting adverse outcome overall.[125,126]

## Ultrasound Evaluation

After a positive second trimester serum screen, patients are routinely offered invasive testing for definitive genetic diagnosis. All patients with a positive screen should undergo a targeted genetic sonogram evaluating for major fetal anomalies as well as minor markers of aneuploidy. Common major anomalies seen in trisomy 21, 13, and 18 are listed in Table 9.3. Less-specific sonographic findings have been described in association with fetal aneuploidy, especially trisomy 21. These findings have become known as sonographic markers as the entities are nonspecific, often found in normal fetuses. The sonographic markers are listed in Table 9.4. Using these markers, an LR for fetal aneuploidy has been reported by several authors (Table 9.5).

In patients with a normal karyotype, consideration to the above-mentioned abnormalities and pregnancy complications should be given. Elevated inhibin-A levels ≥2.0 MoMs have been associated with multicystic dysplastic kidney disease and two-vessel umbilical cord.[84] These structural abnormalities should be readily apparent on routine fetal anatomic survey. As discussed earlier, patients with an extremely low unconjugated estriol level should be evaluated for SLO. The following ultrasound findings in conjunction with a low maternal serum estriol level are highly suggestive of SLO: syndactyly of two or three toes, growth restriction, microcephaly, and cleft palate. Cardiac defects, central nervous system malformations, and ambiguous genitalia can also be observed in cases of SLO.[127]

As in the case of first-trimester serum screening, the addition of uterine artery Doppler studies has been proposed to increase the detection rate of adverse outcome in patients with abnormal levels of second-trimester serum analytes. The combination of

---

**Table 9.3  Common Features of Major Trisomies**

|  | Trisomy 21 | Trisomy 18 | Trisomy 13 |
| --- | --- | --- | --- |
| Major features | Cardiac defects, duodenal atresia, cystic hygroma, hydrops | Cardiac defects, spina bifida, cerebellar dysgenesis, micrognathia, diaphragmatic hernia, omphalocele, clenched hands/wrists, radial aplasia, clubfeet, cystic hygroma | Cardiac defects, central nervous system abnormalities, facial anomalies, cleft lip/palate, urogenital anomalies/echogenic kidneys, omphalocele, polydactyly, rocker-bottom feet, cystic hygroma |
| Markers or subtle findings | Nuchal thickening, hyperechoic bowel, EIF, shortened limbs, pyelectasis, mild ventriculomegaly, widened pelvic angle, shortened frontal lobe, clinodactyly, widened sandal gap, hypoplastic or absent nasal bone | Choroid cysts, brachycephaly, shortened limbs, IUGR, single umbilical artery | EIF, mild ventriculomegaly, pyelectasis, IUGR, single umbilical artery |

EIF, echogenic intracardiac focus; IUGR, intrauterine growth restriction.

From Nyberg DA, Souter VL. Chromosomal abnormalities. In: Nyberg DA, McGahan JP, Pretorius DH, et al, eds. *Diagnostic Imaging of Fetal Anomalies.* Philadelphia, PA: Lippincott Williams & Wilkins; 2003:864.

---

**Table 9.4  Sonographic Markers of Aneuploidy**

Choroid plexus cysts
Strawberry-shaped head
Mild cerebral ventricular dilatation
Nuchal thickening
Hyperechoic bowel
Intraabdominal findings such as hepatic calcification
Shortened limbs or other skeletal anomalies
Echogenic intracardiac focus
Renal pyelectasis
Widened pelvic angle
Intrauterine growth restriction
Single umbilical artery/umbilical cord anomalies
Umbilical cord cysts/pseudocysts
Placental abnormalities, especially cystic changes
Abnormal amniotic fluid volume

---

**Table 9.5  Comparison of Likelihood Ratios Reported for Sonographic Markers of Fetal Aneuploidy**

| Sonographic marker | Likelihood ratio (95% confidence interval) | | |
| --- | --- | --- | --- |
|  | Nyberg et al. | Bromley et al. | Smith-Bindman et al. |
| Nuchal thickening | 11.0 (5.5–22.0) | 12 | 17 (8–38) |
| Hyperechoic bowel | 6.7 (2.7–16.8) | — | 6.1 (3.0–12.6) |
| Short humerus | 5.1 (1.6–16.5) | 6 | 7.5 (4.7–12.0) |
| short femur | 1.5 (0.8–2.8) | 1 | 2.7 (1.2–6.0) |
| Echogenic intra-cardiac focus | 1.8 (1.0–3.0) | 1.2 | 2.8 (1.5–5.5) |
| Pyelectasis | 1.5 (0.6–3.6) | 1.3 | 1.9 (0.7–5.1) |
| Normal ultrasound | 0.36 | 0.2 | — |

From Nyberg DA, Souter VL. Chromosomal abnormalities. In: Nyberg DA, McGahan JP, Pretorius DH, et al, eds. *Diagnostic Imaging of Fetal Anomalies.* Philadelphia, PA: Lippincott Williams & Wilkins; 2003:894; Bromley B, Liebermann E, Shipp T, Bernacerraf BF. The genetic sonogram: a method of risk assessment for Down syndrome: in the second trimester. *J ultrasound Med* 2002; 1087–1096.

second-trimester uterine artery Doppler with elevated levels of inhibin-A appears to provide the best prediction for preeclampsia, especially preeclampsia requiring early delivery.[128–130] Aquilina and colleagues[128] demonstrated that the sensitivity for preeclampsia improved from 27% to 60% when adding abnormal values of inhibin-A to bilateral uterine artery notching, which was a statistically significant increase. Alternatively, Ay and colleagues[124] demonstrated that although the sensitivity and specificity of uterine artery Doppler for the prediction of preeclampsia increases in the setting of abnormal inhibin-A levels, this increase was not clinically significant. Most recently, Filippi and colleagues demonstrated that abnormal second-trimester uterine artery Doppler studies conferred a high risk of adverse pregnancy outcome; however, *normal* uterine artery Doppler studies did not necessarily equate to *normal* pregnancy outcome. In that study, women with extreme levels of serum analytes but normal uterine artery Doppler studies still had a 26% risk of adverse pregnancy outcome.[131] The decision to perform second-trimester uterine artery Doppler studies in patients with unexplained abnormal serum analyte levels remains individualized.

## NONINVASIVE PRENATAL TESTING AND CELL-FREE FETAL DNA

### Noninvasive Prenatal Testing (NIPT)/Cell-Free Fetal DNA (cffDNA)

In late 2011, NIPT via analysis of cffDNA in maternal plasma was first offered to obstetricians and maternal fetal medicine specialists in the United States as a screening test for high-risk pregnancies.[132] Initially, NIPT was performed exclusively to screen for Down syndrome, trisomy 18, and trisomy 13. Since then its uses have expanded, and it is likely that other indications for this procedure will continue to grow. For example, some laboratories now offer NIPT to screen for sex chromosome abnormalities, triploidy, and even some microdeletion syndromes.[133]

This noninvasive screening method relies on the fact that cffDNA fragments from both the fetus and the pregnant woman are present in the mother's bloodstream during pregnancy. Cell-free fetal DNA fragments, mostly of trophoblast origin, cross the placental barrier and enter the maternal circulation. These cells clear from the maternal system within hours, so fetal DNA detected during a pregnancy represents DNA from the current gestation. The fetal fraction of cell-free DNA is approximately 11% of all cell-free DNA circulating in the maternal plasma.[134] The risk of aneuploidy for a particular chromosome can be assessed by comparing the amount of cffDNA of the chromosome of interest to the cell-free DNA counts of other chromosomes. The laboratory method and sensitivity of NIPT varies between testing sites and by the genetic abnormality that is being screened. Most laboratories report detection rates of 99% for Down syndrome, 97% to 99% for trisomy 18, 80% to 92% for trisomy 13, and over 90% for most sex chromosome abnormalities.[135]

There are several advantages to the NIPT screening method. First, it can be done as early as 10 weeks in pregnancy and throughout the remainder of pregnancy, unlike other maternal serum screens which require testing over specific time windows during the pregnancy. Second, it has a higher detection rate and lower FPR than any of the other first- or second-trimester screening modalities for Down syndrome, trisomy 18, and trisomy 13. This ultimately leads to fewer women choosing to pursue invasive testing through CVS or amniocentesis, both of which carry some negative risk to the pregnancy.[136] Last, it can screen for other genetic abnormalities for which historically there has been an absence of noninvasive maternal serum screening. These disorders include triploidy, sex chromosome abnormalities, and some microdeletion syndromes.

Despite many advantages, there are limitations to NIPT. First, NIPT is a screening test, not a diagnostic test. It is not as reliable as CVS or amniocentesis in detecting chromosome abnormalities. Its scope of use is also smaller. Many genetic anomalies such as mosaicism, partial trisomies, translocations, and single gene disorders, cannot yet be screened with NIPT. Second, NIPT is dependent on a sufficient fetal fraction of cell-free DNA. Approximately 0.5% to 1% of women will receive an inconclusive test result owing to insufficient fetal fraction.[135] Fetal fraction decreases with increasing maternal weight, for example, so women who are overweight (esp. >200 lb) are more likely to receive an uninterpretable result.[137] Lastly, although studies are currently being performed on low-risk populations, NIPT has to date been validated only in the high-risk (e.g., advanced maternal age, abnormal serum screen, personal or family history of aneuploidy, and abnormal ultrasound) patient population. In addition, it has not been validated in triplet or higher multiple pregnancies, or in pregnancies conceived using egg donation.[135] However, its use has dramatically changed the paradigm for prenatal screening and testing in the high-risk population, and should future studies validate similar results for other populations, it is likely to become the primary screening option for all pregnant patients.

In summary, NIPT is an effective first-line screening tool for high-risk pregnant women who are >10 weeks gestational age. NIPT should be offered in concert with proven diagnostic tests such as CVS and amniocentesis that have the ability to detect genetic conditions missed by NIPT. Genetic counselors should be consulted to explain the complexities of this screening modality to patients and their families.[138]

## REFERENCES

1. Main DM, Mennuti MT. Neural tube defects: issues in prenatal diagnosis and counseling. *Obstet Gynecol.* 1986;67:1–16.
2. Habib ZA. Maternal serum alpha-fetoprotein: its value in antenatal diagnosis of genetic disease and in obstetrical-gynecological care. *Acta Obstet Gynecol Scand Suppl.* 1977;61:1–92.
3. Norton ME. Genetics and prenatal diagnosis. In: Callen PW, ed. *Ultrasonography in Obstetrics and Gynecology.* 5th ed. Philadelphia, PA: Saunders Elsevier; 2008:26–59.
4. Brock DJH, Sutcliffe RG. Alpha-fetoprotein in the antenatal diagnosis of anencephaly and spina bifida. *Lancet.* 1972;2:197–199.
5. UK Collaborative Study on alpha-fetoprotein in relation to neural-tube defects: amniotic fluid alpha-fetoprotein measurements in antenatal diagnosis of anencephaly and open spina bifida in early pregnancy. *Lancet.* 1979;2:651–662.
6. Milunsky A. Prenatal detection of neural tube defects, VI: experience with 20,000 pregnancies. *JAMA.* 1980;244:2731–2735.
7. Crandall BF, Matsumoto M. Routine amniotic fluid alpha-fetoprotein measurement in 34,000 pregnancies. *Am J Obstet Gynecol.* 1984;149:744–747.
8. Wald NJ, Cuckle H, Brock JH, et al. Maternal serum-alpha-fetoprotein measurement in antenatal screening for anencephaly and spina bifida in early pregnancy: report of U.K. collaborative study on alpha-fetoprotein in relation to neural tube defects. *Lancet.* 1977;1:1323–1332.
9. American College of Obstetricians and Gynecologists. *Neural Tube Defects.* Washington, DC: American College of Obstetricians and Gynecologists; 2003. ACOG practice bulletin no 44.
10. Haddow JE, Kloza EM, Smith DE, et al. Data from an alpha-fetoprotein pilot screening program in Maine. *Obstet Gynecol.* 1983;62:556–560.
11. Burton BK, Sowers ST, Nelson LH. Maternal serum alpha-fetoprotein screening in North Carolina: experience with more than twelve thousand pregnancies. *Am J Obstet Gynecol.* 1983;146:439–444.

12. Loft AG, Hogdall E, Larsen SO, et al. A comparison of amniotic fluid alpha-fetoprotein and acetylcholinesterase in the prenatal diagnosis of open neural tube defects and anterior abdominal wall defects. *Prenat Diagn.* 1993;13:93–109.

13. Kelly JC, Petrocik E, Wassman ER. Amniotic fluid acetylcholinesterase ratios in prenatal diagnosis of fetal abnormalities. *Am J Obstet Gynecol.* 1989;161:703–705.

14. Drugan A, Zador IE, Syner FN, et al. A normal ultrasound does not obviate the need for amniocentesis in patients with elevated serum alpha-fetoprotein. *Obstet Gynecol.* 1988;72:627–630.

15. Lindfors KK, McGahan JP, Tennant FP, et al. Midtrimester screening for open neural tube defects: correlation of sonography with amniocentesis results. *AJR Am J Roentgenol.* 1987;149:141–145.

16. Platt LD, Feuchtbaum L, Filly R, et al. The California Maternal Serum Alpha-Fetoprotein Screening Program: the role of ultrasonography in the detection of spina bifida. *Am J Obstet Gynecol.* 1992;166:1328–1329.

17. Lennon CA, Gray DL. Sensitivity and specificity of ultrasound for the detection of neural tube and ventral wall defects in a high-risk population. *Obstet Gynecol.* 1999;94:562–566.

18. Nadel A, Green JK, Holmes L, et al. Absence of need for amniocentesis in patients with elevated levels of maternal serum alpha-fetoprotein and normal sonographic examinations. *N Engl J Med.* 1990;323:557–561.

19. Nicolaides KH, Gabbe SG, Campbell S, et al. Ultrasound screening for spina bifida: cranial and cerebellar signs. *Lancet.* 1986;1:72–74.

20. Watson WJ, Chescheir NC, Katz VL, et al. The role of ultrasound in evaluation of patients with elevated maternal serum alpha-fetoprotein. *Obstet Gynecol.* 1991;78:123–128.

21. Norem CT, Schoen EJ, Walter DL, et al. Routine ultrasonography compared with maternal serum alpha-fetoprotein for neural tube defect screening. *Obstet Gynecol.* 2005;106:747–752.

22. Chaoui R, Benoit B, Mitkowska-Wozniak H, et al. Assessment of intracranial translucency (IT) in the detection of spina bifida at the 11–13-week scan. *Ultrasound Obstet Gynecol.* 2009;34:249–252.

23. Chaoui R, Benoit B, Heling KS, et al. Prospective detection of open spina bifida at 11–13 weeks by assessing intracranial translucency and posterior brain. *Ultrasound Obstet Gynecol.* 2011;38:722–726.

24. Bernard JP, Cuckle HS, Stirnemann JJ, et al. Screening for fetal spina bifida by ultrasound examination in the first trimester of pregnancy using fetal biparietal diameter. *Am J Obstet Gynecol.* 2012;207:306.e1–306.e5.

25. Karl K, Benoit B, Entezami M, et al. Small biparietal diameter in fetuses with spina bifida on 11–13-week and mid-gestation ultrasound. *Ultrasound Obstet Gynecol.* 2012;40:140–144.

26. O'Brien JE, Dvorin E, Drugan A, et al. Race-ethnicity-specific variation in multiple-marker biochemical screening: alpha-fetoprotein, hCG, and estriol. *Obstet Gynecol.* 1997;89:355–358.

27. Benn PA, Clive JM, Collins R. Medians for second-trimester maternal serum α-fetoprotein, human chorionic gonadotropin, and unconjugated estriol: differences between races or ethnic groups. *Clin Chem.* 1997;43:333–337.

28. Johnson AM, Palomaki GE, Haddow JE. The effect of adjusting maternal serum alpha-fetoprotein levels for maternal weight in pregnancies with fetal open spina bifida. A United States Collaborative Study. *Am J Obstet Gynecol.* 1990;163:9–11.

29. Wald NJ, Cuckle H, Boreham J, et al. Maternal serum alpha-fetoprotein and diabetes mellitus. *BJOG.* 1979;86:101–105.

30. Baumgarten A, Robinson J. Prospective study of an inverse relationship between maternal glycosylated hemoglobin and serum alpha-fetoprotein concentrations in pregnant women with diabetes. *Am J Obstet Gynecol.* 1988;159:77–81.

31. Evans MI, Harrison HH, O'Brien JE, et al. Correction for insulin-dependent diabetes in maternal serum alpha-fetoprotein testing has outlived its usefulness. *Am J Obstet Gynecol.* 2002;187:1084–1086.

32. Sprawka N, Lambert-Messerlian G, Palomaki GE, et al. Adjustment of maternal serum alpha-fetoprotein levels in women with pregestational diabetes. *Prenat Diagn.* 2011;31:282–285.

33. Grau P, Robinson L, Tabsch K, et al. Elevated maternal serum alpha-fetoprotein and amniotic fluid alpha-fetoprotein after multifetal pregnancy reduction. *Obstet Gynecol.* 1990;76:1042–1045.

34. Cuckle H, Wald N, Stevenson JD, et al. Maternal serum alpha-fetoprotein screening for open neural tube defects in twin pregnancies. *Prenat Diagn.* 1990;10:71–77.

35. Kumbak B, Sahin L. Elevated maternal serum alpha-fetoprotein levels in patients with subchorionic hematoma. *J Matern Fetal Neonatal Med.* 2010;23:717–719.

36. Kuo PL, Lin CC, Lin YH, et al. Placental sonolucency and pregnancy outcome in women with elevated second trimester serum alpha-fetoprotein levels. *J Formos Med Assoc.* 2003;102:319–325.

37. Zelop C, Nadel A, Frigoletto FD, et al. Placenta accreta/percreta/increta: a cause of elevated maternal serum alpha-fetoprotein. *Obstet Gynecol.* 1992;80:693–694.

38. Kupferminc MJ, Tamura RK, Wigton TR, et al. Placenta accreta is associated with elevated maternal serum alpha-fetoprotein. *Obstet Gynecol.* 1993;82:266–269.

39. Fleischer AC, Kurtz AB, Wapner RJ, et al. Elevated alpha-fetoprotein and a normal fetal sonogram: association with placental abnormalities. *AJR Am J Roentgenol.* 1988;150:881–882.

40. Jauniaux E, Moscoso G, Campbell S, et al. Correlation of ultrasound and pathologic findings of placental anomalies in pregnancies with elevated maternal serum alpha-fetoprotein. *Eur J Obstet Gynecol Reprod Biol.* 1990;37:219–230.

41. Saller DN, Canick JA, Palomaki GE, et al. Second-trimester maternal serum alpha-fetoprotein, unconjugated estriol, and hCG levels in pregnancies with ventral wall defects. *Obstet Gynecol.* 1994;84:852–855.

42. Palomaki GE, Hill LE, Knight GJ, et al. Second trimester maternal serum alpha-fetoprotein levels in pregnancies associated with gastroschisis and omphalocele. *Obstet Gynecol.* 1988;71:906–909.

43. Hogge WA, Hogge JS, Schnatterly PT, et al. Congenital nephrosis: detection of index cases through maternal serum alpha-fetoprotein screening. *Am J Obstet Gynecol.* 1992;167:1330–1333.

44. Heinonen S, Ryynanen M, Kirkinen P, et al. Prenatal screening for congenital nephrosis in east Finland: results and impact on the birth prevalence of the disease. *Prenat Diagn.* 1996;16:207–213.

45. Ghidini A, Alvarez M, Silverberg G, et al. Congenital nephrosis in low-risk pregnancies. *Prenat Diagn.* 1994;14:599–602.

46. Wapner RJ, Jenkins TM, Silverman N, et al. Prenatal diagnosis of congenital nephrosis by in utero kidney biopsy. *Prenat Diagn.* 2001;21:256–261.

47. Milunsky A, Jick SS, Bruell CL, et al. Predictive values, relative risks, and overall benefits of high and low maternal serum alpha-fetoprotein screening in singleton pregnancies: new epidemiologic data. *Am J Obstet Gynecol.* 1989;161:291–297.

48. Burton BK. Outcome of pregnancy in patients with unexplained elevated or low levels of maternal serum alpha-fetoprotein. *Obstet Gynecol.* 1988;72:709–713.

49. Huerta-Enochian G, Katz V, Erfurth S. The association of abnormal alpha-fetoprotein and adverse pregnancy outcome: does increased fetal surveillance affect pregnancy outcome? *Am J Obstet Gynecol.* 2001;184:1549–1553.

50. Waller DK, Lustig LS, Cunningham GC, et al. Second-trimester maternal serum alpha-fetoprotein levels and the risk of subsequent fetal death. *N Engl J Med.* 1991;325:6–10.

51. Smith GC, Wood AM, Pell JP, et al. Second-trimester maternal serum levels of alpha-fetoprotein and the subsequent risk of sudden infant death syndrome. *N Engl J Med.* 2004;351:978–986.

52. Campbell S, Pearce MF, Hackett G, et al. Qualitative assessment of uteroplacental blood flow: early screening test for high-risk pregnancies. *Obstet Gynecol.* 1986;68:649–653.

53. Bewley S, Cooper D, Campbell S. Doppler investigation of uteroplacental blood flow resistance in the second trimester: a screening study for pre-eclampsia and intrauterine growth retardation. *Br J Obstet Gynecol.* 1991;98:871–879.

54. Bower S, Bewley S, Campbell S. Improved prediction of preeclampsia by two-stage screening of uterine arteries using the early diastolic notch and color Doppler imaging. *Obstet Gynecol.* 1993;82:78–83.

55. Cnossen JS, Morris RK, ter Riet G, et al. Use of uterine artery Doppler ultrasonography to predict pre-eclampsia and fetal growth restriction: a systematic review and bi-variable meta-analysis. *CMAJ.* 2008;178:701–711.

56. Aristidou A, Van den Hof MC, Campbell S, et al. Uterine artery Doppler in the investigation of pregnancies with raised maternal serum alpha-fetoprotein. *BJOG.* 1990;97:431–435.

57. Bromley B, Frigoletto FD, Harlow BL, et al. The role of Doppler velocimetry in the structurally normal second-trimester fetus with elevated levels of maternal serum alpha-fetoprotein. *Ultrasound Obstet Gynecol.* 1994;4:377–380.

58. Konchak PS, Bernstein IM, Capeless EL. Uterine artery Doppler velocimetry in the detection of adverse obstetric outcomes in women with unexplained elevated maternal serum alpha-fetoprotein levels. *Am J Obstet Gynecol.* 1995;173:1115–1119.

59. Toal M, Chaddha V, Windrim R, et al. Ultrasound detection of placental insufficiency in women with elevated second trimester serum alpha-fetoprotein or human chorionic gonadotropin. *J Obstet Gynaecol Can.* 2008;30:198–206.

60. Haddow JE, Palomaki GE, Knight GJ, et al. Screening of maternal serum for fetal Down's syndrome in the first trimester. *N Engl J Med.* 1998;338:955–961.

61. Brambati B, Macintosh MCM, Teisner B, et al. Low maternal serum levels of pregnancy-associated plasma protein A (PAPP-A) in the first trimester in association with abnormal fetal karyotype. *BJOG.* 1993;100:324–326.

62. Krantz DA, Larsen JW, Buchanan PK, et al. First-trimester Down syndrome screening: free β-human chorionic gonadotropin and pregnancy-associated plasma protein A. *Am J Obstet Gynecol.* 1996;174:612–616.

63. Cuckle HS, van Lith JMM. Appropriate biochemical parameters in first-trimester screening for Down syndrome. *Prenat Diagn.* 1999;19:505–512.

64. Evans MI, Krantz DA, Hallahan TW, et al. Meta-analysis of first trimester Down syndrome screening studies: free β-human chorionic gonadotropin significantly outperforms intact human chorionic gonadotropin in a multimarker protocol. *Am J Obstet Gynecol.* 2007;196:198–205.

65. Nicolaides KH, Snijders RJ, Gosden CM, et al. Ultrasonographically detectable markers of fetal chromosomal abnormalities. *Lancet.* 1992;340:704–707.

66. Malone F, Canick JA, Ball RH, et al. First-trimester or second-trimester screening, or both, for Down's syndrome. First-and Second-Trimester Evaluation of Risk (FASTER) Research Consortium. *N Engl J Med.* 2005;353:2001–2011.

67. Tul N, Spencer K, Noble P, et al. Screening for trisomy 18 by fetal nuchal translucency and maternal serum free β-hCG and PAPP-A at 10–14 weeks of gestation. *Prenat Diagn.* 1999;19:1035–1042.

68. Spencer K, Ong C, Skentou H, et al. Screening for trisomy 13 by fetal nuchal translucency and maternal serum free β-hCG and PAPP-A at 10–14 weeks of gestation. *Prenat Diagn.* 2000;20:411–416.

69. Wapner R, Thom E, Simpson JL, et al. First trimester screening for trisomy 21 and 18. *N Engl J Med.* 2003;349:1405–1413.

70. Kagan KO, Wright D, Valencia C, et al. Screening for trisomies 21, 18 and 13 by maternal age, fetal nuchal translucency, fetal heart rate, free beta-hCG and pregnancy-associated plasma protein A. *Hum Reprod.* 2008;23:1968–1975.

71. Dugoff L, Hobbins JC, Malone FD, et al. First-trimester maternal serum PAPP-A and free-beta subunit human chorionic gonadotropin concentrations and nuchal translucency are associated with obstetric complications: a population-based screening study (The FASTER Trial). *Am J Obstet Gynecol.* 2004;191:1446–1451.

72. Lawrence JB, Oxvig C, Overgaard MT, et al. The insulin-like growth factor (IGF)-dependent IGF binding protein-4 protease secreted by human fibroblasts is pregnancy-associated plasma protein-A. *Proc Natl Acad Sci.* 1999;96:3149–3153.

73. Clemmons DR. Role of insulin-like growth factor binding proteins in controlling IGF actions. *Mol Cell Endocrinol.* 1998;140:19–24.

74. Irwin JC, Suen LF, Martina NA, et al. Role of the IGF system in trophoblast invasion and preeclampsia. *Hum Reprod.* 1999;14:S90–S96.

75. Krantz D, Goetzl L, Simpson JL, et al. Association of extreme first-trimester free human chorionic gonadotropin-β, pregnancy-associated plasma protein A, and nuchal translucency with intrauterine growth restriction and other adverse pregnancy outcomes. *Am J Obstet Gynecol.* 2004;191:1452–1458.

76. Pihl K, Sorensen TL, Norgaard-Petersen B, et al. First-trimester combined screening for Down syndrome: prediction of low birth weight, small for gestational age and pre-term delivery in a cohort of non-selected women. *Prenat Diagn.* 2008;28:247–253.

77. Smith GCS, Stenhouse J, Crossley JA, et al. Early pregnancy levels of pregnancy-associated plasma protein A and the risk of intrauterine growth restriction, premature birth, preeclampsia, and stillbirth. *J Clin Endocrinol Metab.* 2002;87:1762–1767.

78. Ong CYT, Liao AW, Spencer K, et al. First trimester maternal serum free β human chorionic gonadotropin and pregnancy associated plasma protein A as predictors of pregnancy complications. *BJOG.* 2000;107:1265–1270.

79. Goetzinger KR, Singla A, Gerkowicz S, et al. Predicting the risk of pre-eclampsia between 11 and 13 weeks' gestation by combining maternal characteristics and serum analytes, PAPP-A and free β-hCG. *Prenat Diagn.* 2010;30:1138–1142.

80. Smith GCS, Shah I, Crossley JA, et al. Pregnancy-associated plasma protein A and alpha-fetoprotein and prediction of adverse perinatal outcome. *Obstet Gynecol.* 2006;107:161–166.

81. Dugoff L, Cuckle HS, Hobbins JC, et al. Prediction of patient-specific risk for fetal loss using maternal characteristics and first- and second-trimester maternal serum Down syndrome markers. *Am J Obstet Gynecol.* 2008;199:290.e1–290.e6.

82. Peterson SE, Simhan HN. First-trimester pregnancy-associated plasma protein A and subsequent abnormalities of fetal growth. *Am J Obstet Gynecol.* 2008;198:e43–e45.

83. Goetzl L, Krantz D, Simpson JL, et al. Pregnancy-associated plasma protein A, free beta-hCG, nuchal translucency, and risk of pregnancy loss. *Obstet Gynecol.* 2004;104:30–36.

84. Hoffman JD, Bianchi DW, Sullivan LM, et al. Down syndrome screening also identifies an increased risk for multicystic dysplastic kidney, two-vessel cord, and hydrocele. *Prenat Diagn.* 2008;28:1204–1208.

85. Poon LCY, Stratieva V, Piras S, et al. Hypertensive disorders in pregnancy: combined screening by uterine artery Doppler, blood pressure and serum PAPP-A at 11–13 weeks. *Prenat Diagn.* 2010;30:216–223.

86. Pilalis A, Souka AP, Antsaklis P, et al. Screening for pre-eclampsia and fetal growth restriction by uterine artery Doppler and PAPP-A at 11–14 weeks' gestation. *Ultrasound Obstet Gynecol.* 2007;29:135–140.

87. Spencer K, Yu CKH, Cowans NJ, et al. Prediction of pregnancy complications by first-trimester maternal serum PAPP-A and free β-hCG and with second-trimester uterine artery Doppler. *Prenat Diagn.* 2005;25:949–953.

88. Cooper S, Johnson JM, Metcalfe A, et al. The predictive value of 18 and 22 week uterine artery Doppler in patients with low first trimester maternal serum PAPP-A. *Prenat Diagn.* 2009;29:248–252.

89. Merkatz IR, Nitowsky HM, Macri JN. An association between low maternal serum alpha-fetoprotein and fetal chromosomal abnormalities. *Am J Obstet Gynecol.* 1984;148:886–894.

90. Cuckle HS, Wald NJ, Lindenbaum RH. Maternal serum alpha-fetoprotein measurement: a screening test for Down syndrome. *Lancet.* 1984;1:926–929.

91. Bogart MH, Pandian MR, Jones OW. Abnormal maternal serum chorionic gonadotropin levels in pregnancies with fetal chromosome abnormalities. *Prenat Diagn.* 1987;7:623–630.

92. Wald NJ, Cuckle HS, Densem JW, et al. Maternal serum unconjugated oestriol as an antenatal screening test for Down's syndrome. *BJOG.* 1988;95:334–341.

93. Haddow JE, Palmoki GE, Knight GJ, et al. Prenatal screening for Down's syndrome with the use of maternal serum markers. *N Engl J Med.* 1992;327:588–593.

94. Haddow JE, Palmaki GE, Knight GJ, et al. Reducing the need for amniocentesis in women 35 years of age or older with serum markers for screening. *N Engl J Med.* 1994;330:1114–1118.

95. Canick JA, Palmaki GE, Osathanondh R. Prenatal screening for trisomy 18 in the second trimester. *Prenat Diagn.* 1990;10:546–548.

96. Reiner MA, Vereecken A, Van Herck E, et al. Second trimester maternal dimeric inhibin-A in the multiple marker screening test for Down's syndrome. *Hum Reprod.* 1998;13:744–748.

97. Spencer K, Wallace EM, Ritoe S. Second-trimester dimeric inhibin-A in Down's syndrome screening. *Prenat Diagn.* 1996;16:1101–1110.

98. American College of Obstetricians and Gynecologists. *Screening for Fetal Chromosomal Abnormalities.* Washington, DC: American College of Obstetricians and Gynecologists; 2007. ACOG practice bulletin no 77.

99. Watt HC, Wald NJ, Smith K, et al. Effect of allowing for ethnic group in prenatal screening for Down's syndrome. *Prenat Diagn.* 1996;16:691–698.

100. Wald NJ, Cuckle HS, Densem JW, et al. Maternal serum unconjugated oetriol and human chorionic gonadotropin levels in pregnancies with insulin-dependent diabetes: implications for screening for Down's syndrome. *BJOG.* 1992;99:51–53.

101. Huttly W, Rudnicka A, Walk NJ. Second-trimester prenatal screening markers for Down syndrome in women with insulin-dependent diabetes mellitus. *Prenat Diagn.* 2004;24:804–807.

102. Wald NJ, Rish S. Prenatal screening for Down syndrome and neural tube defects in twin pregnancies. *Prenat Diagn.* 2005;25:740–745.

103. Cole LA, Shahabi S, Oz UA, et al. Hyperglycosylated human chorionic gonadotropin (invasive trophoblast antigen) immunoassay: a new basis for gestational Down syndrome screening. *Clin Chem.* 1999;45:2109–2119.

104. Cuckle HS, Shahabi S, Sehmi IK, et al. Maternal urine hyperglycosylated hCG in pregnancies with Down syndrome. *Prenat Diagn.* 1999;19:918–920.

105. Palomaki GE, Neveux LM, Knight GJ, et al. Maternal serum invasive trophoblast antigen (hyperglycosylated hCG) as a screening marker for Down syndrome during the second trimester. *Clin Chem.* 2004;50:1804–1808.

106. Wald NJ, Cuckle HS, Boreham J, et al. Maternal serum alpha-fetoprotein and birth weight. *BJOG.* 1980;87:860–863.

107. Davenport DM, Macri JN. The clinical significance of low maternal serum alpha-fetoprotein. *Am J Obstet Gynecol.* 1983;146:657–661.

108. Simpson JL, Baum LD, Depp R, et al. Low maternal serum alpha-fetoprotein and perinatal outcome. *Am J Obstet Gynecol.* 1987;156:852–862.

109. Yaron Y, Cherry M, Kramer RL, et al. Second-trimester maternal serum marker screening: maternal serum alpha-fetoprotein, beta-human chorionic gonadotropin, estriol, and their various combinations as predictors of pregnancy outcome. *Am J Obstet Gynecol.* 1999;181:968–974.

110. Lepage N, Chitayat D, Kingdom J, et al. Association between second-trimester isolated high maternal serum human chorionic gonadotropin levels and obstetric complications. *Am J Obstet Gynecol.* 2003;188:1354–1359.

111. Chandra S, Scott H, Dodds L, et al. Unexplained elevated maternal serum α-fetoprotein and/or human chorionic gonadotropin and the risk of adverse outcomes. *Am J Obstet Gynecol.* 2003;189:775–781.

112. Fox H. Effect of hypoxia on trophoblast in organ culture: a morphologic and autoradiographic study. *Am J Obstet Gynecol.* 1970;107:1058–1064.

113. Kowalcyzyk TD, Cabaniss ML, Cusmano L. Association of low unconjugated estriol in the second trimester and adverse pregnancy outcome. *Obstet Gynecol.* 1998;91:396–400.

114. Ilagan JH, Stamilio DM, Ural SH, et al. Abnormal multiple marker screens are associated with adverse perinatal outcomes in cases of intrauterine growth restriction. *Am J Obstet Gynecol.* 2004;191:1465–1469.

115. Smith DW, Lemli L, Opitz JM. A newly recognized syndrome of multiple congenital anomalies. *J Pediatr.* 1964;64:210–217.

116. Bradley LA, Palomaki GE, Knight GJ, et al. Levels of unconjugated estriol and other maternal serum markers in pregnancies with Smith-Lemli-Opitz (RSH) syndrome fetuses. *Am J Med Genet.* 1999;82:355–358.

117. Schoen E, Norem C, O'Keefe J, et al. Maternal serum unconjugated estriol as a predictor for Smith-Lemli-Opitz syndrome and other fetal conditions. *Obstet Gynecol.* 2003;102:167–172.

118. Craig WY, Haddow JE, Palomaki GE, et al. Identifying Smith-Lemli-Opitz syndrome in conjunction with prenatal screening for Down syndrome. *Prenat Diagn.* 2006;26:842–849.

119. Rossiter JP, Hofman KJ, Kelley RI. Smith-Lemli-Opitz syndrome: prenatal diagnosis by quantification of cholesterol precursors in amniotic fluid. *Am J Med Genet.* 1995;56:272–275.

120. Bradley LA, Canick JA, Palomaki GE. Undetectable maternal serum unconjugated estriol levels in the second trimester: risk of perinatal complications associated with placental sulfatase deficiency. *Am J Obstet Gynecol.* 1997;176:531–535.

121. Cuckle H, Sehmi I, Jones R. Maternal serum inhibin A can predict pre-eclampsia. *BJOG.* 1998;105:1101–1103.

122. Lambert-Messerlin GM, Silver HM, Petraglia F, et al. Second-trimester levels of maternal serum human chorionic gonadotropin and inhibin A as predictors of pre-eclampsia in the third trimester of pregnancy. *J Soc Gynecol Invest.* 2000;7:170–174.

123. Aquilina J, Maplethorpe R, Ellis P, et al. Correlation between second trimester maternal serum inhibin-A and human chorionic gonadotropin for the prediction of pre-eclampsia. *Placenta.* 2000;21:487–492.

124. Ay E, Kavak ZN, Elter K, et al. Screening for pre-eclampsia by using maternal serum inhibin A, activin A, human chorionic gonadotropin, unconjugated estriol, and alpha-fetoprotein levels and uterine artery Doppler in the second trimester of pregnancy. *Aust N Z J Obstet Gynaecol.* 2005;45:283–288.

125. Dugoff L, Hobbins JC, Malone FD, et al. Quad screen as a predictor of adverse pregnancy outcome. *Obstet Gynecol.* 2005;106:260–267.

126. Huang T, Hoffman B, Meschino W, et al. Prediction of adverse pregnancy outcomes by combinations of first and second trimester biochemistry

markers used in the routine prenatal screening of Down syndrome. *Prenat Diagn.* 2010;30:471–477.

127. Bradshaw R, Odibo AO. Smith-Lemli-Opitzs syndrome. In: Copel JA, ed. Obstetric Imaging. Philadelphia, PA: Saunders; 2012:656–657.

128. Aquilina J, Thompson O, Thilaganathan B, et al. Improved early prediction of pre-eclampsia by combining second-trimester maternal serum inhibin-A and uterine artery Doppler. *Ultrasound Obstet Gynecol.* 2001;17:477–484.

129. Florio P, Reis FM, Pezzani I, et al. The addition of activin A and inhibin A measurement to uterine artery Doppler velocimetry to improve the early prediction of pre-eclampsia. *Ultrasound Obstet Gynecol.* 2003;21:165–169.

130. Spencer K, Yu CK, Savvidou M, et al. Prediction of pre-eclampsia by uterine artery Doppler ultrasonography and maternal serum pregnancy-associated plasma protein-A, free beta-human chorionic gonadotropin, activin A and inhibin A at 22 + 0 to 24+6 weeks' gestation. *Ultrasound Obstet Gynecol.* 2006;27:658–663.

131. Filippi E, Staughton J, Peregrine E, et al. Uterine artery Doppler and adverse pregnancy outcome in women with extreme levels of fetoplacental proteins used for Down syndrome screening. *Ultrasound Obstet Gynecol.* 2011;37:520–527.

132. Bianchi DW, Parker RL, Wentworth J, et al. DNA sequencing versus standard prenatal aneuploidy screening. *N Engl J Med.* 2014;370:799–808.

133. Nicolaides KH, Syngelaki A, Gil MM, et al. Prenatal detection of fetal triploidy from cell-free DNA testing in maternal blood. *Fetal Diagn Ther.* 2014;35:212–217.

134. Norton ME, Brar H, Weiss J, et al. Non-Invasive Chromosomal Evaluation (NICE) Study: results of a multicenter prospective cohort study for detection of fetal trisomy 21 and 18. *Am J Obstet Gynecol.* 2012;207:137.e1–e137.e8.

135. National Coalition for Health Professionals in Genetics (HPEG) and National Society of Genetic Counselors (NSGC). *Noninvasive Prenatal Screening (NIPT) Factsheet.* 2012. Available at http://www.nchpeg.org/index.php?option=com_content&view=article&id=384&Itemid=255. Accessed May 12, 2014.

136. Cheddy S, Garabedian NJ, Norton ME. Update of noninvasive prenatal testing (NIPT) in women following positive aneuploidy screening. *Prenat Diagn.* 2013;33(6):542–546.

137. Ashoor G, Poon L, Syngelaki A, et al. Fetal fraction in maternal plasma cell-free DNA at 11–13 weeks' gestation: effect of maternal and fetal factors. *Fetal Diagn Ther.* 2012;31(4):237–243.

138. Devers PL, Cronister A, Ormond KE, et al. Noninvasive prenatal testing/noninvasive prenatal diagnosis: the position of the National Society of Genetic Counselors. *J Genetic Counsel.* 2013;22:291–295.

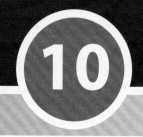
Sonia S. Hassan • Tinnakorn Chaiworapongsa • Jennifer Lam-Rachlin • Amy E. Whitten • Edgar Hernandez-Andrade • Roberto Romero

The uterine cervix plays a central role in the maintenance of pregnancy; its function is critical to normal and pathologic (preterm delivery, arrest of dilation) labor and delivery. During most of normal gestation, the cervix remains firm and closed, despite a progressive increase in the size of the fetus and uterine distention. At the end of pregnancy and during labor, the cervix softens, shortens, and dilates to allow delivery of the fetus. Labor, delivery, and the postpartum period are accompanied by dramatic changes in the uterine cervix.[1-13] Early activation of parturition can often be visualized in the form of a prematurely shortened cervix. Cervical disorders have been implicated in common obstetrical complications, such as "cervical insufficiency,"[14] preterm labor and delivery,[15-18] and abnormal term parturition.[19] Progress has been made toward decreasing the rate of preterm birth with the use of progestogens.[20-24] Yet, preterm parturition is a syndrome with many etiologies, and further investigation is needed. It is well established that a sonographic short cervix is the most powerful predictor of spontaneous preterm birth.[15-18,25-41] This chapter will focus on the role of sonographic cervical length in the prediction and prevention of preterm birth. Diagnostic and therapeutic techniques will be presented. Although the chapter will not emphasize fetal magnetic resonance imaging (MRI) in the evaluation of the cervix, it is imperative that the configuration and competency of the cervix is assessed on every MR exam, especially in the presence of polyhydramnios and twin gestation.

## THE ROLE OF THE CERVIX IN PRETERM PARTURITION

Preterm birth is the leading cause of perinatal morbidity and infant mortality worldwide;[42] In 2005, 12.9 million preterm births were born globally, with over 500,000 in the United States alone.[42] The consequences of preterm birth include respiratory distress syndrome (RDS), necrotizing enterocolitis, neonatal sepsis, cerebral palsy, cognitive disability, and neonatal death.[43]

We have proposed that parturition has a common terminal pathway characterized by increased myometrial contractility, cervical ripening, and membrane/decidual activation.[44] These processes are required for both term and preterm parturition. Normal labor at term is characterized by coordinated activation of these three mechanisms, while premature activation is observed in patients with preterm labor with progressive cervical dilation leading to preterm delivery. Premature cervical ripening may result in a spectrum of disease ranging from midtrimester abortion, preterm labor with or without preterm delivery, and precipitous labor at term.

Importantly, sonographic cervical length is more informative for the prediction of preterm birth than a history of previous preterm birth.[15-18,25-41,45] Sonographic cervical length is not a screening test for spontaneous preterm delivery, because only some patients who will have a spontaneous preterm birth have a short cervix in the midtrimester. However, sonographic cervical length is a method for risk assessment for spontaneous preterm delivery. Furthermore, its importance derives from the observation that patients with or without a history of previous preterm birth, and a short cervix, benefit from treatment.[22-24,46-49]

## SONOGRAPHIC EVALUATION

Assessment of the cervix includes sonographic imaging as well as digital examination. Sonographic imaging of the cervix is a less invasive, more precise and objective method of assessing the cervical status when compared with digital examination.[50]

### Which Method Should Be Used to Examine the Cervix?

The cervix can be evaluated by ultrasound using a transabdominal, transvaginal, and transperineal approach. The transvaginal technique is the preferred method for optimal assessment of the cervix owing to the limitations in image acquisition by the other approaches. Transabdominal sonography requires a full bladder for adequate visualization of the cervix; as a result, bladder distension can compress and artificially lengthen the cervix.[26,51,52] In contrast, transvaginal ultrasound does not require a distended bladder. Cervical length measurements are longer (by 5.2 mm on average) when assessed by transabdominal ultrasound when compared with transvaginal ultrasound.[26] Furthermore, transabdominal ultrasound does not detect a short cervical length in 57% of the cases.[53]

The transperineal technique, introduced prior to the development of the transvaginal transducer, can be used when a transvaginal transducer is not available, and does not require a full bladder[54-59]; yet the presence of air in the vagina or bowel gas may obscure the image obtained by transperineal ultrasound, and a clear image of the cervix cannot be obtained in 30% of patients in the midtrimester and 19% of patients in the third trimester.[59] In summary, transvaginal ultrasound is the recommended technique for evaluation of the uterine cervix in pregnancy.

### Technique

Patients are asked to empty their bladder before conducting a transvaginal ultrasound. During the procedure, the patient lies in the supine position with flexed knees and hips. The probe is covered with either a glove or an appropriate sheath. Gel is placed between the transducer and the cover as well as on the surface sheath. The operator introduces the vaginal probe into the anterior fornix until a midline sagittal view of the cervix and lower uterine segment are seen. The internal os, external os, cervical canal, and endocervical mucosa should be clearly identified (Fig. 10.1). The endocervical mucosa is used to define the upper edge of the cervix. Otherwise, cervical length may erroneously include part of the lower uterine segment.

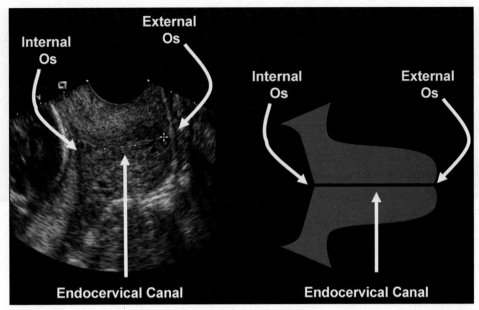

**FIGURE 10.1:** Transvaginal sonographic appearance of a normal uterine cervix; the *internal os*, the *external os*, and the *endocervical canal* are easily visualized. (From Gomez R, Galasso M, Romero R, et al. Ultrasonographic examination of the uterine cervix is better than cervical digital examination as a predictor of the likelihood of premature delivery in patients with preterm labor and intact membranes. *Am J Obstet Gynecol.* 1994;171(4):956–964, copyright © 1994 with permission from Elsevier.)

Excessive pressure with the probe may elongate the cervix. To avoid this pitfall, the probe is slowly withdrawn until the image blurs and pressure is subsequently reapplied to restore the image. This can be avoided by confirming equal cervical width and density of the anterior and posterior lips of the endocervical canal (Fig. 10.2).[60,61]

Cervical length is measured on three separate images. The optimal length of examination ranges from 5 to 10 minutes. If the duration of the examination is too short and the patient has dynamic cervical change during the examination, the cervical length may not represent the true length of the cervix. This may account for some observations in which patients seem to gain cervical length over time. The contours of the anterior and posterior lips of the ectocervix are usually clearly defined. For clinical purposes, the shortest cervical length is reported provided that the image is adequate.

When the cervical canal is curved, the cervical length can be determined by tracing along the canal or by adding the sum of two straight sections. To et al.[62] concluded from a prospective study conducted in 301 women at 23 weeks of gestation that the question of whether to measure the cervix as a straight line or along the cervical canal might not have any clinical significance because a short cervix (<16 mm) is always straight.

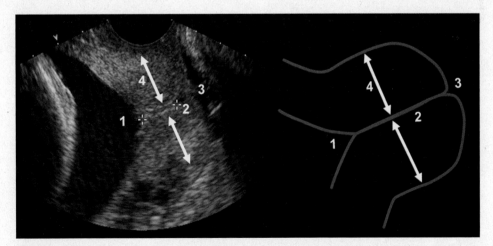

**FIGURE 10.2:** Transvaginal sonographic appearance of a cervix with a schematic to display common pitfalls and landmarks: *(1)*, internal os; *(2)*, visualization of entire endocervical canal; *(3)*, external os; *(4)*, the distance between the anterior lip of the cervix to the cervical canal and the posterior lip of the cervix and the cervical canal are equal. (Reproduced with permission from Burger M, Weber-Rossler T, Willmann M. Measurement of the pregnant cervix by transvaginal sonography: an interobserver study and new standards to improve the interobserver variability. *Ultrasound Obstet Gynecol.* 1997;9(3):188–193.)

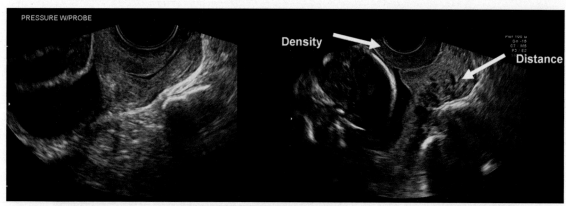

**FIGURE 10.3:** This transvaginal sonographic image of the cervix demonstrates two pitfalls that can occur when assessing cervical length. **A:** Excessive probe pressure (can cause the cervical length to appear falsely long). **B:** Suboptimal image, which displays unequal size and density of the anterior and posterior lips of the cervix. (Reproduced with permission from Hassan SS, Chaiworapongsa T, Vaisbuch E, et al. Sonographic examination of the uterine cervix. In: Fleischer AC, Toy CT, Lee W, et al, eds. *Sonography in Obstetrics and Gynecology: Principles and Practice.* 7th ed. New York, NY: McGraw-Hill Medical; 2011:816–847.)

Although cervical examination may appear simple to the experienced sonographer, certain patients may present significant challenges. The presence of a large cervical polyp can affect the identification of the correct cervical plane.[63] In addition, a cervix with an unusual orientation may be difficult to find. Therefore, several potential pitfalls should be avoided. These include: (1) excessive probe pressure (falsely long measurement; Fig. 10.3A); (2) short examination time (miss true cervical shortening); (3) recognition of a poorly developed lower uterine segment (avoid falsely long measurement); (4) unequal size and density of the anterior and posterior lips (Fig. 10.3B); and (5) recognition of amniotic fluid "sludge" (Fig. 10.4) (the

clinical significance of amniotic fluid "sludge" is reviewed later in this chapter).

Specific recommendations for standardization of each cervical exam within the ultrasound unit can improve the quality of the image acquired (see Fig. 10.2).[61] These include obtaining the following criteria on each image of the cervix:

- Flat internal os or isosceles triangle,
- Entire length of the cervical canal,
- Symmetric image of external os, and
- Equal size and density of the anterior and posterior lips of the cervix.

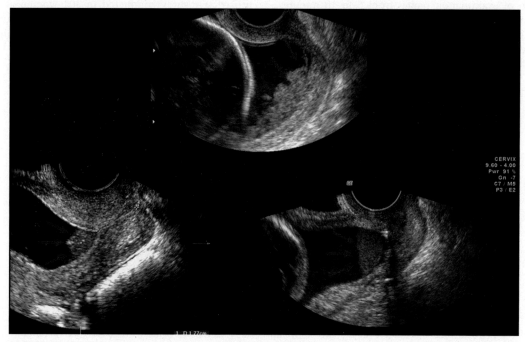

**FIGURE 10.4:** Transvaginal sonographic images of three patients with short cervices. The *arrows* illustrate the presence of dense aggregates of particulate matter in close proximity to the internal cervical os, termed amniotic fluid "sludge." (Reproduced with permission from Hassan SS, Chaiworapongsa T, Vaisbuch E, et al. Sonographic examination of the uterine cervix. In: Fleischer AC, Toy CT, Lee W, et al, eds. *Sonography in Obstetrics and Gynecology: Principles and Practice.* 7th ed. New York, NY: McGraw-Hill Medical; 2011:816–847.)

## First Trimester Cervical Sonography for Risk Assessment

The identification of a short cervix, and therefore a patient at risk of preterm birth, early in pregnancy would allow for more timely identification and treatment (if such an intervention is proven) of women destined to have a midtrimester loss prior to the typical midgestation cervical length examination. The accurate measurement of cervical length in the first trimester can be technically difficult as the lower uterine segment may not be distended and can appear to be part of the cervix. Several authors have evaluated the use of first trimester cervical length to predict preterm birth.[64–70]

Several independent studies concluded that cervical length obtained by first trimester ultrasound does not reliably predict preterm birth.[64–67] However, some have described a modified technique to identify the true cervical length and exclude the lower uterine isthmus.[68,71] Endocervical length at 11 to 13 weeks was shorter in women who delivered before 34 weeks compared with those who delivered after 34 weeks. The use of sonographic cervical length at 11 to 13 weeks' gestational age in combination with maternal characteristics such as ethnicity and obstetrical history to predict preterm birth; approximately, 55% of preterm deliveries before 34 weeks could be predicted with a false-positive rate of 10%.[68–70]

## Midtrimester Cervical Sonography for Preterm Birth Risk Assessment

The optimal gestational age to examine the cervix for preterm birth risk assessment is in the midtrimester of pregnancy. The predictive value of cervical length is greater at 19 to 24 weeks when compared with earlier in gestation (i.e., 14 to 24 weeks).[17,18,64–70] Furthermore, effective interventions have been demonstrated in trials that have evaluated the uterine cervix at 19 to 25 weeks' gestation.[22–24]

## PREDICTING PRETERM BIRTH

Cervical length is generally stable in the first 30 weeks of an uncomplicated pregnancy in nulliparous and in multiparous women, and a progressive (although not substantial) shortening of the cervix occurs in the third trimester of pregnancy.[15,25,27,72–75] Because transvaginal ultrasound is the most reliable method to assess cervical length, cervical sonography has been used to assess the risk for preterm birth in three groups: (1) asymptomatic low-risk patients; (2) asymptomatic patients with risk factors identifying them as high risk for preterm birth and/or midtrimester loss; and (3) patients presenting with symptoms of preterm labor. This section will highlight some of the studies that have contributed to establishing the value of cervical sonography in the risk assessment for spontaneous preterm birth. Emerging strategies for risk assessment will also be discussed.

## Cervical Length for the Prediction of Preterm Delivery

### Low-Risk, Asymptomatic Patients

Andersen et al.[15] conducted one of the first studies to evaluate the relationship between a sonographic short cervix and the risk of spontaneous preterm birth in a cohort of 113 women who were evaluated by transabdominal and transvaginal sonography, along with manual assessment of the cervix on one occasion before 30 weeks' gestation. The patient population, with an overall prematurity rate of 15%, was not separated into low-risk and high-risk categories. The authors reported that a cervical length of <39 mm is associated with a 25% risk of preterm delivery, while a long cervix (defined as a cervical length ≥39 mm) decreases the risk of preterm birth (6.7%).[15] Furthermore, the risk of spontaneous preterm birth was inversely related to the cervical length. These findings have been confirmed by other investigators, both in low-risk[15,17,18,25,27–32,35,37,39,41,75–79] and in high-risk asymptomatic patients.[33,36,38,40,60,80–82] Table 10.1 describes the details of some of the studies with adequate information to allow calculation of diagnostic indices and predictive values.

In a prospective cohort study, patients were examined at 24 and 28 weeks of gestation by transvaginal sonography to evaluate the cervix and calculate the risk of delivery prior to 35 weeks.[30] There was an exponential increase in the relative risk of delivering <35 weeks as cervical length shortened (Fig. 10.5). This study confirmed the results of Andersen et al.,[15] indicating

| Table 10.1 | Diagnostic Indices of Sonographic Cervical Length in Low-Risk, Asymptomatic Pregnant Women According to Different Cervical Length Cutoffs | | | | | | | | |
|---|---|---|---|---|---|---|---|---|---|
| **Reference** | **Year** | **N** | **Gestation (wk)** | **Cutoff (mm)** | **Definition of PTD (wk)** | **Prevalence of PTD (%)** | **Sensitivity (%)** | **Specificity (%)** | **PPV (%)** | **NPV (%)** |
| Andersen et al.[15] | 1990 | 113 | <30 | <39 | <37 | 15 | 76 | 59 | 25 | 93 |
| Tongsong et al.[77] | 1995 | 730 | 28–30 | ≤35 | <37 | 12 | 66 | 62 | 20 | 93 |
| Iams et al.[30] | 1996 | 2,915 | 24 | <20 | <35 | 4 | 23 | 97 | 26 | 97 |
| Taipale and Hiilesmaa[34] | 1998 | 3,694 | 18–22 | ≤25 | <37 | 2 | 6 | 100 | 39 | 99 |
| Heath et al.[17] | 1998 | 2,702 | 23 | ≤15 | ≤32 | 1.5 | 58 | 99 | 52 | 99 |
| Hassan et al.[18] | 2000 | 6,877 | 14–24 | ≤15 | ≤32 | 3.6 | 8 | 99 | 47 | 97 |

PTD, preterm delivery; PPV, positive predictive value; NPV, negative predictive value.
Reproduced with permission from Gervasi M-T, Romero R, Maymon E, et al. Ultrasound examination of the uterine cervix during pregnancy. In: Fleischer AC, Manning FA, Jeanty P, et al, eds. *Sonography in Obstetrics and Gynecology: Principles and Practice*. 6th ed. New York, NY: McGraw-Hill; 2001:821–841.

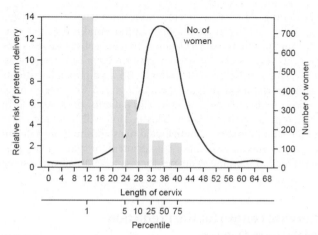

**FIGURE 10.5:** Distribution of subjects among percentiles for cervical length measured by transvaginal ultrasonography at 24 weeks of gestation (*solid line*) and relative risk of spontaneous preterm delivery before 35 weeks of gestation according to percentiles for cervical length (*bars*). (Reproduced with permission from Iams JD, Goldenberg RL, Meis PJ, et al. The length of the cervix and the risk of spontaneous premature delivery. *N Engl J Med.* 1996;334(9):567–572, copyright © 1996, Massachusetts Medical Society.)

that a short cervix increases the risk for preterm delivery, while the risk is reduced as the cervical length increases.[30]

In a population of 2,567 women,[17] patients with a history of preterm birth, Afro-Caribbean origin, low maternal age (<20 years), and with low body mass index had a shorter cervix than those without such risk factors. When logistic regression analysis was used to examine the contribution of all these parameters to the prediction of preterm birth (≤32 weeks), a transvaginal sonographic short cervix was the best predictor of outcome.[17] Our group evaluated 6,877 women with cervical sonography performed between 14 and 24 weeks. Based on the clinical practice of the ultrasound unit at the time of this study, examinations were initially performed transabdominally and, in cases of cervical length <30 mm or suboptimal visualization, cervical length was evaluated by transvaginal ultrasound.[18] (Currently, our unit evaluates the uterine cervix by transvaginal ultrasound); a cervical length of 15 mm or less was associated with preterm delivery at <32 weeks in almost 50% of cases. A history of preterm delivery and African American ethnicity were also associated with the occurrence of spontaneous preterm birth, although the odds ratio was considerably lower than that of a short cervix.[18]

Thus, several studies have confirmed and extended the observations of Andersen et al.[15] in asymptomatic patients at low risk for preterm delivery.[15,17,18,25,27,29–32,34–37,39,41,72,77–79,83–85] While the studies evaluating the predictive ability of a short cervix for preterm birth are difficult to compare directly because of differences in study design (i.e., gestational age at cervical length measurement and assessed outcomes), these data have consistently shown that the shorter the cervical length measurement, the higher the risk for preterm birth. Of note, at least one-third of patients who deliver preterm (<32 weeks) will not have a short cervix in the midtrimester; hence, cervical length measurement with ultrasound is not a screening tool but rather a method for risk assessment. The high positive predictive value of a short cervix (nearly 50% for spontaneous preterm birth <32 weeks for cervical length ≤15 mm) has justified trials of

intervention (progesterone, cerclage, and pessary to prevent preterm birth).[22–24,46–49]

### High-Risk Singleton Gestations

Several authors have evaluated the utility of cervical length in assessing the risk of preterm birth in women with a history of preterm birth, excisional cervical procedure, known uterine anomaly, or second trimester dilation and evacuation surgery.[33,38,72,80,82,86–93]

Guzman et al.[33] enrolled 469 high-risk patients between 15 and 24 weeks of gestation. High risk was defined as the presence of a history of spontaneous preterm birth before 37 weeks of gestation, prior midtrimester loss, more than two terminations of pregnancy, cone biopsy, uterine malformation, previous cerclage, and exposure to diethylstilbestrol (DES) exposure. Transvaginal cervical sonography and transfundal pressure were performed, and the shortest cervical length, funnel width, funnel length, and cervical index were recorded serially. Cervical length was the best parameter in the prediction of preterm birth in women with prior midtrimester losses.

Owen conducted an observational study that included 183 patients with a history of spontaneous preterm birth before 32 weeks of gestation.[38] Patients were enrolled between 16 and 19 weeks of gestation and followed every 2 weeks until 24 weeks of gestation. Forty-eight (26%) women delivered before 35 weeks of gestation. A short cervix (<25 mm) at the first scan was associated with a relative risk of 3.3 (95% CI, 2.1 to 5.0) for spontaneous preterm birth (<35 weeks). The sensitivity, specificity, and positive predictive values were 19%, 98%, and 75%, respectively. After controlling for cervical length, neither funneling nor dynamic shortening were independent predictors of spontaneous preterm birth.

A systematic review of 14 studies evaluating the use of sonographic cervical length to predict preterm birth in patients at high risk for preterm birth demonstrated that patients with a history of spontaneous preterm delivery and a cervical length of <25 mm at <20 weeks had a positive likelihood ratio (LR) of 11.30 (95% CI, 3.59 to 35.57) and at 20 to 24 weeks an LR of 2.86 (95% CI, 2.12 to 3.87), respectively, for delivery at <35 weeks.[91]

A sonographic short cervix is also predictive of preterm birth in other high-risk populations such as patients with uterine anomalies[81] or those with multiple, prior-induced abortions.[82]

The hypothesis that cervical competence or sufficiency represents a spectrum was studied by Parikh and Mehta,[94] who used digital examination of the cervix to assess sufficiency. The authors, however, concluded that degrees of cervical competence did not exist. In contrast, Iams et al.,[28] using sonographic examination of the cervix, demonstrated that cervical sufficiency/insufficiency is a continuum. The authors reported a strong relationship between cervical length and previous obstetrical history. This relationship was nearly linear, and patients with a typical history of an "insufficient" cervix did not constitute a separate group from those who delivered preterm.[28] Similar results have been reported by Guzman et al.[95] Collectively, these studies suggest that there is a relationship between a history of preterm delivery and the cervical length in a subsequent pregnancy. Considering that patients with a short cervix are at increased risk for a midtrimester pregnancy loss (clinically referred to as "cervical insufficiency" by some physicians) or spontaneous preterm delivery with intact or rupture of membranes,[15–18,25–30,33,34,36–41,77–80,95] a short cervix can be considered to be the expression of a spectrum of cervical diseases or abnormal function. It is noteworthy that some women with a short cervix have an adverse pregnancy outcome, while others have an uncomplicated term delivery.[15,17,25–28,30,33,39,95–98] Indeed, approximately 50% of women with a cervix of 15 mm or less deliver after 32 weeks.[17,18] This indicates that cervical length may be only one of the factors determining the degree of cervical strength, and that a short cervix should not be equated with "cervical insufficiency."

The rate of change in cervical length is associated with spontaneous preterm birth <36 weeks among women with a sonographic short cervix <25 mm.[99] Two thousand six hundred ninety-five (2,695) women with a singleton gestation from the general population had a transvaginal cervical length ultrasound performed at 24 weeks (range, 21 to 28 weeks) and a repeat evaluation at 28 weeks (range, 25 to 33 weeks). The change in cervical length (the difference between cervical length at 24 and 28 weeks) was the primary variable of interest. Loss of cervical length between 24 and 28 weeks was represented as a negative value for change in cervical length, while gain in cervical length resulted in a positive value. Calculation of the rate of change was done by dividing the difference in cervical length by the number of days between measurements. The relationships between change in cervical length, average daily change in cervical length, and spontaneous preterm birth <36 weeks were evaluated using logistic regression. The results demonstrate that among women with a sonographic short cervix (<25 mm), change in cervical length between the two visits was significantly associated with a probability of spontaneous preterm birth <36 weeks (odds ratio 0.97; 95% confidence interval, 0.96 to 0.98). In other words, an increase in cervical length between the two visits resulted in decreased risk of spontaneous preterm birth, and conversely, a decrease in cervical length between the two visits resulted in increased risk of spontaneous preterm birth.

Celik et al. proposed the use of an individualized risk assessment for the prediction of preterm birth. The authors conducted a large, prospective observational study of over 58,000 patients.[45] Transvaginal sonographic cervical length screening was performed between 20 and 24 6/7 weeks. All patients received routine antenatal care and were given the option to participate in one of two randomized clinical trials of intervention (cerclage or progesterone) if they had a sonographic cervical length of 15 mm or less. Patients who had received the active intervention of either trial were excluded from the risk assessment study. Obstetrical history was subdivided into five groups: (1) primigravida or only pregnancy losses prior to 16 weeks; previous preterm delivery (defined by earliest preterm birth) at (2) 16 to 23 weeks; (3) 24 to 33 weeks; (4) 34 to 36 weeks; or (5) term (>36 weeks). Adjusted odds ratios were calculated for spontaneous delivery at <28 weeks (extreme), 28 to 30 weeks (early), 31 to 33 weeks (moderate), and 34 to 36 weeks (mild) using logistic regression analysis. The authors concluded that cervical length was the best predictor of spontaneous preterm birth. The risk estimation was improved by the addition of obstetric history, but not any maternal characteristics or other interactions. This important study includes tables that provide LRs to allow for the risk assessment of spontaneous preterm birth. The detection rates of extreme, early, moderate, and mild spontaneous preterm birth, by combining

the obstetric history and cervical length, were 80.6%, 58.5%, 53.0%, and 28.6%, respectively, with a 10% screen-positive rate.[45] This model provides for a higher detection rate than obstetric history or cervical length alone, and allows for population-based screening, which in a setting of potential effective interventions, may have great value.

## Repeat Sonographic Evaluation of Cervix

Carvalho et al.[65] evaluated the utility of serial cervical length measurements obtained at 11 to 14, and at 22 to 24 weeks of gestation in an unselected group of pregnant women. The authors found that cervical length at 11 to 14 weeks was not significantly different between women who delivered preterm and term, but that the cervical length assessments obtained in the second trimester were predictive of preterm delivery; the shortening between the first and the second exam was more pronounced in the group that delivered preterm. Ozdemir et al.[100] subsequently confirmed the observation of a more rapid cervical change between the first and the second trimesters in women destined to deliver preterm.

Several other groups have evaluated repeated measurements in the second trimester and the rate of change in cervical length associated with the risk of preterm birth in high- and low-risk patients.[33,99,101–105] Cervical Length was measured serially in high-risk women between 15 and 24 weeks' gestation. The rate of change in women who did not develop cervical insufficiency was nonsignificant, while those women destined to develop a cervix <2 cm in length, defined as "insufficient," had a significant rate of cervical length change of −0.52 cm per week.[33] Serial evaluation of cervical length in women who were found to have a short cervix between 1 and 25 mm on an initial scan between 16 and 28 weeks,[102] demonstrated that the women whose cervix underwent further shortening on the second measurement delivered at an earlier gestational age (36 + 4 vs. 38 + 2 weeks, P = .031). These data collectively indicate that cervical shortening is a part of the activation of the parturition process. This shortening occurs as a continuum, and subsequent cervical length measurements in women at risk may help to differentiate those with a short cervix who will deliver at term, and those who will have a preterm delivery. Moroz and Simhan[99] evaluated the difference in cervical length between 24 and 28 weeks in a cohort of women from the general obstetric population. Within the group of women with an initial cervical length <25 mm, additional shortening was associated with an increased risk of preterm birth. The authors also suggest a lower risk of preterm birth in women with an initially identified short cervix if the cervix remained stable or increased in length. As the interval for repeat exam reported in the literature varies from 1 to 8 weeks,[102] the optimal timing of a repeat measurement and how clinical management should be adjusted is yet to be determined.

In practice, most algorithms for the management of patients at risk for preterm birth include serial ultrasound evaluation of the uterine cervix; however, there is no consensus on the time interval between measurements, patient population requiring serial ultrasound evaluation, and whether serial evaluations improve pregnancy outcomes.

## Cervical Length in Multiple Gestations

### Twin Pregnancies

Twin gestations occur in 1% of all pregnancies and are at increased risk of preterm birth. Several studies have examined the value of transvaginal sonography for the prediction of preterm delivery in twin pregnancies, and reported an increased risk for preterm birth in patients with a sonographic short cervix.[106–121]

The sensitivity of a short cervix defined as a length of 25 mm or less at 23 weeks' gestation in the prediction of spontaneous preterm delivery at 28, 30, 32, and 34 weeks is 100%, 80%, 47%, and 35%, respectively (Table 10.2).[111] The rate of spontaneous delivery at or before 32 weeks increases exponentially with decreasing cervical length measured at 23 weeks. The risk of preterm delivery for patients with a cervical length of 25 mm or less in twin pregnancies is similar to the risk in singleton pregnancies with a cervical length of 15 mm or less (52%).[17,18] Thus, the cervical length required in twin gestations to provide assurance against the occurrence of preterm delivery is greater than that of singleton gestations. Furthermore, ninety-seven percent of twin gestations with a cervical length of 35 mm or more deliver after 34 weeks of gestation.[110]

The median cervical length for twins at 23 weeks' gestation is similar to singletons (36 mm).[114] However, a greater proportion of twin pregnancies have a cervical length of 25 mm or less (12.9%[114]) when compared with singletons (8.4%[122]). The same holds true for patients with a cervical length of 15 mm or less (4.5% in twins[114] vs. 1.5% in singletons[122]).

Fox et al. reported the utility of a repeat cervical exam 2 to 6 weeks after obtaining a baseline exam at 18 to 24 weeks. Among twin pregnancies in which the cervical length decreased by 20% or more, there was an increased risk of preterm birth, even in the setting of a normal cervical length (36.8% rate of preterm birth at <34 weeks vs. 12.9% with stable exam, $P = .018$).[123]

Conde-Agudelo et al. performed a systematic review and meta-analysis of the predictive test accuracy for cervical length in asymptomatic twin pregnancies. Among asymptomatic women, a cervical length ≤20 mm at 20 to 24 weeks' gestation had a pooled positive LR of 10.1 and a negative LR of 0.64 to predict preterm birth <32 weeks. A cervical length ≤25 mm at 20 to 24 weeks' gestation had a pooled positive LR of 9.6 to predict preterm birth <28 weeks of gestation.[124]

Sonographic cervical length is predictive of preterm birth in twin gestations in acute preterm labor and can predict those who will deliver within 7 days from those who will not.[118] In a study of 87 twin pregnancies presenting in preterm labor, 80% (4 of 5) of patients with a cervical length of 1 to 5 mm delivered within 7 days, in contrast to 0% (0 of 21) of patients with a cervical length of >25 mm.[118] A cutoff of 25 mm (≤25) has

been proposed for the risk assessment of preterm birth in twin pregnancies.[118,120]

The utility of preoperative sonographic cervical length in predicting preterm birth in 137 cases of twin-to-twin transfusion syndrome (TTTS) undergoing laser coagulation of placental anastomoses before 26 weeks' gestation has been examined.[119] The risk of delivery prior to 34 weeks was 74% in patients with a cervical length <30 mm. In addition, logistic regression analysis identified cervical length <30 mm (OR 3.53 [1.55 to 8.03]) and being multiparous (OR 2.27 [1.09 to 4.74]) as independent risk factors for preterm birth at <34 weeks.[119]

### Triplet Pregnancies

Cervical length is also predictive of preterm delivery in triplet gestations.[125–127] The sensitivity, specificity, positive predictive value, and negative predictive value of a short cervical length measured between 21 and 24 weeks and between 25 and 28 weeks are 86%, 79%, 40%, 97%, and 100%, 57%, 18%, 100%, respectively. A short cervix identifies triplet pregnancies at risk for preterm birth and, for an equal cervical length measurement in a singleton pregnancy; the risk of preterm delivery in a triplet pregnancy is higher.[125–127] The identification of patients at risk of preterm birth with triplet gestations may be improved with the combination of cervical length assessment and fetal fibronectin (fFN) testing. In a retrospective study, Fox et al.,[128] evaluated the combination of fFN and cervical length as predictors of preterm birth in triplet pregnancies. A historical cohort of 39 consecutive women with triplet pregnancies managed in one maternal–fetal medicine practice from 2005 to 2011 were included into the analysis for this study. A positive fFN was significantly associated with spontaneous preterm birth <28, <30, <32, and <34 weeks, while a sonographic short cervix was significantly associated with spontaneous preterm birth <32 weeks gestation. Combined screening of fFN and cervical length assessment in asymptomatic triple pregnancy and positive results in both tests were associated with the highest likelihood of spontaneous preterm birth at all gestational ages. For example, a positive fFN with a short cervix had a sensitivity of 62.5%, specificity of 90%, positive predictive value of 62.5%, and negative predictive value of 90% for the prediction of spontaneous preterm birth <32 weeks' gestation. The authors suggest that the combination of fFN and cervical length assessment in the screening of asymptomatic triplet pregnancies for the prediction of spontaneous preterm birth is useful.

| Table 10.2 | Rate of Indicated and Spontaneous Delivery at Different Gestations and Sensitivity for Spontaneous Delivery According to Cervical Length in Twin Pregnancies |

| Gestation (wk) | N | Iatrogenic Delivery | Spontaneous Delivery | Cervical Length | | | |
|---|---|---|---|---|---|---|---|
| | | | | ≤15 mm | ≤25 mm | ≤35 mm | ≤45 mm |
| ≤28 | 10 | 2 (0.9%) | 8 (3.8%) | 4 (50%) | 8 (100%) | 8 (100%) | 8 (100%) |
| ≤30 | 13 | 3 (1.4%) | 10 (4.7%) | 4 (40%) | 8 (80%) | 9 (90%) | 10 (100%) |
| ≤32 | 25 | 8 (3.8%) | 17 (8.0%) | 4 (24%) | 8 (47%) | 12 (71%) | 16 (94%) |
| ≤34 | 59 | 22 (10.4%) | 37 (17.5%) | 4 (11%) | 13 (35%) | 21 (57%) | 34 (92%) |

Reproduced with permission from Souka AP, Heath V, Flint S, et al. Cervical length at 23 weeks in twins in predicting spontaneous preterm delivery. *Obstet Gynecol.* 1999;94(3):450–454.

## Cervical Examination in Patients Presenting with Preterm Labor

Forty-seven percent (47%) of women presenting in preterm labor who are treated with a placebo deliver at term.[129] Differentiating those patients who are in true preterm labor is often a challenge.

Sonographic examination of the cervix in patients presenting with preterm labor can assist in the risk assessment for preterm delivery. In a study of 60 singleton and twin pregnancies presenting with preterm labor, all patients with a cervix >30 mm delivered at term.[16] The high negative predictive value for preterm birth associated with a long cervix provides important clinical information in symptomatic patients.[16,50,130–144]

The observation that a sonographic short cervix is a powerful predictor of preterm birth in patients presenting with symptoms of preterm labor has been confirmed and extended in several other studies. Gomez et al.[145] reported the use of sonographic cervical length and fFN test to predict spontaneous preterm delivery within 48 hours, 7 days, and 14 days of admission as well as delivery at <32 weeks and <35 weeks of gestation. A cervical length of <15 mm was the most powerful predictor of preterm birth within 48 hours (OR 9.7, $P < .05$). Both cervical length and fFN were predictive of preterm birth within 7 and 14 days. When fFN test results were added to a cervical length cutoff of <30 mm, there was significant improvement in the prediction of preterm delivery.[145]

A systematic review of seven studies evaluating the use of transvaginal ultrasound and cervical dilation in patients in preterm labor was conducted by Leitich et al.[146] The authors subdivided patients into three groups: (1) patients with preterm labor, and (2) low-risk asymptomatic patients with early (20 to 24 weeks) or (3) late (27 to 32 weeks) sonographic cervical length. The optimal cutoff values for cervical length in patients in preterm labor ranged between 18 and 30 mm, with sensitivity between 68% and 100%, and specificity was between 44% and 79%.[146] Several studies have demonstrated that the use of sonographic cervical length in labor and delivery can improve the management of patients in preterm labor by decreasing the number of unnecessary interventions. In addition, by applying specific management schemes that utilize a cervical length cutoff, hospital stay and health care costs have been reduced.[135,138,139,142,143,145,147–150] The utility of hospitalization in patients with a short cervix[151] or repeat sonographic evaluation of the cervix after the completion of tocolysis has been questioned.[152]

A randomized controlled trial[141] was conducted in 41 women with threatened preterm labor. Patients underwent a sonographic evaluation of the cervix or received the planned treatment (tocolytics and steroids). Treatment was withheld among patients in the ultrasound group with cervical length >15 mm. A higher proportion of patients in the control group received steroid treatment despite remaining undelivered for more than a week when compared with those in the ultrasound group (90% [18 of 20] vs. 14% [3 of 21], RR 0.16; 95% CI, 0.05 to 0.39). In addition, there was a significant difference in the duration of hospital stay between the two groups (median [range]; 0 hours [0 to 24] in the ultrasound group vs. 24 hours [0 to 67], $P < .0001$).[141] Larger studies are needed to assess the impact of the use of this management scheme on neonatal outcome.

Table 10.3 summarizes the results of some of the studies published to date that evaluated the use of sonographic cervical length in patients presenting with preterm labor. Although the studies have utilized different cervical length cutoffs, gestational age, and populations, there is agreement that the shorter the cervix, the higher the risk for preterm delivery.

Patients with preterm labor and a short cervix are also at an increased risk for intrauterine infection/inflammation. Gomez et al.[153] conducted a study in 401 patients presenting with preterm labor and cervical dilation of <3 cm (as assessed by digital examination). All patients underwent amniocentesis. The prevalence of microbial invasion of the amniotic cavity (MIAC) was 7% (28 of 401). Patients with a short cervix (<15 mm) had a higher rate of MIAC and preterm delivery at <35 weeks compared with those with a long cervix. (MIAC: short cervix, 26.3% [15 of 57] vs. long cervix 3.8% [13 of 344], $P < .05$; and for preterm delivery <35 weeks: short cervix, 66.7% [38 of 57] vs. long cervix, 13.5% [44 of 327], $P < .01$.) Furthermore, the rate of infection was higher in patients presenting at 30 weeks or less with a cervical length <15 mm when compared with those 15 mm or greater (43% [9 of 21] vs. 3.9% [3 of 76], $P < .05$). The authors provided an estimated risk of MIAC in patients in preterm labor according to gestational age and cervical length (Table 10.4).

In summary, cervical sonography is a powerful method to assess the risk of preterm delivery in patients presenting with preterm labor. Clinicians and patients can be reassured with the finding of a long cervix and avoid unnecessary intervention. Patients in preterm labor who are diagnosed with a short cervix are at increased risk for intrauterine infection/inflammation as well as a higher rate of preterm delivery, and thus may benefit from targeted interventions (i.e., antibiotic and/or steroid administration and transfer to a center with a neonatal intensive care unit). Further investigation into the most efficacious algorithm of management for these patients is still needed.

## Cervical Length and Fetal Fibronectin for the Prediction of Preterm Birth

Fetal fibronectin in cervicovaginal fluid has been used in conjunction with sonographic cervical length measurement to identify patients at risk for preterm delivery.

A systematic review demonstrated improved accuracy of the combination of fFN with ultrasound assessment of cervical length as screening tools for preterm labor and preterm birth prediction compared with the traditional clinical method of digital cervical examination.[154] The authors demonstrated that classic clinical criteria correctly identified 30.2% of women presenting with symptoms of preterm labor and delivered preterm at <37 weeks of gestation. The combination of fFN and ultrasound assessment of cervical length had a modest positive predictive value for preterm birth <37 weeks of 49.4%; however, this was higher than that of clinical diagnostic criteria alone. The diagnostic accuracy of the combination of fFN with sonographic cervical length assessment was significantly higher when predicting preterm birth risk within short periods of time (<7 days) and at earlier gestational ages (<28 weeks). For example, the sensitivity for delivery <7days with the combination method was 71.4%, with negative predictive value of 98.9%. Thus, the combined screening approach of sonographic cervical length assessment with fFN sampling may be useful for predicting short-term risks and may be used to guide acute

| Table 10.3 | | | | **Measurement of Cervical Length by Transvaginal Ultrasound in Women with Symptoms of Preterm Labor** | | | | | | |

| Reference | Year | N | Gestation (wk) | Cervical Length Cutoff[a] (mm) | Outcome[a] | Prevalence of Outcome[a] (%) | Sensitivity (%) | Specificity (%) | PPV (%) | NPV (%) |
|---|---|---|---|---|---|---|---|---|---|---|
| Murakawa et al.[130] | 1993 | 32 | 18–37 | <20 | 34 | <37 wk | 27 | 100 | 100 | 72 |
| | | | | | | | 100 | 71 | 65 | 100 |
| Iams et al.[16] | 1994 | 60 | 24–35 | <30 | 40 | <36 wk | 100 | 44 | 55 | 100 |
| Gomez et al.[50] | 1994 | 59 | 20–35 | ≤18 | 37 | <36 wk | 73 | 78 | 67 | 83 |
| Rizzo et al.[131] | 1996 | 108 | 24–36 | ≤20 | 43 | <37 wk | 68 | 79 | 71 | 76 |
| Rozenberg et al.[271] | 1997 | 76 | 24–34 | ≤26 | 26 | <37 wk | 75 | 73 | 50 | 89 |
| Tsoi et al.[132] | 2003 | 216 | 24–36 | <15 | 37 | Delivery within 7 d | 94 | 86 | 37.2 | 99.4 |
| Tsoi et al.[138] | 2005 | 510 | 24–33 6/7 | ≤15 | 14.9 | <35 wk | 71.1 | 90.6 | 56.8 | 94.7 |
| Daskalakis et al.[137] | 2005 | 172 | 24–34 | <20 | 37 | <34 wk | 60 | 97.7 | 93.7 | 81.4 |
| | | | | | 35.7 | Nulliparas | 53.8 | 95.2 | 87.5 | 76.9 |
| | | | | | 38.2 | Multiparas | | | | |
| Palacio et al.[143] | 2007 | 116 | 24–31 6/7 | <15 | 3.4 | Delivery within 7 d <34 wk | 0 | 97.3 | 0 | 96.5 |
| | | | | <20 | 10.3 | | 25 | 92 | 10 | 97.2 |
| | | | | <25 | | | 75 | 85.7 | 15.8 | 99 |
| | | | | <15 | | | 8.3 | 98.1 | 33.3 | 90.3 |
| | | | | <20 | | | 16.7 | 92.3 | 20 | 90.6 |
| | | | | <25 | | | 50 | 87.5 | 31.6 | 93.8 |
| Eroglu et al.[142] | 2007 | 51 | 24–35 | <20 | 19.6 | <35 wk | 60 | 100 | 100 | 91.1 |
| | | | | <25 | | | 60 | 92.7 | 66.7 | 90.5 |
| Schmitz et al.[144] | 2008 | 395 | 24–34 6/7 | ≤30 | 4.3 | Delivery within 48 h | 88 | 40 | 6 | 99 |
| | | | | | 8.1 | Delivery within 7 d | 94 | 42 | 12 | 99 |

[a]Calculated from the published data.

PPV, positive predictive value; NPV, negative predictive value.

Reproduced with permission from Hassan SS, Chaiworapongsa T, Vaisbuch E, et al. Sonographic examination of the uterine cervix. In: Fleischer AC, Toy CT, Lee W, et al, eds. *Sonography in Obstetrics and Gynecology: Principles and Practice.* 7th ed. New York, NY: McGraw-Hill Medical; 2011:816–847.

| Table 10.4 | | | | |
|---|---|---|---|---|
| **Risk of MIAC According to Cervical Length and Gestational Age** | | | | |

| | Gestational Age (wk) | | | |
|---|---|---|---|---|
| Cervical Length (mm) | <35 | <32 | <30 | <28 |
| <15 | 26.3% (15/57) | 33.3% (10/30) | 42.9% (9/21) | 45.5% (5/11) |
| 15–29 | 5.5% (10/183) | 4.8% (4/84) | 6.3% (2/32) | 11.8% (2/17) |
| >30 | 1.9% (3/161) | 2.5% (2/79) | 2.3% (1/44) | 0% (0/24) |
| Prevalence of MIAC | 7.0% (28/401) | 8.3% (16/193) | 12.4% (12/97) | 13.5% (7/52) |

$P < .001$ for all categories of gestational age ($\chi^2$ for trend).

From Gomez R, Romero R, Nien JK, et al. A short cervix in women with preterm labor and intact membranes: a risk factor for microbial invasion of the amniotic cavity. *Am J Obstet Gynecol.* 2005;192(3):678–689, copyright © 2005, with permission from Elsevier.

management of patients presenting with symptoms of preterm labor.

## Emerging Imaging Modalities to Evaluate the Cervix

Although cervical length is the most powerful predictor of preterm birth, there is a need to determine if the degree of cervical softening can be evaluated. Emerging imaging modalities seek to evaluate these changes in the cervix in a more objective fashion than the subjective digital assessment of cervical "softness or firmness."

### Elastography

Ultrasound-derived elastography evaluates tissue strain or stiffness of tissue by assessing the displacement of moving tissues when pressure is applied.[155,156] Specialized software produces a color code to express softness and stiffness (Fig. 10.6). Strain can also be expressed numerically as a percentage of tissue displaced when pressure is applied within a region of interest.[157]

Molina et al.[158] reported a reproducibility study that assessed agreement in ultrasound-elastography assessment of the cervix at a gestational age range of 12 and 40 weeks. The reported intraclass correlation coefficients between 0.16 and 0.8 for different regions of interest within the cervix but concluded that with the exception of the external, superior portion of the cervix, the measurements were reproducible. Of note, the authors suggested that although the part of the cervix nearest to the probe appeared to be the most soft, the measurement may merely be a reflection of the pressure applied by the transducer.

Elastography has been used to evaluate cervical stiffness in a cohort of 262 women with 1,557 strain estimations between 8 and 40 weeks' gestational age.[159] Using regions-of-interest at preselected anatomic locations within the cervix, the endocervical canal strain was on average 33% greater (softer) than that obtained for the entire cervix. Cervical tissue strain was greater for multiparous women than for nulliparous women, and was greater among women with a cervical length between 25 and 30 mm compared with those having cervical lengths >30 mm. Overall, a continuous reduction in cervical stiffness with decreasing cervical length and advancing gestational age was seen;

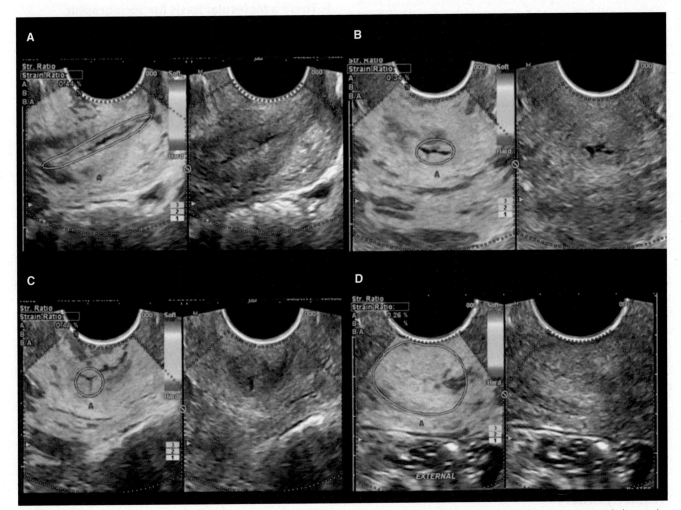

**FIGURE 10.6:** Cervical strain calculation performed in: **A.** endocervical canal in a sagittal plane; **B.** endocervical canal in a cross-sectional plane at the level of the internal os; **C.** endocervical canal in a cross-sectional plane at the level of the external cervical os; and **D.** complete cervix in a cross-sectional plane at the level of the external cervical os. (Reproduced with permission from Hernandez-Andrade E, Hassan SS, Ahn H, et al. Evaluation of cervical stiffness during pregnancy using semiquantitative ultrasound elastography. *Ultrasound Obstet Gynecol.* 2013;41(2):152–161.)

which is in keeping with the known physiologic remodeling changes in the cervix during pregnancy.

Ultrasound-derived cervical elastography may have utility in the identification of women with cervical ripening who do not have a short cervix but are destined to deliver preterm, or in a complementary way to cervical length assessment. However, the use of elastography in clinical practice is not routine. Future research is needed to confirm that the changes in strain correlate with changes in cervical remodeling and to evaluate the best use of this technology in the risk assessment for preterm birth.

### *Acoustic Attenuation*

Cervical tissue hydration increases as a function of cervical ripening and advancing gestational age.[1–4,160] The loss of energy as an ultrasonic wave propagates through tissue, acoustic attenuation, has been noted to be related to tissue stiffness, collagen concentration, and water concentration.[161] Forty women underwent transvaginal ultrasound using a system that allowed access to radiofrequency image data. Radiofrequency data were analyzed using an attenuation coefficient derived from a tissue phantom. Regression analysis revealed that attenuation of the cervix was predictive of the exam-to-delivery interval ($\beta = .43$, $P = .011$) but not predictive of gestational age at the time of the exam ($\beta = -.23$, $P = .15$) or cervical length ($\beta = .077$, $P = .65$). Interestingly, two women in the study had a short cervical length in the midtrimester but moderate or high attenuation values (un-ripe cervix). Both of these women delivered at >34 weeks and remained pregnant for at least 11 weeks after the cervical length measurement. However, a limitation of this technique is the high variation in attenuation values between subjects and operator chosen regions-of-interest for evaluation. Furthermore, cervical tissue is nonhomogeneous, which may limit the application of an attenuation algorithm, which relies on tissue homogeneity.[162]

## CAUSES OF A SONOGRAPHIC SHORT CERVIX

A short cervix often occurs when there is cervical ripening; however, not all short cervices are ripe, hence the observation that some women with a short cervix deliver at term. We have proposed that a short cervix is syndromic in nature and can be caused by multiple etiologies,[14,163–165] such as (1) the loss of connective tissue after a cervical operation such as conization[166–170] or loop electrosurgical excision procedure (LEEP)[171,172]; (2) a congenital disorder such as cervical hypoplasia after DES exposure[168,173–175]; (3) intrauterine infection[153,176,177]; (4) an alteration in progesterone action[178]; and/or (5) a cervical disorder that manifests itself with the clinical presentation of premature cervical dilation. Each of these different causes of the syndrome could be affected by genetic or environmental factors; more than one mechanism of disease may be at work in a specific patient. The possibility of novel and yet undiscovered mechanisms of disease playing a role must also be considered.

### Pregnancy History

Several authors have documented a relationship between a previous obstetrical history of preterm birth and cervical length.[28,95] Iams et al.[28] reported a study of cervical length in patients with

(1) a previous history of "cervical insufficiency"; (2) a previous preterm delivery at <26 weeks; (3) a previous preterm delivery at 27 to 32 weeks; (4) a previous preterm delivery at 33 to 35 weeks; and (5) a control group of women with previous term delivery. A strong relationship was established between cervical length in the index pregnancy and previous obstetric history. This relationship appears to be linear, and patients considered to have a typical history of an incompetent cervix did not constitute a unique group.[28]

Similar results have been reported by Guzman et al.[95] who described a strong relationship between previous obstetric history and cervical length in the subsequent pregnancy. Specifically, the authors observed that the frequency of a short cervix (cervical length <20 mm) or progressive shortening of the cervix to a length of <20 mm was associated with the gestational age at delivery in the previous pregnancy.[95] Collectively, these studies suggest a relationship between a history of preterm delivery and cervical length in a subsequent pregnancy. A short cervical length in the subsequent pregnancy may reflect the result of genetic and environmental factors predisposing to preterm delivery, which can express themselves in changes in cervical structure.

### Is There a Molecular Basis for Sonographic Shortening?

We have demonstrated that sonographic cervical shortening prior to the onset of labor is associated with changes in the transcriptome of the human uterine cervix.[13] A study was conducted in 19 women at term, not in labor, with a ripe cervix (Bishop score >5); sonographic cervical length was measured, and biopsies were obtained. Changes in the transcriptome of the uterine cervix were evaluated as a function of each 1 cm decrease in cervical length. Microarray analysis, pathway analysis, and quantitative real-time polymerase chain reaction (qRT-PCR) analysis were employed. Cervical length shortening was associated with: (1) differential expression of 687 genes; (2) enrichment of 54 biologic processes, 22 molecular functions, and 9 pathways; and (3) bone morphogenetic protein-7 (BMP-7), claudin 1, integrin beta-6, and endometrial progesterone-induced protein (EPIP) messenger ribonucleic acid (mRNA) and protein expressions were down-regulated with cervical shortening. Changes in expression included genes involved in epithelial cell function, signal transduction, and the epithelial–mesenchymal transition. The biologic processes, molecular functions, and pathway analyses further demonstrated a role for the inflammatory response, immune system response, transmembrane receptor activity, and the pathways involved in antigen processing and presentation in cervical shortening at term.

### A Sonographic Short Cervix as the Only Clinical Manifestation of Intra-amniotic Infection and/or Inflammation

Premature cervical ripening in response to a pathologic stimulus such as infection may result in a sonographic short cervix. Gray et al.[179] reported that all women with a positive amniotic fluid culture for *Ureaplasma urealyticum* at the time of genetic amniocentesis delivered a preterm neonate with histologic evidence of chorioamnionitis. This study, however, did not contain information about cervical length. We have established that 9% (5 of 57) of asymptomatic women in the midtrimester with a cervical length <25 mm without cervical dilation had microbiologically proven intra-amniotic infection.[177] The isolated microorganisms included *Ureaplasma urealyticum* and *Fusobacterium*. Patients with amniotic fluid cultures positive for Ureaplasma received intravenous antibiotics (azithromycin) for 7 days and underwent a test-of-cure amniocentesis. Three of the four patients had a negative amniocentesis, thus demonstrating eradication of the Ureaplasma, and subsequently delivered at term. Kiefer et al.[180] reported an association between a cervical length ≤5 mm in the midtrimester and increased amniotic fluid concentrations of inflammatory cytokines such as monocyte chemotactic protein-1 (MCP-1) and interleukin-6 (IL-6). In a subsequent study of 44 patients in the midtrimester with a cervical length ≤25 mm, in which those with intra-amniotic infection and/or preterm labor were not excluded, amniotic fluid MCP-1 was predictive for spontaneous preterm delivery.[181] Vaisbuch et al.[182] noted that intra-amniotic inflammation (defined as an amniotic fluid matrix metalloproteinase-8 concentration >23 ng per mL) was present in 22% of asymptomatic patients (10 of 45) with a cervical length ≤15 mm in the midtrimester of pregnancy; an occurrence that was associated with adverse pregnancy outcomes. Indeed, women with intra-amniotic inflammation had a shorter median diagnosis-to-delivery interval than those without this condition. Furthermore, 40% of patients with intra-amniotic inflammation delivered within one week of the amniocentesis.

Previous studies have indicated that up to 50% of patients presenting with painless cervical dilation before 24 weeks of gestation have a positive amniotic fluid culture for microorganisms.[176,183] In these cases, infection can be a cause of premature cervical dilation, or may be secondary to prolonged exposure of chorioamniotic membranes to the microbial flora present in the lower genital tract.[176]

## ADDITIONAL PARAMETERS TO ASSESS THE RISK OF PRETERM BIRTH DURING TRANSVAGINAL SONOGRAPHY

Several parameters are often noted on transvaginal ultrasound to assess a patient's risk for preterm birth. These include the presence or absence of a funnel, dynamic cervical change, and amniotic fluid "sludge." The presence or absence of a funnel and dynamic change do not increase the predictive value of preterm birth beyond that provided by cervical length; however, the finding of amniotic fluid "sludge" has been found to be useful in the risk assessment for preterm birth.[38,62,96]

### Amniotic Fluid "Sludge"

Particulate matter in the amniotic fluid is present in about 4% of pregnancies during transvaginal ultrasound in the first and early second trimesters.[184] The prevalence of this sonographic finding increases with gestational age, reaching 88% by 35 weeks.[185] Particulate matter in the first two trimesters of pregnancy has been associated with intra-amniotic bleeding[186–188] and the acrania-anencephaly sequence[189] and has been observed in women with high concentrations of maternal serum α-fetoprotein.[190] In contrast, in the last trimester of pregnancy, particulate matter and "echogenic amniotic fluid" have been attributed to the presence of vernix caseosa and/or meconium,[191–194] and with a

lecithin–sphingomyelin ratio indicative of lung maturity.[195,196] Congenital anomalies associated with particulate matter in the amniotic fluid include harlequin ichtiosis[197] and epidermolysis bullosa letalis.[198] Amniotic fluid "sludge" is defined as particulate matter seen in the proximity of the internal cervical os during a transvaginal sonographic examination of the cervix, and occurs in 1% of uncomplicated pregnancies (see Fig. 10.4).[199]

The first description of amniotic fluid "sludge" was in patients in preterm labor. Espinoza et al.[199] conducted a retrospective study of 84 patients in preterm labor with intact membranes. The prevalence of amniotic fluid "sludge" was 22.6% (19 of 84) in patients with preterm labor. Patients with amniotic fluid "sludge" had a higher frequency of positive amniotic fluid cultures, histologic chorioamnionitis, a higher rate of spontaneous preterm delivery within 48 hours, within 7 days, <32 weeks (75% [9 of 12] vs. 25.8% [8 of 31], P = .005), and <35 weeks (92.9% [13 of 14] vs. 37.8% [17 of 45], P < .001) than those without amniotic fluid "sludge." Stepwise logistic regression analysis indicated that the presence of "sludge" was an independent factor associated with the likelihood of spontaneous delivery within 48 hours and 7 days, but not <32 or <35 weeks. The diagnostic indices of the amniotic fluid "sludge" are displayed in Table 10.5. Survival analysis demonstrated that patients with amniotic fluid "sludge" had a shorter examination-to-delivery interval compared with those without "sludge" (sludge median: 1 day [interquartile range: 1 to 5 days] vs. no sludge median: 33 days [interquartile range: 18 to 58 days]; P < .001) (Fig. 10.7). These results indicate that amniotic fluid "sludge" during transvaginal examination of the cervix is a risk factor for MIAC, histologic chorioamnionitis, and impending preterm delivery.[199]

The presence of amniotic fluid "sludge" on transvaginal examination in asymptomatic patients is also associated with delivery within 14 days of ultrasound and preterm delivery at <32 and <34 weeks.[200–203] Bujold et al.[200] conducted a retrospective study of 89 women at 18 to 32 weeks who were at high risk for preterm delivery. Logistic regression analyses revealed that a cervical length <25 mm and light or dense amniotic fluid "sludge" were independent predictors of delivery within 14 days and <34 weeks.[200] In a retrospective case control study, Kusanovic et al.[201] included 281 patients with (n = 66) or without (n = 215) amniotic fluid "sludge" at 13 to 29 weeks of gestation. Patients were at high risk for preterm birth based upon the presence of one or more of the following: a history of spontaneous preterm delivery, previous midtrimester loss, short cervix (<25 mm), Müllerian duct anomalies, and a history of cone biopsy. The prevalence of amniotic fluid "sludge" was 23.5% in this population. Amniotic fluid "sludge" was identified as an independent risk factor for spontaneous preterm delivery at <28, <32, and <35 weeks of gestation; preterm premature rupture of membranes (pPROM); MIAC; and histologic chorioamnionitis. Furthermore, asymptomatic patients with amniotic fluid "sludge" had shorter ultrasound-to-delivery and ultrasound-to-preterm PROM intervals than those without sludge.

Amniotic fluid "sludge" represents a biofilm.[204,205] A sample of sludge was retrieved by transvaginal amniotomy under ultrasound guidance from a patient at 28 weeks with spontaneous labor and clinical chorioamnionitis. Grossly, the sludge had a "pus-like" appearance, and the Gram stain showed gram-positive bacteria. The amniotic fluid culture was positive for *Streptococcus mutans*, *Mycoplasma hominis*, and *Aspergillus flavus*. Of interest, the results of the amniocentesis performed at the time of admission for preterm labor were negative for

| Table 10.5 | Diagnostic Indices and Predictive Value of Amniotic Fluid "Sludge" | | | | | | |

| Outcome Variable | Prevalence, % (Number) | Sensitivity (%) | Specificity (%) | PPV (%) | NPV (%) | LR (+) | LR (−) |
|---|---|---|---|---|---|---|---|
| Positive amniotic fluid cultures | 12.1 (7/58) | 86 | 76 | 33 | 98 | 3.3 | 0.19 |
| Histologic chorioamnionitis | 32.9 (25/76) | 56 | 92 | 78 | 81 | 7.1 | 0.48 |
| *Spontaneous delivery* | | | | | | | |
| Within 48 h | 13.6 (8/59) | 75 | 84 | 43 | 96 | 4.8 | 0.30 |
| Within 7 d | 28.8 (17/59) | 59 | 90 | 71 | 84 | 6.2 | 0.46 |

PPV, positive predictive value; NPV, negative predictive value; LR, likelihood ratio.

Reproduced with permission from Espinoza J, Goncalves LF, Romero R, et al. The prevalence and clinical significance of amniotic fluid "sludge" in patients with preterm labor and intact membranes. *Ultrasound Obstet Gynecol.* 2005;25(4):346–352.

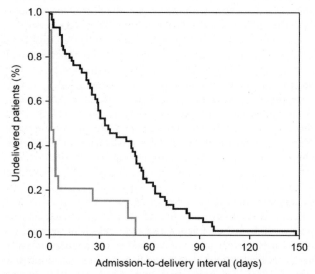

**FIGURE 10.7:** Results of survival analysis in patients in preterm labor with and without the presence of amniotic fluid "sludge." Patients with amniotic fluid "sludge" *(blue line)* had a shorter examination-to-delivery interval compared with those without "sludge" *(red line)*. (Sludge median: 1 day [interquartile range: 1 to 5 days] vs. no sludge, median: 33 days [interquartile range: 18 to 58 days]; *P* < .001.) (Adapted with permission from Espinoza J, Goncalves LF, Romero R, et al. The prevalence and clinical significance of amniotic fluid "sludge" in patients with preterm labor and intact membranes. *Ultrasound Obstet Gynecol.* 2005;25(4):346–352.)

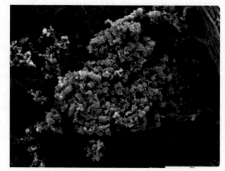

**FIGURE 10.8:** Scanning electron micrograph of a floc of amniotic fluid "sludge." Bacterial cells and the exopolymeric matrix material that constitute a biofilm are shown. (From Romero R, Schaudinn C, Kusanovic JP, et al. Detection of a microbial biofilm in intraamniotic infection. *Am J Obstet Gynecol.* 2008;198(1):135, copyright © 2008, with permission from Elsevier.)

intra-amniotic infection.[204,205] The clinical significance of this relates to the challenges with diagnosis and treatment. The diagnosis of microbial invasion in the presence of biofilms is challenging, and the use of conventional antibiotics may not be effective (Fig. 10.8).

## PREVENTING PRETERM BIRTH IN PATIENTS WITH A SONOGRAPHIC SHORT CERVIX

### Vaginal Progesterone

There is now substantial evidence to support the use of vaginal progesterone for the prevention of preterm birth in patients with sonographic short cervix regardless of pregnancy history.[21–24]

Two randomized clinical trials have demonstrated that cervical length can identify the patient who will benefit from vaginal progesterone administration.[22,23] Fonseca et al.[22] reported a randomized clinical trail in which vaginal progesterone reduced the rate of preterm birth by 44% (from 34.4% in the placebo group to 19.2% in the progesterone treatment group) in women with a sonographic short cervix. A randomized double blind placebo-controlled trial by Hassan et al.[23] demonstrated that administration of vaginal progesterone (8% gel) from 20 to 36 6/7 weeks' gestation significantly reduced the rate of preterm birth by 45% in women with an asymptomatic sonographic short cervix between 10 and 20 mm.

The trail by Fonseca et al.[22] was a randomized, double blind, placebo-controlled trial in which women with a short cervix (≤15 mm), between 20 and 25 weeks of gestation, were allocated to daily vaginal administration of 200 mg of micronized progesterone or placebo (safflower oil) from 24 to 34 weeks. The frequency of spontaneous preterm delivery at <34 weeks (primary end point for the trial) was significantly lower in the progesterone group than that in the placebo group (19.2% [24 of 125] vs. 34.4% [43 of 125]; *P* = .007). A secondary analysis of this trial indicated that among women without a history of delivery before 34 weeks, the incidence of preterm birth was significantly lower in women receiving progesterone than in those allocated to placebo (17.9% [20 of 112] vs. 31.2% [34 of 109]; RR 0.57; 95% CI, 0.35 to 0.93; P = .03). The trial was not designed to test whether progesterone administration could reduce neonatal morbidity, and such a reduction was not observed.[22]

DeFranco et al.[21] reported a secondary analysis of the effect of vaginal progesterone on pregnancy outcome (preterm birth and infant outcome) as a function of cervical length. The authors explored the effect of vaginal progesterone as a function of cervical length <30 mm and <28 mm.[21] For patients with a cervical length <30 mm, there was a trend for a longer randomization-to-delivery interval in women allocated to progesterone than those allocated to placebo (Wilcoxon P = .043, log-rank P = .057). However, no difference in the frequency of preterm delivery <32 weeks was observed.

Patients with cervical length <28 mm, who received vaginal progesterone, had a lower rate of spontaneous preterm delivery <32 weeks of gestation, though the prevalence of preterm delivery <35 and <37 weeks did not differ among women receiving progesterone or placebo. Of note, the frequency of NICU admission and duration of stay was lower in women with short cervix (<30 and <28 mm) receiving vaginal progesterone.[21] This analysis provided the first evidence that vaginal progesterone administration may improve infant outcome. However, these conclusions were considered tentative as they were derived from a secondary analysis, which was intended to be hypothesis-generating[21]; therefore, further investigation was necessary.

Hassan et al.[23] conducted a multicenter, randomized, double-blind, placebo-controlled trial (PREGNANT trial) evaluating the efficacy of vaginal progesterone gel (90 mg daily) for the prevention of preterm delivery in patients with a sonographic short cervix (10 to 20 mm) between 19 and 23 6/7 weeks of gestation regardless of pregnancy history. A total of 465 patients were randomized to receive 90 mg of vaginal progesterone gel or placebo starting from 20 to 23 6/7 weeks until 36 6/7 weeks, rupture of membranes or delivery, whichever occurred first. The study demonstrated a significant 45% reduction in the risk of preterm delivery prior to 33 weeks' gestation in the group treated with vaginal progesterone when compared with those receiving placebo. There was also a significant reduction in the risk of preterm delivery <28 and <35 weeks' gestation (50% and 38%, respectively). Most notably, there was a significant decrease in the risk of neonatal RDS (61%), any neonatal morbidity/mortality (43%), and birth weight <1,500 g (53%).

Following the PREGNANT trial, Romero et al.[24] performed an individual patient data meta-analysis of patients enrolled in five randomized controlled trials of vaginal progesterone in women with a sonographic short cervix. Data for 775 women (93% singleton and 6.7% twin pregnancies) and 827 fetuses/infants met inclusion criteria. Treatment with vaginal progesterone was associated with a significant reduction in the risk of preterm birth prior to 33 (42% reduction), 35 (31% reduction), and 28 (50% reduction) weeks' gestation in patients with a cervical length ≤25 mm in the midtrimester. Vaginal progesterone treatment in patients with a cervical length ≤25 mm was also associated with a significant reduction in neonatal morbidity such as RDS, composite neonatal morbidity and mortality, admission to the NICU, requirement for mechanical ventilation, and birth weight <1,500 g. Subgroup analysis of twin pregnancies did not demonstrate a significant reduction in preterm birth; however, vaginal progesterone treatment was associated with a significant reduction in composite neonatal morbidity/

mortality, which suggests that this study may not have had sufficient power to evaluate the effect of vaginal progesterone in twin gestations with midtrimester short cervix. Based on these studies, we recommend vaginal progesterone treatment for patients with a sonographic short cervix (≤25 mm), regardless of pregnancy history. The individual data meta-analysis showed that the number of patients needed to treat with vaginal progesterone to prevent one case of preterm birth prior to 34 weeks is 9, and 15 to prevent one case of RDS.[24]

Intramuscular injections of 17 alpha-hydroxyprogesterone caproate (17-OHPC) are not effective in preventing spontaneous delivery in women with a sonographic short cervix. A multicenter randomized controlled trial (SCAN trial) conducted by Grobman et al.[206] failed to demonstrate a significant improvement in the prevention of preterm delivery in nulliparous patients with a short cervix (cervical length <30 mm) with weekly administration of intramuscular 17-OHPC. Subgroup analysis of patients with a cervical length <15 mm did not result in a significant reduction in preterm delivery. Based on these findings, 17-OHPC is not recommended for the treatment of women with a short cervix and singleton gestations for prevention of preterm birth.

In the study of Meis et al.,[20] weekly administration of 17-OHPC was done in women with previous spontaneous preterm birth; however, the cervical length was not evaluated; therefore, a common clinical challenge occurs when a patient with a prior spontaneous preterm birth is receiving weekly 17-OHPC and found to have a short cervix. In addition, currently there are no randomized trials evaluating the potential additive effect of cerclage placement in patients receiving 17-OHPC who subsequently develop a short cervix. A secondary analysis of a large randomized trial investigating the use of ultrasound-indicated cerclage for the prevention of preterm birth in high-risk women demonstrated that cerclage did not offer additional benefit for the prevention of recurrent preterm birth in women with a subsequent short cervix who have received at least one dose of 17-OHPC.[207,208] Therefore, there are still unanswered questions regarding the management of patients currently receiving 17-OHPC secondary to history of preterm delivery and subsequent development of a short cervix. In view of the lack of a safety signal or adverse effects with the use of vaginal progesterone, some have advocated the administration of vaginal progesterone to such patients.

## Cervical Cerclage

Several randomized controlled trials[46,47,209–213] to assess the clinical value of cerclage placement in women with a sonographic short cervix have been performed.

The clinical value of cervical cerclage has been the subject of many observational and randomized clinical trials,[46,47,209–241] and the studies have been the topic of several systematic reviews.[49,242–246] The evidence suggests the following conclusions:

1. Cervical cerclage in women with a sonographic short cervix (15 mm or less) and no history of preterm delivery does not reduce the rate of preterm birth.[213]
2. Cervical cerclage is a therapeutic option in women with a sonographic short cervix and a history of preterm delivery for the prevention of preterm birth.[46,210,211,245–249]
3. The role of prophylactic cerclage in high-risk patients without a sonographic short cervix for the prevention of preterm

delivery/midtrimester abortion (by history) is unclear. While the largest trial conducted prior to the introduction of ultrasound evaluation of the cervix suggested a modest beneficial effect,[221] other trials[219,220] and systematic reviews[244] prior to the use of ultrasound have indicated that the evidence of effectiveness is either weak or nonexistent.

In patients at risk for preterm delivery, serial sonographic examination of the cervix followed by cerclage in those who shortened the cervix is a reasonable alternative to prophylactic placement of a cerclage based on uncontrolled studies.[46,226,234,245,246,250,251]

### Cerclage Versus Vaginal Progesterone

There are no prospective randomized trials that directly compare vaginal progesterone and cervical cerclage for the prevention of recurrent preterm birth in women with a sonographic short cervix in the midtrimester and previous spontaneous preterm birth. Conde-Agudelo et al.[49] performed an adjusted indirect meta-analysis of randomized trials available to compare the two treatments. Randomized controlled trials in which asymptomatic women with a sonographic short cervix (<25 mm) in the midtrimester were randomized to receive vaginal progesterone versus placebo/no treatment or cerclage versus no cerclage were included in this indirect individual patient data meta-analysis comparing the two treatment options. Four studies evaluating vaginal progesterone (158 patients) and five studies evaluating cerclage (504 patients) met inclusion criteria. Indirect meta-analysis demonstrated no significant difference in the reduction of preterm birth <32 weeks' gestation with either treatment group. Patients with a history of spontaneous preterm birth and current short cervix (<25 mm) can be offered either cerclage or vaginal progesterone. However, despite the fact that both interventions appear to be effective, cerclage has inherent risks that are greater than vaginal progesterone; thus, a discussion and consideration of treatment should include risks associated with treatment (surgical vs. medical) as well as cost and patient/clinician preference.

### Universal Cervical Length Screening

There is evidence to support the role of universal transvaginal cervical length screening in the identification of patients at risk for preterm delivery.[249,252–256] The policy of universal cervical length screening and treatment with vaginal progesterone with the identification of a midtrimester short cervix is in compliance with the 10 general principles that the World Health Organization outlined for a good screening test.[255,257] Werner et al.[254] developed a decision analysis model to compare the cost-effectiveness of two strategies for identifying pregnancies at risk for preterm birth in an otherwise low-risk singleton pregnancy. The two models were (1) no routine cervical length screening vs. (2) a single routine transvaginal cervical length, and patients with a short cervix were offered vaginal progesterone treatment. The results of the decision analysis model predicted that routine cervical length screening when coupled with the use of vaginal progesterone treatment has a potential savings of $19,603,380 for every 100,000 women screened by ultrasound.

Below is a summary of recommendations and facts regarding the use of progesterone for the prevention of preterm birth:

1. Women with a sonographic short cervix (≤25 mm) diagnosed in the midtrimester should be offered daily vaginal progesterone treatment for the prevention of preterm birth.[22–24]

2. The use of vaginal progesterone for the prevention of recurrent preterm birth in a high-risk population has been shown to be effective.[24,258,259]
3. Weekly injection of 17-OHPC is not effective for the prevention of preterm delivery in patients with a sonographic short cervix.[206]
4. Universal cervical length screening and vaginal progesterone treatment (90-mg vaginal gel or 100-mg micronized vaginal suppositories) for patients with a cervical length ≤25 mm is effective and is a cost-saving for the prevention of preterm birth.[249,252–255]
5. Patients with a midtrimester short cervix ≤25 mm and a previous history of spontaneous preterm delivery can be offered either cervical cerclage or vaginal progesterone. Treatment choice should be based upon consideration of the risks of both treatments and patient/clinician preference. An amniocentesis for the evaluation of subclinical intra-amniotic infection/inflammation is recommended especially prior to placement of cervical cerclage.[177,183,260]
6. Currently, there is not enough evidence to support the use of vaginal progesterone or 17-OHPC for the prevention of preterm delivery in multiple gestations, regardless of cervical length; however, larger randomized trials are needed to evaluate the efficacy of vaginal progesterone for the prevention of preterm birth in multiple gestations with a midtrimester short cervix.[261–263]

### Cervical Pessary

Cervical pessaries have been proposed as a method of treatment for cervical insufficiency since 1959[264]; however, their use as an alternative to cervical cerclage has been considered only in recent years.[48,265–269] Goya et al.[48] conducted an open-label randomized controlled trial (PECEP trial) in women with a midtrimester short cervix (≤25 mm) treated with a pessary placement versus expectant management group. The authors demonstrated a significant 78% reduction in the risk of spontaneous preterm delivery <34 weeks of gestation in patients who received a pessary (Fig. 10.9) when compared with the control group. This reduction in preterm birth suggests that

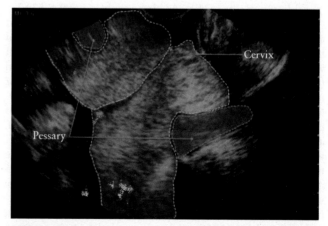

**FIGURE 10.9:** (Reproduced with permission Goya M, Pratcorona L, Higueras T, et al. Sonographic cervical length measurement in a pregnant women with a cervical pessary. *Ultrasound Obstet Gynecol.* 2011;38(2):205–209.)

cervical pessary placement may be effective. However, some have raised concern regarding the generalizability of treatment given the high preterm delivery rate (<34 weeks) of 27% in the expectant management group. In addition, these results were not reproduced in a similar but smaller randomized trial by Hui et al.[268] Hui et al. randomized 108 patients with midtrimester short cervix (<25 mm) to pessary versus expectant management and did not find a significant reduction in preterm birth between groups (5.5% vs. 9.4%). The ability for cervical pessary to prevent preterm birth in patients with a midtrimester short cervix remains controversial owing to these conflicting results.

## FUTURE CHALLENGES

An important challenge is the development of a model to refine the current method for the prediction of spontaneous preterm birth. The following outstanding questions remain:

1. Can serum markers provide further individualized risk assessment for preterm delivery when combined with cervical length?
2. Does noninvasive assessment of collagen content able to provide prognostic information? (Quantitative ultrasonic tissue characterization of the cervix)
3. Does the use of cervical artery Doppler velocimetry and/or cervical gland evaluation have predictive value?
4. Is vaginal progesterone treatment in the prevention of preterm birth effective in twin gestations with a midtrimester sonographic short cervix?

In summary, a large body of literature has examined the nature of cervical change during pregnancy in both human and animal studies. Cervical disease is one of the etiologies of the preterm parturition syndrome. The success of the available treatments such as progesterone or cerclage requires the adequate identification of women with cervical disease. Progesterone or cerclage may benefit some patients who have a primary cervical process and are in the reversible phase of parturition. It is clear that obstetrical history is insufficient to identify such a patient; thus, cervical sonography represents an important tool for the identification of the patient with premature cervical ripening. Additional studies such as the biochemical definition of the short cervix in preterm gestations may contribute to the ability to differentiate the patient with a short cervix who will deliver a preterm neonate from the one who will deliver a term infant, as well as the patient who may benefit from a cerclage or progesterone therapy.

## ACKNOWLEDGMENTS

This research was supported, in part, by the Perinatology Research Branch, Division of Intramural Research, *Eunice Kennedy Shriver* National Institute of Child Health and Human Development, National Institutes of Health, Department of Health and Human Services (NICHD/NIH); and, in part, with Federal funds from NICHD, NIH under Contract No. HHSN275201300006C.

This work is based on several review articles and chapters published previously by the authors in other publications. This work has been modified and adapted for this textbook. The original chapters are referenced and contain a more extensive discussion of the subject. Excerpts from this chapter have been published previously in Hassan SS, Chaiworapongsa T, Vaisbuch E, et al. Sonographic examination of the uterine cervix. In: Fleischer AC, Manning FA, Jeanty P, et al, eds. *Sonography in Obstetrics and Gynecology: Principles and Practice.* 7th ed. New York, NY; McGraw-Hill; 2011:816–847.

## REFERENCES

1. Maillot KV, Zimmermann BK. The solubility of collagen of the uterine cervix during pregnancy and labour. *Arch Gynakol.* 1976;220:275–280.
2. Kleissl HP, van der Rest M, Naftolin F, et al. Collagen changes in the human uterine cervix at parturition. *Am J Obstet Gynecol.* 1978;130:748–753.
3. Junqueira LC, Zugaib M, Montes GS, et al. Morphologic and histochemical evidence for the occurrence of collagenolysis and for the role of neutrophilic polymorphonuclear leukocytes during cervical dilation. *Am J Obstet Gynecol.* 1980;138:273–281.
4. Rajabi MR, Dodge GR, Solomon S, et al. Immunochemical and immunohistochemical evidence of estrogen-mediated collagenolysis as a mechanism of cervical dilatation in the guinea pig at parturition. *Endocrinology.* 1991;128:371–378.
5. Osmers RG, Blaser J, Kuhn W, et al. Interleukin-8 synthesis and the onset of labor. *Obstet Gynecol.* 1995;86:223–229.
6. Osman I, Young A, Ledingham MA, et al. Leukocyte density and pro-inflammatory cytokine expression in human fetal membranes, decidua, cervix and myometrium before and during labour at term. *Mol Hum Reprod.* 2003;9:41–45.
7. Sakamoto Y, Moran P, Searle RF, et al. Interleukin-8 is involved in cervical dilatation but not in prelabour cervical ripening. *Clin Exp Immunol.* 2004;138:151–157.
8. Word RA, Landrum CP, Timmons BC, et al. Transgene insertion on mouse chromosome 6 impairs function of the uterine cervix and causes failure of parturition. *Biol Reprod.* 2005;73:1046–1056.
9. Hassan SS, Romero R, Haddad R, et al. The transcriptome of the uterine cervix before and after spontaneous term parturition. *Am J Obstet Gynecol.* 2006;195:778–786.
10. Hassan SS, Romero R, Tarca AL, et al. Signature pathways identified from gene expression profiles in the human uterine cervix before and after spontaneous term parturition. *Am J Obstet Gynecol.* 2007;197:250.e1–250.e7.
11. Hassan SS, Romero R, Tarca AL, et al. The transcriptome of cervical ripening in human pregnancy before the onset of labor at term: identification of novel molecular functions involved in this process. *J Matern Fetal Neonatal Med.* 2009;22:1183–1193.
12. Hassan SS, Romero R, Pineles B, et al. MicroRNA expression profiling of the human uterine cervix after term labor and delivery. *Am J Obstet Gynecol.* 2010;202:80.e1–80.e8.
13. Hassan SS, Romero R, Tarca AL, et al. The molecular basis for sonographic cervical shortening at term: identification of differentially expressed genes and the epithelial-mesenchymal transition as a function of cervical length. *Am J Obstet Gynecol.* 2010;203:472.e1–472.e14.
14. Romero R, Espinoza J, Erez O, et al. The role of cervical cerclage in obstetric practice: can the patient who could benefit from this procedure be identified? *Am J Obstet Gynecol.* 2006;194:1–9.
15. Andersen HF, Nugent CE, Wanty SD, et al. Prediction of risk for preterm delivery by ultrasonographic measurement of cervical length. *Am J Obstet Gynecol.* 1990;163:859–867.
16. Iams JD, Paraskos J, Landon MB, et al. Cervical sonography in preterm labor. *Obstet Gynecol.* 1994;84:40–46.
17. Heath VC, Southall TR, Souka AP, et al. Cervical length at 23 weeks of gestation: prediction of spontaneous preterm delivery. *Ultrasound Obstet Gynecol.* 1998;12:312–317.
18. Hassan SS, Romero R, Berry SM, et al. Patients with an ultrasonographic cervical length < or = 15 mm have nearly a 50% risk of early spontaneous preterm delivery. *Am J Obstet Gynecol.* 2000;182:1458–1467.
19. Huszar G, Naftolin F. The myometrium and uterine cervix in normal and preterm labor. *N Engl J Med.* 1984;311:571–581.
20. Meis PJ, Klebanoff M, Thom E, et al. Prevention of recurrent preterm delivery by 17 alpha-hydroxyprogesterone caproate. *N Engl J Med.* 2003;348:2379–2385.
21. DeFranco EA, O'Brien JM, Adair CD, et al. Vaginal progesterone is associated with a decrease in risk for early preterm birth and improved neonatal outcome in women with a short cervix: a secondary analysis from a randomized, double-blind, placebo-controlled trial. *Ultrasound Obstet Gynecol.* 2007;30:697–705.
22. Fonseca EB, Celik E, Parra M, et al. Progesterone and the risk of preterm birth among women with a short cervix. *N Engl J Med.* 2007;357:462–469.
23. Hassan SS, Romero R, Vidyadhari D, et al. Vaginal progesterone reduces the rate of preterm birth in women with a sonographic short cervix: a multicenter, randomized, double-blind, placebo-controlled trial. *Ultrasound Obstet Gynecol.* 2011;38:18–31.
24. Romero R, Nicolaides K, Conde-Agudelo A, et al. Vaginal progesterone in women with an asymptomatic sonographic short cervix in the midtrimester

decreases preterm delivery and neonatal morbidity: a systematic review and metaanalysis of individual patient data. *Am J Obstet Gynecol.* 2012;206: 124.e1–124.e19.

25. Kushnir O, Vigil DA, Izquierdo L, et al. Vaginal ultrasonographic assessment of cervical length changes during normal pregnancy. *Am J Obstet Gynecol.* 1990;162:991–993.

26. Andersen HF. Transvaginal and transabdominal ultrasonography of the uterine cervix during pregnancy. *J Clin Ultrasound.* 1991;19:77–83.

27. Okitsu O, Mimura T, Nakayama T, et al. Early prediction of preterm delivery by transvaginal ultrasonography. *Ultrasound Obstet Gynecol.* 1992;2:402–409.

28. Iams JD, Johnson FF, Sonek J, et al. Cervical competence as a continuum: a study of ultrasonographic cervical length and obstetric performance. *Am J Obstet Gynecol.* 1995;172:1097–1103.

29. Hasegawa I, Tanaka K, Takahashi K, et al. Transvaginal ultrasonographic cervical assessment for the prediction of preterm delivery. *J Matern Fetal Med.* 1996;5:305–309.

30. Iams JD, Goldenberg RL, Meis PJ, et al. The length of the cervix and the risk of spontaneous premature delivery. *N Engl J Med.* 1996;334:567–572.

31. Berghella V, Kuhlman K, Weiner S, et al. Cervical funneling: sonographic criteria predictive of preterm delivery. *Ultrasound Obstet Gynecol.* 1997;10:161–166.

32. Goldenberg RL, Iams JD, Mercer BM, et al. The Preterm Prediction Study: the value of new vs standard risk factors in predicting early and all spontaneous preterm births. NICHD MFMU Network. *Am J Public Health.* 1998;88:233–238.

33. Guzman ER, Mellon C, Vintzileos AM, et al. Longitudinal assessment of endocervical canal length between 15 and 24 weeks' gestation in women at risk for pregnancy loss or preterm birth. *Obstet Gynecol.* 1998;92:31–37.

34. Taipale P, Hiilesmaa V. Sonographic measurement of uterine cervix at 18–22 weeks' gestation and the risk of preterm delivery. *Obstet Gynecol.* 1998;92:902–907.

35. Watson WJ, Stevens D, Welter S, et al. Observations on the sonographic measurement of cervical length and the risk of premature birth. *J Matern Fetal Med.* 1999;8:17–19.

36. Andrews WW, Copper R, Hauth JC, et al. Second-trimester cervical ultrasound: associations with increased risk for recurrent early spontaneous delivery. *Obstet Gynecol.* 2000;95:222–226.

37. Hibbard JU, Tart M, Moawad AH. Cervical length at 16–22 weeks' gestation and risk for preterm delivery. *Obstet Gynecol.* 2000;96:972–978.

38. Owen J, Yost N, Berghella V, et al. Mid-trimester endovaginal sonography in women at high risk for spontaneous preterm birth. *JAMA.* 2001;286: 1340–1348.

39. To MS, Skentou C, Liao AW, et al. Cervical length and funneling at 23 weeks of gestation in the prediction of spontaneous early preterm delivery. *Ultrasound Obstet Gynecol.* 2001;18:200–203.

40. Durnwald CP, Walker H, Lundy JC, et al. Rates of recurrent preterm birth by obstetrical history and cervical length. *Am J Obstet Gynecol.* 2005;193:1170–1174.

41. Matijevic R, Grgic O, Vasilj O. Is sonographic assessment of cervical length better than digital examination in screening for preterm delivery in a low-risk population? *Acta Obstet Gynecol Scand.* 2006;85:1342–1347.

42. Committee on Understanding Premature Birth and Assuring Healthy Outcomes, Board on Health Sciences Policy, Institute of Medicine. *Preterm Birth: Causes, Consequences, and Prevention.* Washington, DC: The National Academies Press; 2007.

43. Bos AF, Roze E. Neurodevelopmental outcome in preterm infants. *Dev Med Child Neurol.* 2011;53(suppl 4):35–39.

44. Romero R, Espinoza J, Mazor M, et al. The preterm parturition syndrome. In: Critchley H, Bennett P, Thornton S, eds. *Preterm Birth.* London, UK: RCOG Press; 2004.

45. Celik E, To M, Gajewska K, et al. Cervical length and obstetric history predict spontaneous preterm birth: development and validation of a model to provide individualized risk assessment. *Ultrasound Obstet Gynecol.* 2008;31: 549–554.

46. Althuisius SM, Dekker GA, Hummel P, et al. Final results of the Cervical Incompetence Prevention Randomized Cerclage Trial (CIPRACT): therapeutic cerclage with bed rest versus bed rest alone. *Am J Obstet Gynecol.* 2001;185:1106–1112.

47. Owen J, Hankins G, Iams JD, et al. Multicenter randomized trial of cerclage for preterm birth prevention in high-risk women with shortened midtrimester cervical length. *Am J Obstet Gynecol.* 2009;201:375.e1–375.e8.

48. Goya M, Pratcorona L, Merced C, et al. Cervical pessary in pregnant women with a short cervix (PECEP): an open-label randomised controlled trial. *Lancet.* 2012;379:1800–1806.

49. Conde-Agudelo A, Romero R, Nicolaides K, et al. Vaginal progesterone vs cervical cerclage for the prevention of preterm birth in women with a sonographic short cervix, previous preterm birth, and singleton gestation: a systematic review and indirect comparison metaanalysis. *Am J Obstet Gynecol.* 2013;208:42. e1–42.e18.

50. Gomez R, Galasso M, Romero R, et al. Ultrasonographic examination of the uterine cervix is better than cervical digital examination as a predictor of the likelihood of premature delivery in patients with preterm labor and intact membranes. *Am J Obstet Gynecol.* 1994;171:956–964.

51. Mason GC, Maresh MJ. Alterations in bladder volume and the ultrasound appearance of the cervix. *Br J Obstet Gynaecol.* 1990;97:457–458.

52. To MS, Skentou C, Cicero S, et al. Cervical assessment at the routine 23-weeks' scan: problems with transabdominal sonography. *Ultrasound Obstet Gynecol.* 2000;15:292–296.

53. Hernandez-Andrade E, Romero R, Ahn H, et al. Transabdominal evaluation of uterine cervical length during pregnancy fails to identify a substantial number of women with a short cervix. *J Matern Fetal Neonatal Med.* 2012;25:1682–1689.

54. Jeanty P, d'Alton M, Romero R, et al. Perineal scanning. *Am J Perinatol.* 1986;3:289–295.

55. Zilianti M, Azuaga A, Calderon F, et al. Monitoring the effacement of the uterine cervix by transperineal sonography: a new perspective. *J Ultrasound Med.* 1995;14:719–724.

56. Cicero S, Skentou C, Souka A, et al. Cervical length at 22–24 weeks of gestation: comparison of transvaginal and transperineal-translabial ultrasonography. *Ultrasound Obstet Gynecol.* 2001;17:335–340.

57. Hertzberg BS, Livingston E, DeLong DM, et al. Ultrasonographic evaluation of the cervix: transperineal versus endovaginal imaging. *J Ultrasound Med.* 2001;20:1071–1078.

58. Yazici G, Yildiz A, Tiras MB, et al. Comparison of transperineal and transvaginal sonography in predicting preterm delivery. *J Clin Ultrasound.* 2004;32:225–230.

59. Meijer-Hoogeveen M, Stoutenbeek P, Visser GH. Transperineal versus transvaginal sonographic cervical length measurement in second- and third-trimester pregnancies. *Ultrasound Obstet Gynecol.* 2008;32:657–662.

60. Sonek JD, Iams JD, Blumenfeld M, et al. Measurement of cervical length in pregnancy: comparison between vaginal ultrasonography and digital examination. *Obstet Gynecol.* 1990;76:172–175.

61. Burger M, Weber-Rossler T, Willmann M. Measurement of the pregnant cervix by transvaginal sonography: an interobserver study and new standards to improve the interobserver variability. *Ultrasound Obstet Gynecol.* 1997;9:188–193.

62. To MS, Skentou C, Chan C, et al. Cervical assessment at the routine 23-week scan: standardizing techniques. *Ultrasound Obstet Gynecol.* 2001;17:217–219.

63. Yost NP, Bloom SL, Twickler DM, et al. Pitfalls in ultrasonic cervical length measurement for predicting preterm birth. *Obstet Gynecol.* 1999;93:510–516.

64. Berghella V, Talucci M, Desai A. Does transvaginal sonographic measurement of cervical length before 14 weeks predict preterm delivery in high-risk pregnancies? *Ultrasound Obstet Gynecol.* 2003;21:140–144.

65. Carvalho MH, Bittar RE, Brizot ML, et al. Cervical length at 11–14 weeks' and 22–24 weeks' gestation evaluated by transvaginal sonography, and gestational age at delivery. *Ultrasound Obstet Gynecol.* 2003;21:135–139.

66. Conoscenti G, Meir YJ, D'Ottavio G, et al. Does cervical length at 13–15 weeks' gestation predict preterm delivery in an unselected population? *Ultrasound Obstet Gynecol.* 2003;21:128–134.

67. Antsaklis P, Daskalakis G, Pilalis A, et al. The role of cervical length measurement at 11–14 weeks for the prediction of preterm delivery. *J Matern Fetal Neonatal Med.* 2011;24:465–470.

68. Greco E, Lange A, Ushakov F, et al. Prediction of spontaneous preterm delivery from endocervical length at 11 to 13 weeks. *Prenat Diagn.* 2011;31:84–89.

69. Souka AP, Papastefanou I, Michalitsi V, et al. Cervical length changes from the first to second trimester of pregnancy, and prediction of preterm birth by first-trimester sonographic cervical measurement. *J Ultrasound Med.* 2011;30:997–1002.

70. Greco E, Gupta R, Syngelaki A, et al. First-trimester screening for spontaneous preterm delivery with maternal characteristics and cervical length. *Fetal Diagn Ther.* 2012;31:154–161.

71. Sonek J, Shellhaas C. Cervical sonography: a review. *Ultrasound Obstet Gynecol.* 1998;11:71–78.

72. Zorzoli A, Soliani A, Perra M, et al. Cervical changes throughout pregnancy as assessed by transvaginal sonography. *Obstet Gynecol.* 1994;84:960–964.

73. Cook CM, Ellwood DA. A longitudinal study of the cervix in pregnancy using transvaginal ultrasound. *Br J Obstet Gynaecol.* 1996;103:16–18.

74. Bergelin I, Valentin L. Patterns of normal change in cervical length and width during pregnancy in nulliparous women: a prospective, longitudinal ultrasound study. *Ultrasound Obstet Gynecol.* 2001;18:217–222.

75. Theron G, Schabort C, Norman K, et al. Centile charts of cervical length between 18 and 32 weeks of gestation. *Int J Gynaecol Obstet.* 2008;103:144–148.

76. Riley L, Frigoletto FD Jr, Benacerraf BR. The implications of sonographically identified cervical changes in patients not necessarily at risk for preterm birth. *J Ultrasound Med.* 1992;11:75–79.

77. Tongsong T, Kamprapanth P, Srisomboon J, et al. Single transvaginal sonographic measurement of cervical length early in the third trimester as a predictor of preterm delivery. *Obstet Gynecol.* 1995;86:184–187.

78. De Carvalho MH, Bittar RE, Brizot ML, et al. Prediction of preterm delivery in the second trimester. *Obstet Gynecol.* 2005;105:532–536.

79. Leung TN, Pang MW, Leung TY, et al. Cervical length at 18–22 weeks of gestation for prediction of spontaneous preterm delivery in Hong Kong Chinese women. *Ultrasound Obstet Gynecol.* 2005;26:713–717.

80. Owen J, Yost N, Berghella V, et al. Can shortened midtrimester cervical length predict very early spontaneous preterm birth? *Am J Obstet Gynecol.* 2004;191:298–303.

81. Airoldi J, Berghella V, Sehdev H, et al. Transvaginal ultrasonography of the cervix to predict preterm birth in women with uterine anomalies. *Obstet Gynecol.* 2005;106:553–556.

82. Visintine J, Berghella V, Henning D, et al. Cervical length for prediction of preterm birth in women with multiple prior induced abortions. *Ultrasound Obstet Gynecol.* 2008;31:198–200.

83. Rozenberg P, Gillet A, Ville Y. Transvaginal sonographic examination of the cervix in asymptomatic pregnant women: review of the literature. *Ultrasound Obstet Gynecol.* 2002;19:302–311.

84. Welsh A, Nicolaides K. Cervical screening for preterm delivery. *Curr Opin Obstet Gynecol.* 2002;14:195–202.

85. Erasmus I, Nicolaou E, van Gelderen CJ, et al. Cervical length at 23 weeks' gestation—relation to demographic characteristics and previous obstetric history in South African women. *S Afr Med J.* 2005;95:691–695.

86. Cook CM, Ellwood DA. The cervix as a predictor of preterm delivery in "at-risk" women. *Ultrasound Obstet Gynecol.* 2000;15:109–113.

87. Mercer BM, Goldenberg RL, Meis PJ, et al. The Preterm Prediction Study: prediction of preterm premature rupture of membranes through clinical findings and ancillary testing. The National Institute of Child Health and Human Development Maternal-Fetal Medicine Units Network. *Am J Obstet Gynecol.* 2000;183:738–745.

88. Odibo AO, Berghella V, Reddy U, et al. Does transvaginal ultrasound of the cervix predict preterm premature rupture of membranes in a high-risk population? *Ultrasound Obstet Gynecol.* 2001;18:223–227.

89. Kishida T, Yamada H, Furuta I, et al. Increased levels of interleukin-6 in cervical secretions and assessment of the uterine cervix by transvaginal ultrasonography predict preterm premature rupture of the membranes. *Fetal Diagn Ther.* 2003;18:98–104.

90. Yost NP, Owen J, Berghella V, et al. Number and gestational age of prior preterm births does not modify the predictive value of a short cervix. *Am J Obstet Gynecol.* 2004;191:241–246.

91. Crane JM, Hutchens D. Transvaginal sonographic measurement of cervical length to predict preterm birth in asymptomatic women at increased risk: a systematic review. *Ultrasound Obstet Gynecol.* 2008;31:579–587.

92. Vaisbuch E, Romero R, Erez O, et al. Clinical significance of early (<20 weeks) vs. late (20–24 weeks) detection of sonographic short cervix in asymptomatic women in the mid-trimester. *Ultrasound Obstet Gynecol.* 2010;36:471–481.

93. Poon LC, Savvas M, Zamblera D, et al. Large loop excision of transformation zone and cervical length in the prediction of spontaneous preterm delivery. *BJOG.* 2012;119:692–698.

94. Parikh MN, Mehta AC. Internal cervical os during the second half of pregnancy. *J Obstet Gynaecol Br Emp.* 1961;68:818–821.

95. Guzman ER, Mellon C, Vintzileos AM, et al. Relationship between endocervical canal length between 15–24 weeks gestation and obstetric history. *J Matern Fetal Med.* 1998;7:269–272.

96. Guzman ER, Pisatowski DM, Vintzileos AM, et al. A comparison of ultrasonographically detected cervical changes in response to transfundal pressure, coughing, and standing in predicting cervical incompetence. *Am J Obstet Gynecol.* 1997;177:660–665.

97. Guzman ER, Vintzileos AM, McLean DA, et al. The natural history of a positive response to transfundal pressure in women at risk for cervical incompetence. *Am J Obstet Gynecol.* 1997;176:634–638.

98. Macdonald R, Smith P, Vyas S. Cervical incompetence: the use of transvaginal sonography to provide an objective diagnosis. *Ultrasound Obstet Gynecol.* 2001;18:211–216.

99. Moroz LA, Simhan HN. Rate of sonographic cervical shortening and the risk of spontaneous preterm birth. *Am J Obstet Gynecol.* 2012;206:234.e1–234.e5.

100. Ozdemir I, Demirci F, Yucel O, et al. Ultrasonographic cervical length measurement at 10–14 and 20–24 weeks gestation and the risk of preterm delivery. *Eur J Obstet Gynecol Reprod Biol.* 2007;130:176–179.

101. Dilek TU, Yazici G, Gurbuz A, et al. Progressive cervical length changes versus single cervical length measurement by transvaginal ultrasound for prediction of preterm delivery. *Gynecol Obstet Invest.* 2007;64:175–179.

102. Fox NS, Jean-Pierre C, Predanic M, et al. Short cervix: is a follow-up measurement useful? *Ultrasound Obstet Gynecol.* 2007;29:44–46.

103. Hofmeister C, Brizot Mde L, Liao A, et al. Two-stage transvaginal cervical length screening for preterm birth in twin pregnancies. *J Perinat Med.* 2010;38:479–484.

104. Crane JM, Hutchens D. Follow-up cervical length in asymptomatic high-risk women and the risk of spontaneous preterm birth. *J Perinatol.* 2011;31: 318–323.

105. Iams JD, Cebrik D, Lynch C, et al. The rate of cervical change and the phenotype of spontaneous preterm birth. *Am J Obstet Gynecol.* 2011;205:130.e1–130.e6.

106. Michaels WH, Schreiber FR, Padgett RJ, et al. Ultrasound surveillance of the cervix in twin gestations: management of cervical incompetency. *Obstet Gynecol.* 1991;78:739–744.

107. Kushnir O, Izquierdo LA, Smith JF, et al. Transvaginal sonographic measurement of cervical length: evaluation of twin pregnancies. *J Reprod Med.* 1995;40:380–382.

108. Goldenberg RL, Iams JD, Miodovnik M, et al. The Preterm Prediction Study: risk factors in twin gestations. National Institute of Child Health and Human Development Maternal-Fetal Medicine Units Network. *Am J Obstet Gynecol.* 1996;175:1047–1053.

109. Crane JM, Van den Hof M, Armson BA, et al. Transvaginal ultrasound in the prediction of preterm delivery: singleton and twin gestations. *Obstet Gynecol.* 1997;90:357–363.

110. Imseis HM, Albert TA, Iams JD. Identifying twin gestations at low risk for preterm birth with a transvaginal ultrasonographic cervical measurement at 24 to 26 weeks' gestation. *Am J Obstet Gynecol.* 1997;177:1149–1155.

111. Souka AP, Heath V, Flint S, et al. Cervical length at 23 weeks in twins in predicting spontaneous preterm delivery. *Obstet Gynecol.* 1999;94:450–454.

112. Guzman ER, Walters C, O'Reilly-Green C, et al. Use of cervical ultrasonography in prediction of spontaneous preterm birth in twin gestations. *Am J Obstet Gynecol.* 2000;183:1103–1107.

113. Yang JH, Kuhlman K, Daly S, et al. Prediction of preterm birth by second trimester cervical sonography in twin pregnancies. *Ultrasound Obstet Gynecol.* 2000;15:288–291.

114. Skentou C, Souka AP, To MS, et al. Prediction of preterm delivery in twins by cervical assessment at 23 weeks. *Ultrasound Obstet Gynecol.* 2001;17:7–10.

115. Soriano D, Weisz B, Seidman DS, et al. The role of sonographic assessment of cervical length in the prediction of preterm birth in primigravidae with twin gestation conceived after infertility treatment. *Acta Obstet Gynecol Scand.* 2002;81:39–43.

116. Vayssiere C, Favre R, Audibert F, et al. Cervical length and funneling at 22 and 27 weeks to predict spontaneous birth before 32 weeks in twin pregnancies: a French prospective multicenter study. *Am J Obstet Gynecol.* 2002;187: 1596–1604.

117. Bergelin I, Valentin L. Cervical changes in twin pregnancies observed by transvaginal ultrasound during the latter half of pregnancy: a longitudinal, observational study. *Ultrasound Obstet Gynecol.* 2003;21:556–563.

118. Fuchs I, Tsoi E, Henrich W, et al. Sonographic measurement of cervical length in twin pregnancies in threatened preterm labor. *Ultrasound Obstet Gynecol.* 2004;23:42–45.

119. Robyr R, Boulvain M, Lewi L, et al. Cervical length as a prognostic factor for preterm delivery in twin-to-twin transfusion syndrome treated by fetoscopic laser coagulation of chorionic plate anastomoses. *Ultrasound Obstet Gynecol.* 2005;25:37–41.

120. Sperling L, Kiil C, Larsen LU, et al. How to identify twins at low risk of spontaneous preterm delivery. *Ultrasound Obstet Gynecol.* 2005;26:138–144.

121. Vayssiere C, Favre R, Audibert F, et al. Cervical assessment at 22 and 27 weeks for the prediction of spontaneous birth before 34 weeks in twin pregnancies: is transvaginal sonography more accurate than digital examination? *Ultrasound Obstet Gynecol.* 2005;26:707–712.

122. Heath VC, Daskalakis G, Zagaliki A, et al. Cervicovaginal fibronectin and cervical length at 23 weeks of gestation: relative risk of early preterm delivery. *BJOG.* 2000;107:1276–1281.

123. Fox NS, Rebarber A, Klauser CK, et al. Prediction of spontaneous preterm birth in asymptomatic twin pregnancies using the change in cervical length over time. *Am J Obstet Gynecol.* 2010;202:155.e1–155.e4.

124. Conde-Agudelo A, Romero R, Hassan SS, et al. Transvaginal sonographic cervical length for the prediction of spontaneous preterm birth in twin pregnancies: a systematic review and metaanalysis. *Am J Obstet Gynecol.* 2010;203:128. e1–128.e12.

125. Ramin KD, Ogburn PL Jr, Mulholland TA, et al. Ultrasonographic assessment of cervical length in triplet pregnancies. *Am J Obstet Gynecol.* 1999;180: 1442–1445.

126. Guzman ER, Walters C, O'Reilly-Green C, et al. Use of cervical ultrasonography in prediction of spontaneous preterm birth in triplet gestations. *Am J Obstet Gynecol.* 2000;183:1108–1113.

127. To MS, Skentou C, Cicero S, et al. Cervical length at 23 weeks in triplets: prediction of spontaneous preterm delivery. *Ultrasound Obstet Gynecol.* 2000;16:515–518.

128. Fox NS, Rebarber A, Roman AS, et al. Combined fetal fibronectin and cervical length and spontaneous preterm birth in asymptomatic triplet pregnancies. *J Matern Fetal Neonatal Med.* 2012;25:2308–2311.

129. King JF, Grant A, Keirse MJ, et al. Beta-mimetics in preterm labour: an overview of the randomized controlled trials. *Br J Obstet Gynaecol.* 1988;95:211–222.

130. Murakawa H, Utumi T, Hasegawa I, et al. Evaluation of threatened preterm delivery by transvaginal ultrasonographic measurement of cervical length. *Obstet Gynecol.* 1993;82:829–832.

131. Rizzo G, Capponi A, Arduini D, et al. The value of fetal fibronectin in cervical and vaginal secretions and of ultrasonographic examination of the uterine cervix in predicting premature delivery for patients with preterm labor and intact membranes. *Am J Obstet Gynecol.* 1996;175:1146–1151.

132. Tsoi E, Akmal S, Rane S, et al. Ultrasound assessment of cervical length in threatened preterm labor. *Ultrasound Obstet Gynecol.* 2003;21:552–555.

133. Fuchs IB, Henrich W, Osthues K, et al. Sonographic cervical length in singleton pregnancies with intact membranes presenting with threatened preterm labor. *Ultrasound Obstet Gynecol.* 2004;24:554–557.

134. Sanin-Blair J, Palacio M, Delgado J, et al. Impact of ultrasound cervical length assessment on duration of hospital stay in the clinical management of threatened preterm labor. *Ultrasound Obstet Gynecol.* 2004;24:756–760.

135. Tsoi E, Geerts L, Jeffery B, et al. Sonographic cervical length in threatened preterm labor in a South African population. *Ultrasound Obstet Gynecol.* 2004;24:644–646.

136. Botsis D, Papagianni V, Vitoratos N, et al. Prediction of preterm delivery by sonographic estimation of cervical length. *Biol Neonate.* 2005;88:42–45.

137. Daskalakis G, Thomakos N, Hatziioannou L, et al. Cervical assessment in women with threatened preterm labor. *J Matern Fetal Neonatal Med.* 2005;17:309–312.

138. Tsoi E, Fuchs IB, Rane S, et al. Sonographic measurement of cervical length in threatened preterm labor in singleton pregnancies with intact membranes. *Ultrasound Obstet Gynecol.* 2005;25:353–356.

139. Botsis D, Makrakis E, Papagianni V, et al. The value of cervical length and plasma proMMP-9 levels for the prediction of preterm delivery in pregnant women presenting with threatened preterm labor. *Eur J Obstet Gynecol Reprod Biol.* 2006;128:108–112.

140. Tsoi E, Akmal S, Geerts L, et al. Sonographic measurement of cervical length and fetal fibronectin testing in threatened preterm labor. *Ultrasound Obstet Gynecol.* 2006;27:368–372.

141. Alfirevic Z, Allen-Coward H, Molina F, et al. Targeted therapy for threatened preterm labor based on sonographic measurement of the cervical length: a randomized controlled trial. *Ultrasound Obstet Gynecol.* 2007;29:47–50.

142. Eroglu D, Yanik F, Oktem M, et al. Prediction of preterm delivery among women with threatened preterm labor. *Gynecol Obstet Invest.* 2007;64:109–116.

143. Palacio M, Sanin-Blair J, Sanchez M, et al. The use of a variable cut-off value of cervical length in women admitted for preterm labor before and after 32 weeks. *Ultrasound Obstet Gynecol.* 2007;29:421–426.

144. Schmitz T, Kayem G, Maillard F, et al. Selective use of sonographic cervical length measurement for predicting imminent preterm delivery in women with preterm labor and intact membranes. *Ultrasound Obstet Gynecol.* 2008;31:421–426.

145. Gomez R, Romero R, Medina L, et al. Cervicovaginal fibronectin improves the prediction of preterm delivery based on sonographic cervical length in patients with preterm uterine contractions and intact membranes. *Am J Obstet Gynecol.* 2005;192:350–359.

146. Leitich H, Brunbauer M, Kaider A, et al. Cervical length and dilatation of the internal cervical os detected by vaginal ultrasonography as markers for preterm delivery: a systematic review. *Am J Obstet Gynecol.* 1999;181:1465–1472.

147. Zalar RW Jr. Transvaginal ultrasound and preterm prelabor: a nonrandomized intervention study. *Obstet Gynecol.* 1996;88:20–23.

148. Rageth JC, Kernen B, Saurenmann E, et al. Premature contractions: possible influence of sonographic measurement of cervical length on clinical management. *Ultrasound Obstet Gynecol.* 1997;9:183–187.

149. Mozurkewich EL, Naglie G, Krahn MD, et al. Predicting preterm birth: a cost-effectiveness analysis. *Am J Obstet Gynecol.* 2000;182:1589–1598.

150. Berghella V, Ness A, Bega G, et al. Cervical sonography in women with symptoms of preterm labor. *Obstet Gynecol Clin North Am.* 2005;32:383–396.

151. Fox NS, Jean-Pierre C, Predanic M, et al. Does hospitalization prevent preterm delivery in the patient with a short cervix? *Am J Perinatol.* 2007;24:49–53.

152. Rozenberg P, Rudant J, Chevret S, et al. Repeat measurement of cervical length after successful tocolysis. *Obstet Gynecol.* 2004;104:995–999.

153. Gomez R, Romero R, Nien JK, et al. A short cervix in women with preterm labor and intact membranes: a risk factor for microbial invasion of the amniotic cavity. *Am J Obstet Gynecol.* 2005;192:678–689.

154. DeFranco EA, Lewis DF, Odibo AO. Improving the screening accuracy for preterm labor: is the combination of fetal fibronectin and cervical length in symptomatic patients a useful predictor of preterm birth? A systematic review. *Am J Obstet Gynecol.* 2013;208:233.e1–233.e6.

155. Ophir J, Cespedes I, Ponnekanti H, et al. Elastography: a quantitative method for imaging the elasticity of biological tissues. *Ultrason Imaging.* 1991;13:111–134.

156. Cespedes I, Ophir J, Ponnekanti H, et al. Elastography: elasticity imaging using ultrasound with application to muscle and breast in vivo. *Ultrason Imaging.* 1993;15:73–88.

157. Garra BS. Elastography: current status, future prospects, and making it work for you. *Ultrasound Q.* 2011;27:177–186.

158. Molina FS, Gomez LF, Florido J, et al. Quantification of cervical elastography: a reproducibility study. *Ultrasound Obstet Gynecol.* 2012;39:685–689.

159. Hernandez-Andrade E, Hassan SS, Ahn H, et al. Evaluation of cervical stiffness during pregnancy using semiquantitative ultrasound elastography. *Ultrasound Obstet Gynecol.* 2013;41(2):152–161.

160. Leppert PC. Anatomy and physiology of cervical ripening. *Clin Obstet Gynecol.* 1995;38:267–279.

161. McFarlin BL, Bigelow TA, Laybed Y, et al. Ultrasonic attenuation estimation of the pregnant cervix: a preliminary report. *Ultrasound Obstet Gynecol.* 2010;36:218–225.

162. Feltovich H, Hall TJ, Berghella V. Beyond cervical length: emerging technologies for assessing the pregnant cervix. *Am J Obstet Gynecol.* 2012;207:345–354.

163. Romero R, Avila C, Sepulveda W. The role of systemic and intrauterine infection in preterm labor. In: Fuchs A, Fuchs F, Stubblefield P, eds. *Preterm Birth: Causes, Prevention, and Management.* New York, NY: McGraw-Hill; 1993.

164. Romero R, Gomez R, Mazor M, et al. The preterm labor syndrome. In: Elder M, Romero R, Lamont R, eds. *Preterm Labor.* New York, NY: Churchill Livingstone; 1997.

165. Romero R, Espinoza J, Kusanovic JP, et al. The preterm parturition syndrome. *BJOG.* 2006;113(suppl 3):17–42.

166. Moinian M, Andersch B. Does cervix conization increase the risk of complications in subsequent pregnancies? *Acta Obstet Gynecol Scand.* 1982;61:101–103.

167. Kristensen J, Langhoff-Roos J, Wittrup M, et al. Cervical conization and preterm delivery/low birth weight: a systematic review of the literature. *Acta Obstet Gynecol Scand.* 1993;72:640–644.

168. Levine RU, Berkowitz KM. Conservative management and pregnancy outcome in diethylstilbestrol-exposed women with and without gross genital tract abnormalities. *Am J Obstet Gynecol.* 1993;169:1125–1129.

169. Romero R. Prenatal medicine: the child is the father of the man. *Prenat Neonatal Med.* 1996;1:8–11.

170. Raio L, Ghezzi F, Di NE, et al. Duration of pregnancy after carbon dioxide laser conization of the cervix: influence of cone height. *Obstet Gynecol.* 1997;90:978–982.

171. Jakobsson M, Gissler M, Paavonen J, et al. Loop electrosurgical excision procedure and the risk for preterm birth. *Obstet Gynecol.* 2009;114:504–510.

172. Noehr B, Jensen A, Frederiksen K, et al. Depth of cervical cone removed by loop electrosurgical excision procedure and subsequent risk of spontaneous preterm delivery. *Obstet Gynecol.* 2009;114:1232–1238.

173. Craig CJ. Congenital abnormalities of the uterus and foetal wastage. *S Afr Med J.* 1973;47:2000–2005.

174. Mangan CE, Borow L, Burtnett-Rubin MM, et al. Pregnancy outcome in 98 women exposed to diethylstilbestrol in utero, their mothers, and unexposed siblings. *Obstet Gynecol.* 1982;59:315–319.

175. Ludmir J, Landon MB, Gabbe SG, et al. Management of the diethylstilbestrol-exposed pregnant patient: a prospective study. *Am J Obstet Gynecol.* 1987;157:665–669.

176. Romero R, Gonzalez R, Sepulveda W, et al. Infection and labor, VIII: microbial invasion of the amniotic cavity in patients with suspected cervical incompetence: prevalence and clinical significance. *Am J Obstet Gynecol.* 1992;167:1086–1091.

177. Hassan S, Romero R, Hendler I, et al. A sonographic short cervix as the only clinical manifestation of intra-amniotic infection. *J Perinat Med.* 2006;34:13–19.

178. Stys SJ, Clewell WH, Meschia G. Changes in cervical compliance at parturition independent of uterine activity. *Am J Obstet Gynecol.* 1978;130:414–418.

179. Gray DJ, Robinson HB, Malone J, et al. Adverse outcome in pregnancy following amniotic fluid isolation of *Ureaplasma urealyticum. Prenat Diagn.* 1992;12:111–117.

180. Kiefer DG, Keeler SM, Rust OA, et al. Is midtrimester short cervix a sign of intraamniotic inflammation? *Am J Obstet Gynecol.* 2009;200:374.e1–374.e5.

181. Keeler SM, Kiefer DG, Rust OA, et al. Comprehensive amniotic fluid cytokine profile evaluation in women with a short cervix: which cytokine(s) correlates best with outcome? *Am J Obstet Gynecol.* 2009;201:276.e1–276.e6.

182. Vaisbuch E, Hassan SS, Mazaki-Tovi S, et al. Patients with an asymptomatic short cervix (< or =15 mm) have a high rate of subclinical intraamniotic inflammation: implications for patient counseling. *Am J Obstet Gynecol.* 2010;202:433.e1–433.e8.

183. Mays JK, Figueroa R, Shah J, et al. Amniocentesis for selection before rescue cerclage. *Obstet Gynecol.* 2000;95:652–655.

184. Zimmer EZ, Bronshtein M. Ultrasonic features of intra-amniotic "unidentified debris" at 14–16 weeks' gestation. *Ultrasound Obstet Gynecol.* 1996;7:178–181.

185. Parulekar SG. Ultrasonographic demonstration of floating particles in amniotic fluid. *J Ultrasound Med.* 1983;2:107–110.

186. Sepulveda W, Reid R, Nicolaidis P, et al. Second-trimester echogenic bowel and intraamniotic bleeding: association between fetal bowel echogenicity and amniotic fluid spectrophotometry at 410 nm. *Am J Obstet Gynecol.* 1996;174:839–842.

187. Vengalil S, Santolaya-Forgas J, Meyer W, et al. Ultrasonically dense amniotic fluid in early pregnancy in asymptomatic women without vaginal bleeding: a report of two cases. *J Reprod Med.* 1998;43:462–464.

188. Tskitishvili E, Tomimatsu T, Kanagawa T, et al. Amniotic fluid "sludge" detected in patients with subchorionic hematoma: a report of two cases. *Ultrasound Obstet Gynecol.* 2009;33:484–486.

189. Cafici D, Sepulveda W. First-trimester echogenic amniotic fluid in the acrania-anencephaly sequence. *J Ultrasound Med.* 2003;22:1075–1079.

190. Hallak M, Zador IE, Garcia EM, et al. Ultrasound-detected free-floating particles in amniotic fluid: correlation with maternal serum alpha-fetoprotein. *Fetal Diagn Ther.* 1993;8:402–406.

191. Benacerraf BR, Gatter MA, Ginsburgh F. Ultrasound diagnosis of meconium-stained amniotic fluid. *Am J Obstet Gynecol.* 1984;149:570–572.

192. DeVore GR, Platt LD. Ultrasound appearance of particulate matter in amniotic cavity: vernix or meconium? *J Clin Ultrasound.* 1986;14:229–230.

193. Sepulveda WH, Quiroz VH. Sonographic detection of echogenic amniotic fluid and its clinical significance. *J Perinat Med.* 1989;17:333–335.

194. Sherer DM, Abramowicz JS, Smith SA, et al. Sonographically homogeneous echogenic amniotic fluid in detecting meconium-stained amniotic fluid. *Obstet Gynecol.* 1991;78:819–822.

195. Gross TL, Wolfson RN, Kuhnert PM, et al. Sonographically detected free-floating particles in amniotic fluid predict a mature lecithin-sphingomyelin ratio. *J Clin Ultrasound.* 1985;13:405–409.

196. Mullin TJ, Gross TL, Wolfson RN. Ultrasound screening for free-floating particles and fetal lung maturity. *Obstet Gynecol.* 1985;66:50–54.

197. Vohra N, Rochelson B, Smith-Levitin M. Three-dimensional sonographic findings in congenital (harlequin) ichthyosis. *J Ultrasound Med.* 2003;22:737–739.

198. Dolan CR, Smith LT, Sybert VP. Prenatal detection of epidermolysis bullosa letalis with pyloric atresia in a fetus by abnormal ultrasound and elevated alpha-fetoprotein. *Am J Med Genet.* 1993;47:395–400.

199. Espinoza J, Goncalves LF, Romero R, et al. The prevalence and clinical significance of amniotic fluid "sludge" in patients with preterm labor and intact membranes. *Ultrasound Obstet Gynecol.* 2005;25:346–352.

200. Bujold E, Pasquier JC, Simoneau J, et al. Intra-amniotic sludge, short cervix, and risk of preterm delivery. *J Obstet Gynaecol Can.* 2006;28:198–202.

201. Kusanovic JP, Espinoza J, Romero R, et al. Clinical significance of the presence of amniotic fluid "sludge" in asymptomatic patients at high risk for spontaneous preterm delivery. *Ultrasound Obstet Gynecol.* 2007;30:706–714.

202. Himaya E, Rhalmi N, Girard M, et al. Midtrimester intra-amniotic sludge and the risk of spontaneous preterm birth. *Am J Perinatol.* 2011;28:815–820.

203. Ventura W, Nazario C, Ingar J, et al. Risk of impending preterm delivery associated with the presence of amniotic fluid sludge in women in preterm labor with intact membranes. *Fetal Diagn Ther.* 2011;30:116–121.

204. Romero R, Kusanovic JP, Espinoza J, et al. What is amniotic fluid "sludge"? *Ultrasound Obstet Gynecol.* 2007;30:793–798.

205. Romero R, Schaudinn C, Kusanovic JP, et al. Detection of a microbial biofilm in intraamniotic infection. *Am J Obstet Gynecol.* 2008;198:135.e1–135.e5.

206. Grobman WA, Thom EA, Spong CY, et al. 17 Alpha-hydroxyprogesterone caproate to prevent prematurity in nulliparas with cervical length less than 30 mm. *Am J Obstet Gynecol.* 2012;207:390.e1–390.e8.

207. O'Brien JM. The safety of progesterone and 17-hydroxyprogesterone caproate administration for the prevention of preterm birth: an evidence-based assessment. *Am J Perinatol.* 2012;29:665–672.

208. Szychowski JM, Berghella V, Owen J, et al. Cerclage for the prevention of preterm birth in high risk women receiving intramuscular 17-alpha-hydroxyprogesterone caproate. *J Matern Fetal Neonatal Med.* 2012;25:2686–2689.

209. Althuisius SM, Dekker GA, van Geijn HP, et al. Cervical incompetence prevention randomized cerclage trial (CIPRACT): study design and preliminary results. *Am J Obstet Gynecol.* 2000;183:823–829.

210. Rust OA, Atlas RO, Jones KJ, et al. A randomized trial of cerclage versus no cerclage among patients with ultrasonographically detected second-trimester preterm dilatation of the internal os. *Am J Obstet Gynecol.* 2000;183:830–835.

211. Rust OA, Atlas RO, Reed J, et al. Revisiting the short cervix detected by transvaginal ultrasound in the second trimester: why cerclage therapy may not help. *Am J Obstet Gynecol.* 2001;185:1098–1105.

212. Berghella V, Odibo AO, Tolosa JE. Cerclage for prevention of preterm birth in women with a short cervix found on transvaginal ultrasound examination: a randomized trial. *Am J Obstet Gynecol.* 2004;191:1311–1317.

213. To MS, Alfirevic Z, Heath VC, et al. Cervical cerclage for prevention of preterm delivery in women with short cervix: randomised controlled trial. *Lancet.* 2004;363:1849–1853.

214. Briggs RM, Thompson WB Jr. Treatment of the incompetent cervix. *Obstet Gynecol.* 1960;16:414–418.

215. Seppala M, Vara P. Cervical cerclage in the treatment of incompetent cervix: a retrospective analysis of the indications and results of 164 operations. *Acta Obstet Gynecol Scand.* 1970;49:343–346.

216. Robboy MS. The management of cervical incompetence. UCLA experience with cerclage procedures. *Obstet Gynecol.* 1973;41:108–112.

217. Dor J, Shalev J, Mashiach S, et al. Elective cervical suture of twin pregnancies diagnosed ultrasonically in the first trimester following induced ovulation. *Gynecol Obstet Invest.* 1982;13:55–60.

218. Crombleholme WR, Minkoff HL, Delke I, et al. Cervical cerclage: an aggressive approach to threatened or recurrent pregnancy wastage. *Am J Obstet Gynecol.* 1983;146:168–174.

219. Lazar P, Gueguen S, Dreyfus J, et al. Multicentred controlled trial of cervical cerclage in women at moderate risk of preterm delivery. *Br J Obstet Gynaecol.* 1984;91:731–735.

220. Rush RW, Isaacs S, McPherson K, et al. A randomized controlled trial of cervical cerclage in women at high risk of spontaneous preterm delivery. *Br J Obstet Gynaecol.* 1984;91:724–730.

221. MRC/RCOG Working Party on Cervical Cerclage; Macnaughton MC, Chalmers IG, Dubowitz V, et al. Final report of the Medical Research Council/Royal College of Obstetricians and Gynaecologists multicentre randomised trial of cervical cerclage. *Br J Obstet Gynaecol.* 1993;100:516–523.

222. Ayhan A, Mercan R, Tuncer ZS, et al. Postconceptional cervical cerclage. *Int J Gynaecol Obstet.* 1993;42:243–246.

223. Golan A, Wolman I, Arieli S, et al. Cervical cerclage for the incompetent cervical os: improving the fetal salvage rate. *J Reprod Med.* 1995;40:367–370.

224. Olatunbosun OA, al-Nuaim L, Turnell RW. Emergency cerclage compared with bed rest for advanced cervical dilatation in pregnancy. *Int Surg.* 1995;80:170–174.

225. Guzman ER, Houlihan C, Vintzileos A, et al. The significance of transvaginal ultrasonographic evaluation of the cervix in women treated with emergency cerclage. *Am J Obstet Gynecol.* 1996;175:471–476.

226. Guzman ER, Forster JK, Vintzileos AM, et al. Pregnancy outcomes in women treated with elective versus ultrasound-indicated cervical cerclage. *Ultrasound Obstet Gynecol.* 1998;12:323–327.

227. Heath VC, Souka AP, Erasmus I, et al. Cervical length at 23 weeks of gestation: the value of Shirodkar suture for the short cervix. *Ultrasound Obstet Gynecol.* 1998;12:318–322.

228. Berghella V, Daly SF, Tolosa JE, et al. Prediction of preterm delivery with transvaginal ultrasonography of the cervix in patients with high-risk pregnancies: does cerclage prevent prematurity? *Am J Obstet Gynecol.* 1999;181:809–815.

229. Kurup M, Goldkrand JW. Cervical incompetence: elective, emergent, or urgent cerclage. *Am J Obstet Gynecol.* 1999;181:240–246.

230. Hibbard JU, Snow J, Moawad AH. Short cervical length by ultrasound and cerclage. *J Perinatol.* 2000;20:161–165.

231. Seki H, Kuromaki K, Takeda S, et al. Prophylactic cervical cerclage for the prevention of early premature delivery in nulliparous women with twin pregnancies. *J Obstet Gynaecol Res.* 2000;26:151–152.

232. Guzman ER, Ananth CV. Cervical length and spontaneous prematurity: laying the foundation for future interventional randomized trials for the short cervix. *Ultrasound Obstet Gynecol.* 2001;18:195–199.

233. Hassan SS, Romero R, Maymon E, et al. Does cervical cerclage prevent preterm delivery in patients with a short cervix? *Am J Obstet Gynecol.* 2001;184:1325–1329.

234. Novy MJ, Gupta A, Wothe DD, et al. Cervical cerclage in the second trimester of pregnancy: a historical cohort study. *Am J Obstet Gynecol.* 2001;184:1447–1454.

235. Berghella V, Haas S, Chervoneva I, et al. Patients with prior second-trimester loss: prophylactic cerclage or serial transvaginal sonograms? *Am J Obstet Gynecol.* 2002;187:747–751.

236. Newman RB, Krombach RS, Myers MC, et al. Effect of cerclage on obstetrical outcome in twin gestations with a shortened cervical length. *Am J Obstet Gynecol.* 2002;186:634–640.

237. To MS, Palaniappan V, Skentou C, et al. Elective cerclage vs. ultrasound-indicated cerclage in high-risk pregnancies. *Ultrasound Obstet Gynecol.* 2002;19:475–477.

238. Althuisius SM, Dekker GA, Hummel P, et al. Cervical incompetence prevention randomized cerclage trial: emergency cerclage with bed rest versus bed rest alone. *Am J Obstet Gynecol.* 2003;189:907–910.

239. Odibo AO, Farrell C, Macones GA, et al. Development of a scoring system for predicting the risk of preterm birth in women receiving cervical cerclage. *J Perinatol.* 2003;23:664–667.

240. Williams M, Iams JD. Cervical length measurement and cervical cerclage to prevent preterm birth. *Clin Obstet Gynecol.* 2004;47:775–783.

241. Althuisius SM. The short and funneling cervix: when to use cerclage? *Curr Opin Obstet Gynecol.* 2005;17:574–578.

242. Belej-Rak T, Okun N, Windrim R, et al. Effectiveness of cervical cerclage for a sonographically shortened cervix: a systematic review and meta-analysis. *Am J Obstet Gynecol.* 2003;189:1679–1687.

243. Drakeley AJ, Roberts D, Alfirevic Z. Cervical cerclage for prevention of preterm delivery: meta-analysis of randomized trials. *Obstet Gynecol.* 2003;102:621–627.

244. Drakeley AJ, Roberts D, Alfirevic Z. Cervical stitch (cerclage) for preventing pregnancy loss in women. *Cochrane Database Syst Rev.* 2003;(1):CD003253. doi:10.1002/14651858.CD003253.

245. Berghella V, Rafael TJ, Szychowski JM, et al. Cerclage for short cervix on ultrasonography in women with singleton gestations and previous preterm birth: a meta-analysis. *Obstet Gynecol.* 2011;117:663–671.

246. Berghella V, Mackeen AD. Cervical length screening with ultrasound-indicated cerclage compared with history-indicated cerclage for prevention of preterm birth: a meta-analysis. *Obstet Gynecol.* 2011;118:148–155.

247. American College of Obstetricians Gynecologists, Committee on Practice Bulletins-Obstetrics. ACOG practice bulletin no 127: management of preterm labor. *Obstet Gynecol.* 2012;119:1308–1317.

248. Society for Maternal-Fetal Medicine Publications Committee, with assistance of Vincenzo Berghella. Progesterone and preterm birth prevention: translating clinical trials data into clinical practice. *Am J Obstet Gynecol.* 2012;206:376–386.

249. Berghella V. Universal cervical length screening for prediction and prevention of preterm birth. *Obstet Gynecol Surv.* 2012;67:653–658.

250. Higgins SP, Kornman LH, Bell RJ, et al. Cervical surveillance as an alternative to elective cervical cerclage for pregnancy management of suspected cervical incompetence. *Aust N Z J Obstet Gynaecol.* 2004;44:228–232.

251. Simcox R, Seed PT, Bennett P, et al. A randomized controlled trial of cervical scanning vs history to determine cerclage in women at high risk of preterm birth (CIRCLE trial). *Am J Obstet Gynecol.* 2009;200:623.e1–623.e6.

252. Cahill AG, Odibo AO, Caughey AB, et al. Universal cervical length screening and treatment with vaginal progesterone to prevent preterm birth: a decision and economic analysis. *Am J Obstet Gynecol.* 2010;202:548.e1–548.e8.

253. Campbell S. Universal cervical-length screening and vaginal progesterone prevents early preterm births, reduces neonatal morbidity and is cost saving: doing nothing is no longer an option. *Ultrasound Obstet Gynecol.* 2011;38:1–9.

254. Werner EF, Han CS, Pettker CM, et al. Universal cervical length screening to prevent preterm birth: a cost-effectiveness analysis. *Ultrasound Obstet Gynecol.* 2011;38:32–37.

255. Combs CA. Vaginal progesterone for asymptomatic cervical shortening and the case for universal screening of cervical length. *Am J Obstet Gynecol.* 2012;206:101–103.

256. Miller ES, Grobman WA. Cost-effectiveness of transabdominal ultrasound for cervical length screening for preterm birth prevention. *Am J Obstet Gynecol.* 2013;209:546.e1–546.e6.

257. Wilson JMG, Jungner G. *Principles and Practice of Screening for Disease.* Geneva, Switzerland: World Health Organization; 1968. Public Health Papers, No 34.

258. Da Fonseca EB, Bittar RE, Carvalho MH, et al. Prophylactic administration of progesterone by vaginal suppository to reduce the incidence of spontaneous preterm birth in women at increased risk: a randomized placebo-controlled double-blind study. *Am J Obstet Gynecol.* 2003;188:419–424.

259. Maher MA, Abdelaziz A, Ellaithy M, et al. Prevention of preterm birth: a randomized trial of vaginal compared with intramuscular progesterone. *Acta Obstet Gynecol Scand.* 2013;92:215–222.

260. Aguin E, Aguin T, Cordoba M, et al. Amniotic fluid inflammation with negative culture and outcome after cervical cerclage. *J Matern Fetal Neonatal Med.* 2012;25:1990–1994.

261. Klein K, Rode L, Nicolaides K, et al. Vaginal micronized progesterone and risk of preterm delivery in high-risk twin pregnancies: secondary analysis of a placebo-controlled randomized trial and meta-analysis. *Ultrasound Obstet Gynecol.* 2011;38:281–287.

262. Rode L, Klein K, Nicolaides K, et al. Prevention of preterm delivery in twin gestations (PREDICT): a multicenter, randomized, placebo-controlled trial on the effect of vaginal micronized progesterone. *Ultrasound Obstet Gynecol.* 2011;38:272–280.

263. Serra V, Perales A, Meseguer J, et al. Increased doses of vaginal progesterone for the prevention of preterm birth in twin pregnancies: a randomised controlled double-blind multicentre trial. *BJOG.* 2013;120:50–57.

264. Cross R. Treatment of habitual abortion due to cervical incompetence. *Lancet.* 1959;274:127.

265. Newcomer J. Pessaries for the treatment of incompetent cervix and premature delivery. *Obstet Gynecol Surv.* 2000;55:443–448.

266. Arabin B, Halbesma JR, Vork F, et al. Is treatment with vaginal pessaries an option in patients with a sonographically detected short cervix? *J Perinat Med.* 2003;31:122–133.

267. Khan AM, Dawlatly B, Khan D, et al. Is cervical pessary an answer to preterm delivery? *J Obstet Gynaecol.* 2004;24:176–177.

268. Hui SY, Chor CM, Lau TK, et al. Cerclage pessary for preventing preterm birth in women with a singleton pregnancy and a short cervix at 20 to 24 weeks: a randomized controlled trial. *Am J Perinatol.* 2013;30:283–288.

269. Ting YH, Lao TT, Wa Law L, et al. Arabin cerclage pessary in the management of cervical insufficiency. *J Matern Fetal Neonatal Med.* 2012;25:2693–2695.

270. Heath VC, Southall TR, Souka AP, et al. Cervical length at 23 weeks of gestation: relation to demographic characteristics and previous obstetric history. *Ultrasound Obstet Gynecol.* 1998;12:304–311.

271. Rozenberg P, Goffinet F, Malagrida L, et al. Evaluating the risk of preterm delivery: a comparison of fetal fibronectin and transvaginal ultrasonographic measurement of cervical length. *Am J Obstet Gynecol.* 1997;176:196–199.

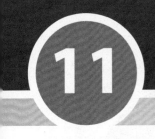

# 11 Multiple Gestation

Mounira Habli

Multiple gestations, of which 98% are twins, are associated with a higher risk of morbidity and mortality than singleton pregnancies. During the past three decades, the rate of twin births has skyrocketed, increasing by 70% from 1980 to 2004.[1] After 2005, this rate slowed to 0.5% annually, and in 2011, the rate actually declined by 1% from the previous year.[1] According to the Centers for Disease Control and Prevention, 33 of every 1,000 births are twin deliveries. In 2011, this totaled 131,269 twins births.[1] Increases in twin births are largely attributed to two factors: delayed childbearing and the increased use of assisted reproductive technology (ART), which includes fertility drugs to superovulate the ovaries and the transfer of multiple embryos. Compared with younger mothers, spontaneously conceived pregnancies in older mothers are prone to twinning because of the different actions of follicle-stimulating hormones.[2] Multiple gestations are a well-known possibility in ART.[3] The use of more selective procedures, such as single embryo transfer, can decrease the risk of twinning[4]; whereas other procedures that decrease the risk of higher multiples actually contribute to more twin gestations.[5] A spontaneously conceived infant has a 1 in 90 chance of being a twin and a tiny chance of being triplet or more.[6] However, an ART infant has 20 to 30 times more likelihood of being a twin and a 400-fold increased risk of triplets. In a recent US review, 47% of ART infants were multiple gestations compared with 3.3% of all births.[7] In that review, 43% of ART pregnancies were twins versus 3.3% of all births, and 3.6% of ART infants were triplets or higher order multiples compared with 0.2% of all infants.[7] Through regulation, European countries have been able to reduce multiple gestations with ART to a rate of 22.7%, whereas the United States, owing to lack of regulation, has been unable to reduce the number below 32%.[6]

In this chapter, the management and outcomes for twin pregnancies, the unique challenges in prenatal screening and diagnosis, the importance of early diagnosis of chorionicity, prenatal genetic testing, and maternal and fetal complications will be discussed. The outcomes of twin pregnancies are largely based on chorionicity, with complication rates lower in dichorionic twins and higher in monochorionic twins. Given the higher infant mortality, with twins being five times more likely to die in infancy than a singleton,[8] and higher maternal risks, including death,[9] this chapter reviews contemporary strategies of care for the mother and twins.

## IMAGING

Ultrasonography has been the imaging modality of choice for diagnosing fetal anomalies for decades. It is relatively inexpensive, has real-time capability, and is considered safe, making it the standard in the evaluation of the fetus.[10] However, ultrasound performance depends highly on the skill and experience of the sonographer, resulting in detection rates of abnormalities that vary from 13% to 82%.[10,11] The sensitivity and specificity of ultrasound depends on the fetal position, presence of oligohydramnios, degree of ossification, and maternal body habitus.[10,11]

Recently, MRI has emerged as a technique to image fetuses when ultrasound findings are inconclusive. Several authors agree that MRI is as good as ultrasound in prenatal diagnosis and in some cases superior, particularly for defining intracranial anatomy. When ultrasound is inconclusive, MRI has been effective in defining both the type of acardiac twinning and the extent of conjoined twins. MRI will likely be utilized more in the future and in conjunction with ultrasound to aid when diagnosis by ultrasound is not definitive and when maternal habitus is not conducive to ultrasound. Several studies have shown that a higher detection rates is achieved by MRI imaging for abnormalities of the central nervous system (CNS), thorax, abdomen, and skeleton[12] and that additional anatomical information can be provided in 45% of cases.[13] Recently, in a case series of complicated multifetal pregnancies, MRI was superior to ultrasound in 64% of cases.[14] Improved diagnosis occurred mainly in CNS abnormalities, abdominal organs, and conjoined twin. In this case series, diagnosis as well as counseling and management were affected.

## EMBRYOLOGY OF TWINNING/ PLACENTATION/AMNION

The embryology of twinning is fascinating. Timing of cell division by one day earlier or later greatly affects the twin outcome. In a normally developing pregnancy, the placenta (or chorion) develops on day 3. Although most sources agree on the timing of embryogenesis, there are several hypotheses that explain why twinning occurs. From a genetics standpoint, a portion of dizygotic twins can be linked to dominant inheritance on chromosome 3.[15–17]

### Zygosity

Twins can be either monozygotic (identical) or dizygotic (fraternal) (Fig. 11.1).

#### Definition/Incidence
*Monozygotic twins*, approximately one-third of twin gestations, result from ovulation and fertilization of single oocyte and subsequent division of the zygote into two fetuses with either mono- or dichorionic placentation (Fig. 11.2). During embryogenesis, dichorionic diamniotic twins split on days 2 to 3, monochorionic diamniotic twinning occurs between days 3 and 7, monochorionic monoamnitoic twinning occurs from days 7 to 14, and conjoined twinning occurs between days 14 and 15.[18] The incidence of monozygotic birth is fairly constant, accounting for 1 in 330 of spontaneous live births, or about 1 in 160 babies.[19–21] Of these, 70% are concordant healthy monozygotic twins and 30% are dizygotic[19–21] (Fig. 11.3). Monzygotic twins have increased risks of complications such as twin reverse arterial perfusion syndrome (TRAP), conjoined twins, and twin-to-twin transfusion.

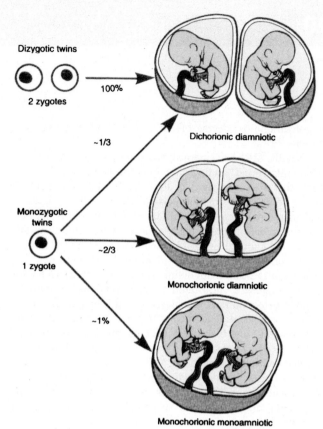

**FIGURE 11.1:** Monozygotic versus dizygotic twins. All dizygotic twins have dichorionic–diamniotic placentation. Monozygotic twins may form dichorionic–diamniotic, monochorionic–diamniotic, or monochorionic–monoamniotic placentation.

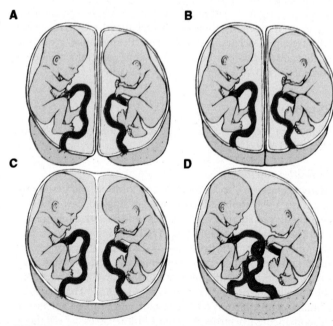

**FIGURE 11.2:** Position of the placenta in dichorionic and monochorionic placentation. **A:** Dichorionic–diamniotic placentation with two separate placentas. **B:** Dichorionic–diamniotic placentation with a fused placenta. **C:** Monochorionic–diamniotic placentation with a single placenta. **D:** Monochorionic–monoamniotic placentation with a single placenta.

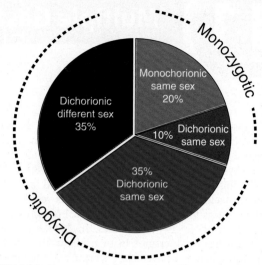

**FIGURE 11.3:** Frequency of dichorionic and monochorionic placentation with regard to zygosity and fetal sex.

*Dizygotic twins* represent two-thirds of twin gestations, and occur from ovulation and fertilization of two oocytes (see Fig. 11.1), almost always resulting in a dichorionic placentation (see Fig. 11.2). Dizygotic twinning is a type of superfecundation in which more than one fertilized egg is present in the uterus. The spontaneous prevalence of live-born dizygotic twinning in North America and Britain is 1 in 100 births,[20] but incidence varies widely by region (see Fig. 11.3). Hereditary tendency may increase the risk three times normal population.

### Diagnosis

Zygosity can be determined by placentation or biochemical testing such as blood types, enzyme polymorphisms, and HLA types.[22–25] Regarding placentation, a monochorionic placenta is monozygotic until proven otherwise. On the other hand, DNA typing is considered the most useful and reliable way of defining zygosity.[26] However, because 70% of monozygotic twins share vascular placental connections, DNA in blood cells may appear to be identical even if the twin pair are genetically or epigenetically discordant.[25,26]

### Classification

Twins can be classified clinically via chorionicity or genetically based on zygosity. Controversy persists on whether outcomes of twin gestations are best assessed by zygosity or chorionicity. In the United Kingdom, a prospective observational study was conducted to compare fetal outcome based on chorionicity or zygosity. The authors, Carroll et al., used umbilical cord blood with microsatellite markers and placenta histology to determine zygosity and chorionicity, respectively. Carroll et al.[27] reported that fetal outcomes in twin pregnancies are better predicted by chorionicity rather than zyosity. Caroll et al. also reported misclassification between genetic testing and clinical diagnosis of chorionicity. Similarly, Spiegler et al.[28] reported significantly higher rates of clinical misclassification in monozygotic twins when compared with dizygotic twins (37% and 11%, respectively). Several studies have reported perinatal outcomes based on both clinical and genetic zygosity (Table 11.1).[28,29] When defining outcomes based on chorionicity, monochorionic monoamniotic pregnancies have the highest mortality rate at 50%, followed by monochorionic diamniotic at 26%, and finally dichorionic diamniotic at 9%.

| Table 11.1 | Perinatal Outcomes in Multiple Gestation Based on Zygosity |
|---|---|

| Author, Year, Country | Study Design | Sample Size (n Cases) | Control Cases (n) | Zygosity Clinical + Genetic | Preterm Delivery Mono vs. Di | Intrauterine Infection Mono vs. Di | Cesarean Mono vs. Di | Comments |
|---|---|---|---|---|---|---|---|---|
| Spiegler, 2012, Germany | Case-control study | 165 twins 87 (monozygotic) 78 (dizygotic) | 2,535 singletons | Yes | 44% vs. 46% ($P > .05$) | 20% vs. 33% ($P = .012$) | 94% vs. 92% ($P > .05$) | Neonatal outcomes as respiratory or brain abnormalities no difference among groups. |
| Gao, 2011, China | Retrospective study | 295 twins 70 (monozygotic) 225 (dizygotic) | NA | Yes | | | | Monozygosity was a risk factor for fetal growth restriction (FGR) (OR was 1.747, 95% CI, 1.164–2.621). Dizygosity was a preventive factor for FGR (OR was 0.815, 95% CI, 0.685–0.971). |

## Determining Chorionicity

Early sonographic documentation of the number of placentas, or chorionicity, is important for optimal management of twin gestations. Evaluating the number of sacs and amniotic membrane also provides clues to chorionicity. In a dichorionic gestation, the amniotic membrane is thick as it is composed of two layers of amnion and two interposed layers of chorion. In monochorionic twins, the membrane is thin, composed only of amnions from each gestational sac. As the pregnancy continues, images of the placenta, sacs, and membranes become more difficult to obtain.[30-32] Some authors have reported that the chorionicity, fetuses, and amnions can be documented by 5, 6, and 8 weeks, respectively.[33] Most attest that accuracy is highest if the assessment of chorionicity is undertaken before 14 weeks' gestation.[34] In a study of 131 twin pregnancies, Stenhouse et al.[34] reported ultrasound sensitivity of 77% for monochorionicity and 90% for dichorionicity after 14 weeks, whereas 99% accuracy was achieved for both groups before 14 weeks. With a composite of second trimester ultrasound markers (i.e., number of placentas, fetal phenotype, membrane thickness, and twin peak sign), the sensitivity and specificity for correct identification of monochorionic pregnancies is reported at 91.7% and 97.3%, respectively.[35] Sometimes, there are cases of twin pregnancies where chorionicity can be difficult to determine. In these mothers, the pregnancy can be diagnosed as dichorionic without other ultrasound parameters if the fetuses *differ in sex*.[33] Providers are cautioned against diagnosing a dichorionic pregnancy based on visualization of two placentas, especially during the second and third trimesters, because the "second" placenta could represent a succenturiate lobe.[33] When chorionicity cannot be determined even with available diagnostics, the provider should consider sending the placenta to pathology after delivery.

### Diagnosis
#### Imaging
##### Before 10 Weeks
Markers for chorionicity include the number of **gestational sacs**, **amniotic sacs within chorioinic cavity**, and **yolk sacs**. A strong relationship exists between the number of gestational sacs and chorionicity. Two gestational sacs and two embryo poles with fetal cardiac activity are suggestive of a dichorioinic twin pregnancy, whereas one sac with two embryo poles is most consistent with monochorionicity (Fig. 11.4).[36] Use of transvaginal ultrasound is helpful before 10 weeks to identify the number of amniotic sacs. Similarly, the number of yolk sacs may help in the diagnosis of amnionicity: for example, two yolk sacs are suggestive of a diamniotic pregnancy (Fig. 11.5).[37] When these findings are no longer present after 10 weeks, later sonographic findings become standard.

#### After 10 Weeks
**Lambda sign:** The lambda sign is a histologic feature of dichorionicity, representing extension of placental tissue into the base of the intertwine membrane (Fig. 11.6). The presence of a lambda or twin peak sign is diagnostic of a dichorionic pregnancy (Fig. 11.7).[33] The lambda sign, which refers to the shape of the lateral edges of the membranes, was first described by Bessis and Papernik[35] in 1981 and later by Finberg[38] in 1992. In the second trimester, the twin peak sign becomes more difficult to visualize and disappears in about 7% of dichorionic pregnancies between 16 and 20 weeks.[39-41] Therefore, the absence of this sign in the second or third trimester cannot exclude dichorionicity.[39]

**T sign:** In contrast, monochorionic placentation is characterized as a single placental mass and a thin separating membrane, which is optimally detected when the membrane is oriented perpendicular to the ultrasound beam (see Fig. 11.6). This membrane intersects the placental junction with a "T" sign (Fig. 11.8). Although the T-sign generally indicates a monochorionic/diamniotic pregnancy,[33] other instances can occur when this sign is not diagnostic. For example, as a dichorionic pregnancy progresses, the hallmark lambda sign may not be visible and can simulate a T configuration. This reiterates the importance of early ultrasound diagnosis of chorionicity.

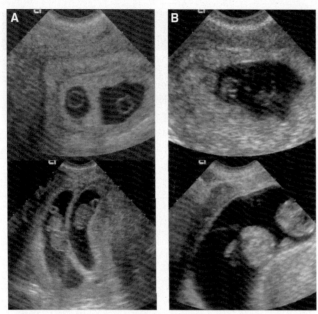

**FIGURE 11.4:** Dichorionic and monochorionic twins, first trimester. First-trimester examples of dichorionic **(A)** and monochorionic **(B)** twin gestations. Note the thick separating membranes of dichorionic placentation.

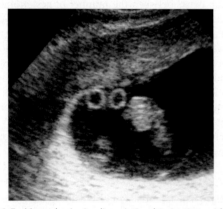

**FIGURE 11.5:** Monochorionic–diamniotic placentation with two yolk sacs. Ultrasound image of a monochorionic twin pregnancy in which there was difficulty in identification of the intertwin membrane shows two discrete yolk sacs, confirming a diamniotic gestation.

***Thickness of intertwin membrane:*** Several authors have measured the thickness of the intertwin membrane as a tool for diagnosing chorionicity.[33] In 1989, Winn et al.[42] reported that during second trimester, the mean thickness of the intertwin membrane was 2.4 mm for dichorionic pregnancies and 1.4 mm for monochorionic pregnancies with an accuracy in predicting monochorionic or dichorionic twinning of 82% and 95%, respectively. Clinically, however, this has been difficult to apply as while the mean for dichorionic and monochorionic pregnancies differs, these dimensions can overlap for each type of placentation. Because it is not universally applicable, this measurement is not routinely used in clinical practice. In general, an intertwin membrane thickness of >2 mm indicates dichorionicity with a positive predictive value of 95%, whereas a thickness ≤2 mm indicates monochorionicity with a positive predictive value of 90% (Fig. 11.9).[32] On fetal MRI, differences in membrane thickness may also provide clues to chronicity (Fig. 11.10).

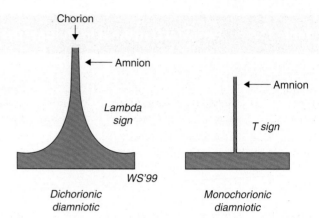

**FIGURE 11.6:** Schematic illustrating the lambda, or twin peak, and T signs observed in dichorionic and monochorionic twin pregnancies, respectively. In a dichorionic pregnancy with fused placentas, both the amnions and the chorions reflect away from the placental surface, creating a potential space into which villi can grow. This is called the lambda or twin peak sign. Monochorionic–diamniotic pregnancies have a single layer of continuous chorion limiting villous growth. This is called the T sign.

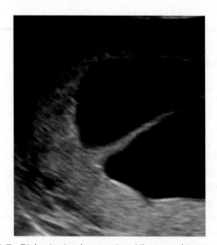

**FIGURE 11.7:** Dichorionic placentation. Ultrasound image of intertwin membrane–placental junction in a dichorionic twin gestation shows extension of the placental tissue into the base of the intertwin membrane (the lambda sign).

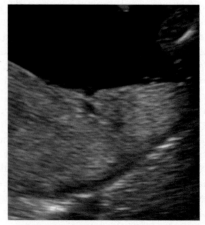

**FIGURE 11.8:** Monochorionic placentation. Transabdominal ultrasound of a monochorionic twin pregnancy shows absence of the lambda sign and the presence of the T sign with the intertwin membrane abruptly joining the placental surface with no intervening chorion.

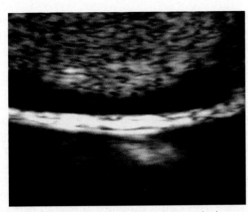

**FIGURE 11.9:** Dichorionic twin. In this ultrasound photograph of a section of intertwin membrane in a dichorionic twin pregnancy, the intertwin membrane is thick and echogenic and three layers are seen, confirming dichorionicity.

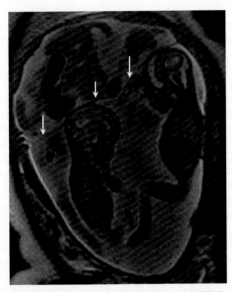

**FIGURE 11.10:** Membranes on Fetal MRI. Coronal SSFSE T2 image in a dichorionic triamniotic triplet gestation. The membrane separating the chorions is thick *(white arrows)* versus that separating the twins which share a placenta *(black arrows).*

*Layers of intertwin membrane:* In the second trimester, the number of membranes may be counted to determine chorionicity, and if there are >2, then dichorionicity is strongly suggested (see Fig. 11.9).[33,43] This technique requires high-powered ultrasound technology that is not routinely available in clinical practice. Using this technique, researchers noted that visualization of four membranes indicated a dichorionic pregnancy, and two membranes a monochorionic pregnancy.

**Prenatal Diagnosis:** Prenatal diagnosis evolved tremendously in the past century in response to increasing pregnancies with higher maternal ages and thus an associated increased risk of Down syndrome. Prenatal diagnosis shifted from a risk assessment based solely on the mother's age (i.e., medical history) to a quantitative risk assessment that evolved from the measurement of maternal alpha-fetoprotein (AFP) to that of human chorionic

gonadotropin levels later during that decade.[44] In the 1990s, nuchal translucency (NT) was introduced as another first trimester screening tool.[45] In 1997, Lo et al.[46] revolutionized prenatal screening and diagnosis with their discovery of cell-free fetal DNA, which is now commercially available. Each of these diagnostic markers has been validated first in singletons and then extrapolated to include twins and other higher order multiples. Twin and multiple gestations present unique challenges in prenatal screening and diagnosis.

## MULTIPLE GESTATIONS AND CONGENITAL MALFORMATION

Anomalies that occur with increased frequency in monozygotic twins include hydrocephalus, anencephaly, holoprosencephaly, and sacrococcygeal teratoma. For any given defect, the pregnancy may be concordant or discordant in terms of the presence, type, and severity of the abnormality. However, the majority (80% to 90%) of structural defects are discordant regardless of zygosity.

### Incidence

The overall prevalence of structural defects is 1.2 to 2.0 times higher in fetuses from twin pregnancies compared with singletons, with most of the excess risk due to increased rates in monochorionic twins.[47] Monozygotic twins have two to three times higher rates of congenital anomalies than singletons or dizygotic twins.

### Pathogenesis/Risk

*Zygosity,* rather than chorionicity, determines the risk of chromosomal abnormalities and whether or not the fetuses may be concordant or discordant for the anomaly. In dizygotic pregnancies, each twin has an independent risk for aneuploidy with the maternal age-related risk for chromosomal abnormalities for each twin being the same as in singleton pregnancies. Therefore, the chance of at least one fetus in a dizygotic twin gestation being affected by a chromosomal defect is twice as high as in singleton pregnancies (if zygosity is unknown, multiply singleton risk by 5/3). For these twins, the pregnancy-specific risk is based on the sum of the individual risk estimates for each fetus. In monozygotic twins, the risk for chromosomal abnormalities in each fetus is the same as in singleton pregnancies.[48]

Given the higher rates of congenital abnormalities in twins and also higher order pregnancies, understanding how multiples affect the sensitivity and specificity of the various prenatal screening and diagnostic tests is crucial. Clinicians should consider that although there are prenatal diagnostic options for twins and multiple gestations, screening accuracy is lower than for a single pregnancy.[49]

Risk for fetal aneuploidy is associated with *advancing maternal age.*[50] In patients with singletons, advanced maternal age is defined as older than 35 years on the expected date of delivery.[51] This designation is applied to women with a singleton or monochorionic twins. However, defining advanced maternal age is far more complex in women with dizygotic twins, triplets, and high-order multiples. In dizygotic twins, the risk of one fetus having an aneuploidy is twice that for a woman of the same age with a singleton.[52]

## Diagnosis

### First Trimester Screening

**Ultrasound:** In a retrospective study to evaluate the accuracy of antenatal ultrasound in the detection of fetal anomalies in 245 twin pregnancies, Edwards et al.[51] reported overall prevalence rates of 4.9%. Antepartum ultrasound had a sensitivity of 88% and a specificity of 100% for the detection of anomalies in these patients, with a positive predictive value of 100% and a negative predictive value of 99%. Despite these findings, data are insufficient to make recommendations about frequency of anatomical ultrasound in multiple gestations.

Nuchal translucency is a noninvasive ultrasound technique that can be used between 11.0 and 13.6 weeks to detect aneuploidy. Although biochemical results vary according to the number of gestations, gestational age, and other factors, NT is an effective choice because it provides direct visualization of the embryo.[51,53] Screening can be technically challenging in multiple gestations; however, if the nuchal region is visible for each fetus, the test can be effective. In evaluating NT in 448 twin pregnancies (both dichorionic and monochorionic), Sebire et al.[54] reported that 7.3% of normal fetuses had an elevated NT above the 95th percentile. In 88.4% of twin pregnancies, both fetuses had a normal NT. The overall sensitivity of 88% was comparable with the singleton detection rate. The screen false positive rate was higher in monochorionic twins at 8.4% than in dichorionic twins at 5.4%. In multiples, risk assessment using first trimester methods can be calculated for each fetus or for the entire pregnancy. In monochorionic twins, each fetus has the same risk of being affected with Down syndrome. Thus, a single risk estimate for the duration of pregnancy is based on the average of the NT measurements. Each fetus in a dichorionic twin pregnancy is treated as a separate individual, and the risk for each fetus is calculated by using published NT values for singletons.[55,56]

Another interesting application of NT in monochorionic twins is the ability to predict twin-to-twin transfusion syndrome (TTTS).[57,58] A NT threshold at the 95th percentile had a positive and a negative predictive value of 43% and 91%, respectively.[57]

### Biochemical Markers

**Pregnancy-Associated Placental Protein (PAPP-A):** One screening tool for aneuploidy is the PAPP-A, a molecule that is secreted by the placenta. In singleton pregnancies, low levels of PAPP-A occur in fetuses with Down syndrome. However, compared with singleton pregnancies, PAPP-A levels are nearly double in normal twin pregnancies.[59] The magnitude of the value depends on chorionicity so that PAPP-A is higher in dichorionic than in monochorionic twins.[60] In general, maternal analyte levels can be adjusted for twin pregnancy; however, the detection rate for Down syndrome is lower than in singleton pregnancy (e.g., 93% detection in MC twins, 78% detection in DC twins, and 95% detection in singletons).[61] In addition, maternal analyte levels for Down syndrome screening in twin pregnancy may be affected by early loss of one embryo of a triplet gestation.[62,63]

**Beta-Human Chorionic Gonadotropin (β-hCG):** It is a hormone that is also secreted from the placental trophoblast. Compared with singletons, β-hCG levels are approximately double in twins compared with singletons.[59] Similar to PAPP-A, levels of β-hCG are lower in monochorionic than in dichorionic pregnancies.[60] These values are also affected by the mode of conception, whether spontaneous or ART.

**Combined Screening Using Ultrasound and Serum Analyte:** In singletons, first trimester combined screening, which includes maternal age, NT, and maternal serum-free β-hCG and PAPP-A levels, has been shown to detect approximately 82% of cases of Down syndrome, with a 5% false positive rate.[64] Wald et al.[56] reported the detection with a 5% false positive rate for Down syndrome in monochorionic, dichorionic, and all twins as 73%, 68%, and 69% for NT alone and 84%, 70%, and 72% for combined tests, respectively. The accuracy of combined testing in the detection of Down syndrome approximated to singleton rates.

**Karyotyping/Invasive Procedures:** Screening detection rates for twin pregnancies are estimated to be 15% less than for singleton pregnancies.[59] This can be explained at least in part as being due to the chemicals produced by the chromosomally normal fetus and abnormal fetus being averaged; thus, a total reported number may cause a normal test result. For these reasons, both fetuses of a dizygotic pair should undergo karyotyping unlike monozygotic twins.

**Chorionic villus sampling:** Chorionic villus sampling is a diagnostic test performed at 10 to 12 weeks of gestation to obtain placental cells for prenatal diagnosis. The procedure can be performed transcervically or transabdominally. Before samples are collected, an ultrasound is obtained to confirm the number of placentas and fetuses and determine chorionicity. In a transcervical technique, the patient is prepped, a sterile speculum is placed, and a small catheter is placed through the cervix under direct ultrasound visualization to obtain chorionic villi. Although some surgeons prefer biopsy forceps rather than a catheter under negative pressure, either technique can be used. In an abdominal approach, the abdomen is prepped, and a needle is inserted through the abdominal wall into the placenta, cells are aspirated, and then the needle is withdrawn. Only one chorionic villus sample is traditionally needed for monochorionic pregnancies. However, there are case reports of genetically discordant monochorionic twins, and thus two samples can be required. For dichorionic pregnancies, two separate placental samples are needed. If access to both placentas can be achieved via a transcervical approach without contamination, one could choose this method. However, if the second placenta is not accessible through a cervical approach, sampling in this twin pregnancy may be achieved using both cervical and abdominal approaches.

As with any invasive procedure, there are risks and benefits associated with chorionic villus sampling. Many patients opt for this test because it can be performed earlier than an amniocentesis. Reported complications of chorionic villus sampling include placental mosaicism, bleeding, infection, maternal–fetal hemorrhage, limb reduction defects, insufficient sample for analysis, and oromandibular hypogenesis.[65–67] Moreover, any Rh-negative patient should receive Rhogam to prevent isoimmunization.

### Second Trimester Screening

**US/MRI:** Ultrasound in discordant twins can define multiple anomalies, which may provide clues to chromosomal anomaly or genetic syndrome (Fig. 11.11A). MRI is sometimes utilized to exclude additional anomalies (Fig. 11.11B) and confirm diagnosis, particularly in the case of complicated monochorionic gestations (Fig. 11.12).

**Biochemical Markers:** In singletons, the second trimester quad test that combines maternal age with second trimester serum AFP, β-hCG, unconjugated estriol, and inhibin-A detects

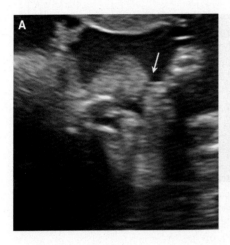
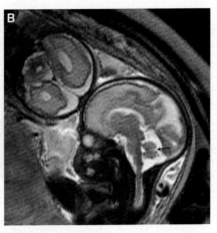

**FIGURE 11.11:** Dichorionic twin gestation with discordant anomalies. **A:** Ultrasound of discordant dichorionic twin gestation at 32 weeks showed cleft lip *(arrow)* and palate and complex cardiac anomalies (not shown) in one twin. **B:** SSFSE T2 sagittal imaging of the brain shows primary fissure *(arrow)* equally separating lobes of the vermis, consistent with small vermis inferiorly. The fetus also had micropthalmia. Postnatally, the twin was found to have trisomy 13.

approximately 75% of cases of Down syndrome with a 5% false positive rate.[68] Many medical centers do not routinely offer this quad screening to patients with multiple fetuses owing to the paucity of data related to the efficacy of second trimester maternal serum screening for aneuploidy in twins. Additionally, reports in the literature reflect the inconsistencies in both sensitivity and detection rates of these analytes and the difficulty in interpreting the variability. On average, maternal serum biochemical markers are twice as high in twins as in singletons of the same gestational age.[69] Recently, Muller et al.[70] evaluated second trimester maternal serum screening for Down syndrome in 3,292 twin pregnancies, and reported that median AFP levels were similar between dichorionic and monochorionic twins and that free β-hCG levels were higher in monochorionic pregnancies. Rates for Down syndrome detection and screen positivity, respectively, were 27.3% and 6.6% using maternal age alone, 54.5% and 24.6% using maternal age corrected for chorionicity, 54.5% and 7.75% using AFP and free β-hCG divided by 2, 54.5% and 8.05% using median values observed from the global twin population, and 54.5% and 7.75% using median values specific to monochorionic and dichorionic twins. The authors concluded that maternal serum screening is better than maternal age alone but still yields low detection rates. In another study[71] of second trimester serum screening, high false positive rates led to an 18.3% amniocentesis rate for twins versus 7.5% rate in singletons. Thus, first trimester ultrasound screening has been suggested to be optimal for detection of Down syndrome.

***Cell-Free Fetal DNA (cff DNA):*** In 1997, Dr. Lo and his coworkers discovered Cff DNA, an innovation that revolutionized prenatal screening. Cff DNA is released into the maternal bloodstream after placental cells undergo apoptosis.[67] It

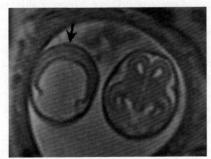

**FIGURE 11.12:** Discordant Monochorionic Twins Axial SSFSE T2 imaging in an 18-week monochorionic gestation with twin-to-twin transfusion syndrome. One twin with alobar holoprosencephaly *(arrow)*. Fetal MRI confirmed normal brain in the co-twin.

constitutes approximately 10% of the total DNA in maternal plasma and is rapidly cleared from maternal blood, within 2 hours of delivery.[72,73] The half-life of fetal DNA is short at approximately 16 minutes, but it has recently been found that the entire fetal genome, in the form of cell-free DNA, is present in maternal blood.[74] Cell-free fetal DNA has been demonstrated as early as prior to the seventh week of gestation.[75] Therefore, cff DNA has become the focus of research for the development of noninvasive prenatal testing (NIPT).

Of the several types, including digital polymerase chain reaction (PCR), massively parallel DNA sequencing (MPS) of the whole genome, and target sequencing of the selected genomic loci on the chromosome of interest, utilized for NIPT for detection of Down syndrome, the primary methods applied in the United States, Asia, and parts of Europe are MPS and target sequencing.[76] The first approach, MPS, uses the whole genome and requires sequencing of many millions of DNA fragments to generate sufficient reads to detect differences in the level of chromosome 21, which constitutes 1.5% of sequenced fragments. The second alternative targets sequencing the select genomic loci on the chromosome of interest, for example, chromosome 21 for NIPT for Down syndrome.[77–83] In a series of validation studies in singletons, the MPS technique demonstrated high accuracy with sensitivity rates between 79% and 100%, and <1% false positive rates for diagnosis of Down syndrome[84–86]; 97% to 100% for trisomy 18[85–87]; and 75% to 79% for trisomy 13.[86,87] Of note, cell-free DNA should be timed appropriately, typically after the 9th week.

In twin pregnancies, recently, Huang et al.[88] reported the use of Cff DNA in 189 twin pregnancies with sensitivity and specificity using maternal plasma sequencing for fetal trisomy 21 being both 100% and for fetal trisomy 18 at 50% and 100%, respectively. This study further supported that sequencing-based NIPT of trisomy 21 in twin pregnancies could be achieved with a high accuracy. However, additional studies are needed to validate NIPT in multiple gestations.

### Karyotype/Invasive Procedures

***Amniocentesis:*** Amniocentesis is the gold standard for prenatal diagnosis. The procedure is typically performed in the second trimester to obtain amniotic fluid for genetic analysis by a needle inserted through a prepped abdominal wall under continuous ultrasound guidance. Complications of amniocentesis include infection, bleeding, and maternal–fetal hemorrhage. As in chorionic villus sampling, an Rh negative patient should receive rhogam. Like most procedures, amniocentesis in twins presents unique diagnostic challenges. After correctly identifying placental location and the intended twin to be tested first, the needle is inserted into the amniotic sac of the first twin, followed by injection of indigo carmine before removing the needle. Methylene blue should not be used because of the risk of atresia of the fetal small bowel, staining of the skin, and methemoglobinemia in the infant. Next, the needle is inserted into the second twin's amniotic sac. If the fluid aspirated appears blue tinged, the first sac is reentered and the physician should remove the needle and try again.[89–91]

ACOG reports the procedure-related loss rate from 1 per 300 to 500 performed.[92] Several studies agree that the loss rate for twins exceeds this, but by what extent is controversial. Loss rates have approximated 1%[93] in some studies, but others were inconclusive because of the heterogeneity of the populations studied and inconsistencies in the definition of procedure-related loss.[49]

## Management

Management of the pregnancy is individualized and mainly expectant or termination. Selective termination is relatively safe in dichorionic twins but can be fraught with danger in monochorionic gestations, putting both twins at risk for demise.

## Recurrence Risk

Recurrence risk is dependent on type of genetic transmission.

## PRETERM DELIVERY

### Definition/Incidence

Preterm delivery, defined as delivery before 37.0 weeks' gestation, affects approximately 12% of singleton births in the United States[1] and approximately 11% worldwide.[94] Over half of twin deliveries occur before 37.0 weeks, and about one-tenth of twin deliveries before 32 weeks.[1] Preterm delivery is the most significant cause of morbidity and mortality in twin gestations.

### Pathogenesis

It is not surprising that multiple gestations are at risk for preterm labor given greater uterine distention, which can initiate labor and cause earlier cervical changes.

### Diagnosis/Surveillance

Sonographic measurement of cervical length (Fig. 11.13) and biochemical testing of fetal fibronectin are the two main screening tools used to predict preterm birth.

#### Imaging

A shortened cervical length (Fig. 11.14) indicates a higher risk of preterm delivery for the twin pregnancy. Among 464 twin pregnancies seen for routine care, Skentou et al.[95] found that the median cervical length at 23 weeks was 36 mm. The rate of spontaneous delivery before 33 weeks was inversely related to cervical length at 23 weeks. It increased gradually from approximately 2.5% at 60 mm to 5% at 40 mm, and to 12% at 25 mm, and exponentially below this length to 17% at 20 mm and to 80% at 8 mm (Fig. 11.15). A meta-analysis of studies that measured cervical length by transvaginal ultrasound to predict spontaneous preterm birth in twin pregnancies found that the test was most useful when performed in asymptomatic women at 20 to 24 weeks of gestation.[96] In establishing a cutoff of 20 mm, the authors found that the positive likelihood ratios for preterm

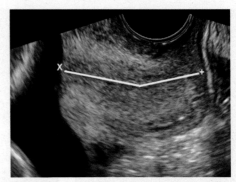

**FIGURE 11.13:** Ultrasound of normal cervix with equal thickness of anterior and posterior cervical lips. *X* marks the internal cervical os; + marks the external cervical os; the echodense line connecting the two points is the endocervical canal.

birth were 5.2 and 10.1, respectively, in the 35% of pregnancies delivered before 28 weeks and 39% before 32 weeks.[96] The usefulness of screening cervical length is limited by high frequency of short cervices in women not at imminent risk of delivery and by the lack of effective interventions to prevent preterm birth. Consequently, universal screening in this population is controversial because there are no known treatments.

In contrast, for women with signs and symptoms of preterm labor between 23 and 33 weeks, cervical length was a better predictor of preterm delivery than funneling or digital examination.[97] In symptomatic twin pregnancies, Crane et al.[97] found rates of delivery were 44% for cervical lengths <15 mm as compared with no delivery within a week if cervical length was >25 mm.

#### Biochemical

Fetal fibronectin is a protein found between the fetal sac and the uterine lining that can be used to predict preterm birth in singleton and twin pregnancies. In the largest prospective study of 147 women expecting twins, fibronectin testing was done at 2-week intervals between weeks 24 and 30.[98] Using fibronectin levels at 28 gestational weeks, Goldenberg et al.,[98] reported deliveries prior to 32 weeks in 30% of women with a positive test (≥50 ng per mL) and 4% of women with a negative result. Although these data support the feasibility of fibronectin in predicting preterm twin birth, this testing is not routinely performed in asymptomatic twin pregnancies in the absence of other prematurity risk factors.

### Management/Prevention

Progesterone has been the biggest advancement in the prevention of preterm birth in singleton pregnancies for women with a history of preterm delivery. However, this therapy does not extrapolate to twin gestations.[99] Furthermore, in a recent meta-analysis, Sotiriadis et al.[99] reported that progesterone use for prevention of preterm delivery in twin pregnancy was associated with increased rates of perinatal death. At this time, there are no effective methods of preventing preterm delivery in twins, even with a history of a preterm delivery.[100]

For women who have a short cervix, vaginal progesterone results are promising, but do not reach statistical significance in reducing preterm twin birth.[101] Similarly, intramuscular injection of 17 hydroxyprogesterone does not reduce the risk for twin pregnancies complicated with a shortened cervix.[102] Although cerclage has proven beneficial in preventing preterm birth in singleton gestations for women with a history of preterm delivery and short cervix, this benefit does not appear to be true for

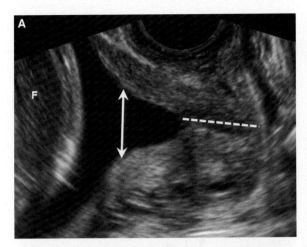

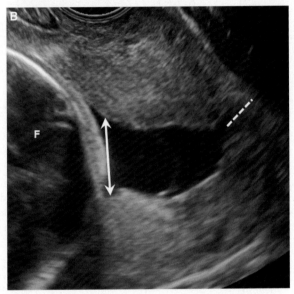

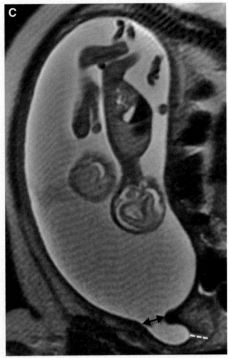

**FIGURE 11.14:** Shortened cervix by US and MRI. **A:** A transvaginal scan at 23 weeks in twin pregnancy shows dilatation and funneling of the internal cervical os (line with end arrows). The closed cervical length (dotted line) measures 2.5 cm with funneling cervix, with walls of funnel in a Y-shaped configuration. F is fetus. **B:** Transvaginal ultrasound with nearly completely effaced cervix, with U-shaped funnel. Same annotations in A. **C:** MRI imaging of U-shaped funneling and shortened cervical length. The *black arrows* show internal os, *dotted lines* show shortened closed cervix.

twin gestations. In fact, a 2005 meta-analysis showed a higher incidence of preterm birth in twin gestations with cerclage.[103]

Recently, there has been a report of cervical incompetence treated with a cerclage and pessary[104] in a monochorionic monoamniotic twin pregnancy. Some authors have also proposed pessaries to prevent preterm birth in severe TTTS treated by laser.[105] However, pessary use in preventing preterm birth in twins remains unclear.

Unfortunately, no intervention has been shown to improve outcomes in twins when the mother's ultrasound has identified a short cervix or there is a history of preterm delivery.[106] Since higher rates of preterm delivery occur in twins conceived by ART than those conceived naturally, the most effective strategy against morbidity and mortality associated with preterm delivery is the prevention of multiple gestations in the ART setting.

## FETAL DEATH

Single intrauterine fetal death (sIUFD) in multiple gestation pregnancies occurs in roughly 3.7% to 6.8% of twin pregnancies.[107–109] In 2006, a systematic review of 19 studies demonstrated that the increased risk of death of a co-surviving twin after the death of 1 twin was 12% for monochorionic pregnancies and 4% for dichorionic pregnancies. The odds ratio for monochorionic co-twin intrauterine death was six times that of

dichorionic twins.[110] Moreover, the studies reinforced that fetal death can occur at any time.

## Single Twin Gestation Demise Before 14 Weeks (Vanishing Twin Syndrome)

This syndrome usually occurs in the first trimester with the identification of a single fetus weeks after confirmation and diagnosis of any twin pregnancy (Fig. 11.16). The true incidence of vanishing twins is unknown but may be as high as 29%.[111] In vanishing twin syndrome, outcomes based on chorionicity are yet unknown. As for long-term outcome, Anand et al.[112] reported no developmental delays in children up to age 1 year when comparing surviving twins from a vanishing twin pregnancy and children from singleton pregnancies.[112]

## Single Twin Demise After 14 Weeks

### Incidence
The overall incidence of single twin death after 20 weeks of pregnancy is estimated between 2.6% and 6.2%.[113]

### Pathogenesis
In primarily *monochorionic* twins, the morbidity and mortality in the surviving twin has been explained by two theories:

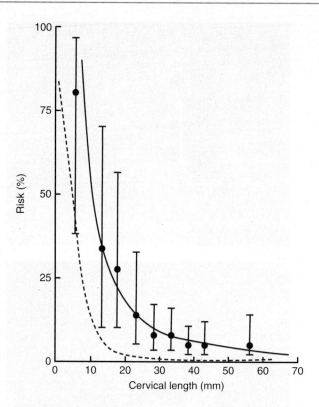

**FIGURE 11.15:** Risk of preterm delivery before 33 weeks' gestation compared with closed cervical length at 23 weeks in twin pregnancies. The rate of spontaneous delivery before 33 weeks is inversely related to cervical length measured at 23 weeks. It increased gradually from approximately 2.5% at 6 cm to 5% at 4 cm, and 12% at 2.5 cm. (Adapted from Skentou C, Souka AP, To MSW, et al. Prediction of preterm delivery in twins by cervical assessment at 23 weeks. *Ultrasound Obstet Gynecol.* 2001;17:7–10.)

transchorionic embolization and coagulopathy or transient hemodynamic fluctuations between the twins. In the first theory, passage of thrombotic materials from the dead twin occurs along the placental vascular anastomoses, resulting in disseminated intravascular coagulopathy in the initially healthy surviving twin.[111] The resulting disseminated intravascular coagulopathy may result in infarcts and cystic degenerative changes in the survivor's renal, pulmonary, hepatic, splenic, and neurologic organs.[114] However, data have demonstrated normal coagulation in the surviving twin after intrauterine death of the co-twin, refuting this hypothesis.[115]

The alternative theory is based on rapid and profound hemodynamic alteration that occurs when one twin dies. Specifically, an acute shift of blood from the surviving twin flows into the dead fetus along the superficial anastomotic channels.[115,116] There has been in utero demonstration of severe fetal anemia in the surviving twin after death of co-twin supporting this hypothesis.[115,117]

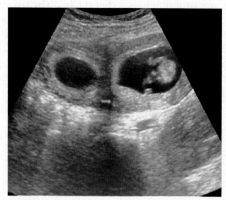

**FIGURE 11.16:** Vanishing twin syndrome in dichorionic pregnancy. A transvaginal scan at 9 weeks showing dichorionic twin pregnancy with thick separation *(green arrow)*. Left sac is empty (representing vanishing twin), and right sac shows an embryonic pole.

### Etiology

The multiple causes for fetal death in twin pregnancy include fetal chromosomal or congenital malformations, and maternal diseases (e.g., diabetes, placenta diseases). Twin pregnancies complicated by a fetal death are at increased risk for both preterm delivery and death of the co-twin.

### Diagnosis/Surveillance

**Imaging:** Regardless of chorionicity, management after a single fetal death is challenging. Expert opinions recommend ultrasound assessment of fetal growth every 2 to 4 weeks. In some cases of single fetal death in a multifetal pregnancy, prenatal ultrasound can detect intracranial abnormalities in the surviving twin.[118] Patten et al.[119] have demonstrated that a normal initial scan cannot rule out damage and that sonographic evidence of intracranial abnormalities in the surviving twin may manifest as early as 7 days after the death of its co-twin. Structural abnormalities observed in survivors include neural tube defects, optic nerve hypoplasia, hypoxic ischemic lesions of the white matter (multicystic encephalomalacia), microcephaly, hydranencephaly, porencephaly, hemorrhagic lesions (Fig. 11.17A), posthemorrhagic hydrocephalus, bilateral renal cortical necrosis, unilateral absence of a kidney, gastrointestinal tract atresia, gastroschisis, hemifacial microsomia, and aplasia cutis of the scalp, trunk, or limbs.[120] Sonographic scan might be complemented with MRI.[121] If time permits, the best timing for MRI is at 32 weeks or later, when white matter is developed and minor (yet clinically important) lesions in the white matter can be visualized. Some physicians advocate fetal MRI at least 3 weeks after single twin demise to assess brain injury in the surviving twin. Three patterns of brain pathology have been described in the surviving twin.[111] First, hypoxic ischemic lesions of white matter usually occur in the area supplied by the middle cerebral artery, which may evolve to porencephaly, multicystic encephalomalacia, microcephaly, and hydrancephaly (Fig. 11.17B). Second, hemorrhagic lesions, either isolated or in combination

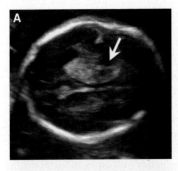

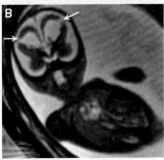

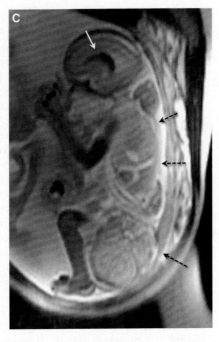

**FIGURE 11.17:** Twin Demise in Three Different Monochorionic Pregnancies with Intracranial Injury in the Surviving Twin. **A:** Axial cranial US of surviving twin after demise in a monochorioinc gestation demonstrates increased echogenicity in the ventricle, suggestive of hemorrhage *(arrow)*. **B:** Coronal SSFP image in a monochorionic gestation at 21 weeks, 3 weeks after demise of co-twin shows moderate ventriculomegaly and areas of porencephaly/multicystic encephalomalacia *(arrows)* in the surviving twin. Fetus sent for MRI as US demonstrated increasing ventricular dilatation. **C:** Monochorionic twin gestation at 20 weeks with recent demise of co-twin *(dotted arrows)*. The SSFSE T2 image demonstrates a large germinal matrix hemorrhage in the surviving twin *(solid arrow)*.

with ischemic lesions, may lead to posthemorrhagic hydrocephalus (Fig. 11.17C). Third, anomalies secondary to a vascular disturbance can occur; these include neural tube defects, limb reduction anomalies, and optic nerve hypoplasia.

### Prognosis

Timing of fetal death and chorionicity are important factors that impact management, counseling, short-term, and long-term outcomes. In studies examining neurologic outcome after one fetal death in twin pregnancies,[111] reports noted rates of cerebral palsy were 6.3% in surviving twins and 1.8% higher in monozygotic twin pregnancies. Nelson and Ellenberg[122] also reported an increased rate of nonfebrile seizures in the surviving twin (5%) after fetal death versus 0.8% when both twins survive. In terms of IQ testing, no significant differences have been observed between survivors after their co-twin's death and surviving twins.[122]

### Management

Several factors impact management and outcome of the surviving co-twin. These include chorionicity, gestational age at time of fetal death, and maternal and placental diseases.

#### Monochorionic

*Previable Pregnancy (<24 Weeks):* Because of the lack of predictive investigation on long-term outcome at this gestational age, regardless of chronicity, most patients are managed conservatively during that period. Despite sparse data, some patients consider termination as another treatment option.[123]

*Viable Pregnancy (≥24 Weeks):* The prevalence of monochorionic twinning after a single fetal death ranges from 50% to 70%.[124] Fetal death increases 1% to 2% per week in monochorionic gestations after 32 weeks.[125] The surviving twin faces increased risk of fetal and neonatal morbidity and mortality, most often fetal death, neurologic morbidities, and prematurity. In a 2006 meta-analysis[110] that assessed the risk of co-twin mortality and neurologic morbidity following the death of one twin after 14 weeks' gestation, researchers reported a 12% risk of

death and 18% neurologic abnormality for the monochorionic surviving twin.

*Timing of Delivery:* Based on the 2011 NICHD workshop, the proceedings recommended delivery if fetal death occurs at or after 34 weeks, and to consider delivery in cases before 34 weeks based on concurrent maternal and fetal conditions.[125]

*Dichorionic:* In the presence of single fetal death, the main risk in the surviving dichorionic diamniotic twin is preterm delivery. In 2006, a meta-analysis[110] reported an estimated risk of both iatrogenic and spontaneous preterm delivery after single fetal death as being 68% and 57% in monochorionic and dichorionic pregnancies, respectively. Based on the NICHD workshop, management strategy for dichorionic diamniotic twin pregnancies is directed similarly to monochorionic diamniotic twin pregnancies.[125] However, expert opinion recommends a conservative approach for dichorionic diamniotic twin pregnancies that includes regular fetal and maternal surveillance and delivery between 37 and 38 weeks.[125] The mode of delivery should be based on the obstetrical indications for either vaginal birth or cesarean section. For maternal monitoring after fetal death, rhesus-negative women should undergo a Kleihauer test, and regular blood pressure monitoring because of the increased risk of preeclampsia.[108]

## FETAL GROWTH ABNORMALITIES

### Incidence

Patients with multifetal pregnancies are at risk for growth abnormalities, along with their associated increased risks of obstetric complications, and perinatal morbidity and mortality.[121]

### Pathogenesis/Etiology

Growth discordance can occur secondary to multiple known risk factors classified as fetal (monochorionic, infections), placental (placenta previa, abruption, velamantous cord insertion), and maternal (maternal age >30 years, nulliparity, tobacco use, no prenatal care).[126]

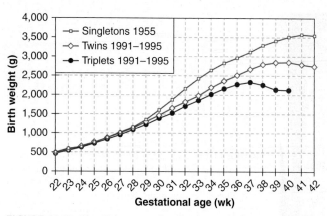

**FIGURE 11.18:** The 50th percentile of birth weight for gestational age was approximately similar among singletons, twins, and triplets before 28 weeks of gestation.

## Diagnosis/Surveillance

### Normal Growth

The normal fetal growth trajectory of a twin gestation diverges around 8 weeks, slowing to a rate lower than for singletons.[127–129] This rate persists until 30 to 32 weeks, at which time a second diversion in slower growth occurs. The slower growth rate in twins has been attributed to placental crowding and the more frequent anomalous umbilical cord insertion (Fig. 11.18). These findings have led to an emerging paradigm, explaining that events early in twin gestation, perhaps at the time of conception, play a critical role in determining intrauterine growth trajectories and size at birth. The American Congress of Obstetricians and Gynecologists (ACOG) technical bulletin on assessment of growth suggests that centers should use growth tables derived from twin gestations.[127] However, most studies of twin growth curves are derived from a small sample size and do not take into account chorionicity, race, or sex, or represent singleton curves applied to multiple gestation.[128,129]

### Growth Discordance:

In trying to improve the assessment of fetal weight in multiple gestations, several investigators have focused on individual biometric parameters. For example, an abdominal circumference ratio of <0.93 has a 3.8 likelihood ratio for twin 25% discordant weight, and a higher head circumference/abdominal circumference has increased rates of adverse pregnancy outcome. Another important assessment is growth discordance, with studies showing an association between significant differences in twin birth weights and increased mortality and morbidity.[130–133]

Growth discordance is defined as estimated fetal weight (EFW) of larger twin – EFW of smaller twin/EFW of larger twin

×100. The ACOG considers growth discordance from 15% to 25% as significant (Fig. 11.19). Growth discordance >20% occurs in 16% of twin pairs and >30% occurs in 5% of twin gestations, regardless of chronicity.[126]

Most patients with twin pregnancies will undergo several ultrasound assessments beginning in the early first trimester. Regardless of chorionicity, first trimester ultrasound cannot predict growth discordance. However, Lewi et al.[134] reported that monochorionic twin pregnancies with early onset discordance (i.e., difference in crown rump length at ≥90th percentile) had higher rates of adverse pregnancy outcomes and fetal death compared with those with late onset discordance in the second trimester (i.e., EFW difference >20%). There are few published studies to indicate how often routine reassessment should be done in twin pregnancies in such instances.

In general, ultrasound scans in monochorionic twin pregnancies are performed every 2 weeks, starting at 16 to 18 weeks, to better ascertain early evidence of TTTS. This is followed by an anatomy comprehensive ultrasound between 18 and 22 weeks.[135] In contrast, ultrasound scans in dichorionic twin pregnancies are recommended every 3 to 4 weeks.[135] Fetal surveillance should be increased when there is either growth restriction observed in one twin or significant growth discordance. Available data show no benefit for routine surveillance by umbilical artery Doppler waveforms in twin pregnancy, regardless of chorionicity, unless there is a complication such as fetal growth restriction.

## Prognosis

Several factors may increase adverse pregnancy outcomes in twin pregnancies regardless of chorionicity. Discordance of >20% compared with the presenting twin and a delivery interval <15 minutes and between 15 and 30 minutes (1.3 and 2.3 times, respectively) have been implicated as risk factors for adverse perinatal outcome.[126] Because of the lack of consensus definition about growth discordance in twin pregnancy based on chorionicity, controversial and conflicting results persist regarding perinatal morbidity and mortality.

## Management

Data are too limited to establish optimal timing of delivery of twin pregnancy complicated with growth discordance. Experts suggest that in the absence of clinical indications for delivery after 34 weeks, delivery for monochorionic twins is recommended at 36 to 37 weeks and for dichorionic gestations at 37 to 38 weeks to avoid late preterm delivery complications.[125]

Recommendations for mode of delivery are based mainly on presenting twin and weight difference relative to the presenting

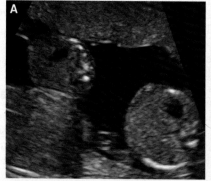
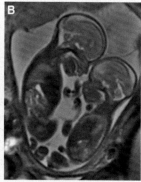

**FIGURE 11.19:** Growth discordance in twin pregnancies. **A:** Ultrasound manifestation of abdominal circumference discordant size in a monochorionic diamniotic twin pregnancy. **B:** MRI showing discordant size in monochorionic diamniotic pregnancy.

twin.[136] The ACOG recommends caesarean delivery if the presenting twin is nonvertex or breech extraction of the second twin if the presenting twin is vertex. If the presenting twin is vertex, the possible route for delivery includes vaginal, planned Cesarean, or combined delivery (vaginal delivery for twin A and emergency cesarean for twin B).[127] The risk of combined delivery is 4%, regardless of weight discordance.[137]

## Recurrence

This is controversial and not well documented.

## TWIN-TO-TWIN TRANSFUSION SYNDROME

Almost all monochorionic twins share a single placenta with intertwin vascular anastomoses that allows blood to transfer from one fetus to the other and vice versa.[138] Unbalanced net intertwin blood transfusion may lead to various complications; the best-known of these is twin twin transfusion syndrome (TTTS).[139]

## Incidence

TTTS is a chronic form of fetofetal transfusion that affects approximately 9% of monochorionic twins.[133]

## Pathogenesis/Etiology

TTTS is a complex and dynamic pathologic condition that involves placental intertwin vascular anastomoses, unequal placental sharing, fetal humoral, biochemical and functional changes, and fetal hemodynamic imbalance (Fig. 11.20). This fetal hemodynamic imbalance creates a hydrostatic difference between the recipient and the donor twins manifested as hyperdynamic, hypervolumic recipient state and hypovolumic, hypodymanic donor state.[139] Due to these volume imbalances, the recipient twin is at risk for cardiac dysfunction while the donor twin may experience placental insufficiency and growth restriction. These changes appear to be responsible for the progression and outcome of this syndrome. Almost all monochorionic twins are believed to have intertwin vascular anastomoses.[140]

These anastomses can be either direct and superficial between the twins' umbilical cord branch vessels on the chorionic plate

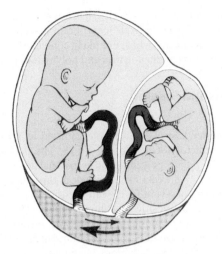

**FIGURE 11.20:** Diagram illustrates monochorionic gestation with twin-to-twin transfusion syndrome. The recipient twin is larger and in a polyhydramniotic sac. The donor twin is smaller and in an oligohydramniotic sac.

surface or deep, in which case the arterial vessels from one twin's cord pierce the chorionic plate to supply a placental cotyledon that is drained by the venous system of its co-twin (Fig. 11.21). Considering the type of anastomoses, vascular communications between the recipient and the donor twin may be from artery to artery, from vein to vein, or from artery to vein within a placental cotyledon. Depending on the number and type of anastomoses present, the exchange of blood may be balanced or unbalanced. Based on pathologic examination and/or fetoscopic studies, the percentage of each of the three types of vascular anastomoses ranges from 20% to 90%.[141,142] The relationship of vascular anastomoses and perinatal outcome in monochorionic twins and TTTS have been reported in several studies. In a retrospective study of placental angioarchitecture in relation to survival in monochorionic twins, fetal survival was higher in pregnancies with artery–artery anastomoses than in those with vein–vein anastomoses.[143,144]

In addition to placental vascular changes in TTTS, the unbalanced blood shunting from donor to recipient has been reported to cause hormonal, hemodynamic, and biochemical fetal changes. Vasoactive hormonal changes include an increase in

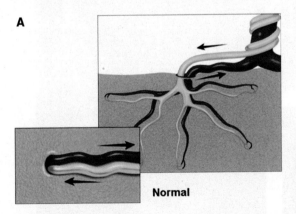

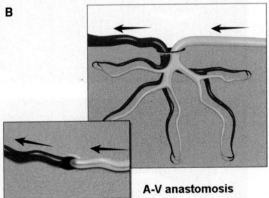

**FIGURE 11.21:** Placental anastomoses. Schematic representation of placental vessels shows the artery depicted in *blue* and the vein in *red*. *Arrows* indicate the direction of blood flow. The *superimposed drawing*, at the lower left of each diagram, shows the vascular structures as viewed from the fetal surface of the placenta. **A:** Normal artery and vein pair emanating from and returning to the fetal cord insertion site. **B:** Arteriovenous (*A-V*) anastomosis. As shown, the artery and vein each travel unaccompanied along the placental surface and traverse a common, shared foramen to perfuse the placenta. (Reproduced with permission from Machin GA, Feldstein VA, Van Gemert MJC, et al. Doppler sonographic demonstrations of arteriovenous anastomosis in monochorionic twin gestation. *Ultrasound Obstet Gynecol.* 2000;16:214–217.)

vasopressin, endothelin-1 (ET-1),[145] natriuretic peptides, mainly atrial natriuretic peptide (ANP), and brain natriuretic peptide (BNP) in the recipient, which are likely contributing factors in worsening hypervolemia polyuria and polyhydramnios.

## Diagnosis and Staging

### *Imaging*

**First Trimester US:** NT is a marker utilized as an early first trimester predictor for developing TTTS. The presence of an increased NT >95th percentile for gestational age assessed between 11.0 and 13.6 weeks in at least one of the fetuses predicted the development of severe TTTS with a sensitivity of 0.32, a specificity of 0.88, and a positive likelihood ratio of 1.45.[146] Another ultrasound marker is folding of the intertwin membrane, which reflects a decreased amount of amniotic fluid in one sac. In a prospective study of 83 monochorionic diamniotic pregnancies that presented for routine NT screening, Sebire et al.[147] reported that 52% of those with membrane folding developed severe TTTS.

**Second Trimester US/MRI:** The main diagnostic criterion for TTTS is the presence of oligohydramnios in the donor twin and polyhydramnios in the recipient twin (Fig. 11.22).[139] In European centers, the gestational age is taken into consideration with polyhydramnios consisting of a deepest vertical pocket of >8 cm before 20 weeks of gestation and >10 cm after 20 weeks.[139]

Diagnosis of TTTS is one of exclusion based on ultrasound findings. Although not all of the following sonographic criteria are necessary for a diagnosis of TTTS, these findings are suggestive of disorder (Table 11.2): (1) monochorionicity, (2) discrepancy in amniotic fluid between the amniotic sacs with polyhydramnios of one twin (largest vertical pocket >8 cm) and oligohydramnios of the other (largest vertical pocket <2 cm). In conjunction, the bladders are often discrepant with the donor small or absent and recipient large and constantly cycling (Fig. 11.23) (3) discrepancy in size of the umbilical cords (Fig. 11.24), (4) presence of cardiac dysfunction in the polyhydramniotic twin (Fig. 11.25), (5) characteristically abnormal umbilical artery or ductus venosus Doppler velocimetry (Fig. 11.26), and (6) less specifically, significant growth discordance of often ≥20% (see Fig. 11.19). Abnormal Doppler waveform is defined as at least one: absent or reverse end-diastolic flow in the umbilical artery, reverse flow in the ductus venosus, or pulsatile umbilical venous flow. The recipient which is at risk for cardiomyopathy tends to show venous Doppler abnormalities while the hypovolemic donor may demonstrate abnormal umbilical arterial Doppler.

There are at least four staging systems available to define TTTS: the Quintero (1- oligo-poly sequence, 2- no bladder in donor, 3-Doppler abnormalities in either twin, 4- hydrops or ascites in either, 5- demise of either), Cincinnati staging system (Table 11.3),[148] the Children's Hospital of Philadelphia (CHOP) system (scores based on 1-ventricular function, 2-valve function, 3-venous doppler, 4-great vessel findings, and 5-donor twin umbilical artery Doppler), and the cardiovascular profile scoring system (CVPS) (scores based on 1-hydrops fetalis, 2-venous and arterial Doppler, and 3-cardiac function).[148] Some of these staging systems include recipient echocardiographic changes (CVPS, CHOP, and Cincinnati system).[148] Cardiovascular compromise occurs in most recipient twins, is a major cause of death for these fetuses, and contributes to morbidity and mortality in the donor co-twin.[149] The most common recipient cardiovascular abnormalities in TTTS are unilateral or bilateral ventricular hypertrophy (18% to 49%), increased

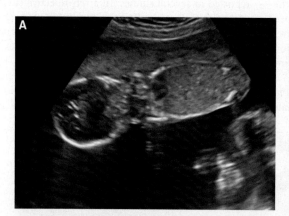

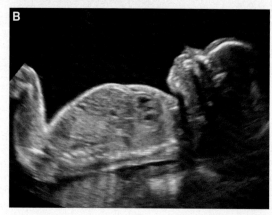

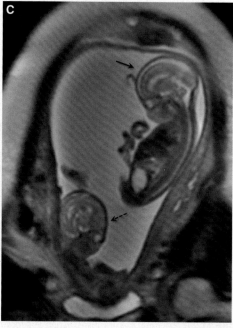

**FIGURE 11.22:** TTTS **A:** Oligohydramnios in donor sac stuck to the uterine wall. **B:** Polyhydramnios in recipient sac. **C:** Fetal MRI also shows decreased fluid around the donor *(dotted arrow)*, stuck to the wall of the myometrium and increased fluid around the recipient *(solid arrow)*.

| Table 11.2 | Twin-to-Twin Transfusion Features | |
|---|---|---|
| **Features** | **Donor Twin** | **Recipient Twin** |
| Size | Small | Large |
| Fluid | Oligohydramnios | Polyhydramnios |
| Bladder | Small to absent | Normal to distended |
| Umbilical cord | Small to normal | Normal to enlarged |
| Blood volume | Hypodynamic hypovolemia | Hyperdynamic hypervolemia |
| Cardiac dysfunction | Normal with minimal changes | Normal to abnormal |
| Doppler changes | Normal to abnormal | Normal to abnormal |
| Complications | Stuck twin, intrauterine growth restriction, hydrops, death | Cardiac dysfunction, hydrops, death |

cardiothoracic ratio as high as 47%, ventricular dilation (17% to 31%), tricuspid regurgitation (35% to 52%), and mitral regurgitation (13% to 15%).[149–151] These abnormalities are more common with advanced stages of disease. Finally, several cases of acquired pulmonary atresia/stenosis with intact ventricular septum have been described in the recipient twin.[149,152]

Given the risk for cerebral injury, fetal MRI is utilized in some centers to exclude neurologic sequalae of the syndrome. The prenatal incidence of cerebral abnormalities in TTTS is reported at 8%.[153] Quarello et al.[153] reported that in 22 cases of TTTS complicated with central nervous system abnormalities, fetal MRI was discordant from ultrasound in 45% of cases. Similarly, Kline-Fath et al.,[154] in a retrospective chart review of 25 fetal MRI exams in TTTS, reported additional findings when compared with ultrasound consisting of renal collecting system dilation in 63% of recipients, lung lesions in 4% (Fig. 11.27), cerebral ischemia or hemorrhage in 8% (Fig. 11.28), and cerebral venous sinus dilation in 13%. A higher incidence of congenital anomalies of the donor brain was also detected. In addition, thinning of the cerebral brain mantle and cerebellar volume loss is noted in the hypovolemic donor.[155] Thus, despite the need for further studies, fetal MRI may be helpful in TTTS for screening

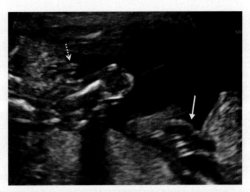

**FIGURE 11.24:** Axial ultrasound of both donor and recipient abdominal cord insertions. Notice small cord (dotted arrow) for the donor due to diminished flow. The recipient cord is large (solid arrow). Edema of the cord can be present.

of brain lesions and may be an important component in counseling prior to intervention.

## Differential Diagnosis

The differential diagnosis of TTTS includes uteroplacental insufficiency, growth disturbances caused by abnormal cord insertions, discordant manifestation of intrauterine infection, preterm premature rupture of membranes (PROM) of one twin, and discordant chromosomal or structural anomalies of one twin.[156,157]

## Prognosis

### Short-Term Outcome

In the absence of therapy, the perinatal mortality rate is high at 60–100%. With therapy, typically laser photocoagulation, survival is significantly improved being 64–68% for both twins.[148] Despite improved survival after fetoscopic laser treatment, neonates of TTTS pregnancies, compared with non-TTTS monochorionic gestations, still suffer severe neonatal morbidities secondary to prematurity and TTTS-related conditions. The reported miscarriage rate ranges between 3.5% and 17%, 1% and 13% PPROM <24 weeks, 5% and 9.8% PPROM >24 weeks with a preterm labor (<33 weeks) rate of 27% to 44%.[158–163] Furthermore, TTTS neonates in neonatal intensive care unit have a 4.8% to 7% rate of acute renal failure, 3% to 4% rate of necrotizing enterocolitis (NEC), 27% to 62% respiratory

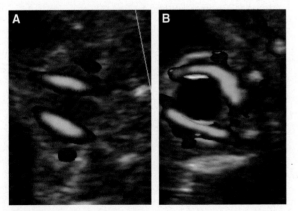

**FIGURE 11.23:** Bladder Discrepancy in TTTS. **A:** A donor twin in monochorioinc pregnancy with TTTS shows small bladder. **B:** Recipient twin demonstrated large and cycling bladder in same pregnancy.

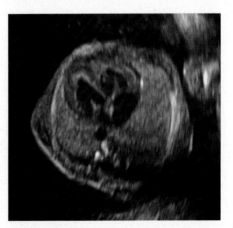

**FIGURE 11.25:** Recipient twin with TTTS cardiomyopathy. The heart is enlarged, and there is biventricular hypertrophy.

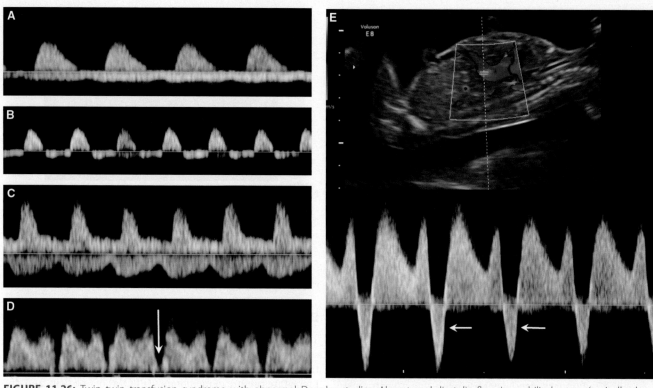

**FIGURE 11.26:** Twin twin transfusion syndrome with abnormal Doppler studies. Absent end-diastolic flow in umbilical artery (typically donor) **(A)**; reversed end-diastolic flow of umbilical artery (typically donor) **(B)**; pulsatile umbilical vein (typically recipient) **(C)**; absent "a" wave *(arrow)* of ductus venosus (typically recipient) **(D)**; and reversed "a" wave *(arrows)* of ductus venosus (typically recipient) **(E)**.

distress syndrome (RDS) rate with 4% to 34% prevalence of intraventricular hemorrhage (IVH) grade 3 to 4. There are also some reported cases of persistent pulmonary hypertension (3%) in pregnancies complicated with TTTS. This wide range

in frequency of neonatal morbidity is mainly because of inadequate sample size, different outcome measure definitions, different centers' experience, and diverse treatment modalities between centers.[158–164]

| Table 11.3 | Cincinnati Staging System | | |
|---|---|---|---|
| Stage | Donor | Recipient | Recipient Cardiomyopathy |
| I | Oligohydramnios (DVP < 2 cm) | Polyhydramnios (DVP > 8 cm) | No |
| II | Absent bladder | Bladder seen | No |
| III | Abnormal Doppler | Abnormal Doppler | None |
| IIIa | | | Mild |
| IIIb | | | Moderate |
| IIIc | | | Severe |
| IV | Hydrops | Hydrops | |
| V | Death | Death | |
| Variables/cardiomyopathy | Mild | Moderate | Severe |
| AV regurgitation | Mild | Moderate | Severe |
| RV/LV thickness | >+2 Z-score | >3+ Z-score | >4+ Z-score |
| MPI     Normal RV MPI is 0.32 ± 0.08     Normal LV MPI is 0.33 ± 0.05 | >+2 Z-score | >3+ Z-score | Severe biventricular dysfunction |

AV, atrioventricular valve; RV/LV, right ventricular/left ventricular; MPI, myocardial performance index.

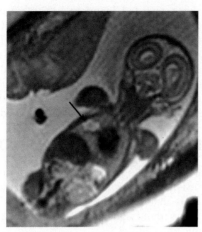

**FIGURE 11.27:** Lung Lesion in TTTS. Coronal SSFSE T2 image demonstrates a small T2 hyperintense lesion *(arrow)* in the right midlung of a recipient. The lesion was not delineated via ultrasound.

### Long-Term Outcome

**Neurodevelopmental Outcome:** In multifetal pregnancies, the risk of developing white matter necrosis in monochorionic twin pregnancy is 10-fold as compared with dichorionic twin pregnancies (33% vs. 3%).[165] In TTTS, the reported incidence of neurologic developmental abnormalities ranges between 7% and 16% after laser photocoagulation.[166] Further, Merhar et al.[167] did a prospective study of 22 premature TTTS cases

with prenatal brain injury. The author reported that postnatal brain injury correlated with severity of Quintero stage but not gestational age at delivery or birth weight. Lastly, Lopriore et al.[168] published a detailed neurologic, mental, and psychomotor follow-up of 115 laser-treated TTTS survivors at 2 years of age corrected for prematurity. The incidence of neurodevelopmental impairment was 17% with etiologies including cerebral palsy, mental developmental delay, psychomotor developmental delay, and deafness. Perinatal factors, including gestational age at delivery and Apgar score, correlated with adverse outcome.

**Cardiovascular Outcome:** There is a paucity of information concerning the long-term cardiovascular implications of TTTS. Herberg et al.[169] reported long-term cardiac function in a prospective study of 89 survivors (38 donor, 51 recipient) at 21 months of age after fetoscopic laser photocoagulation for 73 cases of severe TTTS pregnancies. The author reported a 11.2% incidence of structural heart disease and, specifically, a 7.8% pulmonary stenosis rate, which are higher than the general population. Eighty-seven percent of the survivors had a normal cardiac examination. Despite the high rate and severity of prenatal cardiac impairment in recipients, systolic or diastolic ventricular function completely normalized over the long term.

### Management

Numerous treatments for TTTS have been proposed, including selective feticide, cord coagulation, sectio parva (removing one fetus), placental bloodletting, maternal digitalis, maternal

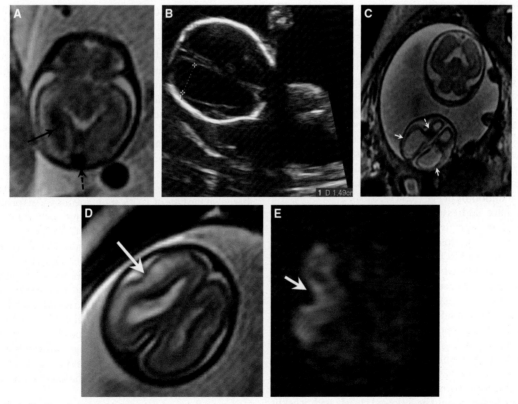

**FIGURE 11.28:** Brain Findings in TTTS. **A:** SSFSE T2 axial image shows hemorrhage along the germinal matrix *(solid arrow)* and enlarged venous sinuses *(dotted arrow)*. **B:** Axial ultrasound demonstrates ventriculomegaly in donor twin. **C:** Axial SSFSE T2 image of same fetus in B demonstrates extensive cerebral parenchymal thinning *(solid arrows)* and abnormal decreased signal in the basal ganglia *(dotted arrow)* consistent with severe encephaloclastic event. **D:** Axial SSFSE T2 in a recipient twin shows abnormal bright signal *(arrow)* in the anatomic area of the right middle cerebral artery. **E:** Diffusion imaging of same fetus in D confirms restricted diffusion *(arrow)* consistent with acute ischemia. The fetal cerebral ultrasound was normal.

indomethacin, serial amnioreduction, microseptostomy of the intertwin membrane, and nonselective or selective fetoscopic laser photocoagulation (SFLP). Microseptostomy has fallen out of favor given the possibility of creating a monoamniotic gestation with risk for cord entanglement. Selective cord coagulation is center dependent but may be considered when a twin is irretrievably compromised. For decades in the United States, serial amnioreduction was the most prevalent therapy for TTTS. However, in recent years, SFLP has become more widely accepted and is the primary treatment offered in many centers today.

### Amnioreduction

Amnioreduction was used initially for maternal comfort and as a means to control polyhydramnios in the hope of prolonging the pregnancy until the risk of extreme prematurity lessened. In addition, amnioreduction has been shown to improve uteroplacental blood flow, likely by reducing intra-amniotic pressure from polyhydramnios. In a review of 26 reports dating from the 1930s of 252 fetuses, Moise[170] found an overall survival of 49% in twins treated with amnioreduction. In more recent series with more consistently aggressive serial amnioreduction to normalize amniotic fluid volumes, survival ranged from as low as 37% to as high as 83%.[171,172]

### Fetoscopic Laser Photocoagulation

The first therapy for TTTS that attempted to treat the anatomic basis for the syndrome was reported by De Lia et al.,[173] who described nonselective fetoscopic laser photocoagulation of all vessels crossing the intertwin membrane. Today, SFLP, laser of only vascular anastomoses across the intertwin membrane, is the standard of care for TTTS between 18 and 26 weeks with Quintero stage II and higher. The turning point in its usage was the 2004 Eurofetus multicenter randomized controlled trial that compared serial amnioreduction with SFLP in 142 women with monochorionic diamniotic twins and TTTS between January 1999 and March 2002.[174] The laser therapy group, compared with the amnioreduction group, reached a significantly higher gestational age at delivery (mean 33 vs. 29 weeks) and had increased survival of at least one fetus to 28 days of age (76% vs. 56%). Although postnatal follow-up was only 6 months in duration, the laser therapy group showed improved neurologic outcomes with decreased risk of periventricular leukomalacia (6% vs. 14%) and a higher likelihood of being free of neurologic complications at 6 months of age (52% vs. 31%).[174]

Few studies have addressed laser complications in TTTS pregnancies. In a retrospective study of 175 TTTS pregnancies treated with laser, Yamamoto et al.[175] reported that the most frequent complication was PROM, which occurred in 28% of the cases. 12% developed PROM in the first three weeks after laser, with the remaining 17% occurred thereafter. The entry of the trocar, which was transplacental in 48 cases (27%), was not associated with adverse outcome.

Few case series have reported late complications of laser photocoagulation, including monoamniotic gestation, amniotic band syndrome, ischemic limb, and bowel atresia related to vascular accidents. However, these complications can also occur in monochorionic twins without TTTS.

All laser-treated cases should be followed closely with weekly US surveillance to detect any late complications. In a large cohort of 151 cases, Robyr et al.[176] demonstrated that progression of the disease occurred in 14% of cases, while another 13% had reversal of TTTS, with the recipient behaving like the donor and vice versa. In addition, twin anemia-polycythemia sequence

(TAPS) has been reported in up to 13% of cases following TTTS. In a 2008 report of early and late complication rates in a cohort of 139 consecutively treated cases with SFLP from the Fetal Care Center of Cincinnati, Habli et al.[159] noted progression or persistence of TTTS in only 2 cases (1.4%) and TAPS in 3 cases (2.2%). The low rate of complications was suggested to be due to infrequent missed vascular connections in the presence of a stringent mapping protocol used by this group during SFLP.

## TWIN ANEMIA-POLYCYTHEMIA SEQUENCE

In 2007, Lopriore et al.[177] reported a new form of chronic fetofetal transfusion termed twin anemia-polycythemia sequence (TAPS). TAPS is characterized by large intertwin hemoglobin (Hb) differences without signs of TTTS (oligopoly sequence) in monochorionic pregnancies.[177]

### Incidence

The incidence of TAPS varies according to definition, type, and diagnostic criteria, such as whether it is antenatal only or both antenatal and postnatal. TAPS can occur spontaneously or postlaser for TTTS. The spontaneous form complicates 3% to 5% of monochorionic twin pregnancies,[139,178] whereas the postlaser form occurs in 2% to 13% of TTTS cases.[159,176] In a report on late complications of 101 TTTS cases treated with fetoscopic laser surgery, Robyr et al.[176] found a 13% incidence of postlaser TAPS, whereas, Habli et al.[159] reported a lower than 2% incidence.

### Pathogenesis

The pathogenesis of TAPS is based on a unique placental angioarchitecture characterized by the presence of only few arteriovenous (AV) vascular anastomoses. These minuscule anastomoses allow a slow transfusion of blood from the donor to the recipient, leading gradually to highly discordant Hb levels without hormonal imbalance.[179] In addition to very few and small unidirectional AV anastomoses, twins with TAPS have less arterioarterio anastomoses, 11% cited in cases of spontaneous TAPS.[180] Importantly, the diameter of these arterio anastomoses are very small.[181,182] In comparison, the incidence of artery–artery anastomoses in uncomplicated monochorionic pregnancies and TTTS pregnancies is 80% and 25%, respectively.[181,182]

Several studies report different placental angioarchitecture based on the type of TAPS, spontaneous versus postlaser. Recently, in a placental injection study of 43 monochorionic twin pregnancies complicated by spontaneous TAPS ($N = 16$) and postlaser TAPS ($n = 27$), Villiers et al.[181] noted that all 43 had AV anastomosis and nearly 96% had AV anastomosis with small diameter localized at placental margins. As compared with twins with postlaser TAPS, spontaneous TAPS had a higher number of anastomosis (4 vs. 2) with increased arterio–arterio anastomosis (18% vs. 14%). Velamentous or marginal cord insertion was found in 43% and 57% of spontaneous and postlaser TAPS, respectively.[181]

The pathogenesis of absent oligo–polyhydramnios sequelae in TAPS is likely related to very slow intertwin blood transfusion, allowing more time for hemodynamic compensatory mechanisms to take place.[180]

### Diagnosis

Given that TAPS has just recently been described, uniform criteria are yet to be clearly established. Diagnosis is based on either antenatal or postnatal findings or both.

Antenatal diagnosis of TAPS can be defined by both grayscale and Doppler findings. In TAPS, there is absence of oligopoly sequence, and there is an increased peak systolic velocity (PSV) in the middle cerebral artery (MCA) in the donor twin, suggestive of fetal anemia and a decreased MCA-PSV in the recipient twin, suggestive of polycythemia. Robyr et al.[176] proposed the use of a MCA-PSV >1.5 multiples of the median (MoM) for the donor twin and <0.8 MoM in the recipient (Fig. 11.29). None of these criteria are validated despite their use by most physicians.

Postnatal criteria include 1-Intertwin Hb difference >8.0 g per dL *with* at least one of the following: reticulocyte count ratio >1.7 or a placenta with only small (diameter <1 mm) vascular anastomoses at pathologic examination.

### Differential Diagnosis

The differential diagnosis of TAPS includes uteroplacental insufficiency, discordant manifestation of intrauterine infection, and any cause of fetal anemia.

### Prognosis

Perinatal outcome in TAPS is not well known, but has varied from mild hematologic complications to severe cerebral injury and perinatal death.[183] Perinatal survival rates vary depending on treatment but are cited from 50% to 100%, with the average gestational age at diagnosis ranging from 19 to 24 weeks and delivery from 28 to 34 weeks.[184]

Data are sparse for short- and long-term neurologic outcomes. In a case-control study of twins with TAPS paired with two monochorionic twin pairs without TAPS, Lopriore et al.[183] found no differences in risk of severe cerebral injury among groups; however, long-term outcomes were not reported. In several case reports, evidence of MRI changes in the anemic fetus was manifested by numerous large cysts in the basal ganglia, bilateral white matter injury, multiple microhemorrhages, and parenchymal hemorrhage in the right occipital lobe.[185] These findings were seen in both postlaser and spontaneous TAPS.[186] In a large multicenter study of long-term follow-up for 212 TTTS pregnancies treated with laser surgery, 16 pregnancies (4%) were affected by TAPS, of which 4 were treated with

intrauterine transfusion.[187] Perinatal survival was 75% for the postlaser surgery TAPS cases. In all 12 surviving TAPS infants, evaluation at 2 years of age, which included a Bayley developmental test, showed that none of these infants had long-term neurodevelopmental impairment. In conclusion, cerebral injury in TAPS cases, treated with or without intrauterine transfusion, may be less common than initially thought. Therefore, large multicenter follow-up studies are urgently needed.

### Management

The treatment options by case reports and small series include expectant management, induction of labor, selective feticide, fetoscopic laser surgery, or intrauterine transfusion. Intrauterine transfusion is considered to be a temporary option, most commonly to treat the anemic donor. Potentially, transfusing the donor may worsen the polycythemia in the other twin. Choosing which modality is the best treatment is difficult given the limited experience in both the intravenous and/or the intraperitoneal transfusion in TAPS cases. Spontaneous resolution of antenatal TAPS has also been reported.

### Recurrence

Risk of recurrence is unknown.

## TWIN-REVERSED ARTERIAL PERFUSION

Acardiac anomaly or twin-reversed arterial perfusion (TRAP) refers to a complication unique to monochorionic twins. The lack of a well-formed cardiac structure is found in one fetus (acardiac), which is abnormally perfused by a structurally normal co-twin (pump twin) through a superficial artery-to-artery placental anastomosis (Fig. 11.30). This anomaly can be recognized antenatally from the first trimester and a range of in-utero interventions have been attempted.[188–190]

### Incidence

TRAP sequence affects around 1 in 35,000 to 40,000 pregnancies, representing around 1% of monochorionic twins.[188–190]

### Pathogenesis

Two conditions are necessary for TRAP development. First, abnormal cardiac embryogenesis occurs between 8 to 12 weeks in

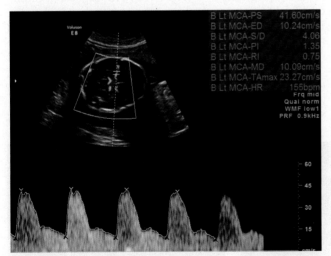

**FIGURE 11.29:** TAPS. Monochorionic–diamniotic twin pregnancy with postlaser twin anemia polycythemia syndrome. Middle cerebral artery peak systolic velocity Doppler of donor twin is >1.5 MOM. Doppler in the recipient with <0.8 MOM (not shown).

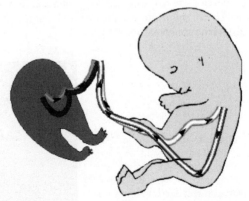

**FIGURE 11.30:** In twin-reversed arterial perfusion syndrome, the acardiac twin receives retrograde perfusion with poorly oxygenated blood.

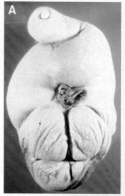
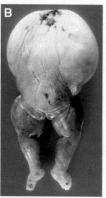
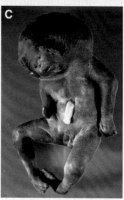

**FIGURE 11.31:** Acardiac Twin in TRAP. **A–C:** Pathologic photographs showing variable development of acardiac twins.

| Table 11.4 | Description of Acardiac Twins |
| --- | --- |
| **Malformation** | **Description** |
| Acephalus | No cephalic structure present |
| Anceps | Some cranial structure or neural tissue present |
| Acormus | Cephalic structure but no truncal structures |
| Amorphus | No distinguishable rostral-to-caudal structure |

| Table 11.5 | Features Associated with Acardiac Twin |
| --- | --- |
| Biometric discordance between the twins | |
| Absence of identifiable cardiac pulsation in one twin | |
| Due to preferential arterial perfusion of lower body, poor definition of the head, trunk, and upper extremities and usually deformed lower extremities | |
| Marked and diffuse subcutaneous edema and abnormal cystic areas in the upper part of the body of the affected twin | |
| An abnormal two-vessel cord is found in more than two-thirds of cases | |

one of the two twins of a monochorionic pregnancy.[191] Second, a specific abnormal placental angioarchitecture defined by an arterio-arterial and a veno-venous intertwin anastomosis supports the development of an abnormal twin (acardiac twin).[191–193] Furthermore, heterokaryotypic monozygotism, such as aneuploidy, which arises after splitting of the fertilized ovum, has been discussed as a possible etiologic factor in TRAP.[194]

In acardiac twin development, all organs are affected, resulting in variable presentation and size. Most commonly, acardiac twins are acephalic with absent upper extremities as deoxygenated blood from the umbilical artery preferentially supplies the lower rather than the upper part of the body. Other structures that are often absent include the heart (less than 20% of fetuses have identifiable cardiac tissue), pancreas, lungs, liver, and small intestines (Fig. 11.31). A two-vessel cord is found in more than two-thirds of cases.[195] Because of the lack of communication between the lymphatic and the vascular systems, the acardiac twin frequently develops severe subcutaneous edema and cystic hygromas, which can significantly increase the size of the fetus and further distort the abnormal anatomy.

A detailed classification system of the acardiac twin had been suggested on the basis of morphology (Table 11.4). The simplest classification system of acardiac twins differentiates between two types: pseudoacardius, with evidence of a rudimentary cardiac structure, and holoacardius, without cardiac structure present. These classifications do not correlate with outcome.

### Diagnosis

Common features in TRAP are described in Table 11.5. The prenatal diagnosis of acardiac twins should be suspected when a grossly malformed fetus is seen in the setting of a monochorionic twin pregnancy[196,197] (Fig. 11.32). The diagnosis is further established by retrograde flow of the umbilical artery by color Doppler ultrasound. Specifically, arterial blood flows toward rather than away from the acardiac twin and in a caudal-to-cranial direction in the abdominal aorta (Fig. 11.33).[198]

Although the pump twin is structurally normal in most cases, associated anomalies reported include prune belly, renal agenesis and dysplasia, renal tubular dysgenesis, anal atresia, gastroschisis, and pulmonary artery calcification.[199] Further karyotyping

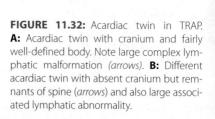

**FIGURE 11.32:** Acardiac twin in TRAP. **A:** Acardiac twin with cranium and fairly well-defined body. Note large complex lymphatic malformation (arrows). **B:** Different acardiac twin with absent cranium but remnants of spine (arrows) and also large associated lymphatic abnormality.

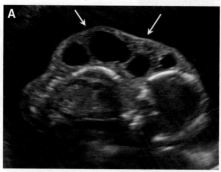
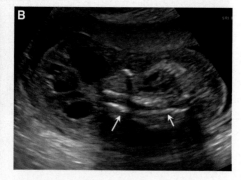

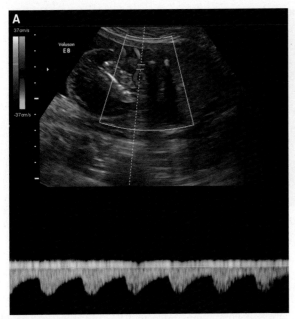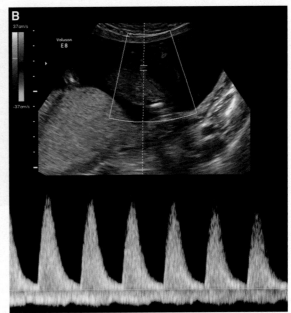

**FIGURE 11.33:** Doppler in TRAP. **A:** Reverse flow on Doppler image in acardiac twin: arterial flow going in (*under the baseline*) and venous flow going out (*above the baseline*). **B:** Normal umbilical artery Doppler flow in pump twin.

of the pump twin should be offered because as many as 9% of pump twins have an abnormal karyotype, including monosomy, trisomy, deletions, mosaicism, and polyploidy.[195]

Fetal MRI has been used to evaluate complications in TRAP syndrome. Guimaraes et al.[200] reported fetal MRI findings in 35 cases diagnosed with TRAP. The author reported 91% correct diagnosis by ultrasound. However, fetal MRI identified 14% associated abnormalities in the pump twin not related to cardiac etiology (Fig. 11.34). Despite this, MRI is considered an adjunct to fetal ultrasound, and further studies are needed.

## Differential Diagnosis

Fetal death in a monochorionic twin pregnancy and teratoma arising from the placenta or umbilical cord may mimic an acardiac twin.

## Prognosis

As the acardiac twin depends on the pump twin for growth, the healthy pump twin's survival is threatened by the risk of

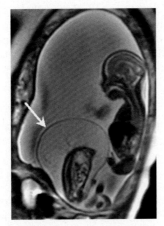

**FIGURE 11.34:** Fetal MRI in TRAP. Coronal SSFSE T2 image demonstrating hydropic acardiac *twin (arrow)* and pump twin.

congestive heart failure, polyhydramnios, intrauterine fetal death, PROM, and preterm labor and delivery. The primary contributors of perinatal death in TRAP are congestive heart failure and preterm delivery. Perinatal mortality of the pump twin ranges from 35% to 55%.[191,192]

In attempting to improve outcome and define optimal management of TRAP, several authors reported prenatal prognostic factors that affect pump twin outcome. Moore et al.[192] reported the percentage of pump twin weight as a prognostic factor. The authors developed a regression model to estimate acardiac twin weight as follows: weight (g) = 1.21 × length (cm)$^2$ − (1.66 × length [cm]) (Fig. 11.35A) with the length of the parabiotic twin representing the longest linear dimension. They reported that if the ratio exceeded 70%, the incidence of preterm delivery was 90%, polyhydramnios was 40%, and pump twin congestive heart failure was 30%, whereas if a ratio was less than 70%, rates were 75%, 30%, and 10%, respectively.

Some have used Doppler ultrasound of the umbilical artery to determine impact on the pump twin. In analyzing the ratio of the umbilical artery pulsatility index between the acardiac and the pump twins, Brassard et al.[201] noted a low acardiac pulsatility index. This value represented a high diastolic velocity in the acardiac twin compared with the pulsatility index of the pump twin and was found to correlate with poor prognosis because it reflected substantial flow into the acardiac twin. Dashe et al.[202] noted that pump twin outcomes varied by differences in resistance index between the twins. Resistance index difference of <0.05 was associated with poor outcome, whereas >0.2 resulted in favorable outcomes.

In a 2013 retrospective chart review, Oliver et al.[203] correlated sonographic findings associated with the pump twin's adverse outcome with acardiac twin mass size by using the formula of a prolate ellipsoid (Fig. 11.35B). Acardiac twin mass, which was estimated by summing body and extremity volumes, was calculated using the equation (width × height × length × 0.523). The total volume was then converted to mass by assuming soft tissue density was similar to water (1 g per mL). After the

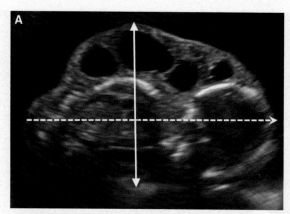
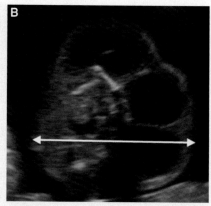

**FIGURE 11.35:** Acardiac measurements. **A:** The total length (*dotted line*) of the acardiac twin used in Moore regression formula to assess estimated weight of acardiac twin: weight (g) = 1.21 × length (cm)$^2$ − (1.66 × length [cm]). AP dimension (*solid line with arrows*) is obtained for the Oliver technique. **B:** Transverse dimension of the acardiac twin. Orthogonal measurement of acardiac twin including hydropic tissues for Oliver technique (length, AP, and transverse).

volume was converted, a percentage of the acardiac to pump twin (i.e., acardiac/pump twin weight ratio) was obtained. Two groups were classified: acardiac/pump twin weight ratio that was either greater than 70% or less than 70%. The author reported that acardiac twin size exceeding 70% of the pump twin correlated with an increased risk of pump twin compromise if using the prolate ellipsoid formula ($P$ = .002) but not the sonographic Moore method ($P$ = .09).

To further assess the impact of the acardiac twin on the cardiovascular status of the pump twin, two-dimensional (2D) ultrasound can detect physical signs of early cardiovascular deterioration of the pump twin, specifically polyhydramnios, cardiomegaly, and pericardial effusion. A fetal echocardiography can also assess cardiac function and provide evidence of congestive heart failure by comparing with cardiac output appropriate for gestational age. Color Doppler ultrasound should be used to look for tricuspid regurgitation, reverse flow in the ductus venosus, pulsation in the umbilical vein, and high peak velocity of middle cerebral artery flow secondary to fetal anemia. The presence of any one of these ultrasound features predicts a poor prognosis.

## Management

The goal of treating acardiac anomaly is to maximize the likelihood of term delivery and survival of the pump twin in a safe and effective manner. The goal of surgery is to interrupt the vascularization of the acardiac twin. There are several techniques described that include ultrasound-guided fetal cord ligation or compression,[204] bipolar coagulation, laser coagulation, trans-section with harmonic ultrasound scalpel,[205] thermocoagulation,[206] and radiofrequency ablation (RFA).[207]

RFA is becoming more popular as a safe and reliable treatment method for TRAP. In a systematic review of the literature reporting seven studies using RFA as treatment choice for TRAP sequence, Cabassa et al.[208] found a total of 85 TRAP cases that included twin and triplets ($n$ = 3) who underwent RFA. Average gestational ages were 18.6 weeks at the time of the procedure and 36.4 weeks at delivery. Neonatal survival rate of the pump twin was 85%. In this review, the rate of preterm delivery/PROM <37 weeks was 28%; fetal death 3.5%; and maternal complications, mainly thermal injury at grounding pads, 2.4%. Neonatal survival rates for cord coagulation ranged between

70% and 80%, comparable to RFA, but were associated with higher rate of preterm delivery (58%).

Other fetoscopic techniques, such as intrafetal laser therapy, have been proposed to prevent the demise of the pump twin. Pagani et al.[209] in 2013 reported outcome data for intrafetal laser therapy of TRAP by systemic review and meta-analysis of 11 studies. Pagani et al. included 51 cases consisting of 5 triplets (dichorionic triamniotic) and 46 (monochorionic twins). Average gestational ages were 17.2 weeks at the time of the procedure, with delivery at 37 weeks and neonatal survival of 82%. Rates of preterm birth were 7% at <32 weeks, 21% at <34 weeks, and 40% at <37 weeks. Rates of adverse pregnancy outcome (i.e., intrauterine death or preterm birth before 37 weeks) were related to gestational age at the procedure with a significantly lower rate at 19% when treatment was undertaken before 16 weeks compared with 66% for pregnancies treated ≥16 weeks. These findings suggest that intrafetal laser therapy could be a good and safe option when performed before 16 weeks.

## MONOCHORIONIC/MONAMNIOTIC TWIN

Monochorionic/monoamniotic twin pregnancies have a single placenta and sac, and occur after splitting of single blastocyst on day 8 to 13 post fertilization.[210] Although the umbilical cords typically insert close to one another (within 6 cm of each other) and are generally located centrally, one-third are either marginal or velamentous.[211] Intertwin vascular anastomoses are always present, but twin-to-twin transfusion is less common than in monochorionic–diamniotic twins.[212]

### Incidence

Monoamniotic twin pregnancies occur in 1% of monozygotic twin pregnancies.[210]

### Diagnosis

Rodis et al.[213] defined the criteria for diagnosis of monoamniotic twin pregnancies as one placenta, same sex fetuses, adequate fluid around both fetuses, and the absence of a dividing membrane (Fig. 11.36). However, a first-trimester transvaginal ultrasound that shows one sac and two embryo poles before 8 weeks

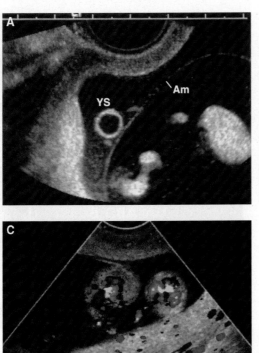

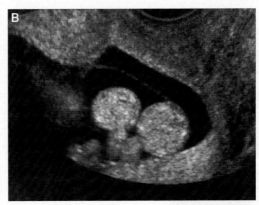

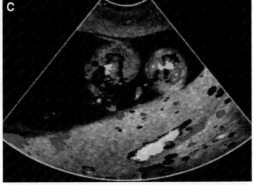

**FIGURE 11.36:** Monoamniotic gestation with single yolk sac at 10.5 weeks. **A:** Yolk sac (*YS*) and single amnion (*Am*). **B:** Two adjacent fetuses are nearly touching. **C:** Color-flow Doppler image shows two adjacent umbilical cords. (Courtesy of Gerald Mulligan, MD.)

is not always diagnostic of monochorionic–monoamniotic twin. Several reported cases actually turned out to be triplets or di-amniotic–dichorionic twins. Thus, late first trimester and early second trimester ultrasound are recommended for accurate diagnosis. Cord entanglement is diagnostic for a monochorionic–monoamniotic twin pregnancy.

## Prognosis

Monoamniotic twin pregnancies suffer from a high perinatal mortality rate that ranges from 10% to 47%, malformation rate of 10%, and cord entanglement up to 70%.[214,215] Cause of death is typically attributed to cord entanglement (50%) with other etiologies including premature deliveries, intrauterine growth restriction, and congenital anomalies. In a Japanese study, the prospective risk of fetal death was 13.9% for women who reached gestational week 22. This rate gradually decreased to the range of 4.5% to 8.0% between gestational weeks 30.0 and 36.0.[216] Most studies show, however, that fetal loss can occur after 32 weeks in monoamniotic twin gestations.

## Management

Antepartum management of a monoamniotic twin pregnancy is challenging. These patients should be offered first trimester screening, an anatomy scan between 18 and 20 weeks, and fetal echocardiography because of the increased risk of congenital malformation. Antepartum fetal surveillance and delivery early in the third trimester are indicated because of the high rate of perinatal mortality, often due to cord entanglement. Data from observational studies to define the value of intensive fetal monitoring are insufficient but suggest that inpatient monitoring provided a better perinatal outcome. In a retrospective study of 87 mono/mono twin pregnancies ≥24 weeks' gestation with two surviving fetuses, Heyborne et al.[217] reported that 43 patients

were hospitalized electively (mean 26.5 weeks) and 28 were hospitalized for specific indications (mean 30.1 weeks). No fetal deaths occurred in the 43 hospitalized patients who were monitored for at least 2 hours daily, whereas 13 intrauterine fetal deaths occurred in 8 of 16 outpatients monitored one to three times weekly. Compared with indicated admissions, the authors found elective inpatient management achieved a lower rate of composite neonatal morbidity (29% vs. 50%), significant improvement in birth weight (3,750 vs. 3,470 g), higher gestational age at delivery (33 vs. 31 weeks), and no difference in NICU days.

Timing of delivery is not well established for monochorionic/monoamniotic twin pregnancies of uncertain or precarious fetal status. In view of increased risk of sudden death after 32 weeks, which is 5% to 10%, the recommended delivery is Cesarean section between 32 and 34 weeks after administration of steroids for fetal lung maturity.[125]

## CORD ENTANGLEMENT

High rates of perinatal loss in monochorionic–monoamniotic twin pregnancies are mostly attributed to cord entanglement and cord knotting.[218]

### Incidence

Current prevalence of umbilical cord entanglement is estimated between 70% and 91% of cases at birth with 22% sonographically diagnosed.[217,219]

### Diagnosis

Although 2D color and power Doppler sonography are usually most helpful for prenatal diagnosis of cord entanglement (Fig. 11.37A,B), this method does not easily visualize the exact location or continuity of the cord or define spatial relationships

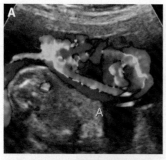
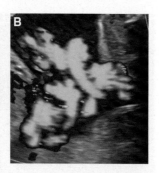
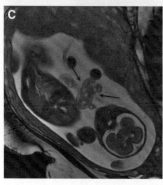

**FIGURE 11.37:** Cord entanglement. **A:** Color Doppler of monochorionic–monoamniotic twin pregnancy with cord entanglement. **B:** Power Doppler flow studies confirming cord entanglement. **C:** MRI of monochorionic–monoamniotic twin pregnancy with cord entanglement (*arrows*).

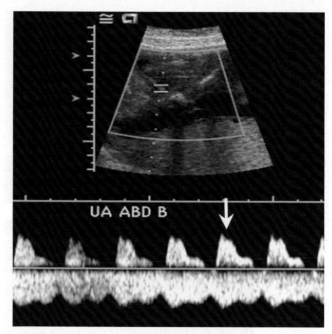

**FIGURE 11.38:** Doppler in the umbilical cord of a twin with a tangled cord. Notch in the umbilical artery denoted with *arrow*. There is also absent end-diastolic flow in the umbilical artery and a pulsatile waveform in the umbilical vein.

related to cord entanglement, twin pairs, and placenta as effectively as 3D ultrasound. When imaging twins, MRI can also define cord entanglement (Fig. 11.37C).

Another indirect sonographic diagnosis of cord entanglement can be achieved by Doppler flow velocimetry. This method reflects hemodynamic alterations in the fetal–placental circulation secondary to narrowing of the umbilical vessels involved in cord entanglement. These Doppler findings include high blood velocity in the umbilical vein,[220,221] a notch in the umbilical artery waveform,[222] or persistent absent end-diastolic flow (Fig. 11.38).[223]

### Prognosis/Management

A recent systematic review and meta-analysis[224] of 114 monochorionic–monoamniotic twin pregnancies with cord entanglement reported overall survival at birth at 89%. In this study, 11% perinatal deaths occurred, of which 65% resulted in utero and 35% neonatal. Gestational age at fetal death ranged between 14 and 33 weeks. Thus, no consensus was reached in this review about the optimal antenatal management of these patients.

## CONJOINED TWINS

The most striking anomaly, conjoined twins, occurs when monozygotic twins fail to separate into two individuals.[225] The extent of conjunction ranges from a simple joining of ectodermal tissues to an extreme case of one twin contained within the other.

### Incidence

The incidence ranges from 1 in 50,000 to 100,000 live births with a female:male ratio of 3:1.[225]

### Pathogenesis/Etiology

Conjoined twins have been reported to arise at around 12 or 13 days post conception from a single blastocyst that had undergone incomplete division of the embryonic cell mass at one pole or at the point between the poles.[226] More recently, embryologic studies of conjoined twinning have indicated that this developmental anomaly could originate from the secondary union of two separate embryonic discs.[226] Thus, two hypotheses exist on the origin of conjoined twins: the fission theory, in which a fertilized ovum divides incompletely, and the fusion theory, explaining secondary fusion of two originally distinct monovular embryos. The recent finding of a monochorionic diamniotic conjoined twin pregnancy may further contribute to the fusion theory.[226,227] Others are in favor of the fission theory, maintained by the observation that the incidence of mirror imaging is higher in conjoined twins than in monozygotic twins.[227,228]

### Diagnosis

Conjoined twins are classified by the site of their most prominent union, which is ventral or dorsal in 87% and 13%, respectively (Fig. 11.39).[229] The abnormality is named with the suffix pagus, which means fixed (Table 11.6).

The diagnosis of conjoined twins is often made on prenatal ultrasound scan as early as week 12 of gestation. Typical features include a fixed position of the fetal heads, an inability to detect separate bodies or skin contours, and the lack of separating membranes.[225] Detailed ultrasonography and echocardiography should be performed at 18 to 20 weeks to characterize the anatomy of shared organs and the structure and function of the heart or hearts (Fig. 11.40 & 11.41). Other malformations are often associated and complicate management. Doppler ultrasound provides another tool to assess prognosis of vital organs, especially the liver and heart (see Fig. 11.40B), which may be shared between the twins. MRI in conjoined twins (Fig. 11.40 & 11.41) can show more accurate diagnosis of shared organs and other associated anomalies that are essential in prognosis, counseling, and management.

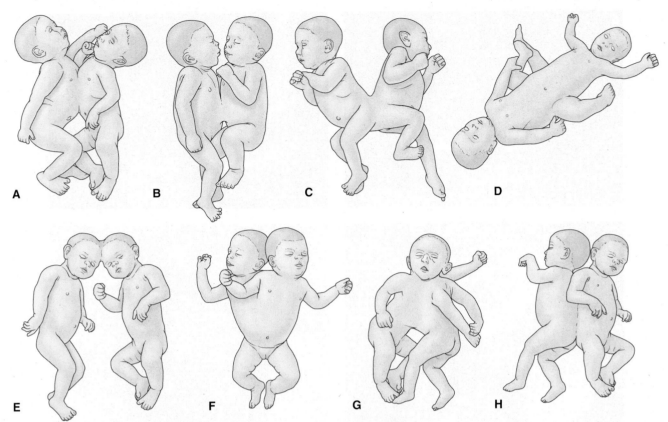

**FIGURE 11.39:** Different types of conjoined twins: thoracopagus **(A)**, omphalopagus **(B)**, pygopagus **(C)**, ischiopagus **(D)**, craniopagus **(E)**, parapagus **(F)**, cephalopagus **(G)**, rachipagus **(H)**. Same as Figure 11.30 Nyberg multiple gestations.

## Prognosis/Management

Little is known about the antenatal natural history of conjoined twins. Around 20% to 40% of conjoined twins are stillborn, and more than half of those born alive die during the neonatal period before any surgical procedure can be attempted.[230] Overall, the prognosis depends on the type of fusion and presence of associated structural defects. As soon as the diagnosis of conjoined twins is made, management of the pregnancy begins. Elective termination is usually offered if severe deformities are anticipated or when there is a cardiac or cerebral fusion in which separation is not possible.[225] If the pregnancy is continued, elective cesarean delivery is planned at a center where appropriate obstetric, neonatal, and pediatric surgical facilities are available.

| Table 11.6 | Conjoined Twin Classification Based on Union Distribution[225–231] | |
| --- | --- | --- |
| **Type** | **Area of Union** | **Percentage/Viability** |
| Cephalopagus | Head to umbilicus fusion | 11%, nonviable and nonseparable |
| Thoracopagus | Thorax to umbilicus fusion | 19%, nonviable and nonseparable |
| Omphalopagus | At the umbilicus | 18%, viable and separable |
| Ischiopagus | Lower abdomen and pelvis | 11%, viable and separable |
| Parapagus | Pelvis and variable trunk | 28%, viable but unlikely separable |
| Dorsal | | Less frequent, viable but unlikely separable |
| Craniopagus | Brain | 5% |
| Rachiopagus | Vertebral column | 2% |
| Pygopagus | Sacrum | 6% |

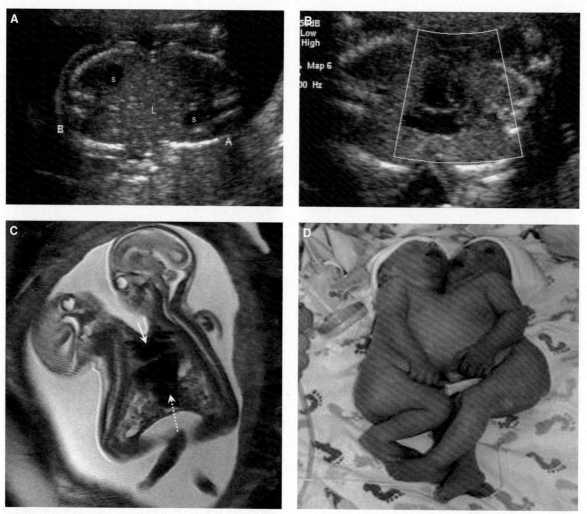

**FIGURE 11.40:** Conjoined thoracopagus twins at 20 weeks. **A:** On axial US, A single liver *(L)* is identified in the midline. Note two stomachs *(s)*. A and B represent twins. **B:** Color Doppler demonstrating a single heart shared between the two twins. **C:** T2 SSFSE image confirms single heart *(solid arrow)* and fused liver *(dotted arrow)*.. **D:** Color photo of the twins at birth..

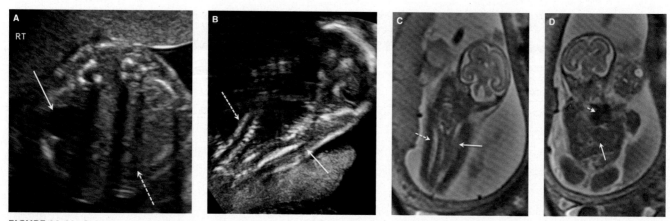

**FIGURE 11.41:** Parapagus conjoined twins at 22 weeks. **A:** Axial US shows a single stomach *(solid arrow)* and fused liver *(dotted arrow)*. **B:** Two spines side by side are identified *(solid and dotted arrow)*. **C:** Coronal T2 MR image confirms separate spinal canals *(solid and dotted arrows)*. **D:** Coronal T2 MR image through anterior chest and abdomen demonstrates fused heart *(dotted arrow)* and single liver *(solid arrow)*.

# ACKNOWLEDGMENT

I thank Dr. Rachel Sinky for the help she provided in the introduction of this chapter.

# REFERENCES

1. Martin JA, Hamilton BE, Ventura SJ, et al. Births: final data for 2010. *Natl Vital Stat Rep.* 2012;61(1):1–72.
2. Lambalk CB, Boomsma DI, DeBoer L, et al. Increased levels and pulsatility of follicle-stimulating hormone in mothers of hereditary dizygotic twins. *J Clin Endocrinol Metab.* 1998;83:481–486.
3. Ananth CV, Chauhan SP. Epidemiology of twinning in developed countries. *Semin Perinatol.* 2012;36(3):156–161.
4. Dickey RP. The relative contribution of assisted reproductive technologies and ovulation induction to multiple births in the United States 5 years after the Society for Assisted Reproductive Technology/American Society for Reproductive Medicine recommendation to limit the number of embryos transferred. *Fertil Steril.* 2007;88(6):1554–1561.
5. Chauhan SP, Scardo JA, Hayes E, et al. Twins: prevalence, problems and preterm births. *Am J Obstet Gynecol.* 2010;203:305–315.
6. Velikonja U. The cost of multiple gestation pregnancies in assisted reproduction. *Harv J Law Gend.* 2009;32:462–504.
7. Sunderam S, Kissin D, Flowers L, et al. Assisted reproductive technology surveillance—United States 2009. *MMWR Morb Mortal Wkly Rep.* 2012;61(SS7):1–23.
8. Mathews TJ, MacDorman MF. Infant mortality statistics from the 2008 period linked birth/infant death data set. *Natl Vital Stat Rep.* 2012;60(5):1–28.
9. Kinzler WL, Ananth CV, Vintzileos AM. Medical and economic effects of twin gestations. *J Soc Gynecol Invest.* 2000;7(6):321–327.
10. Chasen ST, Chervenak FA. What is the relationship between the universal use of ultrasound, the rate of detection of twins, and outcome differences? *Clin Obstet Gynecol.* 1998;41:66–77.
11. Sherer DM. Is less intensive fetal surveillance of dichorionic twin gestations justified? *Ultrasound Obstet Gynecol.* 2000;15:167–173.
12. Vimercati A, Greco P, Vera L, et al. The diagnostic role of in-utero magnetic resonance imaging. *J Perinat Med.* 1999;27:303–308.
13. Bekkar M, van Vught JM. The role of magnetic resonance in the prenatal diagnosis of fetal anomalies. *Eur J Obstet Gynecol Reprod Biol.* 2001;96:173–178.
14. Bekiesinska-Figatowska M, Herman-Sucharska I, Romaniuk-Doroszewska A, et al. Diagnostic problems in case of twin pregnancies: US vs. MRI study. *J Perinat Med.* 2013;41(5):535–541.
15. Lewis CM, Healy SC, Martin NG. Genetic contribution to dizygotic twinning. *Am J Med Genet.* 1996;61:237–246.
16. Meulemans WJ, Lewis CM, Boomsma DI, et al. Genetic modeling of dizygotic twinning in pedigrees of spontaneous dizygotic twins. *Am J Med Genet.* 1996;61:258–263.
17. Busjahn A, Knoblauch H, Faulhaber H-D, et al. A region on chromosome 3 is linked to dizygotic twinning. *Nat Genet.* 2000;26:398–399.
18. Hall JG. Twinning. *Lancet.* 2003;362(9385):735–743.
19. Nylander PPS. Frequency of multiple births. In: MacGillivray I, Nylander PPS, Corney G, eds. *Human Multiple Reproduction.* London, UK: WB Saunders; 1975:87–98.
20. Kiely JL, Kiely B. Epidemiological trends in multiple births in the United States, 1971–1998. *Twin Res.* 2001;4:131–133.
21. Murphy M, Hey K. Twinning rates. *Lancet.* 1997;349:1398–1399.
22. Benirschke K. Accurate recording of twin placentation: a plea to the obstetrician. *Obstet Gynecol.* 1961;18:334–347.
23. Benirschke K, Kim CK. Multiple pregnancy 1. *N Engl J Med.* 1973;288:1276–1284.
24. Benirschke K, Kim CK. Multiple pregnancy 2. *N Engl J Med.* 1973;288:1329–1336.
25. Burn J, Corney G. Zygosity determination and the types of twinning. In: MacGillivray I, Campbell DM, Thompson B, eds. *Twinning and Twins.* Chichester, UK: John Wiley and Sons; 1988:7–25.
26. Machin GA, Keith LG, Bamforth F. *An Atlas of Multiple Pregnancy: Biology and Pathology.* New York, NY: Parthenon; 1999.
27. Carroll SG, Tyfield L, Reeve L, et al. Is zygosity or chorionicity the main determinant of fetal outcome in twin pregnancies? *Am J Obstet Gynecol.* 2005;193(3, pt 1):757.
28. Spiegler J, Härtel C, Schulz L, et al; German Neonatal Network (GNN). Causes of delivery and outcomes of very preterm twins stratified to zygosity. *Twin Res Hum Genet.* 2012;15(4):532–536.
29. Gao Y, He Z, Luo Y, et al. Selective and non-selective intrauterine growth restriction in twin pregnancies: high-risk factors and perinatal outcome. *Arch Gynecol Obstet.* 2012;285(4):973–978.
30. Monteagudo A, Timor-Tritsch IE, Sharma S. Early and simple determination of chorionic and amniotic type in multiple gestation in the first 14 weeks by high frequency transvaginal ultrasonography. *Am J Obstet Gynecol.* 1994;170:824–829.
31. Hill LM, Chenevey P, Hecker J, et al. Sonographic determination of first trimester twin chorionicity and amnionicity. *J Clin Ultrasound.* 1996;24:305–308.
32. Sepulveda W, Sebire NJ, Hughes K, et al. The lambda sign at 10–14 weeks of gestations as a predictor of chorionicity in twin pregnancies. *Ultrasound Obstet Gynecol.* 1996;7:421–423.
33. Shetty A, Smith AP. The sonographic diagnosis of chorionicity. *Prenat Diagn.* 2005;25(9):735–739.
34. Stenhouse E, Hardwick C, Maharaj S, et al. Chorionicity determination in twin pregnancies: how accurate are we? *Ultrasound Obstet Gynecol.* 2002;19:350–352.
35. Bessis R, Papernik E. Echographic imagery of amniotic membranes in twin pregnancies. In: Gedda L, Parisi P, eds. *Twin Research 3: Twin Biology and Multiple Pregnancy.* New York, NY: Alan R Liss; 1981:183–187.
36. Monteagudo A, Roman AS. Ultrasound in multiple gestations: twins and other multifetal pregnancies. *Clin Perinatol.* 2005;32:329–354, vi.
37. Bromley B, Benacerraf B. Using the number of yolk sacs to determine amnionicity in early first trimester monochorionic twins. *J Ultrasound Med.* 1995;14:415–419.
38. Finberg HJ. The twin peak sign: reliable evidence of dichorionic twinning. *J Ultrasound Med.* 1992;11:571–577.
39. Scardo JA, Ellings JM, Newman RB. Prospective determination of chorionicity, amnionicity, and zygosity in twin gestations. *Am J Obstet Gynecol.* 1995;173:1376–1380.
40. Sepulveda W. Chorionicity determination in twin pregnancies: double trouble. *Ultrasound Obstet Gynecol.* 1997;10:79–81.
41. Chervenak FA, Skupski DW, Romero R, et al. How accurate is fetal biometry in the assessment of fetal age? *Am J Obstet Gynecol.* 1998;178:678–687.
42. Winn HN, Gabrielli S, Reece EA, et al. Ultrasonographic criteria for the prenatal diagnosis of placental chorionicity in twin gestations. *Am J Obstet Gynecol.* 1989;161:1540–1542.
43. D'Alton ME, Dudley DK. The ultrasonographic prediction of chorionicity in twin gestation. *Am J Obstet Gynecol.* 1989;160:557–561.
44. Powell KH, Grudzinskas JG. Screening for Down syndrome in the first trimester. *Reprod Fertil Dev.* 1995;7(6):1413–1417.
45. Jackson M, Rose NC. Diagnosis and management of fetal nuchal translucency. *Semin Roentgenol.* 1998;33(4):333–338.
46. Lo YM, Corbetta N, Chamberlain PF, et al. Presence of fetal DNA in maternal plasma and serum. *Lancet.* 1997;350(9076):485–487.
47. Baldwin VJ. Anomalous development of twins. In: Baldwin VJ, ed. *Pathology of Multiple Pregnancy.* New York, NY: Springer-Verlag; 1994:169–197.
48. Jenkins TM, Wapner RJ. The challenge of prenatal diagnosis in twin pregnancies. *Curr Opin Obstet Gynecol.* 2000;12(2):87–92.
49. Vink J, Wapner R, D'Alton ME. Prenatal diagnosis in twin gestations. *Semin Perinatol.* 2012;36(3):169–174.
50. Cleary-Goldman J, Malone FD, Vidaver J, et al. Impact of maternal age on obstetric outcome. *Obstet Gynecol.* 2005;105:983–990.
51. Edwards MS, Ellings JM, Newman RB, et al. Predictive value of antepartum ultrasound examination for anomalies in twin gestations. *Ultrasound Obstet Gynecol.* 1995;6(1):43–49.
52. Nicolaides KH. Screening for fetal chromosomal abnormalities: need to change the rules. *Ultrasound Obstet Gynecol.* 1994;4:353–354.
53. Sebire NJ, Noble PL, Psarra A, et al. Fetal karyotyping in twin pregnancies: selection of technique by measurement of fetal nuchal translucency. *Br J Obstet Gynaecol.* 1996;103:887–890.
54. Sebire NJ, Snijders RJ, Hughes K, et al. Screening for trisomy 21 in twin pregnancies by maternal age and fetal nuchal translucency thickness at 10–14 weeks of gestation. *Br J Obstet Gynaecol.* 1996;103:999–1003.
55. Maymon R, Jauniaux E, Herman A. Down's syndrome screening in twin pregnancies by nuchal translucency measurement current concept. *Minerva Ginecol.* 2002;54:211–215.
56. Wald NJ, Rish S, Hackshaw AK. Combining nuchal translucency and serum markers in prenatal screening for Down syndrome in twin pregnancies. *Prenat Diagn.* 2003;23:588–592.
57. Sebire NJ, D'Ercole C, Hughes K, et al. Increased nuchal translucency thickness at 10–14 weeks of gestation as a predictor of severe twin-to-twin transfusion syndrome. *Ultrasound Obstet Gynecol.* 1997;10:86–89.
58. Kagan KO, Gazzoni A, Sepulveda-Gonzalez G, et al. Discordance in nuchal translucency thickness in the prediction of severe twin-to-twin transfusion syndrome. *Ultrasound Obstet Gynecol.* 2007;29:527–532.
59. Bush MC, Malone FD. Down syndrome screening in twins. *Clin Perinatol.* 2005;32:373–386, vi
60. Linskens IH, Spreeuwenberg MD, Blankenstein MA, et al. Early first-trimester free beta-hcg and PAPP-A serum distributions in monochorionic and dichorionic twins. *Prenat Diagn.* 2009;29:74–78.
61. Wald NJ, Rish S. Prenatal screening for Down syndrome and neural tube defects in twin pregnancies. *Prenat Diagn.* 2005;25(9):740.
62. Spencer K, Staboulidou I, Nicolaides KH. First trimester aneuploidy screening in the presence of a vanishing twin: implications for maternal serum markers. *Prenat Diagn.* 2010;30(3):235.
63. Chasen ST, Perni SC, Predanic M, et al. Does a "vanishing twin" affect first-trimester biochemistry in Down syndrome risk assessment? *Am J Obstet Gynecol.* 2006;195(1):236.
64. Malone FD, D'Alton ME; Society for Maternal-Fetal Medicine. First-trimester sonographic screening for Down syndrome. *Obstet Gynecol.* 2003;102:1066–1079.
65. Olney RS, Khoury MJ, Alo CJ, et al. Increased risk for transverse digital deficiency after chorionic villus sampling: results of the United States Multistate Case-Control Study, 1988–1992. *Teratology.* 1995;51(1):20.

66. Firth HV, Boyd PA, Chamberlain PF, et al. Analysis of limb reduction defects in babies exposed to chorionic villus sampling. *Lancet.* 1994;343:1069–1071.

67. Van der Zee DC, Bax KM, Vermeij-Keers C. Maternoembryonic transfusion and congenital malformations. *Prenat Diagn.* 1997;17:59–69.

68. Wald NJ, Huttly WJ, Hackshaw AK. Antenatal screening for Down's syndrome with the quadruple test. *Lancet.* 2003;361:835–836.

69. Graham G, Simpson LL. Diagnosis and management of obstetrical complications unique to multiple gestations. *Clin Obstet Gynecol.* 2004;47:163–180.

70. Muller F, Dreux S, Dupoizat H, et al. Second-trimester Down syndrome maternal serum screening in twin pregnancies: impact of chorionicity. *Prenat Diagn.* 2001;23:331–335.

71. Lo YM, Lo ES, Watson N, et al. Two-way cell traffic between mother and fetus: biologic and clinical implications. *Blood.* 1996;88(11):4390–4395.

72. Lun FM, Chiu RW, Allen Chan KC, et al. Microfluidics digital PCR reveals a higher than expected fraction of fetal DNA in maternal plasma. *Clin Chem.* 2008;54:1664–1672.

73. Lo YM, Zhang J, Leung TN, et al. Rapid clearance of fetal DNA from maternal plasma. *Am J Hum Genet.* 1999;64:218–224.

74. Lo YM, Chan KC, Sun H, et al. Maternal plasma DNA sequencing reveals the genome-wide genetic and mutational profile of the fetus. *Sci Transl Med.* 2010;2:61.

75. Devaney SA, Palomaki GE, Scott JA, et al. Noninvasive fetal sex determination using cell-free fetal DNA: a systematic review and meta-analysis. *JAMA.* 2011;306(6):627–636.

76. Boon EM, Faas BH. Benefits and limitations of whole genome versus targeted approaches for noninvasive prenatal testing for fetal aneuploidies. *Prenat Diagn.* 2013;33:563–568.

77. Sparks AB, Wang ET, Struble CA, et al. Selective analysis of cell-free DNA in maternal blood for evaluation of fetal trisomy. *Prenat Diagn.* 2012;32:3–9.

78. Sparks AB, Struble CA, Wang ET, et al. Non-invasive prenatal detection and selective analysis of cell-free DNA obtained from maternal blood: evaluation for trisomy 21 and trisomy 18. *Am J Obstet Gynecol.* 2012;206:319.e1–319.e9.

79. Ashoor G, Syngelaki A, Wagner M, et al. Chromosome-selective sequencing of maternal plasma cell-free DNA for first-trimester detection of trisomy 21 and trisomy 18. *Am J Obstet Gynecol.* 2012;206:322.e1–322.e5.

80. Norton E, Brar H, Weiss J, et al. Non-Invasive Chromosomal Evaluation (NICE) Study: results of a multicenter prospective cohort study for detection of fetal trisomy 21 and trisomy 18. *Am J Obstet Gynecol.* 2012;207:137.e1–137.e8.

81. Nicolaides KH, Syngelaki A, Ashoor G, et al. Non-invasive prenatal testing for fetal trisomies in a routinely screened first-trimester population. *Am J Obstet Gynecol.* 2012;207:374.e1–374.e6.

82. Zimmermann B, Hill M, Gemelos G, et al. Non-invasive prenatal aneuploidy testing of chromosomes 13, 18, 21, X, and Y, using targeted sequencing of polymorphic loci. *Prenat Diagn.* 2012;32:1233–1241.

83. Nicolaides H, Syngelaki A, Gil M, et al. Validation of targeted sequencing of single-nucleotide polymorphisms for non-invasive prenatal detection of aneuploidy of chromosomes 13, 18, 21, X, and Y. *Prenat Diagn.* 2013;33:575–579.

84. Garfield SS, Armstrong SO. Clinical and cost consequences of incorporating a novel non-invasive prenatal test into the diagnostic pathway for fetal trisomies. *J Manag Care Med.* 2012;15:34–41.

85. Song K, Musci TJ, Caughey AB. Clinical utility and cost of non-invasive prenatal testing with cfDNA analysis in high-risk women based on a US population. *J Matern Fetal Neonatal Med.* 2013;26:1180–1185.

86. Ohno M, Caughey AB. The role of noninvasive prenatal testing as a diagnostic versus a screening tool—a cost-effectiveness analysis. *Prenat Diagn.* 2013;33:630–635.

87. Cuckle H, Benn P, Pergament E. Maternal cfDNA screening for Down syndrome—a cost sensitivity analysis. *Prenat Diagn.* 2013;33:636–642.

88. Huang X, Zheng J, Chen M, et al. Noninvasive prenatal testing of trisomies 21 and 18 by massively parallel sequencing of maternal plasma DNA in twin pregnancies. *Prenat Diagn.* 2014;34:335–340.

89. Weisz B, Rodeck CH. Invasive diagnostic procedures in twin pregnancies. *Prenat Diagn.* 2005;25:751–758.

90. Jeanty P, Shah D, Roussis P. Single-needle insertion in twin amniocentesis. *J Ultrasound Med.* 1990;9:511–517.

91. Van Vugt JM, Nieuwint A, van Geijn HP. Single-needle insertion: an alternative technique for early second-trimester genetic twin amniocentesis. *Fetal Diagn Ther.* 1995;10:178–181.

92. ACOG practice bulletin No 88

93. Agarwal K, Alfirevic Z. Pregnancy loss after chorionic villus sampling and genetic amniocentesis in twin pregnancies: a systematic review. *Ultrasound Obstet Gynecol.* 2012;40:128–134.

94. WHO, March of Dimes, Partnership for Maternal, Newborn & Child Health, Save the Children. *Born Too Soon: The Global Action Report on Preterm Birth.* www.who.int/maternal_child_adolescent/documents/born_too_soon/en/. Accessed May 4, 2012.

95. Skentou C, Souka AP, To MS, et al. Prediction of preterm delivery in twins by cervical assessment at 23 weeks. *Ultrasound Obstet Gynecol.* 2001;17(1):7–10.

96. Conde-Agudelo A, Romero R, Hassan SS, et al. Transvaginal sonographic cervical length for the prediction of spontaneous preterm birth in twin pregnancies: a systematic review and metaanalysis. *Am J Obstet Gynecol.* 2010; 203(2):128.e1.

97. Crane JM, Van den Hof M, Armson BA, et al. Transvaginal ultrasound in the prediction of preterm delivery: singleton and twin gestations. *Obstet Gynecol.* 1997;90:357–363.

98. Goldenberg RL, Iams JD, Miodovnik M, et al. The preterm prediction study: risk factors in twin gestations. National Institute of Child Health and Human Development Maternal-Fetal Medicine Units Network. *Am J Obstet Gynecol.* 1996;175(4, pt 1):1047.

99. Sotiriadis A, Papatheodorou S, Makrydimas G. Perinatal outcome in women treated with progesterone for the prevention of preterm birth: a meta-analysis. *Ultrasound Obstet Gynecol.* 2012;40(3):257–266.

100. Durnwald CP. 17 OHPC for prevention of preterm birth in twins: back to the drawing board? *Am J Obstet Gynecol.* 2013;208(3):167–168.

101. Romero R, Nicolaides K, Conde-Agudelo A, et al. Vaginal progesterone in women with an asymptomatic sonographic short cervix in the midtrimester decreases preterm delivery and neonatal morbidity: a systematic review and metaanalysis of individual patient data. *Am J Obstet Gynecol.* 2012;206(2):124. e1–124.e19.

102. Senat MV, Porcher R, Winer N, et al; Groupe de Recherche en Obstétrique et Gynécologie. Prevention of preterm delivery by 17 alpha-hydroxyprogesterone caproate in asymptomatic twin pregnancies with a short cervix: a randomized controlled trial. *Am J Obstet Gynecol.* 2013;208(3):194.e1–194.e8.

103. Berghella V, Odibo AO, To MS, et al. Cerclage for short cervix on ultrasonography: meta-analysis of trials using individual patient-level data. *Obstet Gynecol.* 2005;106(1):181–189.

104. Kosińska-Kaczyńska K, Szymusik I, Bomba-Opoń D, et al. Effective treatment of cervical incompetence in a monochorionic monoamniotic twin pregnancy with a rescue cervical cerclage and pessary—a case report and review of the literature. *Ginekol Pol.* 2012;83(12):946–949.

105. Carreras E, Arévalo S, Bello-Muñoz JC, et al. Arabin cervical pessary to prevent preterm birth in severe twin-to-twin transfusion syndrome treated by laser surgery. *Prenat Diagn.* 2012;32(12):1181–1185.

106. Prevention and prediction of preterm birth. number 130 october 2012. Replaces Practice Bulletin Number 31, October 2001 and Committee Opinion No. 419, October 2008.

107. Enbom JA. Twin pregnancy with intrauterine death of one twin. *Am J Obstet Gynecol.* 1985;152:424–429.

108. Kilby MD, Govind A, O'Brien PM. Outcome of twin pregnancies complicated by a single intrauterine death: a comparison with viable twin pregnancies. *Obstet Gynecol.* 1994;84:107–109.

109. Woo HH, Sin SY, Tang LC. Single foetal death in twin pregnancies: review of the maternal and neonatal outcomes and management. *Hong Kong Med J.* 2000;6:293–300.

110. Ong SS, Zamora J, Khan KS, et al. Prognosis for the co-twin following single-twin death: a systematic review. *BJOG.* 2006;113:992–998.

111. Murphy KW. Intrauterine death in a twin: implications for the survivor. In: Ward RH, Whittle M, eds. *Multiple Pregnancy.* London, UK: RCOG Press; 1995:218–230.

112. Anand D, Platt MJ, Pharoah POD. Comparative development of surviving co-twins of vanishing twin conceptions, twins and singletons. *Twin Res Hum Genet.* 2007;10:210–215.

113. Carlson NJ, Towers CV. Multiple gestation complicated by the death of one fetus. *Obstet Gynecol.* 1989;73:685–689.

114. Cleary-Goldman J, D'Alton M. Management of single fetal demise in a multiple gestation. *Obstet Gynecol Surv.* 2004;59:285–298.

115. Okamura K, Murotsuki J, Tanigawara S, et al. Funipuncture for evaluation of hematologic and coagulation indices in the surviving twin following co-twin's death. *Obstet Gynecol.* 1994;83:975–978.

116. Fusi L, McParland P, Fisk N, et al. Acute twin-twin transfusion: a possible mechanism for brain-damaged survivors after intrauterine death of a monochorionic twin. *Obstet Gynecol.* 1991;78(3, pt 2):517–520.

117. Nicolini U, Pisoni MP, Cela E, et al. Fetal blood sampling immediately before and within 24 hours of death in monochorionic twin pregnancies complicated by single intrauterine death. *Am J Obstet Gynecol.* 1998;179(3, pt 1):800–803.

118. Jelin AC, Norton ME, Bartha AI, et al. Intracranial magnetic resonance imaging findings in the surviving fetus after spontaneous monochorionic co-twin demise. *Am J Obstet Gynecol.* 2008;199(4):398.e1–398.e5.

119. Patten RM, Mack LA, Nyberg DA, et al. Twin embolization syndrome: prenatal sonographic detection and significance. *Radiology.* 1989;173:685–689.

120. Karl WM. Intrauterine death in a twin: implications for the survivor. In: Ward RH, Whittle M, eds. *Multiple Pregnancy.* London, UK: RCOG Press; 1995:218–230.

121. De Laveaucoupet J, Audibert F, Guis F, et al. Fetal magnetic resonance imaging (MRI) of ischemic brain injury. *Prenat Diagn.* 2001;21:729–736.

122. Nelson KB, Ellenberg JH. Childhood neurological disorders in twins. *Paediatr Perinat Epidemiol.* 1995;9:135–145.

123. Ong S, Zamora J, Khan K, et al. Single twin demise; consequences to the survivor. In: Kilby MD, Baker P, Critchley H, eds. *Multiple Pregnancy.* London, UK: RCOG Press; 2006.

124. Santema JG, Swaak AM, Wallenburg HC. Expectant management of twin pregnancy with single fetal death. *Br J Obstet Gynaecol.* 1995;102:26–30.

125. Spong CY, Mercer BM, D'alton M, et al. Timing of indicated late-preterm and early-term birth. *Obstet Gynecol.* 2011;118(2, pt 1):323–333.

126. Miller J, Chauhan SP, Abuhamad AZ. Discordant twins: diagnosis, evaluation and management. *Am J Obstet Gynecol.* 2012;206(1):10–20.

127. American College of Obstetricians and Gynecologists. *Multiple Gestation: Complicated Twin, Triplet, and High-Order Multifetal Pregnancy.* Washington, DC: American College of Obstetricians and Gynecologists; 2004. ACOG practice bulletin no 56.

128. Caravello JW, Chauhan SP, Morrison JC, et al. Sonographic examination does not predict growth discordance accurately. *Obstet Gynecol.* 1997;89:529–533.

129. Grobman WA, Parilla BV. Positive predictive value of suspected growth aberration in twin gestations. *Am J Obstet Gynecol.* 1999;181:1139–1141.

130. Alam Machado Rde C, Brizot Mde L, Liao AW, et al. Early neonatal morbidity and mortality in growth-discordant twins. *Acta Obstet Gynecol Scand.* 2009;88:167–171.

131. Kato N, Matsuda T. The relationship between birthweight discordance and perinatal mortality of one of the twins in a twin pair. *Twin Res Hum Genet.* 2006;9:292–297.

132. Branum AM, Schoendorf KC. The effect of birth weight discordance on twin neonatal mortality. *Obstet Gynecol.* 2003;101:570–574.

133. Hollier LM, McIntire DD, Leveno KJ. Outcome of twin pregnancies according to intrapair birth weight differences. *Obstet Gynecol.* 1999;94:1006–1010.

134. Lewi L, Gucciardo L, Huber A, et al. Clinical outcome and placental characteristics of mono chorionic diamniotic twin pairs with early- and ate-onset discordant growth. *Am J Obstet Gynecol.* 2008;199:511.e1–511.e7.

135. Barrett J, Bocking A. Management of twin pregnancies. SOGC consensus statement: part 1, no 91, July 2000. *J Soc Obstet Gynaecol Can.* 2000;22:519–529.

136. Chervenak FA, Johnson RE, Youcha S, et al. Intrapartum management of twin gestation. *Obstet Gynecol.* 1985;65:119–124.

137. Persad VL, Baskett TF, O'Connell CM, et al. Combined vaginal-cesarean delivery of twin pregnancies. *Obstet Gynecol.* 2001;8:1032–1037.

138. Robertson EG, Neer KJ. Placental injection studies in twin gestation. *Am J Obstet Gynecol.* 1983;147:170–174.

139. Lewi L, Jani J, Blickstein I, et al. The outcome of monochorionic diamniotic twin gestations in the era of invasive fetal therapy: a prospective cohort study. *Am J Obstet Gynecol.* 2008;199:514–518.

140. Denbow ML, Cox P, Taylor M, et al. Placental angioarchitecture in monochorionic twin pregnancies: relationship to fetal growth, fetofetal transfusion syndrome, and pregnancy outcome. *Am J Obstet Gynecol.* 2000;182:417–426.

141. Umur A, van Gemert MJ, Nikkels PG, et al. Monochorionic twins and twin-twin transfusion syndrome: the protective role of arterio-arterial anastomoses. *Placenta.* 2002;23:201–209.

142. Crombleholme TM, Shera D, Lee H, et al. A prospective, randomized, multicenter trial of amnioreduction vs selective fetoscopic laser photocoagulation for the treatment of severe twin-twin transfusion syndrome. *Am J Obstet Gynecol.* 2007;197:396.e1–396.e9.

143. De Paepe ME, Burke S, Luks FI, et al. Demonstration of placental vascular anatomy in monochorionic twin gestations. *Pediatr Dev Pathol.* 2002;5:37–44.

144. Bajoria R, Wee LY, Anwar S, et al. Outcome of twin pregnancies complicated by single intrauterine death in relation to vascular anatomy of the monochorionic placenta. *Hum Reprod.* 1999;14(8):2124–2130.

145. Cameron VA, Ellmers LJ. Minireview: natriuretic peptides during development of the fetal heart and circulation. *Endocrinology.* 2003;144(6):2191–2194.

146. Sebire NJ, Souka A, Skentou H, et al. Early prediction of severe twin-to-twin transfusion syndrome. *Hum Reprod.* 2000;15(9):2008–2010.

147. Sebire NJ, D'Ercole C, Carvelho M, et al. Inter-twin membrane folding in monochorionic pregnancies. *Ultrasound Obstet Gynecol.* 1998;11(5):324–327.

148. Habli M, Lim FY, Crombleholme T. Twin-to-twin transfusion syndrome: a comprehensive update. *Clin Perinatol.* 2009;36(2):391–416.

149. Barrea C, Alkazaleh F, Ryan, et al. Prenatal cardiovascular manifestations in the twin-to-twin transfusion syndrome recipients and the impact of therapeutic amnioreduction. *Am J Obstet Gynecol.* 2005;192:892–902.

150. Sueters M, Middeldorp JM, Vandenbussche FP, et al. The effect of fetoscopic laser therapy on fetal cardiac size in twin-twin transfusion syndrome. *Ultrasound Obstet Gynecol.* 2008;31(2):158–163.

151. Habli M, Michelfelder E, Livingston J, et al. Acute effects of selective fetoscopic laser photocoagulation on recipient cardiac function in twin-twin transfusion syndrome. *Am J Obstet Gynecol.* 2008;199(4):412.e1–412.e6.

152. Lougheed J, Sinclair BG, Fung KFK, et al. Acquired right ventricular outflow tract obstruction in the recipient twin in twin-twin transfusion syndrome. *J Am Coll Cardiol.* 2001;38:1533–1538.

153. Quarello E, Molho M, Ville Y. Incidence, mechanisms, and patterns of fetal cerebral lesions in twin-to-twin transfusion syndrome. *J Matern Fetal Neonatal Med.* 2007;20(8):589–597.

154. Kline-Fath BM, Calvo-Garcia MA, O'Hara SM, et al. Twin-twin transfusion syndrome: cerebral ischemia is not the only fetal MR imaging finding. *Pediatr Radiol.* 2007;37(1):47–56.

155. Tarui T, Khwaja O, Estroff J, et al. Altered fetal cerebral and cerebellar development in twin-twin transfusion syndrome. *AJNR Am J Neuroradiol.* 2012;33:1121–1126.

156. Brennan JN, Diwan RV, Rosen MG, et al. Fetofetal transfusion syndrome: prenatal ultrasonographic diagnosis. *Radiology.* 1982;143(2):535–536.

157. Uotila J, Tammela O. Acute intrapartum fetoplacental transfusion in monochorionic twin pregnancy. *Obstet Gynecol.* 1999;5:819–821.

158. Umur A, van Gemert MJ, Nikkels PG. Monoamniotic-versus diamniotic-monochorionic twin placentas: anastomoses and twin-twin transfusion syndrome. *Am J Obstet Gynecol.* 2003;189:1325–1329.

159. Habli M, Bombrys A, Lewis D, Lim FY, Polzin W, Maxwell R, Crombleholme T. Incidence of complications in twin-twin transfusion syndrome after selective fetoscopic laser photocoagulation: a single-center experience. *Am J Obstet Gynecol.* 2009 Oct;201(4):417.

160. Duncombe GJ, Dickinson JE, Evans SF. Perinatal characteristics and outcomes of pregnancies complicated by twin-twin transfusion syndrome. *Obstet Gynecol.* 2003;101(6):1190–1196.

161. Lopriore E, Sueters M, Middeldorp JM, et al. Neonatal outcome in twin-to-twin transfusion syndrome treated with fetoscopic laser occlusion of vascular anastomoses. *J Pediatr.* 2005;147(5):597–602.

162. Lutfi S, Allen VM, Fahey J, et al. Twin-twin transfusion syndrome: a population-based study. *Obstet Gynecol.* 2004;104(6):1289–1297. Erratum in: *Obstet Gynecol.* 2005;105(2):451.

163. Acosta-Rojas R, Becker J, Munoz-Abellana B, et al; for the Catalunya and Balears Monochorionic Network. Twin chorionicity and the risk of adverse perinatal outcome. *Int J Gynaecol Obstet.* 2007;96(2):98–102.

164. Lenclen R, Paupe A, Ciarlo G, et al. Neonatal outcome in preterm monochorionic twins with twin-to-twin transfusion syndrome after intrauterine treatment with amnioreduction or fetoscopic laser surgery: comparison with dichorionic twins. *Am J Obstet Gynecol.* 2007;196(5):450.e1–450.e7.

165. Bejar R, Vigliocco G, Gramajo H, et al. Antenatal origin of neurologic damage in newborn infants, II: multiple gestations. *Am J Obstet Gynecol.* 1990;162(5):1230–1236.

166. Graef C, Ellenrieder B, Hecher K, et al. Long-term neurodevelopmental outcome of 167 children after intrauterine laser treatment for severe twin–twin transfusion syndrome. *Am J Obstet Gynecol.* 2006;194:303–308.

167. Merhar SL, Kline-Fath BM, Meinzen-Derr J, et al. Fetal and postnatal brain MRI in premature infants with twin-twin transfusion syndrome. *J Perinatol.* 2013;33(2):112–118.

168. Lopriore E, Nagel HT, Vandenbussche FP, et al. Longterm neurodevelopmental outcome in twin-to-twin transfusion syndrome. *Am J Obstet Gynecol.* 2003;189:1314–1319.

169. Herberg U, Gross W, Bartmann P, et al. Long term cardiac follow up of severe twin to twin transfusion syndrome after intrauterine laser coagulation. *Heart.* 2006;92(1):95–100.

170. Moise KJ Jr. Polyhydramnios: problems and treatment. *Semin Perinatol.* 1993;17:197–209.

171. Rodestal A, Thomassen PA. Acute polyhydramnios in twin pregnancy. A retrospective study with special reference to therapeutic amniocentesis. *Acta Obstet Gynecol Scand.* 1990;69:297–300.

172. Mari G, Roberts A, Detti L, et al. Perinatal morbidity and mortality rates in severe twin-twin transfusion syndrome: results of the International Amnioreduction Registry. *Am J Obstet Gynecol.* 2001;185:708–715.

173. De Lia JE, Cruikshank DP, Keye WR Jr. Fetoscopic neodymium: YAG laser occlusion of placental vessels in severe twin-twin transfusion syndrome. *Obstet Gynecol.* 1990;75:1046–1053.

174. Senat MV, Deprest J, Boulvain M, et al. Endoscopic laser surgery versus serial amnioreduction for severe twin-to-twin transfusion syndrome. *N Engl J Med.* 2004;351(2):136–144.

175. Yamamoto M, El Murr L, Robyr R, et al. Incidence and impact of perioperative complications in 175 fetoscopy-guided laser coagulations of chorionic plate anastomoses in fetofetal transfusion syndrome before 26 weeks of gestation. *Am J Obstet Gynecol.* 2005;193(3, pt 2):1110–1116.

176. Robyr R, Lewi L, Salomon LJ. Prevalence and management of late fetal complications following successful selective laser coagulation of chorionic plate anastomoses in twin-to-twin transfusion syndrome. *Am J Obstet Gynecol.* 2006;194(3):796.

177. Lopriore E, Middeldorp JM, Oepkes D, et al. Twin anemia-polycythemia sequence in two monochorionic twin pairs without oligo-polyhydramnios sequence. *Placenta.* 2007;28:47–51.

178. Lopriore E, Slaghekke F, Middeldorp JM, et al. Residual anastomoses in twin-to-twin transfusion syndrome treated with selective fetoscopic laser surgery: localization, size, and consequences. *Am J Obstet Gynecol.* 2009;201:66.e1–66.e4.

179. Van den Wijngaard JP, Lewi L, Lopriore E, et al. Modeling severely discordant hematocrits and normal amniotic fluids after incomplete laser therapy in twin-to-twin transfusion syndrome. *Placenta.* 2007;28:611–615.

180. Lopriore E, Deprest J, Slaghekke F, et al. Placental characteristics in monochorionic twins with and without twin anemia-polycythemia sequence. *Obstet Gynecol.* 2008;112:753–758.

181. De Villiers S, Slaghekke F, Middeldorp JM, et al. Arterio-arterial vascular anastomoses in monochorionic twin placentas with and without twin anemia-polycythemia sequence. *Placenta.* 2012;33(3):227–229.

182. De Villiers SF, Slaghekke F, Middeldorp JM, et al. Placental characteristics in monochorionic twins with spontaneous versus post-laser twin anemia-polycythemia sequence. *Placenta.* 2013;34(5):456–459.

183. Lopriore E, Slaghekke F, Oepkes D, et al. Clinical outcome in neonates with twin anemia-polycythemia sequence. *Am J Obstet Gynecol.* 2010;203(1):54.e1–54.e5.

184. Slaghekke F, Kist WJ, Oepkes D, et al. Twin anemia-polycythemia sequence: diagnostic criteria, classification, perinatal management and outcome. *Fetal Diagn Ther.* 2010;27(4):181–190.

185. Genova L, Slaghekke F, Klumper FJ, et al. Management of twin anemia-polycythemia sequence using intrauterine blood transfusion for the donor and partial exchange transfusion for the recipient. *Fetal Diagn Ther.* 2013;34:121–126. doi:10.1159/000346413.

186. Lopriore E, Slaghekke F, Kersbergen K, et al. Severe cerebral injury in a recipient with twin anemia-polycythemia sequence. *Ultrasound Obstet Gynecol.* 2013;41(6):702–706.

187. Lopriore E, Ortibus E, Acosta-Rojas R, et al. Risk factors for neurodevelopment impairment in twin-twin transfusion syndrome treated with fetoscopic laser surgery. *Obstet Gynecol.* 2009;113(2, pt 1):361–366.

188. Chmait RH, Quintero RA. Operative fetoscopy in complicated monochorionic twins: current status and future direction. *Curr Opin Obstet Gynecol.* 2008;20:169–174.

189. Jelin E, Hirose S, Rand L, et al. Perinatal outcome of conservative management versus fetal intervention for twin reversed arterial perfusion sequence with a small acardiac twin. *Fetal Diagn Ther.* 2010;27:138–141.

190. Sebire NJ. Anomalous development in twins (including monozygotic duplication). In: Kilby M, Baker P, Critchley H, et al, eds. *Multiple Pregnancy.* London, UK: RCOG Press; 2006:59–88.

191. De Groot R, Van Den Wijngaard JP, Umur A, et al. Modeling acardiac twin pregnancies. *Ann N Y Acad Sci.* 2007;1101:235–249.

192. Moore TR, Gale S, Benirschke K. Perinatal outcome of forty nine pregnancies complicated by acardiac twinning. *Am J Obstet Gynecol.* 1990;163:907–912.

193. Van Allen MI, Smith DW, Shepard TH. Twin reversed arterial perfusion (TRAP) sequence: a study of 14 twin pregnancies with acardius. *Semin Perinatol.* 1983;7:285–293.

194. Chaliha C, Schwarzler P, Booker M, et al. Trisomy 2 in an acardiac twin in a triplet in-vitro fertilization pregnancy. *Hum Reprod.* 1999;14:1378–1380.

195. Healey MG. Acardia: predictive risk factors for the co-twin's survival. *Teratology.* 1994;50:205–213.

196. Sepulveda WH, Quiroz VH, Giuliano A, et al. Prenatal ultrasonographic diagnosis of acardiac twin. *J Perinat Med.* 1993;21:241–246.

197. Sebire NJ, Sepulveda W, Jeanty P, et al. Multiple gestations. In: Nyberg DA, McGahan JP, Pretorius DH, et al, eds. *Diagnostic Imaging of Fetal Anomalies.* Philadelphia, PA: Lippincott Williams & Wilkins; 2003:777–813.

198. Fouron JC, Leduc L, Grignon A, et al. Importance of meticulous ultrasonographic investigation of the acardiac twin. *J Ultrasound Med.* 1994;14:1001–1004.

199. Buntinx IM, Bourgeois N, Buytaert PM, et al. Acardiac amorphous twin with prune belly sequence in the co-twin. *Am J Med Genet.* 1991;39:453–457.

200. Guimaraes CV, Kline-Fath BM, Linam LE, et al. MRI findings in multifetal pregnancies complicated by twin reversed arterial perfusion sequence (TRAP). *Pediatr Radiol.* 2011;41(6):694–701.

201. Brassard M, Fouron JC, Leduc L, et al. Prognostic markers in twin pregnancies with an acardiac fetus. *Obstet Gynecol.* 1999;94:409–414.

202. Dashe JS, Fernandez CO, Twickler DM. Utility of Doppler velocimetry in predicting outcome in twin reversed-arterial perfusion sequence. *Am J Obstet Gynecol.* 2001;185:135–139.

203. Oliver ER, Coleman BG, Goff DA, et al. Twin reversed arterial perfusion sequence: a new method of parabiotic twin mass estimation correlated with pump twin compromise. *J Ultrasound Med.* 2013;32(12):2115–2123.

204. Gallot D, Laurichesse H, Lemery D. Selective feticide in monochorionic twin pregnancies by ultrasound-guided umbilical cord occlusion. *Ultrasound Obstet Gynecol.* 2003;22:484–488.

205. Lopoo JB, Paek PW, Maichin GA, et al. Cord ultrasonic transection procedure for selective termination of a monochorionic twin. *Fetal Diagn Ther.* 2000;15:177–179.

206. Rodeck C, Deans A, Jauniaux E. Thermocoagulation for the early treatment of pregnancy with an acardiac twin. *N Engl J Med.* 1998;339:1293–1295.

207. Tsao K, Feldstein VA, Albanese CT, et al. Selective reduction of acardiac twin by radiofrequency ablation. *Am J Obstet Gynecol.* 2002;187:635–640.

208. Cabassa P, Fichera A, Prefumo F, et al. The use of radiofrequency in the treatment of twin reversed arterial perfusion sequence: a case series and review of the literature. *Eur J Obstet Gynecol Reprod Biol.* 2013;166(2):127–132.

209. Pagani G, D'Antonio F, Khalil A, et al. Intrafetal laser treatment for twin reversed arterial perfusion sequence: cohort study and meta-analysis. *Ultrasound Obstet Gynecol.* 2013;42(1):6–14.

210. Pauls F. Monoamniotic twin pregnancy: a review of the world literature and a report of two new cases. *Can Med Assoc J.* 1969;100:254–256.

211. Baldwin V. Twinning mechanisms and zygosity determination. In: *Pathology of Multiple Gestation.* New York, NY: Springer-Verlag; 1994:201.

212. Bajoria R. Abundant vascular anastomoses in monoamniotic versus diamniotic monochorionic placentas. *Am J Obstet Gynecol.* 1998;179(3, pt 1):788.

213. Rodis JF, Vintzileos AM, Campbell WA, et al. Antenatal diagnosis and management of monoamniotic twins. *Am J Obstet Gynecol.* 1987;157:1255–1257.

214. Lumme RH, Saarikoski SV. Monoamniotic twin pregnancy. *Acta Genet Med Gemellol (Roma).* 1986;35:99–105.

215. Allen VM, Windrin R, Barrett J, et al. Management of monoamniotic twin pregnancies: a case series and systemic review of the literature. *BJOG.* 2001;108:931.

216. Morikawa M, Yamada T, Yamada T, et al. Prospective risk of intrauterine fetal death in monoamniotic twin pregnancies. *Twin Res Hum Genet.* 2012;15(4):522–526.

217. Heyborne KD, Porreco RP, Garite TJ, et al; for the Obstetrix/Pediatrix Research Study Group. Improved perinatal survival of monoamniotic twins with intensive inpatient monitoring. *Am J Obstet Gynecol.* 2005;192(1):96.

218. Hack KE, Derks JB, Schaap AH, et al. Perinatal outcome of monoamniotic twin pregnancies. *Obstet Gynecol.* 2009;113:353–360.

219. Dias T, Mahsud-Dornan S, Bhide A, et al. Cord entanglement and perinatal outcome in monoamniotic twin pregnancies. *Ultrasound Obstet Gynecol.* 2010;35:201–204.

220. Belfort MA, Moise KJ Jr, Kirshon B, et al. The use of color flow Doppler ultrasonography to diagnose umbilical cord entanglement in monoamniotic twin gestations. *Am J Obstet Gynecol.* 1993;168(2):601.

221. Gembruch U, Baschat AA. True knot of the umbilical cord: transient constrictive effect to umbilical venous blood flow demonstrated by Doppler sonography. *Ultrasound Obstet Gynecol.* 1996;8(1):53.

222. Abuhamad AZ, Mari G, Copel JA, et al. Umbilical artery flow velocity waveforms in monoamniotic twins with cord entanglement. *Obstet Gynecol.* 1995;86(4, pt 2):674.

223. Rosemond RL, Hinds NE. Persistent abnormal umbilical cord Doppler velocimetry in a monoamniotic twin with cord entanglement. *J Ultrasound Med.* 1998;17(5):337.

224. Rossi AC, Prefumo F. Impact of cord entanglement on perinatal outcome of monoamniotic twins: a systematic review of the literature. *Ultrasound Obstet Gynecol.* 2013;41(2):131–135.

225. Spitz L, Kiely EM. Conjoined twins. *JAMA.* 2003;289(10):130.

226. Spencer R. Theoretical and analytical embryology of conjoined twins, part I: embryogenesis. *Clin Anat.* 2000;13:36–53.

227. Destephano CC, Meena M, Brown DL, et al. Sonographic diagnosis of conjoined diamniotic monochorionic twins. *Am J Obstet Gynecol.* 2010;203(6):e4–e6.

228. Kaufman MH. The embryology of conjoined twins. *Childs Nerv Syst.* 2004;20:508–525.

229. Spencer R. Anatomic description of conjoined twins: a plea for standardized terminology. *J Pediatr Surg.* 1996;31(7):941.

230. Harper RG, Kenigsberg K, Sia CG, et al. Xiphopagus conjoined twins: a 300-year review of the obstetric, morphopathologic, neonatal, and surgical parameters. *Am J Obstet Gynecol.* 1980;137:617.

231. Baken et al. Diagnostic techniques and criteria for first-trimester conjoined twin documentation: a review of the literature illustrated by three recent cases. *Obstet Gynecol Surv.* 2013 Nov;68(11):743–52.

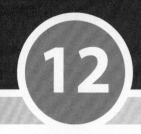

# Central Nervous System

## Supratentorial Anomalies

Beth M. Kline-Fath

The central nervous system (CNS) is frequently abnormal in prenatal malformations. Up to 1 out of 100 neonates are born with a CNS anomaly.[1] CNS malformations vary from minor with little symptomatology to extremely complex causing high morbidity and mortality. Prenatal diagnosis is essential to guide counseling and direct pregnancy decisions including continuation, mode of delivery, and perinatal and postnatal care.

In this chapter, brain malformations are listed in the order of expected embryonic insult. Despite best attempts to understand the timing of insult, classification of the defect can be difficult. Occasionally, the primary event is linked to other pathologies which may make it challenging to define the embryonic stage. In addition, many structures in the brain are developing at the same time, so it is not unusual for multiple malformations to occur simultaneously, thus limiting the ability to classify an anomaly as primary. CNS disorders can also be of different severity, likely because of genetic and environmental factors. Therefore, in general, it is usually best to describe the abnormalities present individually unless the findings reflect a known syndrome. More importantly, when imaging the fetal brain, it is imperative that all anomalies, particularly extra cranial, are identified. When one organ is abnormal, often many body parts are involved. Being able to identify all anomalies may give clues to an underlying genetic syndrome, which can be significant for fetal outcome.

## EMBRYOLOGY/PATHOPHYSIOLOGY

The embryology of the brain is covered in detail in normal imaging of the fetal brain. The stages of development are provided in Table 6.2-2 in Chapter 6.2. Human development is dependent on correct chromosomal complement and organization. Thus, many disorders are related to genetic disorganization. Environmental factors can have an adverse, disruptive effect on the embryo or fetus. Common teratogens include drugs, radiation, and infection, especially viruses. Maternal conditions, especially diabetes mellitus type I, often have an impact on genetic or acquired defects in the fetus. Mechanical disruptions can result from trauma, vascular, amniotic, or extraneous effects.

## IMAGING TECHNIQUES

Sonography has significant advantages over other imaging. There is no radiation, images have high anatomical resolution, real-time capabilities allow dynamic assessment of the fetus, and color Doppler provides excellent interrogation of blood flow. Prenatal sonography is sensitive at detecting the vast majority of primary CNS anomalies through careful examination of the cranium and spine.[2] Ninety-seven percent of CNS anomalies can be identified on one or more of the three standard cranial views.[3] Eighty-eight percent of CNS anomalies are identified on the transventricular view by diagnosis of enlarged cerebral ventricles.[3] Evaluation of the lateral cerebral ventricles is thus very important, especially in the second trimester when head size may be normal or even decreased.[2] Inadequacies of the technique include limited soft tissue contrast and loss in cerebral detail in the near field due to reverberation artifact. In addition, fetal head position, maternal body habitus, the presence of oligohydramnios, and ossification of the fetal skull can degrade cerebral detail. Importantly, ultrasound (US) is dependent on the ability of the person to correctly display anatomy on the imaging and the skill of the reader to diagnose the abnormality.[4]

Fetal magnetic resonance imaging (MRI) is an excellent adjunct to prenatal US. It has multiple advantages, including large field of view that allows evaluation of the fetus in multiple planes and high soft tissue contrast and resolution, both of which allow depiction of the complex normal and abnormal maturation of the developing brain. Neuronal migration, gyration, sulcation, and myelination are accurately depicted. MRI does not suffer from acoustic shadowing of the fetal skull. The posterior fossa, brainstem, and corpus callosum can be easily evaluated, and injury from hemorrhage and ischemia is accurately defined. Multiple authors have demonstrated that fetal MRI is a valuable adjunct to US in the evaluation of fetal brain.[1,4-8] Levine et al found that MRI led to a change in diagnosis in 32% of cases of US detected fetal brain abnormalities, and changed counseling in 50%, and patient management in 19%.[6] MRI also increases confidence in diagnosis, thus reducing patient anxiety.[5] There are, however, limitations to the technique. Fetal MRI is not widely available and high in cost. The study is also operator dependent, and imaging can be suboptimum in the presence of significant fetal and maternal motion and claustrophobia. Imaging early in gestation can be difficult to interpret and less diagnostic because of primitive brain architecture.[6] This may have significant implications if termination of pregnancy is being considered. At this time, restricted sequences and coils are available. Higher MR imaging techniques, such as spectroscopy, functional and diffusion tractography, are more difficult as longer acquisition times are required.

# VENTRICULOMEGALY

Ventriculomegaly (VM) is a descriptive term indicating the presence of excess cerebrospinal fluid (CSF) in the ventricles of the brain. Hydrocephalus is present when there is increased CSF pressure in the ventricles, usually in association with increased head circumference. VM can be isolated (IVM) or associated with other anomalies (AVM). It is important to recognize VM because it may be an indicator or manifestation of additional significant CNS defects.

**Incidence:** The incidence for fetal VM ranges from 1 to 2 cases per 1,000 births.[9–11] It is the most common CNS anomaly identified by prenatal sonography.[12–14] Lateral ventricular enlargement represents the tip of the iceberg in fetal CNS imaging, as it is sensitive for the detection of a wide variety of fetal CNS abnormalities.[15] Reportedly, 70% to 85% of cases with VM have associated anomalies.[10,16–18] IVM is cited in up to 20% of cases VM with an incidence of 0.4 to 0.9 per 1,000.[10,18]

**Pathogenesis:** The pathophysiology underlying the dynamics of normal and abnormal CSF flow is still incompletely understood. The major portion of the CSF is produced by the choroid plexus in the lateral and to a lesser extent third and fourth ventricles.[19] Normal CSF flow is from the lateral ventricles, through the foramen of Monro into the third ventricle, and then by way of the aqueduct of Sylvius to the fourth ventricle, out the foramen of Magendie and Luschka into the subarachnoid space (see Fig. 6.2-5 in Chapter 6.2). The major pathway for CSF reabsorption postnatal is via arachnoid granulations into the blood capillaries and then the cerebral venous sinuses. Minor CSF absorption also occurs via the lymphatic system, at the level of cribriform plate and nasal submucosa, the interstitial and perivascular space and the choroid plexus which drain via capillaries to the vein of Galen.[19,20] In the immature brain, it is favored that the minor pathways are the primary route for CSF reabsorption as the arachnoid granulations are not developed prenatal.[20]

The mechanisms for development of VM are varied (Table 12.1-1). In obstructive VM, there is an imbalance between production and absorption of CSF. Noncommunicating VM does not allow communication between the ventricular system and the subarachnoid space. The lesion can occur internal to the ventricular system, as in maldevelopment of the aqueduct of Sylvius, or external to the ventricular system, such as in Chiari II malformation, or in the presence of an intraparenchymal abnormality effacing ventricle (tumor, mass). Communicating obstructive VM is rare in the fetus but occurs when there is abnormal absorption of the CSF by the cerebral venous sinuses or lymphatics.[21] In the presence of obstructive VM, in which there is increased pressure, there is potential for the ventricular dilatation to cause progressive brain injury. Nonobstructive disorders include ex vacuo dilatation, due to brain injury or dilatation due to abnormal neuronal development. Rarely, increased CSF production can occur in the presence of a choroid plexus papilloma.

The natural history of VM can be difficult to predict. Prenatal, the dilatation can resolve, stabilize, or progress. In a review of nearly 300 cases of IVM, 29% resolved, 57% stabilized, and 14% progressed.[22]

**Etiology:** Given the multiple mechanisms responsible for the development of VM, many etiologies are possible. Chromosomal

| Table 12.1-1 | Mechanisms for Development of Ventriculomegaly |
|---|---|

**Obstructive**

***Noncommunicating***
*Intrinsic—ventricular*
    Aqueductal stenosis
    Posterior fossa malformation
    Posthemorrhagic obstruction
    Postinfectious obstruction
*Extrinsic—parenchymal or mass*
    Tumor or arachnoid cyst
    Hemorrhage or edema
    Malformation (Chiari II)

***Communicating***
    Lack of resorption of CSF by venous sinuses

**Nonobstructive**

***Overproduction of CSF***
    Choroid plexus lesion
***Malformation of cerebral development***
    Holoprosencephaly
    Lissencephaly/schizencephaly
    Agenesis of corpus callosum
    Disorder of proliferation and neuronal migration
    Disorder of organogenesis
        Genetic etiology
            Trisomy 13, 18, 21, and many others
***Destructive-ex vacuo dilatation***
    Vascular
    Infection
    Ischemic

Modified from Levine D, Feldman HA, Kazam Tannus JF, et al. Frequency and cause of disagreements in diagnoses for fetuses referred for ventriculomegaly. *Radiology.* 2008;247:515–527.

anomalies are associated in 2% to 12% of IVM and 10% to 36% of AVM cases.[18] Intrauterine infection is noted in 2% to 5% of all VM cases.[16] Infections, mainly TORCH, are the cause of severe IVM in 10% to 20% of cases.[21] Rarely, intraventricular hemorrhage due to alloiummune thrombocytopenia is the underlying cause.

**Diagnosis:** When VM is identified, a detailed prenatal US should be performed to exclude other anomalies. Fetal echocardiography and MRI may be helpful, especially in the verification of the diagnosis and depiction of associated anomalies. Karyotype testing and TORCH screening is highly recommended.[23] A feto-maternal alloimmune thrombocytopenia screen for anti-HPA (human platelet antigen) antibodies may be considered.[21,24]

**Ultrasound:** The fourth ventricle can be detected earliest on sonograms at 9 menstrual weeks, initially a large anechoic ellipsoid structure compared with the total brain.[15] After brief visibility, the fourth ventricle becomes small. The third ventricle is identified slightly later and demonstrates adult slit-like linear hypoechoic configuration, lying between the thalami.[15] The lateral ventricles are apparent at 13 to 14 menstrual weeks and change dramatically with development of the cerebral hemispheres.[15] Although the volume of the ventricles increases with gestational age (GA), the CSF spaces of the lateral ventricles become less conspicuous during the pregnancy. The choroid plexus can be a helpful landmark, extending from the foramen of Monro to fill the posterior horn of a normal lateral ventricle.[15]

Normal technique and measurements of the lateral ventricles are imperative to avoid false negative and positive diagnosis of VM. The atrium of the lateral ventricle is preferred as a measurable landmark since the size and configuration is essentially stable during the second and the third trimesters, in contrast to the frontal horn, which changes in configuration with gestational age.[25–27] In addition, since the trigone and occipital horn are typically the first areas to dilate in VM, this area of investigation is most important in the diagnosis.[25,26] As the wall of the atrium is perpendicular to the beam in the axial plane, it can be identified easily, and the presence of the choroid plexus aids in localization of the most lateral ventricular wall (Fig. 12.1-1).[3,25,26] VM is one of the most common false positive diagnoses at US screening.[21] Care must be taken to obtain the measurement on a true transventricular plane at the level of the glomus of the choroid.[28] Since the choroid plexus fills the ventricular atrium with only 1 to 2 mm of CSF separating the choroid from the adjacent lateral ventricular wall, the choroid can be utilized as a marker for the most distant ventricular wall.[15,26] The measurement is obtained by placing calipers in the largest part of the lateral ventricles inside the echogenic interface defining the lateral ventricular walls (Fig. 12.1-1).[15,27] Ventricle asymmetry of at least 2 mm without dilatation can be present physiologically as a normal variant.[29,30]

Measurements are subject to error because of off-axis image plane, angled measurement, or improper choice of ventricular boundary.[31] In an attempt to decrease these possible deficiencies, it has been further suggested that the axial view should be strictly assessed by demonstrating that the proximal and distal calvarial margins are equidistant, that anterior landmarks include the cavum septi pellucidi or fornix and posterior landmark, the fluid-filled V shape of the ambient cistern (Fig. 12.1-2). The measurement should be opposite the internal parieto-occipital sulcus and placed at the junction of the ventricular lumen and wall perpendicular to the inner and outer border of the ventricle.[31]

Limitations of the technique include visualization of only one lateral ventricle in the distal hemisphere because of near field artifacts. Angled views through the brain may be helpful to overcome this shortcoming.[32] In addition, it can be difficult to visualize the entire ventricle because of fetal position or calvarial ossification. If the true transverse axial plane cannot be

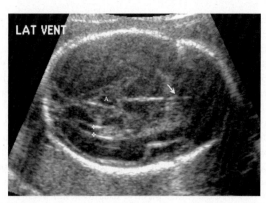

**FIGURE 12.1-2:** Transventricular plane with atrial measurements at the level of the cavum septi pellucidi *(arrow)* and ambient *(A)* cistern.

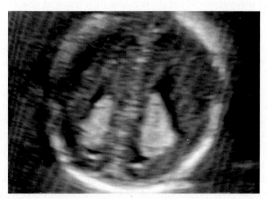

**FIGURE 12.1-3:** Coronal plane of both atria with echogenic choroid.

obtained, then a coronal image at the level of the atria should be utilized for the measurement (Fig. 12.1-3).[27]

The normal mean diameter of the atrium of the lateral ventricle midgestation is 7.6 ± 0.6 mm from 14 to 38 weeks with excellent interobserver reliability.[25] The atrial width of one or both ventricles >10 mm is more than 2.5 to 4 standard deviations above the mean and is thus considered VM midgestation irrespective of gender.[12,25–27] When the ventricle enlarges, the choroid hangs in a dependent location and separates from the nondependent wall. This appearance of a "dangling choroid" will often provide clues to the presence of VM (Fig. 12.1-4).[33]

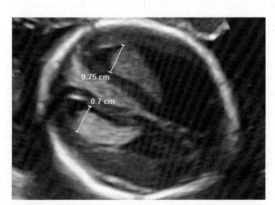

**FIGURE: 12.1-1:** Measurements of the atrium of the lateral ventricles. Note echogenic choroid plexus. Ventricular measurements are also obtained inside the echogenic interface.

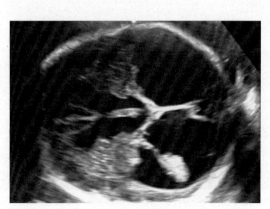

**FIGURE 12.1-4:** Axial transventricular view with dangling choroid in a fetus with ventriculomegaly because of aqueductal stenosis.

VM can also be diagnosed when there is choroid plexus separation from the medial ventricular wall of >3 mm.[34]

In the past, borderline or mild VM has been defined as atrial measurements of 10 to 15 mm, and severe VM when atrial width is >15 mm. Recently, VM has been further segregated such that mild represents measurements between 10 and 12 mm, moderate >12 to 15 mm, and severe >15 mm.[21,35]

Sensitivity of diagnosis is controversial. Previous studies have reported a sensitivity of 88% to 93.5% in the presence of a ventricular dilatation to or greater than 10 mm.[3,36] However, before 24 weeks, the sensitivity drops to 35%.[9] In fact, a recent study noted that only 57% of cases of severe VM were diagnosed prior to 24 weeks.[35] False positive diagnosis has been reported between 10% and 33%, with the most common disagreement being in the diagnosis of mild VM.[4,37,38] Causes for the false positive prenatal diagnosis include regression of VM during fetal life, measurement variability, and difference in criteria with regard to the presence of VM close to 10 mm.[4,21]

Although diagnosis of lateral VM is extremely important, the third and fourth ventricles should also be closely assessed as they may provide clues to the underlying diagnosis. Enlarged third and fourth ventricles are documented when the transverse dimensions are ≥3.5 and ≥4.8 mm, respectively.[10] This may be possible on routine axial imaging, but a complete neurosonographic examination should include both coronal and sagittal views through the fetal brain (Fig. 12.1-5).[39,40] A midsagittal image can be very helpful with a positive predictive value of 93%, improving detection of anomalies of the posterior fossa and corpus callosum.[41] If these planes are difficult to perform because of fetal positioning, transvaginal, and/or 3D imaging can assist with fetal anatomy.[39-41] Transvaginal imaging, especially if the head is in cephalic positioning, uses the fetal fontanelles as an acoustic window allowing visualization of both hemispheres and ventricles without artifact related to fetal skull or maternal obesity.[42]

It is very important to determine whether the VM is isolated or associated with other CNS or non-CNS anomalies. Evaluation of the morphology and borders of the lateral ventricle can provide important clues. In the presence of angular lateral ventricles, a neural

tube defect should be sought (see Fig. 15.2-3C in Chapter 15.2). With a pattern of colpocephaly, agenesis of the corpus callosum (ACC) may be suggested (Fig. 12.1-20A).[43] Evaluation of the ventricular wall for increased echogenicity, thickening or irregularity should be performed to exclude hemorrhage or periventricular heterotopia. Internal ventricular debris, fluid–fluid level, or enlargement of a heterogeneous choroid plexus would indicate hemorrhage. Septation of the ventricles raise the suspicion of infection. The septum pellucidum, germinal matrix area, and cerebral parenchyma should be closely examined. Head circumference and biparietal diameter should be assessed to evaluate for volume loss versus hydrocephalus; however, early in gestation, these measurements may not be helpful. Finally, the entire fetus should be evaluated for extra-CNS anomalies. Most studies indicate that it matters little whether the associated anomaly is CNS or of another organ system in predicting an unfavorable outcome.[15] Up to 30% may develop polyhydramnios, and 33% will be breech presentation at birth.[44] Although a high-quality ultrasound is essential, even in the most experienced hands, anomalies can be difficult to detect on US with a false negative rate reported between 10% and 40%.[14,15,33]

*MRI:* Fetal MRI can be a helpful adjunct to US and has been shown to improve the detection of additional abnormalities in up to 50% of US diagnosed VM.[45] MRI when performed because of abnormal CNS findings on US, may change the referral diagnosis in as high as 35% of cases.[6] Aside from the technical limitations of US, some anomalies in cortical migration, hemorrhage, and parenchymal damage have been noted to be too subtle to be defined by US.[46] In addition, even when an US anomaly is confirmed on MR, many times additional anomalies are seen that are important in determining prognosis.[47] As it is important to separate cases of IVM from AVM, additional imaging with MRI may be considered.

On fetal MRI, precise measurements of the lateral, third, aqueduct of Sylvius, and fourth ventricles can be defined (see Chapter 6.2). Some authors have found that measurements of the lateral ventricles on MRI are slightly larger than on US by an average of 0.6 mm.[4] However, most conclude that there is a 90% agreement between the atrial dimensions on US when compared with MRI.[48] Rarely, measurements defined as VM on US are found to be normal on fetal MRI.[48]

With fetal MRI, many prefer measuring the lateral ventricles on a coronal plane parallel to the brainstem, including the choroid, as it is more reliable than the axial.[10] On a coronal plane, the third ventricle should be below 4 mm, and on sagittal imaging, the fourth below 7 mm.[10]

Below 24 weeks and sometimes beyond, the ventricles may demonstrate a primitive configuration in which the occipital horns are mildly disproportionate to the frontal horns (see Chapter 6.2).[49] If the ventricles are angular, a neural tube defect is almost always present (see Fig. 15.2-2C in Chapter 15.2).[43,49] Colpocephaly, marked dilatation of the posterior horn with abnormal frontal horns, should raise concern for a corpus callosum abnormality (Fig. 12.1-24C).[43,49] The ventricular wall should be evaluated for irregularity, thickening or nodularity that would suggest heterotopia. Septations would support infection. The germinal matrix should be symmetric and of appropriate size for gestational age. T1-weighted imaging and gradient echo may be helpful to confirm hemorrhage. Cystic lesions in the germinal matrix may suggest old insult. The septum pellucidum, corpus callosum, posterior fossa, and aqueduct of Sylvius should

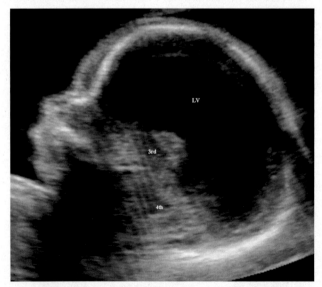

**FIGURE 12.1-5:** Sagittal US in a fetus with aqueductal stenosis. There is severe lateral ventriculomegaly *(LV)*. The third *(3rd)* is mildly enlarged and the fourth *(4th)* is normal.

be closely examined. Parenchymal signal and sulcation should be correlated with gestational age. Measurements of the fronto-occipital and biparietal diameter and evaluation of the sub-arachnoid spaces may be clues to hydrocephalus or volume loss. The entire fetus should be examined for extracranial anomalies.

Fetal MRI in the presence of VM has been shown to demonstrate a higher percentage of associated anomalies (43%) versus US (32%).[50] However, it is important to remember that migrational abnormalities may not be apparent early in gestation. MRI has been shown to be more likely to find additional anomalies at GA >25 weeks when brain development is more advanced.[48] It should also be remembered that there is often a lag in development of the sulci and gyri when a fetus has VM or other CNS abnormalities.[51]

**Associated Anomalies:** VM is often the tip of the iceberg, representing the first and only sign of associated multisystem fetal abnormalities.[15,25,28] Associated anomalies are present in 70% to 85% of fetuses with VM, and 60% of those malformations may be extracranial.[15,17] In AVM, the most common CNS anomalies include aqueductal stenosis (AS) (30% to 40%), Chiari II malformation (25% to 30%), dysgenesis of corpus callosum (20% to 30%), and posterior fossa defects (7% to 10%).[10,16,17] There is a clear relationship between the degree of VM and the risk of other brain abnormalities.[48] Severe VM is 10 times more likely to be associated with a brain anomaly than mild or moderate VM.[48] Those cases with borderline or mild VM have structural anomalies in 41% whereas the moderate VM group cite anomalies in 75%.[35]

The overall frequency of chromosomal anomalies in the presence of VM has been quoted from 2% to 29%.[35,52] The incidence of chromosomal anomalies is strongly related to the presence of multisystem malformations.[52] In a fetus with AVM, chromosomal anomalies are higher at 25% to 36% whereas in IVM, the risk falls to 3% to 6%.[17,21,52]

**Differential Diagnosis:** Misinterpretation of the anechoic brain can sometimes result in incorrect atrial measurements leading to the false diagnosis of VM. A cystic lesion, such as arachnoid or dermoid cyst, or an enlarged extraaxial fluid space can be misinterpreted as VM.

**Prognosis:** Review of the literature suggests that fetal VM is not associated with outcome in a simple or consistent way. VM has many causes and can evolve during gestation. Therefore, counseling should always be performed with a certain degree of caution.[53] Although many studies have been performed in an attempt to improve counseling, one should review the literature carefully. There are variations in outcome and standards between many studies, and this, unfortunately, is because of small sample sizes, variable techniques in the evaluation of VM, variable ages at assessment of development, and lack of standardized methods to assess development. Therefore, prognosticators of outcome are sometimes inconsistent.

The prognosis of VM overall has been stated to be guarded with mortality of 70% to 80% and only half of surviving children developing normally.[15,54] When attempting to determine which VM cases will have a worse outcome, there is agreement in the literature that some factors can guide prognosis. The cause of VM plays an important role in the prognosis for the fetus.[17] The presence of associated intracranial and extracranial malformations decreases the likelihood of a good outcome.[17,55] There is a 56% increased morbidity and mortality in AVM versus 6%

with IVM.[56] Neurologic delay in IVM ranges from 9% to 36% as compared with 84% with AVM.[22,57]

The association of chromosomal abnormality is another negative prognostic indicator.[17] In the presence of VM due to chromosomal/genetic defects, a normal outcome is present in 28% of cases with severe VM and 87% in fetus with VM between 10 and 15 mm.[21] Those cases in which VM is present with viral infection tend to have poor outcomes.[23]

Most support that the severity of the VM is another negative indicator for outcome.[16,17,58,59] In the presence of mild VM, normal outcome has been noted in 93% versus 75% in those with moderate VM and 62.5% in severe.[35] Survival greater than 24 months in fetuses with IVM is 98% when mild, 80% with moderate, and 33.3% with severe VM.[35] Most confirm progression of VM in utero as a poor prognosticator with 80% demonstrating neurodevelopmental delay.[10,16] When VM improves or resolves, 70% to 80% of fetuses have a good outcome.[21] Stable or nonprogressive IVM tends to have a favorable prognosis.[16]

Multiple debated patterns have been described. The early appearance of the VM in pregnancy is controversial but has been associated with a poor prognosis.[10,23,59] It is questioned whether unilateral VM has a better outcome than bilateral VM.[10,59] Asymmetrical VM has been most commonly described with severe VM, which tends to have a worse prognosis.[16,54,60,61] Controversial data suggest that a male fetus with VM has a better outcome than female.[10,21]

**Management:** Depending on gestational age at identification, management options include termination or expectant management at delivery.[62] Counseling should be directed to known findings and potential outcomes. If continuation of the pregnancy is decided, cesarean delivery is recommended for those fetuses with enlarged cranium.[62] In this case, delivery must be delayed until the fetus is mature enough to survive. Dilemma occurs in the presence of progressive hydrocephalus, as increasing ventricular dilatation can result in brain damage.[62] The current recommendation is early shunt placement after induced delivery as soon as lung maturity permits.[53]

Postnatal treatment is directed to cause. In cases of VM due to cerebral malformation or destruction, no surgical intervention is typically warranted. Neurologic consultation and directed neurodevelopmental therapy should be considered to improve outcome. In the presence of open neural tube defect or hydrocephalus, surgical intervention is often necessary. With increased intracranial pressure, ventricular peritoneal shunt is the first line of therapy.

**Recurrence:** Recurrence risk depends on the etiology. The overall recurrence risk for VM without associated anomalies is less than 2%.[63] In the presence of a chromosomal syndrome, the risk may increase.

## MILD, MODERATE, AND UNILATERAL VENTRICULOMEGALY

In the literature, there is lack of standardization in the terms mild and borderline VM. In the past, mild or borderline VM has been described as lateral ventricular dilatation between 10 and 15 mm and a choroid lateral ventricular separation of greater than or equal to 3 mm and less than or equal to 8 mm. However, more recently, VM has been further refined into borderline or mild VM when ventricle dilatation is between 10 and 12 mm and moderate when dilatation is noted between >12 and 15 mm. This section will utilize these new standards, and it is hoped that subsequent research will apply this methodology to homogenize terminology to allow improved counseling.

**Incidence:** Mild-to-moderate VM (10 to 15 mm) represents 15% to 20% of all VM and occurs bilaterally in 0.15% to 0.7% and unilaterally in 0.07% of pregnancies.[14,15,55,56,64]

**Pathogenesis:** Mild-to-moderate IVM is overall less well defined probably because it can be a dynamic process in utero.[22] It typically is not associated with increased intracranial pressure as most cases are nonprogressive. The head circumference is usually normal. Mild-to-moderate IVM may resolve in 41%, remain stable in 43%, and progress in 16%.[57] Progression of VM may suggest underlying disorder that can prevent normal development.[65]

Mild or borderline IVM is a diagnostic dilemma as there is research that suggests it may represent a variation of normal.[25,48] Prior US imaging studies have shown that atrial diameters above 10 mm can include fetuses that are healthy.[66] Studies have suggested that the lateral ventricles are larger in boys than in girls, with a difference of approximately 0.4 to 0.6 mm.[10,66,67] Because of the difference in gender ventricular size, 0.28% of males and 0.06% of healthy girls will have measurements equal to or above 10 mm atrial size.[66] These authors, however, still support that the 10-mm value should be maintained regardless of gender.[66–68]

Other studies have questioned the 10-mm value. Salomon et al.[12] noted that a ventricular width greater than 10 mm can be found in 1% of normal fetuses throughout gestation. In the third trimester, the mean diameter of the lateral ventricles has been found slightly larger, with upper range at 10.2 mm, representing 2 SD at term, and another study demonstrated that the 95% confidence interval exceeded 10 mm from 34 weeks to term.[26,69] Additional research has demonstrated that isolated choroid plexus separation in the presence of normal-sized ventricles is usually temporary, resolving in 70% within 4 weeks of diagnosis, with 80% to 94% normal outcome postnatal.[70] The lesion in these cases may represent an alteration in size or configuration of the choroid plexus or ventricle owing to a variation in the shape of the fetal head.[70]

In support of these findings, some studies have shown that the rate of male fetuses with ventricular size <12 mm is higher than that in the case of females and correlates with a good prognosis, probably because of inclusion of normal fetuses.[58,59,71] This type of VM also tends to be present in large for gestational age fetuses and those near term.[72] Unilateral ventriculomegaly (UVM) has also demonstrated a higher incidence in males or fetuses with birth weight of >90 percentile.[73]

UVM is uncommon and has been hypothesized to result from atresia, maldevelopment, or obstruction of the foramen of Monro by neoplasm, infection, or vascular anomaly or unilateral degenerative changes of the adjacent hemisphere.[73] UVM may also represent a normal variant when mild and nonprogressive.[64]

**Etiology:** Chromosomal anomalies for mild-to-moderate VM are reported between 3% and 12.6% with mean of 9%.[22] The majority of fetuses with mild-to-moderate VM and abnormal karyotype will have additional sonographic abnormalities.[22] With IVM between 10 and 15 mm, positive chromosomal anomaly is defined in 3% to 5%, and in mild IVM, aneuploidy is detected in 3%.[24,61,72] Therefore, karyotype testing is recommended.

Fetal infection is found in 1% to 5% of cases of mild-to-moderate VM.[58,74] If the VM is isolated and between 10 and 15 mm and between 10 and 12 mm, positive infection is 1.5% and 0.4%, respectively.[24,61,72] Cerebral VM is one of the more common prenatal US abnormalities in fetuses with cytomegalovirus (CMV), present in 18% of cases, half of which are isolated.[24] TORCH screen would thus also be prudent.[24]

**Diagnosis**
*Ultrasound:* When VM is identified, the opposite ventricle should be evaluated to exclude unilateral VM (Fig. 12.1-6). Detailed neurosonography with multiplanar imaging should be obtained to exclude additional anomalies.[24] Transvaginal with high-resolution probe usually results in the greatest detail. However, if this is not possible, 3D imaging should be attempted.[24] The false negative rate in detection of anomalies with IVM is equivalent to 11%.[56] IVM is a diagnosis of exclusion.

As progression is possible and 13% of anomalies are detected on sequential ultrasound, follow-up US examination is

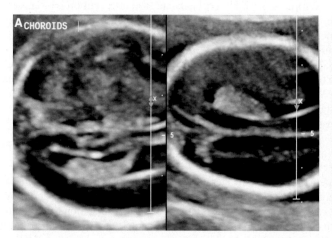
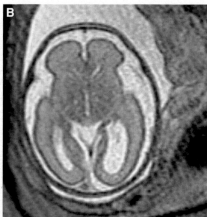

**FIGURE 12.1-6:** Unilateral ventriculomegaly in a fetus at 25 weeks, gestation. **A:** Axial ultrasound of both right and left ventricles demonstrating asymmetric enlargement of the left lateral ventricle. **B:** Axial SSFSE T2 image from same fetus demonstrating asymmetric ventricles without associated anomalies.

suggested.[24] At least one additional detailed US should be performed between 28 and 34 weeks to search for other cerebral and extracerebral anomalies.[24] Some advocate for monthly US to determine whether the ventricles return to normal, remain stable, or progress.[74]

**MRI:** Fetal MRI is helpful in cases in which US is inadequate. Many also support the modality when there is suspicion of cerebral anomaly or in the case of moderate VM or AVM (Fig. 12.1-7). In the presence of IVM, fetal MRI can improve detection in 17%.[75] This leads to an improvement in counseling, as another recent study demonstrated that fetuses with MRI confirmed IVM had normal developmental outcome in 94% of mild and 85% of moderate VM.[59]

However, the contribution of fetal MRI in cases of mild isolated VM remains controversial.[76] MRI performed in the presence of mild IVM provided information that modified obstetric management in 6% of cases and was reassuring to families in the presence of isolation.[77] Another study suggested that in fetuses with mild IVM, MRI diagnosed major cerebral anomalies in 9%.[54] However, a recent study found additional findings on MRI in 20%, but noted that the imaging only changed clinical diagnosis in 1.1% of cases, raising the question of the need for the additional test.[76] There is also no consensus on the optimal time for imaging; but most suggest that later gestation imaging, particularly after 25 weeks, will provide better detail of cortical development.

**Associated Anomalies:** The rate of associated anomalies in mild-to-moderate VM ranged between 10% and 76% with an average of 41%.[9,56] Those with mild VM had a lower rate of associated anomalies than those with moderate VM.

**Differential Diagnosis:** False positive diagnosis may occur with incorrect imaging plane, incorrect placement of calipers, and differences in measurement interpretation for the presence of VM.

**Prognosis:** Outcome in mild-to-moderate VM is also dependent on the presence of associated anomalies, genetic/chromosomal anomalies, or positive titers. Being able to prove that VM is isolated is therefore important for prognosis.[55,56] Moderate VM, when compared with mild VM, is more likely to demonstrate associated anomalies, 56% versus 6%.[24,56] Mild-to-moderate IVM has a reported survival of 85% with normal outcome in 85%.[54] In those with mild-to-moderate AVM, perinatal or early childhood death increased to an average of 37%.[55] Fetuses with mild-to-moderate IVM have abnormal neurologic outcome in 10% to 20%, while those with AVM are abnormal in up to 40% to 50%.[1,56]

The degree of VM is also an important prognosticator, with neurodevelopmental delay being an average of 14% to 17% when the IVM is moderate versus 3% to 11.8% when mild.[9] Therefore, fetuses with mild IVM approach the general population in which neurodevelopmental delay has been noted in 2.5%.[24,56] These numbers have also been supported by a recent study that utilized fetal MRI, in which mild IVM had 94% excellent outcome and those with moderate IVM had 85% good outcome.[59] It is also interesting that fetuses with mild IVM have higher rates of stable or even regressive diameters of the ventricular system, with 90% of cases resolving, decreasing, or stable, but less than 10% increasing over the course of pregnancy.[55]

The overall risk of neurologic sequelae in stable VM is significantly lower than in progressive VM.[54–56,61] Sixteen percent of fetuses with mild to moderate VM have progression, and the neurodevelopmental outcome is worse, 44% versus 7% without progression.[24] There is also a higher incidence of chromosomal anomalies in progressive VM, 22% compared to 1% without progression.[24] Cases of mild to moderate IVM that resolve before birth tend to have a normal outcome.[15]

Because males have a more generous ventricular size, mild IVM is more commonly depicted in males.[56] In support of normal larger ventricles in males, some have found that the risk for abnormal outcome in male fetuses with IVM and normal karyoptype is 5% versus 23% for female.[55,56,72] However, several studies have demonstrated that there is no difference in outcome when comparing male and female fetuses.[24,59] Signorelli et al.[78] have shown that all cases of mild VM had a normal outcome up to 10 years after birth. Therefore, many believe that mild IVM may be a variation of normal.[72,78,79]

There is a controversy in the literature as to whether UVM has a better prognosis than bilateral.[59,72] It is most important to understand that UVM follows the same rules as bilateral in determining outcome. Although many believe UVM tends to be

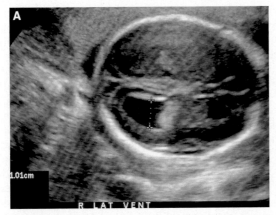
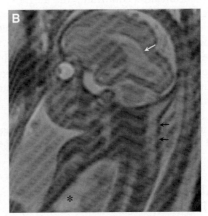

**FIGURE 12.1-7:** Fetus with trisomy 21 at 29 weeks. **A:** Axial ultrasound demonstrating mild VM. **B:** Sagittal T2 MR of the same fetus demonstrating mild lateral ventriculomegaly (*white arrow*), but also moderate pleural effusion (*asterisk*) and nuchal thickening (*black arrows*). Imaging was performed to assess lung compression and exclude mediastinal mass.

benign as it is less likely to have a clinically significant associated anomaly, there is still a 3% risk for chromosomal aberration, with risk for developmental delay ranging from 6% to 15%.[30,55] In a review of 366 cases, 97% had normal development with unilateral VM versus 90% with mild bilateral IVM.[54] Another study reported developmental delay in mild bilateral IVM and unilateral as being very similar at 6% and 7.4%, respectively.[24] Good neurologic outcome has been noted in UVM when it is isolated without genetic disorder or infectious etiology.[10,80] The prognosis is also excellent in the presence of dilatation that is nonprogressive and less than 12 mm.[55,79]

Finally, sometimes although the diagnosis of IVM is made, the VM is in fact not really isolated.[24] Current evidence suggests that even with prenatal workup and fetal MRI, additional anomalies can be discovered at birth, including white matter signal abnormalities, which may not be detected until after birth, some of which were not visible on MRI until 1 year of age.[59] Recent data have shown that prenatal VM is associated with postnatal VM.[81] Neonates with prenatal mild VM have higher cortical volume and reduced white matter volume, suggesting altered cortical development and either delayed or abnormal white matter development.[81] Bloom found a significant linear relationship between ventricle width and decreased mental development index.[82] In recent studies, fetuses with mild VM and postnatal neurologic follow-up showed abnormal, mostly motor disabilities in 12% to 28% of cases and intellective retardation in 5%.[24,83] In addition, studies have demonstrated that up to one-third of cases of moderate IVM have additional findings detected later in pregnancy or postnatally that had a negative impact on neurologic outcome.[66] Therefore, IVM may not be normal, and the physiologic development of the brain should be taken into account.

**Management:** Counseling should be performed after all testing has been obtained with knowledge of associated anomalies, genetic abnormalities, and positive infection titers. In the presence of IVM, the counseling can still be difficult. A physician should advise the family that nonprogressive IVM can be confidently diagnosed only after birth. And, although some children appear normal at birth, a 10-point deficit when compared with normal controls can be documented.[82] There is also limited developmental follow-up of children with prenatal diagnosis of IVM beyond 30 months to guide counseling for long-term outcome.[61]

Most cases of isolated mild VM can be delivered vaginally. Postnatal management includes confirming the diagnosis and checking for associated disorders that were undetected prenatally. Long-term postnatal follow-up may be helpful.[24] Follow-up should continue until development is established as normal. If delay occurs, neurologic consultation and therapeutic intervention should be considered as this can improve outcome.[73] MRI, especially after 1 year of life, may be helpful to evaluate for white matter lesions.[59,81]

**Recurrence:** Recurrence is rare in isolation but is dependent on the cause and the presence of a genetic or chromosomal aberration.

# AQUEDUCTAL STENOSIS/ SEVERE VENTRICULOMEGALY

**Incidence:** The overall incidence of aqueductal stenosis (AS) is 0.5 to 1 per 1,000 births.[84] After Chiari malformation, AS is the second most common cause for fetal VM, accounting for 20%

to 40% of cases.[17] X-linked hydrocephalus is the most common hereditary hydrocephalus with an incidence of 1 in 30,000, accounting for 2% to 25% of primary idiopathic hydrocephalus in newborn males.[84–86]

**Pathogenesis:** There is evidence that suggests AS may develop because of early fetal hydrocephalus. In the presence of massive lateral ventricular enlargement, the midbrain may be compressed laterally, resulting in aqueductal narrowing.[87] Others suggest that the aqueduct may inherently become narrowed, particularly at the superior colliculus or intercollicular sulcus. In some cases, the aqueduct can be "forked," with branching dorsal and ventral channels.[17] Less commonly, a web can develop along the most inferior recess of the aqueduct. Acquired AS has many etiologies, including infection, bleeding, or other pathologies that cause gliosis and then obliterate the aqueduct.[17]

Recent research has found that rhombencephalosynapsis (RES), which is fusion of the cerebellar hemispheres in conjunction with absence of the cerebellar vermis, is identified in 9% of patients with AS.[88] In those patients with RES, up to 50% of cases have associated AS.[88] The anomaly may be related to a defect in dorsal midline signaling leading to malformation of the brainstem and cerebellum.[88] The correlation makes sense as both the aqueduct and the vermis originate from the mesencephalon.

In the presence of AS, increased CSF pressure occurs consistent with hydrocephalus. When hydrocephalus develops, there is pressure on the developing brain from the ventricular system, but there is also uterine amniotic pressure restraining the expansion of the overlying skull.[11] This increased pressure causes alteration in neuronal proliferation, migration, and delayed maturation.[89] With pressure in the ventricles, there is flattening of the ependyma and interruption of the CSF–brain barrier with ependymal rupture, edema in the periventricular white matter, and axonal swelling. In the late phase, destruction of nerve fibers, demyelination, gliosis, and volume loss in the white matter and corpus callosum occur.[62]

**Etiology:** A multifactorial pattern of inheritance or postinflammatory insult is probably likely in most cases. Increased risk of congenital hydrocephalus has been described in males, primogeniture, older maternal age, maternal insulin-dependent diabetes, maternal alcohol abuse, and lower social class of the father.[58,84,90]

In 5% of all cases, an X-linked transmission, known as Bickers–Adams syndrome may be the etiology. This genetic disorder, which is also known as X-linked hydrocephalus and hereditary stenosis of the aqueduct of Sylvius (HSAS), is related to mutation of the *L1CAM* gene on chromosome Xq28.[86] The gene encodes a neural cell adhesion molecule L1, which is involved in neuronal migration, fasciculation, outgrowth, and regeneration. L1 is essential to the formation of the pyramids and corticospinal tracts. Because many diseases have been associated with this gene mutation, the syndrome is now known as CRASH, representing *c*orpus callosum hypoplasia, *r*etardation, *a*dducted thumbs, *s*pastic paraplegia, and *h*ydrocephalus.[86] The mutation primarily affects males, but females are carriers, and there is a 5% risk for a female to develop mild manifestations of the disorder.[44] In X-linked AS, the aqueduct is stenosed in only 40% of cases, and thus some suggest that the aqueduct is narrowed by lateral ventricular compression rather than primary maldevelopment.[85,91]

**Diagnosis:** In the presence of severe VM, it is important to perform karyotype and infectious testing for TORCH. If X-linked AS is suspected, screening should be performed for *L1CAM* gene mutations, as the detection rate can be as high as 93%.[15,86]

***Ultrasound:*** There is often moderate to severe lateral VM and typically a mild-to-moderately dilated third ventricle with disruption of the septum pellucidum (Fig. 12.1-8A,B). Measurements are usually not necessary to define the lateral VM, but can be useful to monitor the progression of ventricular dilatation. The aqueduct of Sylvius obstruction is typically difficult to identify via US. The fourth ventricle should be normal in size. At 18 to 20 weeks, the subarachnoid spaces are large, and with increasing gestation, there is progressive decrease in their size. In the presence of severe VM, the supratentorial parenchyma may be compressed between the skull and the dilated ventricles (Fig. 12.1-9A). With increasing ventricular dilatation, disruption of the cortical mantle can occur due to damage from the intraventricular pressure.[11] Evaluation of the brain and extracranial structures is essential to exclude other anomalies. A search of the hands for adducted thumbs may support X-linked AS.

***MRI:*** On fetal MRI, the aqueduct of Sylvius is well depicted. With obstruction to CSF flow, there can be complete or partial obliteration of the CSF space in the aqueduct (Fig. 12.1-8C,D).[90] The tectum may be deformed or thickened (Fig. 12.1-9B). The lateral and third ventricles are dilated. Ventricular disruption is sometimes depicted in the posterior mesial aspects of the brain, the location of the choroidal fissure and weakest part of the ventricular wall (Fig. 12.1-9C).[87] This results in a focal ventricular diverticulum and thinning of the adjacent brain parenchymal mantle. Most disruptions are lined with white matter and are thus not consistent with schizencephaly. The septum pellucidum can be partially or completely absent. Although MRI can visualize the corpus callosum, in the presence of severe VM, it is often displaced, severely stretched, or partially absent (Fig. 12.1-8C). The subarachnoid spaces may be normal or absent depending on gestational age, and sulcation is typically delayed. The posterior fossa may be small owing to mass effect.

Other anomalies, such as RES or Z-shaped brainstem in the presence of congenital muscular dystrophy, are seen in association with AS (Fig. 12.1-8).[88] In the presence of X-lined AS, corpus callosum agenesis, absent septum pellucidum, fusion of

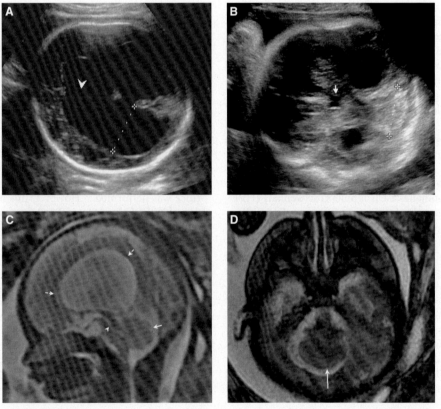

**FIGURE 12.1-8:** Fetus at 36 weeks with aqueductal stenosis and rhomboencephalosynapsis. **A:** Axial US demonstrates severe ventriculomegaly with atrium measuring 34 mm and septum pellucidum absent *(arrowhead)*. **B:** Axial US demonstrating dilated third ventricle *(arrow)*. The cerebellum measured small, appropriate for a 28-week fetus. Notice the continuous foliation of the superior cerebellum. **C:** Sagittal SSFSE T2 image demonstrates obstruction of the aqueduct of Sylvius distally *(arrowhead)*. Notice that the vermis does not appear normal as the deepest fissure is the horizontal fissure *(solid arrow)*, typical for the cerebellar hemispheres. The corpus callosum is thin *(dashed arrows)* due to the hydrocephalus. **D:** Axial SSFP image confirms absence of cerebellar vermis with continuous foliation across midline *(arrow)* consistent with fusion of the cerebellar hemispheres in rhomboencephalosynapsis.

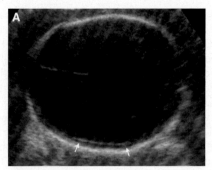
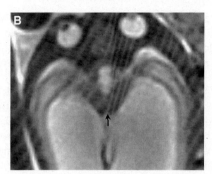
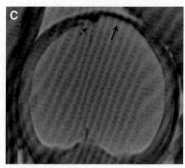

**FIGURE 12.1-9:** Fetus at 34 weeks with AS secondary to TORCH. **A:** Axial US demonstrates severely dilated ventricles and subtle suggestion of brain parenchyma *(arrows)* compressed along the calvarium. It would be difficult to exclude hydranencephaly. **B:** Axial SSFSE T2 image demonstrates heart-shaped midbrain and deformity of tectum *(arrow)*, typical of AS. **C:** Coronal SSFSE T2 image demonstrates ventricular rupture of the left lateral ventricle with destruction of adjacent brain parenchyma *(solid arrow)*. The ventricular wall is ballooned on the right with thinning of the adjacent brain *(dotted arrow)*. The sulcation is significantly delayed for age of 34 weeks.

thalami, small brainstem, hypoplasia of the corticospinal tracts, and absence of the pyramidal tract may be present.[85,86] Fifty percent of fetuses with X-lined AS demonstrate adduction of the thumbs.[44]

**Associated Anomalies:** Associated abnormalities have been diagnosed in approximately 60% to 65% of severe VM.[14,45,92] Chromosomal anomalies are reported to be as high as 15%.[9] The rate of associated infection in severe VM is 10% to 20%.[14]

In a study directed at AS, 60-87% of the cases were associated with a genetic syndrome, chromosomal anomaly or maternal exposure.[90] Chromosomal abnormalities were detected in 8%. The most common genetic syndromes were Walker–Warburg, VATER, and Peter Plus.[90] RES was a common associated anomaly. Environmental exposures, including insulin-dependent maternal diabetes, fetal alcohol and TORCH, were present in 16%.[90]

**Differential Diagnosis:** Severe VM can be seen in association with other known anomalies, such as holoprosencephaly (HPE), hydranencephaly, agenesis of the corpus callosum, Chiari II, or other posterior fossa malformations.

**Prognosis:** Outcome in fetuses with AS is guarded. Overall mortality is 40%, perinatal mortality of 23% and of those that survive only 10% have normal development.[90,93] Normal development in severe AS with associated anomalies is only 5% but increases to 50% when isolated[90]. Although IVM in AS carries the least severe prognosis, it is not common, accounting for only 10% of cases.[90] Those patients with X-linked hydrocephalus have variable clinical symptomatology.[94] Some die in utero or early infancy. If a child with X-linked AS survives, severe mental retardation and spastic diplegia can occur; however, some live into adulthood.[44,94]

A recent study of nonspecific severe IVM showed major morbidity in 50%, minor in 40%, and normal outcome in 10%.[95] Prognosis has been shown to depend on age at diagnosis as progressive increased intracranial pressure can result in further insult to the brain.[91,95] The presence of additional anomalies, karyotype abnormality, and in utero progression result in a negative outcome.[91] When additional anomalies were present, only 23.5% survived and only 15% of the survivors were normal, with the majority having cerebral palsy, seizures, and impaired motor capabilities.[16,17]

**Management:** In the presence of AS or severe VM, termination may be considered, depending on severity of dilatation and presence of associated anomalies. As it is known that progressive injury can occur to the brain throughout the gestational period, in the past, decompression of the ventricular system was attempted by performing cephalocentesis and/or the placement of in-utero shunts.[62,96] However, the ventriculo-amniotic shunts, due to high pressure in the amniotic cavity, sometimes did not allow drainage of fetal CSF and often the catheters migrated or obstructed.[88] The main problem, more importantly, became overall case selection as many of these fetuses had associated anomalies. Because of controversial results and the lack of the ability to define a group of fetuses that would benefit, the procedure was mostly abandoned in 1986.[96] With improved understanding of the natural history of the disease in utero and improved shunt technology, revisitation of the intervention may be entertained.[62]

In the past when the prognosis was poor, cephalocentesis with 90% rate of perinatal death or vaginal delivery with fetal sacrifice was performed.[95] However, this has been virtually abandoned in the United States. Most fetuses with enlarged cranium require delivery by C-section. Postnatally, most infants require ventricular shunting.

**Recurrence:** The recurrence risk for sporadic cases in subsequent siblings is 0.5% to 4%.[77] However, in the presence of X-linked AS, the risk of recurrence is 50% in a male fetus and in the case of a girl, 50% risk for carrier with low (<5%) risk for manifesting clinical features.[28,44]

# DISORDERS OF VENTRAL INDUCTION

## Holoprosencephaly

Holoprosencephaly is a group of complex congenital malformations of the brain and face in which there is impaired or incomplete cleavage of the prosencephalon.

**Incidence:** HPE is considered the most frequent CNS defect in humans, occurring at a prevalence of 1:250 conceptions.[97] However, as only 3% of fetuses with HPE survive to delivery, the incidence decreases to 1 in 10,000 to 20,000 live newborns.[97] There is a female preponderance, being 3:1 in the alobar type.[97,98]

**Pathogenesis:** HPE occurs due to failed diverticulation of the embryonic prosencephalon in the first 4 weeks of embryogenesis. The primary disorder results from failure of migration of the prechordal mesoderm, which is responsible for induction of ventral forebrain, nasofrontal process, and median facial structures.[99] HPE represents a defect in dorsoventral patterning, beginning in the area of the hypothalamus but contiguous along cortex, striatum, midline ventricles, thalamus, and mesencephalon.[100]

HPE is subdivided based on site and degree of failed cleavage; however, no precise boundaries are present and intermediate cases may occur.[101,102] Classically, DeMyer divided HPE into three subcategories from severe to mild including alobar, semilobar, and lobar; however, a milder form known as middle interhemispheric fusion has recently been described (Fig. 12.1-10).[100] Of the three classic forms, alobar is the most frequent type, occurring between 40% and 75% of cases, with semilobar second, followed by lobar.[97]

In classic HPE, the ventral forebrain or embryonic floor plate, in the region of the hypothalamus and subcallosal cortex, is most severely affected. Common possible associated midline anomalies include undivided hypothalamus and thalami, undivided deep gray structures, absent or dysgenetic corpus callosum, absent septum pellucidum, and absent or hypoplastic olfactory bulbs and tracts, and optic bulbs and tracts (Table 12.1-2).

In *alobar* HPE, there is a single midline forebrain ventricle and cerebral holosphere with absent midline structures and thalamic fusion. The monoventricle is continuous with a cyst, hypothesized to represent remnant third ventricle, velum interpositum, or primitive prosencephalic vesicle, demarcated from the ventricular cavity by ridge of cerebral tissue representing hippocampal fornix.[103,104] In *semilobar*, the defect is localized anteriorly with some posterior interhemispheric fissure, rudimentary lateral ventricles but absent frontal horns, partial fusion of thalami, and variable corpus callosum, usually splenium. The *lobar* type

has noncleavage of the frontal basal lobes and separation of most of the cerebral hemisphere, rudimentary frontal horns, and absent anterior corpus callosum. A mild variation of the lobar type with fusion of the septal and preoptic area has been termed *septopreoptic HPE*. In the *middle interhemispheric variant (MIH) or syntelencephaly*, there is a defect of the dorsal mesenchyme or the roof plate resulting in failure of separation of the posterior frontal and parietal lobes with the poles of the frontal and occipital well separated.[105,106] The genu and splenium of the corpus callosum are present, but the body is poorly defined. Classification is not well defined in less severe ends of the phenotypic spectrum which include absent olfactory tracts and bulbs (arrhinencephaly) and hypopituitarism.[107] In addition, with recent molecular data, it has been found that the HPE phenotypic spectrum is very large, including a "microform" variety, encompassing facial malformation but normal brain.[107]

HPE is associated with a number of midline anomalies of the face (Table 12.1-3).[108–110] There is an 80% correlation with the severity of the HPE and the extent of the facial malformation; thus in these cases, the "face may predict the brain."[107,111] However, in 10% to 20% of cases, there is no clear correlation between face and brain anomaly subtypes.[97]

**Etiology:** Genetic, environmental, multifactorial, and unknown causes appear to be involved in the development of HPE (Table 12.1-4).[97] Chromosomal anomalies account for 25% to 50% of HPE cases.[108,112] The most common association is trisomy 13, representing 75% of cases, followed by triploidy at 20% and trisomy 18 at 1% to 2%.[113] The incidence of chromosomal abnormalities is strongly related to the presence of multisystem anomalies.[114] About 18% to 25% of HPE are syndromic with a single gene mutation.[102,111]

The nonsyndromic or isolated HPE can be inherited autosomal dominant, autosomal recessive, and X-linked inheritance.[113] In the cases with normal karyotype, genetic mutations

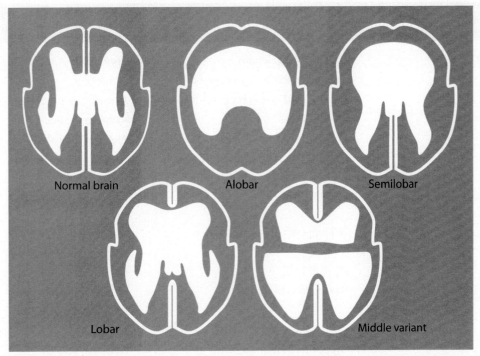

**FIGURE 12.1-10:** Diagram of the four major types of holoprosencephaly. (Modified from Volpe P, Campobasso G, De Robertis V, Rembouskos G. Disorders of prosencephalic development. Prenatal Diagnosis 2009;29:340-354.)

**Table 12.1-2    Findings in HPE**

| Types | Alobar | Semilobar | Lobar | MHF | Septopreoptic |
|---|---|---|---|---|---|
| IHF/falx absent | All | Anterior | Hypoplastic anterior | Midportion | Deep |
| Cerebral nonseparation | All | Frontal | Basal frontal/ cingulate | Posterior frontal/ anterior parietal | Preoptic/ subcallosal |
| Lateral ventricles | Single | Absent anterior Rudimentary occipital | Rudimentary anterior Normal posterior | Fused mid lateral N/hypoplastic anterior | N/small frontal |
| Dorsal cyst | Yes | Variable | Rare | Present 25% | No |
| Third ventricle | Absent | Small | Present | Present | N |
| Septum pellucidum | Absent | Absent | Absent/hypoplastic | Absent/hypoplastic | N/hypoplastic/ absent |
| Thalami | Fused | Partial fusion | Divided | Fused 30%–50% | N |
| Deep gray | Fused | Partial/caudate | Variable | Caudate fused | N |
| Corpus callosum absent | All | Rostrum, genu, body | Rostrum, genu | Body | Rostrum/genu |
| Hypothalamus | Fused | Often fused | Likely fused | Separated | Anterior fused |
| Hippocampal fornix | Fused | Often fused | Fused | Separated | N |
| Olfactory bulbs and neurohypophysis | Absent | Absent/hypoplastic | Absent/hypoplastic/N | N | N |
| Optic tracts | N/fused/absent | Absent/hypoplastic | Present | Present | N |
| Slyvian fissures | Absent | Anterior medial | Anterior medial | Connected over midline | N |
| Cortical dysplasia/ Heterotopia | Broad gyri | Occasional broad gyri | Rare midline/ frontal | Very common | N |
| Cerebral vasculature | No ACA MCA Rete vessels | Azygous ACA | Azygous ACA | Azygous ACA | N/azygous ACA |
| Craniofacial | Severe/mild | Severe/mild | Mild | Hypertelorism | Mild |

Modified from Hahn JS, Plawner LL. Evaluation and management of children with holoprosencephaly. *Pediatr Neurol.* 2004;31:79–88. N, normal; ACA, anterior cerebral artery; MCA, middle cerebral artery

**Table 12.1-3    Facial Anomalies in Association with HPE**

| Facial Defect | Features/Associations | Brain HPE |
|---|---|---|
| Cyclopia | Single eye, arhinia, possible proboscis | Alobar |
| Synophthamia | Partially fused eyes in single eye fissure | Alobar |
| An or micoophthamia | Absent or small eye | Alobar or semilobar |
| Ahrinia | Absent nose | Alobar or semilobar |
| Ethmocephaly | Hypotelorism proboscis between eyes | Alobar or semilobar |
| Cebocephaly | Hypotelorism, single nostril | Alobar or semilobar |
| Median cleft lip/palate (premaxillary agenesis) | Hypotelorism, flat nose | Alobar or semilobar |
| Bilateral cleft lip | Philtrum-premaxillary anlage | Alobar/semilobar/lobar |
| Hypotelorism | | All types/microform |
| Hypertelorism | | All types/microform |
| Eye abnormalities | Iris or retinal coloboma | All types/microform |
| Flat nose | | All types/microform |
| Mild palate | Lateral cleft, high arch, bifid uvula | All types/microform |
| Single central incisor | Hypoplasia piriform aperture | All types/microform |

Modified from Dubourg C, Bendavid C, Pasquier L, et al. Holoprosencephaly. *Orphanet J Rare Dis.* 2007;2:1–14.

| Table 12.1-4 | Causes and Conditions Associated with HPE |
|---|---|

**Chromosomal**
   Trisomy 13
   Trisomy 18
   Triploidy
   Other genetic mutations
      Deletions, duplications, partial monosomy 14q, unbalanced
         aberrations

**Syndromic-monogenetic**
   Autosomal dominant
      Dysgnathia complex
      Pallister–Hall
      Kallmann
      Rubinstein–Taybi
      Steinfeld
      Martin
      Thanatophoric dysplasia type II
   Autosomal recessive
      Spinocerebellar ataxia
      Ivemark (heterotaxy)
      Lambotte
      Meckel
      Genoa
      Hydrolethalus
      Pseudotrisomy 13
      Smith–Lemli–Opitz
      XK aprosencephaly
   X-linked
      Aicardi
      Ectrodactyly
      Fetal hypokinesia/akinesia

**Nonsyndromic**
   Familial
      Inherited autosomal dominant
      Gene mutations, such as *SHH* or *ZIC2*

**Environmental**
   Retinoic acid
   Ethyl alcohol
   Salicylates
   Estrogen/progestin
   Anticonvulsants
   CMV
   Rubella
   Toxoplasma
   Maternal diabetes
   Maternal hypocholesterolemia

Modified from Simon EM, Barkovich AJ. Holoprosencephaly: new concepts. *Magn Reson Imaging Clin N Am.* 2001;9:149–164.

have been identified in 15% to 20% cases.[102] To date, more than 13 genes and mutations thereof have been shown to cause HPE.[113] The four main genes involved in HPE include *SHH*, *ZIC2*, *SIX3*, and *TGIF*. Many of the genes in HPE are linked to sonic hedgehop (*SHH*) signal networks. *SHH* protein appears to be a developmental regulator of the ventral neural tube and thus important for induction and differentiation. The second most common HPE gene is *ZIC2*, which is associated with variable CNS malformations, including MIH and mild facial

anomalies.[107,109] This gene may have a role in editing the response to *SHH* protein signaling but affects the roof plate and dorsal brain structures.[109]

About 10% of individuals with HPE have defects in cholesterol biosynthesis, as cholesterol is required for activation of the *SHH* molecule.[102,112] Environmental factors, most commonly infection (especially cytomegalovirus) and maternal diabetes, are reported in HPE.[108] Infants of diabetic mothers have a 1% risk (200-fold increase) for HPE.[112] Despite these known associations, 70% of HPE have no known molecular basis, and therefore a "multiple hit" from both environment and genetics is likely.[101]

**Diagnosis:** When HPE is identified, karyotyping should always be performed. If karyotype is normal, genetic counseling with molecular testing may be considered. Prenatal history, detailed family history, and focused examination of the parents may help identify microforms of HPE.[102,112] A search for additional anomalies with US, MRI, and echocardiogram should be considered.

***Ultrasound:*** Tranabdominal or transvaginal US can confirm severe HPE as early as 10 weeks.[101,103,115] Coronal and axial imaging of the brain should be performed to verify fusion of hemispheres and thalami and lack of interhemispheric fissure. A helpful marker of alobar HPE is the featureless configuration of the monoventricle and dorsal cyst lacking occipital, temporal, and frontal horns (Fig. 12.1-11).[103] The choroid is prominent at this age, and absence of the normal choroidal "butterfly" configuration may also be a helpful clue[116]

In *alobar HPE*, the cortex of the prosencephalon is displaced rostrally and assumes the shape of a pankcake with the posterior aspect appearing as a horseshoe (Fig. 12.1-12A). When the dorsal cyst is small, the holophere may have a cup- or ball-like appearance.[117] There is complete absence of midline structures and fusion of deep basal ganglia and thalami. If there is absent cleavage of anterior hemisphere with single anterior ventricle, cleavage of the posterior hemispheres with rudimentary occipital horns, partial falx, and incomplete fusion of the thalami, the diagnosis of *semilobar HPE* should be considered (Fig. 12.1-13A,B).[103,118]

Milder degrees of HPE, including *lobar* or *MIH HPE*, are more difficult to detect and differentiate from other anomalies by US.[112,119] In lobar HPE, a midcoronal US image demonstrates

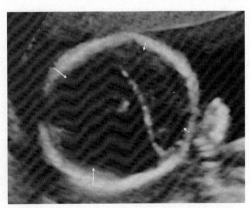

**FIGURE 12.1-11:** Axial US demonstrating large monoventricle *(long arrows)* and pancake mantle of fused brain anteriorly *(short arrows)* in a fetus with alobar HPE.

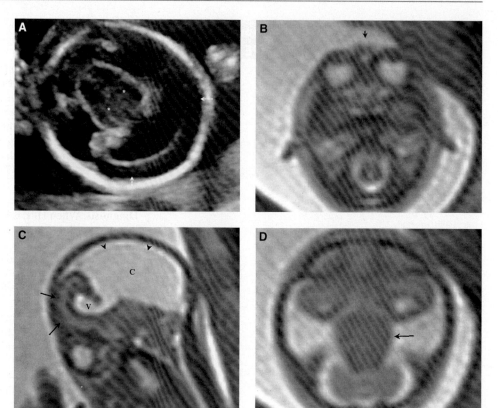

**FIGURE 12.1-12:** Fetus at 21 weeks with alobar HPE. **A:** Axial US demonstrates distorted choroid plexus and cuplike brain *(arrows)*. The thalami *(asterisks)* are fused. **B:** Axial T2 MR image demonstrates hypotelorism and single nostril *(arrow)*. **C:** Sagittal MR image demonstrates cuplike fused cerebral mantle *(arrows)* and monoventricle *(V)* contiguous with dorsal cyst *(C)*. *Arrowheads* denote wall of the cyst. **D:** Axial image demonstrates fused mass of deep gray nuclei, thalami, and midbrain *(arrow)*.

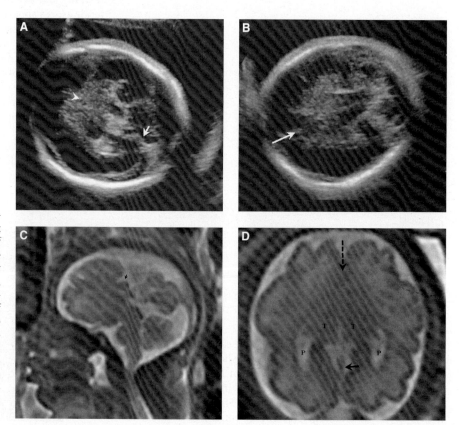

**FIGURE 12.1-13:** Fetus at 34 weeks with semilobar HPE. **A:** Axial image demonstrates falx posteriorly *(arrow)*. There is poor separation of the brain tissue anteriorly *(arrowhead)*. **B:** More inferior axial image verifies fusion of the anterior hemisphere *(arrow)* and partial fusion of thalami. **C:** Sagittal MR image demonstrates fused cerebral hemispheres anterior and small splenium of the corpus callosum *(arrow)*. **D:** Axial T2 image demonstrates separation of hemispheres posteriorly *(arrow)*. The posterior *(P)* horns of the lateral ventricles are normal but frontal horns and septum pellucidum absent owing to fusion of the anterior hemispheres across midline *(dotted arrow)*. The thalami *(T)* are partially fused, and there is fusion of the deep gray nuclei.

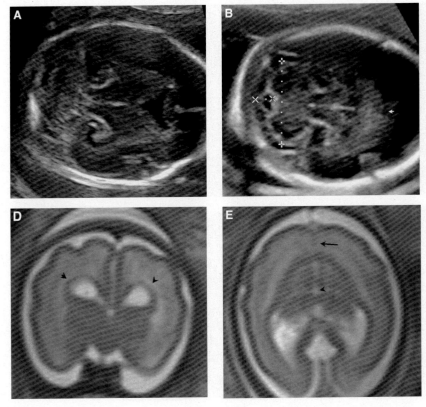

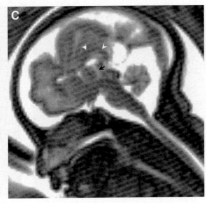

**FIGURE 12.1-14:** Fetus at 29 weeks with lobar HPE. **A:** Axial US demonstrates the typical boxlike configuration of the frontal horns. Thalami did not appear fused. **B:** Axial image through the inferior frontal horns demonstrates fusion of hemispheres and absence of falx (*arrow*). **C:** Sagittal image demonstrates splenium and posterior body of the corpus callosum (*arrowheads*) and small third ventricle (*black arrow*). **D:** Coronal image demonstrates bilateral frontal horns (*arrows*). **E:** Axial image demonstrates third ventricle (*arrowhead*). There is separation of basal ganglia structures, but fusion of the frontal lobes anteriorly (*arrow*).

absence of the cavum septum pellucidum (CSP) and central fusion of the frontal horn appearing as a boxlike squared shape with flattened roof in communication with the third ventricle (Fig. 12.1-14). Absence of the falx can be difficult to identify via US. However, the presence of an echogenic rounded structure variably identified within the third ventricle, representing fused fornices traveling from the anterior to posterior commissure, may help secure diagnosis.[120] An additional sonographic sign on midsagittal view is known as the "snake under the skull," representing a single (azygous) anterior cerebral artery displaced by the abnormal bridging frontal tissue.[121] In MIH, mild-to-moderate ventriculomegaly without CSP is common, but basal ganglia and thalami are normal (Fig. 12.1-15A). Fusion of hemispheres across the convexity can confirm this variant of HPE (Fig. 12.1-15B).

US is limited in diagnosing the HPE type, being inconsistent in 41% of cases.[98] Prenatal diagnosis detection rate of HPE by US has been noted to be as high as 71% but also as low as 22%.[108,117]

Early diagnosis of facial abnormalities may assist in confirmation of HPE.[122,123] Sonographic assessment of the fetal face, especially midline structures, is imperative.[124] The orbits should always be visualized and measured to exclude hypotelorism.[115] Three-dimensional/four-dimensional imaging is extremely helpful in further depiction of these anomalies and facilitates parent's understanding of the abnormality (Fig. 12.1-16).[125,126]

Growth restriction is found in higher than 50% of fetuses with HPE.[98] Microcephaly is noted in 75% of classic HPE and 50% with MIH.[102] As the pregnancy progresses, macrocephaly can develop because of disturbances in CSF dynamics.[114] A fetus with alobar HPE with dorsal cyst and severely nonseparated thalami are the most likely to develop hydrocephalus because of blockage at the third ventricle and aqueduct of Sylvius.[102,127] Exclusion of extracranial anomalies is imperative. In HPE, there is a high incidence of polyhydramnios.[99]

*MRI:* It is important to define the grade of HPE, as the image predicts the function.[102] MRI can identify all forms of HPE by demonstrating areas of cerebral nonseparation, abnormalities of the corpus callosum, and deep gray matter fusion.[128] In addition, MRI may help define subtle but significant facial anomalies (Fig. 12.1-12B).[129] On MRI, the severity of noncleavage of the cerebral hemispheres (grade) correlates with the severity of nonseparation of the deep gray nuclei.[130] The hypothalamus and caudate nuclei, 99% and 96%, respectively, are the most commonly nonseparated deep gray structures.[102,131] The thalami are noncleaved in 67% of HPE, and the degree of thalamic fusion correlates strongly with the presence of dorsal cyst.[100,117]

MR imaging is not typically necessary to diagnose the severe forms of HPE, but fused cerebral mass, monoventricle and dorsal cyst, and absence of septum pellucidum, corpus callosum, and interhemispheric fissure are well delineated (Fig. 12.1-12C). If MRI is obtained for *alobar*, approximately 27% will show nonseparation of the mesencephalon and 11% will demonstrate a single deep gray nuclear mass replacing basal ganglia, thalami, and midbrain (Fig. 12.1-12D).[117]

Differentiation from semilobar and lobar can be difficult as there is no clear boundary between the two types. In *semilobar* HPE, there is fusion anteriorly, presence of falx posteriorly, and partial fusion of the thalami. The splenium of the corpus callosum is present, and deep gray is incompletely separated. The septum pellucidum is absent with poor formation of the frontal horns (Fig. 12.1-13C,D). If the third ventricle is present, thalami are separate, and some frontal horn formation and splenium/posterior body corpus callosum are complete, then HPE variant is considered *lobar* (Fig. 12.1-14C,D). Fusion of the fornices in lobar HPE is better depicted on MRI than on US.[101] In septopreoptic HPE in which there is fusion in the septal (subcallosal) or preoptic region, the septum pellucidum may

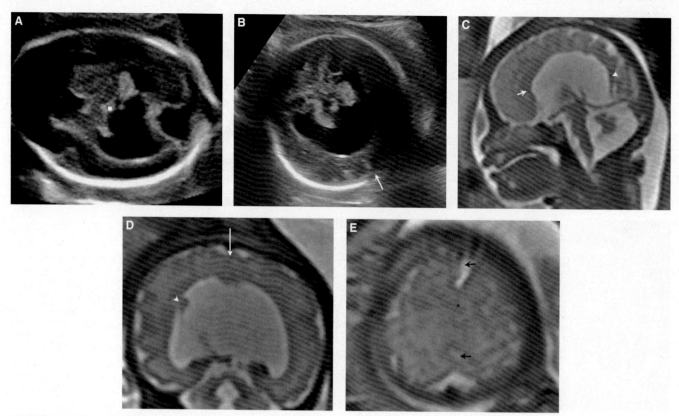

**FIGURE 12.1-15:** Fetus at 34 weeks with middle interhemispheric fusion. **A:** Axial image demonstrates moderate ventriculomegaly and absence of the septum pellucidum. **B:** Coronal image shows absence of interhemispheric fissure and fusion of cerebral hemispheres *(arrow)* at convexity of the brain. **C:** Sagittal T2 MR image demonstrates presence of the genu *(arrow)* and splenium *(arrowhead)*, but lack of visualization of the body. The vermis and brainstem are incidentally small. **D:** Coronal T2 MR image demonstrates fusion across midline *(arrow)*. There is gray matter heterotopia along the right lateral ventricle *(arrowhead)*. **E:** Axial MR T2 image demonstrates interhemispheric fissure anteriorly and posteriorly *(arrows)*, but fusion *(asterisk)* in the posterior frontal anterior parietal area.

be variably abnormal, fornix is dysplastic or thickened, corpus callosum may be thickened or hypoplastic, and azygous artery is usually present.[132,133] In *MIH*, the sylvian fissures are vertical, connected across the midline vertex of the brain in the posterior frontal anterior parietal lobe (Fig. 12.1-15C–E).[134] There is lack of visualization of the body of the corpus callosum, absence of the septum pellucidum with normal basal ganglia and thalami. In MIH, many have mild anomalies of the face, the most common being hypertelorism.[102]

In most forms of HPE, there is a low incidence of sulcation or cortical migrational abnormalities, with broad gyri being seen

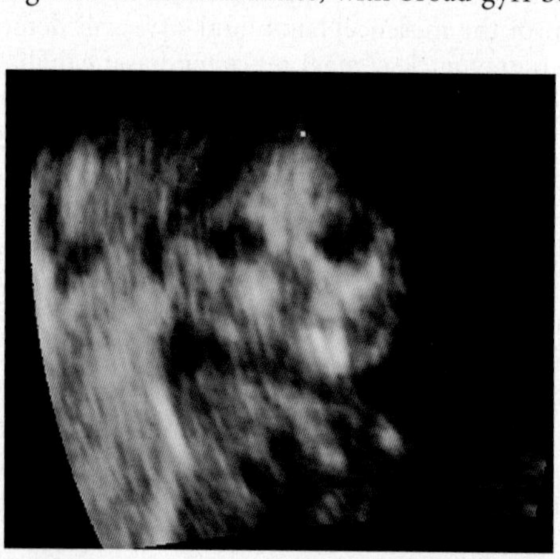

in severe forms, absent sylvian fissures alobar, vertical wide sylvian fissures semilobar and lobar, and rarely cortical abnormalities medial frontal in lobar HPE.[135] The exception is MIH, in which two-third have subcortical heterotopic gray or cortical dysplasia (Fig. 12.1-15D).

**Associated Anomalies:** About 51% to 55% of nonsyndromic HPE have multiple congenital defects.[97] HPE is typically associated with anomalies of the CNS, heart, skeleton, and gastrointestinal tract.[101] Of the CNS, HPE is associated most with neural tube defects and posterior fossa anomalies, including rhomboencephalosynapsis.[136] Of noncraniofacial anomalies, 24% of HPE cases can demonstrate genitourinary defects, 8% postaxial polydactyly, 5% vertebral anomalies, 4% limb reduction, and 4% transposition of the great arteries.[97] Rarely, HPE is seen in the presence of heterotaxy syndromes.[133]

**Differential Diagnosis:** The main differential includes hydrocephalus, midline cerebral defects such as agenesis of corpus callosum (ACC), septo-optic dysplasia (SOD), hydranencephaly, and porencephalic cysts. Hydrocephalus can be differentiated by demonstrating persistence of the interhemipheric fissure, distinct separate ventricles, and splaying of the thalami. In hydranencephaly and porencephaly, thin cerebral cortex, partially present or deviated falx, and lack of fused thalami are noted. HPE is also differentiated from posterior fossa malformations by normal falx, supratentorial structures, and unfused thalami. ACC with interhemispheric cyst is often difficult to

**FIGURE 12.1-16:** 3D reformat in a fetus with semilobar HPE and median cleft, hypotelorism, and trigonencephaly.

distinguish but can be best discriminated by normal cleavage of the brain. Differentiation of lobar HPE from SOD is by identifying the presence of fused fornices and absence of abnormally developed interhemispheric fissure between the anterior hemispheres. MRI in the third trimester may be helpful to exclude optic nerve hypoplasia.[101]

**Prognosis:** There is a natural loss of fetuses with HPE, being as high as 40%, mostly during the first trimester.[108] For the most part, there is a direct correlation with severity of HPE and outcome.[102] The prognosis at birth is much worse for those with severe facial disorders and cytogenetic anomalies, with only 2% surviving beyond 1 year, compared with 30% to 54% with normal karyotype.[102] In those with normal karyotype, an inverse relationship between survival and severity of HPE and facial anomalies is noted.[101] Most with alobar HPE will not survive beyond infancy with 89% perinatal mortality rate.[101,115] Those with milder forms can survive into childhood and beyond, and may only have mild cognitive impairment.[102]

Children with HPE have multiple neurological problems, including mental retardation, motor dysfunction, seizure disorder, and endocrine abnormalities. Motor dysfunction including hypotonia, dystonia, and spasticity are present in all types of HPE, with the classic forms only having involuntary movements.[102] The severity of the brain malformation and the higher degree of nonseparation of gray nuclei correlate with the severity of developmental delay and neurologic deficit.[107,127] Approximately 50% will develop seizure, but only 25% will have chronic epilepsy.[107,127] Feeding problems are common, and the severity of dysfunction correlates with the grade of HPE.[101,107] Seventy-five percent of children with classic HPE have diabetes insipidus correlating with the degree of hypothalamic nonseparation rather than defects of the pituitary gland.[102,127] Dysautonomic dysfunction can also be present with instability of temperature, heart, and/or respiratory rate.[107] Frequent causes of demise include infection, dehydration due to uncontrolled diabetes insipidus, intractable seizures, and brainstem malfunction.[137]

**Management:** Genetic counseling is imperative. In the presence of severe HPE, elective termination of the pregnancy may be considered. Cesarean delivery should be considered only for maternal indications in the absence of fetal macrocephaly.[115] Cephalocentesis may be considered in the presence of macrocephaly. After birth, treatment is based on symptoms and usually requires a multidisciplinary approach. Medical management should focus on endocrine dysfunction, motor and developmental impairments, respiratory issues, seizures, and hydrocephalus. Feeding difficulties are common in neonates with HPE, and about two-thirds of those with lobar and semilobar HPE require gastrostomy tubes.[107] Neurologic management is not specific but may require anticonvulsive, physical, and occupational therapies. Surgery is typically performed to treat hydrocephalus and repair cleft lip and/or palate.[107,112]

**Recurrence:** HPE has a higher recurrence risk than other major malformations, being 6% to 20% after an isolated case, in a fetus with normal karyotype and no syndrome.[108,138] If inherited, the risk is 50% in the dominant form or 25% with recessive transmission.[112] Overall risk to the subsequent child with dominant transmission is 37% for HPE, 27% for HPE microform, and 36% for normal phenotype.[139]

# COMMISSURES/MIDLINE

## Agenesis of Corpus Callosum

The corpus callosum may be completely absent (agenesis), partially lacking (hypogenesis), or globally or partially thin (hypoplastic). Agenesis of the corpus callosum (ACC) can also be associated with meningeal dysplasias such as interhemispheric cysts and lipomas.

**Incidence:** ACC or hypoplasia of the corpus callosum is reported in 2 per 10,000 live births and is seen in approximately 13% of cases referred for VM.[140–142] There is a male preponderance.[141,142] With regard to race, the order of risk is higher for blacks, then whites, and finally Asian descent.[141] Postnatally, the incidence of complete ACC (CACC) and partial ACC (PACC) is equivalent. ACC is isolated in 30% of cases, with the remaining associated with other cerebral or extracranial anomalies.[143]

**Pathogenesis:** The corpus callosum is the largest and most significant of the five midline forebrain commissures, composed of axons which facilitate communication between the cerebral hemispheres. It contains five sections, anterior to posterior: rostrum, genu, body, isthmus, and splenium (see Fig. 6.2-25 in Chapter 6.2). The corpus callosum arises from the lamina terminalis, originates in the area of the massa commisuralis between 7 and 20 weeks of gestation, and reaches adult size by 2 years of age (see section on normal corpus callosum Chapter 6.2).

There are many inciting factors that may result in its absence, with three possible mechanisms described: missing or defective development of the massa commisuralis, failure of the axons to form in the cerebral cortex, or inhibited cellular migration due to the absence of normal chemical attractants or repellants or an interhemispheric lesion. It is suspected that CACC is mostly a primary embryologic disorder with failure of development of the termina laminalis or massa commisuralis, whereas PACC is a malformation or destructive event in which there is partial absence of the commissural plate or lack of normal growth.[144,145] Hypoplasia is likely secondary to a developmental error or insult later in fetal development.

If the axons develop but are unable to cross the midline because of the absence of the massa commisuralis or a lesion in the interhemispheric space, large heterotopic axons that were destined to cross the corpus callosum lie parallel to the interhemispheric fissure along the medial walls of the lateral ventricles, forming the bundles of Probst. If there is a defect in the commissural axons or their parent cell bodies fail to form in the cerebral cortex, the commissures are absent, Probst bundles are absent, and white matter volume is decreased.[146] When the corpus callosum is completely absent, there is associated absence of the hippocampal commissure, and 50% of the time, the anterior commissure is also missing.[146] If the corpus callosum is partially absent, usually the posterior aspect is deficient. ACC is primary when it is the main pathology; however, it can be secondary if it is due to destructive events or when associated with other major malformations, such as encephaloceles and HPE.[146]

In the presence of ACC, there is associated distortion of the intracranial architecture. The cingulate gyrus remains everted, and the sulci of the medial brain extend into the third ventricle, creating a radial or sunburst pattern.[147] When callosal bundles of Probst are present, the lateral ventricles, especially in the frontal area, have a crescentic "steer horn" appearance.[147] The third ventricle is large and high-riding, communicating with the interhemispheric fissure (Fig. 12.1-17). The foramen

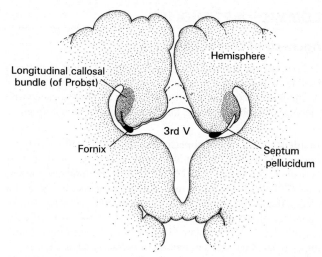

**FIGURE 12.1-17:** Schematic drawing of ACC. The lateral ventricles demonstrate a crescentic shape due to the presence of Probst bundles. The third ventricle is large, extending upward into the interhemispheric fissure. The cingulate gyri are everted, and sulci do not form. (From Barkovich AJ. Apparent atypical callosal dysgenesis: analysis of MR findings in six cases and their relationship to holoprosencephaly. *AJNR Am J Neuroradiol.* 1990;11:333–340, with permission.)

of Monro is enlarged. White matter volume loss is nearly uniform, likely representing a primary dysplasia or hypogenesis. In the case of complete absence, the lateral ventricles maintain a straight parallel configuration with focal dilatation of the temporal, atrial, and occipital horn due to hypogenetic and loose white matter tracts.[148] This ventricular dilatation posteriorly is known as colpocephaly. Abnormalities of the anterior and hippocampal commissures, either being absent or abnormal in size, are common.[149] The hippocampal formations are often incompletely rotated.[148] Malformations in cortical development and delay in sulcation are common, with gray matter heterotopias identified in approximately 29% of cases.[149]

Meningeal dysplasias include cysts and lipomas. Interhemispheric cysts are associated with ACC in 14% to 30% of cases.[149] The cyst can communicate with the ventricles (type 1) or lack ventricular continuity (type 2). *Type 1* lesions represent a single ventricular diverticulation of CSF attenuation which is not typically associated with hemispheric malformations.[145,150] In *type II* cysts, multilocular complex cysts are present, and these children are more likely to be born with hydrocephalus. Associated brain malformations are more common with type II, and in the presence of hemispheric asymmetry and polymicrogyria, Aicardi syndrome should be considered.

Up to 3% of patients with ACC will have interhemispheric lipomas.[149] Pathogenesis of pericallosal lipomas are believed to be because of abnormal resorption of the menix primitiva.[151] Two types are described including the *tubulonodular*, which are round and measuring >2 cm, and the *curvilinear*, which is thin and elongated, measuring <1 cm in diameter. The tubulonodular type is more common, seen with major, usually anterior callosal malformation, often have internal calcification, and may be associated with frontofacial anomalies. The curvilinear is posterior with less severe callosal abnormalities.[145,151] Goldenhar and trisomies have been associated with ACC with lipoma.[151]

**Etiology:** There are innumerable causes of ACC including chromosomal, genetic, infectious, vascular, inborn errors of metabolism, or toxic causes (Table 12.1-5), but the etiology is

| Table 12.1-5 | Common Etiologies for Agenesis of Corpus Callosum (ACC) |
|---|---|

**Genetic Disorders**
*Consistently associated with ACC*
 Aicardi syndrome—chorioretinal lacunae, infantile spasms
 Andermann syndrome—peripheral neuropathy, dementia
 Acrocallosal syndrome—hallux duplication, polydactyly, craniofacial
 Calloso-genital dysplasia—coloboma, amenorrhoea
 Shapiro syndrome—ataxia, drowsiness
 CRASH/L1CAM—hydrocephalus, adducted thumbs
*Inconsistently associated with ACC*
 Meckel–Gruber—encephalocele, polydactyly, polycystic kidneys
 Rubinstein–Taybi—broad thumbs and great toes, microcephaly
 Sotos syndrome—physical overgrowth, craniofacial
 Fryns—congenital diaphragmatic hernia, pulmonary hypoplasia, craniofacial changes

**Inborn errors of metabolism**
 Glutaric aciduria Type II
 Neonatal adrenoleukodystrophy
 Nonketotic hyperglycinemia
 Pyruvate dehydrogenase deficiency

**Chromosomal disorders**
 Trisomy 18, 13, 8

**Teratogens**
 Fetal alcohol syndrome
 Cocaine

Data from Bedeschi MF, Bonaglia MC, Grasso R, et al. Agenesis of corpus callosum: clinical and genetic study in 63 young patients. *Pediatr Neurol.* 2006;34(3):186–193.

unknown in more than 50% of defined cases.[152] For 30% to 45% of individuals with CACC and PACC, the cause is chromosomal (10%) or genetic syndromes (20% to 35%).[153] If only CACC is considered, recognizable syndromes drop to 10% to 15%, with 75% lacking identifiable cause. Aneuploidy is identified in 1 in 10 ACC cases, the most common being trisomy 8, 13, 18, and 21.[154] In the presence of additional structural abnormalities and/or advanced maternal age, ACC is seen at a higher frequency with chromosomal disorders.[141,143]

There are over 175 syndromes in which ACC is a significant finding. A well-known disorder associated with ACC is Aicardi. This X-linked dominant condition seen primarily in females and in males with Klinefelter syndrome (XXY) is due to a balanced translocation of the X chromosome and is characterized by infantile spasms, ACC, and chorioretinal lacunae. The presence of ACC with polymicrogyria, periventricular hetertopia, cysts of the choroid plexus, pineal, and/or interhemispheric region, micropthalmia, asymmetry of the hemispheres, and abnormal EEG is highly suggestive of Aicardia.[155] Another syndrome to consider is CRASH (ACC, retardation, adducted thumbs, spastic paraplegia, and hydrocephalus), which is caused by mutations in the L1 cell adhesion molecule (L1CAM).

Metabolic disorders, fetal infections, or in utero exposure to teratogens, such as fetal alcohol syndrome and maternal diabetes, have been described with ACC. Infants born prematurely have an almost four-fold higher prevalence.[141]

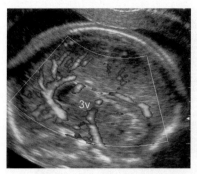

**FIGURE 12.1-18:** Partial agenesis of the corpus callosum. The corpus callosum appears thin but can be positively identified by the pericallosal artery anteriorly.

**Diagnosis:** Fetal karyotyping should be performed to exclude chromosomal anomaly.

***Ultrasound:*** In the first trimester, early ultrasound examination at 11 to 14 weeks can provide clues to the existence of ACC. Normal anatomy of the pericollosal arteries on the sagittal plane demonstrates the vessels arising from the anterior cerebral arteries to curve posteriorly following the normal anatomy of the corpus callosum.[156] Lack of visualization of the normal pericallosal artery raises the suspicion of ACC (Fig. 12.1-18).[156] With ACC, the midbrain diameter is typically increased and falx diameter decreased, yielding a high midbrain-to-falx diameter ratio.[157] These findings are, however, not 100% sensitive or specific and should be confirmed with second-trimester imaging.

In the second trimester, the diagnosis of a callosal abnormality is typically suggested by the presence of mild-to-moderate ventriculomegaly.[158] Direct visualization of the corpus callosum is best via coronal or sagittal imaging but can be difficult prior to 22 weeks (Fig. 12.1-19).[159,160] The sensitivity in identifying ACC by direct visualization is variable in the literature, ranging from 28% to 85%.[161] Three-dimensional reformats of axial images in the sagittal plane are helpful, or in the presence of a cephalic fetus, transvaginal US can increase visualization.

When the corpus callosum cannot be directly visualized, high suspicion for the diagnosis is via indirect signs (Fig. 12.1-20). The indirect signs of ACC include the following[154,158,159,162]:

- Absent septum pellucidum identified as early as 17 to 18 weeks
- Ventriculomegaly with disproportionate dilatation of the occipital horns creating a teardrop configuration (colpocephaly)
- Increased distension of the interhemispheric fissure with separation of the lateral ventricles and both medial and lateral walls aligned parallel to the midline
- Concave appearance of the medial, especially anterior horns of the lateral ventricles, due to protrusion of the cingulate gyrus and Probst bundles
- Upward displacement of a variably dilated third ventricle
- Radial arrangement of medial cerebral sulci
- Abnormal appearance of the pericallosal artery

However, these indirect findings may be absent early in the second trimester with colpocephaly often not apparent until 26 weeks and radial arrangement of the medial sulci until third trimester.[159,160]

Direct diagnosis of CACC can be difficult, and PACC may be technically more difficult because of inconsistent indirect signs.[163,164] In the presence of PACC, the most common finding is colpocephaly, although sometimes a small or absent cavum septi

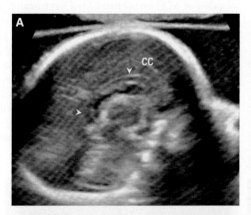

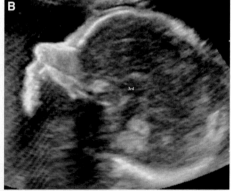

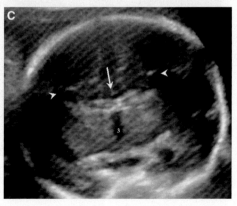

**FIGURE 12.1-19:** Twin gestation at 30 weeks, one with agenesis of the corpus callosum. **A:** Sagittal US in twin with normal corpus callosum *(arrowheads)*. **B:** Sagittal US in twin with ACC showing absent corpus callosum and prominent *3rd* ventricle. **C:** Coronal US demonstrates typical findings of ACC including crescentic frontal horns *(arrowheads)*, lack of corpus callosum across midline *(arrow)*, and enlarged 3rd *(3)* ventricle.

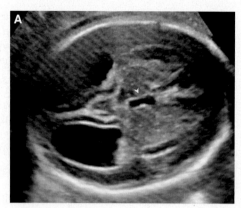
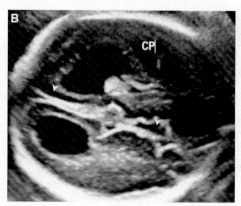

**FIGURE 12.1-20:** Indirect signs of ACC. **A:** Axial image demonstrates colpocephaly and dilatation of the third ventricle *(arrowhead)*. No septum pellucidum was identified. **B:** Axial image through dilated posterior ventricular horns with prominent interhemispheric fluid *(arrows)*. CP represents choroid plexus.

pellucidi is noted. An important pitfall in sonography is that in PACC or CACC, dysplastic or displaced leaflets of the septum pellucidum and fornix may simulate a normal cavum septum pellucidum, and therefore direct visualization of the corpus callosum with sagittal imaging in conjunction with pericallosal color Doppler may be required.[164–166] Using expert sonography with 3D reformation and comparison with normative callosal values, hypogenesis and hypoplasia have been diagnosed.[166,167]

In the presence of interhemispheric cyst, the third ventricle can be mildly dilated or significantly enlarged. The cyst may be simple and communicate with the third or lateral ventricles (Fig. 12.1-21A) or may be complex mulitlocular without ventricular communication (Fig. 12.1-22A). Lipomas are nodular or curvilinear echogenic masses within the interhemispheric fissure. Some large lipomas have spiculated margins with or without extension into the frontal horns or the choroid plexus (Fig. 12.1-23A).[151]

***MRI:*** Fetal MRI is useful in evaluation of the corpus callosum and has high sensitivity in confirming presence or absence as the structure is well defined on axial, sagittal, and coronal images.[161,163] In prior studies, fetal MRI has identified an intact corpus callosum in about 20% of cases referred for ACC.[168,169] Prenatal MRI easily depicts the common intracranial direct and indirect signs that are present with this pathology (Fig. 12.1-24).

MRI has also been shown to identify additional brain anomalies, especially migration anomalies, in 63% to 93% fetuses with ACC that were not apparent on US (Fig. 12.1-25).[168–170]

In a recent study, nearly all cases of ACC have been noted to have abnormalities of sulcation, 50% with disorders of the cerebellum and 33% of the brainstem.[170] Most brainstem abnormalities are present in conjunction with cerebellar anomalies (Fig. 12.1-26).[170] Sulcation delay can be associated with good neurodevelopmental outcome and may reflect white matter dysgenesis. In fact, a recent study notes that sulcation delay is seen at a high frequency in fetuses with ACC in the third trimester, likely because of failed commiseration and not because of additional brain malformations.[171] If delay in sulcation is excluded, only 69% of ACC cases have additional anomalies via fetal MRI.

In the presence of focal abnormal sulcation morphology, 42% of cases of ACC on prenatal MRI have been found to be associated with multiple brain anomalies and a syndrome.[170] In 25% of ACC cases, additional findings identified by fetal MR imaging led to a diagnosis of a specific disorder or syndrome.[169] In 10% of ACC cases, destructive changes suggested acquired injury.[170]

MRI easily defines the presence of associated interhemipheric cyst or lipoma and extent of the lesion. In type 1, the cysts are isotense to CSF and communicate with the ventricle (Fig. 12.1-21B); whereas type II cysts present as multiple cysts demonstrating higher signal than CSF on T1 and heterogeneous

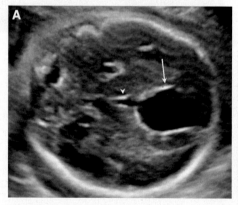
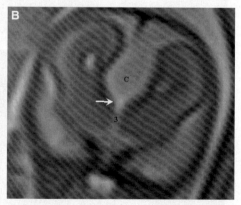

**FIGURE 12.1-21:** Type I interhemispheric cyst in a 20 week-fetus with ACC. **A:** Coronal oblique US image demonstrates simple interhemispheric cyst *(arrow)* in continuity with third ventricle *(arrowhead)*. **B:** Coronal T2 MR image verifies cyst *(C)* and confirms communication *(arrow)* with third ventricle *(3)*.

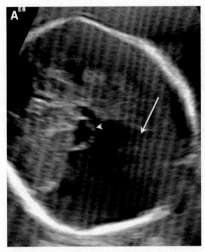 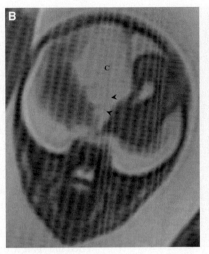 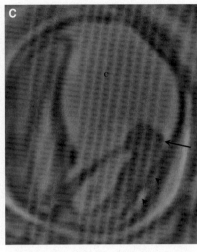

**FIGURE 12.1-22:** Fetus at 23 weeks with ACC and type II interhemispheric cyst. **A:** Axial US demonstrates a large interhemispheric cyst *(arrow)* with septation *(arrowhead)* midline. **B:** Coronal MR SSFP image demonstrates small septated areas *(arrowheads)* deep in the interhemispheric cyst *(C)*. No communication with ventricular system was noted. **C:** Axial T2 image demonstrates large cyst *(C)*. The left hemisphere was abnormally small, and abnormal dark parenchymal signal *(arrow)* and unusual cortical lobulation *(arrowheads)* along the hemisphere were consistent with migrational abnormality.

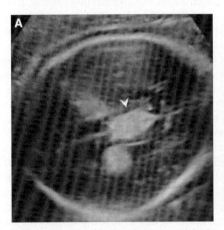 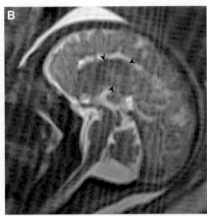 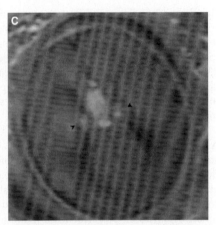

**FIGURE 12.1-23:** ACC and tubulonodular lipoma in a fetus at 35 weeks. **A:** Axial US demonstrates echogenic midline mass *(arrowhead)* with prominent choroid plexus. **B:** Sagittal T2 MR image demonstrates ACC with heterogeneous hypointense *(arrowheads)* mass in the midline. **C:** Axial T1 image demonstrates hyperintense mass in midline and small nodules extending into the choroid *(arrowheads)*.

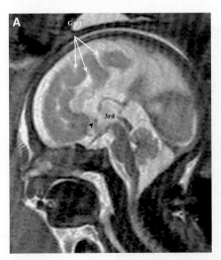 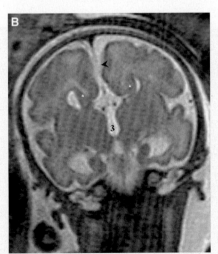 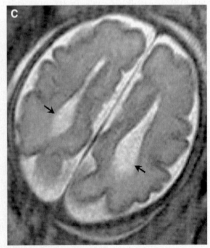

**FIGURE 12.1-24:** MR imaging of fetus at 30 weeks with ACC. **A:** Sagittal T2 shows absence of the corpus callosum and missing hippocampal commissure and fornix. Anterior commissure is present *(arrowhead)*. Notice radial arrangement of gyri and prominent *3rd* ventricle. **B:** Coronal image demonstrates prominent *3rd* ventricle and interhemispheric fluid *(arrowhead)*. Probst bundles are noted *(asterisks)* adjacent to crescentic frontal horns. No cavum septum pellucidum. Hippocampi are incompletely rotated. **C:** Axial image demonstrates parallel configuration of the lateral ventricles consistent with colpocephaly *(arrows)*.

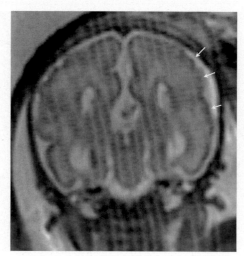

**FIGURE 12.1-25:** Migrational anomaly in fetus at 30 weeks with ACC. Coronal T2 image demonstrates irregularity and poor gray white differentiation left opercula area *(arrows)* consistent with polymicrogyria. Compare with the opposite normal right side.

signal on T2 imaging and do not communicate with the ventricular system (Fig. 12.1-22B,C). Lipomas demonstrate hyperintense signal on T1 and hypointense signal on T2 and when tubulonodular may extend into the choroid plexus (Fig. 12.1-23B,C). Fetal US and MRI are helpful in suggesting the diagnosis of Aicardi by evaluating for choroid plexus cysts (CPCs), microphthamia, asymmetric hemsipheres, and cortical malformations (Fig. 12.1-27).

**Associated Anomalies:** Both intracranial and extracranial anomalies are seen in corpus callosum disorders (Table 12.1-6). Because the corpus callosum development overlaps with complex processes involving neuronal proliferation and migration, common associated CNS anomalies include disorders of neuronal organization, posterior fossa malformations, and neural tube defects.[140,141] The incidence of CNS anomalies in ACC ranges from 50% to 85% in some series.[172] Extra-CNS anomalies are present in approximately 65% of ACC patients.[153] Common organ systems include eyes, heart, and kidneys.[173]

**Differential Diagnosis:** ACC should be differentiated from other causes of VM. In the presence of ACC with an interhemispheric cyst, differential would include enlarged cavum septum pellucidum et vergae, arachnoid cyst, porencephaly, ventricular rupture in obstructive hydrocephalus, and vein of Galen malformation. Interhemipheric cysts may be confused with the dorsal sac of HPE but the morphology of the separated frontal horns helps in differentiation. In the presence of a lipoma, differential diagnosis includes hemorrhage or rare tumor such as craniopharyngioma or choroid plexus papilloma.

**Prognosis:** Outcome is dependent on multiple factors including presence of microcephaly, genetic abnormality, and/or associated anomalies.[152] In the presence of ACC with syndrome or chromosomal abnormalities, the outcome is typically poor.[144] Children with Aicardi have significant developmental delay, seizures, and shortened life span with survival of 76% at 6 years and 40% at 14 years, demise most commonly due to respiratory infection.[155,172] Children with ACC and associated migrational disorder are more likely to have moderate-to-severe developmental delay.[174] It is controversial whether PACC versus CACC has better outcome.[144,164,171,175] When reviewing all patients with ACC, moderate-to-severe developmental delay is described in 80%, epilepsy in 35% to 45.8%, cerebral palsy in 37.5%, microcephaly in 33.3%, and visual and hearing defects and behavioral disorders in many.[152,175,176]

Most believe that an asymptomatic outcome in isolated agenesis can occur; however, it is more likely the exception rather than the rule.[152] Isolated ACC has been shown to have outcomes ranging from normal to severe delay.[142] In addition, even though 5% to 20% of cases have prenatal diagnosis of isolated ACC, additional anomalies have been detected postnatally.[173,177]

Although some research suggests better prognosis in those fetuses with isolated CACC, with small studies quoting 100% normalcy and larger studies noting normal developmental outcomes in two-thirds of cases and literature citing rates between 45% and 85%, the information is still incomplete as these studies include variable number of cases, isolation diagnosed only via fetal MRI and limited follow-up ranging only between 2 and 6 years of age.[140,144,154,178] It has been demonstrated that as age

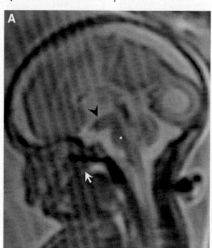

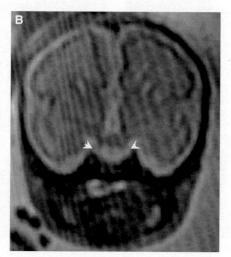

**FIGURE 12.1-26:** Fetus at 30 weeks with ACC and epignathus. **A:** Sagittal T2 image shows ACC with small brainstem *(asterisk)*. Cerebellar vermis also measured small. The hypothalamus is thick *(arrowhead)*. There is heterogeneous tissue in the area of the palate *(white arrow)*. **B:** Coronal T2 image demonstrates two infundibula *(arrowheads)* consistent with duplicated pituitary.

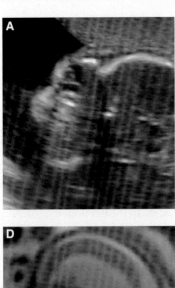
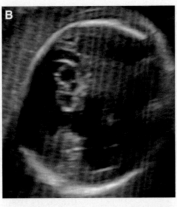
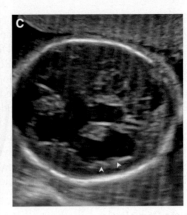
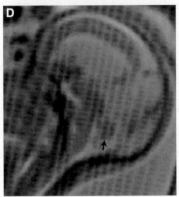
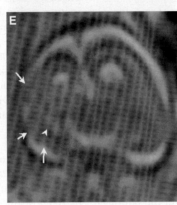

**FIGURE 12.1-27:** Fetus at 20 weeks with suspected Aicardi but lack of confirmation due to termination. **A:** Axial US demonstrates lack of visualization of one globe and small size of other. **B:** Complex choroid plexus cysts were present. **C:** Axial US demonstrates ventriculomegaly and irregularity of the wall (*arrow*) suspect for gray matter heterotopia. **D:** ACC of corpus callosum noted on sagittal T2 MR image. The vermis was also small (*arrow*). **E:** Asymmetric small right hemisphere with gray matter heterotopia (*arrowhead*) and cortical malformation (*arrows*) present.

increases, more delays often become apparent.[178] For example, a recent study demonstrated lower than normal IQ of 19% at 2 years, 33.5% at 4 years, and 43% at 6 years in a series of 17 children with isolated ACC.[178] Another recent study demonstrated that children with isolated ACC may have normal cognitive and neurologic outcome, but lower than expected based on family history and sometimes other subtle to severe defects identified later childhood, including difficulties at school, intellectual impairment, verbal communication defects, sleep disorders, and seizures.[174,178] Prediction of outcome even still must be cautious as some individuals with isolated ACC have deficits in the social and behavioral domain, which may place them in the spectrum of autism, attention deficit disorder, and schizophrenia that usually do not become evident until preteenage years.[174] Recent

epidemiology studies have documented that there is only 27% normal outcome in the presence of isolated ACC.[142]

In ACC with interhemispheric cyst, seizures are noted in less than half of patients. It has been suggested that Type 1 cysts tend to have more developmental delay and neurologic deficits than type II; however, outcome is likely dependent on associated anomalies and the development of hydrocephalus.[150] In the presence of associated lipoma, neurologic status is variable depending on type of lipoma, associated callosal anomalies, and other malformations; however, overall 50% of children with ACC and lipoma have seizures and psychological disorders.[151]

**Management:** Termination of the pregnancy may be considered after complete prenatal workup. At birth, close evaluation for

---

| Table 12.1-6 | CNS and Extra-CNS Abnormalities with Agenesis of Corpus Callosum |
| --- | --- |

| *CNS Abnormalities* | *Extra-CNS Abnormalities* |
| --- | --- |
| Periventricular nodular heterotopia | Cranio facial |
| Pachygyria | Skeletal |
| Hypothalamic, pituitary, and optic hypoplasia | Cardiac |
| Polymicrogyria | Ocular |
| Dandy Walker malformation | Genital |
| Cerebellar vermis agenesis | Renal |
| Pontine hypoplasia | |

Data from Bedeschi MF, Bonaglia MC, Grasso R, et al. Agenesis of corpus callosum: clinical and genetic study in 63 young patients. *Pediatr Neurol.* 2006;34(3):186–193.

extracerebral malformations should be performed to exclude underlying genetic syndrome. If no other abnormalities are detected and the ACC is isolated, close clinical follow-up is suggested. If anomalies are present, postnatal MRI and evaluation by a multidisciplinary team including neonatologists, neuroradiologists, neurologist, and geneticist is indicated. Comorbidities including epilepsy and feeding problems should be addressed.

**Recurrence:** In most cases of ACC, recurrence is moderately increased at 5% to 10%.[160] If the etiology is syndromic, recurrence is dependent on the type of transmission. Risk is high in a family with previous child diagnosed with Aicardi syndrome.

## Septo-optic Dysplasia

Septo-optic dysplasia (SOD), or De Morsier syndrome, is a disorder of midline anomalies that include a triad of findings of complete or partial absence of the septum pellucidum, optic nerve hypoplasia, and hypothalamic pituitary abnormalities.

**Incidence:** SOD is fairly rare with an incidence of 1 per 10,000 live births with equal prevalence in males and females.[179] The disorder is noted at a higher incidence when there is bleeding early in pregnancy or in children born to younger, especially teenage, mothers.[179,180]

**Pathogenesis:** The septum pellucidum is intimately associated with the corpus callosum and is also formed from the lamina terminalis. The structure is bounded by the corpus callosum anteriorly and superiorly, and by the fornix inferiorly and posteriorly. The septum pellucidum forms the medial border of the frontal horns of the lateral ventricles, the posterior margin defined by the foramen Monro. Each leaflet from lateral to medial has a ventricular ependymal lining, thin layer of gray matter, thin layer of white matter, and inner pial layer.

Prosencephalic maldevelopment or destructive insults between 4 and 6 weeks of gestation are suspected to give rise to SOD. This is the time when the septum pellucidum is linked to development of the commissures (see corpus callosum Chapter 6.2). Optic nerve defects are also possible as this is when the optic vesicles and retinal ganglion cells differentiate. Pituitary disorders, particularly in the presence of ectopic posterior lobe, may occur because of ischemic injury to the hypophysis causing necrosis of the infundibulum.[181]

The phenotype of SOD is variable, with the diagnosis obtained by identifying two or more of the triad of findings. Usually, the diagnosis is confirmed by ophthalmology postnatally when hypoplasia of the optic discs is present in conjunction with partial or complete absence of the septum pellucidum. Pituitary dysfunction, commonly in association with structural abnormalities such as ectopic or absent posterior pituitary, truncated or absent infundibulum, and hypoplastic anterior lobe, may be present.[182] Approximately 30% of patients have the triad of findings, 62% have hypopituitarism, and 60% to 75% demonstrate absent septum.[183,184] About 75% to 80% of patients with SOD have optic nerve hypoplasia, which may be unilateral (12%) or more commonly bilateral (88%).[183] SOD can also be associated with absence, hypogenesis, or hypoplasia of the corpus callosum.[185] Isolated absence of the septum pellucidum is rare.

Two distinct groups of SOD are noted. One group has complete or partial absence of the septum pellucidum in conjunction with malformations of cortical development, usually schizencephaly in the frontal lobe area.[186] The term SOD-plus is sometimes utilized to describe these complex cases.[187] The second group has complete absence of the septum, hypoplasia of the cerebral white matter, normal cortex, and often pituitary dysfunction.[188] These findings overlap with HPE, possibly representing a milder form of lobar HPE.

**Etiology:** The etiology of the syndrome is likely multifactorial, related to multiple genetic disorders and environmental factors that result in intrauterine vascular disruption.[184] The condition is primarily sporadic, but rare autosomal recessive and dominant familial cases have been cited.[5] A gene found to cause SOD, documented in familial cases, is the *HESX1* gene, which is produced by tissue adjacent to the developing prosencephalon and is suggested to be important for proper induction of the forebrain and midline.[183] The *HESX1* gene is also one of the earliest markers of the pituitary primordium and may explain the associated hypopituitarism. *SOX2* and *SOX3* genes are also necessary for development of the pituitary, and these genes have been implicated in pituitary anomalies seen in SOD.[183,189] In utero injury causing SOD may be due to viral infections, teratogens such as exposure to alcohol or drugs, or degenerative damage.[183,184]

### Diagnosis

*Ultrasound:* On US, the leaves of the septum pellucidum and interposed cavum can be visualized sonographically as a rectangular or triangular fluid-filled space between the frontal horns in 100% of normal fetuses from at least 18 to 37 weeks.[190] At midgestation, however, if only axial imaging is obtained, an artifact created by US beam crossing, can mimic the septum pellucidum and result in misdiagnosis.[191] Two other causes of false positive include an enlarged cavum septum pellucidum with displaced leaflets laterally and imaging slightly below the plane of the septum pellucidum in which the columns of the fornix, defined as two hypoechoic tubular structures separated by three echogenic interfaces, can be misinterpreted as the cavum.[192] Coronal and sagittal planes either 2D or 3D should be attempted. Transvaginal imaging may also prove helpful.

On US, absence of the septum pellucidum can be diagnosed after 20 weeks and causes the frontal horns to appear fused and squared (Fig. 12.1-28).[187,193] Mild-to-moderate ventriculomegaly

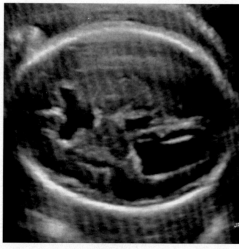

**FIGURE 12.1-28:** Axial image in fetus at 30 weeks with SOD. Note absence of the septum pellucidum, squared frontal horns and mild ventriculomegaly.

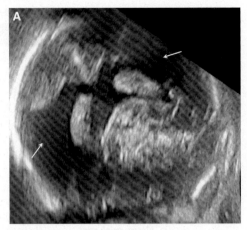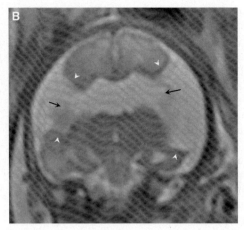

**FIGURE 12.1-29:** Fetus at 36 weeks with SOD with bilateral open-lipped schizencephaly. **A:** Axial oblique US demonstrates absence of the septum pellucidum and large bilateral frontal defects *(arrows)*. **B:** Coronal T2 MR demonstrates open-lipped schizencephaly defects *(arrows)* lined with gray matter *(arrowheads)*. Notice absence of the septum pellucidum. This fetus would be considered in the spectrum of SOD-plus.

may be present, likely because of white matter volume loss. Defects in the brain parenchyma extending from the lateral ventricles to the arachnoid space, especially when bilateral and frontal, are typical findings of open-lipped schizencephaly (Fig. 12.1-29A).

Three-dimensional axial reconstruction of the brain at the level of the circle of Willis can be helpful in confirming normal pituitary tissue and evaluating the optic nerve/tracts.[194,195] Although measurement of the optic tract can be difficult to obtain, recent US data have shown a linear increase in optic tract diameter with gestational age (Table 25B of Appendix A1).[195] Comparing these standards with optic tract diameter, hypoplasia can be diagnosed.[195]

*MRI:* MRI has been shown to be 100% accurate when identifying absence of the septum pellucidum, whereas US has been noted to detect only 70%.[196] On MRI, excellent thin sagittal and coronal view of the midline is important. Similar to US, when the septum pellucidum is absent, the frontal horns will appear square, bat wing, or boxlike (Fig. 12.1-30A). There is usually low position of the fornices, which may be fused, and mild dilatation of the suprasellar cistern and anterior recess of the third ventricle (Fig. 12.1-30B).[197] In the presence of severe hypoplasia of the optic nerves, the imaging may be suggestive, but mild optic nerve hypoplasia is usually difficult to diagnose prenatally, owing to the small size of the nerve, slice thickness, and angle of

the chiasm with regard to the imaging plane.[196] Clinical postnatal opthalmalogic exam remains the standard reference. The pituitary gland can be identified on T2 and T1weighted imaging. In the fetus, both the anterior and the posterior lobe are hyperintense on T1-weighted sequences; therefore, no distinction is typically possible between the anterior and the posterior lobes, unless the posterior is ectopic.[194] Schizencephaly, usually in the frontal lobe area, should be excluded (Fig. 12.1-29B).

**Associated Anomalies:** Up to 75% of patients with SOD have associated brain anomalies, the most common being bilateral polymicrogyria with or without clefting (schizencephaly), followed by cortical heterotopias.[181,185] Fusion of the fornices and thinning or absence of the corpus callosum is often present.[181] Cerebellar hypoplasia, encephaloceles, and cortical dysplasias are frequent. Absence of the olfactory bulbs and tracts is also rarely identified.[198] Dysmorphic features, especially of the head (macrocephaly/microcephaly) and face, are often noted.[185] Genital anomalies and delayed skeletal maturation are usually attributed to pituitary dysfunction.[185] Limb abnormalities such as constriction rings, syndactyly, and reduction deformity of the digits are not uncommonly described.[184,189]

**Differential Diagnosis:** Absence of the septum pellucidum is associated with various malformations, including HPE, ACC,

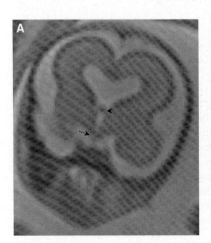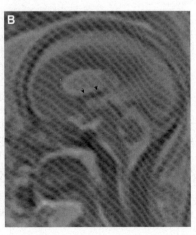

**FIGURE 12.1-30:** Fetus at 23 weeks with SOD. **A:** Coronal T2 image demonstrates absence of the septum pellucidum. The fornix is fused *(arrowhead)*. The optic nerves are identified *(dotted arrow)* but it is difficult to exclude hypopla... **B:** Sagittal T2 image from same fetus again demonstr... low position of fused fornix *(arrows)*. No pituitary a... mality was detected despite T1 imaging. The morp... in this fetus may be considered to be in the spe... lobar HPE. Note also absence of the secondary p...

and predominately basilar encephaloceles.[197] Fusion of the hemispheres and basal ganglia, especially in the presence of facial anomalies, support the diagnosis of HPE. However, some cases of lobar holoprosencephaly overlap and may be difficult to separate from SOD.[199] In ACC, typical findings should be sought, including separated ventricles, colpocephaly, and radial array of medial sulci. Disruption of the septum can occur because of hydrocephalus from AS or Chiari malformations and in an encephaloclastic event, such as hydranencephaly and porencephaly.

**Prognosis:** The outcome for patients with SOD ranges from mild-to-severe endocrine and neurologic dysfunction. Isolated absence of septum is rare and even when present, most if not all have neurologic deficits.[196,200] Patients with complete absence of the septum pellucidum have worse neurological and developmental outcome than those with partial absence. Those with isolated optic nerve findings have good developmental prognosis.[200] However, in the presence of hemisphere abnormalities and posterior pituitary ectopia, the prognosis is more guarded.[200]

Endocrine abnormalities are variable, and 22% with abnormal septum and normal pituitary have endocrine dysfunction, versus 25% with normal septum and abnormal pituitary, and 56% with abnormal septum and pituitary. Overall, in 50% to 90% of patients with SOD, there is associated early or delayed hypothalamic–pituitary dysfunction, usually manifesting at a mean age of 4 to 5 years as growth retardation secondary to decreased levels of growth hormone and thyroid-stimulating hormone.[182,193,201] Rarely, individuals with SOD may exhibit precocious puberty.[201] Diabetes insipidus and hypoglycemia are less commonly associated.[183,201]

Visual symptoms include normal vision, decreased acuity or nystagmus. Neurologic deficits range from global retardation (55% to 78%) to focal deficits such as epilepsy (22%) or hemiparesis.[182,189,201] In addition, over half have behavioral disorders, nearly one-third diagnosed with autism.[189]

**Management:** Prenatal management includes possible termination of the pregnancy or no alteration of standard obstetrical care.[187] Early recognition of pituitary dysfunction is important. Low maternal serum and urinary estriol levels can suggest fetal adrenal insufficiency and aid in the diagnosis of SOD.[193] Hypopituitarism is a serious problem, and failure to recognize carries a risk of adrenal crisis, hypoglycemia, and death.[182] Given the possibility for later development of hormonal deficiencies, long-term follow-up is necessary.[189] Neurologic consultation is important in the presence of seizures or neurologic delay.

**Recurrence:** Most cases are sporadic with low recurrence risk at 2% to 3%.[202] The risk may be increased in the presence of familial transmission.

# DISORDERS OF CORTICAL/CNS DEVELOPMENT

Cortical disorders are classified by the pattern of development, which includes the overlapping phases of cell lineage, proliferation, differentiation, migration, and organization (Table 12.1-7). In humans, cell lineage defines the basic cell type, and then proliferation takes place from 5 - 6 weeks in the ventricular zone after the neural tube is complete. Neuron and glial cells arise

| Table 12.1-7 | Disorders of Cortical (CNS) Formation | |
|---|---|---|
| **Cell Lineage** | *Abnormal* | Hemimegalencephaly Tuberous sclerosis |
| **Proliferation** | *Decreased* | Microcephaly/ microlissencephaly/ simplified gyral |
| | *Increased* | Macrocephaly/ megalencephaly |
| **Differentiation** | *Abnormal* | Cortical dysplasia CNS tumors |
| | ***Leptomeningeal*** | Arachnoid cyst |
| | ***Choroid*** | Choroid plexus cyst |
| | ***Neuroepithelial*** | Glioependymal cyst |
| | ***Vascular*** | Vein of Galen |
| **Migration** | *Undermigration* | Lissencephaly Heterotopia |
| | *Overmigration* | Congenital muscular dystrophy |
| **Organization** | *Deranged* | Polymicrogyria Schizencephaly |

from neuroblast precursors primarily to 15 - 20 weeks (finished 30 weeks) through approximately 35 divisions. Differentiation of the neurons and glial cell into a refined cell type is followed by migration between 6 - 7 weeks to 20 - 24 weeks. Cortical organization starts at 22 weeks and continues until 2 years of age. It should be stressed that disorders of cortical development often present with multiple coexisting anomalies of neuronal transition. In these instances, the cortical disorder is described by the earliest disturbed developmental process.[203]

Pathology related to cortical development is caused by lack of normal gene expression, production of an abnormal gene, or interruption of gene function via infection or ischemia.[204] Unfortunately, the etiology is unknown in about 50% of cases.[203] At the same time as cortical development, differentiation and evolution of the leptomeninges, choroid, and intracranial vasculature is occurring. CNS pathologies in these areas will be inserted for completeness.

## Disorders of Cellular Lineage

### Hemimegalencephaly

**Incidence:** Hemimegalencephaly (HME) is a rare sporadic disorder. It is cited in 1 to 3 cases per 1,000 epileptic children and is equal in sex distribution.[205,206]

**Pathogenesis:** Hemimegalencephaly is a hamartomatous brain malformation characterized by overdevelopment and enlargement of all or part of one cerebral hemisphere (Fig. 12.1-31). In this disorder, cells are altered in their growth and/or differentiation with disorganization of the tissue architecture such that there is an abnormal gyral pattern in the affected hemisphere that may manifest as agyria, pachygyria, polygyria, and polymicrogryia. Hemimegalencephaly is isolated in approximately 53% to 66% of cases. In the remaining, it is seen in

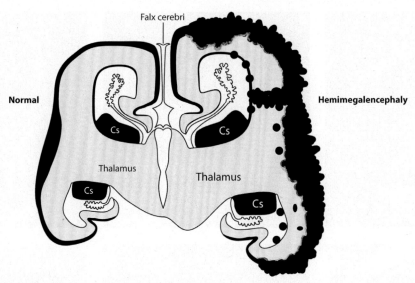

**FIGURE 12.1-31:** Hemimegalencephaly of the left hemisphere showing overgrowth with abnormal migration of gray matter and cortical development.

conjunction with neurocutaneous syndromes including epidermal nevus, Proteus, neurofibromatosis type I, hypomelanosis of Ito, Klippel–Weber–Trenaunay, and tuberous sclerosis.[206,305] In these syndromes, hemicorporal hypertrophy may be present. Total hemimegalencephaly is a rare form described in the presence of ipsilateral enlargement of the cerebral hemisphere, brainstem, and cerebellum.[207]

Current studies suggest that hemimegalencephaly occurs at 3 to 4 weeks' gestation because of a primary disturbance in cellular lineage and cell growth, with secondary effects being disturbed cell migration and organization.[205,208] A recent fetal pathologic evaluation of hemimegalencephaly found a normal number of cells in the proliferative zone.[205] Microscopically, the cells are immature or abnormal with mixed lineage and disturbed morphology, and there is a complete disorganization of the cytoarchitecture and loss of normal lamination with giant immature neurons and glial cells within the cortex and white matter.[205,208] Bizarre glial cells, or balloon cells, myelination delay, and white matter gliosis have been described postnatally.

**Etiology:** It has been hypothesized that genes involving neuraxis or body left right symmetry are involved in the disorder.[209] Advances in recent genetics have shown de novo somatic mutations in components of the phosphatidylinositol 3-kinase (P13K)-AKT mammalian target of rapamycin (mTOR) pathway in HME cases.[210] These genes, which include *AKT3, PIK3CA, PIK3R2,* and *MTOR,* are critical for regulation of cellular proliferation, size, and metabolism.[210] Several of these genes are also linked to overgrowth syndromes and tumors.

### Diagnosis

***Ultrasound:*** Prenatal diagnosis should be suspected in the presence of UVM, with the most commonly dilated area being the posterior horn of the lateral ventricle (Fig. 12.1-32A). The head circumference is increased, usually in the 90th percentile. In conjunction, midline shift, usually in the occipital area, is noted due to asymmetry of the cerebral hemispheres.[211]

Three-dimensional multiplanar reconstruction may be helpful in detecting subtle asymmetry.[212] Sometimes, especially with 3D and transvaginal imaging, abnormal sulcation and cortical thickening along the affected hemisphere can be noted (Fig. 12.1-32B).

***MRI:*** The enlarged hemisphere will have deformity of the lateral ventricle with diffuse dilatation and/or straightening or collapse of the frontal horn and/or disproportionate dilatation of the occipital horn (colpocephaly) (Fig. 12.1-32C,D).[207] The midline is straight or displaced contralaterally, especially in the occipital area. The white matter may be increased in volume and may demonstrate abnormal decreased signal because of heterotopia, gliosis, or abnormal myelination (Fig. 12.1-32D).[213] Sulcation is abnormal for gestational age, demonstrating thick cortex with too many lobulations or not enough, which later will manifest as polymicrogryria, pacygyria, and agyria. The dysplastic gray and white matter is typically heterogeneous, demonstrating increased and decreased T1 and T2 signals, respectively (Fig. 12.1-32E).[214] There typically is loss of normal fetal brain layering and blurring of gray white matter interfaces.[207] The corpus callosum, particularly on the affected side, may be thick (Fig. 12.1-32F).[207] Restricted diffusion can be present, likely owing to increased cellularity in the affected hemisphere.[215] In the presence of a mild case, the distribution may be primarily lobar. In 40% of cases of HME, enlarged deep and/or superficial veins can be seen along the enlarged hemisphere (Fig. 12.1-33).[207,216] The ipsilateral cerebellar hemisphere can be enlarged in 47%, although only 7% will demonstrate ipsilateral brainstem hypertrophy. Abnormal folia of the cerebellum may be identified bilaterally.[216] In 26% of cases, ipsilateral olfactory and in 3% optic nerve enlargement can accompany HME.[216] The opposite hemisphere may be smaller than normal and distorted due to midline shift.

**Associated Anomalies:** Of the neurocutaneous syndromes, epidermal nevus syndrome is the most commonly associated and typically presents with linear nevus, sebaceous nevus, and facial lipoma and hypertrophy typically on the affected

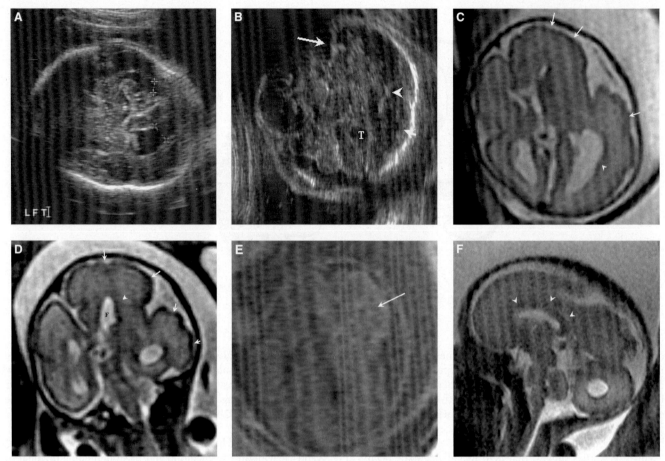

**FIGURE 12.1-32:** Hemimegalencephaly in a 29-week fetus. **A:** Axial US demonstrates mild dilatation of the left lateral ventricle at 11 m versus opposite of 7 mm. Note slight shift of the left occipital lobe across midline. Head circumference was increased. **B:** Coronal US demonstrates subtle asymmetry of sizes of the hemisphere with left larger than right and shift of midline falx *(arrow)*. The left temporal horn *(T)* is prominent. *Arrowheads* point to subtle lobulation along the cortex. **C:** Axial T2 MR demonstrates enlargement of the left hemisphere and dilated occipital horn. Note nodularity *(arrowhead)* along ventricle consistent with heterotopia. The cortex *(arrows)* demonstrates abnormal sulcation (compare with normal opposite side). **D:** Coronal image demonstrates straightened frontal *(F)* horn with abnormal dark signal *(arrowhead)* in the white matter consistent with disorganized neurons. There is again abnormal sulcation with blurring of normal gray white interface *(arrows)*. **E:** Axial T1-weighted image demonstrates increased T1 signal *(arrow)* in the abnormal hemisphere. **F:** Sagittal T2 demonstrates thickening of the corpus callosum *(arrowheads)*.

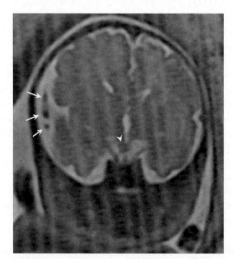

**FIGURE 12.1-33:** Subtle case of right HME in a fetus at 34 weeks. Notice prominent extra-axial space along the abnormal right hemisphere with large dilated veins *(arrows)*. The right optic chiasm is also enlarged *(arrowhead)*.

hemispheric side.[209] Abnormal vascular shunting over the enlarged hemisphere can lead to congestive heart failure.[213]

**Differential Diagnosis:** The main differential is cerebral hemisphere enlargement due to tumor or hemorrhage. Shift of midline structure also may be related to volume loss in one hemisphere.

**Prognosis:** Symptoms are similar in the isolated and syndromic children.[209] The worse developmental outcome has been correlated with the most severe cerebral asymmetry.[210,213] Those with severe HME are at risk of mortality in the first year of life.[207] However, most patients demonstrate developmental delay, psychomotor deficits, progressive hemiparesis, and intractable seizures.[205] The marked hyperexcitability of the dysplastic cortex results in catastrophic epilepsy, with seizures typically beginning in the first 6 months of life.[211] It has been found that the earlier the onset of seizures, the more severe motor and intellectual deficit in children with HME.[209]

**Management:** Therapy is directed to seizure control. Although anticonvulsant drug therapy may be utilized in mild cases, the most common treatment option is surgery. In the past, anatomical total or partial hemispherectomy was performed but at a high morbidity secondary to development of hydrocephalus, intracranial hematomas, and infection.[205,206] Because of fewer complications, the most common surgical approach is now a functional hemispherectomy, a technique which involves disrupting internal capsule and corona radiata with resection and interruption of the mesial temporal structures, section of the corpus callosum, and frontal horizontal fibers.[214] After surgery, approximately 60% to 85% of children have control of their seizures.[210,214] With control of the seizures, there is improved intellectual and physical development.[211,214] For this reason, most advocate surgery as early as possible to preserve neurologic development.[214]

**Recurrence:** Hemimegalencephaly is mostly sporadic with low recurrence risk.

### Tuberous Sclerosis

Tuberous Sclerosis, or Bourneville disease, is the second most common phakomatosis (after neurofibromatosis type 1), representing a neurocutaneous syndrome characterized by the formation of benign hamartomas and low-grade neoplasms in multiple organ systems, most notably the brain, heart, kidneys, and skin.

**Incidence:** Tuberous sclerosis (TS) has an autosomal dominant inheritance with variable expression and incomplete penetrance. The incidence is 1 in 10,000, and prevalence is 1 per 6,000 to 10,000 live births.[217] The disorder occurs equally in all races and both genders.

**Pathogenesis:** TS is characterized by widespread development of hamartomas in many different tissues owing to a disorder of cell lineage. TS is similar to hemimegalencephaly but has pathologically more cellular and nuclear pleomorphism and a potential for neoplastic formation.[208] Almost all patients with TS have cutaneous stigmata, with the most common and earliest being multiple hypopigmented macules known as ashleaf spots. Adenoma sebaceum, a misnomer, is present in 70% of TS patients, representing angiofibromas on the malar region of the face.[218] Brain lesions include subependymal nodules and cortical tubers, seen in infants in 93% and 88%, respectively, and, less commonly, white matter abnormalities and subependymal giant cell astrocytomas.[219] Tubers are hamartomas that exhibit disorganized cortical lamination with atypical giant astrocytes, maloriented neurons, and bizarre giant cells. Subependymal nodules represent dysplastic astrocytic and neuronal cells. White matter lesions are heterotopic neuronal and glial elements arrested in migration. Subependymal giant cell tumors develop in 10% to 15% of patients with TS but are rare prenatal.[220]

Cardiac rhabdomyomas are the most common cardiac tumors prenatally, with 39% to 80% associated with TS.[221,222] Rhabdomyomas usually present during the second or third trimester and are the most common fetal finding in TS.[219] Renal findings, which include cysts and angiomyolipomas (tumors composed of abnormal blood vessels, smooth muscle, and fat) are rare prenatally, usually developing during childhood and adolescence in approximately 61% of patients.[223] Diagnosis of TS is dependent on identification of two major or one major and two minor features in the complex (Table 12.1-8).

| Table 12.1-8 | Criteria for Diagnosis of Tuberous Sclerosis | |
|---|---|---|
| **Major Features** | **Minor Features** | |
| Facial angiofibroma or forehead plaque | Dental pits | |
| Ungual/periungual fibroma | Hamartomatous rectal polyps | |
| Hypomelanotic macules (>3) | Bone cysts | |
| Shagreen patch | Cerebral white matter migratory tracts | |
| Cortical tuber | Gingival fibromas | |
| Subependymal nodule | Nonrenal hamartoma | |
| Subependymal giant cell astrocytoma | Retinal achromic patch | |
| Multiple retinal nodular hamartomas | "Confetti" skin lesions | |
| Cardiac rhabdomyoma | Multiple renal cysts | |
| Lymphangiomyomatosis | | |
| Renal angiomyolipoma | | |

**Diagnosis**

**Definitive:** 2 major or 1 major plus 2 minor
**Probable:** 1 major plus 1 minor
**Possible:** 1 major or 2 or more minor

**Etiology:** TS is caused by mutations of either the *TSC1* or the *TSC2* gene located on chromosomes 9q34 and 16p13, respectively.[220] The gene products hamartin (*TSC1*) and tuberin (*TSC2*) act as tumor suppressors by negative feedback of the mTOR kinase cascade, whose activity is important in regulating cell growth and proliferation. There is high penetrance of the genetic abnormality, but phenotype expression is variable. Approximately 70% to 80% of TS cases are sporadic, resulting from de novo genetic mutations.[220,224] However, there are cases of recurrence in families of unaffected parents, suggesting a germline mosaicism.[225] *TSC2* mutations are more common, lead to a more severe phenotype, and tend to be spontaneous, while, the *TSC1* are less common and more likely to be familial.[218] Polycystic kidney disease is sometimes associated with TS as the gene responsible for this disorder lies adjacent to the *TSC2* gene.[220]

**Diagnosis:** Genetic testing for the *TSC1* and *TSC2* genes from amniotic fluid or chorionic villus sampling can be definitive in about 80% of mutations.[217] However, because of genetic heterogeneity, testing can have a false negative rate of 10% to 20%.[225] Imaging is often helpful for detection and diagnosis.

***Ultrasound:*** About 80% of fetuses with TS have rhabdomyomas, usually presenting during the second or third trimester, as early as 20 weeks.[225] Rhabdomyomas are typically round, homogeneous echogenic intraluminal and sometimes intramural masses, often located in more than one cardiac chamber but usually along ventricular walls or septum (Fig. 12.1-34A).[224,226] Brain lesions may be present but can be inconspicuous on prenatal US. If identifiable, brain lesions present as an echogenic mass along the lateral ventricular wall or a focal area of echogenicity in the brain parenchyma (Fig. 12.1-34B).[227] Renal masses are rarely detected prenatally but include cysts, multiple cysts as in polycystic kidney disease, or focal smooth echogenic lesions in the renal cortex, consistent with angiomyolipomas (Fig. 12.1-34C).[228]

*MRI:* On prenatal MRI, cortical tubers and subependymal nodules are the most common CNS lesions detected with an incidence of 33% to 62%.[220] Other TS lesions, including white matter abnormalities and subependymal astrocytomas, are less frequent. Prenatal imaging is limited by spatial resolution, and small subtle lesions can be missed.[229] However, both T1 and T2 imaging are important as T1 signal abnormality may be most easily seen.[226,229] In the fetus, the tubers are present in the cortex and/or subcortical white matter of primarily the supratentorial brain and demonstrate wedge-shaped or banded areas of increased T1 and decreased T2 signal, opposite of a myelinated child or adult (Fig. 12.1-34D,E).[229,230] Subependymal nodules can be detected prenatally but may not be evident as many develop through the first decade of life. Subependymal nodules, when present, dot the ependymal surface of the lateral ventricles, especially near the caudate and foramen Monro, and are isointense to gray matter being T1 hyperintense and T2 hypointense (Fig. 12.1-34C,F).[229,230] It is important to verify these lesions in two anatomic planes as motion artifact can mimic a lesion. Ninety percent of subependymal lesions do mineralize, but prenatal diagnosis is unlikely as most do not calcify until 1 year of age.[220,225] Subependymal giant cell astrocystomas are rare prenatally but typically arise near the foramen of Monro, measure greater than 5 mm, grow and can obstruct the ventricular system.[220] Associated rhabdomyomas are isointense to cardiac muscle on T1 and T2 images (Fig. 12.1-34G). Renal lesions may be heterogeneous or follow cystic characteristics (dark T1 and bright T2) (Fig. 12.1-34H).

**Associated Anomalies:** Retinal hamartomas occur in 40% to 50% of patients, with one-third bilateral.[231] Harmartomatous gastrointestinal polyps and oral gingival fibromas can develop. Patients with TS are at increased risk for arterial aneurysms, including aorta, peripheral and intracranial. Pulmonary manifestations are present in 1% to 26% of patients, with the most common being lymphangiomyomatosis.[231] Sclerotic and cystic bone lesions and ungal fibromas adjacent to or underneath the nail bed are sometimes noted.

**Differential Diagnosis:** In the presence of a cardiac mass, the most common differential is a fibroma that is typically solitary T2 hypointense and can be seen with orofacial abnormalities and Gorlin syndrome. Intracranial lesions, especially when solitary, should be differentiated from subacute hemorrhage, tumor, congenital infection, ischemia, or cortical dysplasia of other cause. When lesions are defined along the ventricle, germinal matrix hemorrhage or gray matter heterotopia should be considered.

**Prognosis:** TS increases the risk for adverse maternal and perinatal outcomes; thus close surveillance is indicated.[221] Cardiac rhabdomyomas tend to increase in size in utero and regress after delivery, with 80% resolving in infancy or early childhood.[221,224] Most are well tolerated with only a 4% to 6% risk of fetal demise.[224] In the presence of a large lesion >3 cm, fetal dysrythmia and/or compromised fetal cardiac function due to tumor obstruction, prenatal medication, early delivery, and/or surgery

may be indicated. Preterm delivery in TS is as high as 35% and cesarean delivery is reported at 33%.[221]

The clinical triad of TS, *epilepsy, mental retardation,* and *facial angiofibromas,* is actually noted in only 30% to 40% of patients.[220] The most common cause of morbidity is neurologic, with seizures in 90%, mental retardation in 50%, developmental delay, behavioral problems, and autism in 25% to 50%.[220] Postnatally, there is a correlation between number, size, and, importantly, volume of cerebral lesions and neurodevelopmental outcome.[232] However, it is more difficult to predict outcome prenatally, given lower resolution in fetal imaging and the possibility of lesions developing later in pregnancy and postnatal.[222] TS-associated renal disease also increases the risk of perinatal complications, including renal failure, polyhydramnios, and oligohydramnios. Postnatal, renal complications are the most common cause of death, with 10% developing renal failure or hypertension.[220] Angiomyolipomas that are present in 60% to 80% of TS patients are benign but can cause morbidity in about 10% of cases because of catastrophic hemorrhage, either spontaneous or in the presence of minimal trauma.[218] Polycystic renal disease is noted in 5% of TS patients and confers a worse prognosis.[220] Renal carcinomas are seen in 2% to 3% of patients.[220] In female patients postmenarchal, lymphangiomyomatosis of the lung can develop because of smooth muscle cell metastasizes, with 5% progressing to end-stage lung disease.[220]

**Management:** Diagnosis, screening of family members, and appropriate counseling is indicated. Termination may be considered. Close surveillance during the pregnancy is warranted. In the presence of a complicating rhadomyoma, early delivery may be necessary. Brain imaging and abdominal imaging should assess for neoplasm, complicating renal tumors, and vascular malformations, including aneurysms. Anticonvulsants and surgical resection of tubers are treatments for epilepsy. Rapamycin inhibits mTOR pathway and causes regression of giant cell astrocytomas and may be helpful in the treatment of rhabdomyomas, angiomyolipomas, and lymphangiomyomatosis.[218,231] Embolization of symptomatic or large angiomyolipomas may be necessary.

**Recurrence:** The recurrence risk of an unaffected parent having a child with TS is 2% to 3%.[225] In the presence of an affected parent, transmission is 50%.

## Disorders of Cellular Multiplication/Proliferation

### Microcephaly

**Synonyms:** Microcephaly vera, true microcephaly, radial microbrain, microcephaly with simplified gyral pattern, oligogyria, microlissencephaly.

Microcephaly implies a small head size whereas micrencephaly represents a small brain. In the past, microcephaly has been defined when postnatal head circumference was two standard deviations (SD) or more below the mean, being below the third percentile.[233] More recent data suggest that microcephaly should have a cut-off of −3 SD below the mean.[233]

**Incidence:** Birth incidence is estimated at 1 in 5,400 to 8,500 newborns.[234,235] Higher occurrence is noted with parental consanguinity. Microcephaly may present prenatally; however, a significant number of cases develop postnatal.

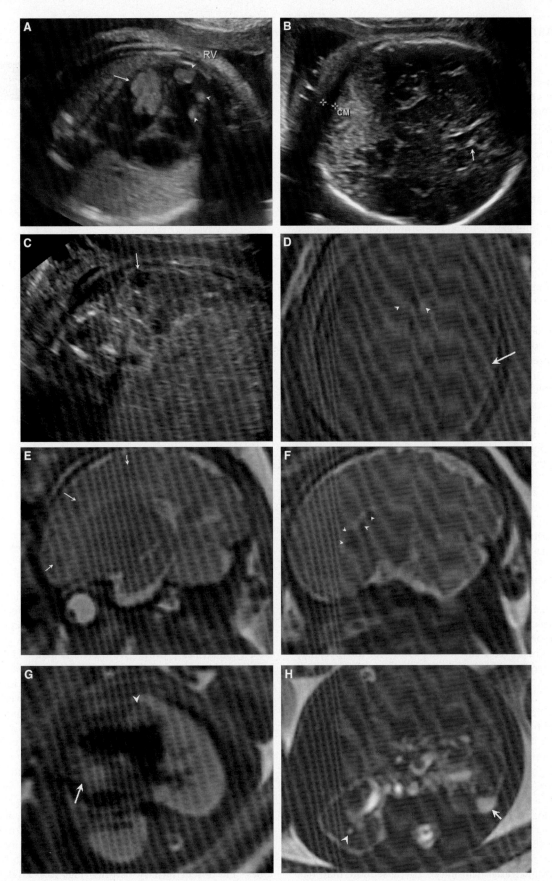

**FIGURE 12.1-34:** Tuberous sclerosis in a fetus at 35 weeks. **A:** Axial US demonstrates multiple homogeneous echogenic masses in the right ventricle *(arrowheads)* and large mass in the left ventricle *(arrow)*. **B:** Axial cranial image shows the area of the foramen Monro with questionable nodularity *(arrow)*. **C:** Axial image of the left kidney demonstrates the presence of a cyst *(arrow)*. **D:** Axial T1 image in the fetal brain demonstrates a band of T1 signal in the left hemisphere consistent with parenchymal tuber *(arrow)*. Also note small hyperintense lesions at the foramen of Monro *(arrowheads)* consistent with small subependymal tubers. **E:** Sagittal T2 image shows focal areas of dark signal *(arrows)* consistent with tubers. **F:** Sagittal T2 demonstrates dark round nodules *(arrowheads)* near the foramen of Monro consistent with subependymal tubers. **G:** Axial T2 image shows T2 hyperintense masses in the left *(arrow)* and right ventricles *(arrowhead)* consistent with rhabdomyomas. **H:** Axial SSFP image through the kidneys confirm left renal cyst *(arrow)* but also defines an additional small right renal lesion *(arrowhead)*.

**Pathogenesis:** Microcephaly results from multiple pathologies that cause either decreased cell production or increased programmed cell death in the germinal zones. Microcephaly can be syndromic, often with other anomalies, or isolated. Primary or congenital microcephaly is typically genetic whereas secondary microcephaly occurs as a result of a destructive insult. Currently, most primary microcephaly pathologies are classified and grouped by the genetic disorder and clinical findings.[203]

In primary or congenital microcephaly, the brain may have a well-preserved gyral pattern or abnormal gyral pattern.[236] Microcephaly without extracerebral malformation in the presence of a small architecturally normal brain and normal gyral pattern is known as true microcephaly or microcephaly vera. Microcephaly with simplified gyral pattern is likely in the continuum of true microcephaly demonstrating reduced gyri, shallow sulci, normal cortical architecture, and normal or reduced thickness cortex. There is a strong correlation between the degree of microcephaly and the presence of a simplified gyral pattern and white matter volume loss.[237] Microlissencephaly is a term that has been utilized previously to describe a brain with abnormal gyration and thickened cortex due to a cortical migrational rather than solely proliferation anomaly. This term is confusing and should be avoided.[237] These pathologies are included here as the earliest insult is abnormal proliferation, which is then associated with disturbed migration. Some currently utilize the term lissencephaly type III to describe a thickened cortex in the presence of severe microcephaly.

**Etiology:** The cause of microcephaly is heterogeneous. Microcephaly may result from chromosomal or genetic disorders or environmental factors that are destructive (Table 12.1-9). Many new loci are being identified, the most common mode of transmission being autosomal recessive.[238] It has been estimated that 20% to 35% of idiopathic microcephaly is hereditary.[239] Genetic associations with microcephaly cannot be completely listed here as more than 500 associations are described in online Mendelian inheritance in man (OMIM). Excluding HPE, in a group of fetuses with microcephaly, 28% have been shown to have abnormal fetal karyotype, 24% genetic syndrome, 28% with complex anomalies, and 20% isolated.[240] The etiology for microcephaly may be detected in only as high as 57%.[241]

### Diagnosis

*Ultrasound:* Prenatal diagnosis may be challenging, particularly in the second trimester, as head measurements may be normal until the third trimester, usually after 27 to 28 weeks.[242,243] Antenatal diagnosis may be lower than 60%.[235] Most concur that fetal microcephaly should only be diagnosed when the head circumference (HC) is smaller than 3 SD below the gestational mean.[242,244] In a recent study by Malinger, there was no deficit in neuropsychological outcome with isolated microcephaly with head circumference −2 to 3 SD below the mean.[244] A biparietal diameter (BPD) and fronto-occipital diameter −3 SD below the mean has also been utilized but can be falsely positive in the presence of calvarial deformity.[243] Because more than half of fetuses with microcephaly are small for gestational age, more than half of HC/abdominal circumference and one-third of HC/femur length ratios are situated within normal range.[240,241]

Sonographic findings that may be helpful include small frontal lobes, sloping forehead, enlarged subarachnoid spaces, and VM due to neuronal loss (Fig. 12.1-35A,B).[233,245] Frontal lobe

| Table 12.1-9 | Causes of Microcephaly |
|---|---|

***Microcephaly with Thin Cortex***
**Genetic**
*Isolated*
 Autosomal recessive, dominant, X linked
*Syndromic*
 Chromosomal
  Trisomy 21, 13, 18
  Gene Deletions
   Wolf-Hirschhorn
   Williams
   Miller-Dieker
 Others
  Smith–Lemli–Opitz
  Cornelia de Lange
  Feingold
  Lymphedema, microcephaly, chorioretinopathy

**Environmental**
 Hypoxic, vascular, intrauterine infection
 Teratogens
  Alcohol
  Hydrantoin
  Radiation
  Maternal phenylketonuria
  Maternal diabetes

***Microcephaly with Thick Cortex (Lissencephaly III)***
 Norman Roberts syndrome
 Barth syndrome
 Seckel syndrome
 Primordial osteodysplastic dwarfism (MOPD 1)

dimensions in the plane of the BPD from the posterior margin of the cavum septum pellucidum to the inner midline fetal skull can identify small frontal lobes and help diagnose microcephaly.[235,246] Sometimes, fetuses with microcephaly have narrow sutures and closed fontanelles providing restricted visibility. However, the brain should be imaged through available windows to exclude abnormal morphology, echos, calcification, and hemorrhage. Poor visualization or smaller caliber of the anterior cerebral circulation when compared with the posterior circulation on Doppler may be helpful.[245] Most cases of microcephaly (83%) are complex; therefore, associated anomalies should be excluded.[240]

*MRI:* A small craniofacial ratio is present, and decreased fronto-occipital and biparietal diameters may be present (Fig. 12.1-35C). In the presence of simplified gyral pattern, MRI early in pregnancy can be diagnostically difficult. Delayed sulcation can be detected after 26 weeks, but confirmation may require imaging after 30 weeks.[247] MRI will identify wide and shallow primary and secondary sulci, especially in the frontal lobes, and absent tertiary fissures (Fig. 12.1-35D).[248,249] The cortex is usually thin (normal 3 to 4 mm), but in some cases can be thick. There is also usually white matter volume loss and mild-to-moderate ventricular dilatation with obliquity of the lateral ventricles. The corpus callosum, brainstem, and cerebellum can be abnormal. Cortical migrational defects should be excluded.

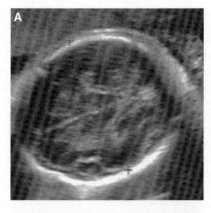
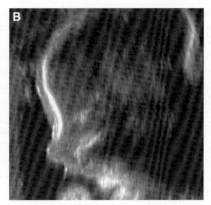
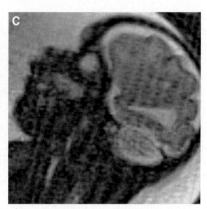
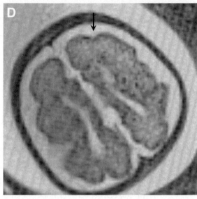

**FIGURE 12.1-35:** Fetus with microcephaly and simplified gyral pattern. **A:** Ultrasound at 28 weeks with BPD measurements (calipers). Head circumference was 3 SD below the mean for age. The frontal lobes appear small. **B:** Sagittal US image demonstrates small head with regard to face and sloping forehead. **C:** Sagittal T2 image from MRI exam performed at 32 weeks showing small brain and prominent face. There is little sulcation along the hemisphere. **D:** Axial T2 image shows small brain and large extra-axial fluid spaces. Only a few sulci are present, and those identified are very shallow *(arrow)*.

**Associated Anomalies:** Microcephaly is often associated with other cortical malformations including agyria, pachygyria, polymicrogyria, and gray matter heterotopia. Agenesis/hypogenesis of corpus callosum, delayed myelination, and dysplasia/hypoplasia of the cerebellum and brainstem may be present.[236,238] In Cohen syndrome, a thick corpus callosum is present with microcephaly.

**Differential Diagnosis:** Holoprosencephaly and lissencephaly have abnormal gyral pattern and often present with microcephaly.[240] Microcephaly can also be seen in conjunction with encephaloceles and craniosynostosis.

**Prognosis:** Prenatal head circumference −3 SD below the mean correlates with microcephaly postnatally; however, those between 2 and 3 SD below may not correspond.[242,244] An occipitofrontal circumference of more than 2 SD below the mean in the past has been considered microcephaly postnatal; however, this value includes 2% of normal individuals with normal cognitive outcome. Evaluation of family head circumference should be considered as small head size may be a normal developmental variant.[236]

Severity of mental delay is related to the severity of microcephaly with median IQ decreasing linearly with head circumference.[244,250] Microcephaly in the presence of abnormal karyotype or intrauterine infection has a poor outcome.[233] The presence of abnormal gyral pattern and/or associated anomalies has also been shown to have a negative impact on outcome.[34,48] Children with microcephaly and preserved gyral pattern demonstrate mild delay in early development, some difficultly with feeding, and limited language skills.[236,238] Those with a simplified or abnormal gyral pattern have a more severe clinical course, including poor feeding, severe developmental delay, intractable epilepsy, and early death.[238] Perinatal mortality for children with microcephaly has been quoted as high as 70%.[240]

**Management:** Microcephaly is not treatable. Evaluation of family head circumference is important as similar small head in the fetus may be a developmental variant. Genetic testing should be performed. Termination of the pregnancy may be considered, depending on chromosomal studies and associated anomalies; however, delayed third trimester diagnosis may limit possibility. Postnatally, children with mild microcephaly usually require special schooling, intensive speech therapy, and early psychomotor support.[247] Children with more severe microcephalies require anticonvulsive therapy and nasogastric tube feeding.[247]

**Recurrence:** Recurrence risk is 25% in the presence of primary microcephaly.[238]

### Macrocephaly/Megalencephaly
Macrocephaly is noted when head circumference is above the 98th percentile or more than 2 standard deviations (SD) above the mean. Megalencephaly indicates a large brain with weight or volume greater than 98th percentile or ≥2 SD above the mean.

**Incidence:** Limited data quote isolated macrocephaly in 0.5% of the population.[251]

**Pathogenesis:** Macrocephaly occurs because of increased neuronal and glial cell proliferation and/or faulty apoptosis. Most cases do not become apparent until the last trimester of pregnancy or postnatally.[252]

**Etiology:** Benign familial macrocephaly accounts for approximately 50% of the cases and is transmitted autosomal dominant.[233,253] Megalencephaly may be associated with over 200 genetic syndromes, many of which are difficult to diagnose prenatally.[252,253] Common genetic disorders with enlarged head size include overgrowth, cutaneous, and polymicrogyria syndromes.[236] Rarely, macrocephaly may be related to chromosomal microdeletions.[252]

### Diagnosis

*Ultrasound:* Prenatal US diagnosis of macrocephaly has been detected as early as 18 weeks.[254] However, most fetuses with macrocephaly have a normal second-trimester head circumference, and diagnosis is not made until late in the pregnancy or postnatally.[252] Fetuses with larger head circumference (HC) and associated anomalies due to associated syndromes will tend to be identified earlier (28 weeks) versus those with isolated macrocephaly (32 weeks).[252] When macrocephaly is identified, head circumference growth will be proportional rather than accelerated.[254] Note should be made that enlarged fetal head circumference has low specificity, with only 67% of children diagnosed prenatally having large head circumference postnatally.[251] Some of this variation is technical, related to limitations in accuracy of HC but also inconsistencies between prenatal and postnatal derived HC growth curves.[251] Most fetuses with macrocephaly will be large for gestational age.[252]

*MRI:* Similar findings are present, including increased craniofacial ratio and head measurements for gestational age. Mild ventriculomegaly and enlarged extra-axial fluid spaces are often present and in isolation are common for benign macrocephaly (Fig. 12.1-36).[252] In syndromic cases, frontal bossing, callosal anomalies, including thick corpus callosum, and cortical migrational abnormalities may be present. A thick corpus callosum has been linked to enlarged white matter, and can be seen in syndromes such as neurofibromatosis type I and macrocephaly–capillary malformation.[255] In the presence of additional white matter signal abnormality and significantly enlarged extraaxial spaces, glutaric aciduria type 1 should be considered.[256]

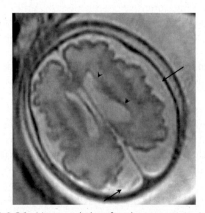

**FIGURE 12.1-36:** Macrocephaly of unknown origin in a fetus at 33 weeks. Head circumference on US was at 3 SD above the mean. MRI biparietal and fronto-occipital dimensions were increased. Axial T2 image demonstrates enlarged extra-axial fluid spaces (*arrows*) and mild asymmetric left lateral ventricular dilatation (*arrowheads*).

**Associated Anomalies:** Macrocephaly is present in the overgrowth syndromes, which include Sotos, Weaver, Simpson–Golabi–Behmel, Gorlin, Macrocephaly-cutis marmorata telangiectatica, and Beckwith Wiedemann. Many of these fetuses are at increased risk for brain, heart, limb, and spine anomalies.[253] Fragile X is also an overgrowth syndrome in white males with facial abnormalities.[257] Cutaneous syndromes, presenting with soft tissue masses, related to mutations in the PTEN (phosphatase and tensin homolog deleted on chromosome TEN) include Bannayan–Riley-Ruvalcaba and Cowden syndrome. Neurofibromatosis type I has cutaneous café au lait lesions and nerve sheath tumors and neuro-cardio-facial-cutaneous syndromes, such as Noonan and LEOPARD, may have heart, face, or soft tissue abnormalities.[257]

**Differential Diagnosis:** Macrocephaly may be secondary to other pathologies, including hydrocephalus, triploidy, and intracranial neoplasms. Disproportionate head size due to intrauterine growth restriction should also be considered.

**Prognosis/Management:** Prognosis is dependent on associated anomalies, etiology, and head size.[252] Prenatal head circumference between 2 and 3 SD above the mean is typically isolated and has a good outcome, while a head circumference >3SD is more likely to be syndromic with developmental delay.[251,252] Children with isolated, particularly familial, macrocephaly usually have normal intelligence with enlarged CSF spaces normalizing by 3 to 4 years of age.[233,251,257] Macrocephaly in the presence of a syndrome is often associated with abnormal development. In 3% to 10% of children with overgrowth syndromes, there is risk for neoplasms.[253]

**Management:** Prenatal evaluation should include family history and parental/sibling head circumference measurements to evaluate for benign familial macrocephaly. Amniocentesis for karyotype and microarray may be considered. Postnatal imaging and evaluation by appropriate pediatrician and clinical geneticist is suggested.[254]

**Recurrence:** Type of genetic transmission guides recurrence risk.

## Disorders of Cellular Differentiation

### CNS Tumors

**Incidence:** The overall incidence of perinatal brain tumors range 1.4 to 3.6 per 100,000.[258] Fetal intracranial tumors are very rare, accounting for approximately 0.5% to 1.9% of intracranial tumors in childhood.[259] Brain tumors represent only 10% of all antenatal tumors.[260]

**Pathogenesis:** Fetal intracranial tumors are "congenital tumors" that have a different pathophysiology than typical pediatric neoplasms. Normal embryonic cells have a high mitotic rate like neoplasms. Fetal tumor development is believed to be due to lack of normal cellular differentiation and maturation of these embryonic cells. In the presence of high mitotic activity, it is not surprising that many of these lesions, whether benign or malignant, grow rapidly and reach enormous proportions. Fetal tumors are also different in prevalence, location, histologic, and biologic behaviors (Table 12.1-10).[259,260] Unlike pediatric tumors, fetal masses tend to be supratentorial, either cerebral

| Table 12.1-10 | Types of Fetal Brain Tumors, Prevalence, and Location[259,260] | |
|---|---|---|
| **Type** | **Prevalence (%)** | **Location** |
| Teratoma | 42 | Cerebral hemisphere, suprasellar, pineal |
| Astryocytoma | 25 | Cerebral hemisphere, basal nuclei |
| Craniopharyngioma | 11 | Suprasellar |
| Primitive neuroectodermal | 10 | Cerebral hemisphere, cerebellum |
| Choroid plexus papilloma | 5 | Intraventricular |
| Meningeal | 4 | Extraaxial |
| Ependymoma | 3 | Ventricular |

hemisphere, suprasellar, or pineal; however, many are undetermined because of size and extent.[260,261] The type of tumor histology is also different, with teratomas being the most common.[259] Fetal tumors often cause demise because of their size and location, inhibiting normal organ development. Large tumors may result in cardiovascular compromise and hydrops.

**Etiology:** *Teratomas* represent abnormal development of pluripotent cells of three germ layers and immature neuroglial elements, can be benign or malignant, and often arise along the midline. There are several forms described: large replacing all intracranial contents, small with hydrocephalus, or as bulky lesions with extension into orbit, oropharynx, or neck.[259] Because many are very large, it is difficult to identify site of origin, but when determined most are in cerebral hemispheres, third or lateral ventricles, and the pineal region. The lesions are complex, containing solid and cystic areas with or without calcification.

*Astrocytomas* are composed of astrocytes of varying degrees of differentiation, from low-grade to high-grade. Unlike pediatric aged tumors, fetal astrocytomas are found supratentorial rather than posterior fossa.[259] Glioblastomas (malignant/high-grade astrocytoma) represent greater than 50% of fetal astrocytomas and are found in the cerebral hemisphere and basal nuclei.[259] Hemorrhage and rapid growth are a common findings.

*Craniopharyngiomas* are epithelial tumors which arise from Rathke pouch, an ectodermal diverticulum important for development of the pituitary gland. Tumors are usually suprasellar and heterogeneous, frequently containing calcification.

*Primitive neuroectodermal tumors* (PNET) are a group of small blue cell malignant lesions which are believed to arise from the neural crest cells of the nervous system and soft tissues. There is overlap of this group with atypical teratoid/rhabdoid tumors (ATRT), with cells mimicking a rhabdomyosarcoma. These tumors may arise in the cerebral hemispheres or cerebellum, are very aggressive, and metastasize early to the cerebral spinal fluid and meninges. Extensive hemorrhage and necrosis in a very large mass is common.

*Choroid plexus papillomas* are composed of mature epithelial cells which line the ventricular choroid plexus. Papillomas are benign and most common prenatally, although carcinomas have rarely been encountered. These lesions are nodular, cauliflower-like lesions typically in the lateral, less likely third or fourth ventricle. The tumor is vascular and secretes CSF, and therefore can cause rapid onset hydrocephalus.

*Meningeal* are benign or malignant mesenchymal tumors arising from the meninges of primarily the middle and less likely anterior or posterior cranial fossa. Hemangiopericytoma is the main histology. The lesion may create a large bulge in the skull with cranial asymmetry.

*Ependymal* lesions arise from the ependymal cells lining the ventricles or spinal cord central canal. Most are very cellular, and ependymoblastomas, which overlap with PNET, are described. These lesions also metastasize to the CSF pathways and tend to have extensive necrosis with location in the lateral and fourth ventricles.

### Diagnosis

***Ultrasound:*** Most fetal tumors present in the third trimester of pregnancy, with 60% diagnosed later than 30 weeks' gestation.[262] US may be obtained because of a sudden increase in maternal uterine size. Polyhydramnios, owing to decreased fetal swallowing, and macrocephaly are the typical presenting signs.[263]

Initial imaging findings include macrocephaly and intracranial mass (Fig. 12.1-37A). The third most common is hydrocephalus (Table 12.1-11). Masses, in general, displace midline structures and distort normal anatomy. In the presence of an enormous lesion, it may not be possible to identify normal cerebrum, midline structures, or ventricles (Fig. 12.1-37B,C).[258,264] The most common etiology for a large mass and undefined origin is teratoma.

Most tumors are heterogeneous rather than homogeneous echogenic. Heterogeneous lesions often have cystic or necrotic areas and the differential of teratoma, craniopharyngiomas, astrocytomas/glial tumors, PNET, and ependymal mass. In the presence of a primarily cystic lesion, teratoma is the prime consideration, but sometimes the mass may be difficult to discern from benign cystic lesions.[264] Calcification in a heterogeneous mass can point to teratoma or craniopharyngioma. A homogeneous vascular echogenic lesion, especially intraventricular with hydrocephalus, would support choroid plexus papilloma (Fig. 12.1-38A).[265] Doppler typically demonstrates vascularization in a mass, although a minor amount may show no Doppler signal, and thus it can be difficult to exclude hematoma.[265] Location may help with diagnosis. The overall accuracy in diagnosis of cell type by US is approximately 57%.[264]

***MRI:*** MRI is ideally suited in the evaluation of fetal tumors and can confirm diagnosis. The internal architecture and extension of the tumor are better assessed by MRI than US.[265] Identification of tumor location and presence of additional lesions may help in definition of cell type. Most lesions are heterogeneous, being isotense on T1-weighted images and hyperintense on T2-weighted images.[265] Choroid plexus papillomas are lobular homogeneous iso-hyperintense on T1 and hypointense on T2 imaging (Fig. 12.1-38B). The solid tissue in PNET and ependymomas may be T1 and T2 isointense to gray matter (Fig. 12.1-39A,B). The presence of hemorrhage, which is described in 3% to 18% of intracranial masses, is most commonly observed in glioblastoma and PNET.[258] Hemorrhage can be detected on T1 sequences as bright signal and gradient echo images with susceptibility artifact (Fig. 12.1-39C).[266] Punctate dark areas on T2, bright areas on T1, or susceptibility artifact on gradient echo may define foci of calcification. Diffusion-weighted

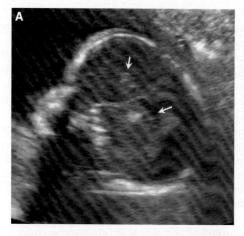

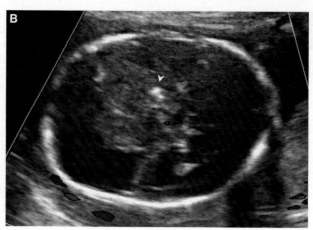

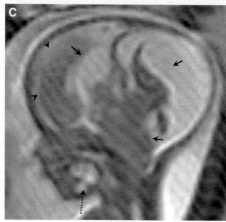

**FIGURE 12.1-37:** Fetus at 21 weeks with intracranial teratoma. **A:** Sagittal US demonstrates macrocephaly and heterogeneous mass replacing most of the brain *(arrows)*. **B:** Axial color US shows a heterogeneous mass with echogenic area *(arrowhead)* that shadowed consistent with calcification. There is some internal blood flow. **C:** Sagittal T2 image of primarily isointense mass containing cystic area anteriorly. The lesion is present in both the supratentorial and the infratentorial location *(arrows)*, replacing most of the normal brain. Small normal brain anteriorly *(arrowheads)*. Fetus also had a sacrococcygeal teratoma, and cystic lesion at the base of the tongue *(dashed arrow)* confirmed to be a teratoma.

imaging is often positive in the presence of PNET and may be helpful in identification of metastasis (Fig. 12.1-39D).[266]

**Associated Anomalies:** Approximately 12.5% of fetal brain tumors have associated anomalies.[261] Many are present in the head or face, with cleft lip or palate being the most frequent.[258] Familial syndromes that have higher incidence of tumors include neurofibromatosis type I (optic glioma/astrocytoma), neurofibromatosis type II (schwannoma, meningioma, astrocytoma, ependymoma), TS (giant cell astrocytoma), von Hippel–Lindau (hemangioblastomas) and Li-Fraumeni (PNET, astrocytoma). Chromosomal studies may show karyotype abnormalities.[262]

**Differential Diagnosis:** Many intracranial masses are missed as they mimic more common conditions such as hemorrhage and hydrocephalus. In the presence of hemorrhage, Doppler shows no flow and MRI may be helpful to exclude mass with or without hemorrhage. Primarily cystic tumors can mimic infarct, porencephaly, arachnoid cyst, or interhemispheric cysts. Other benign lesions to include in the differential are lipomas, hamartomas, intracranial hemangiomas, and vascular malformations. Lipomas are well-defined midline homogeneous echogenic masses often in association with ACC. Hemangiomas are typically extra-axial and appear as a highly vascularized echogenic mass with cysts owing to blood degradation.

| Table 12.1-11 | Prenatal Imaging Findings in Brain Tumors[259,260] |
|---|---|
| Macrocephaly | 58% |
| Intracranial mass | 58% |
| Hydrocephalus | 52% |
| Intrauterine death | 35% |
| Mass filling intracranial cavity | 21% |
| Brain replaced by tumor | 21% |
| Hydramnios | 12% |
| Cephalopelvic disproportion | 11% |
| Breech | 10% |
| Hemorrhage | 8% |
| Fetal hydrops | 6.5% |

**Prognosis:** A fetus with a brain tumor has a poor prognosis.[259] Approximately 35% are stillborn. Overall survival rate is only 15%. Prognosis worsens with increasing tumor size and decreasing gestational age at diagnosis.[259,262] Death of the child shortly after birth is not uncommon.[259] Intracranial teratomas, glioblastomas, and PNET have the lowest survival rate of brain tumors (6% to 8%).[259] A fetus with meningeal tumor has an overall survival rate of 17%, and those with astrocytoma approximately 21%, usually in the presence of low-grade lesions. Craniopharyngiomas have higher survival at 23% and choroid plexus papillomas the best survival at 37.5%.[207] In those cases in which the tumor is resectable postnatally, overall survival is approximately 67%.[259]

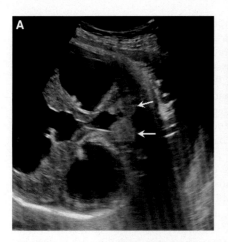

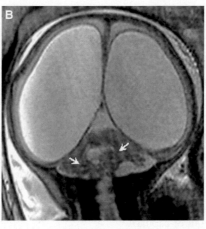

**FIGURE 12.1-38:** Fetus with choroid plexus papilloma. **A:** Axial ultrasound demonstrates severe lateral and third ventricular dilatation with bilobed echogenic mass *(arrows)* filling the fourth ventricle. **B:** Coronal T2 image in same fetus shows primarily T2 hypointense bilobed mass *(arrows)* in the fourth ventricle. Notice severe ventriculomegaly and compressed supratentorial brain. (Courtesy of Chris Cassady, MD.)

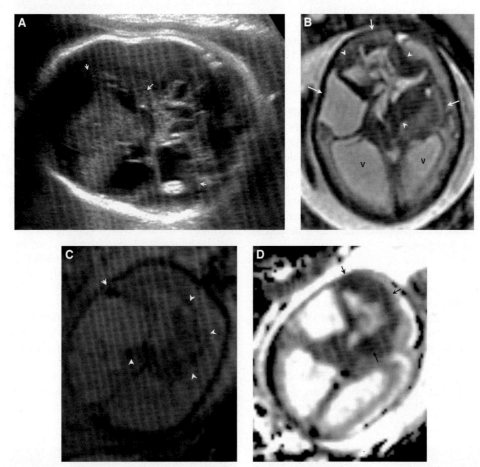

**FIGURE 12.1-39:** Fetus with suspected PNET at 33 weeks with perinatal demise. **A:** Axial US demonstrates heterogeneous echogenic mass with cystic components centered in frontal lobe distorting anatomy. Ultrasound one month prior was normal. **B:** Axial T2 MR image demonstrates a large heterogeneous solid and cystic lesion centered in frontal lobe *(arrows)*. Note rind of tissue that demonstrates hypointense T2 signal *(arrowheads)*. There is bilateral obstructive ventriculomegaly *(V)*. **C:** Gradient echo axial image demonstrates multiple areas of susceptibility artifact *(arrowheads)*, suggesting hemorrhage. **D:** Restricted diffusion *(arrows)* is noted as dark signal on the ADC map. Findings support a high grade cellular lesion.

**Management:** Imaging to identify site and size of the lesion allows an obstetric plan of management to be made prenatally. Many times, the imaging is nonspecific, and histologic diagnosis is obtained after birth. With hydrocephalus, cephalocentesis may be repeated to decrease mass effect on the developing brain.[263] Early delivery, at or even before 34 weeks, may be considered.[263] In the presence of a large mass, cranial decompression or cephalocentesis

may be required for vaginal delivery, but most believe cesarean section should be performed to prevent dystocia.[261,263] Postnatal treatment may be solely supportive care. In the presence of hydrocephalus, a shunt is indicated. Surgical resection of the primary tumor, followed by chemotherapy, is typical therapy. Radiation is contraindicated because of side effects on normal brain development. Survivors often have significant psychomotor deficits.[260,261]

**Recurrence:** Most are sporadic except in the case of familial or genetic predisposition.[262]

## Disorders of Choroid, Leptomeningeal, Neuroepithelial, and Vascular Differentiation

### Choroid Plexus Cyst

**Incidence:** Choroid plexus cysts (CPC) occur in about 0.18% to 3.6% of routine midgestation ultrasounds.[267,268]

**Pathogenesis:** The choroid plexus (CP) first appears as a lobulated protrusion of ependymal epithelium accompanied by mesenchyme and pia mater in the 6th week of gestation. In the 8th week, the CP becomes wavy because of formation of capillary loops, and in the 9th week, the CP produces CSF.[269] Loose mesenchyme stroma, scattered islets of nucleated blood cells, and poorly defined vascular walls become accentuated by spaces and cysts from 9 to 16 weeks. From 17 to 28 weeks, the loose mesenchymal stroma decreases with increase in connective tissue fibers and fully formed vascular walls. After 29 weeks, the CP contains a mature vascular stroma.

**Etiology:** The CPC is actually a pseudocyst with a wall of interconnecting angiomatous irregular capillaries.[269] CPCs are believed to occur in the mesenchymal stroma when CSF is entrapped between the intervillous clefts, hypothesized to develop when there is failure in transformation of the lobulated embryonal capillaries into the wavy fetal pattern.[269] Most cysts form from 13 to 18 weeks when the choroid plexus proliferates. The cysts then regress by week 28 when proliferation and reduction in mesenchymal stroma occur. Approximately 95% of CPCs disappear by 26 weeks' gestation.[270]

#### Diagnosis

*Ultrasound:* The glomus, a focal thickened bulge along the posterior choroid, develops after 13 weeks and is the most common site for a CPC.[270] A CPC is an echolucent, well-circumscribed structure surrounded by echogenic choroid plexus (Fig. 12.1-40A). A true CPC can be diagnosed when the cyst measures 2.5 mm before 22 weeks and at least 2 mm thereafter.[271] CPC may be multiple or bilateral, can contain septations, and protrude into the ventricle (Fig. 12.1-40B). Approximately 86% are detected in the second trimester in isolation as an incidental finding.[272]

When a CPC is identified, however, a careful anatomic survey with attention to heart, brain, and hands should be performed. In approximately 14% of cases, additional anomalies are noted with CPCs, which raises the risk to as high as 48% for aneuploidy (Fig. 12.1-27).[272,273] CPCs that are bilateral and complex do not increase the risk of aneuploidy.[274] However, a large CPC in excess of 10 mm has been suggested to increase risk.[274] If the cyst is isolated, the risk for aneuploidy is low at 0.9% to 6.7%; therefore, other factors such as baseline risk should be considered.[272,274,275]

*MRI:* In the presence of the typical subcentimeter lesion, MRI provides no added advantage, and in fact, most CPCs are not well visualized by MRI. With larger lesions, especially in the presence of complicating factors such as VM, MR imaging can confirm diagnosis of CPC by defining a CSF signal lesion within choroid, evaluating mass effect, and excluding other differentials.[276] In a high-risk pregnancy with CPC or in the presence of multiple other anomalies, MRI may be considered for further information.

**Associated Anomalies:** About 1% to 2% of infants with isolated cysts will have an underlying chromosomal abnormality, the most common being trisomy 18 followed by trisomy 21.[256] Recent evidence suggests that CPCs may also be associated with congenital heart disease and hydronephrosis.[277]

**Differential Diagnosis:** Before 22 weeks, the choroid plexus is heterogeneous, and small anechoic areas measuring <2 mm can mimic a cyst.[271] Partial volume averaging of the striatum and choroid and mild ventriculomegaly may falsely suggest CPC.[271] Choroid plexus papillomas are typically differentiated by solid nature and color Doppler flow. Subacute intraventricular clot adherent to choroid plexus may be difficult to discern from CPC in the absence of other findings. Other intraventricular cysts in the differential include colloid or neuroepithelial cysts, which demonstrate a true epithelial wall.

**Prognosis:** Most CPCs are incidental with no progression of the antenatal cyst after birth.[276] Studies have shown that fetuses with isolated CPC and normal karyotype have normal neurocognitive development after birth.[267,278] In the presence of a large CPC, space-occupying effects can cause obstructive hydrocephalus and/or injury to adjacent tissue that may manifest as focal neurologic deficits or seizure.[276]

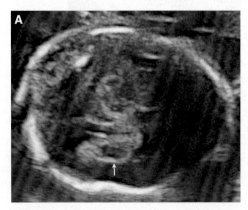
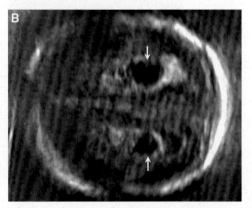

**FIGURE 12.1-40:** Choroid plexus cyst. **A:** Axial image of a single sonolucent lesion *(arrow)* in the choroid of the lateral ventricle. **B:** Axial US image of bilateral cysts *(arrows)* in the choroid of the lateral ventricles.

**Management:** Perinatal surveillance is warranted. Counseling is indicated as increased parental anxiety often occurs as some interpret the finding as a brain anomaly.[267] In the presence of CPC and associated anomalies, advanced maternal age, or abnormal triple screen analysis, most recommend amniocentesis or chorionic villus sampling as risk for aneuploidy is 1 in 3.[271–273,279] Although controversial, many believe testing should not be performed in the presence of only isolated CPC as the likelihood of trisomy 18 is low, risk increased by a factor of 7.[275,280] On the other hand, some perform interventional tests solely in the presence of isolated CPC, knowing that 25% to 30% of cases of trisomy 18 have findings undetectable by US and that the risk of aneuploidy is 0% to 6%, with risk of fetal loss after amniocentesis at 0.5%.[269,271,273] Postnatally, nearly all CPCs resolve, and no further therapy is required. Persistence of a large cyst is extremely rare but could require neurosurgical decompression with fenestration or shunt.[276]

**Recurrence:** Most CPCs are incidental and sporadic.

### Arachnoid Cysts

**Incidence:** Arachnoid cysts (AC) represent 1% of all intracranial masses in newborns.[281]

**Pathogenesis:** The most accepted theory for development of an AC is that early first trimester, at the time of evolution of the meninges, there is an abnormal localized splitting of cell layers in the area between the arachnoid and the pia allowing distension of a potential space with CSF. The wall of the AC is usually composed of a thick layer of collagen and hyperplastic arachnoid cells; however, suprasellar cysts may also contain neuroglial elements.[282] The congenital AC does not typically communicate with the subarachnoid space, whereas a secondary or acquired AC, which develops because of CSF entrapment within arachnoid adhesions following in utero hemorrhage, infection, or trauma, is usually patent with the subarachnoid space. Some cysts enlarge, and this is hypothesized to occur secondary to active secretion of CSF from the cyst membrane, osmotic gradients caused by higher protein in the cyst fluid, or cyst communicating with the subarachnoid space via ball-valve mechanism.[282]

**Etiology:** Intracranial ACs vary in size and location. In the fetus, the majority of ACs are supratentorial (63%), followed by infratentorial (22%), and finally along the incisura (15%).[281,283] Although in children most supratentorial ACs are located in the sylvian fissure or middle cranial fossa, in the fetus the most common location is interhemispheric, followed by skull base, suprasellar, and hemispheric.[281–284]

### Diagnosis

***Ultrasound:*** Most cysts are diagnosed in the third trimester, rarely before a gestational age of 20 weeks.[281,284] ACs are present in the extra-axial fluid space and are uniformly sonolucent (Fig. 12.1-41A). An AC will have thin regular walls and posterior acoustic enhancement. The lesion should be devoid of blood flow on color Doppler. Septation within the cyst is possible. A thorough search for additional anomalies with special attention to the corpus callosum is indicated.[284,285] The ventricles and cerebral parenchyma should be assessed for enlargement and mass effect.[281] Three-dimensional US may be helpful to define the nature of the cyst.[285]

***MRI:*** MRI is helpful in confirming diagnosis by identifying the extra-axial location and CSF signal intensity (Fig. 12.1-41B). MRI can also define the extent of the cyst, compression of adjacent structures, communication with the ventricle, and other associated anomalies, especially of the corpus callosum.[283,286] The technique is helpful in excluding other intracranial cysts that may mimic an AC.

**Associated Anomalies:** ACs are commonly isolated but can be seen with chromosomal abnormalities, especially in the presence of additional anomalies.[281] ACC is the most common association, typically noted in the presence of an interhemispheric cyst. Malformations of the venous system are also possible.[282] Prenatal suprasellar cysts have been seen in association with hypothalamic hamartomas, which are pathologically ectopic benign neural tissue that present as gray matter masses at the floor of the third.[287] Sometimes, ACs are noted in the presence of metabolic diseases such as glutaric aciduria type 1.[285]

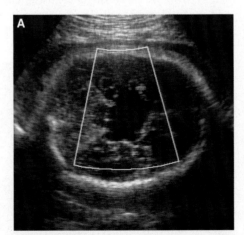
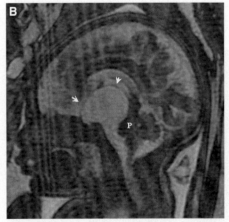

**FIGURE 12.1-41:** Suprasellar arachnoid cyst in a fetus at 34 weeks. **A:** Axial US demonstrating a sonolucent lesion posterior to the frontal lobes with absence of internal color flow. **B:** Sagittal SSFP MR image in same fetus demonstrates a suprasellar cystic lesion (arrows) with thin peripheral wall. There is mass effect on the adjacent pons (P). The cyst continued to grow and postnatal, the child had fenestration of the cyst with good outcome.

**Differential Diagnosis:** Other "cystic" lesions which should be included in the differential are porencephaly, schizencephaly, cystic neoplasms, subacute intracranial hemorrhage, CPCs, and vein of Galen anomalies. In the presence of porencephaly, the margins may have a jagged contour, and in schizencephaly, clefts are lined by gray matter. In both, volume loss, not mass effect, should be present. Cystic neoplasms typically have associated solid tissue. Vein of Galen is documented in the presence of color flow on Doppler. A prominent cavum velum interpositum is a developmental variant which appears as a triangular CSF space below the splenium of the corpus callous, dorsal to the tectum, and bound laterally by the internal cerebral veins.[288] Enlargement of the septum pellucidum and vergae may mimic an interhemispheric cyst. Lesions that may be difficult to separate from AC include glioependymal cysts, neuroepithelial or colloid cysts, usually present in the third ventricle.

**Prognosis:** Prognosis is dependent on the presence of other malformations, the rate of cyst growth, and the progression of VM. Early age at diagnosis, growth of the cyst in utero, and a size of more than 15 mm are unfavorable factors.[289]

In general fetal/neonatal AC have a higher risk for growth than the adult population. Cysts increase in volume in 20% to 24% of fetuses and children; however, cyst volume and location do not determine clinical outcome, with some large lesions being asymptomatic.[281,283] Hydrocephalus has been shown to occur in approximately 17% to 25% of cases.[283,284] Hydrocephalus is more likely to occur with midline ACs, including interhemispheric, incisural (quadrigeminal), or suprasellar cysts which obstruct the aqueduct or third ventricle.[283] Suprasellar ACs also have an increased risk for visual disturbances and pituitary dysfunction.[290]

Approximately 28% (or higher) of AC will require postnatal intervention either because of hydrocephalus or symptoms from mass effect.[283,290] There is a slightly higher risk for subdural hematoma with head trauma, which is thought to be due to tearing of more vulnerable bridging veins by the lesions.[290] Overall, though, an AC without associated chromosomal or structural anomaly has a favorable outcome with behavior, neurological development, and intelligence normal in 88% of cases.[283]

**Management:** Serial prenatal US should be performed to assess the size of the cyst and the ventricles.[281] Close postnatal followup is indicated due to higher risk for growth and secondary complications. In the presence of symptoms from significant mass effect and/or hydrocephalus, current favored therapy is endoscopic cyst fenestration either cystoventriculostomy or cysto-cisternostomy.[281,282] Most do not support shunting of the cyst due to higher risk for secondary complications, including severe CSF overdrainage.[290]

**Recurrence:** Most are isolated without risk for recurrence.

### Cyst of Septum Pellucidum
**Incidence:** Cysts of the cavum septum pellucidum (SPC) are rare, with an incidence of 0.04%.[291]

**Pathogenesis:** The septum pellucidum is related to the development of the commissures, with the leaflets containing glial, neuronal, and ependymal cells. The space in between the leaflets, or the cavum, does not communicate with the ventricles. In 85% of cases, the cavum will disappear in the first 3 to 6 months after birth; however, the cavum septum pellucidum has been cited to persist in 15% to 20% of children and adults.[291]

**Etiology:** Cysts of the septum pellucidum are felt to occur when the septum pellucidum develops the ability to secrete fluid, possibly because of migration of ependymal cells into the leaflets, or as a result of rupture of the cavum, likely secondary to trauma or infection.[292] Increase in intracranial pressure may develop because of obstruction of the interventricular foramina, and the cyst can compress adjacent structures such as the hypothalamus, septal nuclei, and supependymal and internal cerebral veins.[291]

**Ultrasound:** A cavum septum pellucidum greater than 1 cm is considered abnormal.[293,294] Most cysts of the septum pellucidum range in width from 2 to 5 cm, cause collapse of the frontal horns, and extend posteriorly into vergae, to the splenium of the corpus callosum.[295] US will show a dilated CSF cavity, measuring greater than 1 cm, above the thalami and anterior to the third ventricle in the anatomic location of the septum pellucidum (Fig. 12.1-42A).[296]

**MRI:** An SPC appears as a CSF cavity greater than 10 mm between the lateral ventricles with different degrees of bowing of the cyst wall, sometimes collapsing the frontal horns (Fig. 12.1-42B).[293] The lateral ventricles appear more parallel, and ventriculomegaly may occur owing to obstruction of the foramen of Monro.[291,293]

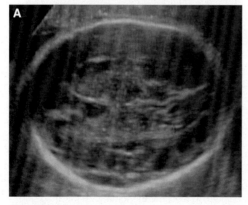
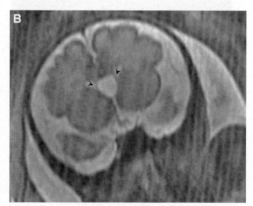

**FIGURE 12.1-42:** Cyst of the septum pellucidum. **A:** Axial US shows a prominent cavum septum pellucidum that measured 11 mm. **B:** Coronal T2 MRI in the same fetus demonstrates enlarged cavum with lateral bowing of the septal leaflets (*arrowheads*).

**Associated Anomalies:** SPCs are typically not associated with intracranial anomalies other than ventriculomegaly.[297]

**Differential Diagnosis:** Differential for a SPC includes a large third ventricle, aneurysm of the vein of Galen, interhemispheric, arachnoid or neuroglial cyst, and an enlarged cavum velum interpositum. A predominately cystic tumor could also mimic an SPC.

**Prognosis:** Some SPCs will resolve spontaneously due to rupture into the lateral or third ventricles.[291,297] Hydrocephalus can occur in up to 32% and is more likely to occur under 5 years of age.[291] Children with SPCs have been shown to have focal deficit in 23%, seizures in 10%, and mental status changes in 42%.[291] A large persistent cavum septum pellucidum, but not cavum vergae, has been noted to be a marker of cerebral dysfunction, being associated with increased risk for mental retardation, developmental delay, and neuropsychiatric disturbances such as schizophrenia.[291]

**Management:** Serial prenatal US should be performed to assess the size of the cyst and ventricles. Symptoms may not be clear, but treatment is usually considered when there are clinical findings from ventricular obstruction or compression of adjacent structures.[291] Neuroendoscopic cyst fenestration is therapy of choice because of high success and low complication rate.[291]

**Recurrence:** Most are isolated without risk for recurrence.

### Glioependymal/Neuroglial Cyst
### (aka Choroidal, Epithelial, Ependymal)
**Incidence:** Glioependymal cysts are uncommon, representing fewer than 1% of all intracranial cysts.[298]

**Pathogenesis/Etiology:** These cysts have a wall composed of neuroepithelium, and are therefore favored to arise from ectopic rests of the primitive neural tube or leptomeningeal neuroglial heterotopy.[299] The wall of the cyst is always lined with epithelium, but the complexing terminology is based on histology, reflecting variable neural, glial, ependymal, and choroidal cells. These cysts can be identified anywhere in the neuroaxis, usually over the cerebral hemisphere but also intraparenchymal.[299] In the fetus, most case reports describe the cyst in the interhemispheric fissure, often in conjunction with ACC.[299–302] Glioependymal cysts have been seen in association with ischemic or hemorrhagic insults.[301]

### Diagnosis
*Ultrasound:* Glioependymal cysts are sonolucent but may be septated or mulitlocular.[300] The lesion will cause mass effect and when interhemispheric is usually associated with agenesis of the corpus callosum. Additional anomalies should be excluded.

*MRI:* The cystic lesion is often similar to CSF but can be slightly hyperintense to CSF on T1 imaging and hypointense on T2 imaging owing to high protein content.[299,301] The lesion may be unilocular, multilocular, or septated. Since these lesions can occur intra-axial or extra-axial, the glioependymal cyst may or may not communicate with the ventricular system.[301] MRI allows depiction of anatomy of the lesion, mass effect, and exclusion of associated anomalies.

**Associated Anomalies:** When present with ACC, other anomalies including heterotopic gray matter, cerebellar hypoplasia, and microgyria should be excluded.[299] When present in the posterior fossa, these cysts can cause obstructive hydrocephalus.[303]

**Differential Diagnosis:** Glioependymal cysts can only be differentiated from an arachnoid cyst by histology. Dorsal cyst with HPE, porencephaly, hydranencephaly, multicystic encephalomalacia, dermoids, epidermoids, and other cystic tumors should be considered.

**Prognosis:** There is a good prognosis in isolated appropriately treated glioependymal cysts.[300,301] A more guarded prognosis may be seen in the presence of associated anomalies.[301]

**Management:** Ideal treatment is complete resection, as the cyst not uncommonly recurs likely due to cellular components in the wall that produce CSF.[301,302] Other therapies include fenestration, shunting, and partial resection.

**Recurrence:** There is no known increased risk for recurrence.

### Arteriovenous Malformations/Vein of Galen
**Incidence:** Most arteriovenous malformations (AVM) in the fetus are vein of Galen malformations (VGM), which represent less than 1% of all intracranial AVM.[304]

**Pathogenesis:** Early in embryology, a primitive sinusoidal vascular network is present with direct connections between arteries and veins. If there is error in normal differentiation of these vascular connections, the arteries and veins remain in direct communication, resulting in an AVM. As AVMs have no intervening capillaries between the artery and the vein, high-flow arteriovenous (AV) shunting develops that can secondarily result in cardiac failure and brain injury.

A "vein of Galen malformation" is a misnomer as the defect is not truly of the vein of Galen. A true VGM is a persistent communication of the primitive choroidal arterial system and the *median prosencephalic vein of Markowski*.[304] During the 5th week, choroidal and quadrigeminal arteries develop. On the roof of the diencephalon, between 6 and 11 weeks, the lateral choroid plexus expands and is drained via choroidal veins into a central primitive vein known as the median prosencephalic vein. In the 12th week, the vein regresses, with the dorsal remnant developing into the vein of Galen. The straight sinus, developing from fusion of multiple small tentorial veins, appears on the 50th day and drains the lateral choroid plexus. A VGM is hypothesized to occur when there is lack of involution of the prosencephalic vein because of either early occlusion or lack of formation of the straight sinus or due to continuous elevated blood flow through persistent abnormal communication of the choroidal arteries and the median prosencephalic vein. The abnormal angioarchitecture of the VGM also prevents normal development of the intracranial venous drainage, resulting in persistence of other embryologic venous sinuses, most commonly the falcine sinus.

Not surprisingly, choroidal arteries, especially the posterior choroidal, are the most common arterial feeders in VGM.[305] This is followed by subependymal perforators of the posterior cerebral arteries and thalamoperforators.[306] Often branches of the pericallosal artery, a vessel arising from the anterior cerebral and an important supply for the choroid plexus in the third ventricle, also supplies the VGM.[305] In approximately half of neonates, a persistent limbic arterial arch, which connects the cortical branches of the anterior choroidal artery with the posterior cerebral artery via the pericallosal artery is noted.[307] Supply from the middle cerebral artery is uncommon. Transmesencephalic branches directly from the basilar can supply an AVM; however, in their presence, the AVM is not a true VGM and are otherwise indicative of a tectal not choroidal malformation.[306]

In a VGM, the primitive vein is arterialized, thick walled, and dilated due to high flow and turbulence from either direct or indirect arteriovenous connections. In over half of cases, the straight sinus is absent or thrombosed. The most common finding is a persistent falcine sinus, which extends from the vein of Galen to the sagittal sinus and ascends in the falx cerebri. Maturation of the jugular bulbs occurs peri and postnatal, and in the presence of a VGM, the maturation process, which includes remodeling of torcula, regression of occipital and marginal sinus, and remodeling of jugular bulbs, may not occur.[306] Occlusions and stenosis of the venous channels can develop, especially the jugular bulbs and sigmoid sinuses, which then increase venous pressure but can improve cardiac function by decreasing overload.[306] Anterior venous collateral drainage through the petrous, cavernous, thalamic, lateral mesencephalic, facial, and ophthalmic veins may develop. As the pacchionian granulations do not function until after the first few months of life, CSF must be absorbed at least partly by medullary veins. In the presence of this pathophysiology and with stenosis of veins leading to venous hypertension, the unbalanced hydrovenous state can lead to hydrocephalus.[306] Cerebral maturation is also dependent on a normal venous system. Intracranial venous hypertension likely in conjunction with cardiac dysfunction (steal phenomenon) results in brain injury, which is reflected by subcortical white matter calcification, white matter lesions, and diffuse brain destruction (melting brain), especially with subependymal atrophy (occipital) and ex vacuo ventricular dilatation.[306]

**Etiology/Types:** VGMs are usually classified by fistula angioarchitecture. The choroidal type is a primitive shunt in the velum interpositum with multiple bilateral feeding arteries, typically choroidal, pericallosal, and thalamoperforators, that converge on a fistula directly into the anterior prosencephalic vein (Fig. 12.1-43).[305,306] This type of VGM leads to a more severe pathology, presenting earlier in life, often with cardiac failure. The mural type is better tolerated and is defined by a single or few feeding typically collicular and posterior choroidal arteries that drain laterally into the wall of the dilated vein. Sometimes, the malformation may be a combination of both types. In all VGMs, the median prosencephalic vein has no connection with the deep venous system.

Although the majority of AVMs in the fetus are VGM, also described antenatally are dural sinus malformations (DSM) and pial arteriovenous fistulas (AVF). DSM are rare, more common in males and represent persistence of an embryonic sinus with or without AV shunt in the wall of a dural lake (see Dural venous thrombosis).[308,309] Pial AVF are typically supratentorial with peripheral pial/cortical feeding arteries draining into an ectatic vein.[106] The pial AVF may secondarily dilate the vein of Galen. Both DSM and pial AVF can result in high-output cardiomegaly and brain injury.[308–310]

### Diagnosis

*Ultrasound:* VGMs are typically diagnosed in the third trimester, with less in the second trimester.[311] The diagnosis is usually suggested when a hypoechogenic less likely heterogeneous

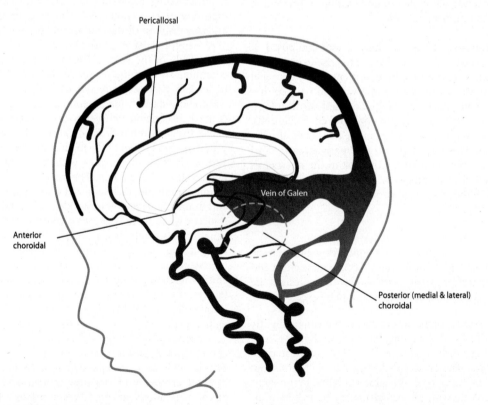

**FIGURE 12.1-43:** Diagram of choroidal type vein of Galen malformation with feeding vessels from the anterior choroidal, posterior choroidal, and pericallosal vessels forming the so-called limbic arterial arch.

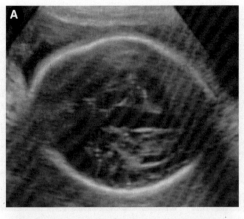
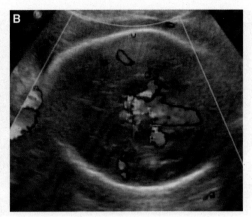
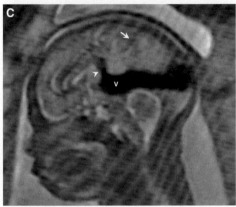

**FIGURE 12.1-44:** Fetus at 33 weeks with vein of Galen malformation. **A:** Axial ultrasound demonstrates a tubular hypoechoic lesion posterior to the third ventricle. **B:** With color, the tubular area demonstrates flow. There is a tangle of vessels and tubulent flow along the anterior aspect of the vein. **C:** Sagittal T2 MR image demonstrates the feeding vessels from the pericallosal artery *(arrowhead)* into persistent prosencephalic vein *(V)*. There is partial visualization of a persistent falcine sinus *(arrow)*.

mass with central color Doppler is identified in the midline of the posterior recess of the third ventricle (Fig. 12.1-44A,B).[304] Doppler will demonstrate bidirectional turbulent flow with very pulsatile "arterialized" veins and high diastolic arterial waveforms (Fig. 12.1-45).[312] If only normal venous Doppler is obtained in the vein of Galen, the dilatation may be related to varicosity or other type of AVM. The sagittal sinus or persistent falcine sinus is often dilated.[312] On 2D US, it can sometimes be difficult to precisely identify the feeders or exclude a parenchymal AVM that drains via the vein of Galen.[305] However, power Doppler, especially with 3D reconstruction, can provide very detailed anatomy of the complex angioarchitecture, allowing depiction of the feeding arteries and venous anatomy (Fig. 12.1-46A,B).[312–314] Limitations of 3D include poor resolution and difficulty in differentiating veins from arteries.[313]

Since brain injury is possible, close evaluation for calcification, hemorrhage, volume loss, and hydrocephalus should be obtained (Fig. 12.1-47).[315] Clues to heart failure include cardiomegaly, tricuspid valve insufficiency, dilated inferior vena cava, retrograde aortic diastolic flow, and tachycardia (>200 bpm).[306,315] Enlarged neck vessels, especially the jugular veins, are pathognomonic and can be seen in approximately one-third of cases (Fig. 12.1-48).[311,315] Elevated cardiac output may be measured and has been suggested to correlate with the magnitude of AV shunt.[316] Polyhydramnios, pericardial and pleural effusion, edema and ascites (hydrops) carry a poor prognosis and suggest intractable high flow.[304,315]

*MRI:* Fetal MRI can aid in confirmation of a VGM and help exclude other arteriovenous anomalies or intracranial anomalies that can mimic a VGM (Figs. 12.1-44C and 12.1-46C). MRI can identify flow void in pathological vessels and can verify the size of the AVM, which may demonstrate flow void or heterogeneous signal due to turbulence.[317] MRI is superior at evaluating for cerebral injury, which may manifest as ventriculomegaly, polymicrogyria, cortical thickening, porencephaly, schizencephaly, periventricular injury, and intraparenchymal hemorrhage in fetuses with VGM (Fig. 12.1-49A).[304,318] T1 imaging is important to exclude acute hemorrhage and/or mineralization

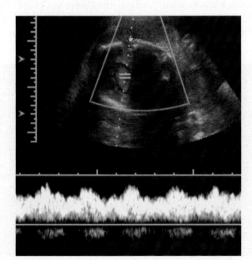

**FIGURE 12.1-45:** Doppler in a vein of Galen demonstrating arterialized waveform.

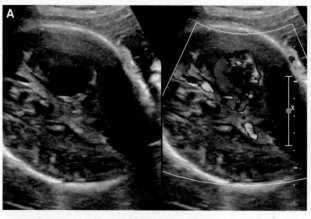

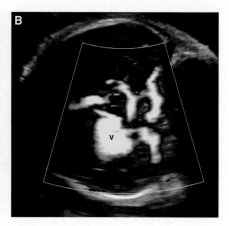

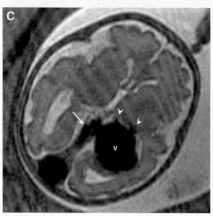

**FIGURE 12.1-46:** Fetus at 33 weeks with AV fistula. **A:** Axial US shows a round hypoechoic lesion in the left choroidal fissure that demonstrates turbulent color flow. **B:** Power Doppler of the same fetus demonstrates the feeding arteries extending to the large choroidal fissure vein (*V*). **C:** Axial T2 MR image shows multiple feeding arteries (*arrowheads*) extending to the large perimesencephalic dilated vein (*V*). The vein of Galen is mildly dilated, acting as secondary drainage (*arrow*).

(Fig. 12.1-49B). Diffusion imaging may provide information about acute ischemia, and gradient echo, in the presence of susceptibility artifact, can define hemosiderin or calcification. MRA, especially 2D time of flight (TOF), which is shorter in scan time than 3D TOF, may be helpful in defining the vascular anatomy of the malformation (Fig. 12.1-49C).[319]

**Associated Anomalies:** VGMs are not associated with chromosomal anomalies. All types of AVM, whether VGM, DVM, or AVF, can cause cardiac failure and brain injury. Sixty to 76%

of fetuses with VGMs will have ventriculomegaly, cardiomegaly, and enlarged neck vessels.[311,316]

**Differential Diagnosis:** Varicose dilatation of the vein of Galen may occur in the absence of AVM. This may be seen in association with heart disease or vascular anomalies that cause venous hypertension.[304] Other differentials include arachnoid cyst, porencephaly, choroid plexus cyst, choroid plexus papilloma, pineal tumor, and intracerebral hematoma. A vascular mass such as hemangioma should also be considered.

**Prognosis:** Fetuses with prenatal diagnosis of VGM and cardiac failure, hydrops, or cerebral anomalies have a poor outcome.[304,306] These fetuses at birth typically suffer from severe

**FIGURE 12.1-47:** Axial ultrasound in a fetus with VGM (*V*). The lateral ventricles are enlarged consistent with brain parenchymal volume loss. The thinned brain parenchyma is increased in echogenicity (*arrows*) concerning for brain injury.

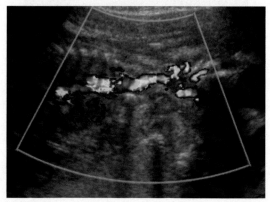

**FIGURE 12.1-48:** Coronal color ultrasound demonstrating enlarged jugular vein in fetus with VGM.

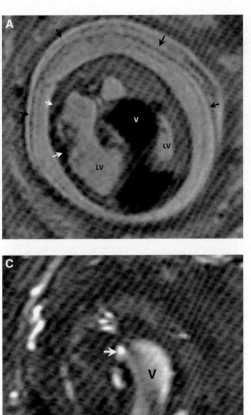

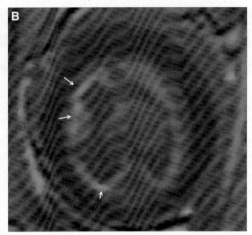

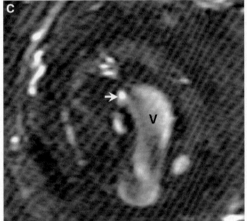

**FIGURE 12.1-49:** Fetus at 35 weeks with VGM, brain ischemia, cardiac compromise, and hydrops. **A:** Axial T2 image demonstrates large prosencephalic vein (*V*) and significant extracalvarial soft tissue swelling (*black arrows*). The ventricles (*LV*) are enlarged consistent with volume loss. The right hemisphere is extremely thin and abnormal dark T2 signal (*white arrows*). **B:** T1-weighted image shows increased signal (*arrows*) along the right hemisphere consistent with hemorrhage or mineralization. **C:** Axial 2D MRA demonstrating large prosencephalic vein (*V*) and small feeding vessels anteriorly (*arrow*).

irreversible multiorgan failure.[306] Those with isolated VGM have a more favorable prognosis; however, the type of AVM and the number and size of the arterial feeders and draining vein reflect the severity of shunt and have implications for outcome.[304,315] In cases with prenatal diagnosis, overall mortality for VGM has been reported at 22% to 25% with normal neurologic outcome in 67%.[305,320] However, a recent review suggested a much higher perinatal death rate of 54%.[304] In this study, 32% of prenatally diagnosed VGM were alive and well, whereas 14% were alive with mental retardation. Without embolization, mortality in VGM is as high as 90%. With embolization, outcomes for VGM prenatal and postnatal have been recorded at 10% demise, 10% severe disability, 16% moderate delay, and 74% neurologically normal.[306]

**Management:** Rarely, mirror syndrome can develop in the mother; therefore, close fetal and maternal monitoring is warranted.[321] Patient selection for therapy is usually dependent on the severity of heart failure and degree of brain injury.[305] Termination or no postnatal intervention may be considered on the basis of these factors.[306] Antenatal diagnosis is usually not an indication for early delivery or C-section.[306] Delivery should be performed at tertiary centers with neurosurgical, cardiovascular, and interventional radiology expertise.

At birth, cardiac failure can worsen after delivery because of removal of the low-resistance placenta, facilitating more flow through the foramen ovale. Medical therapy is directed at cardiac dysfunction and includes administration of diuretics to decrease preload. The main intent is to address feeding so that

weight gain occurs in the first few months. MRI of the brain should be obtained to assess the degree of brain injury.

In a VGM, clinical and laboratory evaluation regarding cardiac, cerebral, respiratory, renal and liver function are utilized in a scoring system (Bicetre) to determine need and timing for therapy (Table 12.1-12). A score of 8 and below is a decision not to treat, and that between 8 and 12 is considered an emergency endovascular intervention.[307] In the presence of cardiac decompensation or with development of hydrocephalus, immediate embolization therapy is warranted to decrease shunt and venous hypertension in an attempt to reverse pathology.[306,322] If the patient is stable and neonatal score is between 13 and 20, therapy is often scheduled at 5 months of age.

The first line of therapy for VGM is embolization, usually transarterial, with the transvenous (femoral or transtorcular) route being utilized as a second choice because of higher morbidity.[306,322] Surgical treatment is dangerous, difficult, and often incomplete. The goal of therapy is not always to obliterate the AVM, but to balance therapy to allow the brain to mature and develop normally by either improving cardiac status or preventing the development of neurologic symptoms.[306] Several sessions of embolization may be required to safely treat, either completely or incompletely, the vascular anastomosis. Spontaneous thrombosis can occur rarely in VGM (2.5%) and is typically associated with 50% neurologic impairment.[306,307] Complications from the lesion and/or therapy include hemorrhage, stroke, and continued brain injury, which can lead to neurologic deficits and seizures. Macrocrania and

| Table 12.1-12 | Bicetre Neonatal Evaluation Score | | | | |
|---|---|---|---|---|---|
| **Points** | **Cardiac Function** | **Cerebral Function** | **Respiratory Function** | **Hepatic Function** | **Renal Function** |
| 5 | Normal | Normal | Normal | — | — |
| 4 | Overload, no medical treatment | Subclinical isolated EEG abnormalities | Tachypnea, finishes bottle | — | — |
| 3 | Failure, stable with medical treatment | Nonconvulsive intermittent neurologic signs | Tachypnea, does not finish bottle | No hepatomegaly, normal function | Normal |
| 2 | Failure, not stable with medical treatment | Isolated convulsion | Assisted ventilation, normal saturation $FIO_2 < 25\%$ | Hepatomegaly, normal function | Transient anuria |
| 1 | Ventilation necessary | Seizures | Assisted ventilation, normal saturation $FIO_2 > 25\%$ | Moderate or transient hepatic insufficiency | Unstable diuresis with treatment |
| 0 | Resistant to medical treatment | Permanent neurologic signs | Assisted ventilation, desaturation | Abnormal coagulation, elevated enzymes | Anuria |

Maximal score = 5 (cardiac) + 5 (cerebral) + 5 (respiratory) + 3 (hepatic) + 3 (renal) = 21.

From Lasjaunias PL, Chng SM, Sachet M, et al. The management of vein of Galen aneurysmal malformation. *Neurosurgery.* 2006;59:S3.184–S3.194.

hydrocephalus that does not respond to therapy can be managed with endoscopic ventriculostomy or shunting.[307] With therapy, venous thrombosis and cerebellar tonsillar herniation due to venous congestion may occur.[103] Facial venous distension can cause epistaxis.

Both DVM and pial AVF have the same complications as VGM.[308–310] Pial AVF, in contradistinction to VGMs, are treated with embolotherapy at birth to prevent brain injury.[310] Spontaneous thrombosis of DVM has been documented; however, close monitoring and embolization may also be required.[308,309]

**Recurrence:** There is no increased risk of recurrence.

## Disorders of Cellular Migration

### Lissencephaly: Agyria, Pachygyria, and Subcortical Band Heterotopia (aka Classic or Type I Lissencephaly)

Agyria represents a thick cortex with lack of gyri, also consistent with complete lissencephaly (smooth brain). Incomplete lissencephaly exists in the presence of pachygyria or band heterotopia. Broad, shallow, and flat gyri with thickened cortex are diagnostic of pachygyria. Subcortical band heterotopia represents a band of heterotopic gray matter beneath the cortex, separated by a thin layer of white matter. Often, there is a combination of these anomalies.

**Incidence:** The estimated incidence of classic or previously denoted type 1 lissencephaly is 1.2 per 100,000 births.[323]

**Pathogenesis:** Lissencephaly is a severe malformation of the fetal brain that occurs because of impaired neuronal migration during the 3rd to 4th month of gestation.[324] The prime defect is a genetic flaw that results in dysfunctional proteins which are necessary for the normal neural migration.[323] A normal brain contains six cortical layers. In both agyria and pachygyria, the cortex is abnormally thick, remodeled and has only four layers. Despite deficient layers, the cortex is thick as the

cells arrested lie in disorganized radial columns.[325] On histology, the two most superficial layers, a cell dense marginal zone and superficial cortical gray zone are formed by neurons that have migrated normal early in gestation. The third layer is cell sparse, with only a few dysplastic neurons. The fourth layer is densely cellular with radial orientated neurons with no lamination (Fig. 12.1-50). Because of the lack of development of axonal and dendritic connections, the subcortical white matter is thin and lacks gray white matter interdigitation.[325] Subcortical band heterotopia demonstrates normal cortical and subcortical white matter architecture with a band of heterotopic columnar neurons.[326]

**Etiology:** Lissencephaly may be isolated or associated with a syndrome, the most common being Miller–Dieker syndrome (MDS). Miller–Dieker syndrome is seen in the presence of severe lissencephaly and facial dysmorphism that includes prominent forehead, bitemporal hollowing, short upturned nose, thickened upper lip, low set ears, and small jaw. Baraitser–Winter syndrome is characterized by lissencephaly, trigonocephaly, shallow orbits, ptosis, and colobomas.[326] Multiple genes have been associated with lissencephaly (Table 12.1-13).[324,326] *LIS1* and *DCX* account for approximately 85% of isolated lissencephaly, whereas *DCX* is associated with 90% of cases of subcortical heterotopia.[327] The topography of the malformation is dependent on the gene which is affected.

The *LIS1* gene mutation is equally seen in males and females, with gyral abnormalities more severe posteriorly, demonstrating agyria parieto-occipital and pachygyria frontal and temporal.[326,328] Rarely, the *LIS1* gene causes subcortical band heterotopia, mostly in the parieto-occipital area. The *DCX* gene is present on the X chromosome, affects the anterior aspect of the brain more than the posterior and in males causes lissencephaly whereas in females a milder phenotype with subcortical band heterotopia is noted.[329] *ARX* causes an X-linked lissencephaly, and therefore is phenotypically more severe in males than in females, and is seen in association with abnormal genitalia, facial

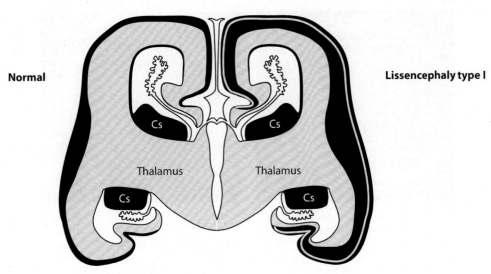

**FIGURE 12.1-50:** Diagram of the layered pattern in lissencephaly type I.

dysmorphism, and ACC. *RELN* causes lissencephaly in association with cerebellar hypoplasia and often brainstem abnormalities.[323] Both *RELN* and *ARX* demonstrate a thickened cortex but no cell-sparse zone in the area of agyria.

**Diagnosis:** When there is a concern for lissencephaly by imaging, karyotype is suggested, as FISH analysis of 17p13.3 deletions and sequencing for abnormalities of the *LIS1* and *DCX* genes can be diagnostic.[327]

***Ultrasound:*** Severe forms of lissencephaly are likely to be more easily detected than milder incomplete forms.[330] Agyria/pachygria can be suggested as early as 23 to 24 weeks when

| Table 12.1-13 | Genes/Syndromes in Association with Lissencephaly | |
|---|---|---|
| ***Genetics/Type*** | ***Gene*** | ***Locus*** |
| Isolated lissencephaly | *LIS1, TUBA1A, PAFAH1B1* | 17p13.3, 12q12–14 |
| Miller-Dieker syndrome | *LIS1, YWHAE, CRK, PAFAH1B1* | 17p13.3 |
| X-linked lissencephaly | *DCX* | Xq22.3–q23 |
| Lissencephaly, cerebellum and brainstem abnormal | *RELN, TUBA1A, VLDLR* | 7q22, 12q12–14 |
| Lissencephaly, ACC, ambiguous genitalia | *ARX* | Xp22.13 |
| Subcortical heterotopia | *DCX, TUBA1A* | Xq22.3–q23, 12q12–14 |
| Paracentral pachygyria Baraitser-Winter syndrome Autosomal recessive frontotemporal pachygyria | | |

there is a smooth thick cerebral surface with absence of parieto-occipital and calcarine fissure and wide sylvian fissures due to abnormal opercular formatin.[330] After 28 weeks, in the presence of a smooth brain, diagnosis of lissencephaly can be confirmed (Fig. 12.1-51A).[330] Three-dimensional imaging may demonstrate sulci better than 2D.[331]

Lamination of the fetal brain can normally be detected as early as 17 weeks, present to 28 weeks' gestation, and disappearing by 34 weeks.[332] The subplate should be anechoic and the intermediate zone homogeneously more echogenic.[332] When lissencephaly is present, no laminar pattern, prominent increased echogenicity in the intermediate zone representing thick disorganized neurons, or persistence of lamination pattern after 33 weeks can be noted.[332] Mild ventriculomegaly and enlarged subarachnoid spaces are often present (Fig. 12.1-52A).[324,333] Immature sulcation with wide and thick gyri is typical.[333] In the presence of other intracranial and extracranial findings, a diagnosis of MDS may be suggested (Table 12.1-14). The most common findings that should raise suspicion of MDS are polyhydramnios (66%), intrauterine growth restriction (62%), and ventriculomegaly (59%).[329] Ultrasound diagnosis for MDS has been noted to be as high as 41% prenatal, mostly third trimester.[329]

**MRI:** Diagnosis prior to 20 weeks is difficult as the brain is normally smooth at this gestational age. At 23 to 24 weeks, absence of normal parieto-occipital and calcarine sulcus with wide sylvian fissures can be noted.[330] On MRI, the cortex is thick, smooth, or shallow, and the normal ratio of gray to white matter is reversed (Fig. 12.1-51B).[325] A normal cortical thickness is 3 to 4 mm, and in lissencephaly the thickness is often 12 to 20 mm.[326] In the thickened cortex, there is often a band of hypertense T2 signal, usually in the parieto-occipital area, which represents the cell-sparse layer with high water content. This may mimic the normal subplate, which should be disappearing between 25 and 28 weeks. A figure 8 configuration of the brain is due to lack of development of the sylvian fissures, also known as opcular dysplasia. Cavitations in the ganglionic eminences have been described.[334] Mild ventriculomegaly, especially colpocephaly, is often present owing to

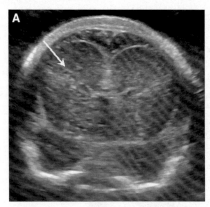
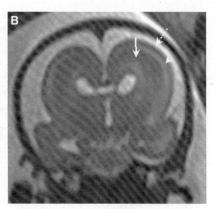

**FIGURE 12.1-51:** Fetus at 36 weeks gestation with type I lissencephaly. **A:** Coronal US image demonstrates abnormal smooth appearance of the cortex. There is increased echogenicity in the area of the intermediate zone *(arrow)*. **B:** Coronal T2 image in same fetus demonstrates thin peripheral cortex *(dotted arrow)*, cell sparse zone *(arrowhead)*, and deep thick disorganized neurons *(arrow)*. Notice abnormal smooth architecture of the brain for gestational age. (Courtesy of Dorothy Bulas, MD.)

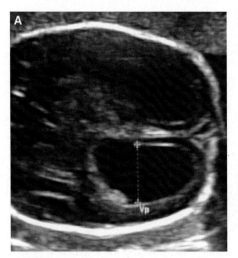
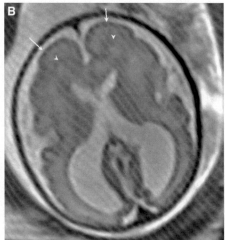

**FIGURE 12.1-52:** Fetus at 33 weeks with confirmed pachygyria and band heterotopia. **A:** Axial US demonstrates moderate ventriculomegaly. **B:** Axial T2 image shows abnormal lack of sulci *(arrows)* in the frontal lobes bilaterally. Notice dark band of signal in the white matter *(arrowheads)*, which is abnormal for gestational age and represented band heterotopia postnatal.

| Table 12.1-14 | Findings in Miller-Dieker Syndrome |
|---|---|

**Common**
Diffuse agyria
Abnormal sylvian fissure and insula
Ventriculomegaly
Corpus callosum dysgenesis
Microcephaly
Intrauterine growth restriction
Hydramnios

**Less common**
Micrognathia
Congenital heart disease
Genitourinary anomalies
Omphalocele
Duodenal atresia

lack of development of the calcarine sulcus.[335] Large temporal horns likely represent arrest in hippocampal maturation and invagination.[335]

MRI is more likely to detect subtle areas of pachygyria or band heterotopia.[330] In pachygria, the cortex is thick with a smooth gray white matter junction and deficient sulci that follow a normal pattern of the primary fissures (Fig. 12.1-52B). With subcortical band heterotopia, there is a band of abnormal gray matter separated from the normal cortex by normal white matter. The band tends to be more pronounced and focal than the dark signal of the intermediate zone that is present from 20 to 28 weeks. Beyond 28 weeks, a band of gray matter signal in the white matter is diagnostic of neuronal band heterotopia. MRI is also excellent at excluding associated anomalies of the corpus callosum, brainstem, and cerebellum.

**Associated Anomalies:** Associated intracranial anomalies are common. The cerebellum, brainstem, and corpus callosum are often abnormal. Extracerebral anomalies may point to the diagnosis of MDS and other genetic disorders.

**Differential Diagnosis:** Understanding normal brain development is imperative as early in gestation the brain is normally smooth, and this should not be interpreted as lissencephaly. Diagnosis for delayed sulcation should not be considered until after 20 weeks, and it must be remembered that there can be a 2-week difference in visualization of a fissure.[324] In the presence of other intracranial anomalies, sulcation may be delayed more than 2 weeks owing to the primary CNS abnormality. Abnormal operculization of the Sylvian fissure does not necessarily support a migration abnormality as it may be related to extracortical factors and can be a normal variant, particularly when only the anterior portion is suggested to be abnormal.[336]

**Prognosis:** In the presence of isolated lissencephaly and MDS, similar neurologic and developmental disabilities are noted.[326] Newborns have hypotonia, poor feeding, and often transient elevations in bilirubin. The head circumference tends to be normal at birth, but is small by 1 year of age. Seizures develop by 6 months in more than 90% of children, and infantile spasms are seen in 80%.[326] With the onset of infantile spasms, there is a rapid decline in function. Most children develop milestones to about 3 to 5 months. Children have poor control of their airway, predisposing to aspiration pneumonia, the most common cause for demise. In children with MDS, death is typically in the first 2 years, whereas in isolated lissencephaly about 50% live to age 10.[326] Milder forms or incomplete lissencephaly tend to have less severe symptomatology. In subcortical heterotopia, the person is predisposed to seizures and intellectual disability, but usually lives into adulthood.[326]

**Management:** Delayed prenatal US and MR imaging in the third trimester may be necessary to confirm diagnosis. Termination may be considered but may not be possible in all countries, depending on time of diagnosis. With knowledge of the anomaly, decisions can be made with regard to site of delivery and management/support at the time of birth. Genetic counseling is indicated both prenatally and postnatally. Parental testing should be considered as up to 20% of fetuses with MDS will inherit the genetic deletion from a parent.[324] This may have implications for recurrence risk in future pregnancy.[330] In X-linked lissencephaly, genetic testing may be performed in the mother to exclude inherited mutation. Discussion of prognosis with decisions on limitations of care should be communicated.[326]

Most children with lissencephaly require feeding via enteric or gastrostomy tubes. Aggressive management of seizures is imperative to prevent rapid decline in function.[326]

**Recurrence:** Most cases of isolated lissencephaly and MDS (80% de novo) are sporadic, and the risk of recurrence is negligible.[326,329]

### Gray Matter Heterotopia

**Incidence:** Prevalence in the general population is unknown, but gray matter heterotopias have been described to occur in 11% to 20% of patients with epilepsy.[337]

**Pathogenesis:** Gray matter heterotopias are normal neurons present in an abnormal location, usually situated anywhere from the subependymal surface to the cerebral cortex (Fig. 12.1-53). Recent evidence suggests that periventricular nodular heterotopia (PVH) is likely due to a disruption in the neuroependyma, which prevents postmitotic neurons from attaching to the radial glial cells, thus impairing migration.[338] Periventricular (subependymal) heterotopias are the most common form of gray matter heterotopia. The heterotopia is located adjacent to the ventricular wall, usually along the trigone or occipital horns of the lateral ventricles.[339] PVH may be nodular or laminar and are commonly described as focal, unilateral, bilateral focal, or bilateral diffuse.[328,340] Histologically, the nodules show rudimentary lamination, similar to that in the cortex.

Subcortical heterotopia (SCH), also due to premature arrest of neurons, is less common but can have many appearances. Some are transmantle, composed of linear columns of neurons continuous from the ependymal surface to cortex. Others may be nodular, curvilinear, or mixed, often solely present in the subcortical white matter.[341] SCH can present as a small, large, sublobar, or regional mass in an otherwise normal hemisphere.

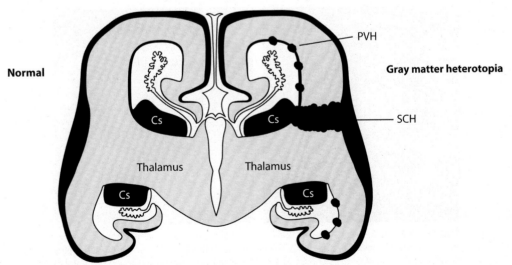

**FIGURE 12.1-53:** Types of gray matter heterotopia. PVH, periventricular heterotopia; SCH, subcortical heterotopia.

**Etiology:** Genetic and nongenetic causes for gray matter heterotopia include single gene disorders, chromosomal anomalies, and disruptive events.[338] Unilateral or sparsely scattered PVH is typically sporadic. Bilateral PVH is present in 54% of cases, and in this group, genetic syndromes and associated intracranial anomalies are more likely.[342]

Many cases of PVH are X-linked caused by mutation of the *FLNA* gene localized at the Xq28 loci.[343] Lack of production of the encoding filamin protein arrests neuronal migration. Since the disorder is X-linked, the phenotype in males results in death or severe neurologic deficit, whereas females are only mildly affected with normal or slightly impaired intelligence and late onset seizures in the second or third decade.[343] *FLNA* genetic mutations may be present in up to 49% of all patients with PVH, and as high as 93% of females with PVH.[342] Females with this disorder typically show bilateral symmetric continuous PVH along the walls of the lateral ventricles, sparing the temporal horns. These patients may also have a mega cistern magna and cerebellar hypoplasia.[338] Cardiovascular defects including patent ductus arteriosus and valvular disorders are more common.[339] *FLNA* mutations are also described in patients with Erlos Danlos syndrome and otopalatodigital (OPD) syndromes.[342]

A rare autosomal recessive defect in the *ARFGEF2* gene is characterized by microcephaly and delayed myelination with PVH.[134] Williams syndrome and chromosomal 5p anomalies may demonstrate PVH.[337] Gray matter heterotopia is often seen in association with other CNS malformations, present in up to 19% of cases of ACC.[337] With posterior distributed PVH, cerebral cortical and midbrain/hindbrain anomalies are more common.[338]

### Diagnosis

*Ultrasound:* On ultrasound, PVH tends to be underdiagnosed, with targeted neurosonography missing 36% detected by MRI.[336,337] PVH can be identified as irregular ventricular margins and/or hyperechoic or intermediate echogenic bands or nodules, sometimes bulging along the ventricle surface or in periventricular area (Fig. 12.1-54A; see Fig. 12.1-38).[333,337,344] Dedicated axial and coronal images of the ventricles allow improved detection.[337] Mild ventriculomegaly is often noted, sometimes in association with a squared appearance of the frontal horns and bodies of the lateral ventricles.[337,339]

*MRI:* Most cases of gray matter heterotopia are detected on a fetal MRI being performed for another indication. On MRI, PVH appears as round or oval nodules which are isointense to the cortex, being dark on T2 and hyperintense on T1 (Fig. 12.1-54B; see Fig. 12.1-38). The nodules are typically within the wall of the ventricle, projecting into the ventricle and/or periventricular area.[328,339] Mild ventricular dilatation, thinning of the overlying cortex, and shallow sulci may be present. In a recent review, fetal MRI was only 67% sensitive for detection of heterotopia, but had 100% specificity when the abnormality was verified on two imaging planes.[345] The detection of heterotopia is often difficult in view of the small size of heterotopia and similar signal to the germinal matrix, and is especially diminished at less than 24 weeks, due to more fetal motion and small size of the brain.[345]

SCH will show gray matter signal extending from the ventricular surface to the cortex or manifest as a focal mass in the white matter (Fig. 12.1-55). The overlying cortex tends to be thin and deficient in sulcation, and the affected area of the brain is small.[340] If large, blood vessels and prominent undulations with CSF signal can be seen in the ectopic gray tissue. Dysgenesis of the corpus callosum is noted in greater than 70% of patients.[340]

**Associated Anomalies:** Other intracranial anomalies are common with PVH and include pachygyria, polymicrogyria, ACC, Chiari II malformation, posterior fossa anomalies, schizencephaly, encephaloceles, and metabolic disorders such as Zellwegers.[339,340]. Limb and frontonasal disorders can be seen with PVH.[342] SCH is often associated with areas of polymicrogyria and callosal anomalies.[203]

**Differential Diagnosis:** The normal germinal matrix, especially the area of the ganglionic eminences, is prominent early in gestation and should not be confused with nodular heterotopia. Differential for PVH includes TS and early subacute subependymal hemorrhage. Nodules of TS appear similar to PVH; however, family history and presence of cardiac or renal

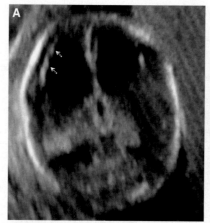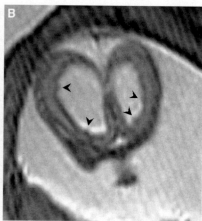

**FIGURE 12.1-54:** Fetus at 21 weeks with aqueductal stenosis. **A:** Axial ultrasound demonstrates irregularity *(dotted arrows)* of the ventricular wall. **B:** Coronal T2 image in same fetus shows dark nodular areas *(arrowheads)* along the wall of the frontal horns proven postnatal to represent gray matter heterotopia.

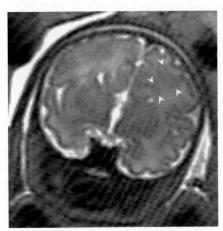

**FIGURE 12.1-55:** Fetus at 35 weeks with ACC and proven subcortical heterotopia. Coronal T2 image demonstrates a nodular band of gray matter signal (*arrowheads*) extending from the ventricular surface to the cortex.

findings may help differentiate. Subacute hemorrhage usually occurs in the presence of intraventricular hemorrhage and ventriculomegaly, and will evolve over time. SCH should be differentiated from tumor or schizencephaly, which demonstrates a central cleft.

**Prognosis:** In the presence of associated anomalies, the outcome is worse for both PVH and SCH with developmental delay of variable severity and early seizure onset.[338,339] Males with X-linked PVH have a worse prognosis than females, with high incidence of neurodevelopmental disorders and seizures.[328,339,340] Disorders of cognition are less likely in the unilateral focal PVH group but more likely in those affected with bilateral diffuse PVH.[338,340] In some patients with PVH, the lesion is incidental as no symptoms are present. Approximately

80% of patients with PVH develop epilepsy, usually in the second decade of life.[338,339] Patients with SCH nearly all develop seizures in the second decade of life.[340] Variable motor and intellectual deficiencies occur, depending on the site and size of the SCH.[340]

**Management:** With epilepsy, treatment with antiepileptic drugs is the first line of therapy. If seizures are refractory, surgical resection of SCH may be considered.[340]

**Recurrence:** Recurrence is dependent on whether the lesion is sporadic or associated with a syndrome/genetic disorder.

### Cobblestone Lissencephaly/Walker-Warburg (aka Lissencephaly Type II; Cerebroocular Dysgenesis; Cerebroocular Dysplasia; Muscular Dystrophy; Chemke, Pagon and HARD Syndrome)

**Incidence:** Cobblestone or type II lissencephaly is rare with unknown worldwide distribution.[346]

**Pathogenesis:** For normal neuronal migration, a normal interaction must occur between the radial glial cells and the outermost pial–glial membrane known as the glia limitans.[347] In cobblestone lissencephaly, typically between the 6th to 7th week of gestation, the neurons move too far past the glia limitans into the subpial space. Pathologically, this is caused by impaired linkage of the radial glia to the pial basement membrane leading to a disruption of the pial barrier, which results in lack of normal cortical plate lamination and neuroglial ectopia in the subarachnoid space (Fig. 12.1-56).[203,347] The cerebellum is affected similar to the supratentorial brain; however, in the cerebellum there is disrupted adhesion of the developing granule cells to the pial basement membrane.[347] Cobblestone lissencephaly is most commonly associated with the congenital muscular dystrophies, which are a group of heterogeneous disorders some

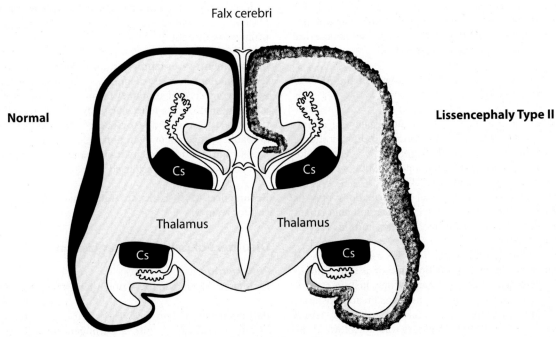

**FIGURE 12.1-56:** Diagram of imaging findings in lissencephaly type II.

primarily affecting muscle and others with muscle and CNS involvement.[348] Those with CNS abnormalities have abnormal O-glycosylation of α-dystroglycan, which in its absence results in defective formation of the basement membrane of the brain, muscle, and retina.[203]

**Etiology:** Multiple genes, all thus far inherited autosomal recessive, have been linked to cobblestone lissencephaly. These include *POMT1*, *POMT2*, *FKTN*, *FKRP*, *LARGE*, *POMgnT1*, and *GPR56*.[203,323] The gene type and mutation abnormality have an impact on the severity of the pathology.[203,347] In general, the *POMT1*, *POMT2*, and *FKRP* are associated with severe phenotype, *LARGE* with moderate, and *POMgnT1* with milder disorders.[347] Congenital muscular dystrophies include Walker–Warburg, muscle-eye-brain disease (initially described in the Finnish), and Fukuyama (described in Japanese descent). The most common and severe phenotype is Walker–Warburg syndrome (WWS) also known as hydrocephalus, agyria, retinal dysplasia with or without encephalocele (HARD+E).[324,349] WWS has been associated with multiple identified and many yet unknown genetic abnormalities. The syndrome is typically caused by *POMT2*, *POMT2*, *FRKP*, and fukutin genes, but only 10% to 20% of cases have been diagnosed with these genetic markers.[346]

Diagnosis of WWS includes type II lissencephaly, cerebellar malformation, retinal malformation, and congenital muscular dystrophy.[324,350] Ventriculomegaly may be present with or without hydrocephalus. Brainstem abnormalities are common and include fused colliculi, small pons, and dysmorphic mesencephalon with a dorsal pontomedullary kink that is characteristic of primitive hindbrain morphology.[351] Ocular abnormalities may or may not be present and include microophthalmia, anterior and posterior segment anomalies, persistent fetal vasculature, retinal dysplasia, retinal detachment, coloboma, and optic nerve hypoplasia.[349] Muscle changes often do not occur till late fetal period or postnatal. The brain malformations of WWS are most severe, followed by muscle-eye-brain (MEB) and, finally, Fukuyama (FMD) on the milder end of the spectrum.[352] MEB disease findings are similar to WWS, with eye findings milder, including progressive myopia and retinal detachment.[346,352] In FMD, frontal or occipital temporal lissencephaly, cerebellar polymicrogyria and hypogenesis, often in the presence of subcortical cerebellar cysts and simple myopia, are noted.[348,352]

**Diagnosis:** Amniocentesis with DNA analysis of the *POMT1* gene may be performed.[346]

**Ultrasound:** In the presence of ventriculomegaly and abnormalities of the posterior fossa, cobblestone lissencephaly should be considered for early prenatal diagnosis.[324,353] Ventriculomegaly is the most common finding, noted in 90% of cases followed by cerebellar abnormalities in 33% (Fig. 12.1-57A).[324,353] Smooth brain, cerebellar, and retinal malformations may be visualized by US in only 25% of cases.[353] Sulcation abnormalities are difficult to diagnose prior to 24 weeks, and this may be even more problematic in the presence of ventriculomegaly, which effaces subarachnoid spaces.[351,353] US may show loss of normal brain parenchymal lamination and/or a thin smooth cortex.[332,333] Transvaginal and 3D imaging may help in evaluation, allowing better detail of the corpus callosum and posterior fossa.[351,353] Ocular anomalies such as bilateral echogenic lenses and conical structures within both globes with apex toward the

retina representing primary hyperplastic vitreous with retinal detachment may be detected (Fig. 12.1-57B).[349]

***MRI:*** On MRI, the supratentorial brain may be smooth, but often demonstrates a pebbled appearance of polymicrogyria (Fig. 12.1-57C).[324] There is an irregular gray white matter differentiation, and the white matter can demonstrate increased T2 signal due to edema or dysmyelination.[352] The normal pattern of lamination is absent.[354] The cerebellum, especially vermis, is usually hypoplastic with abnormal foliation.[348] An enlarged superior cerebellar cistern is commonly present.[355] Brainstem hypoplasia with a kink at the pontomesencephalic junction or Z-shaped configuration can be appreciated by MRI (Fig. 12.1-57D).[324,348] The pons may have a central cleft. The tectum may be thick, and aqueductal stenosis can be present, which is often the cause for the ventriculomegaly. The extraaxiaal fluid spaces are small owing to neuronal and glial heterotopia.[352] Ocular abnormalities can also be detected (Fig. 12.1-57E).[324]

**Associated Anomalies:** Intracranial anomalies of the brainstem, cerebellum, white matter, and corpus callosum are common. Encephaloceles are often present in WWS.[347] Extracranial anomalies are possible and are listed in Table 12.1-15.

**Differential Diagnosis:** Congenital infection may mimic findings of the cobblestone lissencephaly. Classic lissencephaly will also demonstrate abnormal sulcation but a thick smooth cortex. Chromosomal anomalies such as trisomy 13 and 18 and Fryns syndrome may have ventriculomegaly and other brain anomalies. Meckel Gruber can present with posterior fossa encephalocele but is usually seen in conjunction with large polycystic kidneys.

**Prognosis:** Children with WWS never reach any developmental milestones, have severe hypotonia, ocular abnormalities, muscle weakness, occasional seizures, and usually die in the first year of life because of respiratory illness.[346] MEB is less severe and children with FMD, although typically with severe mental retardation, can live to 4 to 6 years of age, though usually with progressive myopathy.[352]

**Management:** With family history of WWS, ultrasound in the first trimester can verify diagnosis.[356] Termination of pregnancy may be considered. Laboratory testing will demonstrate elevated creatine kinase and a muscular dystrophy characterized by hypoglycosylation of α-dystroglycan.[346] No specific treatment is available. Management is supportive.[346] Control of seizures with medication, shunting for hydrocephalus, and surgical repair of encephaloceles may be required.

**Recurrence:** Most forms are autosomal recessive with a 25% risk for recurrence.[346]

## Disorders of Cellular Organization

### Polymicrogyria
**Incidence:** The incidence of polymicrogyria is unknown.[357]

**Pathogenesis:** Polymicrogyria (PMG) is heterogenous in histology and cause, with a pathogenesis still incompletely

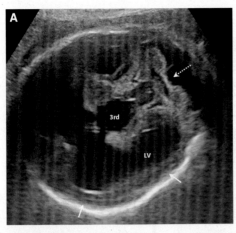
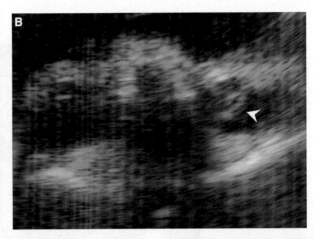
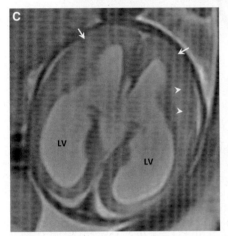
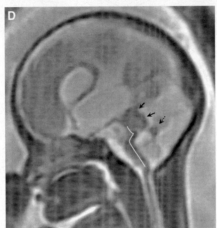
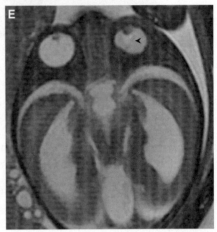

**FIGURE 12.1-57:** Fetus at 33 weeks with Walker–Warburg syndrome. **A:** Axial US demonstrates moderately severe lateral *(LV)* and third *(3rd)* ventriculo-megaly. The visualized cortex is smooth *(solid arrows)*. The cerebellar vermis is small *(dashed arrow)*. **B:** Left globe demonstrates abnormal echogenic tissue extending vertically through the orbit consistent with primary hyperplastic vitreous *(arrowhead)*. **C:** Axial T2 MR image demonstrates smooth mildly irregular cortex *(arrow)* with irregular nodular interface with white matter *(arrowheads)*. The white matter appears hyperintense. The lateral ventricles *(LV)*, are enlarged. **D:** Sagittal T2 image demonstrates the Z- or cobra-shaped configuration of the brainstem *(curved line)*. The tecum is thick *(solid arrows)*, and vermis is dysgenetic *(dashed arrow)*. **E:** Axial SSFP image demonstrates small left globe with abnormal tissue *(arrowhead)* extending from the lens to the retina.

| Table 12.1-15 | Findings of Walker-Warburg Syndrome |
| --- | --- |

**Common**

Widespread agyria, pachygyria, polymicrogyria
Ventriculomegaly
Cerebellar hypoplasia and dysplasia, especially vermis
Occipital encephalocele
Abnormal brainstem, Z-shaped
Heterotopias
Aqueductal stenosis
Abnormalities of the corpus callosum
Disorganized myelination
Eye abnormalities
Muscular disease

**Less common**

Cleft lip
Microtia
Genital abnormalities
Intrauterine growth retardation

understood. The current hypothesis is that PMG results from a genetic disorder or injury that occurs between 16 and 24 weeks, toward the end of neuronal migration or early in cortical organization.[357] Histologically, two types are described. The unlayered PMG is believed to represent an early disruption in cortical migration and organization, and demonstrates a continuous external molecular layer covering neurons that have no laminar organization.[357,358] In the second type, the insult is favored to occur later and the PMG histologically appears as a four-layered cortex with a marginal layer, outer cellular zone of cortical layers II, III, and IV, cell sparse layer V due to laminar necrosis, and an inner cellular layer of VI.[357,358] Both types may be present simultaneously, and both result in numerous 2- to 3-mm gyri, some separated by shallow sulci, others with fusion of the molecular layer, excessive cortical folding, and abnormal cortical cellular architecture (Fig. 12.1-58). PMG may be bilateral, unilateral, focal, multifocal, or diffuse. There is a strong tendency for PMG to develop in the sylvian fissures, seen in up to 80% of patients.[358,359] Other areas include frontal lobe (70%), parietal (64%), temporal (38%), and occipital (7%).[359]

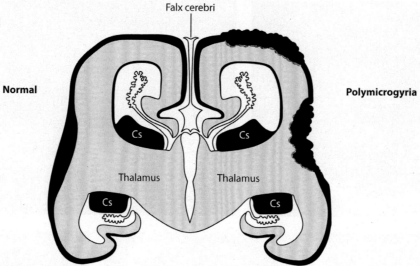

**FIGURE 12.1-58:** Diagram of polymicrogyria.

**Etiology:** Cytotoxic, hypoperfusion, or genetic disturbances are possible etiologies for PMG (Table 12.1-16).[357] Bilateral PMG is favored to represent an early insult which may be sporadic but should raise suspicion for genetic abnormalities, many of which are yet defined. Cytotoxic and hypoperfusion injuries typically result in asymmetrical or focal PMG and likely occur later in cortical development.[357] Numerous prenatal insults, including those from infection, toxins, hypoxic ischemic injury, and maternal trauma, can cause PMG.[203,360,361] The etiology is often idiopathic.[221]

Genetic disorders include bilateral frontoparietal PMG, which is an autosomal recessive disorder on chromosome 16q12.2 to 21 with mutations in the *GPR56* gene, and is seen in conjunction with myelination abnormalities and dysplasia of the brainstem and cerebellum.[357] Familial perisylvian bilateral PMG is located primarily at Xq28 with transmission X linked in 75%, the remaining autosomal recessive or dominant.[357] Perisylvian polymicrogyria (unilateral and bilateral) can be seen in chromosomal aneuploidies, the most common being deletion of chromosome 22q11.2 as in velocardiofacial or DiGeorge syndrome.[362] Polymicrogyria with PVH in frontal perisylvian and temporoparietal areas are likely undiagnosed genetic disorders.[363]

Some syndromes have a high association with PMG. Sturge Weber, which is a leptomeningeal vascular dysplasia causing impaired brain perfusion due to blood stasis in abnormal small veins, should be considered when there is PMG along one hemisphere.[364] Temporal lobe enlargement and PMG are present in nearly all cases of thanatophoric dysplasia, identified by multiple deep fissures along the inferomedial temporal and occipital surfaces.[365] Zellweger syndrome or cerebrohepatorenal syndrome is a peroxisomal metabolic disorder caused by a defect of the *PEX* gene family, transmitted autosomal recessive. In Zellwegers, cortical malformations in the perisylvian and perirolandic region occur that appear similar to PMG and pachygyria but actually represent too numerous and too small gyri.[366] Germinolytic cysts, severe hypomyelination, hepatosplenomegaly due to hepatic dysfunction, and renal cystic disease help diagnose this syndrome.[366,367]

**Diagnosis:** Infectious workup may be considered. FISH analysis for deletions of chromosome 22q11 and 1p35 should be deliberated in the presence of PMG, dysmorphic features, and cardiac defect.[357] *PEX* gene molecular testing or biochemical testing for very long chain fatty acids in the amniotic fluid may be considered if there is concern for Zellwegers.[367]

**Ultrasound:** Polymicrogyria may be suggested in the presence of abnormal overfolded sulci and gyri, overdeveloped often with respect to the gestational age (Fig. 12.1-59).[333,368] Hyperechogenicity of the cerebral cortex has also been described, representing subcortical necrosis or the excessive infolding (Fig. 12.1-60A).[361,369] Sometimes, the sulcation may be immature.[133] Enlargement of the subarachnoid space overlying the PMG is often present.[368] It is likely easier to diagnose PMG in the second trimester than later in the third due to development of the secondary sulci.[368]

**MRI:** PMG leads to accelerated development in gyration with patterns including multiple irregular small bulging and invaginating areas, presence of a major sulcus not yet expected for gestational age, sawtooth pattern, or single to multiple bumps (Figs. 12.1-60B and 12.1-61A).[370,371] There is burring and reduced thickness in the subplate and intermediate zone in 80% of cases (Fig. 12.1-61B).[371] Volume loss, especially white matter, and enlarged subarachnoid spaces have been described.[358,369] Venous anomalies in the area of abnormal gyration are present in more than half of cases.[358] Early in gestation, detection may be more difficult, especially less than 24 weeks, but attention to the normal signal of the cortical ribbon, presence of sulci that are not expected for gestational age, and irregular surface of the brain should raise suspicion.[221,344] Fetal MRI has an overall 85% sensitivity and 100% specificity in detection of PMG.[344]

**Associated Anomalies:** PMG may be isolated but is often present with other intracranial pathologies such as schizencephaly, SOD, periventricular nodular heterotopia, subcortical heterotopia, and ACC.[359] Imaging findings of encephaloclastic insult

| Table 12.1-16 | Causes of Polymicrogyria |
| --- | --- |

**Post insult**
*Infection*
  CMV
  Toxoplasmosis
  Parvovirus
*Toxins*
  Fetal alcohol
  Maternal drug ingestion
*Hypoxic ischemic*
  Monochorionic twin pathologies
  Demise of a co-twin
  Twin-to-twin transfusion syndrome
  Maternal hypotension
*Trauma*

**Malformations with PMG**
  Schizencephaly
  Septo-optic dysplasia
  Bandlike calcification (pseudo-TORCH)
  Periventricular nodular heterotopia

**Genetic**
  Velocardiofacial/DiGeorge syndrome—deletion of chromosome 22q11
  Deletion of 1p36
  Bilateral perisylvian PMG—X-linked, autosomal recessive or dominant at Xq28
  Bilateral frontoparietal PMG—autosomal recessive at 16q12.2–21
  Generalized PMG—autosomal recessive

**Syndromes**
*Vascular*
  Sturge-Weber
  Megalencephaly, PMG and postaxial polydactyly, midface capillary malformations
*Skeletal dysplasias*
  Thanatophoric dysplasia
  Osteosclerosis, cleft palate, and bilateral PMG
*Metabolic*
  Zellwegers
  Neonatal adrenoleukodystrophy
  Congenital muscular dystrophy Walker–Warburg
*Others*
  Aicardi
  Adams–Oliver
  Delleman (oculo-cerebral-cutaneous syndrome)
  Joubert
  Pena–Shokeir

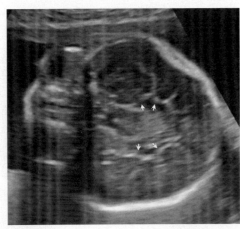

**FIGURE 12.1-59:** Polymicrogyria in thanatophoric dysplasia at 21 weeks. Axial US demonstrates abnormal advanced sulci along the bilateral medial temporal lobes *(arrows)*.

**Prognosis:** Outcome depends on the location and extent of the PMG and the presence of associated anomalies.[371,372] Children with PMG may have developmental delay, focal neurologic deficits, and epilepsy. Bilateral or diffuse PMG or PMG of more than half of a single hemisphere are poor prognostic factors, with these children having moderate to severe developmental delay and significant motor dysfunction.[371]

Sporadic cases of bilateral perisylvian polymicrogyria have 100% oropharyngeal dysfunction and dysarthria, epilepsy in 80% to 90%, mental retardation in 50% to 80%, and sometimes congenital arthrogryposis.[371] Familial perisylvian PMG tend to be less symptomatic.[362] Frontoparietal PMG has developmental delay, mild spastic quadriparesis, impaired language, disconjugate gaze, cerebellar signs and epilepsy.[371] Zellwegers has a poor prognosis with death in the 1st month of life.[367]

**Management:** Depending on the severity of the defect and associated anomalies, termination of the pregnancy may be considered. Postnatal therapy is primarily supportive and includes treatment of epilepsy and physical therapy for neurologic deficits.

**Recurrence:** In the sporadic form, there is no risk of recurrence. In genetic forms, the recurrence is dependent on type of the transmission.

### Schizencephaly
Schizencephaly (SZ), also known as agenetic porencephaly or true porencephaly, represents a transcerebral cleft with a pial ependymal seam, defined as a cleft lined by gray matter from the ependymal lining of the ventricles to the pial covering of the cortex.[373]

**Incidence:** Prevalence is approximately 1.5 in 100,000 births.[374,375] There is a high association with young maternal age.[374,375]

**Pathogenesis:** SZ occurs when there is injury of the entire thickness of the hemisphere. Pathologically, there may be a primary insult to the germinal matrix, failure in induction of neuronal migration, or focal ischemic necrosis with destruction of the radial glial fibers during neuronal migration.[374,376,377]

may be noted. Genetic and chromosomal syndromes that are associated with PMG often present with additional intracranial and extracranial anomalies.

**Differential Diagnosis:** Normal sulcation anatomy should not be confused with PMG. Encephaloclastic insults such as hemorrhage and ischemia may mimic cortical ribbon abnormalities. Schizencephaly is often associated with PMG, but is present with a central cleft.

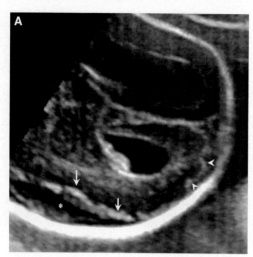
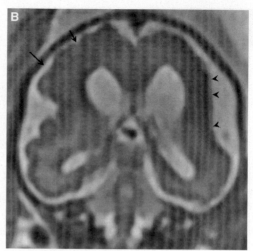

**FIGURE 12.1-60:** Polymicrogyria in a fetus at 27 weeks. **A:** Axial ultrasound demonstrates increased echogenicity of the cortex *(arrows)*, irregularity of the cortex *(arrowheads)*, and enlarged extra-axial fluid space *(asterisk)*. **B:** Coronal T2 MR demonstrates multiple small lobulations along the right hemisphere *(arrows)* and sawtooth pattern along the left *(arrowheads)*. Notice loss of gray white differentiation and lamination with reduced thickness of the brain parenchyma in the left hemisphere.

There has been extensive debate on whether SZ results from a developmental versus destructive insult, though increasing evidence suggests that a vascular disruptive process is likely before 24 weeks' gestation.[374,375] As the perisylvian area is typically abnormal, many believe that SZ may represent a small vessel vascular insult in the watershed zone.

SZ can be bilateral, unilateral, symmetrical, asymmetrical, small, or large. Two type of SZ are described (Fig. 12.1-62). Type I represents a cleft that is closed with gray matter lined lips in contact with each other.[373] Type II is an open defect with CSF separating the gray matter lined clefts. Approximately 49% of SZ are bilateral, 51% unilateral, and 83% are open lipped with remaining fused.[377] Most SZ are frontal or perisylvian with temporal and parietal less likely and occipital least.[377] Approximately 66% of SZ cases are associated with other CNS anomalies.[374]

**Etiology:** The causes for SZ are heterogeneous. Over half can be attributed to a vascular disruptive event in utero, including infection, teratogen, hypoperfusion injury in twins, inherited thrombophilia or trauma in the first or second trimester.[374] Familial cases are reported.[378] Adams-Oliver syndrome with limb reduction and encephaloclastic changes in the brain, and ectrodactyly are two known genetic associations.[374]

**Diagnosis**

***Ultrasound:*** There are no US reports of SZ prior to 20 weeks, with most cases identified after 28 weeks gestation.[375,379] It is suggested that the damaging process in SZ may occur early in pregnancy but continue to evolve and not be apparent until later.[375,380,381] Therefore, it is possible that an early second-trimester scan will miss the abnormality.[375] Ventriculomegaly is often the first sign detected.[381] Wide clefts of CSF communicating between the lateral ventricles and subarachnoid spaces often lined by echogenic tissue should raise suspicion (Fig. 12.1-63A).[333,382] 3D and transvaginal imaging may prove helpful in characterizing the cleft and demonstrating the connection with the ventricle and subarachnoid space.[380,383]

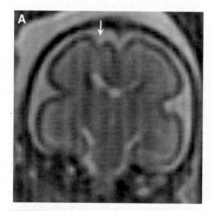
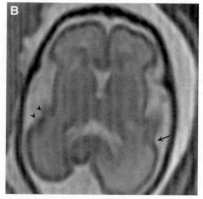

**FIGURE 12.1-61:** Polymicrogyria in two fetuses. **A:** Fetus at 24 weeks with abnormal bump *(arrow)* focally within the right frontal cortex. **B:** Fetus at 28 weeks with arthrogryposis and focal sawtooth appearance to the right sylvian cortex *(arrowheads)*. The opposite demonstrates abnormal lobulation *(arrow)*. Postnatally, the child was proven to have perislyvian syndrome.

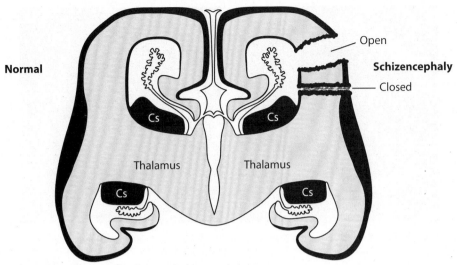

**FIGURE 12.1-62:** Diagram of types of schizencephaly.

Small open- or closed-lipped cleft can be more difficult to detect with antenatal US but may be suggested in the presence of parallel echogenic tissue extending from the lateral ventricle to extraaxial fluid space (Figs. 12.1-64A).[381] Linear echogenic structures in the white matter may represent normal veins or fetal white matter tracts, so care should be taken not to misinterpret them falsely as clefts.[380]

*MRI:* Gray matter lining a cleft extending from the ventricular surface to the subarachnoid space is necessary for diagnosing SZ (Fig. 12.1-63B).[376,382] A fine membrane, likely representing remnant of the pia mater or ependyma, can sometimes be detected (Fig. 12.1-63C).[379] A CSF signal tented area may also be identified extending from the wall of the ventricle, pointing to the defect (Fig. 12.1-64B).[378] SSFP imaging is excellent at defining edges of CSF and soft tissue and may be helpful in verifying the CSF cleft.[382] Gradient echo may demonstrate hemosiderin staining along the defect, seen in as high as 83% (Fig. 12.1-65).[379]

Most clefts identified in the prenatal time are open lipped; however, nearly 50% will close postnatally.[379] Sensitivity in detection of SZ on MRI has been cited at 100% sensitivity and 99% specificity.[345] Anomalies can be detected which include absence or partial absence of the cavum septum pellucidum or corpus callosum.[381] PMG tends not to be detected in the cleft prenatally, and PMG and PVH outside the area of SZ are not commonly defined prenatal.[379] Optic hypoplasia is very limited in visualization owing to lower resolution limits of fetal MR.[379]

Cerebellar clefts may be identified prenatally.[384] Some of these clefts extend from the cerebellar surface to the fourth ventricle, often in association with loss of normal architecture, maloriented cerebellar foliation, and irregular gray white matter junction (Fig. 12.1-66). These clefts may also have similar pathogenesis to SZ.[384]

**Associated Anomalies:** SZ is often associated with PMG (66%), PVH (50%), thin or absent corpus callosum (42%), white matter volume loss, white matter signal abnormalities (20%), optic

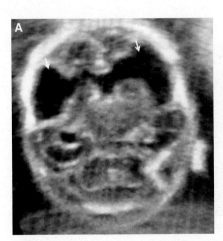 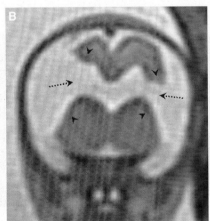 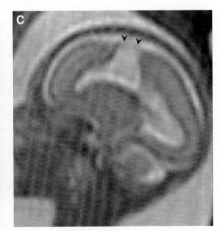

**FIGURE 12.1-63:** Axial image of fetus at 23 weeks with SOD. **A:** US showing absence of the septum pellucidum and large bilateral frontal defects *(arrows)* proved to represent open-lipped schizencephaly. **B:** Coronal image demonstrates open-lipped schizencephaly defects *(dotted arrows)* lined with gray matter *(arrowheads).* Notice absence of the septum pellucidum. **C:** Sagittal T2 image of open-lipped defect with thin membrane *(arrowheads).*

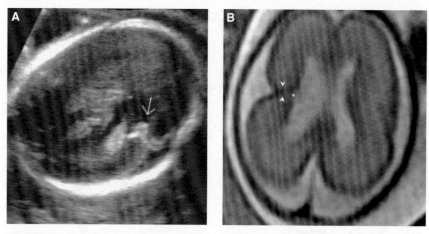

**FIGURE 12.1-64:** Fetus at 22 weeks with closed-lipped schizencepahly. **A:** Axial ultrasound demonstrates parallel echogenic lines *(arrow)* extending from ventricular to extra-axial fluid space. **B:** Axial T2 MR image shows the closed defect lined with gray matter *(arrowheads)*. Notice tenting or nipple *(asterisk)* extending from the ventricle.

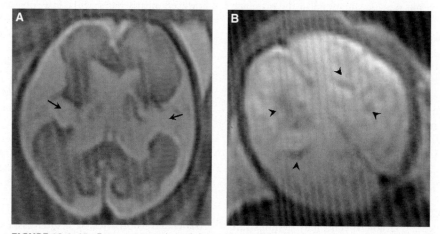

**FIGURE 12.1-65:** Fetus at 32 weeks with bilateral open-lipped schizencephaly. **A:** Axial T2 image demonstrates the gray matter lined open clefts *(arrows)*. **B:** Gradient echo imaging demonstrates susceptibility artifact along the margins of the cleft *(arrowheads)*.

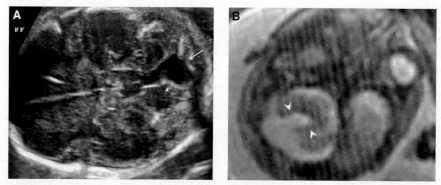

**FIGURE 12.1-66:** Cerebellar cleft in a fetus at 24 weeks. **A:** Axial US demonstrates a prominent CSF defect in the cerebellum *(arrow)* with mild increased echogenicity of the parenchyma along the defect *(arrowhead)*. Vermian abnormality was questioned. **B:** Axial T2 MR image shows gray matter *(arrowheads)* lined defect through right cerebellar hemisphere. Fetus also had a closed-lipped schizencephaly in the occipital lobe (not shown).

nerve hypoplasia (20%), and absence of the septum pellucidum (35% to 50%).[374,377,385] The septum pellucidum is often absent when the defect is bilateral, open lipped, or in the frontal lobe.[385] Ventriculomegaly is seen in 70% of cases and is more likely to be associated with open defects.[377,383] Posterior fossa anomalies are also reported.[382] SZ can be associated with other extracranial vascular insults including amniotic band, arthrogryposis, gastroschisis, cleft palate and lip.[374]

**Differential Diagnosis:** Porencephaly, glioependymal cysts, and arachnoid cysts should be considered but are not lined by gray matter. In the presence of large open defects, hydranencephaly and holoprosencephaly can be excluded by detection of normal basal ganglia structures and midline falx.

**Prognosis:** The size and location of the SZ as well as associated cerebral anomalies have implications on outcome.[376] Bilateral and open clefts as well as SZ with additional anomalies adversely affect outcome.[376] Motor dysfunction tends to correspond to clefts in the frontal lobe. Prenatal diagnosed cases tend to be bilateral, often associated with other CNS anomalies such as absence of the septum pellucidum. These children have a more guarded prognosis.[378] However, when counseling, it should be remembered that an apparently open cleft prenatally may become closed postnatally.[379,380]

Approximately 81% of patients with SZ experience seizures; however, surprisingly, unilateral SZ is more likely than bilateral, but bilateral is more likely to present earlier in life and be more severe.[386] Patients with bilateral SZ have severe developmental delay with language impairment and spastic quadriparesis. Children with unilateral SZ experience variable hemiplegia and mild intellectual deficiencies likely due to the plasticity of the brain at the time of injury.[376]

**Management:** When counseling, it is important to remember that clefts open prenatally may be closed on postnatal imaging. Termination of the pregnancy may be discussed. Management is supportive with therapy directed at seizure control and rehabilitation of motor deficits.

**Recurrence:** No increased risk of recurrence is known in the absence of familial history or known syndrome.

# DESTRUCTIVE INSULTS

## Germinolytic/Subependymal Cysts

**Incidence:** Subependymal cysts (SC) are found in 0.5% to 5% of all neonates, being more common in the preterm.[387–389] The prevalence of in utero subependymal cysts is not known, but they are described less frequently in the fetal literature.[390]

**Pathogenesis:** Histologically, SCs are pseudocysts given that the cavities lack an epithelial wall and are instead limited by a pseudocapsule aggregate of germinal cells and glial tissue encircling fluid containing macrophages with rare iron staining.[391] Two types are suggested, one of which is congenital and the other germinolytic due to injury.[392] The congenital is believed to be due to regression of remnant germinal matrix, as an acellular area exists between the germinal zone and the ependyma, which may normally become cystic with growth of the fetus.[387,388] However, the more commonly entertained etiology is that a SC develops from prenatal lysis of undifferentiated germinal matrix cells, likely due to ischemia, inflammation, or hemorrhage.[387,389,392] It is not surprising that these cysts are found most commonly at the caudothalamic groove, inferior frontal by caudate nucleus or, rarely, adjacent to the temporal horn, representing areas of the ganglionic eminences which persist late in gestation.[387,389] When a SC is found in other areas, it may suggest an earlier insult.[393] The cysts are bilateral in 49% of cases, unilateral, simple or complex; however, when unilateral, the left side tends to be more common.[389]

**Etiology:** Simple pseudocysts are found in up to 50% of cases as isolated cysts, often bilateral and symmetrical in the common locations.[387] In the presence of bilateral simple SC, however, there is still a 20% to 25% chance of the cysts being related to a congenital infection or genetic anomaly.[394] Atypical SCs appear irregular, multilocular, large, along uncommon areas of the ventricle, or different in echotecture or signal from CSF and are very suggestive of an insult.[393,395] A single cyst has lower risk for injury.[394] In the presence of other CNS abnormalities and SC, an insult is more likely.

Subependymal cysts can be caused by vascular disorders, toxic exposures, including cocaine abuse, infection, most notably rubella and CMV, and metabolic, or chromosomal anomalies. Up to 63% of cases of subependymal cysts will have a positive antenatal history predisposing the fetus to hypoperfusion injury.[389] The incidence for infection and SC is as high as 35%.[387] Chromosomal abnormalities associated with SC include DEL q 6 and Del q 4, which impair neuronal migration.[387] Genetic disorders noted with SC include Aicardi-Goutieres transmitted autosomal recessive, with imaging that mimics viral infection.[396] Metabolic disorders associated with SCs include Zellwegers, mitochondrial, Canavans, congenital disorders of glycosylation, organic aciduria, and holocarboxylase synthetase deficiency.[387,390]

### Diagnosis

*Ultrasound:* SCs may be seen as early as 12 weeks.[390] However, most are detected in the third trimester.[390] The type of SC is usually difficult to differentiate sonographically.[6] Most SCs are simple, anechoic well-defined cavities adjacent to the frontal horns, often with a tear-shaped configuration on sagittal imaging (Fig. 12.1-67A).[387,397] The cyst may become increased in echotecture, mimicking hemorrhage.[390] With evolution, SCs can be multiseptated and may increase or decrease in size (Fig. 12.1-68).[390]

*MRI:* Simple SCs are high signal on T2 imaging and low signal on T1 sequences, usually present below the external angle of the ventricle near caudate or posterior to the foramen of Monro at the caudothalamic groove (Fig. 12.1-67B).[387,392] Hemorrhage may be suggested by high T1 signal, low T2 signal, and susceptibility artifact on gradient echo imaging. If the wall of the cyst is very thin or the lesion is less than 5 mm, the cyst may not be apparent.[388] SSFP or heavily weighted T2 imaging may be considered in the presence of an US abnormality. MRI is helpful to confirm the topography of the cyst and exclude additional cerebral pathology.[390]

**Associated Anomalies:** Associated anomalies depend on etiology, though many SCs are isolated.

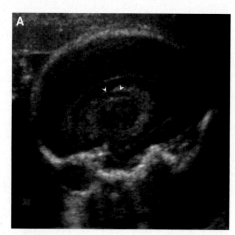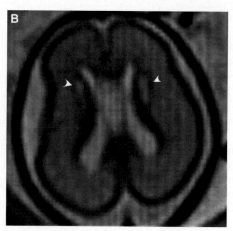

**FIGURE 12.1-67:** Fetus at 36 weeks with bilateral subependymal cysts. **A:** Sagittal US demonstrates teardrop cystic structures at the caudothalamic groove *(arrowheads)*. **B:** Axial T2 image demonstrates small bilateral cysts *(arrowheads)* adjacent to the caudate heads.

**Differential Diagnosis:** SCs should be differentiated from choroid plexus cysts that are intraventricular in location. There are three additional cystic lesions that can lie by the ventricle: coarctation, cystic white matter disease, and porencephaly (Fig. 12.1-69). Coarctation of the lateral ventricle manifests as a cystic area anterior to the foramen of Monro and adjacent to the superolateral margin of the body and frontal horn of the lateral ventricles. These cystic areas represent approximation of the walls of the ventricle and are a normal variant.[392] Injury in the white matter may become cystic and simulate a SC. However, cystic degeneration in the white matter is above the angle of the ventricle; whereas a SC is below.[392] A porencephalic cyst typically communicates with the ventricle and extends into the adjacent white matter.

**Prognosis:** When isolated, 93.5% of SCs regress spontaneously within 1 to 12 months after birth, and in absence of abnormal CMV titers, normal neurologic outcome is expected.[393] In the presence of a positive CMV titer and SC, 50% have neurologic deficit.[389] Atypical cysts are more guarded in outcome, usually dependent on the etiology and associated anomalies.[387,390] In the presence of a history of IUGR, fetal infection, malformation, and chromosomal anomalies, or if the cyst does not resolve postnatally, there is a higher risk of neurodevelopmental impairment.[393]

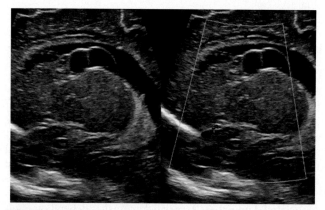

**FIGURE 12.1-68:** Neonatal US showing complex cysts at the caudothalamic groove. The child had positive CMV titers.

**Management:** Infection titers or genetic testing may be considered based on the presence of associated anomalies. If the lesion is isolated, no intervention is necessary.

**Recurrence:** There is no risk of recurrence for isolated SC.

## Hypoxic Ischemic Injury

**Incidence:** The incidence of perinatal stroke, defined as injury between 28 weeks gestation and 28 days postnatal, is reported to occur in 1 in 4,000 live births.[398] The incidence for fetal intracranial hemorrhage and stroke is not clearly known but has been suggested in 1 per 10,000 pregnancies.[399] Many patients remain undiagnosed perinatally as symptomatology is not evident until the first year of life.[398]

**Pathogenesis:** The severity, type, and distribution of the injury depend on numerous factors that include the duration of the hypoperfusion and the fetal gestational age. In contrast to the neonate, an acute response to hypoxia in the fetus is not common. Most fetal hypoxic injuries are chronic. Therefore, chronic imaging findings or a combination of acute and chronic insults may be observed.[400,401] Acute injury to the basal ganglia and cortex are uncommon in the fetus due to greater resistance of neurons to hypoxia earlier in gestation and also the less acute in utero event.[401] White matter injury is also less common in the fetus when compared to the neonate.[401] Germinal matrix hemorrhage, however, is widely described.

Ischemic and hemorrhagic parenchymal injuries are often mixed as after ischemia, reperfusion of a lesion may result in hemorrhage. Hemorrhage can occur anywhere in the fetal brain: germinal matrix, ventricles, cortex, subarachnoid, or subdural spaces. Approximately 80% to 90% of cases of hypoxic ischemic disease cause intracerebral hemorrhage and the remaining 20% subdural hemorrhage.[402,403] In the presence of intracerebral hemorrhage, nearly 90% are supratentorial, and the remaining infratentorial.[398] Germinal matrix hemorrhage is more common than intraparenchymal bleed.[399]

**Etiology:** Injury in the fetal brain may be due to hemorrhage, ischemia, or thrombosis. In the majority of cases of fetal brain injury, there is no identified etiology.[398] A cause may

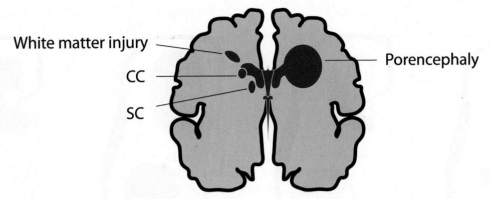

**FIGURE 12.1-69:** Diagram of different types of cysts and their locations: white matter injury, coarctation cyst *(CC)*, subependymal cyst *(SC)*, and porencephaly.

be detected in to 45% of cases, with many etiologies listed in Table 12.1-17.[398,402] The most frequently identified factors are hematologic or maternal trauma.[398,402] Of those with a cause, hemorrhage due to alloimmune thrombocytopenia has been cited in up to 15% of cases.[402] Fetomaternal alloimmune thrombocytopenia (FAT) occurs in 1 to 2 of 50,000 pregnancies, can affect the first born child, and results from maternal fetal platelet antigen incompatibility, the most common being the Pl(A1).[404,405] Fetal platelets carrying specific paternal derived antigens gain access to the maternal system through the placenta, causing alloimmunization. After sensitization, maternal IGG platelet-specific antibody is produced, which then crosses the placenta and results in fetal platelet destruction. The risk of intracranial hemorrhage with this disorder is 10% to 30%, with 25% to 50% of hemorrhages occurring in utero.[404,405]

Other causes for bleeding include drugs such as warfarin and fetal inherited and acquired coagulopathies. Maternal trauma is another leading cause, often secondary to placental hemorrhage and abruption.[403] Placental thrombosis or vasculopathy in the presence of infection is noted in 11% of case.[403] Intrauterine hypoxia and fetal anemia may result in antenatal hemorrhage, especially in monochorionic twin gestations.[402,403] Fetal anemia is believed to cause ischemia and hemorrhage by disruption of vessels due to hyperdynamic circulation. Metabolic disorders can be as high as 22% of cases and include pyruvate carboxylase deficiency, postulated to cause chronic ischemia due to metabolite depletion in the germinal matrix.[403]

### Diagnosis

*Ultrasound:* Ultrasound criteria for fetal hypoxia include intrauterine growth restriction, abnormal Dopplers, especially umbilical artery and cerebral, and later a bad biophysical profile score which reflects abnormalities in fetal heart rate, amniotic fluid volume, fetal breathing, gross body movements, and fetal tone.[406] Imaging may be initiated by decreased fetal movements and low amniotic fluid.[407] Fetal heart changes including smooth baseline variability and late decelerations with sinusoidal pattern may represent the first sign of brain injury.[398,408] In some cases, fetal anemia may be detected by elevated peak systolic velocity in the middle cerebral artery (MCA).[398] Increased resistance in the MCA may be a sign of increase in intracranial pressure related to a hemorrhage.[404] Absent or reversed diastolic flow in the MCA has been associated with poor outcome.[408–410]

| Table 12.1-17 | Predisposing Factors for Antenatal Fetal Intracranial Hemorrhage/Ischemia |
| --- | --- |

**Maternal**

Alloimmune thrombocytopenia
Idiopathic thrombocytopenia purpura
Von Willebrand disease
Vitamin K deficiency
Rh alloimmunization
Drugs including warfarin, cholestyramine, and antiepileptic medications
Toxic exposure alcohol, cocaine, carbon monoxide
Trauma
Iatrogenic—amniocentesis, cordocentesis, blood sampling
Hypoxia related to stroke, hemorrhage, seizure, preeclampsia, or cardiac arrest
Cholestasis of pregnancy
Febrile disease
Diabetic ketoacidosis

**Pregnancy**

Chorioamnionitis
Prolonged rupture of membranes
Placenta previa
Placental hemorrhage
Placental thrombosis
Abruptio placenta
Monochorionic vascular anastomosis
    Twin-to-twin transfusion syndrome
    Demise of the cotwin
Cord accident

**Fetal**

Fetal alloimmune thrombocytopenia
Congenital factor V deficiency
Congenital factor X deficiency
Metabolic disorders—mitochondrial, pyruvate carboxylase deficiency, non-ketotic hyperglycemia, amino acid metabolism, and peroxisomal disorders
Protein C deficiency
Infection—TORCH and non-A, non-B hepatitis
Space-occupying lesions—tumors and cysts

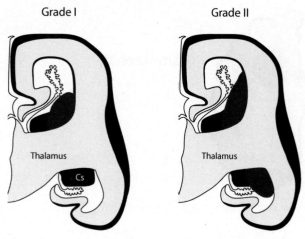
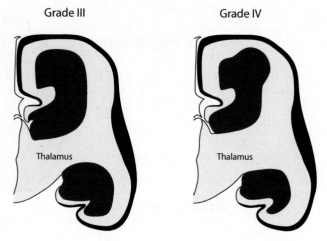

**FIGURE 12.1-70:** The grade of the germinal matrix hemorrhages.

*MRI:* MRI is valuable to confirm the presence of hemorrhage or ischemia and to evaluate for parenchymal abnormalities that may not be apparent via US.[411] In utero hypoxia tends to depict chronic imaging finding of injury (67%) rather than acute (33%).[401] MRI may define cerebral abnormalities in up to 67% of cases of hypoxic ischemic injury. The most common findings are ventricular dilatation (77%), hemorrhage (15%), or brain destruction (35%).[401]

## Germinal Matrix Hemorrhage

Between 24 and 32 weeks, the germinal matrix is highly proliferative and metabolically active, and contains a thin multilayer, highly vascular network which is particularly sensitive to variations in blood pressure, hypoxia, acidosis, and anoxia. Germinal matrix hemorrhages occur due to sudden changes in the cerebral blood pressure and hypoxia which cause bleeding in the fragile premature capillary bed, likely due to a hypoperfusion–reperfusion cycle.[398] Rupture of the ependyma may then result in intraventricular hemorrhage.

A modified grading system denoted by Burstein and Papile can be used to stage fetal germinal matrix injuries (Fig. 12.1-70, Table 12.1-18).[398,402,412]

Periventricular hemorrhagic infarction or Grade IV has been shown to occur as the result of a venous infarct that develops if a large intraventricular hemorrhage compresses or obstructs terminal veins along the surface of the ventricle.[413] Hydrocephalus

| Grade | Description |
|-------|-------------|
| I | Subependymal hemorrhage |
| II | Intraventricular hemorrhage, filling less than 50% of the ventricle with ventricle size 15 mm or less |
| III | Intraventricular with more than 50% of the ventricle with ventriculomegaly >15 mm |
| IV | I–III with intraparenchymal periventricular hemorrhage |

**Table 12.1-18    Burstein and Papile Modified Grading System to Stage Fetal Germinal Matrix Injuries[402,412]**

may develop if the intraventricular hemorrhage incites an inflammatory ependymitis or obstructs the aqueduct of Sylvius or fourth ventricle with clot. Cerebellar hemorrhage has also been described prenatally and is likely the result of germinal matrix hemorrhage in the cells of the external granular layer.

Before 20 to 21 weeks, insults in the brain result in parenchymal necrosis without gliosis, with the most common appearance being a porencephalic cavity. After 26 weeks, there is astrocyte proliferation, and glial septated cavities, known as cystic encephalomalacia, develop. Later in gestation, the insult will usually result in pure gliosis with no cyst.[414]

*Ultrasound:* Most cases of intracranial hemorrhage are detected between 26 and 33 weeks, but cases have been described as early as 20 weeks.[408] Intracranial hemorrhage appears different, depending on the time of imaging after the initial insult. Acutely in the first 3 to 8 days, the clot is hyperechoic (Fig. 12.1-71A). If there is significant intraventricular component, the choroid plexus may appear large and irregular.[411] Choroid plexus is not present anterior to the foramen of Monro, and therefore in the presence of echogenic tissue in the frontal horns, hemorrhage should be suspected.[411] After 3 to 8 days, the liquefying clot appears heterogeneous in echotecture, often with an external echogenic lining and an internal echolucent core (Fig. 12.1-71B). From 7 to 28 days, the clot has completely liquefied, begins to decrease in size, and appears as a cystic hypoechoic mass (Fig. 12.1-71C).[408]

Unilateral hemorrahge is more likely to occur in the left than right hemisphere, possibly because of less susceptibility of right hemisphere vessels to hypoperfusion.[398] Echogenicity of the ventriclular wall due to ventriculitis may be noted. With complete resolution, the brain and ventricles may be normal.[408] Sometimes, a transient ventriculomegaly occurs, which resolves over time as the blood products degrade, relieving obstruction at the foramen of Monro.[402] In grade III and IV, ventricular dilatation is more likely to develop and persist (Fig. 12.1-71D).[415] Ventriculomegaly has been detected in as high as 60%, and some may progress to hydrocephalus due to aqueductal stenosis or ventricular obstruction.[402,403]

Intraparenchymal hemorrhage is seen acutely as a densely echogenic mass, frequently extending from the subependymal layer of the ventricle (Fig. 12.1-71E).[402] As the clot degrades, these lesions often become hypoechoic and then progress to a

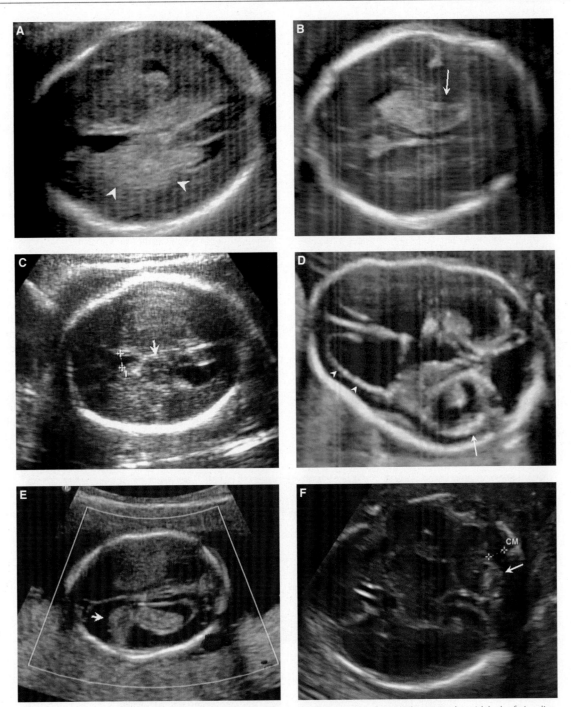

**FIGURE 12.1-71:** Intracranial hemorrhage on US. **A:** Axial image demonstrates large echogenic choroid, lack of visualization of ventricular wall and abnormal echogenicity extending into the adjacent brain parenchyma *(arrowheads)*, consistent with an acute Grade IV hemorrhage. **B:** Evolving subacute hemorrhage depicted by a large heterogeneous choroid with internal echolucent area *(arrow)*. **C:** Axial ultrasound of same fetus in **A** 2 weeks later. There is a hypoechoic cystic structure *(arrow)* in the area of the choroid and lateral ventricle consistent with chronic clot. Calipers represent septum pellucidum. **D:** Axial image in a fetus diagnosed previously with bilateral Grade III hemorrhages. There is significant ventriculomegaly and residual layering blood in the lateral ventricle *(arrow)*. Increased echogenicity of the ependymal surface *(arrowheads)* is consistent with ventriculitis. **E:** Axial view of focal hemorrhage in the frontal lobe *(arrow)*. Notice lack of color flow. The choroid is large, and there is increased echogenicity along the ventricular wall. **F:** Axial view of posterior fossa demonstrates abnormal echogenicity *(arrow)* in the left cerebellum proven to represent hemorrhage. Calipers denote cisterna magna (CM).

porencephalic cyst.[402] Cerebellar hemorrhages have similar imaging, but clues to the presence include an irregular cerebellum and obliterated cistern magna (Fig. 12.1-71F).[416] Because of limited contrast resolution of US in solid tissues, small clots within the cerebral and cerebellar parenchyma may be missed.[416]

*MRI:* The appearance of hemorrhage changes on MRI with degradation of the clot; however, signal changes via hemorrhage age have not been fully studied in the fetus. In general, acute hemorrhage is intermediate on T1 and hypointense on T2, subacute blood is hyperintense on T1 and hypointense on

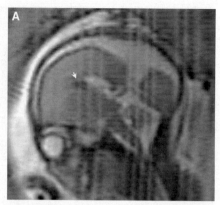
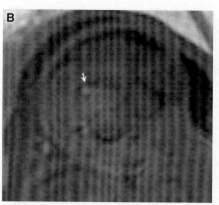

**FIGURE 12.1-72:** Germinal matrix hemorrhage on MRI at 20 weeks in a monochorionic twin gestation. **A:** Sagittal T2 demonstrates a focal area of decreased signal *(arrow)* at the caudothalamic groove. **B:** Sagittal T1 image confirms small bleed by demonstrating high T1 signal *(arrow)*.

T2, and chronic hemorrhage is heterogeneous but with areas of hypointense signal on T1 and T2 (Fig. 12.1-72). The grade of germinal matrix hemorrhage is defined by identifying hemorrhage along the ventricular wall, intraventricular or parenchymal (Fig. 12.1-73).[398,400] As hemorrhage has the same signal as the germinal matrix, symmetry of the brain and knowledge of normal is imperative. Hemorrhages tend to be larger and more irregular than the germinal matrix, often with ventricular enlargement. Gradient echo imaging can aid in defining hemorrhage by demonstrating susceptibility artifact (Fig. 12.1-74).[400]

MRI is more accurate than US with regard to grading germinal matrix hemorrhages and is more sensitive in the detection of either acute or small ischemic lesions.[398,403] Gradient echo and T1-weighted images are helpful in depiction of calcifications.[414] In the presence of ventriculomegaly, evaluation of the aqueduct is important to exclude obstruction.[417]

Hemorrhage and edema may be transient and resolve. However, chronic changes of volume loss, which include unilateral or bilateral large, sometimes distorted ventricles with enlarged subarachnoid spaces, can be noted when injury is permanent.[400]

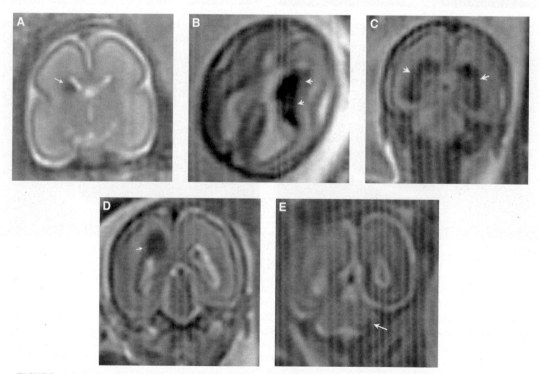

**FIGURE 12.1-73:** Grades of germinal matrix hemorrhages on fetal MRI in twin monochorionic gestations. **A:** Grade I: Coronal image shows small focus of low signal *(arrow)* along the right caudothalamic groove. **B:** Grade II: Axial image shows abnormal dark signal along the wall of the left lateral ventricle *(arrows)*. **C:** Grade III: Coronal image shows abnormal dark signal *(arrows)*, distending the posterior horns of the lateral ventricles. **D:** Grade IV: Coronal image demonstrates abnormal dark signal extending into the right parietal white matter *(arrow)*. **E:** Cerebellar germinal matrix in a fetus with anhydramnios. Coronal image demonstrates crescentic abnormal low signal in the left cerebellum peripherally *(arrow)*.

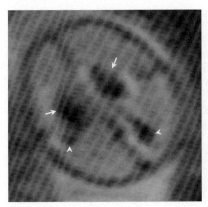

**FIGURE 12.1-74:** Fetus with bilateral grade IV hemorrhages. Gradient echo imaging confirms hemorrhage with susceptibility artifact in the lateral ventricles *(arrows)* and in the adjacent brain *(arrowheads)*.

Irregularity of the ventricular wall or premature loss of the germinal matrix is consistent with germinal matrix injury (Fig. 12.1-75).[417] Parenchymal defects, some appearing cystic or septated, can develop. Supependymal cysts may be seen. Laminar necrosis refers to selective destruction of distinct cortical layers, being most susceptible beginning at 28 weeks. Calcification with laminar necrosis appears as a linear cortical signal abnormality that is hyperintense signal on T1 and hypointense on gradient echo imaging.[414,417] The corpus callosum may be thin or deficient. The sulcation is often abnormal, with PMG developing in 2% of hypoxia cases.[401]

## Extra-axial Hemorrhage

Subdural and, less commonly, epidural hemorrhage have been described in the fetus, occurring most commonly over the cerebral convexity but also in the posterior fossa.[409] Subdural hemorrhages typically develop from tearing of loose draining veins. Epidural and subdural hemorrhages tend to be related

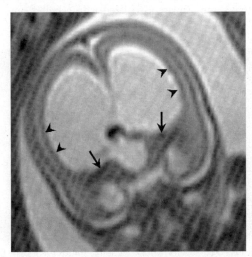

**FIGURE 12.1-75:** Coronal T2 image of a fetus with ventriculomegaly after germinal matrix hemorrhage. There is irregularity of the germinal matrix *(arrowheads)* and dark heterogeneous signal along the basal ganglia *(arrows)*.

to maternal trauma, maternal coagulopathy, or rarely hypoxic ischemic injury.[409,410,416]

***Ultrasound:*** Subdural hematomas appear as echogenic, heterogenous, or hypoechoic collections that displace the brain parenchyma away from the calvarium, usually over the hemispheres, though posterior fossa tentorial collections have also been described (Fig. 12.1-76A).[404,410,418] With organization of the clot, there may be echogenic layering debris in a cyst, an echogenic rim, or development of new collections over time.[418] Macrocephaly is often present. Cerebral edema may result in acoustic enhancement adjacent to the collection.[419]

***MRI:*** This technique is excellent at defining extra-axial hemorrhage in the subdural or epidural space (Fig. 12.1-76B). Even small collections of hemorrhage are easily identified.[418] MRI also can depict mass effect and injury to the adjacent brain.

## White Matter Injury/Parenchymal Ischemia

White matter injury is most common below 32 weeks. The pathogenesis is suggested to be due to incomplete development of the vascular supply in the white matter, lack of regulation in blood flow early in gestation, and immaturity of the oligodendrocyte cell, especially when exposed to glutamate. In the presence of neuronal hypoxia, subsequent cell death results in release of glutamate, which has cytoxic effects on neurons.[420] Microglial cells present in the white matter aggravate the process with inflammatory cytokines. Astrocytes attempt to repair the injury and reduce glutamate which eventually leads to cell membrane swelling and cytotoxic edema. Eventually, there is lysis of the cell membrane and increase in water in the extracellular space with loss of blood-brain barrier and vasogenic edema.

Ischemic infarcts have rarely been noted in the fetus, with most occurring secondary to abnormalities of the middle cerebral artery or venous thrombosis.[420]

***Ultrasound:*** White matter injury is more difficult to detect on US but has been described in the presence of periventricular echodensities that result in loss of normal brain parenchymal lamination.[421] If followed over greater than 2 weeks, cystic areas may become apparent in the periventricular white matter.[404] In the presence of diffuse injury, multiple cystic spaces consistent with multicystic encephalomalacia may be seen.

***MRI:*** In the fetus, white matter injury is different than postnatal. Most cases show increased T2 and decreased T1 signal in the subcortical white matter rather than areas of T1 high and dark T2 in the periventricular area (Fig. 12.1-77).[401] Injury in the white matter will cause loss of normal laminar pattern, especially in the intermediate zone.[400] Sometimes, these lesions are harder to detect on fetal MRI due to lower signal to noise and the high water content of the brain. In general, MRI is more accurate in the detection of small focal lesions than diffuse white matter abnormalities.[414] In some cases diffusion imaging may be helpful by identifying restricted diffusion, though care should be made to ensure delineation from the normal germinal matrix.[417] In the presence of vasogenic edema and astrogylosis, the apparent diffusion coefficient (ADC) value is increased, which can confirm white matter injury.[420]

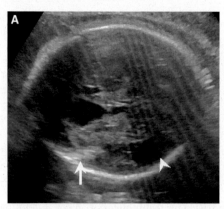
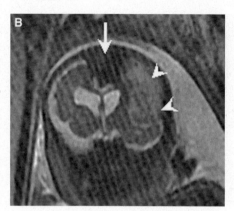

**FIGURE 12.1-76:** Subdural in a fetus with venous thrombosis. **A:** Axial US demonstrates heterogeneous tissue in the extraaxial space displacing the adjacent brain. More anterior, the subdural is echogenic (arrow) and posterior hypoechoic (arrowhead). **B:** Coronal T2 MR image shows heterogeneous T2 hyperintense subdural along the left hemisphere (arrowheads). The sagittal sinus is enlarged and heterogeneous (arrow) consistent with venous congestion. (Courtesy of Dorothy Bulas, MD.)

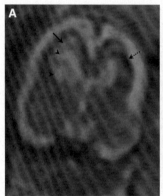
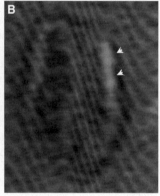

**FIGURE 12.1-77:** White matter injury and laminar necrosis in a fetus at 28 weeks with anhydrmanios. **A:** Coronal T2 image shows white matter hyperintense signal (solid arrow) and small cystic areas of degeneration (arrowheads). Notice that the cortex is thin and extremely dark T2 signal (dashed arrow). There is lack of normal lamination of the brain. **B:** Axial T1 image shows linear hyperintense signal in the cortex of the left hemisphere (arrows) and, to a lesser extent, the right hemisphere. Findings are consistent with lamninar necrosis.

Parenchymal ischemic lesions cause edema which tends to be dark on T1 and high signal on T2 (Fig. 12.1-78A). There may be loss of the normal lamination of the brain.[417] In the presence of acute ischemia, restricted diffusion is noted as high signal on the T2 trace and low on the ADC map (Fig. 12.1-78B).[417] Acute response in the fetal brain is not common, so many of these areas of signal abnormality will not show diffusion restriction.[401] Proton spectroscopy may have a role in the future for evaluation of ischemic lesions, though it is technically more difficult in the fetus.[401,417]

**Associated Anomalies:** Extracerebral findings may be seen in the presence of hypoxic ischemic disease. The most common is intrauterine growth restriction.[417] Infection and ischemia may affect the kidneys, liver, and heart. Fetal hydrops may be present. Evaluation of the placenta for pathology may yield important clues to the cause of intracranial injury.

**Differential Diagnosis:** Tumor should be considered in the presence of a heterogeneous echogenic mass, but unlike a hemorrhage, which decreases in size, a tumor will remain stable or grow. Hemorrhage may result from vascular malformations such as vein of Galen, dural sinus malformations, or cavernoma. In late stages, hemorrhage liquefies and appears cystic. Differential would include cystic lesions such as choroid plexus cyst, arachnoid cyst and if in the posterior fossa, malformations of Blake pouch may be considered.

**Prognosis:** Neurodevelopmental outcome can range from normal to neurologic deficits such as seizure, mental retardation, psychomotor delays, and cerebral palsy. Extreme cases may result in fetal or neonatal death.[398] Prognosis is dependent on the etiology and extent and location of the hemorrhage. In prenatally diagnosed intracranial hemorrhages, 40% to 55% of fetuses die in utero or within the 1st month of life.[402,403] Among survivors, approximately 45% to 50% can be expected to be neurologically normal.[402]

In the presence of a germinal matrix hemorrhage, perinatal mortality and neurologic outcome are dependent on the grade of injury.[402] Lower grade of germinal matrix hemorrhage and those bleeds that disappear are associated with a better outcome.[398]

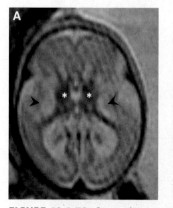
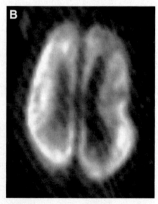

**FIGURE 12.1-78:** Severe hypoxic ischemic injury secondary to twin-to-twin transfusion syndrome. **A:** Axial T2 image demonstrates abnormal hyperintense signal in the white matter (arrowheads), but the basal ganglia also demonstrated abnormal dark T2 signal (astericks) similar to ischemic disease in the newborn. **B:** Axial T2 trace shows diffuse hyperintense signal consistent with diffuse ischemia.

Intrauterine progression of a bleed is associated with a worse neurological outcome.[398] Grade III–IV hemorrhages are associated with a poorer postnatal status.[398] Up to 60% of surviving infants will develop hydrocephalus requiring CSF diversion.[403]

Subdural hemorrhage may be fatal or may resolve completely without therapy, though some require surgical intervention.[418] About two-thirds of fetuses with subdural lesions have normal neurologic outcome.[402] Poor prognosis is more likely if the subdural is in the presence of hydrocephalus, cerebral infarction, or cerebral atrophy leading to microcephaly.[419]

White matter injury may lead to significant neurologic deficits, but prognosis is dependent on the extent and persistent area of abnormality.[416] Associated anomalies or genetic syndromes have a more guarded outcome.[398]

**Management:** Laboratory testing for fetal platelet disorder may be considered. Treatment of alloimmune thrombocytopenia is debatable.[402] However, if there is concern for recurrent thrombocytopenia, fetal blood sampling at 20 weeks may be performed to evaluate fetal platelet phenotype and platelet count. If the fetus is positive for alloimmune thrombocytopienia, maternal treatment with high-dose intravenous immunoglobuluin weekly and oral corticosteroids may be considered.[405,422] Second blood sampling at 24 weeks may be obtained to evaluate for efficacy of treatment. Platelet transfusion may be necessary in the presence of low counts; however, transfusion alone is difficult as the life span for a platelet is only 8 to 10 days, and repeat fetal blood sampling is also associated with increased risk for hemorrhage and exsanguination.[405] Near delivery, fetal sampling may help determine the mode of delivery. If above 50,000 per µL, vaginal delivery is considered safe. Below this level, intrauterine transfusion prior to vaginal delivery or cesarean section may be considered.[405]

Depending on severity of the lesion, termination or supportive care may be solely provided.[402] In the presence of a subdural collection or large hematoma, close monitoring intrauterine is recommended to check for increase in bleeding, hydrocephalus, or hydrops secondary to fetal anemia. The optimum mode of delivery is uncertain and likely case-dependent.[402]

Some infants require surgical evacuation of hematoma postnatally.[418] Hydrocephalus can develop from obstruction at the aqueduct of Sylvius or as a result of mass effect from a large hematoma. In those children, ventricular shunting may be required.

**Recurrence:** The risk of recurrence is low, being between 3% and 5%.[402] With a history of alloimmune thrombocytopenia, the recurrence risk is 75% to 100%, with increased severity of symptoms with sequential pregnancies.[404,419]

## Porencephaly

Porencephaly represents a cavitary fluid-filled area within the brain that usually communicates with the ventricles, subarachnoid spaces, or both.

**Incidence:** Porencephaly is found in 1 per 9,000 births.[416]

**Pathogenesis:** Porencephaly is a cystic lesion replacing cerebral substance, which is smooth and lacks adjacent glial reaction, as the inciting event occurs typically before 27 weeks, prior to the acquisition of mature astroglial response.[414] Two types of porencephaly have been described. Type I or encephaloclastic

porencephaly is the most common. These cases are usually related to a venous medullary infarct or less likely, an arterial insult.[423,424] Type II or developmental porencephaly is believed to arise because of a primary defect in the germinal matrix with abnormal migration of neurons.[425]

**Etiology:** The most common cause for porencephaly is an intraparenchymal hemorrhage occurring between 24 and 32 weeks secondary to medullary vein thrombosis in the presence of an intraventricular hemorrhage.[426] Hereditary porencephaly with hemiplegia has been described in families, usually presenting with frontal porencephaly, hemiparesis, and seizures.[423,427]

**Diagnosis**

*Ultrasound:* Initially, an echogenic clot is identified usually periventricular arising from the germinal matrix. As the clot retracts, the hyperechoic area is replaced by a lesion that is centrally anechoic but with a peripheral echogenic border. Up to 6 weeks later, the area of porencephaly becomes completely anechoic and usually communicates with the lateral ventricle.[426] Coronal and sagittal imaging is often helpful. Sometimes, the septum pellucidum may be partially or completely absent.[426] The cleft of the porencephalic cavity chronically is lined by white matter, and therefore when mature, should not have an echogenic lining. Asymmetrical enlargement of the lateral ventricle with midline shift to the affected side is common (Fig. 12.1-79A).[426] There is no blood flow within the lesion.[425] Microcephaly or macrocephaly may be present.

*MRI:* Centrally, CSF signal on T1- and T2-weighted images extends from the white matter typically in continuity with the ventricle (Fig. 12.1-79B). MRI will often demonstrate evolving hemorrhage or hemosiderin staining along the defect (Fig. 12.1-79C).[416]

**Associated Anomalies:** In the presence of an associated syndrome, intracranial and extracranial anomalies may be noted. Hippocampal and amygdala volume loss are often present.[428]

**Differential Diagnosis:** The main differential diagnosis is schizencephaly. In schizencephaly, the malformation extends form the ventricle to the subarachnoid space and is lined by gray matter. Porencephaly is lined by white matter. In addition, schizencephaly is often bilateral, whereas porencephaly tends to be unilateral.

**Prognosis:** Outcome is related to underlying etiology, timing of the insult, lesion size, and location.[426] Neurologic deficits are typical.[424] The child may have spastic hemi- or quadiparesis and infantile spasms.[423] Many children with porencephaly suffer from epilepsy and cognitive deficits. Seizures tend to correlate with abnormalities in the temporal lobes rather than the porencephalic defect.[428]

**Management:** Epilepsy is treated with antiepileptic drugs, though some children may become refractory to the drugs and require surgical resection.[416]

**Recurrence:** In the absence of genetic syndrome, the risk of recurrence is low.

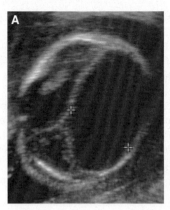 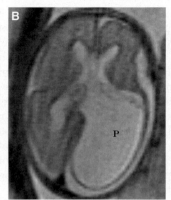 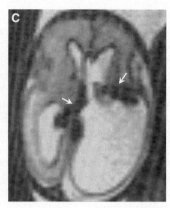

**FIGURE 12.1-79:** Fetus at 26 weeks with diagnosis of porencephaly. **A:** Coronal ultrasound demonstrated asymmetric severe dilatation *(calipers)* of the posterior horn of the left lateral ventricle. **B:** Axial T2 image demonstrates posterior horn of the lateral ventricle contiguous with porencephalic cyst *(P)* replacing most of the left posterior hemisphere. **C:** Gradient echo axial image demonstrates susceptibility artifact *(arrows)* consistent with hemosiderin staining along the defect.

## Hydranencephaly

Hydanencephaly is characterized by complete or near complete absence of cerebral cortex.

**Incidence:** Nearly all cases of hydranencephaly are sporadic, with an incidence of approximately 1 in 5,000 continuing pregnancies or 1 in 10,000 births.[429,430]

**Pathogenesis:** Hydanencephaly occurs when there is a liquefaction necrosis and resorption of most of the cerebral brain. There is complete or near complete absence of the cerebral cortex in the location of the anterior circulation, with most of the brain replaced by large CSF fluid collections. Cortical layers are not present, and the empty CSF spaces are covered by leptomeninges, connective tissue and a layer of ectopic glioneuronal tissue.[423] The occipital and small portions of the frontal and temporal lobes are often present because of collateral flow from the posterior circulations.[431] The basal ganglia and thalami are hypoplastic but present. The cerebellum and brainstem are intact but often are hypoplastic. Rarely, cerebellar hemisphere liquefaction has been noted.[430] Choroid plexus is present but freely floating as the lateral ventricles are destroyed. The falx is usually present but may be partially or completely absent. Hydrocephalus may develop due to aqueduct stenosis or poor CSF absorption.[423]

**Etiology:** The etiology is heterogeneous but destructive. The most commonly proposed mechanism is bilateral occlusion of the internal carotid arteries probably between late first to second trimester, after the brain and ventricles have been formed but before glial response is present.[432,433] However, in hydranencephaly cases, normal and hypoplastic anterior cerebral circulation has been detected. Thus, hydranencephaly is likely due to a nonspecific devastating hypoperfusion, thromboembolic or vascular insult in the area of the anterior circulation, which leads to diffuse extensive intracranial hemorrhage and necrosis.[433–435] Numerous prenatal cases have been described in association with monochorionic twin gestations, fetal infection, ischemia, hemorrhage, or vasculopathies.[434,435] Infrequently, hydranencephaly has been associated with chromosomal aberrations, including trisomy 13 and triploidy.[433,436]

Fowler syndrome, also known as proliferative vasculopathy and hydranencephaly–hydrocephaly or encephaloclastic proliferative vasculopathy, is a genetic syndrome that results in a glomeruloid vascular proliferation which impedes development of the neocortex during the first trimester at the time of vascular invasion of the cerebral mantle.[423] The result is ischemic lesions and progressive destruction of the nervous tissue. Brain injury most commonly presents as hydrocephalus, though hydranencephaly is also possible.[437] The syndrome has an autosomal recessive inheritance.[437,438]

### Diagnosis

*Ultrasound:* Diagnosis of hydranencephaly has been made in both early and late gestation, but usually between 12 and 30 weeks.[431,439] In hydranencephaly, a cerebral falx, although at times partially or rarely absent, is typically identified, and though the supratentorial brain is abnormal, there is usually a brainstem and cerebellum with measurements small owing to hypoplasia.[439,440] The US appearance is dependent on etiology and the stage of evolution. In the phase of vascular insult, homogeneous hyperechoic or diffuse uniform low level echogenic material may replace the supratentorial brain, and no ventricles or cortical structures can be defined. The abnormal echotecture likely represents liquefied brain and hemorrhage (Fig. 12.1-80).[440] In the second phase, the echogenic material

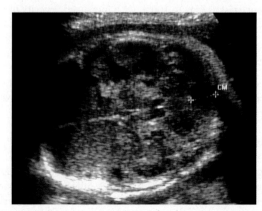

**FIGURE 12.1-80:** Fetus with hydranencephaly at 24 weeks. The supratentorial brain demonstrates diffuse low-level echogenicity.

becomes more hypoechoic with identification of falx and thalami. The final phase demonstrate anechoic fluid surrounding the thalami and midbrain, absence of cortical tissue, and enlargement of the cranial vault (Fig. 12.1-81A,B).[434,439] The head size may be normal, large or small, depending on the development of hydrocephalus. Color Doppler of the circle of Willis is often normal.[440] Usually, polyhydramnios is present because of lack of fetal swallowing.

In Fowler syndrome, fetal akinesia deformation sequence may be detected in the first trimester. In conjunction with hydrocephalus or hydranencephaly, there is often arthrogryposis, pterygia, cystic hygroma, and polyhydramnios.[434,437,438,441] Calcification and necrosis of the white matter, basal ganglia, brainstem, and cerebellum may be present.[437]

*MRI:* There is complete or near complete absence of the cerebral hemispheres with remnants of occipital, temporal and frontal lobes and basal ganglia, and preservation of the thalami, brainstem, and cerebellum (Fig. 12.1-81C,D).[442] Hemorrhage may be detected by high signal on T1, dark signal on T2, or susceptibility artifact on gradient echo images.

**Associated Anomalies:** With Fowler syndrome, additional anomalies may be apparent as described above.

**Differential Diagnosis:** The presence of the falx in hydranencephaly is important to differentiate it from HPE. HPE also usually demonstrates persistent tissue in the frontal lobe region, which is commonly fused. Facial abnormalities in HPE may also help secure the diagnosis. Hydrocephalus should also be considered, but the presence of cerebral tissue, though sometimes quite thin, should help differentiate. In the presence of a dilated third ventricle, aqueductal stenosis should be considered. Severe porencephaly or schizencephaly may be considered, but these cases can be distinguished by areas of preserved supratentorial brain.

**Prognosis:** Although rare cases of prolonged survival have been recorded, prognosis is typically poor with reduced life expectancy, most being either stillborn or dying within the first few weeks of life.[429] Severe retardation is uniform among survivors.[429,443] Survival is possible but complicated by spastic quadriplegia, impossibility of oral feeding, and episodic

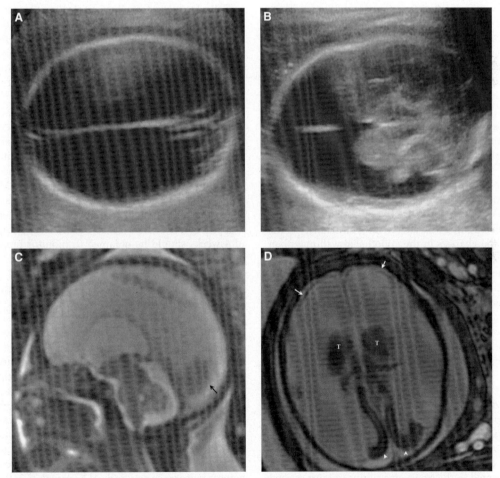

**FIGURE 12.1-81:** Fetus at 25 weeks with hydranencephaly. **A:** Axial US demonstrates persistence of the falx but lack of visualization of normal brain parenchyma. **B:** Axial transthalamic image shows presence of thalami and posterior fossa structures. **C:** Sagittal T2 MR shows lack of supratentorial brain other than small remnants of the occipital lobe *(arrow)*. The posterior fossa anatomy is normal. **D:** Axial SSFP image demonstrates thin remnants of frontal lobe brain mantle *(arrows)*. Small occipital lobes are present *(arrowheads)*, and thalami (T) are small but present.

dysthermoregulation.[423] Some consciousness, mainly auditory, is possible.[423] Seizures are common and pituitary dysfunction can occur. Fowler syndrome is lethal.[438,441]

**Management:** Termination of pregnancy may be discussed given poor outcome. At birth, supportive care may be provided. Some children with hydranencephaly develop hydrocephalus, and shunting may be considered.

**Recurrence:** In the absence of genetic anomalies, the recurrence risk is negligible.

## Dural Sinus Thrombosis

Incidence: Dural venous sinus thrombosis is rare.[444]

**Pathogenesis:** During the 3rd gestational month, the dural venous sinuses and galenic sinuses begin to develop. The sagittal sinus forms via fusion of bilateral marginal sinuses, which initially are separate, draining into each respective transverse sinus. From the 4th to the 5th month, there is ballooning of the occipital sinus, and from the 4th to the 6th month, the lateral then medial transverse and sometimes the posterior sagittal sinus dilate.[445] In the 6th fetal month, with fusion of the marginal sinuses, the venous confluence or torcula develops with its many variations in anatomy. In the 7th month, the ballooning of the sinuses resolves. At birth, the torcula typically demonstrates a plexiform pattern.[446] The venous drainage further develops after birth as a result of further differentiation of the jugular and cavernous sinuses.[446]

Ectasia of the venous sinus is therefore a variant of dural sinus development. It is hypothesized that if a dilated disorganized sinus persists after the time of expected reduction, two secondary events may occur which include development of an AV shunt and/or disruption of the venous drainage, leading to thrombosis.[447] With persistent ballooning of the sinus, it is suspected that the dilated sinus causes elevated venous pressure and secondary dural fistulae, resulting in a dural venous malformation (DVM).[448] In the presence of both or either of these mechanisms, a dilated sinus with altered flow, immaturity of the venous channel, and changes in the endothelial wall may then incite thrombosis.[446,448] Most cases of thrombosis on prenatal imaging are in the area of the torcula Herophili or venous confluence.[444,448] The majority of cases of dural venous thrombosis and ectasia resolve spontaneously, possibly because of the presence of multiple anastomotic channels. However, when there are limited anastomoses or spontaneous thrombosis of a giant sinus, cerebral ischemia, hemorrhage, and hydrocephalus can occur owing to venous hypertension.[446,448,449]

**Etiology:** Unlike the neonate in which common causes for thrombosis include prothrombotic states such as dehydration, shock, hypoxia, polycythemia, leukemia, and congenital deficiency of anticoagulants, the cause of dural venous sinus thrombosis in the fetus is unknown.[444,450] In some cases of venous thrombosis, only ectasia of the veins is identified with the dural lake usually located in the transverse sinus, superior sagittal sinus, or torcular herophili. In other lesions, DVM are detected in association with clot.

DVM are classified into two types: midline giant pouches involving the torcula, transverse sinuses, and posterior sagittal sinus with a more guarded prognosis, or lateral, involving the jugular bulbs, with a benign course and good outcome.[451] Arteriovenous shunting in a DVM is typically via multiple feeding vessels in the wall of the sinus, suspected to be a secondary event. However, dilated veins have been noted to develop after an AV fistula is identified.[452] These arteriovenous shunts are characterized by low flow, rarely causing systemic hemodynamic complications, though disruption in the venous drainage may result in venous thrombosis and intracranial venous hypertension.[453] The thrombus can cause maturation of the sinus with favorable outcome, or the clot may extend into normal cerebral veins causing cerebral injury.[453]

### Diagnosis

***Ultrasound:*** Thrombosis tends to be detected in the second trimester, as early as 18 weeks.[448] Imaging findings are variable depending on the size and stage of the thrombus.[446,448] Typical imaging includes a well-defined triangular or rounded anechoic collection above the cerebellum between the cerebral hemispheres containing an echogenic structure, consistent with acute clot (Fig. 12.1-82A).[450,454] As the clot matures, the lesion becomes more heterogeneous with concentric rings (Fig. 12.1-83A).[446,450] The clot may extend into one or both transverse sinuses. 2D with 3D and transvaginal imaging may be helpful to define clot location.[455]

Color Doppler is excellent at assessing the intracranial venous system with a more continuous waveform noted in vein of Galen and straight sinus, whereas triphasic pulsatile flow is normally noted in the transverse and sagittal.[456] In most cases with ectatic veins, with or without dural thrombus, due to low-flow velocity, color Doppler confirms lack of blood flow centrally even in the presence of AV shunting (Fig. 12.1-82A).[44,448,450,457] Flow around thrombus is rarely apparent on color Doppler.[454] Pulsatile venous flow before thrombus development has been described.[446] In some cases of AV shunting, high-velocity arterial flow may be identified along the periphery of the dilated veins.[450,453,458]

The brain should be evaluated for hemorrhage, infarct, and ventriculomegaly. Macracrania may develop. Most clots show a slow and late decrease in size with stasis around the clot. There may be recanalization of the clot, best depicted on color Doppler before birth.[444] Serial US and color Doppler at intervals of 4 weeks should be obtained to monitor biparietal diameter and decreasing thrombus size.

***MRI:*** MRI is useful in the evaluation of dural venous sinus thrombosis because it is able to confirm venous sinus pathology, exclude other masses, and identify acute and subacute thrombus.[448] MRI will detect a well-defined rounded or triangular lesion in the extra-axial space, conforming to a dilated venous confluence with variable extension into other dural sinuses (Figs. 12.1-82B and 12.1-83B).[448] The sinus is typically isointense to hypointense to gray matter containing eccentric areas of low T2 signal that are T1 hyperintense, likely reflecting acute–subacute thrombus (Fig. 12.1-83C).[444,448–450] With progression, the signal becomes progressively more heterogeneous often with a rim of T2 hyper- or hypointensity, and T1 hyperintensity.[446,449] On diffusion imaging, the intralesional thrombus can demonstrate hyperintense trace and dark ADC signal.[459] MRI can define the location, size, number, and extent of thrombi.[444]

There is usually mass effect and displacement of the adjacent brain. MRI is extremely helpful to exclude brain parenchymal findings including infarction, hemorrhage, or gyration abnormalities.[444] Diffusion imaging can also assist in exclusion of brain

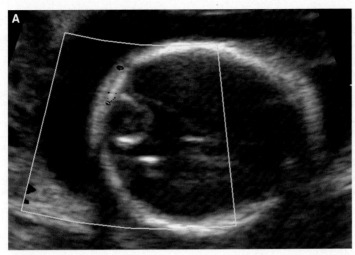
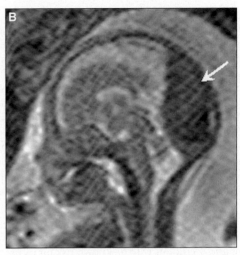

**FIGURE 12.1-82:** Fetus with dural ectasia and venous thrombosis. **A:** Axial US with color Doppler demonstrates avascular triangular structure posteriorly containing a heterogeneous round lesion with peripheral increased echogenicity, consistent with clot. **B:** Sagittal T2 MR image shows enlargement of the torcular and posterior sagittal sinus *(arrow)*. Notice that the sinus has heterogeneous signal. (Courtesy of Chris Cassady.)

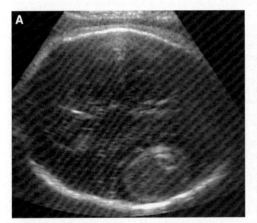
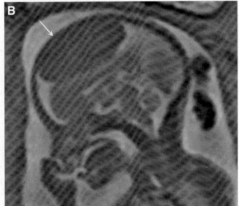
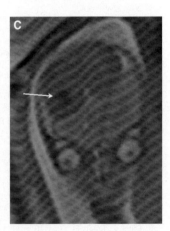

**FIGURE 12.1-83:** Fetus at 22 weeks with dural venous sinus malformation and clot. **A:** Axial US demonstrates echogenic area containing concentric rings consistent with clot. **B:** Sagittal T2 image of the same fetus shows abnormal enlargement and isointense signal of the anterior sagittal sinus *(arrow)*. **C:** Coronal T2 image shows a focal area of decreased T2 signal *(arrow)* in the dilated vein corresponding to the echogenic clot seen in **A**. Note mass effect on the adjacent frontal lobe. The child did well postnatally, with spontaneous resolution of the defect.

ischemia.[448,459] After diagnosis, follow-up MRI may be considered to exclude development of intraparenchymal hemorrhage or infarction and monitor resolution of the thrombus.[444,448]

**Associated Anomalies:** Edema and parenchymal hemorrhages may occur due to venous infarctions. Hydrocephalus may also develop in the presence of venous hypertension and poorly developed arachnoid villi in the fetus. Rarely, a DVM may cause cardiac failure.

**Differential Diagnosis:** The most common mimicking lesions include tumors, cystic lesions such as arachnoid, glioependymal or dermoid cysts, and malformations of the posterior fossa. Tumors are heterogeneous intraparenchymal lesions, whereas cysts tend to be fluid attenuated in the extra-axial space. Other differentials include subdural or large intraparenchymal hematomas that should be differentiated by location. Vein of Galen malformations demonstrate an oblong midline lesion with turbulent flow.

**Prognosis:** Prognosis ranges from normal outcome to mental retardation and death.[61] Review of a small number of cases in the literature show a good neurological outcome in up to 70% to 80% of antenatal detected cases.[446,450,451] If the fetus has a normal biparietal diameter and the malformation undergoes spontaneous regression in utero (55%), a better outcome has been noted.[446,450,460] Prognosis is not dependent on size of the clot, venous dilatation, or number of thrombi.[444] Often the torcula demonstrates thrombosis but with good outcome, likely because of fetal anastomoses which allow redirection of venous blood flow.[444] Outcome is most dependent on lack of other fetal anomalies and the presence of a normal brain.[444] Associated cerebral findings such as hemorrhage, infarct, hydrocephalus, distortion of cerebral anatomy, increasing size of thrombus, or clinical factors such as prematurity, thrombosis due to preexisting conditions, and signs of cardiac decompensation are poor prognostic factors.[64] A fetus with thrombosis and these complications may have intrauterine or postnatal demise or neurologic deficits.[449]

**Management:** Management is variable and includes termination of pregnancy, surgical intervention after birth, or expectant management in hopes of spontaneous regression with favorable outcome. Vaginal delivery does not seem to be contraindicated with normal head size.[453] After birth, the child should be evaluated for cardiac failure, anemia, and coagulopathy with appropriate medical management.[447] Imaging should include an MRI and MR venogram to assess venous ectasia, thrombus, DVM, and brain parenchymal injury. An arteriogram at 4 to 5 months of age is indicated, especially if spontaneous resolution has not occurred.[451,460] Surgery is not recommended because of risk of bleeding and the high likelihood of spontaneous regression.[461] Embolization or hematoma evacuation may be required in some cases.[450,451]

**Recurrence:** Dural thrombosis and dural venous malformations are sporadic conditions with no known risk for recurrence.[444,449]

# REFERENCES

1. Huisman TAGM. Fetal magnetic resonance imaging of the brain: is ventriculomegaly the tip of the syndromal iceberg? *Semin Ultrasound CT MR.* 2011;32:491–509.
2. Nyberg DA. Recommendations for obstetric sonography in the evaluation of the fetal cranium. *Radiology.* 1989;172:309–311.
3. Filly RA, Cardoza JD, Goldstein RB, et al. Detection of fetal central nervous system anomalies: a practical level of effort for a routine sonogram. *Radiology.* 1989;172:403–408.
4. Levine D, Feldman HA, Kazam Tannus JF, et al. Frequency and cause of disagreements in diagnoses for fetuses referred for ventriculomegaly. *Radiology.* 2008;247:515–527.
5. Whitby EH, Paley MNJ, Sprigg A, et al. Comparison of ultrasound magnetic resonance imaging in 100 singleton pregnancies with suspected brain abnormalities. *BJOG.* 2004;111:784–792.
6. Levine D, Barnes PD, Robertson RR, et al. Fast MR imaging of fetal central nervous system abnormalities. *Radiology.* 2003;229:51–61.
7. Sonigo PC, Rypens FF, Carteret M, et al. MR imaging of fetal cerebral anomalies. *Pediatr Radiol.* 1998;28:212–222.
8. Simon EM, Goldstein RB, Coakley FV, et al. Fast MR imaging of fetal CNS anomalies in utero. *AJNR Am J Neuroradiol.* 2000;21:1688–1698.
9. D'Addario V, Rossi AC. Neuroimaging of ventriculomegaly in the fetal period. *Semin Fetal Neonatal Med.* 2012;17:310–318.
10. Garel C, Luton D, Oury JF, et al. Ventricular dilatations. *Childs Nerv Syst.* 2003;19:517–523.
11. Zimmerman RA, Bilaniuk LT. Magnetic resonance evaluation of fetal ventriculomegaly-associated congenital malformations and lesions. *Semin Fetal Neonatal Med.* 2005;10:429–443.
12. Salomon LJ, Bernard JP, Ville Y. Reference ranges for fetal ventricular width: a non-normal approach. *Ultrasound Obstet Gynecol.* 2007;30:61–66.
13. Achiron R, Schimmel M, Achiron A, et al. Fetal mild idiopathic lateral ventriculomegaly: is there a correlation with fetal trisomy? *Ultrasound Obstet Gynecol.* 1993;3:89–92.
14. Goldstein RB, Pidus AS, Filly RA, et al. Mild lateral cerebral ventricular dilatation in utero: clinical significance and prognosis. *Radiology.* 1990;176:237–242.
15. Filly RA, Goldstein RB, Callen PW. Fetal ventricle: importance in routine obstetric sonography. *Radiology.* 1991;181:1–7.
16. Weichert J, Hartge D, Krapp M, et al. Prevalence, characteristics and perinatal outcome of fetal ventriculomegaly in 29,000 pregnancies followed at a single institution. *Fetal Diagn Ther.* 2010;27:142–148.
17. D'Addario V, Pinto V, Di Cagno L, et al. Sonographic diagnosis of fetal cerebral ventriculomegaly: an update. *J Matern Fetal Neonatal Med.* 2007;20:7–14.
18. Nyberg DA, Mack LA, Hirsch J, et al. Fetal hydrocephalus: sonographic detection and clinical significance of associated anomalies. *Radiology.* 1987;163:187–191.
19. Brodbelt A, Stoodley M. CSF pathways: a review. *Br J Neurosurg.* 2007;21:510–520.
20. Oi S, Di Rocco C. Proposal of "evolution theory in cerebrospinal fluid dynamics" and minor pathway hydrocephalus in developing immature brain. *Childs Nerv Syst.* 2006;22:662–669.
21. Gaglioti P, Oberto M, Todros T. The significance of fetal ventriculomegaly: etiology, short- and long-term outcomes. *Prenat Diagn.* 2009;29:381–388.
22. Kelly EN, Allen VM, Seaward G, et al. Mild ventriculomegaly in the fetus, natural history, associated findings and outcome of isolated mild ventriculomegaly: a literature review. *Prenat Diagn.* 2001;21:697–700.
23. Yamaski M, Nonaka M, Bamba Y, et al. Diagnosis, treatment, and long-term outcomes of fetal hydrocephalus. *Semin Fetal Neonatal Med.* 2012;17:330–335.
24. Melchiorre K, Bhide A, Gika AD, et al. Counseling in isolated mild fetal ventriculomegaly. *Ultrasound Obstet Gynecol.* 2009;34:212–224.
25. Cardoza JD, Goldstein RB, Filly RA. Exclusion of fetal ventriculomegaly with a single measurement: the width of the lateral ventricular atrium. *Radiology.* 1988;169:711–714.
26. Alagappan R, Browning PD, Laorr A, et al. Distal lateral ventricular atrium: reevaluation of normal range. *Radiology.* 1994;193:405–408.
27. Paladini D, Malinger G, Monteagudo A, et al. Sonographic examination of the fetal central nervous system: guidelines for performing the "basic examination" and the "fetal neurosonogram." *Ultrasound Obstet Gynecol.* 2007;29:109–116.
28. Heiserman J, Filly RA, Goldstein RB. Effect of measurement errors on sonographic evaluation of ventriculomegaly. *J Ultrasound Med.* 1991;10:121–124.
29. Achiron R, Yagel S, Rotstein Z, et al. Cerebral lateral ventricular asymmetry: is this a normal ultrasonographic findings in the fetal brain? *Obstet Gynecol.* 1997;89:233–237.
30. Sadan S, Malinger G, Schweiger A, et al. Neuropsychological outcome of children with asymmetric ventricles or unilateral mild ventriculomegaly identified in utero. *BJOG.* 2007;114:596–602.
31. Guibaud L. Fetal cerebral ventricular measurement and ventriculomegaly: time for procedure standardization. *Ultrasound Obstet Gynecol.* 2009;34:127–130.
32. Mahony BS, Nyberg DA, Hirsch JH, et al. Mild idiopathic lateral cerebral ventricular dilatation in utero: sonographic evaluation. *Radiology.* 1988;169:715–721.
33. Cardoza JD, Filly RA, Podrasky AE. The dangling choroid plexus: a sonographic observation of value in excluding ventriculomegaly. *AJR Am J Roentgenol.* 1988;151:767–770.
34. Hertzberg BS, Lile R, Foosaner DE, et al. Choroid plexus-ventricular wall separation in fetuses with normal-sized cerebral ventricles at sonography: postnatal outcome. *AJR Am J Roentgenol.* 1994;163:405–410.
35. Gaglioti P, Danelon D, Bontempo S, et al. Fetal cerebral ventriculomegaly: outcome in 176 cases. *Ultrasound Obstet Gynecol.* 2005;25:372–377.
36. Grandjean H, Larroque D, Levi S; and the Eurofetus Study Group. The performance of routine ultrasonographic screening of pregnancies in the Eurofetus study. *Am J Obstet Gynecol.* 1999;181:446–454.
37. Martinez-Zamora MA, Borrell A, Borobio V, et al. False positives in the prenatal ultrasound screening of fetal structural anomalies. *Prenat Diagn.* 2007;27:18–22.
38. Richmond S, Atkins J. A population-based study of the prenatal diagnosis of congenital malformation over 16 years. *BJOG.* 2005;112:1349–1357.
39. Timor-Tritsch IE, Monteagudo A. Transvaginal fetal neurosonography: standardization of the planes and sections by anatomic landmarks. *Ultrasound Obstet Gynecol.* 1996;8:42–47.
40. Malinger G, Ben-Sira L, Lev D, et al. Fetal brain imaging: a comparison between magnetic resonance imaging and dedicated neurosonography. *Ultrasound Obstet Gynecol.* 2004;23:333–340.
41. D'Addario V, Pinto V, Di Cagno L, et al. The midsagittal view of the fetal brain: a useful landmark in recognizing the cause of fetal cerebral ventriculomegaly. *J Perinatal Med.* 2005;33:423–427.
42. Monteagudo A, Timor-Tritsch IE, Moomjy M. Nomograms of the fetal lateral ventricles using transvaginal sonography. *J Ultrasound Med.* 1993;5:265–269.
43. Rickard S, Morris J, Paley M, et al. In utero magnetic resonance of the non-isolated ventriculomegaly: does ventricular size or morphology reflect pathology. *Clin Radiol.* 2006;61:844–853.
44. Schrander-Stumpel C, Fryns JP. Congenital hydrocephalus: nosology and guidelines for clinical approach and genetic counseling. *Eur J Pediatr.* 1998;157:355–362.
45. Morris JE, Rickard S, Paley MNJ, et al. The value of in-utero magnetic resonance imaging in ultrasound diagnosed foetal isolated cerebral ventriculomegaly. *Clin Radiol.* 2007;62:140–144.
46. Li Y, Estroff JA, Mehta TS, et al. Ultrasound and MRI of fetuses with ventriculomegaly: can cortical development be used to predict postnatal outcome. *AJR Am J Roentgenol.* 2011;196:1457–1467.
47. Mehta TS, Levine D. Imaging of fetal cerebral ventriculomegaly: a guide to management and outcome. *Semin Fetal Neonatal Med.* 2005;10:421–428.
48. Griffiths PD, Reeves MJ, Morris JE, et al. A prospective study of fetuses with isolated ventriculomegaly investigated by antenatal sonography and in utero MR imaging. *AJNR Am J Neuroradiol.* 2010;31:106–111.
49. Levine D, Trop I, Mehta TS, et al. MR imaging appearance of fetal cerebral ventricular morphology. *Radiology.* 2002;223:652–660.
50. Manganaro L, Savelli S, Francioso A, et al. Role of fetal MRI in the diagnosis of cerebral ventriculomegaly assessed by ultrasonography. *Radiol Med.* 2009;114:1013–1023.
51. Levine D, Barnes PD. Cortical maturation in normal and abnormal fetuses as assessed with prenatal MR imaging. *Radiology.* 1999;210:751–758.
52. Nicolaides KH, Berry S, Snijders RJM, et al. Fetal lateral cerebral ventriculomegaly: associated malformations and chromosomal defects. *Fetal Diagn Ther.* 1990;5:5–14.
53. Lee SB, Hong SH, Wang KY, et al. Fetal ventriculomegaly: prognosis in cases in which prenatal neurosurgical consultation was sought. *J Neurosurg.* 2006;105:265–270.
54. Quahba J, Luton D, Vuillard E, et al. Prenatal isolated mild ventriculomegaly: outcome in 167 cases. *BJOG.* 2006;113:1072–1079.

55. Wax JR, Bookman L, Cartin A, et al. Mild fetal cerebral ventriculomegaly: diagnosis, clinical associations, and outcomes. *Obstet Gynecol Surv.* 2003;58:407–414.

56. Vergani P, Locatelli A, Strobelt N, et al. Clinical outcome of mild fetal ventriculomegaly. *Am J Obstet Gynecol.* 1998;178:218–222.

57. Parilla BV, Endres LK, Dinsmoor MJ, et al. In utero progression of mild fetal ventriculomegaly. *Int J Gynaecol Obstet.* 2006;93:106–109.

58. Pilu G, Hobbins JC. Sonography of fetal cerebrospinal anomalies. *Prenat Diagn.* 2002;22:321–330.

59. Falip C, Blanc N, Maes E, et al. Postnatal clinical and imaging follow-up of infants with prenatal isolated mild ventriculomegaly: a series of 101 cases. *Pediatr Radiol.* 2007;37:981–989.

60. Durfee SM, Kim FM, Benson CB. Postnatal outcome of fetuses with the prenatal diagnosis of asymmetric hydrocephalus. *J Ultrasound Med.* 2001;20:263–268.

61. Devaseelan P, Cardwell C, Bell B, et al. Prognosis of isolated mild to moderate fetal cerebral ventriculomegaly: a systematic review. *J Perinat Med.* 2010;38:401–409.

62. Davis GH. Fetal hydrocephalus. *Clin Perinatol.* 2003;30:531–539.

63. Chervenak FA, Berkowitz RL, Romero R, et al. The diagnosis of fetal hydrocephalus. *Am J Obstet Gynecol.* 1983;147:703–716.

64. Kinzler WL, Smulian JC, McLean DA, et al. Outcome of prenatally diagnosed mild unilateral cerebral ventriculomegaly. *J Ultrasound Med.* 2001;20:257–262.

65. Breeze ACG, Dey PK, Lees CC, et al. Obstetric and neonatal outcomes in apparently isolated mild fetal ventriculomegaly. *J Perinat Med.* 2005;33:236–240.

66. Patel MD, Goldstein RB, Tung S, et al. Fetal cerebral ventricular atrium: difference in size according to sex. *Radiology.* 1995;194:713–715.

67. Nadel AS, Benacerraf BR. Lateral ventricular atrium: larger in male than female fetuses. *Int J Gynaecol Obstet.* 1995;51:123–126.

68. Almog B, Gamzu R, Achiron R, et al. Fetal lateral ventricular width: what should be its upper limit? A prospective cohort study and reanalysis of the current and previous data. *J Ultrasound Med.* 2003;22:39–43.

69. Snijders RJM, Nicolaides KH. Fetal biometry at 14–40 weeks' gestation. *Ultrasound Obstet Gynecol.* 1994;4:34–48.

70. Bronsteen R, Lee W, Vettraino I, et al. Isolated choroid plexus separation on second-trimester sonography: natural history and postnatal importance. *J Ultrasound Med.* 2006;25:343–347.

71. Patel MD, Filly AL, Hersh DR, et al. Isolated mild fetal cerebral ventriculomegaly: clinical course and outcome. *Radiology.* 1994;192:759–764.

72. Pilu G, Falco P, Gabrielli S, et al. The clinical significance of fetal isolated cerebral borderline ventriculomegaly: report of 31 cases and review of the literature. *Ultrasound Obstet Gynecol.* 1999;14:320–326.

73. Senat MV, Bernard JP, Schwarzler P, et al. Prenatal diagnosis and follow-up of 14 cases of unilateral ventriculomegaly. *Ultrasound Obstet Gynecol.* 1999;14:327–332.

74. Wyldes M, Watkinson M. Isolated mild fetal ventriculomegaly. *Arch Dis Child Fetal Neonatal ED.* 2004;89:F9–F13.

75. Griffiths PD, Reeves MJ, Morris JE, et al. A prospective study of fetuses with isolated ventriculomegaly investigated by antenatal sonography and in utero MR imaging. *AJNR Am J Neuroradiol.* 2010;31:106–111.

76. Parazzini C, Righini A, Doneda C, et al. Is fetal magnetic resonance imaging indicated when ultrasound isolated mild ventriculomegaly is present in pregnancies with no risk factors. *Prenat Diagn.* 2012;32:752–757.

77. Salomon LJ, Ouahba J, Delezoide AL, et al. Third-trimester fetal MRI in isolated 10- to 12-mm ventriculomegaly: is it worth it? *BJOG.* 2006;113:942–947.

78. Signorelli M, Tiberti A, Valseriath D, et al. Width of the fetal lateral ventricular atrium between 10 and 12 mm: a simple variation of the norm? *Ultrasound Obstet Gynecol.* 2004;23:14–18.

79. Leitner Y, Stolar O, Rotstein M, et al. The neurocognitive outcome of mild isolated fetal ventriculomegaly verified by prenatal magnetic resonance imaging. *Am J Obstet Gynecol.* 2009;201:215.e1–215.e6.

80. Lipitz S, Yagel S, Malinger G, et al. Outcome of fetuses with isolated borderline unilateral ventriculomegaly diagnosed at mid-gestation. *Ultrasound Obstet Gynecol.* 1998;12:23–26.

81. Gilmore JH, Smith LC, Wolfe HM, et al. Prenatal mild ventriculomegaly predicts abnormal development of the neonatal brain. *Biol Psychiatry.* 2008;64:1069–1076.

82. Bloom SL, Bloom DD, Dellanebbia C, et al. The developmental outcome of children with antenatal mild isolated ventriculomegaly. *Obstet Gynecol.* 1997;90:93–97.

83. Gomez-Arriaga P, Herraiz I, Puente JM, et al. Mid-term neurodevelopmental outcome in isolated mild ventriculomegaly diagnosed in fetal life. *Fetal Diagn Ther.* 2012;31:12–18.

84. Verhagen WIM, Bartels RHAM, Fransen E, et al. Familial congenital hydrocephalus and aqueduct stenosis with probably autosomal dominant inheritance and variable expression. *J Neurol Sci.* 1998;158:101–105.

85. Kenwrick S, Jouet M, Donnai D. X-linked hydrocephalus and MASA syndrome. *J Med Genet.* 1996;33:59–65.

86. Weller S, Gartner J. Genetic and clinical aspects of x-linked hydrocephalus (L1 disease): mutations in the L1CAM gene. *Hum Mutat.* 2001;18:1–12.

87. Humphreys P, Muzumdar DP, Sly LE, et al. Focal cerebral mantle disruption in fetal hydrocephalus. *Pediatr Neurol.* 2007;36:236–243.

88. Ishak GE, Dempsey JC, Shaw DWW, et al. Rhombencephalosynapsis: a hindbrain malformation associated with incomplete separation of midbrain and forebrain hydrocephalus and a broad spectrum of severity. *Brain.* 2012;135:1370–1386.

89. Oi S, Honda U, Hidaka M, et al. Intrauterine high resolution magnetic resonance imaging in fetal hydrocephalus and prenatal estimation of postnatal outcomes with "perspective classification." *J Neurosurg.* 1998;88:685–694.

90. Rieley MB, Kline-Fath BM, Peach EE, et al. Aqueductal stenosis diagnosed with fetal MRI: etiology, medical and developmental outcomes The David Smith Workshop on Dysmorphology and Morphogenesis, Montremblant, Canada August 2008.

91. Varadi V, Csecsei K, Szeifert GT, et al. Prenatal diagnosis of X linked hydrocephalus without aqueductal stenosis. *J Med Genet.* 1987;24:207–209.

92. Breeze ACG, Alexander PMA, Murdoch EM, et al. Obstetric and neonatal outcomes in severe fetal ventriculomegaly. *Prenat Diagn.* 2007;27:124–129.

93. Levitsky DB, Mack LA, Nyberg DA, et al. Fetal aqueductal stenosis diagnosed sonographically: how grave is the prognosis? *AJR Am J Roentgenol.* 1995;164:725–730.

94. Holmes LB, Nash A, ZuRhein GM, et al. X-linked aqueductal stenosis: clinical and neuropathological findings in two families. *Pediatrics.* 1973;51:697–704.

95. Kennelly MM, Cooley SM, McFarland PJ. Natural history of apparently isolated severe fetal ventriculomegaly: perinatal survival and neurodevelopmental outcomes. *Prenat Diagn.* 2009;29:1135–1140.

96. Cavalheiro S, Fernandes Moron A, Zymberg ST, et al. Fetal hydrocephalus—prenatal treatment. *Childs Nerv Syst.* 2003;19:561–573.

97. Orioli IM, Castilla EE. Epidemiology of holoprosencephaly: prevalence and risk factors. *Am J Med Genet C Semin Med Genet.* 2010;154C:13–21.

98. Wenghoefer M, Ettema AM, Sina F, et al. Prenatal ultrasound diagnosis in 51 cases of holoprosencephaly: craniofacial anatomy, associated malformations, and genetics. *Cleft Palate Craniofac J.* 2010;47:15–21.

99. Joo GJ, Beke A, Papp C, et al. Prenatal diagnosis, phenotypic and obstetric characteristics of holoprosencephaly. *Fetal Diagn Ther.* 2005;20:161–166.

100. Simon EM, Barkovich AJ. Holoprosencephaly: new concepts. *Magn Reson Imaging Clin N Am.* 2001;9:149–164.

101. Volpe P, Campobasso G, De Robertis V, et al. Disorders of prosencephalic development. *Prenat Diagn.* 2009;29:340–354.

102. Hahn JS, Plawner LL. Evaluation and management of children with holoprosencephaly. *Pediatr Neurol.* 2004;31:79–88.

103. Nyberg DA, Mack LA, Bronstein A, et al. Holoprosencephaly: prenatal sonographic diagnosis. *AJR Am J Roentgenol.* 1987;149:1051–1058.

104. Filly RA, Chinn DH, Callen PW. Alobar holoprosencephaly: ultrasonographic prenatal diagnosis. *Radiology.* 1984;151:455–459.

105. Barkovich AJ, Quint DJ. Middle interhemispheric fusion: an unusual variant of holoprosencephaly. *AJNR Am J Neuroradiol.* 1993;14:431–440.

106. Simon EM, Hevner RF, Pinter JD, et al. The middle interhemispheric variant of holoprosencephaly. *AJNR Am J Neuroradiol.* 2002;23:151–155.

107. Dubourg C, Bendavid C, Pasquier L, et al. Holoprosencephaly. *Orphanet J Rare Dis.* 2007;2:1–14.

108. Bullen PJ, Rankin JM, Robson SC. Investigation of the epidemiology and prenatal diagnosis of holoprosencephaly in the north of England. *Am J Obstet Gynecol.* 2001;184:1256–1262.

109. Yamada S. Embryonic holoprosencephaly: pathology and phenotypic variability. *Congenit Anom.* 2006;46:164–171.

110. DeMyer W, Zeman W, Palmer CG. The face predicts the brain: diagnostic significance of median facial anomalies for holoprosencephaly (arhinencephaly). *Pediatrics.* 1964;34:256–263.

111. Johnson CY, Rasmusen SA. Non-genetic risk factors for holoprosencephaly. *Am J Med Genet C Semin Med Genet.* 2010;154C:73–85.

112. Solomon BD, Gropman A, Muenke M. Holoprosencephaly overview. In: Pagon RA, Adam MP, Bird TD, et al, eds. *GeneReviews™* [Internet]. Seattle, WA: University of Washington; 1993–2013, December 27, 2000. [Updated November 3, 2011].

113. Huang J, Wah IY, Pooh RK, et al. Molecular genetics in fetal neurology. *Semin Fetal Neonatal Med.* 2012;17:341–346.

114. Berry SM, Gosden C, Snijders RJM, et al. Fetal holoprosencephaly: associated malformations and chromosomal defects. *Fetal Diagn Ther.* 1990;5:92–99.

115. Bianchi D, Crombleholme T, D'Alton M, et al. *Fetology: Diagnosis and Management of the Fetal Patient.* 2nd ed. New York, NY: McGraw-Hill Medical; 2010:121–129.

116. Sepulveda W, Dezerega V, Be C. First-trimester sonographic diagnosis of holoprosencephaly: value of the "Butterfly" sign. *J Ultrasound Med.* 2004;23:761–765.

117. Hahn JS, Barnes PD. Neuroimaging advances in holoprosencephaly: refining the spectrum of the midline malformation. *Am J Med Genet C Semin Med Genet.* 2010;154C:120–132.

118. Cayea PD, Balcar I, Alberti O Jr, et al. Prenatal diagnosis of semilobar holoprosencephaly. *AJR Am J Roentgenol.* 1984;142:401–402.

119. Pilu G, Sandri F, Perolo A, et al. Prenatal diagnosis of lobar holoprosencephaly. *Ultrasound Obstet Gynecol.* 1992;2:88–94.

120. Pilu G, Ambrosetto P, Sandri F, et al. Intraventricular fused fornices: a specific sign of fetal lobar holoprosencephaly. *Ultrasound Obstet Gynecol.* 1994;4:65–67.

121. Bernard JP, Drummond CL, Zaarour P, et al. A new clue to the prenatal diagnosis of lobar holoprosencephaly: the abnormal pathway of the anterior cerebral artery crawling under the skull. *Ultrasound Obstet Gynecol.* 2002;19:605–607.

122. Wong HS, Lam YH, Tang MHY, et al. First-trimester ultrasound diagnosis of holoprosencephaly: three case reports. *Ultrasound Obstet Gynecol.* 1999;13:356–359.

123. Tongsong T, Wanapirak C, Chanprapaph P, et al. First trimester sonographic diagnosis of holoprosencephaly. *Int J Gynaecol Obstet.* 1999;66:165–169.

124. McGahan JP, Nyberg DA, Mack LA. Sonography of facial features of alobar and semilobar holoprosencephaly. *AJR Am J Roetgenol.* 1990;154:143–148.

125. Chen CP, Shih JC, Hsu CY, et al. Prenatal three-dimensional/four dimensional sonographic demonstration of facial dysmorphisms associated with holoprosencephaly. *J Clin Ultrasound.* 2005;33:312–318.

126. Lee YY, Lin MT, Lee MS, et al. Holoprosencephaly and cyclopia visualized by two- and three-dimensional prenatal ultrasound. *Chang Gung Med J.* 2002;25:207–210.

127. Plawner LL, Delgado MR, Miller VS, et al. Neuroanatomy of holoprosencephaly as predictor of function, beyond the face predicting the brain. *Neurology.* 2002;59:1058–1066.

128. Wong AMC, Bilaniuk LT, Ng KK, et al. Lobar holoprosencephaly: prenatal MR diagnosis with postnatal MR correlation. *Prenat Diagn.* 2005;25:295–299.

129. Johnson N, Windrim R, Chong K, et al. Prenatal diagnosis of solitary median maxillary central incisor syndrome by magnetic resonance imaging. *Ultrasound Obstet Gynecol.* 2008;32:120–122.

130. Hahn JS, Barkovich AJ, Stashinko EE, et al. Factor analysis of neuroanatomical and clinical characteristics of holoprosencephaly. *Brain Dev.* 2006;28:413–419.

131. Simon EM, Hevner R, Pinter JD, et al. Assessment of the deep gray nuclei in holoprosencephaly. *AJNR Am J Neuroradiol.* 2000;21:1955–1961.

132. Hahn JS, Barnes PD, Clegg NJ, et al. Septopreoptic holoprosencephaly: a mild subtype associated with midline craniofacial anomalies. *AJNR Am J Neuroradiol.* 2010;31:1596–1601.

133. Koob M, Weingertner AS, Gasser B, et al. Thick corpus callosum: a clue to the diagnosis of fetal septopreoptic holoprosencephaly? *Pediatr Radiol.* 2012;42:886–890.

134. Pulitzer SB, Simon EM, Crombleholme TM, et al. Prenatal MR findings of the middle interhemispheric variant of holoprosencephaly. *AJNR Am J Neuroradiol.* 2004;25:1034–1036.

135. Barkovich AJ, Simon EM, Clegg NJ, et al. Analysis of the cerebral cortex in holoprosencephaly with attention to the Sylvian fissures. *AJNR Am J Neuroradiol.* 2002;23:143–150.

136. Cohen MM Jr. Holoprosencephaly: clinical, anatomic and molecular dimensions. *Birth Defects Res A Clin Mol Teratol.* 2006;76:658–673.

137. Raam MS, Solomon BD, Muenke M. Holoprosencephaly: a guide to diagnosis and clinical management. *Indian Pediatr.* 2011;48:457–466.

138. David AL, Gowda V, Turnbull C, et al. The risk of recurrence of holoprosencephaly in euploid fetuses. *Obstet Gynecol.* 2007;110:658–662.

139. Dill P, Poretti A, Boltshauser E, et al. Fetal magnetic resonance imaging in midline malformations of the central nervous system and review of the literature. *J Neuroradiol.* 2009;36:138–146.

140. Li Y, Estroff JA, Khwaja O, et al. Callosal dysgenesis in fetuses with ventriculomegaly: levels of agreement between imaging modalities and postnatal outcome. *Ultrasound Obstet Gynecol.* 2012;40:522–529.

141. Glass HC, Shaw GM, Ma C, et al. Agenesis of the corpus callosum in California 1983–2003: a population-based study. *Am J Med Genet.* 2008;146A:2495–2500.

142. Szabo N, Gergev G, Kobor J, et al. Corpus callosum anomalies: birth prevalence and clinical spectrum in Hungary. *Pediatr Neurol.* 2011;44:420–426.

143. Fratelli N, Papageorghiou AT, Prefuno F, et al. Outcome of prenatally diagnosed agenesis of the corpus callosum. *Prenat Diagn.* 2007;27:512–517.

144. Vasudevan C, McKechnie L, Levene M. Long-term outcome of antenatally diagnosed agenesis of the corpus callosum and cerebellar malformations. *Semin Fetal Neonatal Med.* 2012;17:292–300.

145. Raybaud C. The corpus callosum, the other great forebrain commissures, and the septum pellucidum: anatomy, development and malformation. *Neuroradiology.* 2010;52:447–477.

146. Dobyns WB. Absence makes the search grow longer. *Am J Hum Genet.* 1996;58:7–16.

147. Barkovich AJ, Norman D. Anomalies of the corpus callosum: correlation with further anomalies of the brain. *AJR Am J Roentgenol.* 1988;151:171–179.

148. Atlas SW, Zimmerman RA, Bilaniuk LT, et al. Corpus callosum and limbic system: neuroanatomic MR evaluation of developmental anomalies. *Radiology.* 1986;160:355–362.

149. Hetts SW, Sherr EH, Chao S, et al. Anomalies of the corpus callosum: an MR analysis of the phenotypic spectrum of associated malformations. *AJR Am J Roentgenol.* 2006;187:1343–1348.

150. Barkovich AJ, Simon EM, Walsh CA. Callosal agenesis with cyst: a better understanding and new classification. *Neurology.* 2001;56:220–227.

151. Ickowitz V, Eurin D, Rypens F, et al. Prenatal diagnosis and postnatal follow-up of pericallosal lipoma: report of seven new cases. *AJNR Am J Neuroradiol.* 2001;22:767–772.

152. Shevell MI. Clinical and diagnostic profile of agenesis of the corpus callosum. *J Child Neurol.* 2002;17:895–899.

153. Bedeschi MF, Bonaglia MC, Grasso R, et al. Agenesis of the corpus callosum: clinical and genetic study in 63 young patients. *Pediatr Neurol.* 2006;34:186–193.

154. Gupta JK, Lilford RJ. Assessment and management of fetal agenesis of the corpus callosum. *Prenat Diagn.* 1995;15:301–312.

155. Aicardi J. Aicardi syndrome. *Brain Dev.* 2005;27:164–171.

156. Diaz-Guerrero L, Giugni-Chalbaud G, Sosa-Olavarria A. Assessment of pericallosal arteries by color Doppler ultrasonography at 11–14 weeks: an early marker of fetal corpus callosum development in normal fetuses and agenesis in cases with chromosomal anomalies. *Fetal Diagn Ther.* 2013;34:85–89.

157. Lachmann R, Sodre D, Barmpas M, et al. Midbrain and falx in fetuses with absent corpus callosum at 11–13 weeks. *Fetal Diagn Ther.* 2013;33:41–46.

158. Pilu G, Sandri F, Perolo A, et al. Sonography of fetal agenesis of the corpus callosum: a survey of 35 cases. *Ultrasound Obstet Gynecol.* 1993;3:318–329.

159. Bennett GL, Bromley B, Benacerraf BR. Agenesis of the corpus callosum: prenatal detection usually is not possible before 22 weeks of gestation. *Radiology.* 1996;199:447–450.

160. Blum A, Andre M, Droulle P, et al. Prenatal echographic diagnosis of the corpus callosum agenesis: the Nancy experience 1982–1989. *Genet Couns.* 1990;38:115–126.

161. Manfredi R, Tognolini A, Bruno C, et al. Agenesis of the corpus callosum in fetuses with mild ventriculomegaly: role of MR imaging. *Radiol Med.* 2010;115:301–312.

162. Bertino RE, Nyberg DA, Cyr DR, et al. Prenatal diagnosis of agenesis of the corpus callosum. *J Ultrasound Med.* 1988;7:251–260.

163. Blaicher W, Prayer D, Mittermayer C, et al. Magnetic resonance imaging in fetuses with bilateral moderate ventriculomegaly and suspected anomaly of the corpus callosum on ultrasound scan. *Ultraschall Med.* 2003;24:255–260.

164. Volpe P, Paladini D, Resta M, et al. Characteristics, associations and outcome of partial agenesis of the corpus callosum in the fetus. *Ultrasound Obstet Gynecol.* 2006;27:509–516.

165. Griffiths PD, Batty R, Connolly DAJ, et al. Effects of failed commissuration on the septum pellucidum and fornix: implications for fetal imaging. *Neuroradiology.* 2009;51:347–356.

166. Ghi T, Carletti A, Contro E, et al. Prenatal diagnosis and outcome of partial agenesis and hypoplasia of the corpus callosum. *Ultrasound Obstet Gynecol.* 2010;35:35–41.

167. Harreld JH, Bhore R, Chason DP, et al. Corpus callosum length by gestational age as evaluated by fetal MR imaging. *AJNR Am J Neuroradiol.* 2011;32:490–494.

168. Glenn OA. MR imaging of the fetal brain. *Pediatr Radiol.* 2010;40:68–81.

169. Glenn OA, Goldstein RB, Li KC, et al. Fetal magnetic resonance imaging in the evaluation of fetuses referred for sonographically suspected abnormalities of the corpus callosum. *J Ultrasound Med.* 2005;24:791–804.

170. Tang PH, Bartha AI, Norton ME, et al. Agenesis of the corpus callosum: an MR imaging analysis of associated abnormalities in the fetus. *AJNR Am J Neuroradiol.* 2009;30:257–263.

171. Warren DJ, Connolly DJA, Griffiths PD. Assessment of sulcation of the fetal brain in cases of isolated agenesis of the corpus callosum using in utero MR imaging. *AJNR Am J Neuroradiol.* 2010;31:1085–1090.

172. Parrish ML, Roessmann U, Livinsohn MW. Agenesis of the corpus callosum: a study of the frequency of associated malformations. *Ann Neurol.* 1979;6:349–354.

173. Goodyear PWA, Bannister CM, Russell S, et al. Outcome in prenatally diagnosed fetal agenesis of the corpus callosum. *Fetal Diagn Ther.* 2001;16:139–145.

174. Rosser TL, Acosta MT, Packer RJ. Aicardi syndrome: spectrum of disease and long-term prognosis in 77 females. *Pediatr Neurol.* 2002;27:343–346.

175. Paul LK, Brown WS, Adolphs R, et al. Agenesis of the corpus callosum: genetic, developmental and functional aspects of connectivity. *Neuroscience.* 2007;8:287–299.

176. Moes P, Schilmoeller K, Schmilmoeller G. Physical, motor, sensory and developmental features associated with agenesis of the corpus callosum. *Child Care Health Dev.* 2009;35:656–672.

177. Doherty D, Tu S, Schilmoeller K, et al. Health-related issues in individuals with agenesis of the corpus callosum. *Child Care Health Dev.* 2006;32:333–342.

178. Mangione R, Fries N, Godard P, et al. Neurodevelopmental outcome following prenatal diagnosis of an isolated anomaly of the corpus callosum. *Ultrasound Obstet Gynecol.* 2011;37:290–295.

179. Patel L, McNally RJQ, Harrison E, et al. Geographical distribution of optic nerve hypoplasia and septo-optic dysplasia in Northwest England. *J Pediatr.* 2006;148:85–88.

180. Atapattu N, Ainsworth J, Willshaw H, et al. Septo-optic dysplasia: antenatal risk factors and clinical features in a regional study. *Horm Res Paediatr.* 2012;78:81–87.

181. Brodsky MC, Glasier CM. Optic nerve hypoplasia: clinical significance of associated central nervous system abnormalities on magnetic resonance imaging. *Arch Ophthalmol.* 1993;111:66–74.

182. Birkebaek NH, Patel L, Wright NB, et al. Endocrine status in patients with optic nerve hypoplasia: relationship to midline central nervous system abnormalities and appearance of the hypothalamic-pituitary axis on magnetic resonance imaging. *J Clin Endocrinol Metab.* 2003;88:5281–5286.

183. Kelberman D, Dattani MT. Septo-optic dysplasia—novel insights into the aetiology. *Horm Res.* 2008;69:257–265.

184. Stevens CA, Dobyns WB. Septo-optic dysplasia and amniotic bands: further evidence for a vascular pathogenesis. *Am J Med Genet.* 2004;125A:12–16.

185. Polizzi A, Pavone P, Iannetti P, et al. Septo-optic dysplasia complex: a heterogeneous malformation syndrome. *Pediatr Neurol.* 2006;34:66–71.

186. Raybaud C, Girard N, Levrier O, et al. Schizencephaly: correlation between the lobar topography of the cleft(s) and absence of the septum pellucidum. *Childs Nerv Syst.* 2001;17:217–222.

187. Leonhardt EE, Tann-Sinn PA. Septo-optic dysplasia: a neurosonographic review. *J Diagn Med Sonogr.* 2005;21:479–486.

188. Barkovich AJ, Fram EK, Norman D. Sept-optic dysplasia: MR imaging. *Radiology.* 1989;171:189–192.

189. McCabe MJ, Alatzoglou KS, Dattani MT. Septo-optic dysplasia and other midline defects: the role of transcription factors: HESX1 and beyond. *Best Pract Res Clin Endocrinol Metab.* 2011;25:115–124.

190. Falco P, Gabrielli S, Visentin A, et al. Transabdominal sonography of the cavum septum pellucidum in normal fetuses in the second and third trimesters of pregnancy. *Ultrasound Obstet Gynecol.* 2000;16:549–553.

191. Pilu G, Tani G, Carletti A, et al. Difficult early sonographic diagnosis of absence of the fetal septum pellucidum. *Ultrasound Obstet Gynecol.* 2005;25:70–72.

192. Callen PW, Callen AL, Glenn OA, et al. Columns of the fornix, not be mistaken for the cavum septi pellucidi on prenatal sonography. *J Ultrasound Med.* 2008;27:25–31.

193. Lepinard C, Coutant R, Boussion F, et al. Prenatal diagnosis of absence of the septum pellucidum associated with septo-optic dysplaia. *Ultrasound Obstet Gynecol.* 2005;25:73–75.

194. Katorza E, Bault JP, Gilboa Y, et al. Prenatal visualization of the pituitary gland using 2- and 3-dimensional sonography: comparison to prenatal magnetic resonance imaging. *J Ultrasound Med.* 2012;31:1675–1680.

195. Bault JP, Salomon LJ, Guibaud L, et al. Role of three-dimensional ultrasound measurement of the optic tract in fetuses with agenesis of the septum pellucidum. *Ultrasound Obstet Gynecol.* 2011;37:570–575.

196. Li Y, Sansgiri R, Estroff JA, et al. Outcome of fetuses with cerebral ventriculomegaly and septum pellucidum leaflet abnormalities. *AJR Am J Roentgenol.* 2011;196:W83–W92.

197. Barkovich AJ, Norman D. Absence of the septum pellucidum: a useful sign in the diagnosis of congenital brain malformations. *AJR Am J Roentgenol.* 1989;152:353–360.

198. Levine LM, Bhatti MT, Mancuso AA. Septo-optic dysplasia with olfactory tract and bulb hypoplasia. *J AAPOS.* 2001;5:398–399.

199. Pilu G, Sandri F, Cerisoli M, et al. Sonographic findings in septo-optic dysplasia in the fetus and newborn infant. *Am J Perinatol.* 1990;7:337–339.

200. Belhocine O, Andre C, Kalifa G, et al. Does asymptomatic septal agenesis exist? A review of 34 cases. *Pediatr Radiol.* 2005;35:410–418.

201. Antonini SRR, Filho AG, Elias LLK, et al. Cerebral midline developmental anomalies: endocrine, neuroradiographic and opthalmological features. *J Pediatr Endocrinol Metab.* 2002;15:1525–1530.

202. Wales JKH, Quarrell OWJ. Evidence for possible Mendelian inheritance of septo-optic dysplasia. *Acta Paediatr.* 1996;85:391–392.

203. Barkovich AJ, Guerrini R, Kuzniecky RI, et al. A developmental and genetic classification for malformations of cortical development: update 2012. *Brain.* 2012;135(5):1348–1369.

204. Razek AAKA, Kandell AY, Elsorogy LG, et al. Disorders of cortical formation: MR imaging features. *AJNR Am J Neuroradiol.* 2009;30:4–11.

205. Manoranjan B, Provias JP. Hemimegalencephaly: a fetal case with neuropathological confirmation and review of the literature. *Acta Neuropathol.* 2010;120:117–130.

206. Tinkle BT, Schorry EK, Franz DN, et al. Epidemiology of hemimegalencephaly: a case series and review. *Am J Med Genet.* 2005;139A:204–211.

207. Flores-Sarnat L. Hemimegalencepahy, part I: genetic, clinical and imaging aspects. *J Child Neurol.* 2002;17:373–384.

208. Flores-Sarnat L, Sarnat HB, Davila-Gutierrez G, et al. Hemimegalencepahy, part 2: neuropathology suggests a disorder of cellular lineage. *J Child Neurol.* 2003;18:776–785.

209. Sasaki M, Hashimoto T, Furushima W, et al. Clinical aspects of hemimegalencephaly by means of a nationwide survey. *J Child Neurol.* 2005;20:337–341.

210. Baek ST, Gibbs EM, Gleeson JG, et al. *Curr Opin Neurol.* 2013;26:122–127.

211. Alvarez RM, Garcia-Diaz L, Marquez J, et al. Hemimegalencephaly: prenatal diagnosis and outcome. *Fetal Diagn Ther.* 2011;30:234–238.

212. Hafner E, Bock W, Zoder G, et al. Prenatal diagnosis of unilateral megalencephaly by 2D and 3D ultrasound: a case report. *Prenat Diagn.* 1999;19:159–162.

213. Barkovich AJ, Chuang SH. Unilateral megalencephaly: correlation of MR imaging and pathologic characteristics. *AJNR Am J Neuroradiol.* 1990;11:523–531.

214. Di Rocco C, Battaglia D, Pietrini D, et al. Hemimegalencephaly: clinical implications and surgical treatment. *Childs Nerv Syst.* 2006;22:852–866.

215. Agid R, Liberman S, Nadjari M, et al. Prenatal MR diffusion-weighted imaging in a fetus with hemimegalencephaly. *Pediatr Radiol.* 2006;36:138–140.

216. Sato N, Yagishita A, Oba H, et al. Hemimegalencephaly: a study of abnormalities occurring outside the involved hemisphere. *AJNR Am J Neuroradiol.* 2007;28:678–682.

217. Milunsky A, Ito M, Maher TA, et al. Prenatal molecular diagnosis of tuberous sclerosis complex. *Am J Obstet Gynecol.* 2009;200:321.e1–321.e6.

218. Baskin HJ Jr. The pathogenesis and imaging of the tuberous sclerosis complex. *Pediatr Radiol.* 2008;38:936–952.

219. Gusman M, Servaes S, Feygin T, et al. Multimodal imaging in the prenatal diagnosis of tuberous sclerosis complex. *Case Rep Pediatr.* 2012;2012:925646.

220. Curatiolo P, Bombardieri R, Jozwiak S. Tuberous sclerosis. *Lancet.* 2008;372:657–668.

221. King JA, Stamilio DM. Maternal and fetal tuberous sclerosis complicating pregnancy: a case report and overview of the literature. *Am J Perinatol.* 2005;22:103–108.

222. Saada J, Rabia SH, Fermont L, et al. Prenatal diagnosis of cardiac rhabdomyomas: incidence of associated cerebral lesions of tuberous sclerosis complex. *Ultrasound Obstet Gynecol.* 2009;34:155–159.

223. Gedikbasi A, Oztarhan K, Ulker V, et al. Prenatal sonographic diagnosis of tuberous sclerosis complex. *J Clin Ultrasound.* 2011;39:427–430.

224. Bader RS, Chitayat D, Kelly E, et al. Fetal rhabdomyoma: prenatal diagnosis, clinical outcome, and incidence of associated tuberous sclerosis complex. *J Pediatr.* 2003;143:620–624.

225. Muhler MR, Rake A, Schwabe M, et al. Value of fetal cerebral MRI in sonographically proven cardiac rhabdomyoma. *Pediatr Radiol.* 2007;37:467–474.

226. Werner H Jr, Mirleese V, Jacquemard F, et al. Prenatal diagnosis of tuberous sclerosis use of magnetic resonance imaging and its implications for prognosis. *Prenat Diagn.* 1994;14:1151–1154.

227. Sgro M, Barozzimo T, Toi A, et al. Prenatal detection of cerebral lesions in a fetus with tuberous sclerosis. *Ultrasound Obstet Gynecol.* 1999;14:356–359.

228. Zhang YX, Meng H, Zhong DR, et al. Cardiac rhabdomyoma and renal cyst in a fetus: early onset of tuberous sclerosis with renal cystic disease. *J Ultrasound Med.* 2008;27:979–982.

229. Sonigo P, Elmaleh A, Fermont L, et al. Prenatal MRI diagnosis of fetal cerebral tuberous sclerosis. *Pediatr Radiol.* 1996;26:1–4.

230. Baron Y, Barkovich A. MR imaging of tuberous sclerosis in neonates and young infants. *AJNR Am J Neuroradiol.* 1999;20:907–916.

231. Rosser T, Panigrahy A, McClintock W. The diverse clinical manifestations of tuberous sclerosis complex: a review. *Semin Pediatr Neurol.* 2006;13:27–36.

232. Jansen FE, Vincken KL, Algra A, et al. Cognitive impairment in tuberous sclerosis complex is a multifactorial condition. *Neurology.* 2008;70:916–923.

233. Malinger G, Lev D, Lerman-Sagie T. Assessment of fetal intracranial pathologies first demonstrated late in pregnancy: cell proliferation disorders [review]. *Reprod Biol Endocrinol.* 2003;1(1):110.

234. Szabo N, Pap C, Kobor J, et al. Primary microcephaly in Hungary: epidemiology and clinical features. *Acta Paediatr.* 2010;99:690–693.

235. Goldstein I, Reece A, Pilu G, et al. Sonographic assessment of the fetal frontal lobe: a potential tool for prenatal diagnosis of microcephaly. *Am J Obstet Gynecol.* 1988;158:1057–1062.

236. Sztriha L, Dawodu A, Gururaj A, et al. Microcephaly associated with abnormal gyral pattern. *Neuropediatrics.* 2004;35:346–352.

237. Adachi Y, Poduri A, Kawaguch A, et al. Congenital microcephaly with a simplified gyral pattern: associated findings and their significance. *AJNR Am J Neuroradiol.* 2011;32:1123–1129.

238. Dobyns WB. Primary microcephaly: new approaches for an old disorder. *Am J Med Genet.* 2002;112:315–317.

239. Jaffe M, Tirosh E, Oren S. The dilemma in prenatal diagnosis of idiopathic microcephaly. *Dev Med Child Neurol.* 1987;29:187–189.

240. Den Hollander NS, Wessel MW, Los FJ, et al. Congenital microcephaly detected by prenatal ultrasound: genetic aspects and clinical significance. *Ultrasound Obstet Gynecol.* 2000;15:282–287.

241. Dahlgren L, Wilson RD. Prenatally diagnosed microcephaly: a review of etiologies. *Fetal Diagn Ther.* 2001;16:323–326.

242. Malinger G, Lerman-Sagie T, Watemberg N, et al. A normal second-trimester ultrasound does not exclude intracranial structural pathology. *Ultrasound Obstet Gynecol.* 2002;20:51–56.

243. Bromley B, Benacerraf BR. Difficulties in the prenatal diagnosis of microcephaly. *J Ultrasound Med.* 1995;14:303–305.

244. Stoler-Poria S, Lev D, Schweiger A, et al. Developmental outcome of the isolated fetal microcephaly. *Ultrasound Obstet Gynecol.* 2010;36:154–158.

245. Pilu G, Falco P, Milano V, et al. Prenatal diagnosis of microcephaly assisted by vaginal sonography and power Doppler. *Ultrasound Obstet Gynecol.* 1998;11:357–360.

246. Persutte WH, Coury A, Hobbins JC. Correlation of fetal frontal lobe transcerebellar diameter measurements: the utility of a new prenatal sonographic technique. *Ultrasound Obstet Gynecol.* 1997;10:94–97.

247. Verloes A. Microcephalia vera and microcephaly with simplified gyral pattern. *Orphanet Encyclopedia.* 2004;1–5. http://www.orpha.net/data/patho/GB/uk-MVMSG.pdf.

248. Tao G, Yew DT. Magnetic resonance imaging of fetal brain abnormalities. *Neuroembryol Aging.* 2008;5:49–55.

249. Fogliarini C, Chaumoitre K, Chapon F, et al. Assessment of cortical maturation with prenatal MRI, part II: abnormalities of cortical maturation. *Eur Radiol.* 2005;15:1781–1789.

250. Abuelo D. Microcephaly syndromes. *Semin Pediatr Neurol.* 2007;14:118–127.

251. Biran-Gol Y, Malinger G, Cohen H, et al. Developmental outcome of isolated fetal macrocephaly. *Ultrasound Obstet Gynecol.* 2010;36:147–153.

252. Malinger G, Lev D, Ben-Sira L, et al. Can syndromic macrocephaly be diagnosed in utero? *Ultrasound Obstet Gynecol.* 2011;37:72–81.

253. Toi A, Chitayat D, Blaser S. Abnormalities of the foetal cerebral cortex. *Prenat Diagn.* 2009;29:355–371.

254. Saleh-Gargari S, Omrani MD, Hantoushzadeh S. Prenatal diagnosis of benign familial fetal macrocephaly. *Ultrasound Obstet Gynecol.* 2007;30:547–653.

255. Lerman-Sagie T, Ben-Sira L, Achiron R, et al. Thick fetal corpus callosum: an ominous gin? *Ultra Obstet Gynecol.* 2009;34:55–61.

256. Mallerio C, Marignier S, Roth P, et al. Prenatal cerebral ultrasound and MRI findings in glutaric aciduria Type 1: a de novo case. *Ultrasound Obstet Gynecol.* 2008;31:712–714.

257. Williams CA. Macrocephaly syndromes. In: Stalker HJ, ed. *RC Philips Research and Education Unit Newsletter.* 2008;20(1). http://www.peds.ufl.edu/divisions/genetics/newsletters/macrocephaly.pdf.

258. Isaacs H Jr. I: perinatal brain tumors: a review of 250 cases. *Pediatr Neurol.* 2002;27:249–261.

259. Isaacs H Jr. Fetal brain tumors: a review of 154 cases. *Am J Perinatol.* 2009;26:453–466.

260. Woodward PJ, Sohaey R, Kennedy A, et al. From the archives of the AFIP: a comprehensive review of fetal tumors with pathologic correlation. *Radiographics.* 2005;25:215–242.

261. Schlembach D, Bornemann A, Rupprecht T, et al. Fetal intracranial tumors detected by ultrasound: a report of two cases and review of the literature. *Ultrasound Obstet Gynecol.* 1999;14:407–418.

262. Rickert CH. Neuropathology and prognosis of foetal brain tumours. *Acta Neuropathol.* 1999;98:567–576.

263. Cavalheiro S, Moron AF, Hisaba W, et al. Fetal brain tumors. *Childs Nerv Syst.* 2003;19:529–536.

264. D'Addario V, Pinto V, Meo F, et al. The specificity of ultrasound in the detection of fetal intracranial tumors. *J Perinat Med.* 1998;26:480–485.

265. Cassart M, Bosson N, Garel C, et al. Fetal intracranial tumors: a review of 27 cases. *Eur Radiol.* 2008;18:2060–2066.

266. Vazquez E, Castellote A, Mayolas N, et al. Congenital tumours involving the head, neck and central nervous system. *Pediatr Radiol.* 2009;39:1158–1172.

267. DiPietro JA, Cristofalo EA, Voegtline KM, et al. Isolated prenatal choroid plexus cysts do not affect child development. *Prenat Diagn.* 2011;31:745–749.

268. Achiron R, Barkai G, Katznelson BM, et al. Fetal lateral ventricle choroid plexus cysts: the dilemma of amniocentesis. *Obstet Gynecol.* 1991;78:815–818.

269. Kraus I, Jirasek JE. Some observations of the structure of the choroid plexus and its cysts. *Prenat Diagn.* 2002;22:1223–1228.

270. Zafar HM, Ankola A, Coleman B. Ultrasound pitfalls and artifacts related to six common fetal findings. *Ultrasound Q.* 2012;28:105–124.

271. Turner SR, Samei E, Hertzberg BS, et al. Sonography of fetal choroid plexus cysts. *J Ultrasound Med.* 2003;22:1219–1227.

272. Morcos CL, Platt LD, Carlson DE, et al. The isolated choroid plexus cyst. *Obstet Gynecol.* 1998;92:232–236.

273. Sullivan A, Giudice T, Vavelidis F, et al. Choroid plexus cysts: is biochemical testing a valuable adjunct to targeted ultrasonography. *Am J Obstet Gynecol.* 1999;181:260–265.

274. Lopez JA, Reich D. Choroid plexus cysts. *J Am Board Fam Med.* 2006;19:422–425.

275. Ghidini A, Strobelt N, Locatelli A, et al. Isolated fetal choroid plexus cysts: role of ultrasonography in establishment of the risk of trisomy 18. *Am J Obstet Gynecol.* 2000;812:972–977.

276. Becker S, Niemann G, Schoning M, et al. Clinically significant persistence and enlargement of an antenatally diagnosed isolated choroid plexus cyst. *Ultrasound Obstet Gynecol.* 2002;20:620–622.

277. Norton KI, Rai B, Desai H, et al. Prevalence of choroid plexus cysts in term and near-term infants with congenital heart disease. *AJR Am J Roentgenol.* 2011;196:W326–W329.

278. Bernier FP, Crawford SG, Dewey D. Developmental outcome of children who had choroid plexus cysts detected prenatally. *Prenat Diagn.* 2005;25:322–326.

279. Gupta JK, Cave M, Lilford RJ, et al. Clinical significance of fetal choroid plexus cysts. *Lancet.* 1995;346:724–729.

280. Reinsch RC. Choroid plexus cysts—association with trisomy: prospective review of 16,059 patients. *Am J Obstet Gynecol.* 1997;176:1381–1383.

281. Chen CP. Prenatal diagnosis of arachnoid cysts. *Taiwan J Obstet Gynecol.* 2007;46:187–198.

282. Pradilla G, Jallo G. Arachnoid cysts: case series and review of the literature. *Neurosurg Focus.* 2007;22:1–4.

283. Pierre-Kahn A, Hanlo P, Sonigo P, et al. The contribution of prenatal diagnosis to the understanding of malformative intracranial cysts: state of the art. *Child Nerv Syst.* 2000;16:618–626.

284. Pilu G, Falco P, Perolo A, et al. Differential diagnosis and outcome of fetal intracranial hypoechoic lesions: report of 21 cases. *Ultrasound Obstet Gynecol.* 1997;9:229–236.

285. Gedikbasi A, Palabiyik F, Oztarhan A, et al. Prenatal diagnosis of a suprasellar arachnoid cyst with 2- and 3-dimensional sonography and fetal magnetic resonane imaging: difficulties in management and review of the literature. *J Ultrasound Med.* 2010;29:1487–1493.

286. Blaicher W, Prayer D, Kuhle S, et al. Combined prenatal ultrasound and magnetic resonance imaging in two fetuses with suspected arachnoid cysts. *Ultrasound Obstet Gynecol.* 2001;18:166–168.

287. Booth TN, Timmons C, Shapiro K, et al. Pre- and postnatal MR imaging of hypothalamic hamartomas associated with arachnoid cysts. *AJNR Am J Neuroradiol.* 2004;25:1283–1285.

288. Blasi I, Henrich W, Argento C, et al. Prenatal diagnosis of a cavum veli interpositi. *J Ultrasound Med.* 2009;28:683–687.

289. Barjot P, von Theobald P, Refahi N, et al. Diagnosis of arachnoid cysts on prenatal ultrasound. *Fetal Diagn Ther.* 1999;14:306–309.

290. Hayward R. Postnatal management and outcome for fetal-diagnosed intracerebral cystic masses and tumours. *Prenat Diagn.* 2009;29:396–401.

291. Borha A, Ponte KF, Emery E. Cavum septum pellucidum cyst in children: a case-based update. *Childs Nerv Syst.* 2012;28:813–819.

292. Scoffings DJ, Kurian KM. Congenital and acquired lesions of the septum pellucidum. *Clin Radiol.* 2008;63:210–219.

293. Sarwar M. The septum pellucidum: normal and abnormal. *AJNR Am J Neuroradiol.* 1989;10:989–1005.

294. Mott SH, Bodensteiner JB, Allan WC. The cavum septi pellucidi in term and preterm newborn infants. *J Child Neurol.* 1992;7:35–38.

295. Hicdonmez T, Suslu HT, Butuc R, et al. Treatment of a large and symptomatic septum pellicidum cyst with endoscopic fenestration in a child: case report and review of the literature. *Clin Neurol Neurosurg.* 2012;114:1052–1056.

296. Bronshtein M, Weiner Z. Prenatal diagnosis of dilated cava septi pellucidi et vergae: associated anomalies, differential diagnosis, and pregnancy outome. *Obstet Gynecol.* 1992;80:838–842.

297. Vergani P, Locatelli A, Piccoli MG, et al. Ultrasonographic differential diagnosis of fetal intracranial interhemispheric cysts. *Am J Obstet Gynecol.* 1999;180:423–428.

298. Osborn AG, Preece MT. Intracranial cysts: radiologic-pathologic correlation and imaging approach. *Radiology.* 2006;239:650–664.

299. Tange Y, Aoki A, Mori K, et al. Interhemispheric glioependymal cyst associated with agenesis of the corpus callosum, case report. *Neurol Med Chir (Tokyo).* 2000;40:536–542.

300. Moriyama E, Nishida A, Sonobe H. Interhemispheric multilocated ependymal cyst with dysgenesis of the corpus callosum: a case in a preterm fetus. *Childs Nerv Syst.* 2007;23:807–813.

301. Muhler MR, Hartmann C, Werner W, et al. Fetal MRI demonstrates glioependymal cyst in a case of sonographic unilateral ventriculomegaly. *Pediatr Radiol.* 2007;37:391–395.

302. Uematsu Y, Kubo K, Nishibayashi T, et al. Interhemispheric neuroepithelial cyst associated with agenesis of the corpus callosum. *Pediatr Neurosurg.* 2000;33:31–36.

303. Pelkey TJ, Ferguson JE, Veille JC, et al. Giant glioependymal cyst resembling holoprosencephaly on prenatal ultrasound: case report and review of the literature. *Ultrasound Obstet Gynecol.* 1997;9:200–203.

304. Deloison B, Chalouhi GE, Sonigo P, et al. Hidden mortality of prenatally diagnosed vein of Galen aneurysmal malformation: retrospective study and review of the literature. *Ultrasound Obstet Gynecol.* 2012;40:652–658.

305. Brunelle F. Arteriovenous malformation of the vein of Galen malformation in children. *Pediatr Radiol.* 1997;27:501–513.

306. Alvarez H, Garcia Monaco R, Rodesch G, et al. Vein of Galen aneurysmal malformation. *Neuroimaging Clin N Am.* 2007;17:189–206.

307. Lasjaunias PL, Chng SM, Sachet M, et al. The management of Vein of Galen aneurysmal malformation. *Neurosurgery.* 2006;59(5)(suppl 3):S184–S194.

308. Barbosa M, Mahadevan J, Weon YC, et al. Dural sinus malformations (DSM) with giant lakes, in neonates and infants, review of 30 consecutive cases. *Interv Neuroradiol.* 2003;9:407–424.

309. Komiyama M, Ishiguro T, Kitano S, et al. Serial antenatal sonographic observation of cerebra dural sinus malformation. *AJNR Am J Neuroradiol.* 2004;25:1446–1448.

310. Garel C, Azarian M, Lasajaunias P, et al. Pial arteriovenous fistulas: dilemmas in prenatal diagnosis, counseling and postnatal treatment. Report of three cases. *Ultrasound Obstet Gynecol.* 2005;26:293–296.

311. Sepulveda W, Platt CC, Fisk NM. Prenatal diagnosis of cerebra arteriovenous malformation using color Doppler ultrasonography: case report and review of the literature. *Ultrasound Obstet Gynecol.* 1995;6:282–286.

312. Heling KS, Chaoui R, Bollmann R. Prenatal diagnosis of an aneurysm of the vein of Galen with three-dimensional color power angiography. *Ultrasound Obstet Gynecol.* 2000;15:333–336.

313. Ruano R, Benachi A, Aubry MC, et al. Perinatal three-dimensional color power Doppler ultrasonography of vein of Galen of aneurysms. *J Ultrasound Med.* 2003;22:1357–1362.

314. Lee TH, Shih JC, Peng SSF, et al. Prenatal depiction of angioarchitecture of an aneurysm of the vein of Galen with three-dimensional color power angiography. *Ultrasound Obstet Gynecol.* 2000;15:337–340.

315. Yuval Y, Lerner A, Lipitz S, et al. Prenatal diagnosis of vein of Galen aneurysmal malformation: report of two cases with proposal for prognostic indices. *Prenat Diagn.* 1997;17:972–977.

316. Patermoster DM, Manganelli F, Moroder W, et al. Prenatal diagnosis of vein of Galen aneurysmal malformations. *Fetal Diagn Ther.* 2003;18:408–411.

317. Kosla K, Majos M, Polguj M, et al. Prenatal diagnosis of a vein of Galen aneurysmal malformation with MR imaging, report of two cases. *Pol J Radiol.* 2013;78:88–92.

318. Heuer GG, Gabel B, Beslow LA, et al. Diagnosis and treatment of vein of Galen aneurysmal malformations. *Childs Nerv Syst.* 2010;26:879–887.

319. Kurihara N, Tokieda K, Ikeda K, et al. Prenatal MR findings in a case of aneurysm of the vein of Galen. *Pediatr Radiol.* 2001;31:160–162.

320. Rodesch G, Hui F, Alvarez H, et al. Prognosis of antenatally diagnosed vein of Galen aneurysmal malformations. *Childs Nerv Syst.* 1994;10:79–83.

321. Kush ML, Weiner CP, Harman CR, et al. Lethal progression of a fetal intracranial arteriovenous malformation. *J Ultrasound Med.* 2003;22:645–648.

322. Mitchell PJ, Rosenfeld JV, Dargaville P, et al. Endovascular management of vein of Galen aneurysmal malformations presenting in the neonatal period. *AJNR Am J Neuroradiol.* 2001;22:1403–1409.

323. Huang J, Wah IYM, Pooh RK, et al. Molecular genetics in fetal neurology. *Semin Fetal Neonatal Med.* 2012;17:341–346.

324. Ghai S, Fong KW, Toi A, et al. Prenatal US and MR imaging findings of lissencephaly: review of fetal cerebral sulcal development. *Radiographics.* 2006;26:389–405.

325. Barkovich AJ, Chuang SH, Norman D. MR of neuronal migration anomalies. *AJR Am J Roentgenol.* 1988;150:179–187.

326. Dobyns WB, Das S. LIS1-associated lissencephaly/subcortical band heterotopia. In: Pagon RA, Adam MP, Bird TD, et al, eds. *GeneReviews® [Internet].* Seattle, WA: University of Washington; 1993–2014.

327. Haverfield EV, Whited AJ, Petras KS, et al. Intragenic deletions and duplications of the LIS1 and DCX genes: a major disease-causing mechanism in lissencephaly and subcortical band heterotopia. *Eur J Hum Genet.* 2009;17:911–918.

328. Abdel Razek AAK, Kandell AY, et al. Disorders of cortical formation: MR imaging features. *AJNR Am J Neuroradiol.* 2009;30:4–11.

329. Chen C-P, Chang T-Y, Guo W-Y, et al. Chromosome 17p13.3 deletion syndrome: aCGH characterization, prenatal findings and diagnosis, and literature review. *Gene.* 2013;532:152–159.

330. Fong KW, Ghai S, Toi A, et al. Prenatal ultrasound findings of lissencephaly associated with Miller-Dieker syndrome and comparison with pre- and postnatal magnetic resonance imaging. *Ultrasound Obstet Gynecol.* 2004;24:716–723.

331. Rolo LC, Araujo E Jr, Nardozza LMM, et al. Development of fetal brain sulci and gyri: assessment through two and three-dimensional ultrasound and magnetic resonance imaging. *Arch Gynecol Obstet.* 2011;283:149–158.

332. Pugash D, Hendson G, Dunham CP, et al. Sonographic assessment of normal and abnormal patterns of fetal cerebral lamination. *Ultrasound Obstet Gynecol.* 2012;40:642–651.

333. Malinger G, Kidron D, Schreiber L, et al. Prenatal diagnosis of malformations of cortical development by dedicated neurosonography. *Ultrasound Obstet Gynecol.* 2007;29:178–191.

334. Righini A, Frassoni C, Inverardi F, et al. Bilateral cavitations of ganglionic eminence: a fetal MR imaging sign of halted brain development. *AJNR Am J Neuroradiol.* 2013;34:1841–1845.

335. Barkovich AJ, Koch TK, Carrol CL. The spectrum of lissencephaly: report of ten patients analyzed by magnetic resonance imaging. *Ann Neurol.* 1991;30:139–146.

336. Guibaud L, Selleret L, Larroche JC, et al. Abnormal Sylvian fissure on prenatal cerebral imaging: significance and correlation with neuropathological and postnatal data. *Ultrasound Obstet Gynecol.* 2008;32:50–60.

337. Bloundiaux E, Sileo C, Nahama-Allouche C, et al. Periventricular nodular heterotopia on prenatal ultrasound and magnetic resonance imaging. *Ultrasound Obstet Gynecol.* 2013;42:149–155.

338. Gonzalez G, Vedolin L, Barry B, et al. Location of periventricular nodular heterotopia is related to the malformation phenotype on MRI. *AJNR Am J Neuroradiol.* 2013;34:877–889.

339. Manganaro L, Saldari M, Bernardo S, et al. Bilateral subependymal heterotopia, ventriculomegaly and cerebellar asymmetry: fetal MRI findings of a rare association of brain anomalieis. *J Radiol Case Rep.* 2013;7:38–45.

340. Barkovich AJ, Kuzniecky RI. Gray matter heterotopia. *Neurology.* 2000;55:1603–1608.

341. Barkovich AJ. Morphologic characteristics of subcortical heterotopia: MR imaging study. *AJNR Am J Neuroradiol.* 2000;21:290–295.

342. Parrini E, Ramazzotti A, Dobyns WB, et al. Periventricular heterotopia: phenotypic heterogeneity and correlation with Filamin A mutations. *Brain.* 2006;129:1892–1906.

343. Poussaint TY, Fox JW, Dobyns WB, et al. Periventricular nodular heterotopia in patients with filamin-1 gene mutations: neuroimaging findings. *Pediatr Radiol.* 2000;30:748–755.

344. Mitchell LA, Simon EM, Filly RA, et al. Antenatal diagnosis of subependymal heterotopia. *AJNR Am J Neuroradiol.* 2000;21:296–300.

345. Glenn OA, Cuneo AA, Barkovich AJ, et al. Malformations of cortical development: diagnostic accuracy of fetal MR imaging. *Radiology.* 2012;263:843–855.

346. Vajsar J, Schacter H. Walker-Warburg syndrome. *Orphanet J Rare Dis.* 2006;1:29–33.

347. Devisme L, Bouchet C, Gonzales M, et al. Cobblestone lissencephaly: neuropathological subtypes and correlations with genes of dystroglycanopathies. *Brain.* 2012;135:469–482.

348. Barkovich AJ. Neuroimaging manifestations and classification of congenital muscular dystrophies. *AJNR Am J Neuroradiol.* 1998;19:1389–1396.

349. Brasseur-Daudruy M, Vivier PH, Ickowicz V, et al. Walker-Warburg syndrome diagnosed by findings of typical ocular abnormalities on prenatal ultrasound. *Pediatr Radiol.* 2012;42:488–490.

350. Dobyns WB, Pagon RA, Armstrong D, et al. Diagnostic criteria for Walker-Warburg syndrome. *Am J Med Genet.* 1989;32:195–210.

351. Stroustrup Smith A, Levine D, Barnes PD, et al. Magnetic resonance imaging of the kinked fetal brain stem, a sign of severe dysgenesis. *J Ultrasound Med.* 2005;24:1697–1709.

352. Pabuscu Y, Baulakbasy N, Kocaoglu M, et al. Walker-Warburg syndrome variant. *Comput Med Imaging Graph.* 2002;26:453–458.

353. Low ASC, Lee SL, Tan ASA, et al. Difficulties with prenatal diagnosis of the Walker-Warburg syndrome. *Acta Radiol.* 2005;46:645–651.

354. Widjaja E, Geibprasert S, Blaser S, et al. Abnormal fetal cerebral laminar organization in cobblestone complex as seen on post-mortem MRI and DTI. *Pediatr Radiol.* 2009;39:860–864.

355. Strigini F, Valleriani A, Cecchi M, et al. Prenatal ultrasound and magnetic resonance imaging features in a fetus with Walker-Warburg syndrome [letter]. *Ultrasound Obstet Gynecol.* 2009;33:363–368.

356. Monteagudo A, Alayon A, Mayberry P. Walker-Warburg syndrome: case report and review of the literature. *J Ultrasound Med.* 2001;20:419–426.

357. Jansen A, Andermann E. Genetics of the polymicrogyria syndromes. *J Med Genet.* 2005;42:369–378.

358. Hayashi N, Tsutsumi Y, Barkovich AJ. Polymicrogyria without porencephaly/schizencephaly: MRI analysis of the spectrum and the prevalence of macroscopic findings in the clinical population. *Neuroradiology.* 2002;44:647–655.

359. Barkovich AJ. Current concepts of polymicrogyria. *Neuroradiology.* 2010;52:479–487.

360. Glenn OA, Norton ME, Goldstein RB, et al. Prenatal diagnosis of polymicrogyria by fetal magnetic resonance imaging in monochorionic co-twin death. *J Ultrasound Med.* 2005;24:711–716.

361. Simonazzi G, Segata M, Ghi T, et al. Accurate neurosonographic prediction of a brain injury in the surviving fetus after the death of a monochorionic co-twin. *Ultrasound Obstet Gynecol.* 2006;27:517–521.

362. Barkovich AJ. Magnetic resonance imaging: role in the understanding of cerebral malformations. *Brain Dev.* 2002;24:2–12.

363. Wieck G, Leventer RJ, Squier WM, et al. Periventricular nodular heterotopia with overlying polymicrogyria. *Brain.* 2005;128:2811–2821.

364. Cagneaux M, Paoli V, Blanchard G, et al. Pre- and postnatal imaging of early cerebral damage in Sturge-Weber syndrome. *Pediatr Radiol.* 2013;43:1536–1539.

365. Fink AM, Hingston T, Sampson A, et al. Malformation of the fetal brain in thanatophoric dysplasia: US and MRI findings. *Pediatr Radiol.* 2010;40(suppl 1):S134–S137.

366. Barkovich AJ, Peck WW. MR of Zellweger syndrome. *AJNR Am J Neuroradiol.* 1997;18:1163–1170.

367. Mochel F, Grebille AG, Benachi A, et al. Contribution of fetal MR imaging in the prenatal diagnosis of Zellweger syndrome. *AJNR Am J Neuroradiol.* 2006;27:333–336.

368. Dhombres F, Nahama-Allouche C, Gelot A, et al. Prenatal ultrasonographic diagnosis of polymicrogyria. *Ultrasound Obstet Gynecol.* 2008;32:951–954.

369. Urban LABD, Righini A, Rustico M, et al. Prenatal ultrasound detection of bilateral focal polymicrogyria. *Prenat Diagn.* 2004;24:808–811.

370. Righini A, Parazzini C, Doneda C, et al. Early formative stage of human focal cortical gyration anomalies: fetal MRI. *AJR Am J Roentgenol.* 2012;198:439–447.

371. Righini A, Zirpoli S, Mrakic F, et al. Early prenatal MR imaging diagnosis of polymicrogyria. *AJNR Am J Neuroradiol.* 2004;25:343–346.

372. Barkovich AJ, Hevner R, Guerrini R. Syndromes of bilateral symmetrical polymicrogyria. *AJNR Am J Neuroradiol.* 1999;20:1814–1821.

373. Yakovlev PI, Wadsworth RC. Schizencephalies: a study of the congenital clefts in the cerebral mantle, II: clefts with hydrocephalus and lips separated. *J Neuropathol Exp Neurol.* 1946;5(3):169–206.

374. Curry CJ, Lammer EJ, Nelson V, et al. Schizencephaly: heterogeneous etiologies in a population of 4 million California births. *Am J Med Genet.* 2005;137A:181–189.

375. Howe DT, Rankin J, Draper ES. Schizencephaly prevalence, prenatal diagnosis and clues to etiology: a register-based study. *Ultrasound Obstet Gynecol.* 2012;39:75–82.

376. Barkovich AJ, Kjos BO. Schizencephaly: correlation of clinical findings with MR characteristics. *AJNR Am J Neuroradiol.* 1992;13:85–94.

377. Hayashi N, Tsutsumi Y, Barkovich AJ. Morphological features and associated anomalies of schizencephaly in the clinical population: detailed analysis of MR images. *Neuroradiology.* 2002;44:418–427.

378. Oh KY, Kennedy AM, Frias AE Jr, et al. Fetal schizencephaly: pre- and postnatal imaging with a review of the clinical manifestations. *Radiographics.* 2005;25:647–657.

379. Nabavizadeh SA, Zarnow D, Bilaniuk LT, et al. Correlation of prenatal and postnatal MRI findings in schizencephaly. *AJNR Am J Neuroradiol.* 2014. doi:10.3174/ajnr.A3872.

380. Lee W, Comstock CH, Kazmierczak C, et al. Prenatal diagnostic challenges and pitfalls for schizencephaly. *J Ultrasound Med.* 2009;28:1379–1384.

381. Denis D, Maugey-Laulom B, Carles D, et al. Prenatal diagnosis of schizencephaly by fetal magnetic resonance imaging. *Fetal Diagn Ther.* 2001;16:354–359.

382. Edris F, Kielar A, Fung KFK, et al. Ultrasound and MRI in the antenatal diagnosis of schizencephaly. *J Obstet Gynaecol Can.* 2005;27:864–868.

383. Rios LTM Jr, Araujo E, Nardozza LMM, et al. Prenatal and postnatal schizencephaly findings by 2D and 3D ultrasound: pictorial essay. *J Clin Imaging Sci.* 2012;2:30.

384. Poretti A, Leventer RJ, Cowan FM, et al. Cerebellar cleft: a form of prenatal cerebellar disruption. *Neuropediatrics*. 2008;39:106–112.

385. Raybaud C, Girard N, Levrier O, et al. Schizencephaly: correlation between the lobar topography of the cleft(s) and absence of the septum pellucidum. *Childs Nerv Syst*. 2001;17:217–222.

386. Hung J-H, Shen S-H, Guo W-Y, et al. Prenatal diagnosis of schizencephaly with septo-optic dysplasia by ultrasound and magnetic resonance imaging. *J Obstet Gynaecol Res*. 2008;34:674–679.

387. Bats AS, Molho M, Senat MV, et al. Subependymal pseudocysts in the fetal brain: prenatal diagnosis of two cases and review of the literature. *Ultrasound Obstet Gynecol*. 2002;20:502–505.

388. Malinger G, Lev D, Sira LB, et al. Congenital periventricular pseudocysts: prenatal sonographic appearance and clinical implications. *Ultrasound Obstet Gynecol*. 2002;20:447–451.

389. Cevey-Macherel M, Forcada M, Bickle Graz M, et al. Neurodevelopment outcome of newborns with cerebral subependymal pseudocysts at 18 and 46 months: a prospective study. *Arch Dis Child*. 2013;98:497–502.

390. Correa F, Lara C, Carreras E, et al. Evolution of fetal subependymal cysts throughout gestation. *Fetal Diagn Ther*. 2013;34:127–130.

391. Shackelford GD, Fulling KH, Glasier CM. Cysts of the subependymal germinal matrix: sonographic demonstration with pathologic correlation. *Radiology*. 1983;149:117–121.

392. Epelman M, Daneman A, Blaser SI, et al. Differential diagnosis of intracranial cystic lesions at head US: correlation with CT and MR imaging. *Radiographics*. 2006;26:173–196.

393. Makhoul IR, Zmora O, Tamir A, et al. Congenital subependymal pseudocysts: own data and meta-analysis of the literature. *Isr Med Assoc J*. 2001;3:178–183.

394. Fernandez Alvarez JR, Arness PN, et al. Diagnostic value of subependymal pseudocysts and choroid plexus cysts on neonatal cerebral ultrasound: a meta-analysis. *Arch Dis Child Fetal Neonatal Ed*. 2009;94:F443–F446.

395. Larcos G, Gruenewald SM, Lui K. Neonatal subependymal cysts detected by sonography: prevalence, sonographic findings, and clinical significance. *AJR Am J Roentgenol*. 1994;162:953–956.

396. Rossler L, Ludwig-Seibold C, Thiels CH, et al. Aicardi-Goutieres syndrome with emphasis on sonographic features of infancy. *Pediatr Radiol*. 2012;42:932–940.

397. Ramenghi LA, Domizio S, Quartulli L, et al. Prenatal pseudocysts of the germinal matrix in preterm infants. *J Clin Ultrasound*. 1997;25:169–173.

398. Elchalal U, Yagel S, Gomori JM, et al. Fetal intracranial hemorrhage (fetal stroke): does grade matter. *Ultrasound Obstet Gynecol*. 2005;26:233–243.

399. Vergani P, Strobelt N, Locatelli A, et al. Clinical significance of fetal intracranial hemorrhage. *Am J Obstet Gynecol*. 1996;175:536–543.

400. Brunel H, Girard N, Confort-Gouny S, et al. Fetal brain injury. *J Neuroradiol*. 2004;31:123–137.

401. Girard N, Gire C, Sigaudy S, et al. MR imaging of acquired fetal brain disorders. *Childs Nerv Syst*. 2003;19:490–500.

402. Ghi T, Simonazzi G, Perolo A, et al. Outcome of antenatally diagnosed intracranial hemorrhage: case series and review of the literature. *Ultrasound Obstet Gynecol*. 2003;22:121–130.

403. Ozduman K, Pober BR, Barnes P, et al. Fetal stroke. *Pediatr Neurol*. 2004;30:151–162.

404. Sherer DM, Anyaebunam A, Onyeije C. Antepartum fetal intracranial hemorrhage, predisposing factors and prenatal sonography: a review. *Am J Perinatol*. 1998;15:431–441.

405. Sharif I, Kuban K. Prenatal intracranial hemorrhage and neurologic complications in alloimmune thrombocytopenia. *J Child Neurol*. 2001;16:838–842.

406. Dubinsky T, Lau M, Powell F, et al. Predicting poor neonatal outcome: a comparative study of noninvasive antenatal testing methods. *AJR Am J Roentgenol*. 1997;168:827–831.

407. de Laveaucoupet J, Audibert F, Guis F, et al. Fetal magnetic resonance imaging (MRI) of ischemic brain injury. *Prenat Diagn*. 2001;21:729–736.

408. Huang Y-F, Chen W-C, Tseng J-J, et al. Fetal intracranial hemorrhage (fetal stroke): report of four antenatally diagnosed cases and review of the literature. *Taiwan J Obstet Gynecol*. 2006;45:135–141.

409. Muench MV, Zheng M, Bilica PM, et al. Prenatal diagnosis of a fetal epidural hematoma using 2- and 3-dimensional sonography and magnetic resonance imaging. *J Ultrasound Med*. 2008;27:1369–1373.

410. De Spirlet M, Goffinet F, Philippe HJ, et al. Prenatal diagnosis of a subdual hematoma associated with reverse flow in the middle cerebral artery: case report and literature review. *Ultrasound Obstet Gynecol*. 2000;16:72–76.

411. Hines N, Mehta T, Romero J, et al. What is the clinical importance of echogenic material in the fetal frontal horns? *J Ultrasound Med*. 2009;28:1629–1637.

412. Burstein J, Papile L-A, Burstein R. Intraventricular hemorrhage and hydrocephalus in premature newborns: a prospective study with CT. *AJR Am J Roentgenol*. 1979;132:621–635.

413. Groothuis AMC, de Kleine MJK, Guid Oei S. Intraventricular haemorrhage in utero: a case report and review of the literature. *Eur J Obstet Gynecol Reprod Biol*. 2000;89:207–211.

414. Garel C, Delezoide A-L, Elmaleh-Berges M, et al. Contribution of fetal MR imaging in the evaluation of cerebral ischemic lesions. *AJNR Am J Neuroradiol*. 2004;25:1563–1568.

415. Fleischer AC, Hutchison AA, Bundy AL, et al. Serial sonography of posthemorrhagic ventricular dilatation and porencephaly after intracranial hemorrhage in the preterm neonate. *AJNR Am J Neuroradiol*. 1983;4:971–975.

416. Lituania M, Passamonti U. Prenatal ultrasound: brain. In: Raybaud C, Paolo T-D, Rossi A, eds. *Pediatric Neuroradiology*. Heidelberg, Germany: Springer Berlin; 2005:1157–1218.

417. Prayer D, Brugger PC, Kasprian G, et al. MRI of fetal acquired brain lesions. *Eur J Radiol*. 2006;57:233–249.

418. Folkerth RD, McLaughlin ME, Levine D. Organizing posterior fossa hematomas simulating developmental cysts on prenatal imaging, report of three cases. *J Ultrasound Med*. 2001;20:1233–1240.

419. Rios LTM, Araujo E Jr, Nardozza LMM, et al. Hidden maternal autoimmune thrombocytopenia complicated by fetal subdural hematoma, case report and review of the literature. *Childs Nerv Syst*. 2012;28:1113–1116.

420. Guimiot F, Garel C, Fallet-Bianco C, et al. Contribution of diffusion-weighted imaging in the evaluation of diffuse white matter ischemic lesions in fetuses: correlation with fetopathologic findings. *AJNR Am J Neuroradiol*. 2008;29:110–115.

421. Strigini FAL, Cioni G, Canapicchi R, et al. Fetal intracranial hemorrhage: is minor maternal trauma a possible pathogenetic factor? *Ultrasound Obstet Gynecol*. 2001;18:335–342.

422. Bussel JB, Berkowitz RL, McFarland JG, et al. Antenatal treatment of neonatal alloimmune thrombocytopenia. *N Engl J Med*. 1988;319:1374–1378.

423. Govaert P. Prenatal stroke. *Semin Fetal Neonatal Med*. 2009;14:250–266.

424. Grant EG, Kerner M, Schellinger D, et al. Evolution of porencephalic cysts from intraparenchymal hemorrhage in neonates: sonographic evidence. *AJR Am J Roentgenol*. 1982;138:467–470.

425. Gul A, Gungorduk K, Yildirim G, et al. Prenatal diagnosis of porencephaly secondary to maternal carbon monoxide poisoning. *Arch Gynecol Obstet*. 2009;279:697–700.

426. Eiler KM, Kuller JA. Fetal porencephaly: a review of the etiology, diagnosis and prognosis. *Obstet Gynecol Surv*. 1995;50:684–687.

427. Berg RA, Aleck KA, Kaplan AM. Familial porencephaly. *Arch Neurol*. 1983;40:567–569.

428. Ho SS, Kuzniecky RI, Gilliam F, et al. Congenital porencephaly: MR features and relationship to hippocampal sclerosis. *AJNR Am J Neuroradiol*. 1998;19:135–141.

429. Quek Y-W, Su P-H, Tsao T-F, et al. Hydranencephaly associated with interruption of bilateral internal carotid arteries. *Pediatr Neonatol*. 2008;49:43–47.

430. Taori KB, Sargar KM, Disawal A, et al. Hydranencephaly associated with cerebellar involvement and bilateral microphthalmia and colobomas. *Pediatr Radiol*. 2011;41:270–273.

431. Byers BD, Barth WH, Stewart TL, et al. Ultrasound and MRI appearance and evolution of hydranencephaly in utero. *J Reprod Med*. 2005;50:53–56.

432. Myers RE. Brain pathology following fetal vascular occlusion: an experimental study. *Invest Ophthalmol*. 1969;8:41–50.

433. Cecchetto G, Milanese L, Giordano R, et al. Looking at the missing brain: hydranencephaly case series and literature review. *Pediatr Neurol*. 2013;48:152–158.

434. Greene MF, Benacerraf B, Crawford JM. Hydranencephaly: US appearance during in utero evolution. *Radiology*. 1985;156:779–780.

435. Edmondson SR, Hallak M, Carpenter RJ Jr, et al. Evolution of hydranencephaly following intracerebral hemorrhage. *Obstet Gynecol*. 1992;79:870–871.

436. Dixon A. Hydranencephaly. *Radiography*. 1998;54:12–13.

437. Williams D, Patel C, Fallet-Bianco C, et al. Fowler syndrome: a clinical, radiological, and pathological study of 14 cases. *Am J Med Genet Am*. 2009;152A:153–160.

438. Laurichesse-Delmas H, Beaufrere AM, Martin A, et al. First-trimester features of Fowler syndrome (hydrocephaly-hydranencephaly proliferative vasculopathy). *Ultrasound Obstet Gynecol*. 2002;20:612–615.

439. Lam YH, Tang HY. Serial sonographic features of a fetus with hydranencephaly from 11 weeks to term. *Ultrasound Obstet Gynecol*. 2000;16:77–79.

440. Sepulveda W, Cortes-Yepes H, Wong AE, et al. Prenatal sonography in hydranencephaly, findings during the early stages of disease. *J Ultrasound Med*. 2012;31:799–804.

441. Usta IM, AbuMusa AA, Khoury NG, et al. Early ultrasonographic changes in Fowler syndrome features and review of the literature. *Prenat Diagn*. 2005;25:1019–1023.

442. Aguirre Vila-Coro A, Dominguez R. Intrauterine diagnosis of hydranencephaly by magnetic resonance. *Magn Reson Imaging*. 1989;7:105–107.

443. Merker B. Editorial: life expectancy in hydranencephaly. *Clin Neurol Neurosurg*. 2008;110:213–214.

444. Laurichesse Delmas H, Winer N, Gallot D, et al. Prenatal diagnosis of thrombosis of the dural sinuses: report of six cases, review of the literature and suggested management. *Ultrasound Obstet Gynecol*. 2008;32:188–198.

445. Okudera T, Peng Huang Y, Ohta T, et al. Development of posterior fossa dural sinuses, emissary veins, and jugular bulb: morphological and radiologic study. *AJNR Am J Neuroradiol*. 1994;15:1871–1883.

446. Merzoug V, Flunder S, Drissi C, et al. Dural sinus malformation (DSM) in fetuses: diagnostic value of prenatal MRI and followup. *Eur Radiol*. 2008;18:692–699.

447. Pandey V, Dummula K, Parimi P. Antenatal thrombosis of torcular herophili presenting with anemia, consumption coagulopathy and high-output cardiac failure in a preterm infant. *J Perinatol*. 2013;32:728–730.

448. Fanou EM, Reeves MJ, Howe DT, et al. In utero magnetic resonance imaging for diagnosis of dural venous sinus ectasia with thrombosis in the fetus. *Pediatr Radiol.* 2013;43:1591–1598.

449. Byrd S, Abramowicz J, Kent P, et al. Fetal MR imaging of posterior intracranial dural sinus thrombosis: a report of three cases with variable outcomes. *Pediatr Radiol.* 2012;42:536–543.

450. Has R, Esmer AC, Kalelioglu I, et al. Prenatal diagnosis of torcular herophili thrombosis, report of two cases and review of the literature. *J Ultrasound Med.* 2013;32:2205–2211.

451. Barbosa M, Mahadevan J, Weon YC, et al. Dural sinus malformations (DSM) with giant lakes, in neonates and infants, review of 30 consecutive cases. *Interv Neuroradiol.* 2003;9:407–424.

452. McInnes M, Fong K, Grin A, et al. Malformations of the fetal dural sinuses. *Can J Neurol Sci.* 2009;36:72–77.

453. Legendre G, Picone O, Levaillant JM, et al. Prenatal diagnosis of a spontaneous dural sinus thrombosis. *Prenat Diagn.* 2009;29:808–813.

454. Grange G, LeTohic A, Merzoug V, et al. Prenatal demonstration of afferent vessels and progressive thrombosis in a torcular malformation. *Prenat Diagn.* 2007;27:670–673.

455. Schwartz N, Monteagudo A, Bornstein E, et al. Thrombosis of an ectatic torcular herophili: anatomic localization using fetal neurosonography [letter]. *J Ultrasound Med.* 2008;27:989–992.

456. Laurichesse-Delmas Grimaud O, Moscoso G, Ville Y. Color Doppler study of the venous circulation in the fetal brain and hemodynamic study of the cerebral transverse sinus. *Ultrasound Obstet Gynecol.* 1999;13:34–42.

457. Visentin A, Falco P, Pilu G, et al. Prenatal diagnosis of thrombosis of the dural sinuses with real-time and color Doppler ultrasound. *Ultrasound Obstet Gynecol.* 2001;17:322–325.

458. Rossi A, De Biasio P, Scarso E, et al. Prenatal MR imaging of dural sinus malformation: a case report. *Prenat Diagn.* 2006;26:11–16.

459. Ebert M, Esenkaya A, Huisman T, et al. Multimodality, anatomical and diffusion weighted fetal imaging of a spontaneously thrombosing congenital dural sinus malformation. *Neuropediatrics.* 2012;43:279–282.

460. Spampinato MV, Hardin V, Davis M, et al. Thrombosed fetal dural sinus malformation diagnosed with magnetic resonance imaging. *Obstet Gynecol.* 2008;111:569–572.

461. Jenny B, Zerah M, Swift D, et al. Giant dural venous sinus ectasia in neonates, report of four cases. *J Neurosurg Pediatr.* 2010;5:523–528.

Fetal central nervous system (CNS) infections include perinatally acquired infections, ascending infections from chorioamnionitis, and transplacental spread of prenatally acquired infection.

Chorioamnionitis from prolonged rupture of membranes (PROM) can lead to infections with traditional bacteria such as streptococcus, *Escherichia coli,* and *Candida.* PROM is a risk factor for intraventricular hemorrhage (IVH), leukomalacia, and developmental delay. Humoral factors may be responsible for the IVH.[1]

Intrauterine infections of the fetal CNS were made famous by the acronym TORCH. It stands for *Toxoplasma gondii*, rubella, cytomegalovirus (CMV), herpes viruses, and others (including syphilis). The ranges of pathogens that are known to cause CNS infections have since expanded. The imaging findings, however, remain similar and nonspecific.

**Incidence/Etiology:** The incidence of fetal CNS infections is not well known. Many of the maternal infections remain subclinical and under recognized. Currently, CMV infection is the most commonly documented with an incidence of 0.2% to 2.2% of infants at birth. About 2.2% of pregnant women develop a primary infection during conception. Most infants remain asymptomatic. Urine polymerase chain reaction (PCR) or blood spot Guthrie card PCR is used to identify neonatal infection. A urine/salivary viral culture is deemed to be the gold standard. CMV-specific IgM in the neonatal serum can also establish diagnosis. Past the neonatal phase, beyond 4 weeks, infection may be acquired after birth and does not confirm fetal infection.[2]

Congenital toxoplasmosis is the second most commonly recognized infection. *Toxoplasma gondii*, a ubiquitous parasite, infects pregnant women most commonly from a feline fecal source or food contamination. The incidence of congenital infection ranges from 0.1 to 1 per 1,000 live births. Infection is confirmed by specific serum IgM detection in neonates. Conversely, the presence of IgG in maternal serum eliminates the possibility of current fetal infection.[2]

The incidence of congenital rubella has decreased significantly in the developed world following the institution of vaccination of young children and varies from 0% to 0.1%. Also rare is congenital syphilis in the developed world, with an overall incidence of 0.01%. Syphilis, a sexually transmitted disease, is obtained by contact with infected human secretions and is caused by *Treponema pallidum.* There is 50% transmission of infection to fetus in maternal infections.[2]

Less commonly recognized sources of infection with incidence rates below 0.001% include varicella zoster virus, herpes simplex viruses, lymphocytic choriomeningitis virus, Chagas disease from *Trypanosoma cruzi,* West Nile virus, and human parechovirus.

**Pathogenesis:** The exact mechanisms of fetal infection are not known. Most agents causing liver damage are known to infest hepatocytes and cause hepatic dysfunction. Similarly, marrow infection in association with autoimmune destruction of platelets, hypersplenism, and consumption coagulopathy is postulated to cause thrombocytopenia. Hemolysis and marrow infection lead to anemia.

The systemic signs and symptoms of infection alert the neonatologist to the diagnosis of a congenital infection and are summarized in Table 12.2-1.

CNS manifestations depend on maternal immunity, time of infection during the gestation, infectious agent and its cellular tropism as well as less well-understood genetic factors. Rubella infection between the 8th and 20th weeks leads to more severe fetal manifestations. Given the propensity for CMV to cause neuronal migrational anomalies, it is postulated that infection before 20 weeks would likely produce more severe outcomes. Congenital varicella syndrome is also more likely to occur with maternal infection between 5 and 24 weeks of gestation.

Most transmissible agents infect the placenta and travel via the placenta to cause disseminated fetal infection. Leptomeningeal proliferation of virus in rubella is known. The pathogenesis of migrational anomalies in CMV and lymphocytic choriomeningitis likely involves associated genetic factors. The similarity of these infections in the fetus to the much rarer familial noninfective pseudo-TORCH syndrome is unexplained at present.

### Diagnosis

*Ultrasound:* Ultrasound remains the screening modality for detection of prenatal CNS abnormalities. Findings associated with intrauterine CMV infection include microcephaly, intraparenchymal echogenic foci representing calcifications (Fig. 12.2-1A), and in some cases cerebellar or vermian hypoplasia (Fig. 12.2-1B).[4] Cortical sulcation abnormalities may be visualized (Fig. 12.2-1C). Periventricular hyperechogenic foci and pseudocysts (Fig. 12.2-2) can be present. Ventriculomegaly and hydrocephalus may be seen with echogenic ependyma and septations (Fig. 12.2-3). Polar temporal cysts, subcortical cysts, and porencephaly in congenital toxoplasmosis can be seen. The middle cerebral artery peak systolic velocity can be elevated, supporting anemia related to the infection.

*MRI:* Fetal MRI is increasingly playing an important role in investigating presumed cases of fetal infection. Approximately 53% of fetal MRIs demonstrate an abnormality in suspected CMV infection and provide information in addition to the US imaging.[5] The most useful sequence remains a T2-weighted sequence such as a half Fourier single-shot or single-shot fast spin echo (SSFSE) sequence. The T1-weighted spoiled gradient sequences take a longer time, but convey important information in suspected intracranial calcification, laminar necrosis, and hemorrhage. Diffusion-weighted images can detect infarcts, and echo planar gradient echo images can detect old hemorrhage.

Early gestational infection results in more congenital malformations as the fetal CNS develops between 8 and 23 weeks

| Table 12.2-1 | Systemic Symptoms of Common Agents Causing Neonatal Infections[2,3] | |
|---|---|---|

| Agent | Diagnostic Method | Systemic Symptoms and Lab Markers |
|---|---|---|
| CMV | Urine or serum PCR/culture, specific IgM | *Jaundice, HSM,* purpuric or petechial rash, blueberry muffin rash, microcephaly, meningitic features, growth retardation, *sensorineural hearing loss,* chorioretinitis (less common) |
| | | Elevated serum transaminase, hepatitis |
| | | Thrombocytopenia (15–50,000/µL) |
| | | Anemia |
| *Toxoplasma gondii* | Specific IgM | Jaundice, hepatosplenomegaly, petechial rash, macrocephaly and hydrocephalus, *chorioretinitis* (may be isolated), sensorineural hearing loss (less common) |
| | | Transient hepatic dysfunction, thrombocytopenia, anemia |
| Rubella (German measles) | Specific serum IgM; RT-PCR | *Cataracts, pigmentary retinopathy and microphthalmia, sensorineural hearing loss, patent ductus arteriosus, congenital heart diseases,* petechial rash, blueberry muffin rash, microcephaly, HSM (less common), meningoencephalitis, late-onset postrubella panencephalitis |
| *Treponema pallidum* | CSF, serum VDRL | HSM, petechial rash |
| | | Late onset of Hutchinson triad of hearing loss, interstitial keratitis, peg-shaped incisors; saber shin, saddle nose, mulberry molar, rhagades, frontal bossing |
| Varicella zoster virus | Specific IgM; CSF PCR | *Vesicular rash, zigzag dermatomal cicatrix rash,* microcephaly, cataracts, chorioretinitis |
| Herpes simplex virus | PCR (serum, CSF, vesicle) | Vesicular rash (in mucocutaneous form of disease), microcephaly, hydranencephaly, meningoencephalitis, cataracts, chorioretinitis, hydrops |
| | | Neonatal forms more common (localized, encephalitic, disseminated) |
| West Nile virus | Specific IgM in serum or CSF | |
| Lymphocytic choriomeningitis virus | Specific IgM | *Chorioretinitis,* bullous skin lesions, either microcephaly or hydrocephalus, cataract |
| Trypanosoma cruzi | | Jaundice, HSM |
| Human parechovirus, polio and coxsackie viruses | CSF PCR | Encephalitis, developmental delay, and epilepsy |
| Parvovirus B19 | Specific IgM | *Fetal hydrops,* encephalitis, meningitis and vasculitis, myocarditis, intrauterine fetal death |
| | | Congenital anemia |
| Human immunodeficiency virus (HIV) | PCR-based HIV nucleic acid amplification tests | *Craniofacial dysmorphism (nonspecific),* often asymptomatic, intrauterine growth retardation, hepatosplenomegaly, lymphadenopathy |
| | | <2% (perinatal transmission rate) |

Note: More common symptoms are italicized.
HSM, hepatosplenomegaly; CSF, cerebrospinal fluid; PCR, polymerase chain reaction; RT-PCR, reverse transcription polymerase chain reaction.

of gestation (Fig. 12.2-4). Late infections manifest mainly as destructive lesions (Figs. 12.2-5 and 12.2-6). Acute effects of infection may lead to focal necrosis, edema, and hemorrhage (esp. CMV). These, however, may be difficult to see if not imaged at the appropriate time interval. The chronic results of infection are more often imaged postnatally (Figs. 12.2-7 and 12.2-8) and are summarized in Table 12.2-2.

**Differential Diagnosis:** Aicardi–Goutiere syndrome, Cree encephalitis, and pseudo-TORCH or Baraitser–Reardon syndrome are now postulated to be closely related autosomal recessive conditions characterized by increased interferon-alpha (IFN-α) in the CSF. CSF IFN-α is also raised in infections, including TORCH and autoimmune conditions such as lupus. They are characterized by cerebral and basal ganglia

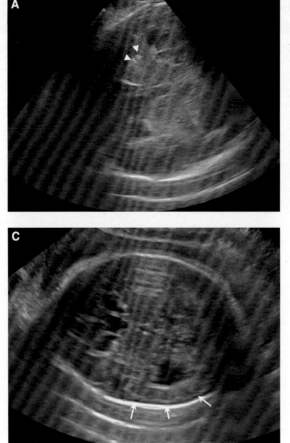

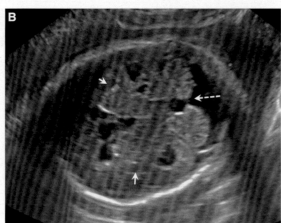

**FIGURE 12.2-1:** Fetus at 33 weeks diagnosed postnatally with CMV. **A:** Axial ultrasound demonstrates echogenic foci *(arrowheads)* consistent with calcifications. **B:** Central bilateral basal ganglia echogenic foci *(arrows)*. Mild ventriculomegaly and inferior vermian abnormality detected *(dotted arrow)*. The fetus also had microcephaly and an elevated peak systolic velocity (PSV) in the middle cerebral artery. **C:** Axial ultrasound demonstrating abnormal wavy nodular configuration of the fetal cortex *(arrows)* suspicious for migration anomaly.

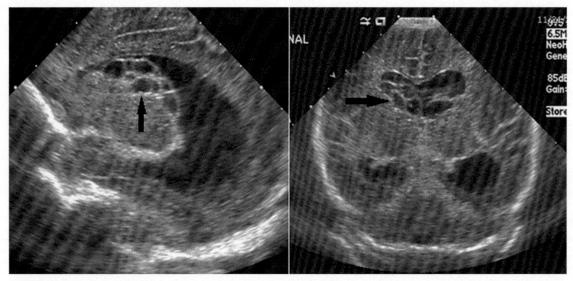

**FIGURE 12.2-2:** Neonatal ultrasound demonstrates periventricular pseudocysts *(arrows)*.

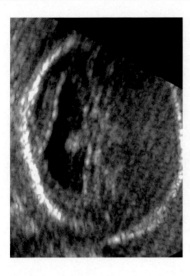

**FIGURE 12.2-3:** Ventricular enlargement with echogenic ependyma in a fetus. A nonspecific sign of fetal infection.

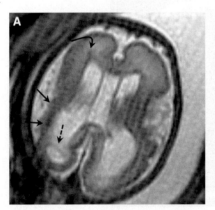
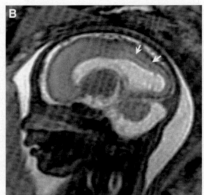
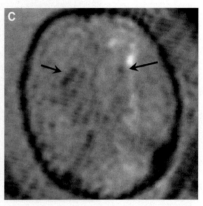

**FIGURE 12.2-4:** Same fetus as in Figure 12.2-1 found to be CMV positive. **A:** Axial SSFSE T2 demonstrates abnormal dark t2 signal in the periventricular white matter *(curved arrow)*. The cortex of the right posterior temporal and occipital lobe demonstrates nodular appearance consistent with polymicrogyria *(arrows)*. The sulcation is abnormally delayed for 33 weeks consistent with diffuse migrational abnormalities. There is a septation in the right posterior horn of the dilated lateral ventricles *(dotted arrow)*. **B:** Sagittal T2 image shows a dark band in the central white matter *(arrows)* consistent with band heterotopia (was present bilaterally). **C:** On axial gradient echo imaging, dark susceptible areas *(arrows)* are present in the basal ganglia.

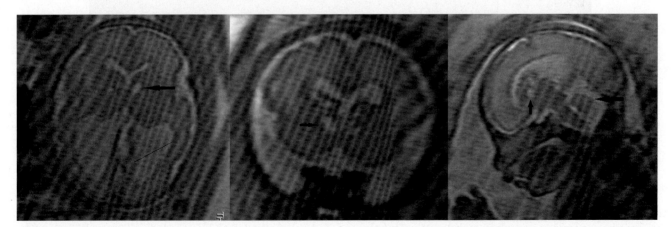

**FIGURE 12.2-5:** T2-weighted images from a fetal MRI demonstrate ventriculomegaly and periventricular cysts *(arrows)* with cerebellar hypoplasia *(large thick arrow* on sagittal image). Neonatal ultrasound in Figure 12.2-2 is the same patient confirming the antenatal findings.

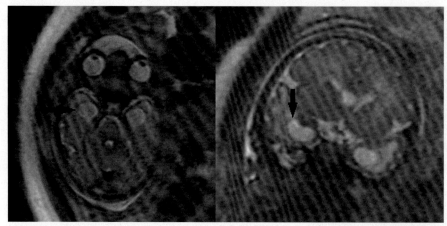

**FIGURE 12.2-6:** Polar temporal white matter cystic change *(arrows)* in a fetus with CMV infection.

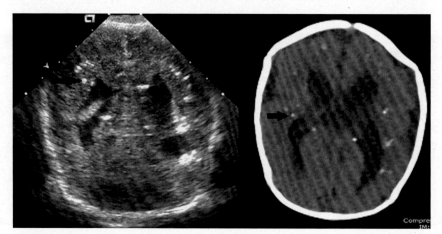

**FIGURE 12.2-7:** Periventricular and diffuse parenchymal calcifications *(arrows)* on neonatal ultrasound and CT in a patient with positive CMV serology.

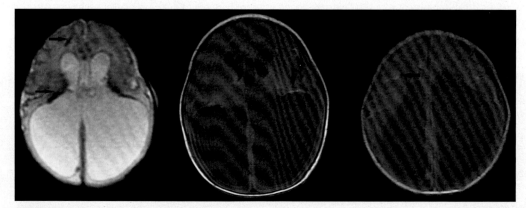

**FIGURE 12.2-8:** Hydrocephalus, periventricular, and cortical calcification *(arrows)* with areas of necrosis in a neonate with toxoplasmosis.

calcifications, gyral simplification, microcephaly, hepatomegaly, thrombocytopenia, and leukoencephalopathy. Mutations in AGS1-4 and TREX 1 genes may be associated.[6] Clinical presentation at birth suggests an infectious etiology with CSF lymphocytosis; however, extensive testing for infection, including TORCH titers, is negative. Parental consanguinity is a risk factor.

**Prognosis:** Infected infants are at high risk for permanent neurodevelopmental disabilities, including hearing loss, visual dysfunction, cerebral palsy, developmental delays, and epilepsy.

**Management:** Prevention remains the most effective way of combating morbidity. Rubella vaccination has helped in eradicating congenital rubella in many countries. There are potential

| Table 12.2-2 | **Common Intracranial Manifestations of Fetal CNS Infections** |
|---|---|

| *Agent* | *CNS Inflammation* | *Calcification* | *Anomalies of Central Nervous System* |
|---|---|---|---|
| CMV | Meningoencephalitis (predilection for periventricular white matter) | Typically periventricular or diffuse | Polymicrogyria, lissencephaly, pachygyria, heterotopia, microcephaly, polar temporal white matter signal abnormality, porencephaly, hydrocephalus, hydranencephaly, focal subcortical cysts, impaired myelination, cerebellar hypoplasia |
| *Toxoplasma gondii* | Meningoencephalitis (multifocal necrotizing granulomas), perivascular infiltrates | Diffuse | Cortical dysplasia (possible), hydrocephalus, hydranencephaly, porencephaly, multifocal and diffuse necrosis of parenchyma |
| Rubella | Meningoencephalitis (necrosis of brain parenchyma) | Diffuse, periventricular and parenchymal | Vasculopathy with focal ischemic necrosis. Delayed myelination |
| Herpes simplex | Meningoencephalitis (multifocal parenchymal necrosis, occasionally hemorrhagic) | Periventricular, thalamic and basal ganglia, cerebral cortex | Neuronal migration disorder (reported in some cases of fetally acquired HSV-1), brain swelling, multicystic encephalomalacia |
| HIV | Meningoencephalitis (multinucleated giant cells) | Basal ganglia, white matter, cerebral cortex | Atrophy (neuronal and myelin loss), spinal cord myelin loss, CNS lymphoma, opportunistic infections, infarcts |
| *Treponema pallidum* | Acute or subacute meningitis (mononuclear inflammation), chronic meningitis, esp. in basal meninges | | Vasculitis with cerebral infarction, hydrocephalus |
| Varicella | Meningoencephalitis (predilection for periventricular white matter) | Yes | Polymicrogyria, focal lissencephaly, ventricular dilation, porencephalic cysts, vasculitis with ischemic lesions |
| Lymphocytic choriomeningitis virus (LCMV) | Ependymitis | Periventricular, ependymal and parenchymal calcifications | Lissencephaly, cortical dysplasia, schizencephaly, polymicrogyria, cerebellar hypoplasia, chorioretinitis, microcephaly, hydrocephalus |
| Parvovirus B19 | Meningoencephalitis and vasculitis | | |
| Pseudo-TORCH syndrome | Familial autosomal recessive inheritance | Cortical band-like calcifications | Simplified gyration and polymicrogyria |

benefits to varicella zoster immunization as well. Identifying women with syphilis and early treatment can prevent fetal infection. Avoiding cat litter in pregnancy is recommended to thwart toxoplasmosis. Avoiding contact with mice and hamsters can potentially reduce lymphocytic choriomeningitis virus (LCMV) infection. Chagas disease can be prevented by vector control of Triatominae insects in Latin America. Prevention of HSV, which is often under recognized in pregnant women, is difficult.

After birth, early postnatal treatment with antivirals and appropriate antibiotics is beneficial in CMV, congenital toxoplasmosis, and congenital syphilis. There are no documented benefits of therapy for herpes, varicella, or rubella. Chagas disease is treated; however, benefit is unknown.

**Recurrence:** There is no known recurrence risk for fetal infections. However, disorders mimicking TORCH infections such as Aicardi–Goutiere and pseudo-TORCH syndromes are postulated to have autosomal recessive inheritance and hence are known to recur in subsequent pregnancies.

## REFERENCES

1. Barkovich AJ, Girard N. Fetal brain infections. *Childs Nerv Syst*. 2003;19:501–507.
2. Bale JF. Fetal neurology fetal infections and brain development. *Clin Perinatol*. 2009;36(3):639–653.
3. Remington JS, Klein JO, Wilson CB, et al, eds. *Infectious Diseases of the Fetus and Newborn Infant*. 7th ed. Philadelphia, PA: Elsevier; 2010.
4. Malinger G, Lev D, Zahalka N, et al. Fetal cytomegalovirus infection of the brain: the spectrum of sonographic findings. *AJNR Am J Neuroradiol*. 2003;24(1):28–32.
5. Doneda C, Parazzini C, Righini A, et al. Early cerebral lesions in cytomegalovirus infection: prenatal MR imaging. *Radiology*. 2010;255:613–621.
6. Stephenson JBP. Aicardi-Goutières syndrome (AGS). *Eur J Pediatr Neurol*. 2007;12:355–358.

# Posterior Fossa Anomalies

Ashley James Robinson

## INTRODUCTION

Evaluation of the posterior fossa is an essential part of routine fetal sonography, as defined by guidelines from the American College of Radiology, American Institute of Ultrasound in Medicine and American College of Obstetricians and Gynecologists, and also the Society of Obstetricians and Gynaecologists of Canada, and Canadian Association of Radiologists, which state that views of the cerebellum and cisterna magna should be specifically included.[1-3] Normal measurements of the cisterna magna (between 2 and 11 mm) and ventricular atrium (<10 mm) confer a very high negative predictive value (P < .005%) for abnormal CNS and spinal cord development.[4]

When an abnormality is found, however, there are a variety of pathologies that can look similar and even identical by standard axial ultrasonography, including Dandy-Walker continuum and other vermian hypoplasia syndromes, mega cisterna magna, persistent Blake pouch, and posterior fossa arachnoid cyst. Differentiation is difficult, and although direct sagittal and coronal views of the posterior fossa are possible,[5-8] they can often be technically difficult. For this reason, in the past considerable attention has been paid to the more readily obtained axial sonographic views, and while most of the aforementioned disorders can be demonstrated, so can a variety of false-positive vermian pathologies.[9-11] For example, imaging the posterior fossa in the semicoronal plane can give a false appearance of an enlarged cisterna magna or even partial vermian agenesis.[12]

The advent of 3D (3-dimensional) ultrasound and fetal MR (magnetic resonance) has provided new tools in the imaging armamentarium that is proving to be extremely useful in difficult cases, because those orthogonal views are more readily obtainable, and because other limitations of ultrasonography such as maternal obesity, fetal skull ossification, and oligohydramnios, can frequently be overcome by MRI. These newer techniques therefore allow additional further assessment of the fourth ventricle, brainstem, cisterna magna, and cerebellum that was not previously possible.

### Important Embryology Milestones

At around 8 to 10 weeks' gestation, a focal dilatation of the neural tube is seen in the dorsal aspect of the developing hindbrain, which is the rhombencephalic vesicle, the predecessor to the fourth ventricle (Fig. 12.3-1A,B). At this level in the brainstem, which is known as the open medulla, the two alar laminae do not touch in the midline dorsally, and the gap is bridged by a layer of tela choroidea,[13] known as the area membranacea, which forms the roof of the rhombencephalic vesicle (Fig. 12.3-1C). The hindbrain develops a kink, known as the dorsal pontine flexure, which causes a transverse crease to form in the area membranacea, dividing it into anterior (rostral) and posterior (caudal) membranous areas (Fig. 12.3-2A,B). The cerebellum develops from the rhombic lips at the cranial end of the area membranacea, and the vermis and cerebellum grow

exophytically, inferiorly, and laterally to cover it. Because of its thinness, this layer of tela choroidea has until recently been nonresoluble by in vivo imaging, thus giving the false impression that the fourth ventricle is initially open to the developing subarachnoid space, and then appears to close owing to caudal growth of the overlying vermis.[14,15] This developmental appearance is therefore often referred to in the literature as "closure" of the fourth ventricle. This process is usually complete by around 18 weeks' gestation; however, physiologic variation may give the appearance that the vermis is incomplete at the time of initial midtrimester assessment.[16]

The vermis does not completely cover the roof of the fourth ventricle, and a part of the posterior membranous area evaginates beneath the vermis into the overlying meninx primitiva.[17,18] This evagination occurs through a space that is delimited by the vermis superiorly, nucleus gracilis inferiorly, and the developing cerebellar hemispheres laterally, also known in the mature state as the cerebellar vallecula (Fig. 12.3-2C). This evagination was first described in 1900 and is known as Blake pouch,[13] and where it constricts to pass through the cerebellar vallecula, it is known as Blake metapore (Fig. 12.3-2D,E). Normal linear echoes (the cisterna magna septa), which are typically seen in the fetal and neonatal cisterna magna and which are most often described as bridging arachnoid septations,[19] have recently been shown to represent the walls of Blake pouch, a normal and persistent structure in the posterior fossa. The cisterna magna septa or Blake pouch walls are a potential marker for normal development (Fig. 12.3-3).[18]

The future cisterna magna therefore forms in two compartments, a mesial compartment between the cisterna magna septa, which is derived from the rhombencephalic vesicle (Blake pouch), and compartments lateral to the cisterna magna septa that develop through cavitation of the meninx primitiva overlying the surface of the brain, forming the subarachnoid space proper.

Blake pouch usually, but not always, fenestrates to a variable degree[13,20] down to the obex (the inferior recess of the fourth ventricle), which leads to communication between the mesial ventricular-derived compartment and the true subarachnoid space of the cisterna magna. Fenestration and disappearance of Blake pouch thus leaves an opening at Blake metapore,[18,20,21] which is the predecessor to the foramen of Magendie, allowing free communication between the fourth ventricle and the cisterna magna. Imaging the posterior fossa in the semicoronal plane will show this normal opening,[14,18,22] but can give a false appearance of partial vermian agenesis[12] (Fig. 12.3-4). This error can be avoided by making sure that the cavum septi pellucidi is included in the image, thus ensuring that the scan plane is truly axial or modified axial. Thus, the foramen of Magendie does not demarcate the actual junction between the fourth ventricle and the true subarachnoid space of the cisterna magna. A *small* communication beneath the vermis, between the fourth ventricle and the "cisterna magna," often shown in the literature by sonography[14,15,18,22,23] and sometimes subsequently "confirmed" on midsagittal images, is therefore the normal Blake metapore. Unfortunately, it is often wrongly ascribed to "Dandy-Walker variant" (*vide infra*).

In the literature, the phrase "a posterior fossa cyst communicating with the 4th ventricle" is often used to describe cystic malformations of the posterior fossa; however, this is actually a description of the normal anatomy. What is abnormal is the size of the posterior fossa "cyst," not the fact that it communicates

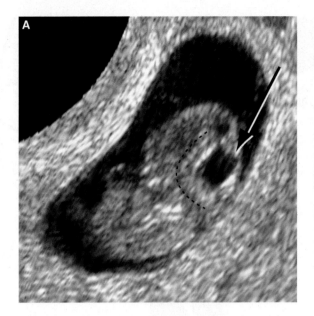

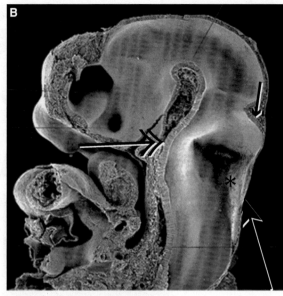

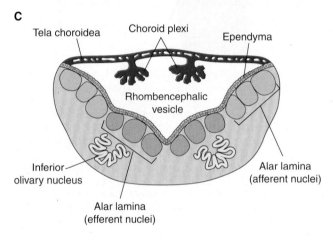

**FIGURE 12.3-1:** Embryology of the Posterior Fossa **A:** Sagittal sonogram of the cranial end of the fetal pole at 8 to 10 weeks' gestation demonstrating the rhombencephalic vesicle (*long arrow*) and the dorsal pontine flexure (*dotted line*). **B:** Electron micrograph of the embryo. Rhombencephalic vesicle (*asterisk*), rhombic lips (*small arrow*), rhombencephalic roof (*long arrow*), and dorsal flexure of pons (*double arrow*). **C:** Diagram of section through open medulla. The roof of the rhombencephalic vesicle comprises tela choroidea, which comprises an inner layer of ependyma continuous with the lining of the neural tube, outer layer of pia-arachnoid continuous with over surface of the brain, and intervening attenuated neuroglial tissue. (**A**, from Robinson AJ, Goldstein R. The cisterna magna septa: vestigial remnants of Blake's pouch and a potential new marker for normal development of the rhombencephalon. *J Ultrasound Med.* 2007;26: 83–95, with permission of the American Institute of Ultrasound in Medicine. **B, C**, from Sadler TW. *Langman's Essential Medical Embryology.* Baltimore, MD: Lippincott Williams & Wilkins; 2005, with permission of Lippincott Williams & Wilkins.)

with the fourth ventricle. The Dandy-Walker "cyst" is in fact Blake pouch, which expands to fill the subarachnoid space of the cisterna magna.[18] The cisterna magna septa are not typically seen in cystic malformations of the posterior fossa[24] because as Blake pouch expands, its walls, that is the septa, are displaced laterally and can become indistinguishable from the walls of the cisterna magna, although often the true subarachnoid space of the cisterna magna is still visible very laterally beyond the septa. Additionally seen in the literature is the description of the fourth ventricle "widely communicating with the cisterna magna." Again, it is not actually the cisterna magna with which the fourth ventricle is in communication; it is in communication with Blake pouch, which in turn is itself contained within the cisterna magna.

## CYSTIC ANOMALIES

### Blake Pouch Cyst and Persistent Blake Pouch

**Incidence:** This is a rare diagnosis. The largest study to date of all posterior fossa collections (including Blake pouch cyst, mega cisterna magna, Dandy-Walker continuum, posterior fossa arachnoid cysts) had a total of 105 fetuses over a 10-year period in two referral centers for prenatal diagnosis.[25]

**Embryology and Genetics:** In persistent Blake pouch (Fig. 12.3-5), there is thought to be inadequate fenestration of both Blake pouch and the foramen of Luschka, leading to imbalance of CSF egress into the subarachnoid space of the cisterna magna with consequent dilatation of the fourth ventricle.[21] Although the pouch communicates freely with the fourth ventricle, there is a failure of communication between the pouch and the perimedullary subarachnoid spaces.[20,26] Unfortunately, the consequent elevation of the vermis often leads to the false-positive diagnosis of inferior vermian hypoplasia (*vide infra*).This explains why there has historically been poor correlation of ultrasound and autopsy findings in apparent cystic malformations of the posterior fossa.[11]

**Etiology and Pathogenesis:** The *lateral* recesses of the rhombencephalic vesicle are in direct contact with the developing

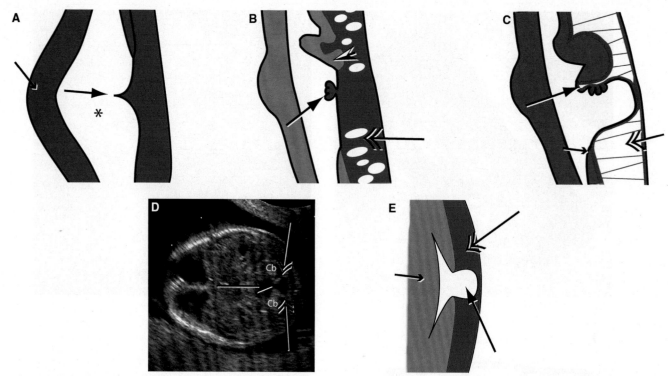

**FIGURE 12.3-2:** Blake Pouch **A:** Diagrammatic representation demonstrating the formation of the dorsal pontine flexure *(white tipped arrow)* and the consequent crease that develops in the roof of the rhombencephalic vesicle *(solid black arrow)*. The vesicle *(asterisk)* is the predecessor to the fourth ventricle. **B:** Choroid plexus forms as the wedge of meninx primitiva within the transverse crease that becomes vascularized *(long arrow)*. The overlying meninx primitiva starts to cavitate *(double arrow)*. Cerebellum starts to develop in area membranacea anterior *(short arrow)*. **C:** The posterior membranous area evaginates below the developing vermis *(long arrow)* and the nucleus gracilis *(short arrow)*. Coalescence of the cavities within the meninx primitiva leads to development of the subarachnoid space, which is trabeculated in random planes by multiple pia-arachnoid septations *(double arrow)*. **D:** Axial fetal sonogram at 13 weeks' gestation demonstrating Blake pouch evaginating into the cavitating meninx primitiva, between the developing cerebellar hemispheres *(Cb)*. The walls of the pouch are visible as linear echoes *(double arrows)*. Blake metapore *(single arrow)* is the predecessor of the foramen of Magendie. **E:** Diagrammatic representation showing the meninx primitiva *(double arrow)*, Blake pouch *(long arrow)*, and tegmentum of the brainstem *(short arrow)*. (**A–D**, from Robinson AJ, Goldstein R. The cisterna magna septa: vestigial remnants of Blake's pouch and a potential new marker for normal development of the rhombencephalon. *J Ultrasound Med.* 2007;26:83–95, with permission of the American Institute of Ultrasound in Medicine. **E**, from Robinson AJ. Inferior vermian hypoplasia: preconception, misconception. *Ultrasound Obstet Gynecol.* 2014;43:123–136, with permission of John Wiley & Sons Ltd.)

subarachnoid space and fenestrate to form the foramen of Luschka. If fenestration of Blake pouch does not occur, it is the later fenestration of the foramen of Luschka that leads to

equilibration of CSF between the ventricular system and the subarachnoid space,[27] and therefore in lower species, where it is normal for Blake pouch not to fenestrate, the foramen of

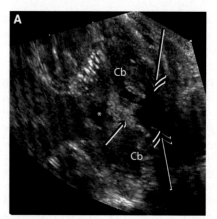
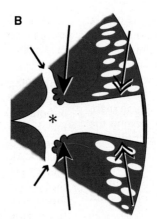
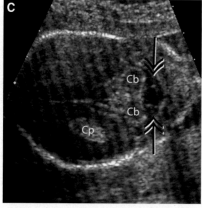

**FIGURE 12.3-3:** Development of Fourth Ventricle **A:** Above vallecula, the 4th ventricle *(asterick)* and septa *(double arrows)* are separated by the inferior vermis *(small arrow)*. **B:** Diagrammatic representation demonstrating the relationship between the fourth ventricle *(asterisk)* and the space between the septa *(double arrows)*. The foramen of Luschka *(short arrows)* forms at the lateral recesses of the fourth ventricle. Lateral caudal extensions of the choroid plexus form on each side *(long arrows)*. **C:** Semicoronal fetal sonogram at 20 weeks' gestation. The CSF between the septa *(double arrows)* is completely anechoic because it forms as an evagination of the neural tube, whereas the CSF lateral to the septa is slightly echogenic because it forms through cavitation of the meninx primitiva. Cerebellar hemispheres *(Cb)*. Choroid plexus of the lateral ventricle *(Cp)*. (From Robinson AJ, Goldstein R. The cisterna magna septa: vestigial remnants of Blake's pouch and a potential new marker for normal development of the rhombencephalon. *J Ultrasound Med.* 2007;26:83–95, with permission of the American Institute of Ultrasound in Medicine.)

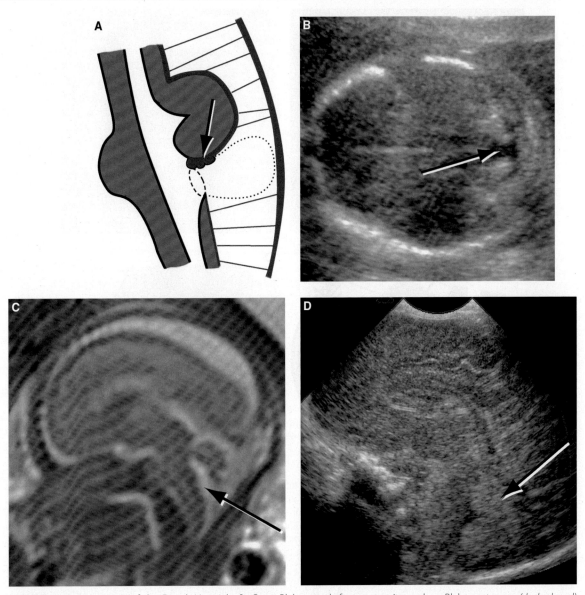

**FIGURE 12.3-4:** Imaging of the Fourth Ventricle **A:** Once Blake pouch fenestrates, its neck or Blake metapore *(dashed oval)* becomes the foramen of Magendie. The choroid plexus in the roof of the fourth ventricle *(short arrow)* now appears to be "in the cisterna magna." **B:** On sonography at 19 weeks, fetus having an apparently normal vermis was seen superiorly (not shown). Modified axial sonogram in the same fetus demonstrating normal appearances of the communication between the fourth ventricle and the subarachnoid space *(arrow)*, in keeping with the foramen of Magendie. **C:** Sagittal fetal MRI study at 21 weeks' gestation in the same fetus showing a small "defect" *(arrow)* gap between the inferior vermis and the brainstem. **D:** Follow-up sonography at 26 weeks showed normal appearances of the posterior fossa with an intact vermis. Postnatal sagittal sonography on day 1 of life demonstrates an apparently complete vermis *(arrow)* with no evidence of an increased tegmento-vermian angle. This baby had normal development at 2 years of age. (**A**, from Robinson AJ, Goldstein R. The cisterna magna septa: vestigial remnants of Blake's pouch and a potential new marker for normal development of the rhombencephalon. *J Ultrasound Med.* 2007;26:83–95, with permission of the American Institute of Ultrasound in Medicine. **B–D**, from Robinson AJ, Blaser S, Toi A, et al. The fetal cerebellar vermis: assessment for abnormal development by ultrasonography and magnetic resonance imaging. *Ultrasound Q.* 2007;23:211–223, with permission of Wolters Kluwer Health.)

Luschka are correspondingly larger than in humans. In humans, therefore, the foramen of Luschka are not large enough to compensate for the lack of fenestration of Blake pouch at the foramen of Magendie, and so equilibration of CSF might only be achieved with the ventricles persistently enlarged.[28] Even at the foramen of Luschka, the degree of fenestration can be variable.[29] The variable degrees of fenestration at both Blake pouch and the foramen of Luschka and the balance of CSF production and egress into the subarachnoid space probably explain why outward bowing of the cisterna magna septa is often normally seen giving the impression of a posterior fossa cyst[19] (Fig. 12.3-6),

which subsequently may resolve as fenestration progresses, depending on degree and timing of fenestration.[25] In one study, Blake pouch cyst was seen to resolve by 26 weeks,[30] which corresponds exactly with the timing of opening of the foramen of Luschka by another author.[31]

It has also been suggested by several cases in the literature that persistent Blake pouch phenotype can be "acquired" if the balance of CSF egress is upset by the presence of fetal intraventricular hemorrhage[25,28] and fetal infection,[32,33] which result in tetraventricular dilatation and enlargement of the "cisterna magna" (Blake pouch). Presumably, the obstruction occurs

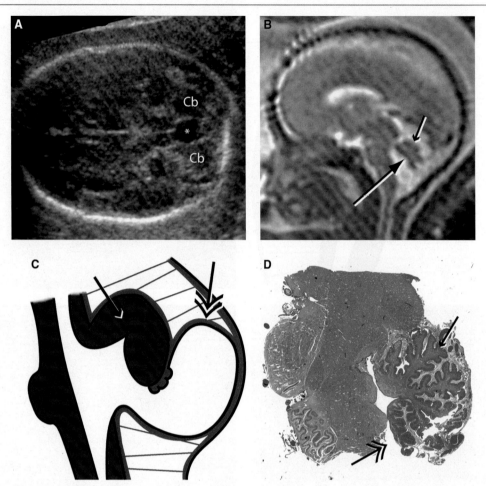

**FIGURE 12.3-5:** Blake Pouch Cyst **A:** Modified axial fetal sonogram at 23 weeks' gestation demonstrating a distended and misshapen fourth ventricle *(asterisk)* with mass effect on the adjacent cerebellar hemispheres *(Cb)*. **B:** Sagittal fetal MRI scan of the same fetus demonstrating that the vermis is morphologically normal; its craniocaudal diameter was gestation-appropriate, and the major landmarks comprising the primary fissure *(short arrow)* and fastigial point *(long arrow)* are present. **C:** Diagrammatic representation Blake pouch cyst. In this condition, there is inadequate fenestration of the pouch *(double arrow)* and coexistent inadequate fenestration of the foramen of Lushcka leading to elevation of the vermis *(short arrow)* and hydrocephalus. **D:** Histopathologic specimen of the same fetus showing that the vermis *(short arrow)* is normal and that the pouch *(double arrow)* has decompressed. (**A, C, D**, from Robinson AJ, Blaser S, Toi A, et al. The fetal cerebellar vermis: assessment for abnormal development by ultrasonography and magnetic resonance imaging. *Ultrasound Q.* 2007;23:211–223, with permission of Wolters Kluwer Health.)

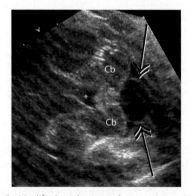

**FIGURE 12.3-6:** Modified axial neonatal sonogram at 24 weeks' gestation demonstrating outward bowing of the cisterna magna septa *(double arrows)* giving the impression of a posterior fossa cyst. 4th ventricle *(asterick)* and cerebellar hemispheres (Cb). (From Robinson AJ, Goldstein R. The cisterna magna septa: vestigial remnants of Blake's pouch and a potential new marker for normal development of the rhombencephalon. *J Ultrasound Med.* 2007;26:83–95, with permission of the American Institute of Ultrasound in Medicine.)

through resultant debris within the ventricular system causing obstruction of the fenestrations in both the foramen of Luschka and Blake pouch, in much the same way as can be demonstrated postnatally (Fig. 12.3-7), recognizing that depending on the nature and timing of the insult, injury to the brain parenchyma itself can also occur because of endotoxins, free radicals, and inflammatory cytokines.[34–36] Consequently, a compensated Blake pouch cyst may never be diagnosed even in adults until such a precipitating event tips the balance of CSF egress in favour of hydrocephalus and the patient becomes symptomatic.

**Diagnosis:** The wall of Blake pouch can be seen by ultrasound but with more difficulty by MRI. The Blake pouch elevates/rotates the vermis away from the brainstem. This has been described as an increased tegmento-vermian angle (*vide infra*).[15] Importantly, the vermis is intrinsically normal, that is, this is an isolated abnormality of the posterior membranous area, and there is no associated abnormality of the anterior membranous area structures (vermis). Thus, the essential task is to ensure that the vermis is normal, and the problem is our ability to distinguish an isolated persistent Blake pouch from vermian hypoplasia (vide infra), which have different outcomes.

**Differential Diagnosis:** Other causes of cystic malformations of the posterior fossa include vermian hypoplasia (Dandy-Walker continuum), mega cisterna magna, and posterior fossa arachnoid cyst.

**Prognosis:** Isolated elevation/rotation of the vermis due to a persistent Blake pouch does not necessarily indicate an adverse outcome.[14,18,37-42] In one study, one-third of cases of Blake pouch cyst or mega cisterna magna underwent spontaneous resolution in utero, and 90% of survivors with no associated anomalies had normal developmental outcome at 1 to 5 years once the initial referral misdiagnosis of vermian hypoplasia had been excluded.[25]

In another large retrospective study of 19 cases of Blake pouch cyst, associated anomalies were seen in 8. There were two neonatal deaths. In nine survivors, one had trisomy 21, and the other eight were neurodevelopmentally normal, although one developed obstructive hydrocephalus.[30]

In adults with Blake pouch cyst, after ventricular shunting, subtotal or total re-expansion of the cerebellar hemispheres and vermis can be seen. Sometimes, these structures may appear to be hypoplastic because of mass effect of the cyst; however, there is actually no intrinsic hypoplasia, and these patients are neurologically normal.[27]

**Management:** Blake pouch cyst often regresses in utero.[25] Expectant management is indicated, provided vermian hypoplasia and other associated abnormalities can be excluded.

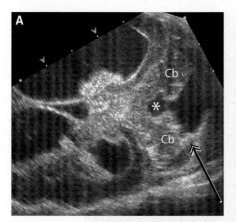
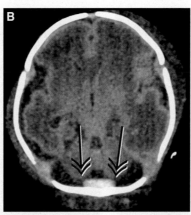
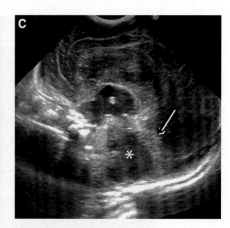
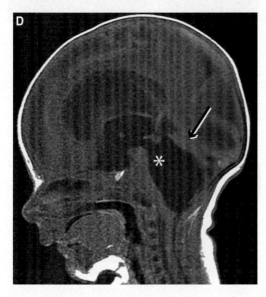
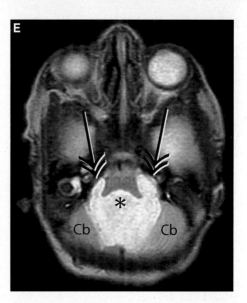

**FIGURE 12.3-7:** Acquired Blake Pouch Phenotype **A:** Axial neonatal sonogram at 31 weeks' gestation. There is blood apparently "within the cisterna magna" *(double arrow)* with hydrocephalus. Fourth ventricle *(asterisk),* cerebellar hemispheres *(Cb).* Closer inspection shows that the blood is limited in its lateral extent; the more dependent subarachnoid space over the cerebellar hemisphere does not contain blood but is slightly more echogenic because of the pia-arachnoid trabeculations. **B:** Axial neonatal CT in a different patient again showing blood "within the cisterna magna." Closer inspection shows that the blood is limited in its lateral extent by invisible walls *(double arrows)* and is most likely contained within Blake pouch. **C:** Sagittal US in a neonate showing a normal vermis on the first ultrasound. Follow-up ultrasound postintraventricular hemorrhage showing fourth ventricular dilatation *(asterick)* and an abnormal (compressed) vermis *(arrow)* similar in appearance to Dandy-Walker continuum. **D:** Sagittal MRI in the same neonate. The vermis is elevated *(arrow)* by the distended Blake pouch, and there is wide communication with the fourth ventricle *(asterisk).* **E:** Axial MRI in the same neonate demonstrating a distended Blake pouch and fourth ventricle *(asterisk).* The cerebellar hemispheres *(Cb)* are displaced laterally. It also appears as though the fenestrae at the foramen of Luschka are also blocked, causing their evagination *(double arrows)* into the perimedullary subarachnoid space. (**A, B**, from Robinson AJ, Goldstein R. The cisterna magna septa: vestigial remnants of Blake's pouch and a potential new marker for normal development of the rhombencephalon. *J Ultrasound Med.* 2007;26:83–95, with permission of the American Institute of Ultrasound in Medicine.)

**Recurrence Risk:** This is unknown. Full evaluation of any subsequent pregnancies is suggested.

## Mega Cisterna Magna

**Incidence:** This is a rare diagnosis. The largest study to date of all posterior fossa collections (including Blake pouch cyst, mega cisterna magna, Dandy-Walker continuum, posterior fossa arachnoid cysts) had a total of 105 fetuses over a 10-year period in two referral centers for prenatal diagnosis.[25]

**Embryology and Genetics:** In mega cisterna magna, the vermis is fully formed, but fenestration of Blake pouch and the foramen of Luschka is mildly deficient, thus allowing sufficient CSF equilibration for Blake pouch to cause mild

expansion of the cisterna magna but not sufficient to cause elevation of the vermis or obstructive hydrocephalus.[18] In this sense, mega cisterna magna may be more accurately termed "mega Blake pouch" (Fig. 12.3-8). Partial fenestration would explain the communication seen between the fourth ventricle and the subarachnoid space that can be demonstrated on cisternography.[21]

**Etiology and Pathogenesis:** Mega cisterna magna is thought to result from a defect of the posterior membranous area during embryogenesis.[21]

**Diagnosis:** The definition of mega cisterna magna is an enlargement of the cisterna magna >10 mm (see Fig. 12.3-8). The vermis should be intact and in a normal position, and the

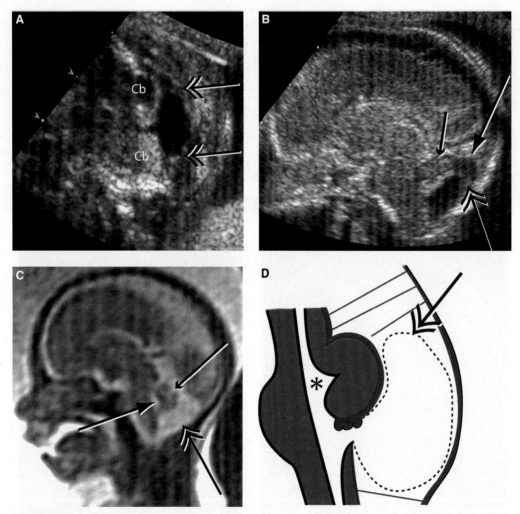

**FIGURE 12.3-8:** Mega Cisterna Magna **A:** Modified axial fetal sonogram at 19 weeks' gestation showing a prominent "cisterna magna" with the septa displaced laterally *(double arrows)*. The cerebellar hemispheres *(Cb)* appear normal. **B:** Direct sagittal fetal sonogram of the same fetus demonstrates the anechoic CSF contained within Blake pouch *(double arrow)*, the echogenic true subarachnoid space below the falx cerebelli *(long arrow)*, and slight mass effect on the underside of the cerebellar vermis *(small arrow)*. **C:** Sagittal fetal MRI of the same fetus showing that the vermis has the normal morphologic features of the primary fissure *(long arrow)* and the fastigial point *(short arrow)*. The "cisterna magna" appears large *(double arrow)*, but the walls of Blake pouch are not resoluble. **D:** Diagrammatic representation of mega cisterna magna. In this condition, the pouch expands within the subarachnoid space of the cisterna magna *(double arrow)*, but later there is sufficient fenestration to allow communication with the fourth ventricle *(asterisk)* by contrast cisternography. (From Robinson AJ, Goldstein R. The cisterna magna septa: vestigial remnants of Blake's pouch and a potential new marker for normal development of the rhombencephalon. *J Ultrasound Med.* 2007;26:83–95, with permission of the American Institute of Ultrasound in Medicine.)

cerebellar hemispheres should be normal. No associated abnormalities should be present.

**Differential Diagnosis:** Other causes of cystic malformations of the posterior fossa include the vermian hypoplasia (Dandy-Walker continuum), persistent Blake pouch, and posterior fossa arachnoid cyst. This differential is further discussed in the section on Blake pouch cyst (*vide supra*).

**Prognosis:** Mega cisterna magna often regresses in utero.[25] It is associated with overall normal cognitive function, but subjects may score inferior to controls on some parameters of memory and verbal fluency.[43]

**Management:** This often regresses in utero.[25] Expectant management is indicated, provided vermian hypoplasia and other associated abnormalities can be excluded.

**Recurrence Risk:** This is unknown. Full evaluation of any subsequent pregnancies is suggested.

## Arachnoid Cyst

**Incidence:** This is a rare diagnosis. The largest study to date of all posterior fossa collections (including Blake pouch cyst, mega cisterna magna, Dandy-Walker continuum, and posterior fossa arachnoid cysts) had a total of 105 fetuses over a 10-year period in two referral centers for prenatal diagnosis.[25]

**Embryology and Genetics:** Embryologically, the pia-arachnoid is initially a solid condensation of mesenchyme over the brain, known as the meninx primitiva. Small fluid-filled cavities form within the meninx primitiva, which then coalesce to form a sponge-like network of cavities over the surface of the brain (Fig. 12.3-9). The inner membrane directly in contact with the surface of the brain is the pia mater, and the outer is the arachnoid mater. The subarachnoid space is therefore trabeculated by numerous pia-arachnoid septations,[19] which make it diffusely echogenic by ultrasound compared with the CSF in the ventricular system. This relative echogenicity decreases throughout gestation as cavitation increases.[18]

**Etiology and Pathogenesis:** If coalescence is incomplete, a cavity may not communicate with its neighbors and remains isolated from the surrounding subarachnoid space.

**Diagnosis:** Because of its embryology, an arachnoid cyst, in contradistinction to a Blake pouch cyst, does not communicate with the fourth ventricle. Sometimes, a thin septum can be seen separating the two. Because of the fact that it has to arise in the subarachnoid space, its continued enlargement can cause mass effect on the vermis and cerebellar hemispheres, but it cannot elevate the vermis like a Blake pouch cyst (Fig. 12.3-10).

**Differential Diagnosis:** Other causes of cystic malformations of the posterior fossa include vermian hypoplasia (Dandy-Walker continuum), persistent Blake pouch, and posterior fossa arachnoid cyst.

**Prognosis:** If not associated with brain insult or karyotype anomalies, these have an excellent prognosis. Most either stabilize or regress, and prenatal hydrocephalus is rare. Those who develop hydrocephalus postnatally tend not to have hydrocephalus prenatally, and therefore postnatal surveillance is advised, especially in the first few months of life.[44,45]

**Management:** Neurosurgical consultation is advised because postnatal surveillance imaging and surgical intervention may be necessary.

**Recurrence Risk:** There is no recurrence risk.

## Vermian Hypoplasia and Dandy-Walker Continuum

The Dandy-Walker continuum (DWC), the preferred nomenclature, includes classic Dandy-Walker malformation (DWM), Dandy-Walker variant, and possibly also mega cisterna magna and persistent Blake pouch cyst.[18,27]

Classic DWM comprises complete or partial vermian agenesis, cystic dilatation of the fourth ventricle, and enlargement of the posterior fossa with elevation of transverse sinus, tentorium, and torcula ("torcula-lambdoid inversion")[46] (Fig. 12.3-11). The problem with the nomenclature arises in that the vermis can be variably abnormal, the size of the fourth ventricle and retrocerebellar CSF inconsistent, and defining whether the tentorium is high enough to be inverted with regard to the lambdoid impossible by fetal imaging. In addition, some authors also include hydrocephalus[47]; however, hydrocephalus is a frequent complication of, but not actually a part of the malformation,[46] and is not usually present at birth.[48]

Dandy-Walker "variant" is a terminology that should probably be abandoned, possibly in favor of Dandy-Walker "continuum," or "complex"[49] as abnormalities of the posterior fossa remain unclear from a prognostic perspective and the term "continuum" more clearly refers to the variable degrees of vermian hypoplasia,

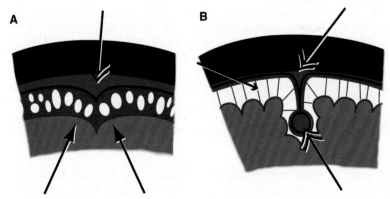

**FIGURE 12.3-9:** Development of Subarachnoid Space **A:** The meninx primitiva starts to cavitate *(red with white bubbles)* and the lateral neural tissues overgrow the midline structures *(long arrows)* trapping a wedge of conjunctive tissue containing rich vascular plexi in the midline *(double arrow)*. **B:** The rich vascular plexi coalesce to form the dural venous sinuses, for example, the superior sagittal sinus *(double superior arrow)* and inferior sagittal sinus *(inferior double arrow)*. Subarachnoid space is single arrow. (From Robinson AJ, Goldstein R. The cisterna magna septa: vestigial remnants of Blake's pouch and a potential new marker for normal development of the rhombencephalon. *J Ultrasound Med.* 2007;26:83–95, with permission of the American Institute of Ultrasound in Medicine.)

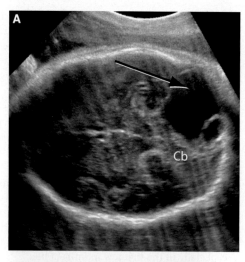

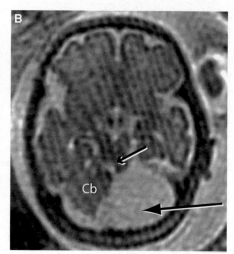

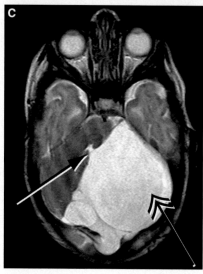

**FIGURE 12.3-10:** Arachnoid Cyst **A:** Modified axial view of a fetus showing a large cyst in the posterior fossa *(arrow)*. **B:** Axial fetal MRI study of the same fetus demonstrating the cyst *(long arrow)* with displacement of the brainstem, fourth ventricle *(short arrow)*, and cerebellum *(Cb)*. **C:** Axial neonatal MRI of the same fetus demonstrates that the cyst *(double arrow)* and the fourth ventricle are definitely separated by a thin septum *(long arrow)*.

fenestration of the fourth ventricular outlet foramen, and associated anomalies that are seen in these cases.[15,48] The term inferior vermian hypoplasia is growing in usage apparently as an alternative to the nomenclature "Dandy-Walker variant."[10,50–52] However, despite the confusing terminology, in the absence of a known genetic syndrome, it is probably more important for counseling to identify the anomalies present than to provide a "defined name."

Although still controversial, an attempt at summarizing this is demonstrated in Table 12.3-1.

**Incidence:** The reported incidence of DWM is 1:30,000.[48]

**Embryology and Genetics:** The Dandy-Walker continuum is associated with single-gene disorders such as Walker-Warburg, Meckel–Gruber syndromes, and chromosomal abnormalities.[53]

**Etiology and Pathogenesis:** Classic DWM was initially described in infants with hydrocephalus and was thought to be the sequelae of atresia of foramina of Luschka and Magendie[54–56]; however, current theories suggest that it is a more global developmental defect affecting the roof of the rhombencephalon[18,49] leading to variable degrees of vermian hypoplasia, variable fenestration of the fourth ventricular outlet foramen, and variable associated anomalies.[48]

Current theories suggest that the spectrum of findings with respect to the posterior fossa "cyst" in Dandy-Walker continuum might result from two potential processes: either arrest of vermian development so it does not cover the fourth ventricle, or failure of adequate fenestration of the fourth ventricular outflow foramen, leading to an enlarged Blake pouch with secondary elevation and compression of the vermis. Often, these two processes are seen together as in classic DWM.

**Diagnosis**

***Assessment for Presence of the Vermis Using Its Major Landmarks:*** Various biometric and morphologic criteria for assessment of vermian hypoplasia have been described.[14,41,57] By 17.5 weeks, one should be able to identify whether the vermis is present by assessing for the major landmarks that should be present by this gestation as determined by in vitro studies. This includes whether the fastigial point is present and has a normal acute angle, or whether it is deficient (i.e., absent or obtuse angle) and whether the primary fissure is identifiable (Fig. 12.3-12).

***Assessment of Vermian Maturity:*** Having determined that the vermis is present, one must evaluate its developmental maturity, because this has been demonstrated to correlate

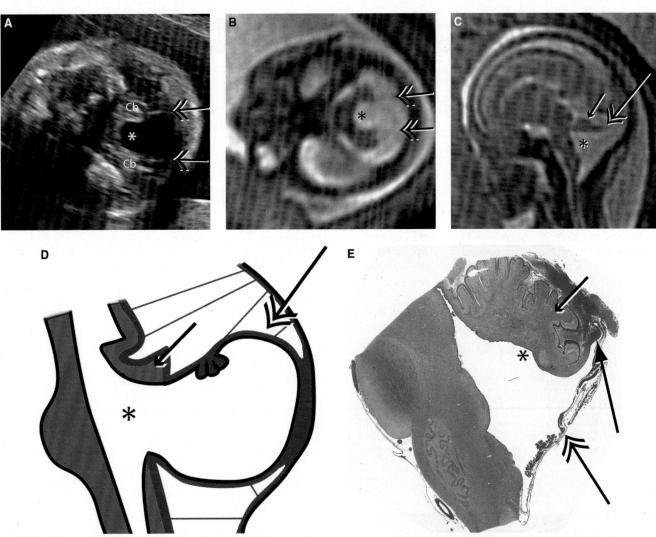

**FIGURE 12.3-11:** Dandy Walker Continuum/Anomaly of Vermian Development **A:** Modified axial fetal sonogram showing "a posterior fossa cyst communicating with the fourth ventricle." The cisterna magna septa (walls of Blake pouch) are displaced laterally *(double arrows)*. The pia-arachnoid trabeculations can be seen lateral to the septa. The space between the septa is continuous with the fourth ventricle *(asterisk)*. **B:** Axial fetal MRI scan of the same fetus showing the cisterna magna septa *(double arrows)* and fourth ventricle *(asterisk)*. The septa are very rarely visible on fetal MRI. **C:** Sagittal fetal MRI scan of the same fetus showing the vermis *(small arrow)* is elevated by the distended Blake pouch. Displaced germinal matrix can be seen *(double arrow)* at the superior aspect of the pouch. There is wide communication between the pouch and the fourth ventricle *(asterisk)*. **D:** Diagrammatic representation of Dandy-Walker continuum. There is variable vermian hypoplasia *(small arrow)*, and variable fenestration of Blake pouch *(double arrow)* and the foramen of Lushcka. Position of fourth ventricle *(asterisk)*. **E:** Sagittal histopathologic specimen of a different fetus, akin to Dandy-Walker continuum. It can be seen that there is mild vermian dysmorphology with deficient lobulation *(small arrow)* and a flattened fastigial point *(asterisk)*. Blake pouch *(double arrow)* is intact. The germinal matrix is displaced *(long arrow)*. (**C, D**, from Robinson AJ, Goldstein R. The cisterna magna septa: vestigial remnants of Blake's pouch and a potential new marker for normal development of the rhombencephalon. *J Ultrasound Med.* 2007;26:83–95, with permission of the American Institute of Ultrasound in Medicine. **E**, courtesy of William Halliday, Department of Pathology, Hospital for Sick Children, Toronto, Canada; from Robinson AJ. Inferior vermian hypoplasia: preconception, misconception. *Ultrasound Obstet Gynecol.* 2014;43:123–136, with permission of John Wiley & Sons Ltd.)

with prognosis.[37] In addition to the fastigial point and the primary fissure, we can assess for vermian lobulation, biometry including the craniocaudal diameter of the vermis and the relative growth of the anterior versus posterior lobes, and the tegmento-vermian angle.

*Lobulation:* By 21 weeks, the prepyramidal fissure can be seen between the tuber and the pyramis, and by 21 to 22 weeks, the preculminate fissure can be seen between the central lobule and the culmen. By 24 weeks, the secondary fissure can be seen between the pyramis and the uvula, and from 27 weeks, all the vermian lobules and fissures become visible (Fig. 12.3-13).[58–61] Therefore, prior to 24 weeks' gestation, a

critical time in many jurisdictions with respect to considering termination of pregnancy, it can be difficult to determine whether vermian lobulation is complete because the declive, folium and tuber are not normally separately distinguishable at that stage of development because they are the last to develop and differentiate. Also, all three are united by a single white matter core to the arbor vitae, whereas all the other named lobules have their own individual white matter cores (see Fig. 12.3-13F). Therefore, it will appear as if only seven lobules out of nine are present.

*Biometry: The craniocaudal and anteroposterior diameters and surface area of the vermis* By 18 weeks, the fastigial point

## Table 12.3-1    Categorization of "Cystic" Posterior Fossa Malformations

| Findings | Vermis | | Cisterna Magna Septa | Choroid Plexus Position | Diagnosis |
|---|---|---|---|---|---|
| | Rotation/ Elevation | Hypoplasia | | | |
| Enlarged Blake pouch, **enlarged** posterior fossa, elevated torcula (often hydrocephalus) | Yes—greater than 40°–45° | Yes—variable—may be severe | Invisible—apposed to side walls of cisterna magna | Inferior margin of Blake pouch | Vermian hypoplasia—a.k.a. Dandy-Walker *malformation* |
| Enlarged Blake pouch, **normal**-sized posterior fossa, normal torcula | Yes—usually between 30° and 45° | Yes—variable—intermediate | Invisible—apposed to side walls of cisterna magna | Inferior margin of Blake pouch | Vermian hypoplasia—a.k.a. Dandy-Walker *variant* or "inferior vermian hypoplasia" |
| Enlarged Blake pouch, **normal**-sized posterior fossa, normal torcula | Yes—mild to moderate (usually <30°) | **No**—may be misdiagnosed as "inferior vermian hypoplasia" | Visible—bowed laterally | Superior margin of Blake pouch | Blake pouch cyst—a.k.a. persistent Blake pouch |
| Enlarged Blake pouch, **enlarged** posterior fossa (cisterna magna >10 mm) | **No** | **No** | Visible—bowed laterally | Superior margin of Blake pouch | Mega cisterna magna (= mega Blake pouch) |
| True cyst that does *not* communicate with the fourth ventricle (not Blake pouch) | **No** | **No**—may have extrinsic compression | Normal—but may be distorted by mass effect | Superior margin of Blake pouch | Posterior fossa arachnoid cyst |

N.B. Dandy-Walker variant is a term seen in the literature that referred to cases that resembled classic Dandy-Walker malformation but did not have an enlarged posterior fossa, hydrocephalus, and was often seen with associated anomalies and syndromes. Inferior vermian hypoplasia is now the latest nomenclature in the literature for the spectrum of abnormalities between classic Dandy-Walker and Blake pouch cyst, although this terminology is also debatable, and simply "vermian hypoplasia" may be more appropriate until it can be demonstrated precisely which part of the vermis is deficient.

Reproduced from Robinson AJ. Inferior vermian hypoplasia: preconception, misconception. *Ultrasound Obstet Gynecol.* 2014;43:123–136, with permission of John Wiley & Sons Ltd.

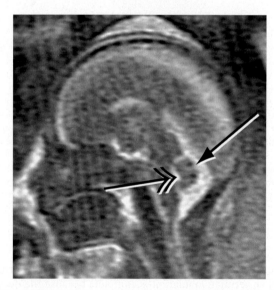

**FIGURE 12.3-12:** Primary Fissure at 17.5 weeks. The primary fissure *(single arrow)* is the first major vermian fissure to appear and marks the boundary between the superior (anterior) and inferior (posterior) vermis. By MR, it is seen as a high-signal indentation on the posterosuperior aspect of the vermis. The fastigial point *(double arrow)* is the posterosuperior recess of the fourth ventricle and should form an acute angle, giving it a diamond shape. (From Robinson AJ, Blaser S, Toi A, et al. The fetal cerebellar vermis: assessment for abnormal development by ultrasonography and magnetic resonance imaging. *Ultrasound Q.* 2007;23:211–223, with permission of Wolters Kluwer Health.)

and primary fissure should always be visible. The declive is seen immediately below the primary fissure. A line can usually therefore be drawn through the fastigial point and declive (the fastigium-declive line). The craniocaudal diameter of the vermis should be measured perpendicular to this line, and this measurement is therefore independent of any tegmentovermian angulation (Fig. 12.3-14B). According to this method of measurement,[59,62] growth of the craniocaudal diameter is linear, and this has been confirmed ultrasonographically. From this we can predict expected craniocaudal diameter at any gestational age. Similar data have been derived for anteroposterior diameter and surface area by both modalities.[7,8,63–68] The most contemporary data published include measurements of the craniocaudal diameter, anteroposterior diameter and surface area of the vermis and pons, and surface area of the brainstem by ultrasound (Table 23 in Appendix A1). Similar data by MRI are also provided (Tables 12.3-2 and 12.3-3).

*The ratio of Vermian tissue above and below the fastigial point* A second measurement that can be made from the same fastigium-declive line is the relative growth of the superior and inferior lobes. Instead of measuring the entire vermis, it is measured above and below this line, and the values are compared (Fig. 12.3-14A). This is useful to determine whether the anterior or posterior lobes are primarily affected, for example, in cases of Joubert syndrome where the anterior lobe is typically smaller, or "inferior vermian hypoplasia" where the inferior vermis is smaller.

There should be linear and symmetrical growth of the vermis throughout gestation. The average height above and below the

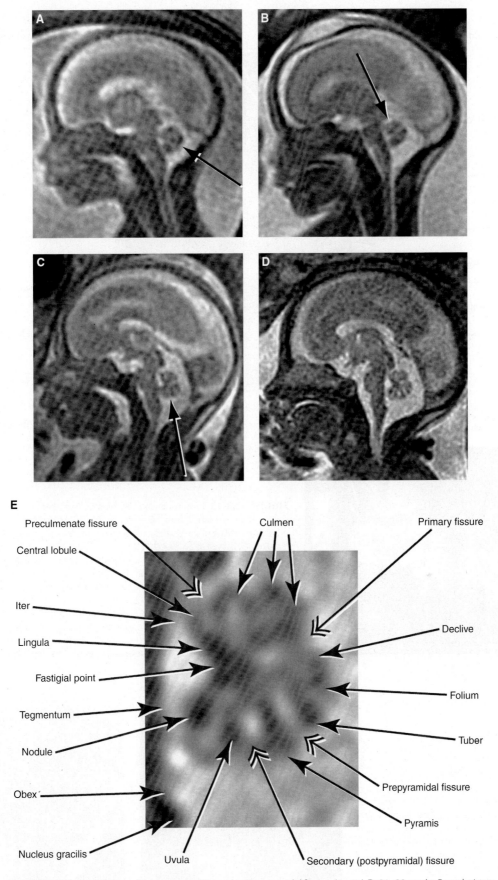

**FIGURE 12.3-13:** Fissures of the Vermis **A:** 21 weeks. Prepyramidal fissure *(arrow)*. **B:** 21–22 weeks. Preculminate fissure *(arrow)*. **C:** 24 weeks. Secondary (postpyramidal) fissure *(arrow)*. **D:** 27 weeks. All lobules visible. **E:** Detail of **D**.

*(continued)*

**F**

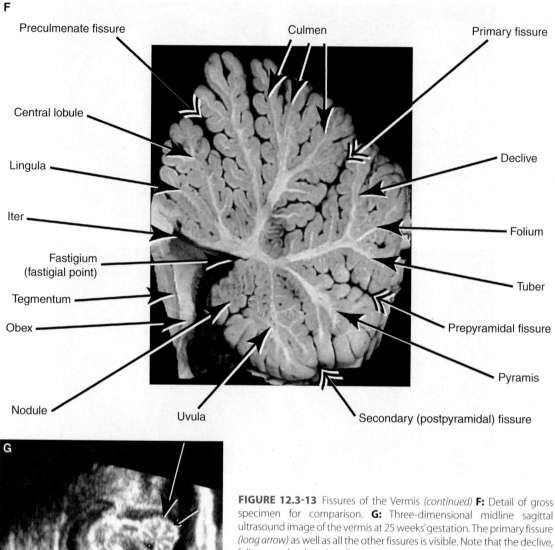

Preculmenate fissure

Culmen

Primary fissure

Central lobule

Lingula

Declive

Iter

Folium

Fastigium (fastigial point)

Tuber

Tegmentum

Obex

Prepyramidal fissure

Pyramis

Nodule

Uvula

Secondary (postpyramidal) fissure

**G**

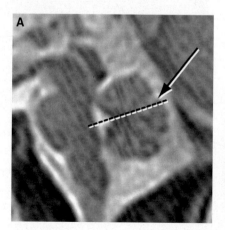

**FIGURE 12.3-13** Fissures of the Vermis *(continued)* **F:** Detail of gross specimen for comparison. **G:** Three-dimensional midline sagittal ultrasound image of the vermis at 25 weeks' gestation. The primary fissure *(long arrow)* as well as all the other fissures is visible. Note that the declive, folium, and tuber *(small arrow)* are barely differentiated. (**A–F**, from Robinson AJ, Blaser S, Toi A, et al. The fetal cerebellar vermis: assessment for abnormal development by ultrasonography and magnetic resonance imaging. *Ultrasound Q.* 2007;23:211–223, with permission of Wolters Kluwer Health. **G**, courtesy of Ants Toi, Department of Medical Imaging, University of Toronto, Canada; from Robinson AJ. Inferior vermian hypoplasia: preconception, misconception. *Ultrasound Obstet Gynecol.* 2014;43:123–136, with permission of John Wiley & Sons Ltd.)

**FIGURE 12.3-14:** Vermian Biometry (may also be done by ultrasound). **A:** Fastigial point-declive line *(dotted line)*. The declive is the first lobule posterior to the primary fissure, seen as a low-signal focus *(arrow)*. **B:** Cranio caudal diameter (perpendicular to fastigial point-declive line). (From Robinson AJ, Blaser S, Toi A, et al. The fetal cerebellar vermis: assessment for abnormal development by ultrasonography and magnetic resonance imaging. *Ultrasound Q.* 2007;23:211–223, with permission of Wolters Kluwer Health.)

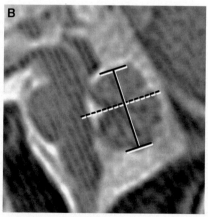

**A**

**B**

| Table 12.3-2 | Predicted Cerebellar Vermian Craniocaudal Diameter by MRI |
|---|---|
| **Gestational Age (wk)** | **Mean Diameter (mm)** |
| 14 | 4.6 |
| 15 | 5.3 |
| 16 | 6.1 |
| 17 | 6.8 |
| 18 | 7.5 |
| 19 | 8.3 |
| 20 | 9.0 |
| 21 | 9.7 |
| 22 | 10.4 |
| 23 | 11.2 |
| 24 | 11.9 |
| 25 | 12.6 |
| 26 | 13.4 |
| 27 | 14.1 |
| 28 | 14.8 |
| 29 | 15.6 |
| 30 | 16.3 |
| 31 | 17.0 |
| 32 | 17.7 |
| 33 | 18.5 |
| 34 | 19.2 |
| 35 | 19.9 |
| 36 | 20.7 |
| 37 | 21.4 |
| 38 | 22.1 |
| 39 | 22.9 |
| 40 | 23.6 |

Reproduced from Robinson AJ, Blaser S, Toi A, et al. The fetal cerebellar vermis: assessment for abnormal development by ultrasonography and magnetic resonance imaging. *Ultrasound Q.* 2007;23:211–223, permission of Wolters Kluwer Health.

fastigial point should increase linearly, with average percentages above and below 47% and 53%, respectively, and no significant change in this ratio with gestational age.[59,62]

*The tegmento-vermian angle* The tegmento-vermian angle is a way of measuring "closure" of the fourth ventricle.[59,62] This angle is measured by drawing a line along the dorsal surface of the brainstem parallel to the tegmentum, which should transect the nucleus gracilis at the obex. A second line is drawn along the ventral surface of the vermis. The angle between them is the tegmento-vermian angle (Fig. 12.3-15A). The normal fetal tegmento-vermian angle is usually <18°, and a significantly elevated tegmento-vermian angle (>45° approximately) is typically associated with classic Dandy-Walker.[69,70] Angles in between are less clearly pathologic, and the main differential is between Blake pouch cyst (normal vermis) and inferior vermian hypoplasia (Fig. 12.3-15B).

Utilizing these important measurements and landmarks, diagnosis of vermian and fourth ventricle anomalies can be obtained (Figs. 12.3-16 to 12.3-18).

**Differential Diagnosis:** Other causes of a cystic appearance of the posterior fossa are often confused with the more severe entities within DWC, particularly on axial sonographic images. Such appearances can be seen with persistent Blake pouch and mega cisterna magna (*vide supra*).[18] The latter can have normal outcomes; therefore, differentiation from true vermian pathology is imperative. Unfortunately, it is likely in the literature that owing to the subtleties of distinguishing between Blake pouch cyst and a true inferior vermian hypoplasia, these two groups of patients have been included together.

One suggested useful landmark is that if the choroid plexus is in its normal position on the inferior surface of the vermis, then this is compatible with Blake pouch cyst because it indicates that the anterior membranous area formed normally, whereas if the choroid plexus is on the inferior margin of the cyst, then it indicates that the anterior membranous area formed abnormally,[21,39] and thus warrants further evaluation of the vermis.

Another suggested way of distinguishing between inferior vermian hypoplasia and persistent Blake pouch is the overall morphology of the fourth ventricle and Blake pouch. In true cerebellovermian pathology, the posterior fossa "cyst" appears either oval or trapezoidal with the walls of Blake pouch apposed to and indistinguishable from the walls of the posterior fossa on axial views, whereas in persistent Blake pouch more of a keyhole (trefoil) shape is seen where the walls of the pouch may still be visible[22] (see Figs. 12.3-11, 12.3-16 to 12.3-18).

Other causes of severe pontocerebellar hypoplasia include the congenital muscular dystrophies and similar-appearing abnormalities such as microlissencephaly with pontocerebellar hypoplasia (Fig. 12.3-19). In these conditions, the brainstem typically retains its primitive dorsal pontine flexure seen in early embryogenesis, and may have a Z-shape,[71] and in the congenital muscular dystrophies there may be additional structural eye and CNS abnormalities, typically cobblestone lissencephaly

| Table 12.3-3 | Cerebello-Vermian Biometry by MRI | | | | | | | | | | | | |
|---|---|---|---|---|---|---|---|---|---|---|---|---|---|
| | **Gestational Age (wk)** | | | | | | | | | | | | |
| | **19** | **20** | **21** | **22** | **23** | **24** | **25** | **27/28** | **29/30** | **31/32** | **33** | **34/35** | **36/37** |
| Transverse diameter of both cerebellar hemispheres (mm) | 17 | 19.5 | 21.5 | 21.5 | 24 | 25 | 25 | 31.5 | 37 | 39 | 40 | 48.5 | 47.5 |
| Anteroposterior diameter of the vermis (mm) | 6 | 6.5 | 7 | 7 | 8 | 8 | 9.5 | 11.5 | 12.5 | 13 | 13 | 14.5 | 18.5 |
| Height of the vermis (mm) | 7.5 | 8.5 | 10 | 11 | 11 | 11 | 11.5 | 15.5 | 17 | 19 | 21 | 24 | 24 |

Reproduced from Triulzi F, Parazzini C, Righini A. MRI of fetal and neonatal cerebellar development. *Semin Fetal Neonatal Med.* 2005;10:411–420, with permission.

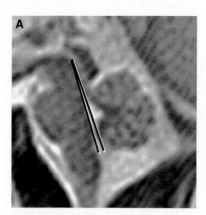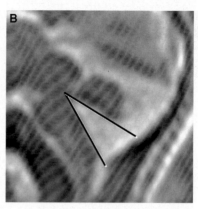

**FIGURE 12.3-15:** Construction of lines used to assess the tegmento-vermian angle (may also be done by ultrasound). **A:** Normal tegmento-vermian angle. **B:** Abnormal tegmento-vermian angle. (From Robinson AJ, Blaser S, Toi A, et al. The fetal cerebellar vermis: assessment for abnormal development by ultrasonography and magnetic resonance imaging. *Ultrasound Q.* 2007;23:211–223, with permission of Wolters Kluwer Health.)

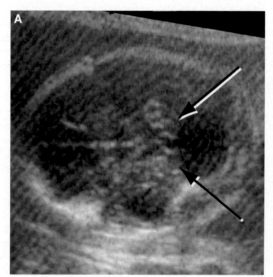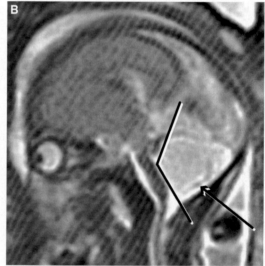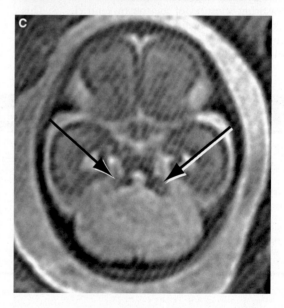

**FIGURE 12.3-16:** Cerebellar Anomaly with Abnormal Tegmento-vermian angle **A:** In this 22-week fetus, a large cystic posterior fossa is seen on axial sonography with small cerebellar hemispheres on either side of the midline *(arrows)*. No midline vermian tissue is identified. **B:** On sagittal MR, the tegmento-vermian angle is increased *(lines)* with the fourth ventricle uncovered *(arrow)*. The vermis is very small; there is no primary fissure or fastigial point, again in keeping with a primitive configuration. **C:** On axial MR, the cerebellar hemispheres are small *(arrows)*. The ventricular system is dilated, resulting in large temporal horns. (From Robinson AJ, Blaser S, Toi A, et al. The fetal cerebellar vermis: assessment for abnormal development by ultrasonography and magnetic resonance imaging. *Ultrasound Q.* 2007;23:211–223, with permission of Wolters Kluwer Health.)

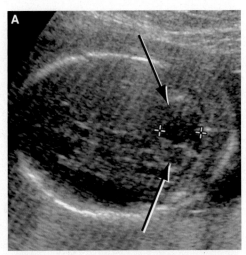
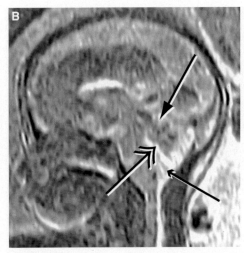

**FIGURE 12.3-17:** Vermian Anomaly/Dandy Walker Continuum **A:** In this 21-week fetus, there is a trapezoid shape to Blake pouch, and the cerebellar hemispheres *(arrows)* are larger than in the prior case. **B:** By fetal MRI, the tegmento-vermian angle is increased. The fastigial point is visible, and vermian lobulation is seen. Again, this would fall into the Dandy-Walker continuum, but this fetus had other facial, visceral, and skeletal anomalies. The autopsy diagnosis was Wolf–Hirschhorn syndrome, characterized by multiple congenital anomalies, including midline fusion defects, associated with a chromosomal deletion of the short arm of chromosome 4.[125] Thus even though the cerebellar hemispheres are larger and vermian morphology is better than in the prior case, the presence of associated abnormalities gives a worse prognosis. (From Robinson AJ, Blaser S, Toi A, et al. The fetal cerebellar vermis: assessment for abnormal development by ultrasonography and magnetic resonance imaging. *Ultrasound Q.* 2007;23:211–223, with permission of Wolters Kluwer Health.)

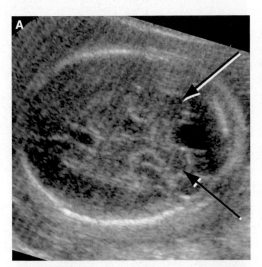
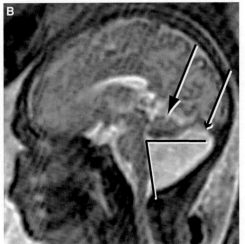

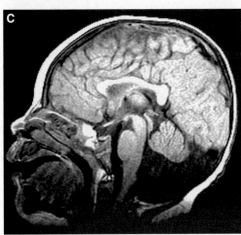

**FIGURE 12.3-18:** Vermian Hypoplasia **A:** In this fetus, at 34 weeks by axial sonography, the cerebellar hemispheres are approaching normal size *(arrows)*, and proportionally more midline vermian tissue is seen than in Figures 12.3-16 and 12.3-17. **B:** On sagittal MR, the tegmento-vermian angle is increased *(lines)*, with elevation of the torcula *(small arrow)*. The vermis is less hypoplastic than in the previous examples, and the primary fissure is seen *(single arrow)*. The fastigial point is less flattened. **C:** Postnatal MR at 8 months of age shows good vermian lobulation. (From Robinson AJ, Blaser S, Toi A, et al. The fetal cerebellar vermis: assessment for abnormal development by ultrasonography and magnetic resonance imaging. *Ultrasound Q.* 2007;23:211–223, with permission of Wolters Kluwer Health.)

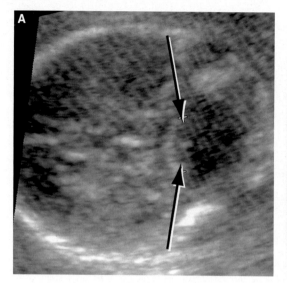

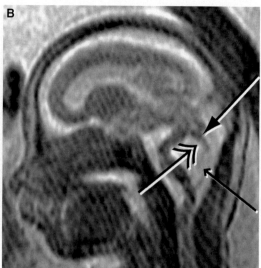

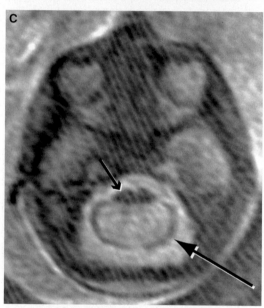

**FIGURE 12.3-19:** Severe Pontocerebellar Hypoplasia **A:** In this fetus at 20 weeks' gestation, the axial sonogram shows a large posterior fossa cystic space and two tiny cerebellar hemispheres either side of the midline *(arrows)*. Biometric measurements were abnormally small. **B:** On sagittal MR, we see that the vermis is incomplete, and there is no fastigial point *(double arrow)* or primary fissure *(single arrow)*. The fourth ventricle is uncovered *(small arrow)*. There is a thin cerebral cortex with a prominent subarachnoid space, and the brainstem has a primitive "Z-shaped" configuration owing to a retained embryonic dorsal pontine flexure. There is complete agenesis of the corpus callosum that cannot be seen at all on this midline section. **C:** On axial MR, there are shell-like cerebellar hemispheres *(arrow)* and a hypoplastic brainstem *(small arrow)*. (From Robinson AJ, Blaser S, Toi A, et al. The fetal cerebellar vermis: assessment for abnormal development by ultrasonography and magnetic resonance imaging. *Ultrasound Q.* 2007;23: 211–223, with permission of Wolters Kluwer Health.)

and microphthalmia.[72] It is difficult to differentiate microlissencephaly from congenital muscular dystrophy prenatally without genetic studies; however, in the latter, one would expect a normal head size and other features such as asymmetric orbits and ventricular dilatation. In either case, the outcome is dismal. Vermian hypoplasia can also be associated with an occipital cephalocele (Fig. 12.3-20) and also dorsal traction of the brainstem in tectocerebellar dysraphia.[73]

**Prognosis:** Specifically, out of the three original morphologic criteria for DWM (vermian dysgenesis, cystic dilatation of the fourth ventricle with enlargement of the posterior fossa, elevation of the transverse sinus, tentorium, and torcula),[46] only vermian and regional cerebellar morphology has so far been demonstrated to correlate with prognosis.[37,74,75] Hydrocephalus is seen in 80% and, although also correlating with prognosis, was not part of the original criteria, and other associated abnormalities (see below) also have a much more significant prognostic value.

Dandy-Walker continuum is often associated with an abnormal karyotype in 29%,[9,10] CNS abnormalities in 50% to 70%, including ventriculomegaly, brainstem dysgenesis, callosal dysgenesis, migrational disorders, encephaloceles, neural tube defects[48,53,76–80] and in 47% with concurrent non-CNS anomalies,[9] including heart defects,[48,53,78,81] polydactyly and syndactyly,[48,78,82] and facial anomalies.[53,78] Dandy-Walker continuum with additional findings, especially brainstem dysgenesis, has an associated poorer outcome.[20,83] Seizures, hearing or visual difficulties, systemic abnormalities, and other CNS abnormalities are associated with poor intellectual development; the presence of two of these four risk factors identifies patients with borderline or lower intelligence 94% of the time.[84]

The term "isolated inferior vermian hypoplasia" has been used to describe that subset in which there are no known underlying or associated abnormalities,[38,85,86] and this group generally has a better outcome.[87–92] However, it can often be impossible to tell prenatally whether vermian hypoplasia is isolated since associated abnormalities, for example, genetic or chromosomal, may be undetectable.[93] In one study, 50% of Dandy-Walker and inferior vermian hypoplasia patients were abnormal even if the

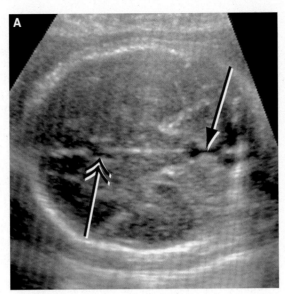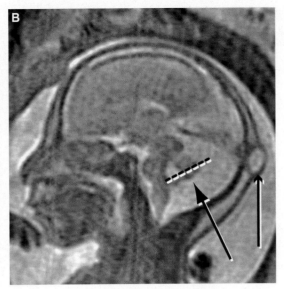

**FIGURE 12.3-20:** Vermian Hypoplasia and Occipital Cephalocele **A:** In this 25-week fetus, the axial sonogram demonstrates a defect in the vermis with a communication between the fourth ventricle and the cisterna magna *(arrow)*. Notice that the *cavum septi pellucidi* is included in this axial plane *(double arrow)*, thereby suggesting that this finding is not an artifact that is caused by imaging the posterior fossa in too coronal a plane. **B:** On sagittal MR, the tegmento-vermian angle is normal (fourth ventricle is closed); the vermis is small overall, especially inferiorly *(arrow)*. Dotted line represents fastigial point-declive line. The cisterna magna appears large because of an ex-vacuo effect. Note an occipital cephalocele *(small arrow)*. (From Robinson AJ, Blaser S, Toi A, et al. The fetal cerebellar vermis: assessment for abnormal development by ultrasonography and magnetic resonance imaging. *Ultrasound Q.* 2007;23:211–223, with permission of Wolters Kluwer Health.)

abnormality appeared to be isolated.[25] In another study, postnatal imaging and follow-up was normal in 6 out of 19 cases of isolated inferior vermian hypoplasia, and those 13 with postnatal confirmation had good overall outcome with only mild developmental delays in a subset of infants.[38]

**Recurrence Risk:** Because of the autosomal recessive nature of many of the causes of vermian hypoplasia, there is a 25% recurrence risk (Table 12.3-4).

## Rhombencephalosynapsis

Rhombencephalosynapsis is a disorder in which the vermis is severely deficient and the cerebellar hemispheric folia are continuous across the midline (Fig. 12.3-21). The nomenclature does nothing to improve the understanding of the condition or cerebellar development in general. The etymology of "synapsis" is from Greek, meaning "fusion." Consequently, the description of the abnormalities seen in this condition includes "fusion" of the fastigial nuclei, "apposition" of deep cerebellar nuclei, "fusion" of the middle cerebellar peduncles, and folia "fused" across the midline. For this reason, it would probably be more accurate to rename rhombencephalosynapsis as holo*rhomb*encephaly, although "holo*pros*encephaly of the hindbrain" has also been suggested.[85] The frequent association of holo*pros*encephaly with rhombencephalosynapsis then becomes conceptually more logical.

In contradistinction to Dandy-Walker continuum, it is the anterior vermis that is usually absent, with the posterior vermis demonstrating variable deficiency, and, interestingly, the most inferior lobule, the nodulus, is typically preserved.[94]

**Incidence:** The incidence is rare.

**Embryology and Genetics:** The cerebellar primordium is a single but bilobed structure that is continuous across the midline, and the vermis grows from proliferation of the cerebellar primordium, not through fusion of the cerebellar hemispheres. The fact that in rhombencephalosynapsis the posterior vermis and most inferior lobule can sometimes be present in the absence of the anterior vermis[95] demonstrates that the posterior part of the vermis develops independently from its own primordium, and not as a result of craniocaudal growth of a single midline primordium. This concept is backed up from experimental evidence, which shows that granule cells arising from the lateral upper rhombic lip migrate medially into the posterior cerebellum, whereas granule cells arising in the median upper rhombic lip are confined to an anterior cerebellar distribution.[96]

Rhombencephalosynapsis has been seen together with VACTERL-H association (vertebral, anorectal, cardiac, tracheo-esophageal fistula, renal, limb, hydrocephalus), with Gomez-Lopez-Hernandez syndrome[97–100] (trigeminal anesthesia, bilateral temporal alopecia, short stature, mental retardation, midface hypoplasia, oxycephaly secondary to bilateral lambdoid suture synostosis, low set ears, fifth finger clinodactyly), and with polycystic kidney disease.[101]

**Etiology and Pathogenesis:** Unknown, however, the association with holoprosencephaly is suggestive of defective dorsoventral patterning.[102]

**Diagnosis:** The key feature is that of the cerebellar folia crossing the midline from one cerebellar hemisphere to the other with no intervening vermis.[103] The normal dumbbell shape of the cerebellum on axial views is not present because the central

| Table 12.3-4 | Associations with Cerebellar Hypoplasia | |
|---|---|---|
| **Etiology** | **Disorder** | |
| Chromosomal | 45,X | |
| | Trisomies 18, 13, 21, and 9 | |
| | Triploidy | |
| | Unbalanced translocation | |
| | Subtelomeric deletion | |
| Genetic | | |
| Congenital muscular dystrophies | Walker–Warburg | |
| | Muscle-eye brain | |
| | Fukuyama | |
| Ciliopathies (AR) | | |
| Confirmed | Joubert syndrome | |
| | Meckel–Gruber | |
| | COACH | |
| | CORS | |
| | Arima (cerebro-oculo-hepato-renal) | |
| | Oral facial digital syndrome | |
| | Senior Loken | |
| | Bardet–Biedl | |
| | Leber congenital amaurosis | |
| | Cogan-type congenital oculomotor apraxia | |
| | Nephronophthisis | |
| | Jeune asphyxiating thoracic dystrophy | |
| | Ellis van Creveld | |
| Suspected | Neural tube defects | |
| | Polysyndactyly | |
| | Callosal dysgenesis | |
| | Congenital heart disease | |
| Metabolic | Congenital disorders of glycosylation | |
| | Mitochondrial disorders | |
| | Infantile neuroaxonal dystrophy | |
| Other | Aase-Smith arthrogryposis (AD) | |
| | Ruvalcaba syndrome (AR) | |
| | Aicardi syndrome (X-linked & XXY males) | |
| | Fraser cryptophthalmos (AR) | |
| | Opitz | |
| | PHACE (associated with facial hemangioma) | |
| | Klippel-Feil | |
| | Cornelia de Lange | |
| Teratogenic | Diabetes | |
| | Alcohol | |
| | Coumadin | |
| | Isotretinoin | |
| Infectious | CMV | |
| | Rubella | |
| Hemorrhagic | Intraventricular hemorrhage | |
| | Cerebellar hemorrhage | |
| Syndromic | Goldenhar | |
| | Holoprosencephaly | |
| Unknown | Cleft lip/palate | |
| | polymicrogyria | |
| | Gray matter heterotopias | |

Reproduced from Robinson AJ. Inferior vermian hypoplasia: preconception, misconception. *Ultrasound Obstet Gynecol.* 2014;43:123–136, with permission.

"stem" of the dumbbell that represents the vermis is missing. There may be dorsal pointing of the fourth ventricle.

On midline sagittal views, the normal vermian landmarks cannot be seen. The craniocaudal diameter in the midline is larger than expected, because the normal vermis, which is absent in this condition, always has a smaller craniocaudal diameter than the adjacent cerebellar hemispheres (see Fig. 12.3-21).

Other midline structures may also be deficient, including the cavum septi pellucidi, corpus callosum, aqueduct of Sylvius leading to hydrocephalus, optic nerves, chiasm, tracts, posterior pituitary, quadrigeminal plate, or features of holoprosencephaly.[104]

**Differential Diagnosis:** Other forms of vermian hyoplasia are in the differential, although the continuous cerebellar folia without intervening vermis are a pathognomonic feature.

**Prognosis:** A wide range of clinical features have been reported,[105] and presentation correlates with the presence and degree of supratentorial abnormalities, most commonly in the spectrum of holoprosencephaly.

Clinical presentation after birth ranges from mild truncal ataxia and normal cognition to severe cerebral palsy with epilepsy and mental retardation. Most patients have some degree of cognitive dysfunction, often associated with attention deficit and hyperactivity. Motor milestones are often delayed.[102,106,107]

**Management:** Thorough evaluation for coexistent anomalies is necessary as these severely impact prognosis. Presence of more severe forms of holoprosencephaly is incompatible with life.

**Recurrence Risk:** All cases are sporadic.

## Joubert Syndrome and Related Disorders (Molar Tooth Malformations)

It has recently been shown that this brainstem and cerebellar malformation is seen with many associated anomalies that encompass many syndromes, and these are collectively known as Joubert syndrome and related disorders (JSRD).[108–110] These disorders are unified by a common abnormality of ciliary function that in general are characterized by a combination of ocular, cerebral, hepatic, renal, and skeletal manifestations.

The classification of JSRD has recently been revised and divided into four distinct disorders[111]: Joubert syndrome, COACH (Cerebellar vermis hypoplasia, Oligophrenia, Ataxia, Ocular Coloboma, Hepatic fibrosis) syndrome, CORS (cerebro-oculo-renal syndrome), and oculo-facial-digital syndrome type VI (OFD-VI syndrome).

**Incidence:** Initially thought to be rare, but as our understanding expands around this group of conditions, it is apparent that many previously unclassified forms of vermian hypoplasia fall into the category of ciliopathies.

**Embryology and Genetics:** Most of the related syndromes seem to be the result of mutations to genes encoding ciliary proteins, which are important in a wide range of functions, including ciliogenesis, body axis formation, renal function, brain development, and ocular development.[112–115]

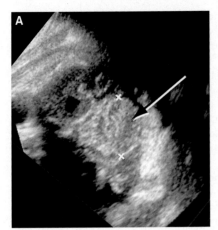
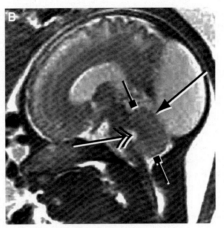
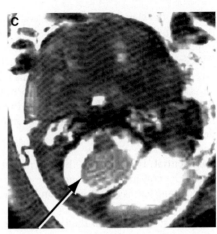

**FIGURE 12.3-21:** Rhomboencephalosynapsis **A:** In this fetus case at 30 weeks' gestation, sonography showed several abnormalities, including schizencephaly and polymicrogyria. Axial sonography demonstrates an abnormal cerebellum with transverse folia that are seen to be continuous between the hemispheres across the midline *(arrow)*. The transcerebellar diameter was 3.02 cm, which would be normal for 26 weeks' gestational age. **B:** On sagittal MR, the fastigial point is rounded off *(double arrow)* rather than triangular. There is no primary fissure *(single arrow)*. The craniocaudal diameter *(square callipers)* of the "vermis" is much larger than expected, because it is actually the "fused" cerebellar hemispheres that are being measured (see below for vermian craniocaudal diameter measurement). This could lead to false reassurance that the vermis is present. A large left-sided CSF collection is also present and included on the slightly off-axis sagittal image. **C:** On axial MR views, the cerebellar folia are again seen to be continuous across the midline *(arrow)*. (Courtesy of A. Michelle Fink, Department of Medical Imaging, Royal Children's Hospital, Melbourne, Australia; from Robinson AJ, Blaser S, Toi A, et al. The fetal cerebellar vermis: assessment for abnormal development by ultrasonography and magnetic resonance imaging. *Ultrasound Q.* 2007;23:211–223, with permission of Wolters Kluwer Health.)

**Etiology and Pathogenesis:** It is at present unknown how the defective ciliary proteins have such wide-ranging effects, but they are known to play a role in normal cellular function in many cell types and are necessary for perceptory input such as sight, hearing, and smell.

**Diagnosis:** The classic finding is that of a "molar tooth" configuration of the mesencephalon, which can be demonstrated both sonographically[116] and by MRI.[15,117–120] This feature is seen on axial sections and is caused by thickened superior cerebellar peduncles (representing the roots of the molar tooth) and a deep interpeduncular cistern owing to the absence of decussation of the superior cerebellar peduncles.[121] The fourth ventricle has a bat-wing configuration and has a midline point posteriorly where the two cerebellar hemispheres touch each other in the midline. The vermis is abnormally lobulated (Fig. 12.3-22).

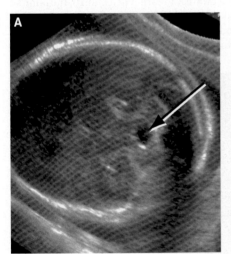
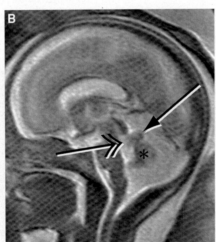
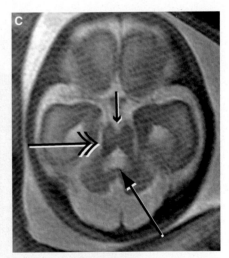

**FIGURE 12.3-22:** Molar Tooth Malformation **A:** In this fetus at 20 weeks' gestation, axial sonography shows an enlarged cisterna magna measuring 15 mm in the standard AP direction. There is an abnormally shaped fourth ventricle *(arrow)*, which is rounded rather than the normal diamond shape. Some apparent tissue is seen to separate the fourth ventricle and cisterna magna, but this is actually the two cerebellar hemispheres touching in the midline. This has been referred to as the "buttocks" sign. **B:** On sagittal MR, we see a small amount of midline tissue between the cerebellar hemispheres consistent with vermian tissue. On this view, most of what looks to be midline tissue is actually partial volume averaging of adjacent cerebellar hemispheres *(asterisk)*. The vermis is only the superior part, and there is no fastigial point *(double arrow)* or primary fissure *(single arrow)*. The roof of the fourth ventricle appears squared-off. **C:** On the axial MR, there is a "molar tooth" shape to the brainstem because of thickened horizontally oriented superior cerebellar peduncles *(double arrow)* and a deep interpeduncular cistern *(small arrow)* secondary to nondecussation, and the fourth ventricle has an abnormal "batwing" shape *(large arrrow)*. (**A**, courtesy of Dr. Phyllis Glanc, Department of Medical Imaging, Women's College Hospital, Toronto, Canada. **A–C**, from Robinson AJ, Blaser S, Toi A, et al. The fetal cerebellar vermis: assessment for abnormal development by ultrasonography and magnetic resonance imaging. *Ultrasound Q.* 2007;23:211–223, with permission of Wolters Kluwer Health.)

On sagittal views, the vermis is elevated, and the anterior lobe is generally the most hypoplastic. The fourth ventricle has a trapezoidal configuration. Often, partial volume effect from the adjacent cerebellar hemispheres that touch in the midline can give the false impression that the vermis is larger.

Associated retinopathy, hepatic fibrosis, renal cysts, polydactyly, facial clefting, hamartomas of the tuber cinereum, and tongue tumours[122] can help with the diagnosis; these may not be detectable antenatally.

**Differential Diagnosis:** Other forms of vermian hyoplasia should be considered, although the molar tooth configuration of the brainstem is a pathognomonic feature.

**Prognosis:** Patients with the JSRD syndromes have hypotonia, ataxia, developmental delay (cognitive and motor), oculomotor apraxia, and the "molar tooth sign." Other features include episodic neonatal hyperpnea and rhythmic tongue protrusion, mental retardation, postaxial polydactyly, mild retinopathy, and polymicrogyria.[123]

**Management:** Genetic counseling is recommended. Infants and children with abnormal breathing may require stimulatory medications (e.g., caffeine); supplemental oxygen; mechanical support; or tracheostomy in rare cases. Other interventions may include speech therapy for oromotor dysfunction; occupational and physical therapy; educational support, including special programs for the visually impaired; and feedings by gastrostomy tube. Surgery may be required for polydactyly and symptomatic ptosis and/or strabismus. Nephronophthisis, end-stage renal disease, liver failure, and/or fibrosis are treated with standard approaches.[124]

**Recurrence Risk:** Joubert is transmitted autosomal recessive, so the recurrence risk is 25%.

## Pontocerebellar Hypoplasia

**Incidence:** Pontocerebellar hypoplasia (PCH) is very rare.[126]

**Embryology and Genetics:** PCH is a neurodegenerative process with early prenatal onset.[127] Changes typical of PCH include volume loss in the ventral pons and cerebellum and to a lesser extent cerebral cortex.[126] During gestation, especially third trimester and postnatal, there is progressive degeneration of the cerebellar cortex with loss of Purkinje cells, fragmentation of the dentate nuclei and often neuronal loss and degeneration of the inferior olivary nucleus.[126] Cerebellar hemispheres are typically more severely affected than vermis. In the pons, there is progressive loss of ventral nuclei and transverse fibers.[126]

**Etiology and Pathogenesis:** Previously two classical types of pontocerebellar hypoplasia were described: type 1 in which cases had accompanying spinal anterior horn disease with prenatal onset of contractures and polyhydramnios and type 2 with chorea and dyskinesia. Currently there are at least 7 subtypes described.[126] Most cases are inherited autosomal recessive. PCH3 has been linked to chromosome 7q11. However, PCH2, PCH4, and PCH5 have been linked to the *TSEN* gene and PCH6 to *RARS2* gene. Mutations of *TSEN*, *RARS2* and *VRK1* have been described in PCH1. PCH2 is the most common type, and the most encountered gene mutation is *TSEN54*.[128] These three genes are essential for general protein synthesis and both *TSEN* and *RARS2* for RNA transfer which are vital for maturing neurons.[126,128]

**Diagnosis:** Molecular genetic testing for known mutations in PCH may confirm diagnosis in the presence of positive family history. Prenatal diagnosis via US is often not possible in the first and second trimester as findings of volume loss manifested by decreased transverse cerebellar diameter are detected primarily in the third trimester, usually after 30 weeks gestation.[127,129] Head circumference is typically normal prenatal since microcephaly tends to develop after birth.[129] Concern for PCH may be raised by intrauterine contractures, seizures or development of polyhydramnios.

Fetal MRI may hold promise in earlier detection of the pontine and cerebellar volume loss as the technique allows excellent definition of brainstem hypoplasia and cerebellar pathology.[130] In addition, diffusion tensor imaging may be able to demonstrate

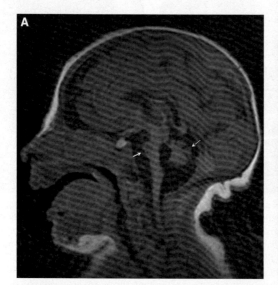
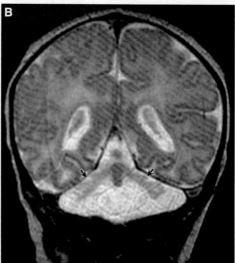

**FIGURE 12.3-23:** 5 day old with Pontocerebellar Hypoplasia Type 2 and TSEN54 mutation. **A:** Sagittal T1 image demonstrates small pons *(arrow)* and volume loss in the cerebellar vermis *(dotted arrow)*. **B:** Coronal T2 image demonstrates small bilateral cerebellar hemisphere *(arrows)*, appearing like a dragonfly.

absent crossing fibers at the level of the pons.[127] On postnatal MRI, the most common findings described in PCH are flat and severely reduced cerebellar hemispheres (dragonfly appearing) and small pons (Fig. 12.3-23).[128]

**Differential Diagnosis:** Brainstem abnormalities are often seen in conjunction with cerebellar hypoplasia and dysplasia as the germinal matrix in the rhombic lips are responsible for the formation of the ventral pons.[131] Other disorders seen with cerebellar and brainstem anomalies include the congenital muscular dystrophies, most notably Walker Warburg syndrome.

**Prognosis:** In all cases of PCH, children experience severe intellectual deficit, global developmental delay, swallowing problems, and seizures.[126] Most patients with PCH die during infancy or childhood due to primary respiratory insufficiency.[126,128]

**Management:** Termination of pregnancy may be considered if diagnosis can be confirmed. Management is primarily supportive after birth with nutrition obtained via gastrostomy tube.

**Recurrence Risk:** Most cases are transmitted autosomal recessive with 25% risk for recurrence.

## ACKNOWLEDGMENTS

Portions of the text are reproduced from the following previous publications by the author:

Robinson AJ, Blaser S, Toi A, et al. The fetal cerebellar vermis: assessment for abnormal development by ultrasonography and magnetic resonance imaging. *Ultrasound Q.* 2007;23:211–223, with permission from Wolters Kluwer Health.

Robinson AJ, Goldstein R. The cisterna magna septa: vestigial remnants of Blake's pouch and a potential new marker for normal development of the rhombencephalon. *J Ultrasound Med.* 2007;26:83–95, with permission from the American Institute of Ultrasound in Medicine.

Robinson AJ. Inferior vermian hypoplasia: preconception, misconception. *Ultrasound Obstet Gynecol.* 2014;43:123–136, with permission from John Wiley and Sons Ltd.

## REFERENCES

1. *AIUM Practice Guideline for the Performance of an Antepartum Obstetric Ultrasound Examination.* American Institute of Ultrasound in Medicine; 2003. http://www.aium.org/publications/clinical/obstetrical.pdf.
2. *SOGC Clinical Practice Guidelines. Antenatal Fetal Assessment.* Society of Obstetricians and Gynaecologists of Canada. No 90; June 2000. http://www.sogc.org/guidelines/pdf/ps90.pdf.
3. *CAR Standards for Performing and Interpreting Diagnostic Antepartum Obstetric Ultrasound Examination.* Canadian Association of Radiologists; September 2001. http://www.car.ca/ethics/standards/antepartum.htm.
4. Filly RA, Cardoza JD, Goldstein RB, et al. Detection of fetal central nervous system anomalies: a practical level of effort for a routine sonogram. *Radiology.* 1989;172:403–408.
5. Visentin A, Pilu G, Falco P, et al. The transfrontal view: a new approach to the visualization of the fetal midline cerebral structures. *J Ultrasound Med.* 2001;20:329–333.
6. Zalel Y, Seidman DS, Brand N, et al. The development of the fetal vermis: an in-vivo sonographic evaluation. *Ultrasound Obstet Gynecol.* 2002;19:136–139.
7. Achiron R, Kivilevitch Z, Lipitz S, et al. Development of the human fetal pons: in utero ultrasonographic study. *Ultrasound Obstet Gynecol.* 2004;24:506–510.
8. Malinger G, Ginath S, Lerman-Sagie T, et al. The fetal cerebellar vermis: normal development as shown by transvaginal ultrasound. *Prenat Diagn.* 2001;21:687–692.
9. Estroff JA, Scott MR, Benacerraf BR. Dandy-Walker variant: prenatal sonographic features and clinical outcome. *Radiology.* 1992;185:755–758.
10. Chang MC, Russell SA, Callen PW, et al. Sonographic detection of inferior vermian agenesis in Dandy-Walker malformations: prognostic implications. *Radiology.* 1994;193:765–770.
11. Carroll SG, Porter H, Abdel-Fattah S, et al. Correlation of prenatal ultrasound diagnosis and pathologic findings in fetal brain abnormalities. *Ultrasound Obstet Gynecol.* 2000;16:149–153.
12. Laing FC, Frates MC, Brown DL, et al. Sonography of the fetal posterior fossa: false appearance of mega-cisterna magna and Dandy-Walker variant. *Radiology.* 1994;192:247–251.
13. Blake JA. The roof and lateral recesses of the fourth ventricle considered morphologically and embryologically. *J Comp Neurol.* 1900;10:79–108.
14. Ben-Amin M, Perlitz Y, Peleg D. Transvaginal sonographic appearance of the cerebellar vermis at 14–16 weeks' gestation. *Ultrasound Obstet Gynecol.* 2002;19:208–209.
15. Robinson AJ, Blaser S, Toi A, et al. The fetal cerebellar vermis: assessment for abnormal development by ultrasonography and magnetic resonance imaging. *Ultrasound Q.* 2007;23:211–223.
16. Bromley B, Nadel AS, Pauker S, et al. Closure of the cerebellar vermis: evaluation with second trimester US. *Radiology.* 1994;193:761–763.
17. Strand RD, Barnes PD, Poussaint TY, et al. Cystic retrocerebellar malformations: unification of the Dandy-Walker complex and the Blake's pouch. *Pediatr Radiol.* 1993;23:258–260.
18. Robinson AJ, Goldstein R. The cisterna magna septa: vestigial remnants of Blake's pouch and a potential new marker for normal development of the rhombencephalon. *J Ultrasound Med.* 2007;26:83–95.
19. Knutzon RK, McGahan JP, Salamat MS, et al. Fetal cisterna magna septa: a normal anatomic finding. *Radiology.* 1991;180:799–801.
20. Raybaud C. Cystic malformations of the posterior fossa: abnormalities associated with the development of the roof of the fourth ventricle and adjacent meningeal structures. *J Neuroradiol.* 1982;9:103–133.
21. Tortori-Donati P, Fondelli MP, Rossi A, et al. Cystic malformations of the posterior cranial fossa originating from a defect of the posterior membranous area. Mega cisterna magna and persisting Blake's pouch: two separate entities. *Childs Nerv Syst.* 1996;12:303–308.
22. Phillips JJ, Mahony BS, Siebert JR, et al. Dandy-Walker malformation complex: correlation between ultrasonographic diagnosis and postmortem neuropathology. *Obstet Gynecol.* 2006;107:685–693.
23. Oh KY, Rassner UA, Frias AE Jr, et al. The fetal posterior fossa: clinical correlation of findings on prenatal ultrasound and fetal magnetic resonance imaging. *Ultrasound Q.* 2007;23:203–210.
24. Pretorius DH, Kallman CE, Grafe MR, et al. Linear echoes in the fetal cisterna magna. *J Ultrasound Med.* 1992;11:125–128.
25. Gandolfi Colleoni G, Contro E, Carletti A, et al. Prenatal diagnosis and outcome of fetal posterior fossa fluid collections. *Ultrasound Obstet Gynecol.* 2012;39:625–631.
26. Arai H, Sato K. Posterior fossa cysts: clinical, neuroradiological and surgical features. *Childs Nerv Syst.* 1991;7:156–164.
27. Calabro F, Arcuri T, Jinkins JR. Blake's pouch: an entity within the Dandy-Walker continuum. *Neuroradiology.* 2000;42:290–295.
28. Cornips EM, Overvliet GM, Weber JW, et al. The clinical spectrum of Blake's pouch cyst: report of six illustrative cases. *Childs Nerv Syst.* 2010;26:1057–1064.
29. ten Donkelaar HJ, Lammens M, Wesseling P, et al. Development and developmental disorders of the human cerebellum. *J Neurol.* 2003;250:1025–1036.
30. Paladini D, Quarantelli M, Pastore G, et al. Abnormal or delayed development of the posterior membranous area of the brain: anatomy, ultrasound diagnosis, natural history and outcome of Blake's pouch cyst in the fetus. *Ultrasound Obstet Gynecol.* 2012;39:279–287.
31. Brocklehurst G. The development of the human cerebrospinal fluid pathway with particular reference to the roof of the fourth ventricle. *J Anat.* 1969;105:467–475.
32. Malinger G, Lev D, Zahalka N, et al. Fetal cytomegalovirus infection of the brain: the spectrum of sonographic findings. *AJNR Am J Neuroradiol.* 2003;24:28–32.
33. Dogan Y, Yuksel A, Kalelioglu IH, et al. Intracranial ultrasound abnormalities and fetal cytomegalovirus infection: report of 8 cases and review of the literature. *Fetal Diagn Ther.* 2011;30:141–149.
34. Tam EW, Ferriero DM, Xu D, et al. Cerebellar development in the preterm neonate: effect of supratentorial brain injury. *Pediatr Res.* 2009;66:102–106.
35. Volpe JJ. Neurobiology of periventricular leukomalacia in the premature infant. *Pediatr Res.* 2001;50:553–562.
36. Duncan JR, Cock ML, Scheerlinck JP, et al. White matter injury after repeated endotoxin exposure in the preterm ovine fetus. *Pediatr Res.* 2002;52:941–949.
37. Klein O, Pierre-Kahn A, Boddaert N, et al. Dandy-Walker malformation: prenatal diagnosis and prognosis. *Childs Nerv Syst.* 2003;19:484–489.
38. Limperopoulos C, Robertson RL, Estroff JA, et al. Diagnosis of inferior vermian hypoplasia by fetal magnetic resonance imaging: potential pitfalls and neurodevelopmental outcome. *Am J Obstet Gynecol.* 2006;194:1070–1076.
39. Nelson MD Jr, Maher K, Gilles FH. A different approach to cysts of the posterior fossa. *Pediatr Radiol.* 2004;34:720–732.
40. Zalel Y, Gilboa Y, Gabis L, et al. Rotation of the vermis as a cause of enlarged cisterna magna on prenatal imaging. *Ultrasound Obstet Gynecol.* 2006;27:490–493.
41. Triulzi F, Parazzini C, Righini A. Magnetic resonance imaging of fetal cerebellar development. *Cerebellum.* 2006;5:199–205.

42. Barkovich AJ, Kjos BO, Norman D, et al. Revised classification of posterior fossa cysts and cystlike malformations based on the results of multiplanar MR imaging. *AJR Am J Roentgenol.* 1989;153:1289–1300.

43. Zimmer EZ, Lowenstein L, Bronshtein M, et al. Clinical significance of isolated mega cisterna magna. *Arch Gynecol Obstet.* 2007;276:487–490.

44. Pierre-Kahn A, Sonigo P. Malformative intracranial cysts: diagnosis and outcome. *Childs Nerv Syst.* 2003;19:477–483.

45. Pierre-Kahn A, Hanlo P, Sonigo P, et al. The contribution of prenatal diagnosis to the understanding of malformative intracranial cysts: state of the art. *Childs Nerv Syst.* 2000;16:619–626.

46. Kollias SS, Ball WS Jr, Prenger EC. Cystic malformations of the posterior fossa: differential diagnosis clarified through embryologic analysis. *Radiographics.* 1993;13:1211–1231.

47. Bordarier C, Aicardi J. Dandy-Walker syndrome and agenesis of the cerebellar vermis: diagnostic problems and genetic counselling. *Dev Med Child Neurol.* 1990;32:285–294.

48. Hirsch JF, Pierre-Kahn A, Renier D, et al. The Dandy-Walker malformation: a review of 40 cases. *J Neurosurg.* 1984;61:515–522.

49. Barkovich AJ. *Pediatric Neuroimaging.* 3rd ed. Philadelphia, PA: Lippincott Williams & Wilkins; 2000:337–341.

50. Limperopoulos C, du Plessis AJ. Disorders of cerebellar growth and development. *Curr Opin Pediatr.* 2006;18:621–627.

51. Ko SF, Wang HS, Lui TN, et al. Neurocutaneous melanosis associated with inferior vermian hypoplasia: MR findings. *J Comput Assist Tomogr.* 1993;17:691–695.

52. Aynaci FM, Mocan H, Bahadir S, et al. A case of Menkes' syndrome associated with deafness and inferior cerebellar vermian hypoplasia. *Acta Paediatr.* 1997;86:121–123.

53. Murray JC, Johnson JA, Bird TD. Dandy-Walker malformation: etiologic heterogeneity and empiric recurrence risks. *Clin Genet.* 1985;28:272–283.

54. Dandy WE, Blackfan KD. Internal hydrocephalus: an experimental, clinical, and pathological study. *Am J Dis Child.* 1914;8:406–482.

55. Dandy WE. The diagnosis and treatment of hydrocephalus due to occlusion of the foramina of Magendie and Luschka. *Surg Gynecol Obstet.* 1921;32:112–124.

56. Taggart JK, Walker AE. Congenital atresias of the foramens of Luschka and Magendie. *Arch Neurol Psychiatr.* 1942;48:583–612.

57. Garel C. *MRI of the Fetal Brain: Normal Development and Cerebral Pathologies.* 2nd ed. Berlin, Germany: Springer-Verlag; 2004:30–31.

58. Adamsbaum C, Moutard ML, Andre C, et al. MR of the fetal posterior fossa. *Pediatr Radiol.* 2005;35:124–140.

59. Robinson AJ, Blaser S. In-utero MR imaging of developmental abnormalities of the fetal cerebellar vermis. In: Griffiths PD, Paley MNJ, Whitby EH, eds. *Imaging the Central Nervous System of the Fetus and Neonate.* New York, NY: Taylor & Francis; 2006.

60. Stazzone MM, Hubbard AM, Bilaniuk LT, et al. Ultrafast MR imaging of the normal posterior fossa in fetuses. *AJR Am J Roentgenol.* 2000;175:835–839.

61. Guibaud L. Practical approach to prenatal posterior fossa abnormalities using MR. *Pediatr Radiol.* 2004;34:700–711.

62. Robinson AJ, Blaser S, Toi A, et al. MR imaging of the fetal cerebellar vermis in utero: description of some useful anatomical criteria for normal and abnormal development. In: *Radiological Society of North America Scientific Assembly and Annual Meeting Program.* Oak Brook, IL: Radiological Society of North America; 2003.

63. Smith PA, Johansson D, Tzannatos C, et al. Prenatal measurement of the fetal cerebellum and cisterna cerebellomedullaris by ultrasound. *Prenat Diagn.* 1986;6:133–141.

64. Chang CH, Chang FM, Yu CH, et al. Three-dimensional ultrasound in the assessment of fetal cerebellar transverse and antero-posterior diameters. *Ultrasound Med Biol.* 2000;26:175–182.

65. Garel C. *MR of the Fetal Brain: Normal Development and Cerebral Pathologies.* 2nd ed. (English translation). Berlin, Germany: Springer-Verlag; 2004:95.

66. Triulzi F, Parazzini C, Righini A. MR of fetal and neonatal cerebellar development. *Semin Fetal Neonatal Med.* 2005;10:411–420.

67. Bertucci E, Gindes L, Mazza V, et al. Vermian biometric parameters in the normal and abnormal fetal posterior fossa: three-dimensional sonographic study. *J Ultrasound Med.* 2011;30:1403–1410.

68. Tilea B, Alberti C, Adamsbaum C, et al. Cerebral biometry in fetal magnetic resonance imaging: new reference data. *Ultrasound Obstet Gynecol.* 2009;33:173–181.

69. Robinson AJ, Blaser S, Toi A, et al. MR imaging of the fetal cerebellar vermis in utero: criteria for abnormal development, with ultrasonographic and clinicopathologic correlation. *Pediatr Radiol.* 2004;32:Supplement 2:page S135.

70. Volpe P, Contro E, De Musso F, et al. Brainstem-vermis and brainstem-tentorium angles allow accurate categorization of fetal upward rotation of cerebellar vermis. *Ultrasound Obstet Gynecol.* 2012;39:632–635.

71. Smith AS, Levine D, Barnes PD, et al. Magnetic resonance imaging of the kinked fetal brain stem: a sign of severe dysgenesis. *J Ultrasound Med.* 2005;24:1697–1709.

72. Barkovich AJ. *Pediatric Neuroimaging.* 3rd ed. Philadelphia, PA: Lippincott Williams & Wilkins; 2000:297–301.

73. Krishnamurthy S, Kapoor S, Sharma V, et al. Tectocerebellar dysraphia and occipital encephalocele: an unusual association with abdominal situs inversus and congenital heart disease. *Indian J Pediatr.* 2008;75:1178–1180.

74. Boddaert N, Klein O, Ferguson N, et al. Intellectual prognosis of the Dandy-Walker malformation in children: the importance of vermian lobulation. *Neuroradiology.* 2003;45:320–324.

75. Bolduc ME, du Plessis AJ, Sullivan N, et al. Regional cerebellar volumes predict functional outcome in children with cerebellar malformations. *Cerebellum.* 2012;11:531–542.

76. Toi A. The fetal head and brain. In: Rumack CM, Wilson SR, Charbonneau JW, eds. *Diagnostic Ultrasound.* 3rd ed. St Louis, MS: Elsevier Mosby; 2005.

77. Sawaya R, McLaurin RL. Dandy-Walker syndrome: clinical analysis of 23 cases. *J Neurosurg.* 1981;55:89–98.

78. Nyberg DA, Cyr DR, Mack LA, et al. The Dandy-Walker malformation prenatal sonographic diagnosis and its clinical significance. *J Ultrasound Med.* 1988;7:65–71.

79. Cohen MM Jr, Lemire RJ. Syndromes with cephaloceles. *Teratology.* 1982;25:161–172.

80. Pilu G, Romero R, De Palma L et al. Antenatal diagnosis and obstetric management of Dandy-Walker syndrome. *J Reprod Med.* 1986;31:1017–1022.

81. Olson GS, Halpe DC, Kaplan AM, et al. Dandy-Walker malformation and associated cardiac anomalies. *Childs Brain.* 1981;8:173–180.

82. Hart MN, Malamud N, Ellis WG. The Dandy-Walker syndrome: a clinicopathological study based on 28 cases. *Neurology.* 1972;22:771–780.

83. Blazer S, Berant M, Sujov PO, et al. Prenatal sonographic diagnosis of vermal agenesis. *Prenat Diagn.* 1997;17:907–911.

84. Bindal AK, Storrs BB, McLone DG. Management of the Dandy-Walker syndrome. *Pediatr Neurosurg.* 1990–1991;16:163–169.

85. Alkan O, Kizilkilic O, Yildirim T. Malformations of the midbrain and hindbrain: a retrospective study and review of the literature. *Cerebellum.* 2009;8:355–365.

86. Keogan MT, DeAtkine AB, Hertzberg BS. Cerebellar vermian defects: antenatal sonographic appearance and clinical significance. *J Ultrasound Med.* 1994;13:607–611.

87. Fenichel GM, Phillips JA. Familial aplasia of the cerebellar vermis: possible X-linked dominant inheritance. *Arch Neurol.* 1989;46:582–583.

88. Imamura S, Tachi N, Oya K. Dominantly inherited early-onset non-progressive cerebellar ataxia syndrome. *Brain Dev.* 1993;15:372–376.

89. Sasaki-Adams D, Elbabaa SK, Jewells V, et al. The Dandy-Walker variant: a case series of 24 pediatric patients and evaluation of associated anomalies, incidence of hydrocephalus, and developmental outcomes. *J Neurosurg Pediatr.* 2008;2:194–199.

90. Long A, Moran P, Robson S. Outcome of fetal cerebral posterior fossa anomalies. *Prenat Diagn.* 2006;26:707–710.

91. Bolduc ME, Limperopoulos C. Neurodevelopmental outcomes in children with cerebellar malformations: a systematic review. *Dev Med Child Neurol.* 2009;51:256–267.

92. Patek KJ, Kline-Fath BM, Hopkin RJ, et al. Posterior fossa anomalies diagnosed with fetal MRI: associated anomalies and neurodevelopmental outcomes. *Prenat Diagn.* 2012;32:75–82.

93. Guibaud L, Larroque A, Ville D, et al. Prenatal diagnosis of "isolated" Dandy-Walker malformation: imaging findings and prenatal counselling. *Prenat Diagn.* 2012;32:185–193.

94. Utsunomiya H, Takano K, Ogasawara T, et al. Rhombencephalosynapsis: cerebellar embryogenesis. *AJNR Am J Neuroradiol.* 1998;19:547–549.

95. Pasquier L, Marcorelles P, Loget P, et al. Rhombencephalosynapsis and related anomalies: a neuropathological study of 40 fetal cases. *Acta Neuropathol.* 2009;117:185–200.

96. Sgaier SK, Millet S, Villanueva MP, et al. Morphogenetic and cellular movements that shape the mouse cerebellum; insights from genetic fate mapping. *Neuron.* 2005;45:27–40.

97. Tan TY, McGillivray G, Goergen SK, et al. Prenatal magnetic resonance imaging in Gomez-Lopez-Hernandez syndrome and review of the literature. *Am J Med Genet.* 2005;138A:369–373.

98. Brocks D, Irons M, Sadeghi-Najad A, et al. Gomez-Lopez-Hernandez syndrome: expansion of the phenotype. *Am J Med Genet.* 2000;94:405–408.

99. Gomez MR. Cerebellotrigeminal and focal dermal dysplasia: a newly recognized neurocutaneous syndrome. *Brain Dev.* 1979;1:253–256.

100. Gomy I, Heck B, Santos AC, et al. Two new Brazilian patients with Gomez-Lopez-Hernandez syndrome. *Am J Med Genet.* 2008;146A:649–657.

101. Elliott R, Harter DH. Rhombencephalosynapsis associated with autosomal dominant polycystic kidney disease Type 1. *J Neurosurg Pediatr.* 2008;2:435–437.

102. Barkovich AJ, Raybaud CA. Congenital malformations of the brain and skull. In: Barkovich AJ, ed. *Pediatric Neuroimaging.* Lippincott Williams & Wilkins; 2000; 473–476.

103. Napolitano M, Righini A, Zirpoli S, et al. Prenatal magnetic resonance imaging of rhombencephalosynapsis and associated brain anomalies: report of 3 cases. *J Comput Assist Tomogr.* 2004;28:762–765.

104. Sergi C, Hentze S, Sohn C, et al. Telencephalosynapsis (synencephaly) and rhombencephalosynapsis with posterior fossa ventriculocele ("Dandy-Walker cyst"): an unusual aberrant syngenetic complex. *Brain Dev.* 1997;19:426–432.

105. Barkovich AJ. *Pediatric Neuroimaging.* 3rd ed. Philadelphia, PA: Lippincott Williams & Wilkins; 2000:346–350.

106. Toelle S, Yalcinkaya C, Kocer N, et al. Rhombencephalosynapsis: clinical findings and neuroimaging in 9 children. *Neuropediatrics.* 2002;33:209–214.

107. Poretti A, Alber FD, Bürki S, et al. Cognitive outcome in children with rhombencephalosynapsis. *Eur J Paediatr Neurol.* 2009;13:28–33.

108. Gleeson J, Keeler L, Parisi M, et al. Molar tooth sign of the midbrain-hindbrain junction: occurrence in multiple distinct syndromes. *Am J Med Genet A.* 2004;125A:125–134.

109. Satran D, Pierpont MEM, Dobyns WB. Cerebello-Oculo-Renal syndromes including Arima, Senior-Löken and COACH syndromes: more than just variants of Joubert syndrome. *Am J Med Genet.* 1999;86:459–469.

110. Louie CM, Gleeson JG. Genetic basis of Joubert syndrome and related disorders of cerebellar development. *Hum Mol Genet.* 2005;14:R235–R242.

111. Zaki MS, Abdel-Aleem A, Abdel-Salam GMH, et al. The molar tooth sign: a new Joubert syndrome and related cerebellar disorders classification system tested in Egyptian families. *Neurology.* 2008;70:556–565.

112. Badano JL, Mitsuma N, Beales PL, et al. The ciliopathies: an emerging class of human genetic disorders. *Annu Rev Genomics Hum Genet.* 2006;7:125–148.

113. Valente EM, Brancati F, Silhavy JL, et al. AHI1 gene mutations cause specific forms of Joubert syndrome-related disorders. *Ann Neurol.* 2006;59:527–534.

114. Valente EM, Silhavy JL, Brancati F, et al. Mutations in CEP290, which encodes a centrosomal protein, cause pleiotropic forms of Joubert syndrome. *Nat Genet.* 2006;38:623–625.

115. Cantagrel V, Silhavy J, Bielas S, et al. Mutations in the cilia gene ARL13B lead to the classical form of Joubert syndrome. *Am J Hum Genet.* 2008;83:170–179.

116. Pugash D, Oh T, Godwin K, et al. Sonographic "molar tooth" sign in the diagnosis of Joubert syndrome. *Ultrasound Obstet Gynecol.* 2011;38:598–602.

117. Saleem SN, Zaki MS. Role of MR imaging in prenatal diagnosis of pregnancies at risk for Joubert syndrome and related cerebellar disorders. *AJNR Am J Neuroradiol.* 2010;31:424–429.

118. Aslan H, Ulker V, Gulcan EM, et al. Prenatal diagnosis of Joubert syndrome: a case report. *Prenat Diagn.* 2002;22:13–16.

119. Doherty D, Glass IA, Siebert JR, et al. Prenatal diagnosis in pregnancies at risk for Joubert syndrome by ultrasound and MRI. *Prenat Diagn.* 2005;25:442–447.

120. Fluss J, Blaser S, Chitayat D, et al. Molar tooth sign in fetal brain magnetic resonance imaging leading to the prenatal diagnosis of Joubert syndrome and related disorders. *J Child Neurol.* 2006;21:320–324.

121. Widjaja E, Blaser S, Raybaud C. Diffusion tensor imaging of midline posterior fossa malformations. *Pediatr Radiol.* 2006;36:510–517.

122. Barkovich AJ, Raybaud CA. Congenital malformations of the brain and skull. In: Barkovich AJ, ed. *Pediatric Neuroimaging.* Philadelphia, PA: Lippincott Williams & Wilkins; 2000;481–483.

123. Joubert M, Eisenring JJ, Robb JP, et al. Familial agenesis of the cerebellar vermis: a syndrome of episodic hyperpnea, abnormal eye movements, ataxia, and retardation. *Neurology.* 1969;19:813–825.

124. Parisi M, Glass I. Joubert syndrome and related disorders: 2003 Jul 9 [Updated 2013 Apr 11]. In: Pagon RA, Adam MP, Bird TD, et al, eds. *GeneReviews™* [Internet]. Seattle, WA: University of Washington, Seattle; 1993–2014. Available from http://www.ncbi.nlm.nih.gov/books/NBK1325/.

125. Zollino M, Di Stefano C, Zampino G, et al. Genotype-phenotype correlations and clinical diagnostic criteria in Wolf-Hirschhorn syndrome. *Am J Med Genet.* 2000;94:254–261.

126. Namavar Y, Barth P, Tien Poll-The B, Baas F. Classification, diagnosis and potential mechanisms in pontocerebellar hypoplasia. *Ophanet Journal of Rare Diseases.* 2001;6:1–50.

127. Graham J, Spencer A, Brinberg I, Niesen C, et al. Molecular and neuroimaging findings in pontocerebellar hypoplasia Type 2 (PCH2): Is prenatal diagnosis possible? *American Journal of medical genetics.* 2010;152A:2268–2276.

128. Namavar Y, Barth P, Kasher P, van Ruissen F, Brockmann K, et al. Clinical, neuroradiological and genetic findings in pontocerebellar hypoplasia. *Brain.* 2011;134:143–156.

129. Malinger G, Lev K, Lerman-Sagle T. The fetal cerebellum. Pitfalls in diagnosis and management. *Prenatal Diagnosis.* 2009. 10.1002/pd.2196.

130. Tilea B, Delezoide A, Khung-Savatovshi S, Guimiot F, et al. Comparison between magnetic resonance imaging and fetopathology in the evaluation of fetal posterior fossa non-cystic abnormalities. *Ultrasound in Obstetrics Gynecology.* 2007;29:651–659.

131. Patel S, Barkovich A. Analysis and classification of cerebellar malformations. *American Journal of Neuroradiology.* 2002;23;1074–1087.

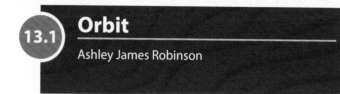

# 13 Face

## 13.1 Orbit

Ashley James Robinson

## EVALUATION

Sonographic assessment of the fetal eyes is not a requirement for routine prenatal sonography according to the amalgamated guidelines from the (American Institute of Ultrasound in Medicine, American Congress of Obstetricians and Gynecologists, American College of Radiology) AIUM, ACOG, and ACR.[1] Assessment of orbital biometry is a reasonable expectation as part of a detailed anatomy scan, particularly in the setting of suspected central nervous system (CNS) malformation. However, evaluation of the globe itself can be far more challenging.

Complete ocular evaluation comprises ocular biometry, assessment for the presence of the globes, and examination of the morphology of the lens, vitreous, and optic nerves.[2] There is a necessity for a working knowledge of ocular pathologies because syndromes involving the eyes can go unrecognized without a systematic approach.

### Embryology

At 22 days' gestation, the optic vesicles start to develop as bilateral outpouchings from the inner wall of the forebrain. When the vesicles contact the surface ectoderm, this induces the lens placode, which then starts to invaginate into the optic vesicles that become the optic cups. By 5 to 7 weeks, the lens placode loses contact with the surface ectoderm to form the lens vesicle. Elongation of the cells within the lens vesicle fills the lumen of the lens vesicle to form the solid lens. With growth, the optic cups envelop the lens circumferentially to form the globe. The hyaloid artery, the primary supply of nutrients to the developing lens, is contained within the optic stalk, which extends from the optic disc through the vitreous humor to the lens. After the tenth week, the lens grows independent of blood supply and the hyaloid artery regresses leaving a clear central zone, known as the hyaloid canal or Cloquet canal.

### Imaging/Biometry

Growth charts for the fetal lens and orbit,[3,4] as well as the measurements of binocular (BOD) and interocular (IOD) distances have been determined sonographically (see Table 25A in Appendix A1).[5–7] The latter are measured according to the bony landmarks of the medial and lateral orbital walls. The orbital measurements are ideally made in the axial plane, with both orbits of equal and largest possible diameter.[8] The binocular distance is measured between the two malar margins, and the interocular distance between the two ethmoidal margins of the *bony orbits* (Fig. 13.1-1).

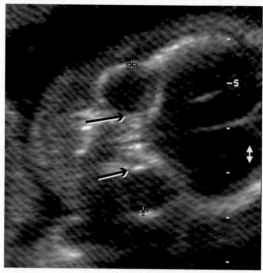

**FIGURE 13.1-1:** Orbital Measurements by US. Transorbital view of the fetal face shows the measurement of the BOD with the calipers on the malar margins of the orbit. The IOD is measured between the two ethmoidal margins of the orbit (arrows).

These bony landmarks are difficult to see by fetal magnetic resonance imaging (MRI), and therefore standard sonographic growth charts cannot accurately be applied to fetal MR studies.

On T2-weighted MRI, the whole lens is low signal compared with the high signal of the vitreous. The BOD and IOD measurements can be made in any plane from true axial to true coronal, provided both eyes can be seen in the same image and have the most equal and largest possible transverse diameters. The binocular and interocular distances are, respectively, measured between the two malar or ethmoidal margins of each *vitreous* (Fig. 13.1-2). These measurements can be plotted against gestational age (see Table 26 in Appendix A1).[2] Other available nomograms additionally include measurements of the transverse diameter of the lens[9] and anteroposterior diameter of the globe.[10] It has been noted that the globe is ellipsoid earlier in gestation. This is thought to be attributable to the presence of the hyaloid artery initially tethering the lens to the optic disc. With involution of the hyaloid artery, the globe is increased in anteroposterior diameter.

## ANOPHTHALMIA/MICROPHTHALMIA

Anophthalmia and microphthalmia can really only be differentiated pathologically. Anophthalmia is complete absence of the globe but in the presence of the ocular adnexa (eyelids, conjunctiva, and lacrimal apparatus). Microphthalmia by definition means small globe. It should be differentiated from cyptophthalmos, that is a failure of separation of the eyelids, which should occur by 24 weeks, but in the presence of normal intraorbital contents. Cryptophthalmos is usually bilateral, and when it occurs with multiple other abnormalities,

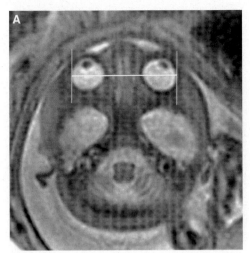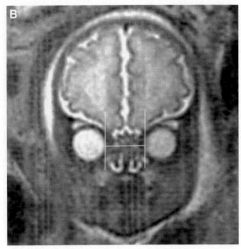

**FIGURE 13.1-2:** Orbital Measurements by MRI. **A:** The BOD is measured between the two malar margins of each high-signal vitreous. The measurements can be made in any plane orthogonal to the sagittal plane. **B:** Here, the IOD is measured in the coronal plane between the two orbital margins of each high-signal vitreous. (Reproduced from Robinson AJ, Blaser S, Toi A, et al. Magnetic resonance imaging of the fetal eyes: morphologic and biometric assessment for abnormal development with ultrasonographic and clinicopathologic correlation. *Pediatr Radiol.* 2008;38:971–981, with permission of Springer-Verlag.)

Fraser syndrome, which has an autosomal recessive inheritance, should be considered.

**Incidence:** Anophthalmia is seen in approximately 1:2,400 pregnancies.

**Pathogenesis/Etiology:** *Primary* anophthalmia/microphthalmia occurs when one or both eyes never form. It is usually associated with chromosomal abnormalities such as trisomy 13, genetic abnormalities such as CHARGE (Coloboma, Heart defects, Choanal atresia, Growth retardation, Genital, and Ear abnormalities) syndrome (CHD7), incontinentia pigmenti (IKBKG), Norrie disease (NDP), SOX2-related eye disorders, Walker–Warburg syndrome (POMT1),[11–16] and over 180 syndromes.

In *secondary* anophthalmia/microphthalmia, the development of the eyes is initially normal but is disrupted by an insult. Etiologies include infection such as TORCH (toxoplasmosis, other, rubella, cytomegalovirus, and herpes), syphilis, Eppstein-Barr virus (EBV), parvovirus, a vascular event (e.g., Goldenhar syndrome [oculo-auriculo-vertebral spectrum]), or a toxic or metabolic event, for example, low or high vitamin A, ethanol, and retinoic acid. Table 13.1 summarizes the ocular disorder and its primary and secondary causes.

**Imaging:** On ultrasound (US) and MRI, microphthalmia or anophthalmia may be present when the orbital diameter is below the 5th percentile.[8] Walker–Warburg syndrome, a type of congenital muscular dystrophy, comprises a Z-shaped brainstem on midline sagittal views, an occipital cephalocele, and ocular asymmetry (Fig. 13.1-3). Matthew Wood syndrome, i.e., Spear syndrome, comprises Pulmonary agenesis, Microphthalmia, and Diaphragmatic defect (PMD) or Pulmonary agenesis, Diaphragmatic defect, Anopthalmia and Cardiac anomalies (PDAC). (Fig. 13.1-4).[17] Aicardi syndrome is a rare genetic malformation syndrome that can be diagnosed antenatally by the association of partial or complete absence of the corpus callosum, ocular abnormalities, and posterior fossa cyst (Fig. 13.1-5).

| Table 13.1-1 | Ocular Abnormalities and Associations | |
|---|---|---|
| **Anophthalmia/ Microphthalmia** | Primary | Trisomy 13 |
| | | CHARGE syndrome |
| | | Incontinentia pigmenti |
| | | Norrie disease |
| | | Sox2 |
| | | Walker–Warburg syndrome |
| | Secondary | TORCH infections |
| | | Syphilis |
| | | EBV |
| | | Parvovirus |
| | | Goldenhar syndrome |
| | | Hypervitaminosis A |
| | | Hypovitaminosis A |
| | | Ethanol |
| | | Retinoic acid |
| **Hypotelorism** | Primary | Trisomy 13 |
| | Secondary | Plagiocephaly |
| | | Microcephaly |
| **Hypertelorism** | Primary | Median facial cleft syndrome |
| | Secondary | Frontal cephalocele |
| | | Craniosynostosis |

## HYPOTELORISM

**Pathogenesis/Etiology:** The craniofacial skeleton is derived from both mesoderm and neural crest cells of the mesencephalon. Its development is intimately related to forebrain development and has a similar induction mechanism. For this reason, facial skeletal abnormalities are often associated with underlying cerebral malformations (the face predicts the brain[18]). Typically, the craniofacial abnormalities are actually secondary to a

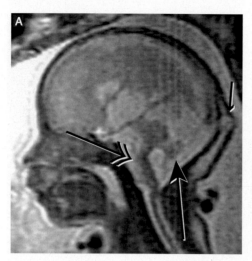
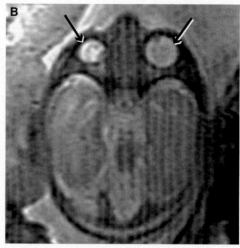

**FIGURE 13.1-3:** Walker–Warburg syndrome **A:** Sagittal T2 MRI demonstrates Z-shaped brainstem *(double-headed arrow)*, small vermis *(large arrow)*, and occipital cephalocele *(small arrow)*. **B:** Axial MRI shows asymmetric globes *(arrows)*. (Reproduced from Robinson AJ, Blaser S, Toi A, et al. The fetal cerebellar vermis: assessment for abnormal development by ultrasonography and magnetic resonance imaging. *Ultrasound Q.* 2007;23(3):211–223.)

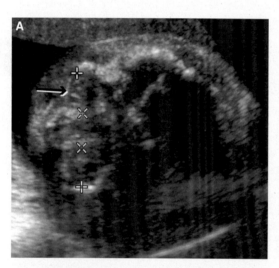
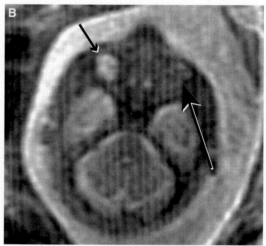
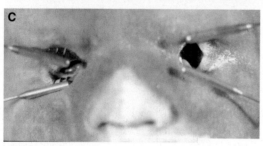

**FIGURE 13.1-4:** Matthew Wood syndrome. **A:** US biometry was delayed and there was an abnormal appearance to lens and globe, which appear echogenic *(arrow)*. **B:** MRI demonstrates apparent anophthalmia *(large arrow)* and microphthalmia *(small arrow)*. **C:** Postmortem showed absent globes. (Reproduced from Robinson AJ, Blaser S, Toi A, et al. Magnetic resonance imaging of the fetal eyes: morphologic and biometric assessment for abnormal development with ultrasonographic and clinicopathologic correlation. *Pediatr Radiol.* 2008;38:971–981, with permission of Springer-Verlag.)

more caudal expression of an abnormal genetic gradient that exists within the neural crest, and therefore it is actually the brain abnormality that affects the development of the craniofacial skeleton, that is, the brain predicts the face (H. Sarnat, personal communication, 2012).

During normal embryologic development, the opening for the eye forms during development of the face, when the paired nasal swellings on either side migrate medially and inferiorly and fuse with the midline frontal swelling to form the nose. If there is deficient forebrain development, with deficient development of the midline frontal swelling, the paired nasal swellings migrate

more medially, and this results in ***primary*** hypotelorism. The corresponding underlying brain anomaly is often in the spectrum of holoprosencephaly,[8,19] with approximately 55% of cases associated with chromosomal abnormalities, most commonly trisomy 13.[5,8]

In ***secondary*** hypotelorism, the defect is most frequently the result of abnormalities of the bony skull, for example, microcephaly and plagiocephaly.[8]

**Imaging:** Hypotelorism is defined as an interocular distance below the 5th percentile on US and MRI.[8] Close inspection of the brain for imaging findings of holoprosencephaly is indicated (Fig. 13.1-6).

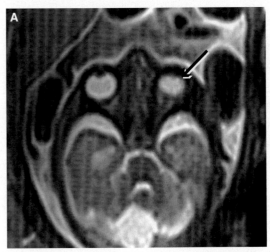
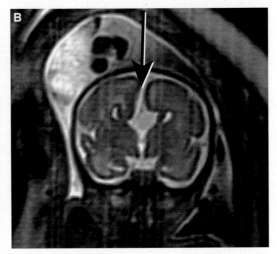

**FIGURE 13.1-5:** Aicardi syndrome. **A:** Unilateral microphthalmia *(arrow)*. **B:** Callosal dysgenesis with "high-riding" third ventricle continuous with interhemispheric fissure *(arrow)*.

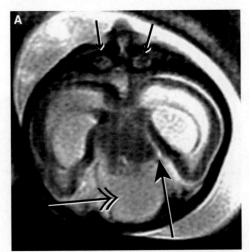
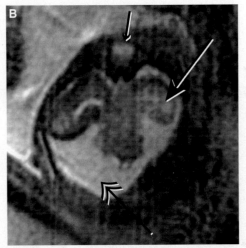

**FIGURE 13.1-6:** Holoprosencephaly. **A:** Axial MR image shows severe hypotelorism and microphthalmia *(small arrows)*. There is a dorsal interhemispheric cyst *(double-headed arrow)*, and the hippocampus touches the brainstem at the ambient cistern *(large arrow)*, in keeping with lobar holoprosencephaly. **B:** Axial MR image shows a single small midline globe *(small arrow)*. The hippocampus is not touching the brainstem *(large arrow)*, and there is wide communication of the ambient cistern with the dorsal interhemispheric cyst *(double-headed arrow)*, in keeping with alobar holoprosencephaly. (Reproduced from Robinson AJ, Blaser S, Toi A, et al. Magnetic resonance imaging of the fetal eyes: morphologic and biometric assessment for abnormal development with ultrasonographic and clinicopathologic correlation. *Pediatr Radiol.* 2008;38:971–981, with permission of Springer-Verlag.)

## HYPERTELORISM

**Pathogenesis/Etiology:** In *primary* hypertelorism, the defect is due to deficient migration of the neural crest cells in the lamina terminalis of the prosencephalon. When this occurs, there is deficient formation of a structure known as the medial canthal ligament, and the eyes stay in their early embryonic position on the side of the face similar to lesser mammals, fish, and birds (except owls). The deficient migration of neural crest cells also typically results in associated callosal dysgenesis. Hypertelorism can result from many chromosomal anomalies and genetic syndromes,[11] including median facial cleft syndrome, otherwise known as frontonasal dysplasia, which comprises hypertelorism, facial clefting, and callosal agenesis.

In *secondary* hypertelorism, the defect typically results from abnormalities of the skull; the most common being anterior cephalocele and craniosynostoses.[11,19,20] Although typically used to describe the appearance of the skull in type II thanatophoric dysplasia, the term "cloverleaf skull" has also been used to describe the dysmorphic appearance of the skull in craniosynostosis,[21,22] and several case reports have described the utility of fetal MRI in antenatal diagnosis.[23–25]

**Imaging:** Hypertelorism is defined as an interocular distance above the 95th percentile on US and MRI.[8] Interocular distance may be the most reliable for making the diagnosis of hypertelorism, as by US this measurement is usually more than two standard deviations from the mean, whereas the

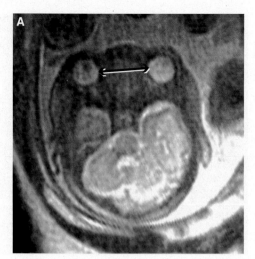
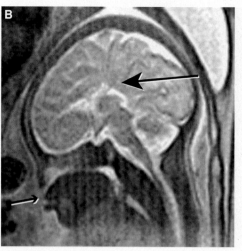

**FIGURE 13.1-7:** Frontonasal Dysplasia **A:** Axial MR image shows hypertelorism *(double-headed arrow)*. The BOD and IOD were both greater than the 95th centile for gestational age. **B:** Absence of the corpus callosum *(large arrow)* and facial defect with absence of the hard palate separating the nasal and oral cavities with the tongue protruding through the defect *(small arrow)*. (**A**, reproduced from Robinson AJ, Blaser S, Toi A, et al. Magnetic resonance imaging of the fetal eyes: morphologic and biometric assessment for abnormal development with ultrasonographic and clinicopathologic correlation. *Pediatr Radiol.* 2008;38:971–981, with permission of Springer-Verlag.)

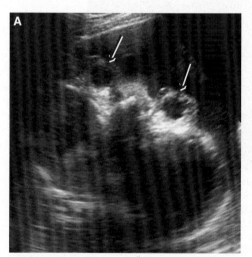
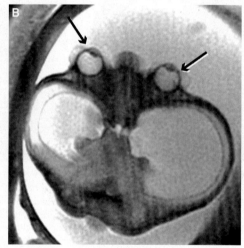
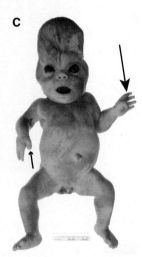

**FIGURE 13.1-8:** Craniosynostosis in Pfeiffer Syndrome. **A:** Axial transorbital US image shows severe hypertelorism, exorbitism *(arrows)*. **B:** Fetal MRI. Severe ventriculomegaly, exorbitism *(arrows)*, and hypertelorism. **C:** Gross pathologic specimen shows hypertelorism, broad thumbs *(small arrow)*, and syndactyly *(long arrow)*. (Reproduced from Robinson AJ, Blaser S, Toi A, et al. Magnetic resonance imaging of the fetal eyes: morphologic and biometric assessment for abnormal development with ultrasonographic and clinicopathologic correlation. *Pediatr Radiol.* 2008;38:971–981, with permission of Springer-Verlag.)

binocular distance remains at the upper limit of normal.[8] In primary hypertelorism, other anomalies are commonly identified (Fig. 13.1-7). In the presence of craniosynostosis or cephaloceles, hypertelorism may be secondary (Fig. 13.1-8).

## MORPHOLOGY OF THE LENS, VITREOUS, AND OPTIC NERVES

### Cataract

**Pathogenesis/Etiology:** Cataracts represent clouding of the lens and are seen in a variety of metabolic, infectious, genetic, and chromosomal abnormalities that affect the fetus, including toxoplasmosis, X-irradiation, in-vitro fertilization, persistent hyperplastic primary vitreous, Nance–Horan, Adams–Oliver, Walker–Warburg, and Neu-Laxova syndromes, rhizomelic chondrodysplasia punctata, trisomy 17 mosaicism, and trisomy 21.[14,26–35]

**Imaging:** By endovaginal US, the normal lens is visible by 14 weeks anteriorly within the globe as a thin echogenic rim with an anechoic center (Fig. 13.1-9A). Typically, however, the only reflection from the lens is from the surfaces perpendicular to the insonating beam, and it can therefore be difficult to visualize. On MRI, the normal lens is homogeneous low signal on T2-weighted images compared with the high signal of the

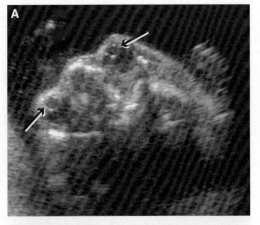

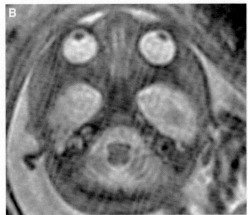

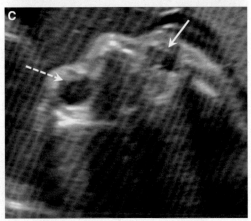

**FIGURE 13.1-9:** Normal Lens and vitreous **(A, B)** and Cataract **(C)**. **A:** Ultrasound. The surfaces of the lenses are seen as faint curvilinear echoes in the anterior globe *(arrows)*. **B:** MRI. The whole lens is in low signal compared with the high signal of the vitreous. **C:** Axial ultrasound showing normal lens *(arrow)* in a small globe and echogenic lens *(dashed arrow)* in the opposite globe in this fetus with trisomy 13. (**A** and **B**, reproduced from Robinson AJ, Blaser S, Toi A, et al. Magnetic resonance imaging of the fetal eyes: morphologic and biometric assessment for abnormal development with ultrasonographic and clinicopathologic correlation. *Pediatr Radiol.* 2008;38:971–981, with permission of Springer-Verlag.)

adjacent anterior chamber and vitreous (Fig. 13.1-9B). A cataract is seen as abnormal echogenicity by US (Fig. 13.1-9C) or abnormal signal on MRI in the position of the lens. Sometimes, it can be difficult to determine whether only the lens is abnormal. If the vitreous is also abnormal, then persistent hyperplastic primary vitreous and coloboma should be considered in the differential.

## Persistent Hyperplastic Primary Vitreous

**Pathogenesis/Etiology:** Failure of involution of the hyaloid artery results in a spectrum of abnormalities known as persistent hyperplastic primary vitreous. The characteristic findings are a persistent hyaloid artery and a cone-shaped retrolental density. Other findings include a small irregular triangular-shaped lens with the apex pointing posteriorly and a shallow anterior chamber. Calcification is unusual. It is frequently seen with trisomy syndromes and other forms of abnormal brain development.[36,37]

**Imaging:** By US, the normal vitreous is hypoechoic, and on T2-weighted MRI, it is high signal compared with the low signal of the lens. The hyaloid artery can be seen on US as an echogenic line bisecting the vitreous (Fig. 13.1-10A), which during conversion of the primary vitreous to mature secondary vitreous, gradually becomes beaded as it involutes, a process which should be completed by 30 weeks gestational age.[38,39] Therefore, the hyaloid artery should not be identified via US past 30 weeks gestation. The remnant channel through the vitreous is known as Cloquet canal.

The normal hyaloid artery should not usually be detectable on MRI, and a corresponding abnormal low-signal linear plaque extending from the posterior part of the lens to the optic nerve head through the central vitreous in the position of Cloquet canal is considered to be pathologic[2] (Fig. 13.1-10B–D).

## Coloboma

**Pathogenesis/Etiology:** Coloboma is one of three types of excavation of the optic disc that can significantly impair visual function.[40] The other types, peripapillary staphyloma and morning glory disc, cannot be easily distinguished antenatally. Coloboma can be a unilateral or bilateral condition. During embryological development after the optic cup invaginates, it normally grows circumferentially to surround the lens vesicle and hyaloid artery, and once surrounded, the two sides close along the choroidal fissure to form the globe. If this envelopment is incomplete, the choroidal fissure stays open, resulting in a cleft anywhere along the length of the optic cup from the iris to the optic nerve.

In the majority of cases, coloboma is a feature of a syndrome; especially common associations are CHARGE and Aicardi syndrome.

**Imaging:** On US, associated ocular findings such as microphthalmia, an orbital cyst (outside the globe), or a persistent hyaloid artery may prompt the diagnosis (Fig. 13.1-11A). Because of the difficulties in depicting the posterior orbit sonographically, the diagnostic feature detectable antenatally is a deeply excavated optic disc on MRI (Fig. 13.1-11B, C).[41] Differential diagnosis includes persistent hyperplastic primary vitreous and cataract.

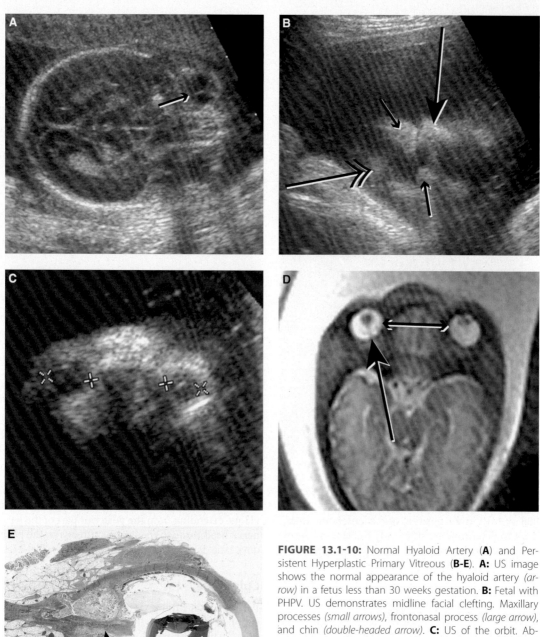

**FIGURE 13.1-10:** Normal Hyaloid Artery (**A**) and Persistent Hyperplastic Primary Vitreous (**B-E**). **A:** US image shows the normal appearance of the hyaloid artery (arrow) in a fetus less than 30 weeks gestation. **B:** Fetal with PHPV. US demonstrates midline facial clefting. Maxillary processes (small arrows), frontonasal process (large arrow), and chin (double-headed arrow). **C:** US of the orbit. Absence of normal anatomy and ocular hyperechogenicity. **D:** Fetal MRI. Hypertelorism (double-headed arrow) plus persistent hyaloid artery (large arrow) and triangular-shaped lens. **E:** Histopathologic specimen confirms persistence of hyaloid artery (arrow). (**C** and **D**, reproduced from Robinson AJ, Blaser S, Toi A, et al. Magnetic resonance imaging of the fetal eyes: morphologic and biometric assessment for abnormal development with ultrasonographic and clinicopathologic correlation. *Pediatr Radiol.* 2008;38: 971–981, with permission of Springer-Verlag.)

## Optic Nerve Hypoplasia

**Pathogenesis/Etiology:** Optic nerve hypoplasia is usually sporadic and difficult to detect prenatally; however, it has a number of associations that can potentially be diagnosed intrauterine (Table 13.1-2). Evaluation of the optic nerves is usually necessary in the setting of absence of the cavum septi pellucidi, which can be an isolated finding or can be associated with severe neurological abnormalities such as holoprosencephaly or septo-optic dysplasia.[42]

**Imaging:** With US, optic tract hypoplasia can be assessed by fetal sonography,[43–45] by measurement of the transverse diameter of the optic chiasm and optic nerves (Fig. 13.1-12A, B), normal and abnormal growth of which has been described (Table 25B in Appendix A1).

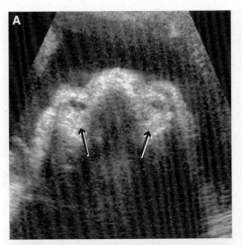

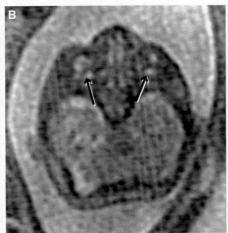

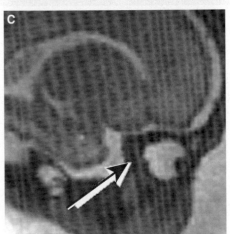

**FIGURE 13.1-11:** Coloboma. **A:** US image demonstrates an abnormal echogenicity of the globes *(arrows)*, but the lenses appear relatively normal. **B:** Axial MR image in the same fetus shows bilateral symmetrical abnormal globes with mixed low- and high-signal vitreous *(arrows)*, and no definite lens structures. **C:** Parasagittal MR image through the globe shows deep excavation of the optic disc *(arrow)* in posterior coloboma in a different fetus. (**A** and **B**, reproduced from Robinson AJ, Blaser S, Toi A, et al. Magnetic resonance imaging of the fetal eyes: morphologic and biometric assessment for abnormal development with ultrasonographic and clinicopathologic correlation. *Pediatr Radiol.* 2008;38:971–981, with permission of Springer-Verlag. **C**, reproduced from Righini A, Avagliano L, Doneda C, et al. Prenatal magnetic resonance imaging of optic nerve head coloboma. *Prenat Diagn.* 2008;28:242–246, with permission of John Wiley & Sons Ltd.)

| Table 13.1-2 | Associations with Optic Nerve Hypoplasia |
|---|---|

Aicardi syndrome
Anticonvulsants
CHARGE association
Congenital muscular dystrophy
Dominant inheritance
Duane retraction syndrome
Chromosome 5q distal deletion syndrome
Chromosome 6p partial deletion
Chromosome 7(q22–q34) and 7(q32–34) interstitial duplication
Chromosome 17 interstitial deletion
Ethanol toxicity
Frontonasal dysplasia
Goldenhar–Gorlin syndrome
Idiopathic growth hormone deficiency
Isotretinoin toxicity
Nevus sebaceous of Jadassohn
Maternal diabetes mellitus
Orbital haemangioma
Periventricular leukomalacia
Septo-optic dysplasia
Suprasellar teratoma
Valproic acid toxicity

Modified from Dutton GN. Congenital disorders of the optic nerve: excavations and hypoplasia. *Eye (Lond).* 2004;18:1038–1048.

The same anatomy can be assessed with some difficulty by fetal MRI[46]; however, a relatively crude assessment can be made by ensuring that the optic nerves are symmetric in size and approximately the same size as the adjacent carotid arteries and pituitary gland. The overall configuration is reminiscent of the Olympic rings (Fig. 13.1-12C).

## ORBITAL ABNORMALITIES

### Dacrocystocele

**Incidence:** The incidence on prenatal MRI studies has been reported between 0.7% and 2.7%, depending on definition, and only 50% of affected eyes are symptomatic postnatally.

**Pathogenesis/Etiology:** Congenital dacrocystocele is a distension of the nasolacrimal duct usually due to obstruction at its distal end at the valve of Hasner.

**Imaging:** Prenatal US and MRI can be used to make the diagnosis.[47,48] It is not expected to be seen prior to 24 weeks gestation, because nasolacrimal duct canalization is incomplete, and even normal fluid-filled nasolacrimal ducts can be seen only by MRI after 24 weeks gestation. Dacrocystoceles can also spontaneously resolve prior to delivery owing to rupture of the valve of Hasner[49,50] (Fig. 13.1-13).

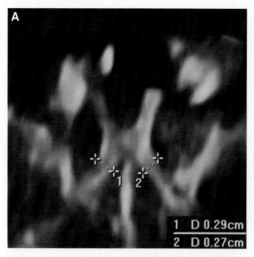
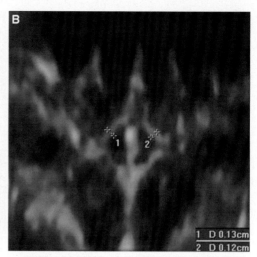
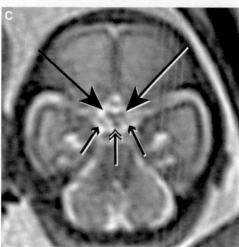

**FIGURE 13.1-12:** Normal Optic Nerves **(A, C)** and Optic nerve hypoplasia/SOD **(B)**. **A:** Measurement of optic tract diameter using a transabdominal approach in a (normal) 28-week fetus. **B:** Hypoplastic optic tract in a 31-week fetus with agenesis of the septum pellucidum. **C:** "Olympic rings" sign on fetal MRI. Normal Optic nerves *(large arrows)* and carotid arteries *(small arrows)*. Pituitary stalk *(double-headed arrow)*. (**A** and **B**, reproduced from Bault JP, Salomon LJ, Guibaud L, et al. Role of three-dimensional ultrasound measurement of the optic tract in fetuses with agenesis of the septum pellucidum. *Ultrasound Obstet Gynecol.* 2011;37(5):570–575, with permission of John Wiley & Sons Ltd.)

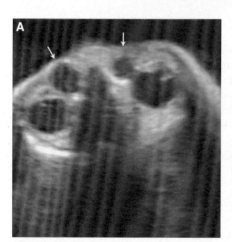
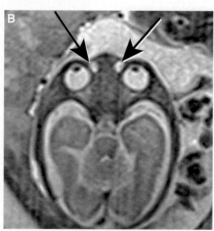
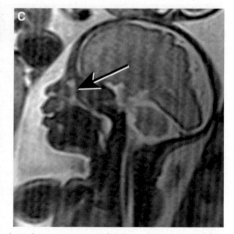

**FIGURE 13.1-13:** Dacrocystocele. **A:** Axial ultrasound demonstrates bilateral cysts *(arrows)* medial to the orbit consistent with bilateral dacrocystoceles. **B:** Fetal MRI showing bilateral cysts in the medial canthi *(arrows)*. **C:** Fetal MRI showing dilated nasolacrimal duct *(arrow)*.

## Orbital Masses

**Incidence:** Orbital masses are sporadic and very uncommon, and usually incidentally detected later in pregnancy, but most commonly detected postnatally.

**Pathogenesis:** The most common mass in the fetal head and neck is teratoma, and they can be large enough to interfere with

labor and delivery. They can damage not only the globe because of mass effect but also the surrounding bony structures. They may be detectable because of proptosis or via polyhydramnios by interfering with fetal swallowing.[51]

**Imaging:** The typical appearance of teratoma by US and MRI is a mixed solid and cystic mass with scattered amorphous calcifications.

**Differential:** The main differential is hemangioma, but other rarer tumors such as congenital fibrosarcoma and vascular malformations should also be considered.[52]

**Management:** Ideally, the eye should be preserved postnatally, but there is often secondary damage due to ocular exposure or optic nerve atrophy.[53]

## ACKNOWLEDGMENT

Portions of this chapter are from Robinson AJ, Blaser S, Toi A, et al. Magnetic resonance imaging of the fetal eyes: morphologic and biometric assessment for abnormal development with ultrasonographic and clinicopathologic correlation. *Pediatr Radiol.* 2008;38:971–981, with permission of Springer-Verlag.

## REFERENCES

1. *AIUM Practice Guideline for the Performance of an Antepartum Obstetric Ultrasound Examination.* American Institute of Ultrasound in Medicine. http://www.aium.org/loginRequired/membersOnly/guidelinesEnhanced/obstetric.aspx. Accessed March 17, 2013.
2. Robinson AJ, Blaser S, Toi A, et al. Magnetic resonance imaging of the fetal eyes: morphologic and biometric assessment for abnormal development with ultrasonographic and clinicopathologic correlation. *Pediatr Radiol.* 2008;38:971–981.
3. Dilmen G, Köktener A, Turhan NO, et al. Growth of the fetal lens and orbit. *Int J Gynaecol Obstet.* 2002;76:267–271.
4. Goldstein I, Tamir A, Zimmer EZ, et al. Growth of the fetal orbit and lens in normal pregnancies. *Ultrasound Obstet Gynecol.* 1998;12:175–179.
5. Rosati P, Guariglia L. Early transvaginal fetal orbital measurements: a screening tool for aneuploidy? *J Ultrasound Med.* 2003;22:1201–1205.
6. Trout T, Budorick NE, Pretorius DH, et al. Significance of orbital measurements in the fetus. *J Ultrasound Med.* 1994;13:937–943.
7. Mayden KL, Tortora M, Berkowitz RL, et al. Orbital diameters: a new parameter for prenatal diagnosis and dating. *Am J Obstet Gynecol.* 1982;144:289–297.
8. Babcook C. The fetal face and neck. In: Callen P, ed. *Ultrasonography in Obstetrics and Gynecology.* Philadelphia, PA: WB Saunders; 2000:307–315.
9. Paquette LB, Jackson HA, Tavare CJ, et al. In utero eye development documented by fetal MR imaging. *Am J Neuroradiol.* 2009;30:1787–1791.
10. Li XB, Kasprian G, Hodge JC, et al. Fetal ocular measurements by MRI. *Prenat Diagn.* 2010;30:1064–1071.
11. Robson CD, Barnewolt CE. MR imaging of fetal head and neck anomalies. *Neuroimaging Clin N Am.* 2004;14:273–291.
12. Berg C, Geipel A, Germer U, et al. Prenatal detection of Fraser syndrome without cryptophthalmos: case report and review of the literature. *Ultrasound Obstet Gynecol.* 2001;18:76–80.
13. Fryns JP, van Schoubroeck D, Vandenberghe K, et al. Diagnostic echographic findings in cryptophthalmos syndrome (Fraser syndrome). *Prenat Diagn.* 1997;17:582–584.
14. Bardakjian T, Weiss A, Schneider A. *Anophthalmia/Microphthalmia Overview.* NCBI. http://http://www.ncbi.nlm.nih.gov/books/NBK1378/. Accessed March 17, 2013.
15. Strigini F, Valleriani A, Cecchi M, et al. Prenatal ultrasound and magnetic resonance imaging features in a fetus with Walker-Warburg syndrome. *Ultrasound Obstet Gynecol.* 2009;33(3):363–365.
16. Castori M, Brancati F, Rinaldi R, et al. Antenatal presentation of the oculo-auriculo-vertebral spectrum (OAVS). *Am J Med Genet A.* 2006;140(14):1573–1579.
17. Chitayat D, Sroka H, Keating S, et al. The PDAC syndrome (pulmonary hypoplasia/agenesis, diaphragmatic hernia/eventration, anophthalmia/microphthalmia, and cardiac defect) (Spear syndrome, Matthew-Wood syndrome): report of eight cases including a living child and further evidence for autosomal recessive inheritance. *Am J Med Genet A.* 2007;143:1268–1281.
18. Demyer W, Zeman W, Palmer CG. The face predicts the brain: diagnostic significance of median facial anomalies for holoprosencephaly (arrhinencephaly). *Pediatrics.* 1964;34:256–263.
19. Stroustrup A, Levine D. MR imaging of the fetal skull, face and neck. In: Levine D, ed. *Atlas of Fetal MRI.* Boca Raton, FL: Taylor & Francis; 2005:73–90.
20. Cohen MM Jr, Richieri-Costa A, Guion-Almeida ML, et al. Hypertelorism: interorbital growth, measurements, and pathogenetic considerations. *Int J Oral Maxillofac Surg.* 1995;24(6):387–395.
21. Nazzaro A, Della Monica M, Lonardo F, et al. Prenatal ultrasound diagnosis of a case of Pfeiffer syndrome without cloverleaf skull and review of the literature. *Prenat Diagn.* 2004;24(11):918–922.
22. David DJ, Cooter RD, Edwards TJ. Crouzon twins with cloverleaf skull malformations. *J Craniofac Surg.* 1991;2:56–60.
23. Tonni G, Panteghini M, Rossi A, et al. Craniosynostosis: prenatal diagnosis by means of ultrasound and SSSE-MRI: family series with report of neurodevelopmental outcome and review of the literature. *Arch Gynecol Obstet.* 2011;283:909–916.
24. Weber B, Schwabegger AH, Vodopiutz J, et al. Prenatal diagnosis of apert syndrome with cloverleaf skull deformity using ultrasound, fetal magnetic resonance imaging and genetic analysis. *Fetal Diagn Ther.* 2010;27:51–56.
25. Itoh S, Nojima M, Yoshida K. Usefulness of magnetic resonance imaging for accurate diagnosis of Pfeiffer syndrome type II in utero. *Fetal Diagn Ther.* 2006;21:168–171.
26. Reches A, Yaron Y, Burdon K, et al. Prenatal detection of congenital bilateral cataract leading to the diagnosis of Nance-Horan syndrome in the extended family. *Prenat Diagn.* 2007;27:662–664.
27. Fayol L, Garcia P, Denis D, et al. Adams-Oliver syndrome associated with cutis marmorata telangiectatica congenita and congenital cataract: a case report. *Am J Perinatol.* 2006;23:197–200.
28. Başbuğ M, Serin IS, Özçelik B, et al. Prenatal ultrasonographic diagnosis of rhizomelic chondrodysplasia punctata by detection of rhizomelic shortening and bilateral cataracts. *Fetal Diagn Ther.* 2005;20:171–174.
29. Terhal P, Sakkers R, Hochstenbach R, et al. Cerebellar hypoplasia, zonular cataract, and peripheral neuropathy in trisomy 17 mosaicism. *Am J Med Genet A.* 2004;130:410–414.
30. Vutova K, Peicheva Z, Popova A, et al. Congenital toxoplasmosis: eye manifestations in infants and children. *Ann Trop Paediatr.* 2002;22:213–218.
31. Cengiz B, Baxi L. Congenital cataract in triplet pregnancy after ivf with frozen embryos: prenatal diagnosis and management. *Fetal Diagn Ther.* 2001;16:234–236.
32. Romain M, Awoust J, Dugauquier C, et al. Prenatal ultrasound detection of congenital cataract in trisomy 21. *Prenat Diagn.* 1999;19:780–782.
33. Beinder EJ, Pfeiffer RA, Bornemann A, et al. Second-trimester diagnosis of fetal cataract in a fetus with Walker-Warburg syndrome. *Fetal Diagn Ther.* 1997;12:197–199.
34. Shapiro I, Borochowitz Z, Degani S, et al. Neu-Laxova syndrome: prenatal ultrasonographic diagnosis, clinical and pathological studies, and new manifestations. *Am J Med Genet.* 1992;43:602–605.
35. Brent RL. The effects of ionizing radiation, microwaves, and ultrasound on the developing embryo: clinical interpretations and applications of the data. *Curr Probl Pediatr.* 1984;14:1–87.
36. Milic A, Blaser S, Robinson A, et al. Prenatal detection of microtia by MRI in a fetus with trisomy 22. *Pediatr Radiol.* 2006;36(7):706–710.
37. Ramji FG, Slovis TL, Baker JD. Orbital sonography in children. *Pediatr Radiol.* 1996;26:245–258.
38. Achiron R, Kreiser D, Achiron A. Axial growth of the fetal eye and evaluation of the hyaloid artery: in utero ultrasonographic study. *Prenat Diagn.* 2000;20:894–899.
39. Birnholz JC, Farrell EE. Fetal hyaloid artery: timing of regression with US. *Radiology.* 1988;166:781–783.
40. Dutton GN. Congenital disorders of the optic nerve: excavations and hypoplasia. *Eye.* 2004;18:1038–1048.
41. Righini A, Avagliano L, Doneda C, et al. Prenatal magnetic resonance imaging of optic nerve head coloboma. *Prenat Diagn.* 2008;28:242–246.
42. Bault JP, Salomon LJ, Guibaud L, et al. Role of three-dimensional ultrasound measurement of the optic tract in fetuses with agenesis of the septum pellucidum. *Ultrasound Obstet Gynecol.* 2011;37(5):570–575.
43. Kusanovic J, Mittal P, Goncalves L, et al. 3D ultrasound evaluation of the fetal optic chiasma potential parameter for the differential diagnosis of developmental midline brain anomalies. *Ultrasound Obstet Gynecol.* 2005;26:311.
44. Bault, JP. Prognostic value of fetal optic chiasm measurements in foetuses with septal agenesis. *Ultrasound Obstet Gynecol.* 2007;30:367–455.
45. Bault JP, Salomon LJ. Fetal optic chiasm measurements: reference range at 22–36 weeks of gestation. *Ultrasound Obstet Gynecol.* 2007;30:547–653.
46. Whitby E. In utero magnetic resonance imaging of developmental abnormalities of the fetal CNS. In: Griffiths P, Paley M, Whitby E, eds. *Imaging the Central Nervous System of the Fetus and Neonate.* New York, NY: Taylor & Francis; 2006:99–110.
47. Goldberg H, Sebire NJ, Holwell D, et al. Prenatal diagnosis of bilateral dacrocystoceles. *Ultrasound Obstet Gynecol.* 2000;15:448–449.
48. Davis WK, Mahony BS, Carroll BA, et al. Prenatal sonographic detection of benign dacryocystoceles (lacrimal duct cysts). *J Ultrasound Med.* 1987;6:461–465.
49. Yazici Z, Kline-Fath BM, Yazici B, et al. Congenital dacryocystocele: prenatal MRI findings. *Pediatr Radiol.* 2010;40:1868–1873.
50. Brugger PC, Weber M, Prayer D. Magnetic resonance imaging of the fetal efferent lacrimal pathways. *Eur Radiol.* 2010;20:1965–1973.
51. Smirniotopoulos JG, Chiechi MV. Teratomas, dermoids, and epidermoids of the head and neck. *Radiographics.* 1995;15(6):1437–1455.
52. Yoshida S, Kikuchi A, Naito S, et al. Giant hemangioma of the fetal neck, mimicking a teratoma. *J Obstet Gynaecol Res.* 2006;32(1):47–54.
53. Gnanaraj L, Skibell BC, Coret-Simon J, et al. Massive congenital orbital teratoma. *Ophthal Plast Reconstr Surg.* 2005;21(6):445–447.

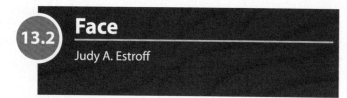

# Face

Judy A. Estroff

Craniofacial abnormalities are among the most common human malformations (Table 13.2-1),[1] which may occur in isolation or associated with other anomalies, chromosomal aberrations, genetic and nongenetic syndromes, and physical- or toxin-induced injury. Identification of a craniofacial abnormality on fetal imaging should prompt a thorough search for abnormalities in all other organ systems. When associated with part of a syndrome of multiple anomalies, craniofacial defects are sometimes easier to identify sonographically than more subtle abnormalities in other organs. After the face, the most frequently observed malformations are cardiovascular system, CNS, and skeletal.[2]

Facial abnormalities are important themselves but may also indicate an underlying problem, particularly a chromosome abnormality or syndromic condition (Table 13.2-2).[3] Therefore, it is important to evaluate the face when other anomalies are demonstrated and, conversely, search for additional anomalies when facial abnormalities are evident. The frequency of chromosome abnormalities varies with reasons for referral, patient population, and the sensitivity of detecting isolated facial abnormalities.

Sonographic craniofacial evaluation has been technically feasible only since the early 1980s.[4,5] Reports of cohorts undergoing routine sonographic screening suggest that sensitivity for

| Table 13.2-1 | Examples of Most Common Craniofacial Anomalies |
| --- | --- |

| Anomaly | Prevalence at Birth per 10,000 |
| --- | --- |
| Cleft lip ± palate | |
|   Caucasian | 10 |
|   Japanese | 20 |
|   Native (North) American | 36 |
|   African American population | 3 |
| Cleft palate | |
|   Averaged across races | 5 |
| Craniosynostosis | 3 |
|   Crouzon syndrome | 0.4 |
|   Apert syndrome | 0.15 |
| Otomandibular anomalies | 1.2 |
|   Treacher Collins syndrome | 0.2 |
| CHARGE association | 1 |
| Holoprosencephaly | 1.2 |
| Stickler syndrome | 1 |
| Fetal alcohol syndrome | 2 |

From Shaw W. Global strategies to reduce the health care burden of craniofacial anomalies: report of WHO meetings on international collaborative research on craniofacial anomalies. *Cleft Palate Craniofac J.* 2004;41(3):238–243; © Allen Press Publishing Services.

| Table 13.2-2 | Common Craniofacial Syndromes |
| --- | --- |
| Trisomy 21 Down syndrome | Flat facial profile Up-slanted palpebral fissures Small nose Small, dysplastic ears |
| Trisomy 13 Patau syndrome | Holoprosencephaly associated with midline facial anomalies, cyclopia, hypotelorism and clefts, scalp defects, microcephaly with sloping forehead, hypotelorism, micropthalmia with iris colobomas, dysplastic ears, premaxillary agenesis, cleft lip, micrognathia, cleft palate |
| Trisomy 18 Edward syndrome | Prominent occiput, bifrontal narrowing, low-set dysplastic ears, small mouth plus micrognathia |
| 4p minus Wolf–Hirshhorn syndrome | Cleft lip/palate "Greek-warrior helmet" facies: prominent sloped forehead, hypertelorism, high arched eyebrows, low-set ears with pre-auricular pit, short philtrum, downturned angles of the mouth, and micrognathia, ± microthalmia, and colobomas |
| 5p minus Cri-du-chat syndrome | Round face, down-slanting palpebral fissures, hypertelorism, low-set dysplastic and posteriorly rotated ears, downturned angles of mouth |
| Mosaic trisomy 8 | Low-set dysplastic ears Micrognathia |
| 22q II deletion syndrome | Hypertelorism, low-set ears, micrognathia, cleft palate |
| Beckwith–Wiedemann syndrome | Macroglossia Abnormal ears, ear lobe creases Capillary hemangiomas over forehead Coarse facial features |
| Campomelic dysplasia | Robin sequence, macrocephaly, large anterior fontanelle, flat nasal bridge, low-set ears, micrognathia, short neck |
| Stickler syndrome | Prominent eyes, midface hypoplasia, small nose, cataracts |
| Smith-Lemli-Opitz syndrome | Microcephaly, cleft palate, small anteverted nose, low-set ears, bifrontal narrowing, micrognathia |
| De Lange syndrome | Microbrachycephaly, excessive hair over face, single eyebrow (synophrys), small anteverted nose, hairy dysplastic and low-set ears, long philtrum, thin upper lip, downturned angles of the mouth, micrognathia |
| Apert syndrome | Turribrachycephaly, hypertelorism with proptosis, beaked nose, low-set ears, high-arched cleft palate |

Adapted from Suri M. Craniofacial syndromes. *Semin Fetal Neonatal Med.* 2005;10(3):243–257.

detection of craniofacial anomalies, such as cleft lip and palate is very low, under 20%.[6,7] Tertiary referral centers appear to have a significantly higher detection rate, as high as 70%.[8] This implies that although detection may be feasible, routine screening of the otherwise normal appearing fetus may not always include complete evaluation of the fetal face and head.

The American Institute of Ultrasound and Medicine (AIUM) standard of 2003 did not include routine fetal face evaluation, and only added this requirement to its guidelines for second- and third-trimester fetal sonography in its revised statement in 2007, on the basis of the consensus that it is extremely important to demonstrate that evaluable craniofacial aspects of the fetus are normal or to characterize the abnormality in an anomalous fetus.[9] Imaging of the fetal face in three planes, whenever possible, adds very little time and increases the likelihood of anomaly detection from 20% to 30% when only two planes are evaluated to nearly 90% when all three planes are used and the anatomy is understood.[10] Especially in the era of high-resolution three-dimensional (3D) sonography, many craniofacial anomalies are detected when the sonographer attempts to take a keepsake 3D frontal or profile image of the fetus for the parents and notes an aberration.[11]

Fetal diagnosis of craniofacial anomalies, especially orofacial clefts, is even possible in the first trimester, at or before the time of first trimester nuchal translucency measurement.[12–16] Timmerman et al.,[17] found a strong association between increased nuchal translucency and orofacial clefts in chromosomally normal fetuses.

## EMBRYOLOGY OF THE FACE

Facial morphology is established between weeks 4 and 10 after conception. Formation is based on the fusion of the midline frontonasal prominence (FNP) and three other paired prominences: maxillary processes (MXP), lateral nasal processes (LNP), and mandibular nasal processes (MNP). These prominences are filled with neural crest cells. The FNP leads to formation of the forehead, midline of the nose, philtrum, middle portion of the upper lip, and primary palate. The LNP gives rise to the nasal alae. The MXP forms the upper jaw, the sides of the face, the sides of the upper lip, and the secondary palate (Fig. 13.2-1).

The four branchial arches appear at 4 to 5 weeks of development, and represent bars of mesenchymal tissue that are separated by clefts. They appear between days 22 and 29 and give rise to skeletal, visceral, arterial, muscular, and neurologic components of the head and neck. At the end of week 4, the stomodeum (rudimentary mouth) forms in the center of the face and is surrounded by the first pair of branchial arches. Branchial arches have a mesenchymal core covered on the outside by ectoderm and on the inside by epithelium (endodermal in origin). Branchial arches contain neural crest cells that contribute to the skeletal development of the face. The mesoderm develops

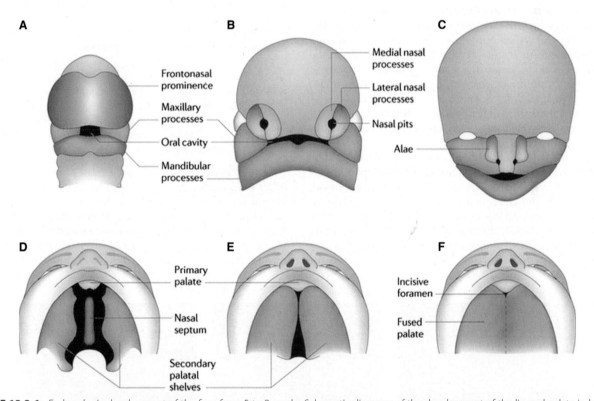

**FIGURE 13.2-1:** Embryologic development of the face from 5 to 8 weeks. Schematic diagrams of the development of the lip and palate in humans. **A:** The developing frontonasal prominence, paired maxillary processes, and paired mandibular processes surround the primitive oral cavity by the 4th week of embryonic development. **B:** By the 5th week, the nasal pits have formed, which leads to the formation of the paired medial and lateral nasal processes. **C:** The medial nasal processes have merged with the maxillary processes to form the upper lip and primary palate by the end of the 6th week. The lateral nasal processes form the nasal alae. Similarly, the mandibular processes fuse to form the lower jaw. **D:** During the 6th week of embryogenesis, the secondary palate develops as bilateral outgrowths from the maxillary processes, which grow vertically down the side of the tongue. **E:** Subsequently, the palatal shelves elevate to a horizontal position above the tongue, contact one another, and commence fusion. **F:** Fusion of the palatal shelves ultimately divides the oronasal space into separate oral and nasal cavities. (Reproduced with permission from Dixon MJ, Marazita ML, Beaty TH, et al. Cleft lip and palate: understanding genetic and environmental influences. *Nat Rev Genet.* 2011;12.)

into the muscles of the face and the neck. The first branchial arch gives rise to the maxilla and the mandible (including the premaxilla, zygoma) and part of the temporal bone.

The nasal placodes evaginate to form the nasal pits. The resulting ridges, the FNP, form the upper boundary of the stomodeum. Coming from the first branchial arch, the paired MXP form the lateral boundaries of the stomodeum. The paired MNP (also from the first branchial arch) form the caudal boundary. Between weeks 5 and 8, the MXP grow medially, obliterating the grooves between the nasal FNP and the MXP. The upper lip is formed by the fusion of the MXP and medial nasal prominences. The mandibular prominences (MNP) merge to form the lower lip, chin, and mandible.

The nose is formed by five prominences. The FNP forms the bridge of the nose, and the two medial nasal swellings that fuse together to form the intermaxillary segment are responsible in forming the crest, tip, and central portion and philtrum of the upper lip, the incisor teeth, and the front triangular portion of the palate (primary palate). The LNP form the sides, or the alae. The secondary palate is formed by shelf-like outgrowth from the maxillary prominences. These palatine shelves appear in the 6th week and in the 7th week ascend in a horizontal position above the tongue, fusing to form the secondary palate. The triangular primary palate is separated from the secondary by the incisive foramen (see Fig. 13.2-1).

The partial or complete lack of fusion of one or both of the prominences with the medial nasal swellings and maxillary prominences results in a unilateral or bilateral cleft lip and palate, which may involve the primary and/or secondary palate. A split in the primary palate occurs between the lateral incisors and the canine teeth and along the side of the upper lip in the paramedian position. If only the secondary palate is abnormal, a cleft behind the incisive foramen or bifid uvula may result. The rare median cleft lip is caused by incomplete merging of the two medial nasal swellings, or intermaxillary segment, and is more often associated with severe congenital anomalies such as holoprosencephaly.

The primitive nasal cavity begins as a single chamber. The nasal septum has both a cartilaginous and a bony stage of development. At about 5 weeks, the septum forms anteriorly from the enlarging frontonasal process and continues to grow posteriorly until it meets with the horizontal palatine processes in the midline (see Fig. 13.2-1). Eventually, by the 9th or 10th week, the embryo has distinct and separate respiratory and digestive openings.

First branchial arch anomalies are from an insufficiency of neural crest cells. Malformations resulting from this defect include Treacher Collins syndrome (mandibulofacial dysostosis) and Robin association. Because neural crest cells also contribute to the formation of the aortic and pulmonary arteries, some first arch syndromes can be accompanied by congenital heart defects.[18]

## TECHNIQUE FOR EXAMINATION

For those charged with the task of identifying and classifying fetal cleft lip/palate and other craniofacial anomalies, a comprehensive routine 2D and 3D sonographic protocol should be in place and would ideally include the option for additional evaluation of the secondary palate and brain by fetal MRI. The imager should have familiarity with craniofacial embryology and with the most common systems for classifying craniofacial anomalies (Table 13.2-3). There is great value in fostering a close and collaborative working relationship with regional craniofacial surgeons and their team, and in understanding what these clinicians wish to know about the fetus to accurately counsel parents and prepare for postnatal evaluation and treatment.[19–22]

Ultrasound can optimally demonstrate the external contour of the face when it is outlined by fluid. Most imagers evaluate the fetal face subjectively using three orthogonal views (Table 13.2-4):

- **Coronal**: from the most superficial, "en face" view of the face, looking first at the soft tissues of the eyes, cheeks, nose, and mouth (Fig. 13.2-2A), from the outermost surface of the tip of the nose, then inward to deeper bony and soft tissue structures of the nasal vomer, tooth-bearing bony alveolus and tongue, and finally into the primary bony palate and orbits
- **Axial**: viewing the mandible, maxilla, tongue (Fig. 13.2-2B), tooth buds, and orbits
- **Sagittal**: evaluating the facial profile (Fig. 13.2-2C), including the nasal bridge, frontal bone, maxilla, mandible, and position of the tongue

Facial features can also be seen from a unique perspective using 3D sonography (Figs. 13.2-3 to 13.2-5), which is often helpful for clinicians and parents, but can be of limited use in the setting of oligohydramnios, fetal crowding, or unfavorable fetal position. Three-dimensional ultrasound often adds detail to the evaluation of fetal craniofacial malformations, including cleft lip, with or without cleft lip and/or palate (CLP).[11,23,24]

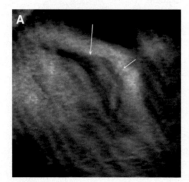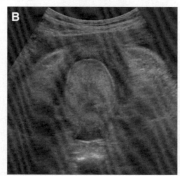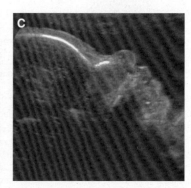

**FIGURE 13.2-2: A:** Normal lip. 2D sonogram of a normal fetal lip at 31 weeks showing the white roll, vermillion border *(long arrow)*, and Cupid's bow *(short arrow)*. **B:** Normal tongue. 2D sonogram of a normal fetal tongue in axial view at 36 weeks' gestation. **C:** Normal 2D sagittal face profile.

| Table 13.2-3 | Glossary of Craniofacial Terms |
|---|---|
| Aglossia | Absent tongue |
| Agnathia | Absent mandible |
| Ala or alar | Tissue comprising the lateral boundary of the nose |
| Alveolus/alveolar ridge/ alveolar process/alveolar arches | Bony arches of the maxilla (upper jaw) and mandible (lower jaw) that contain teeth |
| Anotia | Absent ears |
| Canthus | Corner of the eyelids |
| Cebocephaly | Orbital hypotelorism associated with a single nostril nose |
| Choanal atresia | Unilateral or bilateral obstruction of the posterior choanae of the nose |
| Coloboma | Congenital malformation of the eye causing defects in the lens, iris, or retina |
| Columella | Fleshy lower margin of the nasal septum, between the nostrils; the strip of skin running from the tip of the nose to the upper lip, which separates the nostrils |
| Craniosynostosis | Premature closure of the skull sutures |
| Ethmoid bone | Bone between the eyes; forms upper part of nasal septum, sidewalls of eye socket |
| Exorbitism | Abnormal protrusion of the eyeball secondary to a shallow or small orbit |
| Frontal bone | Forehead, including brow and top of eye socket |
| Frenulum | Folds of mucous membrane connecting the inside of the lips to the gums, and the tongue to the floor of the mouth |
| Glabella | Bony part between the eyebrows |
| Globe | Eyeball |
| Glossoptosis | Downward and posterior displacement of the tongue |
| Glossopexy | Surgical anterior pexy of the tongue to prevent airway obstruction |
| Hypertelorism | Abnormally increased orbital distance |
| Hypotelorism | Abnormally decreased orbital distance |
| IOD (inner orbital distance) | Distance from inner to inner bony margins of the orbits |
| Incisive foramen | Opening in incisive fossa of the hard palate |
|  | Primary palate = anterior to incisive foramen |
|  | Secondary palate = posterior to incisive foramen |
| Macroglossia | Enlarged tongue |
| Macrostomia | Large or wide mouth |
| Malar | Cheekbone just below the eyes |
| Mandible | Lower jaw |
| Maxilla | Upper jaw |
| Microform cleft lip | Vermillion cutaneous notch less than 3 mm above the normal peak |
| Micrognathia | Having an unusually small upper or lower jaw |
| Microstomia | Small mouth |
| Microtia | Small ears |
| Midface retrusion | Posterior positioning and/or vertical shortening of the infraorbital and perialar regionsIncreased concavity of the face |
| Mini-microform cleft lip | Disrupted vermillion-cutaneous junction without elevation of the bow peak |
| Minor-form cleft lip | Defect extending 3 mm or more above the normal Cupid's bow peak |
| Nasal bone | Bridge of the nose |
| Nares | Openings in the nasal cavity; nostrils |
| OOD (outer orbital distance) | Distance between bony margins of the outer lateral orbital walls |
| Otocephaly | Absent or hypoplastic mandible, microstomia, hypo or aglossia, posteriorly rotated and low-set ears |
| Perpendicular plate of the ethmoid | Upper part of the nasal septum |
| Philtrum | Vertical groove in median portion of upper lip |
| Premaxilla | Front middle portion of the upper jaw containing front teeth (incisors) |
| Prolabium | Prominent central part of the upper lip overlying the premaxilla |
| Proptosis | Forward projection or displacement of the eyeball |
| Retrognathia | Posteriorly positioned lower jaw, set back from plane of the face |
| Robin sequence | Includes cleft soft palate, small mouth, micrognathia/retrognathia, and glossoptosis |
| Sphenoid bone | Central part of the cranial floor. Forms part of the floor and sidewalls of the eye socket |
| Submucous cleft palate | Cleft of the muscle layer of the soft palate with an intact layer of mucosa lying over the defect |
| Tissue band | Thin bridge of tissue connecting the lateral and medial sides of a cleft lip |
| Vermillion border | Pink/purple lip tissue outlining the upper lip; "Cupid's bow" of upper lip |
| Vomer | Back and bottom part of the nasal septum |
| Zygomatic arch | The cheekbone that connects to the temple, a continuation of the malar bone |

| Table 13.2-4 | Sonographic Protocol for Evaluation of Fetal Face and Neck: 2D + 3D in the Axial, Coronal, and Sagittal Planes |
|---|---|
| Skull and brain | Skull shape: normal, dolichocephalic, brachycephalic, unusual |
| | Sutures: open, no defects |
| | Normal underlying brain |
| | Measurements: normal head size compared with long bone and abdominal biometry for given gestational age (BPD/OFD/HC vs. GA, AD, FL, HL) |
| | Skin around head: normal, thickened, mass |
| Face | Mouth: vermillion border intact |
| | Nares: symmetric, not flattened or cleft |
| | Vomer: straight, midline |
| | OOD/IOD, OD, orbital shape, symmetry: two orbits with normal size globes and normal interocular distance |
| | Maxilla: normal intact arc-shaped alveolus |
| | Mandible: normal intact arc-shaped alveolus |
| | Tongue: position, size |
| | Ears: size, shape, position |
| | Forehead: normal, sloped, bulging |
| | Midface: normal, retruded |
| | Chin: normal vs. small (micrognathia), retruded (retrognathia) or both |
| Neck and spine | Head position |
| | Length of spine, curvature |
| | Presence of nuchal cord, skin thickening |
| | Integrity of vertebrae, lamina, and spinous processes |
| | Position of trachea, thyroid, strap muscles |
| | Evaluate vallecula and pyriform sinuses, glottis, subglottic trachea, carina |

BPD, biparietal diameter; OFD, occipitofrontal diameter; HC, head circumference; GA, gestational age; AD, abdominal diameter; FL, femur length; HL, humeral length; OOD, outer orbital distance; IOD, inner orbital distance; OD, ocular diameter.

New techniques using 3D ultrasound have been described to visualize the secondary palate, including the "3D reverse view," described by Campbell et al.[25] in 2005, the "flipped face view" described by Platt et al.[26] in 2006, and the "oblique face view" described by Pilu and Segata[27] in 2007. All of these views require software manipulation and add to the length of the study, although the patient may be discharged as these images are created. In expert hands, the manipulation may take only a few minutes. A study comparing the accuracy of reverse, flipped, and oblique face methods for visualization of the hard and soft palate by Martinez Ten et al. demonstrated accuracy of all three methods to visualize the upper lip and alveolar ridge (71%, 86%, and 100%, respectively). However, soft (secondary) palate involvement was diagnosed correctly in only one of seven fetuses in the flipped face and oblique face views. The reverse face view could not identify the secondary palate.[28]

Because of its unique display, 3D ultrasound aids parents and referring physicians to understanding the extent of the defects. Parental decisions may be affected in evaluation of CL/P, because they can view the abnormality on a recognizable image.

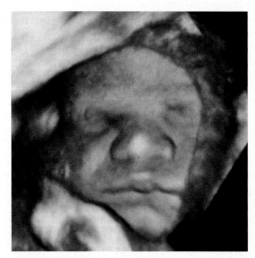

**FIGURE 13.2-3:** The normal fetal face. 3D sonogram at 34 weeks' gestation.

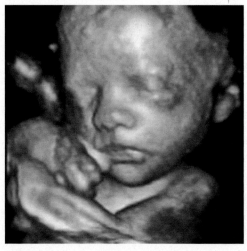

**FIGURE 13.2-4:** The normal fetal face. 3D sonogram at 28 weeks' gestation.

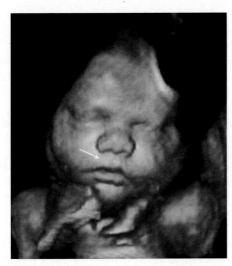

**FIGURE 13.2-5:** The normal fetal nose. 3D sonogram of a third-trimester fetus showing normal nasal structures: bridge, tip, nostrils, ala, alar base, philtral columns *(arrow)*, and philtral dimple *(asterisk)*.

Three-dimesional ultrasonographic imaging of fetal tooth buds can aid in the accurate classification of clefts,[11,27–29] but accurate detection of accompanying or isolated cleft secondary palate is often possible only by the addition of fetal MRI.

Fetal magnetic resonance imaging (MRI) has the potential to better visualize the palate as well as internal craniofacial, brain, and body anatomy. MRI is now routinely used to evaluate the fetal brain and chest, and is increasingly being used to evaluate the fetal face. Fetal MRI has an advantage over fetal sonography in its ability to demonstrate the secondary palate, which is mainly soft tissue (Fig. 13.2-6). Assessment of the secondary palate is limited on sonography because of the proximity of normal bony structures, which block ultrasound waves.

Nomograms for the proportions of the fetal face have been published, including frontomaxillary angle, nasal bone length, chin length, and tongue dimensions. Identification of tooth buds within the normal arc-shaped maxillary and mandibular alveoli is extremely helpful in assessing facial features and in excluding facial clefts (Fig. 13.2-6C). Maxillary and mandibular shapes are readily assessed with 2D and 3D sonography as well

as with fetal MRI. An abnormally shaped maxilla can be seen in various chromosomal anomalies, such as trisomy 21, in the setting of cleft lip ± palate, and in many syndromes.[30]

Fetal nose evaluation is often subjective. However, normal biometric measurements for nasal bone width and length between 14 and 40 weeks are available, and there is a linear growth relationship between those measurements and gestational age.[31–33] Measurement of nasal bone length is now a standard part of the first trimester (between 11 and 13 weeks) fetal sonogram, along with measurement of the nuchal translucency. A short or absent nasal bone raises the likelihood of trisomy 21. Very recent transition from imaging findings to routine first trimester maternal serum screening by measurement of free fetal DNA (ffDNA) will likely make first trimester nasal bone measurement less important, and has already significantly reduced the use of second trimester amniocentesis for advanced maternal age or the presence of "soft markers" for Down Syndrome on sonography, including echogenic bowel, pyelectasis, and echogenic intracardiac focus (EIF).[34]

Evaluating fetal jaw position and morphology is also usually subjective. However, mandibular measurements may be obtained in several different ways (see Chapter 20, Syndromes characterized by Mandibular/Auricular Anomalies). Chitty advocates measuring the length of the mandibular rami and provides normative data between 12 and 28 weeks.[35]

The orbits are routinely assessed on sonography in an axial or a coronal view of the face, but are often seen to advantage on fetal MR. Two equal-sized orbits should be present. The distance between the orbits (interorbital distance) should be slightly greater than the diameter of one globe. If these measurements are abnormal, the rest of the fetal face and body must be scrutinized because of the high number of associated systemic abnormalities.[36,37] It is important to note that MR and US orbit nomograms are different and should not be interchanged.

## Holoprosencephaly

As De Meyer et al.[38] pointed out in 1964, "The face predicts the brain." Certain facial anomalies predictably have associated brain anomalies, such as cyclopia with a proboscis seen in association with holoprosencephaly. Other facial anomalies seen in holoprosencephaly (Fig. 13.2-7) include cebocephaly, in

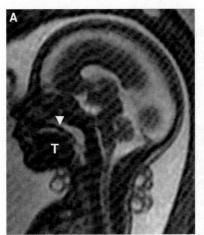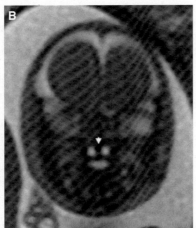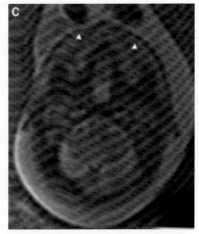

**FIGURE 13.2-6:** 23-Week fetus with normal palate. **A:** Sagittal plane shows secondary palate *(arrowhead)*. T, tongue. **B:** Coronal plane shows vomer *(arrowhead)* and palatal shelves. **C:** Axial plane shows tooth-bearing alveolus *(arrowheads)* and ear anatomy.

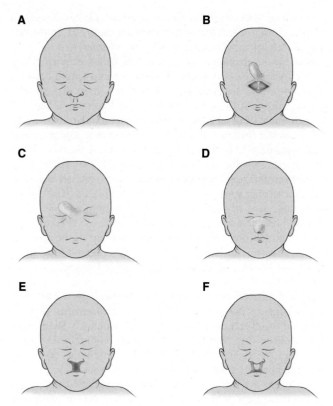

**FIGURE 13.2-7:** The many faces of holoprosencephaly: normal **(A)**, cyclopia **(B)**, ethmocephaly **(C)**, cebocephaly **(D)**, median cleft lip and palate **(E)**, bilateral cleft lip and palate **(F)**.

which the eyes are close together and the nose has a single nostril (Fig. 13.2-8); ethmocephaly, in which there is absence of the nose (arhinia) and a blind-ending tubular structure (proboscis) between the eyes; or median cleft lip and palate.[39–42]

# NOSE

The nose is well seen on fetal sonography (see Fig. 13.2-5), and is visible but often less well seen on fetal MRI. Contour anomalies of the nose can include asymmetry and flattening, as is seen in cleft lip, especially in severe unilateral complete CLP, frontonasal dysplasia, and arhinia. The nose may be abnormally prominent, as is seen when there is a nasal mass, such as a dermoid, frontal encephalocele, or a duplicated nostril. The intermaxillary segment in bilateral CLP can be confused for a nasal mass. The normal regions of the nose include the bridge, nares, alae, and alar base.

## Arhinia

**Definition/Incidence:** Absence of the nose, arhinia, is a rare anomaly with a poorly understood pathogenesis, likely occurring between weeks 3 and 10 of life.[43,44]

**Pathogenesis/Etiology:** The formation of the nose and sinuses is an intricate process that progresses through three distinct phases: the preskeletal phase, the chondrocranial stage, and the stage of ossification. In the preskeletal phase, mesenchymal swellings develop around the olfactory placodes. The primary nasal cavity appears at about 4 weeks,

heralding the chondrocranial stage, in which the cartilaginous nasal framework develops. The bony structures of the nose and sinuses are well along in development by the end of the first trimester. Arhinia may develop from failure of the nasal epithelial plugs to reabsorb during the 13th to 15th weeks of gestation.

**Imaging:** In the fetus, arhinia can be suspected when on sonography, the imager cannot identify the nostrils or nasal bone, and the fetal profile shows severe midface flattening (Fig. 13.2-9). The upper lip can be mistaken for the nose. On fetal MRI, there will be absence of the nasal cavity and vomer. Multiple anomalies are associated with arhinia, including holoprosencephaly, CLP, and micro- or anopthalmia.

**Management:** Infants who are born with arhinia have difficulty breathing and eating, as newborns are obligate nose-breathers. The condition is associated with cleft lip and palate, and anomalies affecting the eyes and brain, as well as anomalies related to chromosome 9. The diagnosis is obvious at birth, with an absent nose, hypoplastic maxilla, and a high-arched palate. Some reports indicate that the infant with arhinia can adapt to oral breathing, with nutritional support given directly into the stomach. If the child survives, definitive repair is usually undertaken during the preschool years.[44]

## Proboscis

**Definition/Incidence:** Proboscis lateralis, or congenital tubular nose, is a rare anomaly in which the external nose fails to develop on one side and is replaced by a small-caliber elephant trunk-like soft tissue structure hanging from the inner canthus of the eye. It has no nasal cavity but may connect to deeper structures such as the dura or skull base. This peculiar abnormality is often associated with holoprosencephaly.

**Imaging:** A proboscis appears as a soft tissue protrusion in the middle of the face, usually between the eyes (Fig. 13.2-10). As it is fully formed of soft tissue, it is often seen best on sonography, especially early in gestation.

**Management:** Treatment involves excision of the proboscis at an early age and re-routing of the nasolacrimal duct.[44]

## Choanal Atresia

**Definition/Incidence:** Unilateral or bilateral obstruction of the posterior choanae of the nose occurs in approximately 1 in 7,000 to 1 in 8,000 live births. The condition occurs more often in females and on the right side.

**Pathogenesis/Etiology:** Choanal atresia is associated with other anomalies in up to 50% of cases, with the most common being the CHARGE association (see Chapter 20) (Fig. 13.2-11). The CHARGE association occurs in approximately 1 in 10,000 to 1 in 15,000 births. **CHARGE** is an acronym standing for the following components: *c*oloboma; *h*eart (ASD, conotruncal lesions); *a*tresia, membranous or bony of the choanae; *r*etardation in growth and development; *g*enitourinary, involving undescended testes, microphallus, hydronephrosis; and *e*ar, involving external, middle, and inner ear defects.[44] The criteria

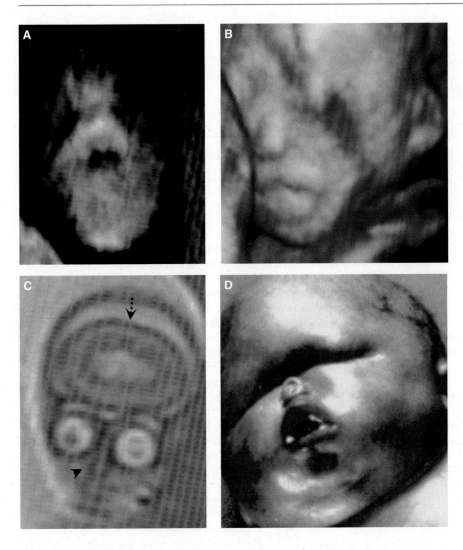

**FIGURE 13.2-8:** 21-Week fetus with alobar holoprosencephaly. **A:** Coronal US showing single nostril. **B:** 3D demonstrating single nostril and closely spaced eyes. **C:** Coronal MRI also depicts single nostril *(arrowhead)*, hypotelorism and fused cerebral hemispheres *(dotted arrow)*. **D:** A different infant with cebocephaly and holoprosencephaly. Images courtesy of Beth Kline-Fath.

for the diagnosis of CHARGE syndrome have been expanded to include any newborn with four major or three major and three minor criteria. Major criteria include coloboma, choanal atresia, external, middle or inner ear anomalies, and cranial nerve dysfunction. Minor criteria include genital hypoplasia, developmental delay, cardiovascular anomalies, short stature, cleft lip or palate, tracheoesophageal defects, and characteristic facial features.[3]

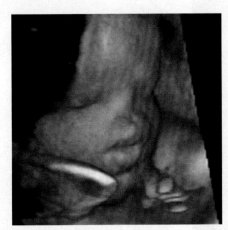

**FIGURE 13.2-9** 34-Week gestation fetus with arhinia (absent nose) and microphthalmia. After birth, the diagnosis of Bosma arhinia syndrome was made.

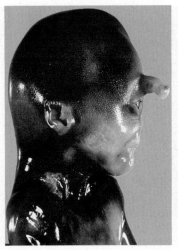

**FIGURE 13.2-10:** Proboscis. Pathologic photograph of a fetus with proboscis and cyclopia.

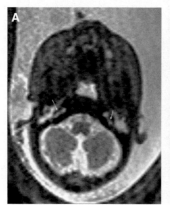
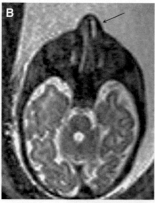

**FIGURE 13.2-11:** CHARGE syndrome: Fetal MR at 34 weeks shows multiple anomalies in keeping with CHARGE syndrome, including bilateral inner ear anomalies *(arrows)* **(A)**, left choanal atresia *(black arrow)* **(B)**. The fetus also had left coloboma, esophageal atresia, and inferior vermian hypoplasia (not shown).

**Imaging:** On US, the nasal cavity is filled with fluid. On MRI, the posterionasal cavity is closed, either by bone or by soft tissue (see Fig. 13.2-11B).

**Prognosis/Management:** Most choanal atresia is bony (90%). Bilateral choanal atresia is a neonatal emergency as the infant, an obligate nose breather, presents with respiratory distress at rest, relieved only by crying. Immediate treatment is by placement of an oral airway. Definitive treatment involves surgically creating new posterior choanae.[44] Isolated choanal atresia can present as the only anomaly in otherwise normal fetuses, or may be part of a syndrome.

## Nasal Masses

Nasal masses are uncommon but are frequently seen in specialized pediatric centers and are often recognized in utero. The most common congenital nasal masses are nasal dermoids, nasopharyngeal teratomas, gliomas (Fig. 13.2-12), encephaloceles, and lacrimal duct cysts. Nasal duplication is a rare

anomaly. Nasal dermoids and lacrimal duct cysts are benign, and most are treated fairly easily after birth. Teratomas, gliomas, and encephaloceles are much more concerning lesions as they often invade or distort adjacent tissues or craniofacial structures.

## MOUTH AND LIP

### Cleft Lip and/or Palate (CLP)

Sonographic detection of facial clefts has been possible only since the early 1980s. Since then, advances in 2D, 3D, and 4D imaging have been startling, with continuous improvements in resolution and technique from year to year. It is now possible to detect even the most subtle surface anomalies, such as preauricular skin tags and microform incomplete cleft lip, and to observe fetal facial expression and behavior.[24]

The value of detecting fetal craniofacial anomalies has been controversial, proponents arguing that fetal detection allows parents to prepare, both psychologically and practically, for the birth of a child with a facial anomaly, and that detection of a craniofacial anomaly allows the obstetric specialist the opportunity to search for other or associated anomalies, and to refer the family to a craniofacial specialist. Opponents of fetal craniofacial screening argue that (1) facial clefts alone do not threaten fetal survival; (2) there is currently no practical fetal treatment; and that (3) postnatal remedies are well established and have a very favorable outcome. However, both parents and specialists maintain that knowledge of the fetal anomaly is of great benefit and eases the transition into treatment after birth.[22]

**Epidemiology/Incidence:** Cleft L/P is the most common congenital anomaly aside from congenital heart disease, and occurs more frequently in aborted fetuses and stillborns than in live births. Cleft L/P incidence is estimated at 1:500 to 1:1,000 live births.[1,4,13,29,45] The risk of genetic syndromes is increased if the alveolus or secondary palate is involved. There are racial differences in the incidence of clefts, highest in the Asian population (0.79 to 3.74 per 1,000), lower for Caucasians (0.91 to 2.7/1,000), and lowest for blacks (0.18 to 1.67/1,000). Males are more frequently affected than females for CL/P by approximately 1.4:1.0.

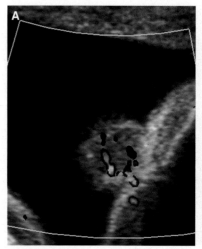
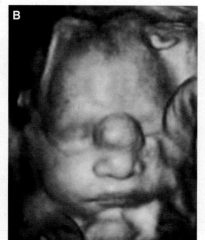
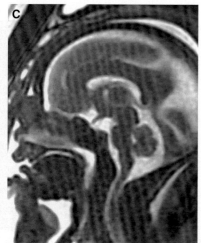

**FIGURE 13.2-12:** Nasal glioma. Fetal US **(A and B)** and MRI **(C)** at 28-week 5-day gestation showing vascular soft tissue mass in the midline, above the bridge of the nose.

Females more frequently have isolated CP. Males and females are equally affected by isolated cleft lip.[46]

**Pathogenesis/Types:** Knowledge of normal embryology is important for understanding the pathogenesis of facial clefts. Nonfusion of the normal medial nasal swelling and maxillary prominence is the etiology for most cleft lip and/or palate. If the facial abnormality does not follow a normal embryologic pattern, then an amniotic band syndrome should be considered.

The array of possible types of facial clefts is vast (Fig. 13.2-13). In a recent large series of 782 patients by Nagase et al., in Japan, the most frequent type of cleft was cleft lip and palate (40.8%) (Fig. 13.2-14). Cleft lip and palate occurred more often in males; isolated cleft palate occurred more often in females. Cleft lip (55.3%) and cleft lip and palate (50.7%) occurred more often on the left side. A total of 44 cleft patterns were diagnosed, including 9 patterns seen in only one patient each.[47] Cleft lip can be unilateral (Fig. 13.2-15) or bilateral and each side can be completely cleft or incompletely cleft. If the cleft is bilateral, the sides may be symmetric or asymmetric (Fig. 13.2-16).

Mulliken defined three subgroups of incomplete cleft lip, and placed them in a spectrum termed "lesser-form" cleft lip, depending upon how far above the vermillion border of the lip

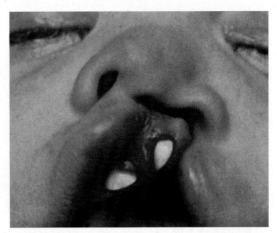

**FIGURE 13.2-14:** Unilateral cleft lip and palate. Infant at time of surgical repair showing unilateral cleft lip and palate with depression of nose on side of cleft.

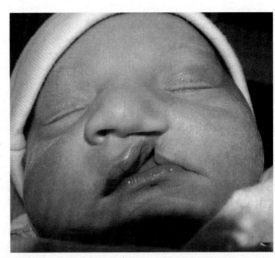

**FIGURE 13.2-15:** Incomplete cleft lip. Photograph of newborn with left unilateral incomplete cleft lip, intact alveolus, and secondary palate. Note flattening and widening of the ipsilateral nostril and ala.

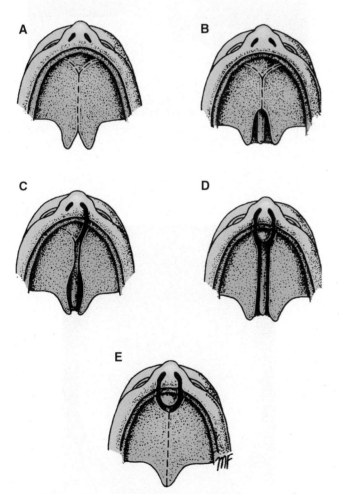

**FIGURE 13.2-13:** Types of cleft lip and palate. Inferior view of various types of cleft lip and palate. **A:** Bifid uvula. **B:** Cleft soft palate. **C:** Unilateral complete cleft lip and palate. **D:** Bilateral complete cleft lip and palate. **E:** Bilateral cleft lip. (From Snell RS. The head and neck. In: *Clinical Anatomy by Regions*. Philadelphia, PA: Lippincott Williams & Wilkins; 2011.)

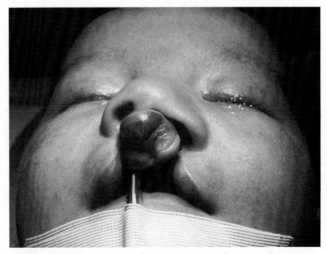

**FIGURE 13.2-16:** Bilateral cleft lip and palate with premaxillary protrusion. Photograph at time of surgical repair shows bilateral cleft lip and palate with prominent premaxillary protrusion.

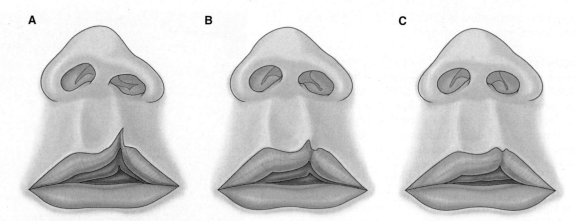

**FIGURE 13.2-17:** Microform cleft lip. **A:** Minor-form cleft lip. **B:** Microform cleft lip. **C:** Mini-microform cleft lip. (Adapted from Yuzuriha S, Mulliken JB. Minor-form, microform, and mini-microform cleft lip: anatomical features, operative techniques, and revisions. *Plast Reconstr Surg.* 2008;122:1485–1493.)

they extend.[48] "Minor-form" cleft extends equal to or greater than 3 mm above the normal Cupid's bow peak; "microform" cleft has a notch less than 3 mm above the normal side, and "mini-microform" clefts have a discontinuity in the vermillion border (Fig. 13.2-17).

In patients with bilateral cleft lip, there is also a wide variation in presentation. Bilateral symmetric complete cleft lip with an uplifted, protruding premaxillary segment, is the most common (Figs. 13.2-18 and 13.2-19; see Fig. 13.2-16). Bilateral symmetric incomplete cleft lip is less common. In this form, there may be notches in the tooth-bearing maxillary alveolus, and the secondary palate is intact. The least common form of bilateral cleft lip is complete or incomplete on the more severe side, and incomplete or lesser-form on the contralateral side.[49]

Median cleft lip and palate occur rarely, typically associated with other anomalies or syndromes such as holoprosencephaly (Figs. 13.2-20). Asymmetric or slash-like defects in the lip or palate should raise suspicion for amniotic band syndrome.

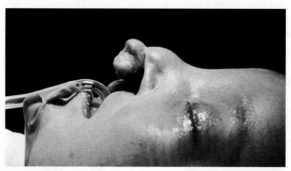

**FIGURE 13.2-19:** Premaxillary protrusion. Photograph of an infant with bilateral cleft lip and palate showing prominent premaxillary protrusion.

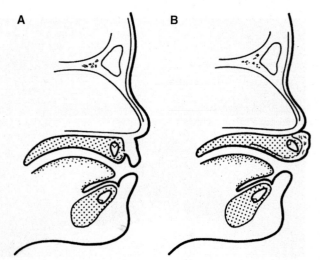

**FIGURE 13.2-18:** Development of premaxillary protrusion with bilateral cleft lip and palate. **A:** Normal sagittal view. **B:** Bilateral cleft lip and palate permits forward migration of the premaxillary segment.

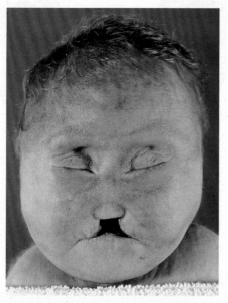

**FIGURE 13.2-20:** Holoprosencephaly with central cleft lip. Postmortem photograph of infant with hypotelorism, holoprosencephaly, and a midline cleft lip and palate.

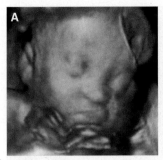
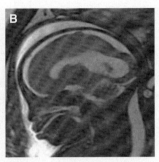

**FIGURE 13.2-21:** Midface hypoplasia. 28w3d fetus with midface hypoplasia secondary trisomy 21. **A:** 3D ultrasound. **B:** Sagittal MRI.

## Imaging

***Ultrasound:*** The ability to detect a cleft lip is dependent upon the technical resolution of the individual sonographic unit, and upon the knowledge and skill of the sonographer. In the early 1980s, the diagnosis was made by 2D US, which was supplemented by the additional capabilities of 3D technology in the late nineties, and 4D sonography in the decade following. 3D US technology, when optimal conditions are present (adequate amniotic fluid, favorable fetal position, and maternal habitus), is astonishingly detailed. The evolution of 4D US has allowed the evaluation of fetal behavior through the observation of fetal expressions. Using the intrinsic capability of 3D US, the imager can be certain when the rendered profile is midline, leading to increased accuracy and reproducibility of such diagnoses as micrognathia and midface hypoplasia (Fig. 13.2-21).[24]

Although the major events in facial development have all occurred by 8 weeks' gestation, anomalies are difficult to see sonographically at that age. However, by the end of the first trimester, fortuitously corresponding to the ideal timepoint for first trimester screening and measurement of the nuchal translucency, the fetal craniofacial structures are large enough to be evaluable in many patients.

In the first and second trimesters, evaluation by sonography involves both surface renderings and evaluation of deeper bony structures. Coronal and axial imaging are very helpful and an axial view of the tooth-bearing aveolar ridge can determine if a cleft palate is present. Sonography is ideal for assessing the fetal lip and nose, and even subtle clefts of the lip can often be detected (Fig. 13.2-22). Although fetal MRI can be used for evaluation of the fetal lip, resolution of these tissues is better on US, especially in the second trimester. For evaluating the structures posterior to the lip, sonography may be exceptionally accurate for bone detail, if fetal position and amniotic fluid volume are favorable. Unilateral cleft lip and palate is most common (Fig. 13.2-23). Bilateral cleft lip and palate may be suggested by prominent echogenic soft tissue below the nose, representing the protuberant premaxillary segment (Fig. 13.2-24); sometimes, however, bilateral cleft lip and palate is not associated with a protuberant premaxillary segment. Although there are secondary clues to the presence of a cleft palate on sonography, the secondary palate itself cannot easily or reliably be visualized (Table 13.2-5).

Clefts are more common in some populations than in others, and certain types of clefts are more common than others. Some specialized centers and practices have high rates of cleft detection on sonography, often using particular 2D- and 3D-enhanced views, which may not easily be transferable to screening practices.[50] A recent meta-analysis of cleft detection rate in 27 studies including both low- and high-risk populations showed rates of 9% to 100% for detection of cleft lip without cleft palate, 0% to 22% for cleft palate only, and 0% to 73% for all clefts.[51]

Differing levels of expertise and use of a range of advanced and more basic or older US equipment likely led to this range of detection rates, but this variation may reflect the reality of contemporary screening. This study also pointed out that, while 3D US did well in predicting cleft palate in the presence of cleft lip, 3D US is not reliable for the detection of isolated cleft palate.

Most screening for cleft lip and other anomalies takes place at centers relying on 2D sonography. The routine use of 3D sonography for screening has not been validated, as it is time consuming and is not cost-effective. Analyzing 3D and 4D images as a primary screen often introduces artifacts that decrease the accuracy of cleft detection.[24,52–54]

However, several authors have reported a higher sensitivity for facial clefts using various 3D sonographic techniques.[25,28,55–62] Even in the best of hands, the secondary palate cannot be well delineated on 2D or 3D sonography. In a study by Ramos et al.,[63] cleft palate accuracy in the setting of cleft lip ranged from 33% to 63%, and the specificity ranged from 84% to 95%. These authors concluded that their observed low sensitivity was mainly due to artifacts, shadowing, and suboptimal fetal position. In many studies, the sonographic detection rate for an isolated cleft secondary palate approaches 0%.[55,64]

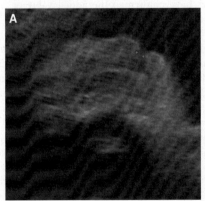
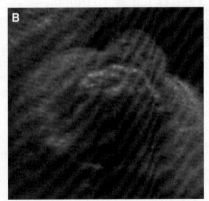
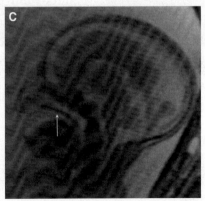

**FIGURE 13.2-22:** Microform cleft lip. 26-Week gestation fetus. **A:** 2D sonogram demonstrates a very small width cleft *(markers)* in the fetal lip. **B:** Intact maxillary alveolus. **C:** The secondary palate *(arrow)* was normal on MRI.

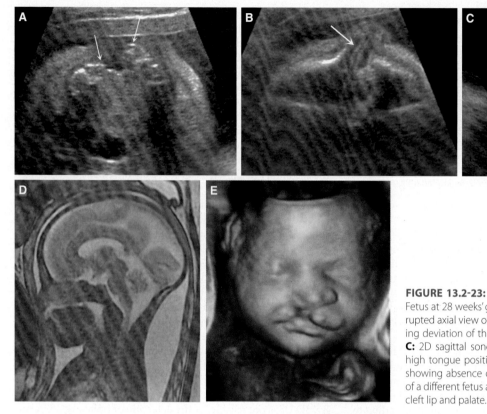

**FIGURE 13.2-23:** Unilateral complete cleft lip and palate. Fetus at 28 weeks' gestation. **A:** 2D sonogram showing interrupted axial view of alveolus *(arrows)*. **B:** 2D sonogram showing deviation of the vomer *(arrow)* away from the cleft side. **C:** 2D sagittal sonogram showing midface hypoplasia and high tongue position *(T)*. **D:** Sagittal MRI of the same fetus showing absence of the secondary palate. **E:** 3D sonogram of a different fetus at 32w2d showing left unilateral complete cleft lip and palate.

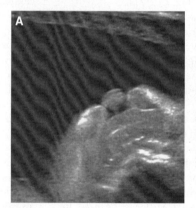
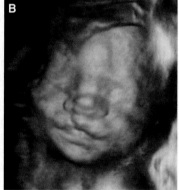

**FIGURE 13.2-24:** Bilateral incomplete cleft lip, intact palate. 2D **(A)** and 3D **(B)** sonogram in a 22w5d fetus with bilateral incomplete cleft lip, intact palate.

| Table 13.2-5 | Associated Signs of Cleft Palate in Presence of Cleft Lip on US and MRI |
|---|---|
| **Axial/Coronal Views** | |
| Lips | Cleft |
| Nares | Flattened or deformed |
| Vomer | Deviated away from side of cleft; often midline if bilateral cleft lip and palate |
| Maxilla | Interrupted alveolus, wide gap |
| Orbits | Hypertelorism |
| **Sagittal View** | |
| Profile | Midface retrusion |
| Position of tongue | High |

*MRI:* Recent studies have confirmed the added value of fetal MRI to sonography in the detection of cleft secondary palate[65–74] in the setting of cleft lip. Using T2 SSFSE and/or SSFP in the axial, coronal, and sagittal planes, excellent imaging of the lip and palate can be obtained. Although fetal MRI has limitations including excessive fetal motion and fetal crowding, the technique can usually detect deeper structures such as the tooth-bearing alveolus, which is part of the primary palate, areas anterior to the incisive foramen, and anomalies of the secondary hard or soft palate, posterior to the incisive foramen (Figs. 13.2-25 and 13.2-26). In a series of 49 fetuses between 24 and 37 weeks' gestation with either a family history of cleft secondary palate or a facial cleft seen on screening sonography, the positive predictive value of fetal MRI for detection of cleft secondary palate was 96%, and the negative predictive value was 80%.[69] Although isolated cleft secondary palate is often seen in the setting of other

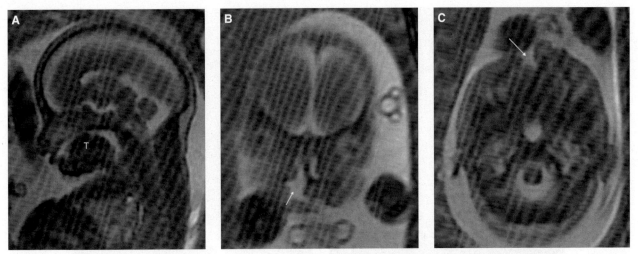

**FIGURE 13.2-25:** Unilateral complete cleft lip and palate. Sagittal **(A)**, coronal **(B)**, and axial **(C)** fetal MR in a 21-week fetus with complete right cleft lip and palate *(arrows)*. Note high-riding tongue *(T)*.

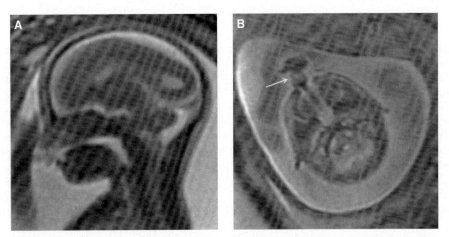

**FIGURE 13.2-26:** Bilateral complete cleft lip and palate. Sagittal **(A)** and axial **(B)** fetal MRI at 21 weeks' gestation showing absence of the secondary palate and two tooth buds *(arrow)* within the intermaxillary protrusion.

anomalies, such as micrognathia, fetal MRI may currently be the only way to accurately detect fetal cleft secondary palate when cleft lip is not present (Fig. 13.2-27).

Small series studies have all shown that additional information about fetal facial clefts can be obtained by fetal MRI. Manganaro et al.[72] studied 27 fetuses at a mean gestational age of 24 weeks. Descamps et al.[69] studied 49 fetuses between 24 and 37 weeks and found a positive predictive value (PPV) for palatal involvement of 96% and a negative predictive value (NPV) of 80%, and noted that accuracy increased with experience during the study. A third study by Mailath-Pokorny et al.[71] in 34 Austrian women between 24 and 27 weeks' gestation also showed an advantage of MRI for evaluation of the fetal secondary palate.

**Detection Rates:** Detection rates vary depending upon the type of cleft, and certain cleft types have more associated anomalies than do other cleft types. In a large series by Paterson et al.[75] in Scotland in 2010, isolated cleft lip occurred in 20%; cleft lip with

cleft alveolus was seen in 6%; cleft lip, cleft alveolus, and cleft palate were seen in 75%; and isolated cleft palate was seen in 1%. In this series, detection rate was low overall (15%), but did improve over the 10 years of the study.

A large prospective series from Norway covering the period from 1987 to 2004 detected 101 facial clefts in fetuses or newborns in a population of 49,314 (incidence 1 in 500 to 1 in 1,000).[64] Isolated cleft lip was detected prenatally in 4.5%; cleft lip and palate in 43%, and cleft palate alone in 0%. Associated anomalies were seen in 43% who had cleft lip and palate, and in 58% who had cleft palate only. Twelve percent had chromosomal anomalies; 18% were part of a syndrome or sequence.

Another recent large series from Ireland studied 851 cases of facial clefts over 25 years from 1984 to 2008 in over 500,000 births.[76] Four hundred eighty-three (51%) had cleft lip and palate; 413 (48.5%) had cleft palate. This population differed somewhat from the other European populations in that mothers were older, abortions were less frequent, and the birth rate was high. The prevalence of all types of facial clefts was 16 per 10,000

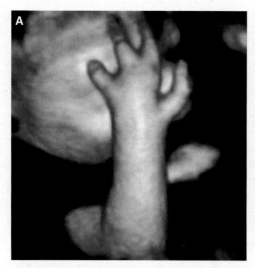
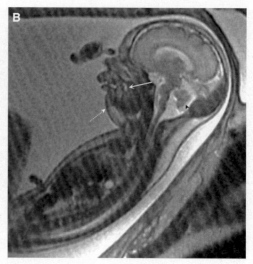

**FIGURE 13.2-27:** Cleft palate and micrognathia. Fetal images at 33 weeks' gestation. **A:** 3D fetal sonogram showing cleft hand and oligodactyly. **B:** Sagittal MR showing micrognathia *(dotted arrow)* and cleft secondary palate *(arrow)*. There is inferior vermian hypogenesis *(arrowhead)*. The fetus also had congenital diaphragmatic hernia (not shown).

births in this population over 25 years, which is similar to other studies.

In a study by Johnson et al.[77] in 2009, the frequencies for accurate prenatal diagnosis for cleft lip and palate were as follows: Cleft lip and palate, 33.3%; cleft lip only, 20.3%, and cleft palate only, 0.3%, concluding that a prenatal diagnosis was made in only one-fifth of live-born infants with orofacial clefts. In this study, other factors were also at play, including the observation that higher-income mothers were much more likely to receive a prenatal diagnosis than mothers with lower incomes. Other studies showed higher detection rates for clefts when they were accompanied by multiple other fetal malformations.

**Associated Anomalies:** Anomalies are present in 3% to 7% of all live births. Seventy-five percent of these involve head, face, or neck. In a recent series of patients with cleft palate alone or cleft lip and palate,[2] 20% to 25% of associated malformations were also in the face, including:

- Nasal anomalies: bifid nose, frontonasal dysplasia, hypoplastic malar eminence, median cleft nose, and choanal atresia.
- Ear anomalies: bifid ear lobe, ear pits, Mondini malformation, periauriculur sinus or fistula, preauricular skin tags, or cysts.
- Eye malformations: anterior segment dysgenesis, coloboma, congenital cataract, congenital eyelid fistula, hypertelorism, microphthalmia, and lacrimal duct atresia.

A recent study in Minnesota found that congenital malformations are more frequently seen in cleft palate without cleft lip (38.7%) than in cleft lip and palate (26.4%). Of associated anomalies, 63.1% were chromosomal or syndromic, and 36.9% were nonchromosomal/syndromic.[2]

Although imagers, obstetricians, parents, and craniofacial surgeons all acknowledge that accurate detection of craniofacial anomalies is important so that prospective parents may be accurately counseled, there is no consensus about best imaging practices. A recent review of prenatal diagnosis and assessment of facial clefts by To[29] summarizes the current state of imaging and counseling, including the uses of sonography and MRI.

This review discusses the increasing accuracy of cleft lip detection because of new technology, accumulated expertise, and raised expectations for imagers. To points out that in a prospective screening study in Norway between 1987 and 2004, the rate of detection of craniofacial clefts increased significantly from 34% in the first 8 years to 58% in the next 8 years.[64] Most cases (69%) were detected on routine US screening in the second trimester. In this study, associated anomalies were observed either before or after birth in 43% of infants with cleft lip and cleft palate; and in 58% of those with isolated cleft palate. Of those patients with associated anomalies, 12% had chromosomal aberrations, and 18% were part of a syndrome or sequence.[29]

*Syndromic Associated Anomalies:* There are more than 300 syndromes associated with orofacial clefts that affect approximately 10% of all cases (Fig. 13.2-28).[46] Certain genetic loci are more frequently involved, including chromosomes 2p, 4p, 6p, 17q, 19q, and 22q. Some clefts are x-linked, autosomal dominant (AD), or autosomal recessive (AR). Syndromes associated with cleft lip/palate include Robin, Vanderwoude, trisomy 21, Treacher Collins, Apert, Marfan, Turner, Cleidocranial dysostosis, CATCH 22, velocardiofacial syndrome, frontonasal dysplasia, and 4p minus syndrome.[78]

*Nonsyndromic Associated Anomalies:* Nonsyndromic clefts may be secondary to genetic factors, such as a family history of cleft lip; environmental factors such as smoking; exposure to certain drugs, such as retinoic acid and antiepileptic drugs; or lack of other factors such as folate.

**Differential Diagnosis:** It is possible for normal fetal facial structures, such as the philtrim, to simulate a cleft lip. The umbilical cord overlying the lip could mimic a cleft. Amniotic bands, Tessier clefts, intracranial tumors, lip masses such as hemangiomas, or nasal masses could mimic a cleft.

**Prognosis/Classification:** There are more than 40 classification systems for cleft lip and palate[79,80] (Table 13.2-6), and

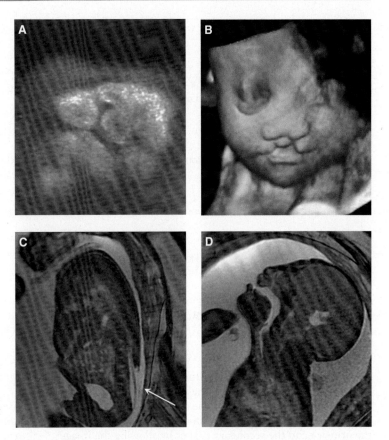

**FIGURE 13.2-28:** Bilateral complete cleft lip and palate, with additional anomalies. **A:** 33-Week fetal 2D sonogram shows bilateral cleft lip. **B:** 3D sonogram of bilateral cleft lip. **C:** Sagittal fetal MRI showing associated open neural tube defect *(arrow)*. **D:** Sagittal fetal MRI showing severe midface retrusion and cleft secondary palate.

flowcharts are available for further definition (Fig. 13.2-29). In 1931, Veau[81] presented a widely accepted system for classifying oral clefts, consisting of four subtypes (Table 13.2-7 and Fig. 13.2-30).

| Table 13.2-6 | Classification of Cleft Lip and Palate: Definitions |
|---|---|
| Cleft, lip/palate | Cleft of primary palate (anterior to incisive foramen) and secondary palate (posterior to incisive foramen) |
| Cleft lip ± alveolus | Cleft of primary palate only (lip ± alveolus) and intact secondary palate |
| Cleft palate | Cleft of secondary palate only (posterior to incisive foramen) |
| Atypical cleft | Examples include: median, oblique, transverse/lateral clefts |
| Incomplete cleft lip | Labial cleft does not extend through nasal floor. Also ± "notch" in alveolus, which does not extend through entire alveolus |
| Complete cleft Lip/alveolus | Cleft involves entire lip and entire alveolus. No tissue connection between alar base, medial labial elements, or premaxilla |
| Tissue band | Small bridge of tissue between the two sides of complete cleft lip/alveolus, which has a vertical height of less than 5 mm |
| Microform | Tiny labial cleft or vertical notch |

Veau I: Cleft of the posterior soft palate
Veau II: Clefts of the soft and hard palate, posterior to the incisive foramen
Veau III: Complete unilateral cleft lip and cleft palate
Veau IV: Complete bilateral cleft lip and cleft palate

In 1971, Kernahan[82] improved upon existing earlier classification systems purely based on anatomy and suggested a pictorial representation using a "striped Y" diagram representing the lip, palate, and maxillary alveolus (Fig. 13.2-31). Kriens developed this classification system further using a right-to-left palindromic labeling system he called "LAHSHAL," which begins on the patient's right and moves to the left, and stands for "Lip, Alveolus, Hard palate, Soft palate, Hard palate, Alveolus, Lip." This system, while complex, is excellent for accurate description in the hands of craniofacial surgeons, and has been fairly widely adopted in international circles and by the large NIDCR-funded studies.[83] In 1976, Tessier[84] published a classification system for unusual facial clefts that do not easily fit into other categories and often involve complex clefts which extend from mouth to facial structures above the nose, such as the eyes and forehead. Tessier clefts involve both superficial facial soft tissues and deeper bony structures (Figs. 13.2-32 and 13.2-33).

Following the lead of our craniofacial surgeons, we use a combination of the modified Kernahan Y drawing, the Veau classification, and the Tessier system in classifying craniofacial clefts, with the goal of imager and surgeon understanding each other as accurately as possible and then presenting a precise description and prognosis for the anomaly to the prospective parents. Studies have shown that prepared parents deal more easily with the appearance of their newborn's face and with the subsequent

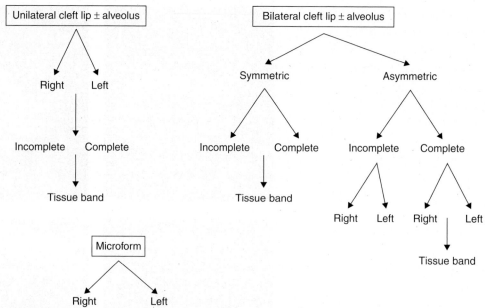

**FIGURE 13.2-29:** Flow chart for classification of cleft lip and alveolus.

series of surgeries predictably in store for the infant and child than those parents who discover the anomaly at birth.[19,22]

We have found the strength of the modified Kernahan Y classification to be the clarity of anatomic demarcation between the primary and the secondary palates by allowing the imager to comprehend the exact location and importance of the incisive foramen. The dividing point between the primary and the

secondary palates, the incisive foramen, is represented symbolically at the junction of the limbs of the Y by a small circle, the incisive foramen. Anterior to the incisive foramen are the three distinct tissues of the primary palate: the lip, the bony tooth-bearing alveolus, and the area of the hard palate extending from the alveolus posteriorly to the incisive foramen. Posterior to the incisive foramen are the three segments of the secondary palate: Two sections of hard palate posterior to the incisive foramen and the palatal shelves, and the most posterior tissues composing the entire soft palate ending in the uvula. The importance of understanding clefting of the primary and secondary palates cannot be overstated: If the secondary palate is cleft, the child will have significant issues with hearing and speech; if the secondary palate is NOT cleft, these serious problems do not occur.[21]

Understanding palatal embryology allows the imager to understand the common forms of both unilateral and bilateral cleft lip and palate. Bilateral facial clefts may be suggested by the visualization of an anterior projection of the intermaxillary segment in combination with the nose, forming a mass that projects anteriorly and superiorly above the normal level of the lip, following embryologic lines of fusion (see Figs. 13.2-24, 13.2-26, 13.2-28). In bilateral facial clefts, the tooth-bearing maxillary alveolus is cleft between the lateral incisors and the canine teeth. This fact explains why there are often two tooth buds in the intermaxillary segment in complete bilateral cleft lip.

Isolated cleft secondary palate without an associated cleft lip is very difficult to detect on fetal sonography, but is readily detected on best-technique fetal MRI. Thin slices and cinegraphic imaging has increased cleft palate detection. Most cases of isolated cleft palate involve the secondary soft palate but not the hard portions of the primary palate, Veau Type II. There is a strong association of isolated cleft secondary palate with micrognathia and the Robin sequence (see Fig. 13.2-27). Indirect imaging features of isolated cleft secondary palate may include a small or nonvisualized fetal stomach and polyhydramnios, because of the fetus's difficulty in swallowing normally.

| Table 13.2-7 | Cleft Palate: Veau Classification and corresponding Modified Kernahan Y drawing |
|---|---|
| **Veau Classification Shown in Fig. 13.2-30** | **Description and corresponding Y drawing position numbers labelled in Fig. 13.2-31** |
| Type I | Cleft of the soft palate (#11) |
| Type II | Complete cleft secondary palate with both soft and hard palate involvement (#9-11) |
| Type III<br>Greater segment = side opposite cleft<br>Lesser segment = same side of cleft | Unilateral complete cleft lip and palate<br>(Right-sided cleft: #1-4 and #9-11)<br>(Left-sided cleft: #5-8 and #9-11) |
| Type IV | Bilateral complete cleft lip and palate (#1-11) |
| Submucous cleft<br>Location:<br>Hard palate<br>Soft palate | Cleft palate covered by mucosa. Features include bifid uvula, palatal muscle diastasis, midline blue mucosal lining, and notch in posterior hard palate |

(Modified by Mulliken, JB, data from Marrinan EM, LaBrie RA, Mulliken JB. Velopharyngeal function in nonsyndromic cleft palate: relevance of surgical technique, age at repair, and cleft type. *Cleft Palate Craniofac J*. 1998 Mar;35(2):95–100).

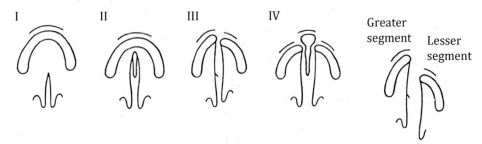

**FIGURE 13.2-30:** Veau classification of cleft palate. **I,** cleft soft palate, **II,** complete cleft secondary palate; **III,** unilateral complete cleft lip/palate; **IV,** bilateral cleft lip/palate. (Modified by Mulliken JB, data from Marrinan EM, LaBrie RA, Mulliken JB. Velopharyngeal function in nonsyndromic cleft palate: relevance of surgical technique, age at repair, and cleft type. *Cleft Palate Craniofac J.* 1998;35(2):95–100.)

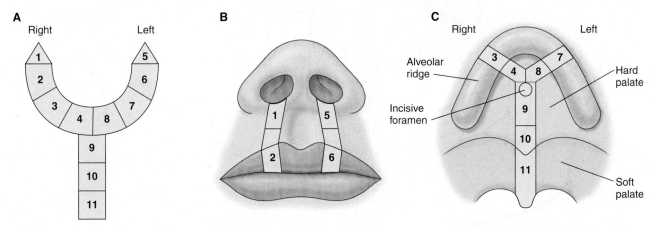

**FIGURE 13.2-31:  A–C:** Modified Kernahan Y drawing. Algorithm for comprehensive characterization of cleft lip and palate. (Modified by Mulliken JB, from Kernahan DA. The striped Y—a symbolic classification for cleft lip and palate. *Plast Reconstr Surg.* 1971;47(5):469–470.)

**Management/Treatment:** Infants with a cleft of the secondary palate, particularly those with Robin sequence, may have respiratory distress at birth, and the airway must be secured. All infants with cleft lip and palate will need assistance in feeding, because they cannot generate adequate pressure during sucking and swallowing. Those with cleft palate risk aspiration of liquids unless specialized nipples and bottle are used.[85] Unilateral cleft lip is usually repaired in the first year of life. Dentofacial orthodontic appliances are often used before definitive surgery to bring the cleft segments closer together. The goal of all types of cleft surgery is nasolabial symmetry and repair of alveolar and palate deficiency. Three-dimensional photography is often used by the surgeon. Cleft palate repair is usually performed between 12 and 18 months of age, with the goal of attaining normal speech, hearing, dental occlusion, and facial and palatal growth. Staged repairs are then performed as needed in childhood and adolescence until skeletal maturity is reached. The psychosocial journey can be difficult for both the child and the parents.

## TONGUE

Fetal tongue evaluation is subjective, though tables exist for the normal size of the tongue between 14 and 26 weeks.[86] The fetal tongue is often well seen on sonography when fetal position is optimal and amniotic fluid is adequate (see Fig. 13.2-2B). It can also be seen on fetal MRI in all three planes and during real-time cine-mode imaging, especially if the fetus swallows during imaging (see Fig. 13.2-6A).[87]

## Macroglossia

**Incidence:** There is a known association with trisomy 21, Beckwith-Wiedemann syndrome (BWS), and hypothyroidism. Adding up the incidences of trisomy 21, BWS, and hypothyroidism and the 1% of individuals with each of these conditions who have macroglossia, overall incidence is approximately 1:11,000 to 1:25,000 live births.[87]

**Etiology/Management:** Macroglossia may be congenital or acquired. Abnormal enlargement of the tongue may be because of overgrowth, as in BWS or Down Syndrome, or be due to the presence of benign or malignant tumors.[85] Masses known to involve the tongue include lymphatic malformations (Fig. 13.2-34), teratomas, and foregut duplication cysts (Fig. 13.2-35). An enlarged tongue may cause airway obstruction and prevent normal swallowing. Portions of the tongue can be surgically removed (glossectomy) to make the tongue fit properly into the closed oral cavity.

## JAW AND MANDIBLE

### Micrognathia

Micrognathia is usually characterized by a small mandible and a receding chin (retrognathia). This diagnosis is most often made subjectively, and is not difficult to make when the condition is severe. In normal craniofacial anthropometry, the chin

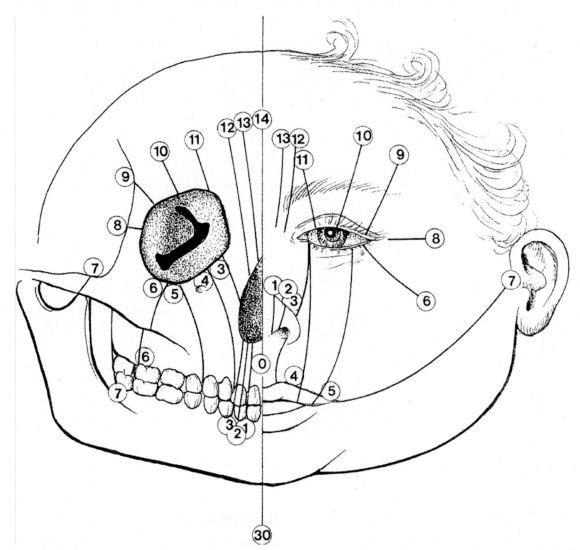

**FIGURE 13.2-32:** Classification of Tessier clefts. The left half *(right side of face)* depicts the various clefts relative to the skeletal landmarks, and the right half *(left side of face)* outlines the locations based on soft tissue landmarks. Facial clefts = numbers 0 through number 7 and cranial clefts = numbers 8 through number 14. Mandibular midline facial cleft number 30 is also seen. (From Kawamoto H Jr, Bradley JP. Craniofacial clefts and hypertelorbitism. In: Thorne CH, Bartlett SP, Beasley RW, et al. *Grabb and Smith's Plastic Surgery.* 6th ed. Philadelphia, PA: Lippincott Williams & Wilkins; 2006.)

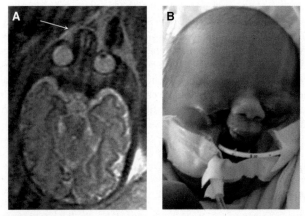

**FIGURE 13.2-33:** Tessier Cleft. **A:** Fetal MR at 35 weeks shows hypotelorism and an unusual configuration of the nose *(arrow)*. **B:** Newborn photograph showing bilateral deep clefts of soft tissue and bone extending from the mouth to the eyes.

is usually on or close to the same vertical plane as the forehead, and the nose protrudes beyond this plane. In micrognathia, the height of the mandible is reduced and the mandible is posteriorly positioned. Nomograms for the fetal mandible have been published.[35]

**Incidence:** Micrognathia is a relatively rare condition, occurring in approximately 1 in 1,600 fetuses, which characteristically has obligatory mandibular hypoplasia and a small, posteriorly positioned chin in which the tongue falls backward and blocks the airway.

**Pathogenesis:** Micrognathia is often associated with chromosomal anomalies and syndromes (Fig. 13.2-36), varying from 38% to 66% in several series.[88–90]

**Imaging:** Fetal micrognathia is associated with polyhydramnios, and most fetuses have associated anomalies. The diagnosis is often

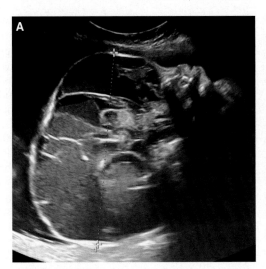
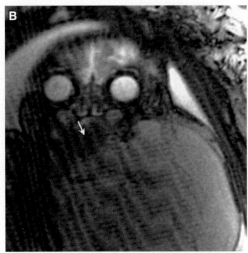

**FIGURE 13.2-34:** Lymphatic malformation invading tongue base. Third-trimester 34-week fetal sonograms **(A)** and MRI **(B)**, prior to EXIT delivery showing very large, multiseptated fluid-filled mass *(markers)* that invades the face and tongue *(arrow)*.

made subjectively, though several authors have published nomograms for mandibular size and growth.[35,91,92] Three-dimensional US and fetal MRI aid greatly in assuring assessment is made on a midline sagittal view. In addition, fetal MRI can detect associated cleft palate. Cleft of the uvula as a marker for the secondary palate can sometimes be seen on 2D fetal sonography and more reliably on fetal MRI.[93]

**Associated Malformations/Conditions:** Multiple chromosomal, neuromuscular, genetic, and teratogenic causes are associated with micrognathia, including trisomies 8, 9, 13, 18, and triploidy, Pena Shokeir and fetal akinesia syndromes, Sticker,

Treacher–Collins, diastrophic and camptomelic dysplasias, Nager acrofacial dysostosis, Saethre–Chotzen Syndrome and Isotretinoin exposure.

**Recurrence Risk:** Recurrence depends on the cause. If it is genetic, the recurrence risk is 25% if autosomal recessive or 50% if autosomal dominant.

## Robin Sequence

Formerly called Robin or Pierre Robin syndrome, anomalad or complex, it is now called the Robin sequence because most

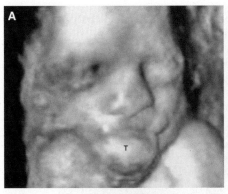
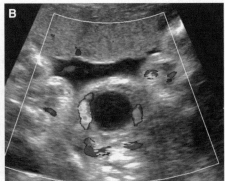
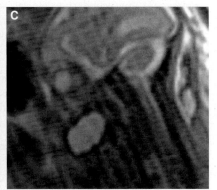
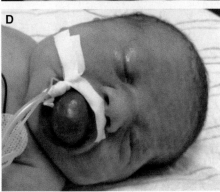

**FIGURE 13.2-35:** Macroglossia secondary to foregut duplication cyst of the tongue. **A:** 3D fetal sonogram at 28w5d gestation showing macroglossia *(T)*. **B:** Color Doppler sonogram showing no flow in the cystic tongue mass. **C:** Sagittal fetal MR of cystic tongue mass. **D:** Photograph of the newborn in the delivery room. After complete surgical resection, the pathologic diagnosis was a GI duplication cyst.

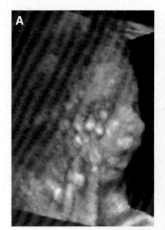
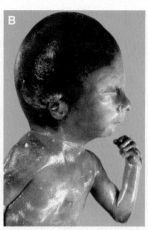

**FIGURE 13.2-36:** Micrognathia with trisomy 18. **A:** 3D sonogram shows micrognathia. **B:** Pathologic photograph of another case of trisomy 18 shows micrognathia and clenched hand.

specialists consider the abnormality to be caused by a series of developmental events causing the triad of micrognathia, glossoptosis, and cleft palate.

**Incidence:** 1:8,500 to 1:14,000 births.[94]

**Pathogenesis:** The etiology of Robin sequence is uncertain. Some authors posit that a small embryonic mandible causes the tongue to be displaced posteriorly and superiorly, thereby preventing closure of the secondary palate.

**Imaging:** The Robin sequence is a clinical diagnosis when there is micrognathia, cleft secondary palate, and glossoptosis, when the tongue falls posteriorly and obstructs the oral and nasal airway (Fig. 13.2-37). Glossoptosis can be seen in some fetuses on sonography and more often on fetal MRI. Cleft of the uvula as a marker for the secondary palate can sometimes be seen on 2D fetal sonography and more reliably on fetal MRI.[93] Cleft palate is not usually detected sonographically, although it is readily detectable on fetal MRI.

**Differential Diagnosis:** Agnathia, in which the mandible is absent and the mouth is small (Fig. 13.2-38), may resemble Robin sequence. In mild micrognathia, the fetus may subjectively be normal.

**Prognosis and Management:** When the anomaly is known prenatally, ideally, delivery should take place at a specialized center with neonatal, plastic surgical, and otolaryngology specialists in attendance to manage the airway. A surgical tongue tie may be necessary to prevent airway obstruction. Tracheostomy may also be necessary. If the airway can be managed in the neonatal period, there is often catch-up growth of the small mandible, which allows improvement in respiratory status. The mandible often does catch up in growth during infancy and childhood, once the tongue has been pexed anteriorly. Children with Robin sequence have difficulty breathing and eating, and some have temporary or permanent tracheostomies. Palatal repair can be performed once the mandibular size has increased, but airway compromise remains a risk. Surgical mandibular distraction osteogenesis may also be used to accelerate mandibular growth. Approximately, 60% to 90% of infants with Robin sequence have cleft palate and many have other anomalies, most frequently cardiac and renal.[95] Prone or lateral positioning of the infant may keep the airway open for many affected infants. A nasopharyngeal tube may be used to keep the airway open. Infants may need to be gavage fed to save energy and to gain weight.[96]

**Recurrence Risk:** Robin sequence recurrence is unknown but infrequent, though there is some data to suggest that there may be a genetic component involved. If it is genetic, the recurrence risk is 25% if autosomal recessive or 50% if autosomal dominant.

## Otocephaly

**Definition:** Otocephaly is a rare and lethal malformation involving a defect in the ventral portion of the first branchial arch. Affected fetuses have microstomia (small mouth), aglossia (absent tongue), agnathia (absent mandible), and synotia (medially positioned, low and malformed ears).

Synonyms for otocephaly are agnathia–microstomia–synotia syndrome and synotia.

**Incidence:** Otocephaly is rare and sporadic, occurring in less than 1 in 70,000 births.[97]

**Pathogenesis/Etiology:** In otocephaly, there is failure of the ascent of the developing auricles, resulting in low-set to markedly displaced ears positioned along the anterior lower neck. It is always associated with agnathia (see Fig. 13.2-38) or micrognathia.[97]

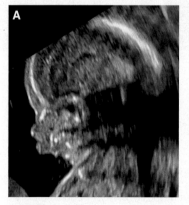
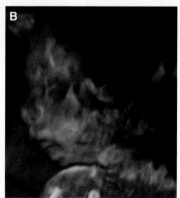
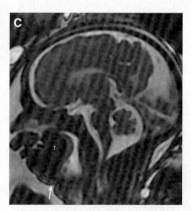

**FIGURE 13.2-37:** Robin sequence. **A:** Sagittal 2D ultrasound at 21 weeks demonstrates foreshortened mandible that is confirmed on 3D US. **B, C:** Sagittal SSFP at 33 weeks demonstrates micrognathia *(arrow)* and tongue *(T)* obstructing the airway. There is absence of the secondary palate. Images courtesy of Beth Kline-Fath.

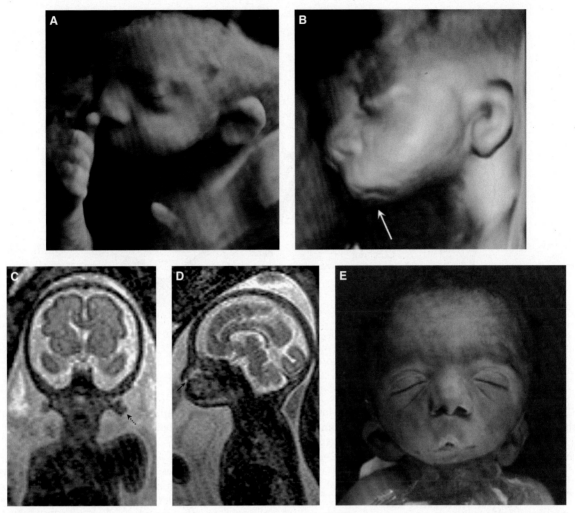

**FIGURE 13.2-38:** Otocephaly. 25-Week gestation 3D fetal sonograms **(A, B)**, and coronal and sagittal MRI **(C, D)** show small mouth (microstomia) *(solid arrow)*, severe micrognathia/absent mandible and low-set ears *(dotted arrow)*. **E:** Postmortem photograph at 29 weeks after unsuccessful intubation.

**Diagnosis:** On imaging, the mandible and lower jaw cannot be seen and the ears are extremely low (Fig. 13.2-38). The mouth is often small.

**Associated Anomalies:** Otocephaly can be associated with brain anomalies, such as holopresencephaly and cephalocele; choanal atresia and tracheoesophogeal fistula; cardiac, renal, and vertebral anomalies; and a two-vessel umbilical cord.[98–102]

**Prognosis/Management:** This is a lethal malformation.

**Recurrence Risk:** No recurrence risk is known.

# EARS

Malformations of the ear can affect the external, middle, or inner ear, or any combination of these regions. External ear malformations can involve abnormal shape, size, and position of the pinna. Ear pits, sinuses, and skin tags can be seen anterior to the pinna. The external auditory canal can be small or atretic. Middle ear anomalies can affect the presence, position, and configuration of the ossicles.

**Incidence:** Incidence of all ear malformations: 1:3,800 newborns. Incidence of outer ear malformations is between 1:6,000 and 1:6,830 newborns. Incidence of microtia is 3:10,000 newborns.

**Embryology:** The external and middle ear share a common embryology, developing between the 40th and the 45th day from mesenchymal hillocks 1 through 6 from the first and second branchial arches and the first branchial groove. By 16 weeks, pinna development is complete. By 22 weeks, the middle ear bones have grown to adult size. The inner ear develops differently, from the ectodermal layer. By 12 weeks of gestation, the semicircular canals and cochlea are present. Development of the inner ear is complete by 25 weeks. For normal anatomy of the inner and middle ear and external canal, see Figure 13.2-39. Figure 13.2-40 depicts the normal external ear landmarks.

**Imaging:** 3D ultrasound has been exceptionally helpful in evaluation of the position, orientation, and structure of the fetal ear (Fig. 13.2-41A). It is often difficult to appreciate the relationship of the ear to other craniofacial landmarks. For instance, the normal top of the external ear helix should be at the level of the inner canthus of the eye. Malformations of the external ear are readily

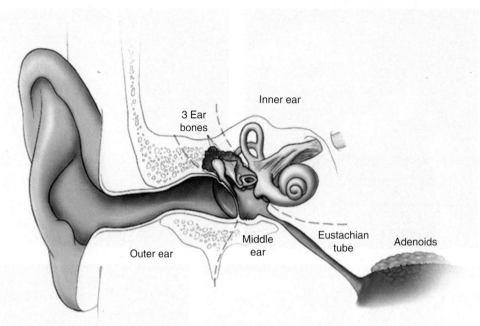

**FIGURE 13.2-39:** The normal ear. Schematic drawing of the normal auditory apparatus. (From Hill MA, ed. Normal ear. 2009. Image source: UNSW Embryology, modified from NIH image. http://embryology. med.unsw.edu.au/embryology/index.php?title=File:Hearing_cartoon.jpg.)

seen on 2D and 3D sonography, unless amniotic fluid is low or fetal position is unfavorable. Middle and inner ear anomalies are often visible on fetal MRI, unless excessive fetal movement or maternal body habitus prevents visualization (Fig. 13.2-41B).

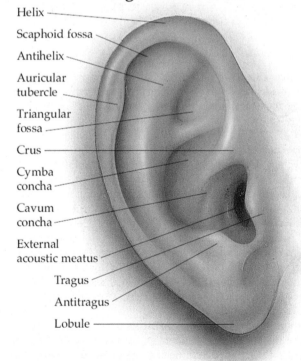

**FIGURE 13.2-40:** Normal external ear landmarks. (From Anatomical Chart Company. *Anatomy of the Inner Ear Anatomical Chart.* 2004.)

Knowledge of the normal configuration and position of the external ear is important, and 3D sonography may be extremely helpful.

**Associated Anomalies:** Malformed or low-set ears are associated with many syndromes and genetic conditions listed in Table 13.2-2 and include trisomies 13 and 18, Wolf Hirschhorn syndrome, Cri-du-Chat syndrome and mosaic trisomy 8 (Fig. 13.2-42). Ear anomalies are also seen in approximately 2% of individuals with CLP. The most common anomalies were microtia, prominent ears, and skin tags. A full discussion of the middle and inner ear anomalies is beyond the scope of this chapter, but there are many

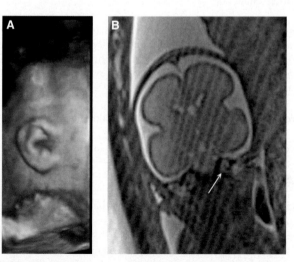

**FIGURE 13.2-41:** Normal external ear on sonography and cochlea on MRI. **A:** 3D sonogram of a normal fetal ear at 29 weeks' gestation. **B:** Coronal MR at 25 weeks showing the normal fetal cochlea *(arrow)*.

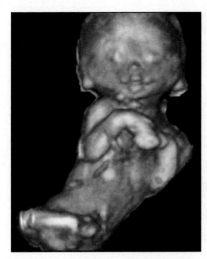

**FIGURE 13.2-42:** Low-set ears. 3D sonogram of 18w4d gestation fetus referred with multiple anomalies, clubfeet, two-vessel cord, and absent stomach. Other findings after Fetal Center evaluation included low-set ears, clubbed hands and feet, pectus deformity of chest, "windswept" deformity with dislocated hips, and micrognathia. Brain abnormalities (not shown) included cortical defects, absent corpus callosum, and ventriculomegaly. The karyotype was abnormal: 46, XY, del (13) (q33) dn.ish del (13) (scp13+, LAMP1~, D135327).

detailed classification systems for anomalies in this region.[103] See Chapter 20 for further genetic anomalies.

## Microtia

**Incidence:** Incidence varies between ethnic groups, ranging from 1:7,000 to 1:8,000 births in the Western world to 1:4,000 in Japan. Males are twice as often affected as females. Microtia can occur as a sporadic event or can be inherited. Microtia is associated with almost too many syndromes to count, and can also be associated with preauricular skin tags or pits, atresia of the external auditory canal, and abnormal middle and inner ear structure.

**Pathogenesis/Types:** Congenital anomalies of the external ear, or pinna, are generally of three types: microtia, constricted ears,

and prominent ears.[104] Microtia (Fig. 13.2-43) describes a spectrum of anomalies of the pinna, which ranges from anotia, in which there is complete absence of the soft tissue of the ear, to a small but otherwise well-formed ear. The clinical classification of microtia by Marx (1911)[105] includes three types:

Type I: Auricle is small: different structures of each part of the ear are recognizable.
Type II: Ear is smaller than normal; auricular remnant retains some structural resemblance to a helix in its configuration
Type III: Auricular configuration is absent; only a narrow remnant or irregular ridge of tissue is present

### Hemifacial Microsomia

Hemifacial microsomia was first described in 1964 by Gorlin and Pindborg[106] as a condition in which one ear was small, the mouth was large and the mandibular ramus and condyle failed to fully develop. It is now viewed as part of a spectrum of disorders also known as oculoauricular-vertebral (OAV) anomaly, in so far as conditions causing one side of the face to be affected are associated with anomalies in other organ systems, such as eyes, ears, heart, spine, and kidneys. The term "Goldenhar Syndrome" is also used, originally described by Goldenhar in 1952 to elucidate an association between hemifacial microsomia, ear anomalies, and epibulbar dermoid malformation of the eye.

**Incidence:** Reported as 1:3,000 to 1:5,000 live births if all minor forms are considered[107]; 1:45,000 if only the most severe forms are included.[108] Most cases are unilateral (67%), occurring more often on the right side.

**Pathogenesis/Etiology:** Predominantly unilateral craniofacial malformation developing from the first and second branchial arches in which there is hypoplasia of the malar, maxillary, and/or mandibular regions with associated anomalies of ears and vertebra.[109] The condition may be caused by an embryonic vascular accident or teratogens affecting cranial neural crest derivatives.

**Imaging:** On sonography, there may be associated polyhydramnios secondary to ineffective fetal swallowing. There will often be some combination of facial asymmetry and ear anomaly (Fig. 13.2-45). Scoliosis secondary to abnormal

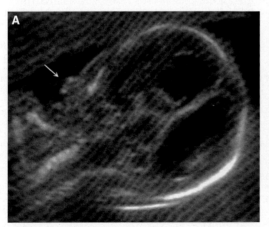
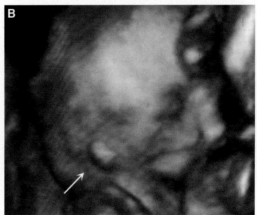

**FIGURE 13.2-43:** Microtia. 2D **(A)** and 3D **(B)** fetal sonograms at 18 weeks' gestation showing an abnormally small and malformed ear (arrows).

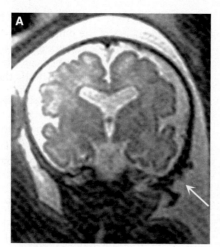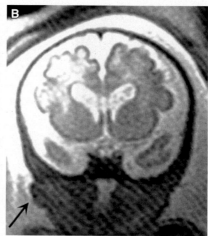

**FIGURE 13.2-44:** Hemifacial microsomia. Goldenhar syndrome. Coronal MR images of 35 week fetus showing absent cavum septum pellucidum and mild ventriculomegaly. The left ear is normal *(white arrow);* the right ear is severely hypoplastic *(black arrow).*

spine segmentation may be present. The diagnosis should be considered whenever a cleft lip and palate is accompanied by other facial anomalies, such as facial asymmetry; ear and eye abnormalities (like absent or misshaped ears, small or absent eyes, orbital coloboma, epibulbar dermoids); and vertebral anomalies, especially of the cervical and upper thoracic spine. Cardiac defects are often associated, including tetralogy of Fallot, double outlet right ventricle (DORV), ventriculoseptal defect (VSD), and total anomalous pulmonary venous return (TAPVR). Heterotaxy may also be associated.[110] The presence of cardiac anomalies can adversely affect survival. There are also associated genitourinary anomalies, including ectopic or fused kidneys, absent kidneys, vesicoureteral reflux, ureteropelvic junction obstruction, duplex ureter, and multicystic dysplastic kidney. Given the range of anomalies, a detailed fetal survey is needed, with particular attention to the craniofacial structure, especially superficial structures such as skin tags and external ear formation.[111]

**Associated Anomalies:** According to Rollnick,[112] many chromosomal anomalies can be associated with OAV anomaly, including chromosome 5p deletion, monosomy 6q, mosaic trisomy 7, duplication of 7q and 8q, mosaic trisomy 9, chromosome 18q deletion, trisomy 18, Recombinant chromosome 18, and deletion chromosome 22q 13.31, 47, XXY (Klinefelter syndrome) and 49, XXXXY.

**Prognosis/Management:** Depends on the presence of associated anomalies. After birth, the face should be closely inspected, a spine radiograph and a postnatal echocardiogram should be performed, and renal sonography and a detailed hearing evaluation is warranted. Karyotyping is suggested. Treatment is directed toward attaining facial symmetry, usually by staged surgery to address mandibular deformities and ear anomalies. The long-term outcome is favorable, as the majority of affected individuals have normal intelligence.

**Recurrence Risk:** The risk is not known, but it is obviously increased in families of affected individuals who have a karyotypic anomaly, such as chromosome 5p deletion, monosomy 6q,

mosaic trisomy 7, mosaic trisomy 9, chromosome 18q deletion, trisomy 18, ring chromosome 21, deletion 22q13.31, and others. If no one else in the family is affected, the recurrence risk is likely low, 2% to 3%.[109,112,113]

## REFERENCES

1. Shaw W. Global strategies to reduce the health care burden of craniofacial anomalies: report of WHO meetings on international collaborative research on craniofacial anomalies. *Cleft Palate Craniofac J.* 2004;41:238–243.
2. Beriaghi S, Myers SL, Jensen SA, et al. Cleft lip and palate: association with other congenital malformations. *J Clin Pediatr Dent.* 2009;33:207–210.
3. Suri M. Craniofacial syndromes. *Semin Fetal Neonatal Med.* 2005;10:243–257.
4. Seeds JW. The routine or screening obstetrical ultrasound examination. *Clin Obstet Gynecol.* 1996;39:814–830.
5. Benacerraf BR, Frigoletto FD Jr, Bieber FR. The fetal face: ultrasound examination. *Radiology.* 1984;153:495–497.
6. Shaikh D, Mercer NS, Sohan K, et al. Prenatal diagnosis of cleft lip and palate. *Br J Plast Surg.* 2001;54:288–289.
7. Russell KA, Allen VM, MacDonald ME, et al. A population-based evaluation of antenatal diagnosis of orofacial clefts. *Cleft Palate Craniofac J.* 2008;45:148–153.
8. Vial Y, Tran C, Addor MC, et al. Screening for foetal malformations: performance of routine ultrasonography in the population of the Swiss Canton of Vaud. *Swiss Med Wkly.* 2001;131:490–494.
9. American Institute of Ultrasound in Medicine. AIUM practice guideline for the performance of obstetric ultrasound examinations. *J Ultrasound Med.* 2010;29:157–166.
10. Babcook CJ, McGahan JP, Chong BW, et al. Evaluation of fetal midface anatomy related to facial clefts: use of US. *Radiology.* 1996;201:113–118.
11. Rotten D, Levaillant J-M. Prenatal diagnosis of facial clefts. In: Losee JE, Kirschner RE, eds. *Comprehensive Cleft Care.* New York, NY: McGraw-Hill Professional; 2008:44–70.
12. Gillham JC, Anand S, Bullen PJ. Antenatal detection of cleft lip with or without cleft palate: incidence of associated chromosomal and structural anomalies. *Ultrasound Obstet Gynecol.* 2009;34:410–415.
13. Tonni G, Grisolia G, Sepulveda W. Early prenatal diagnosis of orofacial clefts: evaluation of the retronasal triangle using a new three-dimensional reslicing technique. *Fetal Diagn Ther.* 2013;34:31–37.
14. Sepulveda W, Wong AE, Martinez-Ten P, et al. Retronasal triangle: a sonographic landmark for the screening of cleft palate in the first trimester. *Ultrasound Obstet Gynecol.* 2010;35:7–13.
15. Sepulveda W, Cafici D, Bartholomew J, et al. First-trimester assessment of the fetal palate: a novel application of the volume NT algorithm. *J Ultrasound Med.* 2012;31:1443–1448.
16. Martinez-Ten P, Adiego B, Illescas T, et al. First-trimester diagnosis of cleft lip and palate using three-dimensional ultrasound. *Ultrasound Obstet Gynecol.* 2012;40:40–46.
17. Timmerman E, Pajkrt E, Maas SM, et al. Enlarged nuchal translucency in chromosomally normal fetuses: strong association with orofacial clefts. *Ultrasound Obstet Gynecol.* 2010;36:427–432.
18. Rodriguez ED, Neligan PC, Losee JE. *Plastic Surgery: Craniofacial, Head and Neck Surgery and Pediatric Plastic Surgery.* Philadelphia, PA: Elsevier Saunders; 2012.

19. Mulliken JB. The changing faces of children with cleft lip and palate. *N Engl J Med*. 2004;351:745–747.

20. Mulliken JB. Microform cleft lip. In: Losee JE, Kirschner RE, eds. *Comprehensive Cleft Care*. New York, NY: McGraw-Hill Professional; 2008: 273–283.

21. Mulliken JB, Benacerraf BR. Prenatal diagnosis of cleft lip: what the sonologist needs to tell the surgeon. *J Ultrasound Med*. 2001;20:1159–1164.

22. Costello BJ, Edwards SP, Clemens M. Fetal diagnosis and treatment of craniomaxillofacial anomalies. *J Oral Maxillofac Surg*. 2008;66:1985–1995.

23. Rotten D, Levaillant JM. Two- and three-dimensional sonographic assessment of the fetal face, 1: a systematic analysis of the normal face. *Ultrasound Obstet Gynecol*. 2004;23:224–231.

24. Kurjak A, Azumendi G, Andonotopo W, et al. Three- and four-dimensional ultrasonography for the structural and functional evaluation of the fetal face. *Am J Obstet Gynecol*. 2007;196:16–28.

25. Campbell S, Lees C, Moscoso G, et al. Ultrasound antenatal diagnosis of cleft palate by a new technique: the 3D "reverse face" view. *Ultrasound Obstet Gynecol*. 2005;25:12–18.

26. Platt LD, Devore GR, Pretorius DH. Improving cleft palate/cleft lip antenatal diagnosis by 3-dimensional sonography: the "flipped face" view. *J Ultrasound Med*. 2006;25:1423–1430.

27. Pilu G, Segata M. A novel technique for visualization of the normal and cleft fetal secondary palate: angled insonation and three-dimensional ultrasound. *Ultrasound Obstet Gynecol*. 2007;29:166–169.

28. Martinez Ten P, Perez Pedregosa J, Santacruz B, et al. Three-dimensional ultrasound diagnosis of cleft palate: "reverse face", "flipped face" or "oblique face"—which method is best? *Ultrasound Obstet Gynecol*. 2009;33:399–406.

29. To WW. Prenatal diagnosis and assessment of facial clefts: where are we now? *Hong Kong Med J*. 2012;18:146–152.

30. Ulm MR, Chalubinski K, Ulm C, et al. Sonographic depiction of fetal tooth germs. *Prenat Diagn*. 1995;15:368–372.

31. Guis F, Ville Y, Vincent Y, et al. Ultrasound evaluation of the length of the fetal nasal bones throughout gestation. *Ultrasound Obstet Gynecol*. 1995;5:304–307.

32. Pinette MG, Blackstone J, Pan Y, et al. Measurement of fetal nasal width by ultrasonography. *Am J Obstet Gynecol*. 1997;177:842–845.

33. Sonek JD, Cicero S, Neiger R, et al. Nasal bone assessment in prenatal screening for trisomy 21. *Am J Obstet Gynecol*. 2006;195:1219–1230.

34. Morain S, Greene MF, Mello MM. A new era in noninvasive prenatal testing. *N Engl J Med*. 2013;369:499–501.

35. Chitty LS, Campbell S, Altman DG. Measurement of the fetal mandible—feasibility and construction of a centile chart. *Prenat Diagn*. 1993;13:749–756.

36. Goldstein I, Tamir A, Zimmer EZ, et al. Growth of the fetal orbit and lens in normal pregnancies. *Ultrasound Obstet Gynecol*. 1998;12:175–179.

37. Robinson AJ, Blaser S, Toi A, et al. MRI of the fetal eyes: morphologic and biometric assessment for abnormal development with ultrasonographic and clinicopathologic correlation. *Pediatr Radiol*. 2008;38:971–981.

38. De Meyer W, Zeman W, Palmer CG. The face predicts the brain: diagnostic significance of median facial anomalies for holoprosencephaly (arhinencephaly). *Pediatrics*. 1964;34:256–263.

39. Bundy AL, Lidov H, Soliman M, et al. Antenatal sonographic diagnosis of cebocephaly. *J Ultrasound Med*. 1988;7:395–398.

40. Rolland M, Sarramon MF, Bloom MC. Astomia-agnathia-holoprosencephaly association: prenatal diagnosis of a new case. *Prenat Diagn*. 1991;11:199–203.

41. Greene MF, Benacerraf BR, Frigoletto FD Jr. Reliable criteria for the prenatal sonographic diagnosis of alobar holoprosencephaly. *Am J Obstet Gynecol*. 1987;156:687–689.

42. McGahan JP, Nyberg DA, Mack LA. Sonography of facial features of alobar and semilobar holoprosencephaly. *AJR Am J Roentgenol*. 1990;154:143–148.

43. Albernaz VS, Castillo M, Mukherji SK, et al. Congenital arhinia. *AJNR Am J Neuroradiol*. 1996;17:1312–1314.

44. Tewfik TL, Der Kaloustian VM. *Congenital Anomalies of the Ear, Nose, and Throat*. New York, NY: Oxford University Press; 1997.

45. Cash C, Set P, Coleman N. The accuracy of antenatal ultrasound in the detection of facial clefts in a low-risk screening population. *Ultrasound Obstet Gynecol*. 2001;18:432–436.

46. Wantia N, Rettinger G. The current understanding of cleft lip malformations. *Facial Plast Surg*. 2002;18:147–153.

47. Nagase Y, Natsume N, Kato T, et al. Epidemiological analysis of cleft lip and/or palate by cleft pattern. *J Maxillofac Oral Surg*. 2010;9:389–395.

48. Yuzuriha S, Mulliken JB. Minor-form, microform, and mini-microform cleft lip: anatomical features, operative techniques, and revisions. *Plast Reconstr Surg*. 2008;122:1485–1493.

49. Yuzuriha S, Oh AK, Mulliken JB. Asymmetrical bilateral cleft lip: complete or incomplete and contralateral lesser defect (minor-form, microform, or mini-microform). *Plast Reconstr Surg*. 2008;122:1494–1504.

50. Demircioglu M, Kangesu L, Ismail A, et al. Increasing accuracy of antenatal ultrasound diagnosis of cleft lip with or without cleft palate, in cases referred to the North Thames London Region. *Ultrasound Obstet Gynecol*. 2008;31:647–651.

51. Maarse W, Berge SJ, Pistorius L, et al. Diagnostic accuracy of transabdominal ultrasound in detecting prenatal cleft lip and palate: a systematic review. *Ultrasound Obstet Gynecol*. 2010;35:495–502.

52. Leung KY, Ngai CS, Tang MH. Facial cleft or shadowing artifact? *Ultrasound Obstet Gynecol*. 2006;27:231–232.

53. Timor-Tritsch IE, Platt LD. Three-dimensional ultrasound experience in obstetrics. *Curr Opin Obstet Gynecol*. 2002;14:569–575.

54. Zajicek M, Achiron R, Weisz B, et al. Sonographic assessment of fetal secondary palate between 12 and 16 weeks of gestation using three-dimensional ultrasound. *Prenat Diagn*. 2013;33:1256–1259.

55. Baumler M, Faure JM, Bigorre M, et al. Accuracy of prenatal three-dimensional ultrasound in the diagnosis of cleft hard palate when cleft lip is present. *Ultrasound Obstet Gynecol*. 2011;38:440–444.

56. Campbell S. Prenatal ultrasound examination of the secondary palate. *Ultrasound Obstet Gynecol*. 2007;29:124–127.

57. Chmait R, Pretorius D, Jones M, et al. Prenatal evaluation of facial clefts with two-dimensional and adjunctive three-dimensional ultrasonography: a prospective trial. *Am J Obstet Gynecol*. 2002;187:946–949.

58. Faure JM, Baumler M, Boulot P, et al. Prenatal assessment of the normal fetal soft palate by three-dimensional ultrasound examination: is there an objective technique? *Ultrasound Obstet Gynecol*. 2008;31:652–656.

59. Faure JM, Captier G, Baumler M, et al. Sonographic assessment of normal fetal palate using three-dimensional imaging: a new technique. *Ultrasound Obstet Gynecol*. 2007;29:159–165.

60. McGahan MC, Ramos GA, Landry C, et al. Multislice display of the fetal face using 3-dimensional ultrasonography. *J Ultrasound Med*. 2008;27:1573–1581.

61. Wong HS, Tait J, Pringle KC. Viewing of the soft and the hard palate on routine 3-D ultrasound sweep of the fetal face—a feasibility study. *Fetal Diagn Ther*. 2008;24:146–154.

62. Hata T, Yonehara T, Aoki S, et al. Three-dimensional sonographic visualization of the fetal face. *AJR Am J Roentgenol*. 1998;170:481–483.

63. Ramos GA, Romine LE, Gindes L, et al. Evaluation of the fetal secondary palate by 3-dimensional ultrasonography. *J Ultrasound Med*. 2010;29:357–364.

64. Offerdal K, Jebens N, Syvertsen T, et al. Prenatal ultrasound detection of facial clefts: a prospective study of 49,314 deliveries in a non-selected population in Norway. *Ultrasound Obstet Gynecol*. 2008;31:639–646.

65. Stroustrup Smith A, Estroff JA, Barnewolt CE, et al. Prenatal diagnosis of cleft lip and cleft palate using MRI. *AJR Am J Roentgenol*. 2004;183:229–235.

66. Salomon LJ, Sonigo P, Ou P, et al. Real-time fetal magnetic resonance imaging for the dynamic visualization of the pouch in esophageal atresia. *Ultrasound Obstet Gynecol*. 2009;34:471–474.

67. Kazan-Tannus JF, Levine D, McKenzie C, et al. Real-time magnetic resonance imaging aids prenatal diagnosis of isolated cleft palate. *J Ultrasound Med*. 2005;24:1533–1540.

68. Shen SH, Guo WY, Hung JH. Two-dimensional fast imaging employing steady-state acquisition (FIESTA) cine acquisition of fetal non-central nervous system abnormalities. *J Magn Reson Imaging*. 2007;26:672–677.

69. Descamps MJ, Golding SJ, Sibley J, et al. MRI for definitive in utero diagnosis of cleft palate: a useful adjunct to antenatal care? *Cleft Palate Craniofac J*. 2010;47:578–585.

70. Tonni G, Panteghini M, Pattacini P, et al. Integrating 3D sonography with targeted MRI in the prenatal diagnosis of posterior cleft palate plus cleft lip. *J Diagn Med Sonogr*. 2006;22:367–372.

71. Mailath-Pokorny M, Worda C, Krampl-Bettelheim E, et al. What does magnetic resonance imaging add to the prenatal ultrasound diagnosis of facial clefts? *Ultrasound Obstet Gynecol*. 2010;36:445–451.

72. Manganaro L, Tomei A, Fierro F, et al. Fetal MRI as a complement to US in the evaluation of cleft lip and palate. *La Radiologia Medica*. 2011;116:1134–1148.

73. Moreira NC, Ribeiro V, Teixeira J, et al. Visualization of the fetal lip and palate: is brain-targeted MRI reliable? *Cleft Palate Craniofac J*. 2013;50:513–519.

74. Wang Y, Shan R, Zhao L, et al. Fetal cleft lip with and without cleft palate: comparison between MR imaging and US for prenatal diagnosis. *Eur J Radiol*. 2011;79:437–442.

75. Paterson P, Sher H, Wylie F, et al. Cleft lip/palate: incidence of prenatal diagnosis in Glasgow, Scotland, and comparison with other centers in the United Kingdom. *Cleft Palate Craniofac J*. 2011;48:608–613.

76. McDonnell R, Owens M, Delany C, et al. Epidemiology of orofacial clefts in the east of Ireland in the 25-year period 1984–2008. *Cleft Palate Craniofac J*. 2013.

77. Johnson CY, Honein MA, Hobbs CA, et al. Prenatal diagnosis of orofacial clefts, National Birth Defects Prevention Study, 1998–2004. *Prenat Diagn*. 2009;29:833–839.

78. Gorlin RJ, Cohen MM, Levin LS. *Syndromes of the Head and Neck*. New York, NY: Oxford University Press; 1990.

79. Wang BC, Hakimi M, Martin MC. Use of two cleft lip and palate classification systems by nonsubspecialized health care providers. *Cleft Palate Craniofac J*. 2013.

80. Mooney M. Classification of orofacial clefting. In: Losee JE, Kirschner RE, eds. *Comprehensive Cleft Care*. New York, NY: McGraw-Hill Professional; 2008:21–23.

81. Veau V. *Division Palatine*. Paris: Masson; 1931.

82. Kernahan DA. The striped Y—a symbolic classification for cleft lip and palate. *Plast Reconstr Surg*. 1971;47:469–470.

83. Kriens O. *What Is a Cleft Lip and Palate?: A Multidisciplinary Update*. Stuttgart, Germany: Thieme; 1989.

84. Tessier P. Anatomical classification of facial, cranio-facial and latero-facial clefts. *J Maxillofac Surg*. 1976;4:69–92.

85. Tewfik TL, Karsan N. Congenital malformations, mouth and pharynx. Emedicine from WebMD http://emedicine.medscape.com/article/837347-print Accessed 1/13/2009. Medscape, USA; 2008.

86. Achiron R, Ben Arie A, Gabbay U, et al. Development of the fetal tongue between 14 and 26 weeks of gestation: in utero ultrasonographic measurements. *Ultrasound Obstet Gynecol.* 1997;9:39–41.

87. Bianchi D, Crombleholme T, D'Alton M, et al. Macroglossia. In: Bianchi D, Crombleholme T, D' Alton M, et al, eds. *Fetology: Diagnosis and Management of the Fetal Patient.* New York, NY: McGraw-Hill Professional; 2010:207–213.

88. Bromley B, Benacerraf BR. Fetal micrognathia: associated anomalies and outcome. *J Ultrasound Med.* 1994;13:529–533.

89. Nicolaides KH, Salvesen DR, Snijders RJ, et al. Fetal facial defects: associated malformations and chromosomal abnormalities. *Fetal Diagn Ther.* 1993;8:1–9.

90. Turner GM, Twining P. The facial profile in the diagnosis of fetal abnormalities. *Clin Radiol.* 1993;47:389–395.

91. Otto C, Platt LD. The fetal mandible measurement: an objective determination of fetal jaw size. *Ultrasound Obstet Gynecol.* 1991;1:12–17.

92. Paladini D, Morra T, Teodoro A, et al. Objective diagnosis of micrognathia in the fetus: the jaw index. *Obstet Gynecol.* 1999;93:382–386.

93. Wilhelm L, Borgers H. The "equals sign": a novel marker in the diagnosis of fetal isolated cleft palate. *Ultrasound Obstet Gynecol.* 2010;36:439–444.

94. Vettraino IM, Lee W, Bronsteen RA, et al. Clinical outcome of fetuses with sonographic diagnosis of isolated micrognathia. *Obstet Gynecol.* 2003;102:801–805.

95. Hoffman WY. Cleft palate. In: Rodriguez ED, Losee JE, Neligan PC, eds. *Plastic Surgery, Volume 3: Craniofacial, Head and Neck Surgery and Pediatric Plastic Surgery.* Philadelphia, PA: Saunders; 2012.

96. Gangopadhyay N, Mendonca DA, Woo AS. Pierre robin sequence. *Semin Plast Surg.* 2012;26:76–82.

97. Agarwal S, Sen J, Jain S, et al. Otocephaly: prenatal and postnatal imaging findings. *J Pediatr Neurosci.* 2011;6:94–95.

98. Hersh JH, McChane RH, Rosenberg EM, et al. Otocephaly-midline malformation association. *Am J Med Genet.* 1989;34:246–249.

99. Lawrence DL, Bersu ET. An anatomical study of human otocephaly. *Teratology.* 1984;30:155–165.

100. Persutte WH, Lenke RR, DeRosa RT. Prenatal ultrasonographic appearance of the agnathia malformation complex. *J Ultrasound Med.* 1990;9:725–728.

101. Cayea PD, Bieber FR, Ross MJ, et al. Sonographic findings in otocephaly (synotia). *J Ultrasound Med.* 1985;4:377–379.

102. Rahmani R, Dixon M, Chitayat D, et al. Otocephaly: prenatal sonographic diagnosis. *J Ultrasound Med.* 1998;17:595–598.

103. Suutaria S, Rautio J, Klockars T. Cleft lip and/or palate and auricular malformations. *Cleft Palate Craniofac J.* 2014.

104. Lin KYK, Gampper TJ. Congenital anomalies of the pinna: surgical management. In: Tewfik TL, Der Kaloustian VM, eds. *Congenital Anomalies of the Ear, Nose, and Throat.* New York, NY: Oxford University Press; 1997:107–117.

105. Marx H. *Die Missbildungen des Ohres.* Jena, Germany: Gustav Fischer; 1911.

106. Gorlin RJ, Pindborg JJ. *Syndromes of the Head and Neck.* New York, NY: McGrawHill; 1964.

107. Benacerraf BR, Frigoletto FD Jr. Prenatal ultrasonographic recognition of Goldenhar's syndrome. *Am J Obstet Gynecol.* 1988;159:950–952.

108. Morrison PJ, Mulholland HC, Craig BG, et al. Cardiovascular abnormalities in the oculo-auriculo-vertebral spectrum (Goldenhar syndrome). *Am J Med Genet.* 1992;44:425–428.

109. Burck U. Genetic aspects of hemifacial microsomia. *Hum Genet.* 1983;64:291–296.

110. Bianchi D, Crombleholme T, D'Alton M, et al. Hemifacial microsomia. In: Bianchi D, Crombleholme T, D'Alton M, et al, eds. *Fetology: Diagnosis and Management of the Fetal Patient.* New York, NY: McGraw-Hill Professional; 2010:193–198.

111. McKusick-Nathans Institute of Genetic Medicine. *Online Mendelian Inheritance in Man, OMIM®.* Johns Hopkins University; Baltimore, MD. 2013. http://omim.org/

112. Rollnick BR. Oculoauriculovertebral anomaly: variability and causal heterogeneity. *Am J Med Genet Suppl.* 1988;4:41–53.

113. Rollnick BR, Kaye CI. Hemifacial microsomia and variants: pedigree data. *Am J Med Genet.* 1983;15:233–253.

## EMBRYOLOGY

The basic tissues of the head and neck become organized in the branchial apparatus and, therefore, the origin of many fetal neck lesions reside in this embryologic structure. The branchial apparatus contains five pairs of mesenchymal condensations, which develop on both sides of the pharyngeal foregut on day 22, equivalent to branchial arches 1, 2, 3, 4, and 6. The fifth arch is very small and essentially regresses. The mesodermal arches are separated externally by ectodermal grooves notated as clefts and internally by endoderm-lined pouches (Figs. 14.1 and 14.2). The core of each arch contains its own arterial element and crest cells that contribute to skeletal structures. The mesodermal component will give rise to musculature of the face and neck, and carry their own nerve and cranial nerve component.

There are four ectoderm-lined clefts along the arches. In the 5th to 6th week, the second arch grows and elongates inferiorly to meet the enlarging fifth arch or developing epipericardial ridge (see Fig. 14.1A). As a result, an ectoderm-lined cavity forms enclosing the second, third, and fourth branchial clefts. This temporary cavity, known as the "Sinus of His," usually obliterates secondary to fusion of its walls. However, failure of complete wall fusion can result in branchial cleft cyst, sinus, or fistula and, depending on the area of the branchial arch, can be classified into type 1, 2, 3, or 4 (see Fig. 14.1B). The first branchial is the only cleft that will become a definitive structure, eventually giving rise to the epithelium of the external auditory canal.

There are five pharyngeal or branchial pouches lined by endoderm, though the fifth evolves late and is usually considered part of the fourth. The first pouch gives rise to the pharyngotympanic tube that develops into the middle ear cavity and tympanic membrane (see Fig. 14.2). The second becomes the palatine tonsil. The third and fourth branchial pouches give rise to the thymus, parathyroid glands, and ultimobranchial body, representing parafollicular calcitonin secreting cells that are incorporated into the thyroid gland. With branchial pouch maldevelopment, there is lack of or erroneous formation of structures to which each pouch contributes. For example, incomplete obliteration of the thymopharyngeal duct may result in thymopharyngeal duct cyst or ectopic thymus, persisting along the tract of the migrating tissue (Fig. 14.3).

Table 14.1 summarizes the different structures arising from the branchial arches, clefts, and pouches. First arch syndrome includes anomalies secondary to abnormal development or absence of various components of the first pharyngeal arch. Examples include Treacher Collins Syndrome and Pierre Robin sequence.[1]

The thyroid gland arises during the 4th week as a small mass of proliferating endoderm at the apex of the foramen cecum in the developing tongue. It descends as a bilobed structure in the soft tissues of the neck attached to the thyroglossal duct that extends from the tongue, anterior to the hyoid and laryngeal cartilage to the lower neck. The thyroid reaches its final location in front of the trachea by the 7th week. At this time, the

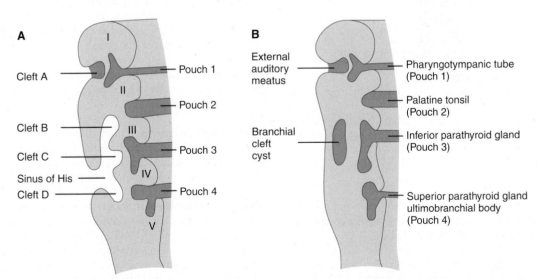

**FIGURE 14.1: A:** Differentiation of the pharyngeal clefts and pouches. There is elongation and growth of the second and fifth arches forming the sinus of His. **B:** Further maturation of the epithelium in the walls of the pharyngeal pouches. (Adapted from Benson MT, Dalen K, Mancuso AA, et al. Congenital anomalies of the branchial apparatus: embryology and pathologic anatomy. *Radiographics*. 1992;12(5):943–960.)

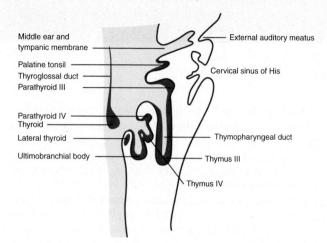

**FIGURE 14.2:** The structures that develop from the branchial clefts and pouches, particularly origin of the thymus, parathyroids, and ultimobranchial body. (Adapted from Benson MT, Dalen K, Mancuso AA, et al. Congenital anomalies of the branchial apparatus: embryology and pathologic anatomy. *Radiographics.* 1992;12(5):943–960.)

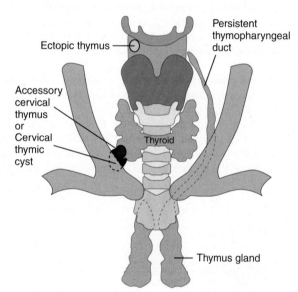

**FIGURE 14.3:** The course of the thymopharyngeal duct and possible locations for ectopic thymic tissue and/or thymic cyst. (Adapted from Benson MT, Dalen K, Mancuso AA, et al. Congenital anomalies of the branchial apparatus: embryology and pathologic anatomy. *Radiographics.* 1992;12(5):943–960.)

thyroglossal duct involutes, although if any portion persists, a thyroglossal cyst or sinus may remain. Infrequently, ectopic thyroid tissue can be found in the path of descent.

The lymphatic sacs begin to develop at the end of the 5th week of gestation, approximately 2 weeks after the cardiovascular system. There are six primary lymphatic sacs: paired jugular lymphatic sacs, cisterna chili, retroperitoneal (mesenteric) lymph sac, and paired iliac lymph sacs that will eventually evolve into groups of lymph nodes (Fig. 14.4). Lymphatic sacs develop alongside vessels and later make connections with the venous system. Lymphatic malformations may evolve secondary to incomplete or inadequate venous connections with stasis of lymphatic fluid causing dilated lymphatic channels.

## CONGENITAL LESIONS OF THE NECK

Congenital neck lesions detected during the fetal period are very rare with unknown incidence. A list of congenital lesions of the neck is shown in Table 14.2.

### Branchial Anomalies

**Incidence:** Prenatal diagnosis of branchial apparatus anomalies is very rare with few cases described in the literature.[2–5]

**Pathogenesis/Etiology:** Defects in the embryogenesis of the branchial apparatus include branchial, parathyroid, and thymic anomalies, which may manifest as sinuses, fistulas, or cysts. These anomalies can be further classified according to their branchial pouch or cleft of origin; branchial "cleft" cyst or branchial "pouch" cyst. Histologic evaluation of the epithelium lining the fistulas, sinuses, or cysts can define the pouch or cleft derivation.

The etiology of these lesions is poorly understood. The most accepted theory proposes that branchial anomalies are vestigial remnants resulting from incomplete obliteration of the branchial apparatus or buried epithelial cell rests.[6] The most common lesion is a branchial cleft cyst type 2, which arises because of persistence of the cervical sinus of His. These lesions can be present in many anatomic locations, but the most common type 2 is a cyst in the anterolateral neck, most often on the left, lying anterior to the sternocleidomastoid, posterior to the submandibular gland, and lateral to the carotid sheath.[2]

**Diagnosis:** By ultrasound (US), branchial cysts are round or ovoid anechoic or hypoechoic thin-walled cysts (Fig. 14.5). Real-time imaging can demonstrate movement of internal echoes differentiating from a solid lesion. On MRI, the cysts are hypointense on T1-weighted sequences and hyperintense on T2-weighted sequences (Fig. 14.6).

**Associated Anomalies:** Branchial cleft cysts are usually isolated lesions; however, they have been reported with branchio-oto-renal syndrome.[7]

**Differential Diagnosis:** Differential diagnosis includes thymic cyst, lymphatic malformation, and thyroglossal duct cyst, though branchial cysts are typically lateral, whereas thyroglossal duct lesions are predominately midline.

**Prognosis/Management:** Rarely, branchial cleft cyst can cause airway or esophageal obstruction and necessitate an ex utero intrapartum treatment (EXIT).[2] Given susceptibility to hemorrhage, infection, and questionable predisposition to cancer, surgical resection, and marsupialization of the tract is curative. The prognosis is excellent following complete resection.

### Cervical Thymic Cyst

**Incidence:** Thymic cysts are very rare and infrequently diagnosed in utero.

| Table 14.1 | Derivatives of the Branchial Apparatus | | |
|---|---|---|---|
| Level | Derivative of Branchial Pouch (Endoderm) | Derivative of Branchial Arch (Mesoderm) | Derivative of Branchial Cleft (Ectoderm) |
| 1 | Eustachian tube, tympanum, mastoid air cells | Mandible, muscles of mastication, ear ossicles, CN V | External ear canal |
| 2 | Palatine tonsils | Muscles of facial expression, lesser horn of the hyoid bone, CN VII and VIII | Sinus of His |
| 3 | Inferior parathyroid, thymus and pyriform fossa | Superior constrictor muscle, ICA, greater horn of the hyoid bone, CN IX | Sinus of His |
| 4 | Superior parathyroid gland, apex of pyriform sinus | Most pharyngeal constrictors, laryngeal muscles, thyroid, aortic arch, right subclavian artery, CN X | None |
| 5 and 6 | Parafollicular C cells of thyroid | Laryngeal and pharyngeal muscles, CN XI | None |

CN, cranial nerve; ICA, internal carotid artery.

**Pathogenesis/Etiology:** Thymic cysts may be encountered in the neck, thoracic inlet, or mediastinum because of persistence of the thymopharyngeal tracts.[8] The thymus is derived from the ventral division of the paired third and fourth pharyngeal pouches around 6 weeks of gestation. The thymic buds at each side migrate inferiorly, forming the thymopharyngeal ducts, extending from the angle of the mandible, along the carotid sheath to the superior mediastinum owing to attachment to the pericardium. During the 7th to 9th week, there is obliteration of the proximal ducts that then separate from the pharynx. Epithelial proliferation within the distal ducts gives rise to bilateral thymic tissue that fuse in the anterior mediastinum. Rests of thymic tissue, known as ectopic thymus, can be found along the normal path of descent.[9]

**Diagnosis:** Cervical thymic cysts are commonly multilocular, but may be unilocular and vary in size from 1.4 to 8 cm.

| Table 14.2 | Fetal Cervical Lesions | |
|---|---|---|
| Cystic | Solid | Mixed Cystic and Solid |
| Branchial cleft cyst | Ectopic thymus | Neuroblastoma |
| Cervical meningocele | Goiter | Teratoma |
| Cervical thymic cyst | Hemangioma | |
| Esophageal atresia | Neuroblastoma | |
| Esophageal duplication cyst | Rhabdomyosarcoma | |
| Laryngocele | Sarcoma | |
| Lymphatic malformations | Teratoma | |
| Neuroenteric cyst | Metastasis (rare) | |
| Thyroglossal duct cyst | | |
| Thyroid cyst | | |

They are intimately associated with the carotid space, splaying the carotid artery and jugular vein.[9] Thymic cysts are more common on the left, and up to 50% have a mediastinal connection. By US, they are anechoic but may have internal debris (Fig. 14.7). On MRI, the lesions are hypointense on T1-weighted images and hyperintense on T2 (Fig. 14.8). If they are complicated by hemorrhage, the internal signal will be heterogeneous.[10]

**Differential Diagnosis:** The differential diagnoses include lymphatic malformation, thyroid cyst, thyroglossal duct cyst, and branchial cleft cyst.

**Prognosis/Management:** Thymic cysts are usually asymptomatic, although respiratory distress, dysphagia, and vocal cord

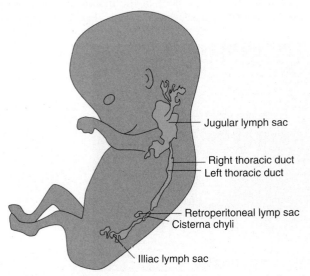

**FIGURE 14.4:** Seven-week embryo shows lymphatic sacs before the venous connections are formed.

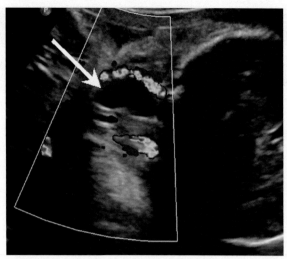

**FIGURE 14.5:** Branchial Cyst. Coronal Doppler US image shows an anechoic avascular cervical lesion *(arrow)* with acoustic enhancement in the lateral neck diagnosed as branchial cyst postnatal.

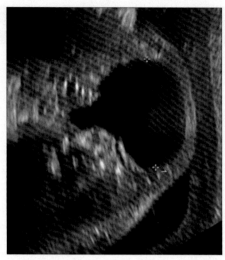

**FIGURE 14.7:** Thymic Cyst. Axial US image demonstrates lobulated anechoic lesion designated by *calipers* centered in the lateral neck diagnosed as thymic cyst postnatal.

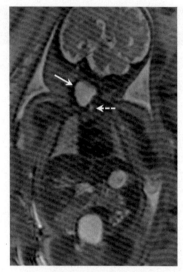

**FIGURE 14.6:** Branchial Cyst. Same fetus as in Figure 14.5. Coronal SSFSE T2 image shows hyperintense lesion *(solid arrow)* in the lateral fetal neck. The airway is partially visualized in this image *(dotted arrow)*.

paralysis have been described.[11] Treatment consists of surgical excision of the cyst and residual tract although spontaneous resolution has been reported.[11]

## Ranula

**Incidence:** The incidence of congenital ranula is estimated to be 0.7%. Prenatal diagnosis is very rare.[12]

**Pathogenesis/Etiology:** A ranula is a sublingual or minor salivary gland retention cyst located at the floor of the mouth. They are classified by location into simple (intraoral) or plunging (oral/cervical) types. Congenital ranulas are thought to arise secondary to atresia of the salivary gland ducts or ostial adhesion.[12] The histopathology is distinctive with salivary duct epithelium lining the walls of the cyst, distinguishing from lymphatic malformation.

**Diagnosis:** By US, ranulas are well-defined anechoic or hypoechoic cysts in the floor of the mouth that may extend into the submandibular/cervical region (Fig. 14.9). No Color

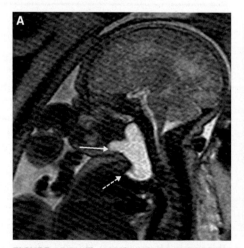
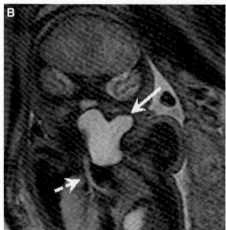

**FIGURE 14.8:** Thymic Cyst. **A:** Sagittal T2 SSFSE image of same fetus in Figure 14.7. Lobular lesion is T2 hyperintense *(solid arrow)* and extends the length of neck but is also present in the mediastinum *(dotted arrow)*, contiguous with thymic tissue. **B:** Coronal T2 SSFSE image in the same fetus demonstrates lesion *(solid arrow)* and patency of the airway *(dotted arrow)*.

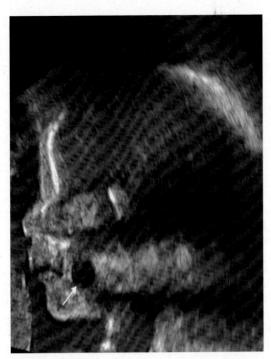

**FIGURE 14.9:** Ranula. Sagittal gray-scale US image demonstrates a round anechoic lesion *(arrow)* in the floor of the mouth, noted to represent ranula postnatal.

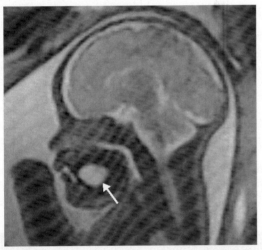

**FIGURE 14.10:** Ranula. Sagittal T2 SSFSE image shows a T2 hyperintense cystic lesion *(arrow)* in the floor of the mouth, below the tongue.

Doppler is usually observed. Well-delineated borders are seen on MRI with low T1 and high T2 signals (Fig. 14.10).

**Differential Diagnosis:** Differential diagnosis includes lymphatic malformation, thyroglossal duct cyst, and dermoid because of its midline/paramidline positioning.

**Prognosis/Management:** Congenital ranulas may present as cystic structures in the oral cavity and can rarely grow to completely fill the oral cavity, possibly obstructing the upper airway at birth.[13] They elevate the floor of the mouth and cause the tongue to be superiorly and anteriorly displaced. Infrequently, giant congenital ranula may result in airway obstruction, necessitating EXIT procedure at birth to secure the airway.[12,13] Treatments of congenital ranula include marsupialization, aspiration of the ranula, and resection of the sublingual salivary gland, all

of which showed no recurrence except for marsupialization with 61% recurrence.[14] Spontaneous resolution in the neonatal period has also been described.[12]

## Thyroglossal Duct Cyst

**Incidence:** Prenatal diagnosis of thyroglossal duct cyst is rare.[15] However, the cysts are the most common midline cervical anomaly, representing 70% of all congenital neck masses.[16] The exact incidence is unknown, but 7% of the population has been shown to have a thyroglossal duct remnant.[16]

**Pathogenesis/Etiology:** The anatomy of the thyroglossal duct follows the pathway of embryology from the foramen cecum of the tongue, along the anterior surface of the hyoid to the pyramidal lobe of the thyroid. Persistence of the duct results in cyst or sinus formation at any point of descent. The majority of duct remnants are midline or parasagittal, adjacent to the hyoid bone.[17] Rarely, these cysts are found within the tongue or the floor of the mouth.[15] The lesion can be occasionally associated with Cowden syndrome.

**Diagnosis:** On US, the classic appearance of a thyroglossal duct cyst is a thin-walled anechoic unilocular lesion. However, because of high protein content, these lesions may be hypoechoic or heterogeneous echotexture, some appearing pseudosolid and mimicking ectopic tissue.[18] Posterior acoustic enhancement is present in the majority of lesions, and absence of color Doppler flow can be helpful. Demonstration of a normal thyroid gland is recommended to exclude the diagnosis of ectopic tissue. On MRI, signal depends on protein content, but most are typically bright on T1 and T2 sequences.[19]

**Differential Diagnosis:** Other cystic lesions in the midline/paramidline include dermoid, esophageal duplication cyst, or ranula. Branchial and thymic cysts tend to be lateral neck. Lymphatic malformations and teratomas are typically complex cystic and solid.

**Prognosis/Management:** Up to one-third of patients with thyroglossal duct cyst will develop superimposed infection.[18] There is a 1% increased risk of cancer, primarily of the papillary type.[20] Rarely, the cyst may be within the tongue or floor of the mouth and can cause airway obstruction.[15] In the presence of large cyst obstructing airway, an EXIT procedure may be necessary. Postnatal therapy is surgical resection with the Sistrunk procedure, which involves excision of cyst, remnant tract, and a portion of the hyoid bone.[20]

## Dermoid/Epidermoid

**Incidence:** Prenatal diagnosis is rare, but overall these lesions represent 7% of head and neck lesions and 25% of midline cervical anomalies.[20]

**Pathogenesis/Etiology:** Dermoid/epidermoids develop when there is inclusion of ectodermal tissue during the fusion of the branchial arches. Dermoid cysts contain two germ layers, both ectoderm and mesoderm, whereas epidermoid cysts consist of only one germ layer, the ectoderm.[21] Although the majority of these masses are found around the orbit or adjacent to the nose, approximately 11% of these cysts will present in the midline in the floor of the mouth in the submandibular space.[20] These lesions can be associated with Gardner syndrome.[19]

**Diagnosis:** US of these lesions demonstrate a well-circumscribed, thin-walled unilocular mass with internal echos and little posterior echo enhancement. MRI depicts these lesions as T1 hyperintense to isointense, T2 hyperintense, and with a few lesions having fat–fluid or fluid–fluid levels. These are the only cystic lesions to restrict diffusion, which can confirm diagnosis.[19]

**Prognosis/Management:** Rarely, lesions in the floor of the mouth may cause airway obstruction, and EXIT may be considered. Surgical resection is the treatment of choice since these anomalies are at risk for rupture or infection, and 5% will undergo malignant degeneration to squamous cell neoplasms.[20]

## INFLAMMATORY LESIONS

### Thyroid Goiter

Thyroid goiter manifests as diffuse enlargement of the thyroid gland and may be associated with decreased, increased, or normal (euthyroid) function.

**Incidence:** Fetal goiter is very rare and can present with fetal hypothyroidism or hyperthyroidism. Hypothyroid goiter is more common than hyperthyroid, with incidence of 1 in 3,000 to 4,000 births worldwide.[22] The incidence of hyperthyroid goiter is unknown. Graves disease is seen in 1% of pregnant women, and 2% to 12% of those fetuses will develop hyper- or hypothyroidism in utero or in the neonatal period.

**Pathogenesis/Etiology:** Fetal thyroid function begins in the late first trimester, approximately by week 12.[23] The fetal thyroid slowly increases in size until week 32, after which a rapid growth pattern ensues. Several published nomograms compare gestational age and biparietal diameter to thyroid gland size to aid in the diagnosis of thyroid gland enlargement[24–26] (see Tables 30 and 31 in Appendix A1).

Fetal goiter associated with hypothyroidism is primarily due to transplacental passage of maternal antithyroid treatment drugs (propylthiouracil, metimazole) or antithyroid antibodies, maternal iodine deficiency, or congenital thyroid dyshormogenesis. Maternal iodine intoxication by seaweed and iodine-containing vitamins are rare causes. Maternal thyroid function can be normal despite fetal goiter and should not deter monitoring and treatment of fetal thyroid dysfunction. In the absence of maternal thyroid disease, fetal goiter is likely due to congenital dyshormonogenesis. If untreated in the first 3 months of life, congenital hypothyroidism can cause severe irreversible mental retardation with impairment in speech and hearing.

Fetal goiter associated with hyperthyroid goiter is secondary to transplacental passage of maternal thyroid-stimulating IgG antibody, usually in women with Graves disease. It is not detected in the fetus before 20 to 24 weeks' gestational age as the fetal thyroid is not mature enough to respond to antibody stimulation.

**Diagnosis:** Maternal thyroid function tests, including antithyroid antibody titers, should be obtained. However, maternal thyroid status does not reflect fetal thyroid state, and, therefore, fetal blood sampling may be required. The definitive diagnosis of fetal thyroid dysfunction is made by cordocentesis, with a risk for fetal loss of 0.5% to 1.4%.[27] Historically, amniotic fluid analysis of fetal thyroid function is considered unreliable as there is poor correlation between amniotic fluid thyroid hormone levels and fetal serum levels.[28] Fetal blood will show elevated TSH and low thyroxine in cases of hypothyroidism and low TSH in cases of hyperthyroidism.

**Ultrasound:** Fetal goiter is diagnosed by US at an average gestational age of 26 weeks.[29] The thyroid is symmetrically enlarged with bilobed configuration and varying echogenicity, either homogeneous or heterogeneous with multiple cysts. Enlargement of the thyroid may result in neck hyperextension seen via 2D and 3D ultrasound. The airway and esophagus may be compressed by the enlarged gland; polyhydramnios ensues if swallowing is impaired. Color Doppler shows increased vascular flow within the enlarged thyroid (Fig. 14.11). The pattern of increased central flow has been associated with hyperthyroid goiter, and peripherally increased flow with hypothyroid goiter.[30] In fetuses with hyperthyroid goiter with high-output cardiac failure, Doppler may show increased velocities in the common carotid artery and descending aorta (~200 cm per second) and dilatation of the superior vena cava. Cardiomegaly and pleural effusions have been reported.

In fetuses with hyperthyroid goiter, additional US findings include tachycardia, advanced bone age, hydrops, intrauterine growth restriction, and hepatosplenomegaly. In those with hypothyroid goiter, ultrasound may reveal cardiac dysfunction and delayed bone age.

**MRI:** On MRI, the normal thyroid gland is hyperintense on T1-weighted images and isointense on T2-weighted images, relative to muscle. With fetal goiter, there is symmetric thyroid enlargement with increased T1 and intermediate T2 signals[31] (Fig. 14.12). Thyroid enlargement with T2 signal greater than muscle suggests thyroid dysfunction, either hypo- or hyperthyroid state. Intrinsic thyroid T1 hyperintensity persists despite hypo- or hyperthyroid state.[32] MRI is useful in evaluation of tracheal and esophageal compression by the goiter as well as degree of neck hyperextension. MRI is particularly helpful in delivery planning as the most severe cases may require cesarean section or EXIT procedure to secure the airway at delivery. In this instance, MRI performed closer to delivery will best depict the airway.

**Differential Diagnosis:** The differential diagnosis for fetal thyroid enlargement includes other fetal neck masses (cystic or solid), notably lymphatic malformation, hemangioma,

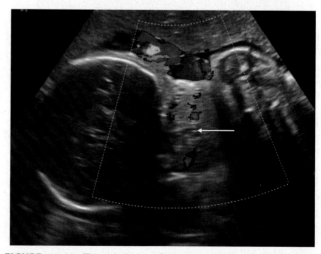

**FIGURE 14.11:** Thyroid Goiter. Coronal Doppler US image shows vascular enlargement of the thyroid. There is questionable mass effect on the airway (*arrow*).

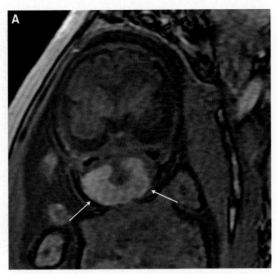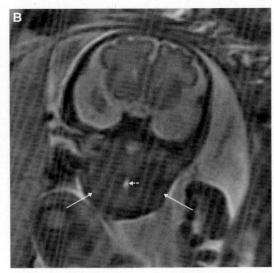

**FIGURE 14.12:** Thyroid Goiter. **A:** Coronal T1-weighted image demonstrates enlargement and hyperintensity of the thyroid gland *(arrows)*. **B:** Coronal T2-weighted image shows isointense signal (with regard to muscle) of enlarged thyroid *(solid arrows)*, which encircles narrowed but patent airway *(dotted short arrow)*.

and cervical teratoma. Cervical teratomas are usually midline, mixed cystic and solid, show rapid growth, and cause greater degree of mass effect upon the airway and esophagus and secondary polyhydramnios when compared with goiter. Lymphatic malformations are usually lateral rather than medial and are predominantly cystic. Hemangiomas characteristically have high vessel density and flow. Thyroglossal duct cyst, thyroid cyst, branchial cleft cyst, cervical neuroblastoma, cervical rhabdomyosarcoma, and ectopic thymus are much less common.

**Associated Anomalies:** Rarely, fetal goiter with hypothyroidism has been associated with other congenital anomalies, such as Prader–Willi syndrome.[33]

**Prognosis:** Fetal goiter is usually self-limited and has good prognosis. In many cases, the thyroid decreases in size prenatally or soon after birth once treatment has been established. In fetuses born to mothers with Graves disease, the hyperthyroid goiter will resolve as circulating maternal thyroid-stimulating antibodies abate. The prognosis for newborns with congenital hypothyroidism depends on timely levothyroxine treatment.

**Management:** Treatment of fetal goiter depends on maternal thyroid state and medications, as well as fetal thyroid function. In fetal hypothyroid goiter, single or multiple intra-amniotic and fetal intramuscular injections of levothyroxine have been successful in treating hypothyroidism.[27,34–37] If cordocentesis reveals increased high thyroid-stimulating autoantibody titers, then administration of antithyroid drugs, such as propylthiouracil or methimazole, to the mother is recommended. Repeated cordocentesis can demonstrate normalization of fetal thyroid function. Ultrasound can aid in monitoring the fetal thyroid state by assessing the thyroid size, degree of neck hyperextension, polyhydramnios, and pleural effusions. Doppler US will show decreased vascular flow within the goiter.

Independent of fetal thyroid function, goiter may cause mass effect upon the airway and esophagus, leading to polyhydramnios, which could prompt preterm labor. Neck hyperextension may necessitate cesarean section owing to risk of dystocia. Rarely, if the goiter causes severe airway compression, EXIT procedure may be necessary to rapidly secure the fetal airway upon delivery.

**Recurrence:** The recurrence risk of fetal goiter in subsequent pregnancies is a concern in women with thyroid dysfunction. Of the estimated 1% of pregnant women with Graves disease,[38] the incidence of fetal hypo- or hyperthyroidism is 2% to 12%.[34,38] In mothers with hyperthyroidism taking propylthiouracil, 1% of their fetuses will have hypothyroidism.[28] Thyroid dyshormonogenesis, although rare, is transmitted as an autosomal recessive trait; therefore, the recurrence risk is 25%.

## VASCULAR MALFORMATIONS

Vascular anomaly is an all-encompassing term that includes both vascular malformations and vascular tumors. Vascular malformations are classified according to hemodynamics into high-flow and low-flow malformations, and are further classified according to the type of vessel present (arteries, veins, or lymphatics). Low-flow vascular malformations include pure or combined malformations of capillary, lymphatic, and venous channels. High-flow vascular malformations include both arteriovenous malformations and fistulas. Vascular tumors include hemangiomas, which are classified into congenital or infantile types.

### Lymphatic Malformations

Lymphatic malformations (LM) contain dysplastic but mature lymphatic channels. The fetal literature frequently refers to macrocystic lesions as cystic hygroma (if in the neck) or microcystic lesions as lymphangioma. This nomenclature has largely been replaced since 1982 by Mulliken and Glowacki in that all these lesions are now referred to as lymphatic malformations.[39] Therefore, for the purposes of this chapter, we will refer to these as nuchal and nonnuchal lymphatic malformations, respectively.

**Incidence:** Seventy-five percent of LM occur in the neck, and the majority originate in the posterior triangle (nuchal) or oral cavity, left side greater than right.[40] The incidence of nuchal LM between 10 and 14 weeks of gestation is approximately 0.35%.[41] Less is known about the incidence of nonnuchal LM (lymphangiomas); however, they have been reported to be approximately one-fifth as common as nuchal LM.[42] LM when large are often diagnosed prenatally, but the majority present by age 2 years.

**Pathogenesis:** The communication between jugular lymphatic sacs and jugular veins is formed at 40 days' conceptional age.[43] A failure in this communication results in dilated jugular lymphatic sacs. Nonnuchal LM may result from noncommunication at any portion of the lymphatic or lymphovenous system. LM are well-defined, multicystic lesions with numerous internal septa and may be infiltrative and cross fascial planes. They are classified into microcystic, macrocystic, and combined lesions. LMs often coexist with venous malformations, termed venolymphatic malformations. Pathologic biomarkers for LM include the VEGFR-3 and PROX1 antibodies[44] and D2-40 monoclonal antibody.[45]

**Etiology:** Nuchal LM diagnosed during the first trimester are highly associated with chromosomal abnormalities (51%), the most common being trisomy 21. Other aneuploidies include Turner syndrome, trisomies 13 and 18, and deletions such as 13q and 18p.[41] Additionally, cardiac and skeletal malformations are seen in 34% of cases.[41]

Nonnuchal LM are usually isolated, yet can be associated with syndromes such as Gorham–Stout disease, Klippel–Trenaunay syndrome, and Generalized Lymphatic Anomaly syndrome.[46]

**Diagnosis**

*Ultrasound:* LM are multilocular cystic masses with posterior acoustic enhancement and vascular flow limited to the internal septations (Fig. 14.13). Vascular flow is not seen in pure LM; however, venous flow will be present in a combined (venolymphatic) malformation. Macrocystic LM are anechoic centrally when simple, yet may appear complex related to internal hemorrhage or protein. Fluid–fluid levels are not uncommon. Microscystic LM appear hyperechoic on account of innumerable interfaces created by multiple small cysts, often too small to resolve.

*MRI:* MRI demonstrates a multilocular cystic transspatial mass. The cystic component is typically isointense to muscle on T1 and hyperintense on T2-weighted images, unless complicated by protein or hemorrhage, in which case there may be fluid–fluid levels (Fig. 14.14). Nonnuchal LM may cause airway compromise. The deep component of the malformation is often not well delineated by ultrasound, particularly if microcystic. Thus, dedicated fetal MRI should be considered to evaluate deep extent and airway involvement to guide perinatal management, in particular the decision for EXIT procedure (Fig. 14.15).[46]

**Differential Diagnosis:** The main differential diagnosis for nuchal LM is increased nuchal translucency. The presence of multiple septations and the posterolateral involvement of the neck seen in LM should aid in the diagnosis. Neural tube defect, encephalocele, and cystic teratoma should also be kept in the

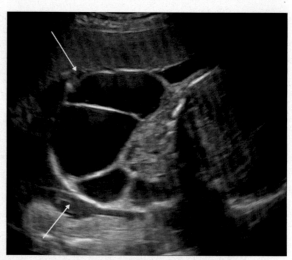

**FIGURE 14.13:** Lymphatic Malformation. First trimester axial US imaging showing a septated fluid-filled lesion in the anterolateral neck consistent with a lymphatic malformation *(arrows)*.

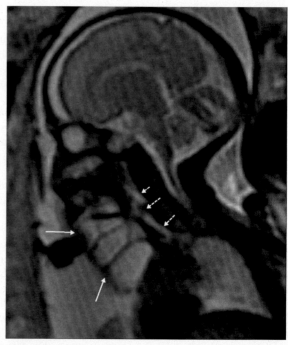

**FIGURE 14.14:** Lymphatic Malformation. Sagittal T2 Haste image of the head and neck shows the same patient as Figure 14.16 with multiseptated LM *(solid arrows)*. Note the patent hypopharynx, glottis, and hypoglottic region *(dotted arrows)*.

differential. For nonnuchal lymphatic malformation, the differential diagnosis includes cystic teratoma, hemangioma, venous malformation, arteriovenous malformation, and soft tissue sarcoma.

**Prognosis:** Nearly 50% of fetuses with the US diagnosis of nuchal LM in the first trimester will have a chromosomal abnormality and therefore poor prognosis, with up to 25% risk of fetal or perinatal death. Only 17% will result in a healthy newborn. However, if the fetus has a nuchal LM but has no aneuploidy, no cardiac anomalies and has a normal anatomic sonographic evaluation at 16 to 20 weeks gestation, there is a 95% chance of

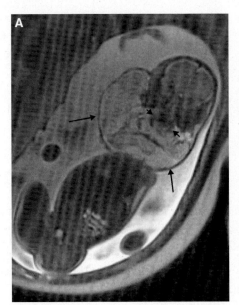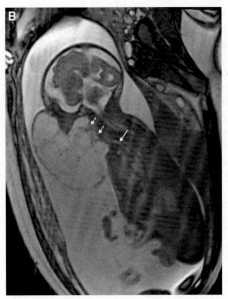

**FIGURE 14.15:** Lymphatic Malformation. **A:** Coronal T2 image of a fetus with a large multiseptated cystic lesion in the anterolateral neck *(long black arrows)* with suspicion for airway compromise as the lesion invades oral cavity/tongue *(short arrows)*. **B:** Sagittal T2 image in the same patient showing poor delineation of the hypopharynx and proximal trachea *(dotted arrows)*. Note the patent thoracic trachea *(solid arrow)*.

normal pediatric outcome.[41] Spontaneous regression of nuchal LM has been reported in utero, usually between 2 and 7 months of age.[44]

The outcome for isolated nonnuchal LM is favorable, depending on the extent and treatment response of the lesion. Approximately 3% to 10% of infants with LM have respiratory compromise due to airway obstruction or mediastinal extension.[40]

**Management:** Prenatal aspiration of lymphatic fluid in macrocystic lesions is rarely performed but considered when there is rapid fluid reaccumulation, infection, and intralesional hemorrhage.[47] Few cases have been described in the literature where aspiration of macrocystic lesions immediately prior to delivery has allowed normal vaginal delivery.[48] In the presence of airway obstruction, delivery via the EXIT procedure may be imperative. Surgical resection is the treatment of choice, but can be difficult in the presence of neural, vascular, or muscular invasion. Macrocystic LM are often successfully treated postnatal with sclerotherapy, but other treatment strategies include radiofrequency ablation and laser.

Small, focal LM have excellent prognosis both with percutaneous sclerosis and with surgical resection. Large, infiltrating lesions can be difficult to treat fully; recurrence is seen in 17% of complete and 40% of incomplete excisions.[49]

## Venous Malformations

**Incidence:** Venous malformations occur in approximately 1% of the general population. Of these, approximately 40% occur in the head and neck.[50]

**Pathogenesis/Etiology:** Venous malformations contain dysplastic but mature venous channels. They may be purely venous, venolymphatic (most common) or arteriovenous. Venous malformations may occur at any time during angiogenesis. Similar to LM, these lesions are often infiltrative and cross fascial planes, usually subcutaneous tissue and muscle. Venous malformations can be associated with Blue Rubber Bleb Nevus Syndrome, Maffucci syndrome, and Klippel–Trenaunay and Parkes–Weber syndrome.[50]

**Diagnosis:** With US, Doppler is helpful to differentiate venous from other vascular malformations. Pulsed Doppler shows slow velocity with monophasic to biphasic waveforms. On occasion, flow within the vessels is so slow; no color flow can be seen. Fluid–fluid levels and acoustic shadowing related to phleboliths may be present. On MRI, these malformations are typically isointense to muscle on T1 and hyperintense on T2-weighted images, but appear heterogeneous if thrombus or hemorrhage is present. T2* GRE images are useful to demonstrate blooming artifact from phleboliths or hemorrhage.

**Differential Diagnosis:** Differential diagnosis includes lymphatic malformation, arteriovenous malformation, hemangioma, and soft tissue sarcoma.

**Prognosis:** Many, if not all, venous malformations are present at birth; however, most are small and often go unrecognized on prenatal imaging. After birth, they tend to grow proportional to the growth of the child. Some lesions may enlarge suddenly because of hemorrhage, infection, thrombosis, or hormonal changes.

**Treatment:** Most venous malformations are treated conservatively, either with elastic compression, sclerotherapy, or surgical excision.[51]

## Arterial Venous Fistula or Malformation

**Incidence:** Arterial malformations are most common in the head and neck, yet the true incidence is unknown.

**Pathogenesis/Etiology:** An arterial venous malformation is a tangle of abnormal thin-walled vessels connecting dilated high-flow feeding arteries vessels to a draining vein (which is often enlarged related to the increased pressures and high flow). Arteriovenous fistulas are similar; however, these lesions lack the tangle of dysplastic vessels that are present in the malformations and are more often acquired rather than congenital. It is believed that arteriovenous malformations arise in the fetus from failure of regression of arteriovenous channels in the primitive retiform plexus.[52]

They can be associated with phosphatase and tensin (PTEN) homolog gene mutations, such as Cowden and Bannayan–Riley–Ruvalcaba syndrome, RASA (angiogenic) gene mutations (which includes some forms of Parkes–Weber syndrome), and hereditary hemorrhagic telangiectasia (HHT).[50]

**Diagnosis:** In the literature, the arterial venous malformations are typically described as a vascular lesion without soft tissue mass. In the fetus, in our experience, a soft tissue mass is often seen in conjunction with high-flow lesions. On US, multiple hypoechoic channels with or without soft tissue mass are noted (Fig. 14.16A). Doppler demonstrates high systolic and high diastolic flow in the arteries. Arterialized venous waveforms with spectral broadening is also noted (Fig. 14.16B).

MRI may show multiple tubular structures with flow void and heterogeneous T2 signal intensity (Fig. 14.16C). A single or multiple large vessels can be seen coursing through the mass. Cardiac failure and hydrops may develop in the presence of high AV shunting.

**Management:** These lesions are treated with transarterial embolization or surgery.

## NEOPLASMS

### Cervical Hemangioma

**Incidence:** Hemangioma is the most common vascular tumor in infancy, affecting approximately 10% of infants. Greater than 50% of hemangiomas involve the head and neck region.[53] They commonly appear in the neonatal period, though some present at birth and are known as congenital hemangioma. There is a high female predilection.

**Pathogenesis/Etiology:** Hemangiomas arise from abnormal cellular proliferation of vascular endothelial cells. Boon et al. introduced a new classification for hemangiomas and showed a clear histologic distinction between infantile hemangiomas

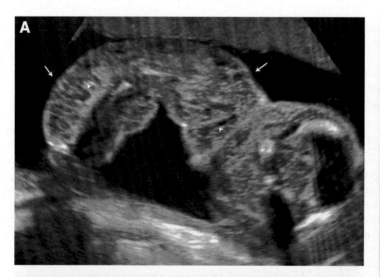

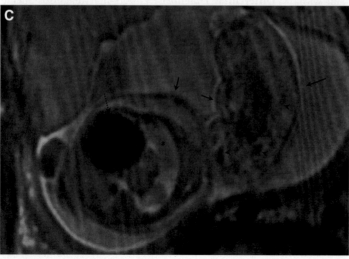

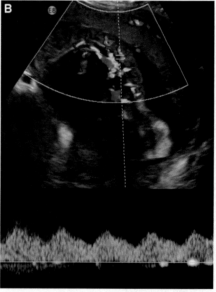

**FIGURE 14.16:** High Flow Combined Lesion. Fetus at 21 weeks with diagnosis of Parkes–Weber syndrome. **A:** Axial US demonstrates heterogeneous mass along upper extremity *(arrows)* containing multiple tubular hypoechoic enlarged vessels *(arrowheads)*. **B:** With color Doppler, there are large arterial feeders demonstrating spectral broadening and low-impedance arterial waveform. **C:** Axial image from fetal MRI demonstrates heterogeneous lesion along the upper extremity and chest *(arrows)* containing multiple flow voids *(arrowheads)*. There is mild cardiomegaly *(dotted arrow)* and pleural effusion *(star)*.

and congenital hemangiomas (CH) by demonstrating that CH are glut-1 (glucose-1 transporter 1) negative and infantile hemangiomas are glut-1 positive. Congenital hemangiomas were further divided into rapidly involuting congenital hemangiomas (RICH) and noninvoluting congenital hemangiomas (NICH).[54] Most CH are solitary as opposed to infantile hemangiomas in which 20% are multiple. Congenital hemangiomas have a steady growth in utero until the third trimester, when they stabilize in size.

**Diagnosis:** Congenital hemangiomas have been diagnosed as early as 12 weeks' gestation and usually involve the posterolateral neck.[55] There is no apparent imaging differentiation between rapidly involuting and noninvoluting congenital hemangiomas. They share location, size, and similar imaging features. On US, CH are heterogeneous, solid, and vascular masses with high vessel density and high flow velocity, and low-resistance index and broadening of spectrum on Doppler ultrasound (Figs. 14.17A and 14.17B). MRI will show a well-defined heterogeneous solid mass in the head and neck region with intermediate signal intensity on T1-weighted images and increased signal intensity on T2-weighted images (Fig. 14.17C). High T2 signal intensity is likely secondary to slow vascular flow through small vascular spaces of the hemangioma. Flow void signal can

be seen in high-flow vessels within the mass. Additional imaging findings, including polyhydramnios, neck hyperextension, or lateral head tilting will depend on the location and size of the hemangioma and the amount of airway and esophageal compression. Congestive heart failure secondary to arteriovenous shunting can also be seen. Unlike infantile hemangiomas, CH may contain vascular aneurysms, intravascular thrombi, and arteriovenous shunting.[56]

**Associated Anomalies:** Several studies have reported association of brain cortical malformations with arterial anomalies; therefore, careful scrutiny of the brain should be sought.[55,57] Hemangiomas can also be seen as part of the PHACES syndrome (*p*osterior fossa malformations, *h*emangiomas, *a*rterial anomalies, *c*ardiac defects, *e*ye abnormalities, and *s*ternal cleft).

**Differential Diagnosis:** The imaging features of hemangiomas may be difficult to distinguish from congenital fibrosarcoma. A well-defined heterogeneous mass with flow voids and increased flow will be seen in ultrasound and MR images[55,58] in both entities. When located in the posterior neck, hemangiomas can mimic an occipital cephalocele in prenatal ultrasound.[59] Fetal MRI imaging is a valuable tool to evaluate associated

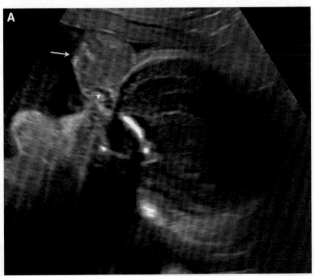

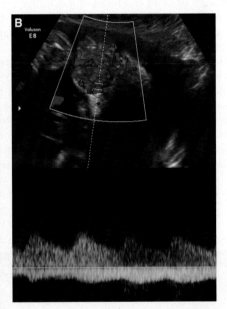

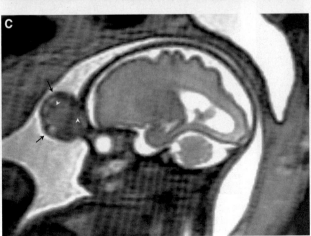

**FIGURE 14.17:** Congenital Hemangioma. Fetus at 31 weeks. **A:** Sagittal ultrasound demonstrates echogenic mass *(arrows)* arising from the subcutaneous tissues of the forehead with prominent feeding vessels *(arrowhead)*. **B:** Doppler of lesion demonstrates arterial waveform with high diastolic flow and pulsatile vein. **C:** Sagittal T2 MR image demonstrates heterogeneous hyperintense subcutaneous lesion *(black arrows)* above the orbit containing prominent flow voids *(white arrowheads)*. There is no intracranial extension.

intracranial anomalies and help distinguish hemangiomas from other entities.

**Prognosis/Management:** Rapidly involuting hemangiomas usually regress by 14 months of age and may leave behind atrophic skin or large veins in the region of prior hemangiomas. NICH usually require surgical treatment. Unfortunately, there are no distinguishing imaging characteristics to predict postnatal course. Maternal administration of steroid may accelerate involution of the hemangioma, and if there is compression upon the airway, delivery by cesarean section or EXIT procedure to secure the airway should be performed.

## Cervical Teratoma

Teratomas are germ cell tumors that contain tissue from each of the three embryonic layers, the ectoderm, mesoderm, and endoderm.

**Incidence:** Cervical teratomas occur in approximately 1 in 20,000 to 40,000 live births.[60] They represent 3% to 5% of all teratomas, and approximately 300 cases have been described in the literature.[60,61] Compared with other teratomas, cervical teratomas show no female predominance.[62]

**Pathogenesis/Etiology:** Cervical teratomas arise from totipotential germ cells or as an end result of a defective twin pregnancy with fetus in fetu.[28,63] These masses likely originate in the thyroid gland, based on the presence of a thin pseudocapsule in continuity between the mass and the thyroid.[61]

Cervical teratomas are mixed cystic and solid lesions arising in the anterior midline neck. They are composed of a combination of skin, skin appendages, cartilage, muscle, and respiratory and gastrointestinal epithelium. Teratomas can be further classified into mature and immature types. The immature type contains embryonic cells, usually neural, and occur more commonly in the cervical region (>50%)[64] compared with other extragonadal teratomas. Importantly, most immature teratomas are not malignant; however, the presence of yolk sac tumor cells carries a higher association with malignancy and recurrence.[65]

**Diagnosis:** Amniotic fluid alpha-fetoprotein (AFP) has been suggested to help in the differential diagnosis of a cervical mass. However, the dilemma is that both maternal and fetal AFP levels can be elevated or normal as only 30% of fetal cervical teratomas produce AFP. Therefore, this test is not always helpful in the prenatal diagnosis of cervical teratoma.[28] Postnatal AFP levels are, however, often useful to evaluate for recurrence after resection.

**Ultrasound:** Ultrasound can detect cervical teratomas as early as 15 to 17 weeks' gestational age, although the majority is diagnosed in the late second to third trimester. They differ from LM and branchial cleft cysts in location as these lesions predominantly occur in the posterolateral neck, whereas cervical teratomas occur anteriorly. They are usually large tumors varying in size from 4 to 12 cm in diameter. Ultrasound shows a complex mass with multiloculated cystic and solid components. Hyperechoic adipose tissue and calcification with posterior acoustic shadowing may be seen. The presence of calcifications is fairly specific for the diagnosis of teratoma (Fig. 14.18). Teratomas are less pliable tumors compared with LM and may cause mass effect with compression of the neck vasculature and hypopharynx. If vasculature compression is severe, high-output cardiac failure can result, as well as nonimmune hydrops with potential intrauterine fetal demise. Polyhydramnios can also occur if swallowing is impaired.

**MRI:** MRI is valuable in confirming the diagnosis of cervical teratomas as well as aiding in perinatal planning. It can demonstrate the internal architecture and extent of the mass as well as the degree of compression of the airway and esophagus. Imaging shows a well-defined complex mass with multiloculated cystic and solid components (Fig. 14.19). Intratumoral hemorrhage can be seen as dark signal on gradient echo images and bright signal on T1-weighted images. In large cervical teratomas, polyhydramnios and a small stomach may be seen because of impaired swallowing from esophageal compression. MRI may also show pulmonary hypoplasia, a severe complication in large cervical teratomas secondary to severe distortion of the airway by the mass. In these cases, the carina is retracted superiorly, resulting in compression of the lungs in the upper thorax with resultant poor lung development (Fig. 14.20).[66]

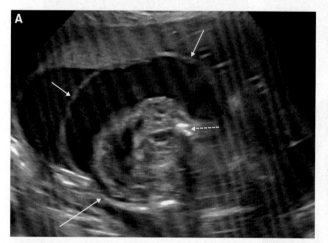
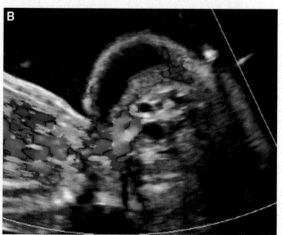

**FIGURE 14.18:** Cervical Teratoma. **A:** Axial US gray-scale image shows a complex solid and cystic mass *(solid arrows)* with areas of calcification *(dotted arrow)* and posterior acoustic shadowing in the fetal neck. **B:** Coronal Doppler US image of the same patient shows increased vascular supply to the mass.

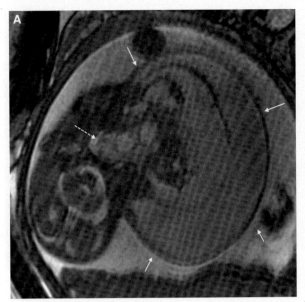
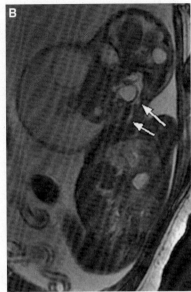

**FIGURE 14.19:** Cervical Teratoma in a 23 week gestation fetus. **A:** Axial T2 image shows a large complex mass *(solid arrows)* arising from the neck and extending into the oropharynx *(dotted arrows)*. **B:** Coronal T2 image shows a patent left piriform sinus and infraglottic airways *(white arrows)*.

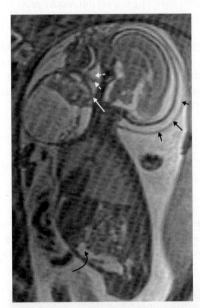

**FIGURE 14.20:** Cervical Teratoma. Sagittal T2 shows cervical mass causing hyperextension of the neck known as "flying fetus" position. There is obstruction of the oropharynx *(solid short and long arrows)* with fluid distention of the proximal airway *(dotted arrow)*. Hydrops with scalp edema *(black arrows)* and intraabdominal ascites *(curved black arrow)* is noted.

**Associated Anomalies:** Anomalies associated with cervical teratoma include agenesis of the corpus callosum, imperforate anus, hypoplastic left heart, trisomy 13, and mandibular hypoplasia.[28]

**Differential Diagnosis:** Vascular anomalies, including lymphatic, venous malformations and mixed venolymphatic lesions, and hemangioma are the primary differential diagnosis for cervical teratoma. Macrocystic lymphatic malformation may mimic teratomas because of their multiloculated cystic appearance and hemorrhagic potential. However, LM are usually located in the posterolateral neck and cause less mass effect upon the airway, esophagus, and neck vessels. Venous malformations have internal flow on color Doppler and may contain calcified phleboliths. Hemangiomas are highly vascular, and color Doppler will demonstrate increased intralesional flow.

**Prognosis/Management/Recurrence:** Cervical teratomas have a poor prognosis and near 100% mortality in the presence of airway obstruction as it can be difficult to secure an airway at delivery. Therefore, accurate prenatal diagnosis and perinatal planning is essential as delay may lead to hypoxic ischemic brain injury. The EXIT procedure has been successful in securing the airway and may be combined with surgical resection of the teratoma while on placental support (operation on placental support, OOPS). Postnatal morbidity depends on degree of pulmonary hypoplasia and other associated anomalies.

Fetuses with large cervical teratomas are at increased risk for preterm labor because of polyhydramnios and premature rupture of membranes. Hyperextension of the neck can lead to dystocia requiring cesarean section. Hypothyroidism and hypoparathyroidism may result as the thyroid may be hypoplastic and the parathyroid glands may not be easily discernible during resection and may be removed. In these cases, calcium and vitamin D supplementation with or without thyroid hormone replacement may be needed.

While the majority of cervical teratomas are histologically benign, they may grow quickly and recur. Most recurrences occur within 7 months of resection. The presence of yolk sac tumor cells appears to be the only valid predictor of increased risk of malignancy and recurrence rather than the histologic immaturity of the tumor. A 4% risk of death at 2 to 6 years has been reported secondary to development of yolk sac tumor; therefore, close follow-up with serum AFP after resection can aid in early detection of recurrences or malignant transformation.[28,64] Malignant teratomas as well as fetal metastatic lesions have rarely been reported.[67,68]

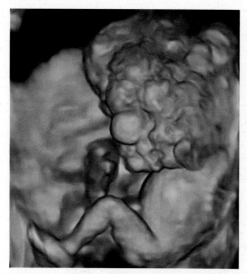

**FIGURE 14.21:** Epignathus. Three-dimensional US of a 22-week fetus shows a large lobulated mass arising from the face.

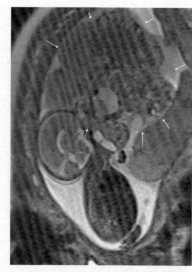

**FIGURE 14.22:** Epignathus. Sagittal T2 Haste image of same fetus with a very large lobulated heterogeneous mass *(solid arrows)* arising from the oral cavity *(dotted arrow)*. Note the cystic and solid components of the mass.

## Epignathus

**Incidence:** The incidence of epignathus is reported as 1 in 35,000 to 200,000 live births, representing 2% to 9% of all teratomas.[69,70] They are more common in females with a 3:1 ratio.[71]

**Pathogenesis/Etiology:** Epignathus (also known as oral teratomas or oropharyngeal teratomas) are rare oral tumors with components of all three germ layers with similarities to teratomas arising in the neck. Oral teratomas arise from the soft or hard palate and are believed to derive from pluripotential cells in Rathke pouch that grow in a disorganized manner.[70] Approximately 6% of patients with oral teratomas have associated anomalies, including cleft palate, branchial cleft cyst, duplicated pituitary gland, agenesis of the corpus callosum, and congenital heart disease.[71,72] They usually present during the second trimester as unidirectional or bidirectional masses, involving only the oral cavity and protruding forward but may extend intracranially.

**Diagnosis:** On US and MRI, epignathus has similar characteristics as those described for cervical teratomas (Figs. 14.21 and 14.22).

These tumors can vary in size: from a few centimeters to as large as the fetal head or body. Epignathus can rapidly grow and cause swallowing dysfunction leading to polyhydramnios or airway obstruction

**Prognosis/Management:** Because of the high degree of airway obstruction, operation while on placental support (OOPS) or EXIT procedures are required to secure the airway (Fig. 14.23). The prognosis is very poor in cases of intracranial extension with rare surviving cases.[69]

## Epulis

**Incidence:** Congenital epulis is rare, occurring almost exclusively in females.[69]

**Pathogenesis/Etiology:** Congenital epulis (also known as congenital gingival granular cell tumors) is a benign tumor arising from the gingival mucosa of the alveolar ridge of the maxilla and less commonly the mandible. It is usually solitary, although few

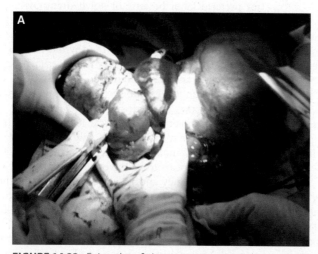
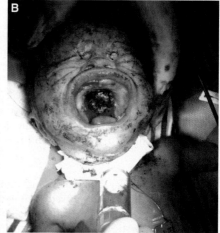

**FIGURE 14.23:** Epignathus. **A:** Intra-operative image during an EXIT procedure of a fetus with epignathus. Note the size of the oral teratoma *(right)* compared with the size of the baby's head *(left)*. **B:** Same patient after resection of the epignathus showing the origin of the mass from the hard palate.

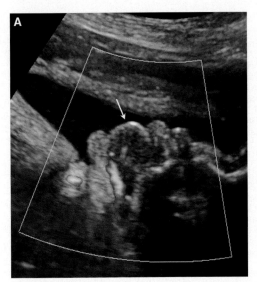
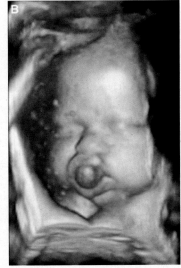

**FIGURE 14.24:** Congenital Epulis. **A:** Sagittal Doppler US image shows a rounded lesion protruding through the fetal mouth *(arrow)* with a vascular pedicle. **B:** Three-dimensional volume rendering image of the same fetus shows the fetal profile and mass protruding through the mouth.

cases of synchronous epulides have been described.[73,74] Its etiology is unknown and controversial. The term epulis and congenital gingival granular cell tumor have been synonymously used in the literature, but their histology and epidemiology are different. Epulis are gingival tumors of infancy, while granular cell tumors occur in adulthood.[73,75]

**Diagnosis:** Congenital epulis is a well-defined pedunculated mass protruding through the fetal mouth. On US, an epulis demonstrates a solid mass with internal blood flow with a vascular pedicle from the mouth (Fig. 14.24). Usually, fetal swallowing is not affected, but if the lesion becomes large it may impair fetal swallowing, leading to polyhydramnios and/or airway obstruction.[73] By MRI, epulis are hypointense on T2-weighted images, and the origin from the maxilla or mandibular alveolar ridge can infrequently be seen (Fig. 14.25).

**Differential Diagnosis:** Differential diagnoses include epignathus, oropharyngeal rhabdomyosarcoma, and hemangioma.

**Prognosis/Management:** Surgical excision is curative with no reported recurrence in the literature.[76] Small lesions may regress spontaneously.[73]

## Neuroblastoma

**Incidence:** Congenital cervical neuroblastoma is rarely encountered, accounting for 4.4% of congenital neuroblastomas (most common location in the adrenal gland).[77]

**Diagnosis:** Prenatal US findings include a solid or mixed solid and cystic mass in the lateral aspect of the neck with or without calcification. Fetal MRI shows a mass with low signal intensity on T1 and high signal intensity on T2-weighted images. Extension to the brain and metastasis are extremely rare but have been reported.[78]

**Prognosis/Management:** As with other neck masses, neuroblastomas may cause compression upon the airway and esophagus and neck hyperextension. Maternal elevation of catecholamine metabolites is present in >90% of the cases and can lead to maternal hypertension. Furthermore, fetal urinary catecholamine metabolites (VMA–HVA) may also be elevated. Congenital neuroblastoma, especially purely cystic, has a better prognosis than those occurring during childhood.[77] Disappearance of the tumor before birth has been reported.[79]

## Rhabdomyosarcoma

**Incidence:** Congenital rhabdomyosarcoma is extremely rare with little information published regarding prenatal diagnosis.

**Pathogenesis/Etiology:** Congenital rhabdomyosarcoma is often associated with chromosomal translocations; therefore, amniocentesis for fetal karyotype should be performed. Association with Robert syndrome, Beckwith–Wiedemann syndrome, and Neurofibromatosis has been reported.[80] Prenatal metastases to the sacral region have been reported.[81]

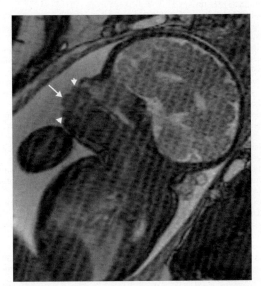

**FIGURE 14.25:** Congenital Epulis. Sagittal T2 SSFP image of the same fetus in 14.24 illustrates the mass *(arrow)* protruding through the lips *(arrowheads)*, anterior to the tongue.

# REFERENCES

1. Sadler TW. *Langman's Medical Embryology*. Philadelphia, PA United States: Wolters Kluwer Health; 2011.
2. Lind RC, Hulscher JB, van der Wal JE, et al. A very rare case of a giant third branchial pouch remnant discovered in utero. *Eur J Pediatr Surg*. 2010;20(5):349–351.
3. Robichaud J, Papsin BC, Forte V. Third branchial cleft anomaly detected in utero. *J Otolaryngol*. 2000;29(3):185–187.
4. Suchet IB. Ultrasonography of the fetal neck in the second and third trimesters, part 3: anomalies of the anterior and anterolateral nuchal region. *Can Assoc Radiol J*. 1995;46(6):426–433.
5. Tsai PY, Chang CH, Chang FM. Prenatal imaging of the fetal branchial cleft cyst by three-dimensional ultrasound. *Prenat Diagn*. 2003;23(7):605–606.
6. Benson MT, Dalen K, Mancuso AA, et al. Congenital anomalies of the branchial apparatus: embryology and pathologic anatomy. *Radiographics*. 1992;12(5):943–960.
7. Smith RJH. Branchiootorenal spectrum disorders. In: Pagon RA, Adam MP, Bird TD, et al, eds. *GeneReviews*. Seattle, WA: University of Washington, Seattle; 1993.
8. Nguyen Q, deTar M, Wells W, et al. Cervical thymic cyst: case reports and review of the literature. *Laryngoscope*. 1996;106(3, pt 1):247–252.
9. Cigliano B, Baltogiannis N, De Marco M, et al. Cervical thymic cysts. *Pediatr Surg Int*. 2007;23(12):1219–1225.
10. De Miguel Campos E, Casanova A, Urbano J, et al. Congenital thymic cyst: prenatal sonographic and postnatal magnetic resonance findings. *J Ultrasound Med*. 1997;16(5):365–367.
11. McEwing R, Chaoui R. Fetal thymic cyst: prenatal diagnosis. *J Ultrasound Med*. 2005;24(1):127–130.
12. Gul A, Gungorduk K, Yildirim G, et al. Prenatal diagnosis and management of a ranula. *J Obstet Gynaecol Res*. 2008;34(2):262–265.
13. Chan DF, Lee CH, Fung TY, et al. Ex utero intrapartum treatment (EXIT) for congenital giant ranula. *Acta Paediatr*. 2006;95(10):1303–1305.
14. Crysdale WS, Mendelsohn JD, Conley S. Ranulas—mucoceles of the oral cavity: experience in 26 children. *Laryngoscope*. 1988;98(3):296–298.
15. Lindstrom DR, Conley SF, Arvedson JC, et al. Anterior lingual thyroglossal cyst: antenatal diagnosis, management, and long-term outcome. *Int J Pediatr Otorhinolaryngol*. 2003;67(9):1031–1034.
16. Keizer AL, Deurloo KL, van Vugt JM, et al. A prenatal diagnosis of a thyroglossal duct cyst in the fetal anterior neck. *Prenat Diagn*. 2011;31(13):1311–1312.
17. Hsieh YY, Hsueh S, Hsueh C, et al. Pathological analysis of congenital cervical cysts in children: 20 years of experience at Chang Gung Memorial Hospital. *Chang Gung Med J*. 2003;26(2):107–113.
18. Kutuya N, Kurosaki Y. Sonographic assessment of thyroglossal duct cysts in children. *J Ultrasound Med*. 2008;27(8):1211–1219.
19. Mossa-Basha M, Yousem DM. Congenital cystic lesions of the neck. *Appl Radiol*. 2013;42(1):8–22.
20. Masters F, Given CA. Cystic neck masses: a pictorial review of unusual presentations and complicating features. *Appl Radiol*. 2008;37(9):26–32.
21. Lev S, Lev MH. Imaging of cystic lesions. *Radiol Clin North Am*. 2000;38(5):1013–1027.
22. Koyuncu FM, Tamay AG, Bugday S. Intrauterine diagnosis and management of fetal goiter: a case report. *J Clin Ultrasound*. 2010;38(9):503–505.
23. Bromley B, Frigoletto FD, Cramer D, et al. The fetal thyroid: normal and abnormal sonographic measurements. *J Ultrasound Med*. 1992;11(1):25–28.
24. Ho SS, Metreweli C. Normal fetal thyroid volume. *Ultrasound Obstet Gynecol*. 1998;11(2):118–122.
25. Ranzini AC, Ananth CV, Smulian JC, et al. Ultrasonography of the fetal thyroid: nomograms based on biparietal diameter and gestational age. *J Ultrasound Med*. 2001;20(6):613–617.
26. Gietka-Czernel M, Debska M, Kretowicz P, et al. Fetal thyroid in two-dimensional ultrasonography: nomograms according to gestational age and biparietal diameter. *Eur J Obstet Gynecol Reprod Biol*. 2012;162(2):131–138.
27. Francois A, Hindryckx A, Vandecruys H, et al. Fetal treatment for early dyshormonogenetic goiter. *Prenat Diagn*. 2009;29(5):543–545.
28. Bianchi DW. *Fetology: Diagnosis and Management of the Fetal Patient*. 2nd ed. New York, NY: McGraw-Hill Medical; 2010.
29. Agrawal P, Ogilvy-Stuart A, Lees C. Intrauterine diagnosis and management of congenital goitrous hypothyroidism. *Ultrasound Obstet Gynecol*. 2002;19(5):501–505.
30. Huel C, Guibourdenche J, Vuillard E, et al. Use of ultrasound to distinguish between fetal hyperthyroidism and hypothyroidism on discovery of a goiter. *Ultrasound Obstet Gynecol*. 2009;33(4):412–420.
31. Karabulut N, Martin DR, Yang M, et al. MR imaging findings in fetal goiter caused by maternal graves disease. *J Comput Assist Tomogr*. 2002;26(4):538–540.
32. Kondoh M, Miyazaki O, Imanishi Y, et al. Neonatal goiter with congenital thyroid dysfunction in two infants diagnosed by MRI. *Pediatr Radiol*. 2004;34(7):570–573.
33. Insoft RM, Hurvitz J, Estrella E, et al. Prader-Willi syndrome associated with fetal goiter: a case report. *Am J Perinatol*. 1999;16(1):29–31.
34. Friedland DR, Rothschild MA. Rapid resolution of fetal goiter associated with maternal Grave's disease: a case report. *Int J Pediatr Otorhinolaryngol*. 2000;54(1):59–62.
35. Hanono A, Shah B, David R, et al. Antenatal treatment of fetal goiter: a therapeutic challenge. *J Matern Fetal Neonatal Med*. 2009;22(1):76–80.
36. Ribault V, Castanet M, Bertrand AM, et al. Experience with intraamniotic thyroxine treatment in nonimmune fetal goitrous hypothyroidism in 12 cases. *J Clin Endocrinol Metab*. 2009;94(10):3731–3739.
37. Corral E, Reascos M, Preiss Y, et al. Treatment of fetal goitrous hypothyroidism: value of direct intramuscular L-thyroxine therapy. *Prenat Diagn*. 2010;30(9):899–901.
38. Hatjis CG. Diagnosis and successful treatment of fetal goitrous hyperthyroidism caused by maternal Graves disease. *Obstet Gynecol*. 1993;81(5, pt 2):837–839.
39. Donnelly LF, Adams DM, Bisset GS. Vascular malformations and hemangiomas: a practical approach in a multidisciplinary clinic. *AJR Am J Roentgenol*. 2000;174(3):597–608.
40. Fordham LA, Chung CJ, Donnelly LF. Imaging of congenital vascular and lymphatic anomalies of the head and neck. *Neuroimaging Clin N Am*. 2000;10(1):117–136, viii.
41. Malone FD, Ball RH, Nyberg DA, et al. First-trimester septated cystic hygroma: prevalence, natural history, and pediatric outcome. *Obstet Gynecol*. 2005;106(2):288–294.
42. Woodward P, Kennedy A, Sohaey R. *Diagnostic Imaging Obstetrics*. Vol I. 2nd ed. Canada: Amirsys; 2011.
43. Chervenak FA, Isaacson G, Blakemore KJ, et al. Fetal cystic hygroma: cause and natural history. *N Engl J Med*. 1983;309(14):822–825.
44. Perkins JA, Manning SC, Tempero RM, et al. Lymphatic malformations: review of current treatment. *Otolaryngol Head Neck Surg*. 2010;142(6):795–803, 803.e1.
45. Sherer DM, Perenyi AR, Glick SA, et al. Prenatal sonographic findings of extensive low-flow mixed lymphatic and venous malformations. *J Ultrasound Med*. 2006;25(11):1469–1473.
46. Kathary N, Bulas DI, Newman KD, et al. MRI imaging of fetal neck masses with airway compromise: utility in delivery planning. *Pediatr Radiol*. 2001;31(10):727–731.
47. Oosthuizen JC, Burns P, Russell JD. Lymphatic malformations: a proposed management algorithm. *Int J Pediatr Otorhinolaryngol*. 2010;74(4):398–403.
48. Kaufman GE, D'Alton ME, Crombleholme TM. Decompression of fetal axillary lymphangioma to prevent dystocia. *Fetal Diagn Ther*. 1996;11(3):218–220.
49. Alqahtani A, Nguyen LT, Flageole H, et al. 25 years' experience with lymphangiomas in children. *J Pediatr Surg*. 1999;34(7):1164–1168.
50. Donnelly LF, Jones B, O'Hara S, et al. Diagnostic imaging: pediatrics. *Radiol Med*. 2006;111:1168–1169.
51. Dubois J, Alison M. Vascular anomalies: what a radiologist needs to know. *Pediatr Radiol*. 2010;40(6):895–905.
52. Kohout MP, Hansen M, Pribaz JJ, et al. Arteriovenous malformations of the head and neck: natural history and management. *Plast Reconstr Surg*. 1998;102(3):643–654.
53. Tseng JJ, Chou MM, Chen WH. Prenatal 3- and 4-dimensional ultrasonographic findings of giant fetal nuchal hemangioma. *J Chin Med Assoc*. 2007;70:460–463.
54. Boon LM, Enjolras O, Mulliken JB. Congenital hemangioma: evidence of accelerated involution. *J Pediatr*. 1996;128:329–335.
55. Robson CD, Barnewolt CE. MR imaging of fetal head and neck anomalies. *Neuroimaging Clin N Am*. 2004;14:273–291, viii.
56. Alamo L, Beck-Popovic M, Gudinchet F, et al. Congenital tumors: imaging when life just begins. *Insights Imaging*. 2011;2:297–308.
57. O'Connor SC, Rooks VJ, Smith AB. Magnetic resonance imaging of the fetal central nervous system, head, neck, and chest. *Semin Ultrasound CT MR*. 2012;33(1):86–101.
58. Boon LM, Fishman SJ, Lund DP, et al. Congenital fibrosarcoma masquerading as congenital hemangioma: report of two cases. *J Pediatr Surg*. 1995;30:1378–1381.
59. Miyakoshi K, Tanaka M, Matsumoto T, et al. Occipital scalp hemangioma: prenatal sonographic and magnetic resonance images. *J Obstet Gynaecol Res*. 2008;34:666–669.
60. Tonni G, De Felice C, Centini G, et al. Cervical and oral teratoma in the fetus: a systematic review of etiology, pathology, diagnosis, treatment and prognosis. *Arch Gynecol Obstet*. 2010;282(4):355–361.
61. Riedlinger WF, Lack EE, Robson CD, et al. Primary thyroid teratomas in children: a report of 11 cases with a proposal of criteria for their diagnosis. *Am J Surg Pathol*. 2005;29:700–706.
62. Garmel SH, Crombleholme TM, Semple JP, et al. Prenatal diagnosis and management of fetal tumors. *Semin Perinatol*. 1994;18(4):350–365.
63. Hitchcock A, Sears RT, O'Neill T. Immature cervical teratoma arising in one fetus of a twin pregnancy: case report and review of the literature. *Acta Obstet Gynecol Scand*. 1987;66(4):377–379.
64. Bianchi B, Ferri A, Silini EM, et al. Congenital cervical teratoma: a case report. *J Oral Maxillofac Surg*. 2010;68:667–670.
65. Isaacs H Jr. Perinatal (fetal and neonatal) germ cell tumors. *J Pediatr Surg*. 2004;39:1003–1013.
66. Liechty KW, Hedrick HL, Hubbard AM, et al. Severe pulmonary hypoplasia associated with giant cervical teratomas. *J Pediatr Surg*. 2006;41(1):230–233.
67. Baumann FR, Nerlich A. Metastasizing cervical teratoma of the fetus. *Pediatr Pathol*. 1993;13(1):21–27.
68. Shoenfeld A, Ovadia J, Edelstein T, et al. Malignant cervical teratoma of the fetus. *Acta Obstet Gynecol Scand*. 1982;61(1):7–12.

69. Clement K, Chamberlain P, Boyd P, et al. Prenatal diagnosis of an epignathus: a case report and review of the literature. *Ultrasound Obstet Gynecol.* 2001;18(2):178–181.

70. Sumiyoshi S, Machida J, Yamamoto T, et al. Massive immature teratoma in a neonate. *Int J Oral Maxillofac Surg.* 2010;39(10):1020–1023.

71. Kaido Y, Kikuchi A, Oyama R, et al. Prenatal ultrasound and magnetic resonance imaging findings of a hypovascular epignathus with a favorable prognosis. *J Med Ultrason.* 2013;40(1):61–64.

72. Vazquez E, Castellote A, Mayolas N, et al. Congenital tumours involving the head, neck and central nervous system. *Pediatr Radiol.* 2009;39(11): 1158–1172.

73. Koch BL, Myer C III, Egelhoff JC. Congenital epulis. *AJNR Am J Neuroradiol.* 1997;18(4):739–741.

74. Roy S, Sinsky A, Williams B, et al. Congenital epulis: prenatal imaging with MRI and ultrasound. *Pediatr Radiol.* 2003;33(11):800–803.

75. Lopez de Lacalle JM, Aguirre I, Irizabal JC, et al. Congenital epulis: prenatal diagnosis by ultrasound. *Pediatr Radiol.* 2001;31(6):453–454.

76. Jiang L, Hu B, Guo Q. Prenatal sonographic diagnosis of congenital epulis. *J Clin Ultrasound.* 2011;39(4):217–220.

77. Isaacs H Jr. Fetal and neonatal neuroblastoma: retrospective review of 271 cases. *Fetal Pediatr Pathol.* 2007;26:177–184.

78. Guzelmansur I, Aksoy HT, Hakverdi S, et al. Fetal cervical neuroblastoma: prenatal diagnosis. *Case Rep Med.* 2011;2011:529749.

79. Moore SW, Satge D, Sasco AJ, et al. The epidemiology of neonatal tumours: report of an international working group. *Pediatr Surg Int.* 2003;19(7):509–519.

80. Onderoglu LS, Yucel A, Yuce K. Prenatal sonographic features of embryonal rhabdomyosarcoma. *Ultrasound Obstet Gynecol.* 1999;13(3):210–212.

81. Yoshino K, Takeuchi M, Nakayama M, et al. Congenital cervical rhabdomyosarcoma arising in one fetus of a twin pregnancy. *Fetal Diagn Ther.* 2005;20(4): 291–295.

## 15.1 Cranium

Beth M. Kline-Fath and Dorothy I. Bulas

Neural tube defects (NTDs) encompass a heterogeneous group of congenital brain and spine anomalies that result from the defective closure of the neural tube early in gestation.[1–4] The most common anomalies include myelomeningoceles, encephaloceles, and anencephaly. Anencephaly and spinal dysraphism are equal in prevalence, accounting for 95% of cases, whereas encephaloceles account for the remaining 5%.[8] After a review of epidemiology and embryology, these malformations will be discussed by their primary location, either cranial or spinal.

## EPIDEMIOLOGY

NTDs are one of the most common fetal malformations, second only to cardiac anomalies. The lesions are present in 1 to 5 of 1,000 live births and occur due to failure of primary neurulation in the first 3 to 4 weeks postconception.[5] Causes are heterogeneous and include chromosomal or genetic abnormalities, teratogens, environmental, and maternal predisposing factors. Approximately 85% of NTDs have been related to a combined influence of environmental and genetic factors. The incidence varies with race, geography, and family history. NTD risk is highest among relatives of most severely affected patients. If one child is affected, the risk for subsequent siblings is around 3%, with two affected siblings 10%, and with three affected siblings 20%.[5a] There is marked geographical variation between countries, with the highest rates in the United Kingdom and the United States and the lowest in Japan.[6] Other significant factors include valproic acid, folic acid antagonists (methotrexate and aminopterin), vitamin A, maternal diabetes, maternal obesity, hyperthermia, and folate deficiency.[6] Despite these risk factors, 90% of children with NTDs are born to women with no identifiable risk factor.

In the past few decades, the number of births with NTDs worldwide has declined because of primary prevention with folic acid supplementation in pregnancy and early ultrasound (US) diagnosis followed by therapeutic termination.[7] Women are advised to consume food high in folate or take folate supplements at least 3 months prior to pregnancy.[7] There has been a 27% decline in NTDs in the United States with folic acid fortification in grains.[7]

## EMBRYOLOGY

Dysraphism is the result of defective closure of the neural tube and is reserved for defects of primary neurulation, or dorsal induction, which involves tubulation of the neural plate and disjunction of superficial from neural ectoderm.[1–3]

The neural tube forms from infolding of the embryonic ectoderm—the neural plate. The fusion of the neural groove starts in the middorsal aspect, usually the cervical area, and proceeds anteriorly to the lamina terminalis, also known as the anterior neuropore (cranial), and posteriorly in the sacral area, also known as the posterior neuropore (spinal). The anterior neuropore closes at day 24, and posterior at day 26. The neural tube separates from the ectoderm, and the mesoderm proliferates laterally to form the axial skeleton and dura (Fig. 15.1-1). If this process is interrupted, a defect in the neural tube results. At times, the process is interrupted on both ends, resulting in cranial defects such as anencephaly with myelomeningoceles.

## ACRANIA/EXENCEPHALY-ANENCEPHALY

**Description:** *Acrania* is a defect that occurs due to complete or partial absence in the development of the cranial vault above the orbits, with absence of parietal, squamousal, occipital, temporal, and frontal bones above the supraciliary ridge.[9] *Exencephaly* is acrania with protrusion of substantial brain into the amniotic cavity.[10–12] *Anencephaly* represents absence of forebrain, midbrain, and skull. The cerebral hemispheres are replaced with residual covering of hemorrhagic, fibrotic, degenerated neurons and glia with little definable structure (Fig. 15.1-2).

**Incidence:** The incidence of anencephaly is difficult to assess, but in the United States, frequency is estimated at 1 in 1,000 pregnancies.[13] A progressive decline is suspected with periconceptional folate fortification and termination.[14,15] Anencephaly has a higher rate in countries such as Egypt, Lebanon, Ireland, Scotland, and New Zealand. In the United States, fetuses of Caucasian and Hispanic ethnicity are more frequently affected than those of African descent.[16] Twin gestations also have a higher risk for anencephaly. There is a female preponderance of 3:1.[15,16] Ninety-five percent of infants born with anencephaly are in families with no prior history for a NTD.[15]

**Pathogenesis:** Exencephaly–anencephaly sequence is the most severe NTD and results from failed closure of the rostral end of the neural tube. The severity of the bone defect is variable and may result in absent brain or rudimentary disorganized brain. Exencephaly pathologically demonstrates a highly vascular layer of epithelium with two relatively equivalent disorganized, dysplastic cerebral hemispheres.[12,13,17] With progression to anencephaly, the cerebral hemispheres are replaced by a mass of connective and vascular tissue with scattered islands of brain tissue, so-called angiomatous stroma or area cerebrovasculosa.[17,18]

Acrania is a developmental anomaly that is characterized by partial or complete absence of the cranium with complete but abnormal development of the cerebral tissue. This disorder is hypothesized to occur at the beginning of the 4th week at the

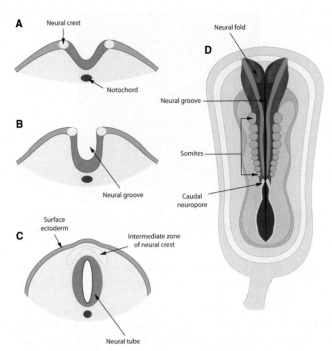

**FIGURE 15.1-1:** Embryology of primary neurulation in which neural plate develops **(A)** and then infolds to become a groove **(B)** and with closure a neural tube **(C)**. **D:** Diagram of the dorsal aspect of the developing craniospinal area in the embryo.

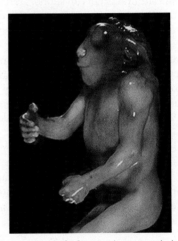

**FIGURE 15.1-2:** Postmortem of a fetus with anencephaly.

same time the anterior neuropore closes, but is related to failure of the mesenchyme to migrate under the ectoderm and superficial to the cerebral hemispheres.[8] The cerebral hemispheres are present but disorganized, and the brain is covered only by a thin membrane.

The major insult in acrania, exencephaly, and anencephy is due to lack of cranial development. The cerebral tissue is not protected by meninges, skull, and skin, and is progressively destroyed through exposure to amniotic fluid and mechanical trauma.[17] As a result, the brain disappears from 14 weeks onward.[19,20] Prior animal and US reports have demonstrated that there typically is progression of acrania-exencephaly to anencephaly (AEA).[7,17,21] In some cases, residual disorganized brain may persist late in gestation or even postnatal.

**Etiology:** AEA appears to be multifactorial in origin, being from both genetic and environmental causes.[9] Associated chromosomal syndromes have been reported in 5% to 10% of these cases and include trisomy, triploidy, mosaic trisomy 11 and 20, and a number of deletions and duplications or single gene disorders.[7] Hyperthermia, deficiency in zinc and copper, and occupation solvent exposure have been associated with a higher risk of anencephaly.[14,20] Most relevant is inadequate dietary consumption of folates prior to conception.[7,13,14]

**Diagnosis:** Preliminary screening for high maternal serum alpha-fetoprotein (AFP) at 10 to 15 weeks may disclose evidence of leakage from the fetal neural tube in 90% of cases.[22] The combination of elevated AFP and low estriol levels is highly predictive for anencephaly.[22,23] However, screening can be falsely positive and may require confirmation with amniocentesis or US.

*Ultrasound:* Sonography can identify almost 100% of anencephalic fetuses.[6,9,21,24] The disorder can be diagnosed transvaginally prior to 10 weeks' gestation by the presence of a widened cranial pole, altered brain echotexture, variable asymmetric or lobulated disorganized tissue, and decreased head-to-trunk ratio.[24,25] However, confirmation is usually obtained after 11 to 12 weeks' gestation when calvarial ossification defined as a hyperechogenic structure compared with the underlying soft tissues is noted to be absent.[6,21,24,25] Detection may also improve after 14 weeks when the brain has completely formed, although in AEA a moderate to large amount of disorganized cranial tissue may be present early in gestation as it has not yet been destroyed by amniotic fluid.[19] From 10 to 14 weeks, the "Mickey Mouse" sign can be seen on coronal images, as cerebral lobes floating in amniotic fluid above the orbits (Fig. 15.1-3).[26] AEA may result in a reduced crown rump length or chin length-to-crown rump length ratio, but in some cases the measurement is normal and can lead to a false negative study below 14 weeks.[19,26–28] Echogenic amniotic fluid, believed to represent particles of degenerated brain, has also been described in the first trimester.[20]

In the second trimester, the diagnosis is easier as less brain tissue is present. The typical "frog eyes" sign on coronal plane is due to prominent orbits in conjunction with the symmetric absence of a normally formed calvarium and brain (Fig. 15.1-4).[18] Exposed residual neural tissue may be echogenic, cystic, or normally formed with pseudosulcations.[12,18]

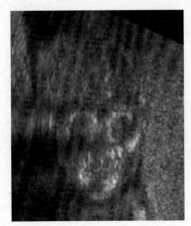

**FIGURE 15.1-3:** Coronal US of acrania/exencephaly with absent calvarium and protruding brain above orbits giving rise to Mickey Mouse appearance.

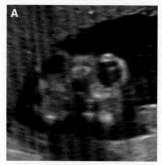
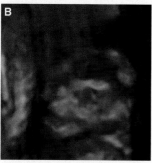

**FIGURE 15.1-4:** Anencephaly **A:** Coronal 2D image shows prominent "frog eye" appearance. **B:** 3D image demonstrating lack of skull above the orbits.

The cerebellar hemispheres may be absent, and spinal segmentation anomalies are common, especially in the cervical area. In the second or third trimester, as many as 30% to 50% of cases have associated polyhydramnios from impaired fetal swallowing, excess CSF across the meninges, or increased fetal urine output due to absent antidiuretic hormone.[18]

*MRI:* Fetal MRI is usually not required to confirm the diagnosis of anencephaly. MRI may be utilized when there is limitation in US imaging (obesity) or in the case of medical, legal, or ethical issues.[29] It can be helpful to exclude other pathologies mimicking AEA and useful in multiple gestations when it is necessary to confirm normal development of the co-twin.

The calvarium is absent, and there may be disorganized brain tissue in the area of the cerebral hemispheres in the presence of acrania or exencephaly (Fig. 15.1-5). With anencephaly, the orbits are prominent, no brain tissue is seen, and a cervical spine defect with absence of brainstem and spinal cord can be identified (Fig. 15.1-6).

**Associated Anomalies:** Associated spinal lesions can be found in up to 50% of cases. Other common anomalies include cleft lip/palate, cardiac, gastrointestinal, clubfoot, and omphalocele.[8,9,30]

**Differential Diagnosis:** Differential includes large cephaloceles, osteogenesis imperfecta (OI), and hypophosphatasia. In

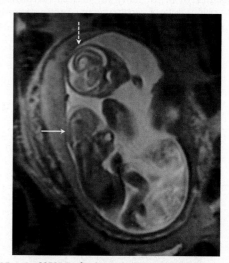

**FIGURE 15.1-5:** SSFSE T2 fetal MR showing lack of calvarium and dysmorphic brain in acrania/exencephaly *(solid arrow)* and normal brain and calvarium in co-twin *(dashed arrow).*

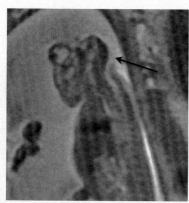

**FIGURE 15.1-6:** SSFSE T2 sagittal image of fetus with anencephaly demonstrating cervical spine defect and absent brainstem and cervical cord *(arrow).*

both OI and hypophosphatasia, the bones are present but poorly mineralized, and other fractures, bone shortening, and/or bowing are typically present.

This disorder should be distinguished from amniotic band syndrome, in which there is an asymmetric brain defect, multiple limb or digit amputations, asymmetric ventral wall defects, and unusual craniofacial or spinal defects.[11] Amniotic band is often associated with oligohydramnios, which is rare in anencephaly.[18]

**Prognosis:** Approximately 65% of pregnancies with anencephaly die in utero.[20] Affected fetuses born alive have a rudimentary brainstem. The brainstem can support reflex actions such as breathing and sometimes responses to sound and touch. Children with AEA are not viable and have only short-term survival.[13]

**Management:** Elective termination is often considered. In the United States, prenatal diagnosis and pregnancy termination have decreased the prevalence of anencephaly at birth by 60% to 70%. In Europe, America, and Asia, the overall frequency for termination of anencephaly pregnancy is 83%, ranging from 59% to 100%.[30,31]

Labor and delivery are commonly associated with unstable fetal lie, dysfunctional labor, shoulder dystocia, and postpartum hemorrhage.[32] Up to 35% of anencephalic infants will die during labor. For the 45% that are born alive, supportive care is typically provided for minutes to days.[32] The potential for neonatal organ donation has raised both legal and ethical issues.

**Recurrence Risk:** There is a 2% to 5% recurrence risk.[9,15] Increased risk also exists for those with relatives affected by anencephaly or those with genetic predisposition.

## CEPHALOCELES

**Description:** A cephalocele is a defect in the skull and dura with extracalvarial extension of intracranial structures enclosed by overlying skin.

There are four major types.[33,34] *Meningoencephaloceles,* the most common, are herniations of cerebrospinal fluid (CSF), brain, and meninges through a calvarial defect. If an encephalocele includes part of a ventricle and choroid plexus, it is termed *meningoencephalocystocele. Meningoceles* are herniations of only meninges and CSF. An *atretic cephalocele* is typically parieto-occipital and consists of a tract and small defect of dura, fibrous tissue, and degenerated brain. *Glioceles* are glial-lined CSF defects.

**Incidence:** Cephaloceles account for 10% to 20% of craniospinal dysraphisms. Estimated prevalence is 0.8 to 4 per 10,000 live births.[39] The actual incidence may be higher as many of these malformations result in termination, in utero demise, and stillbirth.[40] There is a difference in incidence geographically. The Western hemisphere reports 1 to 3 per 10,000 births, whereas Southeast Asia reports 1 in 5,000 births.[28] In the West, occipital encephaloceles are most common (80%), while midline frontal and parietal are evenly divided between the remaining 20%.[41] Females are affected twice as commonly as males in the occipital location.[39,42] In Southeast Asia and Russia, frontal cephaloceles are most prevalent.[43]

**Pathogenesis:** Cephaloceles occur early in embryogenesis, at between 24 and 60 days.[40,44] Several theories have been suggested. Many believe that a cephalocele occurs because of a failure of neural tube closure.[44,45] Occipital and parietal cephaloceles, sometimes associated with other craniospinal defects, are more likely to develop from this pathophysiology.[34,39] However, the presence of skin over the defect raises the question of a mesodermal insufficiency, with herniation of brain and meninges due to a primary defect in the bone and dura.[35,36,43,46,47] Anterior cephaloceles may be mesodermal in origin as they are not commonly associated with other NTDs.[36] A third theory emphasizes the guidance of genes, stating that variation in the pattern of cranial neural tube closure is a genetically determined factor.[48]

**Etiology:** Cephaloceles have been associated with both genetic and environmental teratogens. The defect can develop owing to exposure to trypan blue, irradiation, excess vitamin A, folic acid antagonists, triamcinolone, warfarin exposure, hyperthermia,

| Table 15.1-1 | Syndromes/Association in Cephaloceles |
|---|---|
| **Syndrome/Association** | **Genetic Transmission** |
| **Occipital** | |
| Meckel–Gruber | Autosomal recessive |
| Knobloch | Autosomal recessive |
| Walker–Warburg (Chemke, HARD ± E) | Autosomal recessive |
| Cryptophthalmos | Autosomal recessive |
| Dyssegmental dwarfism | Autosomal recessive |
| Von Voss | Autosomal recessive |
| Joubert | Primary autosomal recessive |
| Klippel–Feil | Variable |
| Craniostenosis | Variable syndrome |
| Hemifacial microsomia (oculoauriculovertebral) | Sporadic |
| Ectrodactyly–ectodermal dysplasia | Sporadic and familial |
| Warfarin embryopathy | |
| Dandy–Walker | |
| Arnold–Chiari | |
| Iniencephaly | |
| Myelomeningocele | |
| **Parietal** | |
| Absent corpus callosum | |
| Atretic form | |
| **Frontal** | |
| Roberts syndrome | Autosomal recessive |
| Frontonasal dysplasia | Autosomal recessive |
| Cleft lip/palate | |
| Absent corpus callosum | |
| **Basal/transphenoidal** | |
| Cleft palate/lip | |
| Hypothalamic pituitary dysfunction | |
| Absent corpus callosum | |

and malnutrition.[35,47] Cephaloceles are seen at a higher rate with increased maternal age, maternal diabetes mellitus, rubella, and consanguineous marriages.[47] Geographic differences in the distribution of encephaloceles suggest racial and other environmental effects.[39] Although most cephaloceles are sporadic, some are part of recognized genetic and nongenetic syndromes (Table 15.1-1).[43,49]

**Diagnosis:** An elevated antenatal AFP can be present if the lesion is incompletely covered.[50] However, many cephaloceles are covered with normal or dysplastic skin and show no elevation in AFP.[39,47] Because of inconsistency, prenatal diagnosis is typically dependent on US. Most cephalocele defects are found midline or paramidline and named for their location. The most common types are occipital, frontoethmoidal, parietal, and basal.

■ *Occipital:* The defect is between the lambda and the foramen magnum, can include the infratentorial and supratentorial brain, and may demonstrate venous sinus extension into the lesion[33,35] (Fig. 15.1-7).
■ *Frontoethmoidal:* The defect is at the foramen cecum, anterior to the crista galli where the frontal and ethmoidal bones meet. Failure of involution can lead to a nasal dermal sinus, nasal glioma, or encephalocele.[35–37] A nasal dermal sinus occurs when there is incomplete separation of the dura from the skin, resulting in dermal inclusion cysts anywhere along the tract, including intracranial. Nasal gliomas are heterotopic glial tissue without intracranial connection that can be found

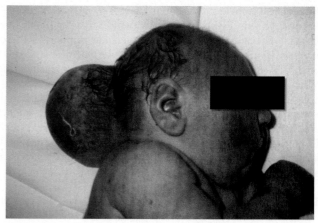

**FIGURE 15.1-7:** Postnatal image of a child with large occipital encephalocele.

in the nose or, more commonly, above the nose (glabella) (Fig. 15.1-8). The cephalocele defect can be at the foramen cecum or through other sites along the midline frontal bone (Fig. 15.1-9).[28] Hypertelorism is a common association.[39]

■ *Parietal:* The defect is between the intersection of coronal sutures and the lambda. Atretic cephaloceles are commonly found in this location and have a good prognosis. The atretic lesion is typically identified in the presence of a vertical straight sinus (falcine sinus), minimal dysplastic extracranial

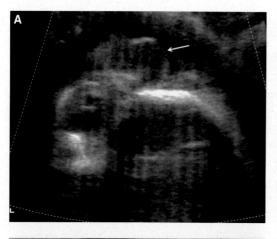

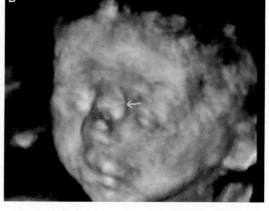

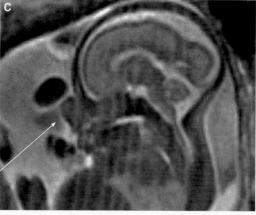

**FIGURE 15.1-8:** Nasal glioma **A:** Axial US at level of the orbits with mass at the glabella with central hypoechogenicity and well-defined hyperechoeic wall *(arrow)*. **B:** 3D image of the fetus is provided. Arrow denotes mass. **C:** SSFSE sagittal T2 image of same fetus shows homogeneous mass along nasal bridge *(arrow)*.

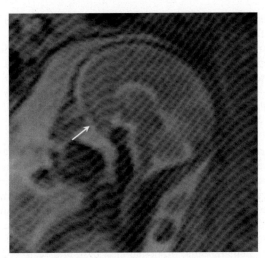

**FIGURE 15.1-9:** Sagittal SSFSE T2 MR image demonstrating large fronto-ethmoidal encephalocele with herniation of brain and CSF *(arrow)* through defect. The child was diagnosed with Roberts syndrome after birth.

tissue, and CSF cigar-shaped tract within the posterior interhemispheric fissure[38] (Fig. 15.1-10).

- *Basal:* This rare defect is in the skull base at the junction of the sphenoid and ethmoid, and may present as a mass in the mouth or posterior pharynx.[33]

*Ultrasound:* Prenatal US detects approximately 80% to 100% of cephaloceles.[51,52] The diagnosis can be confidently made during the second and often in the first trimester.[51] Transvaginal imaging can improve diagnosis and identify sac contents as early as 12 weeks.[50,53] The utilization of three-dimensional (3D) US can improve detection of small lesions and provide assistance in the first trimester.[51,54]

Cephaloceles are variable in size, shape, and echotexture and may enlarge or change over time.[34] To diagnose a cephalocele, a defect in the cranial vault and continuity between the defect contents and the intracranial structures must be demonstrated[50] (Fig. 15.1-11). However, care must be taken to ensure that the

calvarial defect is not an artifact related to angle dropout or the normal posterior fontanel.[41,52] If the skull defect is small (up to 20% of cases), diagnosis can be difficult.[41]

Cephaloceles may be solid, cystic, or mixed[41] (Fig. 15.1-12). Detection of fetal brain with a gyral pattern within the sac is helpful, although the US appearance may change throughout gestation with solid tissue becoming more cystic with time[51,55] (Fig. 15.1-13). Thus, it can sometimes be difficult to discriminate a cranial meningocele from an encephalocele.[47] A cephalocele can be differentiated from an extracranial lesion by the acute angle with the surface of the fetal head.[47,50] Vascular flow into and around the lesion can indicate venous sinus extension and may be helpful in securing diagnosis of a cephalocele (Fig. 15.1-14). Factors on US that can help to predict a good outcome include: a sac containing only CSF or a nubbin of neural tissue, no associated anomalies, normal-sized brain, and absence of ventriculomegaly.[56] If more than 50% of the intracranial contents are exteriorized, survival and outcome are poor.[50]

Associated anomalies commonly identified on US include ventriculomegaly, microcephaly, loss of normal cerebral landmarks, lemon skull, Chiari II, obliteration of cisterna magna, and flattened basiocciput[43,50] (Fig. 15.1-15). Evaluation of extracranial structures should be performed with special attention to the kidneys and spine.[57] The presence of oligohydramnios, polycystic kidneys and occipital cephalocele should raise suspicion for Meckel–Gruber syndrome.[50] Although prenatal US can diagnose cephaloceles, assessment can be difficult because of low amniotic fluid, maternal obesity, or fetal head positioning.[41,50]

*MRI:* Given high soft tissue contrast and large field of view, MRI can diagnose 100% of cranial dysraphisms.[29] In the presence of a NTD, fetal MR has been shown to detect new findings that change US diagnosis in 15% of cases and discern new findings that were not defined on US in 42% of cases. MRI has the ability to influence management decisions such as continuation of pregnancy or mode of delivery in 21%.[29] Multiplanar imaging allows sharp delineation of the calvarial defect and can define the varying amounts of brain tissue, venous sinus

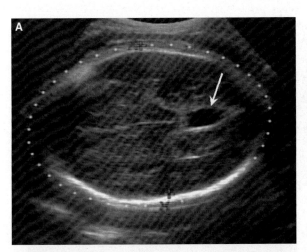
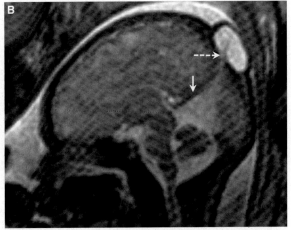

**FIGURE 15.1-10:** Atretic Parietal Cephalocele **A:** Axial US shows cigar-shaped interhemispheric CSF collection *(arrow)* in a fetus in third trimester. **B:** On sagittal SSFSE T2 image, the same fetus shows vertical straight sinus *(solid arrow)*, small parietal calvarial defect, and CSF extracranial *(dotted arrow)*.

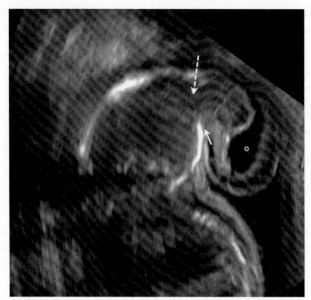

**FIGURE 15.1-11:** Sagittal ultrasound images in fetus with meningo-encephalocystocele. There is a defect in the calvarium *(solid arrow)* and continuity of intracranial brain extending into sac *(dotted arrow).* Cystic dilatation in extracranial tissue represents dilated ventricle *(circle).*

extension, and CSF in the cephalocele sac, thus providing important information with regard to prognosis (Fig. 15.1-16).[29,58] SSFP imaging demonstrates good contrast between water and soft tissue and can be helpful at defining borders of the defect (Fig. 15.1-17). Diffusion imaging can exclude ischemia or lesions such as dermoids, which show restricted diffusion.

Fetal MR is also extremely useful in identifying additional CNS anomalies, such as hindbrain malformations, corpus callosum dysgenesis, and cerebral parenchymal abnormalities[29] (Fig. 15.1-18). Because of its ability to define other anomalies, fetal MR can aid in the diagnosis of syndromes.

**Associated Anomalies:** Both intracranial and extracranial anomalies have been cited in up to 50% of children with cephaloceles.[40] Associated extracranial anomalies include facial,

cardiovascular, gastrointestinal, genitourinary, limb, heterotaxy, and other NTDs.[40,59]

Complications of intracranial malformation include hydrocephalus and microcephaly. Ventriculomegaly has been reported in 65% of occipital cephaloceles and 15% of frontal encephaloceles.[60] Spinal defects are noted in 7% to 15% of all cephaloceles.[60] Microcephaly has been observed in 20% of postnatal studies.

**Differential Diagnosis:** Demonstration of a calvarial bone defect confirms the diagnosis of cephalocele. However, if the fetus has an asymmetric cephalocele and constriction deformities, findings are more consistent with amniotic band syndrome. In the presence of a small skull defect, extracranial lesions can mimic cephaloceles. The differential diagnosis of a mass adjacent to the fetal skull includes teratoma, vascular malformation or hemangioma, branchial cleft cyst, and scalp edema.[61] A lesion arising from the skin surface should have an obtuse angle with the skull on US.[50] Rarely, fetal hair mimicking a thin membrane on US may be misinterpreted as a defect.[61] A frontal encephalocele should be differentiated from simple dermoid cyst and dacrocystotcele.[62] Basal encephaloceles must be differentiated from epignathus and congenital granular epulis tumors.[63]

**Prognosis:** Predictors of poor outcome include associated intracranial abnormalities, development of hydrocephalus, seizure disorder, microcephaly, and presence of brain tissue in the malformation.[42,64,65] Occipital lesions in some series do worse than anterior or parietal lesions.[39,42] In the presence of hydrocephalus, other intracranial abnormalities or genetic syndrome, the prognosis is poor.[56] The overall mortality rate is 5% to 29%.[40,64] The disability rate is approximately 52%.[61] Up to 20% will have seizures and 50% hydrocephalus.[31,65]

**Management:** In the presence of a cephalocele, karyotyping should be considered as 44% have a chromosomal abnormality.[41] If the encephalocele is large, with severe microcephaly and/or association with other anomalies, termination of the pregnancy may be considered.[51] A caesarean section is recommended to minimize trauma to the brain if the defect is

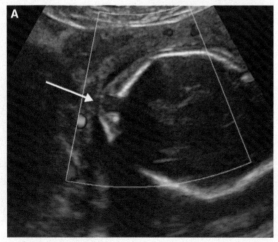
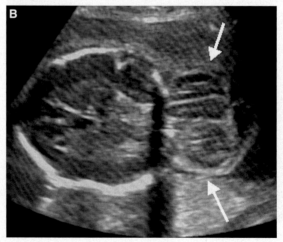

**FIGURE 15.1-12:** Variable appearance of cephaloceles **A:** Axial color US shows small defect in calvarium in association with cystic appearance of sac *(arrow).* **B:** Axial US shows sac containing mainly solid, brain parenchymal tissue *(arrows).*

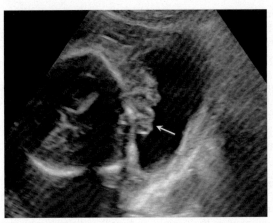

**FIGURE 15.1-13:** Axial US of meningoencephalocele showing pseudo-sulcation of herniated brain tissue *(arrow)*.

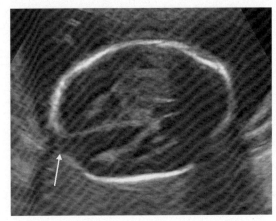

**FIGURE 15.1-15:** Axial US demonstrating lemon configuration and ventriculomegaly *(arrow)* in fetus with cephalocele.

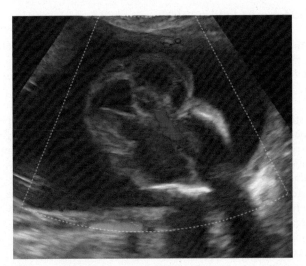

**FIGURE 15.1-14:** Axial color US with sagittal sinus extending into meningoencephalocele.

large.[51,61] If the cephalocele is small, vaginal delivery may be considered. Most cephaloceles are treated with surgery because of risk of injury to displaced brain, leakage of CSF, or facial maldevelopment.[55] As the lesion is covered with skin, timing of surgery is typically elective. A staged procedure may be indicated in complex cases.[33,42] Postoperatively, children with cephaloceles are at risk for hydrocephalus, CSF leak, infection, and lesion recurrence.

**Recurrence:** The sporadic cases do not have an increased risk of recurrence.[28] In the presence of a genetic syndrome, recurrence can be increased.

## AMNIOTIC BAND SYNDROME

**Synonyms:** Adhesions, amniotic disruption complex, amniotic bands, constricting bands.

**Description:** Amniotic band syndrome is a collection of malformations thought to be secondary to fetal entanglement in

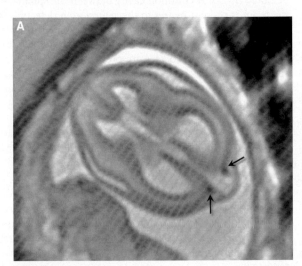

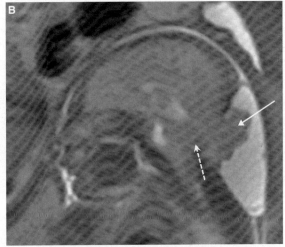

**FIGURE 15.1-16:** Cephalocele imaging on MRI **A:** Axial SSFSE T2 MRI showing meningocele containing CSF and venous sinuses as dark flow voids *(arrows)* along either side of the occipital skull defect, corresponding with US in Figure 15.1-12A. **B:** Sagittal SSFSE T2 image in occipital meningoencephalocele, corresponding to US in Figure 15.1-13, with sac containing supratentorial *(solid arrow)* and infratentorial *(dotted arrow)* brain.

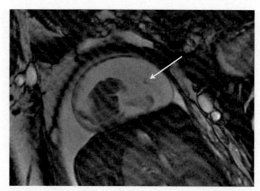

**FIGURE 15.1-17:** Coronal SSFP in same fetus as Figures 15.1-13 and 15.1-16B, showing membrane from herniated meninges *(arrow)*.

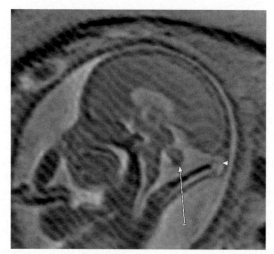

**FIGURE 15.1-18:** Sagittal SSFSE T2 image from fetus in Figure 15.1-12A, demonstrating occipital defect and sac *(arrowhead)* but also vermian hypogenesis *(arrow)*.

bands resulting in asymmetric defects that can involve the spine or the cranium.[66]

**Incidence:** 1 in 1,200 to 15,000 live births.[67]

**Pathogenesis:** Etiology is unknown. The exogenous theory suggests early amnion rupture leading to fibrous bands, which entrap the fetal body.[66] There is asymmetric amputation of fetal parts. If it occurs early, cranial or spinal defects may develop. The endogenous theory suggests lesions are secondary to vascular compromise. Neither mechanism explains all anomalies seen in this syndrome.

**Diagnosis:** Whenever unusual clefts are noted by US or MRI, such as asymmetric spine defects, cephaloceles, extremity amputation, or facial defects, the diagnosis should be considered. Clefts involving more than one region are also suggestive of the diagnosis.[67] Diagnosis has been made in the first trimester with nuchal translucency reported.[68]

**Differential Diagnosis:** Open NTD, anencephaly, encephalocele, limb body wall complex, and body stalk anomaly can look similar.

**Associated Anomalies:** Variable anomalies have been associated including major cranial, facial, thorax, abdomen, or spine anomalies. Limb constriction, clubfeet, scoliosis, and single digits are often noted.

**Prognosis:** Outcome depends on location size and number of defects.[69–72] Termination is considered if severe craniofacial and visceral abnormalities are present.

**Recurrence:** Most cases are sporadic.

## INIENCEPHALY

**Description:** *Inion* is Greek for the nape of the neck. Iniencephaly involves the occiput and inion with rachischisis of the cervical and thoracic spine with fixed extension of the head. Iniencephaly apertus is associated with an encephalocele, while iniencephaly clausus has no encephalocele.[73–75]

**Incidence:** 0.1 to 10 in 10,000.

**Etiology:** Etiology is likely similar to other open NTD. Folic acid supplements may decrease the risk of iniencephaly. Antiepileptic drugs, diuretics, and sulfa drugs have all been associated with increased risk for NTD.[75,76]

**Pathogenesis:** Onset is likely a few days later than anencephaly. Features include deficit of the occipital bone with enlarged foramen magnum and partial or total absence of cervical and thoracic vertebra with lack of segmentation and irregular vertebral archfusion. Shortening of the spinal column with hyperextension of the cervical thoracic spine is present. The face is upturned with the mandibular skin continuous with the chest because of the short neck.

**Diagnosis:** AFP is typically elevated.[77]

**Ultrasound:** Fixed dorsal flexion of the head "star gazing," short cervical and thoracic spine, and irregular vertebrae can be noted by US. A common cavity between the spinal cord and the brain is present owing to the neural arch defects. The skin of the chest directly connects to the face, while the scalp is directly connected to the back[78–80] (Fig. 15.1-19). Polyhydramnios is often noted. Cephaloceles are present in the open form. Associated anomalies such as arthrogryposis can be identified. Three-dimensional sonography has been used to further assess this complex anomaly.[81]

**MRI:** MRI is a useful adjunct in confirming the diagnosis and is superior in the delineation of the complex brain and spinal cord anomalies.[74,76]

**Associated Anomalies:** Associated anomalies include cleft palate, anencephaly, cephaloceles, omphalocele, gastroschisis, congenital diaphragmatic hernia, cardiac malformations, renal anomalies, arthrogryposis, and clubfoot. Polymicrogyria, heterotopias, holoprosencephaly, and vermian agenesis have been reported.[73,78]

**Differential Diagnosis:** Differential diagnosis includes Klippel–Feil syndrome, which also has a short neck because of fusion of

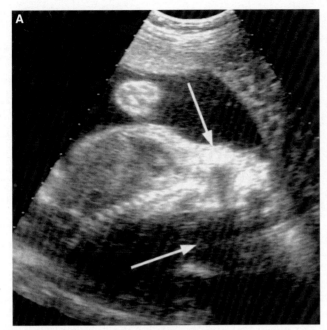 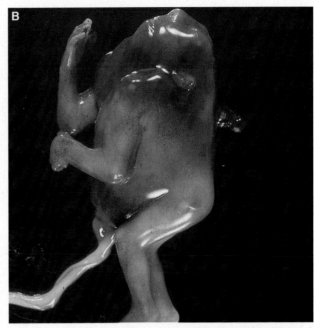

**FIGURE 15.1-19:** Iniencephaly. **A:** Sonogram shows the anterior neck *(top arrow)* is contiguous with the chest and the chin without the normal protrusion of the mandible. Note the retroflexion of the neck *(bottom arrow)*. **B:** Postnatal photograph of a similar case shows anencephaly with marked retroflexion of the neck. (From McGahan JP, Pilu G, Nyberg DA. Neural tube defects and the spine. In: Nyberg DA, McGahan DP, Pretorius DH, et al. *Diagnostic Imaging of Fetal Anomalies*. Philadelphia, PA: Lippincott Williams & Wilkins; 2003:291–334.)

cervical vertebrae and scapular anomalies. However, retroflexion of the head is typically not as severe, and AFP is normal. Anencephaly, cervical myelomeningocele, and encephaloceles should also be considered in the differential. In these cases, the cervical spine is typically normal.

**Prognosis:** Iniencephaly of both types are typically lethal. Cases of stillbirth or death within hours of delivery have been described.[79,82]

**Management:** Decisions regarding termination of pregnancy or providing supportive care at delivery should be discussed. Dystocia has been reported, and thus avoidance of a ceasarean section may require early induction.[82]

**Recurrence Risk:** The risk of recurrence increases to 1% to 5%.[76]

# REFERENCES

1. Naidich T, Blaser SI, Delman BN, et al. Congenital anomalies of the spine and spinal cord-embryology and malformations. In: Atlas S, ed. *Magnetic Resonance Imaging of the Brain and Spine*. Vol. 3. Philadelphia, PA: Lippincott Williams & Wilkins; 2002:1527–1631.
2. Tortori-Donati P, Rossi A, Cama A. Spinal dysraphism: a review of neuroradiological features with embryological correlations and proposal for a new classification. *Neuroradiology*. 2000;42:471–491.
3. Barkovich A. Congenital anomalies of the spine. In: Barkovich A, ed. *Pediatric Neuroimaging*. 3rd ed. Philadelphia, PA: Lippincott Williams & Wilkins; 2000:621–683.
4. Finnell RH, Gould A, Spiegelstein O. Pathobiology and genetics of neural tube defects. *Epilepsia*. 2003;44(suppl 3):14–23.
5. Frey L, Hauser WA. Epidemiology of neural tube defects. *Epilepsia*. 2003;44 (suppl 3):4–13.
5a. Seller MJ. Risks in spina bifida. *Dev Med Child Neurol*. 1994;36:1021–1025.
6. Cameron M, Moran P. Prenatal screening and diagnosis of neural tube defects. *Prenat Diagn*. 2009;29:402–411.
7. Williams LJ, Rasmussen SA, Flores A, et al. Decline in the prevalence of spina bifida and anencephaly by race/ethnicity: 1995–2002. *Pediatrics*. 2005;116:580–586.

8. Nicolaides KH, Campbell S. Diagnosis and management of fetal malformations. *Baillieres Clin Obstet Gynaecol*. 1987;1:591–622.
9. Cook RJ, Erdman JN, Hevia M, et al. Prenatal management of anencephaly. *Int J Gynaecol Obstet*. 2008;102:304–308.
10. Cox GC, Rosenthal SJ, Holsapple JW. Exencephaly: sonographic findings and radiologic-pathologic correlation. *Radiology*. 1985;155:755–756.
11. Hendricks SK, Cyr DR, Nyberg DA, et al. Exencephaly—clinical and ultrasonic correlation to anencephaly. *Obstet Gynecol*. 1988;72:898–900.
12. Weissman A, Diukman R, Auslender R. Fetal acrania: five new cases and review of the literature. *J Clin Ultrasound*. 1997;25:511–514.
13. Gupta P, Nain P, Singh J. Anencephaly: a neural tube defect—a review. *Am J Pharm Tech Res*. 2012;2:227–235.
14. Stumpf DA, Cranford RE, Elias S, et al. The infant with anencephaly. *N Engl J Med*. 1990;322:669–674.
15. Mitchell LE. Epidemiology of neural tube defects. *Am J Med Genet*. 2005;135: 88–94.
16. Wilkins-Haug L, Freedman W. Progression of exencephaly to anencephaly in the human fetus: an ultrasound perspective. *Prenat Diagn*. 1991;11:227–233.
17. Goldstein RB, Filly RA. Prenatal diagnosis of anencephaly: spectrum of sonographic appearances and distinction from the amniotic band syndrome. *AJR Am J Roentgenol*. 1988;151:547–550.
18. Goldstein RB, Filly RA, Callen PW. Sonography of anencephaly: pitfalls in early diagnosis. *J Clin Ultrasound*. 1989;17:397–402.
19. Cafici D, Sepulveda W. First-trimester echogenic amniotic fluid in the acrania-anencephaly sequence. *J Ultrasound Med*. 2003;22:1075–1079.
20. Souka AP, Nicolaides KH. Diagnosis of fetal abnormalities at the 10–14 week scan. *Ultrasound Obstet Gynecol*. 1997;10:429–442.
21. Gorgal R, Ramalho C, Brandao O, et al. *Fetal Diagn Ther*. 2011;29:164–168.
22. Yaron Y, Hamby DD, O'Brien JE, et al. Combination of elevated maternal serum alpha-fetoprotein (MSAFP) and low estriol is highly predictive of anencephaly. *Am J Med Genet*. 1998;75:297–299.
23. Campbell S, Holt EM, Johnstone FD, et al. Anencephaly: early ultrasonic diagnosis and active management. *Lancet*. 1972;9:1226–1227.
24. Machado RA, Brizot ML, Carvalho MH, et al. Sonographic markers of exencephaly below 10 weeks' gestation. *Prenat Diagn*. 2005;25:31–33.
25. Becker R, Mende B, Stiemer B, et al. Sonographic markers of exencephaly at 9 + 3 weeks of gestation. *Ultrasound Obstet Gynecol*. 2000;16:582–584.
26. Chatzipapas IK, Whitlow BJ, Economides DL. The Mickey Mouse sign and the diagnosis of anencephaly in early pregnancy. *Ultrasound Obstet Gynecol*. 1999;13:196–199.
27. Johnson SP, Sebire NJ, Snijders RJM, et al. Ultrasound screening for anencephaly at 10–14 weeks of gestation. *Ultrasound Obstet Gynecol*. 1997;9:14–16.
28. Sepulveda W, Sebire NJ, Fung TY, et al. Crown-chin length in normal and anencephalic fetuses at 10–14 weeks' gestation. *Am J Obstet Gynecol*. 1997;176: 852–855.

29. Saleem SN, Said A-H, Abdel-Raouf M, et al. Fetal MRI in the evaluation of fetuses referred for sonographically suspected neural tube defects (NTDs): impact on diagnosis and management decision. *Neuroradiology.* 2009;51:761–772.

30. Cragan JD, Roberts HE, Edmonds LKD, et al. Surveillance for anencephaly and spina bifida and the impact of prenatal diagnosis: United States, 1985–1994. *MMWR CDC Surveill Summ.* 1995;44:1–13.

31. Johnson CY, Honein MA, Flanders WD, et al. Pregnancy termination following prenatal diagnosis of anencephaly or spina bifida: a systematic review of the literature. *Birth Defects Res.* 2012;94:857–863.

32. Obeidi N, Russell N, Higgins JR, et al. The natural history of anencephaly. *Prenat Diagn.* 2010;30:357–360.

33. David DJ, Proudman TW. Cephaloceles: classification, pathology and management. *World J Surg.* 1989;13:349–357.

34. Naidich TP, Altman NR, Braffman BH, et al. Cephaloceles and related malformations. *AJNR Am J Neuroradiol.* 1992;13:655–690.

35. Diebler C, Dulac O. Cephaloceles: clinical and neuroradiological appearances. *Neuroradiology.* 1983;25:199–216.

36. Hedlund G. Congenital frontonasal masses: developmental anatomy, malformations, and MR imaging. *Pediatr Radiol.* 2006;36:647–662.

37. Grzegorczyk V, Brasseur-Daudruy M, Labadie G, et al. Prenatal diagnosis of a nasal glioma. *Pediatr Radiol.* 2010;40:1706–1709.

38. Patterson RJ, Egehoff JC, Crone KR, et al. Atretic parietal cephaloceles revisited: an enlarging clinical and imaging spectrum? *AJNR Am J Neuroradiol.* 1998;19:791–795.

39. Simpson DA, David D, White J. Cephaloceles: treatment, outcome and antenatal diagnosis. *Neurosurgery.* 1984;15:14–21.

40. Brown MS, Sheridan-Pereira M. Outlook for the child with a cephalocele. *Pediatrics.* 1992;90:914–919.

41. Goldstein RB, LaPidus AS, Filly RA. Fetal cephaloceles: diagnosis with US. *Radiology.* 1991;180:803–808.

42. Hockley AD, Goldin JH, Wake MJC. Management of anterior encephalocele. *Childs Nerv Syst.* 1990;6:444–446.

43. Rapport RL, Dunn RC Jr, Alhady F. Anterior encephalocele. *J Neurosurg.* 1981;54:213–219.

44. Van Allen MI, Kalousek DK, Chernoff GF, et al. Evidence for multi-site closure of the neural tube in humans. *Am J Med Genet.* 1993;47:723–743.

45. O'Rahilly R, Muller F. The two sites of fusion of the neural folds and the two neuropores in the human embryo. *Teratology.* 2002;65:162–170.

46. Gluckman TJ, George TM, McLone DG. Postneurulation rapid brain growth represents a critical time for encephalocele formation: a chick model. *Pediatr Neurosurg.* 1996;25:130–136.

47. Martinez-Lage JF, Poza M, Sola J, et al. The child with a cephalocele: etiology, neuroimaging and outcome. *Childs Nerv Syst.* 1996;12:540–550.

48. Fleming A, Copp AJ. A genetic risk factor for mouse neural tube defects: defining the embryonic basis. *Hum Mol Genet.* 2000;9:575–581.

49. Cohen MM, Lemire RL. Syndromes with cephaloceles. *Teratology.* 1992;25:161–172.

50. Budorick NE, Pretorius DH, McGahan JP, et al. Cephalocele detection in utero: sonographic and clinical features. *Ultrasound Obstet Gynecol.* 1995;5:77–85.

51. Liao SL, Tsai PY, Chen YC, et al. Prenatal diagnosis of fetal encephalocele using three dimensional ultrasound. *J Ultrasound Med.* 2012;20:150–154.

52. Jeanty P, Shah D, Zaleski W, et al. Prenatal diagnosis of fetal cephalocele: a sonographic spectrum. *Am J Perinatol.* 1991;8:144–149.

53. Bromshtein M, Zimmer EZ. Transvaginal sonographic followup on the formation of fetal cephalocele at 13–19 weeks' gestation. *Obstet Gynecol.* 1991;78:528.

54. Tsai PY, Chang CH, Chang FM. Prenatal diagnosis of fetal frontal encephalocele by three-dimensional ultrasound. *Prenat Diagn.* 2006;26:373–394.

55. Radulescu M, Ulmeanu EM, Nedelea M, et al. Prenatal ultrasound of diagnosis of neural tube defects: pictorial essay. *Med Ultrason.* 2012;14:147–153.

56. Bannister CM, Russell SA, Rimmer S, et al. Can prognostic indicators be identified in a fetus with an encephalocele? *Eur J Pediatr Surg.* 2000;10:20–23.

57. Graham D, Johnson RB Jr, Winn K, et al. The role of sonography in prenatal diagnosis and management of encephalocele. *J Ultrasound Med.* 1982;1:111–115.

58. Kojima K, Suzuki Y, Miyajima S, et al. Antenatal evaluation of an encephalocele in a dizygotic twin pregnancy using fast magnetic resonance imaging. *Fetal Diagn Ther.* 2003;18:338–341.

59. Wininger SJ, Donnenfeld AE. Syndromes identified in fetuses with prenatally diagnosed cephaloceles. *Prenat Diagn.* 1994;14:839–843.

60. Fitz CR. Midline anomalies of the brain and spine. *Radiol Clin North Am.* 1982;20:95–104.

61. Noriega CA, Fleming AD, Bonebrake RG. A false-positive diagnosis of a prenatal encephalocele on transvaginal ultrasonography. *J Ultrasound Med.* 2001;20:925–927.

62. Shahabi S, Busine A. Prenatal diagnosis of an epidermal scalp cyst simulating an encephalocele. *Prenat Diagn.* 1998;18:373–377.

63. Carlan SJ, Angel JL, Leo J, et al. Cephalocele involving the oral cavity. *Obstet Gynecol.* 1990;75:494–495.

64. Chervenak FA, Isaacson G, Mahoney MJ, et al. Diagnosis and management of fetal cephalocele. *Obstet Gynecol.* 1984;64:86–90.

65. Lo BWY, Kulkarni AV, Rutka JT, et al. Clinical predictors of developmental outcome in patients with cephaloceles. *J Neurosurg Pediatr.* 2008;2:254–257.

66. Sentilhes L, Verspyck E, Patrier S, et al Amniotic band syndrome: pathogenesis, prenatal diagnosis and neonatal management. *J Gynecol Obstet Biol Reprod.* 2003;32:693–704.

67. Burton KJ, Jilly RA. Sonographic diagnosis of the amniotic band syndrome. *AJR Am J Roentgenol.* 1991;156:555.

68. Higuchi T, Tanaka M, Kuroda K, et al. Abnormal first-trimester fetal nuchal translucency and amniotic band syndrome. *J Med Ultrason.* 2012;39(3):177–180.

69. Moran SL, Jensen M, Bravo C. Amniotic band syndrome of the upper extremity: diagnosis and management. *J Am Acad Orthop Surg.* 2007;15(7):397–407.

70. Hudgins RJ, Edwards MS, Ousterhout DK, et al. Pediatric neurosurgical implications of the amniotic band disruption complex: case reports and review of the literature. *Pediatr Neurosci.* 1985–1986;12(4–5):232–239.

71. Richter J, Wergeland H, DeKoninck P, et al. Fetoscopic release of an amniotic band with risk of amputation: case report and review of the literature. *Fetal Diagn Ther.* 2012;31(2):134–137.

72. Hüsler MR, Wilson RD, Horii SC, et al. When is fetoscopic release of amniotic bands indicated? Review of outcome of cases treated in utero and selection criteria for fetal surgery. *Prenat Diagn.* 2009;29(5):457–463.

73. Aleksic S, Budzilovich G, Greco MA, et al. Iniencephaly a neuropathologic study. *Clin Neuropathol.* 1983;2:55–61.

74. Gadodia A, Gupta P, Sharma R, et al. Antenatal sonography and MRI of iniencephaly apertus and clausus. *Fetal Diagn Ther.* 2010;27(3):178–180.

75. Kulkarni PR, Rao RV, Alur MB, et al. Iniencephaly: a case report with review of literature. *J Pediatr Neurosci.* 2011;6(2):121–123.

76. Pungavkar SA, Sainani NI, Karnik AS, et al Antenatal diagnosis of iniencephaly: sonographic and MR correlation: a case report. *Korean J Radiol.* 2007;8(4):351–355.

77. Mórocz I, Szeifert GT, Molnár P, et al. Prenatal diagnosis and pathoanatomy of iniencephaly. *Clin Genet.* 1986;30(2):81–86.

78. Tugrul S, Uludoğan M, Pekin O, et al. Iniencephaly: prenatal diagnosis with postmortem findings. *J Obstet Gynaecol Res.* 2007;33(4):566–569.

79. Balci S, Aypar E, Altinok G, et al. Prenatal diagnosis in three cases of iniencephaly with unusual postmortem findings. *Prenat Diagn.* 2001;21(7):558–562.

80. Sahid S, Sepulveda W, Dezerega V, et al. Iniencephaly: prenatal diagnosis and management. *Prenat Diagn.* 2000;20;202–205.

81. Sepulveda W. Three-dimensional sonography of fetal iniencephaly. *J Ultrasound Med.* 2012;31(8):1296–1298.

82. Katz VL, Aylsworth AS, Albright SG. Iniencephaly is not uniformly fatal. *Prenat Diagn.* 1989;9(8):595–599.

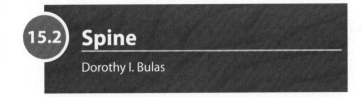

## 15.2 Spine

Dorothy I. Bulas

## CLASSIFICATION

A clinical-neuroradiological classification system described by Tortori-Donati et al.[1] helps organize the imaging features of the various forms of spinal dysraphism. This classification divides spinal dysraphism into open or closed defects (Fig. 15.2-1). An open neural tube defect (ONTD; open spinal dysraphism) is present when neural elements and/or membrane are exposed via a boney defect and lack skin covering. The most common forms include myelomeningocele and myelocele (myeloschisis), which are commonly associated with the Chiari II malformation. A closed neural tube defect (CNTD; closed spinal dysraphism) is covered by skin and includes anomalies such as meningocele, lipomeningocele, and diastomatomyelia. These are not commonly associated with the Chiari II malformation but can be associated with a subcutaneous mass or cyst, hemangioma, or overlying hairy patch.[2–4]

## OPEN NEURAL TUBE DEFECTS

**Synonyms:** Spinal dysraphism, myelomeningoceles, myeloceles, myeloschisis.

**Description:** ONTDs are abnormalities in neurulation that result in the meninges and neural tissue being exposed to the intrauterine environment.[5] In the spine, ONTDs can be subdivided into myelomeningoceles and myeloceles (myeloschisis). The position of the neural placode with respect to the level of the skin surface differentiates myelomeningocele from myelocele. When there is elevation due to expansion of the subarachnoid space, the lesion is called a *myelomeningocele* (MMC) with an overlying thin-walled membrane. When the subarachnoid space is not expanded and the placode remains flat to the surface within the confines of the dysraphic spinal canal, the lesion is called a myelocele or myeloschisis (see Fig. 15.2-1). Each can occur with or without spinal cord splitting.[3,4]

**Incidence:** Incidence currently is reported to be between 0.5 and 1 in 1,000 live births.[6] Infants of Hispanic mothers have a significantly higher birth prevalence of ONTD as compared with African American and Caucasian mothers.[7,8]

The reported incidence has decreased due to the increased use of periconceptional folic acid and rate of elective termination.[7] Women who take at least 0.4 mg of folic acid a day for at least 3 months before conception decrease the risk of ONTD by 70% to 80%.[9]

Most cases of ONTDs are sporadic with multifactor etiologies. About 1.6% of isolated ONTDs are associated with a defined chromosomal or single gene disorder.[10,11] That number goes up to 24% if there are additional fetal anomalies noted.[12] Fifty-three percent of spontaneously aborted fetuses with ONTDs have an abnormal karyotype, including trisomy, triploidy, tetraploidy, or deletions. The most common aneuploidy is trisomy 18. Syndromes which have MMC as a feature include autosomal dominant conditions such as Lehman syndrome, and recessive inheritance such as Meckel Gruber syndrome.[7,10–12]

Environmental and maternal factors may play a role as well. Medications such as valproic acid and carbamazepine increase the chance of ONTD to as high as 1% to 2%.[13] Warfarin and vitamin A also are risk factors.[7,14] Obesity and diabetes are also associated with increased risk of neural tube defect (NTD). Women with a BMI greater than 29 kg per m$^2$ have a 1.5 to 3.5 times greater chance of conceiving a child with ONTD and may not be ameliorated by taking folic acid.[15–18] Maternal hyperthermia has also been implicated, possibly doubling the rate.[18]

Having a previous pregnancy with ONTD or a family history increases the odds of recurrence. Risks increase to 2% to 3% if one pregnancy has been affected, and to 10% if two pregnancies have been affected.[7,19,20]

**Embryology/Pathogenesis:** Open NTD of the spine occurs during the formation of the primitive neural tube (neurulation) in the third week of gestation when there is a localized failure of neural tube closure. This can occur anywhere along the length of the spinal cord, but it is most common in the lumbar region. A lack of signaling between the neural tissue and overlying mesoderm and ectoderm may be what leads to defects in the bones overlying the unfused portions of the neural tube. The resulting lesion is an open spinal canal with a flat neural placode instead of a cylindrical spinal cord, associated with a posterior osseous as well as skin defect. Tethering of the spinal cord secondary to adhesions leads to tension on the neural axis.

The association with Chiari II malformation is proposed to be due to the leakage of cerebrospinal fluid (CSF) via the spinal defect which collapses the primitive ventricular system and prevents expansion of the rhombencephalic vesicle.[21] This may result in a small posterior fossa with medulla, vermian, and cerebellar tonsil herniation. There can be elongation and kinking of the medulla, caudal displacement of the cervical spinal cord and medulla, and obliteration of the cisterna magna (Fig. 15.2-2). Hindbrain herniation can lead to brain stem compression, a leading cause of mortality.[21,22]

Progressive hindbrain herniation has been demonstrated in animal models. Cases of low lumbosacral MMC have been noted to have minimal hindbrain herniation early in pregnancy.[23]

Associated abnormalities of the brain include herniation of the cerebellar tonsils and vermis through the foramen magnum; "beaking" of the tectum; an enlarged massa intermedia of the thalami; partial or complete callosal dysgenesis; hypoplastic falx; and structural changes in the skull. Migrational abnormalities, particularly subependymal gray matter heterotopia, are often present.

Theories as to why hydrocephalus develops include mechanical obstruction secondary to the Chiari II malformation and/or dysfunctional CSF absorption.[21] At times, hydrocephalus develops only after postnatal closure of the skin opening.

**Diagnosis:** Alpha-fetoprotein (AFP) is increased with ONTD in both maternal blood and amniotic fluid. Maternal serum AFP at 16 weeks' gestation, amniotic fluid testing of AFP, and acetylcholinesterase (ACHE) have been the main method of screening for ONTD. The maternal serum AFP level varies with gestation, so it needs to be expressed as multiples of the median (MoM). Using 2.5 MoM as screen positive in singleton pregnancies, the detection rate for ONTD ranges between 65% and 80%. False-positive rates range between 1% and 3%. An increased serum AFP can be associated with ventral wall defects, congenital nephrosis, and fetal demise. It is important to remember that skin-covered closed NTD will have a normal AFP.[24,25]

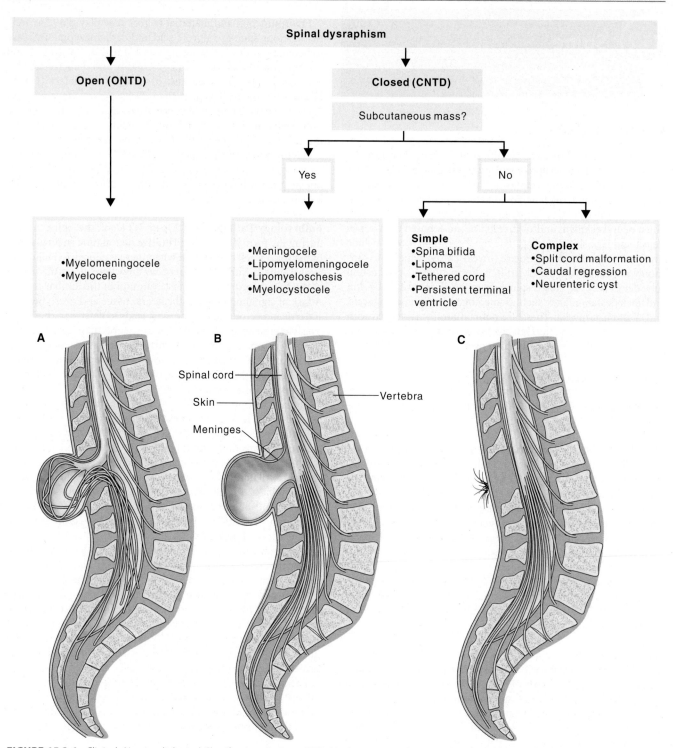

**Spinal dysraphism**

**Open (ONTD)**

**Closed (CNTD)**

Subcutaneous mass?

Yes

No

•Myelomeningocele
•Myelocele

•Meningocele
•Lipomyelomeningocele
•Lipomyeloschesis
•Myelocystocele

**Simple**
•Spina bifida
•Lipoma
•Tethered cord
•Persistent terminal
 ventricle

**Complex**
•Split cord malformation
•Caudal regression
•Neurenteric cyst

A    B    C

Spinal cord

Skin

Meninges

Vertebra

**FIGURE 15.2-1:** Clinical- Neuroradiological Classification. **A:** Open NTD; Myelomeningocele - neural elements and meninges protrude through the spine defect into a membrane covered sac. **B:** Closed NTD with mass; Meningocele with skin covered sac. **C:** Closed NTD, no mass. Cord may be normal or tethered.

*Ultrasound:* The accuracy of identifying spinal anomalies during a nontargeted screening ultrasound (US), is variable and depends on operator experience, fetal lie, and maternal body habitus. When a referral is made to an experienced center for suspected ONTD due to elevated maternal serum AFP and ACHE, accuracy of detailed targeted exams have been reported to be as high as 100%.[26] With ONTD, even when spine visualization is limited due to fetal lie or maternal obesity, cranial findings of Chiari II are usually well visualized sonographically.

The fetal brain, including skull shape, ventricular size, and cerebellar contour, should be evaluated carefully (Table 15.2-1). A small cisterna magna with rounded small cerebellum, the "banana sign" is 99% sensitive in diagnosing Chiari II malformations (Fig. 15.2-3A,B) and is present in most cases of open NTD.

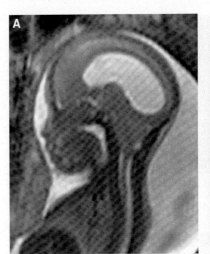
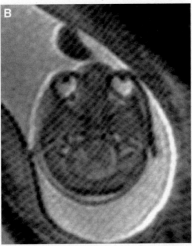
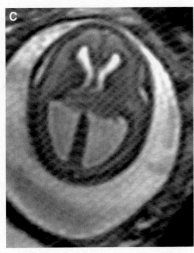

**FIGURE 15.2-2:** Chiari II malformation MRI at 21 weeks' gestation. **A:** Sagittal T2w image demonstrates herniation of the cerebellar tonsils and vermis through the foramen magnum with obliteration of the cisterna magna and fourth ventricle. **B:** Axial T2w image of the posterior fossa demonstrates obliterated cisterna magna, fourth ventricle with a small rounded cerebellum. **C:** Axial image through the ventricles demonstrates decreased subarachnoid space with dilated occipital horns.

Concavity of the frontal bones, the "lemon sign" (Fig. 15.2-3A,C) can be seen in 98% of cases before 24 weeks.[27–29] It has been described as early as 13 weeks' gestation. The "lemon sign" is present in up to 1% to 2% of normal fetuses and typically resolves by the third trimester of fetuses with ONTD (present in only 13% of affected fetuses after 24 weeks). Biparietal diameter (BPD) and head circumference (HC) measurements can be below 5% in the early second trimester. Microcephaly has been described in up to 69% of cases between 16 and 24 weeks.[30,31] Both of these measurements typically normalize by the later second trimester. If ventriculomegaly develops, macrocephaly may develop. While hydrocephalus may develop early in the second trimester, it may not develop until postnatally after the defect is closed. Filly et al.[32] described the "Too-Far-Back Ventricle" in cases of Chiari II malformation in which the occipital horn is closer to the occipital bone compared to normal fetuses due to hind-brain herniation.

Ossification of vertebral bodies progresses through the second trimester with the L5 arch ossified by 16 weeks' gestation, S1 by 19 weeks' gestation and S2 by 22 weeks' gestation[33] (Fig. 15.2-4). One can count the vertebral level using the lowest rib as T12 or the superior aspect of the iliac crest as L5. The axial plane is most helpful in evaluation of the three ossification centers and overlying skin. Evaluation of the fetal spine by US requires imaging of all three planes. Transverse planes are most useful in demonstrating the three ossification centers with splayed pedicles and overlying sac or skin defect.[34] It is important to assess the thickness of the sac: thin when membrane covered, thick when skin covered. High frequency linear transducers can demonstrate cord tethering and placode contents. The level of the defect, conus, presence of scoliosis, and additional vertebral anomalies should be searched for (Figs. 15.2-5 and 15.2-6).

3D ultrasound can help evaluate spine lesions by examination of structures in planes other than the original acquisition plane. The various rendering algorithms allow visualization of various characteristics: skeletal mode highlights bony structures, surface mode highlights the sac or overlying skin (Figs. 15.2-7 and 15.2-8).[35,36] 3D views are best obtained with the fetal spine up in the sagittal plane. Surface rendering requires sufficient overlying amniotic fluid.

Once the spine anomaly is identified, the lower extremities should be reviewed for possible equinovarus deformity. Leg function, defined as flexion and extension at the hips, knees, and ankles, should be commented upon. Additional anomalies should be searched for.[37,38] When spine findings are equivocal, correlation with AFP, ACHE, and fetal MRI are helpful in further assessment.[21]

First trimester sonography may be an opportunity to diagnose open NTD during the 11- to 13-week screening scan. It has been noted that on the mid-sagittal plane of the fetal face used to measure the nuchal translucency (NT) and nasal bone, an intracranial translucency (IT) that is parallel to the nuchal translucency can be seen normally. This intracranial lucency represents the fourth ventricle. In fetuses with open NTD the fourth ventricle is small and thus the IT is absent.[39] Prospective large studies will determine if this sign can provide an effective screening method for early first trimester accurate diagnosis.[40]

***MRI:*** MRI is a useful adjunct to confirm the diagnosis of ONTD, and search for additional cranial and extracranial anomalies.[41–49] MRI has become particularly important in the age of fetal surgery, where accurate diagnosis is critical in determining appropriateness of therapy.[43,47,48] Small field of view

| Table 15.2-1 | Sonographic Features of Open NTD |
|---|---|

Small BPD and HC

Frontal concavity (lemon sign)

Small/absent cisternal magna

Rounded small cerebellum (banana sign)

Lateral ventriculomegaly

Dorsal vertebra splayed

No skin covering

Overlying sac with thin membrane

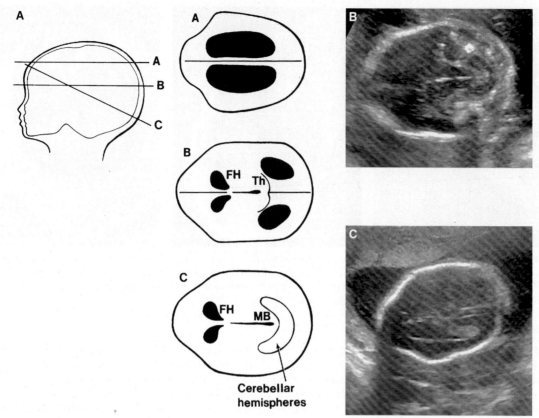

**FIGURE 15.2-3:** Cranial US findings associated with Chiari malformation. **A:** Diagram demonstrates the cranial findings associated with MMC. Lemon-shaped calvaria, dilatation of the lateral cerebral ventricles, obliteration of the cisterna magna with herniation of the cerebellum resulting in the banana sign. FH, frontal horn; MB, midbrain; Th, thalamus. **B:** Axial US of the posterior fossa demonstrates compression of the cerebellum with obliterated cisterna magna—the "banana sign." **C:** Axial US of the fetal head demonstrates bifrontal convexity of the calvaria—the "lemon sign."

in orthogonal planes with respect to the should be obtained, each adjusted from the preceding series.[49] T2w images half-Fourier acquisition single-shot rapid accelertion with relaxation enhancement (RARE)—ultrafast T2w echo planar spine echo sequences at thin slice thickness (2 to 4 mm) are most useful in assessing spine and cranial anomalies. Balanced steady-state free precession (bSSFP), known as TrueFISP (Siemens Medical Solutions) and FIESTA (GE Healthcare), produces T2w images for high signal fluid and soft tissue contrast.[50] Fast T1w gradient echo imaging can be used to assess for fat and blood. Rapid gradient echo, echo planar imaging (EPI), with high sensitivity to paramagnetic susceptibility can be useful for skeletal and vascular structures.

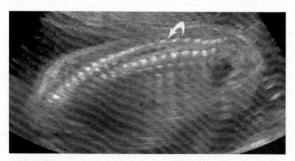

**FIGURE 15.2-4:** Oblique US of a normal spine at 22 weeks' gestation. Note conus at L3 (arrow).

Small field of view 2 to 4 mm thickness slices in all three planes should be obtained of the brain to evaluate hindbrain herniation as well as associated anomalies such as subependymal heterotopias, collosal agenesis, hypoplastic falx, small subarachnoid space, and tectal beaking, all better visualized by MRI (see Fig. 15.2-2).

The axial plane of the spine is important for the assessment of cord tethering and location of the placode (Figs. 15.2-5 to 15.2-7). Sagittal and coronal abdominal planes are useful in the evaluation of scoliosis as well as associated gastrointestinal and urologic anomalies such as cloaca. Sagittal views of the limbs can be used to evaluate for equinovarus, with cine images able to review lower extremity movement.[51]

With post-processing, MR sequences can be used to create models either virtual or using various materials such as paper (Figs. 15.2-8 and 15.2-9).[52]

**Associated Anomalies:** ONTD are associated with Chiari II malformation, equinovarus deformity of the feet, and hip dislocation due to spasticity as well as more complex anomalies such as OEIS complex (omphalocele–extrophy–imperforate anus–spinal defects).

**Differential Diagnosis:** Several spinal masses need to be differentiated from ONTD. Cystic exophytic sacrococcygeal teratomas lack the Chiari II changes and typically have no spinal dysraphism or cord tethering. Closed NTD such as

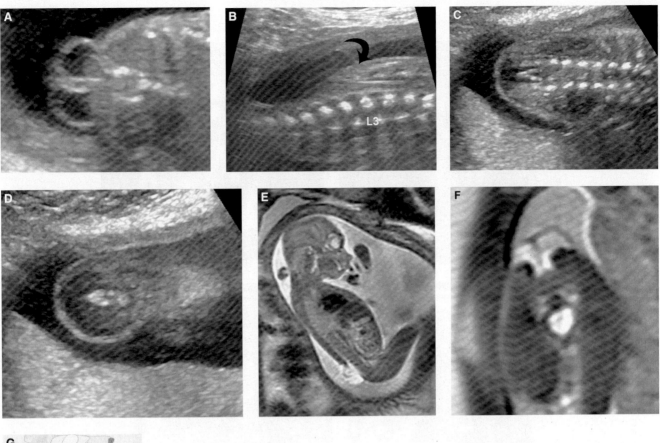

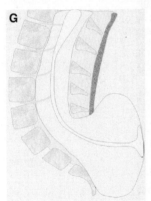

**FIGURE 15.2-5:** Myelomeningocele at 22 weeks' gestation. **A:** Axial US image of the lumbar spine demonstrates spinal dysraphism with overlying thin-walled sac containing nerve roots and placode. **B:** Sagittal US demonstrates cord tethering *(arrow)*. **C and D:** Coronal images of the thin walled sac. Sagittal **(E)** and axial **(F)** T2w MR images confirm the presence of a MMC. Notice the cranial findings of Chiari II in figure **E**. **G:** Sagittal diagram of myelomeningocele. (**G** from Zugazaga Cortazar A, Martín Martinez C, Duran Feliubadalo C, et al. Magnetic resonance imaging in the prenatal diagnosis of neural tube defects. *Insights Imaging*. 2013;4:225–237. doi:10.1007/s13244-013-0223-2.)

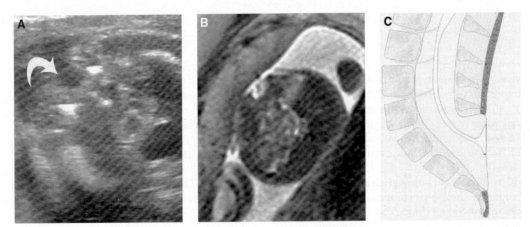

**FIGURE 15.2-6:** Myeloschisis at 19 weeks' gestation. **A:** Axial US demonstrates spinal dysraphism with skin defect and no overlying sac *(arrow)*. **B:** Axial SSFSE T2w MRI demonstrates cord tethering with skin defect and no overlying sac. Cord remains within the spinal canal. **C:** Sagittal diagram of myelochisis. (**C** from Zugazaga Cortazar A, Martín Martinez C, Duran Feliubadalo C, et al. Magnetic resonance imaging in the prenatal diagnosis of neural tube defects. *Insights Imaging*. 2013;4:225–237. doi:10.1007/s13244-013-0223-2.)

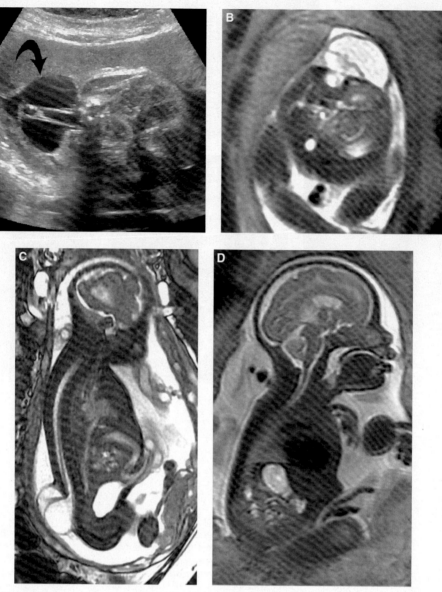

**FIGURE 15.2-7:** Myelomeningocele at 28 weeks' gestation. **A:** Axial US demonstrates a thin-walled sac *(arrow)* containing placode. Axial **(B)** and sagittal **(C)** T2w MRI confirm the presence of spinal dysraphism and cord tethering. **D:** Only mild hindbrain herniation is present.

lipomyelomeningocele, meningocele, and myelocystoceles have thicker skin-covered defects and typically no Chiari II changes. However, it is important to remember that meningoceles and myelocystoceles can have transitional findings of hindbrain herniation, as well as nerve roots in the sac. It becomes critical in these cases to assess for skin versus membrane coverage. Correlation with AFP may be useful in these cases.[23]

**Prognosis:** MMC is associated with significant lifelong morbidity affecting cognitive function, orthopedic disabilities, and bowel and bladder dysfunction. Lifelong coordinated care is required from neurosurgery, urology, orthopedics, neurodevelopmental pediatrics, nutrition, and rehabilitation.[7,53]

Outcome is variable around the world, dependent on access to medical, surgical, and community resources.[54,55] Up to 14% of MMC neonates do not survive past 5 years of age, with

mortality increasing to 35% in those with brainstem dysfunction from the Chiari II malformation.[56] Seventy-five percent of patients are estimated to reach adulthood with aggressive support but suffer from various degrees of neurological deficits depending on the level of the lesion.

Efforts to predict prognosis have had limited success. Factors that appear to influence prognosis include level of the lesion, degree of ventriculomegaly, and amount of cerebellar tonsillar herniation. The degree of cerebellar herniation is associated with childhood seizure activity, bladder dysfunction, and decreased independent ambulation.[55] The larger and higher the lesion, the increased risk of dysphagia and full-time wheelchair use.[54] Individuals with an L3 lesion or higher are not expected to walk.[7,57] Urinary and fecal incontinence are common at all levels. It remains unclear whether the absence or presence of a covering membrane results in a worse prognosis. Chao et al.[54]

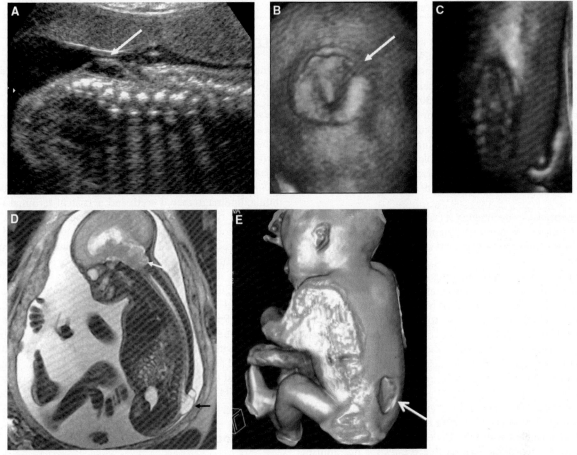

**FIGURE 15.2-8:** Myelomeningocele at 26 weeks' gestation. **A:** Sagittal US demonstrates overlying thin-walled sac *(arrow)* with cord tethering. 3D US images of the sac in surface mode **(B)** and spinal dyraphism in skeletal mode **(C)**. **D:** Sagittal MRI demonstrates the Chiari malformation *(white arrow)* and MMC sac containing neural elements *(black arrow)*. **E:** 3D MR surface model demonstrates skin defect *(arrow)*. (Courtesy of Heron Werner.)

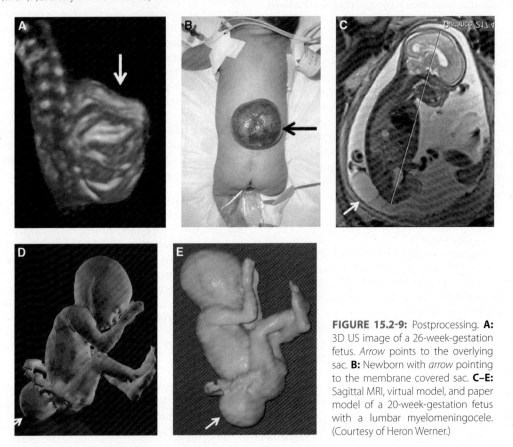

**FIGURE 15.2-9:** Postprocessing. **A:** 3D US image of a 26-week-gestation fetus. *Arrow* points to the overlying sac. **B:** Newborn with *arrow* pointing to the membrane covered sac. **C–E:** Sagittal MRI, virtual model, and paper model of a 20-week-gestation fetus with a lumbar myelomeningocele. (Courtesy of Heron Werner.)

noted that a lack of a membrane was associated with scoliosis and higher risk of bladder dysfunction. Wilson et al.,[58] however, suggested that a sac resulted in decreased leg function though this data did reach statistical significance. An estimated 20% require special education classes and 30% have an IQ below 80 secondary to hydrocephalus and complications with shunting and infection.[7,59,60] Hydrocephalus occurs in up to 85% of patients, with up to 80% requiring shunting. Up to 45% have shunt complications within the first year of placement.[60–62] Complications following shunt placement underscore the shortcoming of prenatal assessment of future morbidity and mortality.

**Management:** Accurate imaging is critical toward making well-informed decisions regarding the management of the pregnancy, labor, delivery, the possibility of fetal surgery, or interruption of the pregnancy.[38]

In the presence of a myelomeningocele, karyotyping should be considered particularly if additional anomalies are identified. A cesarean section is recommended to minimize trauma to the spine.[63] Postnatally, the defect needs to be closed as soon as possible to prevent infection. The need for a ventriculo-peritoneal shunt is determined by the progression of hydrocephalus and is typically required in 80% of cases. Postoperatively children with ONTD are at risk for shunt failure, CSF leak, and infection.

In utero repair of ONTDs is now being performed in selected patients and offers an alternative for a mother carrying a fetus with MMC.[53] Fetuses with ONTD develop neurologic deficits by the primary neurulation defect that creates the dysraphism and associated myelodysplasia. It is thought that further injury occurs from chemical and/or physical trauma to the neural tissue as a result of exposure to amniotic fluid. Fetal surgery could theoretically reduce this later injury by covering the exposed spinal cord.[64]

In fetal sheep experiments, surgically-created MMCs were repaired inutero.[64] At birth, these sheep demonstrated near-normal motor function and sensation and were continent unlike the unrepaired control group. Early studies on human fetuses suggested some improvement in distal sensorimotor function. In addition, it was noted that there was reversal of hindbrain herniation with decreased need for ventricular shunting in some cases.[65–70] A multicenter randomized prospective National Institute of Health trial (MOMS) convincingly showed that open fetal surgery could improve neurologic outcome with a decreased need for shunting.[71] The surgery, however, is associated with iatrogenic maternal and fetal risks, including premature rupture of membranes, amnio infection, and preterm delivery.[72,73] Fetal endoscopic MMC closure may provide a less invasive method of in utero repair.[74,75]

Due to the risk of surgery to the fetus and mother, accurate diagnosis is critical and should include US, MRI, and amniocentesis to exclude additional anomalies. A thick-walled sac, absence of hindbrain herniation, and lack of elevation of maternal or amniotic fluid AFP should raise suspicion of a CNTD such as meningocele, lipomyelomeningocele or myelocystocele and thus not a candidate for fetal surgery.

**Recurrence Risk:** Both genetic and micronutrient causes can increase in the risk of open NTD. For women at increased risk, it is recommended to take folic acid supplement on a daily basis and to increase the supplementation when they are planning a pregnancy.[76]

# CLOSED NEURAL TUBE DEFECTS

**Synonyms:** Skin-covered neural tube defects, closed neural tube defects, closed spinal dyraphism.

**Description:** CNTDs are a group of neural arch defects covered with intact skin. These account for up to 15% of neural tube defects. Closed dysraphism can be further divided into two subsets based on the presence or absence of a subcutaneous mass.

*Simple CNTDs* that are not associated with a mass include spina bifida, lipoma, tethered cord, and persistent terminal ventricle. These are typically not diagnosed prenatally. *Complex CNTDs* that are not associated with a mass include split cord malformations, caudal regression, intradural lipomas, and neurenteric cysts.[1–4] Cutaneous signs are present in up to 50% of cases.[77]

*CNTDs associated with a subcutaneous mass* include meningocele, lipomyelomeningocele, lipomeningocele, and myelocystoceles.[1–4] These may be identified prenatally but can be mistaken for an ONTD if not carefully evaluated. It is important to remember that these skin-covered lesions are usually not associated with Chiari II malformations, often have a better prognosis, and are not candidates for prenatal surgery. Thus, in the era of fetal surgery for MMC, it has become critical to distinguish CNTD from ONTD prenatally for appropriate counseling and management.

## Meningocele

**Description:** Spinal meningoceles are skin-covered sacs of spinal meninges protruding through a posterior spinal defect with the spinal cord remaining confined to the vertebral canal. They can be associated with cord tethering or hydromyelia.[78,79] The sac contains meninges and CSF but nerve and spinal cord are typically not involved. Meningoceles occur most commonly at the thoracic level (Fig. 15.2-10) and can also be cervical in location.[80] Typically there is no associated Chiari II.

It is important to remember that exceptions occur and transitional meningoceles can be associated with hindbrain herniation, placodes, and ventriculomegaly.[23]

**Incidence:** 10% of patients with spinal bifida have a meningocele.[81] Anterior lateral or anterolateral defects are less common. An anterior sacral mass with an associated sacral defect when present with an anorectal anomaly is known as Currarino triad.[82–84]

**Embryology/Pathogenesis:** During gastrulation (weeks 2 to 3), the embryo undergoes conversion from a bilaminar to a trilaminar structure with establishment of the nuchal cord. This is followed during gestational weeks 3 and 4 by primary neurulation where the upper 9th/10th of the spinal cord is formed. Finally secondary neurulation and retrogressive differentiation occur in weeks 5 to 6 with formation of the conus medullaris and filum terminale. Lumbar meningoceles are believed to occur as a disorder of secondary neurulation.[2,3]

**Diagnosis:** AFP levels are typically normal, as the lesions are skin-covered.

*Ultrasound:* Typically there is no association with Chiari II malformation. With no cranial findings to suggest a spinal lesion, US may miss an isolated spinal defect if the spine lies adjacent to the uterus or not carefully searched for.

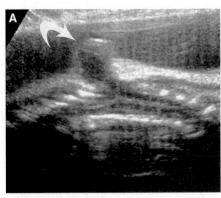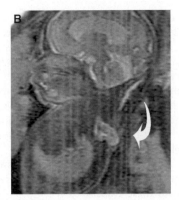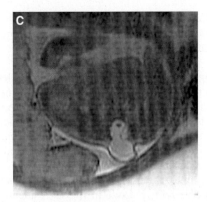

**FIGURE 15.2-10:** Thoracic meningocele. **A:** Sagittal US demonstrates a thick-walled cyst *(arrow)* overlying a thoracic spinal dysraphism. Sagittal **(B)** and axial **(C)** T2w MRI images confirm the presence of a thoracic MC with skin-covered fluid filled-sac *(arrow)*. There was no Chiari malformation.

The spine should be evaluated in both sagittal and axial planes. The overlying fluid-filled sac is typically thick as it is covered by skin (Fig. 15.2-11A,B). US can evaluate the level of cord tethering and the presence or absence of a placode.[47]

**MRI:** MRI can be a useful adjunct in evaluating the skin-covered sac, contents of the sac, and conus level. It is particularly useful in confirming that the hindbrain is normal (Fig. 15.2-11C,D).[43,47,85]

**Associations:** 90% of patients with meningocele have associated occult spinal lesions such as tight filum terminale, split cord malformation, and epidermoid. Subsequent tethering of the spinal cord may lead to progressive neurological deficit.[86]

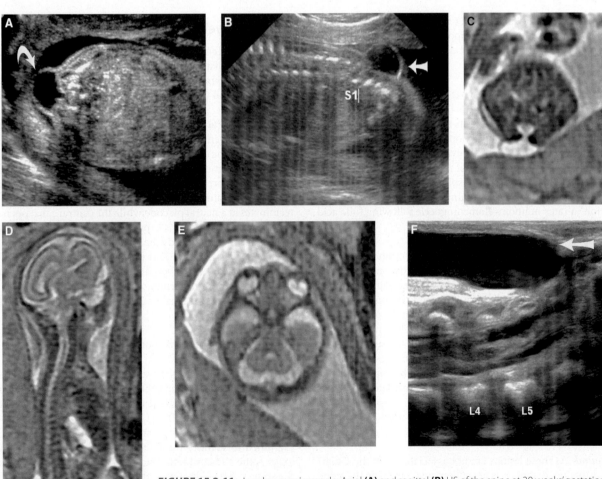

**FIGURE 15.2-11:** Lumbar meningocele. Axial **(A)** and sagittal **(B)** US of the spine at 20 weeks' gestation demonstrate a thick-walled sac containing fluid and no neural elements *(arrow)*. Axial **(C)** and saggital **(D)** T2w MRIs at 20 weeks confirm the lack of nerve roots or placode in the thick-walled sac. **E:** Axial MRI of the brain demonstrates normal cerebellum and cisterna magna with no Chiari malformation. **F:** Post-natal US demonstrates cord tethering with skin covered fluid filled sac *(arrow)*. **S1** - first sacral vertebra, **L4** - fourth lumbar vertebra, **L5** - fifth lumbar vertebra.

**Differential Diagnosis:** Differential includes myelomeningocele, sacrococcygeal teratoma, myelocystocele, and lipomyelomeningocele.

**Prognosis and Management:** Meningoceles are skin covered and typically not associated with Chiari II malformation. Thus, they are not candidates for fetal surgery. As the neuroglial tissue is covered by the thick layer of skin, the neurological exam is often normal or near normal after delivery. Long-term cord tethering may result in impaired bowel and bladder control as well as spasticity.[87,88]

At times, a meningocele may have hindbrain herniation and/or nerve roots/placode in the sac. Patients with these transitional meningoceles may require shunting if hydrocephalus develops with outcomes more similar to that of a patient with a meningomyelocele.[23]

Mode of delivery is dependent on the size of the sac. Large sacs may require caesarian section to prevent rupture at delivery. Following delivery, early repair may be needed to prevent sac injury, CSF leak, and infection.

## Lipomyelomeningocele or Lipomyelocele

**Synonym:** Lipomyeloschisis.

**Description:** Skin-covered CNTD where the neural placode is associated with a lipoma. The lipoma is contiguous with the subcutaneous fat through a spinal defect attaching and tethering the spinal cord.

**Incidence:** Incidence is 0.3 to 0.6 per 10,000 live births. Account for 14% to 20% of skin-covered NTD.[6,89–91] Lipomyelomeningocele has higher reported rates in infants born to mothers in younger and older age groups. Compared with non-Hispanic whites, Hispanics have a higher prevalence of lipomyelomeningocele and lipomeningocele than of myelomeningocele, meningocele, and myelocele subtypes of spinal dysraphisms.[8,91,92]

Familial forms of lipomyelomeningocele are rare. There is no reduction in rates of lipomyelomeningocele following folic acid supplementation.[93,94]

**Embryology/Pathogenesis:** Premature disjunction of the cutaneous ectoderm from the neuroectoderm allows mesenchyme to contact the inner portion of the developing neural tube. As the tube closes, the mesenchyme is induced to become fat which interferes with neurulation.[1–4,90] This results in the formation of a lipomyelomeningocele or lipomyeloceles. A lipomyelomeningocele is a lipomyelocele with enlargement of the subarachnoid space. It is less common than the flatter lipomyelocele. The lipoma covers the neural elements, causing tethering but generally prevents herniation of the cord through the defect.[95]

**Diagnosis:** These skin-covered lesions have normal AFP and acetyl cholinesterase levels.

**Ultrasound:** As these lesions are not associated with the Chiari II malformation, diagnosis is dependent on identifying the spine lesion.[96] The diagnosis can be difficult to make by US if the spine lies adjacent to the uterus with limited visualization of the subcutaneous mass. Axial images are particularly important in identifying splayed pedicles. Coronal views may help identify the tethered cord (Fig. 15.2-12A,B). The brain is typically normal.

**MRI:** MRI can be helpful in documenting cord tethering and the presence of a fatty mass within the sac (Fig. 15.2-12C,D). T1w images can be useful in the assessment of fatty components (Fig. 15.2-12E).[43,47]

**Associations:** Associated anomalies include sacral dysgenesis, segmentation anomalies, anal atresia, genitourinary, split cord malformations, and scoliosis.[97] There is an increase in Chiari I malformation compared with the general population.[97]

**Management:** Because the sac is skin covered, cesarian section can be reserved for those masses that are particularly large.

**Prognosis:** The placode in the lipomyelomeningocele is often deformed, rotated toward the lipoma away from the protruded meninges. This makes postnatal repair difficult as the nerve roots are distorted, with short roots on the lipoma side and elongated roots on the other side which require careful repositioning at surgery.[90,98–100]

Compared with MMC patients, patients with lipomeningocele typically have milder neurologic deficits including retained bowel and bladder continence despite significant dysplasia of the caudal spinal cord.[101,102] Incidence of retethering, however, is 10% to 30%.[95,100,102]

## Terminal Myelocystocele

**Description:** Terminal myelocystocele (MCC) is a rare CNTD in which the distal central canal dilates and herniates through a posterior lumbosacral spinal defect. The leptomeninges may herniate around the distal cord as well.

**Embryology/Pathogenesis:** MCC may represent a large persistent terminal ventricle. It is thought that CSF may not be able to escape from the neural tube during its formation[103] with progressive herniation of the cord through the skin-covered spine defect. It can present as a large, epithelialized, cystic lumbosacral mass containing fat, CSF, and neural tissue. The spinal cord terminates at a neural placode while the central canal opens into a CSF-filled cavity that is separate from fluid in the subarachnoid space that surrounds the spinal cord.[104]

As a CNTD, MCC should not be associated with the Chiari II malformation. However, at times, particularly in the third trimester, hindbrain herniation has been described. This may develop as the cord further herniates through the dysraphic defect.[43,23,105]

**Diagnosis:** AFP should be normal.

**Ultrasound:** Findings that suggest MCC by US include the presence of a thick-walled protruding sac (due to skin coverage) with absence of the Chiari II malformation (particularly in the second trimester) (Fig. 15.2-13A,B).

In the early second trimester, the spine should be carefully examined to identify the thick skin-covered sac overlying the lower spine and cord tethering. The diagnosis may be missed if the spine is lying adjacent to the uterus.[106]

In the third trimester, hind-brain herniation may develop. Thus, this anomaly can be particularly difficult to distinguish prenatally from an MMC.[23] By US the main differentiating finding may simply be the thickness of the overlying sac and herniated cord with dilated central canal.

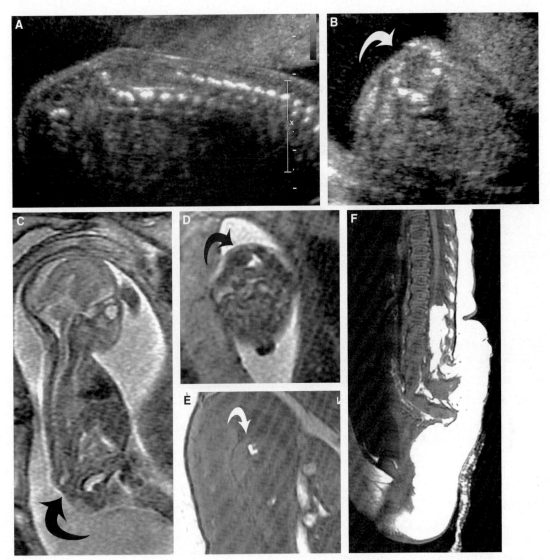

**FIGURE 15.2-12:** Lipomyelomeningocele 21-week gestation. Longitudinal **(A)** and transverse **(B)** US of the spine demonstrate spinal dysraphism with a thick overlying mass *(arrow)*. Sagittal **(C)** and axial **(D)** T2w MRIs demonstrate the presence of a thick-walled sac containing a mass *(arrow)*. There is cord tethering and no Chiari malformation. **E:** Axial T1w MRI confirms the presence of high signal fat in the mass *(arrow)*. **F:** Postnatal MRI confirms the presence of an LMMC.

**MRI:** MRI can help assess contents within the herniated sac, presence of cord tethering, and dilated central canal (Fig. 15.2-13C,D).[107] It is particularly useful in evaluating the hind brain which may demonstrate Chiari II changes in the late second and early third trimesters. It is also useful in the assessment of associated cloacal malformations (Fig. 15.2-13E).[23,105]

**Differential Diagnosis:** It is important to remember that downward displacement of the cerebellar tonsils and decrease of the subarachnoid spaces can develop in the third trimester in myelocystocele, making it difficult, at times, to differentiate from meningomyelocele. In a series by Hüsler et al., four cases of myelocystocele developed hindbrain herniation in late pregnancy. Hüsler et al. also described three cases of low lumbosacral meningomyelocele with only mild hindbrain herniation in the early second trimester. Thus, the presence or absence of hindbrain herniation may be dependent on gestational age for both mild meningomyelocele and severe myelocystocele, important

when evaluating for possible fetal surgery. Skin coverage, contents of sac, and severity of hindbrain herniation must be carefully reviewed in these cases both by US and by MRI.[23]

Other differentials include OEIS (omphalocele, exstrophy, imperforate anus, and spinal anomalies), sacrococcygeal teratomas (skin-covered tumor with no cord tethering and no Chiari) and Currarino triad (sacral agenesis, anal atresia, and either a presacral teratoma or a meningocele).

**Associated Anomalies:** Terminal myelocystocele is often associated with maldevelopment of the lower spine, pelvis, genitalia, bowel, bladder, kidney, and the abdominal wall, including cloacal exstrophy.[104] OEIS complex has been associated with terminal MCC as well.[23]

**Management/Prognosis:** Outcome is dependent on severity of anorectal and other visceral anomalies. Neurologically, patients may be intact but can progressively lose neurologic function.[104]

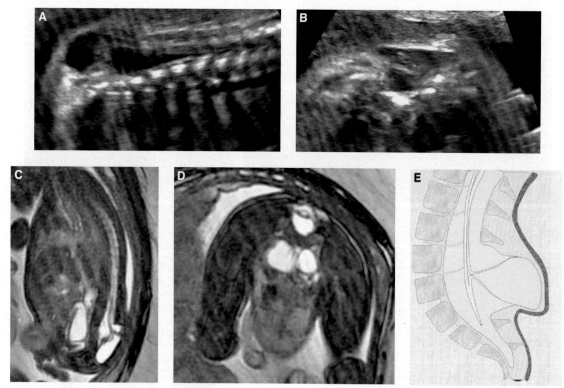

**FIGURE 15.2-13:** Myelocystocele at 27 weeks' gestation. Sagittal **(A)** and axial **(B)** US images demonstrate a skin-covered sac containing dilated distal central canal herniated into the sac. Sagittal **(C)** and axial **(D)** SSFP MRIs confirm the presence of a thick-walled sac and cord tethering. The central canal opens into a CSF-filled cavity in the sac. A cloaca was present as well. **E:** Sagittal diagram of myelocystocele. (**E** from Zugazaga Cortazar A, Martín Martinez C, Duran Feliubadalo C, et al. Magnetic resonance imaging in the prenatal diagnosis of neural tube defects. *Insights Imaging.* 2013;4:225–237. doi:10.1007/s13244-013-0223-2.)

## Split Cord Malformation

**Synonyms:** Diastematomyelia, diplomyelia.

**Description:** Longitudinal clefting of the spinal cord.

**Incidence:** Rarely reported prenatally.

**Pathogenesis:** A bony, fibrous, or cartilaginous septum divides the vertebral canal partially or completely. This results in a cleft of the cord, conus medularus, and/or filum.

Diastematomyelia (spinal cord and canal splitting) and diplomyelia (spinal cord and canal duplication) cannot be distinguished radiologically. Thus, split cord malformation (SCM) is the name most commonly used for both entities.[108,109] SCM can be present in up to 40% of MMC.[3] The spinal cord is divided into two hemicords. Often only a short segment is involved with asymmetry in size of the hemicords. Each hemicord has a central canal, dorsal and ventral horn, and one nerve root. An osseous septum can be present between two dural tubes (type I) or a nonossified fibrous septum can be present within a single dural tube (type II) separating the hemicords. With type II there may not be a septum.[110]

### Diagnosis
*Ultrasound:* SCM can be associated with vertebral body anomalies. With type I SCM, an extra echogenic focus representing the osseous septum may be seen in the spinal canal by US. There may be widening of the spinal canal.[108,111–114] However, a fibrous septum or cord duplication may not be identified by US.[47,115]

*MRI:* Two- to three-mm high-resolution MR axial images of the spine are needed to demonstrate a SMC (Fig. 15.2-14) with two hemicords. In cases of MMC, SCM most commonly involves splitting of the placode, which can be difficult to detect prenatally by an MRI.[112,115] As the spinal cord can remain tethered by the septum following MMC repair, it is important to identify this anomaly prior to surgical repair.[116]

**Associated Anomalies:** ONTD are often associated with SCM. Spinal anomalies associated with SCM include scoliosis, kyphosis, hemivertebra, and butterfly vertebra. Equinovarus deformities are common. Dorsal midline cutaneous lesions can be present, including telangiectasias, hemangiomas, lipomas, and cutaneous nevi.

**Prognosis/Management:** When isolated, prognosis may be favorable depending on neurologic and orthopedic surgical outcome.[111,116]

**Recurrence Risk:** Unknown. Autosomal dominant transmission has been described.

## Hemivertebra

**Synonyms:** Scoliosis, unilateral fusion.

**Incidence:** 5 to 10 per 10,000.

**Pathogenesis:** At 6 weeks' gestation, the two lateral chondrification centers arise. They unite by 8 weeks' gestation to form the

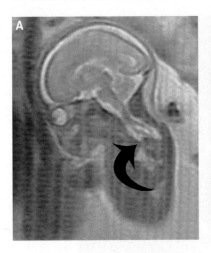

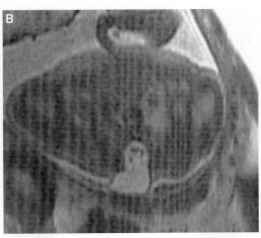

**FIGURE 15.2-14:** Split cord malformation. Sagittal **(A)** and axial **(B)** T2w MRI of the spine demonstrate a type II split cord malformation *(arrow)* at 31 weeks' gestation in a fetus with a thoracic meningocele. No septum is visible between the two hemicords.

primary ossification center of the vertebral body. A hemivertebra is the result of failure of one of the centers to develop.

### Diagnosis

***Ultrasound:*** US findings include irregular shape of the spine, best demonstrated on sagittal and coronal views. A triangular bony structure smaller than the adjacent vertebra may be seen at the site of angulation. When multiple levels are affected, the alignment may be balanced with no significant resultant scoliosis.[117–123]

Three-dimensional US is particularly useful for assessing scoliosis and associated vertebral and rib anomalies (Fig. 15.2-15).[124]

***MRI:*** MRI may be limited in the assessment of an isolated hemivertebra if curvature is minimal. It is useful in evaluating associated anomalies such as cord tethering, cloacal anomalies, and VACTERL (vertebral, anal, cardiac, tracheo esophageal fistula, limb anomalies) anomalies (Fig. 15.2-16).[47]

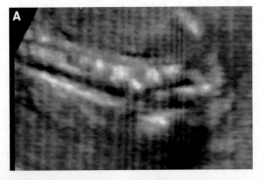

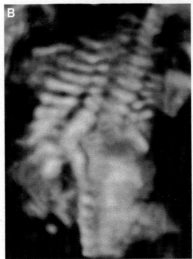

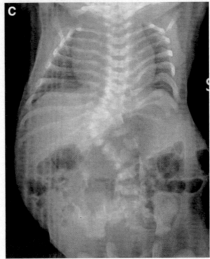

**FIGURE 15.2-15:** Hemivertebra. **A:** Coronal US demonstrates hemivertebra with acute angulation. **B:** 3D US skeletal mode rendering of the spine and ribs confirms the lower thoracic scoliosis. **C:** Postnatal radiograph reveals multiple lower left thoracic rib anomalies in addition to thoracolumbar hemi and butterfly vertebra in this patient with spondylocostal dysplasia.

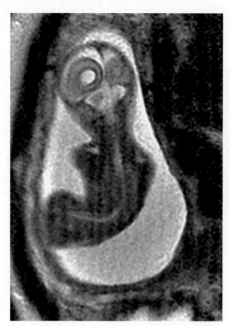

**FIGURE 15.2-16:** Coronal MRI demonstrates severe lower thoracic scoliosis.

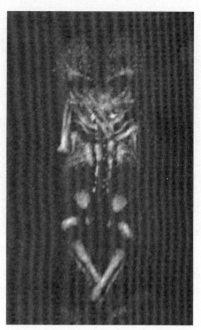

**FIGURE 15.2-17:** Spondylocostal dysplasia. 3DCT at 21 weeks' gestation demonstrates abnormal ribs and vertebra. (Courtesy of Teresa Victoria.)

*CT:* The use of intrauterine three-dimensional computer tomography for the assessment of fetal skeletal anomalies has been described[125,126] (see Chapter 21 for technique description). Spinal anomalies delineated by this technique include platyspondyly, hemivertebrae, decreased intervertebral distance, and vertebral agenesis.

Using a multislice scanner with relatively low mAs (40 to 80) and kVp (80 to 120), the mean CT—dose index has been reported to be approximately 3 mGy per study. The acquisitions are performed during breath hold with the mother supine. Postprocessing 3D reconstruction of the fetal skeleton involves using maximum intensity projection and segmentation with removal of the overlying maternal pelvic bones. Centers using this technique typically perform the exam in the third trimester. Decreased skeletal ossification, increased fetal movement, smaller size of the fetus, and increased radiation sensitivity may limit the use of this technique earlier in pregnancy (Fig. 15.2-17).

**Differential Diagnosis:** Anomalies associated with scoliosis include MMC, OEIS, VACTERL, and Currarino triad (sacral agenesis, anal atresia, and either a presacral teratoma or a meningocele).

**Associated Anomalies:** Hemivertebra can be associated with other musculoskeletal anomalies, including spine, ribs, and limbs. Syndromes including Jarcho-Levin, Klippel Feil, and VACTERL are often associated with hemivertebrae. Chromosomal anomalies are uncommon.[121,122]

**Prognosis:** Prognosis is related to the presence of associated anomalies. Spinal fusion is the treatment of choice with congenital scoliosis that is progressive, which can result in a markedly short spine and low lung volumes.[127]

**Management:** Close evaluation for other anomalies in critical. Vaginal delivery may be appropriate if the anomaly is isolated. Orthopedic follow-up is important.

**Recurrence Risk:** There may be an increased risk of NTD in siblings.[128]

## Sacral Agenesis/Caudal Regression Syndrome

**Synonyms:** Caudal dysplasia, caudal dysgenesis.

**Description:** Caudal regression syndrome is relatively rare. This complex continuum can be associated with infants of diabetic mothers, OEIS, VACTERL, and the Currarino triad. There is a wide spectrum ranging from mild lumbosacral hypogenesis to sirenomelia[129,130] (Fig. 15.2-18).

**Incidence:** Incidence is 0.1 to 0.25 per 10,000 in normal pregnancies and 200 times higher in diabetic pregnancies.[129] Up to 16% of cases are associated with infants of diabetic mothers.

**Pathogenesis:** Hypogenesis or agenesis of the caudal cell mass produces the caudal regression syndrome resulting in dysplasia or absence of the sacrum. The severest form, called type I, has a spine which ends above the first sacral vertebra. It is associated with a high lying blunted conus and severe associated anomalies (Fig. 15.2-19). The less severe type II has a spine ending at or below S2. The conus is often a tethered cord with milder associated malformations such as lipoma. There is a strong association with maternal diabetes. Other metabolic and teratogenic causes have been suggested.

**Diagnosis**

*Ultrasound:* Sonographic findings are variable. There may be complete absence of the sacrum with associated abnormalities of the lumbar spine and lower extremities, including club feet and knee and hip contractions. Absence of several vertebrae, fused iliac wings, and decreased interspace of the femoral heads can be noted. Transverse view of the abdomen may fail to show the normal spine. Decreased motion of the lower extremities may be present. Polyhydramnios has been described.[131–134]

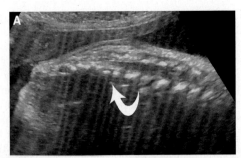

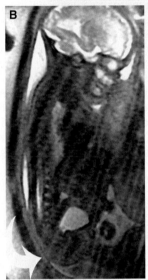 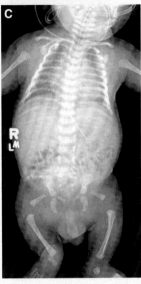

**FIGURE 15.2-18:** Caudal regression syndrome. **A:** Sagittal US of the lower spine at 34 weeks' gestation demonstrates hypoplastic sacral elements *(arrow)*. **B:** Sagittal T2w MRI confirms the hypoplastic sacrum *(arrow)* as well as the presence of short femurs. **C:** Postnatal radiograph demonstrates multiple sacral hemivertebrae and hypoplastic dislocated femurs in this infant of a diabetic mother.

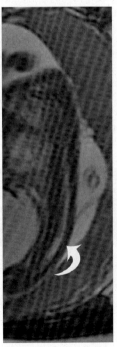

**FIGURE 15.2-19:** Sacral agenesis. Sagittal FIESTA MRI demonstrates a blunted conus *(arrow)*.

Diagnosis has been made in the first trimester with a short crown-rump length.[135]

When only a few sacral elements are missing, the diagnosis can be elusive both by US and MRI. With mild caudal regression, only the tip of the conus is absent and will not be detected prenatally.

***MRI:*** MRI can help confirm the diagnosis of sacral agenesis and identify a blunted conus (see Fig. 15.2-19). Both sagittal and axial views are useful in assessing the number of sacral elements. When oligohydramnios is present due to renal anomalies, MRI is superior to US in the assessment of associated fetal anomalies.

**Associated Anomalies:** Genitourinary and gastrointestinal anomalies have been associated with caudal regression, including renal agenesis, renal dysplaisa, duodenal atresia, and esophageal atresia. Lower extremity anomalies can be present.

**Prognosis and Management:** Prognosis depends on the severity of the defect and associated anomalies. Often urologic and orthopedic long-term care is required.

**Recurrence Risk:** Recurrence risk is thought to be small, though higher in diabetic mothers.

## Sirenomelia

**Synonym:** Mermaid syndrome.

**Description:** Lethal anomaly with fusion or near complete fusion of the lower extremities.

**Incidence:** Incidence is 1 in 60,000 live births, with a male-to-female ratio of 2.7:1.[136] Maternal diabetes is associated with a higher incidence. There is a 100-fold increased incidence in monozygotic twins. Cocaine and high doses of vitamin A and E have been associated with this anomaly.

**Embryology/Pathogenesis:** The cause is thought to be a localized insult to the caudal end of the developing embryo between days 13 and 22 gestation. A persistent vitelline artery has been noted with a dorsal hypoplasic distal aorta.[137,138] Shunting of nutrients away from the caudal structure may result in malrotation, merging, and dysgenesis of the lower extremities.[139] Chromosomes are typically normal. With a high association with monozygotic twinning, a vascular steal phenomenon could explain the high incidence in this group.

In 1987, Stocker and Heifetz classified sirenomelia into seven types: type I (thigh and leg bones present), type II (single fibula), type III (no fibula), type IV (femurs partially fused and fibula completely fused), type V (femurs partially fused), type VI (single femur and single tibia), and type VII (single femur and absent tibia).[140]

**Associated Anomalies:** Associated anomalies include sacral agenesis, anorectal atresia, renal agenesis, bladder agenesis, urethral agenesis, single umbilical artery, and ambiguous genitalia Oligohydramnios is common.[136]

**Diagnosis:** In the first trimester, fused lower limbs may be seen with a nuchal translucency present.[141-146] A single umbilical artery is common. In the second trimester, a single large intraabdominal vessel, the vitelline artery, may be seen coursing to the umbilical cord. Oligohydramnios, renal agenesis, and intrauterine growth retardation are typically present with a single lower extremity. When two femurs are present the diagnosis may be more difficult to make.[144,147] Color Doppler can be useful to search for the presence of renal arteries and the single vitelline artery.[148,149,150]

3D US can delineate the extremity anomalies if amniotic fluid is present.[146] However, with renal anomalies common, oligohydramnios often limits the resolution of US, particularly 3D. When oligohydramnios is present, MRI is a useful adjunct to confirm the diagnosis of renal agenesis and fused lower extremities (Fig. 15.2-20).[133,151,152]

**Differential Diagnosis:** Bilateral renal agenesis. Caudal regression syndrome typically has a normal amount of amniotic fluid.

**Prognosis:** Typically lethal.

**Recurrence Risk:** Families at risk for increased incidence of monozygotic twins may have an increased risk of sirenomelia.

### Limb Body Wall Complex
Findings include severe scoliosis, body wall defects, and craniofacial defects (Chapter 18.2).

## Sacrococcygeal Teratoma

**Description:** Germ cell tumor from the presacral region.

**Incidence:** 1 per 40,000. Female-to-male ratio is 4 to 1. Malignancy is more common in males.[153–155]

**Pathogenesis:** Henson's node is a caudal cell mass of the embryo that migrates anteriorly to the coccyx.[156] Sacrococcygeal

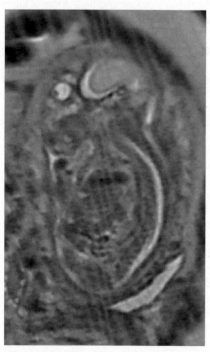

**FIGURE 15.2-20:** Sirenmelia. Sagittal T2w MRI demonstrates severe oligohydramnios secondary to renal agenesis. Lower sacrum was absent. A single femur was present.

teratoma (SCT) is thought to arise from Hensen's node, an aggregate of totipotential cells.

SCT has been classified by the amount of presacral and external components of the mass. The American Academy of Pediatric Surgery Section distinguishes these into four types (Table 15.2-2, Fig. 15.2-21). Type 1 is primarily an external mass and so is typically identified prenatally, is the easiest to resect, and has a low malignant potential (Fig. 15.2-22). Types II and III have intrapelvic as well as external components; so resection may be more difficult (Figs. 15.2-23 to 15.2-25). Type IV is entirely internal; so it is difficult to diagnose prenatally. It may not be identified until its symptoms develop at a later age. Malignant transformation is most common with type IV.

Types I and II represent 80% of cases of cases. About 15% of SCT are entirely cystic, while are 85% mixed or solid. Mature teratomas consist of normal well-developed structures, while immature teratomas contain embryonal tissue. Malignant teratomas are yolk sac or endodermal sinus tumors with increased AFP. Mature and immature teratomas are often cystic, while malignant teratomas are usually solid. Solid tumors can be quite vascular resulting in prenatal complications such as high output failure from hydrops and/or hemorrhage.[157–159]

### Diagnosis
***Ultrasound:*** SCT presents as a skin-covered cystic, solid, or mixed mass protruding from the sacrum without evidence of a spinal dysraphism or Chiari malformation. The pelvic and abdominal extent, however, can be difficult to visualize by US unless the mass is cystic or large enough to displace the bladder[160] (see Fig. 15.2-24). Calcifications, while present microscopically, are usually not visible prenatally. 3D can help outline the mass.[161–163] Doppler is useful in assessing the amount of vascularity.[161,164]

Polyhydramnios and hydrops may develop due to high output shunting or anemia after a hemorrhage. Hepatomegaly and/or placentomegaly may also develop.[159,160] Tumors can increase rapidly in size; so close follow-up is important. The development of heart failure or hydrops is usually a preterminal event unless aggressive intervention is performed.[159]

***MRI:*** Fetal MRI has become an important adjunct in evaluating the external mass and adjacent spine, as well as the presence or absence of an intrapelvic component.[165–169]

MRI can help differentiate a cystic SCT from a meningocele or myelomeningocele.[169] In cases where fetal surgery or immediate postnatal surgery is being considered, MRI provides information critical for emergent operative planning (see Fig. 15.2-25).

| Table 15.2-2 | The American Academy of Pediatric Surgery Staging Classification of Sacrococcygeal Teratomas |
| --- | --- |

| Type | Description |
| --- | --- |
| I | External with minimal presacral component |
| II | External with intrapelvic component |
| III | External and primarily internal component with abdominal extension |
| IV | Entirely internal with no external component |

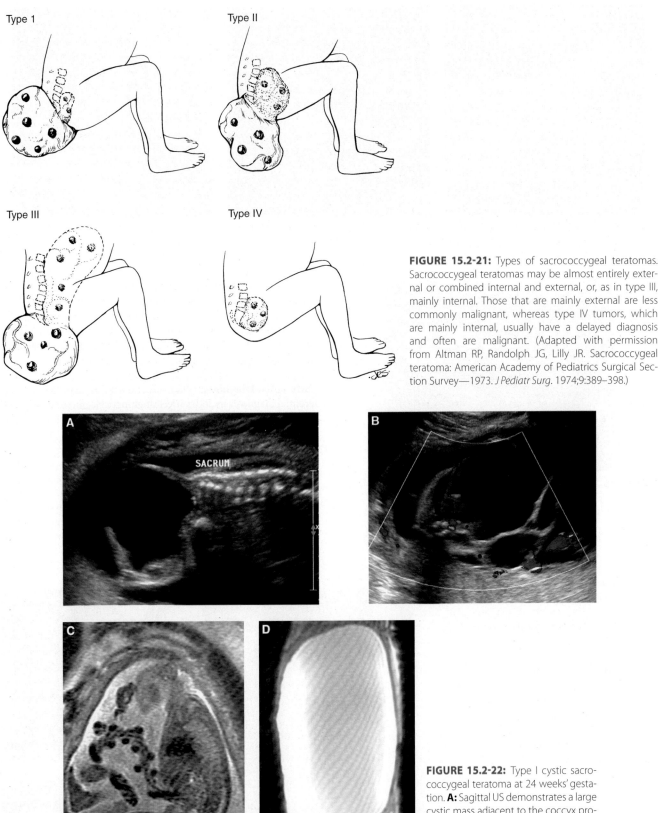

Type 1

Type II

Type III

Type IV

**FIGURE 15.2-21:** Types of sacrococcygeal teratomas. Sacrococcygeal teratomas may be almost entirely external or combined internal and external, or, as in type III, mainly internal. Those that are mainly external are less commonly malignant, whereas type IV tumors, which are mainly internal, usually have a delayed diagnosis and often are malignant. (Adapted with permission from Altman RP, Randolph JG, Lilly JR. Sacrococcygeal teratoma: American Academy of Pediatrics Surgical Section Survey—1973. *J Pediatr Surg.* 1974;9:389–398.)

SACRUM

**FIGURE 15.2-22:** Type I cystic sacrococcygeal teratoma at 24 weeks' gestation. **A:** Sagittal US demonstrates a large cystic mass adjacent to the coccyx protruding externally. **B:** Minimal vascularity is seen by color Doppler. **C:** Sagittal T2w MRI demonstrates the large cystic exophytic mass at the base of the coccyx. There was no internal component. **D:** Postnatal MRI confirms the presence of a large exophytic cystic mass.

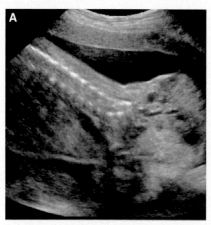
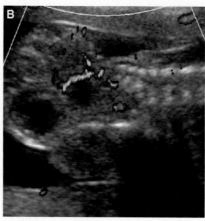
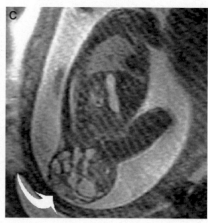

**FIGURE 15.2-23:** Type I cystic and solid sacrococcygeal teratoma at 24-week gestation. **A:** Sagittal US demonstates a mixed external mass adjacent to the coccyx. **B:** Doppler US demonstrates moderate vascularity. **C:** Sagittal T2w image demonstrates the solid and cystic mass at the base of the buttocks with no internal component (arrow).

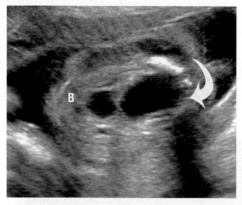

**FIGURE 15.2-24:** Type II sacrococcygeal teratoma. Axial US demonstrates a large cystic mass (arrow) deviating the bladder anteriorly. A large external component was present as well.

**Associated Anomalies:** Whether additional anomalies are associated with SCT remains controversial with incidence reported from 11% to 38%.[170] Aneuploidy is not associated with SCT. Rectovaginal fistula and imperforate anus are sometimes noted, possibly related to tumor growth during fetal development. Currarino triad has been associated with SCT.

**Differential Diagnosis:** When a sacral mass is identified, the differential diagnosis includes myelomeningocele, meningocele, and lipomeningocele. Myelomeningocele are cystic, not skin covered, have cord tethering and cranial findings of Chiari II malformation. AFP may be elevated in both meningomyeloceles and SCT.

Meningoceles and lipomeningoceles may be more difficult to differentiate as they do not have Chiari II findings and are skin covered. In these cases, identification of spinal dysraphism and cord tethering may help exclude SCT from the differential.

Other mimickers of SCT include neuroblastoma, hemangioma, lipoma, as well as other tumors or malformations that grow in the sacrococcygeal region.[171]

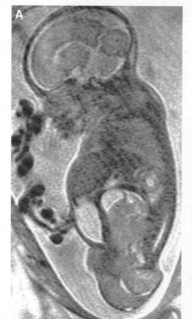
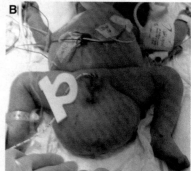
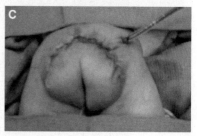

**FIGURE 15.2-25:** Type III sacrococcygeal teratoma. **A:** MRI demonstrates a mixed solid and cystic mass with internal and external components. The bladder is deviated anteriorly by the internal mass. **B:** Newborn with large skin-covered SCT. **C:** The infant was taken to surgery without additional imaging. Postoperative image of the buttock following successful resection.

**Prognosis:** Prognosis is related to development of fetal hydrops, histology, and size of the mass.[172] Hydrops typically develops in large vascular solid tumors. The large size is associated with greater surgical risk as well as hemorrhage at delivery. Outcome is poor if the mass is solid, vascular, and large with an internal component. Good outcome is associated with small lesions, and external cystic masses that are avascular. In these cases, long-term outcome is excellent with complete surgical excision.[173]

**Management:** When an SCT is identified, close follow-up is required to assess for potential rapid growth and development of hydrops.[174] Fetal intervention has been attempted, including resection, radiofrequency ablation, and percutaneous needle drainage of cystic sacrococcygeal teratomas.[175–177]

The recommended mode of delivery is dependent on the size of the tumor. Vaginal delivery may be appropriate for small masses. Rupture and avulsion have been described. Thus, caesarean delivery is often recommended to avoid hemorrhage as well as dystocia. Delivery should be performed at a tertiary care center where neonatologists and pediatric surgeons are available.

**Recurrence Risk:** While typically sporadic, some cases appear to be familial with an autosomal dominant inheritance, particularly type IV.[178] Familial cases are associated with anorectal malformations and Currarino triad (presacral tumor, anorectal malformation, and sacral anomaly). Chromosomal abnormalities are rare but have been described with 10q trisomy.[179]

# REFERENCES

1. Tortori-Donati P, Rossi A, Cama A. Spinal dysraphism: a review of neuroradiological features with embryological correlations and proposal for a new classification. *Neuroradiology.* 2000;42:471–491.
2. Tortori-Donati P, Rossi A, Biancheri R, et al. Magnetic resonance imaging of spinal dysraphism. *Top Magn Reson Imaging.* 2001;12:375–409.
3. Barkovich A. Congenital anomalies of the spine. In: Barkovich A, ed. *Pediatric Neuroimaging.* 3rd ed. Philadelphia, PA: Lippincott Williams & Wilkins; 2000:621–683.
4. Naidich TP, Blaser SI, Delman BD, et al. Congenital anomalies of the spine and spinal cord: embryology and malformations. In: Atlas SW, ed. *Magnetic Resonance Imaging of the Brain and Spine.* 4th ed. Vol 2. Philadelphia, PA: Lippincott-Raven; 2008:1364–1444.
5. Finnell RH, Gould A, Spiegelstein O. Pathobiology and genetics of neural tube defects. *Epilepsia.* 2003;44(suppl 3):14–23.
6. Frey L, Hauser WA. Epidemiology of neural tube defects. *Epilepsia.* 2003;44(suppl 3):4–13.
7. Shaer CM, Chescheir N, Schulkin J. Myelomeningocele: a review of the epidemiology. Genetics, risk factors for conception, prenatal diagnosis, and prognosis for affected individuals. *Obstet Gynecol Surv.* 2007;62:471–479.
8. Agopian AJ, Canfield MA, Olney RS, et al. Spina bifida subtypes and subphenotypes by maternal race/ethnicity in the National Birth Defects Prevention Study. *Am J Med Genet A.* 2012;158A(1):109–115.
9. Williams LJ, Rasmussen SA, Flores A, et al. Decline in the prevalence of spina bifida and anencephaly by race/ethnicity: 1995–2002. *Pediatrics.* 2005;116:580–586.
10. Sepulveda W, Corral E, Ayala C, et al. Chromosomal abnormalities in fetuses with open neural tube defects: prenatal identification with ultrasound. *Ultrasound Obstet Gynecol.* 2004;23:352–356.
11. Harmon JP, Heitt AK, Palmer C, et al. Prenatal US detection of isolated neural tube defect: is cytogenetic evaluation warranted? *Obstet Gynecol.* 1995;86:595–599.
12. Hume R, Drugan A, Reicher A, et al. Aneuploidy among prenatally detected neural tube defects. *Am J Med Gen.* 1996;61:171–173.
13. Jentink J, Dolk H, Loane MA, et al. Intrauterine exposure to carbamazepine and specific congenital malformations: systematic review and case-control study. *BMJ.* 2010;341:c6581.
14. Copp AJ. Prevention of neural tube defects: vitamins, enzymes and genes. *Curr Opin Neurol.* 1998;11(2):97–102.
15. Werler M, Louik C, Shapiro S, et al. Prepregnant weight in relation to risk of neural tube defects. *JAMA.* 1996;275:1089.
16. Shaw GM, Velie EM, Schaffer D. Risk of NTD affect pregnancies among obese women. *JAMA.* 1996;275:1093–1096.
17. Rasmussen SA, Chu SY, Kim SY, et al. Maternal obesity and risk of NTD: a metaanalysis. *Am J Obstet Gynecol.* 2008;198:611–619.
18. Shaw GM, Nelson V, Todoroff K, et al. Maternal periconceptional use of electric bed heating and risk for NTD and orofacial clefts. *Teratology.* 1999;60:124–129.
19. Padmanabhan R. Etiology pathogenesis and prevention of neural tube defects. *Congenit Anom (Kyoto).* 2006;46:55–67.
20. Rasmussen SA, Erickson JD, Reef SE, et al. Teratology: from science to birth defects prevention. *Birth Defects Res A Clin Mol Teratol.* 2009;85:82–92.
21. McLone DG, Knepper PA. The cause of Chiari II malformation: a unified theory. *Pediatr Neurosci.* 1989;15(1):1–12.
22. Oaks W, Gaskill S. Symptomatic Chiari malformations in childhood. In: Park T, ed. *Spinal Dysraphism.* Boston, MA: Blackwell; 1992:104–125.
23. Hüsler MR, Danzer E, Johnson MP, et al. Prenatal diagnosis and postnatal outcome of fetal spinal defects without Arnold-Chiari II malformation. *Prenat Diagn.* 2009;29(11):1050–1057.
24. Cameron M, Moran P. Prenatal screening and diagnosis of neural tube defects. *Prenat Diagn.* 2009;29(4):402–411.
25. Kooper AJ, de Bruijn D, van Ravenwaaif-Arts CM, et al. Fetal anatomy scan potentially will replace routine AFAFP assays for the detection of NTD. *Prenat Diagn.* 2007;27:29–33.
26. Nicolaides K, Campbell J. Neural tube abnormalities. *Clinc Diagn Ultrasound.* 1989;25:55–65.
27. Blaas HG, Eik-Nes SH. Sonoembryology and early prenatal diagnosis of neural anomalies. *Prenat Diagn.* 2009;29(4):312–325.
28. Van den Hov MC, Nicolaides KH, Campbell J, et al. Evaluation of the lemon and banana signs in 130 fetuses with open spina bifida. *Am J Obstet Gynecol.* 1990;162:322–327.
29. D'Addario V, Rossi AC, Pinto V, et al. Comparison of six sonographic signs in the prenatal diagnosis of spina bifida. *J Perinat Med.* 2008;36:330–334.
30. Campbell J, Gilbert WM, Nicolaides KH, et al. US screening for spina bifida, cranial and cerebellar signs in a high risk population. *Obstet Gynecol.* 1987;70:247–250.
31. Thiagarajoh S, Henke J, Hogge WA, et al. Early diagnosis of spina bifida the value of cranial US markers. *Obstet Gynecol.* 1990;76:54–57.
32. Filly MR, Filly RA, Barkovich AJ, et al. Supratentorial abnormalities in the Chiari II malformation, IV: the too-far-back ventricle. *J Ultrasound Med.* 2010;29(2):243–248.
33. Tutschek B, Pilu G. Virtual reality ultrasound imaging of the normal and abnormal fetal central nervous system. *Ultrasound Obstet Gynecol.* 2009;34:259–267.
34. Budorick NE, Pretorius DH, Grafe MR, et al. Ossification of the fetal spine. *Radiology.* 1991;181:561–565.
35. Shekdar K, Feygin T. Fetal neuroimaging. *Neuroimaging Clin N Am.* 2011;21(3):677–703.
36. Benacerraf B, Shipp T, Bromley B. Three dimensional US of the fetus: volume imaging. *Radiology.* 2006;238:988–996.
37. Yazici LE, Malatyalioglu E, Sakinci M, et al. Chromosomal anomalies and additional sonographic findings in fetuses with open neural tube defects. *Arch Gynecol Obstete* 2012;286:1393–1398.
38. Thompson D. Postnatal management and outcome for neural tube defects including spinabifida and encephalocoeles. *Prenat Diagn.* 2009;29:412–419.
39. Chaoui R, Benoit B, Mitkowska-Wozniak H, et al. Assessment of intracranial translucency (IT) in the detection of spina bifida at the 11–13-week scan. *Ultrasound Obstet Gynecol.* 2009;34:249–252.
40. Chaoui R, Nicolaides KH. Detecting open spina bifida at 11–13 week scan by assessing intracranial translucency and the posterior brain region: mid sagittal or axial plane? *Ultrasound Obstet Gynecol.* 2011;38:609–612.
41. Mangels KJ, Tulipan N, Tsao LY, et al. Fetal MRI in the evaluation of intrauterine myelomeningocele. *Pediatr Neurosurg.* 2000;32(3):124–131.
42. Aaronson OS, Hernanz-Schulman M, Bruner JP. Myelomeningocele: prenatal evaluation—comparison between transabdominal US and MR imaging. *Radiology.* 2003;227(3):839–843.
43. Simon EM, Pollock A. Prenatal and postnatal imaging of spinal dysraphism. *Semin Roentgenol.* 2004;39:182–195.
44. Saleem SN, Said AH, Abdel-Raouf M, et al. Fetal MRI in the evaluation of fetuses referred for sonographically suspected neural tube defects (NTDs): impact on diagnosis and management decision. *Neuroradiology.* 2009;51(11):761–772.
45. Blaicher W, Mittermayer C, Messerschmidt A, et al. Fetal skeletal deformities: the diagnostic accuracy of prenatal ultrasonography and fetal magnetic resonance imaging. *Ultraschall Med.* 2004;25(3):195–199.
46. Griffiths PD, Porteous M, Mason G, et al. The use of in utero MRI to supplement ultrasound in the foetus at high risk of developmental brain or spine abnormality. *Br J Radiol.* 2012;85(1019):e1038–e1045.
47. Bulas D. Fetal evaluation of spine dysraphism. *Pediatr Radiol.* 2010;40:1029–1037.
48. Zugazaga Cortazar A, Martín Martinez C, Duran Feliubadalo C, et al. Magnetic resonance imaging in the prenatal diagnosis of neural tube defects. *Insights Imaging.* 2013;4:225–237. doi:10.1007/s13244-013-0223-2.
49. Hibbeln JF, Shors SM, Byrd SE. MRI: is there a role in obstetrics? *Clin Obstet Gynecol.* 2012;55(1):352–366.
50. Abele T, Lee S, Twickler D. MR imaging quantitative analysis of fetal Chiari II malformations and associated open neural tube defects: balanced SSFP vs. half Fourier rare and interobserver reliability. *J Magn Reson Imaging.* 2013;38:786–793.

51. Servaes S, Hernandez A, Gonzalez L, et al. Fetal MRI of clubfoot associated with myelomeningocele. *Pediatr Radiol.* 2010;40(12):1874.
52. Werner H, Dos Sanot J, Fontes R, et al. Virtual bronchoscopy for evaluating cervical tumors of the fetus. *Ultrasound Obstet Gynecol.* 2013;41:90–94.
53. Adzick NS. Fetal myelomeningocele: natural history, pathophysiology, and in-utero intervention. *Semin Fetal Neonatal Med.* 2010;15(1):9–14.
54. Chao TT, Dashe JS, Adams RC, et al. Fetal spine findings on MRI and associated outcomes in children with open neural tube defects. *AJR Am J Roentgenol.* 2011;197(5):W956–W961.
55. Chao TT, Dashe JS, Adams RC, et al. Central nervous system findings on fetal magnetic resonance imaging and outcomes in children with spina bifida. *Obstet Gynecol.* 2010;116:323–329.
56. Oakeshott P, Hunt GM. Long-term outcome in open spina bifida. *Br J Gen Pract.* 2003;3:632–636.
57. Coniglio SJ, Anderson SM, Ferguson JE II. Functional motor outcome in children with myelomeningocele: correlation with anatomic level on prenatal ultrasound. *Dev Med Child Neurol.* 1996;38:675–680.
58. Wilson RD, Johnson MP, Bebbington M, et al. Does a myelomeningocele sac compared to no sac result in decreased postnatal leg function following maternal fetal surgery for spina bifida aperta? *Fetal Diagn Ther.* 2007;22(5):348–351.
59. Fichter MA, Dornseifer U, Henke J, et al. Fetal spina bifida repair: current trends and prospects of intrauterine neurosurgery. *Fetal Diagn Ther.* 2008;23:271–286.
60. Dias MS, McLone DG. Hydrocephalus in the child with dysraphism. *Neurosurg Clin N Am.* 1993;4:715–726.
61. McLone DG. Results of treatment of children born with a myelomeningocele. *Clin Neurosurg.* 1983;30:407–412.
62. Caldarelli M, DiRocco C, LaMarca F. Shunt complications in the first postoperative year in children with meningomyelocele. *Childs Nerv Syst.* 1996;12:748–754.
63. Luthy DA, Wardinsky T, Shurtleff DB, et al. Cesarean section before the onset of labor and subsequent motor function in infants with meningomyelocele diagnosed antenatally. *N Engl J Med.* 1991;324:662–666.
64. Hirose S, Farmer D. Fetal surgery for myelomeningocele. *Clin Perinatol.* 2009;36:431–438.
65. Paek BW, Farmer DL, Wilkinson CC, et al. Hindbrain herniation develops in surgically created myelomeningocele but is absent after repair in fetal lambs. *Am J Obstet Gynecol.* 2000;183(5):1119–1123.
66. Rintoul NE, Sutton LN, Hubbard AM, et al. A new look at myelomeningoceles: functional level, vertebral level, shunting, and the implications for fetal intervention. *Pediatrics.* 2002;109(3):409–413.
67. Johnson MP, Sutton LN, Rintoul N, et al. Fetal myelomeningocele repair: short-term clinical outcomes. *Am J Obstet Gynecol.* 2003;189(2):482–487.
68. Bruner JP, Tulipan N, Paschall RL. Fetal surgery for myelomeningocele and the incidence of shunt-dependent hydrocephalus. *JAMA.* 1999;282(19):1819–1825.
69. Tulipan N, Sutton LN, Bruner JP, et al. The effect of intrauterine myelomeningocele repair on the incidence of shunt-dependent hydrocephalus. *Pediatr Neurosurg.* 2003;38(1):27–33.
70. Grant RA, Heuer GG, Carrión GM, et al. Morphometric analysis of posterior fossa after in utero myelomeningocele repair. *J Neurosurg Pediatr.* 2011;7:362–368.
71. Adzick NS, Thom EA, Spong CY, et al. A randomized trial of prenatal versus postnatal repair of myelomeningocele. *N Engl J Med.* 2011;365:993–1004.
72. Danzer E, Johnson MP, Adzick NS. Fetal surgery for myelomeningocele: progress and perspectives. *Dev Med Child Neurol.* 2011;54:8–14.
73. Gupta N, Farrell JA, Rand L, et al. Open fetal surgery for myelomeningocele. *J Neurosurg Pediatr.* 2012;9(3):265–273.
74. Verbeek RJ, Heep A, Maurits NM, et al. Fetal endoscopic myelomeningocele closure preserves segmental neurological function. *Dev Med Child Neurol.* 2012;54(1):15–22.
75. Shurtleff D. Fetal endoscopic myelomeningocele repair. *Dev Med Child Neurol.* 2012;54(1):4–5.
76. Centers for Disease Control and Prevention. Use of dietary supplements containing folic acid among women of childbearing age—United States, 2005. *MMWR Morb Mortal Wkly Rep.* 2005;54(38):955–958.
77. Rossi A, Biancheri R, Cama A, et al. Imaging in spine and spinal cord malformations. *Eur J Radiol.* 2004;50:177–200.
78. McComb JG, Chen TC. Closed spinal neural tube defects. In: Tindall GT, Cooper PR, Barrow DL, eds. *The Practice of Neurosurgery.* Baltimore, MD: Williams & Wilkins; 1996:2754–2777.
79. Maiuri F, Corriero G, Giampaglia, et al. Lateral thoracic meningocele. *Surg Neurol.* 1986;26:409–412.
80. Steinbok P, Cochrane DD. Cervical meningoceles and myelocystoceles: a unifying hypothesis. *Pediatr Neurosurg.* 1995;23(6):317–322.
81. Marks JD, Khoshnood B. Epidemiology of common neurosurgical diseases in the neonate. *Neurosurg Clin N Am.* 1998;9(1):63–72.
82. Feltes CH, Fountas KN, Dimopoulos VG, et al. Cervical meningocele in association with spinal abnormalities. *Childs Nerv Syst.* 2004;20:357–361.
83. Gocer AI, Tuna M, Gezercan Y, et al. Multiple anterolateral cervical meningoceles associated with neurofibromatosis. *Neurosurg Rev.* 1999;22:124–126.
84. Salomao JF. Cervical meningocele in association with spinal abnormalities. *Childs Nerv Syst.* 2005;21:4–5.
85. Duczkowska A, Bekiesinska-Figatowska M, Herman-Sucharska I, et al. MRI in the evaluation of the fetal spinal canal contents. *Brain Dev.* 2011;33:10–20.
86. Ersahin Y, Barcin E, Mutluer S. Is meningocele really an isolated lesion? *Childs Nerv Syst.* 2001;17:487–490.
87. Pang D, Dias MS. Cervical myelomeningoceles. *Neurosurgery.* 1993;33:363–372.
88. Cornette L, Verpoorten C, Lagae L, et al. Closed spinal dysraphism: a review on diagnosis and treatment in infancy. *Eur J Paediatr Neurol.* 1998;2:179–185.
89. Northrup H, Volcik KA. Spina Bifida and othere neural tube defects. *Curr Probl Pediatr* 200;30:313–332.
90. Pierre-Kahn A, Zerah M, Renier D. Congenital lumbosacral lipomas. *Childs Nerv Syst.* 1997;13(6):298–334.
91. Forrester MB, Merz RD. Descriptive epidemiology of lipomyelomeningocele, Hawaii, 1986–2001. *Birth Defects Res A Clin Mol Teratol.* 2004;70:953–956.
92. Canfield MA, Marengo L, Ramadhani T, et al. The prevalence and predictors of anencephaly and spina bifida in Texas. *Pediatr Perinat Epidemiol* 2009;23:41–50.
93. De Wals P, Van Allen MI, Lowry RB, et al. Impact of folic acid food fortification on the birth prevalence of lipomyelomeningocele in Canada. *Birth Defects Res A Clin Mol Teratol.* 2008;82:106–109.
94. McNeely PD, Howes WJ. Ineffectiveness of dietary folic acid supplementation on the incidence of lipomyelomeningocele: pathogenetic implications. *J Neurosurg.* 2004;100(2 suppl Pediatrics):98–100.
95. Sutton LN. Lipomyelomeningocele. *Neurosurg Clin N Am.* 1995;6:325–338.
96. Kim SY, McGahan JP, Boggan JE, et al. Prenatal diagnosis of lipomyelomeningocele. *J Ultrasound Med.* 2000;19:801–805.
97. Tubbs RS, Bui CJ, Rice WC, et al. Critical analysis of the Chiari malformation type I found in children with lipomyelomeningocele. *J Neurosurg.* 2007;106(3 suppl):196–200.
98. Huang SL, Shi W, Zhang LG. Surgical treatment for lipomyelomeningocele in children. *World J Pediatr.* 2010;6:361–365.
99. Cochrane DD. Cord untethering for lipomyelomeningocele: expectation after surgery. *Neurosurg Focus.* 2007;23(2):E9.
100. Arai H, Sato K, Okuda O, et al. Surgical experience of 120 patients with lumbosacral lipomas. *Acta Neurochir (Wien).* 2001;143:857–864.
101. Atala A, Bauer SB, Dyro FM, et al. Bladder functional changes resulting from lipomyelomeningocele repair. *J Urol.* 1992;148:592–594.
102. Colak A, Pollack IF, Albright AL. Recurrent tethering: a common long-term problem after lipomyelomeningocele repair. *Pediatr Neurosurg.* 1998;29:184–190.
103. Midrio P, Silberstein HJ, Bilaniuk LT, et al. Prenatal diagnosis of terminal myelocystocele in the fetal surgery era: case report. *Neurosurgery.* 2002;50(5):1152–1154.
104. Choi S, McComb JG. Long-term outcome of terminal myelocystocele patients. *Pediatr Neurosurg.* 2000;32(2):86–91.
105. Tandon V, Garg K, Mahapatra AK. Terminal Myelocystocele: a series of 30 cases and review of the literature. *Pediatr Neurosurg* 2012;48:229–235.
106. Bhargava R, Hammond DI, Benzie RJ. Prenatal diagnosis of a fetus with lumbar myelocystocele. *Prenat Diagn.* 1992;12(8):653–659.
107. Kölbe N, Huisman TA, Stallmach T, et al. Prenatal demonstration of a cervical myelocystocele. *Ultrasound Obstet Gynecol.* 2001;18(5):536–539.
108. Allen LM, Silverman RK. Prenatal ultrasound evaluation of fetal diastematomyelia: two cases of type I split cord malformation. *Ultrasound Obstet Gynecol.* 2000;15(1):78–82.
109. Hoffman CH, Dietrich RB, Pais MJ. The split notochord syndrome with dorsal enteric fistula. *AJNR Am J Neuroradiol.* 1993;14(3):622–627.
110. Pang D, Dias MS, Ahab-Barmada M. Split cord malformation, part 1: a unified theory of embryogenesis for double spinal cord malforamtions. *Neurosurgery.* 1992;31:451–480.
111. Sepulveda W, Kyle PM, Hassan J, et al. Prenatal diagnosis of diastematomyelia: case reports and review of the literature. *Prenat Diagn.* 1997;17:161–165.
112. Has R, Yuksel A, Buyukkurt S, et al. Prenatal diagnosis of diastematomyelia: presentation of eight cases and review of the literature. *Ultrasound Obstet Gynecol.* 2007;30(6):845–849.
113. Anderson NG, Jordan S, MacFarlane MR, et al. Diastematomyelia: diagnosis by prenatal sonography. *AJR Am J Roentgenol.* 1994;163(4):911–914.
114. Sonigo-Cohen P, Schmit P, Zerah M, et al. Prenatal diagnosis of diastematomyelia. *Childs Nerv Syst.* 2003;19:555–560.
115. Kutuk MS, Ozgun MT, Tas M, et al. Prenatal diagnosis of split cord malformation by ultrasound and fetal magnetic resonance imaging: case report and review of the literature. *Childs Nerv Syst.* 2012;28(12):2169–2172.
116. Proctor MR, Bauer SB, Scott RM. The effect of surgery for split spinal cord malformation on neurologic and urologic function. *Pediatr Neurosurg.* 2000;32(1):13–19.
117. Abrams SL, Filly RA. Congenital vertebral malformations: prenatal diagnosis using ultrasonography. *Radiology.* 1985;155:762.
118. Benacerraf BR, Greene MF, Barss VA. Prenatal sonographic diagnosis of congenital hemivertebrae. *J Ultrasound Med.* 1986;5:257–259.
119. Goldstein I, Makhoul IR, Weissman A, et al. Hemivertebra: prenatal diagnosis, incidence and characteristics. *Fetal Diagn Ther.* 2005;20:121–126.
120. Harrison LA, Pretorius DH, Budorick NE. Abnormal spinal curvature in the fetus. *J Ultrasound Med.* 1992;11:473–479.
121. Zelop CM, Pretorius DN, Benacerraf BR. Fetal hemivertebrae: associated anomalies significance, and outcome. *Obstet Gynecol.* 1993;81:412–416.
122. Lawson ME, Share J, Benacerraf B. Jarcho-Levin syndrome: prenatal diagnosis, perinatal care, and follow-up of siblings. *J Perinatol.* 1997;17(5):407–409.
123. Cassart M. Suspected fetal skeletal malformations or bone diseases: how to explore. *Pediatr Radiol.* 2010;40:1046–1051.

124. Ruanon R, Molho M, Roume J, et al. Prenatal diagnosis of fetal skeletal dysplasias by combining 2D and 3D ultrasound and intrauterine 3D helical computer tomography. *Ultrasound Obstet Gynecol.* 2004;24:134–140.

125. Cassart M, Massez A, Cos T, et al. Contribution of 3-D computed tomography in the assessment of fetal skeletal dysplasia. *Ultrasound Obstet Gynecol.* 2007;29:537–543.

126. Victoria T, Epelman M, Bebbington M, et al. Low-dose fetal CT for evaluation of severe congenital skeletal anomalies: preliminary experience. *Pediatr Radiol.* 2012;42(suppl):S142–S149.

127. McMaster MF, Ohtuska K. The natural history of congenital scoliosis. *J Bone Joint Surg Br.* 1982;64:1128–1147.

128. Connor JM, Conner AN, Connor RA, et al. Genetic aspects of early childhood scoliosis. *Am J Med Genet.* 1987;27:419–424.

129. Jaffe R, Zeituni M, Fejgin M. Caudal regression syndrome. *Fetus Spinal Anomalies.* 1991;7561:1–3.

130. Nievelstein RA, Valk J, Smit LM, et al. MR of the caudal regression syndrome: embryologic implications. *AJNR Am J Neuroradiol.* 1994;15:1021–1029.

131. Adra A, Cordero D, Mejides A, et al. Caudal regression syndrome: etiopathogenesis, prenatal diagnosis, and perinatal management. *Obstet Gynecol Surv.* 1994;49(7):508–516.

132. Benacerraf BR. *Caudal Regression Syndrome and Sirenmelia in US of Fetal Syndromes.* New York, NY: Churchill Livingstone; 1998:250–254.

133. Twickler D, Budorick N, Pretorius D, et al. Caudal regression versus sirenomelia: sonographic clues. *J Ultrasound Med.* 1993;12:323–330.

134. Sonek JD, Gabbe SG, Landon MB, et al. Antenatal diagnosis of sacral agenesis syndrome in a pregnancy complicated by diabetes mellitus. *Am J Obstet Gynecol.* 1990;162(3):806–808.

135. Das BB, Rajegowda BK, Bainbridge R. Caudal regression syndrome versus sirenomelia: a case report. *J Perinatol.* 2002;22(2):168–170.

136. Valenzano M, Paoletti R, Rossi A, et al. Sirennomelia: pathological features antenatal US clues and a review of current embryogenic theories. *Hum Reprod Update.* 1999;5:82–86.

137. Stevenson RE, Jones KL, Phelan MC, et al. Vascular steal: the pathogenetic mechanism producing sirenomelia and associated defetct of the viscera and soft tissues. *Pediatrics.* 1986;78:451–457.

138. Talamo TS, Macpherson TA, Dominquez R. Sirenomelia: angiographic demonstration of ascular anomalies. *Arch Pathol Lab Med.* 1982;106:347–348.

139. Kapur RP, Mahony BS, Nyberg DA, et al. Sirenomelia associated with a vanishin twin. *Teratology.* 1991;43:103–108.

140. Stocker JR, Heifetz SA. Sirenomelia: a morphological study of 33 cases and review of the literature. *Perspect Pediatr Pathol.* 1987;10:7–50.

141. Schiesser M, Holzgreve W, Lapaire O, et al. Sirenomelia, the mermaid syndrome-detection in the first trimester. *Prenat Diagn.* 2003;23:493–495.

142. Akbayir O, Gungorduk K, Sudolmus S. First trimester diagnosis of sirenomelia: a case report and review of the literature. *Arch Gynecol Obstet.* 2008;278(6):589–592.

143. Blaicher W, Lee A, Deutinger J, et al. Sirenomelia: early prenatal diagnosis with combined two and three dimensional sonography. *Ultrasound Obstet Gynecol.* 2001;17:542–543.

144. Van Keirsbilck J, Cannie M. First trimester diagnosis of sirenomelia. *Prenat Diagn.* 2006;26(8):684–688.

145. Contu R, Zoppi M, Aziana C, et al. First trimester diagnosis of sirenomelia by 2D and 3D US. *Fetal Diagn Ther.* 2009;26:41–44.

146. Monteagudo A, Mayberry P, Rebarber A, et al. Sirenomelia sequence: first-trimester diagnosis with both two and three dimensional sonography. *J Ultrasound Med.* 2002;21:915–920.

147. Chenoweth CK, Kellogg SJ, Abu-Yousef MM. Antenatal sonographic diagnosis of sirenomelia. *J Clin Ultrasound.* 1991;19:167–171.

148. Sepulveda W, Corral E, Sanchez J, et al. Sirenomelia sequence versus reman agenesis: prenatal differentiation with power Doppler ultrasound. *Ultrasound Obstet Gynecol.* 1998;11:445–449.

149. Patel S, Suchet I. The role of color and power Doppler ultrasound in the prenatal diagnosis of sirenomelia. *Ultrasound Obstet Gynecol.* 2004;24:684–691.

150. Van Zalen-Sprock MM, van Vugt JMG, van der Harten JJ, et al. Early second-trimester diagnosis of sirenomelia. *Prenat Diagn.* 1995;15:171–177.

151. Gamez C, DeLeon-Luis J, Gamez F, et al. Fetal MRI as a complementary technique afterprenatal diagnosis of persistent vitelline artery in an otherwise normal fetus. *Magn Reson Imaging* 2013;38:951–954.

152. Fitzmorris-Glass R, Mattrey R, Cantrell C. Magnetic resonance imaging as an adjunct to ultrasound in oligohydramnios: detection of sirenomelia. *J Ultrasound Med.* 1989;8:159–162.

153. Altman RP, Randolph JG, Lilley FU. SCT: American Academy of Pediatrics Surgical Section Survey. *J Pediatr Surg.* 1974;9:389–398.

154. Valdiserri RO, Unis EF. SCT a review of 68 cases. *Cancer.* 1981;48:217–221.

155. Benachi A, Durin L, Maurer SV, et al. Prenatally diagnosed sacrococcygeal teratoma: a prognostic classification. *J Pediatr Surg.* 2006;41:1517–1521.

156. Bale PM. Sacrococcygeal developmental abnormalities and tumors in children. *Perspect Pediatr Pathol.* 1984;8(1):9–56.

157. Grisoni ER, Gauderer MWL, Wolfson RN, et al. Antenatal diagnosis of sacrococcygeal teratomas: prognostic features. *Pediatr Surg Int.* 1988;3:173–175.

158. Sheth S, Nussbaum AR, Sanders RC, et al. Prenatal diagnosis of sacrococcygeal teratomas: sonographic-pathologic correlation. *Radiology.* 1988;169:131–136.

159. Bond SJ, Harrison MR, Schmidt KG, et al. Death due to high-output cardiac failure in fetal sacrococcygeal teratoma. *J Pediatr Surg.* 1990;25:1287–1291.

160. Hendrick NH, Flake AE, Crombleholme TMN, et al. Sacrococcygeal teratoma: prenatal assessment, fetal intervention, and outcome. *J Pediatr Surg.* 2004;39:430–438.

161. Sciaky-Tamir Y, Cohen SM, Hochner-Celnikier D, et al. Three dimensional power Doppler (3DPD) ultrasound in the diagnosis and follow-up of fetal vascular anomalies. *Obstet Gynecol.* 2006;104:274–281.

162. Hogge WA, Thiagaraj S, Barber VG, et al. Cystic sacrococcygeal teratoma: ultrasound diagnosis and perinatal management. *J Ultrasound Med.* 1987;6:707–710.

163. Roman AS, Monteagudo A, Timor-Tristsch I, et al. First-trimester diagnosis of sacrococcygeal teratoma: the role of three dimensional ultrasound. *Ultrasound Obstet Gynecol.* 2004;23:612–614.

164. Schmidt KG, Silverman NH, Harrison MR, et al. High-output cardiac failure in fetuses with large SCT: diagnosis by echocardiography and Doppler ultrasound. *J Pediatr.* 1989;114:1023–1028.

165. Garel C, Mizouni L, Menez F, et al. Prenatal diagnosis of a cystic type IV sacrococcygeal teratoma mimicking a cloacal anomaly: contribution of MR. *Prenat Diagn.* 2005;25:216–219.

166. Quinn TM, Hubbard AM, Adzick NS. Prenatal magnetic resonance imaging enhances fetal diagnosis. *J Pediatr Surg.* 1998;33:553–558.

167. Nassenstein K, Schweiger B, Barkhausen J. Prenatal diagnosis of anasarca in an end-second trimester fetus presenting with sacrococcygeal teratoma by magnetic resonance imaging. *Magn Reson Imaging.* 2006;24:977–978.

168. Avni FE, Guibaud L, Robert Y, et al. MR imaging of fetal sacrococcygeal teratoma: diagnosis and assessment. *AJR Am J Roentgenol.* 2002;178:179–183.

169. Danzer E, Hubbard AM, Hendrick HL, et al. Diagnosis and characterization of fetal sacrococcygeal teratoma with prenatal MRI. *AJR Am J Roentgenol.* 2006;187:W350–W356.

170. Kuhlmann RS, Warsof SL, Levy DL, et al. Fetal sacrococcygeal teratoma. *Fetal Therapy.* 1987;2(2):95–100.

171. Tanaka K, Kanai M, Yosizawa J, et al. A case of neonatal neuroblastoma mimicking Altman type III sacrococcygeal teratoma. *J Pediatr Surg.* 2005;40(3):578–580.

172. Langer JC, Harris MR, Schmidt KG, et al. Fetal hydrops and death from sacrococcygeal teratoma: rationale for fetal surgery. *Am J Obstet Gynecol.* 1989;160:1145–1150.

173. Marina NM, Cushing B, Giller R, et al. Complete surgical excision is effective treatment for children with immature teratomas with or without malignant elements: a Pediatric Oncology Group/Children's Cancer Group Intergroup Study. *J Clin Oncol.* 1999;17:2137–2143.

174. Wilson RD, Hedrick H, Flake AW, et al. Sacrococcygeal teratomas: prenatal surveillance, growth and pregnancy outcome. *Fetal Diagn Ther.* 2009;25(1):15–20.

175. Jouannic JM, Dommergues M, Auber F, et al. Successful intrauterine shunting of a sacrococcygeal teratoma (SCT) causing fetal bladder obstruction. *Prenat Diagn.* 2001;21:824–926.

176. Kay S, Khalife S, Laberge JM, et al. Prenatal percutaneous needle drainage of cystic sacrococcygeal teratomas. *J Pediatr Surg.* 1999;34:1158–1151.

177. Pack BW, Jennings RW, Harrison MR, et al. Radiofrequency ablation of human fetal sacrococcygeal teratoma. *Am J Obstet Gynecol.* 2001;184:503–507.

178. Gopal M, Turnpenny PD, Spicer R. Hereditary sacrococcygeal teratoma—not the same as its sporadic counterpart! *Eur J Pediatr Surg.* 2007;17(3):214–216.

179. Wax JR, Benn P, Steinfeld JD, et al. Prenatally diagnosed sacrococcygeal teratoma: a unique expression of trisomy 10q. *Cancer Genet Cytogenet.* 2000;117:84–86.

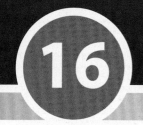

# 16 Cardiac Anomalies

Sarah B. Clauss • Jodi I. Pike • Maria A. Calvo-Garcia • Mary T. Donofrio

Approximately 1% of all children are born with a congenital heart defect (CHD), making cardiac disease the most common congenital malformation. Ventricular septal defects are the most common, comprising 26% of all congenital cardiac lesions, followed by tetralogy of Fallot, atrioventricular septal defects, atrial septal defects (ASDs), pulmonary stenosis, coarctation of the aorta, hypoplastic left heart syndrome, and transposition of the great arteries, all of which occur with a frequency of approximately 5% to 10% (Table 16.1). The percentage of fetuses with heart defects is up to 5-fold higher, many of which are lethal. Cardiac defects account for more than 20% of perinatal deaths from congenital abnormalities. Fetal echocardiography is widely available, and current technology allows for definitive diagnosis or exclusion of congenital heart disease in most patients. This chapter will review diagnostic utility and impact on management of fetal echocardiography.

## TIMING AND INDICATIONS

Fetal echocardiography has been in use since the late 1980s, and current technology allows for diagnostic testing starting at 18 weeks' gestation. Transvaginal transducers are available and can be used early as an adjunct to transabdominal imaging. Ideal imaging usually occurs between 20 and 28 weeks' gestation, but can be performed up to delivery. Third trimester imaging may be limited by a lack of amniotic fluid and limited variability in fetal position. Indications for fetal echocardiography can be related to maternal and/or fetal risk factors (see Chapter 4). The most common reasons for referral are family history of CHD, fetal dysrhythmia, maternal diabetes, and noncardiac fetal defect (i.e., increased nuchal fold). Indications that are most predictive of cardiac disease are an abnormal four-chamber view on routine ultrasound (30% to 50%), fetal dysrhythmia (30%),

hydrops (30%), and polyhydramnios (25%). See Chapter 4 for a detailed discussion of indications.

## CLASSIFICATION OF DEFECTS

### Septal Defects

#### Atrial Septal Defects

**Definition:** An ASD is a defect within the atrial septum that leads to a communication between the right and the left atria.

**Incidence:** In total, ASDs comprise 8% of CHD in live births, though prenatal diagnosis can be challenging owing to the expected opening of the foramen ovale in normal fetal hearts.[1] Both prenatally and within the initial postnatal period, a normal patent foramen ovale (PFO) can be difficult to distinguish from a small secundum ASD.

**Pathology and Hemodynamics:** ASDs are classified by location within the atrial septum. The most common ASD is a secundum ASD, followed by primum, sinus venosus, and coronary sinus defects. A PFO is an opening in the atrial septum and is a normal structure in the fetus (allowing right to left shunting of oxygenated blood from the umbilical vein to the left side of the heart) (Fig. 16.1). An aneurysm of the atrial septum is common, giving the septum a "wind sock" appearance. It is difficult to use fetal echocardiography to predict persistence of the foramen

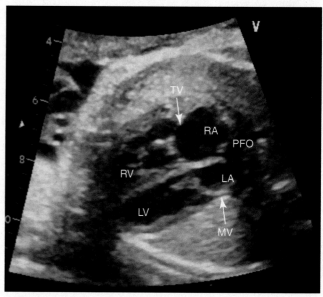

**FIGURE 16.1:** Four-chamber view obtained by cross-sectional imaging of the chest. The four chambers are readily visualized: right atrium (RA), left atrium (LA), right ventricle (RV), left ventricle (LV). In addition, the two atrioventricular valves are seen: tricuspid valve (TV), and mitral valve (MV). The heart is perpendicular to the plan of imaging, and the ventricular septum is well visualized and appears intact. The patent foramen ovale (PFO) is also visualized.

| Table 16.1 | The Baltimore-Washington Infant Study |
| --- | --- |

| Diagnosis | Children with CHD (%) |
| --- | --- |
| Ventricular septal defect | 26 |
| Tetralogy of Fallot | 9 |
| Atrioventricular septal defect | 9 |
| Atrial septal defect | 8 |
| Pulmonary valve stenosis | 7 |
| Coarctation of the aorta | 7 |
| Hypoplastic left heart syndrome | 6 |
| D-Transposition of the great arteries | 5 |
| Other | 23 |

From Ferencz C, Rubin JD, McCarter RJ, et al. Congenital heart disease: prevalence at livebirth. The Baltimore-Washington Infant Study. *Am J Epidemiol.* 1985;121:31–36.

ovale or a small secundum ASD after birth. Secundum ASDs represent a defect within septum primum, often adjacent to the foramen ovale. A primum ASD represents a defect in the endocardial cushion, adjacent to the atrioventricular valves, and is the second most common type of ASD. If a primum ASD is suspected, the presence of an atrioventricular septal defect must be considered, and the ventricular septum and mitral valve should be closely evaluated. Sinus venosus defects are located posteriorly and adjacent to the superior vena cava or inferior vena cava. In cases of a sinus venosus ASD, the pulmonary veins should be carefully imaged as superior sinus venosus defects are often associated with anomalous drainage of the right pulmonary veins. The least common ASD is the coronary sinus ASD, which is located at the coronary sinus ostium within the left atrium. If a coronary sinus defect is suspected, the possibility of a left superior vena cava should be considered.

**Associated Anomalies:** Most major types of CHD can be associated with an ASD, including endocardial cushion defect, anomalous pulmonary venous return, tetralogy of Fallot, double outlet right ventricle, and hypoplastic left heart syndrome. These anomalies will be discussed later in the chapter. Specific genetic defects are also associated with an atrial-level shunt. Holt–Oram syndrome consists of a secundum ASD, hypoplasia of the thumbs and radius, triphalangeal thumbs, abrachia, and phocomelia. Other congenital syndromes in which a secundum ASD may occur include Noonan syndrome, Treacher Collins syndrome, and the thrombocytopenia–absent radii (TAR) syndrome.

**Treatment/Outcome:** Postnatally, small secundum ASDs can be followed clinically as these defects often spontaneously close. Secundum ASDs that do require intervention are often amenable to percutaneous device closure in the cardiac catheterization laboratory, although some require surgical intervention, depending on size and location. All other types of ASDs require surgical closure, although timing is dependent on exact diagnosis, clinical situation, and associated cardiac abnormalities.

### Ventricular Septal Defects

**Definition:** A ventricular septal defect (VSD) is a defect in the ventricular septum that causes a communication between the two ventricles.

**Incidence:** VSDs are the most commonly diagnosed CHD, involving 25% of live births with CHD.[1]

**Pathology and Hemodynamics:** Like ASDs, VSDs are classified by their location within the ventricular septum, though various classification systems exist. VSDs can be classified as muscular, atrioventricular, conoventricular (including membranous/perimembranous and malalignment-type defects), and conoseptal. Muscular VSDs are defects within the muscular septum and are entirely surrounded by muscle. These defects can be further classified by location within the muscular septum, such as apical (below the moderator band), midmuscular, posterior, and anterior. Atrioventricular (AV) (or inlet) defects are defects in the posterior ventricular septum abutting the AV valves. These defects may or may not be associated with an atrioventricular canal defect. Membranous defects involve the membranous septum with the defect bordering the tricuspid valve. Perimembranous defects are around the membranous

septum. Conoventricular VSDs encompass those defects that involve the conal or outlet septum. The malalignment-type VSD is a type of conoventricular VSD. Defects of conal septal position result in malalignment, yielding the potential for outflow tract obstruction. The conal septum can be anteriorly displaced (as in tetralogy of Fallot) or posteriorly displaced (often associated with interrupted aortic arch). Defects of the conal septum resulting in conal hypoplasia are closely associated with the semilunar valves. These defects can lead to aortic insufficiency due to lack of support of the aortic valve and distortion of the right coronary cusp if the valve gets pulled into the defect.

**Associated Anomalies:** Most VSDs are isolated, but they can be found with almost all other CHD. Therefore, when a VSD is identified, all other cardiac structures must be thoroughly evaluated (i.e., to exclude more extensive anomalies, such as tetralogy of Fallot and coarctation of the aorta). VSDs are also seen in fetuses with chromosomal abnormalities, including trisomy 21, 18, and 13.

**Imaging:** VSDs are best seen when the ultrasound beam is perpendicular to the septum, as "false dropout" occurs when the beam is parallel to the septum (Fig. 16.2). Large defects will be easily visible; however, small defects are often missed. Color Doppler demonstrates bidirectional shunting. Perimembranous defects will be wedged under the tricuspid valve; these types of defects are best seen from the short- and long-axis views of the heart. Conal septal defects occur in the outlet septum in the muscle that supports the aortic valve adjacent to the pulmonary valve. These defects are best seen in short axis imaging. Anterior malalignment of the conal septum is typically seen in conjunction with aortic override, making the diagnosis of tetralogy of Fallot. The conal septum may also be posteriorly malaligned, which may be associated with subaortic narrowing, aortic valve stenosis, and coarctation of the aorta or interrupted aortic arch. Atrioventricular canal–type VSDs or inlet defects are well seen in the four-chamber view under the atrioventricular valves.

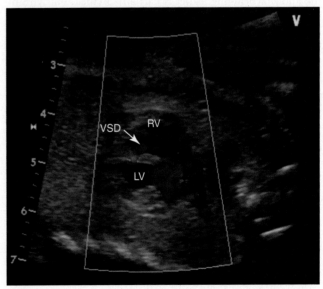

**FIGURE 16.2:** A sagittal image of the heart, sweeping leftward; one can see the anterior right ventricle *(RV)* and the posterior left ventricle *(LV)*. The *red* flow represents a muscular ventricular septal defect *(VSD)*. The *blue* color flow demonstrates the laminar flow in the right ventricular outflow tract.

**Treatment/Outcome:** Postnatally, small VSDs can be followed clinically as perimembranous and muscular defects often close spontaneously (more likely when the defects are smaller than 3 mm in a term infant). Moderate-to-large defects often require surgical closure in the setting of congestive heart failure that cannot be managed medically. In older patients, muscular VSDs are sometimes amenable to percutaneous device closure in the cardiac catheterization laboratory, although most VSDs that require closure necessitate surgical intervention. Malalignment and atrioventricular canal–type defects will not close spontaneously and therefore need surgical closure. Typically, conal septal hypoplasia defects do not close, but the decision to operate depends on the amount of left to right shunting and the effect the defect has on the aortic valve.

### Endocardial Cushion Defects

**Definition:** Endocardial cushion defects include the spectrum of diseases involving the endocardial cushion and include complete atrioventricular canal (CAVC), transitional AVC defects, and isolated primum ASD with cleft mitral valve. These defects can be classified by size/presence of the VSD, the balance of the atrioventricular valve over the ventricles, and the anatomy of the common valve.

**Incidence:** Endocardial cushion defects account for 5% to 7% of all live births with CHD.[1]

**Pathology and Hemodynamics:** A CAVC defect includes defects of the atrial septum (primum ASD) and ventricular septum (atrioventricular VSD) with a common atrioventricular valve. A partial AVC is comprised of a primum ASD and a cleft mitral valve. A transitional AVC is similar to a complete CAVC except that there is a small restrictive VSD. CAVCs can be further classified by the anatomy of the anterior bridging leaflet of the common atrioventricular valve. Using the classification system of Rastelli et al.,[2] in type A defects, the anterior bridging leaflet is divided and has attachments to the crest of the ventricular septum. In type B defects, the anterior bridging leaflet is partially divided, but with no attachments to the ventricular septum. In type C defects, the anterior bridging leaflet is both undivided and unattached to the ventricular septal crest. The Rastelli classification is best determined by short axis imaging of the ventricles, noting the valve en face.

Further classification of endocardial cushion defects must include a description of the absolute and relative size of the ventricles. In a balanced CAVC, both ventricles are approximately equal in size, and the common valve is positioned symmetrically over both ventricles. In an unbalanced CAVC, the atrioventricular canal sits predominantly over either the right or the left ventricle; flow is toward that ventricle, and the contralateral ventricle is usually small.

**Associated Anomalies:** Defects associated with endocardial cushion defects include tetralogy of Fallot, double outlet right ventricle, coarctation of the aorta, subaortic stenosis, pulmonary valve stenosis, and single ventricle. In the cases of multiple defects (i.e., CAVC with double outlet right ventricle and/or with complete heart block [CHB]), heterotaxy syndrome should be considered. When CAVC exists as an isolated lesion, trisomy 21 is present in 60% of the cases.[3] Endocardial cushion defects may also occur with T13, T18, and T21.

**Imaging:** Endocardial cushion defects are easily seen in the four-chamber view, with the components of the ASD, VSD, and common valve easily visible (Figs. 16.3 to 16.5). The details of the common atrioventricular valve (en face view) are best seen in short axis imaging of the ventricle (Fig. 16.6). The cleft of the anterior leaflet refers to the division of the leaflet with the attachment to the left ventricular septal surface. Color Doppler should be performed to evaluate for atrioventricular valve regurgitation in the four-chamber view.

**Treatment/Outcome:** CAVC defects always require surgical correction, although the type of repair can be dependent

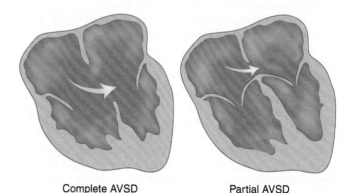

Complete AVSD                      Partial AVSD

**FIGURE 16.3:** Illustration of partial and complete atrioventricular canal. (From Rice MJ, McDonald RW, Pilu G, et al. Cardiac malformations. In: Nyberg DA, McGahan JP, Pretorius DH, et al, eds. *Diagnostic Imaging of Fetal Anomalies.* Philadelphia, PA: Lippincott Williams & Wilkins; 2003:459.)

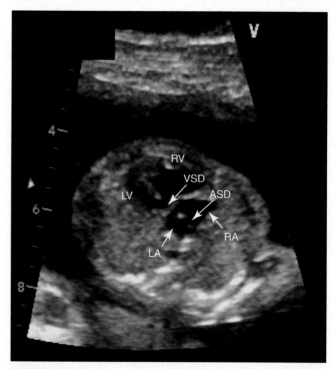

**FIGURE 16.4:** Four-chamber view of a complete atrioventricular canal. The crux of the heart is absent in this view, demonstrating both the inlet ventricular septal defect *(VSD) (arrow)* and the primum atrial septal defect *(ASD) (arrow).* The patent foramen ovale is also present in this image. In this systolic view, the single or common valve is also appreciated. RA, right atrium *(arrow);* LA, left atrium; RV, right ventricle *(arrow);* LV, left ventricle.

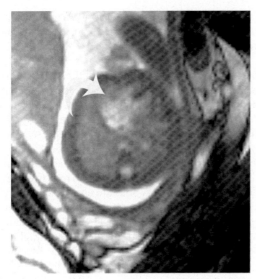

**FIGURE 16.5:** Atrioventricular canal. Axial SSFP MR image of the fetal heart demonstrates a single common valve *(curved arrow)*. A large primum atrial septal defect and ventricular septal defect are also present.

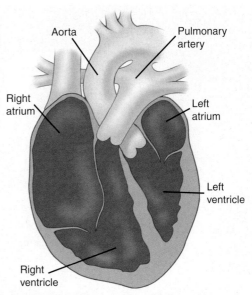

**FIGURE 16.7:** Illustration of Ebstein anomaly of the tricuspid valve. The tricuspid valve is displaced into the right ventricle. (From Rice MJ, McDonald RW, Pilu G, et al. Cardiac malformations. In: Nyberg DA, McGahan JP, Pretorius DH, et al, eds. *Diagnostic Imaging of Fetal Anomalies.* Philadelphia, PA: Lippincott Williams & Wilkins; 2003:461.)

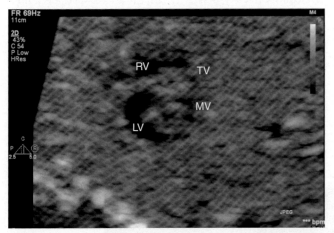

**FIGURE 16.6:** In this short axis view of the fetal heart, the two components of the right and left side of the atrioventricular valves are well seen. This image will aid in determining Rastelli classification and balance of the valves over the ventricles. Here the right-sided atrioventricular valve is labeled as the tricuspid valve *(TV)*, and the left-sided atrioventricular valve is labeled as the mitral valve *(MV)*. RV, right ventricle; LV, left ventricle.

on other anatomic factors (e.g., a significantly unbalanced CAVC may require single ventricle palliation). The technique of the surgical repair of CAVCs can vary widely, and be comprised of a single patch, two-patch, or modified patch technique. Short- and long-term outcomes are greatly dependent on associated cardiac defects, residual atrioventricular valve regurgitation, outflow tract obstruction, and chromosomal anomalies.

## Inflow Defects

### Diseases of the Tricuspid Valve

#### Ebstein Anomaly of the Tricuspid Valve

**Definition:** Ebstein anomaly of the tricuspid valve is defined by specific anatomical features, including apical displacement

of the septal and posterior leaflets of the tricuspid valve within the right ventricle (Fig. 16.7). This creates a displaced tricuspid valve orifice into the body of the ventricle with the proximal right ventricle becoming functionally part of the right atrium.

**Incidence:** Ebstein anomaly accounts for 0.5% of live births with CHD, although it occurs in approximately 3% to 8% of fetal CHD, with a 44% rate of fetal demise.[1]

**Pathology and Hemodynamics:** There is a wide spectrum of disease related to Ebstein anomaly, ranging from minimal displacement of the tricuspid valve to severe apical displacement wherein nearly the entire right ventricle is "atrialized" and there is little to no functional right ventricle. Severe tricuspid regurgitation can be associated with secondary hydrops fetalis and in utero fetal demise. In some cases, there is associated pulmonary stenosis or atresia.

**Associated Anomalies:** Ebstein anomaly may be associated with other CHD, such as severe pulmonary stenosis or pulmonary atresia, ASDs, Wolf–Parkinson–White syndrome and congenitally corrected transposition of the great arteries.[4] Additionally, severe cardiomegaly may contribute to lung hypoplasia, increasing the risk of death.

**Imaging:** Ebstein anomaly is well seen in the four-chamber view (Fig. 16.8). The displacement of the hinge point of the septal leaflet of the tricuspid valve is quantified by measuring the distance between the crux of the heart (from the mitral valve hinge point) and the hinge point of the septal leaflet of the tricuspid valve; this distance should be less than 5 mm at birth. Cardiomegaly secondary to atrial or ventricular dilation may be present. Color Doppler should be used to evaluate the degree of tricuspid regurgitation (Fig. 16.9). Tricuspid regurgitation may progress during fetal life. When severe tricuspid regurgitation

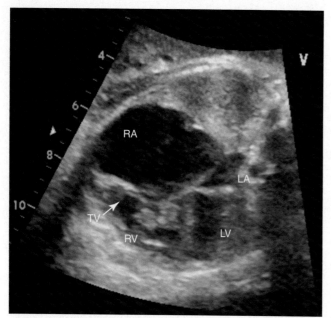

**FIGURE 16.8:** Four-chamber view of Ebstein anomaly of the tricuspid valve in systole. Note the severely enlarged right atrium *(RA)* and the abnormal tricuspid valve *(TV)*. LA, left atrium; RV, right ventricle; LV, left ventricle.

"functional" or anatomical pulmonary atresia is likely present. Finally, the right heart may be dilated, causing the left heart to be compressed and appear hypoplastic.

**Prognosis:** A neonate with significant Ebstein anomaly associated with pulmonary stenosis or atresia will present with cyanosis in the immediate newborn period. Postnatally, when the pulmonary vascular resistance falls, antegrade pulmonary blood flow may improve if the valve is not atretic. If there is pulmonary atresia or a delayed decrease in pulmonary vascular resistance, prostaglandin is often used to maintain ductal patency and pulmonary blood flow. These neonates may need a surgical systemic to pulmonary artery shunt to ensure adequate pulmonary blood flow. Additional surgeries such as right ventricular outflow patch reconstruction or single ventricle palliation may need to be performed, depending on the degree of right ventricular outflow tract obstruction, right ventricular hypoplasia, or tricuspid valve competency. Alternatively, if the tricuspid valve displacement is minimal and the tricuspid valve regurgitation is mild, patients may not be diagnosed until adulthood (often due to associated atrial arrhythmias).

exists, the right ventricle may not be able to generate sufficient pressure to open the pulmonary valve even though it may be patent; this is termed functional pulmonary atresia. The branch pulmonary arteries can be best seen in short axis imaging; these may be normal in size or hypoplastic. The ductus arteriosus flow may be normal or reversed. If flow is reversed, associated

**Tricuspid Valve Dysplasia:** Tricuspid valve dysplasia is a nonspecific term that can include various abnormalities of tricuspid valve anatomy. Unlike Ebstein anomaly, in tricuspid valve dysplasia the tricuspid valve leaflet attachments are at the level of the valve annulus. The leaflets are often thickened with poor coaptation and have abnormal papillary muscle and chordae. Various amounts of tricuspid valve regurgitation will often be present, and the degree of the regurgitation will determine severity and outcome of the disease. Tricuspid valve dysplasia is associated with varying degrees of right ventricular hypoplasia, pulmonary stenosis, or pulmonary atresia.

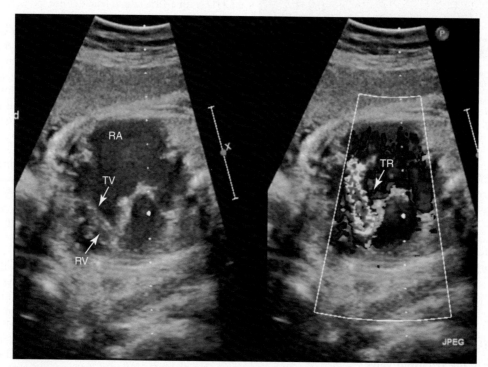

**FIGURE 16.9:** Four-chamber color compare view of Ebstein anomaly of the tricuspid valve in diastole. The apical displacement of the tricuspid valve leaflets *(TV)* into the right ventricle *(RV)* is readily visualized. There is moderate to severe tricuspid insufficiency *(TR)* with severe right atrial *(RA)* enlargement.

**Isolated Tricuspid Valve Regurgitation:** Tricuspid valve regurgitation can vary in severity and clinical significance. An attempt to quantify the regurgitation can be made by evaluating the duration of the insufficiency during systole, the peak velocity of the regurgitant jet, the diameter of the regurgitant jet, and how far back within the right atrium the jet reaches.[5] Trivial tricuspid valve regurgitation may be found in up to 5% of fetuses with structurally normal hearts, and resolution is usually expected.[6] More significant amounts of tricuspid valve regurgitation can be associated with structural heart defects, volume overload states (such as fetal anemia or vein of Galen aneurysms), poor fetal cardiac function, or in fetuses of maternal anti SSA/SSB antibodies (SSA) antibody positive women.[7]

**Cor Triatriatum Dexter:** Cor triatriatum dexter is an extremely rare condition whereby there is a persistence of a right venous valve that results in septation of the smooth and trabeculated portions of the right atrium. Normal venous valves exist to help direct oxygenated blood flow from the placenta across the foramen ovale. Complete persistence of the right venous valve or prominent chiari network may result in cor triatriatum dexter. The physiology and presentation is dependent on the degree of septation of the right atrium. Cor triatriatum dexter can occur in isolation or with other right-sided defects, such as pulmonary stenosis or atresia, tricuspid valve anomalies, ASD, or Ebstein anomaly.

**Tricuspid Stenosis and Tricuspid Atresia:** Tricuspid stenosis and tricuspid atresia are typically associated with varying degrees of right ventricular hypoplasia. Either of these lesions may be associated with a VSD. It is important to evaluate the size of the right ventricle and the source of pulmonary blood flow (antegrade via a pulmonary artery or retrograde via a ductus arteriosus). These lesions are typically classified in the single ventricle lesion and will be discussed further in the single ventricle section.

### Diseases of the Mitral Valve

**Dysplastic Mitral Valve:** A dysplastic mitral valve with primary mitral regurgitation is rare. Mitral regurgitation is more often associated with severe aortic stenosis and left ventricular injury, endocardial cushion defects, or primary left ventricular heart failure. Mitral regurgitation is also seen in fetuses of SSA antibody positive mothers or in those with myocarditis. Often, the left ventricle is dilated, and the endocardium and papillary muscles are echo bright.

**Mitral Stenosis:** Congenital mitral stenosis is a rare condition. Congenital mitral stenosis can occur with other left-sided obstructive lesions. Shone syndrome is a term used for patients with multiple left-sided obstructions. Severe mitral stenosis may lead to progressive aortic and left ventricular hypoplasia in utero. In congenital mitral stenosis, the annulus, leaflets, chordae, and/or the papillary muscles may be abnormal.[8] The chordae may be absent or extremely short so that the valve apparatus attaches directly to the papillary muscles; this is termed a mitral valve arcade. The chordae may attach to a single papillary muscle; this is termed a parachute mitral valve. Imaging of the heart in the short axis will demonstrate the papillary muscles. Imaging from the apical four-chamber view will demonstrate the mitral valve annulus diameter and chords. Color and pulse wave Doppler should be used to identify the degree of stenosis or regurgitation. Ventricular size and function should be assessed, as

should the direction of foramen ovale flow. Reversed foramen ovale flow suggests severe disease. Some patients may be candidates for mitral valvuloplasty postnatally; however, patients are generally managed conservatively, and surgical intervention is delayed as long as possible valve replacement may be needed.

**Cor Triatriatum Sinister:** Cor triatriatum sinister describes a membrane within the body of the left atrium, proximal to the left atrial appendage, which causes a varying degree of obstruction to pulmonary venous return to the left side of the heart. Developmentally, this is thought to be due to incomplete incorporation of the pulmonary veins into the left atrium. There is usually a communication between the superior and the inferior chambers of the left atrium of variable size. There may be an ASD or PFO with the right atrium connecting to the distal chamber, and there may be anomalous pulmonary venous drainage. The physiology of this lesion depends on the degree of restriction between the superior and the inferior chambers caused by the cor triatriatum membrane. If the opening is large, the neonate will be asymptomatic. If the opening is small, there will be venous obstruction with subsequent pulmonary edema, pulmonary hypertension, and decreased cardiac output. The echocardiographic evaluation should include the size of the foramen ovale, the communication between the superior and the inferior chambers, and pulmonary venous return. Color and pulse wave Doppler should be performed to evaluate restriction of the communication. The treatment includes resection of the left atrial membrane if it is restrictive or in patients who are symptomatic or have pulmonary artery hypertension.

**Supravalvar Mitral Ring:** A supravalvar mitral ring consists of a ring of tissue that adheres to the atrial surface of the mitral valve leaflets. This tissue is distal to the left atrial appendage (thus differentiating it from a cor triatriatum membrane). This may be associated with other left-sided defects such as subaortic stenosis, coarctation of the aorta, and VSD. There will be varying degrees of mitral regurgitation and mitral stenosis. The membrane will be best seen in the long axis or posteriorly tipped in four-chamber views adherent to the mitral valve annulus. Surgical resection is the treatment of choice.

## Outflow Defects

### Pulmonary Valve Stenosis

**Definition:** Pulmonary valve stenosis is an abnormality in the pulmonary valve leading to varying degrees of obstruction to the right ventricular outflow tract, often due to fusion of the valve commissures.

**Incidence:** Isolated pulmonary valve stenosis accounts for approximately 7% of live births.[1]

**Pathology and Hemodynamics:** Pulmonary valve stenosis, like stenosis at any valve, can progress during gestation. Interval imaging should be performed as the disease can evolve. Serial fetal echocardiograms will allow for postnatal planning to assess for disease progression. Severe pulmonary stenosis may cause inadequate pulmonary blood flow and require postnatal initiation of prostaglandin to maintain patency of the ductus arteriosus.

**Associated Anomalies:** Complete fetal echocardiogram should include evaluation for commonly associated cardiac anomalies, such as an ASD, tetralogy of Fallot, Ebstein anomaly, and double outlet right ventricle. Associated genetic anomalies and syndromes should be considered, such as Noonan syndrome and Beckwith–Wiedemann. Rubella is a known teratogen causing both pulmonary stenosis and peripheral pulmonic stenosis.

**Imaging:** The pulmonary valve can be visualized from several different views and should be assessed for thickening, doming, and poor excursion of the valve leaflets. The amount and velocity of antegrade blood flow can be assessed with color and pulsed-wave Doppler. Pulse wave Doppler can be used to calculate the gradient across the valve using the modified Bernoulli equation, where the pressure gradient across a discrete stenosis is equal to $4 \times (velocity^2)$, also written as $4v^2$.[3] Right ventricular hypertrophy and/or hypoplasia and tricuspid valve regurgitation may be seen in the four-chamber view. Right ventricular hypertension may develop and right ventricular pressures can be estimated by measuring the velocity of the tricuspid regurgitation and calculating right ventricular pressure by the Bernoulli equation where right ventricular pressure equals $4 \times (tricuspid velocity)^2$.[3] Poststenotic dilatation of the main pulmonary artery may be associated with pulmonary stenosis. In some cases, mild pulmonary stenosis may not be visualized, and the only indicator of valve disease is poststenotic dilation of the main pulmonary artery. In severe or critical pulmonary stenosis, there will be reversed flow in the ductus arteriosus.

**Treatment/Outcome:** The prognosis for pulmonary valve stenosis is dependent on the severity of the outflow tract obstruction and associated defects. Mild or moderate pulmonary stenosis has an excellent prognosis and often requires no immediate postnatal intervention, although percutaneous balloon valvuloplasty may be required in infancy or early childhood. More severe forms of pulmonary stenosis or functional pulmonary atresia may require more urgent neonatal intervention. Reversal of flow in the ductus arteriosus prenatally can be indicative of ductal-dependent pulmonary blood flow and need for early initiation of prostaglandin to maintain ductal patency until balloon valvuloplasty or surgical intervention in the immediate neonatal period can be undertaken.

### Pulmonary Atresia

**Definition:** In pulmonary atresia, no antegrade flow is present across the pulmonary valve leaflets, and the leaflets are often fused (Fig. 16.10). The diagnosis of pulmonary atresia with intact ventricular septum is used to distinguish this disease from tetralogy of Fallot with pulmonary atresia.

**Incidence:** Pulmonary atresia with intact ventricular septum occurs in 1% to 2% of all live births with CHD.

**Pathophysiology and Hemodynamics:** The pulmonary valve is atretic in pulmonary atresia/intact ventricular septum. There are usually varying degrees of tricuspid valve and right ventricular hypoplasia. The pulmonary valve leaflets are often present but fused, and the branch pulmonary arteries are typically small but not severely hypoplastic. Coronary artery fistulous connections to the right ventricle may be present and are related to right ventricular pressure elevation. Some will have associated coronary artery atresia, obstruction, or right ventricular pressure-dependent circulation.

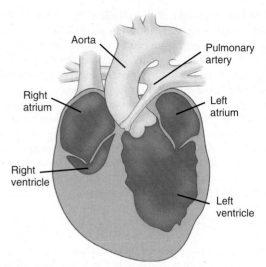

**FIGURE 16.10:** Illustration of pulmonary atresia with intact ventricular septum. (From Rice MJ, McDonald RW, Pilu G, et al. Cardiac malformations. In: Nyberg DA, McGahan JP, Pretorius DH, et al, eds. *Diagnostic Imaging of Fetal Anomalies.* Philadelphia, PA: Lippincott Williams & Wilkins; 2003:464.)

**Imaging:** In the four-chamber view, the tricuspid valve will be patent but is usually small. The right ventricle may be hypoplastic and echogenic (Fig. 16.11). There may be tricuspid insufficiency as there is no other egress from the right ventricle (Fig. 16.12). Use of pulse wave Doppler of the tricuspid insufficiency will allow an estimation of right ventricular pressure, which may be suprasystemic (Fig. 16.13). Imaging from the short axis and ductal views will demonstrate no antegrade flow across the pulmonary valve and reversed flow in the ductus arteriosus. A main pulmonary artery will be present and give rise to continuous though small pulmonary arteries. Finally, coronary fistulae may be present and are best visualized in either the four-chamber view or short axis of the ventricles with color Doppler (Fig. 16.14). Typically, there is a stretched PFO or secundum ASD.

**Treatment/Outcome:** By definition, newborns with pulmonary atresia are ductal dependent, and therefore prostaglandin should be initiated immediately after delivery. In addition to echocardiography, cardiac catheterization is performed to evaluate coronary artery anatomy. Right ventricular–dependent coronary arteries are a significant risk factor for death. A small percentage of patients will have an adequate size tricuspid valve ($>-2$ to $-3$ z-score), a well-developed right ventricle, and normal coronary arteries with flow not dependent on the right ventricle. These patients may be candidates for radiofrequency ablation to open up the right ventricular outflow tract. The remainder of patients will need a systemic to pulmonary artery shunt. Patients are followed over the first year of life, and if the tricuspid valve z-score is $>-2$ and the right ventricle is adequate, a two ventricular repair may be undertaken later. If the right ventricle is small but has some output, a "one and a half ventricular repair" may be performed. This repair includes a Glenn shunt (superior vena cava anastomosis to the pulmonary artery) with the inferior vena cava flow returning to the right ventricle to be pumped to the lungs. Finally, some patients must follow a single ventricle approach to repair. One indication for single ventricle palliation is right ventricular–dependent

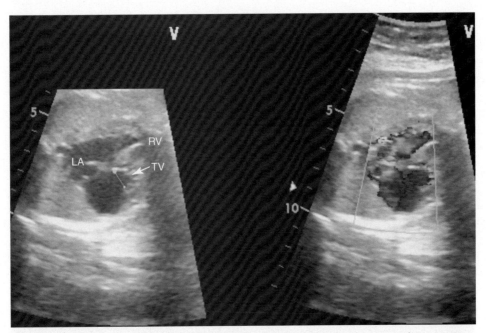

**FIGURE 16.11:** Color compare view of pulmonary atresia with intact ventricular septum demonstrating a hypoplastic tricuspid valve *(TV)* annulus. Note in the color image the foramen ovale is widely patent, allowing unrestrictive right to left atrial flow. LA, left atrium; RV, right ventricle.

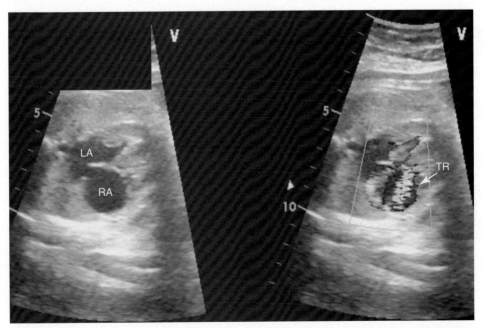

**FIGURE 16.12:** Color compare view of four-chamber view of fetal heart with pulmonary atresia intact ventricular septum. The *blue* color Doppler demonstrates severe tricuspid regurgitation *(TR)*. LA, left atrium; RA, right atrium.

coronary circulation. In these patients, the right ventricle cannot be used as the pulmonary pump because of the high risk of coronary artery ischemia. Other indications for single ventricle palliation is an extremely small tricuspid valve (z-score < −4) or severely hypoplastic right ventricle. In these patients, a systemic to pulmonary artery shunt will be placed in the newborn period. These patients will then ultimately undergo Glenn shunt and Fontan procedure (see hypoplastic left heart syndrome for further discussion of these surgeries).

A small subset of fetuses with pulmonary atresia/intact ventricular septum may be considered for fetal intervention; however, there is debate as to whether intervention should be offered.[9–11] The goal of intervention is to promote right ventricular growth and avoid single ventricle palliation or as a lifesaving measure if severe tricuspid regurgitation and hydrops exists and there is impending fetal demise.[12] The technique for intervention is difficult given the right ventricular cavity is small, hypertrophied, and located behind the sternum.[13]

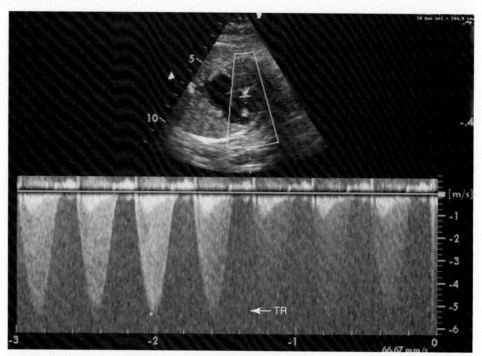

**FIGURE 16.13:** Pulse wave Doppler imaging of the tricuspid regurgitation *(TR)* demonstrates a high velocity, 5.3 m per second, predicting a right ventricular pressure of 112 mm Hg.

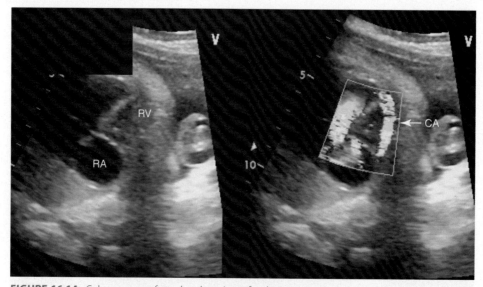

**FIGURE 16.14:** Color compare four-chamber view of pulmonary atresia intact ventricular septum with a fistula from the right ventricle *(RV)* to the coronary artery *(CA)*. Color Doppler is necessary to show this diagnosis. RA, right atrium.

Long-term prognosis for children with pulmonary atresia intact ventricular septum depends on the degree of tricuspid, degree of right ventricular hypoplasia, and the presence of coronary abnormalities. The outcome is good for those that undergo pulmonary valve dilation or right ventricular outflow plasty with a two ventricular repair. In patients that undergo single ventricle palliation, early deaths have been reported secondary to coronary ischemia, but long-term survival is reported to be 83% at 5 years.[14]

### Aortic Stenosis

**Definition:** Aortic stenosis is an abnormality in the aortic valve leading to left-sided outflow tract obstruction at the level of the aortic valve. The valve may be bicuspid, unicuspid, or thickened with fused commissures.

**Incidence:** Aortic stenosis accounts for 5% to 7% of children with cardiac disease. A bicuspid nonstenotic aortic valve may be as common as 3% of the population but does not always present as heart disease in childhood.

**Pathology and Hemodynamics:** The abnormal aortic valve itself may have three leaflets; more commonly, there may be fusion of the leaflets, resulting in unicuspid or bicuspid valve. Aortic stenosis, like stenosis at any valve, can progress during gestation. Interval imaging should be performed as the disease can evolve. Serial fetal echocardiograms will allow for postnatal planning to assess for disease progression. Severe aortic stenosis may cause inadequate systemic blood flow and require postnatal initiation of prostaglandin to maintain patency of the ductus arteriosus.

**Associated Anomalies:** Aortic stenosis is often familial. Bicuspid aortic valve and coarctation of the aorta can be seen in association with Turner syndrome. Supravalvar aortic stenosis can be associated with Williams syndrome. Subvalvar aortic stenosis does not typically present in the fetus. Associated abnormalities include hypoplasia of the left ventricle, mitral valve, or aortic arch (see hypoplastic left heart syndrome section).

**Imaging:** Ultrasound findings vary according to the severity of the disease. The aortic leaflets will be best visualized in a short axis view, and they may appear thickened and fused. Color and pulse Doppler should be performed to accurately determine degree of stenosis (Fig. 16.15). Aortic flow gradient can be calculated by the Bernoulli equation (aortic gradient = $4 \times$ velocity$^2$). In the presence of severe left ventricular dysfunction, the gradient may be minimal. Dilation of the ascending aorta is a subtle clue of mild aortic stenosis and is best seen in the long axis evaluation of the left ventricular outflow tract. Significant mitral regurgitation may be present and is best visualized in the four-chamber view. Severe aortic stenosis may cause left ventricular dysfunction resulting in retrograde aortic arch and foramen flow; this may be a precursor to hypoplastic left heart syndrome.

**Treatment/Outcome:** Postnatal management of aortic stenosis is dependent on severity of the disease. With critical aortic stenosis, there is little to no antegrade blood flow, and prostaglandin is necessary to supply sufficient cardiac output. Balloon aortic valvuloplasty is performed if there is aortic stenosis with ventricular dysfunction, or if the peak gradient is greater than 70 to 80 mm Hg. Balloon angioplasty is typically successful, although most patients will need further procedures and ultimate aortic valve replacement. Morbidity and mortality will be dependent on the degree of stenosis or left ventricular dysfunction.

## Conotruncal Defects

Conotruncal defects encompass a wide spectrum of CHD with abnormalities of the connection between the ventricles and the great vessels, including tetralogy of Fallot, transposition of the great arteries, truncus arteriosus, and double outlet right ventricle. Conotruncal anomalies account for 20% to 30% of all live births with structural CHD.

### Tetralogy of Fallot

**Definition:** The anatomic features of tetralogy of Fallot include infundibular and valvar pulmonary stenosis, a malalignment-type VSD, overriding aorta, and right ventricular hypertrophy (a late sequela of the outflow tract obstruction and not observed in utero) (Fig. 16.16). The aortic valve is in continuity with the right ventricle.

**Incidence:** Tetralogy of Fallot is the most common type of cyanotic CHD, accounting for approximately 9% of CHD live births.[1]

**Pathophysiology and Hemodynamics:** If not diagnosed prenatally, timing of presentation can vary significantly, depending on the severity of the right ventricular outflow tract obstruction. Postnatally, patients with tetralogy of Fallot become cyanotic because of right to left shunting across the VSD in the

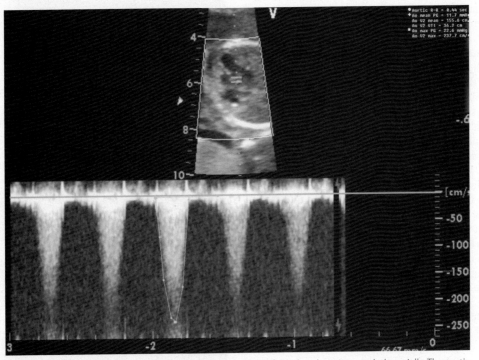

**FIGURE 16.15:** In the upper panel, the heart is imaged in a four-chamber view angled cranially. The aortic valve and left ventricle appear echobright. Pulse wave Doppler demonstrates increased velocity across the aortic valve of 4.1 m per second or a peak gradient of 67 mm Hg.

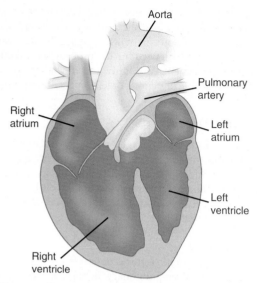

**FIGURE 16.16:** Illustration of tetralogy of Fallot. A large aorta overrides a ventricular septal defect, and the pulmonary outflow tract is hypoplastic. (From Rice MJ, McDonald RW, Pilu G, et al. Cardiac malformations. In: Nyberg DA, McGahan JP, Pretorius DH, et al, eds. *Diagnostic Imaging of Fetal Anomalies*. Philadelphia, PA: Lippincott Williams & Wilkins; 2003:475.)

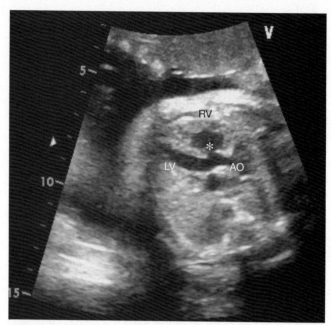

**FIGURE 16.17:** Long axis view of tetralogy of Fallot with an overriding aorta *(AO)*. The *asterisk* denotes the ventricular septal defect. RV, right ventricle; LV, left ventricle.

presence of severe right ventricular outflow tract obstruction. The degree of shunting and cyanosis is secondary to the right ventricular outflow tract obstruction. Newborns with little right to left shunting will be "pink" and will have clinical symptoms of a large VSD. The right ventricular outflow tract obstruction may progress and therefore warrants close observation. During a "tet spell," there is dynamic muscular obstruction of the right ventricular outflow tract, causing severe cyanosis. "Tet spells" may be precipitated by crying, illness, or decreased systemic vascular resistance. Treatment includes oxygen, IV fluids, morphine, knee to chest position, and often emergency surgery.

**Associated Anomalies:** Tetralogy of Fallot is often associated with genetic and extracardiac anomalies such as DiGeorge syndrome, VACTERL (verterbral anomalies, anal atresia, cardiac anomalies, tracheoesophageal fistula, renal anomalies, and limb anomalies) association, and Goldenhar syndrome, among many others. A right aortic arch suggests a deletion on chromosome 22q11. Tetralogy of Fallot can also be found in association with endocardial cushion defects, most commonly in those fetuses diagnosed with trisomy 21. A variation of tetralogy of Fallot with significant hypoplasia of the conal septum is more commonly found in Asian and Native American populations. In some cases, the distinction between tetralogy of Fallot and double outlet right ventricle can be difficult. Double outlet right ventricle can be classified with tetralogy of Fallot-like physiology if the aorta overrides the ventricular septum more than 50% toward the right ventricle with a lack of fibrous continuity between the aortic and the mitral valves.

**Imaging:** The anterior malalignment-type VSD is best viewed in the long axis of the heart where the overriding aorta can be easily appreciated (Fig. 16.17). The VSD will not be seen in the four-chamber view as it is located in the outlet conal septum. The short axis views will demonstrate the VSD and the anterior deviation of the conal septum and allow for assessment of right

ventricular outflow obstruction. The degree of pulmonary stenosis may progress in utero, and therefore serial imaging should be performed. The pulmonary valve, main pulmonary artery, and branch pulmonary arteries should be carefully measured as they may be hypoplastic (Fig. 16.18). The direction of ductus arteriosus flow is important because with severe obstruction there

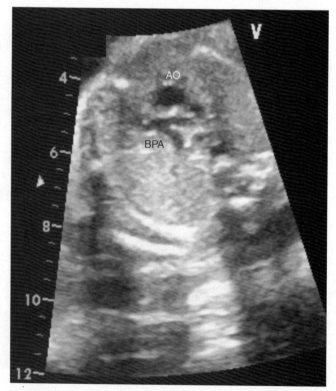

**FIGURE 16.18:** Three-vessel view in tetralogy of Fallot demonstrating hypoplastic branch pulmonary arteries *(BPA)* relative to the aorta *(AO)*.

will be reversed flow and these babies will have significant right to left ventricular-level shunting and will be ductal dependent at birth. There can be varying degrees of abnormalities of the pulmonary valve (see tetralogy of Fallot with pulmonary atresia and tetralogy of flow with absent pulmonary valve).

**Treatment/Outcome:** Surgical repair is necessary in tetralogy of Fallot and usually occurs between 2 and 6 months of age or earlier if cyanosis is present. Surgical repair includes closure of the VSD and relief of the right ventricular outflow tract obstruction. If the pulmonary valve annulus is small, a patch may be placed across the right ventricular outflow tract to relieve valvar obstruction ("transannular patch repair"). If the valve size is within normal limits ($>-2$ SD), an infundibular patch may be considered. Finally, stenosis or discontinuity of the branch pulmonary arteries, if present, is usually also corrected. Outcomes are good, although some patients may need catheter intervention for residual right ventricular outflow tract or branch pulmonary artery stenosis.

**Tetralogy of Fallot with Pulmonary Atresia:** Tetralogy of Fallot with pulmonary atresia (TOF/PA) is a severe form of tetralogy of Fallot in which the pulmonary valve is atretic and there is no antegrade pulmonary blood flow. TOF/PA is typically associated with good-sized branch pulmonary arteries if there is a large patent ductus arterious. However, it may be associated with hypoplastic branch pulmonary arteries and aortopulmonary collateral arteries (MAPCAs) arising from the aorta if the ductus is absent. The type and timing of surgical repair of TOF/PA is dependent on the nature of the pulmonary blood supply. Outcome is typically not as good, especially in the presence of hypoplastic pulmonary arteries.

**Tetralogy of Fallot with Absent Pulmonary Valve:** TOF with absent pulmonary valve (TOF/APV) is a rare variant of TOF. The pulmonary valve is not truly absent, but primitive with underdeveloped leaflets that do not function effectively. This abnormality leads to severe or "wide open" pulmonary insufficiency with severe dilatation of the main pulmonary arteries, branch pulmonary arteries, and the right ventricle (Fig. 16.19 to 16.21). There may be airway compression from the massive dilation of the pulmonary arteries, and the lungs can be hypoplastic[15] (Fig. 16.22). Typically, there is no patent ductus arteriosus. There is a high risk of hydrops and in utero fetal demise, as well as postnatal demise due to respiratory complications.

### *Transposition of the Great Arteries*
### D-Transposition

**Definition:** In D-Transposition of the great arteries (D-TGA), there is a normal atrioventricular relationship with ventricular–arterial discordance; the aorta is connected to the right ventricle, and the pulmonary artery is connected to the left ventricle (Fig. 16.23).

**Incidence:** D-Transposition of the great arteries is the second most common (5% to 7% live births) form of cyanotic heart disease, and the most common cyanotic lesion presenting in the newborn period.

**Pathology and Hemodynamics:** Embryologically, D-TGA results from abnormal neural crest cell migration and failure of normal twisting during truncal septation.[16] Postnatally, the abnormal connection of the aorta and pulmonary artery results in two parallel circulations; with deoxygenated blood circulating to the body and oxygenated blood recirculating to the lungs. Patency of the foramen ovale and ductus arteriosus allows for mixing until surgical repair is performed. Prostaglandin is utilized to ensure the patency of the ductus arteriosus. In most newborns, cyanosis is present, and the foramen ovale needs to be enlarged to promote effective pulmonary blood flow. To enlarge the ASD, a balloon atrial septostomy is performed by introducing an umbilical or venous balloon-tipped catheter into the femoral vein. The balloon is inflated in the left atrium and then pulled across the septum, creating an ASD. This allows mixing between the two parallel circuits. Adequate shunting at the atrial level is the only way to improve arterial oxygenation and maintain hemodynamic stability prior to surgery.

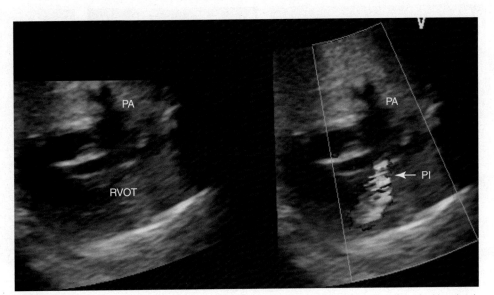

**FIGURE 16.19:** Color compare view of the short axis view of the heart showing significantly dilated pulmonary artery *(PA)*. Color Doppler demonstrates severe pulmonary insufficiency *(PI)*. RVOT, right ventricular outflow tract.

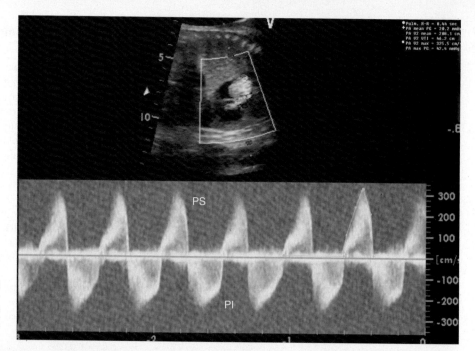

**FIGURE 16.20:** Pulse wave Doppler in the right ventricular outflow tract shows a to-and-fro pattern with systolic pulmonary stenosis *(PS)* with a peak gradient of 32 mm Hg and diastolic pulmonary insufficiency *(PI)*.

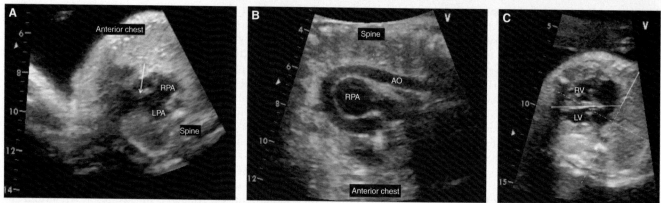

**FIGURE 16.21: A:** Fetal echocardiogram demonstrating severely dilated main and branch pulmonary arteries. *Arrow* indicates rudimentary pulmonary valve leaflets. **B:** Sagittal image showing a dilated right pulmonary artery in cross section. **C:** Transverse image of the fetal chest demonstrating marked left shift of the heart with right lung overexpansion and left lung hypoplasia vs. compression. LV, left ventricle, RV, right ventricle, AO, aorta, LPA, left pulmonary artery, RPA, right pulmonary artery. (From Chelliah A, Berger JT, Blask A, et al. Clinical utility of fetal magnetic resonance imaging in tetralogy of Fallot with absent pulmonary valve. *Circulation*. 2013;127[6]:757–759.)

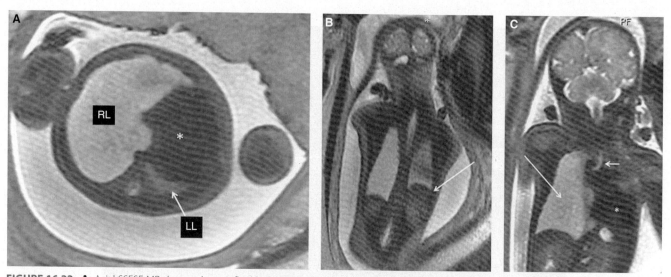

**FIGURE 16.22: A:** Axial SSFSE MR shows a hyperinflated right lung and severe left shift of the cardiac silhouette. LL, left lung, RL, right lung, *, heart. **B:** Coronal SSFSE MRI image demonstrating hyperinflated T2-bright right lung and decreased signal and volume of the left lung volume. *Arrow* points to elevated left hemidiaphragm. **C:** Additional coronal image demonstrates high-signal hyperinflated right lung *(long arrow)*, severe leftward cardiac shift, and compressed trachea *(short arrow)*. (From Chelliah A, Berger JT, Blask A, et al. Clinical utility of fetal magnetic resonance imaging in tetralogy of Fallot with absent pulmonary valve. *Circulation*. 2013;127[6]:757–759.)

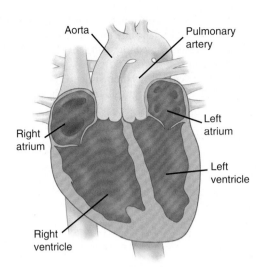

**FIGURE 16.23:** Illustration of complete transposition of the great arteries (D-TGA). (From Rice MJ, McDonald RW, Pilu G, et al. Cardiac malformations. In: Nyberg DA, McGahan JP, Pretorius DH, et al, eds. *Diagnostic Imaging of Fetal Anomalies.* Philadelphia, PA: Lippincott Williams & Wilkins; 2003:481.)

**Imaging:** D-Transposition of the great arteries can be very difficult to identify on routine prenatal ultrasound because the four-chamber view will be normal. In D-TGA with cranial angulation from the four-chamber view, the first great vessel that is visualized will be the pulmonary artery originating from the left ventricle. The second great vessel originating from the right ventricle will be the aorta. In addition, the great vessels rise in a parallel fashion more superiorly instead of the normal crossing orientation (Figs. 16.24 and 16.25). The foramen ovale should be evaluated in the bicaval view or a short axis view. The foramen ovale and anatomy of septum primum should be evaluated to determine the need for urgent septostomy after delivery. Deviation of the atrial septum into the right atrium suggests restriction of the foramen ovale. It is important to evaluate semilunar valvar size and presence of pulmonary or aortic valve stenosis as these may impact surgical repair.

**Associated Anomalies:** D-transposition of the great arteries is more common in males (3:1 ratio). Babies usually have normal chromosomes, and D-TGA is more common in infants of diabetic mothers. D-TGA may be associated with pulmonary stenosis, ASD, VSD (30% to 50%), and left ventricular outflow tract obstruction. If the aorta is hypoplastic, there may be hypoplasia of the arch (with coarctation of the aorta and interrupted aortic arch), or the pulmonary valve may be hypoplastic with associated main pulmonary artery/branch pulmonary artery hypoplasia.

**Treatment/Outcome:** D-transposition of the great arteries is often difficult to diagnose prenatally. Reports suggest that in the United Kingdom there is only a 25% prenatal detection rate without a VSD and a 40% detection rate with a VSD. In the United States, there is only a 19% prenatal detection rate.[17,18] Prenatal diagnosis is important for D-TGA because newborns rely on patency of the foramen ovale for mixing of the oxygenated and deoxygenated blood, and with foramen ovale closure newborns become extremely compromised in the delivery room.[19] Optimally, delivery should be at a tertiary care center with cardiology available if an urgent balloon septostomy

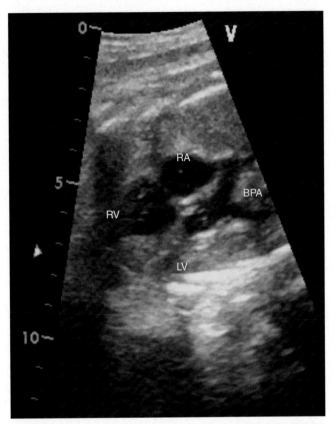

**FIGURE 16.24:** Anteriorly angled four-chamber view of the fetal heart. The first great vessel that is visualized is the pulmonary artery with the branch pulmonary arteries *(BPA)*. RA, right atrium; RV, right ventricle; LV, left ventricle.

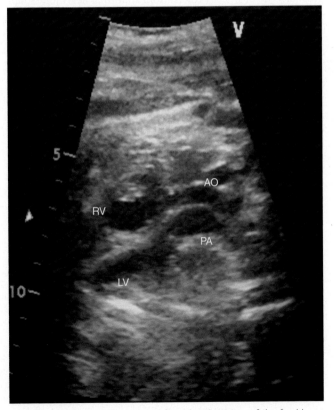

**FIGURE 16.25:** Anteriorly angled four-chamber view of the fetal heart demonstrating parallel great arteries. RV, right ventricle; AO, aorta; LV, left ventricle; PA, pulmonary artery.

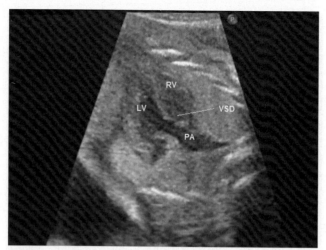

**FIGURE 16.26:** Corrected transposition of the great arteries. Anteriorly angled four chamber image of SLL TGA, demonstrating a trabeculated right sided left ventricle *(LV)* which gives rise to the pulmonary artery *(PA)* and a left sided right ventricle *(RV)*. There is also a ventricular septal defect *(VSD)*.

is needed. The arterial switch is the operation of choice for D-TGA. The great vessels are transected and connected to the appropriate ventricle, and the coronary arteries are translocated to the neoaorta. The operative mortality is low and long-term outcome is good.

**L-Transposition:** Congenitally corrected transposition of the great arteries or L-TGA results from abnormal heart tube looping (L loop) resulting in ventricular inversion and atrioventricular discordance in which the right atrium is connected to the left ventricle to the pulmonary artery, and the left atrium to the right ventricle to the aorta (Fig. 16.26). Atrioventricular discordance is associated with transposition of the great arteries, and therefore the blue blood goes to the lungs, and the red blood to the body. Usually, these babies are not cyanotic unless there are associated defects. Inversion of the ventricles is recognized by identifying a right-sided mitral valve and a left-sided tricuspid valve. In addition, the left-sided ventricle will be coarsely trabeculated and have a moderator band. L-TGA is commonly

associated with a VSD or pulmonary stenosis. Heart block may be associated with L-TGA. The outcome of patients with L-TGA is dependent on the associated anomalies, including VSD, pulmonary stenosis, and heart block. Given that patients with L-TGA have a right ventricle as their systemic pump, over their lifetime significant tricuspid regurgitation and heart failure may develop.[20]

### Truncus Arteriosus

**Definition:** In truncus arteriosus, a single outflow tract originates from the heart, with a conoventricular-type VSD. The single outflow tract gives rise to the systemic, pulmonary, and coronary circulation.

**Incidence:** Truncus arteriosus occurs in 1% to 1.5% of all live births with CHD.[1]

**Pathology and Hemodynamics:** Truncus arteriosus is classified into four subtypes.[21] Type I has a main pulmonary artery segment that gives rise to confluent branch pulmonary arteries with no patent ductus arteriosus; type II has no main pulmonary artery segment, and the branch pulmonary arteries arise from the back of the truncus in close proximity to one another with no PDA; in type III, the branch pulmonary arteries arise separately, and one may originate from the ductus arteriosus; and type IV is associated with coarctation of the aorta and interrupted aortic arch (Fig. 16.27). Type I and II do not require prostaglandin after birth. Newborns with truncus arteriosus will often present with congestive heart failure secondary to pulmonary over circulation and truncal valve insufficiency if not diagnosed prenatally.

**Associated Anomalies:** One-third of babies with truncus arteriosus will have 22q11 deletion.

**Imaging:** The four-chamber view will show four normal chambers; however, with cranial angulation the VSD and single outflow tract will be appreciated (Fig. 16.28). The VSD is large and also seen in short and long axis images. Delineation of the pulmonary arteries is important as they can have variable origins. The truncal valve is best seen in the short axis. Most of the time the truncal valve is tricuspid; however, it can be unicuspid or quadricuspid. The truncal valve may be both stenotic and

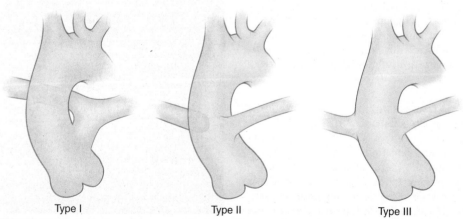

Type I            Type II            Type III

**FIGURE 16.27:** Illustration of the types of truncus arteriosus. (From Rice MJ, McDonald RW, Pilu G, et al. Cardiac malformations. In: Nyberg DA, McGahan JP, Pretorius DH, et al, eds. *Diagnostic Imaging of Fetal Anomalies*. Philadelphia, PA: Lippincott Williams & Wilkins; 2003:479.)

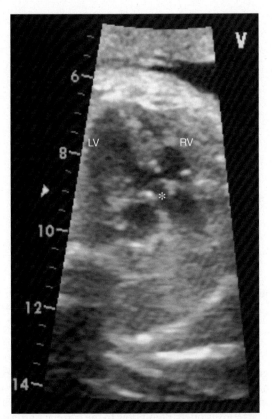

**FIGURE 16.28:** Anteriorly angled four-chamber image of truncus arteriosus with a single large vessel, the common trunk *(asterisk)*, overriding a large ventricular septal defect. RV, right ventricle; LV, left ventricle.

insufficient, and therefore color and pulse wave Doppler interrogation should be performed (Fig. 16.29).

**Treatment/Outcome:** Neonatal repair is typically performed. The repair usually includes closing the VSD to the aortic trunk and placement of a valved homograft from the right ventricle

to the pulmonary arteries; often they are transected from the main trunk. Additional surgeries are needed to replace the right ventricle to pulmonary artery conduit, and possibly repair or replace the truncal valve.

### Double Outlet Right Ventricle

**Definition:** In double outlet right ventricle (DORV), both the aorta and the pulmonary artery arise from the right ventricle (Fig. 16.30). The ventricles can be normal in size and position, or there can be right or left ventricular hypoplasia.

**Incidence:** DORV constitutes 1% to 1.5% of all live births with CHD.[1]

**Pathology and Hemodynamics:** DORV can be classified into subtypes by VSD location and postnatal cardiac physiology. The VSD can be described as subaortic (50%), subpulmonary (30%), doubly committed, or remote. DORV with a subaortic VSD will have similar physiology to a large VSD, although some may be cyanotic ("tetralogy like") if there is associated pulmonary stenosis. DORV with a subpulmonary-type VSD will have similar pathophysiology to D-TGA with large VSD. A Taussing–Bing type of DORV consists of a subpulmonary VSD, no pulmonary stenosis, side-by-side great vessels and bilateral conus. A doubly committed VSD sits below both arterial valves. A remote VSD is typically inlet or muscular and remote from both the aorta and the pulmonary valves. The relationship of the VSD to the great vessels and the presence of outflow tract obstruction determine postnatal hemodynamics and symptoms that may include congestive heart failure or cyanosis.

**Associated Anomalies:** Chromosomal anomalies may be seen including T13, T18, 22q11, and heterotaxy syndrome. There may be varying anomalies of the atrioventricular valves with straddling, atresia, or overriding. Heterotaxy syndrome should be considered, especially if there are associated atrioventricular canal defects or if there are anomalies of abdominal and atrial situs and/or pulmonary and systemic venous return.

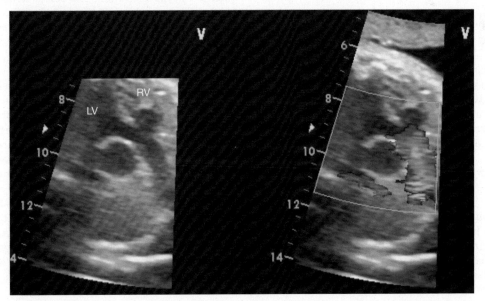

**FIGURE 16.29:** Color compare view of the truncal valve. Color Doppler should be performed to evaluate for truncal stenosis or insufficiency. The origins of the branch pulmonary arteries should be identified. RV, right ventricle; LV, left ventricle.

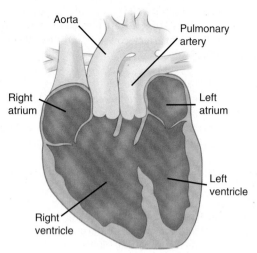

**FIGURE 16.30:** Illustration of double outlet right ventricle. (From Rice MJ, McDonald RW, Pilu G, et al. Cardiac malformations. In: Nyberg DA, McGahan JP, Pretorius DH, et al, eds. *Diagnostic Imaging of Fetal Anomalies.* Philadelphia, PA: Lippincott Williams & Wilkins; 2003:478.)

**Imaging:** Definitive diagnosis is demonstrated by visualizing both great vessels arising from the right ventricle. There may be valvar or subvalvar obstruction of either outflow tract. The four-chamber view may be normal or show hypoplasia of either ventricle. Careful sweeps cranially of the outflow tracts will demonstrate the VSD and that the right ventricle gives rise to both the great vessels. If there is aortic stenosis there may be coarctation of the aorta or interrupted aortic arch. Similarly, with valvar or subvalvar pulmonary obstruction there may be hypoplasia of the branch pulmonary arteries.

**Treatment/Outcome:** These patients most often undergo surgery in the neonatal period, with the ultimate goal of establishing unobstructed flow to both outflow tracts and closure of the VSD. In some cases, associated defects prohibit a two ventricle repair, and single ventricle palliation is warranted.

## Single Ventricle Anomalies

### *Hypoplastic Left Heart Syndrome*

**Definition:** Hypoplastic left heart syndrome (HLHS) is a spectrum of disease in which the left side of the heart cannot support the systemic circulation. HLHS may be secondary to mitral atresia or stenosis, aortic atresia or stenosis, DORV with mitral atresia or stenosis, unbalanced AVC to the right with left ventricular hypoplasia, or critical aortic stenosis with evolving HLHS (Fig. 16.31).

**Incidence:** HLHS accounts for 1.2% to 1.5% of all CHD live births.

**Associated Anomalies:** HLHS may be associated with Turner syndrome (XO), Jacobsen syndrome (deletion of distal 11q), trisomy 13, and trisomy 18.[22,23] However, most children with HLHS do not have a syndrome or significant extracardiac anomalies. HLHS is more common in males than in females.

**Pathology and Hemodynamics:** The most common form of HLHS is due to aortic atresia. Many of these children will also have mitral valve abnormalities (mitral valve hypoplasia, stenosis, or atresia). The ascending aorta will be diminutive with

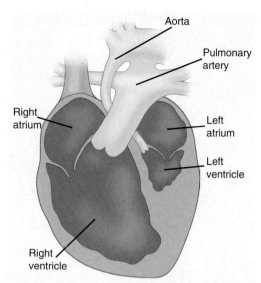

**FIGURE 16.31:** Illustration of hypoplastic left heart syndrome. (From Rice MJ, McDonald RW, Pilu G, et al. Cardiac malformations. In: Nyberg DA, McGahan JP, Pretorius DH, et al, eds. *Diagnostic Imaging of Fetal Anomalies.* Philadelphia, PA: Lippincott Williams & Wilkins; 2003:472.)

retrograde flow. Survival after birth with aortic valve atresia is dependent on patency of the ductus arteriosus. The right ventricle supplies both pulmonary and systemic blood flow with the ductus arteriosus open. Blood flow to the coronary arteries and head and neck vessels is supplied in a retrograde fashion. This is noted as reversed flow in the isthmus and transverse aortic arch. The size and restriction of the foramen ovale will impact both systemic and pulmonary blood flow at delivery.

HLHS with an intact or nearly intact atrial septum is associated with significant morbidity and mortality. This may be in part due to damage to the lung parenchyma in utero from elevated pulmonary venous pressures. If HLHS with a restrictive/intact atrial septum is not diagnosed prenatally, these newborns become severely ill in the delivery room, given that blood is unable to exit the left atrium. This results in hypoxemia, acidosis, and pulmonary edema. Even when identified prenatally and an urgent balloon septostomy is performed, outcomes are poor. Fetal intervention to open the atrial septum with either septoplasty or stent placement to minimize damage to the pulmonary bed has been reported.[24–27]

An important subtype of HLHS is severe aortic stenosis with evolving HLHS.[28–30] HLHS secondary to aortic stenosis is believed to have had a normally formed left ventricle early in gestation.[31,32] As the aortic stenosis becomes more severe, the left ventricle becomes injured with left ventricular dilation, scarring, and reversal of flow at the foramen ovale and transverse arch. With scarring, seen as bright endocardium (endocardial fibroelastosis) on imaging, blood is diverted away from the left ventricular cavity, which ultimately becomes hypoplastic. Some centers perform fetal intervention to prevent the development of HLHS in this disease.[28] In one large experience, of 70 fetuses who had in utero aortic balloon valvuloplasty, the procedure was technically successful in 74%, and greater than 30% of babies went on to have a biventricular repair, and another 8% were converted to a biventricular repair after initial univentricular palliation.[28]

In utero the presence of HLHS is well tolerated as the right ventricle can support the fetal circulation. After delivery, the systemic and the coronary circulation is dependent on the patency of the ductus arteriosus. As the patent ductus arteriosus closes,

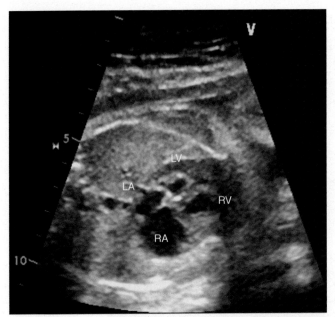

**FIGURE 16.32:** Apical four-chamber view of hypoplastic left heart syndrome. A hypoplastic, echogenic left ventricle *(LV)* is easily visualized. The left atrium *(LA)* appears hypoplastic, and the mitral valve appears bright and abnormal as well. RA, right atrium; RV, right ventricle.

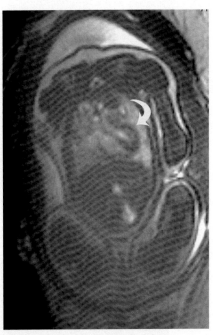

**FIGURE 16.33:** Coronal SSFP MR demonstrates a hypoplastic left ventricle with thick walls *(arrow)*.

infants not prenatally diagnosed may present with lethargy, pallor, difficulty breathing, low cardiac output, and acidosis. Of note, there is usually no heart murmur. Prostaglandin is indicated immediately after delivery to maintain ductal patency. Even this circulation is tenuous as there is a delicate balance between pulmonary and systemic circulation, and therefore, these infants should be cared for by centers with significant experience in pediatric cardiology.

**Imaging:** Left ventricular hypoplasia is recognizable in the four-chamber view, although early in pregnancy if there are patent mitral and aortic valves, left ventricular hypoplasia may be subtle. The left ventricle may appear hyperechoic from endocardial fibroelastosis (Figs. 16.32 and 16.33). The mitral and

aortic annuli usually measure small with decreased leaflet motion. Retrograde flow in the transverse arch suggests that there is inadequate left ventricular outflow (Fig. 16.34). Another important finding is abnormal reversed color Doppler flow across the foramen ovale. Foramen ovale flow and pulmonary venous Doppler should be evaluated to assess degree of foramen ovale obstruction given that an associated restrictive or intact atrial septum is associated with poor outcomes. Pulmonary venous Doppler with reversed flow (f/r < 3) suggests severe restriction and has been shown to be associated with need for intervention (Fig. 16.35).[33–35] The use of color Doppler is also important in the four-chamber view to evaluate for tricuspid insufficiency. Finally, right ventricular function should be assessed. Decreased right ventricular function and significant

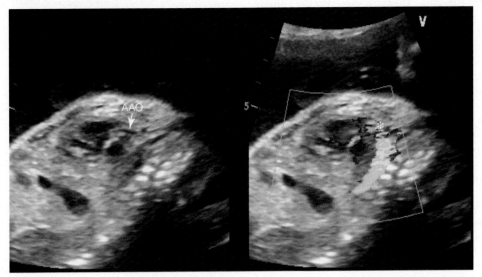

**FIGURE 16.34:** Color compare view of sagittal long axis view of the fetal heart. The ascending aorta *(AAO)* is labeled and may be overlooked given its diminutive size. Color Doppler demonstrates retrograde flow, denoted by the *red* flow and *asterisk*.

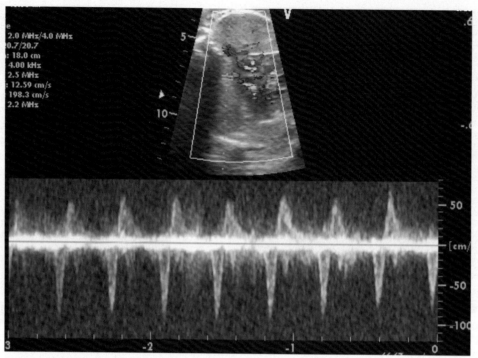

**FIGURE 16.35:** Pulsed Doppler in the pulmonary vein shows no diastolic flow and a biphasic pattern with an f/r < 3, suggesting significant obstruction.

tricuspid insufficiency may be associated with hydrops and poor outcomes.

**Treatment/Outcome:** Surgical repair for HLHS consists of a three-staged palliation. The Norwood operation, introduced in the 1980s, includes reconstruction of the aortic arch using the pulmonary valve and main pulmonary artery and establishment of pulmonary blood flow via a Blalock-Taussing shunt (aortic to pulmonary artery shunt). More recently, the Blalock-Taussing shunt has been replaced by the Sano shunt (RV to PA conduit) in many centers. The second stage is the bidirectional Glenn or hemi-Fontan, which entails connecting the superior vena cava to the pulmonary artery with takedown of the Blalock-Taussing or Sano shunt at 4 to 6 months. The third surgery is the Fontan, which baffles the inferior vena cava and hepatic veins to the branch pulmonary arteries at 2 to 4 years of age. Overall surgical survival is approximately 80%. HLHS with an intact atrial septum has a worse prognosis with early survival at only 33% owing to damage to lung parenchyma and vasculature from left atrial hypertension.[36]

### Tricuspid Atresia

**Definition:** In tricuspid atresia, the tricuspid valve is absent with usually some degree of associated right ventricular hypoplasia.

**Incidence:** Tricuspid atresia occurs in 1% to 3% of all live births with CHD.[1]

**Pathology and Hemodynamics:** Tricuspid atresia is divided into two types, type I with normally related great vessels (70%), and type II with transposition of the great arteries (30%). There may be an associated VSD or ASD, and there is usually some degree of right ventricular hypoplasia (Fig. 16.36). Postnatal presentation depends on the size of VSD if present, the degree

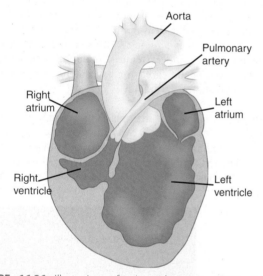

**FIGURE 16.36:** Illustration of tricuspid atresia. (From Rice MJ, McDonald RW, Pilu G, et al. Cardiac malformations. In: Nyberg DA, McGahan JP, Pretorius DH, et al, eds. *Diagnostic Imaging of Fetal Anomalies.* Philadelphia, PA: Lippincott Williams & Wilkins; 2003:484.)

of right outflow tract obstruction, and the position of the great vessels.

**Imaging:** Atresia of the tricuspid valve and hypoplasia of the right ventricle is readily apparent in the four-chamber view. The foramen ovale must be patent with right to left flow to allow egress from the right atrium. A large VSD will be apparent in the four-chamber view. The great vessels should carefully be inspected as they may be normally related or transposed. There will usually be some degree of pulmonary stenosis if the great vessels are normally related; therefore, careful color and pulse Doppler should be performed. Alternatively, there may be aortic stenosis, coarctation of the aorta, or interrupted aortic arch if there is transposition of the great arteries. Reversal of ductal flow suggests ductal-dependent pulmonary circulation. Tricuspid atresia may be associated with ventricular inversion.

**Treatment/Outcome:** Palliation for tricuspid atresia is dependent on additional defects present. Depending on the degree of pulmonary blood flow, infants may have no operation at birth, pulmonary artery banding, or a Blalock-Taussing shunt. If transposition is present, the aortic arch may need repair. Infants will ultimately undergo staged single ventricle repair with a bidirectional Glenn and then Fontan. Outcomes for patients with a Fontan palliation for tricuspid atresia are similar to HLHS with approximately 80% survival at 10 years. Long-term complications include heart failure, arrhythmias, and the need for reoperation.

### Double-Inlet Left Ventricle

**Definition:** Double-inlet left ventricle (DILV) is diagnosed when both atrioventricular valves empty into a single dominant left ventricle with right ventricular outlet chamber giving rise to one or both great arteries originating. The left ventricle is connected to the right ventricle via a VSD or "bulboventricular foramen."

**Incidence:** DILV is an uncommon lesion occurring in 0.01% of CHD live births. It is usually associated with ventricular inversion though it can occur with atrioventricular concordance.

**Diagnosis:** From a four-chamber view, the single left ventricle is seen with two atrioventricular valves emptying into it. The atrioventricular valves may be normal, or one may be stenotic or atretic. Typically, the pulmonary artery arises from the left ventricle and the aorta from an outlet chamber (transposed great vessels). Color and pulse wave Doppler should be performed to determine whether there is associated aorta or pulmonary obstruction. Color Doppler should also be performed to evaluate for atrioventricular valve regurgitation. Significant valve regurgitation may be associated with the development of hydrops. CHB may be present, especially if there is ventricular inversion.

**Treatment/Outcome:** Surgical management and outcome depends on the associated defects. Ultimately, single ventricle palliation with Fontan is performed.

## Arterial Abnormalities

### Coarctation of the Aorta

**Definition:** Coarctation of the aorta is a narrowing of the aorta typically just distal to the origin of the left subclavian artery (juxtaductal).

**Incidence:** Coarctation of the aorta represents 3% to 4% of all live births with CHD.

**Pathophysiology and Hemodynamics:** Coarctation of the aorta typically presents in the first days of life as the ductus arteriosus closes. Ductal tissue is present around the posterior aspect of the aorta and as the ductus constricts the arch narrows. Postnatally, coarctation should be considered if the lower extremity pulses are decreased and there is greater than a 10 mm Hg gradient between the upper and the lower extremity blood pressures. At birth, decreased saturations in the lower extremities indicate right to left shunting at the level of the ductus arteriosus in severe coarctation. Prostaglandin infusion is indicated to maintain ductal flow to ensure adequate perfusion to the lower extremities.

**Associated Anomalies:** Coarctation of the aorta may be associated with many other types of heart disease, most often other left-sided defects. Fifty percent of the cases with coarctation will have a bicuspid aortic valve.[37] Approximately one-third of infants with Turner syndrome will have coarctation. Coarctation of the aorta may also be seen in conjunction with ASDs, VSDs, DORV, or HLHS.

**Imaging:** Coarctation is difficult to diagnose in the fetus. Signs that suggest a coarctation include right ventricular dilation, hypertrophy, or dysfunction, or tricuspid insufficiency. Imaging of the aortic arch may reveal aortic isthmus hypoplasia, aliasing color Doppler, or diastolic runoff. (Fig. 16.37). In addition, in the three-vessel view, a size discrepancy between the transverse aorta and the ductus or abnormal color flow may be noted.

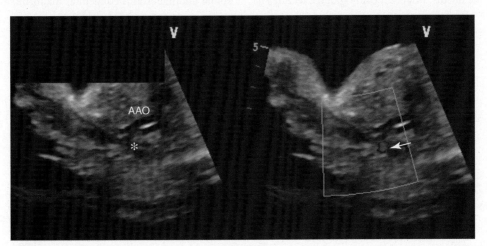

**FIGURE 16.37:** Sagittal long axis imaging of the fetal aortic arch with color compare demonstrates a very hypoplastic aortic isthmus *(asterisk)* in comparison with the ascending aorta *(AAO)*. Color compare denotes diastolic flow, as indicated by the *blue* color and *arrow.*

If coarctation is suspected, other left-sided structures should be closely examined, as there is an increased incidence of aortic and mitral valve anomalies. Color Doppler should also be performed to evaluate for VSDs.

**Treatment/Outcome:** Definitive diagnosis of coarctation of the aorta cannot be made until after delivery. If a significant coarctation is diagnosed at less than 2 years of age, surgical repair is indicated. Older patients may be eligible for catheter-based intervention such as angioplasty or stent placement. Patients with coarctation of the aorta need lifelong monitoring. Patients have increased rates of hypertension and atherosclerotic heart disease, and may have residual or recurrent obstruction. For those patients with recurrent obstruction, catheter-based intervention with angioplasty/stent placement is generally recommended.

### Interrupted Aortic Arch

Interrupted aortic arch is a severe type of coarctation in which the ascending and descending aorta are discontinuous, with the descending aorta supplied by the ductus arteriosus. There are three types of arch interruption. In type A, the interruption occurs distal to the left subclavian artery. In type B, interruption occurs between the left carotid and left subclavian arteries. Type C interruption occurs after the innominate artery and is very rare (Fig. 16.38). Interrupted aortic arch may be overlooked on fetal imaging because there will be a normal four-chamber image, normal crossing outflow tracts, and good heart function. However, there may be right ventricular dilation in the four-chamber view. In the aortic arch views, there will be an inability to connect the ascending and descending aorta. A malalignment-type VSD is usually present with a type B interruption and present in about in half of type A cases. Interrupted aortic arch may be associated with 22q11 deletion. All neonates with interrupted aortic arch will need prostaglandin infusion to maintain ductal patency. Surgical repair is performed in the newborn period.

### Restriction or Closure of the Ductus Arteriosus

A patent ductus arteriosus is a normal fetal structure, and premature closure can lead to right-sided heart failure in utero. Treatment with indomethacin or other nonsteroidal anti-inflammatory drugs for tocolysis may result in premature restriction or closure of the ductus. Fetal echocardiographic features of restrictive or closure of the ductus include right ventricular dilation with right ventricular dysfunction, tricuspid insufficiency, and ductal narrowing with aliasing color Doppler and increased pulse wave Doppler in the ductal arch (Fig. 16.39). Typically, if the causative drug is discontinued, ductal patency is restored and the heart normalizes. However, in some cases premature closure of the ductus in utero is associated with postnatal right ventricular dysfunction and pulmonary artery hypertension.[38]

## Venous Anomalies

### Anomalies of Systemic Venous Connections

A common anomaly of the systemic veins is bilateral superior vena cavae with drainage of the left superior vena cava into the coronary sinus. This defect is usually suspected when an enlarged coronary sinus is noted in the four-chamber view (Fig. 16.40). This anatomy exists in 3% of the normal population; however, it is much more prevalent in patients with CHD.

### Interrupted Inferior Vena Cava

Interruption of the hepatic portion of the inferior vena cava is the most common anomaly of the inferior vena cava. Venous blood from the lower half of the body reaches the heart via the azygous vein, which drains into the superior vena cava. This finding may occur in isolation or can be associated with heterotaxy syndrome. An interrupted inferior vena cava is diagnosed when the hepatic portion of the inferior cava is absent; usually the azygous vein is visualized as a venous vessel posterior to the aorta. Color Doppler interrogation will demonstrate opposite color flow compared with the aorta (Fig. 16.41). If an interrupted inferior vena cava is documented, the heart should be examined to evaluate for complex CHD.

### Absent Ductus Venosus

The ductus venosus connects the portal and umbilical veins with the inferior vena cava. The ductus venosus acts as a sphincter to placental flow to protect the fetus from placental overcirculation. An absent ductus venosus results in umbilical venous flow directly to the inferior vena cava, another venous structure, or the right atrium. An absent ductus venosus may cause congestive heart failure or hydrops fetalis. In addition, with absent ductus venosus there is an increased rate of chromosomal anomalies and congenital malformations.[39] If an absent

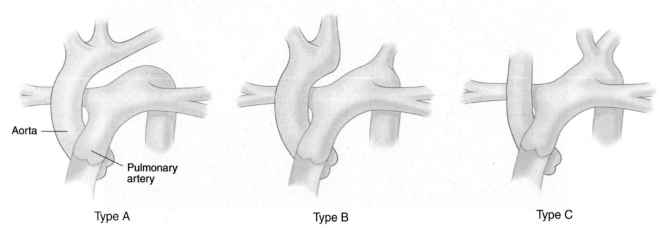

**FIGURE 16.38:** Illustration of the types of interrupted aortic arch. (From Rice MJ, McDonald RW, Pilu G, et al. Cardiac malformations. In: Nyberg DA, McGahan JP, Pretorius DH, et al, eds. *Diagnostic Imaging of Fetal Anomalies.* Philadelphia, PA: Lippincott Williams & Wilkins; 2003:470.)

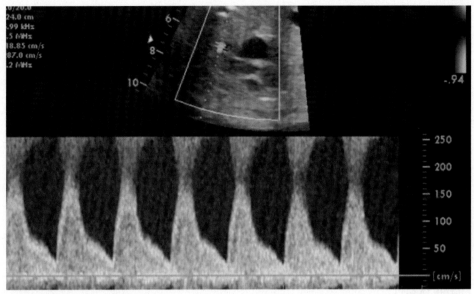

**FIGURE 16.39:** Pulse wave Doppler in a fetus with ductal restriction showing continuous diastolic flow and increased systolic velocity.

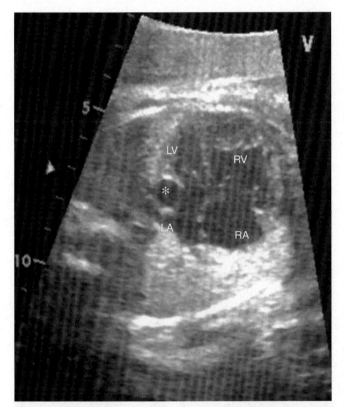

**FIGURE 16.40:** Apical four-chamber view showing a significantly dilated coronary sinus *(asterisk)*, indicating a left-sided superior vena cava. RA, right atrium; LA, left atrium; RV, right ventricle; LV, left ventricle.

ductus venosus is identified, a full cardiac evaluation should be performed (Fig. 16.42).

### Anomalies of Pulmonary Venous Connections

Some or all of the pulmonary veins can drain into the systemic circulation, entering above the heart (usually through a vertical vein into the innominate vein), into the heart (directly into the right atrium or into the coronary sinus), or below the heart (through the liver). If the pulmonary venous drainage becomes obstructed postnatally, infants will be critically ill and require lifesaving surgery in the newborn period. This most often occurs if the drainage is below the diaphragm. Abnormal drainage of all pulmonary veins, total anomalous pulmonary venous return, is suspected on fetal echocardiography when a small left atrium is seen in combination with a large right atrium and right ventricle and the pulmonary venous flow cannot be confirmed entering into the left atrium. In addition, in most fetuses an abnormal venous structure can be identified coursing behind the heart. Anomalous pulmonary venous drainage may be difficult to diagnose in the fetus because of the limited amount of the fetal cardiac output that enters the pulmonary circulation. Surgical repair is the only therapy for this condition. The prognosis is typically good if there is not venous obstruction; however, long-term follow-up is needed.

### Heterotaxy Syndrome

**Definition:** Heterotaxy syndrome (cardiosplenic syndrome, right and left isomerism, and situs ambiguous) is a disorder leading to abnormal arrangement of the abdominal viscera, thoracic organs, and cardiac atria across the left-right axis. In this disease, some organs are in the correct side, while others will be found on the opposite of the expected side, and the cardiac axis can be variable. Cardiac defects are usually present.

**Associated Anomalies:** In addition to right to left axis displacement, organs that typically are asymmetric, such as the lungs and atrial appendages, will develop in a symmetrical or mirror-image way. It is usual to find associated complex congenital heart malformations, and in some forms there are rhythm disturbances, such as CHB. There are also noncardiac abnormalities. The splenic function may be normal, marginal (if polysplenia), or absent (if asplenia), leading to potential immune deficiency. There might be gastrointestinal complications from increased incidence of malrotation, biliary atresia,

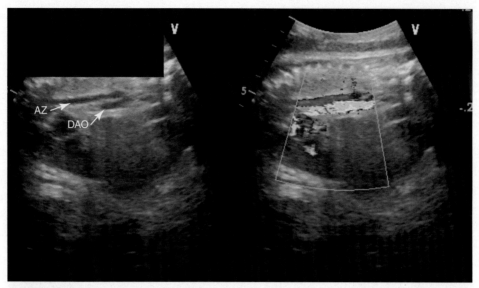

**FIGURE 16.41:** Color compare view of the azygous vein *(AZ)* located more posteriorly to the aorta *(DAO)*. Color Doppler demonstrates *blue*, superiorly directed blood, in the azygous vein compared with descending aortic flow directly inferiorly in *red*.

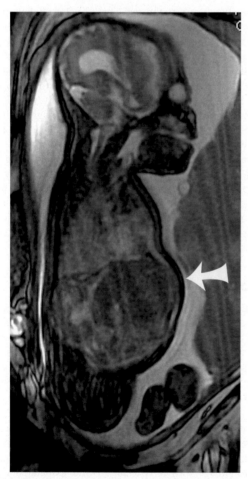

**FIGURE 16.42:** Sagittal SSFP image of the fetal chest and abdomen demonstrates absence of the ductus venosus *(arrow)*.

microgastria, and anorectal malformations. Other systems can also be affected, and craniofacial, renal, and CNS defects as well as musculoskeletal abnormalities have been observed in association with heterotaxy syndrome.[40]

**Diagnosis:** Correct determination of abdominal and cardiac situs is dependent on clear delineation of fetal position. There are two recognized subtypes of heterotaxy syndrome; *heterotaxy syndrome with asplenia* (characterized by isomerism of right atrial appendages) and *heterotaxy syndrome with polysplenia* (associated with isomerism of the left atrial appendages) (Fig. 16.43). However, not all patients show all the expected combinations for each category.

**Imaging:** Prenatal ultrasound and fetal MRI detection of heterotaxy syndrome requires a systematic approach that will start

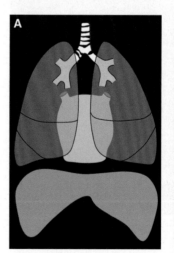
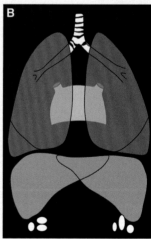

**FIGURE 16.43:** Diagrams of classic features in heterotaxy syndrome. **A:** Heterotaxy syndrome with asplenia, characterized by symmetric development of typical right-sided structures. There are trilobed lungs with bilateral minor fissures, eparterial bronchi (main bronchi superior to the ipsilateral pulmonary artery), bilateral systemic atria, midline liver, absent spleen, and variable position of the stomach. **B:** Heterotaxy syndrome with polysplenia, characterized by symmetric development of typical left-sided structures. There are bilateral bilobed lungs with hyparterial bronchi (main bronchi caudal to ipsilateral pulmonary arteries), bilateral pulmonary atria, midline/right or left-sided liver, variable position of the stomach, and multiple spleens along the greater curvature of the stomach.

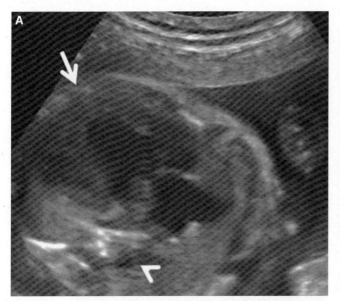 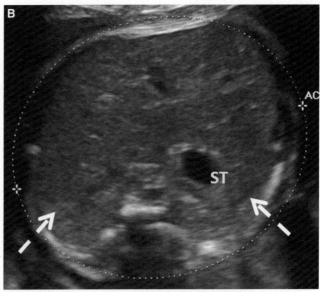

**FIGURE 16.44:** 33-Week gestation.Heterotaxy syndrome with asplenia. US transverse views through the chest **(A)** and abdomen **(B)**. The fetus is in vertex presentation and supine position (fetal spine close to maternal spine). Cardiac apex *(arrow)* is left-sided, and the stomach *(ST)* and descending aorta *(arrowhead)* are on the right. The liver is symmetric *(dashed arrows)*, and posterior/lateral to the stomach there is no splenic tissue. Cardiac findings were consistent with complete atrioventricular canal.

describing the fetal situs. This will be determined by the fetal orientation within the uterus and fetal lie, and should be performed at the beginning of any exam.[41] Then, the position of the organs will be defined. Heterotaxy syndrome should be suspected if there is discordance between the position of the stomach and the cardiac apex and/or if there is a midline symmetric liver (Fig. 16.44). Cardiac malformations are present in 50% to nearly 100% of the cases. Defining the type of atrial appendage helps to identify the subtype of heterotaxy syndrome. This may need to be inferred from the associated cardiac and vascular defects.

In the setting of heterotaxy syndrome with asplenia, typical findings include intact inferior vena cava on the same side of the aorta, bilateral superior vena cavae (70%), total anomalous pulmonary venous return to a systemic vein (58%), CAVC (69%), DORV (82%), and dextrocardia (36%).

Typical features of heterotaxy syndrome with polysplenia include interrupted inferior vena cava with azygous continuation (80%), bilateral superior vena cavae (50%), total anomalous pulmonary venous return (2%), CAVC (33%), DORV (37%), and CHB.[42,43] Abnormal looping of the fetal heart can result in ventricular inversion.

Fetal imaging, including US and fetal MRI, will also be able to provide clues to define the subtype of heterotaxy on the basis of systemic vascular anatomy and noncardiac anomalies. Evaluation of the aorta and inferior vena cava is valuable in particular. In a transverse view of the upper abdomen of a fetus with situs solitus, the descending aorta is to the left and close to the spine, while the inferior vena cava is more anterior and to the right. Any variation from this standard arrangement can raise concern for heterotaxy syndrome, particularly if both vessels are on the same side. Another frequent variation of the venous system seen in heterotaxy syndrome is azygous continuation of the interrupted inferior vena cava. In this specific situation, the azygous vein is dilated, with similar size and parallel to the adjacent thoracic aorta (Fig. 16.45). Careful assessment of the fetal anatomy will be able to define potential associated noncardiac anomalies. In heterotaxy syndrome with asplenia, the spleen is

most frequently absent, and microgastria and imperforate anus have also been described.

In heterotaxy with polysplenia multiple, small, poorly functioning spleens are expected, and biliary atresia (typically represented by a persistently absent gallbladder) is seen in up to 10%. Note is made that in utero, it might not be possible to detect more than one spleen, given the frequent small size of the splenules. However, our assessment should try to be as definitive as possible in regard to presence or absence of the spleen, which would be expected in the area adjacent to the stomach (Fig. 16.46).

In both subtypes, intestinal malrotation is a common association (up to 70%) that could potentially be detected during the third trimester with fetal MRI (Fig. 16.47).[44]

Some preliminary studies have reported the use of fetal cardiac MRI for the characterization of cardiovascular morphology and function.[45,46]

**Treatment/Outcome:** The prognosis is dependent on the type of CHD. The majority of heterotaxy cases, however, are associated with complex heart diseases and therefore have significant morbidity and mortality. Furthermore, the complexity of care for these patients is increased because of comorbid diagnosis such as immune deficiency, malrotation, or other gastrointestinal anomalies.

Recent studies have shown that 42% of patients with CHD and heterotaxy syndrome have ciliary dysfunction.[47] Embryonic cilia are critical in establishing right-left axis, patterning, and location of organ situs. Primary ciliary dysfunction likely plays a role in the development of heterotaxy syndrome and may be implicated in outcomes with increased risk of respiratory complications.

## Fetal Cardiac Tumors

The prevalence of cardiac tumors is approximately 0.14% in pregnancies referred for fetal echocardiography.[48] Rhabdomyomas

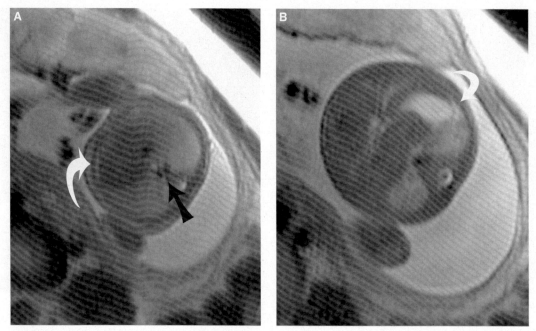

**FIGURE 16.45:** 26-Week gestation. Heterotaxy syndrome with asplenia. Axial T2w MR images demonstrate dextrocardia *(curved arrow)* **(A)** and asplenia *(curved arrow)* **(B)** as well as interrupted inferior vena cava with azygous continuation *(black arrow)*.

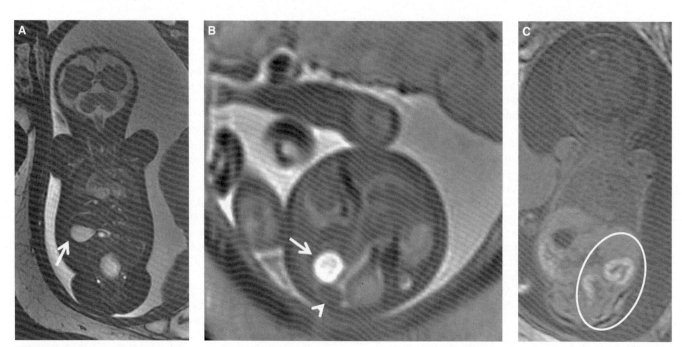

**FIGURE 16.46:** 28-Week gestation. Heterotaxy syndrome with polysplenia. T2w MR images, Coronal 2D SSFP **(A)** and axial SSFSE **(B)** as well as T1-WI coronal FSPGR **(C)**. There is a discordant abdominal situs with a right-sided stomach *(arrow)*. The liver is symmetric. Splenic tissue was noted adjacent and posterior to the greater curvature of the stomach *(arrowhead)*. T1-WI shows meconium-filled colon located only in the left abdomen *(ellipse)*, supporting intestinal malrotation.

are the most common, followed by fibromas and hemangiomas. Associated findings include hydrops fetalis, pericardial effusion, or a family history of tuberous sclerosis.[49–51]

Rhabdomyomas tend to increase in size prenatally and then regress after birth.[52–54] The association of rhabdomyomas with tuberous sclerosis is well documented.[55–58] Tuberous sclerosis has been found in 100% of cases of fetuses with multiple rhabdomyomas, and approximately 50% of fetuses with single

tumors and no family history. Arrhythmias may be seen with rhabdomyomas.[55] Rhabdomyomas are homogeneous and more echogenic than the surrounding myocardium. They may be found in the ventricular septum or free wall and may extend into the cardiac chambers (Fig. 16.48).

Fibromas represent 5% to 7% of all fetal cardiac tumors.[48,59] Fibromas are more likely to be associated with pericardial effusion, hydrops, heart failure, and fetal demise.[59] Fibromas

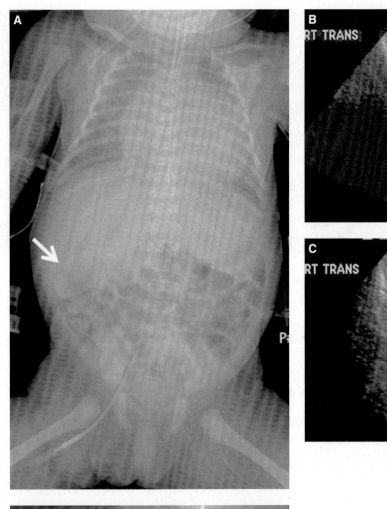

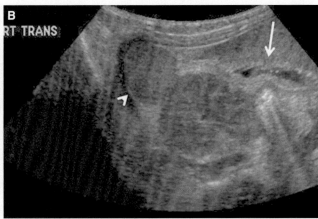

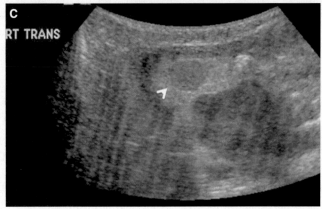

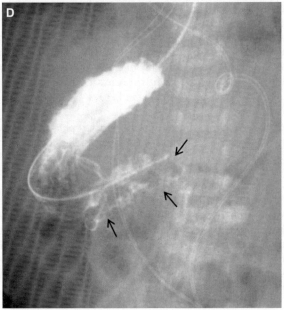

**FIGURE 16.47:** Heterotaxy syndrome with polysplenia. Postnatal assessment of same patient as in Figure 16.46. Chest-abdomen X-ray on 1st day of life (**A**) and axial ultrasound images (**B, C**). Two spleens *(arrowhead)* are noted adjacent to the right-sided stomach *(white arrow).* The most caudal spleen was not detectable in utero. **D:** Frontal view during upper gastrointestinal series (UGI) with contrast in the duodenum *(black arrows),* which never crossed the midline, in concordance with the prenatal concern for malrotation.

are often single and appear homogeneous.[48] Hemangiomas are uncommon in fetuses and children. They typically have mixed echogenicity due to cysts and calcifications.[48] Hemangiomas may also invade the atrioventricular node, and varying degrees of heart block may be seen.[55] Ultimately, hemangiomas may regress after birth.[59] Teratomas are rare as well and are typically extracardiac, intrapericardial, and attached to the aortic root or pulmonary artery.[60] These also have mixed echogenicity secondary to cysts and calcifications.[48] Fibromas and teratomas will not regress and may require surgery.

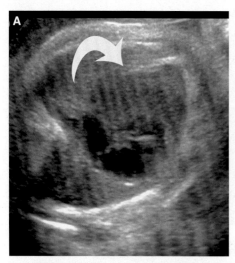
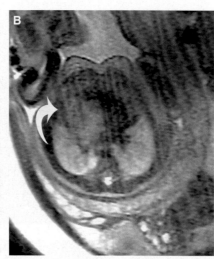
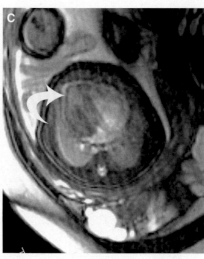

**FIGURE 16.48:** Rhabdomyoma, 35 weeks' gestation. **A:** Axial ultrasound demonstrates a large echogenic homogeneous mass filling the left ventricle *(arrow)*. Axial SSFSE **(B)** and axial SSFS **(C)** MR images confirm the presence of the intraventricular mass *(curved arrows)*, intermediate in signal.

Fetal cardiac tumors can be visualized using the four-chamber view and outflow. Imaging can identify size, location, and hemodynamic significance of the tumor. It is important to image with color Doppler to evaluate for atrioventricular valve regurgitation. Other important measures include assessment of heart function, presence of pericardial or pleural effusion, heart rate, and rhythm.

Echogenic foci are usually found in the left ventricle within a papillary muscle. In one study, 20% of second and third trimester fetuses had echogenic foci.[61] These foci may be distinguished from true tumors in that they are usually smaller and intensely echogenic (Fig. 16.49). Autopsies done on fetuses with abnormal chromosomes (most frequently trisomy 13 and 21) have demonstrated papillary calcification.[62–64] Echogenic foci do not increase in size and do not become clinically significant.[64–66] In a large prospective study of greater than 10,000 fetuses, isolated echogenic foci were benign and did not increase the risk of fetal

aneuploidy. Advanced maternal age (>35 years), abnormal biochemical markers, and/or other ultrasound markers were present in all fetuses found to have aneuploidy.[67]

## Cardiomyopathy

**Definition:** Primary hypertrophic cardiomyopathy is defined as hypertrophy of the ventricles, not in response to a pressure or volume overload. There is often normal systemic function but abnormal diastolic function. Dilated cardiomyopathy refers to primary dilation of the ventricles due to muscle dysfunction.

**Incidence:** Fetal cardiomyopathies are infrequent. Hypertrophic cardiomyopathy can be associated with genetic disorders (i.e., Noonan syndrome, mitochondrial disorders) or familial idiopathic hypertrophic cardiomyopathy. Dilated cardiomyopathies are rarer and are typically due to a myocarditis. The most common causes of myocarditis are coxsackievirus, cytomegalovirus, parvovirus, adenovirus, and herpes.[68,69]

**Imaging:** Imaging of a fetus with hypertrophic cardiomyopathy will demonstrate increased thickness of the septum and free wall. The systolic function will be normal. When hypertrophy is identified, evaluation for outflow tract obstruction should be performed with color and pulse wave Doppler to rule out primary valve disease. Fetuses with hypertrophic cardiomyopathies are at increased risk for arrhythmias. In dilated cardiomyopathy, the ventricles are enlarged, there is decreased function, and the septum and free wall are thin (Fig. 16.50). In both hypertrophic and dilated cardiomyopathies, atrioventricular valve regurgitation may be present and may be a precursor to heart failure and in utero fetal demise.

**Prognosis:** Hypertrophy secondary to maternal diabetes has a good outcome, with spontaneous resolution of the cardiomyopathy by 3 to 6 months of age. After delivery, infants with significant ventricular hypertrophy should have adequate preload as dehydration can result in dynamic outflow tract obstruction. In addition, inotropes should be avoided. Infants can be observed

**FIGURE 16.49:** Four-chamber view demonstrates the hyperechoic echogenic foci *(arrow)*. RA, right atrium; LA, left atrium; RV, right ventricle; LV, left ventricle.

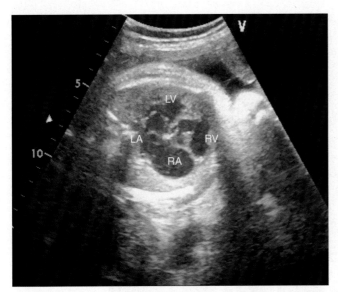

**FIGURE 16.50:** Apical four-chamber view demonstrating a severely dilated right atrium and right ventricle. The left-sided chambers are also dilated. RA, right atrium; LA, left atrium; RV, right ventricle; LV, left ventricle.

for symptoms, and supportive measures should be utilized if needed. Outcomes of the dilated cardiomyopathies are generally associated with a poor outcome, especially in the presence of hydrops or significant atrioventricular valve regurgitation.

## Fetal Arrhythmias

**Definition:** The normal fetal heart rate usually ranges from 120 to 160 bpm. Tachycardia is defined as greater than 180 bpm and bradycardia below 120 bpm.

**Incidence:** Fetal arrhythmia is a common indication for referral for fetal echocardiogram. Premature atrial contractions account for 70% to 80% of fetal arrhythmia, tachycardia for 10% to 15%, and bradycardia 8% to 12%.

**Imaging:** The mechanism of fetal arrhythmia can be determined using several modalities. Simultaneous M-mode echocardiography of the atrial and ventricular wall or semilunar valve can be used to assess the atrial and ventricular contraction and atrial–ventricular synchrony (Fig. 16.51). Alternatively, pulse Doppler can be performed within the left ventricle sampling mitral inflow (EA wave = atrial contraction) and aortic outflow (V = ventricular contraction) (Fig. 16.52). Simultaneous superior vena cava flow and aortic outflow can also be used (Fig. 16.53).

Often, analysis of the initiation and termination of the tachycardia or bradycardia is helpful in determining the mechanism of arrhythmia. A complete evaluation of the fetal heart structures should be performed to evaluate for structural heart disease. There may be ventricular dysfunction or atrioventricular valve insufficiency secondary to persistent arrhythmia. All fetuses with persistent arrhythmias (excluding occasional premature atrial contractions) should be followed for development of hydrops or other signs of fetal distress.

### Premature Atrial Contractions

Premature atrial contractions (PACs) are very common and most often are benign (Fig. 16.54). Frequent PACs in a bigeminy pattern with block will result in a fetal heart rate between 75 to 90 bpm when conduction is a 2:1 pattern.[70] No treatment is required unless supraventricular tachycardia (SVT) occurs. A baseline fetal echocardiogram to assess cardiac structure and auscultation of the fetal heart rate by the obstetrician or maternal fetal medicine specialist is recommended. Close follow-up is recommended to monitor for sustained SVT, which occurs in approximately 10% of fetuses with frequent PACs.

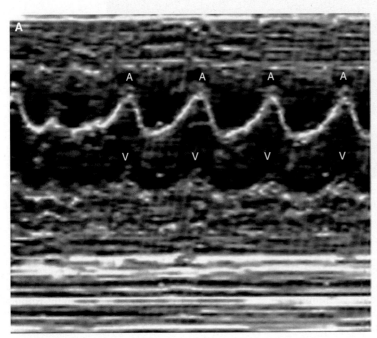

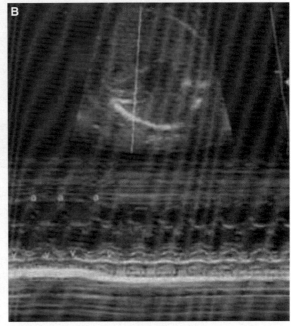

**FIGURE 16.51: A,B:** M-mode image of normal sinus rhythm. Atrial contraction is noted by *A* and ventricular contraction by a *V*.

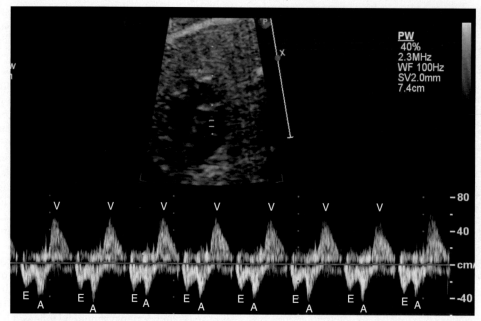

**FIGURE 16.52:** Pulse Doppler obtaining mitral inflow (E/A) and aortic outflow *(V)* demonstrating normal sinus rhythm.

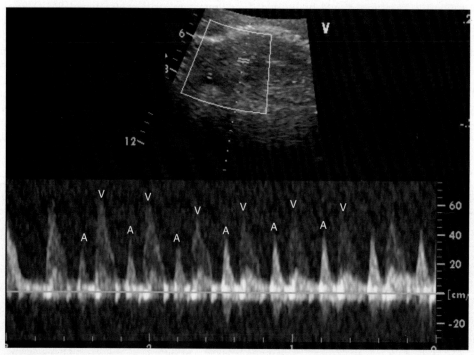

**FIGURE 16.53:** Doppler of superior vena cava flow indicating atrial contraction *(A)* and aortic flow indicating ventricular *(V)* contraction. This image demonstrates normal sinus rhythm.

### Supraventricular Tachycardia

Supraventricular tachycardia is typically due to an accessory conduction pathway between the atrium and the ventricle. The rate is usually 220 to 280 bpm (Fig. 16.55). There is 1:1 conduction between the atrium and the ventricle. Maternal administration of digoxin is often successful as a first-line drug in fetuses with SVT. Second-line drugs include sotalol, flecanide, and amiodarone. Drug initiation requires hospitalization for close monitoring of the mother and fetus.

### Atrial Flutter

Atrial flutter accounts for about 30% of fetal tachyarrhythmias and can be seen with myocarditis, CHD, or SSA/SSB isoimmunization.[71] Atrial flutter is due to a reentry circuit within the atrium. Typically, the atrial rate is greater than 300 bpm. There may be varying levels of block at the atrioventricular node (2:1 or 3:1 AV conduction) (Fig. 16.56). Sotalol is generally recommended as the first-line agent, although digoxin and amiodarone may be used.[72,73] After delivery, transesophageal

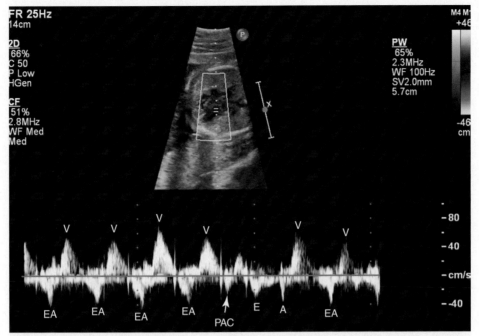

**FIGURE 16.54:** Pulse Doppler pattern of a premature atrial contraction *(PAC)*. The normal E/A wave pattern is disrupted.

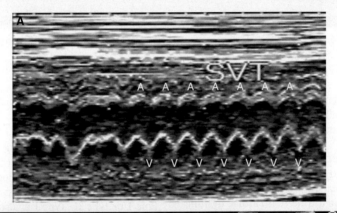

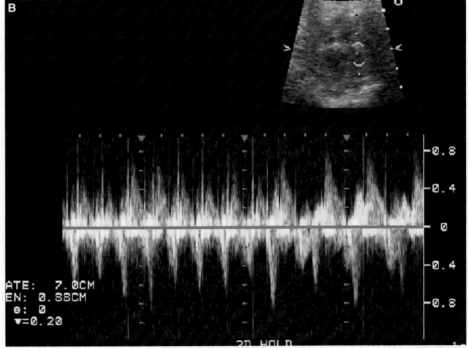

**FIGURE 16.55: A:** M-mode Doppler of supraventricular tachycardia; the heart rate is about 230 bpm. Note that the atrial *(A)* and ventricular *(V)* waves occur in a 1-to-1 pattern. **B:** Left-sided inflow and outflow Doppler demonstrating supraventricular tachycardia.

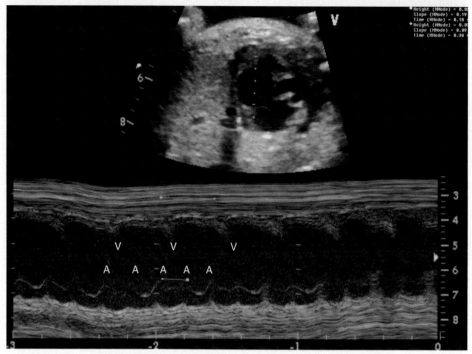

**FIGURE 16.56:** M-mode Doppler of atrial flutter. Note that the atrial rate *(A)* is twice that of the ventricular *(V)* rate.

pacing or synchronized cardioversion will convert the neonate to normal sinus rhythm. Typically, once converted to normal sinus rhythm, postnatal atrial flutter does not reoccur.

### Chaotic or Multifocal Atrial Tachycardia
Chaotic or multifocal atrial tachycardia is rare and is usually seen in the last trimester of pregnancy. The heart rate will be 180 to 220 bpm. Treatment is indicated if there is cardiac dysfunction or if the average HR heart rate is above 200 bpm. These arrhythmias are difficult to treat; however, digoxin, flecainide, or sotolol can be used.

### Ventricular Tachycardia
Ventricular tachycardia is rare in the fetus, and the heart rates are usually 150 to 250 bpm and there is dissociation between the ventricular and the atrial contraction. Ventricular tachycardia secondary to long QT syndrome (LQTS) is usually associated with both tachy and brady arrhythmias. Ventricular tachycardia may also be a complication of atrioventricular block, cardiac tumors, or myocarditis. Treatment is dependent on the etiology of the ventricular tachycardia, and may include dexamethasone, intravenous immunoglobulin (IVIG), magnesium, intravenous (IV) lidocaine, oral propranolol, or mexiletine.[74–79]

## Bradycardia

### Long QT Syndrome
Long QT Syndrome (LQTS) may present with persistent sinus bradycardia.[80,81] Management of the fetus with suspected LQTS includes close observation and postnatal evaluation. Fetal treatment is not recommended for bradycardia; however, torsade de pointes and ventricular tachycardia require treatment if they occur. Maternal electrolyte abnormalities (hypomagnesemia and hypocalcemia) should be avoided as well as drugs/anesthetics that prolong the QT interval.

### Atrioventricular Heart Block
**Definition:** First-degree heart block is defined as a PR interval >150 milliseconds. Second-degree heart block, defined as intermittent atrioventricular dissociation, can be subdivided into type I or type II. Type I is also known as Wenckebach and is characterized by progressive PR prolongation until there is a blocked atrial beat. Type II is an abrupt failure of AV conduction without prior PR prolongation. Type II second-degree heart block may progress to CHB. During second-degree AV block, there may be a repetitive conduction drop between the atrium and the ventricle, whereby there is a regular conduction ratio between the atrial and the ventricular beats (2:1 block, 3:1 block, etc.).

**Incidence:** CHB occurs when there is complete dissociation between the atria and the ventricle. The electrical impulses from the atrium do not signal the ventricle, and the ventricle beats independently. CHB may be due to congenitally malformed conduction system secondary to complex congenital heart disease (50% to 55%), to maternal autoantibodies (SSA/SSB) (40%), or to an undetermined etiology. In mothers with SSA antibodies, there is a 1% to 5% risk of CHB in the fetus if there is no prior affected pregnancy. The recurrence risk is 11% to 19% for women who have had a previously affected pregnancy.[82,83]

**Imaging:** CHB can be diagnosed by M-Mode or Doppler echocardiography. Serial Doppler assessment of the time between atrial and ventricular contraction is used for surveillance in maternal SSA positive patients to measure the PR interval to

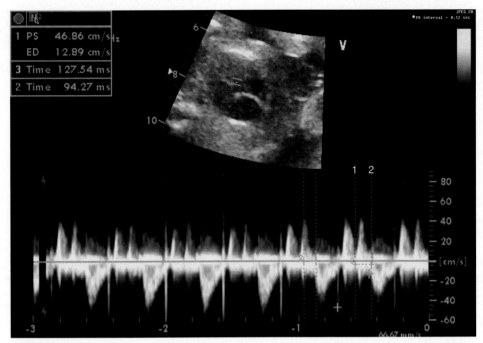

**FIGURE 16.57:** Assessment of the PR interval by mitral valve inflow Doppler and aortic outflow. The PR interval is measured by the time between the occurrence of the A wave *(1)* and the ventricular systole *(2)*.

detect primary heart block (Fig. 16.57).[84] Serial assessment at 1- to 2-week intervals starting at 16 weeks and continuing through 28 weeks' gestation is suggested. For previously affected pregnancies, weekly evaluation is recommended.

**Treatment:** Treatment of the CHB depends on etiology, ventricular rate, and presence and degree of heart failure. Heart rates below 55 to 60 bpm increase fetal risk. Maternal steroid, beta agonist, and IVIG treatment have been used with variable success in these patients, though timing of dosing and efficacy is still controversial.[85–87]

The majority of fetal arrhythmias can be controlled in utero. The prognosis is poor with hydrops. Most tachycardias with the exception of atrial flutter will need postnatal medical therapy. Fetuses with CHB will often ultimately need a pacemaker, and fetuses with LQTS will need continued medical therapy and monitoring.

## DELIVERY PLANNING

Delivery brings a transition from fetal to postnatal circulation. In fetal life, the right and left circulations are functionally connected in parallel; however, with delivery the low-resistance placental circulation is eliminated, and the pulmonary vascular bed and lungs expand. Postnatally, after foramen ovale and ductus arteriosus closure, the circulation functions in series, with the right heart ejecting to the lungs and the left heart to the body. The pulmonary vascular resistance falls, causing increased pulmonary blood flow, which results in a rise in left atrial pressure, which closes the foramen ovale. In addition, smooth muscle cells begin to close the ductus. The parallel circulation in utero allows major cardiac malformations with obstructed outflow to be well tolerated. However, after delivery the change in the circulation may result in inadequate pulmonary or systemic blood flow. Infants may present with cyanosis, hypotension, acidosis, heart failure, and shock.

Most fetuses with CHD will not have ductal or systemic dependent pulmonary blood flow. These babies can be delivered and cared for in local community hospitals. Some babies with significant heart disease can be born at an outlying hospital and stabilized by a neonatologist, and then transferred to a tertiary care center for further care. A small subset will need pediatric cardiology care and intervention immediately after delivery. Babies with defects at risk for compromise in the delivery room include HLHS with restrictive foramen ovale or intact atrial septum, D-TGA, uncontrolled tachycardia, heart block with low ventricular rate, severe Ebstein anomaly, tetralogy of Fallot with absent pulmonary valve, and others with cardiac dysfunction and heart failure. A risk stratification system developed at the Children's National Medical Center to help guide postnatal delivery and management is summarized in Table 16.2.[88] Most infants with CHD are assigned level of care (LOC) 1 and can deliver at an outlying hospital with elective cardiology consultations. Newborns with ductal-dependent pulmonary or systemic circulation are assigned LOC 2. These babies will require initiation of prostaglandin to maintain ductal patency by a neonatologist prior to transfer to the tertiary care center. Babies that need urgent intervention after delivery by a pediatric cardiologist, such as balloon atrial septostomy, are assigned LOC 3 or 4, depending on disease severity. Delivery in these complex cases is planned with a neonatology and cardiology team available to assess and care for the infant immediately after birth. For all CHD, regulation of systemic and pulmonary blood flow is critical to ensure adequate oxygenation and optimal organ perfusion.

Accurate prenatal diagnosis and understanding of the physiology of specific heart defects allow for a safe delivery at a local hospital when possible, or adequate planning for

| Table 16.2 | Definition of Congenital Heart Disease Level of Care Assignment and Coordinating Action Plan | | | |
|---|---|---|---|---|
| **LOC** | **Expected Physiology** | **Example CHD** | **Delivery Recommendations** | **Cardiac DR Recommendations** |
| 1 | No instability expected in first weeks of life | ASD, VSD, AVSD, mild valve disease | Delivery at local hospital | Arrange outpatient follow up |
| 2 | Stability in DR expected though requiring postnatal cath/surgery | Ductal-dependent lesions including HLHS, PA/IVS, severe TOF | Planned vaginal induction at ~39 weeks at local hospital; transport to cardiac center | Neonatalogist in DR; PGE if indicated |
| 3 | Instability requiring immediate specialty care in DR prior to cath/surgery | HLHS or TGA with RFO, CHD, or arrhythmia with decreased heart function | Planned vaginal induction at 38–39 wks close to cardiac center, C/S if necessary | Specialists in DR; medications predetermined by care plan |
| 4 | Instability requiring immediate cath/surgery in DR | HLHS or TGA with severe RFO or IAS, CHD or arrhythmia with hydrops | Planned C/S close to cardiac center at 38 weeks | Multidisciplinary team in DR; medications/equipment predetermined including ECMO if indicated |

LOC, level of care; CHD, congenital heart disease; DR, delivery room; ASD, atrial septal defect; VSD, ventricular septal defect; AVSD, atrioventricular septal defect; HLHS, hypoplastic left heart syndrome; PA/IVS, pulmonary atresia/intact ventricular septum; TOF, tetralogy of Fallot; PGE; TGA, transposition of the great arteries; RFO, restrictive foramen ovale; C/S, cesarean section; IAS, interatrial septum; ECMO, extracorporeal membrane oxygenation.
Revised from Donofrio MT, Levy RJ, Schuette JJ, et al. Specialized delivery room planning for fetuses with critical congenital heart disease. *Am J Cardiol.* 2013;111:737–747.

a multidisciplinary delivery at the tertiary hospital if indicated. Success is ultimately dependent on essential collaborations between the prenatal diagnostic team and the postnatal care team.

# REFERENCES

1. Fyler DC. Report of the New England Regional Infant Cardiac Program. *Pediatrics.* 1980;65:375–461.
2. Rastelli GC, Kirklin JW, Titus JL. Anatomic observations on complete form of persistent common atrioventricular canal with special reference to atrioventricular valves. *Mayo Clin Proc.* 1966;41:296–308.
3. Ferencz C, Rubin JD, McCarter RJ, et al. Congenital heart disease: prevalence at livebirth. The Baltimore-Washington Infant Study. *Am J Epidemiol.* 1985;121:31–36.
4. Sharland GK, Chita SK, Allan LD. Tricuspid valve dysplasia or displacement in intrauterine life. *J Am Coll Cardiol.* 1991;17:944–949.
5. Hornberger LK, Sahn DJ, Kleinman CS, et al. Tricuspid valve disease with significant tricuspid insufficiency in the fetus: diagnosis and outcome. *J Am Coll Cardiol.* 1991;17:167–173.
6. Respondek ML, Kammermeier M, Ludomirsky A, et al. The prevalence and clinical significance of fetal tricuspid valve regurgitation with normal heart anatomy. *Am J Obstet Gynecol.* 1994;171:1265–1270.
7. Krishnan AN, Sable CA, Donofrio MT. Spectrum of fetal echocardiographic findings in fetuses of women with clinical or serologic evidence of systemic lupus erythematosus. *J Matern Fetal Neonatal Med.* 2008;21:776–782.
8. Nakano H, Ueda K, Saito A. Acute hemodynamic effects of nitroprusside in children with isolated mitral regurgitation. *Am J Cardiol.* 1985;56:351–355.
9. Roman KS, Fouron JC, Nii M, et al. Determinants of outcome in fetal pulmonary valve stenosis or atresia with intact ventricular septum. *Am J Cardiol.* 2007;99:699–703.
10. Salvin JW, McElhinney DB, Colan SD, et al. Fetal tricuspid valve size and growth as predictors of outcome in pulmonary atresia with intact ventricular septum. *Pediatrics.* 2006;118:e415–e420.
11. Gardiner HM, Belmar C, Tulzer G, et al. Morphologic and functional predictors of eventual circulation in the fetus with pulmonary atresia or critical pulmonary stenosis with intact septum. *J Am Coll Cardiol.* 2008;51:1299–1308.
12. Tulzer G, Arzt W, Franklin RC, et al. Fetal pulmonary valvuloplasty for critical pulmonary stenosis or atresia with intact septum. *Lancet.* 2002;360:1567–1568.
13. Tworetzky W, McElhinney DB, Marx GR, et al. In utero valvuloplasty for pulmonary atresia with hypoplastic right ventricle: techniques and outcomes. *Pediatrics.* 2009;124:e510–e518.
14. Jahangiri M, Zurakowski D, Bichell D, et al. Improved results with selective management in pulmonary atresia with intact ventricular septum. *J Thorac Cardiovasc Surg.* 1999;118:1046–1055.
15. Chelliah A, Berger JT, Blask A, et al. Clinical utility of fetal magnetic resonance imaging in tetralogy of Fallot with absent pulmonary valve. *Circulation.* 2013;127(6):757–759.
16. Bockman DE, Kirby ML. Dependence of thymus development on derivatives of the neural crest. *Science.* 1984;223:498–500.
17. Blyth M, Howe D, Gnanapragasam J, et al. The hidden mortality of transposition of the great arteries and survival advantage provided by prenatal diagnosis. *BJOG.* 2008;115:1096–1100.
18. Friedberg MK, Silverman NH, Moon-Grady AJ, et al. Prenatal detection of congenital heart disease. *J Pediatr.* 2009;155:26–31.
19. Bonnet D, Coltri A, Butera G, et al. Detection of transposition of the great arteries in fetuses reduces neonatal morbidity and mortality. *Circulation.* 1999;99:916–918.
20. Graham TP Jr, Bernard YD, Mellen BG, et al. Long-term outcome in congenitally corrected transposition of the great arteries: a multi-institutional study. *J Am Coll Cardiol.* 2000;36:255–261.
21. Van Praagh R, Van Praagh S. The anatomy of common aorticopulmonary trunk (truncus arteriosus communis) and its embryologic implications: a study of 57 necropsy cases. *Am J Cardiol.* 1965;16(3):406–402.
22. Allan LD, Sharland GK, Milburn A, et al. Prospective diagnosis of 1,006 consecutive cases of congenital heart disease in the fetus. *J Am Coll Cardiol.* 1994;23:1452–1458.
23. Raymond FL, Simpson JM, Sharland GK, et al. Fetal echocardiography as a predictor of chromosomal abnormality. *Lancet.* 1997;350:930.
24. Marshall AC, Levine J, Morash D, et al. Results of in utero atrial septoplasty in fetuses with hypoplastic left heart syndrome. *Prenat Diagn.* 2008;28:1023–1028.
25. Selamet Tierney ES, Wald RM, McElhinney DB, et al. Changes in left heart hemodynamics after technically successful in-utero aortic valvuloplasty. *Ultrasound Obstet Gynecol.* 2007;30:715–720.
26. Marshall AC, van der Velde ME, Tworetzky W, et al. Creation of an atrial septal defect in utero for fetuses with hypoplastic left heart syndrome and intact or highly restrictive atrial septum. *Circulation.* 2004;110:253–258.
27. Xu Z, Owens G, Gordon D, et al. Noninvasive creation of an atrial septal defect by histotripsy in a canine model. *Circulation.* 2010;121:742–749.
28. McElhinney DB, Marshall AC, Wilkins-Haug LE, et al. Predictors of technical success and postnatal biventricular outcome after in utero aortic valvuloplasty for aortic stenosis with evolving hypoplastic left heart syndrome. *Circulation.* 2009;120:1482–1490.
29. Maxwell D, Allan L, Tynan MJ. Balloon dilatation of the aortic valve in the fetus: a report of two cases. *Br Heart J.* 1991;65:256–258.
30. Mizrahi-Arnaud A, Tworetzky W, Bulich LA, et al. Pathophysiology, management, and outcomes of fetal hemodynamic instability during prenatal cardiac intervention. *Pediatr Res.* 2007;62:325–330.
31. Hornberger LK, Sanders SP, Rein AJ, et al. Left heart obstructive lesions and left ventricular growth in the midtrimester fetus: a longitudinal study. *Circulation.* 1995;92:1531–1538.
32. Hornberger LK, Need L, Benacerraf BR. Development of significant left and right ventricular hypoplasia in the second and third trimester fetus. *J Ultrasound Med.* 1996;15:655–659.

33. Divanovic A, Hor K, Cnota J, et al. Prediction and perinatal management of severely restrictive atrial septum in fetuses with critical left heart obstruction: clinical experience using pulmonary venous doppler analysis. *J Thorac Cardiovasc Surg.* 2011;141:988–994.

34. Chintala K, Tian Z, Du W, et al. Fetal pulmonary venous doppler patterns in hypoplastic left heart syndrome: relationship to atrial septal restriction. *Heart.* 2008;94:1446–1449.

35. Michelfelder E, Gomez C, Border W, et al. Predictive value of fetal pulmonary venous flow patterns in identifying the need for atrial septoplasty in the newborn with hypoplastic left ventricle. *Circulation.* 2005;112:2974–2979.

36. Rychik J, Rome JJ, Collins MH, et al. The hypoplastic left heart syndrome with intact atrial septum: atrial morphology, pulmonary vascular histopathology and outcome. *J Am Coll Cardiol.* 1999;34:554–560.

37. Becker AE, Becker MJ, Edwards JE. Anomalies associated with coarctation of aorta: particular reference to infancy. *Circulation.* 1970;41:1067–1075.

38. Huhta JC, Cohen AW, Wood DC. Premature constriction of the ductus arteriosus. *J Am Soc Echocardiogr.* 1990;3:30–34.

39. Berg C, Kamil D, Geipel A, et al. Absence of ductus venosus-importance of umbilical venous drainage site. *Ultrasound Obstet Gynecol.* 2006;28:275–281.

40. Cohen MS, Anderson RH, Cohen MI, et al. Controversies, genetics, diagnostic assessment, and outcomes relating to the heterotaxy syndrome. *Cardiol Young.* 2007;17(suppl 2):29–43.

41. Barboza JM, Dajani NK, Glenn LG, et al. Prenatal diagnosis of congenital cardiac anomalies: a practical approach using two basic views. *Radiographics.* 2002;22(5):1125–1137.

42. Cohen MS, Schultz AH, Tian ZY, et al. Heterotaxy syndrome with functional single ventricle: does prenatal diagnosis improve survival? *Ann Thorac Surg.* 2006;82(5):1629–1636.

43. Lapierre C, Dery J, Guerin R, et al. Segmental approach to imaging of congenital heart disease. *Radiographics.* 2010;30(2):397–411.

44. Nemec SF, Brugger PC, Nemec U, et al. Situs anomalies on prenatal MRI. *Eur J Radiol.* 2012;81(4):e495–e501.

45. Saleem SN. Feasibility of MRI of the fetal heart with balanced steady-state free precession sequence along fetal body and cardiac planes. *AJR Am J Roentgenol.* 2008;191(4):1208–1215.

46. Yamamura J, Kopp I, Frisch M, et al. Cardiac MRI of the fetal heart using a novel triggering method: initial results in an animal model. *J Magn Reson Imaging.* 2012;35(5):1071–1076.

47. Nakhleh N, Francis R, Giese RA, et al. High prevalence of respiratory ciliary dysfunction in congenital heart disease patients with heterotaxy. *Circulation.* 2012;125(18):2232–2242.

48. Holley DG, Martin GR, Brenner JI, et al. Diagnosis and management of fetal cardiac tumors: a multicenter experience and review of published reports. *J Am Coll Cardiol.* 1995;26:516–520.

49. Gresser CD, Shime J, Rakowski H, et al. Fetal cardiac tumor: a prenatal echocardiographic marker for tuberous sclerosis. *Am J Obstet Gynecol.* 1987;156:689–690.

50. Harding CO, Pagon RA. Incidence of tuberous sclerosis in patients with cardiac rhabdomyoma. *Am J Med Genet.* 1990;37:443–446.

51. Wu CT, Chen MR, Hou SH. Neonatal tuberous sclerosis with cardiac rhabdomyomas presenting as fetal supraventricular tachycardia. *Jpn Heart J.* 1997;38:133–137.

52. Groves AM, Fagg NL, Cook AC, et al. Cardiac tumours in intrauterine life. *Arch Dis Child.* 1992;67:1189–1192.

53. Smythe JF, Dyck JD, Smallhorn JF, et al. Natural history of cardiac rhabdomyoma in infancy and childhood. *Am J Cardiol.* 1990;66:1247–1249.

54. Fesslova V, Villa L, Rizzuti T, et al. Natural history and long-term outcome of cardiac rhabdomyomas detected prenatally. *Prenat Diagn.* 2004;24:241–248.

55. Boxer RA, Seidman S, Singh S, et al. Congenital intracardiac rhabdomyoma: prenatal detection by echocardiography, perinatal management, and surgical treatment. *Am J Perinatol.* 1986;3:303–305.

56. Goh RH, Lappalainen RE, Mohide PT, et al. Multiple cardiac masses diagnosed with prenatal ultrasonography in the fetus of a woman with tuberous sclerosis. *Can Assoc Radiol J.* 1995;46:461–464.

57. Bader RS, Chitayat D, Kelly E, et al. Fetal rhabdomyoma: prenatal diagnosis, clinical outcome, and incidence of associated tuberous sclerosis complex. *J Pediatr.* 2003;143:620–624.

58. Lethor JP, de Moor M. Multiple cardiac tumors in the fetus. *Circulation.* 2001;103:E55.

59. Isaacs H Jr. Fetal and neonatal cardiac tumors. *Pediatr Cardiol.* 2004;25:252–273.

60. De Geeter B, Kretz JG, Nisand I, et al. Intrapericardial teratoma in a newborn infant: use of fetal echocardiography. *Ann Thorac Surg.* 1983;35:664–666.

61. Levy DW, Mintz MC. The left ventricular echogenic focus: a normal finding. *AJR Am J Roentgenol.* 1988;150:85–86.

62. Roberts DJ, Genest D. Cardiac histologic pathology characteristic of trisomies 13 and 21. *Hum Pathol.* 1992;23:1130–1140.

63. Veldtman GR, Blackburn ME, Wharton GA, et al. Dystrophic calcification of the fetal myocardium. *Heart.* 1999;81:92–93.

64. Brown DL, Roberts DJ, Miller WA. Left ventricular echogenic focus in the fetal heart: pathologic correlation. *J Ultrasound Med.* 1994;13:613–616.

65. Petrikovsky B, Klein V, Herrera M. Prenatal diagnosis of intra-atrial cardiac echogenic foci. *Prenat Diagn.* 1998;18:968–970.

66. Petrikovsky B, Challenger M, Gross B. Unusual appearances of echogenic foci within the fetal heart: are they benign? *Ultrasound Obstet Gynecol.* 1996;8:229–231.

67. Bradley KE, Santulli TS, Gregory KD, et al. An isolated intracardiac echogenic focus as a marker for aneuploidy. *Am J Obstet Gynecol.* 2005;192:2021–2026; discussion 2026-2028.

68. Bennet P, Nicolini U. Fetal infections in: Fisk NM, Moise KJ eds. Fetal. Therapy: Invasive and Transplacental. Cambridge, Mass: Cambridge University Press 2002.

69. Wagner HR. Cardiac disease in congenital infections. *Clin Perinatol.* 1981;8:481–497.

70. Eliasson H, Wahren-Herlenius M, Sonesson SE. Mechanisms in fetal bradyarrhythmia: 65 cases in a single center analyzed by doppler flow echocardiographic techniques. *Ultrasound Obstet Gynecol.* 2011;37:172–178.

71. Strasburger JF, Wakai RT. Fetal cardiac arrhythmia detection and in utero therapy. *Nat Rev Cardiol.* 2010;7:277–290.

72. Shah A, Moon-Grady A, Bhogal N, et al. Effectiveness of sotalol as firstline therapy for fetal supraventricular tachyarrhythmias. *Am J Cardiol.* 2012;109:1614–1618.

73. Strasburger JF, Cuneo BF, Michon MM, et al. Amiodarone therapy for drug-refractory fetal tachycardia. *Circulation.* 2004;109:375–379.

74. Cuneo BF, Strasburger JF, Niksch A, et al. An expanded phenotype of maternal ssa/ssb antibody-associated fetal cardiac disease. *J Matern Fetal Neonatal Med.* 2009;22:233–238.

75. Zhao H, Cuneo BF, Strasburger JF, et al. Electrophysiological characteristics of fetal atrioventricular block. *J Am Coll Cardiol.* 2008;51:77–84.

76. Cuneo BF, Ovadia M, Strasburger JF, et al. Prenatal diagnosis and in utero treatment of torsades de pointes associated with congenital long QT syndrome. *Am J Cardiol.* 2003;91:1395–1398.

77. Horigome H, Nagashima M, Sumitomo N, et al. Clinical characteristics and genetic background of congenital long-QT syndrome diagnosed in fetal, neonatal, and infantile life: a nationwide questionnaire survey in japan. *Circ Arrhythm Electrophysiol.* 2010;3:10–17.

78. Simpson JM, Maxwell D, Rosenthal E, et al. Fetal ventricular tachycardia secondary to long QT syndrome treated with maternal intravenous magnesium: case report and review of the literature. *Ultrasound Obstet Gynecol.* 2009;34:475–480.

79. Roberts JFE. *Pregnancy Related Hypertension.* Philadelphia, PA: WB Saunders; 2009.

80. Serra V, Bellver J, Moulden M, et al. Computerized analysis of normal fetal heart rate pattern throughout gestation. *Ultrasound Obstet Gynecol.* 2009;34:74–79.

81. Mitchell JL, Cuneo BF, Etheridge SP, et al. Fetal heart rate predictors of long QT syndrome. *Circulation.* 2012;126:2688–2695.

82. Brucato A, Frassi M, Franceschini F, et al. Risk of congenital complete heart block in newborns of mothers with anti-ro/ssa antibodies detected by counter-immunoelectrophoresis: a prospective study of 100 women. *Arthritis Rheum.* 2001;44:1832–1835.

83. Buyon JP, Hiebert R, Copel J, et al. Autoimmune-associated congenital heart block: demographics, mortality, morbidity and recurrence rates obtained from a national neonatal lupus registry. *J Am Coll Cardiol.* 1998;31:1658–1666.

84. Nii M, Hamilton RM, Fenwick L, et al. Assessment of fetal atrioventricular time intervals by tissue doppler and pulse doppler echocardiography: normal values and correlation with fetal electrocardiography. *Heart.* 2006;92:1831–1837.

85. Cuneo BF, Lee M, Roberson D, et al. A management strategy for fetal immune-mediated atrioventricular block. *J Matern Fetal Neonatal Med.* 2010;23:1400–1405.

86. Eliasson H, Sonesson SE, Sharland G, et al. Isolated atrioventricular block in the fetus: a retrospective, multinational, multicenter study of 175 patients. *Circulation.* 2011;124:1919–1926.

87. Skog A, Wahren-Herlenius M, Sundstrom B, et al. Outcome and growth of infants fetally exposed to heart block-associated maternal anti-ro52/ssa autoantibodies. *Pediatrics.* 2008;121:e803–e809.

88. Donofrio MT, Levy RJ, Schuette JJ, et al. Specialized delivery room planning for fetuses with critical congenital heart disease. *Am J Cardiol.* 2013;111:737–747.

# 17.1 Pulmonary Hypoplasia and Chest Wall Abnormalities

Jennifer H. Johnston

Fetal anomalies of the chest include a heterogeneous group of abnormalities with diverse etiologies, presentations, natural histories, and prognoses. Sonography is a key tool not only for screening and diagnosis of fetal chest disorders, but also for providing potential prognostic indicators and identifying unstable fetuses requiring urgent therapy. With the continued development of ultrafast magnetic resonance imaging (MRI) techniques in the fetus, MRI is increasingly utilized in the evaluation of chest disorders. Because of excellent tissue contrast, MRI is able to provide detailed information about the contents and structure of the fetal chest.

The clinical relevance and prognosis of chest lesions can be generally related to the degree of mass effect on the adjacent structures, including the heart, great vessels, lungs, trachea, and esophagus. While some lesions may be self-resolving, others can result in serious in utero distress with subsequent hydrops and fetal demise. Moreover, fetuses with chest abnormalities who survive may bear the postnatal consequences of lung disease.

## LUNG DEVELOPMENT

### Embryologic Considerations

The salient features required for a functioning pulmonary system include a branching conducting airway, adequate gas-exchange surface area with a thin air–blood barrier, surfactant, and vasculature to supply deoxygenated blood and carry away oxygenated blood.

The development of the lung is divided into five stages: embryologic (26 days to 6 weeks), pseudoglandular (6 to 16 weeks), canalicular (16 to 28 weeks), saccular (28 to 36 weeks), and alveolar (36 weeks to childhood).[1–3] There is significant overlap between these stages owing to differing speeds of maturation between the central and the peripheral lung regions, as well as cephalad and caudal segments.[4]

Lung development begins at 26 days when the respiratory diverticulum arises as an outpouching from the ventral surface of the embryologic foregut.[5] The lung bud initially communicates with the foregut but is eventually separated by two longitudinal ridges (the tracheoesophageal ridges), leaving behind the dorsal portion of the foregut, which is the precursor of the esophagus (Fig. 17.1-1A,B).

The respiratory diverticulum elongates to form the trachea and two lung buds, each of which enlarges to form the main bronchi at the 5th week of gestation. Branching morphogenesis is driven by signals received in the epithelium of the lung bud from the surrounding mesenchyme. The lung buds divide successively in dichotomous fashion, resulting in 10 right segmental bronchi and 8 left by the end of 6 weeks' gestation, the precursors of the bronchopulmonary segments in the adult lung (Fig. 17.1-1C–E). By 16 weeks after additional rounds of branching, the basic conducting architecture of the lung has been established.

The development of the pulmonary vasculature closely mirrors that of the bronchial tree. After their appearance at approximately 5 weeks' gestation, the sixth branchial arches develop into the main pulmonary artery and its right and left branches.[1] The preacinar pulmonary arteries and veins form by vasculogenesis using the budding airways as a scaffold through the 17th week of gestation. Postacinar pulmonary vessels subsequently form by angiogenesis in a network closely associated with the growing alveoli.[6] The bronchial arteries develop later than the pulmonary arteries, arising during the 8th week of gestation from the dorsal aorta and entering the lungs alongside the main bronchi.

The peripheral airways enlarge during the canalicular period, and the capillaries in the surrounding mesenchyme undergo massive proliferation and become closely apposed to the airway epithelium.[6] Type II epithelial cells are derived from the cuboidal epithelium of the bronchial tree and begin to produce surfactant at approximately 22 to 24 weeks. The acinar epithelium also differentiates into type I epithelial cells, which contribute to formation of the first functional gas-exchange surfaces.[5] During the subsequent saccular phase, an increase in the number of terminal sacs (primitive alveoli) results in a rapid expansion of the gas-exchanging surface area. By 26 to 28 weeks' gestation, there is sufficient vascularization of the lungs, surfactant, and terminal sacs to potentially allow survival of a prematurely born infant who receives intensive neonatal care.

Alveolarization commences at 36 weeks' gestation; however, the vast majority of alveoli develop after birth.[2] This process continues until late childhood, approximately 8 years of age.[1] Postnatal growth in the lung is due primarily to an increase in the number of respiratory bronchioles and alveoli as opposed to an increase in alveolar size.

### Factors Affecting Lung Growth

The most important factors needed for normal lung development and growth include amniotic and lung fluid and adequate thoracic space. The formation and clearance of fetal lung fluid is a dynamic process. Lung liquid is formed by active transport across the pulmonary epithelium into the bronchial system, establishing positive transpulmonary pressure. Clearance of this fluid is achieved by fetal breathing movements[7] and by peristaltic airway contractions.[8] Approximately 50% of lung fluid is swallowed by the fetus, the principal mechanism of amniotic fluid resorption, with the other 50% effluxed through the trachea into the amniotic space, comprising 30% of the amniotic fluid.[9] The efflux of lung liquid and intratracheal pressures are carefully regulated by the larynx.

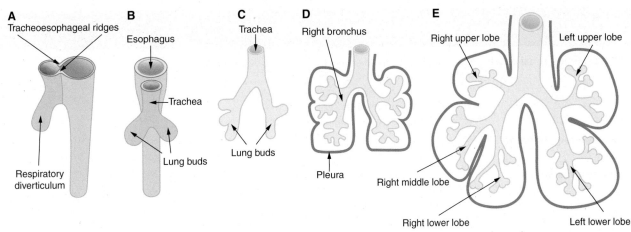

**FIGURE 17.1-1:** Embryologic development of the respiratory diverticulum, lung buds, trachea, and bronchi. **A:** Formation of the respiratory diverticulum from the ventral surface of the embryologic foregut, from which it is eventually separated by two tracheoesophageal ridges. **B:** Elongation of the respiratory diverticulum with subsequent formation of the lung buds. **C–E:** Development of the trachea and lungs at 5 weeks **(C)**, 6 weeks **(D)**, and 8 weeks **(E)**. (Adapted from Sadler TW. *Langman's Medical Embryology.* 12th ed. Philadelphia, PA: Lippincott Williams & Wilkins; 2012.)

Inadequate amniotic fluid is well documented to be associated with pulmonary hypoplasia, although the exact mechanism remains unclear. Proposed mechanisms include physical compression of the thorax by the uterine wall, inhibition of fetal breathing movements, and increased efflux of lung liquid into the amniotic space.[1] Limited intrathoracic space also has a detrimental effect on lung growth and can result in pulmonary hypoplasia, as seen in the case of congenital diaphragmatic hernia (CDH), pulmonary masses, and skeletal malformations. Fetal breathing movements, which appear as early as 11 weeks' gestation, produce changes in intrathoracic pressure, and there is experimental evidence that these movements also contribute to normal lung development.[10,11]

A balance between lung volume and pressure is required for appropriate growth as adequate transpulmonary pressure maintains lung expansion. Lung liquid not only distends the developing airways but also stimulates proliferation of alveolar cells. Disruption of this balance in either direction has significant consequences on lung development, as seen in the opposing examples of pulmonary hypoplasia and congenital high airway obstruction syndrome (CHAOS).

Increased knowledge of fetal lung fluid dynamics has resulted in the development of fetoscopic tracheal occlusion for treatment of CDH and the use of amnioinfusion for pulmonary hypoplasia related to oligohydramnios.

## PULMONARY HYPOPLASIA

Pulmonary hypoplasia can be clinically defined as incomplete development of the pulmonary parenchyma in the presence of a normal tracheobronchial tree. Pulmonary agenesis is a complete failure of airway and parenchymal development, and pulmonary aplasia is defined by incomplete development of lung parenchyma with a rudimentary bronchus. The formal histologic diagnosis of pulmonary hypoplasia is determined by postmortem measurements, including lung weight-to-body weight ratio, radial alveolar count, and DNA estimation,[12] and therefore limited for clinical use. Ultrasound (US) and MRI, however, are noninvasive tools that can aid in the antenatal prediction of

and differentiation between lethal and nonlethal forms of pulmonary hypoplasia.

**Incidence:** Pulmonary hypoplasia is relatively common with a reported incidence of 0.9 to 1.1 per 1,000 live births and 1.4 per 1,000 of all births.[13,14] The prevalence of this condition in autopsies ranges between 4.9% and 22%.[13,15,16]

**Pathogenesis/Etiology:** Bilateral pulmonary hypoplasia may be the result of various congenital abnormalities or complications of pregnancy that inhibit lung development (Table 17.1-1). Pulmonary hypoplasia most commonly occurs in the setting of oligohydramnios due to preterm premature rupture of membranes (PPROM) or fetal renal abnormalities, reportedly occurring with oligohydramnios for as short as 6 days.[12] Intrathoracic masses, including CDH and congenital pulmonary airway malformations (CPAM), also cause pulmonary hypoplasia. Other potential etiologies include skeletal malformations deforming the thoracic cavity, pleural effusions, neuromuscular anomalies, abdominal wall defects, and cardiac lesions. Complete pulmonary agenesis may be due to the failure of the development of bronchial buds or an in utero vascular accident.

Numerous syndromes are associated with primary abnormalities in lung development, including trisomies 13, 18, and 21. Other syndromes associated with pulmonary hypoplasia include fetal akinesia deformation sequence (FADS), cerebrooculofacioskeletal (COFS) syndrome due to hypotonia and decreased fetal breathing, and various skeletal dysplasias that cause restriction of thoracic volume. Primary isolated pulmonary hypoplasia in the absence of an underlying disorder is extremely uncommon, typically sporadic, but may have rare familial occurrence.[17]

Unilateral pulmonary hypoplasia is typically secondary to conditions that limit the thoracic space available for lung growth and is rarely due to a primary embryologic defect.[18] Less common etiologies for congenital unilateral pulmonary hypoplasia include main pulmonary artery atresia or thrombus, lobar agenesis–aplasia complex (including pulmonary venolobar or scimitar syndrome), and accessory diaphragm.[18–20]

| Table 17.1-1 | Anomalies Associated with Pulmonary Hypoplasia |
|---|---|
| **Oligohydramnios, renal or urinary** | Renal agenesis/dysplasia or multicystic dysplastic kidneys<br>Bladder outlet obstruction<br>Autosomal recessive (infantile) polycystic kidney disease<br>Meckel–Gruber syndrome<br>Renal dysplasia-limb defects syndrome |
| **Oligohydramnios, nonrenal** | Prolonged preterm rupture of membranes<br>Idiopathic |
| **Intrathoracic masses** | Congenital diaphragmatic hernia<br>Pulmonary masses (congenital pulmonary airway malformation, bronchopulmonary sequestration, bronchogenic cyst)<br>Pleural effusions or chylothoraces<br>Thoracic neuroblastoma (rare)<br>Chest wall hamartoma (rare) |
| **Skeletal malformations** | Thanatophoric dwarfism<br>Osteogenesis imperfecta<br>Jeune asphyxiating thoracic dystrophy<br>Atelosteogenesis, type II<br>Tetraamelia<br>Other skeletal dysplasias |
| **Neuromuscular and central nervous system anomalies** | Fetal akinesia deformation sequence<br>Cerebrooculofacioskeletal syndrome<br>Intrauterine anoxic or ischemic damage<br>Anencephaly<br>Phrenic nerve abnormalities |
| **Cardiac lesions** | Hypoplastic left or right heart, pulmonary stenosis, and so forth<br>Cardiomyopathy<br>Ebstein anomaly |
| **Abdominal wall defects** | Omphalocele<br>Gastroschisis |
| **Syndromes associated with pulmonary hypoplasia** | Trisomy 13<br>Trisomy 18<br>Trisomy 21<br>Roberts syndrome<br>Matthew–Wood syndrome<br>Familial pulmonary hypoplasia<br>Larson-like syndrome, lethal type<br>Aphalangy with hemivertebrae<br>Fryns syndrome |

Adapted from Goldstein RB. The thorax. In: Nyberg DA, McGahan JP, Pretorius DH, et al, eds. *Diagnostic Imaging of Fetal Anomalies*. Philadelphia, PA: Lippincott Williams & Wilkins; 2002:381–420.

**Diagnosis:** In the setting of pulmonary hypoplasia, a reduction in pulmonary lung volumes will be observed on both US and MRI. A bell-shaped chest is common. Decreased T2 parenchymal signal intensity for gestational age is typically seen on MRI.[21,22] Both US and MR may show ancillary findings that may explain the presence of pulmonary hypoplasia (Fig. 17.1-2). In unilateral pulmonary agenesis or hypoplasia, the affected lung and pulmonary artery are absent or small, and there is shift of mediastinal structures toward that side (Fig. 17.1-3A,B). The contralateral lung may be normal in size but is often hyperdistended. MRI may be helpful to exclude underlying lung mass (Fig. 17.1-3C).

**Prognosticators:** Gray scale US can assess fetal lung size by two-dimensional (2D) sonographic parameters, including thoracic circumference (TC) (Table 33 in Appendix A1), thoracic area, and lung length. The TC is measured by the axial plane, along the outer margin of the thoracic cage at the level of the four chambers of the heart and the atrioventricular valves during fetal diastole (Fig. 17.1-4). Ratios utilizing these parameters may be calculated to adjust for gestational age (GA) or fetal size, including a ratio of TC to abdominal circumference (AC),[23,24] gestational age, or femur length,[25] thoracic area/heart area[26] (Fig. 17.1-5), and (thoracic area-heart area) × 100/thoracic area.[26] Despite their high specificity, 2D sonographic parameters, with the exception being the lung area-to-head circumference ratio (LHR) discussed in the CDH section of this chapter, have been shown to be less sensitive than preferred for clinical practice.[27]

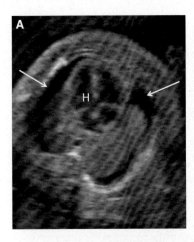

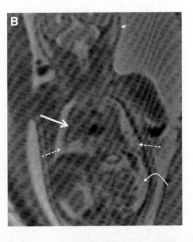

**FIGURE 17.1-2:** Pulmonary hypoplasia and hydrops in a fetus at 27 weeks' GA. **A:** Axial ultrasound image of small lungs and bilateral pleural effusions *(arrows)*. H, Heart. **B:** Coronal T2 MR image of the chest demonstrates marked pulmonary hypoplasia. The lungs are small and dark T2 signal *(solid straight arrow)* and are surrounded by hyperintense pleural fluid *(dashed arrows)*. Ascites *(curved arrow)* and skin thickening *(arrowhead)* are also present.

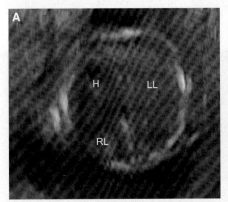

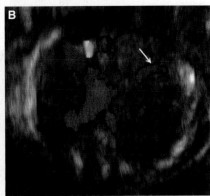

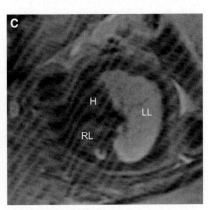

**FIGURE 17.1-3:** Unilateral pulmonary hypoplasia in a fetus at 25 weeks' GA. Gray scale ultrasound **(A)** and color Dopper **(B)** axial images through the chest demonstrate markedly small right lung with rightward mediastinal shift and overexpansion of the left lung. *Arrow* in **B** shows normal-sized left pulmonary vessels but lack of visualization of right. **C:** Axial T2-weighted MR demonstrates diminished signal intensity in the affected right lung. H, heart; LL, left lung; RL, right lung.

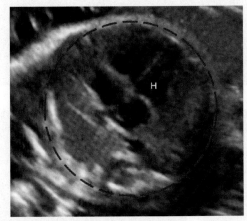

**FIGURE 17.1-4:** Normal thoracic circumference. Axial four chamber view at the level of the atrioventricular valves shows normal thoracic circumference measurement. H, heart.

Three-dimensional (3D) US, which can correct for contour irregularities, has been shown to produce reliable lung volume measurements (Table 34 Appendix A1) and may be useful in the assessment of pulmonary hypoplasia[28–30] (Fig. 17.1-6). There are two main approaches to obtaining lung volume measurements by 3D US. The multiplanar approach involves scrolling through the lungs in one reference plane, while simultaneously displaying three orthogonal planes. Alternatively, virtual organ computer-aided analysis (VOCAL) allows volume calculation around a fixed axis in a sequential number of steps.[31] Nomograms for right and left lung volumes versus estimated fetal weight have been shown to be reliable for prediction of hypoplasia despite differing methodologies and sonographic equipment across studies[29,32] (Tables 35 and 36 in Appendix A1).

Fetal MRI may also be used in the assessment for pulmonary hypoplasia, particularly in fetuses with CDH in which lung and liver parenchyma may be difficult to differentiate sonographically. While 3D US has the advantage of lower cost and quicker volume acquisition, benefits of MRI include increased spatial resolution and greater contrast between the lungs and the adjacent structures. Lung volumes are commonly calculated by planimetric analysis in which the area of the lungs, excluding the mediastinum and hilar vessels, is measured on a series of images through the fetal chest that have little motion and multiplied by the section thickness to obtain the section volume. The sum of the section volumes is then taken as the total lung volume. Lung volumes are also commonly performed on 3D reconstruction software (Fig. 17.1-7). Although there are reports that measurements obtained in the axial plane yield more accurate lung volumes than those obtained in the coronal or sagittal planes,[21,33] other studies have reported that lung volume measurements are independent of imaging plane.[34,35]

Rypens et al.[36] calculated fetal lung volumes in a large cohort of 215 fetuses and constructed a nomogram of lung volumes in relation to gestational age utilizing fast spin-echo T2-weighted

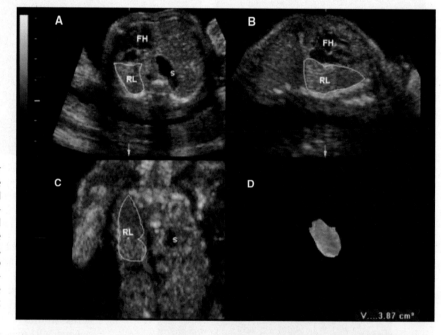

**FIGURE 17.1-5:** Graph illustrating distribution of chest area-to-heart area ratios of 13 fetuses at risk for pulmonary hypoplasia. *Solid triangles,* lethal pulmonary hypoplasia; *open triangles,* no lethal pulmonary hypoplasia. (Reproduced with permission from Vintzileos AM, Campbell WA, Rodis JF, et al. Comparison of six different ultrasonographic methods for predicting lethal fetal pulmonary hypoplasia. *Am J Obstet Gynecol.* 1989;161:606–612.)

**FIGURE 17.1-6:** Three-dimensional multiplanar imaging of the fetal thorax and measurement of the contralateral *(right)* lung volume at 23 gestational weeks in a case of left congenital diaphragmatic hernia. **A:** Transverse plane. **B:** Sagittal plane. **C:** Coronal plane. **D:** 3D rendering of the right lung, the volume of which is 3.87 cm³. FH, fetal heart; RL, right lung; s, stomach. (Reproduced with permission from Ruano R, Aubry M, Barthe B, et al. Three-dimensional sonographic measurement of contralateral lung volume in fetuses with isolated congenital diaphragmatic hernia. *J Clin Ultrasound.* 2009;36:273–278.)

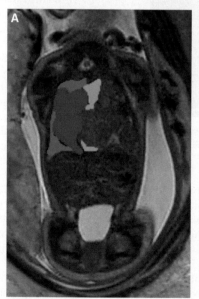

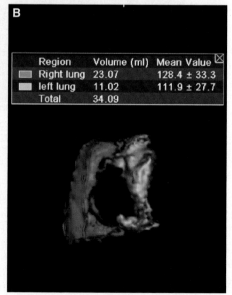

**FIGURE 17.1-7:** Determination of fetal lung volumes by MRI in a fetus at 34 weeks with left-sided congenital diaphragmatic hernia. The boundaries of the lungs, excluding the mediastinum and hilar vessels, are drawn on sequential coronal images through the chest, and the subsequent area of these regions of interest is multiplied by the section thickness to obtain the lung volume. **A:** Right lung, *blue;* left lung, *aquamarine;* mediastinum, *red.* **B:** 3D rendering of the right and left lung volumes.

MRI (Table 37 in Appendix A1). To date, however, significant heterogeneity and overlap exists in MRI-computed normal fetal lung volumes, likely related to nonuniformity in methodologies.[37] Improved standardization of MR image acquisition and measurement of fetal lung volumes will be helpful for further investigations into the role of MR-based evaluation of pulmonary hypoplasia.

*Doppler velocimetry* of fetal pulmonary circulation is another method for evaluation of pulmonary hypoplasia as the maldevelopment of the pulmonary vasculature parallels the development of the pulmonary airways. Peak systolic velocity (PSV) in the proximal pulmonary artery has been shown to be reduced in lethal lung hypoplasia, likely because of high peripheral pulmonary vascular resistance; however, the accuracy of this parameter alone is lower than desirable for clinical use.[23] A reduction of the ratio between acceleration and ejection time in pulmonary artery branches of fetuses with subsequent pulmonary hypoplasia has also been reported.[38] Alternatively, fetal pulmonary artery reactivity to maternal hyperoxygenation has been tested with reaction (20% reduction in the pulsatility index in branches of fetal pulmonary arteries) noted in 92% of survivors[39]; however, further studies are needed to fully assess the clinical reliability of these methods.

Other proposed markers for lethal pulmonary hypoplasia include fetal breathing movements and perinasal flow. Studies on the correlation between pulmonary hypoplasia and the presence or absence of fetal breathing movements have yielded contradictory results, although the prolonged absence of these movements over weeks may be a poor prognostic indicator.[12] Perinasal flow as assessed by color and spectral Doppler was detected in four of five fetuses with CDH who survived and was absent in one fetus who died in the neonatal period with pulmonary hypoplasia; these preliminary results require further investigation with larger cohorts.[40]

It may be that the most accurate prediction of lethal pulmonary hypoplasia requires an approach integrating clinical, biometric, and Doppler parameters. In cases of midtrimester PPROM, gestational age at the time of rupture, amount of amniotic fluid, and latency time between rupture and delivery have been studied extensively with regard to pulmonary hypoplasia. A meta-analysis of 28 studies reporting on the prediction of pulmonary hypoplasia found that gestational age at PPROM performed significantly better than the two other parameters.[41] The predictive value of the degree of oligohydramnios is disputed, with some studies showing it to be an independent prognosticator and others demonstrating no impact on the occurrence of pulmonary hypoplasia.[12] An approach combining clinical (degree and duration of oligohydramnios, and gestational age at PROM), biometric (TC/AC), and Doppler (PSV in the proximal pulmonary arterial branch) parameters yielded positive predictive value of 100%, accuracy of 93%, and sensitivity of 71%.[23]

**Differential Diagnosis:** A small chest circumference may be related to various skeletal dysplasias. When the lungs appear relatively small in comparison with the heart, fetal cardiomegaly should be excluded by careful examination.

**Prognosis:** The perinatal mortality rate related to pulmonary hypoplasia is approximately 70% in most investigative series.[12] Although most cases of pulmonary hypoplasia are lethal, a spectrum of manifestations exists, ranging from neonatal death due to respiratory failure to mild respiratory disease. Mortality is increased in infants with associated anomalies, particularly renal agenesis and CDH.

**Management:** The management of pulmonary hypoplasia depends mainly on the underlying etiology. Large pleural effusions may be treated with thoracentesis or thoracoabdominal shunting in an effort to increase thoracic space available for lung development. Removal of an intrathoracic mass is usually performed soon after birth to permit reexpansion of the lung. In the case of midtrimester PPROM, several studies have evaluated the use of amnioinfusion and amnioplugging with various agents in an attempt to normalize amniotic fluid volume.[42–44] Although late-gestation administration of maternal retinoid acid increased lung volume and stimulated alveologenesis in a rat model of CDH, no significant benefit was demonstrated in an oligohydramnios-induced pulmonary hypoplasia rat model.[45] While fetoscopic tracheal occlusion has shown promise in fetuses with CDH, this procedure would be significantly more technically challenging in cases of oligohydramnios related to PPROM owing to limited access and maneuverability.[46]

**Recurrence Risk:** The recurrence risk of pulmonary hypoplasia depends primarily on the underlying etiology. The reported recurrence of PPROM ranges between 16% and 32%.[47]

# CHEST WALL

Chest wall abnormalities encompass deformities related to anomalies in growth and masses.

## Chest Wall Deformities

Congenital chest wall deformities include pectus excavatum, pectus carinatum, and sternal defects, including ectopic cordis and Pentalogy of Cantrell. Pectus excavatum (funnel chest) is characterized by depression of the sternum and the adjacent costal cartilages. Pectus carinatum refers to outward protrusion of the sternal body and adjacent ribs and may be isolated or occur in combination with pectus excavatum.

The chest wall shape may be deformed in fetuses with skeletal dysplasias such as thanatophoric dysplasia, achondrogenesis, asphyxiating thoracic dysplasia (Jeune syndrome), Ellis Van–Creveld syndrome, and rib-polydactyly syndromes. In osteogenesis imperfecta, multiple rib fractures may be present.

**Incidence:** Pectus excavatum occurs in 1 in 400 to 1,000 live births and is up to five times more common in boys than in girls.[48] Pectus carinatum is the second most common congenital chest wall deformity, with an incidence of approximately 1 in 2,500 live births, also exhibiting a male predominance.[49]

**Pathogenesis:** The thoracic cavity is formed after the establishment of the intraembryonic cavity at approximately the 4th week of gestation. A group of mesenchymal cells pass ventrolaterally from the developing vertebrae to form the ribs and costal cartilages at the beginning of the 5th gestational week; the ribs fuse with the developing sternum 1 week later.[50] The sternum arises from paired mesenchymal bands that are first apparent at 35 days and fuse in the ventral midline by the 10th gestational week.[49]

The current dominant hypotheses regarding the pathogenesis of pectus excavatum and pectus carinatum focus on defective metabolism of the sternocostal cartilage leading to biomechanical weakness and overgrowth.[50]

**Etiology:** The exact genetic basis of pectus excavatum is as yet unclear.[51] The occurrence of pectus excavatum in patients with Marfan syndrome, Ehlers–Danlos syndromes, Sprengle deformity, and scoliosis suggests an association with connective tissue disorders.[52] Reports of familial nonsyndromic inheritance of pectus excavatum exist. Among the numerous other genetic syndromes associated with pectus excavatum and/or pectus carinatum are Noonan syndrome, cardiofaciocutaneous syndrome, Holt–Oram syndrome, and osteogenesis imperfecta.[51]

**Diagnosis:** The contour of the fetal chest wall can be visualized by both US and MRI. Pectus excavatum will be evident by an abnormal fetal contour related to a ventral depression in the thoracic wall (Fig. 17.1-8).[53] In pectus carinatum, the sternum and adjacent ribs protrude anteriorly. In the setting of skeletal dysplasia, a chest wall deformity will be accompanied by other skeletal abnormalities.

**Differential Diagnosis:** Pectus excavatum should be differentiated from depressions in the ventral thoracic wall caused by oligohydramnios, which may deform the fetal contour by uterine wall compression. Umbilical cord loops may also simulate indentations.

**Prognosis:** Depending on the degree of sternal depression and resultant displacement of the heart and diminished pulmonary volume, pectus excavatum may result in measurable pulmonary and cardiac dysfunction. Mitral valve prolapse can be found in up to 25% of patients.[54] Most patients with pectus carinatum are asymptomatic, although some patients with severe deformity may complain of pain.

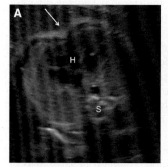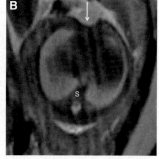

**FIGURE 17.1-8:** Pectus excavatum. Axial images through the lower chest in two different fetuses at GA of 33 weeks demonstrate depression of the sternum *(arrow)* on ultrasound **(A)** and T2-weighted MRI **(B)**. H, heart; S, spine.

**Management:** Pectus excavatum may be surgically repaired postnatally, depending on the severity. Nonoperative management with a brace for patients with pectus carinatum may achieve progressive remodeling; surgical correction is often reserved when conservative management fails.[49]

**Recurrence Risk:** Pectus excavatum may be sporadic; however, a genetic predisposition is likely as positive family history is noted in up to 43% of cases.[50] Recurrence of pectus excavatum or pectus carinatum related to genetic syndromes or chromosomal aberrations depends on the specific genetic abnormality.

## Chest Wall Masses

Soft tissue masses that occur elsewhere in the body may potentially arise in the chest wall, including fibromatosis, myofibromatosis, fibrous hamartoma, and infantile fibrosarcoma. A handful of soft tissue masses, however, are found typically or characteristically in the chest. Mesenchymal hamartomas of the chest wall are relatively rare lesions that always arise from the ribs and comprise benign proliferations of skeletal tissue with a prominent cartilaginous component. Vascular lesions, including hemangiomas, lymphatic, venous and arteriovenous malformations, may also occur within the chest wall.

**Incidence:** Chest wall mesenchymal hamartomas are extremely rare, comprising approximately 1 in 3,000 of primary bone tumors, or less than 1 in 1 million of the general population.[55] Lymphatic malformations, previously known as lymphangiomas, are uncommonly diagnosed prenatally in the chest wall. 75% to 80% of prenatal lymphatic malformations occur in the nuchal region.[56]

**Pathogenesis/Etiology:** Mesenchymal hamartomas are composed of maturing normal skeletal elements with characteristically benign histologic features. Most are nonfamilial, with all but one reported case in the literature having no familial association.[55]

Lymphatic malformations are believed to be related to the abnormal development of the lymphatic system. Although classic cervical lymphatic malformations carry a high risk of associated chromosomal abnormalities and a poor prognosis, those found elsewhere in the body, including the chest wall, may represent a separate entity with a relatively low rate of structural and genetic abnormalities.[56] The small number of reported cases in the literature, however, limits the drawing of definite conclusions at this time.

**Diagnosis:** Mesenchymal hamartomas of the chest wall are typically characterized by prominent aneurysmal bone cystic components. On US, these masses are heterogeneous and typically intrathoracic, centered at one or more ribs (Fig. 17.1-9A).

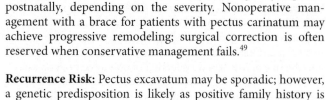

**FIGURE 17.1-9:** Mesenchymal hamartoma. **A:** Axial US of the chest in a fetus at 32 weeks' GA demonstrating a heterogeneous mass with echogenic capsule that appears to be related to the posterior rib *(white arrowheads)*. **B:** Steady-state free precession fetal MR in the coronal plane demonstrates a well-circumscribed mass associated with the lateral chest wall. H, fetal heart; S, spine; M, mass. (Reproduced with permission from Chu L, Seed M, Howse E, et al. Mesenchymal hamartoma: prenatal diagnosis by MRI. *Pediatr Radiol.* 2011;41:781–784.)

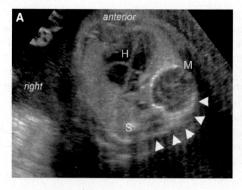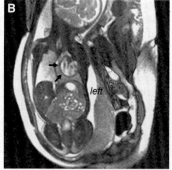

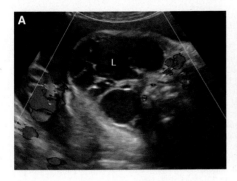
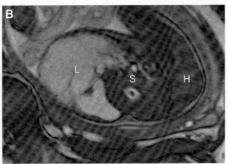

**FIGURE 17.1-10:** Chest wall lymphatic malformation. **A:** Color Doppler US image in the axial plane through a fetus at 26 weeks' GA demonstrates a predominantly cystic structure in the right upper chest wall containing numerous septations without detectable hypervascularity. **B:** Steady-state free precession MR image in the axial plane shows an infiltrating multiloculated cystic lesion superior right chest wall. L, lymphangioma; S, spine; H, humeral head.

MRI demonstrates a heterogeneous mass with mixed T1 and T2 signal intensity (Fig. 17.1-9B). Hemorrhage in the mass as evidenced by focally increased T1 signal intensity is a common finding, and fluid–fluid levels may be seen on both prenatal and postnatal imaging.[57] Depending on the size of the lesion, mediastinal displacement or scoliosis may be present.

Chest wall lymphatic malformations may be unilocular or multilocular and are similar in appearance to those elsewhere in the body (Fig. 17.1-10).

**Differential Diagnosis:** Differential considerations for mesenchymal hamartomas of the chest wall include congenital fibrosarcoma, neuroblastoma, or chondrosarcoma, although the latter is exceedingly uncommon in children. A chest wall mass must also be differentiated from a mass of pulmonary origin.

**Prognosis:** Mesenchymal hamartomas of the chest wall have a benign histology and self-limiting natural history. If not diagnosed prenatally, these masses usually come to light in infancy as a mass or as an incidental finding on chest radiography. Depending on the tumor size, perinatal respiratory distress may result because of pulmonary hypoplasia or mass effect. In the case of chest wall lymphatic malformations, the major risks are dystocia during labor and, in the long-term, infiltration and organ involvement with potential infection and hemorrhage.[56]

**Management:** Mesenchymal hamartomas are sometimes associated with large pleural effusions that may require in utero treatment with thoracoamniotic shunting. Postnatal treatment modalities include surgical removal and thermal radio-ablation, although conservative management with observation may be appropriate in asymptomatic patients.[55] The treatment for chest wall lymphatic malformations is surgical excision.

**Recurrence Risk:** Recurrence of mesenchymal hamartomas has been reported in cases with incomplete resection.[58] Following surgical excision of a chest wall lymphatic malformation, the recurrence risk is 10% to 15%.[56]

## REFERENCES

1. Laudy JA, Wladimiroff JW. The fetal lung, 1: developmental aspects. *Ultrasound Obstet Gynecol.* 2000;16(3):284–290.
2. Burri PH. Structural aspects of postnatal lung development: alveolar formation and growth. *Biol Neonate.* 2006;89(4):313–322.
3. Pringle KC. Human fetal lung development and related animal models. *Clin Obstet Gynecol.* 1986;29(3):502–513.
4. Langston C, Kida K, Reed M, et al. Human lung growth in late gestation and in the neonate. *Am Rev Respir Dis.* 1984;129(4):607–613.
5. Schittny JC, Burri PH. Development and growth of the lung. In: Fishman AP, Elias JA, Fishman JA, et al, eds. *Fishman's Pulmonary Diseases and Disorders.* Vol 1. 4th ed. New York, NY: McGraw-Hill; 2008:91–114.
6. Hislop A. Developmental biology of the pulmonary circulation. *Paediatr Respir Rev.* 2005;6(1):35–43.
7. Harding R, Hooper SB. Regulation of lung expansion and lung growth before birth. *J Appl Physiol.* 1996;81(1):209–224.
8. Schittny JC, Miserocchi G, Sparrow MP. Spontaneous peristaltic airway contractions propel lung liquid through the bronchial tree of intact and fetal lung explants. *Am J Respir Cell Mol Biol.* 2000;23(1):11–18.
9. Brace RA, Wlodek ME, Cock ML, et al. Swallowing of lung liquid and amniotic fluid by the ovine fetus under normoxic and hypoxic conditions. *Am J Obstet Gynecol.* 1994;171(3):764–770.
10. Adzick NS, Harrison MR, Glick PL, et al. Experimental pulmonary hypoplasia and oligohydramnios: relative contributions of lung fluid and fetal breathing movements. *J Pediatr Surg.* 1984;19(6):658–665.
11. Wigglesworth JS, Desai R. Effect on lung growth of cervical cord section in the rabbit fetus. *Early Hum Dev.* 1979;3(1):51–65.
12. Laudy JA, Wladimiroff JW. The fetal lung, 2: pulmonary hypoplasia. *Ultrasound Obstet Gynecol.* 2000;16(5):482–494.
13. Knox WF, Barson AJ. Pulmonary hypoplasia in a regional perinatal unit. *Early Hum Dev.* 1986;14(1):33–42.
14. Moessinger AC, Santiago A, Paneth NS, et al. Time-trends in necropsy prevalence and birth prevalence of lung hypoplasia. *Paediatr Perinat Epidemiol.* 1989;3(4):421–431.
15. Gupta K, Das A, Menon P, et al. Revisiting the histopathologic spectrum of congenital pulmonary developmental disorders. *Fetal Pediatr Pathol.* 2012;31(2):74–86.
16. Husain AN, Hessel RG. Neonatal pulmonary hypoplasia: an autopsy study of 25 cases. *Fetal Pediatr Pathol.* 1993;13(4):475–484.
17. Frey B, Fleischhauer A, Gersbach M. Familial isolated pulmonary hypoplasia: a case report, suggesting autosomal recessive inheritance. *Eur J Pediatr.* 1994;153(6):460–463.
18. Abrams ME, Ackerman VL, Engle WA. Primary unilateral pulmonary hypoplasia: neonate through early childhood—case report, radiographic diagnosis and review of the literature. *J Perinatol.* 2004;24(10):667–670.
19. Van Schendel MP, Visser DH, Rammeloo LA, et al. Left pulmonary artery thrombosis in a neonate with left lung hypoplasia. *Case Rep Pediatr.* 2012; 2012:314256.
20. Currarino G, Williams B. Causes of congenital unilateral pulmonary hypoplasia: a study of 33 cases. *Pediatr Radiol.* 1985;15(1):15–24.
21. Kasprian G, Balassy C, Brugger PC, et al. MRI of normal and pathological fetal lung development. *Eur J Radiol.* 2006;57(2):261–270.
22. Kuwashima S, Nishimura G, Iimura F, et al. Low-intensity fetal lungs on MRI may suggest the diagnosis of pulmonary hypoplasia. *Pediatr Radiol.* 2001;31(9):669–672.
23. Laudy JA, Tibboel D, Robben SG, et al. Prenatal prediction of pulmonary hypoplasia: clinical, biometric, and Doppler velocity correlates. *Pediatrics.* 2002;109(2):250–258.
24. Yoshimura S, Masuzaki H, Gotoh H, et al. Ultrasonographic prediction of lethal pulmonary hypoplasia: comparison of eight different ultrasonographic parameters. *Am J Obstet Gynecol.* 1996;175(2):477–483.
25. Fong K, Ohlsson A, Zalev A. Fetal thoracic circumference: a prospective cross-sectional study with real-time ultrasound. *Am J Obstet Gynecol.* 1988;158(5):1154–1160.
26. Vintzileos AM, Campbell WA, Rodis JF, et al. Comparison of six different ultrasonographic methods for predicting lethal fetal pulmonary hypoplasia. *Am J Obstet Gynecol.* 1989;161(3):606–612.
27. Vergani P. Prenatal diagnosis of pulmonary hypoplasia. *Curr Opin Obstet Gynecol.* 2012;24(2):89–94.
28. Peralta CF, Cavoretto P, Csapo B, et al. Lung and heart volumes by three-dimensional ultrasound in normal fetuses at 12–32 weeks' gestation. *Ultrasound Obstet Gynecol.* 2006;27(2):128–133.
29. Vergani P, Andreani M, Greco M, et al. Two- or three-dimensional ultrasonography: which is the best predictor of pulmonary hypoplasia? *Prenat Diagn.* 2010;30(9):834–838.
30. Gerards FA, Twisk JW, Fetter WP, et al. Predicting pulmonary hypoplasia with 2- or 3-dimensional ultrasonography in complicated pregnancies. *Am J Obstet Gynecol.* 2008;198(1):140.e1–140.e6.

31. Kalache KD, Espinoza J, Chaiworapongsa T, et al. Three-dimensional ultrasound fetal lung volume measurement: a systematic study comparing the multiplanar method with the rotational (VOCAL) technique. *Ultrasound Obstet Gynecol.* 2003;21(2):111–118.

32. Gerards FA, Engels MA, Twisk JW, et al. Normal fetal lung volume measured with three-dimensional ultrasound. *Ultrasound Obstet Gynecol.* 2006;27(2):134–144.

33. Jani J, Breysem L, Maes F, et al. Accuracy of magnetic resonance imaging for measuring fetal sheep lungs and other organs. *Ultrasound Obstet Gynecol.* 2005;25(3):270–276.

34. Busing KA, Kilian AK, Schaible T, et al. Reliability and validity of MR image lung volume measurement in fetuses with congenital diaphragmatic hernia and in vitro lung models. *Radiology.* 2008;246(2):553–561.

35. Ward VL, Nishino M, Hatabu H, et al. Fetal lung volume measurements: determination with MR imaging—effect of various factors. *Radiology.* 2006;240(1):187–193.

36. Rypens F, Metens T, Rocourt N, et al. Fetal lung volume: estimation at MR imaging-initial results. *Radiology.* 2001;219(1):236–241.

37. Deshmukh S, Rubesova E, Barth R. MR assessment of normal fetal lung volumes: a literature review. *AJR Am J Roentgenol.* 2010;194(2):W212–W217.

38. Fuke S, Kanzaki T, Mu J, et al. Antenatal prediction of pulmonary hypoplasia by acceleration time/ejection time ratio of fetal pulmonary arteries by Doppler blood flow velocimetry. *Am J Obstet Gynecol.* 2003;188(1):228–233.

39. Broth RE, Wood DC, Rasanen J, et al. Prenatal prediction of lethal pulmonary hypoplasia: the hyperoxygenation test for pulmonary artery reactivity. *Am J Obstet Gynecol.* 2002;187(4):940–945.

40. Fox HE, Badalian SS, Timor-Tritsch IE, et al. Fetal upper respiratory tract function in cases of antenatally diagnosed congenital diaphragmatic hernia: preliminary observations. *Ultrasound Obstet Gynecol.* 1993;3(3):164–167.

41. Van Teeffelen AS, van der Ham DP, Oei SG, et al. The accuracy of clinical parameters in the prediction of perinatal pulmonary hypoplasia secondary to midtrimester prelabour rupture of fetal membranes: a meta-analysis. *Eur J Obstet Gynecol Reprod Biol.* 2010;148(1):3–12.

42. Hofmeyr GJ, Essilfie-Appiah G, Lawrie TA. Amnioinfusion for preterm premature rupture of membranes. *Cochrane Database Syst Rev.* 2011;(12):CD000942.

43. Tranquilli AL, Giannubilo SR, Bezzeccheri V, et al. Transabdominal amnioinfusion in preterm premature rupture of membranes: a randomised controlled trial. *BJOG.* 2005;112(6):759–763.

44. Nicksa GA, Yu DC, Kalish BT, et al. Serial amnioinfusions prevent fetal pulmonary hypoplasia in a large animal model of oligohydramnios. *J Pediatr Surg.* 2011;46(1):67–71.

45. Chen CM, Chou HC, Wang LF, et al. Retinoic acid fails to reverse oligohydramnios-induced pulmonary hypoplasia in fetal rats. *Pediatr Res.* 2007;62(5):553–558.

46. Williams O, Chou HC, Wang LF, et al. Pulmonary effects of prolonged oligohydramnios following mid-trimester rupture of the membranes—antenatal and postnatal management. *Neonatology.* 2012;101(2):83–90.

47. Lee T, Carpenter MW, Heber WW, et al. Preterm premature rupture of membranes: risks of recurrent complications in the next pregnancy among a population-based sample of gravid women. *Am J Obstet Gynecol.* 2003;188(1):209–213.

48. Fokin AA, Steuerwald NM, Ahrens WA, et al. Anatomical, histologic, and genetic characteristics of congenital chest wall deformities. *Semin Thorac Cardiovasc Surg.* 2009;21(1):44–57.

49. Blanco FC, Elliott ST, Sandler AD. Management of congenital chest wall deformities. *Semin Plast Surg.* 2011;25(1):107–116.

50. Brochhausen C, Turial S, Müller FK, et al. Pectus excavatum: history, hypotheses and treatment options. *Interact Cardiovasc Thorac Surg.* 2012;14(6):801–806.

51. Kotzot D, Schwabegger AH. Etiology of chest wall deformities—a genetic review for the treating physician. *J Pediatr Surg.* 2009;44(10):2004–2011.

52. Kelly RE Jr. Pectus excavatum: historical background, clinical picture, preoperative evaluation and criteria for operation. *Semin Pediatr Surg.* 2008;17(3):181–193.

53. Salamanca A, Girona A, Padilla MC, et al. Prenatal diagnosis of pectus excavatum and its relation to Down's syndrome. *Ultrasound Obstet Gynecol.* 1992;2(6):446–447.

54. Jaroszewski D, Notrica D, McMahon L, et al. Current management of pectus excavatum: a review and update of therapy and treatment recommendations. *J Am Board Fam Med.* 2010;23(2):230–239.

55. Braatz B, Evans R, Kelman A, et al. Perinatal evolution of mesenchymal hamartoma of the chest wall. *J Pediatr Surg.* 2012;45(12):e37–e40.

56. Goldstein I, Leibovitz Z, Noi-Nizri M. Prenatal diagnosis of fetal chest lymphangioma. *J Ultrasound Med.* 2006;25(11):1437–1440.

57. Chu L, Seed M, Howse E, et al. Mesenchymal hamartoma: prenatal diagnosis by MRI. *Pediatr Radiol.* 2011;41(6):781–784.

58. Groom KR, Murphey MD, Howard LM, et al. Mesenchymal hamartoma of the chest wall: radiologic manifestations with emphasis on cross-sectional imaging and histopathologic comparison. *Radiology.* 2002;222(1):205–211.

# Congenital Diaphragmatic Hernia

Beth M. Kline-Fath

Congenital diaphragmatic hernia (CDH) occurs when there is a defect in the fetal diaphragm allowing herniation of intraabdominal structures into the thoracic cavity. The most common type of CDH is posterolateral, known as the *Bochdalek type*; accounting for 90% to 95% of CDH cases.[1] The remaining types will not be discussed but include anterior retrosternal, also known as *Morgagni hernias*, parasternal as found in *pentalogy of Cantrell* and *hiatal hernia*, through the esophageal hiatus. *Eventrations* are extreme elevations of all or part of the diaphragm that occur because of thinning or atrophy of the muscle.

**Incidence:** CDH (Bochdalek) occurs at an incidence of 1 in 2,500 with inclusion of stillborn pregnancies.[2] In the neonatal population, the incidence is 1 in 5,000 live born infants.[2] About 85% to 90% of CDH are left sided, 10% to 15% right sided, and 1% to 2% bilateral. A sac-type CDH, which represents a hernia covered by a membrane, may be present in 10% to 15% of cases.[3] CDH occurs in isolation, in the absence of additional congenital malformations, in about 60% of cases.

**Pathogenesis:** The diaphragm develops between the 4th and the 12th week of gestation. The current understanding is that the diaphragm forms first as a nonmuscular primitive anlage termed the pleuroperitoneal fold.[4] From the 4th to the 10th week of gestation, this mesenchymal substrate originates from the lateral cervical wall to fuse with the esophageal mesentery and ventral septum transversum. Sequentially, cervical neural and myogenic cells then migrate across the fold to form the diaphragm. When there is a "hole" in the primitive mesenchymal anlage, a CDH develops.[3,4] If there is thinning or undermuscularization of the diaphragm, an eventration or sac-type CDH may result.[3] Because the membrane closes later on the left, left-sided CDH are more common.[5] True agenesis of the hemidiaphragm may also rarely occur.[6] In the presence of CDH, a spectrum of complicating diseases is often present that occur secondary to the defect (Table 17.2-1).[1]

The clinical course of patients with CDH is dependent on the timing of the insult, the duration of the herniation, and the amount of viscera displaced intrathoracic. The pathophysiology is believed to result from a "dual hit hypothesis," in which abnormal parenchymal development is followed by compression resulting in injury to both the ipsilateral and the contralateral lung.[5] First, early in gestation (5 to 16 weeks), there is a direct insult to the developing lung which results in decreased bronchial branching and reduction in alveoli. Second, with diminished fetal breathing movements and increasing compression of the growing lung, there is a decrease in airway size, reduced alveoli, increased interstitial tissue, abnormal sacculo–alveolar maturation, and diminished alveolar air space and gas-exchange surface area. At the same time that the lung parenchyma is affected, pulmonary vascular changes, which include reduction in the number of vessels and abnormal extension of the muscular layer into the small intraacinar arterioles, are also occurring. The result of these parenchymal and vascular alterations becomes evident postnatally as pulmonary hypoplasia and hypertension. It is the severity of these changes that has the most impact on postnatal survival.

**Etiology and Detection:** The cause of a CDH is incompletely understood. It is believed that the majority of CDH cases develop secondary to a complex inheritance pattern in which chromosomal aberrations and environmental factors cause a defect in the genes that guide normal diaphragm growth.[3] Familial CDH is rare, comprising 2% of cases.[7] Toxins, such as maternal antiepileptic medication and thalidomide, have been implicated as causative of CDH, but the most important environmental factor known to cause CDH is disturbance in the retinol pathways.[1,8] Vitamin A (retinol) and its derivatives (retinoids) play a central role in embryonic morphogenesis and are important in development of the diaphragm and lung.[1,9] In humans with CDH, vitamin A deficiency and genetic mutations tightly related to retinoid signaling have been noted.[1,9]

Chromosomal anomalies have been described in 10% of affected individuals.[10,11] The most common aneuploidies associated with CDH include trisomy 13, 18, 21, 45 X, and tetrasomy 12p.[1] The most frequently diagnosed syndrome in association with CDH is Fryns, which is a syndrome that is seen in conjunction with coarse facial features, cleft lip and palate, cardiac and cerebral malformations, and hypoplastic finger and toenails.[1] Many syndromes are linked with CDH at higher rates than the general population (Table 17.2-2).[1]

| Table 17.2-1 | Complicating Diseases in CDH |
|---|---|

Pulmonary hypoplasia
Malrotation or incomplete rotation bowel
Patent ductus arteriosus
Patent foramen ovale
Heart hypoplasia and/or dextroposition
Tricuspid/mitral valve regurgitation
Undescended testes
Accessory spleen

| Table 17.2-2 | Genetic Syndromes Associated with CDH | |
|---|---|

| Syndrome | Inheritance |
|---|---|
| Beckwith–Wiedemann | Autosomal dominant |
| CHARGE | Autosomal dominant |
| Cornelia de Lange | Autosomal dominant |
| Craniofrontonasal | X-linked dominant |
| Denys–Drash | Autosomal dominant |
| Donnai–Barrow | Autosomal recessive |
| Fryns | Autosomal recessive |
| Pallister–Killian | Random mosaicism 12p |
| Simpson–Golabi–Behmel | X-linked recessive |
| Thoracoabdominal | X-linked dominant |
| Wolf–Hirschhorn | Random deletion 4p |

### Diagnosis

Because of known genetic associations, amniocentesis with karyotype is imperative in patients with CDH. As routine amniocentesis can miss cryptic deletions and duplications, some believe it to be prudent to obtain higher resolution cytogenetic testing.[1] Diagnosis prenatal is typically via sonography. Additional imaging with fetal MRI and echocardiography are helpful to exclude associated anomalies, assist in predicting prognosis, and guide prenatal counseling.

*US:* US evaluation of the fetal chest should be performed in all three anatomic planes, but the most important view is the axial. Diagnosis of CDH via ultrasound (US) requires detecting direct signs of an intrathoracic mass containing liver, bowel, and/or stomach or indirect evidence such as abnormal cardiac axis and mediastinal shift. Identification of the diaphragm as a thin hypoechoic line on a sagittal or coronal image is helpful but not always sufficient to exclude a hernia as only a portion of the diaphragm may be absent.[12] When diagnosing a CDH, it is important to exclude associated anomalies that may support the presence of an underlying syndrome.

*Left CDH,* representing 85% to 90% of CDH cases, is usually first suspected when the stomach is not observed in the normal intra-abdominal location. In a true transverse plane through the fetal chest, the two cardinal findings of left CDH are (1) identification of a fluid-filled stomach intrathoracic at the level of the heart and (2) displacement of the heart to the right of midline (Fig. 17.2-1). It must be remembered, however, that the stomach is intrathoracic in only 90% of left CDH, with the remaining 10% being intra-abdominal.[13] In these situations, other secondary findings must be utilized to diagnose CDH.

Early in gestation, bowel loops are usually decompressed and echogenic, and can be difficult to separate from lung and liver (Fig. 17.2-2A). However, later in gestation, the small bowel is better discriminated as it is fluid-filled, and in the presence of intrathoracic bowel peristalsis is confirmative of CDH (Fig. 17.2-2B). Primary indirect signs of left CDH, in addition to displacement of the heart and mediastinum, include a scaphoid abdomen and small abdominal circumference due to absence of intra-abdominal structures (Fig. 17.2-3). Polyhydramnios may occur because of impaired fetal swallowing and/or partial gastric outlet obstruction due to kinking of the gastroduodenal junction.[14] Hydrothorax occurs in 5% of left CDH cases, but hydrops rarely develops despite significant heart and vascular compression.[15]

Identification of intrathoracic liver can be difficult because of similar echogenicity to fetal lung and collapsed bowel. When the liver herniates into the left chest in a CDH, the left lobe lies perpendicular to the normal liver axis and adjacent to the heart, in the anterior aspect of the left hemithorax. The position of the stomach can be helpful in supporting the presence of liver herniation. If the stomach is present along the anterior lower thoracic wall, the likelihood of liver herniation is low (Fig. 17.2-4A). If the stomach is displaced posteriorly away from the anterior thoracic wall, liver herniation is probable (Fig. 17.2-4B). The gallbladder, identified separate from the stomach, is often displaced intrathoracic, midline, or left upper quadrant with liver herniation. However, the most accurate way to validate liver positioning is via color Doppler, as displacement and intrathoracic extension of the portal or hepatic venous structures will confirm ectopic liver (Fig. 17.2-5).[16]

*Right CDH* represents 10% to 15% of CDH cases. The right lobe of the liver is displaced with or without the gastrointestinal tract, resulting in a shift of the heart and mediastinum to the left. The fetal stomach is almost always intra-abdominal. Given that right CDH is primarily because of herniated liver, the defect can sometimes be confused with a lung lesion. On gray scale, the easiest structure to evaluate is the gallbladder, which is often displaced high in the right abdomen or intrathoracic. As the right lobe of the liver is typically herniated into the right thorax, gray scale imaging can be utilized to identify portal triads and hepatic vessels (Fig. 17.2-6). However, confirmation is best achieved with color Doppler by demonstrating kinking of the sinus venosus, bowing of the umbilical segment of the portal vein, and/or coursing portal venous structures in the thoracic cavity (Fig. 17.2-7).[16] Right-sided hernias are not uncommonly, approximately 29%, associated with pleural and intraperitoneal

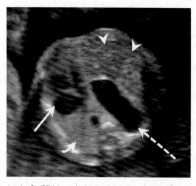

**FIGURE 17.2-1:** Left CDH with Liver Up. Axial US of the chest showing fluid-filled stomach *(dashed arrow)* in left thorax and heart *(straight arrow)* displaced into the right chest. Notice tissue anterior to the heart, consistent with herniated liver *(arrowheads)*, which is decreased echogenicity with regard to normal lung *(curved arrow)*.

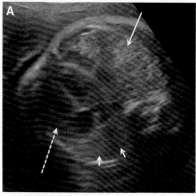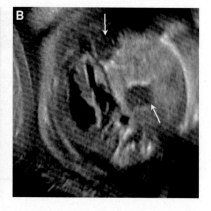

**FIGURE 17.2-2:** Left CDH and Intrathoracic Bowel. **A:** Axial US of chest in a 24-week fetus with left CDH with stomach intra-abdominal. In the left chest, the bowel is heterogeneous increased echogenicity *(long arrow)*. The heart is shifted into the right chest *(dashed arrow)* and normal homogeneous right lung is noted posteriorly *(short arrows)*. **B:** Axial US of the chest in same fetus as in A at 32 weeks. Note fluid-dilated bowel in left thorax *(arrows)*.

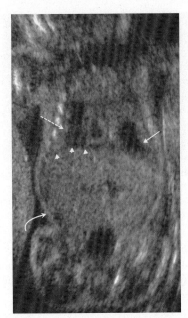

**FIGURE 17.2-3:** Left CDH. Coronal US demonstrates stomach *(straight arrow)* in the left thorax with displacement of the heart into the right chest *(dashed arrow)*. The hypoechoic diaphragm *(arrowheads)* is seen on the right but absent on the left. The abdomen is scaphoid *(curved arrow)*.

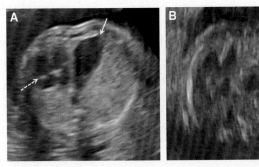

**FIGURE 17.2-4:** Left CDH with and without Liver Up. **A:** Axial thoracic US image of left CDH with liver down. The stomach *(arrow)* is along the anterior thoracic wall. Note heart at the same level in the anterior right chest *(dashed arrow)*. **B:** Axial thoracic US image of fetus with left CDH with liver up. The stomach *(solid arrow)* is displaced from the anterior thoracic wall *(curved arrow)* because of liver herniated anteriorly *(dotted arrow)*. Heart is shifted into the anterior right chest.

fluid, and rarely, hydrops may incur (Fig. 17.2-8).[15] Although sequestrations are rarely seen with hydrothorax, the presence of pleural fluid is more likely to support CDH than lung lesion.

*Bilateral CDH* is rare, occurring in 1% to 2% of all CDH cases. Complete absence of the diaphragm is even more uncommon, but can be considered the most extreme form of bilateral CDH. Diagnosis of bilateral CDH is a challenge as there is typically little to no cardiac or mediastinal shift. Diagnosis relies on visualization of the stomach and bowel in the left thorax and liver in the right and/or both thoraces.[17,18] The ectopic stomach is often present posterior or lateral to the heart, which is often displaced anterior and superior but present close to midline (Fig. 17.2-9).[15,17] Herniation of the liver is demonstrated by verifying intrathoracic hepatic vessels with color or power Doppler.[17] Bilateral CDH has a higher incidence of associated anomalies and chromosomal aberrations and is present in 10% of familial cases.[19,20]

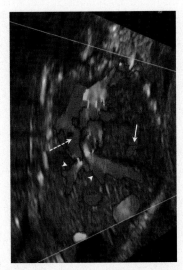

**FIGURE 17.2-5:** Left CDH with Liver Up. Coronal color Doppler US image demonstrates heart displaced into the right thorax *(dashed arrow)*. The right and middle hepatic veins *(arrowheads)* are intra-abominal, but the left hepatic vein *(solid arrow)* projects at the same level as the heart in the herniated intrathoracic liver.

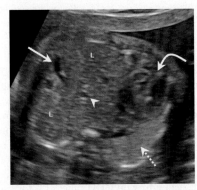

**FIGURE 17.2-6:** Right CDH. Axial US shows that the heart is displaced into the left chest *(curved arrow)*. Tubular anechoic structure consistent with gallbladder *(long arrow)* is within the right thorax, providing a clue to liver herniation *(L)*. The liver is slightly less echogenic when compared with the normal left lung posterior to the heart *(dashed arrow)*. Also note portal triads in the herniated liver *(arrowhead)*.

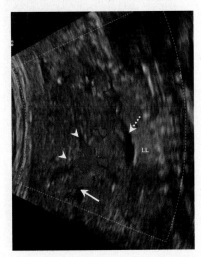

**FIGURE 17.2-7:** Right CDH. Coronal color Doppler US demonstrates kinking of the ductus venosus *(arrow)* and extension of right and middle hepatic veins *(arrowheads)* into the chest. Descending aorta *(dotted arrow)* and left lung *(LL)* are delineated.

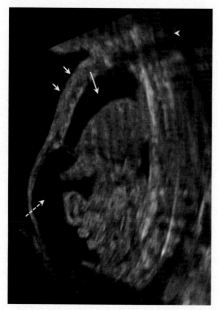

**FIGURE 17.2-8:** Right CDH with Hydrops. Sagittal US of fetus with liver within the thorax. There is large pleural fluid *(long arrow)*, ascites *(dotted arrow)*, chest wall *(short arrows)*, and nuchal *(arrowhead)* edema consistent with hydrops. Despite thoracoamniotic shunting, neonatal demise occurred.

Unless a systematic approach is made when imaging the fetal chest, diagnosis of CDH can be missed. Although Guibaud et al. found prenatal sonography detection rate was 93% at a mean gestational age (GA) of 19 weeks, in the European literature, sonographic screening for CDH resulted in only an overall detection rate in 54% to 59% after average GA of 24 weeks, improving later in gestation and in the presence of associated anomalies.[10,13,21] Prenatal detection rate has also been reported to be different depending on CDH type: 31% for right, 52% for

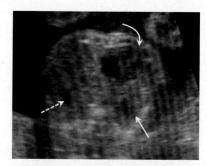

**FIGURE 17.2-9:** Bilateral CDH. Axial US of chest in a fetus with bilateral CDH. The heart is not significantly deviated *(curved arrow)*. There is a fluid-filled stomach *(arrow)* posterior to the heart in left chest, and the gallbladder *(dotted arrow)* is present in right posterior thorax.

left, and 63% in bilateral.[21] In a study that reviewed prenatal US missed CDH diagnosis, the authors found that most significant factors were quality of the imaging, lack of standard views in 55%, and missed findings in 30%.[22]

***MRI:*** In many institutions, fetal MRI is performed at age of diagnosis and late gestation (32 to 36 weeks). Prenatal MRI easily discriminates between lung, herniated liver, other herniated intra-abdominal organs, and mediastinal structures. The early imaging confirms the presence of CDH, identifying herniated tissue, lung distribution, and associated malformations.[23] Late gestation MRI is primarily obtained for lung volumes analysis.

*In left CDH*, the stomach is typically intrathoracic and may be displaced in the lower left chest, anterior to the spine or herniated into the right lower thorax, and can be distended because of impaired emptying.[23] Malrotation of the stomach organoaxial and mesenteric axial is almost always present when the stomach is intrathoracic (Fig. 17.2-10). Typically, all of the small bowel and most of the large bowel, except the left colon, is intrathoracic. Depending on GA, the small bowel will be tubular dark

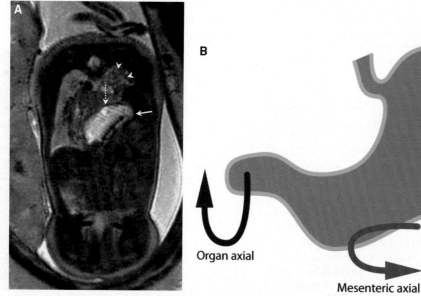

**FIGURE 17.2-10:** Left CDH with Stomach Up. **A:** Coronal T2-weighted SSFSE image in a fetus at 22 weeks. *Dotted arrow* points to the greater curvature of the stomach, superior in location, consistent organ axial malrotation. *Solid arrow* demonstrates the antrum directed to the left consistent with mesenteric axial malrotation. *Arrowheads* show collapsed dark tubular bowel. **B:** Diagram of the stomach demonstrating organ axial and mesenteric axial rotation.

structures or fluid filled (Fig. 17.2-11), and the large bowel will have variable meconium T1 hyperintensity and T2 hypointensity (Fig. 17.2-12). In most cases, the bowel is abnormally rotated and lacks normal anatomy. If the stomach is displaced, the spleen is typically intrathoracic and tends to lie adjacent to the stomach, likely because of gastrosplenic ligaments (Fig. 17.2-13). The liver is herniated in approximately 50% of cases, and the left lobe, contiguous with the liver, will extend for variable degrees into the anterior left thorax and sometimes in the presence of severe herniation, into the right thorax. T1-weighted imaging helps verify liver positioning (Fig. 17.2-14). Additional findings defined on fetal MRI are displacement of adrenal and/or kidney into the hernia (Fig. 17.2-15).

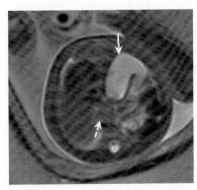

**FIGURE 17.2-13:** Left CDH and Herniated Spleen. Axial SSFSE T2 image. *Solid arrow* indicates herniated stomach. Near the stomach in the prespinal area is T2 hypointense tissue consistent with herniated spleen *(dashed arrow)*.

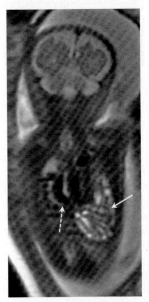

**FIGURE 17.2-11:** Left CDH with Fluid Dilated Bowel. Coronal SSFSE T2 image of fetus at GA of 33 weeks with fluid distended small bowel *(solid arrow)*. Notice dark T2 signal meconium in herniated colon *(dotted arrow)*.

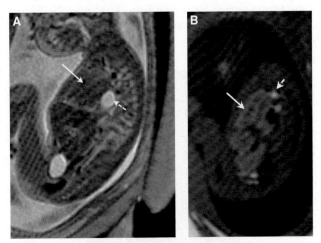

**FIGURE 17.2-14:** Left CDH with Liver Up. **A:** Sagittal SSFSE T2 image. Notice liver herniated in the anterior chest *(solid arrow)*. The stomach *(dashed arrow)* is posterior to the liver. **B:** Sagittal gradient echo T1 image in same fetus as in A. *Solid arrow* indicates herniated liver, mildly hyperintense on the T1 imaging. *Dashed arrow* indicates meconium-filled bowel within the thorax.

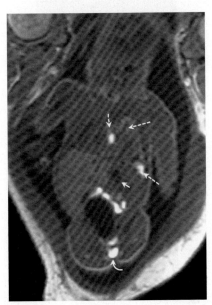

**FIGURE 17.2-12:** Left CDH and Meconium. Coronal T1 SPGR image of fetus at 32 weeks with stomach intra-abdominal *(short arrow)*. Meconium can be seen in multiple bowel loops in the left chest *(dashed arrows)* and in the rectum *(curved arrow)*.

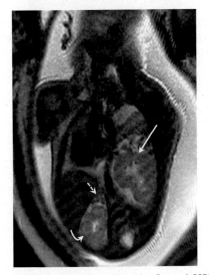

**FIGURE 17.2-15:** Left CDH with Kidney Up. Coronal SSFSE T2 image of a fetus at 32-week gestation with left kidney *(solid arrow)* partly intrathoracic and right adrenal *(dashed arrow)* and right kidney *(curved arrow)* intra-abdominal.

*In Right CDH*, the right lobe of the liver is almost constantly herniated into the anterior right chest. The gallbladder may be displaced into the right lower thorax. Liver herniation in a right CDH can result in Budd-Chiari syndrome or liver lock, in which the herniated liver is constricted by the remaining diaphragm.[23,24] In this instance, hepatic venous obstruction and liver edema develop in the intrathoracic liver. On fetal MRI, this is manifested as increased T2 signal in the intrathoracic liver when compared with the intra-abdominal portion. Small ipsilateral pleural effusions and sometimes ascites, possibly related to venous congestion, are not uncommon in the presence of a right CDH (Fig. 17.2-16).

*Bilateral CDH* are well delineated on fetal MRI as liver is easily discriminated from lung despite the absence of cardiomediastinal shift (Fig. 17.2-17).[25]

*Sac-type hernias,* which have in general a good prognosis, can be suggested by the presence of a well-defined rounded border of the hernia capped by normal lung. A sac may also be supported by pleural or peritoneal fluid lining the membrane of the hernia (Fig. 17.2-18).[24]

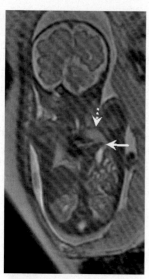

**FIGURE 17.2-18:** Sac Type Left CDH. Coronal SSFSE T2 image demonstrates that superior border of the hernia is rounded and well defined *(solid arrow)*, and there is a normally formed "cap" of left lung tissue *(dotted arrow)* consistent with sac-type hernia.

On fetal MRI, lung signal in the presence of a CDH is typically not as T2 hyperintense as expected for GA because of hypoplasia and compression.[26] If there is a dilated esophageal segment with polyhydramnios, an associated tracheoesophageal fistula may be present. MRI is also helpful in defining associated anomalies, including lung lesions that can be seen in conjunction with CDH (Fig. 17.2-19).[27,28]

**Differential Diagnosis:** Differential diagnosis for a fetal intrathoracic mass includes bronchopulmonary sequestration, congenital pulmonary airway malformations, bronchial airway

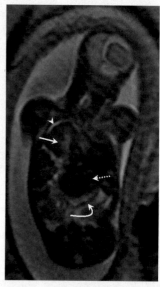

**FIGURE 17.2-16:** Right CDH with Liver Lock. Coronal SSFSE T2 imaging in a 28-week fetus. *Solid arrow* points to liver herniated and thickened edematous portal triad. Notice that the herniated liver demonstrates higher T2 signal than intra-abdominal nonedematous liver *(dotted arrow)*. *Arrowhead* shows small pleural effusion likely related to hepatic venous obstruction. *Curved arrow* is consistent with intra-abdominal stomach.

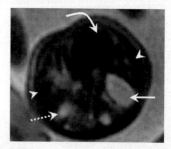

**FIGURE 17.2-17:** Bilateral CDH. Axial SSFSE T2 image of same fetus as in Figure 17.2-11. *Curved arrow* shows a normally positioned heart. In the left thorax, the *solid arrow* represents stomach. In the right thorax, *dotted arrow* indicates gallbladder. *Arrowheads* demarcate bilateral herniated liver.

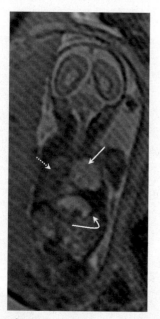

**FIGURE 17.2-19:** Left CDH with Lung Lesion. Coronal SSFSE T2 image of fetus at 23 weeks with left CDH containing stomach and liver *(curved arrow)*. There is a T2 hyperintense lung lesion *(solid arrow)* in the left upper chest that demonstrates higher signal than normal right lung *(dotted arrow)*.

obstruction, bronchopulmonary foregut anomalies, thoracic primary lung mass, and mediastinal mass such as teratoma or neurenteric cyst. Pulmonary agenesis/hypoplasia can present with displacement of the heart into the chest with absent/small lung and may mimic CDH. Diaphragmatic eventrations can also be difficult to distinguish from CDH, particularly when large. In the presence of an eventration, clues to diagnosis include lack of polyhydramnios and normal or slightly small abdominal circumference.[29]

**Associated Anomalies:** Associated anomalies occur commonly in CDH, as high as 40%. In CDH cases associated with stillbirth or intrauterine demise, this figure rises to 95%.[29] Anomalies identified commonly include, in descending order: cardiac, renal, central nervous system, and gastrointestinal.[30] Sequestrations of the lung have been associated in <5% of CDH cases.[24] Cardiac anomalies have been noted in 10% of CDH patients.[31]

**Prognosis:** If a fetus is diagnosed with CDH, the postnatal survival is approximately 25%, whereas in a population-based study, postnatal survival is cited at 52% to 69%.[32,33] Differences in outcome reflect those cases in which the fetus was stillborn or did not make it to transfer to an appropriate referral center. It is therefore important to determine which fetuses are likely to have a poor prognosis and will need immediate support (Table 17.2-3).

The identification of *additional anomalies* is imperative as these fetuses have an overall poor prognosis with survival quoted only at 19%.[21] In the presence of *diaphragmatic agenesis*, a worse outcome has been cited.[34] *Bilateral hernias* have a guarded prognosis with survival at highest 30% to 35%.[18,19,25] Right-sided hernias have been previously suggested to have less,[35] no different,[21] and increased morbidity with regard to left hernias.[36] A sac-type hernia has improved outcome.

The position of the liver is one of the most important prognostic factors, as liver up is associated with survival rates of 45% and liver down with 74%.[37,38] The existence of the *stomach in the chest* in a left CDH patient has a worse outcome, with a survival rate of 90% to 100% when intra-abdominal.[38–41] Hydrothorax and ascites have not shown to affect outcome, but may be a source for worsening pulmonary hypoplasia if large, and in the presence of cardiac/venous compression, can be lethal.[15,30] Several US markers remain controversial, including diagnosis prior to 25 weeks' gestation, polyhydramnios, and left ventricular hypoplasia/disproportion.[38,39,42]

**US Prognostic Tools:** *Pulmonary hypoplasia* is an important factor in the survival of a CDH patient. The *LHR or lung-to-head ratio* is an US tool that was devised to predict pulmonary hypoplasia and fetal outcome. The measurement is obtained by quantifying orthogonal dimensions of the right lung at the level of the cardiac atria and then, to standardize for GA, dividing the product by head circumference in millimeters. In 1996, Metkus et al.[39] described the technique and showed that a fetus with CDH and LHR < 0.6 did not survive despite postnatal therapy. In 2003, Laudy et al.[43] demonstrated that a fetus with CDH and LHR < 1 had 100% mortality, whereas those with a ratio >1.4 predicted 100% survival. Recent studies have suggested that the LHR is most reliable at predicting outcome when performed between 24 and 34 weeks.[44]

Three LHR techniques have been described. Using the University of California San Francisco methodology, the largest

| Table 17.2-3 | Markers of Poor Prognosis |
| --- | --- |

**US/MRI Anatomic Markers**

Additional anomalies
Stomach up in L CDH
Liver up
Bilateral CDH

**Pulmonary Hypoplasia**
**US tools**
*Lung*
  LHR < 1
  o/e LHR < 25%
  3D o/e TFLV < 35%
*Pulmonary artery*
  Low o/e PA ratios
**MRI tools**
*Lung*
  o/e TFLV < 25%
  PPLV < 15%
  Late gestation TLV < 20 mL
*Liver*
  LiTR ≥ 20%

**Pulmonary Hypertension**
**US tools**
*Doppler waveform*
  PI > 1
  PEDRF > 3.5
*Maternal hyperoxygenation*
  HPVR ≤ 20% PI
*Power Doppler*
  <3 divisions PA branching
  3D o/e perfusion indices <25%
  Lower FMBV
**MRI tools**
*Modified McGoon*
  MMG < 1
*Diffusion (?)*

US, ultrasound; MRI, magnetic resonance imaging; L, left; CDH, congenital diaphragmatic hernia; LHR, lung head ratio; o/e, observed-to-expected ratio; 3D, three-dimensional; TFLV, total fetal lung volume; PPLV, percent predicted lung volume; TLV, total lung volume; LiTR, liver to thoracic volume ratio; PI, pulsatility index; PEDRF, peak end diastolic reversed flow; HPVR, hyperoxygenation test for pulmonary vascular reactivity; PA, pulmonary artery; FMBV, fractional moving blood volume; MMG, modified McGoon ratio.

transverse dimension of the right lung is drawn parallel to the sternum at the level of the four-chamber heart. The largest anterior to posterior (AP) measurement is then obtained by drawing a line perpendicular to the transverse (Fig. 17.2-20A). The second technique quantifies the longest transverse measurement, regardless of plane, and then multiplies by longest perpendicular AP dimension (Fig. 17.2-20B). The third method is a tracing technique in which the outline of the right lung is performed at the level of the four-chamber heart (Fig. 17.2-20C). When comparing the three techniques, the lung tracing method has been shown be the most accurate in predicting survival.[36,45]

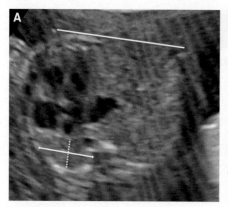 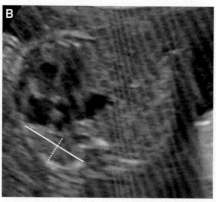 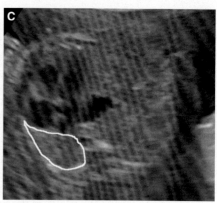

**FIGURE 17.2-20:** LHR Techniques. **A:** San Francisco method: Axial US at level of four-chamber heart in a fetus with left CDH. The *long solid line* represents line drawn parallel to sternum. Transverse right lung dimension demarcated by the *shorter solid line* is parallel to the sternal line. Perpendicular AP measurement is shown with *dotted line*. **B:** Maximum transverse dimension *(solid line)* with AP drawn perpendicular *(dotted line)*. **C:** Trace method: The circumference of the right lung is traced.

Since the lung growth increases between 12 and 32 weeks at a rate of four times the head circumference, it has been suggested that the LHR should be expressed as a ratio divided by the mean LHR of the same lung in a normal fetus for a given GA.[45,46] The expected LHR (eLHR) is obtained by an equation devised for GA, and the observed-to-expected (o/e) LHR ratio is then multiplied by 100 to obtain percentage (Table 17.2-4).[47] Using this technique, it has been demonstrated that a fetus with CDH and o/e LHR < 15% have *extreme* pulmonary hypoplasia with virtually no survivors, those between 15–20% have *severe* pulmonary hypoplasia with survival of 20%, those between 26–35% or 36–45% with liver up are *moderate* with expected survival of 30 to 60%, and those with ratios 36–45% with liver down or >45% have *mild*

| Table 17.2-4 | Important Prognosticator Equations |
| --- | --- |

**Ultrasound**

LHR[45]

Right $e$LHR $= -2.2481 + 0.2712 \times GA - 0.0033 \times GA^2$
Left $e$LHR $= -1.4815 + 0.1824 \times GA - 0.0023 \times GA^2$

3D US TFLV[54]

$e$TFLV (mL) $= \exp(4.72/(1 + \exp(20.32 - GA)/6.05))$

Pulmonary arteries[58]

MPA (mm) $= -2.77 + 0.30 \times GA$
RPA (mm) $= -1.71 + 0.18 \times GA$
LPA (mm) $= -1.95 + 0.19 \times GA$

Doppler waveform

PI: P50th: $Y = 0.537 + 0.246 \times GA - 0.005 \times GA^2$
  SD: 0.57
PEDRF (cm/s): P50th: $Y = -7.465 + 1.049 \times GA - 0.015 \times GA^2$
  SD: $Y = -7.128 + 0.56 \times GA - 0.008 \times GA^2$

**MRI**

TLV or TFLV[72,73]

By GA eFLV (mL) $= 0.0033 \times (GA)^{2.86}$
By FBV eFLV (mL) $= (0.04 \times FBV) + 3.82$

LHR, lung to head circumference ratio; GA, gestational age in weeks; TLV or TFLV, total (fetal) lung volume; MPA, main pulmonary artery; RPA, right pulmonary artery; LPA, left pulmonary artery; PI, pulsatility index; PEDRF, peak end diastolic reversed flow; FBV, fetal body volume.

hypoplasia and a survival of >75%.[48] For simplification, most utilize an o/e LHR of <25% to 26% as a high risk for pulmonary hypoplasia (see Table 17.2-3).[47,49]

The primary measurement for LHR is dependent on obtaining a true transverse plane of the fetal chest at the level of the four-chamber heart. Many question the accuracy, stating that there can be difficulty in reproducibility.[50,51] In addition, the LHR underestimates the actual total lung volume and leaves a significant group of fetuses between the two extremes in the "gray" area. For this reason, some centers do not routinely perform the LHR. Most that do obtain the measurement note that there is definitely a learning curve and that education of the technique is best taught in experienced referral centers.[52]

*Three-dimensional ultrasound (3D US),* described in the pulmonary hypoplasia section, has been utilized in fetuses with CDH. With normograms of normal lung 3D (Table 34 in Appendix A1), an o/e TFLV below 35% has been shown to predict survival, even more accurately than ipsilateral, contralateral 3D volume, or LHR (see Tables 17.2-3 and 17.2-4).[53–55] However, comparative studies have demonstrated that the 3D technique is suboptimal to LHR and MR lung volumes, as in up to 45% of cases, it is difficult to measure ipsilateral lung, and measurements are consistently 25% lower than MRI.[56]

*Prenatal pulmonary artery (PA) measurements* have been performed in the hila at the level of the four-chamber heart. Although intuitively it was thought to reflect pulmonary hypertension, it has been documented that these measurements more likely reflect lung mass.[57] Measuring the main, right, and left pulmonary arteries and comparing with normal fetuses via the o/e ratio showed a significant reduction in fetuses with CDH and pulmonary hypoplasia (see Tables 17.2-3 and 17.2-4).[58,59]

Although predicting pulmonary hypoplasia is important, it is well known that despite adequate lung volumes some infants die of *pulmonary arterial hypertension* (PAH). *Doppler waveform analysis* has proven helpful to further stratify infants, defining the most severe CDH cases at risk for lung hypoplasia and PAH. Increased pulmonary artery pulsatility index (PI) and especially peak early diastolic reversed flow (PEDRF) in the main pulmonary artery branch have been found to correlate with lung growth in fetuses but also reflect high resistance in the pulmonary vascular bed and preferential flow through the ductus arteriosus (Fig. 17.2-21).[60] In the presence of o/e LHR < 26%, PI and PEDRF transformed to z scores

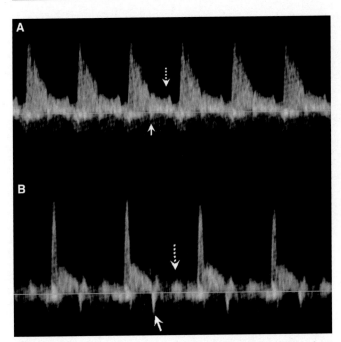

**FIGURE 17.2-21:** Pulmonary Artery Doppler. **A:** Doppler waveform from a normal fetus. There is small PEDRF *(solid arrow)* and positive diastolic flow *(dotted arrow)*. **B:** Doppler waveform from a fetus with left CDH and liver up. The PEDRF is increased *(solid arrow)*. There is intermittent loss in diastolic flow *(dotted arrow)*.

(Z-score = measured fetus − mean$_{GA}$/SD$_{GA}$), documented limited survival after fetoscopic tracheal occlusion (FETO) when the PI > 1 and PEDRF > 3.5.[60,61]

*Maternal hyperoxygenation,* with oxygen provided at 60%, can normally lower fetal pulmonary arterial resistance in the third trimester. The hyperoxygenation test for pulmonary vascular reactivity (HPVR) performed in fetuses with CDH at 31 to 36 weeks and after fetoscopic occlusion therapy demonstrated a good outcome when a reactive test, ≥20% reductions in pulmonary artery pretest PI, was noted.[62,63]

*Power Doppler* may also provide important information about changes in lung tissue perfusion. When the contralateral lung is evaluated at the level of the four-chamber heart, PAH has been predicted if there is visualization of less than three divisions of vascular branching on 2D US or when 3D volume rendered perfusion indices compared with normal were <25%.[64,65] However, these methods are qualitative or limited by lack of correction for attenuation and depth or variation in power Doppler setting.[63] Recently, a quantitative highly accurate method termed *fractional moving blood volume (FMBV)* has been developed. This technique depicts the percentage of moving blood in a specific region of interest (ROI).[66] Currently, there are no commercial systems available to accurately measure blood volume but MATLAB software 7.5 (The MathWorks, Natick, MA, USA) has proven valid at quantitating perfusion.[67] Decreased FMBV has been shown to correlate with decreased lung growth and increased intrapulmonary artery impedance in CDH and has proven helpful in evaluating the potential of survival after tracheal occlusion procedure, with delayed imaging documenting a ≥30% of FMBV, ≥50% LHR change, and 100% survival.[67,68]

**MRI Prognostic Tools:** MRI imaging has become a well-documented technique when evaluating for *pulmonary hypoplasia*. The least validated method is the use of *lung signal intensity,*

as compressed and hypoplastic lung demonstrates decreased signal when compared with normal lung for GA. Fetal lung-to-liver signal intensity ratio, LLSIR, has been shown to increase with GA; however, recent literature has shown that the ratio is not useful when predicting CDH outcome.[69,70]

*Volumetric analysis of the lung* with MRI has become the method of choice to obtain *total fetal lung volume (TLV or TFLV),* has been described since the 1990s, and is utilized to predict severity of hypoplasia in CDH and response to fetoscopic occlusion therapy. Several researchers have developed GA-based normograms of lung volumes with 3D processing (see Table 37 in Appendix A1)[71–73]. When describing fetal lung volume in CDH, the amount of lung present in the fetus with CDH is often related to normal expected lung volumes, most commonly those that reflect normal volumes for GA or fetal body volume.[74,75] Multiple researchers have noted a strong correlation with outcome when utilizing these ratios, known as *relative fetal lung volume (rFLV)* or an *observed to expected total fetal lung volume (O/E TFLV).* Paek found that a rFLV less than 40% suggested poor outcome, whereas Datin-Dorriere et al. noted a rFLV cut-off at 30%.[38,74] Gorincour et al.[75] and Jani et al.[76] noted poor survival in those fetuses in which the O/E TFLV was <25%.

An innovative technique to standardize lung volume includes the *percent predicted lung volume (PPLV),* a calculation that utilizes the total thoracic volume subtracted from the mediastinal volume to estimate expected lung volume (Fig. 17.2-22). The PPLV is obtained by dividing the actual lung volume in the CDH fetus by this estimated lung volume.[77] Barnewolt et al.[77] found that a PPLV of <15% had a 40% survival, whereas a PPLV of 20% had 100% survival.

The rFLV or O/E TFLV ratios have also been compared with TLV, with studies demonstrating that both techniques are equally predictable of survival and morbidity in CDH.[78,79] Because lung growth is accelerated later in gestation, some hypothesized that MRI fetal lung volumes later in gestation, at 34 to 35 weeks, may

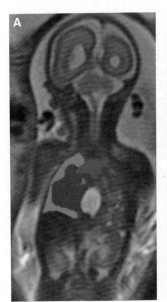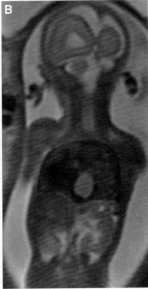

**FIGURE 17.2-22:** Volumes for Percent Predicted Lung Volume. **A:** Coronal SSFSE T2 image with superimposed 3D MRI lung volume of the right lung *(orange)*, left lung *(blue)*, and mediastinal volume *(pink)* in a fetus with left CDH. **B:** Coronal SSFSE T2 image with superimposed 3D MRI total thoracic volume.

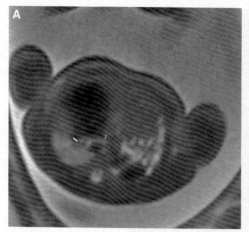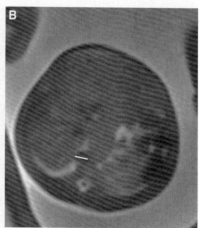

**FIGURE 17.2-23:** Modified McGoon Index. **A:** The right *(solid line)* and left *(dotted line)* pulmonary artery transverse dimensions obtained on an axial SSFSE T2 image in a fetus with left CDH. **B:** The transverse dimension of the descending aorta *(line)* at the level of the diaphragm.

be a better gauge of outcome and need for postnatal support. Lee et al.[80] noted that a late gestation TLV of less than 20 mL was associated with 35% survival and 86% extracorporeal membrane oxygenation (ECMO), whereas those above 40 mL had a survival of 90%, with 10% needing ECMO.

Despite different methodologies and GA at time of assessment, there remain questions regarding the validity of the volumetric analysis. Assessment of normal fetal lung volume literature demonstrates that there is no standardization of the technique, including pulse sequence parameters, plane of imaging to assess volume, and ROI with inclusion or exclusion of mediastinum and pulmonary vessels/hila.[81] In defense, a study directed at obtaining MR lung volumetry in CDH cases demonstrated good interobserver reliability, independent of sequence or imaging plane.[82]

Since MRI easily discriminates liver from lung, the technique is extremely helpful in confirming liver up or down morphology. *Volumetric analysis of the liver* with fetal MRI has been performed and compared as a ratio or percentage with total thoracic volume. This liver-to-thoracic ratio (LiTR) was predictive of postnatal survival in CDH, with neonatal death more likely when ≥20% of fetal thoracic volume was occupied by the liver.[83,84]

Fetal MRI may be helpful in the prediction of *PAH*. The *modified McGoon (MMG) index*, previously described as an US technique, has also been performed on late gestation fetal MRI. On an axial T2 image, maximum diameters are obtained of the right and left pulmonary artery and aorta at the level of the diaphragm (Fig. 17.2-23). Vuletin et al.[85] found that an index of <1 correlated with severe postnatal pulmonary hypertension at 3 weeks postnatally.

*Diffusion imaging* may also hold promise in providing functional information with regard to lung development, since the apparent diffusion coefficient (ADC) measurement reveals capillary perfusion and water diffusion in the extravascular space. In the presence of CDH, however, a difference in the ADC values compared with normal fetuses did not predict survival and did not correlate with fetal lung volume.[86] These findings may reflect the limitations of the technique, which include high sensitivity to fetal motion, lower signal, and longer scan times.

**Management:** Many fetuses with CDH are detected early in gestation with liver herniation and LHR < 1.35. With these parameters, parents may choose to terminate the pregnancy attempt fetal intervention, or continue the pregnancy to term.

Prenatal surgical intervention for CDH has been evaluated for years with first attempts at open repair failing because of kinking of the umbilical vein during liver reduction and preterm labor from uterine irritability. Utilizing fetal sheep with CDH, it was proven that tracheal obstruction accelerated lung growth and pushed viscera back into the abdomen, resulting in significant improvement in outcome (Fig. 17.2-24).[87] Because of these experiments, tracheal occlusion in the human fetus was first attempted open and then via fetoscopic placement of a detachable endoluminal balloon.[88] This early trial, however, was terminated when it was found that the standard care group had as high a survival (77%) as the tracheal occlusion group (73%).

Fetoscopic endotracheal occlusion (FETO) has reemerged and is currently performed via balloon occlusion in Europe and a few centers in the United States (Fig. 17.2-25).[89] The surgery is offered to those CDH fetuses with extreme or severe hypoplasia represented by an LHR < 1 and/or o/e LHR < 27% to 28% with liver herniation. The balloon is inserted at 26 to 28 weeks and then removed at 34 weeks. There is a high risk for premature rupture of membranes, which may require EXIT to balloon retrieval. However, the technique holds promise in the presence of severe CDH, as FETO improved survival rate in left CDH from 24% conventional therapy to 49% with FETO and in right CDH from 0% to 35%, respectively.[90] Another similar study cited 52% survival with FETO and 5% with conservative therapy.[91] Major predictors for survival in FETO include GA at delivery and lung measurements, o/e LHR, pre-FETO.[48,49]

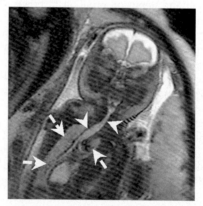

**FIGURE 17.2-24:** Trachael balloon occlusion in CDH. Coronal T2 MRI shows dilatation of the airway *(arrowheads)* and hyperintense lungs *(dashed arrows)* because of balloon trachael occlusion. Image courtesy of Chris Cassady, MD.

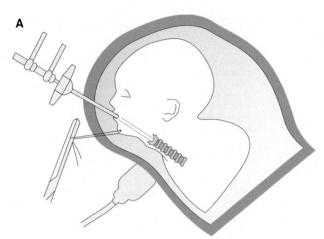
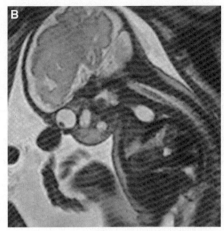

**FIGURE 17.2-25:** Fetoscopic Endotrachael Balloon Occlusion. **A:** The diagram demonstrates placement of the balloon into the trachea under ultrasound guidance. **B:** Corresponding sagittal T2 MR image shows the balloon positioned in the trachea. Image courtesy of Chris Cassady, MD.

An increase in lung volume after FETO was an independent variant for survival, while pulmonary vascular reactivity was a predictor for both survival and PAH.[49]

If the pregnancy is continued without prenatal intervention, US is recommended once a month prior to 32 weeks and at least weekly as term approaches. Close observation late in gestation is necessary to manage developing polyhydramnios and evaluate fetal well-being. In those cases in which there is high risk, especially low lung volume, arrangements should be made for planned delivery at a tertiary care center around 37 to 38 weeks.

Prior to the 1990s, neonatal management of CDH included emergent repair followed by aggressive ventilation. Evidence now suggests that better outcome may be achieved by delivering at an experienced center, delaying surgery until acceptable hemodynamic and respiratory stability has been attained with nonaggressive mechanical ventilation.[92] Nonaggressive ventilation, also known as "gentilation," is aimed at reducing barotrauma and pneumothorax by limiting inflation pressure and preventing hyperventilation. Nitrous oxide is utilized to treat pulmonary hypertension, and prostaglandins are commonly administered to keep the ductus arteriosus patent, especially with severe right ventricular dysfunction.[2] ECMO is utilized in 15% to 54% of neonates with CDH and may be a rescue after birth in those infants with significant pulmonary hypertension, hypoplasia, or ventilator lung injury.[93] In the presence of poor prognosticators, some centers have delivered the infant ex utero intrapartum treatment to extracorporeal membrane oxygenation (EXIT to ECMO); however, recent studies have shown no outcome benefit.[94,95] The decision to utilize ECMO has shifted to early use to achieve lung preservation when medical therapy has failed.

When appropriate respiratory and hemodynamic stability is achieved, surgical repair is currently favored thoracoscopic rather than via thoracotomy.[96] In neonates with a large defect, a patch of synthetic or bioprosthetic material may be necessary to close the defect.

The long-term outcome for these children remains complicated. Approximately, 50% of these children have chronic respiratory disease.[48,96] Gastroesophageal reflux is frequent, and as many as 30% will have failure to thrive between 6 months and 2 years of life.[96] Neurodevelopmental deficits are possible, particularly when ECMO is required, but is also seen in 23% to 46% of children not requiring ECMO.[97] Sensorineural hearing loss is common.[48] Chest asymmetry and vertebral anomalies may originate because of abnormal fetal development.[98]

**Recurrence:** Most cases are sporadic with recurrence risk at 2%, increasing to 10% in a family with two affected siblings.[3,7] Familial CDH inheritance is either multifactorial or autosomal recessive, but in the presence of diaphragmatic agenesis or bilateral CDH, autosomal recessive inheritance is likely.[7,48,98]

## REFERENCES

1. Holder AM, Klaassens M, Tibboel D, et al. Genetic factors in congenital diaphragmatic hernia. *Am J Hum Genet.* 2007;80:825–845.
2. Deprest JA, Gratacos E, Nicolaides K, et al. Changing perspectives on the perinatal management of isolated congenital diaphragmatic hernia in Europe. *Clin Perinatol.* 2009;36:329–347.
3. Pober BR. Genetic aspects of human congenital diaphragmatic hernia. *Clin Genet.* 2008;74:1–15.
4. Babiuk RP, Greer JP. Diaphragm defects occur in a CDH hernia model independently of myogenesis and lung formation. *Am J Physiol Lung Cell Mol Physiol.* 2002;283:L1310–L1314.
5. Ackerman KG, Pober BR. Congenital diaphragmatic hernia and pulmonary hypoplasia: new insights from developmental biology and genetics. *Am J Med Genet C Semin Med Genet.* 2007;145C:105–108.
6. Tovar JA. Congenital diaphragmatic hernia. *Orphanet J Rare Dis.* 2012;7:1–15.
7. Nagase H, Ishikawa H, Kurosawa K, et al. Familial severe congenital diaphragmatic hernia: left herniation in one sibling and bilateral herniation in another. *Congenit Anom.* 2013;53:54–57.
8. Waag KL, Loff S, Zahn K, et al. Congenital diaphragmatic hernia: a modern day approach. *Semin Pediatr Surg.* 2008;17:244–254.
9. Goumy C, Gousas L, Marceau G, et al. Retinoid pathway and congenital diaphragmatic hernia: hypothesis from the analysis of chromosomal abnormalities. *Fetal Diagn Ther.* 2010;28:129–139.
10. Garne E, Haeusler M, Barisic I, et al. Congenital diaphragmatic hernia: evaluation of prenatal diagnosis in 20 European regions. *Ultrasound Obstet Gynecol.* 2002;19:329–333.
11. Howe DT, Kilby MD, Sirry H, et al. Structural chromosome anomalies in congenital diaphragmatic hernia. *Prenat Diagn.* 1996;16:P1003–P1009.
12. Claus F, Sandaite I, Dekoninck P, et al. Prenatal anatomical imaging in fetuses with congenital diaphragmatic hernia. *Fetal Diagn Ther.* 2011;29:88–100.
13. Guibaud L, Filiatrault D, Garel L, et al. Fetal congenital diaphragmatic hernia: accuracy of sonography in the diagnosis and prediction of the outcome after birth. *AJR Am J Roentgenol.* 1996;166:1195–1202.
14. Bianchi DW, Crombleholme TM, D'Alton ME, et al. *Fetology: Diagnosis and Management of the Fetal Patient.* 2nd ed. New York, NY: McGraw Hill Medical; 2010.
15. Mieghem TV, Cruz-Martinez R, Allegaerts K, et al. Outcome of fetuses with congenital diaphragmatic hernia and associated intrafetal fluid effusions managed in the era of fetal surgery. *Ultrasound Obstet Gynecol.* 2012;39:50–55.
16. Bootstaylor BS, Filly RA, Harrison MR. Prenatal sonographic predictors of liver herniation in congenital diaphragmatic hernia. *J Ultrasound Med.* 1995;14:515–520.
17. Song MS, Yoo SJ, Smallhorn JF, et al. Bilateral congenital diaphragmatic hernia: diagnostic clues at fetal sonography. *Ultrasound Obstet Gynecol.* 2001;17:255–258.

18. Kamata S, Sawai T, Usui N, et al. Bilateral diaphragmatic hernia followed by fetal ultrasonography. A report of two cases. *Fetal Diagn Ther.* 2001;16(4):248–50.

19. Eroglu D, Yanik F, Sakallioglu AE, et al. Prenatal diagnosis of bilateral diaphragmatic hernia by fetal sonography. *J Obstet Gynaecol Res.* 2006;32:90–93.

20. Neville HL, Jaksic T, Wilson JM, et al. Bilateral congenital diaphragmatic hernia. *J Pediatr Surg.* 2003;38:522–524.

21. Gallot D, Boda C, Ughetto S, et al. Prenatal detection and outcome of congenital diaphragramtic hernia: a French registry-based study. *Ultrasound Obstet Gynecol.* 2007;29:276–283.

22. Lewis DA, Reickert C, Bowerman R, et al. Prenatal ultrasonography frequently fails to diagnose congenital diaphragmatic hernia. *J Pediatr Surg.* 1997;32:352–356.

23. Leung JWT, Coakley FV, Hricak H, et al. Prenatal MR imaging of congenital diaphragmatic hernia. *AJR Am J Roentgenol.* 2000;174:1607–1612.

24. Mehollin-Ray AR, Cassady CI, Cass DL, et al. Fetal MR imaging of congenital diaphragmatic hernia. *Radiographics.* 2012;32:1067–1084.

25. Hiasa KI, Fujita Y, Fukushima K, et al. Ultrasound and MR images of prenatally diagnosed bilateral congenital diaphragmatic hernia, a rare variation of CDH. *Clin Imaging.* 2012;36:639–642.

26. Barth RA, Rubesova E. Fetal magnetic resonance imaging: anomalies of the neck, chest and abdomen. *Neoreviews.* 2007;8:e313–e335.

27. Hubbard AM, Crombleholme TM, Adzick NS, et al. Prenatal MRI evaluation of congenital diaphragmatic hernia. *Am J Perinatol.* 1999;16:407–413.

28. Hubbard AM, Adzick NS, Crombleholme TM, et al. Congenital chest lesions: diagnosis and characterization with prenatal MR imaging. *Radiology.* 1999;212:43–48.

29. Puri P, Gorman F. Lethal nonpulmonary anomalies associated with congenital diaphragmatic hernia: implications for early intrauterine surgery. *J Pediatr Surg.* 1984;19:29–32.

30. Graham G, Devine PC. Antenatal diagnosis of congenital diaphragmatic hernia. *Semin Perinatol.* 2005;29:69–76.

31. Graziano JN. Cardiac anomalies in patients with congenital diaphragmatic hernia and their prognosis: a report from the Congenital Diaphragmatic Hernia Study Group. *J Pediatr Surg.* 2005;40:1045–1050.

32. Skari H, Bjornland K, Haugen G, et al. Congenital diaphragmatic hernia: a meta-analysis of mortality factors. *J Pediatr Surg.* 2000;35:1187–1197.

33. Mayer S, Klaritsch P, Petersen S, et al. The correlation between lung volume and liver herniation measurements by fetal MRI in isolated congenital diaphragmatic hernia: a systematic review and meta-analysis of observational studies. *Prenat Diagn.* 2011;31:1086–1096.

34. Gibbs DL, Rice HE, Farrell JA, et al. Familial diaphragmatic agenesis: an autosomal-recessive syndrome with a poor prognosis. *J Pediatr Surg.* 1997;32:366–368.

35. Hedrick HL, Crombleholme TM, Flake AW, et al. Right congenital diaphragmatic hernia. *J Pediatr Surg.* 2004;39:319–323.

36. Fisher JC, Jefferson RA, Arkovitz MS, et al. Redefining outcomes in right congenital diaphragmatic hernia. *J Pediatr Surg.* 2008;43:373–379.

37. Mullassery D, Ba'ath ME, Jesudason EC, et al. Value of liver herniation in prediction of outcome in fetal congenital diaphragmatic hernia: a systematic review of meta-analysis. *Ultrasound Obstet Gynecol.* 2010;35:609–614.

38. Datin-Dorriere V, Rouzies S, Taupin P, et al. Prenatal prognosis in isolated congenital diaphragmatic hernia. *Am J Obstet Gynecol.* 2008;198:80.e1–80.e5.

39. Metkus AP, Filly RA, Stringer MD, et al. Sonographic predictors of survival in fetal diaphragmatic hernia. *J Pediatr Surg.* 1996;31:148–152.

40. Hatch EI Jr, Kendall J, Blumhagen J. Stomach position as an in utero predictor of neonatal outcome in left-sided diaphragmatic hernia. *J Pediatr Surg.* 1992;27:776–779.

41. Hedrick HL, Danzer E, Merchant A. Liver position and lung-to-head ratio for prediction of extracorporeal membrane oxygenation and survival in isolated left congenital diaphragmatic hernia. *Am J Obstet Gynecol.* 2007;197:422.e1–422.e4.

42. Thebaud B, Azancot A, de Lagausie P. Congenital diaphragmatic hernia: antenatal prognostic factors: does cardiac ventricular disproportion in utero predict outcome and pulmonary hypoplasia? *Intensive Care Med.* 1997;23:1062–1069.

43. Laudy JAM, Van Gucht M, Dooren MF, et al. Congenital diaphragmatic hernia: an evaluation of the prognostic value of the lung-to-head ratio and other prenatal parameters. *Prenat Diagn.* 2003;23:634–639.

44. Yang SH, Nobuhara KK, Keller RL, et al. Reliability of the lung-to-head ratio as a predictor of outcome in fetuses with isolated left congenital diaphragmatic hernia at gestation outside 24–26 weeks. *Am J Obstet Gynecol.* 2007;197:30.e1–30.e7.

45. Peralta CFA, Cavoretto P, Csapo B, et al. Assessment of lung area in normal fetuses at 12–32 weeks. *Ultrasound Obstet Gynecol.* 2005;26:718–724.

46. Jani JC, Peralta CFA, Ruano R, et al. Comparison of fetal lung area to head circumference ratio with lung volume in the prediction of postnatal outcome in diaphragmatic hernia. *Ultrasound Obstet Gynecol.* 2007;30:850–854.

47. Jani J, Nicolaides KH, Keller RL, et al. Observed to expected lung area to head circumference ratio in the prediction of survival in fetuses with isolated diaphragmatic hernia. *Ultrasound Obstet Gynecol.* 2007;30:67–71.

48. Deprest JA, Flemmer AW, Gratacos E, et al. Antenatal prediction of lung volume and in-utero treatment by fetal endoscopic tracheal occlusion in severe isolated congenital diaphragmatic hernia. *Semin Fetal Neonatal Med.* 2009;14:8–13.

49. Jani JC, Nicolaides KH, Gratacos E, et al. Fetal lung-to-head ratio in the prediction of survival in severe left-sided diaphragmatic hernia treated by fetal endoscopic tracheal occlusion (FETO). *Am J Obstet Gynecol.* 2006;195:1646–1650.

50. Arkovitz MS, Russo M, Devine P. Fetal lung-head ratio is not related to outcome for antenatal diagnosed congenital diaphragmatic hernia. *J Pediatr Surg.* 2007;42:107–111.

51. Ba'ath ME, Jesudason EC, Losty PD. How useful is the lung-to-head ratio in predicting outcome in the fetus with congenital diaphragmatic hernia? A systematic review and meta-analysis. *Ultrasound Obstet Gynecol.* 2007;30:897–906.

52. Cruz-Martinez R, Figueras F, Moreno-Alvarez O. Learning curve for lung area to head circumference ratio measurement in fetuses with congenital diaphragmatic hernia. *Ultrasound Obstet Gynecol.* 2010;36:32–36.

53. Ruano R, Takashi E, Da Silva MM, et al. Prediction and probability of neonatal outcome in isolated congenital diaphragmatic hernia using multiple ultrasound parameters. *Ultrasound Obstet Gynecol.* 2012;39:42–49.

54. Ruano R, Benachi A, Joubin L, et al. Three-dimensional ultrasonographic assessment of fetal lung volume as a prognostic factor in isolated congenital diaphragmatic hernia. *BJOG.* 2004;111:423–429.

55. Ruano R, Aubry MC, Barthe B, et al. Three-dimensional sonographic measurement of contralateral lung volume in fetuses with isolated congenital diaphragmatic hernia. *J Clin Ultrasound.* 2008;36:273–278.

56. Jani JC, Cannie M, Peralta CFA, et al. Lung volumes in fetuses with congenital diaphragmatic hernia: comparison of 3D US and MR imaging assessments. *Radiology.* 2007;244:575–582.

57. Sokol J, Bohn D, Lacro RV, et al. Fetal pulmonary artery diameters and their association with lung hypoplasia and postnatal outcome in congenital diaphragmatic hernia. *Am J Obstet Gynecol.* 2002;186:1085–1090.

58. Ruano R, de Fatima M, Maeda Y, et al. Pulmonary artery diameters in healthy fetuses from 19 to 40 weeks' gestation. *J Ultrasound Med.* 2007;26:309–316.

59. Ruano R, Aubry MC, Barthe B, et al. Predicting perinatal outcome in isolated congenital diaphragmatic hernia using fetal pulmonary artery diameters. *J Pediatr Surg.* 2008;43:606–611.

60. Moreno-Alvarez O, Hernandez-Andrade E, Oros D, et al. Association between intrapulmonary arterial Doppler parameters and degree of lung growth as measured by lung-to-head ratio in fetuses with congenital diaphragmatic hernia. *Ultrasound Obstet Gynecol.* 2008;31:164–170.

61. Cruz-Martinez R, Moreno-Alvarez O, Hernandez-Andrade E, et al. Contribution of intrapulmonary artery Doppler to improve prediction of survival in fetuses with congenital diaphragmatic hernia treated with fetal endoscopic tracheal occlusion. *Ultrasound Obstet Gynecol.* 2010;35:572–577.

62. Broth RE, Wood DC, Rasanen J, et al. Prenatal prediction of lethal pulmonary hypoplasia: the hyperoxygenation test for pulmonary artery reactivity. *Am J Obstet Gynecol.* 2002;187:940–945.

63. Cruz-Martinez R, Hernandez-Andrade E, Moreno-Alvarez O, et al. Prognostic value of pulmonary Doppler to predict response to tracheal occlusion in fetuses with congenital diaphragmatic hernia. *Fetal Diagn Ther.* 2011;29:18–24.

64. Ruano R, Aubry MC, Barthe B, et al. Quantitative analysis of fetal pulmonary vasculature by 3-dimensional power Doppler ultrasonography in isolated congenital diaphragmatic hernia. *Am J Obstet Gynecol.* 2006;195:1720–1728.

65. Mahieu-Caputo D, Aubry MC, El Sayed M, et al. Evaluation of fetal pulmonary vasculature by power Doppler imaging in congenital diaphragmatic hernia. *J Ultrasound Med.* 2004;23:1011–1017.

66. Hernandez-Andrade E, Thuring-Jonsson A, Jasson T, et al. Fractional moving blood volume estimation in the fetal lung using power Doppler ultrasound: a reproducibility study. *Ultrasound Obstet Gynecol.* 2004;23:369–373.

67. Moreno-Alvarez O, Cruz-Martinez R, Hernandez-Andrade E, et al. Lung tissue perfusion in congenital diaphragmatic hernia and association with the lung-to-head ratio and intrapulmonary artery pulsed Doppler. *Ultrasound Obstet Gynecol.* 2010;35:578–582.

68. Cruz-Martinez R, Moreno-Alvarez O, Hernandez-Andrade E, et al. Changes in lung tissue perfusion in the prediction of survival in fetuses with congenital diaphragmatic hernia treated with fetal endoscopic tracheal occlusion. *Fetal Diagn Ther.* 2011;29:101–107.

69. Brewerton LJ, Chair RS, Liang Y, et al. Fetal lung-to-liver signal intensity ratio at MR imaging: development of a normal scale and possible role in predicting pulmonary hypoplasia *in utero.* *Radiology.* 2005;235:1005–1010.

70. Balass C, Kasprian G, Brugger PC, et al. Assessment of lung development in isolated congenital diaphragmatic hernia using signal intensity ratios on fetal imaging. *Eur Radiol.* 2010;20:829–837.

71. Coakley FV, Lopoo JB, Lu Y, et al. Normal and hypoplastic fetal lungs: volumetric assessment with prenatal signal-shot rapid acquisition with relaxation enhancement MR imaging. *Radiology.* 2000;216:107–111.

72. Rypens F, Metens T, Rocourt N, et al. Fetal lung volume: estimation at MR imaging—initial results. *Radiology.* 2001;219:236–241.

73. Cannie M, Jani JC, DeKeyzer F, et al. Fetal body volume: use at MR imaging to quantify relative lung volume in fetuses suspected of having pulmonary hypoplasia. *Radiology.* 2006;241:847–853.

74. Paek BW, Coakley FV, Lu Y, et al. Congenital diaphragmatic hernia: prenatal evaluation with MR lung volumetry: preliminary experience. *Radiology.* 2001;220:63–67.

75. Gorincour G, Bouvenot J, Mourot MG, et al. Prenatal prognosis of congenital diaphragmatic hernia using magnetic resonance imaging measurement of fetal lung volume. *Ultrasound Obstet Gynecol.* 2005;26:738–744.

76. Jani J, Cannie M, Sonigo P, et al. Value of prenatal magnetic resonance imaging in the prediction of postnatal outcome in fetuses with diaphragmatic hernia. *Ultrasound Obstet Gynecol.* 2008;32:791–799.

77. Barnewolt CE, Kunisaki SM, Fauza DO, et al. Percent predicted lung volumes as measured on fetal magnetic resonance imaging: a useful biometric parameter for risk stratification in congenital diaphragmatic hernia. *J Pediatr Surg.* 2007;42:193–197.

78. Busing KA, Killian AK, Schaible T, et al. MR relative fetal lung volume in congenital diaphragmatic hernia: survival and need for extracorporeal membrane oxygenation. *Radiology.* 2008;248:240–246.

79. Killian AK, Schaible T, Hofmann V, et al. Congenital diaphragmatic hernia: predictive value of MRI relative lung-to-head ratio compared with MRI fetal lung volume and sonographic lung-to-head ratio. *AJR Am J Roentgenol.* 2009;192:153–158.

80. Lee TC, Lim FY, Keswani SG, et al. Late gestation fetal magnetic resonance imaging-derived total lung volume predicts postnatal survival and need for extracorporeal membrane oxygenation support in isolated congenital diaphragmatic hernia. *J Pediatr Surg.* 2011;46:1165–1171.

81. Deshmukh S, Rubesova E, Barth R. MR assessment of normal fetal lung volumes: a literature review. *AJR Am J Roentgenol.* 2010;194:W212–W217.

82. Busing KA, Killian AK, Schaible T, et al. Reliability and validity of MR image lung volume measurement in fetuses with congenital diaphragmatic hernia and in vitro lung models. *Radiology.* 2008;246:533–561.

83. Cannie M, Jani J, Chaffiotte C, et al. Quantification of intrathoracic liver herniation by magnetic resonance imaging and prediction of postnatal survival in fetuses with congenital diaphragmatic hernia. *Ultrasound Obstet Gynecol.* 2008;32:627–632.

84. Worley KC, Dashe JS, Barber RG, et al. Fetal magnetic resonance imaging in isolated diaphragmatic hernia: volume of herniated liver and neonatal outcome. *Am J Obstet Gynecol.* 2009;200:318.e1–318.e6.

85. Vuletin JF, Lim FY, Cnota J, et al. Prenatal pulmonary hypertension index: novel prenatal predictor of severe postnatal pulmonary artery hypertension in antenatally diagnosed congenital diaphragmatic hernia. *J Pediatr Surg.* 2010;45:703–708.

86. Cannie M, Janis J, De Keyyzer F, et al. Diffusion-weighted MRI in lungs of normal fetuses and those with congenital diaphragmatic hernia. *Ultrasound Obstet Gynecol.* 2009;34:678–686.

87. Hedrick MH, Estes JM, Sullivan KM, et al. Plug the lung until grows (PLUG): a new method to treat congenital diaphragmatic hernia *in utero. J Pediatr Surg.* 1994;29:612–617.

88. Harrison MR, Keller RL, Hawgood SB, et al. A randomized trial of fetal endoscopic tracheal occlusion for severe fetal congenital diaphragmatic hernia. *N Engl J Med.* 2003;349:1916–1924.

89. Deprest JA, Hyett JA, Flake AW, et al. Current controversies in prenatal diagnosis 4: should fetal surgery be done in all cases of severe diaphragmatic hernia? *Prenat Diagn.* 2009;29:15–19.

90. Jani JC, Nicolaides KH, Gratacos E, et al. Severe diaphragmatic hernia treated by fetal endoscopic tracheal occlusion. *Ultrasound Obstet Gynecol.* 2009;34: 304–310.

91. Ruano R, Yoshisaki CT, Da Silva MM, et al. A randomized controlled trial of fetal endoscopic tracheal occlusion versus postnatal management of severe isolated congenital diaphragmatic hernia. *Ultrasound Obstet Gynecol.* 2012;39: 20–27.

92. Downard CD, Jaksic T, Garza JJ, et al. Analysis of an improved survival rate for congenital diaphragmatic hernia. *J Pediatr Surg.* 2003;38:729–732.

93. Kays DW. Congenital diaphragmatic hernia: real improvements in survival. *Neoreviews.* 2006;7:e428–e439.

94. Rollins MD. Recent advances in the management of congenital diaphragmatic hernia. *Curr Opin Pediatr.* 2012;24:379–385.

95. Hedrick HL. Management of prenatally diagnosed congenital diaphragmatic hernia. *Semin Pediatr Surg.* 2013;22:37–43.

96. Haroon J, Chamberlain RS. An evidence-based review of the current treatment of congenital diaphragmatic hernia. *Clin Pediatr.* 2012;52:115–124.

97. Frisk V, Jakobson LS, Unger S, et al. Long-term neurodevelopmental outcomes of congenital diaphragmatic hernia survivors not treated with extracorporeal membrane oxygenation. *J Pediatr Surg.* 2011;46:1309–1318.

98. Hitch DC, Carson JA, Smith EI, et al. Familial congenital diaphragmatic hernia is an autosomal recessive variant. *J Pediatr Surg.* 1989;24:860–864.

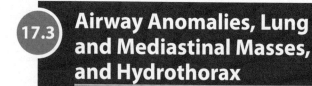

## 17.3 Airway Anomalies, Lung and Mediastinal Masses, and Hydrothorax

Richard A. Barth

## AIRWAY ANOMALIES

### Congenital High Airway Obstruction Syndrome

Congenital high airway obstruction syndrome (CHAOS) is a rare fetal anomaly resulting from airway obstruction secondary to laryngeal atresia, or less commonly a laryngeal cyst, laryngeal web, laryngeal stenosis, or tracheal atresia.[1,2] CHAOS is typically bilateral; however, sporadically can be unilateral secondary to central bronchial atresia.

**Incidence:** The incidence of CHAOS is unknown as only a few cases have been reported in the literature.[3,4]

**Pathogenesis/Associated Anomalies:** The pathogenesis relates to a complete airway obstruction resulting in trapping and accumulation of fluid within the fetal airways and lungs. Pathologic findings include severe distention of the fetal trachea, bronchi, and hyperplastic lungs. The markedly enlarged fetal lungs compress the heart and inferior vena cava decreasing venous return to the heart, which often results in fetal ascites, in-utero heart failure, placentomegaly, and hydrops fetalis.[1] Isolated CHAOS is a sporadic fetal malformation with a low risk for associated anomalies or chromosomal abnormalities. Less-commonly CHAOS can be associated with Fraser syndrome, which is an autosomal recessive disorder characterized by laryngeal atresia secondary to underlying fusion of the false vocal cords. Other associations with Fraser syndrome include renal agenesis, microphthalmia, cryptophtalmos, polydactyly, syndactyly, cleft lip/palate, ear anomalies, ambiguous genitalia, congenital heart disease, and severe oligohydramnios secondary to bilateral renal agenesis.[5,6]

**Diagnosis:** On ultrasound (US), the characteristic findings of CHAOS include hyperechogenic and hyperexpanded lungs resulting in flattening or inversion of the diaphragms (Fig. 17.3-1A,B).[3,6] A dilated fluid-filled trachea and bronchi are often identified below the level of the airway obstruction, which most commonly occurs at the level of the larynx. Color Doppler will allow separation of the dilated airway from adjacent vasculature. Fetal ascites is a common feature of CHAOS resulting from obstructed venous return to the heart.

On magnetic resonance imaging (MRI), T2-weighted sequences show similar findings including hyperinflated high-signal lungs inverting diaphragms and severely dilated bronchi distal to the more proximal airway obstruction (see Fig. 17.3-1C,D).

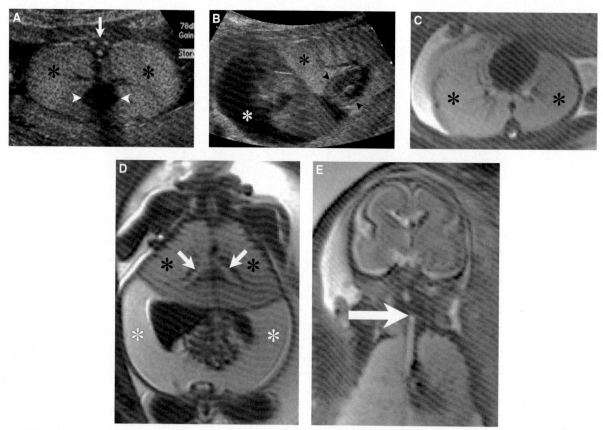

**FIGURE 17.3-1:** CHAOS in 25-week gestational age fetus. Axial **(A)** and sagittal **(B)** plane US images through the fetal chest demonstrate hyperinflated lungs *(black asterisks)*, a compressed heart *(arrowheads)*, and fetal ascites *(B, white asterisk)*. Arrow indicates the spine. Axial **(C)** and coronal **(D)** plane T2-weighted MR images demonstrate enlarged hyperintense lungs *(black asterisks)*, distended airways *(arrows)*, inverted diaphragms, and fetal ascites *(white asterisks)*. **E:** Coronal MRI demonstrates precise level of obstruction at the level of the fetal larynx *(arrow)*.

Fetal ascites is also frequently seen. MRI may compliment US by demonstrating the precise level of airway obstruction in preparation for the mandatory tracheostomy required as a lifesaving intervention during the delivery process (see Fig. 17.3-1E).

**Differential Diagnosis:** Congenital pulmonary airway malformation (CPAM) is the primary differential diagnosis. In distinction to CHAOS, the majority of CPAMs are unilateral lesions; however, the rare case of bilateral-type 3 microcystic CPAM or the even rarer variant of type 0 CPAM composed of acinar dysplasia affecting all lobes may appear similar to CHAOS.[7,8]

**Prognosis:** CHAOS is usually a lethal anomaly with mortality in approximately 80% to 100% of cases.[1] This is especially true when CHAOS is associated with Fraser syndrome. In the absence of additional congenital malformations, prognosis depends on lung size and presence of hydrops. In the absence of hydrops, some cases may be salvageable with proper perinatal management. Rarely, a spontaneous in utero fistula between the obstructed airway and esophagus may develop, improving survival postnatal.

**Management:** In most cases, the natural history of CHAOS includes a progressive enlargement of both lungs with secondary hydrops and a high association with perinatal demise. Termination of pregnancy is a reasonable option to be discussed with the parents. The perinatal outcome of CHAOS is 100% mortality without intervention to secure an airway. Fetuses with CHAOS may benefit from in-utero fetal therapy via a fetoscopic tracheostomy to ameliorate the intrapulmonary hyperexpansion, and to provide mediastinal decompression thereby improving venous return to the heart.[9] The only viable perinatal management option to improve survival is delivery via the ex utero intrapartum treatment (EXIT) procedure.[10,11] Even with tracheostomy and delivery via the EXIT procedure only a few survivors have been reported.[1,10,11]

**Recurrence:** Isolated CHAOS is a sporadic event with no known recurrence risk.

## Emphysema/Overinflation

### *Congenital Lobar Overinflation*

Congenital lobar overinflation (CLO; aka congenital lobar emphysema) is an overinflation of a lung lobe, characterized on microscopic analysis by air space enlargement without maldevelopment.[12] Congenital lung overinflation is likely a better descriptor than congenital lobar overinflation as the abnormality often involves only a lung segment or subsegment. The designation of overinflation is preferred to that of emphysema since the lung is hyperinflated, with intact alveolar walls.

**Incidence:** Overinflation accounts for approximately 20% of all prenatally diagnosed fetal lung malformations (Table 17.3-1).[13]

**Pathogenesis:** Pathologically, CLO is composed of two subgroups. The first group is associated with an overinflated lung lobe caused by an intrinsic cartilage abnormality of the airway, absent bronchial cartilage, or extrinsic compression of the airway by an enlarged pulmonary artery or bronchogenic cyst.[14] The collapsed airway acts as a one-way valve resulting in air

| Table 17.3-1 | Distribution of Pathologically Proven Fetal Lung Lesions (108 Cases) |
|---|---|
| CPAM | 47% |
| Hybrid (CPAM and sequestration) | 25% |
| Overinflation/bronchial atresia | 20% |
| Sequestration | 8% |

Adapted from Epelman M, Kreiger PA, Servaes S, et al. Current imaging of prenatally diagnosed congenital lung lesions. *Semin Ultrasound CT MR.* 2010;31:141–157.

trapping, and historically, the majority of cases presented with respiratory distress in the newborn or infant. This form of CLO, previously known as CLE, occurs most frequently in the left upper lobe followed by the right middle and right upper lobes with the lower lobes involved in less than 1% of cases.[15] A second subgroup of overinflation patients has emerged largely via prenatal diagnosis. This group is characterized by lobar, segmental, or subsegmental overinflation and a high association with bronchial atresia. This subgroup has a predisposition to the lower lobes and lower symptomatology.[16]

**Diagnosis:** On prenatal US, CLO appears as a primarily homogeneous hyperechogenic mass compared with normal lung tissue (Fig. 17.3-2A). A central dilated bronchus distal to an atretic bronchus helps to confirm the diagnosis of associated bronchial atresia/anomaly.[15,16] In addition, mass effect with mediastinal shift may be identified. On color Doppler, CLO demonstrates blood supply from the pulmonary artery and drainage via the pulmonary vein.[17]

On MRI T2-weighted images, CLO typically appears as a homogeneous high-signal lung mass compared with normal lung tissue (see Fig. 17.3-2B,C). On MRI, it is often possible to identify the central dilated mucoid impacted bronchus distal to an atretic or abnormal bronchus (see Fig. 17.3-2D).

**Differential Diagnosis:** The microcystic form of CPAM is the primary differential diagnosis for CLO. Microcystic CPAM appears similar on US and MRI, and is often an incorrect default prenatal diagnosis when an echogenic mass is detected on US. Pacharn et al.[18] reported high accuracy of prenatal MRI for the diagnosis of the specific type of bronchopulmonary malformation (BPM) with postnatal confirmation of the correct diagnosis on pathology or postnatal imaging in 96% of the cases utilizing a designated algorithm (Fig. 17.2-3). On MRI, CPAMs may have a more heterogeneous appearance associated with small cystic areas. Identification of a central dilated bronchus suggests bronchial atresia and favors the diagnosis of CLO. Bronchopulmonary sequestrations (BPSs) may also appear similar to CLO on US and MRI; however, identification of a systemic arterial feeder in a sequestration should allow for accurate diagnosis.

**Prognosis:** Prenatal complications and postnatal sequelae of prenatally diagnosed CLO are rare. The majority of prenatally diagnosed CLO cases are asymptomatic at birth.[16]

**Management:** Prenatal management of CLO consists of serial USs to assess for the infrequent case associated with a large degree of mass effect, which is more likely to be associated with respiratory distress at birth. Fetal intervention is rarely indicated

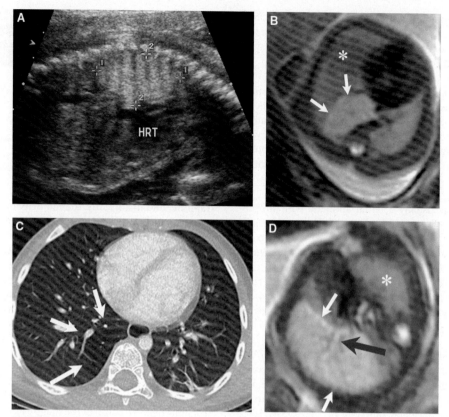

**FIGURE 17.3-2:** CLO in 22-week gestational age fetus. **A:** Sagittal plane US through the fetal chest demonstrates a homogeneous hyperechogenic mass in the right lower lobe *(calipers)*. HRT, heart. **B:** Axial plane T2-weighted MRI demonstrates a homogeneous high-signal intensity mass *(arrows)* in the right lower lung *(asterisk)*. **C:** CT in the same patient as a newborn demonstrates a hyperlucent segment in the right lower lobe *(arrows)* with otherwise normal architecture. **D:** Axial T2-weighted MRI in different fetus with confirmed right lower lobe congenital lung overinflation *(white arrows)* and bronchial atresia. Dilated mucoid impacted bronchus *(red arrow)*. *Asterisk* indicates normal lung.

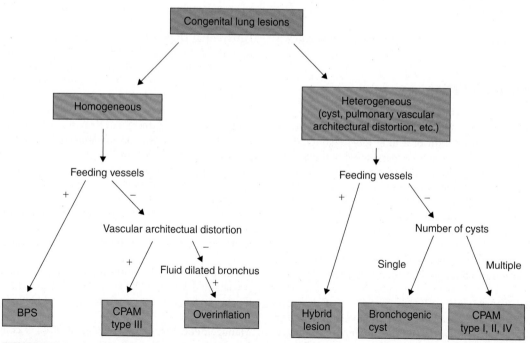

**FIGURE 17.3-3:** Algorithm for diagnosing lung lesions on fetal MRI. (Adapted from Pacharn P, Kline-Fath B, Calvo-Garcia M, et al. Congenital lung lesions: comparison between prenatal magnetic resonance imaging (MRI) and postnatal findings. In: Radiological Society of North America 95th Scientific Assembly & Annual Meeting; November 29–December 4, 2009; Chicago, IL.)

for CLO. Accurate diagnosis of CLO is important since the incidence of fetal and postnatal complications are uncommon compared with CPAM, and the postnatal management of asymptomatic CLO may be conservative without surgical intervention.

**Recurrence:** There is no known recurrence risk for isolated congenital lobar overinflation.

### Esophageal Atresia/Tracheoesophageal Fistula
Esophageal atresia is characterized by interruption of the esophagus, resulting in a blind-ending pouch. Often, there is an associated fistula between the trachea and the esophagus.

**Incidence:** The incidence of esophageal atresia is approximately 1:4,000 live births.[19,20] More than 90% have an associated tracheoesophageal fistula.[21,22]

**Pathogenesis/Associated Anomalies:** Esophageal atresia results when the tracheoesophageal septum of the foregut fails to complete division of the foregut into the ventral respiratory and dorsal digestive portions. Esophageal atresia can be subclassified into five major types (Fig. 17.3-4). Type A is the most common anatomic configuration, representing proximal esophageal atresia with a tracheoesophageal fistula to the distal esophageal segment. The other types of esophageal atresia

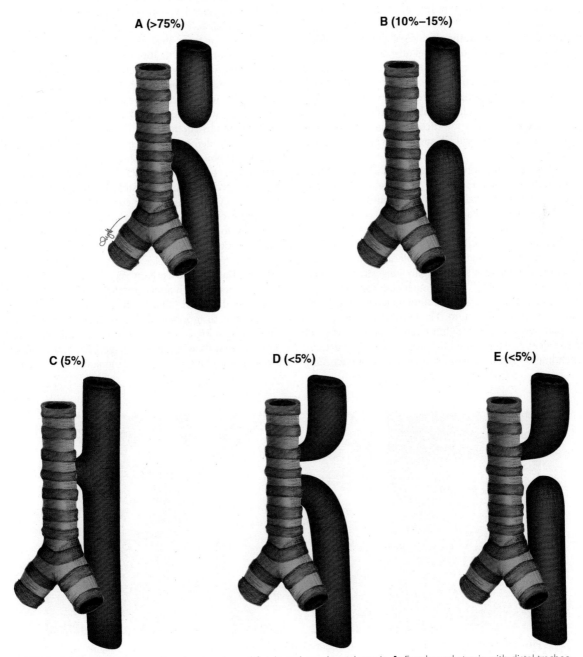

**FIGURE 17.3-4:** Five subtypes of tracheoesophageal fistula and esophageal atresia. **A:** Esophageal atresia with distal tracheoesophageal fistula. **B:** Esophageal atresia with no tracheoesophageal fistula. **C:** H-type tracheoesophageal fistula with no esophageal atresia. **D:** Esophageal atresia with both proximal and distal tracheoesophageal fistulas. **E:** Esophageal atresia with proximal tracheoesophageal fistula.

in decreasing order of frequency are: Type B: Esophageal atresia without tracheoesophageal fistula; Type C: Tracheoesophageal fistula with no esophageal atresia; Type D: Esophageal atresia with tracheoesophageal fistula to both the proximal and the distal esophageal segments; and Type E: Esophageal atresia with tracheoesophageal fistula to the proximal esophageal segment.

Other associated malformations are seen in up to 70% of fetuses with esophageal atresia with the incidence for the most frequent abnormalities as follows: cardiovascular (35%) (most commonly PDA and VSD), gastrointestinal (24%) (most commonly anal atresia and duodenal atresia), genitourinary (20%) (most commonly unilateral renal agenesis or renal dysplasia), skeletal (13%) (most commonly vertebral, rib, or radial ray), and neurologic (10%) (most commonly hydrocephalus).[19,21–24] Esophageal atresia may also occur in association with other gastrointestinal tract atresias.[25,26] The association of esophageal atresia and duodenal atresia in the absence of a tracheoesophageal fistula results in a closed loop bowel obstruction involving the distal esophagus, stomach, and duodenum.[27] Approximately 10% of cases of esophageal atresia are part of the VACTERL association (Vertebral anomalies, Anal atresia, Cardiac anomalies, Tracheoesophageal fistula, Renal anomalies, and Limb anomalies).[28,29] Careful search for these associated anomalies should be performed on prenatal US and MRI when esophageal atresia is suspected.

Aneuploidy, most commonly trisomy 18 and 21, is relatively common in esophageal atresia ranging from 5% to 10% in different series.[28,30] The risk of trisomy 21 is 30 times higher than expected in the general population.[21,31,32]

**Diagnosis:** Prenatal US detection of esophageal atresia is challenging; however, the constellation of a small or absent stomach, polyhydramnios, and a pouch sign is highly suggestive of esophageal atresia (Fig. 17.3-5A).[33,34] The pouch sign represents the proximal fluid-containing esophageal blind pouch located in the neck or the superior mediastinum. The detection of the proximal esophageal pouch is not straightforward because it fills and empties periodically, likely related to fetal swallowing. Furthermore, depending on the nature of the anomaly, the pouch may

be located in the cervical region or superior mediastinum. The sensitivity and accuracy for identifying the proximal esophageal pouch has not been carefully examined. Diagnosis of esophageal atresia with an absent stomach and polyhydramnios is rare prior to 22 weeks' gestation. In fact, a normal appearing stomach and a normal amount of amniotic fluid may be seen earlier in gestation. Overall sensitivity for detecting esophageal atresia associated with tracheoesophageal fistula is low, cited at 30% prenatal detection rate.[35,36] Limited detection may be explained by the fact that in the presence of esophageal atresia with tracheoesophageal fistula, the stomach may fill with fluid via the fistula. It is possible that in many cases of esophageal atresia, the tracheoesophageal fistula maintains flow into the stomach early in pregnancy, but that the fistula progressively narrows as pregnancy continues, resulting in a small or non visualized stomach.

Stringer et al.[35] reported a predictive value for esophageal atresia ranging from 39% with identification of a small stomach and polyhydramnios to 56% for polyhydramnios in the absence of an identifiable fetal stomach. When esophageal atresia without a tracheoesophageal fistula is associated with duodenal atresia, US will typically reveal significant polyhydramnios in association with a severely distended stomach because of the closed loop obstruction.[27,37]

MRI may demonstrate a proximal fluid-filled blind-ending esophageal pouch on T2-weighted sequences, which can be difficult to detect on US (see Fig. 17.3-5B,C). MRI may also rarely identify the tracheoesophageal fistula. Although MRI may increase the accuracy of diagnosis, the current MRI data are mainly from case reports with no large series yet available.[32,36,38] MRI may also be useful to identify associated anomalies not definitively diagnosed on US, including anal atresia and vertebral anomalies.

**Differential Diagnosis:** Non visualization of the fetal stomach has been reported in approximately 0.07% to 0.4% of pregnancies with abnormal outcome in 48% to 100% of the cases.[39,40] In addition to esophageal atresia, lack of visualization of the fluid-filled stomach may be seen in conditions associated with abnormal swallowing and passage of amniotic fluid into the esophagus and stomach, including severe fetal central nervous

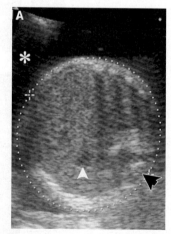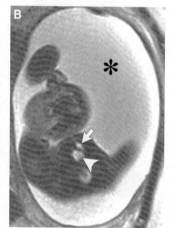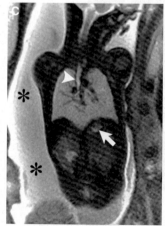

**FIGURE 17.3-5:** Esophageal atresia with tracheoesophageal fistula in 30-week gestational age fetus. **A:** Axial sonogram through the upper abdomen demonstrates a very small fetal stomach *(white arrowhead)* and polyhydramnios *(asterisk).* The spine is indicated by *black arrowhead.* T2-weighted MRI axial scan through the neck **(B)** and coronal view of the chest **(C)** demonstrate the proximal esophageal pouch *(arrowheads),* posterior to the trachea *(arrow in B),* and polyhydramnios *(asterisks).* The *arrow* in C indicates the small stomach.

system disorders, neck masses (particularly anterior neck teratomas or fetal goiter), anatomic disorders of swallowing (such as severe cleft palate), diaphragmatic hernia with an intrathoracic stomach, and any cause of oligohydramnios, which limits the available fluid for swallowing.

A small stomach may also be seen with congenital microgastria, which is an extremely rare anomaly believed to result from impairment of normal foregut development. On sonography, these cases demonstrate a very small stomach on serial scans. Of note, in congenital microgastria, the amniotic fluid may be normal, whereas in esophageal atresia, polyhydramnios is usually present late in gestation.[41–43]

**Prognosis:** The outcome of fetuses and infants with esophageal atresia has been reported as unfavorable with perinatal mortality of 21%, primarily as a result of associated congenital malformations and prematurity.[19,44–46]

Morbidity in survivors depends mostly on the timing of diagnosis and the presence of associated anomalies. Postoperative mortality in infants surviving to undergo primary surgery has been reported at 9%.[19] The prognosis for esophageal atresia without associated anomalies or genetic disorder is good.

**Management:** All patients suspected to have esophageal atresia should undergo genetic counseling and referred for karyotype evaluation given the increased risk for trisomies 18 and 21. In addition, all patients should undergo a fetal cardiac echo to assess for associated cardiac anomalies. Esophageal atresia is usually well managed after birth with surgical correction, and therefore fetal intervention is not indicated.[44]

**Recurrence:** Esophageal atresia can occur as an isolated finding, as part of a genetic syndrome, or as part of a non isolated (but not syndromic) set of findings. Most individuals with esophageal atresia are the only affected member of the family, and when esophageal atresia is the only abnormality without a clear etiology, the recurrence risk for siblings is approximately 1%.[47] When esophageal atresia is associated with an inherited chromosomal abnormality or specific syndrome, genetic counseling for recurrence risk is indicated.[47]

## LUNG LESIONS

### Congenital Pulmonary Airway Malformation (aka Congenital Cystic Adenomatoid Malformation)

Congenital pulmonary airway malformations are part of the bronchopulmonary malformation (BPM) spectrum, which include BPS, hybrid lesions (CPAM and sequestration), and CLO/bronchial atresia.

**Incidence:** CPAMs are the most common lung anomaly diagnosed in the fetus, accounting for approximately half of all lesions (see Table 17.3-1).[13] The estimated incidence for prenatal diagnosis is 1:4,000 to 1:6,000 pregnancies.[48,49]

**Pathogenesis:** The definite etiology is unknown but several mechanisms have been referenced. A gene interaction (Hox B-5; FGF-7; PDGFB Gene) has been a suggested cause of CPAMs.[50,51] Homeobox genes control axial identity and organ-specific patterning during embryogenesis.[52] Abnormal Hox B-5 expression during human lung branching morphogenesis

has been implicated in the development of CPAMs.[50,51] Airway obstruction in the developing fetus has also been cited as the etiology of most BPMs, with the type of malformation depending on the severity and timing of airway obstruction during lung development.[12,53,54] Supporting this conclusion is the associated pathologic diagnosis of bronchial atresia in 70% of CPAMs.[53]

CPAMs represent a benign hamartomatous or dysplastic tumor, which are composed of a mass of abnormal solid or cystic pulmonary tissue in which there is proliferation of bronchial structures at the expense of alveolar development. These lesions are thought to result from abnormal endodermal and mesodermal differentiation between the 5th to 7th week of gestation.

These lesions typically involve one pulmonary lobe and usually communicate with the tracheobronchial tree, although the communication is abnormal. CPAMs receive blood supply from the pulmonary artery and drain via the pulmonary veins with the exception of hybrid lesions (CPAM and sequestration), which also have a systemic arterial blood supply. CPAMs may be predominately cystic, solid, or mixed pathologically.

Stocker et al.[49] has pathologically classified CPAMs into three types according to cyst size and histologic resemblance to the segments of the developing bronchial tree and airspaces (Fig. 17.3-6). Type 1 macrocystic CPAM lesions are characterized by single or multiple cysts greater than 2 cm in diameter lined by ciliated pseudo stratified columnar epithelium.[55] These account for approximately half of all CPAM lesions in postnatal series.[55] Type 2 lesions are characterized by macroscopic cysts ranging from 0.5 to 2.0 cm in diameter and lined with mixed ciliary, columnar, and cuboidal epithelium.[55] Type 3 lesions are predominantly solid with microcystic components and are histologically composed of alveolus-like structures lined by ciliated cuboidal epithelium.[55] Type 3 CPAM comprises approximately 10% of all CPAMs. Type 1 lesions represent an anomaly of the more proximal bronchial tree affecting primarily the bronchioles, whereas type 3 lesions affect the more distal portion of the bronchial tree at the level of the alveoli.[56] Recently, two additional subtypes of CPAM have been added to the classification (types 0 and 4).[55] Type 0 is characterized by acinar dysplasia or agenesis and is very rare, involving all of the lung lobes, and is incompatible with postnatal survival.[55] Type 4 lesions, which cannot be differentiated from Type 1 and 2 lesions by imaging,

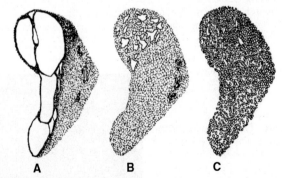

**FIGURE 17.3-6:** The three original types of congenital pulmonary airway malformation of the fetus as described by Stocker et al.[49] **A:** Type I lesions have large cysts of variable sizes. **B:** Type II lesions have smaller cysts. **C:** Type III lesions are microcystic and appear solid on US owing to reflections from numerous microscopically dilated bronchioles. (Redrawn from Stocker JT, Madewell JE, Drake RM. Congenital cystic adenomatoid malformation of the lung: classification and morphologic spectrum. *Hum Pathol.* 1977;8:155–171. Copyright 1977 Elsevier.)

are characterized by large peripheral cysts of the distal acinus lined predominately by alveolar-type cells. With this new classification, Stocker[55] proposed that the prior designation of congenital cystic adenomatoid malformation (CCAM) be changed to CPAM as the lesions are cystic in only three of the five pathological classifications and adenomatoid in one type.

**Diagnosis:** On prenatal US, most CPAMs are detected as an incidental finding. CPAMs may appear as a predominantly macrocystic mass, microcystic hyperechogenic solid mass, or a complex mass with both cystic and echogenic components (Fig. 17.3-7). Solid masses are typically hyperechogenic compared with normal fetal lung in the second trimester, and often become isoechoic with the normal fetal lung and invisible on sonography in the third trimester (Fig. 17.3-8). The decreasing conspicuity relates to both the increasing echogenicity of the normal fetal lungs as pregnancy progresses and the propensity of solid masses to decrease in size as pregnancy progresses. When solid masses are isoechoic to normal lung, the sonographic diagnosis is more challenging and relies on mass effect, including mediastinal shift, altered cardiac position or axis, or an inverted diaphragm to confirm the diagnosis (Fig. 17.3-9A). Color Doppler US is useful in demonstrating pulmonary artery blood supply to the mass and drainage via the pulmonary vein (see Fig. 17.3-9B). Identification of an associated systematic arterial blood supply confirms the diagnosis of a hybrid

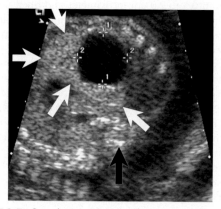

**FIGURE 17.3-7:** Complex cystic lung malformation detected as incidental finding on US at 22 weeks' gestational age. Axial sonogram through the fetal chest shows a complex mass composed of macrocystic (*calipers*) and solid (*white arrows*) components. Fetal spine is indicated by *black arrow*.

BPM composed of both CPAM and sequestration components (Fig. 17.3-10). Adzick[57] suggested a sonographic characterization based on a predominately macrocystic or microcystic appearance of CPAMs as a more clinically useful classification. The macrocystic lesions are composed of single or multiple cysts larger than 5 mm in diameter on US, and microcystic lesions appear as a solid hyperechogenic mass because of the numerous acoustic interfaces created by small cysts measuring less than 5 mm in diameter (Fig. 17.3-11).[57] The presence or absence of macroscopic cysts may be important as these can predispose to rapid growth and complications, and are also important in determining therapy for cases complicated by fetal hydrops. CPAMs are usually unilateral and unilobar with a slight predisposition to the lower lobes. Approximately 40% of CPAMs increase in size during pregnancy, with the most rapid growth occurring between 20 and 26 weeks' gestational age, after which growth peaks and plateaus.[58,59]

MRI may also be useful in the diagnosis and characterization of CPAMs. MRI is reported to provide alternative or additional diagnoses compared with US in 38% to 50% of fetuses with chest anomalies.[38,60] In the second trimester, CPAMs usually appear as a hyperintense mass compared with normal lung tissue on T2-weighted MRI sequences (Fig. 17.3-12A). CPAMs may appear high signal, isosignal, or lower signal compared with lung tissue in the third trimester of pregnancy. The identification of a high-signal mass alone on MRI is not specific for the type of bronchopulmonary malformation; however, identification of a macrocystic component and/or distortion of the vascular architecture is highly suggestive for CPAM (see Fig. 17.3-12B).[38,61] MRI may be useful during the third trimester of pregnancy in evaluating for pulmonary hypoplasia via lung volume measurements and confirming the presence and size of a CPAM when solid masses may not be visualized on US. In our experience, the latter is helpful in planning delivery location (see Fig. 17.3-8B). When the mass is ascertained to be small on MRI, patients can safely deliver in their local community and undergo elective evaluation of the mass after birth.

**Differential Diagnosis:** Differential diagnosis for a solid microcystic CPAM includes hybrid BPMs (CPAM and BPS), congenital lobar or segmental overinflation, and congenital diaphragmatic hernia. Solid hybrid lesions may be differentiated by identification of both pulmonary artery and systemic arterial blood supply to the mass on US or MRI. Lobar or segmental overinflation may appear similar to a CPAM on prenatal imaging.

**FIGURE 17.3-8:** Disappearing fetal lung mass in the third trimester. **A:** Coronal plane sonogram through the fetal chest shows no evidence of a fetal lung mass. Normal lungs are indicated by *asterisks* and the aorta by *arrowheads*. **B:** Axial plane fetal MRI confirms a small high-signal bronchopulmonary malformation (*arrow*). The *arrowhead* indicates the spine.

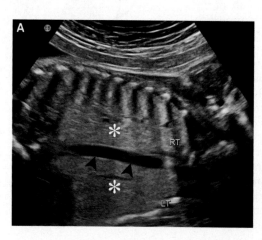
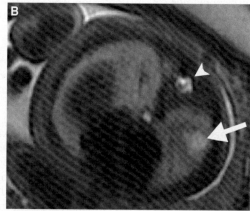

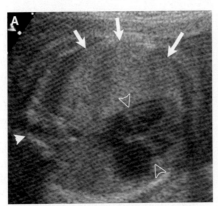 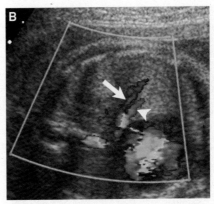

**FIGURE 17.3-9:** Isoechoic lung mass. **A:** Axial sonogram through the fetal chest demonstrates dextroposition of the heart *(open arrowheads)* secondary to an isoechoic lung mass *(arrows)*. The spine is indicated by *closed arrowhead*. **B:** Axial plane Doppler sonogram demonstrates pulmonary artery blood supply to the mass *(arrow)* and drainage via the pulmonary vein *(arrowhead)*. Postnatal surgical resection confirmed congenital pulmonary airway malformation.

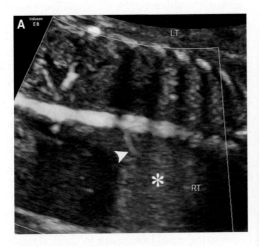 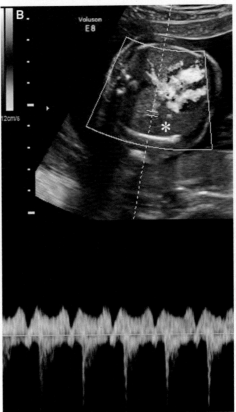

**FIGURE 17.3-10:** Hybrid bronchopulmonary malformation at 22 weeks gestational age. Coronal **(A)** and axial **(B)** plane sonograms through the fetal chest demonstrates a systemic artery *(arrowhead)* arising from the lower thoracic aorta and the pulmonary artery (spectral tracing) supplying the hybrid bronchopulmonary malformation *(asterisks)*. Spectral tracing demonstrates both pulmonary arterial supply and pulmonary venous drainage.

Identification of a dilated central bronchus with mucoid impaction suggests CLO. Congenital diaphragmatic hernia (CDH) can usually be differentiated from CPAM by identification of the fetal stomach in the thorax and observation of peristalsis of herniated intestinal loops in the chest. A right-sided CDH associated with liver herniation may appear similar to a microcystic CPAM presenting as a solid intrathoracic mass. In contrast to CPAMs, the herniated liver does not appear as hyperechogenic on US. Color Doppler US should correctly diagnose the herniated liver by identifying the intrahepatic portal veins and the inferior vena cava within the mass.

Pulmonary hypoplasia or agenesis may also present with ipsilateral mediastinal shift, thereby mimicking an isoechoic mass such as a CPAM on US.[62] MRI can confirm the correct diagnosis by excluding an underlying lung mass as the cause of the mediastinal shift, thereby confirming the presence of a hypoplastic right lung.

An intrapulmonary bronchogenic cyst is the main differential diagnosis for a macrocystic CPAM. Bronchogenic cysts are usually unilocular cystic lesions, which can occur in the pulmonary parenchyma and are unassociated with a solid component. Lymphatic malformations may also mimic a macrocystic

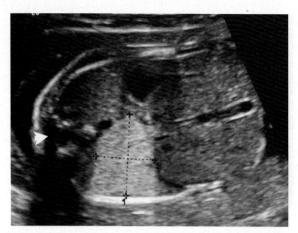

**FIGURE 17.3-11:** Microcystic CPAM at 22 weeks' gestational age. Axial sonogram through the fetal chest demonstrates a hyperechogenic mass *(calipers)* representing a microcystic CPAM. Spine *(arrowhead)*.

CPAM, but these lesions almost always originate in an extrathoracic location with secondary invasion into the thorax. The other differential is the rare case of cystic pleuropulmonary blastoma, which is difficult to differentiate from CPAM on imaging.

**Associated Anomalies:** Isolated CPAMs are not associated with increased risk for chromosomal abnormalities[63,64]; however, prenatal series have reported associated anomalies in 8% to 12% of CPAMs. Associated anomalies include renal abnormalities, CDH, tracheoesophageal fistula, and congenital heart defects.[63,65,66] Genetic counseling for fetal karyotyping should be offered when associated anomalies are identified.[67,68]

**Prognosis:** Imaging plays a key role in predicting the clinical outcome for a fetus diagnosed with a CPAM. Prognosis depends on the size of the mass and the presence or absence of hydrops fetalis. Small isolated fetal lung malformations with no mass effect have excellent outcomes and usually are asymptomatic at birth. A subset of fetuses with large CPAMs have mass effect resulting in mediastinal shift and can develop life-threatening complications including hydrops fetalis or, less-commonly, severe pulmonary hypoplasia. Earlier literature reported that 30% to 50% of fetuses with CPAMs developed hydrops fetalis with an associated mortality approaching 100% without intervention.[69] More recent literature suggests that hydrops is less frequent and occurs in 9% to 21% of cases.[70,71] The pathophysiology for hydrops fetalis is felt to be secondary to compression of the heart and inferior vena cava, obstructing venous return

to the heart. Large masses may also be associated with isolated polyhydramnios secondary to compression of the esophagus obstructing normal passage of amniotic fluid into the gastrointestinal tract. In a prospective series, Crombleholme et al.[58] reported that sonographic measurement of the cystic adenomatoid malformation volume ratio (CVR) predicted the risk of hydrops in fetuses with CPAM (aka CCAM). CVR is the measured CPAM volume divided by the head circumference (Fig. 17.3-13). The CPAM volume is a calculated measurement utilizing the formula for a prolate ellipse (mass length × height × width × 0.52). In Crombleholme series, a CVR greater than 1.6 predicted an increased risk of hydrops fetalis occurring in 75% of cases.[58] A CVR less than or equal to 1.6 in the absence of a dominant cyst was associated with a less than 3% risk of hydrops fetalis. Crombleholme et al. noted that in addition to the absolute size of the mass, the rate of lesion growth, particularly when associated with a macroscopic cyst, is a risk factor for developing hydrops fetalis.

**Management:** The vast majority of CPAMs are managed conservatively with sonographic surveillance every 1 to 2 weeks to assess for the complication of hydrops fetalis. After 30 weeks' gestational age, the risk of developing hydrops fetalis is unlikely, and the frequency of surveillance can be decreased. Recent literature has suggested that maternal administration of betamethasone for fetuses with large CVRs may have a beneficial effect on microcystic CPAMs in preventing or reversing hydrops fetalis.[72–74] The exact mechanism is unknown, but it is postulated that steroids may accelerate lung maturation or mass involution. Reports from three centers have shown resolution of hydrops fetalis in approximately 80% of CPAMs treated with maternal steroids (Table 17.3-2).[74] In addition, Curran et al.[74] reported survival to discharge ranging from 75% to 100% for large microcystic CPAMs managed with maternal betamethasone. Macrocystic CPAMs do not seem to respond as well to treatment with betamethasone.[72] Loh et al. reported a series comparing steroid treatment to surgical treatment for CPAMs associated with fetal hydrops in the second trimester. Improved survival, particularly for microcystic CPAMs, was noted in the steroid treated group compared with the open surgery group (Table 17.3-3).[75] The current consensus in many centers is to administer maternal steroids as the first line of treatment prior to surgical intervention in fetuses at high risk for fetal hydrops. In fetuses with large CPAMs complicated by hydrops fetalis, who are unresponsive to maternal steroid administration, a spectrum of interventional procedures, including cyst aspiration, placement of a thoracoamniotic shunt, percutaneous laser ablation, or surgical resection, may be considered prior to

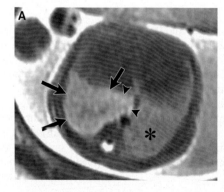
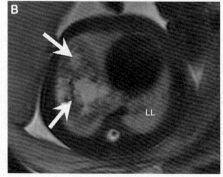

**FIGURE 17.3-12:** MRI appearance of CPAM **A:** Axial T2-weighted MR image of fetus at a gestational age of 22 weeks demonstrates a high-signal intensity CPAM *(arrows)* with small peripheral cysts *(arrowheads)* in the right lower lobe. Normal lung is indicated by *asterisk*. **B:** Axial T2 MRI of fetus at 21 weeks with confirmed CPAM showing complex lesion of mixed signal containing multiple cysts *(arrows)*. LL, normal left lung.

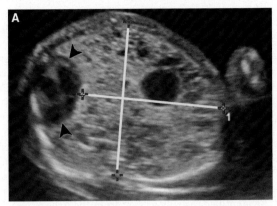 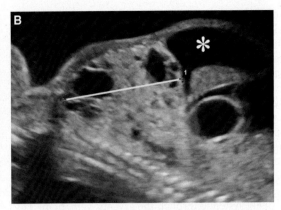

**FIGURE 17.3-13:** CPAM Volume Ratio (CVR): Large CPAM of mixed increased echogenicity and cystic components complicated by early hydrops in a 24-week gestational age pregnancy. CPAM volume ratio (CVR) = 2.6. CVR is calculated as the CPAM volume divided by head circumference. CVR = $L \times H \times W \times 0.52$/head circumference. Axial **(A)** and sagittal **(B)** sonograms demonstrate measurement of the CPAM volume *(calipers)*. Displaced heart is indicated by *arrowheads* and ascites by *asterisk*.

| Table 17.3-2 | Prenatal Steroids for Microcystic CPAM (Data from Three Centers) | | | | |
|---|---|---|---|---|---|
| | *Patients* | *CVR* | *Hydrops* | *Hydrops Resolved* | *Survival* |
| UCSF | 13 | 2.7 | 9 (69%) | 7 (78%) | 11 (85%) |
| CHOP | 10 | 2.2 | 5 (50%) | 4 (80%) | 10 (100%) |
| Cincinnati | 8 | 2.5 | 6 (75%) | 5 (83%) | 6 (75%) |
| **Total** | **31** | **2.5** | **20/31(65%)** | **16/20(80%)** | **27/31(87%)** |

Adapted from Curran PF, Jelin EB, Rand L, et al. Prenatal steroids for microcystic congenital cystic adenomatoid malformations. *J Pediatr Surg.* 2010;45:145–150.

32 weeks gestational age.[76–79] Open surgery with mass resection has been reported to be approximately 50% successful in managing CPAMs; however, it is controversial because of maternal complications related to the procedure, which include increased risk for premature rupture of the membranes, preterm delivery, and fetal demise.[80] Percutaneous laser ablation of microcystic lesions may be an alternative treatment to surgical resection for microcystic lesions, but additional studies are necessary to consider this as a valid therapeutic option.[81] Fetal percutaneous sclerotherapy has also been reported as a minimally invasive and effective palliative strategy to ameliorate hydrops fetalis

| Table 17.3-3 | Steroid Rx vs. Fetal Surgery in 24 Fetuses with CPAM and Fetal Hydrops | |
|---|---|---|
| | *Steroid Rx* | *Surgical Rx* |
| Mean GA age | 23 wk | 24 wk |
| CVR | 2.68 ± 0.29 | 2.95 ± 0.31 |
| Survival to delivery | 12/13 (92%) | 9/11 (82%) |
| Survival to discharge | 10/12 (83%) | 5/9 (56%) |

Adapted from Loh KC, Jelin E, Hirose S, et al. Microcystic congenital pulmonary airway malformation with hydrops fetalis: steroids vs open fetal resection. *J Pediatr Surg.* 2012;47:36–39.

associated with predominately solid types of CPAMs, and may represent an alternative to surgical resection.[82]

**Recurrence:** There is no known recurrence risk for isolated CPAM.

### Bronchopulmonary Sequestration

BPSs represent a cystic developmental lung malformation composed of non functioning pulmonary tissue, which lack communication to the tracheobronchial tree and are supplied by a systemic artery.

**Incidence:** BPS is the second most common cause of a congenital lung mass occurring in approximately 1.1% to 1.8% of all pulmonary resections.[83] In the fetus, BPS occurs primarily as an isolated lesion, but can have associated anomalies in approximately 8% of cases and is associated with a CPAM in 25% of cases (see Table 17.3-1).[13]

**Pathogenesis/Associated Anomalies:** BPS is thought to originate from a supernumerary caudally positioned lung bud and has a preferential location for the left lower thorax in 65% to 90% of cases.[83,84] BPSs are characterized as intralobar sequestration (ILS) or extralobar sequestration (ELS).[85] ELS is completely separated from the adjacent normal lung tissue and invested in its own pleural covering. Late development of the lung bud after formation of the pleura leads to formation of a separate pleural covering surrounding the ELS. ILS shares common pleura with the normal lung tissue. On occasion, ELS and ILS forms of BPS can coexist.[86] ELS accounts for the majority of BPS diagnosed prenatally and approximately 25% to 50% of cases of BPS diagnosed postnatally.[85] Bronchial atresia affecting the lobar, segmental, or subsegmental bronchi has been reported in 100% of ELS and 82% of ILS cases.[53] Approximately 10% to 15% of ELS are found within or below the diaphragm.[84,87] All BPSs receive blood supply from an anomalous systemic feeding artery usually arising from the lower thoracic aorta, upper abdominal aorta, or the celiac artery. Multiple systematic artery feeders may be identified on imaging and at pathology. Venous drainage is via the pulmonary veins in ILS.[88] The venous drainage of ELS is usually systemic through the azygous vein, hemi azygous vein, or the superior vena cava.[83,89] ELS may be associated with other fetal anomalies, most commonly CDH and foregut abnormalities.[84,90]

**Diagnosis:** On US, BPS appears as a homogeneous hyperechogenic mass compared with the normal lung in the vast majority of cases (Fig. 17.3-14).[85] Less commonly, there may be a cystic component, with a high percentage attributed to hybrid lesions. Large masses may result in mass effect with mediastinal shift or compression of the diaphragm. BPS are usually detected in the second trimester as an incidental finding and are most commonly localized in the left lower hemithorax or below the diaphragm in approximately 10% of cases.[84,87] Hybrid lesions composed of both CPAM and ELS components are described in approximately 50% of cases (see Fig. 17.3-10).[91,92] A systematic feeding artery or multiple arteries arising from the lower thoracic or abdominal upper aorta can be identified on color

Doppler US in the majority of cases; thereby confirming the diagnosis.[92] On rare occasions, ELS may be complicated by a large ipsilateral hydrothorax, which is thought to occur secondary to torsion of the sequestration, resulting in obstruction of the efferent venous and lymphatic drainage.[93] ELS may be associated with other congenital anomalies, including CDH, cardiac abnormalities, or foregut duplications.[94]

On MRI, BPSs usually appear as a high-signal mass compared with normal fetal lung on T2-fluid sensitive sequences (see Fig. 17.3-14C). The lesions are typically homogeneous high signal intensity and only slightly less intense than that of amniotic fluid. The presence of an associated cyst suggests a hybrid lesion with a CPAM component. Systematic feeding vessels may be identified, usually arising from the lower thoracic or upper abdominal aorta.

**Differential Diagnosis:** Differential diagnosis for an intrathoracic BPS includes other causes of a solid intrathoracic mass—congenital pulmonary airway malformation, congenital lobar or segmental overinflation, and CDH. The identification of a systematic arterial feeder to the BPS should allow for a specific diagnosis. Differential diagnosis for a subdiaphragmatic suprarenal BPS includes adrenal neuroblastoma and adrenal hemorrhage, and again a systemic feeder to a hyperechogenic mass in a subdiaphragmatic location should allow for accurate diagnosis of BPS. On MRI, congenital neuroblastoma can appear as a predominately cystic or solid mass in a fetus. Solid neuroblastomas tend to be heterogeneous with intermediate signal intensity on T2-weighted sequences in contrast to BPS, which are usually high signal intensity lesions on fluid-sensitive T2-weighted MRI sequences. Adrenal hemorrhage is usually diagnosed in

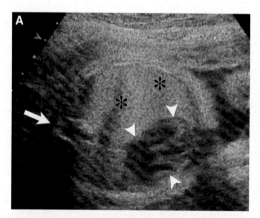

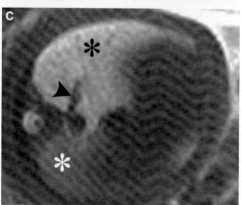

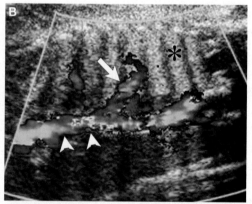

**FIGURE 17.3-14:** Bronchopulmonary sequestration at 22 weeks gestational age. **A:** Axial sonogram through the fetal chest shows a homogeneous hyperechoic left-sided solid chest mass *(asterisks)* displacing the heart *(arrowheads)* to the right. Fetal spine is indicated by *arrow*. **B:** Coronal color Doppler through the fetal chest and abdomen shows a systemic arterial feeder *(arrow)* arising from the lower thoracic aorta *(arrowheads)* supplying the fetal chest mass *(asterisk)*. **C:** Axial plane T2-weighted MRI scan demonstrates a homogeneous high-signal mass *(black asterisk)* compared with normal lung *(white asterisk)*; systemic arterial feeder *(arrowhead)* is seen arising from the lower thoracic aorta.

the subacute phase and appear as intermediate to high signal on both T2- and T1-weighted sequences.

**Prognosis:** Approximately 68% of BPS lesions regress dramatically before birth, and most are generally associated with an outstanding prognosis.[57] Hydrops fetalis is a rare complication of BPS and much less frequent than in CPAM. ELS may be complicated by a large ipsilateral pleural effusion secondary to torsion, which has a very high mortality in the absence of interventional treatment.

**Management:** Prenatal management consists of surveillance via US. No intervention is required in the vast majority of cases. Early delivery may be contemplated after 32 weeks gestation in the rare case complicated by hydrops fetalis. Thoracoamniotic shunt may be considered for treatment of the infrequent case complicated by a large ipsilateral pleural effusion as the associated mortality is very high in the absence of intervention.[76,78] Open fetal surgical resection is considered controversial because of the maternal risks associated with surgery.

**Recurrence:** There is no known recurrence risk for isolated BPS.

## MASSES

### Pleuropulmonary Blastoma

Pleuropulmonary blastoma (PPB) is also known as pulmonary sarcoma and pulmonary rhabdomyosarcoma.

**Incidence:** PPB is a rare tumor but represents the most common cause of a primary lung malignancy in childhood.[95] The incidence of PPB in the fetus is unknown.

**Pathogenesis:** Although rare, PPB occurs predictably in certain clinical and familial circumstances. Approximately 20% of children with PPB have a family history of pediatric neoplasia, most commonly cystic nephroma of the kidney and rhabdomyosarcoma.[96] PPB families may harbor heterozygous germline mutations in the DICER 1 gene, which have been shown to predispose to PPB.[96]

PPB is a dysembryonic malignancy, which is believed to arise from pleuropulmonary germ cells and is composed of both epithelial and mesenchymal components.[95] Mesenchymal cells susceptible to malignant transformation reside within cyst walls and may evolve into sarcomas. Priest et al.[97] subclassified PPB as type 1 (purely cystic), type 2 (cystic and solid), or type 3 (purely solid) lesions. The type 1 (predominately cystic) lesion represents the early form of the disease and is the type most commonly reported in the fetus or young infant.[97,98] The cystic nature of the mass renders it difficult to distinguish from CPAM as it is pathologically deceptive because of its resemblance to developmental lung cysts.[99] PPB may be unilateral or bilateral.

**Diagnosis:** On imaging with prenatal US or MRI, PPB appears as a primarily cystic or a complex mass with cystic and solid components, which are usually indistinguishable from the findings in congenital pulmonary airway malformation (Fig. 17.3-15). Findings which may help differentiate a PPB from a CPAM include a positive family history, multifocal disease, associated pleural effusion, or continued growth late in gestation past the typical plateau of CPAM growth.[95,100]

**Differential Diagnosis:** Congenital pulmonary airway malformation is the primary differential diagnosis and may appear identical to PPB on prenatal imaging. A positive family history, continued interval growth beyond 28 weeks, and the presence of pleural effusion should raise consideration for a PPB.

**Prognosis:** Complete surgical resection of PPB may be curative, particularly for type 1 (cystic) disease. Type 2 and 3 diseases are often progressive and carry a much worse prognosis.

**Management:** PPB is a very rare lesion in the fetus, and most are presumed to represent a CPAM and, therefore, undergo US surveillance to assess for the complication of hydrops fetalis. In the majority of cases, the diagnosis is not confirmed until after birth, when the lesion is surgically resected. No fetal intervention has been reported in PPB. PPB survival statistics suggest that it is vital to diagnose and treat children at an early age, at which time the lesion is more curable.[99]

**Recurrence:** The recurrence risk for PPB is increased in patients with a familial predisposition associated with the DICER1 gene mutation.[96]

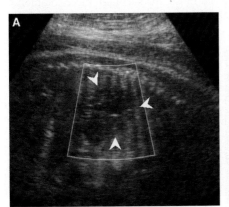
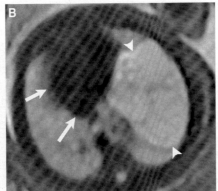
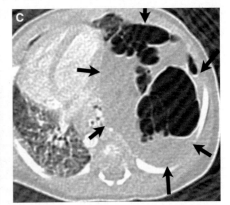

**FIGURE 17.3-15:** Cystic pleuropulmonary blastoma. **A:** Sagittal plane sonogram through the fetal chest demonstrates complex cystic and solid lung mass *(arrowheads)*. **B:** Axial T2-weighted MRI demonstrates high-signal mass *(arrowheads)* within the left chest displacing the heart *(arrows)* to the right. **C:** Axial CT scan after birth demonstrates a solid and air-containing cystic mass *(arrows)*, confirmed on surgical pathology to represent a cystic pleuropulmonary blastoma. Images courtesy of Beth Kline-Fath, MD.

# MEDIASTINUM

## Thymus

The thymus is a normal lymphoid organ, which is important for immune function during both intrauterine and extrauterine life.[101,102]

**Embryology:** The thymus is derived embryologically from the third pharyngeal pouch and the third pharyngeal cleft, which gives rise respectively to the endodermal (cortical) and ectodermal (medullary) components of the thymus. The pouch is anterior to the aorta in the anterior mediastinum.

**Diagnosis:** On prenatal US, the normal thymus gland can be identified in the majority of fetuses in the second and third trimesters. The thymus gland appears as a bilobed structure in the anterior superior mediastinum ventral to the pericardium and great vessels of the heart. The thymus echogenicity is similar or slightly more echogenic than the fetal lungs early in the second trimester and less echogenic than normal fetal lung tissue in the later part of pregnancy (Fig. 17.3-16A).[103] Occasionally, non-shadowing linear or punctate echogenic foci may be seen in the thymus gland, likely corresponding to normal connective tissue septa and blood vessels. Nomograms for normal fetal thymic size have been reported with no substantial size difference between male and female fetuses.[103–106]

On MRI, the thymus gland should be identified in all normal fetuses in the second and third trimesters with the gland appearing bilobed and intermediate signal intensity on T2-weighted sequences (see Fig. 17.3-16B). The thymus gland is higher in signal than adjacent muscle in the chest wall but of lesser signal intensity than that of adjacent lung tissue in the late second and third trimesters. The two lobes of the thymus gland may substantially differ in size. The normal thymus gland is very pliable, and even when appearing large on US or MRI, does not exhibit compression or displacement of adjacent mediastinal structures.

**Differential Diagnosis:** Solid masses in the thymus gland are extremely rare, and the primary consideration for a solid mass in the anterior/superior mediastinum is a teratoma. Teratomas are usually complex masses with cystic and solid components. Ectopic thyroid or fetal goiter may also mimic a thymic region mass. MRI should accurately characterize the tissue as thyroid gland by identifying the typical bilobed appearance and homogeneous bright signal on T1-weighted sequences. Differential

diagnosis for an apparently absent thymus gland includes ectopic thymus. Early in development, the thymus may fail to normally descend from the neck into the mediastinum as part of normal embryogenesis, in which case the thymus gland can be partially or completely ectopic in the cervical region. The latter is important to recognize as a potential explanation for non visualization of the thymus gland in its expected normal location in the superior mediastinum.[107]

**Associated Anomalies:** Prenatal diagnosis of a thymic mass is a rare occurrence. There have been case reports of prenatally diagnosed thymic cysts. Absence of the thymus gland is indicative of thymic aplasia, and a small gland is associated with thymic hypoplasia (Fig. 17.3-17). These findings are of high concern because of the association in various diseases, including DiGeorge syndrome, Ellis–Van Creveld syndrome, and severe combined immunodeficiency.[108–110] Other associations with an underdeveloped or absent thymus include human immunodeficiency virus, infection, intrauterine growth restriction, acute illnesses, and chorioamnioitis.[111–113] Others have reported that an absent or hypoplastic thymus on US is a marker for deletion 22q11.1 associated with fetal cardiac defects.[114,115] Focused imaging of the thymus gland on US or MRI may be indicated in fetuses at risk for a hypoplastic or absent thymus gland.[104]

## Bronchogenic Cyst

A bronchogenic cyst is a cystic duplication of the tracheobronchial tree.

**Incidence:** Bronchogenic cysts are relatively rare but represent the most common cystic lesion of the mediastinum and account for approximately 20% of surgically resected cystic lung lesions.[116] Prevalence may be underestimated because of cases not coming to clinical recognition.[85]

**Pathogenesis:** Bronchogenic cysts result from abnormal budding of the ventral diverticulum of the foregut, which leads to a focal cystic duplication of the tracheobronchial tree.[85] The cyst walls are lined with ciliated columnar epithelium and often contain fibrous tissue and small amounts of cartilage. Cyst contents may vary from a thin watery fluid collection to thicker mucoid material.[85] The majority of bronchogenic cysts (approximately 85%) are located in the mediastinum most commonly adjacent to the distal trachea or proximal main stem bronchi.

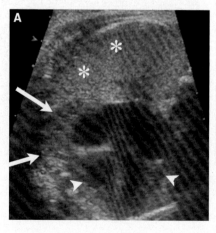
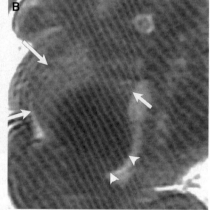

**FIGURE 17.3-16:** Normal thymus gland in third trimester fetus. **A:** Axial sonogram through the chest demonstrates a normal thymus gland (arrows), which is hypoechoic relative to the normal lung (asterisks). Arrowheads indicate the heart. **B:** Coronal T2-weighted MRI through the fetal chest demonstrates the thymus gland as an intermediate signal bilobed structure (arrows). Note normal asymmetry of lobes. Heart is indicated by arrowheads.

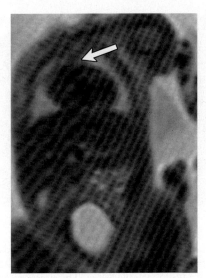

**FIGURE 17.3-17:** Coronal T2-weighted MR image through the fetal chest demonstrates absence of the thymus gland in the superior mediastinum *(arrow)* in a fetus with De George syndrome. (Courtesy of Guillome Gourincour, MD, Marseille, France.)

The remainder of bronchogenic cysts occur within the lung parenchyma. If the budding abnormality occurs early in bronchial development, the cyst is mediastinal in location, and when abnormal budding occurs later in development, the result is usually an intrapulmonary bronchogenic cyst.[117]

**Diagnosis:** On US, bronchogenic cysts usually appear as a well-defined unilocular hypoechoic mass within the fetal mediastinum near the carina of the trachea or, less commonly, within the lung parenchyma (Fig. 17.3-18A). The cysts are typically solitary or, less commonly, manifest as multiple lesions.[117] Large mediastinal bronchogenic cysts may compress the tracheobronchial tree and esophagus, and result in lung overinflation and polyhydramnios.[118]

On MRI, a bronchogenic cyst appears as a high signal intensity fluid containing structure on T2-weighted sequences (Figs. 17.3-18B and 17.3-19).[119,120] MRI may complement US by ascertaining the precise location of the cyst and assessing for any associated lung parenchyma abnormalities.

**Differential Diagnosis:** The differential diagnosis for a mediastinal bronchogenic cyst includes an enteric duplication cyst involving the esophagus. Enteric duplication cysts are rare congenital anomalies that may arise anywhere in the gastrointestinal tract. Approximately one-third of cases involve the foregut, which includes the esophagus, stomach, and proximal duodenum. A large neurenteric cyst may also mimic a bronchogenic cyst; however, accurate localization of the cyst between the esophagus and the trachea should confirm the correct diagnosis of a bronchogenic cyst. The differential diagnosis for an intrapulmonary bronchogenic cyst includes a unilocular CPAM with a single dominant cyst or the very rare case of a cystic PPB.

**Prognosis:** Limited data are available for the prognosis of prenatally diagnosed bronchogenic cysts. Most lesions are small and unassociated with mass effect, and fare well with no significant complications. Some lesions that compress the bronchial tree may cause overinflation of the adjacent lung parenchyma.

**Management:** Most cysts require no fetal intervention and are managed with serial US to assure stability in size. A very large bronchogenic cyst associated with mediastinal shift may have improved outcome with percutaneous drainage, but the experience is very limited.[118,121]

Most are removed postnatally to prevent superimposed infection, hemorrhage, or growth that could impinge on adjacent structures.

**Recurrence:** There is no known recurrence risk.

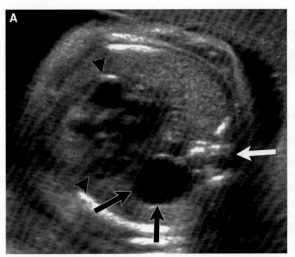
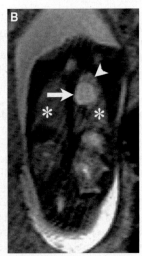
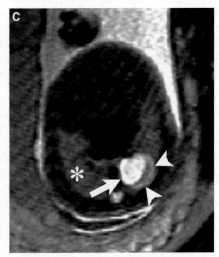

**FIGURE 17.3-18:** Intrapulmonary bronchogenic cyst in 25-week gestational age fetus. **A:** Axial plane sonogram through the fetal chest demonstrates an intrapulmonary unilocular hypoechoic lesion with through transmission *(black arrows)*. The heart is indicated by *arrowheads*, and the spine by *white arrow*. Coronal **(B)** and axial **(C)** plane T2-weighted MR images demonstrate a left-sided high-signal mass *(arrow)* confirmed to be a bronchogenic cyst. High signal intensity lung *(arrowheads)* surrounding the cyst corresponded to fluid trapped in the lung distal to the bronchogenic cyst. Normal lungs are indicated by *asterisks*.

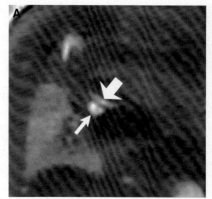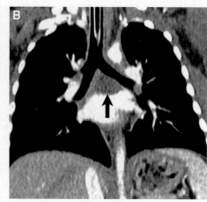

**FIGURE 17.3-19:** Mediastinal bronchogenic cyst causing lung hyperinflation in a 23-week gestational age fetus. **A:** Coronal plane T2-weighted MRI demonstrates a subcarinal bronchogenic cyst *(thin arrow)*. Left main stem bronchus is indicated by *thick arrow*. **B:** Newborn coronal plane CT confirms subcarinal bronchogenic cyst *(arrow)*.

## Neurenteric Cyst

Neurenteric cysts represent enteric remnants, which result from incomplete separation of the notochord from the foregut during early embryogenesis.[122–124]

**Incidence:** Neurenteric cysts are rare lesions, and the incidence in the fetus is not known.

**Pathogenesis:** Neurenteric cysts are felt to occur due to incomplete notochord separation in the presence of a persistent communication between the ectoderm of the spinal cord and the endoderm of the foregut before closure of the neural tube. Neurenteric cysts are characterized by an intraspinal cystic component that is connected to a mediastinal or thoracic cyst.[125] Approximately 90% of all neurenteric cysts are localized to the posterior mediastinal compartment superior to the carina; however, the cysts may occur at any location throughout the spinal column. The most common locations are in the lower cervical and upper thoracic regions. Most are associated with an intradural extamedullary cystic component within the spinal canal. Connections with the gastrointestinal tract may also be identified.[126] Approximately 50% are associated with vertebral body segmentation anomalies and scoliosis.[122,124,127]

Neurenteric cysts are usually unilocular and appear as a round or tubular mediastinal cystic mass with connection to the spinal canal. Large mediastinal neurenteric cysts may result in mass effect on the adjacent lung, airways, heart, and vessels, and when coexisting with intraspinal lesions may result in signs and symptoms of central nervous system abnormalities after birth.

**Diagnosis:** On US, neurenteric cysts appear as a posterior mediastinal unilocular or septated cyst with a thin wall, most commonly superior to the carina (Fig. 17.3-20A,B). Large cysts with mass effect may result in cardiac malposition or hydrops fetalis. Associated spinal findings include vertebral segmentation anomalies (hemivertebra or butterfly vertebra) and scoliosis.[122,124,127]

On MRI, T2-weighted fluid-sensitive sequences demonstrate a high signal intensity well-marginated cyst in the posterior mediastinum (see Fig. 17.3-20B,C). MRI may also show the extent of the lesion into the spinal canal. Neurenteric cysts may be associated with the rare split notochord syndrome characterized by a cleft of the vertebral column. Gastrointestinal and other central nervous system anomalies have been described.[128–130]

**Differential Diagnosis:** Differential diagnosis for a neurenteric cyst includes bronchopulmonary malformations, including a macrocystic CPAM. Other considerations include a bronchogenic cyst, pericardial cyst, CDH with herniated stomach, and cystic pleural pulmonary blastoma. The presence of associated spinal anomalies should confirm the correct diagnosis of neurenteric cyst.

**Prognosis:** The outcome for a neurenteric cyst depends largely on the extent of the mass, mass effect on adjacent organs, and the presence of associated central nervous system abnormalities. Large cysts may compress the developing lung and result in pulmonary hypoplasia or hydrops fetalis. Pulmonary hypoplasia secondary to a neurenteric cyst can be associated with respiratory distress after birth.[64,127]

**Management:** There is minimal literature regarding the role of surgical intervention in fetuses diagnosed with a neurenteric cyst.[125] Prenatal intervention is rarely indicated, although there have been case reports of treatment by aspiration or placement of a shunt if the cystic mass is large enough to raise concern for pulmonary hypoplasia.[125] Postnatal surgical correction is indicated.

**Recurrence:** The lesion is sporadic with no known recurrence risk.

## Masses-Teratoma

Teratomas are a type of germ cell tumor that histologically contains tissue elements of ectodermal, mesodermal, and endodermal origin.

**Incidence:** Prenatal diagnosis of a mediastinal teratoma is a rare occurrence, and pericardial lesions are extremely rare with fewer than 100 cases reported.[131,132] Teratomas are the most common congenital neoplasm in children, and the vast majority of prenatally diagnosed teratomas are sacrococcygeal, accounting for approximately 80% of all teratomas.[131] Approximately 10% of teratomas are localized in the mediastinum, most commonly in the anterior superior compartment, and when large may result in severe compression of adjacent mediastinal structures and the developing lung.[132]

**Pathogenesis:** Teratomas are neoplasms composed of all three germ layers or multiple foreign tissues without organ specificity. Etiology is yet unknown, but hypothesized to result from aberrant twinning, totipotent cells from Hensen node or from

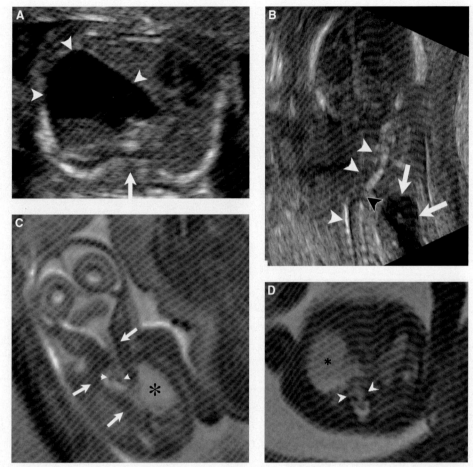

**FIGURE 17.3-20:** Neurenteric cyst. **A:** Axial sonogram shows a large mediastinal cyst *(arrowheads)*. Spine is indicated by *arrow*. **B:** Coronal sonogram demonstrates cyst *(arrows)* communicating with spinal canal *(black arrowhead)*. Scoliotic spine with abnormal curvature *(white arrowheads)*. **C:** Coronal T2-weighted MRI demonstrates split spinal cord *(arrowheads)* and abnormal curvature to the spine *(arrows)*. Neurenteric cyst *(asterisk)*. **D:** Axial plane SSFP MRI demonstrates neurenteric cyst *(asterick)* and open communication of spinal canal with posterior mediastinal cyst *(arrowheads)*. Images courtesy of Beth Kline-Fath.

reproductive gland analog. The majority of teratomas in children are benign.[133]

**Diagnosis:** On US, mediastinal teratomas are localized to the anterior/superior mediastinum and appear as a cystic, solid, or a complex mass with heterogeneous echogenicity (Fig. 17.3-21A). Hyperechogenic foci associated with acoustic shadowing are indicative of internal calcifications and are helpful to confirm diagnosis. Pericardial teratomas may be differentiated from mediastinal teratoma by the association with pericardial effusion in the majority of cases.[133] On T2-weighted MRI sequences, mediastinal and pericardial teratomas appear as cystic, solid, or complex masses in the superior anterior mediastinum (see Fig. 17.3-21B,C). High-signal foci on T1-weighted sequences are indicative of internal fat, calcification, or hemorrhage into the cystic components. The lesion usually displaces the heart inferiorly.

**Differential Diagnosis:** Differential diagnosis for a mediastinal or pericardial teratoma includes mediastinal bronchogenic cyst or enteric duplication cyst. Bronchogenic cysts or enteric duplication cysts tend to be in the middle or posterior mediastinum respectively and are not associated with solid components.

When large, the lesion may mimic a CPAM, but can be differentiated by inferior more than right or leftward displacement of the heart. The anterior mediastinal location of teratomas and the frequent presence of solid components or calcifications should also allow for accurate diagnosis.

**Prognosis:** Complications of teratomas in the fetus are uncommon, and prognosis is expected to be good for small lesions. Large mediastinal or pericardial teratomas may cause significant mass effect on airway, heart, lungs, and esophagus, resulting in airway obstruction, diminished cardiac output, pulmonary hypoplasia, and polyhydramnios.[132,134] In the presence of polyhydramnios, the fetus is at risk for preterm labor. Hydrops fetalis likely results when a large mass inhibits venous return to the heart and is associated with high morbidity and mortality.[131]

**Management:** Management is surveillance with serial USs to assess for the rare complication of airway obstruction, hydrops fetalis, or diminished cardiac output. If hydrops occurs late in gestation >30 weeks, the fetus may be delivered preterm or EXIT to airway if airway compression is noted.[134] If the fetus is less than 30 weeks with large pericardial effusion or dominant lesion cyst, pericardiocentesis and/or cyst aspiration

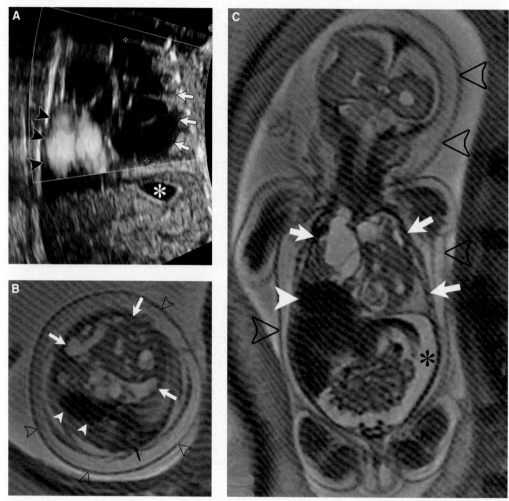

**FIGURE 17.3-21:** Mediastinal teratoma. **A:** Coronal US demonstrates a large complex cystic mediastinal mass *(arrows)* displacing the heart *(arrowheads)*. *Asterisk* indicates the stomach. Axial **(B)** and coronal **(C)** T2-weighted MR images demonstrate a large complex mediastinal teratoma *(white arrows)* displacing the heart *(white arrowheads)* inferiorly into the right chest and associated fetal hydrops. Skin thickening *(black arrowheads)* and fetal ascites *(black asterisk)*. *Black arrow* indicates spine. Images courtesy of Beth Kline-Fath, MD.

may be considered.[135] In the absence of drainable fluid in a severely <30-week hydropic fetus, in utero resection may be attempted. Postnatal resection is mandated because of risk of malignancy.

**Recurrence:** Most cases are sporadic with no recurrence risk; however, there is a small group that is inherited as a familial genetic disturbance.

## Fetal Pleural Effusion (Hydrothorax)

**Incidence:** Fetal pleural effusions are relatively uncommon, manifesting in approximately 1:10,000 to 15,000 pregnancies.[136]

**Pathogenesis:** Fetal pleural effusion may occur as a primary abnormality, usually associated with chylothorax, or as part of hydrops fetalis.[136–140] Most commonly, a pleural effusion in the fetus is associated with hydrops fetalis, which may be caused by numerous conditions, including cardiovascular disease, underlying bronchopulmonary malformations, chromosomal abnormalities (most commonly trisomy 21 and Turner syndrome), CDH, cystic hygroma, or infection.[137–139] Cardiac, pulmonary,

or chromosomal abnormalities are associated in approximately 80% of cases.[137,140]

Maternal parvovirus infection has been associated with transient isolated pleural effusions, which often resolve spontaneously before term and are thought to result from direct pleural inflammation.[141]

Chylothorax is the most common cause of a primary congenital pleural effusion in a fetus and is a diagnosis to be considered after excluding other causes.[142] Chylothorax is commonly due to a primary defect in the lymphatic system, caused either via inflammation or genetic origin or, less likely, as a secondary finding in the presence of an underlying lymphatic malformation. When a primary pleural effusion is large, it may result in mediastinal compression and lead to hydrops fetalisis; thereby, making it difficult to distinguish between primary and secondary effusions.[142–144]

**Diagnosis:** On US, fetal pleural effusion is usually detected as an incidental finding by identifying an intrathoracic fluid collection surrounding the fetal lung, most often on the right side but may be bilateral (Fig. 17.3-22). It is often the first sign of fetal hydrops; therefore, identification of pleural effusion should

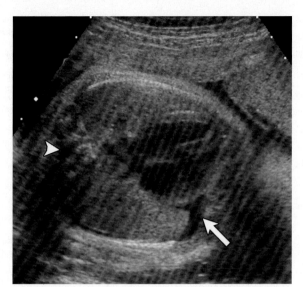

**FIGURE 17.3-22:** Pleural effusion. Axial sonograms demonstrate a right pleural effusion *(arrow)* secondary to maternal parvovirus infection, which resolved spontaneously without postnatal sequelae. *Arrowhead* indicates spine.

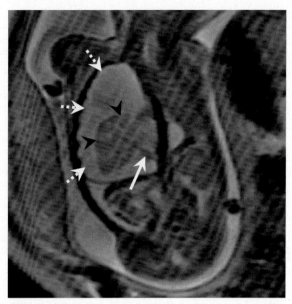

**FIGURE 17.3-23:** A 31-week gestation fetus with large pleural effusion. Coronal T2 MRI identified a heterogeneous lung lesion *(arrowheads)* supplied by a feeding vessel from aorta *(white arrow)* in association with large pleural effusion *(dotted arrows)*. Postnatal confirmed hybrid lesion. Images courtesy of Beth Kline-Fath, MD.

trigger an investigation to exclude the more common causes of fetal hydrops prior to assuming the diagnosis of a chylothorax. A search for additional anomalies, including lymphatic malformation or sequestration, should be performed. When pleural effusions are large, the underlying lung will appear to float freely in the pleural cavity.

On MRI, pleural effusions can also be readily identified, which by itself does not add significant information to that provided by US. The potential value of MRI in the setting of a hydrothorax is to identify an associated underlying mass as the etiology of the effusion. For example, torsion of an extralobar sequestration may present with a large ipsilateral pleural effusion (Fig. 17.3-23).

**Differential Diagnosis:** Diagnosis of pleural effusion is usually straightforward. Occasionally, a massive pericardial effusion may mimic a pleural effusion; however, the appearance of the fluid surrounding the heart should allow for distinction. The main challenge in diagnosis of pleural effusion is to distinguish a primary from a secondary effusion. Careful scrutiny to exclude an underlying mass or other anomalies is important for patient counseling and pregnancy management.

**Prognosis:** The prognosis for pleural effusion in the fetus is variable. Some cases resolve or remain stable throughout pregnancy; whereas, others evolve to severe hydrothorax, which can result in hydrops fetalis. Approximately 10% of isolated hydrothoraces resolve spontaneously with good postnatal outcome. Mild-to-moderate pleural effusions which remain stable throughout pregnancy are associated with good postnatal outcome.[140,142,145] Cases associated with hydrops fetalis have a high mortality rate, reported as greater than 50%.[146] Large bilateral pleural effusions with significant mediastinal compression associated with hydrops fetalis constitute poor prognostic signs with a high likelihood for fatal outcome, reported as greater than 90% in the absence of intervention.[139,143,144,146–151] Large pleural effusions may also compress the underlying lung and result

in pulmonary hypoplasia or compress the esophagus, causing polyhydramnios. Karyotyping to exclude trisomy 21 or Turner syndrome is indicated.

**Management:** Small-to-moderate isolated pleural effusions, which remain stable, can undergo surveillance with serial USs without intervention. Given the high mortality in the presence of large effusions and propensity to develop hydrops, prenatal intervention is typically considered. If the karyotype is normal, maternal diet modification by supplementation with medium-chain triglycerides may decrease or resolve the effusion.[152] If titers are negative for infection and effusion persists, thoracentesis may aid in confirming chylothorax by documenting lymphocyte predominance (>95%).

Thoracoamniotic shunting is the gold standard therapy in the presence of large effusion or hydrops. Shunting may reduce the risk of lung hypoplasia and hydrops and has been reported to improve the outcome.[144,148,149,153,154] With thoracoamniotic shunting, mortality rates are reduced; however, they still remain high at 10% to 30% for non hydropic cases and 50% to 60% for hydropic cases.[142,144,154] Some centers will consider a thoracentesis prior to placing a thoracoamniotic shunt since decompression of fluid may enhance sonographic examination of the fetal heart and the underlying lungs. However, in the majority of cases, the fluid will reaccumulate within 24 hours, and a shunt will need to be placed if prolonged decompression is desired.[142,143,145,155] Recently, pleurodesis with OK-432, a derivative of Group A *Streptococcus pyogenes* treated with penicillin G, has been shown to resolve pleural effusion via inducing sclerosing adhesions. The technique is still investigational and has not yet been proven as effective as thoracoamniotic shunting but may hold promise as an alternative therapy.[152]

**Recurrence:** Risk of recurrence is dependent on the etiology of the effusion. Chylothorax is usually sporadic with low recurrence, although familial cases have been cited.[156]

# REFERENCES

1. Lim FY, Crombleholme TM, Hedrick HL, et al. Congenital high airway obstruction syndrome: natural history and management. *J Pediatr Surg.* 2003;38:940–945.
2. Barth RA. Imaging of fetal chest masses. *Pediatr Radiol.* 2012;42(suppl 1):S62–S73.
3. Gilboa Y, Achiron R, Katorza E, et al. Early sonographic diagnosis of congenital high-airway obstruction syndrome. *Ultrasound Obstet Gynecol.* 2009;33:731–733.
4. Vidaeff AC, Szmuk P, Mastrobattista JM, et al. More or less CHAOS: case report and literature review suggesting the existence of a distinct subtype of congenital high airway obstruction syndrome. *Ultrasound Obstet Gynecol.* 2007;30:114–117.
5. Kassanos D, Christodoulou CN, Agapitos E, et al. Prenatal ultrasonographic detection of the tracheal atresia sequence. *Ultrasound Obstet Gynecol.* 1997;10:133–136.
6. Berg C, Geipel A, Germer U, et al. Prenatal detection of Fraser syndrome without cryptophthalmos: case report and review of the literature. *Ultrasound Obstet Gynecol.* 2001;18:76–80.
7. Mong A, Johnson AM, Kramer SS, et al. Congenital high airway obstruction syndrome: MR/US findings, effect on management, and outcome. *Pediatr Radiol.* 2008;38:1171–1179.
8. Guimaraes CV, Linam LE, Kline-Fath BM, et al. Prenatal MRI findings of fetuses with congenital high airway obstruction sequence. *Korean J Radiol.* 2009;10:129–134.
9. Kohl T, Van de Vondel P, Stressig R, et al. Percutaneous fetoscopic laser decompression of congenital high airway obstruction syndrome (CHAOS) from laryngeal atresia via a single trocar—current technical constraints and potential solutions for future interventions. *Fetal Diagn Ther.* 2009;25:67–71.
10. DeCou JM, Jones DC, Jacobs HD, et al. Successful ex utero intrapartum treatment (EXIT) procedure for congenital high airway obstruction syndrome (CHAOS) owing to laryngeal atresia. *J Pediatr Surg.* 1998;33:1563–1565.
11. Bui TH, Grunewald C, Frenckner B, et al. Successful EXIT (ex utero intrapartum treatment) procedure in a fetus diagnosed prenatally with congenital high-airway obstruction syndrome due to laryngeal atresia. *Eur J Pediatr Surg.* 2000;10:328–333.
12. Langston C. New concepts in the pathology of congenital lung malformations. *Semin Pediatr Surg.* 2003;12:17–37.
13. Epelman M, Kreiger PA, Servaes S, et al. Current imaging of prenatally diagnosed congenital lung lesions. *Semin Ultrasound CT MR.* 2010;31:141–157.
14. Biyyam DR, Chapman T, Ferguson MR, et al. Congenital lung abnormalities: embryologic features, prenatal diagnosis, and postnatal radiologic-pathologic correlation. *Radiographics.* 2010;30:1721–1738.
15. Stigers KB, Woodring JH, Kanga JF. The clinical and imaging spectrum of findings in patients with congenital lobar emphysema. *Pediatr Pulmonol.* 1992;14:160–170.
16. Barth RA, Newman B, Rubesova E, et al. Congenital lobar overinflation (CLO)/congenital lobar emphsysema (CLE)—not an uncommon cause for a fetal chest mass (Paper # PA9). *Pediatr Radiol.* 2009;39:S255 (Suppl 2): S252.
17. Olutoye OO, Coleman BG, Hubbard AM, et al. Prenatal diagnosis and management of congenital lobar emphysema. *J Pediatr Surg.* 2000;35:792–795.
18. Pacharn P, Kline-Fath B, Calvo-Garcia M, et al. Congenital lung lesions: comparison between prenatal magnetic resonance imaging (MRI) and postnatal findings. In: Radiological Society of North America 95th Scientific Assembly & Annual Meeting; November 29–December 4, 2009; McCormick Place, Chicago, IL.
19. Sparey C, Jawaheer G, Barrett AM, et al. Esophageal atresia in the Northern Region Congenital Anomaly Survey, 1985–1997: prenatal diagnosis and outcome. *Am J Obstet Gynecol.* 2000;182:427–431.
20. Depaepe A, Dolk H, Lechat MF. The epidemiology of tracheo-oesophageal fistula and oesophageal atresia in Europe: EUROCAT Working Group. *Arch Dis Child.* 1993;68:743–748.
21. Torfs CP, Curry CJ, Bateson TF. Population-based study of tracheoesophageal fistula and esophageal atresia. *Teratology.* 1995;52:220–232.
22. Forrester MB, Merz RD. Epidemiology of oesophageal atresia and tracheo-oesophageal fistula in Hawaii, 1986–2000. *Public Health.* 2005;119:483–488.
23. Pringle KC. Human fetal lung development and related animal models. *Clin Obstet Gynecol.* 1986;29:502–513.
24. Slovis TL. *Caffey's Pediatric Diagnostic Imaging.* 11th ed. Philadelphia, PA: Mosby Elsevier; 2008.
25. Pameijer CR, Hubbard AM, Coleman B, et al. Combined pure esophageal atresia, duodenal atresia, biliary atresia, and pancreatic ductal atresia: prenatal diagnostic features and review of the literature. *J Pediatr Surg.* 2000;35:745–747.
26. Marquette GP, Skoll MA, Yong SL, et al. First-trimester imaging of combined esophageal and duodenal atresia without a tracheoesophageal fistula. *J Ultrasound Med.* 2004;23:1232.
27. Estroff JA, Parad RB, Share JC, et al. Second trimester prenatal findings in duodenal and esophageal atresia without tracheoesophageal fistula. *J Ultrasound Med.* 1994;13:375–379.
28. Genevieve D, de Pontual L, Amiel J, et al. An overview of isolated and syndromic oesophageal atresia. *Clin Genet.* 2007;71:392–399.
29. Holder TM, Cloud DT, Lewis JE Jr, et al. Esophageal atresia and tracheoesophageal fistula: a survey of its members by the Surgical Section of the American Academy of Pediatrics. *Pediatrics.* 1964;34:542–549.
30. Bundy AL, Saltzman DH, Emerson D, et al. Sonographic features associated with cleft palate. *J Clin Ultrasound.* 1986;14:486–489.
31. Kallen B, Mastroiacovo P, Robert E. Major congenital malformations in Down syndrome. *Am J Med Genet.* 1996;65:160–166.
32. Matsuoka S, Takeuchi K, Yamanaka Y, et al. Comparison of magnetic resonance imaging and ultrasonography in the prenatal diagnosis of congenital thoracic abnormalities. *Fetal Diagn Ther.* 2003;18:447–453.
33. Satoh S, Takashima T, Takeuchi H, et al. Antenatal sonographic detection of the proximal esophageal segment: specific evidence for congenital esophageal atresia. *J Clin Ultrasound.* 1995;23:419–423.
34. Centini G, Rosignoli L, Kenanidis A, et al. Prenatal diagnosis of esophageal atresia with the pouch sign. *Ultrasound Obstet Gynecol.* 2003;21:494–497.
35. Stringer MD, McKenna KM, Goldstein RB, et al. Prenatal diagnosis of esophageal atresia. *J Pediatr Surg.* 1995;30:1258–1263.
36. Langer JC, Hussain H, Khan A, et al. Prenatal diagnosis of esophageal atresia using sonography and magnetic resonance imaging. *J Pediatr Surg.* 2001;36:804–807.
37. Mitani Y, Hasegawa T, Kubota A, et al. Prenatal findings of concomitant duodenal and esophageal atresia without tracheoesophageal fistula (Gross type A). *J Clin Ultrasound.* 2009;37:403–405.
38. Levine D, Barnewolt CE, Mehta TS, et al. Fetal thoracic abnormalities: MR imaging. *Radiology.* 2003;228:379–388.
39. McKenna KM, Goldstein RB, Stringer MD. Small or absent fetal stomach: prognostic significance. *Radiology.* 1995;197:729–733.
40. Brumfield CG, Davis RO, Owen J, et al. Pregnancy outcomes following sonographic nonvisualization of the fetal stomach. *Obstet Gynecol.* 1998;91:905–908.
41. Hill LM. Congenital microgastria: absence of the fetal stomach and normal third trimester amniotic fluid volume. *J Ultrasound Med.* 1994;3:894–896.
42. Kroes EJ, Festen C. Congenital microgastria: a case report and review of literature. *Pediatr Surg Int.* 1998;13:416–418.
43. Menon P, Rao KL, Cutinha HP, et al. Gastric augmentation in isolated congenital microgastria. *J Pediatr Surg.* 2003;38:E4–E6.
44. Spitz L. Oesophageal atresia. *Orphanet J Rare Dis.* 2007;2:24.
45. Lopez PJ, Keys C, Pierro A, et al. Oesophageal atresia: improved outcome in high-risk groups? *J Pediatr Surg.* 2006;41:331–334.
46. Sinha CK, Haider N, Marri RR, et al. Modified prognostic criteria for oesophageal atresia and tracheo-oesophageal fistula. *Eur J Pediatr Surg.* 2007;17:153–157.
47. Scott DA. Esophageal atresia/tracheoesophageal fistula overview. In: *GeneReviews* [Internet]. Seattle, WA: University of Washington, Seattle; 2009.
48. Burge D, Wheeler R. Increasing incidence of detection of congenital lung lesions. *Pediatr Pulmonol.* 2010;45:103; author reply 104.
49. Stocker JT, Madewell JE, Drake RM. Congenital cystic adenomatoid malformation of the lung: classification and morphologic spectrum. *Hum Pathol.* 1977;8:155–171.
50. Simonet WS, DeRose ML, Bucay N, et al. Pulmonary malformation in transgenic mice expressing human keratinocyte growth factor in the lung. *Proc Natl Acad Sci U S A.* 1995;92:12461–12465.
51. Volpe MV, Pham L, Lessin M, et al. Expression of Hoxb-5 during human lung development and in congenital lung malformations. *Birth Defects Res A Clin Mol Teratol.* 2003;67:550–556.
52. Volpe MV, Archavachotikul K, Bhan I, et al. Association of bronchopulmonary sequestration with expression of the homeobox protein Hoxb-5. *J Pediatr Surg.* 2000;35:1817–1819.
53. Riedlinger WF, Vargas SO, Jennings RW, et al. Bronchial atresia is common to extralobar sequestration, intralobar sequestration, congenital cystic adenomatoid malformation, and lobar emphysema. *Pediatr Dev Pathol.* 2006;9:361–373.
54. Kunisaki SM, Fauza DO, Nemes LP, et al. Bronchial atresia: the hidden pathology within a spectrum of prenatally diagnosed lung masses. *J Pediatr Surg.* 2006;41:61–65.
55. Stocker JT. Congenital pulmonary airway malformation: a new name for and an expanded classification of congenital cystic adenomatous malformation of the lung. *Histopathology.* 2002;41:424–431.
56. Stocker JT. The respiratory tract. In: Stocker JT, Dehner LP, eds. *Pediatric Pathology.* Philadelphia, PA: Lippincott Williams & Wilkins; 2001:445.
57. Adzick NS. Management of fetal lung lesions. *Clin Perinatol.* 2003;30:481–492.
58. Crombleholme TM, Coleman B, Hedrick H, et al. Cystic adenomatoid malformation volume ratio predicts outcome in prenatally diagnosed cystic adenomatoid malformation of the lung. *J Pediatr Surg.* 2002;37:331–338.
59. Azizkhan RG, Crombleholme TM. Congenital cystic lung disease: contemporary antenatal and postnatal management. *Pediatr Surg Int.* 2008;24:643–657.
60. Hubbard AM, Adzick NS, Crombleholme TM, et al. Congenital chest lesions: diagnosis and characterization with prenatal MR imaging. *Radiology.* 1999;212:43–48.
61. Hubbard AM. Prenatal magnetic resonance imaging for fetal abnormalities. In: Milunsky A, ed. *Genetic Disorders and the Fetus: Diagnosis, Prevention, and Treatment.* Baltimore and London, UK: Johns Hopkins University Press; 2004:944.
62. Abdullah MM, Lacro RV, Smallhorn J, et al. Fetal cardiac dextroposition in the absence of an intrathoracic mass: sign of significant right lung hypoplasia. *J Ultrasound Med.* 2000;19:669–676.

63. Cavoretto P, Molina F, Poggi S, et al. Prenatal diagnosis and outcome of echogenic fetal lung lesions. *Ultrasound Obstet Gynecol.* 2008;32:769–783.

64. Adzick NS, Harrison MR, Crombleholme TM, et al. Fetal lung lesions: management and outcome. *Am J Obstet Gynecol.* 1998;179:884–889.

65. Wilson RD, Hedrick HL, Liechty KW, et al. Cystic adenomatoid malformation of the lung: review of genetics, prenatal diagnosis, and in utero treatment. *Am J Med Genet A.* 2006;140:151–155.

66. Husler MR, Wilson RD, Rychik J, et al. Prenatally diagnosed fetal lung lesions with associated conotruncal heart defects: is there a genetic association? *Prenat Diagn.* 2007;27:1123–1128.

67. Bromley B, Parad R, Estroff JA, et al. Fetal lung masses: prenatal course and outcome. *J Ultrasound Med.* 1995;14:927–936; quiz p1378.

68. Thorpe-Beeston JG, Nicolaides KH. Cystic adenomatoid malformation of the lung: prenatal diagnosis and outcome. *Prenat Diagn.* 1994;14:677–688.

69. Miller JA, Corteville JE, Langer JC. Congenital cystic adenomatoid malformation in the fetus: natural history and predictors of outcome. *J Pediatr Surg.* 1996;31:805–808.

70. Duncombe GJ, Dickinson JE, Kikiros CS. Prenatal diagnosis and management of congenital cystic adenomatoid malformation of the lung. *Am J Obstet Gynecol.* 2002;187:950–954.

71. Illanes S, Hunter A, Evans M, et al. Prenatal diagnosis of echogenic lung: evolution and outcome. *Ultrasound Obstet Gynecol.* 2005;26:145–149.

72. Morris LM, Lim FY, Livingston JC, et al. High-risk fetal congenital pulmonary airway malformations have a variable response to steroids. *J Pediatr Surg.* 2009;44:60–65.

73. Peranteau WH, Wilson RD, Liechty KW, et al. Effect of maternal betamethasone administration on prenatal congenital cystic adenomatoid malformation growth and fetal survival. *Fetal Diagn Ther.* 2007;22:365–371.

74. Curran PF, Jelin EB, Rand L, et al. Prenatal steroids for microcystic congenital cystic adenomatoid malformations. *J Pediatr Surg.* 2010;45:145–150.

75. Loh KC, Jelin E, Hirose S, et al. Microcystic congenital pulmonary airway malformation with hydrops fetalis: steroids vs open fetal resection. *J Pediatr Surg.* 2012;47:36–39.

76. Brown MF, Lewis D, Brouillette RM, et al. Successful prenatal management of hydrops, caused by congenital cystic adenomatoid malformation, using serial aspirations. *J Pediatr Surg.* 1995;30:1098–1099.

77. Ryo E, Okai T, Namba S, et al. Successful thoracoamniotic shunting using a double-flower catheter in a case of fetal cystic adenomatoid malformation associated with hydrops and polyhydramnios. *Ultrasound Obstet Gynecol.* 1997;10:293–296.

78. Wilson RD, Baxter JK, Johnson MP, et al. Thoracoamniotic shunts: fetal treatment of pleural effusions and congenital cystic adenomatoid malformations. *Fetal Diagn Ther.* 2004;19:413–420.

79. Yokoyama T, Yamashita K, Nishiyama T, et al. A case of thoraco-amniotic shunt for congenital cystic adenomatoid malformation [in Japanese]. *Masui.* 2005;54:287–290.

80. Harrison MR, Adzick NS, Jennings RW, et al. Antenatal intervention for congenital cystic adenomatoid malformation. *Lancet.* 1990;336:965–967.

81. Bruner JP, Jarnagin BK, Reinisch L. Percutaneous laser ablation of fetal congenital cystic adenomatoid malformation: too little, too late? *Fetal Diagn Ther.* 2000;15:359–363.

82. Lee FL, Said N, Grikscheit TC, et al. Treatment of congenital pulmonary airway malformation induced hydrops fetalis via percutaneous sclerotherapy. *Fetal Diagn Ther.* 2012;31:264–268.

83. Rosado-de-Christenson ML, Frazier AA, Stocker JT, et al. From the archives of the AFIP. Extralobar sequestration: radiologic-pathologic correlation. *Radiographics.* 1993;13:425–441.

84. Stocker JT. Sequestrations of the lung. *Semin Diagn Pathol.* 1986;3:106–121.

85. Winters WD, Effmann EL. Congenital masses of the lung: prenatal and postnatal imaging evaluation. *J Thorac Imaging.* 2001;16:196–206.

86. Wesley JR, Heidelberger KP, DiPietro MA, et al. Diagnosis and management of congenital cystic disease of the lung in children. *J Pediatr Surg.* 1986;21:202–207.

87. Lager DJ, Kuper KA, Haake GK. Subdiaphragmatic extralobar pulmonary sequestration. *Arch Pathol Lab Med.* 1991;115:536–538.

88. Johnson AM, Hubbard AM. Congenital anomalies of the fetal/neonatal chest. *Semin Roentgenol.* 2004;39:197–214.

89. Frazier AA, Rosado de Christenson ML, Stocker JT, et al. Intralobar sequestration: radiologic-pathologic correlation. *Radiographics.* 1997;17:725–745.

90. Gerle RD, Jaretzki A III, Ashley CA, et al. Congenital bronchopulmonary-foregut malformation: pulmonary sequestration communicating with the gastrointestinal tract. *N Engl J Med.* 1968;278:1413–1419.

91. Conran RM, Stocker JT. Extralobar sequestration with frequently associated congenital cystic adenomatoid malformation, type 2: report of 50 cases. *Pediatr Dev Pathol.* 1999;2:454–463.

92. Cass DL, Crombleholme TM, Howell LJ, et al. Cystic lung lesions with systemic arterial blood supply: a hybrid of congenital cystic adenomatoid malformation and bronchopulmonary sequestration. *J Pediatr Surg.* 1997;32:986–990.

93. Hernanz-Schulman M, Stein SM, Neblett WW, et al. Pulmonary sequestration: diagnosis with color Doppler sonography and a new theory of associated hydrothorax. *Radiology.* 1991;180:817–821.

94. Newman B. Congenital bronchopulmonary foregut malformations: concepts and controversies. *Pediatr Radiol.* 2006;36:773–791.

95. Priest JR, Williams GM, Hill DA, et al. Pulmonary cysts in early childhood and the risk of malignancy. *Pediatr Pulmonol.* 2009;44:14–30.

96. Hill DA, Ivanovich J, Priest JR, et al. DICER1 mutations in familial pleuropulmonary blastoma. *Science.* 2009;325:965.

97. Priest JR, McDermott MB, Bhatia S, et al. Pleuropulmonary blastoma: a clinicopathologic study of 50 cases. *Cancer.* 1997;80:147–161.

98. Miniati DN, Chintagumpala M, Langston C, et al. Prenatal presentation and outcome of children with pleuropulmonary blastoma. *J Pediatr Surg.* 2006;41:66–71.

99. Hill DA, Jarzembowski JA, Priest JR, et al. Type I pleuropulmonary blastoma: pathology and biology study of 51 cases from the international pleuropulmonary blastoma registry. *Am J Surg Pathol.* 2008;32:282–295.

100. Naffaa LN, Donnelly LF. Imaging findings in pleuropulmonary blastoma. *Pediatr Radiol.* 2005;35:387–391.

101. Haynes BF, Hale LP. The human thymus: a chimeric organ comprised of central and peripheral lymphoid components. *Immunol Res.* 1998;18:175–192.

102. Schwartz RH. Acquisition of immunologic self-tolerance. *Cell.* 1989;57:1073–1081.

103. Cho JY, Min JY, Lee YH, et al. Diameter of the normal fetal thymus on ultrasound. *Ultrasound Obstet Gynecol.* 2007;29:634–638.

104. De Leon-Luis J, Gamez F, Pintado P, et al. Sonographic measurements of the thymus in male and female fetuses. *J Ultrasound Med.* 2009;28:43–48.

105. Felker RE, Cartier MS, Emerson DS, et al. Ultrasound of the fetal thymus. *J Ultrasound Med.* 1989;8:669–673.

106. Li L, Bahtiyar MO, Buhimschi CS, et al. Assessment of the fetal thymus by two- and three-dimensional ultrasound during normal human gestation and in fetuses with congenital heart defects. *Ultrasound Obstet Gynecol.* 2011;37:404–409.

107. Han BK, Yoon HK, Suh YL. Thymic ultrasound, II: diagnosis of aberrant cervical thymus. *Pediatr Radiol.* 2001;31:480–487.

108. Dodson WE, Alexander D, Al-Aish M, et al. The DiGeorge syndrome. *Lancet.* 1969;1:574–575.

109. Ichijima K, Yamabe H, Kobashi Y, et al. An unusual case of metaphyseal chondrodysplasia with an abnormal perilacunar matrix associated with agranulocytosis and hypoplasia of the thymus. *Virchows Arch.* 1981;391:275–289.

110. Martin JP, Aguilar FT. Thymic hypoplasia with severe combined immunodeficiency. *Ann Allergy.* 1977;39:196–200.

111. Hartge R, Jenkins DM, Kohler HG. Low thymic weight in small-for-dates babies. *Eur J Obstet Gynecol Reprod Biol.* 1978;8:153–155.

112. Zalel Y, Gamzu R, Mashiach S, et al. The development of the fetal thymus: an in utero sonographic evaluation. *Prenat Diagn.* 2002;22:114–117.

113. Toti P, De Felice C, Stumpo M, et al. Acute thymic involution in fetuses and neonates with chorioamnionitis. *Hum Pathol.* 2000;31:1121–1128.

114. Chaoui R, Kalache KD, Heling KS, et al. Absent or hypoplastic thymus on ultrasound: a marker for deletion 22q11.2 in fetal cardiac defects. *Ultrasound Obstet Gynecol.* 2002;20:546–552.

115. Barrea C, Yoo SJ, Chitayat D, et al. Assessment of the thymus at echocardiography in fetuses at risk for 22q11.2 deletion. *Prenat Diagn.* 2003;23:9–15.

116. Shanti CM, Klein MD. Cystic lung disease. *Semin Pediatr Surg.* 2008;17:2–8.

117. Young G, L'Heureux PR, Krueckeberg ST, et al. Mediastinal bronchogenic cyst: prenatal sonographic diagnosis. *AJR Am J Roentgenol.* 1989;152:125–127.

118. Barbut J, Fernandez C, Blanc F, et al. Pulmonary sequestration of the left upper lobe associated with a bronchogenic cyst: case report of an exceptional association. *Pediatr Pulmonol.* 2011;46:509–511.

119. Levine D, Jennings R, Barnewolt C, et al. Progressive fetal bronchial obstruction caused by a bronchogenic cyst diagnosed using prenatal MR imaging. *AJR Am J Roentgenol.* 2001;176:49–52.

120. Ward VL. MR imaging in the prenatal diagnosis of fetal chest masses: effects on diagnostic accuracy, clinical decision making, parental understanding, and prediction of neonatal respiratory health outcomes. *Acad Radiol.* 2002;9:1064–1069.

121. Bayar UO, Numanoglu V, Bektas S, et al. Management of fetal bronchogenic lung cysts: a case report and short review of literature. *Case Rep Med.* 2010;2010:751423.

122. Uludag S, Madazli R, Erdogan E, et al. A case of prenatally diagnosed fetal neurenteric cyst. *Ultrasound Obstet Gynecol.* 2001;18:277–279.

123. Reed JC, Sobonya RE. Morphologic analysis of foregut cysts in the thorax. *AJR Am J Roentgenol.* 1974;120:851–860.

124. Strollo DC, Rosado-de-Christenson ML, Jett JR. Primary mediastinal tumors, part II: tumors of the middle and posterior mediastinum. *Chest.* 1997;112:1344–1357.

125. Aydin AL, Sasani M, Ucar B, et al. Prenatal diagnosis of a large, cervical, intraspinal, neurenteric cyst and postnatal outcome. *J Pediatr Surg.* 2009;44:1835–1838.

126. Fernandes ET, Custer MD, Burton EM, et al. Neurenteric cyst: surgery and diagnostic imaging. *J Pediatr Surg.* 1991;26:108–110.

127. Ryckman FC, Rosenkrantz JG. Thoracic surgical problems in infancy and childhood. *Surg Clin North Am.* 1985;65:1423–1454.

128. Perera GB, Milne M. Neurenteric cyst: antenatal diagnosis by ultrasound. *Australas Radiol.* 1997;41:300–302.

129. Almog D, Leibovitch L, Achiron R. Split notochord syndrome—prenatal ultrasonographic diagnosis. *Prenat Diagn.* 2001;21:1159–1162.

130. Agangi A, Paladini D, Bagolan P, et al. Split notochord syndrome variant: prenatal findings and neonatal management. *Prenat Diagn.* 2005;25:23–27.

131. Schild RL, Plath H, Hofstaetter C, et al. Prenatal diagnosis of a fetal mediastinal teratoma. *Ultrasound Obstet Gynecol.* 1998;12:369–370.

132. Liang RI, Wang P, Chang FM, et al. Prenatal sonographic characteristics and Doppler blood flow study in a case of a large fetal mediastinal teratoma. *Ultrasound Obstet Gynecol.* 1998;11:214–218.

133. Tollens M, Grab D, Lang D, et al. Pericardial teratoma: prenatal diagnosis and course. *Fetal Diagn Ther.* 2003;18:432–436.

134. Merchant A, Hedrick H, Johnson M, et al. Management of fetal mediastinal teratoma. *J Pediatr Surg.* 2005;40:228–231.

135. Takayasu H, Yoshihiro K, Kuroda T, et al. Successful management of a large fetal mediastinal teratoma complicated by hydrops fetalis. *J Pediatr Surg.* 2010;45:621–624.

136. Yinon Y, Grisaru-Granovsky S, Chaddha V, et al. Perinatal outcome following fetal chest shunt insertion for pleural effusion. *Ultrasound Obstet Gynecol.* 2010;36:58–64.

137. Ruano R, Ramalho AS, Cardoso AK, et al. Prenatal diagnosis and natural history of fetuses presenting with pleural effusion. *Prenat Diagn.* 2011;31:496–499.

138. Yinon Y, Kelly E, Ryan G. Fetal pleural effusions. *Best Pract Res Clin Obstet Gynaecol.* 2008;22:77–96.

139. Gratacos E. *Medicina Fetal.* Barcelona: Ed Medica Panamericana (ME); 2007.

140. Aubard Y, Derouineau I, Aubard V, et al. Primary fetal hydrothorax: a literature review and proposed antenatal clinical strategy. *Fetal Diagn Ther.* 1998;13:325–333.

141. Parilla BV, Tamura RK, Ginsberg NA. Association of parvovirus infection with isolated fetal effusions. *Am J Perinatol.* 1997;14:357–358.

142. Deurloo KL, Devlieger R, Lopriore E, et al. Isolated fetal hydrothorax with hydrops: a systematic review of prenatal treatment options. *Prenat Diagn.* 2007;27:893–899.

143. Hayashi S, Sago H, Kitano Y, et al. Fetal pleuroamniotic shunting for bronchopulmonary sequestration with hydrops. *Ultrasound Obstet Gynecol.* 2006;28:963–967.

144. Alkazaleh F, Saleem M, Badran E. Intrathoracic displacement of pleuroamniotic shunt after successful in utero treatment of fetal hydrops secondary to hydrothorax: case report and review of the literature. *Fetal Diagn Ther.* 2009;25:40–43.

145. National Institute for Health and Clinical Excellence. *Insertion of Pleuro-amniotic Shunt for Fetal Pleural Effusion.* London, UK: National Institute for Health and Clinical Excellence; 2006.

146. Longaker MT, Laberge JM, Dansereau J, et al. Primary fetal hydrothorax: natural history and management. *J Pediatr Surg.* 1989;24:573–576.

147. Paladini D, Volpe P. *Ultrasound of Congenital Fetal Anomalies: Differential Diagnosis and Prognostic Indicators.* London, UK: Informa Health Care, Informa UK Ltd; 2007.

148. Blott M, Nicolaides KH, Greenough A. Pleuroamniotic shunting for decompression of fetal pleural effusions. *Obstet Gynecol.* 1988;71:798–800.

149. Rodeck CH, Fisk NM, Fraser DI, et al. Long-term in utero drainage of fetal hydrothorax. *N Engl J Med.* 1988;319:1135–1138.

150. Pumberger W, Hörmann M, Deutinger J, et al. Longitudinal observation of antenatally detected congenital lung malformations (CLM): natural history, clinical outcome and long-term follow-up. *Eur J Cardiothorac Surg.* 2003;24:703–711.

151. Knox EM, Kilby MD, Martin WL, et al. In-utero pulmonary drainage in the management of primary hydrothorax and congenital cystic lesion: a systematic review. *Ultrasound Obstet Gynecol.* 2006;28:726–734.

152. Yang Y, Ma G, Shih J, et al. Experimental treatment of bilateral fetal chylothorax using in-utero pleurodesis. *Ultrasound Obstet Gynecol.* 2012;39:56–62.

153. Witlox RS, Lopriore E, Walther FJ, et al. Single-needle laser treatment with drainage of hydrothorax in fetal bronchopulmonary sequestration with hydrops. *Ultrasound Obstet Gynecol.* 2009;34:355–357.

154. Bianchi S, Lista G, Castoldi F, et al. Congenital primary hydrothorax: effect of thoracoamniotic shunting on neonatal clinical outcome. *J Matern Fetal Neonatal Med.* 2010;23:1225–1229.

155. Picone O, Benachi A, Mandelbrot L, et al. Thoracoamniotic shunting for fetal pleural effusions with hydrops. *Am J Obstet Gynecol.* 2004;191:2047–2050.

156. Battin M, Yan J, Aftimos S, et al. Congenital chylothorax in siblings. *Br J Obstet Gynaecol.* 2000;107:1516–1518.

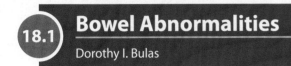

## 18.1 Bowel Abnormalities

Dorothy I. Bulas

Prenatal detection of a wide variety of anomalies and masses of the gastrointestinal tract is possible with ultrasonography and, in selected cases, with magnetic resonance imaging (MRI). Familiarity with the underlying disease process, associated malformation, and outcomes is important for determining the best obstetric management, mode of delivery, and postnatal care.

### EMBRYOLOGY

The primitive gut forms at 20 days postfertilization, with the dorsal yolk sac invaginating into the growing embryonic disc. The foregut, midgut, and hindgut are supplied by the celiac artery, superior mesenteric artery, and inferior mesenteric artery, respectively. The foregut derives the pharynx, respiratory tract, esophagus, stomach, duodenum, liver, and pancreas. The midgut derives the small bowel and proximal large bowel. The hindgut derives the distal colon and rectum as well as portions of the vagina and urinary bladder (Fig. 18.1-1).

The fetal gastrointestinal tract forms and undergoes its rotational process in the first trimester, returning into the abdomen by 11-weeks' gestation. In the first trimester, meconium is produced from secretions of the liver and intestinal glands.

Desquamated intestinal epithelium and amniotic fluid with meconium migrate from the small bowel to the rectum with increasing gestation age.

Fetal swallowing begins at 14 weeks' gestation with the advent of bowel peristalsis. The fetus swallows 2 to 7 mL per day by 16 weeks' gestation, 16 mL per day by 20 weeks, and 450 mL per day by term.[1]

### THE NORMAL ABDOMEN

#### Ultrasound

Physiologic midgut herniation into the umbilical cord can be visualized as early as 8 weeks' gestation with transvaginal scanning (see Fig. 18.2-5 in subchapter 18.2).[2–4]

Because of the greater supply of oxygenated blood to the left lobe of the liver, the left lobe is larger than the right in utero. The spleen may be visualized posterior to the stomach on the left. Normal measurements of the fetal liver, spleen, pancreas, stomach, gallbladder, and intestine are available (see Appendix tables 40–44).

Normally, the collapsed esophagus is not visualized by ultrasound (US).[5] Fluid may be observed within the lumen of the small bowel by 13 weeks' gestation.[6,7] Meconium accumulates in the small and large bowel throughout the second and third trimesters.[8,9] Bowel normally is collapsed and can be variably echogenic, at times similar in echogenicity to adjacent liver, spleen, and kidneys. Higher resolution linear transducers can be helpful in differentiating these organs. Linear transducers can make the bowel look unusually echogenic and must be carefully

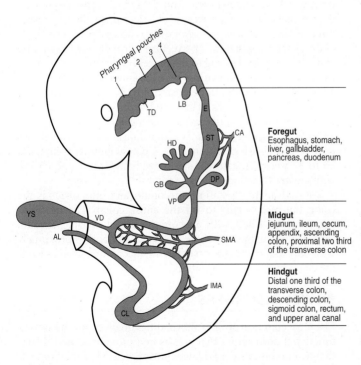

**FIGURE 18.1-1:** Development of gastrointestinal tract showing the foregut, midgut, and hindgut along with the adult derivatives. The entire length of the endodermal gut tube is shown from the mouth to the anus. 1–4, pharyngeal pouches; AL, allantois; CA, celiac artery; CL, cloaca; DP, dorsal pancreas; E, esophagus; GB, gallbladder; HD, hepatic ducts; IMA, inferior mesenteric artery; LB, lung bud; SMA, superior mesenteric artery; ST, stomach; TD, thyroid diverticulum; VD, vitelline duct; VP, ventral pancreas; YS, yolk sac. (From Dudek RW, ed. *High-Yield Systems: Gastrointestinal Tract.* Philadelphia, PA: Lippincott Williams & Wilkins; 2010.)

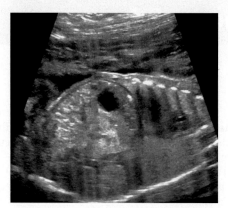

**FIGURE 18.1-2:** Echogenic bowel at 25 weeks of gestation. Coronal US demonstrates abnormally echogenic bowel in a fetus with cystic fibrosis.

differentiated from truly echogenic bowel that can be associated with infections, IUGR, and cystic fibrosis (see section on meconium ileus) (Fig. 18.1-2).

Swallowing occurs by 14 weeks' gestation, so a fluid-filled stomach should always be detectable by the second and third trimesters.[10,11] Echogenic debris can sometimes be seen layering in the stomach and can represent vernix, protein, or intra-amniotic hemorrhage.[12] It is important to confirm situs (see section on heterotaxy in Chapter 16). An absent or small stomach on serial fetal US can suggest a mechanical obstruction such as esophageal atresia or neck mass; CNS anomalies or syndromes in which fetal swallowing is depressed; or oligohydramnios.

Fluid-filled bowel lumen is not seen in the first trimester, but begins to be noted by US by 20 weeks' gestation. Peristalsis may be observed by 18 weeks' gestation. Small bowel should not exceed 5 mm in diameter. The presence of dilated loops (>15 mm in length and 7 mm in diameter) suggests fetal bowel obstruction.[13]

Colon is best seen after 24 weeks' gestation as hypoechoic regions along the periphery of the abdomen.[8] The colon fills with meconium, enlarging throughout gestation measuring 3 to 5 mm at 20 weeks and by term measuring up to 28 mm in diameter.[14] While variable, lumen diameter tables are available for gestational ages.[4,14] At times, normal colon can be mistaken for dilated small bowel or masses.[13]

The prenatal US diagnosis of bowel atresia can be difficult and is dependent on the site of obstruction, presence of associated anomalies, and timing of the study. The prenatal detection rate for obstruction is highest with duodenal obstruction and lowest for esophageal (24%) and anal atresia (6% to 8%).[15–17] There is poor sensitivity in the prenatal US diagnosis of large bowel lesions and misdiagnosis between small and large bowel obstruction.[18] Overall prenatal detection rate of gastrointestinal obstruction by US has varied from 24% to 34%.[16,17] With confounding variables such as maternal obesity; overlying gas and bone; transient normal variant; and late presentation, prenatal diagnosis and assessment of potential prognosis of fetuses with gastrointestinal abnormalities can be difficult by US.

## Magnetic Resonance Imaging

Fetal bowel is well visualized by MRI and can be easily differentiated from adjacent liver, spleen, kidneys, bladder, and gallbladder.[19–24]

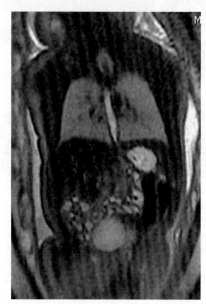

**FIGURE 18.1-3:** Normal esophagus. Coronal T2w MR image of a fluid-filled esophagus at 33 weeks of gestation.

Fluid-filled small bowel loops are high signal on T2w and low signal on T1w, while meconium is low signal on T2w and high signal on T1w. Thus, MRI can be a useful tool to help characterize bowel anomalies.[19,20,23,24]

The gastrointestinal tract is progressively filled by swallowed amniotic fluid that is T2 hyperintense and T1 hypointense. The esophagus may be transiently seen with fluid (Fig. 18.1-3). The stomach and duodenum should always be filled with T2 hyperintense fluid.

The jejunum should normally be high T2 and low T1 signal after 33 weeks' gestation. The distal small bowel has a more variable appearance dependent on gestational age. Before 32 weeks, 50% of distal small bowel remains high signal on T1w owing to slow protein-rich meconium progression.[19,25] T1 high signal may remain in proximal dilated loops because of lack of progression of meconium if bowel atresia is present or there is delayed peristalsis.[23–25]

By 20 weeks' gestation, the rectum normally is of high T1w and low T2w signal owing to the protein and mineral content of the meconium accumulating near the functionally obstructed anus. The rectum should be posterior to the bladder and 1 cm below the bladder neck. The rectal anteroposterior diameter increases with gestational age, measuring 4 to 8 mm at 24 weeks and 9 to 15 mm by 35 weeks.[19] Colonic luminal volume increases exponentially with gestational age. Colonic luminal volumes at 20 to 37 weeks' gestational age range between 1.1 and 65 mL with greater variations later gestation.[23]

With advancing gestation, meconium not only distends the colon but also begins to fill the entire colon. The descending colon is filled with meconium by 24 weeks gestation (Fig. 18.1-4). However, there is greater variability proximally with only half of normal cases having meconium-filled ascending colon by 31 weeks' gestation.[19]

## BOWEL DISORDERS

The most common bowel abnormalities involve a mechanical or functional obstruction that results in a proximal bowel dilatation. Common causes of dilated bowel are listed in Table 18.1-1.

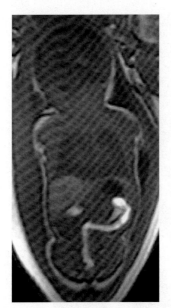

**FIGURE 18.1-4:** Meconium. Coronal T1w MR image demonstrates high signal within the descending colon and rectosigmoid at 33 weeks of gestation.

At times, associated anomalies are present (Table 18.1-2). Dilated bowel loops may contain fluid or meconium. It is important to consider normal bowel in the differential when dilated bowel is thought to be present. Other intra-abdominal cystic masses should also be considered when a dilated loop of bowel is thought to be present. Differentiating dilated ureter from bowel may be difficult as well.

It can take time for bowel dilatation to become apparent. Distal atresias such as anal atresia may never develop dilated bowel because of the absorption of fluid by the multiple proximal bowel loops. Jejunal and ilial atresias secondary to vascular ischemia may not develop until the second trimester, with bowel dilatation progressing only later in gestation. Conversely, proximal obstructions from duodenal atresia may be easily identified in the early second trimester.

Polyhydramnios can develop with bowel obstruction, but its presence is variable and its absence should not exclude the

| Table 18.1-1 | Etiology of Dilated Bowel |
| --- | --- |

Esophagus
  Esophageal atresia
Small bowel
  Jejunal atresia
  Ilial atresia
  Meconium ileus
  Enteric duplication
  Congenital diarrhea
  Hirschsprung disease
Large bowel
  Hirschsprung disease
  Anorectal atresia
Pitfalls
  Hydroureter
  Normal bowel/meconium

| Table 18.1-2 | Abnormalities Associated with Atresias | |
| --- | --- | --- |
| **Abnormality** | **Prenatal Findings** | **Associated Abnormalities** |
| Esophageal atresia/TEF | Absent or small stomach Polyhydramnios | VACTERL |
| Duodenal atresia | Double bubble | Tri 21 |
| Jejunal atresia | Dilated small bowel | Isolated |
| Meconium ileus | Hyperechoic bowel | Cystic fibrosis |
| Anal atresia | Rarely dilated colon | VACTERL |

diagnosis. Esophageal atresias may present with early polyhydramnios, but if a tracheoesophageal fistula (TEF) accompanies the atresia, the presence of a fluid-filled stomach and normal amniotic fluid can result in a missed diagnosis prenatally. Proximal duodenal obstructions may only develop polyhydramnios in 50% of cases owing to the absorption of fluid within the dilated stomach and duodenum. It is common for more distal small and large bowel obstructions to have normal amniotic fluid volumes.[26]

The following sections will discuss the major bowel disorders that can be identified by US. MRI has become a useful adjunct in helping assess meconium location and further defining pathology. Accurate diagnosis allows for improved counseling, appropriate delivery planning, and delivery planning, and postnatal care.[27–30]

## Proximal Gastrointestinal Disorders

### Esophageal Atresia
**Incidence:** Esophageal atresia with or without TEF occurs in 1 in 2,500 to 4,000 live births. Males are slightly more affected than females.[31]

**Embryology and Pathology:** Tracheoesophageal anomalies are the result of incomplete division of the foregut into the ventral respiratory portion and dorsal digestive portion by the tracheoesophageal septum. At the 4th week of gestation, the growth of the ectodermal ridge is interrupted, resulting in a TEF.

There are five types of tracheoesophageal anomalies (see Fig. 17.3-4 in previous chapter):

Type A: Esophageal atresia with a TEF to the distal esophageal segment (>75%)
Type B: Esophageal atresia without TEF (10% to 15%)
Type C: H-type TEF with no esophageal atresia (5%)
Type D: Esophageal atresia with TEF to both the proximal and the distal esophageal segments (<5%)
Type E: Esophageal atresia with a TEF to the proximal esophageal segment (<5%)

**Diagnosis**
*Ultrasound:* Esophageal atresia, with or without a distal fistula, can be difficult to diagnose prenatally with sonographic detection rate for esophageal obstruction ranging from 24% to 30%.[15,32–36] When a TEF is present, the sensitivity of US in prospectively making the diagnosis drops to 12%. Diagnosis relies on indirect sonographic findings including polyhydramnios and a persistently small or absent stomach but can result in a false-positive rate as high as 27%[34] (Fig. 18.1-5).

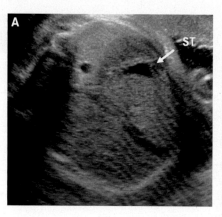

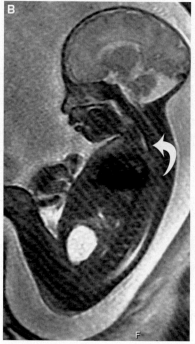

**FIGURE 18.1-5:** Tracheoesophageal fistula in a 32-week-gestation fetus with two-vessel cord. **A:** Axial US demonstrates a small stomach *(arrow)*. Polyhydramnios was present. **B:** Sagittal T2w MRI demonstrates a small amount of fluid in the proximal esophageal pouch *(arrow)*. Following delivery, an esophageal atresia with distal TEF was diagnosed.

Associated anomalies suggesting VACTERL association (vertebral, renal, radial ray, cardiac, two-vessel cord) may help in suspecting this diagnosis prenatally.[35]

Type A isolated esophageal atresias are the most likely to be diagnosed prenatally by US. If there is failure to visualize the fetal stomach over several hours, the diagnosis of esophageal atresia should be considered, particularly in the presence of polyhydramnios. At times, a dilated proximal esophageal pouch may be noted in the neck or upper mediastinum.[36–45]

The high false-negative rate of identifying a TEF is due to the fact that the amniotic fluid from the proximal pouch can pass into the stomach through the tracheo-fistula with a resultant fluid-filled stomach present. Polyhydramnios develops in only one-third of these cases. The proximal pouch is more likely to be missed because of intermittent filling and emptying.[37,39]

If the stomach is small, TEF should be considered, particularly if polyhydramnios is also present. If there is marked polyhydramnios with a visualized stomach, and no additional findings, the diagnosis of TEF should be considered in the differential.

The presence of vertebral, cardiac, renal, limb anomalies, or two-vessel cord is suggestive of VACTERL. Up to 60% of individuals with VACTERL association have either esophageal atresia or TEF.[43] Thus, in cases with one or two of the above findings, careful evaluation for possible TEF should be performed. The presence of polyhydramnios and small stomach in addition to a two-vessel cord is highly suggestive of a TEF and should be counseled appropriately.[35]

*MRI:* MRI can be a useful adjunct in the prenatal diagnosis of esophageal atresia. Dilated proximal esophageal pouches have been identified by MRI.[19,21,46] However, this finding may be transient by both US and MR, and the esophagus can be collapsed throughout each study.

MRI is also useful in the identification of associated VACTERL anomalies such as pulmonary atresia, vertebral anomalies, and at times anal atresia (see later).

**Differential Diagnosis:** The absence of a fluid-filled stomach by US or MRI can be due to multiple etiologies. A repeat scan should be performed to confirm that the stomach has not simply emptied during the study.

If no normal stomach is identified, differential includes displacement of the stomach into the chest, or heterotaxy. Oligohydramnios is the most common cause of an empty stomach, and microgastria is the least common.

Oral and neck masses occluding the pharynx may result in a small or empty stomach. Sonographic observation of swallowing and muscular activity may help exclude a neuromuscular etiology.

**Associated Findings:** Up to 50% of patients with esophageal atresia have other anomalies. Cardiac malformations are the most common (25%) and result in the highest morbidity and mortality.[47] Additional anomalies include gastrointestinal (28%), genitourinary (13%), musculoskeletal (11%), CNS (7%), and facial anomalies (6%).[48]

Gastrointestinal anomalies include malrotation, anorectal atresia, duodenal atresia, and annular pancreas.[48] In Down syndrome, the combination of esophageal and duodenal atresia has been reported.[49–53]

The VACTERL association typically presents with several anomalies, including TEF (see section on VACTERL in Chapter 20).[54]

The risk of aneuploidy includes trisomy 18 and 21. Prenatal series report a wide incidence of aneuplody ranging from 6% to 44%.[32,35,41] In a large postnatal series, however, chromosomal abnormalities were reported to be 5% of cases.[51]

**Management:** If the diagnosis of TEF is suspected, serial USs may be needed to confirm the diagnosis. Careful assessment of potential associated anomalies should be performed, including echocardiography. Karyotype should be performed because of the risk of chromosomal abnormalities, including trisomy 21 and 18.[35]

Polyhydramnios develops in up to 60% of cases of esophageal atresia/TEF, typically in the third trimester.[32] Thus, follow-up studies to assess amniotic fluid volume are important because of the added risk of preterm labor with polyhydramnios. Bed rest, tocolytic agents, and reduction amniocenteses may be required. Betamethasone can be administered to increase fetal lung maturity if preterm labor develops.

Delivery should be planned at a center that has appropriate neonatal support. Caesarian section should be reserved for obstetric indications. If the esophageal atresia is confirmed postnatally, the infant should be transferred to a tertiary care center. Intravenous fluid should be administered. A sump tube should be placed in the proximal esophageal pouch to prevent aspiration.

Abdominal radiographs will demonstrate absent air in the bowel with esophageal atresia and associated spine anomalies. If there is a TEF, air typically will course into the stomach with normal appearing distal bowel.

Surgery is performed depending on the gestational age, birth weight, and presence of other anomalies. A decision is made as to whether a primary repair or a staged repair is to be executed. If the gap is long between the proximal and the distal pouch, a gastrostomy tube is placed for a staged repair. Growth of the two pouches typically occurs over several weeks and often results in successful reconstruction at 10 to 12 weeks' gestation.

**Prognosis:** It is unclear whether the prenatal diagnosis of esophageal atresia/TEF actually improves the prognosis. Early diagnosis allows for appropriate counseling, screening for associated anomalies, and planned delivery at an appropriate center. Immediate supportive management may decrease the risk of aspiration.

Increased perinatal loss rates have been noted in several series because of the high incidence (60%) of associated anomalies.[41,49,51]

The overall prognosis depends on associated anomalies, gestational age, and respiratory complications. When there are no severe cardiac anomalies or chromosomal anomalies, survival is reported to be greater than 95% in infants over 2.5 kg.[54] Infants may require mechanical ventilation, and prolonged hospital stays due to gastrointestinal issues. Short- and long-term follow-up is required after tracheoesophageal repair is performed to monitor possible complications such as leakage at the anastomosis or the development of esophageal strictures and gastrointestinal reflux.

### Hiatal Hernia
**Incidence:** Rare in the prenatal and newborn period.

**Pathology/Embryology:** The gastroesophageal junction slides above the diaphragm through the esophageal hiatus.

**Diagnosis:** A dilated esophagus may be seen in the chest prenatally by both US and MRI.[55–59] The stomach may be small.[60,61] (Fig. 18.1-6).

**Differential Diagnosis:** Esophageal atresia may present with a dilated proximal esophageal pouch and small stomach mimicking a hiatal hernia. Esophageal duplication cyst could be considered in the differential. Hiatal hernia could be mistaken for a congenital diaphragmatic hernia.[62]

**Associated Anomalies:** Hiatal hernias have been associated with heterotaxy and Marfan syndrome.

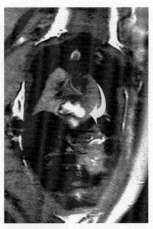

**FIGURE 18.1-6:** Hiatal hernia. Coronal T2w MR image demonstrates a fluid-filled structure above the diaphragm *(curved arrow)* with a small infradiaphragmatic stomach consistent with a hiatal hernia.

**Prognosis and Management:** Isolated hiatal hernias typically have a good prognosis following surgical repair. There is a report of two giant hiatal hernias with associated anomalies having poor outcomes following delivery.[63]

**Recurrence Risk:** Familial cases have be reported rarely.[64]

### Duodenal Atresia/Obstruction
**Incidence:** Duodenal atresia or stenosis is the most common type of intestinal atresia detected in the fetus occurring in 1 in 10,000 live births.[27] Atresia is more common than stenosis occurring in up to 75% of cases.[65] Approximately 30% of infants with duodenal atresia have trisomy 21.

**Embryology/Pathology:** The most common type of obstruction detected in the fetus is duodenal atresia or stenosis, thought to result from a failure of recanalization of the bowel at 8 to 10 weeks' gestation. The blockage may be associated with an annular pancreas.

There are three types of duodenal atresia:

Type 1—Membranous mucosal atresia with an intact muscular wall (most common 69%)
Type 2—Short fibrous cord connecting two ends of the atretic duodenum
Type 3—Complete separation of the two ends associated with biliary tract anomalies[65,66]

Duodenal atresia can be associated with annular pancreas either by extrinsic compression or more commonly complete intrinsic atresia. The remaining 25% of cases are stenosis.

More than half of fetuses with duodenal atresia have associated anomalies. Trisomy 21 is the most frequent, occurring in up to 30% of cases. Increased incidence of duodenal atresia has been reported with gestational and preexisting diabetes, VACTERL association, and malrotation.[67,68]

**Diagnosis**
*Ultrasound.* Sonographic findings suggestive of duodenal atresia include a dilated fluid-filled stomach and proximal duodenum (fetal "double bubble"). The two structures should be contiguous to confirm the diagnosis (Fig. 18.1-7).[69–71] A dilated duodenum that persists is abnormal. Prior to 24 weeks, the duodenum

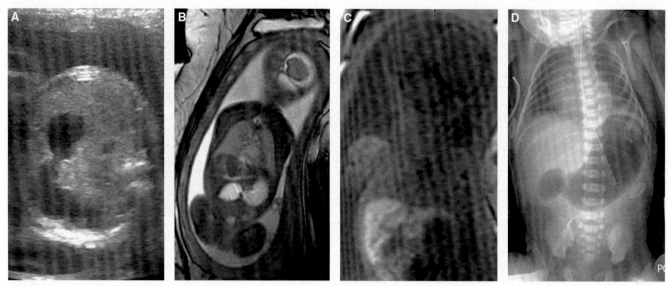

**FIGURE 18.1-7:** Duodenal atresia. **A:** Axial US demonstrates a fluid-filled double bubble at 28-week GA. **B,C:** T2w and T1w MR images, respectively, confirm the presence of a fluid-filled double bubble. **D:** Postnatal radiograph confirms the presence of an air-filled double bubble.

may not be sufficiently dilated to make the diagnosis.[72-74] There are reports of the diagnosis being made in the first trimester.[75] The diagnosis can be made in the early second trimester but is more commonly is made in the third trimester when the duodenum becomes more dilated.[73,74] Polyhydramnios may develop in up to 50% of cases.[69]

In cases of duodenal stenosis or associated esophageal atresia, the diagnosis can be missed prenatally if the duodenum does not become sufficiently dilated to recognize.[76] At times, the stomach becomes extremely dilated, and the duodenal bulb may be difficult to visualize, resulting in a missed diagnosis.[77]

As 30% of fetuses with duodenal atresia have trisomy 21, other sonographic features of Down syndrome need to be searched for.[72,78,79] Anomalies associated with trisomy 21 include small or absent nose, nuchal fold thickening, hypoplastic middle phalanx of the fifth digit, short humerus and femur, echogenic bowel, mild ventriculomegaly, mild pyelectasis, and cardiac anomalies such as AV canal and ventriculoseptal defects (see section on trisomy 21 in Chapter 20).

Duodenal atresia and stenosis can be part of the VACTERL association. In these cases, hemivertebra, radial ray, and renal anomalies may be identified.[79] When a TEF and duodenal atresia are present together, a markedly dilated stomach may develop. If esophageal atresia and duodenal atresia are present together, the stomach may be small with a collapsed duodenum, making the diagnosis difficult to confirm prenatally.[49,50,53,79]

*MRI:* MRI can be used as an adjunct in the diagnosis of duodenal atresias. On T2w, the fluid-filled dilated stomach and duodenum will be of high signal with decompressed bowel loops distally (see Fig. 18.1-7B). The distal normal size small bowel loops of fluid signal and normal size colon and rectum filled with meconium should be easily visualized. Thus, multiple intestinal atresias which may mimic duodenal obstruction can be excluded by MRI if normal distal bowel is identified. The dilated duodenum is easily differentiated from adjacent gallbladder, and duplication cysts by MRI.[18]

Associated anomalies in the brain, spine, limbs, lung, and anal atresia may be confirmed and further evaluated by MRI.[80]

**Differential Diagnosis:** The differential diagnosis includes annular pancreas, malrotation with Ladd's bands, duplication cysts, preduodenal portal vein, and choledochal cyst.[76] Documenting that the fluid-filled structure is contiguous with the stomach can help differentiate duodenal atresia/stenosis from a duplication or choledochal cyst.[81,82]

**Associated Anomalies:** Duodenal atresia is an isolated finding in one-third to one-half of cases. However, it is often associated with other malformations, including cardiac, gastrointestinal (biliary atresia, agenesis of the gall bladder), renal, and vertebral anomalies.[72,78,79]

Thirty percent of newborns with duodenal atresia or stenosis have Down syndrome. Conversely, approximately 2.5% of patients with Down syndrome have duodenal atresia or stenosis.[72]

**Prenatal Management:** If the diagnosis of duodenal atresia or stenosis is suspected, serial USs may be needed to confirm the diagnosis. As 30% of fetuses with duodenal atresia have trisomy 21 and 20% to 30% have congenital heart disease, fetal karyotype analysis and detailed fetal survey, including fetal echocardiography, are indicated.[83]

Amniotic fluid digestion enzyme assays, including gamma glutamyl transpeptidase (GGTP), aminopeptidase (AMP), total alkaline phosphatase (ALP), and intestinal form (iALP) and total protein have been evaluated. Muller et al. correlated elevations of GGTP and iALP with duodenal and small bowel atresias. For duodenal atresia, sensitivity was reported to be 71% with a 100% specificity, while distal bowel sensitivity was 69% and 83% specific.[20,84] Normal values in amniotic fluid do not exclude the diagnosis of obstructions.

As duodenal atresia can be complicated by polyhydramnios in up to 50% of cases[69,83] follow-up sonograms are useful to track amniotic fluid volume. Polyhydramnios can result in preterm labor, so close monitoring is useful. Prenatal pediatric surgical consultation with parents can be helpful in alleviating anxiety and planning postnatal care.

The fetus will usually not need delivery at a high-risk center, and can be safely transported after birth to a pediatric center after enteric tube decompression of the intestinal tract to prevent aspiration of gastric contents. Intravenous fluid should be administered to replace volume with attention to electrolyte imbalance.

Abdominal radiographs will demonstrate the typical air-filled "double bubble" with absent gas distally (see Fig. 18.1-7D). If there is a stenosis or the biliary tree bridges the atresia, air may be traversed distally into the small bowel. A postnatal double bubble radiographic appearance may also be seen in the setting of malrotation of the midgut with or without associated volvulus.

Surgery is typically performed on the day of the delivery after assessment of other associated anomalies, and volume resuscitation and electrolyte imbalances are corrected.

**Prognosis/Outcome:** Several series suggest that prenatal diagnosis does reduce morbidity and shortens hospitalization.[85–87] Survival has improved over the past two decades, with a 95% survival reported.[76,78,88,89] Outcome now is more related to associated anomalies, particularly cardiac defects.[83] Late complications include dysmotility of the proximal duodenum resulting in reflux, gastritis, pancreatitis, and/or cholecystitis.[89]

### Jejunal and Ileal Atresia

**Incidence:** The incidence of small bowel atresia is 1 per 1,500 to 5,000 births.[29,90] Atresias can occur anywhere in the small bowel but most commonly present in the proximal jejunal (30%) and distal ileum (35%) with multiple atresias are found in up to 6% of cases.[28,91]

**Embryology/Pathology:** Jejunal and ileal atresia are a complete obstruction of the bowel lumen and are more common than small bowel stenosis. Small bowel atresias are thought to be caused by vascular ischemia in the second trimester with the ischemic necrosis leading to resorption of the segment or fibrous scarring.[92–94]

Type 1—32%; lumen is obstructed by an intact diaphragm or membrane made of mucosa and submucosa. The muscularis and serosa are intact with continuity of the proximal and distal segments. If the membrane stretches, it takes the shape of a windsock.

Type 2—25%; fibrotic cord connecting two blind-ending bowel segments

Type 3

3a—15%; complete separation of blind-ending loops

3b—11%; mesenteric defect with large gap in small bowel mesentery. The distal small bowel is short and coiled like an apple peel. Terminal ileum is perfused from a single ileocolic artery (can be familial)

Type 4—6%; multiple atresias[95,96]

Lesions can range from a focal atresia to complete atresia of the entire herniated bowel possibly related to constriction/volvulus.[97] In these cases, the necrotic bowel is resorbed with the abdominal wall defect closing as the herniated bowel involutes. The prognosis is poor because of loss of most of the small bowel. Placental vascular abnormalities have also been associated with small bowel atresias.[93] Atresias have been reproduced in experimental animals by ligation of mesenteric blood vessels.[98] Maternal use of vasoconstrictive medications may contribute to interruption of mesenteric blood flow.[99] Inherited thrombophilia leading to spontaneous thrombosis may play a role in some cases.[100]

Gastroschisis have been associated with bowel atresia because of ischemic injury from bowel kinking.[101–104]

The incidence of small bowel atresia secondary to meconium ileus is reported to be 10% of cases. The incidence of associated aneuploidy and extraintestinal anomalies is low.

### Diagnosis

*Ultrasound:* Obstruction of the fetal bowel may be sonographically diagnosed when dilated bowel loops are detected proximal to a point of obstruction. Hyperperistalsis of the proximal bowel may be observed. The diagnosis of obstruction before 18 weeks' gestation is rare and may be difficult to diagnose before 24 weeks' gestation. Bowel loops become progressively more dilated with vigorous peristalsis in the third trimester.

The presence of dilated loops (>15 mm in length and 7 mm in diameter) and/or mural thickness of greater than 3 mm is most suggestive of fetal bowel obstruction.[4,105,106] The abdomen can be distended with asymmetric increase in the abdominal circumference. A proximal or jejunal atresia may show a sonographic fetal "triple bubble" representing the dilated stomach, duodenum, and proximal jejunum (Figs. 18.1-8A and 18.1-9A). The jejunum's capacity to dilate is greater than that of the ileum, and is therefore less likely to be associated with the complications of perforation, such as meconium peritonitis and meconium pseudocyst. Multiple dilated loops of bowel are more suggestive of a distal obstruction such as an ileal atresia. If meconium ileus is present, increased bowel echogenicity may be noted.

Bowel distal to the level of obstruction is difficult to assess by US. Thus, differentiating an isolated atresia from multiple atresias is difficult sonographically.[16,107]

While proximal gastrointestinal obstruction can lead to polyhydramnios, increased amniotic fluid is seen in fewer than 50% of cases with jejunal obstruction and rarely with more distal obstructions.[108,109] Iacobelli et al.[26] suggested that polyhydramnios and dilated bowel loops are markers of more severe obstruction with a longer predicted length of stay when present.

Other clues to sonographic diagnosis include ascites and echogenic bowel.[18] A perforation at the site of ischemia may result in leakage of fluid and meconium. This can result in ascites and meconium peritonitis. Loculated collections of fluid and debris may develop, which calcify, developing into meconium pseudocysts (Fig. 18.1-10). Scattered peritoneal calcifications with posterior acoustical shadowing may be noted[110,111] (Fig. 18.1-11).

US has limitations in the assessment of bowel anomalies. Maternal obesity, overlying gas, and maternal pelvic bones may obscure imaging of the fetus. Expertise of the sonographer is important in the assessment of more complex anomalies. At times, it may be difficult to differentiate dilated small bowel loops from colon or megaureters sonographically. US lacks the specificity to identify the number and location of obstructions, and is limited in assessing the viability of unobstructed distal bowel.

A multicenter retrospective sonographic study from Europe in an unselected study showed an overall detection rate of bowel atresia of 34%, with 40% of those detected at less than 4 weeks gestation.[15,16,107]

*MRI:* MRI has been used as an adjunct in the characterization of bowel obstruction, including the level of obstruction.[9,19,20,22,23,112–117] In a series by Veyrac et al.,[18] MRI provided more accurate findings than US in the assessment of small bowel atresias.

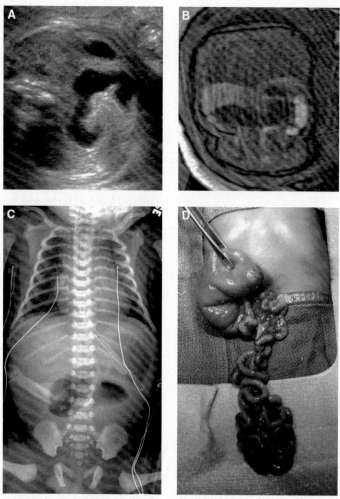

**FIGURE 18.1-8:** Jejunal atresia with fluid-filled dilated jejunal loops. **A:** Axial US image demonstrates a fluid-filled dilated loop of bowel. **B:** Coronal T1w MR image demonstrates a dilated fluid-filled loop of bowel containing no high-signal meconium. **C:** Postnatal radiograph demonstrates air in the stomach and proximal jejunum. **D:** Surgical image of jejunal atresia.

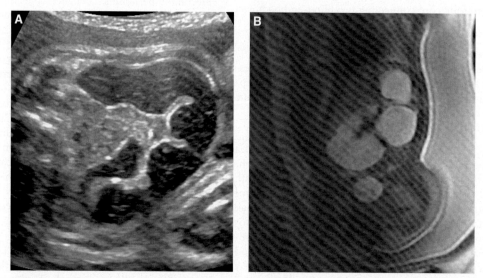

**FIGURE 18.1-9:** Jejunal atresia with meconium-filled dilated jejunal loops. **A:** Axial US image demonstrates a dilated loop of bowel filled with echogenic material. **B:** Coronal T1w MR image demonstrates dilated high-signal meconium-filled loops of small bowel. At surgery, jejunal atresia was confirmed.

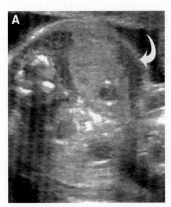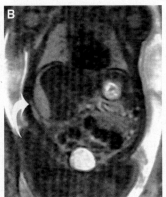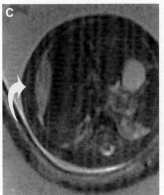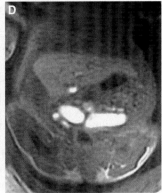

**FIGURE 18.1-10:** Ileal atresia with meconium peritonitis. **A:** Axial US image demonstrates dilated bowel loops, echogenic bowel, and fluid adjacent to the liver *(arrow)* at 32 weeks' gestation. **B,C:** Coronal and axial T2w MR images, respectively, demonstrate a perihepatic collection of fluid consistent with a loculated meconium pseudocyst *(arrow)*. Dilated low-signal bowel loops are present as well. **D:** Coronal T1w images demonstrate high-signal meconium-filled small dilated bowel.

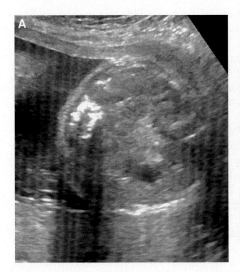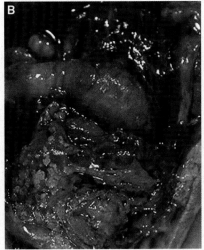

**FIGURE 18.1-11:** Meconium peritonitis. **A:** Axial US at 26 weeks of gestation demonstrates echogenic foci with posterior acoustical shadowing in the anterior abdomen. **B:** Surgical image of a different patient with meconium scattered within the peritoneum.

Bowel loops proximal to the obstruction are dilated (13 to 30 mm). The signal characteristics are variable, depending on the gestational age and location of obstruction. The bowel can be fluid-filled high-signal T2w or meconium-filled high-signal T1w or intermediate in signal (see Figs. 18.1-8 and 18.1-9). Distally, the rectum may contain less meconium and thus decreased in size (2 to 7 mm).[18,23]

The level of obstruction can be suggested by the number of dilated loops as well as nondilated loops proximal to the dilated loops. Assessment of bowel distal to the obstruction is possible as well. The absence of loops distal to the level of obstruction may suggest multiple atresias.[18] Shinmoto and Kuribayashi[115] described dilated loops with two different signals in a case with two levels of atresia. As it takes time for meconium to course into the colon, the presence of T1 high signal in a dilated loop of bowel is not specific for a distal ileal or colonic occlusion (see Fig. 18.1-9). In a series by Colombani et al.,[24] of 11 patients between 23 and 35 weeks' gestation with T1 high signal in dilated bowel, 9 had proximal jejunal atresia (5 with short bowel syndrome), and 2 had meconium ileus at delivery.

**Differential Diagnosis:** The differential for dilated tubular loops within the abdomen includes jejunal or ileal atresia, total colonic aganglionosis, malrotation with volvulus, meconium ileus, and meconium peritonitis. Rarer entities to consider include megacystis–microcolon–intestinal hypoperistasis syndrome, and fetal diarrhea. At times, hydronephrosis duplication cysts and abdominal mesenteric cysts can mimic dilated bowel loops.

**Associated Anomalies:** Other gastrointestinal anomalies can be present in up to 45%. These include malrotation (23%), microcolon (3%), duplication cysts (3%), esophageal atresia (3%), and meconium peritonitis 8%.[118] Some fetuses may have associated chromosomal anomalies, or an underlying syndrome coexisting with multiple other anomalies.

**Management:** Once the diagnosis of small bowel atresia is made, a complete anatomic survey should be performed. If echogenic bowel is present, amniocentesis for fetal karyotype and cystic fibrosis DNA mutation analysis should be performed. As congenital infections have also been associated with echogenic bowel, a close evaluation for additional anomalies as well as TORCH titers may be useful.

Polyhydramnios rarely develops with small bowel atresias, so follow-up sonograms once the diagnosis is confirmed can be spread apart. Amniotic fluid digestion enzymes assays including GGTP, AMP, ALP, and iALP, and total protein have been evaluated, though sensitivity of 69% and specificity of 83% specific limit its usefulness in distal obstructions.[20,84]

Prenatal pediatric surgical consultation with parents is helpful in alleviating anxiety and planning delivery and postnatal care. If meconium peritonitis is present without bowel obstruction, the outcome is typically favorable and may not require surgery. Large meconium pseudocysts with or without associated bowel atresias, however, require surgery.[17,,27,110,119,120]

Delivery of fetuses with bowel obstruction can be at term and vaginal. Delivery should be planned at a center with appropriate neonatal support. Postnatal management of small bowel atresias includes gastric decompression and intravenous fluid to correct fluid and electrolyte imbalances.

Radiographs will document dilated small bowel loops. A water-soluble contrast enema is useful in the assessment of colonic size. If the colon is normal in caliber, a more proximal jejunal atresia is likely present. If microcolon is present, a diagnosis of ileal atresia or meconium ileus should be considered. If the obstruction is secondary to meconium ileus, sequential enemas may help to relieve the obstruction by breaking up the inspissated meconium.

**Prognosis/Outcome:** Surgery is performed after associated anomalies are excluded and the infant is adequately resuscitated. The proximal dilated bowel is typically resected to prevent functional obstruction at the anastomosis.[121] This dilated loop may have poor motility and can develop blind loop syndrome. Short bowel syndrome can occur in cases of multiple atresias or with the apple peel deformity.

In proximal atresias, enteral feedings can begin quickly. More distal atresias may require longer periods of rest until normal gut activity returns.

Long-term outcome is typically excellent with survival of 95%. Most of the mortality occurs in infants with medical conditions such as prematurity, respiratory distress syndrome, associated anomalies, cystic fibrosis, or short gut syndrome. Late complications include recurrent obstruction from strictures, adhesions, and liver abnormalities from prolonged TPN.[122]

**Recurrence Risk:** Most small bowel atresias are sporadic. However, with Type IIIB atresias, apple peel deformity, short bowel, and retrograde perfusion of the distal ileum, there is an 18% recurrence risk, suggesting a genetic component.[123] Type IV also has been described as recurring in families. Hereditary multiple atresias have be noted.[124]

### Meconium Ileus/Cystic Fibrosis

Meconium ileus should always be included in the differential when small bowel obstruction is identified. In these cases, obstruction of the terminal ileum occurs from impacted thick meconium. Perforation with secondary ileal atresia and meconium peritonitis may develop.

**Incidence:** Cystic fibrosis is one of the most common autosomal recessive disorders in the United States. About 1:3,000 newborns have the disease. Up to 15% of fetuses with cystic fibrosis are present with meconium ileus.[125,126] Up to 50% of these cases will be complicated with an atresia, volvulus, perforation, and/ or meconium pseudocysts.

CF is rare in African American and Asian populations.

**Embryology and Pathology:** The fetus with cystic fibrosis may present prenatally with a distal small bowel obstruction due to meconium ileus. The obstruction of the terminal ileum is from the thick viscous meconium that occurs in the fetus and neonate with cystic fibrosis. A microcolon will be present because of the lack of passage of the meconium into the colon.

### Diagnosis

*Ultrasound:* Cystic fibrosis is diagnosed in approximately 3% to 9.9% of fetuses with echogenic bowel.[127–129] Echogenic bowel associated with bowel dilatation is suspicious for meconium ileus (Fig. 18.1-12). There is a high incidence of complications (up to 50%), including small bowel atresia and volvulus.

Perforation in cases of meconium ileus or small bowel atresia can result in leakage of meconium and fluid, with ascites, meconium peritonitis, and occasionally a meconium pseudocyst formation (see Fig. 18.1-11).[130–132] Sonogram may demonstrate scattered calcifications in the fetal abdomen and along the liver margin.

Lack of visualization of the fetal gallbladder may be another clue to the diagnosis.[125,133]

*MRI:* MRI may be useful as an adjunct in the demonstration of meconium distribution. In a series by Carcopino et al.,[116] two cases of meconium ileus were noted to have unusual hyperintense T1 and intermediate T2 signal of the dilated bowel loops.

Meconium peritonitis can be diagnosed by the demonstration of extraluminal fluid collections scattered through the abdomen. MR can more easily distinguish meconium cysts from adjacent bowel because of different signal characteristics (see Fig. 18.1-10). Peritoneal calcifications, however, may be more easily noted by US.[18,130–132]

**Differential Diagnosis:** Prenatal differentiation between distal ileal atresia and meconium ileus may not be possible, because both have a meconium-filled dilated distal ileum and a microcolon.[9]

Echogenic bowel is nonspecific and may also be seen with bleeding in the amniotic cavity, aneuploidy, fetal growth restriction, infection, gastrointestinal obstruction, and biliary atresia.[134–140] Although associated with a higher rate of fetal loss, the majority of neonates with echogenic bowel are normal at delivery. Echogenic bowel is diagnosed in 0.2% to 1.4% of second trimester studies.[141] The diagnosis of fetal echogenic bowel can be made by comparing the echogenicity with adjacent bone or liver (Fig. 18.1-13). Bowel that is as echogenic as adjacent bone has been proposed as an objective marker to decrease the subjectivity of assessing echogenic bowel, particularly when using higher-frequency linear transducers.[135,141]

A rare cause of dilated bowel includes megacystis–microcolon–intestinal hypoperistalsis syndrome.[142]

**Associated Anomalies:** Fetuses with meconium ileus have cystic fibrosis. Long-term complications include pulmonary, pancreatic, and bowel sequelae.

**Prognosis and Management:** If cystic fibrosis is suspected, a sweat chloride test or cystic fibrosis DNA mutation analysis should be performed after delivery if not prenatally.[125,129,137,139]

Polyhydramnios rarely develops with small bowel atresias, so follow-up sonograms once the diagnosis is confirmed can be

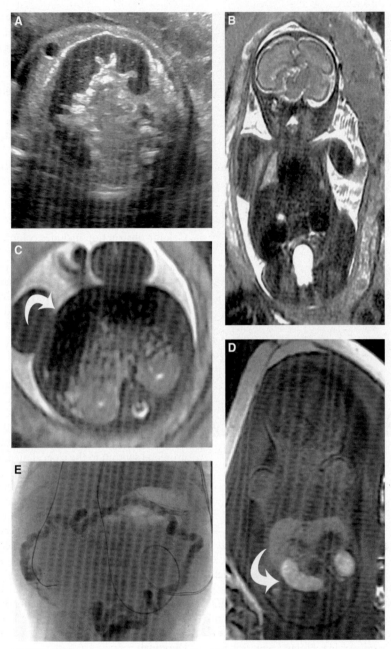

**FIGURE 18.1-12:** Meconium ileus. **A:** US axial image at 28 weeks of gestation demonstrates echogenic bowel with a dilated loop anteriorly. **B,C:** Coronal and axial T2w MR images, respectively, demonstrate that the dilated loop contains low-signal meconium (*arrow*). **D:** T1w Coronal confirms the dilated bowel loop contains meconium (*arrow*), with no meconium in the rectosigmoid. **E:** Enema following delivery demonstrates microcolon. Infant was diagnosed with cystic fibrosis following delivery.

spread apart. Prenatal pediatric surgical consultation with parents is helpful in alleviating anxiety and planning delivery and postnatal care.

Delivery of fetuses with meconium ileus can be at term and vaginal. Delivery should be planned at a center with appropriate neonatal support. Postnatal management of small bowel atresias includes gastric decompression and intravenous fluid to correct fluid and electrolyte imbalances. Radiographs will document dilated small bowel loops. A water-soluble contrast enema is performed in an attempt to unblock the inspissated

meconium. Sequential enemas may be required to relieve the obstruction. If unsuccessful, the infant may require surgery to relieve the obstruction which may be the result of a stenosis/atresia.[143]

**Recurrence Risk:** Cystic fibrosis is autosomal recessive with a 25% risk of recurrence.

Preimplantation genetic diagnosis and DNA prenatal diagnosis are available for future pregnancies if cystic fibrosis is indeed documented.[128,143]

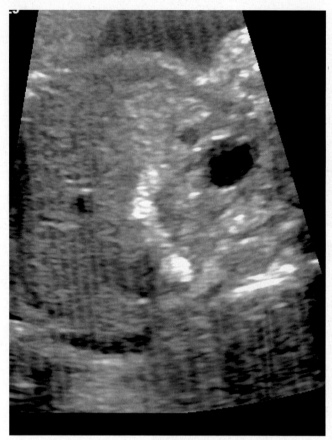

**FIGURE 18.1-13:** Echogenic bowel. Coronal US demonstrates echogenic bowel at 25 weeks of gestation. The fetus died a few days later.

*Congenital Diarrhea*
**Incidence:** Rare case reports in the literature.[144–147]

**Pathology:** Congenital diarrhea is a rare disorder in which the infant has watery diarrhea for which no infectious agent is identified in at least three stool samples, lasting 2 weeks in an infant under 3 months of age. Chloride diarrhea is a rare form caused by an autosomal recessive gene, with a few hundred cases reported primarily in Saudi Arabia, Finland, and Poland. The chloride bicarbonate channels are abnormal with resultant hypochloremia and hypokalemia. Sodium diarrhea is also recessive and causes metabolic disturbances because of sodium loss. Over 30 genetic mutations have been identified, including SCL26A3 on chromosome 7.[144]

**Diagnosis:** Assessment of amniotic fluid reveals normal cytogenetic and microbiologic results. Chloride or sodium levels can be elevated.

*Ultrasound:* Moderate generalized bowel dilatation and polyhydramnios between 24 and 32 weeks' gestation.[144–147]

*MRI:* MRI can play an important role in the diagnosis of this prenatally. In a series of four cases, all four were correctly diagnosed prospectively with MRI.[145] High-signal intraluminal fluid is seen throughout the small and large bowel. In addition, there is absence of T1w meconium in the colon.

**Management:** Close prenatal follow-up is required owing to the potential development of polyhydramnios and risk of premature delivery. Following delivery, aggressive fluid replacement is required. Colostomy may be required.

**Outcome:** Serious fluid loss and electrolyte disorders can be lethal if not properly managed.

The prognosis for sodium diarrhea appears worse than chloride diarrhea with a higher death rate.

**Recurrence Risk:** Autosomal recessive disorders with frequency higher in some countries than others.

## Large Bowel Abnormalities

Colonic obstruction includes colonic atresias, anorectal malformations, and Hirschsprung disease. The presence of anal and colonic obstruction is often missed prenatally. This is due to the fact that fluid is resorbed in the small bowel and colonic loops. Thus, small bowel and colon typically remain normal in caliber despite a distal obstruction. Each diagnosis has its own etiology and outcome, with diagnosis usually only made following delivery.

*Imperforate Anus*
**Incidence:** Anorectal malformations affect 1 in 5,000 live births and range from isolated imperforate anus to persistent cloaca.

**Embryology/Pathology:** Abnormalities of the rectum and anus are thought to be due to an arrest of the caudal descent of the urorectal septum to the cloacal membrane.[148] By 6 weeks' gestation, the cloacal membrane divides into the anterior urogenital sinus and posterior anorectum by the urorectal septum. Fusion of the hindgut mesoderm with the ectoderm occurs at the dentate line. Failure of Rathke folds to develop arrests the inferior urorectal septum, resulting in a rectourethral fistula in males and cloaca in females. Isolated imperforate anus without fistula occurs from failure of the anal pit to form.

Bourdelat studied sphincter development in the fetus by US and noted slow growth from 14 to 19 weeks. There was rapid growth from 19 to 30 weeks. After 30 weeks, contractions were noted with no further growth.[14]

**Diagnosis**
*Ultrasound:* Anorectal malformations are often missed prenatally because fluid is resorbed in the small bowel and colonic loops typically remain normal in caliber.[149–151] Polyhydramnios is rare and, when present, suggest a more proximal obstruction. Perforation with ascites and meconium peritonitis are rare as well.

Transient bowel dilatation and a dilated distal colon are potential prenatal findings.[150,152,153] Colonic dilatation has been described in fetuses greater than 26 weeks' gestation and may have a V- or U-shaped configuration.[150,154] Transiently dilated rectum supportive of the diagnosis has been described at 12 to 13 weeks with a transvaginal scan, and at 16 weeks with transabdominal images.[3,152,153,155]

Vesicorectal fistulas are associated with anorectal malformations. In these cases, urine mixes with meconium and intraluminal calcifications (enterolithiasis) develop. The presence of enterolithiasis can be seen by US as punctuate foci of echogenicity in the rectum mixed with fluid.[156–159] The entire colon

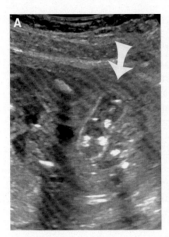
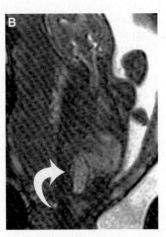

**FIGURE 18.1-14:** Anal atresia with vesicourethral fistula. **A:** Coronal US at 20 weeks of gestation demonstrates dilated rectosigmoid filled with fluid and calcifications—enteroliths *(arrow)*. Two-vessel cord was present. **B:** Coronal T2w MRI confirms fluid-filled rectosigmoid *(arrow)*, enteroliths not as well visualized. Infant was found to have a vesicourethral fistula at delivery and diagnosed with VACTERL sequence.

may become fluid filled and can be mistaken for a dilated small bowel loop[8] (Fig. 18.1-14).

Prenatal diagnosis of anal atresia may increase in the future with careful analysis of the fetal anus with high-resolution sonographic scanning. The rectum can be seen in the normal fetus posterior to the bladder as a hypoechogenic structure with lack of visualization highly suggestive of anal atresia[160–163] (Fig. 18.1-15). Reference values for the in utero development of the fetal anal sphincter are available.[161] Three-dimensional US can further aid in the evaluation of the fetal anal canal.[162,163] The fetal perianal muscular complex (PAMC), which includes the internal and external anal sphincter and puborectalis muscle,[163,164] appears as a hypoechogenic ring in the axial plane (target sign) and two hypoechogenic parallel stripes in the coronal and sagittal plane just posterocephalad to the external genitalia. In a series by Ochoa et al.,[164] absence of the PAMC had a high sensitivity and specificity for the diagnosis of anorectal atresia.

Anal atresia should be suspected when associated abnormalities such as sacral agenesis, hemivertebrae, caudal regression syndrome, and VACTERL sequence are detected. The presence of these anomalies suggest a closer inspection of the anus to determine whether indeed a target sign is absent or the colon appears dilated.

*MRI:* MRI has been used as an adjunct in the assessment of distal colonic obstruction.[18] Dilated meconium-filled rectum has been described by MRI in cases of anal atresia (see Fig. 18.1-15). The detection of abnormal fluid in the rectum has been noted in cases with vesicorectal fistulas (see Fig. 18.1-14B).[165] Assessment of the cul de sac by MRI has allowed for differentiation between a high anorectal malformation and cloaca.[18]

MRI is useful in further assessment of complex associated anomalies including OEIS, cloaca, and VACTERL.[166–170]

**Differential Diagnosis:** The differential for distal obstruction includes colonic atresia, meconium ileus, persistent cloaca, meconium plug syndrome, megacystic–microcolon–hypoperistalsis syndrome. Urachal cysts, ovarian cysts, and hydrometrocolpos should also be considered.

When calcifications are noted, it is important to determine whether they are intraluminal or extraluminal. Intraluminal calcifications suggest a rectovesicle fistula, while extraluminal may be secondary to meconium peritonitis.

**Associated Anomalies:** Anorectal malformations are associated with anomalies in up to 50% to 70% of cases. Anorectal malformations are separated into "high" supralevator lesions that end above the levator sling and are typically associated with fistulas.

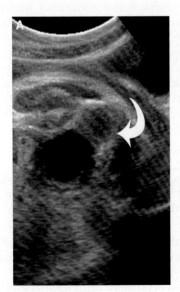
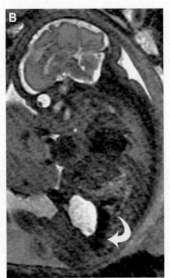
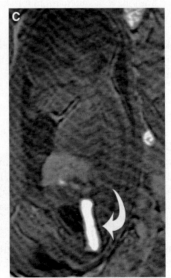

**FIGURE 18.1-15:** Anal atresia in a 31-week-gestation fetus with a two-vessel cord. **A:** Axial US image demonstrates distended rectum *(arrow)* measuring 13 mm *(arrow)* posterior to the bladder at 31 weeks gestation. **B:** Sagittal T2w image confirms presence of distended rectosigmoid *(arrow)*. At delivery, anal atresia was noted in this infant with VACTERL sequence. **C:** Note prominent rectum *(arrow)* in a different 31-week-gestation fetus. This infant was normal at delivery with no anal atresia.

"Low" infralevator lesions end below the levator sling and are not associated with fistulas.

Anal atresia is most commonly associated with the VACTERL association. Cloaca, omphalocele-extrophy-imperforate anus-spinal defects complex (OEIS), and caudal regression syndrome[148,150,152] also are associated with anal atresia. It is also described in trisomy 21.[171–176]

**Management:** If anal atresia is suspected, careful sonographic evaluation for associated anomalies of the spine, skeleton, kidneys, and umbilical cord should be performed. Because of the increased risk of cardiac disease, a fetal echocardiogram should be performed. Karyotype should be reserved for cases with associated anomalies that are linked with chromosome abnormalities such as trisomy 21 and long-segment aganglionosis.

Prenatal pediatric surgical consultation with the parents can be helpful in alleviating anxiety. The diagnosis of a distal colonic obstruction is not typically associated with prematurity or polyhydramnios. If isolated, the diagnosis has no implications for timing or route of delivery. Delivery should be planned at a center with appropriate high-risk obstetric and neonatal support.

Following delivery, the infant will develop abdominal distension and fail to pass meconium. A nasogastric tube should be placed to relieve abdominal distension. An intravenous line should be placed for fluid resuscitation.

If an imperforate anus is present, the diagnosis needs to be further defined into low, intermediate, or high lesions. Low lesions, typically with a perineal fistula, have a perineal anoplasty performed soon after birth. Intermediate and high lesions require a diverting colostomy in the first few days of life.[177] Anorectal reconstruction is then carried out at 4 to 8 weeks of age following MR of the spine and pelvis to assess for associated tethered cord.[178]

**Outcome:** Mortality rate of imperforate anus is because of associated cardiac or renal anomalies.[177–180] Voiding dysfunction, stenosis, and chronic constipation can occur. Continence is a major issue in these cases. While 90% of children with low imperforate anus are continent, those with high or intermediate imperforate anus have a much higher risk of long-term incontinence.[179,180]

**Recurrence Risk:** Recurrence depends on whether the atresia is isolated or syndromic. Isolated cases are thought to be sporadic with rare familial cases reported.[173]

## Cloaca

See Chapter 19.2.

## Hirschsprung Disease

**Incidence:** Hirschsprung disease is one of the most common causes of intestinal obstruction in the newborn. The incidence is 1 in 5,000.[181] Males are more affected than females, 4:1. Up to 25% have associated anomalies with a strong association with trisomy 21.

**Embryology/Pathology:** Aganglionosis of a segment of colon results in a functionally obstructed distal segment with a dilated proximal segment that tapers at a transition zone. As fetuses do not stool, it takes time after delivery for a transition zone with a dilated proximal segment to develop. Thus, prenatal diagnosis is rare with obstructive symptoms and constipation typically developing only after birth.[182,183]

**Diagnosis:** Short-segment Hirschsprung disease typically is not diagnosed prenatally. Echogenic bowel has been described with fetal Hirschsprung disease[184] but is not specific to this diagnosis. Enterolithiasis owing to functional obstruction and precipitation of urates within the lumen may be seen.

Cases of total aganglionosis have been diagnosed in the third trimester with polyhydramnios and small bowel dilatation.[184–186] Total colonic aganglionosis is rare, accounting for only 3% to 12% of cases and can mimic ileal atresia or meconium ileus prenatally as well as postnatally.[187]

**Differential Diagnosis:** Differential for bowel dilatation with polyhydramnios includes colonic atresia, ileal atresia, meconium ileus, meconium plug, small left colon, and imperforate anus.[188–190]

**Associated Anomalies:** Up to 25% have associated anomalies, including heart disease, renal anomalies, imperforate anus, colonic atresia, and hypospadias.[188] About 2% of cases with Hirschsprung disease have trisomy 21. Genetic conditions including Bardot–Biedl, cartilage hair hypoplasia, Riley Day, and Smith Lemli Opitz syndrome have been associated with Hirschsprung disease.[191]

**Prognosis and Management:** If an anus is present but distal obstruction is suspected, an abdominal radiograph can help document the level of the distal obstruction by demonstrating multiple loops of dilated bowel with air fluid levels. A water-soluble contrast enema may document the level of obstruction. However, the colon is often normal in caliber as a transition zone has not yet developed. At times, spasm of the rectum or abnormal sigmoid rectal ratio suggests the diagnosis. If the entire colon is small, total aganglionosis, distal ileal atresia, or meconium ileus should be considered in the differential.[192,193]

If Hirschsprung disease is confirmed with suction biopsy, a pull-through procedure is typically performed. Hirschsprung disease often results in good long-term function.[193,194] However, complications including enterocolitis (23%), fecal incontinence (3% to 10%), and chronic constipation (6% to 34%) can occur. Deaths can be secondary to associated anomalies, or a delay in diagnosis.[193,195–197]

**Recurrence Risk:** Typically sporadic. Four percent to 8% of cases are familial with an increased risk of recurrence in siblings.[198] The association with trisomy 21 and other chromosomal abnormalities suggest a genetic component.[191,199,200]

## Colonic Atresia

**Incidence:** Colonic atresias are a rare cause of intestinal obstruction and account for up to 10% of all bowel atresias.[201] Incidence has been reported to be around 1 in 20,000.[202]

**Embryology/Pathology:** Colonic atresias are thought to be secondary to a vascular or mechanical event (such as intestinal volvulus) similar to jejunal and ileal atresia.[203–207] The majority of colonic atresias occur proximal to the splenic flexure with resultant distal microcolon. In two-thirds of cases, colonic atresia occurs as an isolated defect without associated abnormalities. Colonic atresia may occur in combination with Hirschsprung disease.[208,209]

**Diagnosis:** The US appearance is indistinguishable from other distal obstructions and difficult to make prenatally. Bowel dilatations and polyhydramnios may rarely develop and suggest a more proximal obstruction. Perforation has been reported with the development of ascites and meconium peritonitis.[210]

The lack of meconium in the rectum by MRI may help suggest the diagnosis.

**Associated Anomalies:** Anomalies associated with colonic atresia include gastroschisis, omphalocele, Hirschsprung disease, and ocular and skeletal anomalies.[204,209,211] Cardiac anomalies and genetic defects have rarely been described.

**Management:** Primary repair often is technically feasible in colonic atresia. A suction rectal biopsy prior to the primary repair, to rule out Hirschsprung disease, is recommended.

At times, a colostomy is performed so that the infant can be discharged earlier from the hospital than with a primary repair.[212]

**Prognosis/Outcome:** Colonic atresia typically has an excellent prognosis with survival greater than 90%.

**Recurrence Risk:** Recurrence is rare. Cases of colonic atresia because of genetic or familial occurrence have been reported.[206,207,213]

# REFERENCES

1. Pritchard JA. Fetal swallowing and amniotic fluid volume. *Obstet Gynecol.* 1966;28:606–610.
2. Cyr DR, Mack LA, Schoenecker SA, et al. Bowel migration in the normal fetus: US detection. *Radiology.* 1986;161:119.
3. Lam YH, Shek T, Tang MH. Sonographic features of anal atresia at 12 weeks. *Ultrasound Obstet Gynecol.* 2002;19:523–524.
4. Nyberg DA, Mack LA, Patten RM, et al. Fetal bowel: normal sonographic findings. *J Ultrasound Med.* 1987;6:3–6.
5. Hertzberg BS. The fetal gastrointestinal tract. *Semin Roentgenol.* 1998;33:360–368.
6. Hertzberg BS. Sonography of the fetal gastrointestinal tract: anatomic variants, diagnostic pitfalls, and abnormalities. *AJR Am J Roentgenol.* 1994;162:1175–1182.
7. Parulekar SG. Sonography of normal fetal bowel. *J Ultrasound Med.* 1991;10:211–220.
8. Zalel Y, Perlitz Y, Gamzu R, et al. In-utero development of the fetal colon and rectum: sonographic evaluation. *Ultrasound Obstet Gynecol.* 2003;21:161–164.
9. Rubesova E. Fetal bowel anomalies—US and MR assessment. *Pediatr Radiol.* 2012;42(suppl 1):S101–S106.
10. Sase M, Asada M, Okuda M, et al. Fetal gastric size in normal and abnormal pregnancies. *Ultrasound Obstet Gynecol.* 2002;19:467–470.
11. Goldstein I, Reece EA, Yarkoni S, et al. Growth of the fetal stomach in normal pregnancies. *Obstet Gynecol.* 1987;70:641.
12. Fakry J, Shapiro LR, Schechter A, et al. Fetal gastric pseudomasses. *J Ultrasound Med.* 1987;6:177–180.
13. Karnik TJ, Rubenstein JB, Swayne LC. The fetal presacral pseudomass: a normal sonographic variant. *J Ultrasound Med.* 1991;10:579–581.
14. Bourdelat D, Muller F, Droullé P, et al. Anatomical and sonographical studies of the development of fecal continence and sphincter development in human fetuses. *Eur J Pediatr Surg.* 2001;11:124–130.
15. Haeusler MC, Berghold A, Stoll C, et al; EUROSCAN Study Group. Prenatal ultrasonographic detection of gastrointestinal obstruction: results from 18 European congenital anomaly registries. *Prenat Diagn.* 2002;22(7):616–623.
16. Stoll C, Alembik Y, Dott B, et al. Evaluation of prenatal diagnosis of congenital gastrointestinal atresias. *Eur J Epidemiol.* 1996;12:611–616.
17. Corteville JE, Gray DL, Langer JC. Bowel abnormalities in the fetus—correlation of prenatal ultrasonographic findings with outcome. *Am J Obstet Gynecol.* 1996;175:724–729.
18. Veyrac C, Couture A, Saguintaah M, et al. MRI of fetal GI tract abnormalities. *Abdom Imaging.* 2004;29:411–420.
19. Huisman T, Kellenberger C. MR imaging characteristics of the normal fetal gastrointestinal tract and abdomen. *Eur J Radiol.* 2008;65:170–181.
20. Garel C, Dreux S, Philippe-Chomette P, et al. Contribution of fetal magnetic resonance imaging and amniotic fluid digestive enzyme assays to the evaluations of gastrointestinal tract abnormalities. *Ultrasound Obstet Gynecol.* 2006;28:282–291.
21. Barnewolt CE. Congenital abnormalities of the gastrointestinal tract. *Semin Roentgenol.* 2004;39(2):263–281.
22. Saguintaah M, Couture A, Veyrac C, et al. MRI of the fetal gastrointestinal tract. *Pediatr Radiol.* 2002;32:395–404.
23. Rubesova E, Vance CJ, Ringertz HG, et al. Three-dimensional MRI volumetric measurements of the normal fetal colon. *AJR Am J Roentgenol.* 2009;192(3):761–765.
24. Colombani M, Ferry M, Garel C, et al. Fetal gastrointestinal MRI: all that glitters in T1 is not necessarily colon. *Pediatr Radiol.* 2010;40:1215–1221.
25. Farhatazia N, Engels JE, Ramus RM, et al. Fetal MRI of urine and meconium by gestational age for the diagnosis of genitourinary and gastrointestinal abnormalities. *AJR Am J Roentgenol.* 2005;184(6):1891–1897.
26. Iacobelli BD, Zaccara A, Spirydakis I, et al. Prenatal counseling of small bowel atresia: watch the fluid! *Prenat Diagn.* 2006;26:214–217.
27. Forrester MB, Merz RD. Population-based study of small intestinal atresia and stenosis, Hawaii, 1986–2000. *Public Health.* 2004;118:434–438.
28. Robertson FM, Crombleholme TM, Paidas M, et al. Prenatal diagnosis and management of gastrointestinal anomalies. *Semin Perinatol.* 1994;18:182–195.
29. Rowe MI, O'Neill JA Jr, Grosfeld JL, et al. Intestinal atresia and stenosis. In: Rowe MI, O'Neill JA Jr, Grosfeld JL, et al, eds. *Essentials of Pediatric Surgery.* St Louis, MO: Mosby; 1995:508–514.
30. Aite L, Trucchi A, Nahom A, et al. Antenatal diagnosis of surgically correctable anomalies: effects of repeated consultations on parental anxiety. *J Perinatol.* 2003;23:652–654.
31. Depaepe A, Dolk H, Lechat MF. The epidemiology of TEF and esophageal atresia in Europe EURO-CAT Working Group. *Arch Dis Child.* 1993;68:743–748.
32. Pretorius DH, Drose JA, Dennis MA, et al. Tracheoesophageal fistula in utero: twenty-two cases. *J Ultrasound Med.* 1987;6(9):509–513.
33. Sparey C, Robson SC. Oesophageal atresia. *Prenat Diagn.* 2000;20(3):251–253.
34. Borsellino A, Zaccara A, Nahom A, et al. False-positive rate in prenatal diagnosis of surgical anomalies. *J Pediatr Surg.* 2006;41(4):826–829.
35. Shaw-Smith C. Oesophageal atresia, tracheo-oesophageal fistula, and the VACTERL association: review of genetics and epidemiology. *J Med Genet.* 2006;43:545.
36. Solt I, Rotmensch S, Bronshtein M. The esophageal "pouch sign": a benign transient finding. *Prenat Diagn.* 2010;30(9):845–848.
37. Estroff JA, Parad RB, Share JC, et al. Second trimester prenatal findings in duodenal and esophageal atresia without tracheoesophageal fistula. *J Ultrasound Med.* 1994;13:375.
38. Shulman A, Mazkereth R, Zalel Y, et al. Prenatal identification of esophageal atresia: the role of ultrasonography for evaluation of functional anatomy. *Prenat Diagn.* 2002;22:669–674.
39. Kalache KD, Wauer R, Mau H, et al. Prognostic significance of the pouch sign in fetuses with prenatally diagnosed esophageal atresia. *Am J Obstet Gynecol.* 2000;182:978–981.
40. Mourali M, Essoussi-Chikhaoui J, Fatnassi A, et al. Prenatal diagnosis of esophageal atresia. *Tunis Med.* 2011;89(2):213–214.
41. Stringer MD, McKenna KM, Goldstein RB, et al. Prenatal diagnosis of esophageal atresia. *J Pediatr Surg.* 1995;30:1258–1263.
42. Develay-Morice E, Rathat G, Duyme M, et al. Ultrasonography of fetal esophagus: healthy appearance and prenatal diagnosis of a case of esophagus atresia with esotracheal fistula. *Gynecol Obstet Fertil.* 2007;35:249–257.
43. Botto LD, Khoury MJ, Mastroiacovo P, et al. The spectrum of congenital anomalies of the VATER association: an international study. *Am J Med Genet.* 1997;71(1):8–15.
44. Eyheremendy E, Pfister M. Antenatal real-time diagnosis of esophageal atresias. *J Clin Ultrasound.* 1983;11(7):395–397.
45. Has R, Günay S, Topuz S. Pouch sign in prenatal diagnosis of esophageal atresia. *Ultrasound Obstet Gynecol.* 2004;23(5):523–524.
46. Langer JC, Hussain H, Khan A, et al. Prenatal diagnosis of esophageal atresia using MRI. *J Pediatr Surg.* 2001;36:804–807.
47. Olgun H, Karacan M, Caner I, et al. Congenital cardiac malformations in neonates with apparently isolated gastrointestinal malformations. *Pediatr Int.* 2009;51(2):260–262.
48. Holder TM, Cloud DT, Lewis JE Jr, et al. Esophageal atresia and TEF: a survey of its members by the Surgical Section of the American Academy of Pediatrics. *Pediatrics.* 1964;34:542.
49. Mitani Y, Hasegawa T, Kubota A, et al. Prenatal findings of concomitant duodenal and esophageal atresia without tracheoesophageal fistula (Gross type A). *J Clin Ultrasound.* 2009;37(7):403–405.
50. Dave S, Shi E. The management of combined oesophageal and duodenal atresia. *Pediatr Surg Int.* 2004;20:689–691.
51. Beasley SW, Allen M, Myers N. The effects of Down syndrome and other chromosomal abnormalities on survival and management in esophageal atresia. *Pediatr Surg.* 1997;12:550–551.
52. Pameijer CR, Hubard AM, Colemean B, et al. Combined pure esophageal atresia, duodenal atresia, biliary atresia, and pancreatic ductal atresia: prenatal diagnostic features and review of the literature. *J Pediatr Surg.* 2000;35:745–747.

53. Chitty LS, Goodman J, Seller MF. Esophageal and duodenal atresia in a fetus with Down's syndrome: prenatal sonographic features. *Ultrasound Obstet Gynecol.* 1996;7:450–452.

54. Spitz L. Esophageal atresia: past, present, and future. *J Pediatr Surg.* 1996;31:19.

55. Bahado-Singh RO, Romero R, Vecchio M, et al. Prenatal diagnosis of congenital hiatal hernia. *J Ultrasound Med.* 1992;11:297–300.

56. Ogunyemi D. Serial sonographic findings in a fetus with congenital hiatal hernia. *Ultrasound Obstet Gynecol.* 2001;17:350–353.

57. Chacko J, Ford WD, Furness ME. Antenatal detection of hiatus hernia. *Pediatr Surg Int.* 1998;13:163–164.

58. Ruano R, Benachi A, Aubry MC, et al. Prenatal sonographic diagnosis of congenital hiatal hernia. *Prenat Diagn.* 2004;24(1):26–30.

59. Yamamoto N, Hidaka N, Anami A, et al. Prenatal sonographic diagnosis of a hiatal hernia in a fetus with asplenia syndrome. *J Ultrasound Med.* 2007;26(9):1257–1261.

60. Al-Assiri A, Wiseman N, Bunge M. Prenatal diagnosis of intrathoracic stomach (gastric herniation). *J Pediatr Surg.* 2005;40(2):E15–E17.

61. Parida SK, Driss VM, Hall BD. Hiatus/paraesophageal hernias in neonatal Marfan syndrome. *Am J Med Genet.* 1995;72:156–158.

62. Yadav K, Myers NA. Paraesophageal hernia in the neonatal period another differential diagnosis of esophageal atresia. *Pediatr Surg Int.* 1997;12:420–421.

63. Al-Arfaj AL, Khwaja MS, Upadhyaya P. Massive hiatal hernia in children. *Eur J Surg.* 1991;157:465–468.

64. Baglaj SM, Noblett HR. Paraoesophageal hernia in children: familial occurrence and review of the literature. *Pediatr Surg Int.* 1999;15:85–87.

65. Skandalakis JE, Gray SW, et al. The small intestines. In: Skandalakis JE, Gray SW, eds. *Embryology for Surgeons.* Baltimore, MD: Williams & Wilkins; 1994:184.

66. Boyden EA, Cope JG, Bill AH. Anatomy and embryology of congenital intrinsic obstruction of the duodenum. *Am J Surg.* 1967;114:190–195.

67. Schaefer-Graf UM, Buchanan TA, Xiang A, et al. Patterns of congenital anomalies and relationship to initial maternal fasting glucose levels in pregnancies complicated by type 2 and gestational diabetes. *Am J Obstet Gynecol.* 2000;182(2):313–320.

68. Ben Ahmed Y, Ghorbel S, Chouikh T, et al. Combination of partial situs inversus, polysplenia and annular pancreas with duodenal obstruction and intestinal malrotation. *JBR-BTR.* 2012;95(4):257–260.

69. Farrant P, Dewbury KC, Meire HB. Antenatal diagnosis of duodenal atresia. *Br J Radiol.* 1981;54(643):633–635.

70. Zimmer EZ, Bronshtein M. Early diagnosis of duodenal atresia and possible sonographic pitfalls. *Prenat Diagn.* 1996;16:564–566.

71. Lawrence M, Ford A, Furness M, et al. Congenital duodenal obstruction: early antenatal ultrasound diagnosis. *Pediatr Surg Int.* 2000;16:342–345.

72. Balcar I, Grant DC, Miller WA, et al. Antenatal detection of Down syndrome by sonography. *AJR Am J Roentgenol.* 1984;143(1):29–30.

73. Nelson LH, Clark CE, Fishburn JI, et al. Value of serial sonography in the in utero detection of duodenal atresia. *Obstet Gynecol.* 1982;59:657–661.

74. Bovicelli L, Rizzo N, Orsini LF, et al. Prenatal diagnosis and management of fetal gastrointestinal abnormalities. *Semin Perinatol.* 1983;7(2):109–117.

75. Petrikovsky BM. First trimester diagnosis of duodenal atresia. *Am J Obstet Gynecol.* 1994;171:569–570.

76. Stauffer UG, Schwoebel M. Duodenal atresia and stenosis annular pancreas. In: O'Neill JA, Rowe MI, Grosfeld JL, et al, eds. *Pediatric Surgery.* 5th ed. St Louis, MO: Mosby-Year Book; 1998:1133–1143.

77. Pariente G, Landau D, Aviram M, et al. Prenatal diagnosis of a rare sonographic appearance of duodenal atresia: report of 2 cases and literature review. *J Ultrasound Med.* 2012;31(11):1829–1833.

78. Choudhry MS, Rahman N, Boyd P, et al. Duodenal atresia: associated anomalies, prenatal diagnosis and outcome. *Pediatr Surg Int.* 2009;25(8):727–730.

79. Fujishiro E, Suziki Y, Sato T, et al. Characteristics findings for diagnosis of baby complicated with both VACTERL association and duodenal atresia. *Fetal Diagn Ther.* 2004;19:134–137.

80. Obata-Yasuoka M, Hamada H, Ohara R, et al. Alveolar capillary dysplasia associated with duodenal atresia: ultrasonographic findings of enlarged, highly echogenic lungs and gastric dilatation in a third-trimester fetus. *J Obstet Gynaecol Res.* 2011;37(7):937–939.

81. Gilbertson-Dahdal DL, Dutta S, Varich LJ, et al. Neonatal malrotation with midgut volvulus mimicking duodenal atresia. *AJR Am J Roentgenol.* 2009;192(5):1269–1271.

82. Malone F, Crombleholme TM, Nores J, et al. Pitfalls of the "double bubble" sign: a case of congenital duodenal duplication. *Fetal Diagn Ther.* 1997;12:298–300.

83. Hancock BJ, Wiseman NE. Congenital duodenal obstruction: the impact of an antenatal diagnosis. *J Pediatr Surg.* 1989;24:1027–1031.

84. Muller F, Dommergues M, Ville Y, et al. Amniotic fluid digestive enzymes: diagnostic value in fetal gastrointestinal obstructions. *Prenat Diagn.* 1994;14(10):973–979.

85. Murshed R, Nicholls G, Spitz L. Intrinsic duodenal obstruction: trends in management and outcome over 45 years (1951–1995) with relevance to prenatal counseling. *Br J Obstet Gynaecol.* 1999;106:1197–1199.

86. Bittencourt DG, Barini R, Marba S, et al. Congenital duodenal obstruction does prenatal diagnosis improve the outcome? *Pediatr Surg Int.* 2004;20:582–585.

87. Cohen-Overbeek T, Grijseels E, Niemeijer N, et al. Isolated or nonisolated duodenal obstruction: perinatal outcome following prenatal or postnatal diagnosis. *Ultrasound Obstet Gynecol.* 2008;32:784–792.

88. Grosfeld JL, Rescorla FJ. Duodenal atresia and stenosis: reassessment of treatment and outcome based on antenatal diagnosis, pathologic variances, and long-term follow-up. *World J Surg.* 1993;17:301–309.

89. Escobar MA, Ladd AP, Grosfeld JL, et al. Duodenal atresia and stenosis: long-term follow-up over 30 years. *J Pediatr Surg.* 2004;39(6):867–871.

90. Touloukian RJ. Diagnosis and treatment of jejunoileal atresia. *World J Surg.* 1993;17:310–319.

91. Baglaj M, Carachi R, Lawther S. Multiple atresia of the small intestine: a 20 year review. *Eur J Pediatr Surg.* 2008;18:13–18.

92. Foucade L, Shima H, Miyazaki E, et al. Multiple gastrointestinal atresias result from disturbed morphogenesis. *Pediatr Surg Int.* 2001;17:361–364.

93. Kumuro H, Amagai T, Hori T, et al. Placental vascular compromise in jejunoileal atresia. *J Pediatr Surg.* 2004;39:1701–1705.

94. Sweeney B, Surana R, Puri P. Jejunoileal atresia and associated malformations: correlation with the timing of in utero insult. *J Pediatr Surg.* 2001;35:774–776.

95. Martin LW, Zerella JT. Jejuno-ileal atresia: a proposed classification. *J Pediatr Surg.* 1976;11:399–403.

96. Ahlgren LS. Apple peel jejunal atresia. *J Pediatr Surg.* 1987;22:451–453.

97. Komuro H, Hori T, Amagai T, et al. The etiologic role of intrauterine volvulus and intussusception in jejunoileal atresia. *J Pediatr Surg.* 2004;39:1812–1814.

98. Patricolo M, Noia G, Rossi L. An experimental animal model of intestinal obstruction to simulate in utero therapy for jejunoileal atresia. *Fetal Diagn Ther.* 1998;13(5):298–301.

99. Graham JM Jr, Marin-Padilla M, Hoefnagel D. Jejunal atresia associated with Cafergot ingestion during pregnancy. *Clin Pediatr (Phila).* 1983;22(3):226–228.

100. Lubinsky M. Hypothesis: estrogen related thrombosis explains the pathogenesis and epidemiology of gastroschisis. *Am J Med Genet A.* 2012;158A(4):808–811.

101. Basaran UN, Inan M, Gucer F, et al. Prenatally closed gastroschisis with midgut atresia. *Pediatr Surg Int.* 2002;18:550–552.

102. Ghionzoli M, James CP, David AL, et al. Gastroschisis with intestinal atresia—predictive value of antenatal diagnosis and outcome of postnatal treatment. *J Pediatr Surg.* 2012;47(2):322–328.

103. Kumar T, Vaughan R, Polak M. A proposed classification for the spectrum of vanishing gastroschisis. *Eur J Pediatr Surg.* 2013;23(1):72–75.

104. Ogunyemi D. Gastroschisis complicated by midgut atresia, absorption of bowel, and closure of the abdominal wall defect. *Fetal Diagn Ther.* 2001;16(4):227–230.

105. Langer JC, Adzick NS, Filly RA, et al. Gastrointestinal tract obstruction in the fetus. *Arch Surg.* 1989;124(10):1183–1186.

106. Langer JC, Khanna J, Caco C, et al. Prenatal diagnosis of gastroschisis: development of objective sonographic criteria for predicting outcome. *Obstet Gynecol.* 1993;81(1):53–56.

107. Wax J, Hamilton T, Cartin A, et al. Congenital jejunal and ileal atresia. *J Ultrasound Med.* 2006;25:337–342.

108. Damato N, Filly RA, Goldstein RB, et al. Frequency of fetal anomalies in sonographically detected polyhydramnios. *J Ultrasound Med.* 1993;12:11–15.

109. Touloukian RJ. Composition of amniotic fluid with experimental jejunoileal atresia. *J Pediatr Surg.* 1977;12:397–401.

110. Estroff J, Bromley B, Benecerraf B. Fetal meconium peritonitis without sequelae. *Pediatr Radiol.* 1992;22:277–278.

111. Dirkes K, Crombleholme TM, Craigo SD, et al. The natural history of meconium peritonitis diagnosed in utero. *J Pediatr Surg.* 1995;30:979–982.

112. Benachi A, Sonig P, Jounnic JM, et al. Determination of the anatomical location of an antenatal intestinal occlusion by magnetic resonance imaging. *Ultrasound Obstet Gynecol.* 2001;18:163–165.

113. Kubik-Huch RA, Huisman TA, Wisser J, et al. Ultrafast MR imaging of the fetus. *AJR Am J Roentgenol.* 2000;174:1599–1606.

114. Brugger PC, Prayer D. Fetal abdominal magnetic resonance imaging. *Eur J Radiol.* 2006;57:278–293.

115. Shinmoto H, Kuribayashi S. MRI of fetal abdominal abnormalities. *Abdom Imaging.* 2003;28:877–886.

116. Carcopino X, Chaumoitre K, Shojai R, et al. Use of fetal magnetic resonance imaging in differentiating ileal atresia from meconium ileus. *Ultrasound Obstet Gynecol.* 2006;28(7):976–977.

117. Whitby EH, Paley MN, Sprigg A, et al. Comparison of ultrasound and magnetic resonance imaging in 100 singleton pregnancies with suspected brain abnormalities. *BJOG.* 2004;111:784–792.

118. Nixon HH. Small intestinal atresia. *Proc R Soc Med.* 1971;64(4):372–374.

119. Shawis R, Antao B. Prenatal bowel dilatation and the subsequent postnatal management. *Early Hum Dev.* 2006;82(5):297–303. Epub 2006 Apr 19.

120. Basu R, Burge DM. The effect of antenatal diagnosis on the management of small bowel atresia. *Pediatr Surg Int.* 2004;20:177–179.

121. Ozguner IF, Savas C, Ozguner M, et al. Intestinal atresia with segmental musculature and neural defect. *J Pediatr Surg.* 2005;40(8):1232–1237.

122. DallaVecchia LK, Grosfeld JL, West KW, et al. Intestinal atresia and stenosis: a 25 year experience with 277 cases. *Arch Surg.* 1998;133:490–496.

123. Arnal-Monreal F, Pombo F, Capdevila-Puerta A. Multiple hereditary gastrointestinal atresias: study of a family. *Acta Paediatr.* 1983;72:773–777.

124. Shorter NA, Georges A, Perenyi A, et al. A proposed classification system for familial intestinal atresia and its relevance to the understanding of the etiology of jejunoileal atresia. *J Pediatr Surg.* 2006;41(11):1822–1825.

## Meconium Ileus

125. Muller F, Frot JC, Aubry MC, et al. Meconium ileus in cystic fibrosis fetuses. *Lancet.* 1984;1:223.
126. Caspi B, Elchalal U, Lancet M, et al. Prenatal diagnosis of cystic fibrosis: ultrasonographic appearance of meconium ileus in the fetus. *Prenat Diagn.* 1988;8:379–382.
127. Barki Y, Bar-Ziv J. Meconium ileus: ultrasonic diagnosis of intraluminal inspissated meconium. *J Clin Ultrasound.* 1985;13(7):509–512.
128. Bulas D. Prenatal diagnosis of gastrointestinal atresia and obstruction. In: Basow DS, ed. *UpToDate.* Waltham, MA: Wolters Kluwer Health; 2012.
129. Scotet V, De Braekeleer M, Audrezet M-P, et al. Prenatal detection of cystic fibrosis by ultrasonography: a retrospective study of more than 346,000 pregnancies. *J Med Genet.* 2002;39:443–448.
130. Degnan AJ, Bulas DI, Sze RW. Ileal atresia with meconium peritonitis: fetal MRI evaluation. *J Radiol Case Rep.* 2010;4:15–18.
131. Wong A, Toh CH, Lien R, et al. Prenatal MR imaging of a meconium pseudocyst extending to the right subphrenic space with right lung compression. *Pediatr Radiol.* 2006;36:1208–1211.
132. Simonovsky V, Lisy J. Meconium pseudocyst secondary to ileal atresia complicated by volvulus: antenatal MR demonstration. *Pediatr Radiol.* 2007; 37:305–309.
133. Blazer S, Zimmer EZ, Bronshtein M. Nonvisualization of the fetal gallbladder in early pregnancy: comparison with clinical outcome. *Radiology.* 2002;224(2):379–382.
134. Carcopino X, Chaumoitre K, Shojai R, et al. Foetal magnetic resonance imaging and echogenic bowel. *Prenat Diagn.* 2007;27:272–278.
135. Al-Kouatly HB, Chasen ST, Streltzoff J, et al. The clinical significance of fetal echogenic bowel. *Am J Obstet Gynecol.* 2001;185:1035–1038.
136. Kesrouani AK, Guibourdenche J, Mullr F, et al. Etiology and outcome of fetal echogenic bowel: ten years of experience. *Fetal Diagn Ther.* 2003;18:240–246.
137. Scotet V, Dugueperoux I, Audrezet MP, et al. Focus on cystic fibrosis and other disorders evidenced in fetuses with sonographic finding of echogenic bowel: 16-year report from Brittany, France. *Am J Obstet Gynecol.* 2010;203: 592.e1–592e.6.
138. Sepulveda W, Leung KY, Roberson ME, et al. Prevalence of cystic fibrosis mutations in pregnancies with fetal echogenic bowel. *Obstet Gynecol.* 1996; 87:103–106.
139. Chasen ST. Fetal echogenic bowel. In: Wilkins-Haug L, ed. *UpToDate.* Waltham, MA: Wolters Kluwer Health; 2012.
140. Jackson CR, Orford J, Minutillo C, et al. Dilated and echogenic fetal bowel and postnatal outcomes: a surgical perspective. Case series and literature review. *Eur J Pediatr Surg.* 2010;20(3):191–193.
141. Bashiri A, Burstein E, Hershkowitz R, et al. Fetal echogenic bowel by ultrasound: what is the clinical significance? 2007;146(12):964–969, 996–997.
142. Oka Y, Asabe K, Shirakusa T, et al. An antenatal appearance of megacystismicrocolon-intestinal hypoperistalsis syndrome. *Turk J Pediatr.* 2008;50(3): 269–274.
143. Gaillard D, Bouvier R, Scheiner C, et al. Meconium ileus and intestinal atresia in fetuses and neonates. *Pediatr Pathol Lab Med.* 1996;16:25–40.
144. Kirkinen P, Jouppila P. Prenatal ultrasonic findings in congenital chloride diarrhea. *Pernat Diagn.* 1984;4:457.
145. Colombani M, Ferry M, Toga CV, et al. Magnetic resonance imaging in the prenatal diagnosis of congenital diarrhea. *Ultrasound Obstet Gynecol.* 2010; 35:560–565.
146. Usui N, Kamiyama M, Tani G, et al. Prenatal differential diagnosis of congenital chloride diarrhea: the importance of a dilated fluid-filled rectum. *Eur J Pediatr Surg.* 2011;21(3):193–194.
147. Langer JC, Winthrop AL, Burrows RF. False diagnosis of intestinal obstruction in a fetus with congenital chloride diarrhea. *Pediatr Surg.* 1991;26(11):1282–1284.
148. Hohlschneider AM, Hutson JM. *Anorectal Malformations in Children: Embryology, Diagnosis, Surgical Treatment, Follow-up.* Berlin, Germany: Springer-Verlag; 2006.
149. Bean WJ, Calonje MA, Aprill CN, et al. Anal atresia: a prenatal ultrasound diagnosis. *J Clin Ultrasound.* 1978;6:111–114.
150. Harris RD, Nyberg DA, Mack LA, et al. Anorectal atresia: prenatal sonographic diagnosis. *AJR Am J Roentgenol.* 1987;149:395–400.
151. Brantberg A, Blass HGK, Haugen SE, et al. Imperforate anus: a relatively common anomaly rarely diagnosed prenatally. *Ultrasound Obstet Gynecol.* 2006;28:904–910.
152. Gilbert CE, Hamil J, Metcalfe RF, et al. Changing antenatal sonographic appearance of anorectal atresia from first to third trimesters. *J Ultrasound Med.* 2006;25:781–784.
153. Kaponis A, Paschopoulos M, Parakevaidis E, et al. Fetal anal atresia presenting as transient bowel dilatation at 16 weeks of gestation. *Fetal Diagn Ther.* 2006;21:383–385.
154. Taipale P, Rovamo L, Hiilesmaa V. First-trimester diagnosis of imperforate anus. *Ultrasound Obstet Gynecol.* 2005;25:187–188.
155. Chen M, Meagher S, Simpson I, et al. Sonographic features of anorectal atresia at 12 weeks. *J Matern Fetal Neonatal Med.* 2009;22:931–933.
156. Mandell J, Lillehei C, Greene M, et al. The prenatal diagnosis of imperforate anus with rectourinary fistula: dilated fetal colon with enterolitiasis. *J Pediatr Surg.* 1992;27(1):82–84.

157. Grant T, Newman M, Gould, et al. Intraluminal colonic calcifications associated with anorectal atresia: prenatal sonographic detection. *J Ultrasound Med.* 1990;9:411–413.
158. Sepulveda W, Romero R, Qureshi F, et al. Prenatal diagnosis of enterolithiasis: a sign of fetal large bowel obstruction. *J Ultrasound Med.* 1994;13:581–585.
159. Bergholz R, Wenke K. Enterolithiasis: a case report and review. *J Pediatr Surg.* 2008;44:828–830.

## Anus

160. Vijayaraghavan SB, Prema AS, Suganyadevi P. Sonographic depiction of the fetal anus and its utility in the diagnosis of anorectal malformations. *J Ultrasound Med.* 2011;30:37–45.
161. Moon MH, Cho JY, Kim JH, et al. In utero development of the fetal anal sphincter. *Ultrasound Obstet Gynecol.* 2010;35:556–559.
162. Elchalal U, Yanai N, Valsky DV, et al. Application of 3-dimensional ultrasonography to imaging the fetal anal canal. *J Ultrasound Med.* 2010;29: 1195–1201.
163. Gindes L, Weissmann-Brenner A, Achiron R, et al. 3-Dimensional demonstration of fetal anal canal and sphincter. *Ultraschall Med.* 2012;33(7):E25–E30.
164. Ochoa JH, Chiesa M, Vildoza RP, et al. Evaluation of the perianal muscular complex in the prenatal diagnosis of anorectal atresia in a high-risk population. *Ultrasound Obstet Gynecol.* 2012;39(5):521–527.
165. Lubusky M, Prochazka M, Dhaifalah I, et al. Fetal enterolithiasis: prenatal sonographic and MRI diagnosis in two cases of urorectal septum malformation (URSM) sequence. *Prenat Diagn.* 2006;26(4):345–349.
166. Chen CP, Chang TY, Liu YP, et al. Prenatal 3-dimensional sonographic and MRI findings in omphalocele-exstrophy-imperforate anus-spinal defects complex. *J Clin Ultrasound.* 2008;36(5):308–311.
167. Warne S, Chitty LS, Wilcox DT. Prenatal diagnosis of cloacal anomalies. *BJU Int.* 2002;89:78–81.
168. Witters I, Meylaerts L, Peeters H, et al. Fetal hydrometrocolpos, uterus didelphys with low vaginal and anal atresia: difficulties in differentiation from a complex cloacal malformation: a case report. *Genet Couns.* 2012;23(4):513–517.
169. Goto S, Suzumori N, Obayashi S, et al. Prenatal findings of omphalocele-exstrophy of the bladder-imperforate anus-spinal defects (OEIS) complex. *Congenit Anom (Kyoto).* 2012;52(3):179–181.
170. Vasudevan PC, Cohen MC, Whitby EH, et al. The OEIS complex: two case reports that illustrate the spectrum of abnormalities and a review of the literature. *Prenat Diagn.* 2006;26(3):267.
171. Nour S, Kumor D, Dickson JAS. Anorectal malformations with sacral bony abnormalities. *Arch Dis Child.* 1989;64:1618–1624.
172. Jaramillo D, Lebowitz RL, Hendren WH. The cloacal malformation: radiologic findings and imaging recommendations. *Radiology.* 1990;177:441–448.
173. Boocock GR, Donnai D. Anorectal malformation: familial aspects and associated anomalies. *Arch Dis Child.* 1987;62:576–579.
174. Cuschieri A. EROCAT Working Group: anorectal anomalies associated with or as part of other anomalies. *Am J Med Genet.* 2002;110:122–130.
175. Cho S, Moore SP, Fangman T. One hundred three consecutive patients with anorectal malformations and their associated anomalies. *Arch Pediatr Adolesc Med.* 2001;155:587–591.
176. Stoll C, Alembik Y, Dott B, et al. Associated malformations in patients with anorectal anomalies. *Eur J Med Genet.* 2007;50:281–290.
177. Livingston J, Elicevik M, Crombleholme T, et al. US findings in neonates with anorectal malformations: a review of 95 cases. *Am J Obstet Gynecol.* 2006;195:S63.
178. Pena A, DeVries P. Posterio sagittal anorectoplasty: important technical considerations and new applications. *J Pediatr Surg.* 1982;17:796–802.
179. Kazizoke H. Preexisitng neurogenic voiding dysfunction in children with imperforate anus: problems in management. *J Urol.* 1994;151:1041–1045.
180. Rintala R, Lindahl H, Louchimo I. Anorectal malformations—results of treatment and long-term follow-up in 208 patients. *Pediatr Surg Int.* 1991;6:36–42.
181. Parisi MA, Kapur RP. Genetics of Hirschsprung's disease. *Curr Opin Pediatr.* 2000;12:610–617.
182. Bickler SW. Long-segment Hirschsprung disease. *Oral Surg.* 1992;127:1047–1051.
183. Puri P. Hirschsprung's disease: clinical and experimental observations. *World J Surg.* 1993;17:374–384.
184. Wrobleski D, Wesselhoeft C. US diagnosis of prenatal intestinal obstruction. *J Pediatr Surg.* 1979;14:598–600.
185. Vermesh M, Mayden KL, Confino E, et al. Prenatal sonographic diagnosis of Hirschsprung's disease. *J Ultrasound Med.* 1986;5:37–39.
186. Eliyahu S, Yanai N, Blondheim O, et al. Sonographic presentation of Hirschsprung's disease: a case of an entirely aganglionic colon and ileum. *Prenat Diagn.* 1994;14:1170–1172.
187. Wildhaber BE, Teitelbaum DH, Coran AG. Total colonic Hirschsprung's disease: a 28-year experience. *J Pediatr Surg.* 2005;40:203–207.
188. Cowles RA, Berdon WE, Holt PD, et al. Neonatal intestinal obstruction simulating meconium ileus in infants with long-segment intestinal aganglionosis: radiographic findings that prompt the need for rectal biopsy. *Pediatr Radiol.* 2006;36:133–137.
189. Johnson JF, Dean BL. Hirschsprung's disease co-existing with colonic atresia. *Pediatr Radiol.* 1981;11:97–98.

190. Arbell D, Gross E, Orkin B, et al. Imperforate anus, malrotation, and Hischsprung's disease: a rare and important association. *J Pediatr Surg.* 2006;41: 1335–1337.

191. Kusafuha T, Puri P. Genetic aspects of Hirschsprung's disease. *Semin Pediatr Surg.* 1998;7:148–155.

## Management

192. Bodian M, Carter CO, Ward BCH. Hirschsprung disease (with radiological observations). *Lancet.* 1951;1:302–309.

193. Swenson O, Sherman JO, Fisher JH, et al. The treatment and post-operative complications of congenital megacolon: a twenty-five year follow-up. *Ann Surg.* 1985;182:266–273.

194. Teitelbaum DH, Coran AG, Primary pull-through in the newborn. *Semin Pediatr Surg.* 1998;7:103–107.

195. Craigie RJ, Conway SJ, Cooper L, et al. Primary pull-through for Hirschsprung's disease: comparison of open and laparoscopic assisted procedures. *J Laparoendosc Adv Surg Tech A.* 2007;17:809–812.

196. Rescorla F, Morrison A, Engles D, et al. Hirschsprung's disease: evaluation of mortality and long-term outcome in 260 cases. *Arch Surg.* 1992;127:934–941.

197. Suita S, Taguchi T, Ieiri S, et al. Hirschsprung's disease in Japan: analysis of 3852 patients based on a national wide survey in 30 years. *J Pediatr Surg.* 2005; 40:197–202.

198. Raffefensperger JG, ed. *Swenso's Pediatric Surgery.* 5th ed. Norwalk, CT: Appleton and Lange; 1990.

199. Martucciello G, Biococchi MP, Dodero P, et al. Total colonic aganglionosis associated with interstitial deletion of the long arm of chromosome 10. *Pediatr Surg Int.* 1992;7:300–310.

200. Edery P, Pelet A, Mulligan LM, et al. Long segment and short segment familial Hirschsprung's disease variable clinical expression of the RET locus. *J Med Genet.* 1994;31:602–606.

201. Touloukian RI. Diagnosis and treatment of jejunal ilial atresia. *World J Surg.* 1993;17:310–317.

202. Philippart AI. Atresia stenosis and other obstructions of the colon. In: Welch KI, Randolph IT, eds. *Pediatric Surgery.* Chicago, IL: Year Book Medical Publishers; 1986:984–985.

203. Boweles ET, Vassy LE, Ralston M. Atresia of the colon. *J Pediatr Surg.* 1976; 11:69–75.

204. Etensel B, Temir G, Karkiner A, et al. Atresia of the colon. *J Pediatr Surg.* 2005;40:1258–1268.

205. Sturim HA, Ternberg JL. Congenital atresia of the colon. *Surgery.* 1966; 59:458–464.

206. Guttman FM, Braun P, Garanace PH, et al. Multiple atresias involving the GI tract form the stomach to rectum. *J Pediatr Surg.* 1973;8:633–640.

207. Puri P, Fujimoto T. New observation on the pathogenesis of multiple intestinal atresia. *J Pediatr Surg.* 1988;23:221.

208. Currie ABM, Hemalatha AH, Doraiswomy NV, et al. Colonic atresia in association with Hirschsprung's disease. *J R Coll Surg Edinb.* 1983;28:31–34.

209. Draus JM, Maxfield CM, Bond SJ. Hirschsprung's disease in an infant with colonic atresia and normal fixation of the distal colon. *J Pediatr Surg.* 2007;42:E5–E8.

210. Agrawala G, Predanic M, Perni SC, et al. Isolated fetal ascites caused by bowel perforation due to colonic atresia. *J Matern Fetal Neonatal Med.* 2005;17:291–294.

211. Saxonhouse MA, Kays DW, Burchfield DJ, et al. Gastroschisis with jejunal and colonic atresia, and isolated colonic atresia in dichorionic, diamniotic twins. *Pediatr Surg Int.* 2009;25(5):437–439.

212. Davenport M, Bianchi A, Doig CM, et al. Colonic atresia: current results of treatment. *J R Coll Surg Edinb.* 1990;35:25–28.

213. Benawra R, Puppla BL, Mangurten HH, et al. Familial occurrence of congenital colonic atresia. *J Pediatr.* 1981;99:435–436.

# 18.2 Ventral Wall Defects

Leann E. Linam

Ventral wall defects are commonly occurring malformations, seen in approximately 1 in 2,000 live births. This group of defects range from complex lethal anomalies that develop early in gestation, such as limb body wall complex (LBWC), and include pentalogy of Cantrell, ectopia cordis, bladder exstrophy, omphalocele, cloacal exstrophy, as well as the later occurring gastroschisis. Urachal anomalies can also be included in this classification as well. With appropriate prenatal evaluation, including maternal serum alpha-fetoprotein screening and ultrasound, many of these anomalies are successfully detected prenatally.

When evaluating a fetus sonographically, it is important to obtain views of the anterior abdominal wall and abdominal umbilical cord (UC) insertion (Fig. 18.2-1) and critical in avoiding missing small defects during screening exams.[1] Once identified, the malformation should be further categorized and associated

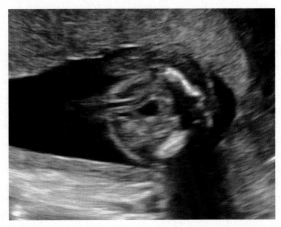

**FIGURE 18.2-1:** Normal cord insertion at 20 weeks, gestation. Transverse sonogram of the abdomen shows a normal insertion of the UC into the anterior abdominal wall.

anomalies searched for (Table 18.2-1). Fetal MRI can be useful in confirming the diagnosis and identifying additional abnormalities. Accurate diagnosis is important for parental counseling, pregnancy management, delivery planning, and prognosis.

| Table 18.2-1 | Typical Features of Ventral Wall Defects and Associated Conditions | | |
|---|---|---|---|
| **Type of Defect** | **Description** | **Sonographic Features** | **Associated Anomalies** |
| Gastroschisis | Paraumbilical defect | Typically, only bowel is eviscerated; occasionally other organs, rarely liver No membrane Defect to the right of cord insertion | Associated anomalies uncommon; low risk of aneuploidy; high rate of bowel-related complications |
| Omphalocele | Midline defect, contained by membrane | Large—extracorporeal liver Small—intracorporeal liver Membrane covered Central cord insertion | High risk of anomalies/aneuploidy; isolated extracorporeal liver—low risk of aneuploidy/high rate of cardiac anomalies; intracorporeal liver—greater than 50% risk of aneuploidy |
| Beckwith–Wiedemann syndrome | Syndromic | Macroglossia, omphalocele typically intracorporeal liver type, visceromegaly | Wilms tumor Hepatoblastoma |
| Pentalogy of Cantrell | (1) Omphalocele, (2) anterior diaphragmatic hernia, (3) distal partial sternal defect, (4) pericardial defect, (5) cardiac defect | High omphalocele; pleural effusion suggestive of diaphragmatic hernia | Cardiac defects |
| Ectopia cordis | Thoracic defect of sternum and skin | Ectopic heart not covered by skin | Cardiac defects; high omphalocele |
| Limb Body Wall Complex | Multiple anomalies | Complex ventral wall defect, close attachment to placenta, short umbilical cord scoliosis | Limb, spine, short umbilical cord, Lethal |

## EMBRYOLOGY

In the 3rd gestational week (menstrual week 5), the embryo is an elongated disc consisting of two cell layers (Fig. 18.2-2A).[2,3] Late in this week, gastrulation converts the two layers into the three germ cell layers (Fig. 18.2-3A): dorsally, the ectoderm will become the central nervous system, skin, and sensory organs; the mesoderm (middle layer) will become the skeletal system, heart and blood vessels, and urogenital system; ventrally, the endoderm becomes abdominal organs, including the gastrointestinal tract.[2] The process of gastrulation begins in the cranial portion of the embryo and proceeds caudally. As a region develops, the mesoderm layer divides into three types: paraxial, intermediate, and lateral plate mesoderm. The lateral plate mesoderm splits into two layers. The parietal mesoderm adheres to the ectoderm and becomes the body wall; the visceral mesoderm covers the gut tube and becomes the smooth muscle, and the visceral and parietal membranes that cover the surfaces of organs (Fig. 18.2-3).[2,3]

The parietal mesoderm, together with the ectoderm, makes up the lateral body folds. These folds grow ventrally (Figs. 18.2-3D and 18.2-4A), eventually fusing to become the ventral body wall.[2] This movement narrows the connection between the yolk sac and the ventral portion of the embryo to form the midgut (Fig. 18.2-4). The body stalk and the yolk stalk come together at 5 to 6 fetal weeks (7 to 8 menstrual weeks) to form the UC.

Development of the midgut is followed by rapid elongation of the gut and its mesentery, forming a primary intestinal loop.

This primary intestinal loop elongates so much that there is no room in the abdominal cavity for the contents, and the intestinal loop herniates into the base of the UC (Fig. 18.2-5).[4] Within the UC, the midgut loop rotates 90° counterclockwise around the axis of the superior mesenteric artery. During the 10th fetal week (12th menstrual week), the bowel begins to return to the abdomen, undergoing another 180° rotation during this return. During this time of physiologic gut herniation, it is possible to mistake this normal process for a ventral wall defect.

## GASTROSCHISIS

Gastroschisis is a full thickness defect in the umbilical wall that occurs lateral to the normally inserted UC (Fig. 18.2-6). This defect is nearly always to the right of the abdominal cord insertion, but left-sided defects have been reported.[5] The small intestine is typically herniated outside the abdominal cavity, and occasionally stomach, colon, and gonads are herniated as well. There is no covering membrane.[6]

**Incidence:** The incidence of gastroschisis is approximately 1 in 2,500 births.[7] Variability of prevalence is seen with maternal age, with the highest incidence being in younger women (1 in approximately 1,100 births for women under 20 years of age).[8] The incidence of gastroschisis has steadily increased worldwide since the first case was described in 1963,[9–12] suggesting a new environmental teratogen combining with behaviors of young mothers to produce the defect.[6]

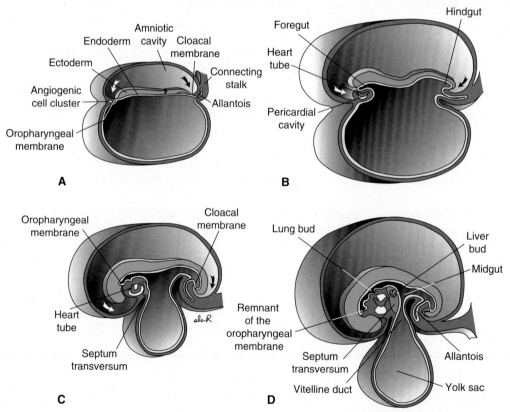

**FIGURE 18.2-2:** Sagittal sections through embryos at various stages of development demonstrating the effect of cephalocaudal and lateral folding on the position of the endoderm-lined cavity. Note formation of the foregut, midgut, and hindgut. **A:** Presomite embryo. **B:** Embryo with 7 somites. **C:** Embryo with 14 somites. **D:** At the end of the first month. (From Sadler TW. *Langman's Medical Embryology*. 12th ed. Philadelphia, PA: Lippincott Williams & Wilkins; 2012:87.)

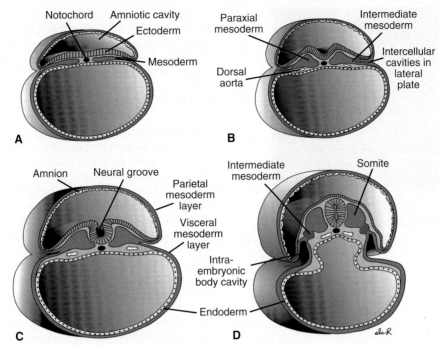

**FIGURE 18.2-3:** Transverse sections showing development of the mesodermal germ layer. **A:** Day 17. **B:** Day 19. **C:** Day 20. **D:** Day 21. The thin mesodermal sheet gives rise to paraxial mesoderm (future somites), intermediate mesoderm (future excretory units), and lateral plate, which is split into parietal and visceral mesoderm layers lining the intraembryonic cavity. (From Sadler TW. *Langman's Medical Embryology.* 12th ed. Philadelphia, PA: Lippincott Williams & Wilkins; 2012:71.)

**Embryology and Pathology:** There are many theories regarding the embryologic origin of gastroschisis. One hypothesis is that one or more of the folds responsible for closure of the abdominal wall fails. This prevents the yolk stalk from merging with the connecting stalk; part of the primary intestinal loop then herniates through this defect.[13] Other theories include the following:

■ Gastroschisis is the result of abnormal involution of the right umbilical vein.[14]
■ Disruption of the omphalomesenteric artery results in infarction of a portion of the abdominal wall.[15]
■ Embryonic mesenchyme fails to differentiate as the result of teratogenic exposure during the 4th week after conception.[16]

■ The amniotic membrane at the base of the UC ruptures as a result of delay in closure of the umbilical ring.[17]

Most cases of gastroschisis are sporadic, but rare cases of familial gastroschisis have been reported.[6] The cause of gastroschisis is unknown. Young maternal age is a risk factor in nearly every epidemiologic study conducted on gastroschisis. Behaviors typically found in younger mothers are also associated such as primigravida and short cohabitation time with the father and change in paternity.[6] Other risk factors include low socioeconomic status, low income, and poor nutrition. Maternal obesity is thought to be protective.

Because of the theory that gastroschisis is the result of vascular disruption, vasoactive drugs have been investigated as potential

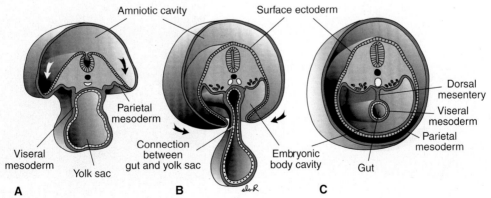

**FIGURE 18.2-4:** Cross sections through embryos at various stages of development to show the effect of lateral folding on the embryonic cavity. **A:** Folding is initiated. **B:** Transverse section through the midgut to show the connection between the gut and the yolk sac. **C:** Section just below the midgut to show the closed ventral abdominal wall and gut suspended from the dorsal abdominal wall by its mesentery. *Arrows,* lateral folds. (From Sadler TW. *Langman's Medical Embryology.* 12th ed. Philadelphia, PA: Lippincott Williams & Wilkins; 2012:79.)

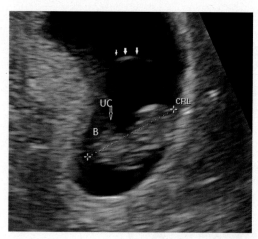

**FIGURE 18.2-5:** Normal gut migration. Longitudinal sonogram shows echogenic bowel *(B)* herniated into the base of the *UC.* The *small arrows* indicate amnion. Crown rump length (CRL) consistent with a 9-week gestation.

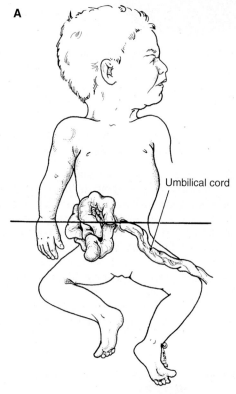

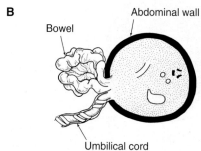

**FIGURE 18.2-6:** Typical features of gastroschisis shown on external examination **(A)** and on cross-sectional view **(B).** (From Hertzberg BS, Nyberg DA, Neilson IA. Ventral wall defects. In: Nyberg DA, McGahan JP, Pretorius DH, et al, eds. *Diagnostic Imaging of Fetal Anomalies.* Philadelphia, PA: Lippincott Williams & Wilkins; 2003:519–512.)

teratogens. However, acetaminophen and pseudoephedrine are the only two legal drugs implicated in the literature.[6] Illicit drugs, on the other hand, have been found to be significant risk factors for the development of gastroschisis, including cocaine, methamphetamines, and marijuana. Maternal smoking and alcohol consumption have been implicated in some studies, but not others.

**Diagnosis:** Although prenatal diagnosis of gastroschisis has not been shown to improve postnatal outcome,[18] accurate prenatal diagnosis allows for physicians to counsel families, adequately monitor the pregnancy, and prepare for transferring the infant to a pediatric specialty center for immediate treatment. Elevated alpha-fetoprotein in the second trimester is a diagnostic clue, which should lead the clinicians to perform a detailed ultrasound looking for specific structural anomalies. However, maternal serum alpha-fetoprotein is now only measured in women who do not undergo first trimester screening.[11] Thus, routine first and second trimester screening sonography has led to the detection of the majority of cases of gastroschisis.[19]

***Ultrasound:*** The classic sonographic appearance of gastroschisis is multiple loops of free-floating bowel herniating through a defect to the right of the UC insertion (Fig. 18.2-7). There is no surrounding membrane. The small bowel is uniformly involved; variable amounts of colon, the stomach, and the urinary bladder may also herniate into the amniotic fluid. The presence of eviscerated solid organs suggests a ruptured omphalocele or diagnosis other than gastroschisis.[20] Gastroschisis tends to be isolated, though a search for additional anomalies should always be performed.

Serial sonographic evaluation with amniotic fluid assessment is important in pregnancies with gastroschisis. These fetuses are at risk of intrauterine growth restriction, although this can be difficult to measure because of the herniated abdominal contents, resulting in a small abdominal circumference. Injury to the exposed bowel can occur. A fibrous peel may develop owing to a sterile inflammatory reaction to amniotic fluid. This causes the bowel to appear echogenic and thick-walled on ultrasound.[19] Sudden increase in echogenicity of the bowel or loss of peristaltic activity should be concerning for bowel ischemia.[21] Polyhydramnios may indicate the development of a bowel atresia.

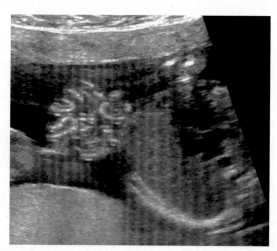

**FIGURE 18.2-7:** Gastroschisis at 19 weeks' GA. Transverse sonogram demonstrates bowel floating outside the abdomen with no covering membrane.

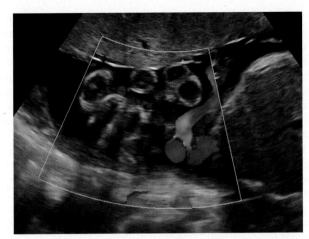

**FIGURE 18.2-8:** Gastroschisis at 32 weeks. Transverse Doppler sonogram shows the cord in color. The bowel is dilated with a thickened wall.

Mild bowel dilatation is commonly seen in gastroschisis and may be related to a difference in transmural pressure when it is outside the abdomen[21] (Fig. 18.2-8). It has been suggested that more severe bowel dilatation is an indicator of poor postnatal outcome, and multiple studies have undertaken to evaluate this further. There is no clear consensus, but recent studies have shown no statistically significant difference in outcome between gastroschisis with and without bowel thickening on prenatal ultrasound.[21–24] However, progressive dilation of the bowel with decreased peristalsis is considered a more reliable indicator of poor prognosis than bowel dilation alone.[25]

Occasionally, in severe cases, the extruded bowel can vanish completely. In these cases, the ventral wall defect may spontaneously close in utero ("vanishing gastroschisis" or "vanishing gut"). Often the remaining bowel within the abdomen is dilated and thickened with atretic portions.[26] It is thought that this vanishing gut and atresia is because of ischemia from a tight defect. These fetuses have an extremely poor prognosis.

*MRI:* As gastroschisis tends to be an isolated GI anomaly and well delineated by sonogram, MRI is not routinely recommended. Prenatal MRI does allow for improved soft tissue contrast and assessment of meconium. In addition, MRI has a larger field of view, allowing more detailed evaluation of complex anomalies. Single-shot rapid acquisition sequence with multiple 180° refocusing echoes should be obtained in the axial and sagittal planes. T1w images can assess for liver and meconium position. MR imaging shows free-floating bowel loops herniating through an abdominal wall defect to the right of an intact UC insertion[20] (Fig. 18.2-9). The abdominal wall defect can be visualized and bowel mucosa assessed.[27]

**Differential Diagnosis:** The major differential diagnosis of gastroschisis is a bowel-containing omphalocele. Other ventral wall defects such as LBWC, cloacal exstrophy, and pentalogy of Cantrell should be excluded. In omphalocele, the bowel has a peritoneal covering and the UC inserts at the base of the defect. LBWC often has herniated liver, characteristic cranial and limb defects, scoliosis and a short UC. Cloacal exstrophy is an infra-umbilical defect, with absent bladder.

**Prognosis:** Long-term prognosis for gastroschisis is generally excellent. Mortality rate has continually decreased, and survival now exceeds 90%.[11,19,28] Improved perinatal care, fetal monitoring, surgical management, and neonatal intensive care all contribute to the improved survival. The major causes of neonatal death in gastroschisis are bowel ischemia, necrotizing enterocolitis, sepsis, and liver failure.[28]

Fetal distress is common in fetuses with gastroschisis, and these pregnancies have a higher rate of third-trimester intrauterine fetal demise.[19] Fetal distress is hypothesized to arise from cord compression by extruded bowel,[29] but may also be related to oligohydramnios. Intrauterine growth restriction (IUGR) has been reported to affect 30% to 70% of fetuses.[11] Bowel dilatation may indicate a poor prognosis, but this is controversial and does not warrant early delivery at this time.

About 10% to 20% of newborns with gastroschisis have associated anomalies, predominantly involving the GI tract.[6] Bowel complications include intestinal atresia, stenosis, necrosis, and perforation. In the past, atresia has been the major determining prognostic factor, but patients with atresias can now do very well as long as the bowel is not irreversibly damaged.[30] Necrosis is usually related to a small abdominal wall defect that cuts off blood supply to the extruded bowel, and often results in short bowel syndrome.[30] Perforation can often be managed by resection and primary anastomosis.[30]

About 60% of infants are preterm (mean 35.7 weeks) and low birth weight (mean 2,492 g).[31] In general, most children with gastroschisis will have no long-term physical complications, and normal physical growth after 5 years of age.[31] Earlier studies suggested that infants with gastroschisis are at risk

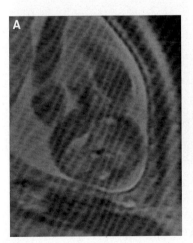
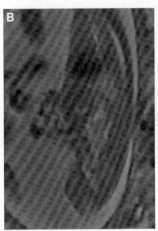

**FIGURE 18.2-9:** Gastroschisis at 26-week fetus. **A:** Axial MRI shows defect lateral to cord insertion. **B:** Sagittal MRI shows bowel outside the abdominal cavity with no covering membrane.

for developmental or neurologic abnormalities. Improved fetal monitoring has probably lowered these complications. Recent studies evaluating the neurodevelopmental outcomes in gastroschisis show increased utilization of early intervention services for neurodevelopmental delay when compared with the general population.[31,32] However, when gastroschisis patients were compared with nonsurgical preterm infants, rates of utilization were similar. Therefore, neurodevelopmental delay may be related to prematurity and low birth weight, not gastroschisis itself.

**Management:** The majority of fetuses with gastroschisis are detected in early second trimester with maternal serum AFP and sonogram. Once diagnosis is established, counseling should be performed by a multidisciplinary team that includes perinatologists, neonatologists, and pediatric surgeons. Assuming the pregnancy is continued, a targeted ultrasound including an echocardiogram should be performed, followed by serial sonograms and evaluation by a perinatologist. At each visit, fetal growth, amniotic fluid volume, bowel dilatation, bowel wall thickness, and peristalsis should be assessed.[25]

Animal research suggests that amnioinfusion with warm saline may reduce bowel inflammation.[33] The potential benefit of amnioinfusion is thought to be related to dilution of GI waste products that cause bowel wall damage. However, a recent study of amnioinfusion performed bimonthly in humans did not prevent bowel injury in gastroschisis.[34] This potential therapeutic option warrants further study.

The mode and timing of delivery for fetuses with gastroschisis is a source of debate. It is thought that much of the bowel injury occurs because of exposure to amniotic fluid in late pregnancy, suggesting that early delivery is beneficial. However, a randomized controlled trial comparing elective delivery at 36 weeks to spontaneous delivery at term showed no significant difference in neonatal outcomes,[35] and later retrospective studies support this finding.[36,37] In addition, preterm infants with gastroschisis are more likely to develop sepsis and have longer hospital courses than full-term infants with gastroschisis.[24] Cesarean section was originally thought to be the optimal mode of delivery of fetuses with gastroschisis, because it was thought that the bowel would undergo further trauma during vaginal delivery. Data have failed to show a difference in outcomes between vaginal delivery and caesarean section. A large proportion (up to 39% in two studies) is delivered via caesarean section because of fetal distress.[11] Immediately following delivery, appropriate fluid resuscitation should be initiated; high water losses can occur from evaporation through the exposed bowel (Fig. 18.2-10). The herniated bowel should be placed in a sterile covering, and the bowel should be placed in the midline of the abdomen to prevent kinking of the mesentery. Once the baby has been assessed and initial resuscitation performed, the abdominal wall defect should be assessed and treatment determined.

Primary closure of the abdominal wall defect has long been the standard of care. In this method, the bowel is reduced into the abdominal cavity, and a primary suture repair of the fascia is performed. When primary repair is performed, intra-abdominal or bladder pressure must be monitored during the procedure, as abdominal compartment syndrome can occur, causing intestinal and renal ischemia, as well as respiratory distress.

With the development of a preformed, spring-loaded silo, staged reduction with delayed primary suture closure has largely supplanted immediate primary closure in the management of gastroschisis.[38] In this method, a prefabricated silo with a circular spring is placed into the abdominal defect at the patient's bedside (Fig. 18.2-10). The bowel is reduced daily into the abdominal cavity, and the silo is sequentially shortened.[30] Multiple studies, predominantly retrospective, have undertaken to determine the most beneficial method of closure; the best level of evidence shows no survival difference between immediate closure and silo placement with delayed closure.[39] In addition, a CAPSnet study showed no difference in ventilation time, length of stay, or length of TPN.[39] One recent retrospective study showed that while preformed silo placement may be associated with decreased ventilation days and shorter time to full enteral feeds, this treatment method has a longer hospital stay.[38]

In 2004, a nonoperative technique was introduced, termed plastic closure. This closure method involves placement of a preformed silo, with sequential reduction of the intestines. Once the intestines are reduced, the defect is covered with the UC, and an occlusive plastic dressing is used. Two retrospective studies evaluating this closure technique[40,41] showed no statistically significant differences between plastic closure and suture closure with regard to length of stay, ventilation days, or time to feeding.

Following closure, infants with gastroschisis have abnormal intestinal motility and nutrient absorption, generally requiring

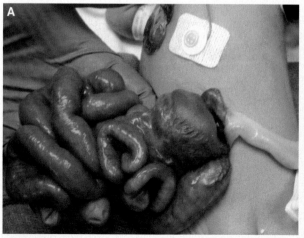
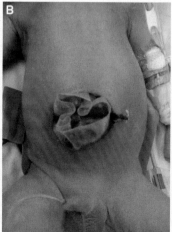
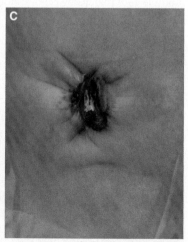

**FIGURE 18.2-10:** Newborn with gastroschisis. **A:** Immediately after birth. **B:** Bowel is completely reduced into the abdomen and suture closure has been performed. **C:** After closure with neo-umbilicus formation.

these infants to remain on total parenteral nutrition until bowel function returns. Although gastrointestinal dysmotility is often treated with prokinetic agents such as erythromycin, evidence in the literature does not support their use.[30] The median time of parenteral nutrition is in the range of 22 to 36 days, time to full oral feeding is 25 to 44 days, and median hospitalization time is 1 to 2 months.[19,35,38,42] However, patients with gastroschisis complicated by intestinal atresia or perforation may take significantly longer to achieve full feeds.

**Recurrence Risk:** Gastroschisis is typically sporadic, although occasional familial cases have been reported. A recent study summarizing all population-based studies of familial recurrence of gastroschisis (412 cases) suggests a 2.4% recurrence risk.[43]

## OMPHALOCELE

Omphalocele is a midline abdominal wall defect containing variable amounts of viscera that is covered by a membrane made up of peritoneum and amnion, and Wharton's jelly between the two layers. The UC inserts directly onto the membrane (Fig. 18.2-11).

**Incidence:** Omphalocele occurs in approximately 1 in 5,000 live births. This incidence increases to 1 in 1,100 if the incidence is based on 14 to 18 week fetuses.[44,45] These defects have a high rate of termination and still birth. The incidence of omphalocele increases with increasing maternal age.[7]

**Embryology and Pathology:** Physiologic herniation of the intestine occurs in the 6th to 10th gestational week; when the intestines fail to return to the abdominal cavity, an omphalocele results. The exact cause of this failure is incompletely understood, but is thought to result from a defect in lateral wall folding. If the defect predominantly involves the cranial folds, an epigastric omphalocele, as seen in pentalogy of Cantrell, results. If the defect involves the caudal fold, the omphalocele may be associated with bladder or cloacal exstrophy.[5]

A specific etiology for omphalocele has not been identified. Most cases are sporadic, but familial cases of omphalocele have been reported.[46] Risk factors for omphalocele include advanced maternal age, African American race, and maternal obesity. Teratogens have not been implicated in the etiology of omphalocele.

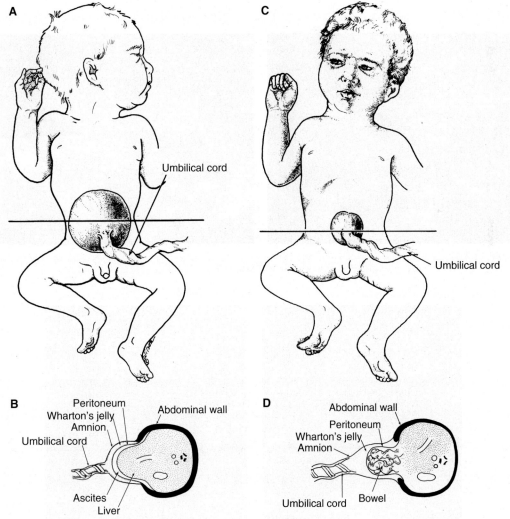

**FIGURE 18.2-11: A,B:** Omphalocele with typical features of extracorporeal liver. **C,D:** Typical features of omphalocele with intracorporeal liver. (From Hertzberg BS, Nyberg DA, Neilson IA. Ventral wall defects. In: Nyberg DA, McGahan JP, Pretorius DH, et al, eds. *Diagnostic Imaging of Fetal Anomalies*. Philadelphia, PA: Lippincott Williams & Wilkins; 2003:519–520.)

Omphalocele is frequently associated with chromosomal anomalies, predominantly trisomy 13, 18, and 21. These chromosomal anomalies are also associated with advanced maternal age. Other genetic variations identified include mutations in the PITX2 protein, which is thought to be responsible for Axenfeld–Rieger syndrome (congenital malformations of the face, teeth, and skeletal system). A mutation in the CDKN1C gene, which encodes a kinase inhibitor, has also been associated with omphalocele; this mutation is often diagnosed in Beckwith–Wiedemann syndrome (macroglossia, macrosomia, midline abdominal wall defects, ear creases or ear pits, and neonatal hypoglycemia). Autosomal dominant and x-linked forms of omphalocele have also been reported.[6]

### Diagnosis

*Ultrasound:* Current sensitivity of prenatal ultrasound in the diagnosis of omphalocele is 75%.[47] The ultrasound appearance of omphalocele is variable. Size can range from a small umbilical hernia to a giant omphalocele greater than 5 cm. Eviscerated organs can vary; ascites may be present, and there is a range of associated anomalies. Therefore, it is important to keep in mind those features that reliably diagnose omphalocele and differentiate omphalocele from gastroschisis.

Omphalocele is a central abdominal wall defect, located at the base of the UC. The cord typically inserts on the apex of the defect.[48] This can be demonstrated in transverse images, but sagittal imaging may also be helpful in demonstrating the cord insertion (Fig. 18.2-12). Observing the intrahepatic umbilical vein coursing through the defect can also be helpful in confirming the central location of the defect.

A surrounding membrane is another characteristic unique to omphalocele. However, the membrane may be difficult to visualize or may rupture in utero. If the membrane is present, but unapparent, its presence can be inferred by the eviscerated organs appearing contained rather than freely floating. The presence of ascites is also a helpful indicator of omphalocele[49] (Fig. 18.2-13). The membrane covering the omphalocele allows fluid to accumulate within the peritoneal cavity; this fluid can also help delineate the covering membrane on ultrasound. However, a large amount of ascites may be confused for amniotic fluid and misdiagnosis of gastroschisis can be made; in distinction to gastroschisis, the bowel within an omphalocele will not be thickened or dilated.

Approximately 80% of prenatally diagnosed omphaloceles contain liver[45] (Fig. 18.2-14). Liver is never seen outside the abdominal cavity during normal development, so omphalocele with extracorporeal liver can be diagnosed at any gestational age.

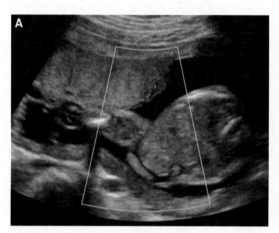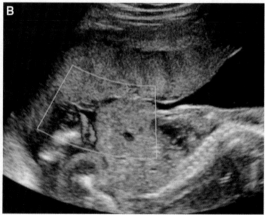

**FIGURE 18.2-12:** Omphalocele. **(A)** Transverse and **(B)** Sagittal color Doppler ultrasound images of 23-week fetus with omphalocele demonstrating cord insertion at the base of the defect *(color)*.

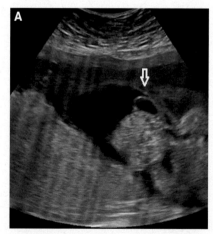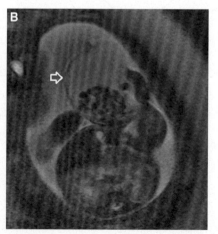

**FIGURE 18.2-13:** Omphalocele with ascites. Transverse ultrasound **(A)** and axial MRI **(B)** of omphalocele with ascites. The membrane *(arrow)* is delineated by the fluid on both sides.

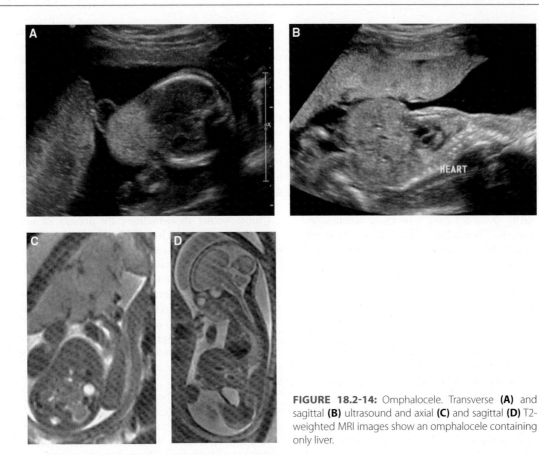

**FIGURE 18.2-14:** Omphalocele. Transverse **(A)** and sagittal **(B)** ultrasound and axial **(C)** and sagittal **(D)** T2-weighted MRI images show an omphalocele containing only liver.

Liver has a homogeneous sonographic appearance, and hepatic vessels can be demonstrated within it. The amount of extruded liver and size of the defect are variable, but an omphalocele is generally termed "giant" when the majority of the liver is extraabdominal.[45] There is no strict definition for giant omphaloceles.

Polyhydramnios has been associated with omphalocele in approximately 10% of cases.[50] Although the etiology is unclear, it is associated with a more complicated postnatal course.[49]

***MRI:*** As omphalocele is frequently associated with other anomalies, MRI may be useful for improved delineation of associated anomalies. On MRI, an omphalocele appears as a central abdominal wall defect. The viscera can be seen herniating into a membrane-covered sac.[20] Liver is easily distinguished from bowel on MRI as opposed to ultrasound (Fig. 18.2-15).

MRI is useful in evaluating the size of the abdominal wall defect. In addition, MRI shows promise as a predictor of pulmonary hypoplasia.[51] A study by Danzer et al. measured total lung volume in fetuses with omphalocele and compared this as a ratio to the expected lung volume based on age-matched nomograms, and found that fetuses with giant omphalocele had significantly lower than expected lung volumes compared with age-matched nomograms. In addition, they found that a ratio less than 50% predicted a more complicated postnatal/postrepair course.[51]

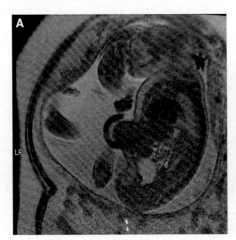
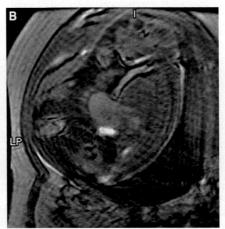

**FIGURE 18.2-15:** Omphalocele Sagittal T2w **(A)** and T1w **(B)** images of a fetus with omphalocele containing liver. The cord inserts onto the base of the defect.

**Differential Diagnosis:** Because the ultrasound appearance of omphalocele is variable, they can be difficult to distinguish from other types of ventral wall defects. When the liver is within the defect, the main differential is LBWC. At least two of the typical findings of LBWC must be present to make the diagnosis. These include anterior body wall defect, limb defect, exencephaly, and/or encephalocele. Additional findings of LBWC that may be seen are kyphoscoliosis, short or single-artery UC, neural tube defects, GU malformations, chest wall, lung, and/or diaphragm abnormalities.[52]

If the liver is not extracorporeal and only bowel is eviscerated, then the differential considerations include gastroschisis and umbilical hernia. The gastroschisis defect is located to the right of the umbilicus, does not have a covering membrane, and ascites is not present.[30] A small omphalocele may be more difficult to distinguish from an umbilical hernia since both defects are located in the midline at the abdominal cord insertion site. An umbilical hernia is a defect only in the abdominal wall muscles; therefore, the intestine protrudes only into the base of the UC, and the defect is covered by skin as well as a membrane.[53] An omphalocele defect is covered only by a membrane.

Simple omphalocele should be differentiated from other complex syndromes, which may include omphalocele. Pentalogy of Cantrell, a defect in the cephalic fold, includes not only omphalocele, but also diaphragmatic defect, sternal cleft, pericardial defect, and cardiovascular malformations (see section on pentalogy of Cantrell later in this chapter). Cloacal exstrophy is a defect of the caudal fold; this includes a low ventral wall defect associated with bladder or cloacal exstrophy.

Occasionally, a false-positive diagnosis of omphalocele, or pseudo-omphalocele, may occur. Two clinical settings may cause this appearance. The first is in the setting of oligohydramnios; the uterine wall causes the fetal abdominal wall to elongate anterior–posterior and narrow transverse, giving the appearance of herniated abdominal contents. The second setting is when the fetal abdomen is wedged in the uterus, in direct contact with the myometrium or placenta. The angle between the abdominal wall and the defect in these two settings should be an obtuse angle, as opposed to an acute angle in a true omphalocele.[54]

**Prognosis:** Prognosis of omphalocele depends on primarily the presence and severity of associated anomalies. Approximately 70% of fetuses with omphalocele have additional malformations.[8] Musculoskeletal malformations are seen in 23%, including clubfoot, polydactyly, limb deficiency, and vertebral anomalies. Urinary anomalies comprise approximately 17% of associated malformations and include renal agenesis, polycystic kidney, hydronephrosis, ureteral anomalies, and vesicoureteral reflux. Approximately 15% of patients with omphalocele have associated heart defects, including ventricular septal defect, tetralogy of Fallot, and dextrocardia. Anomalies of the bowel are less common than gastroschisis, but are seen in approximately 10% of cases. Central nervous system anomalies can also be present. Other less common anomalies include diaphragmatic hernias, facial anomalies, and genital and pulmonary abnormalities.[8]

Chromosomal abnormalities are present in up to 30% of omphalocele cases.[5,8] The most common chromosomal abnormalities are trisomy 18 (68%) and trisomy 13 (20%). The risk of chromosomal abnormalities is increased when the liver is not within the omphalocele sac.[55]

Beckwith–Wiedemann syndrome, a complicated genetic condition that can involve 11p15 deletion or mutations in the CDKN1C gene, is also associated with omphalocele.[56] This is defined as a large-for-gestational-age fetus with omphalocele and macroglossia.[56] These infants also have early hypoglycemia, and increased risk of Wilms tumor, hepatoblastoma, and neuroblastoma in childhood.[5]

Many studies have been performed to evaluate the size of omphalocele and contents of omphalocele sac in relation to prognosis. Small omphaloceles generally have intracorporeal liver. Both of these designations have been found to have a higher association with chromosomal anomalies.[55] However, extracorporeal liver and larger defects are associated with a poorer prognosis.[55,57,58]

Giant omphalocele is generally defined as a defect larger than 5 cm, but there is no universal consensus on this definition (Fig. 18.2-16). In addition, the size can change as the fetus grows in gestation. In a study in 2011, Montero et al.[59] suggested a standard that is based on a ratio of the omphalocele size to the head circumference (O/HC ratio). In this study, they found that an O/HC ratio less than 0.21 predicts inability to achieve primary closure of the defect. In addition, they found that this ratio was a better predictor of prognosis than the measurement of the defect alone.[59] Giant omphalocele is associated with a poorer prognosis, with 75% developing respiratory insufficiency in the first 24 hours of life; these children have narrow chest width and smaller lung areas and can have long-term pulmonary issues

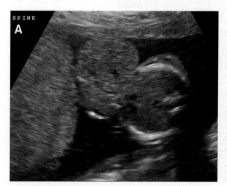
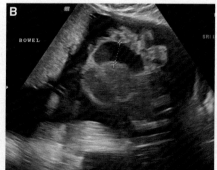
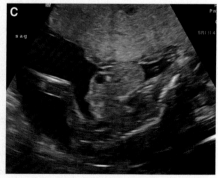

**FIGURE 18.2-16:** Giant omphalocele. Transverse **(A,B)** and sagittal **(C)** ultrasound images of a fetus show a giant omphalocele that contains liver, stomach, and bowel. The bowel is dilated **(B).** Some of the bowel appears free-floating, suggesting rupture of the membrane.

such as asthma.[57] Pregnancies with giant omphalocele can be complicated by polyhydramnios, indicating a more complicated postnatal course.[57]

**Management:** When a diagnosis of omphalocele is made prenatally, further evaluation is required. A detailed ultrasound evaluation should be performed to evaluate other structural abnormalities. Given the frequency of major cardiac defects, a fetal echocardiogram should also be performed. The patient should be offered chromosomal analysis.[5,60] Serial ultrasounds are recommended, as these fetuses can be at increased risk of IUGR and polyhydramnios.[5,30,60]

Delivery at a tertiary care center at or near term is recommended. Mode of delivery is controversial, and neither vaginal delivery nor caesarean section has been shown to be superior.[30,45,60] However, caesarian section is usually performed for large omphaloceles to prevent rupture or dystocia of the omphalocele sac or trauma to the visceral contents of the sac.[60]

Following delivery, cardiopulmonary status should be carefully assessed; these infants may have unsuspected pulmonary hypoplasia or a cardiac defect requiring immediate intubation and ventilation.[30,60] The UC should be cut generously, as abdominal contents may protrude further into the cord than appreciated.[60] The omphalocele should be covered with saline gauze or other nonadherent dressing until the infant is stabilized and further assessment is possible (Fig. 18.2-17).

The method of closure of omphalocele is dependent upon the size of the defect. If the defect is small, primary closure can be performed. However, in large defects, primary closure can cause increased abdominal pressure because of the small size of the peritoneal cavity[30]; this increased pressure, if not relieved, can lead to abdominal compartment syndrome, with bowel necrosis, respiratory compromise, and loss of blood flow to kidneys and liver.[30] When the defect is too large to accomplish primary closure, either a staged or delayed closure can be performed. There are multiple reported staged techniques: reduction using a pressure dressing, prosthetic silo placement with gradual reduction, as in gastroschisis, vacuum-assisted closure,[61] tissue expanders,[62] and other types of mesh to close the defect.

Nonsurgical delayed closure is often employed when the defect is large and the infant is not stable enough to undergo surgical repair of the defect.[60] This technique is referred to as "paint and wait." Several different substances have been employed in this technique: mercurochrome, povidone–iodine,

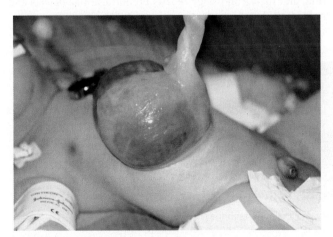

**FIGURE 18.2-17:** Newborn with omphalocele.

silver sulfadiazine, and neomycin–bacitracin ointments. Silver sulfadiazine is currently the most widely used agent. It is inexpensive and requires only daily application, and associated with very little toxicity.[63]

**Recurrence Risk:** Omphalocele is typically sporadic, although occasional familial cases have been reported. Syndromic forms of omphalocele are typically associated with chromosomal abnormalities, including trisomy 13, 18, and 21. Beckwith–Wiedemann syndrome has a mutation in the CDKN1C gene. Isolated omphalocele should be considered to have a low recurrence risk; syndromic omphalocele recurrence is that of the chromosomal abnormality.

## CLEFT STERNUM, ECTOPIA CORDIS, PENTALOGY OF CANTRELL

Cleft sternum, ectopia cordis, and pentalogy of Cantrell share a defect of the sternum. Cleft sternum has partial or absent sternum without ectopia. In true ectopia cordis, only the heart is displaced outside of the thoracic cavity and lacks pericardial coverage.[64] Pentalogy of Cantrell includes a midline, supraumbilical abdominal wall defect; defect of the lower sternum; deficiency of the anterior diaphragm; defect in the diaphragmatic pericardium; and congenital intracardiac defects.[65]

**Incidence:** All are rare. Ectopia cordis occurs in approximately 5.5 to 7.9 per million live births.[66] Pentalogy of Cantrell occurs in fewer than five per million live births.[67]

**Embryology and Pathology:** The embryological defect is poorly understood; the most common theory is that a defect in the maturation of midline mesodermal components causes failure of fusion of the cephalic lateral body folds. These abnormal midline mesodermal components include failure of the transverse septum to develop, causing a diaphragmatic hernia, and abnormal development of myocardium, resulting in heart defects.

Ectopia cordis can also result from amniotic band syndrome.[68] The normal descent of the heart is interrupted by mechanical compression from tissue bands in thoracic ectopia cordis; tethering of the heart to paraumbilical structures is thought to be a cause of thoracoabdominal ectopia cordis.[68]

There is a weak association with trisomy 18, and x-linked recessive cases have been reported.[69] Teratogenesis can occur with amniotic bands.

### Diagnosis
#### Ultrasound
*Pentalogy of Cantrell*: Early prenatal diagnosis of pentalogy of Cantrell is possible. The primary finding on ultrasound is a supraumbilical omphalocele.[70] A pericardial effusion is an indicator of diaphragmatic pericardial defects, and pleural effusion may signal an associated anterior diaphragmatic hernia.[70,71] The pericardial effusion may be transient. Other anomalies associated with pentalogy of Cantrell include cleft lip/palate, encephalocele, hydrocephalus, limb defects, gallbladder agenesis, and polysplenia[71] (Fig. 18.2-18). Echocardiograms are important to assess the complexity of cardiac anomalies.

*Ectopiac ordis:* The heart is identified by ultrasound as either complete or partially displaced outside the thoracic cavity with lack of skin covering. Classification is based on the location of the heart and is divided into cervical, cervicothoracic, thoracic,

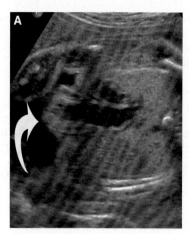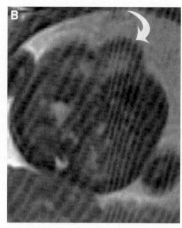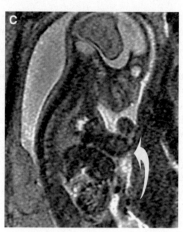

**FIGURE 18.2-18:** Pentalogy of Cantrell. **A:** Ultrasound shows left ventricle protruding through a defect in the sternum *(arrow)*. Axial SSFP **(B)** and sagittal T2w **(C)** MRI demonstrates heart protruding outside the chest *(arrow)*.

and thoracoabdominal. Displacement may be only partial or may be transient[70] (Fig. 18.2-19). Cardiac anomalies can be complex.

*Cleft sternum:* The anterior chest wall is dynamic when the sternum is absent. The heart may appear to protrude through the chest, yet the chest wall is intact.

**MRI:** MRI provides soft tissue differentiation and can delineate the extent of the thoracoabdominal defect.[72] The diaphragmatic defects should be searched for, but may be difficult to detect if small. Lung volumes can be calculated (Figs. 18.2-21).

**Differential Diagnosis:** The major differential consideration for ectopia cordis and pentalogy of Cantrell is amniotic band syndrome. This syndrome is heterogeneous in presentation and can cause a broad range of abnormalities.[73] The characteristic finding in amniotic band syndrome is echogenic bands that attach to the fetus.[73] Other differentials include LBWC and omphalocele.

**Prognosis:** Cervical and cervicothoracic forms of ectopia cordis are considered fatal.[66] Thoracic, or true ectopia cordis is associated with a poor prognosis. Survivors tend to have limited intracardiac defects.[64,66] Abdominal ectopia cordis, or displacement of the heart into the abdomen, has a better prognosis, and often does not require surgery to survive.[66]

Thoracoabdominal ectopia cordis is the classification associated with pentalogy of Cantrell, and is the most common form of cardiac displacement. Overall survival rate is approximately 50%,[66,68] and is dependent on the severity of the cardiac and associated malformations. Cardiac defects include ventricular septal defect (100%), atrial septal defect (53%), tetralogy of Fallot (20%), and left ventricular diverticulum (20%).[66,68] There have been reports of hypoplastic left heart syndrome[74] and tricuspid atresia.[75] A review in 2008 by van Hoorn et al.[71] found that prognosis is worse in complete pentalogy, isolated ectopia cordis, and patients with non–cardiac-associated anomalies. This review did not find cardiac defects to affect prognosis.

**Management:** Following prenatal diagnosis, a detailed ultrasound and echocardiogram should be performed to evaluate for associated anomalies and cardiac defects. Delivery should be performed by caesarean section to avoid compression of the exposed heart during labor.[68] Routine resuscitation of the neonate should be performed, beginning with airway management. These neonates are more likely to have pulmonary hypoplasia because of the chest wall defect and possible diaphragmatic hernia.[68]

Milder cases can be repaired in a single stage, but two- or three-stage repair is common.[66,68] In general, symptomatic cardiac anomalies should be corrected first. The exception is in cases of complete thoracoabdominal ectopia, because of the lack of skin coverage of the heart.[66] In this case, the first stage provides soft tissue coverage of the heart and hemodynamic palliation, and the second stage repairs the intracardiac defects and reduces the heart into the thoracic cavity.[64,66,68]

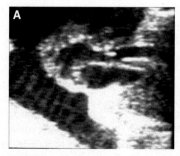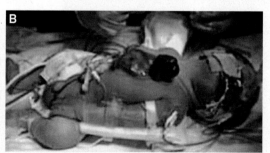

**FIGURE 18.2-19:** Ectopia cordis. **A:** Transverse ultrasound image through the chest demonstrates the heart protruding through a thoracic wall defect. There was no associated omphalocele. **B:** Postnatal image of the infant demonstrating the ectopic heart.

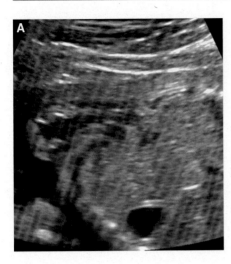
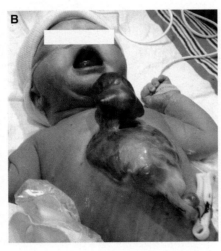

**FIGURE 18.2-20:** Thoracoabdominal ectopia cordis. **A:** Transverse ultrasound image at 25 weeks' gestation demonstrates the heart protruding into the amniotic fluid. **B:** Postnatal image of thoracoabdominal ectopia cordis. (Courtesy of Renee Bornemeier.)

**Recurrence Risk:** Sporadic, there is no known genetic origin, making the recurrence risk low.[68]

## LIMB–BODY WALL COMPLEX, BODY STALK ANOMALY

LBWC is a complex congenital defect that includes at least two of the following three abnormalities: neural tube defect (exencephaly, encephalocele, myelomeningocele); thoraco and/or abdominoschisis; limb anomalies. Body stalk anomaly includes a large abdominal defect, absent or abnormal UC, and severe kyphoscoliosis. These two anomalies overlap and can be considered two points on a spectrum.

**Incidence:** The incidence of LBWC is estimated at 1 in 14,000 to 1 in 31,000 live births.[76] However, in a study of 106,727 cases of 10-to-14-week pregnancies, the prevalence was approximately 1 in 7,500 pregnancies, suggesting a high spontaneous abortion and planned termination rate.

**Embryology and Pathology:** There is no known genetic anomaly. Embryology is poorly understood. Three hypotheses have been proposed, but none of these has been supported in animal studies. These hypotheses include the following:

- The amniotic band theory: In this theory, it is postulated that the amnion ruptures before the obliteration of the celomic cavity. The lower half of the fetal body then passes into the celomic cavity through the defect in the amniotic sac, causing the abdominal and spinal defects.[77–79] However, this theory does not explain the coexistent internal defects seen in the majority of cases.[79]
- The theory of vascular disruption: A vascular disturbance causes a general disruption of blood supply during embryogenesis. This causes failure of closure of ventral abdominal wall and persistence of celomic cavity.[77,79]
- The theory of abnormal embryonic folding: In this theory, LBWC is the result of faulty folding in the cephalic, lateral, and caudal axes.[77]

There have been two cases reported in which the mother abused cocaine.[80] One case has been reported after in vitro fertilization and embryo transfer.[81] A single case has been reported with antiepileptic use during pregnancy.[82]

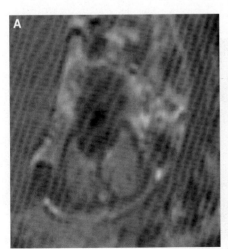
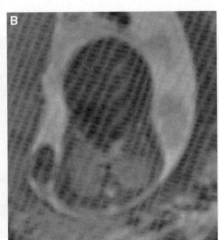
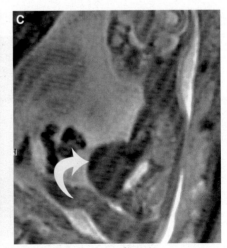

**FIGURE 18.2-21:** Pentalogy of Cantrell. **A.** Axial MR image of the thorax shows thoracic defect with ectopic heart. **B.** Axial MR image at the level of the chest shows the defect with ectopic heart. **C.** Sagittal MR image shows heart and liver protruding through thoracoabdominal defect *(arrow)*.

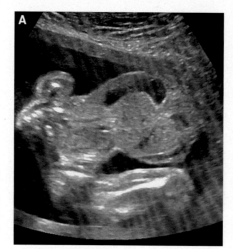
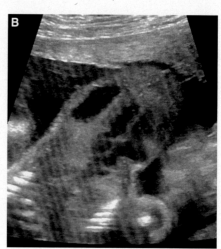

**FIGURE 18.2-22:** Limb Body Wall Complex. **A.** Axial ultrasound images at 23 wks GA show large membrane covered anterior midline thoracoabdominal wall defect containing liver and stomach. **B.** A majority of the heart is external as well. The defect is in close approximation to the placenta.

### Diagnosis

***Ultrasound:*** Prenatal ultrasound findings include abdominal wall defect, scoliosis, attachment of the head or body to the placenta, limb reduction anomalies, and short or two-vessel (or both) UC.[83] The body wall defect is eccentric and typically large; left-sided defects are much more common.[48] Three-dimensional (3D) ultrasound can be helpful in differentiating the abdominal wall defect from other forms of ventral wall defects by showing adjacent structures in relation to the defect[84] (Fig. 18.2-22).

***MRI:*** MRI can be helpful in further delineating the associated anomalies and providing a large field of view. MRI will show an abnormally located placenta often directly adjacent to the fetus.[20] The herniated abdominal organs are well delineated (Fig. 18.2-23). Amniotic bands may be seen.[20]

**Differential Diagnosis:** The major differential consideration is amniotic band syndrome. This syndrome is heterogeneous in presentation and can cause a broad range of abnormalities.[73] The characteristic finding in amniotic band syndrome is echogenic bands that attach to the fetus.[73]

Pentalogy of Cantrell and OEIS (omphaloceles-exstrophy of the bladder-imperforate anus-spinal defects) should be

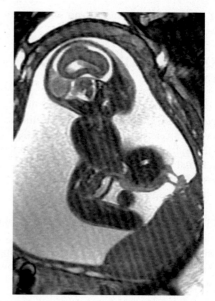

**FIGURE 18.2-23:** LBWC at 23 weeks' gestation. Sagittal T2-weighted T2w MR image demonstrates a large membrane-covered anterior midline thoracoabdominal wall defect containing liver and bowel. There is kyphoscoliosis. The umbilical cord is short.

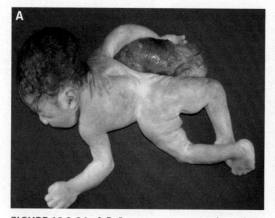
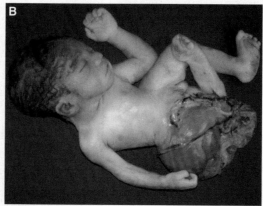

**FIGURE 18.2-24: A,B:** Postmortem images of an infant with LBWC. The ventral wall is plastered to the placenta. Note the limb anomalies and kyphosis.

included in the differential. Bladder exstrophy should be suspected if there is non-visualization of the fetal urinary bladder, and the expected T1-weighted hyperintensity of meconium late in gestation will be absent if a cloacal anomaly allows for mixing of urine and meconium.

**Prognosis and Management:** LBWC is lethal (Fig. 18.2-24). Many pregnancies spontaneously terminate.[77] Many patients choose to terminate electively. Management is supportive following delivery.

**Recurrence Risk:** The majority of cases of LBWC are sporadic. The development of this disorder has been associated with the use of the cigarette smoking, alcohol use, and illicit drug use.[82,85]

## REFERENCES

1. American Institute of Ultrasound Medicine. *AIUM Practice Guideline for the Performance of Obstetric Ultrasound Examinations.* Laurel, MD: American Institute of Ultrasound Medicine; 2007.
2. Sadler TW. The embryologic origin of ventral body wall defects. *Semin Pediatr Surg.* 2010;19(3):209–214.
3. Sadler TW, Feldkamp ML. The embryology of body wall closure: relevance to gastroschisis and other ventral body wall defects. *Am J Med Genet C Semin Med Genet.* 2008;148C(3):180–185.
4. Sadler TW. *Langman's Medical Embryology.* 12th ed. Baltimore, MD: Lippincott Williams & Wilkins; 2012.
5. Ledbetter DJ. Congenital abdominal wall defects and reconstruction in pediatric surgery: gastroschisis and omphalocele. *Surg Clin North Am.* 2012;92(3):713–727.
6. Frolov P, Alali J, Klein MD. Clinical risk factors for gastroschisis and omphalocele in humans: a review of the literature. *Pediatr Surg Int.* 2010;26(12):1135–1148.
7. Bird TM, Robbins JM, Druschel C, et al. Demographic and environmental risk factors for gastroschisis and omphalocele in the National Birth Defects Prevention Study. *J Pediatr Surg.* 2009;44(8):1546–1551.
8. Stoll C, Alembik Y, Dott B, et al. Omphalocele and gastroschisis and associated malformations. *Am J Med Genet A.* 2008;146A(10):1280–1285.
9. Collins SR, Griffin MR, Arbogast PG, et al. The rising prevalence of gastroschisis and omphalocele in Tennessee. *J Pediatr Surg.* 2007;42(7):1221–1224.
10. Fillingham A, Rankin J. Prevalence, prenatal diagnosis and survival of gastroschisis. *Prenat Diagn.* 2008;28(13):1232–1237.
11. Holland AJ, Walker K, Badawi N. Gastroschisis: an update. *Pediatr Surg Int.* 2010;26(9):871–878.
12. Mastroiacovo P, Lisi A, Castilla EE, et al. Gastroschisis and associated defects: an international study. *Am J Med Genet A.* 2007;143(7):660–671.
13. Feldkamp ML, Carey JC, Sadler TW. Development of gastroschisis: review of hypotheses, a novel hypothesis, and implications for research. *Am J Med Genet A.* 2007;143(7):639–652.
14. deVries PA. The pathogenesis of gastroschisis and omphalocele. *J Pediatr Surg.* 1980;15(3):245–251.
15. Hoyme HE, Higginbottom MC, Jones KL. The vascular pathogenesis of gastroschisis: intrauterine interruption of the omphalomesenteric artery. *J Pediatr.* 1981;98(2):228–231.
16. Duhamel B. Embryology of exomphalos and allied malformations. *Arch Dis Child.* 1963;38(198):142–147.
17. Shaw A. The myth of gastroschisis. *J Pediatr Surg.* 1975;10(2):235–244.
18. Murphy FL, Mazlan TA, Tarheen F, et al. Gastroschisis and exomphalos in Ireland 1998–2004: does antenatal diagnosis impact on outcome? *Pediatr Surg Int.* 2007;23(11):1059–1063.
19. David AL, Tan A, Curry J. Gastroschisis: sonographic diagnosis, associations, management and outcome. *Prenat Diagn.* 2008;28(7):633–644.
20. Daltro P, Fricke BL, Kline-Fath BM, et al. Prenatal MRI of congenital abdominal and chest wall defects. *AJR Am J Roentgenol.* 2005;184(3):1010–1016.
21. Badillo AT, Hedrick HL, Wilson RD, et al. Prenatal ultrasonographic gastrointestinal abnormalities in fetuses with gastroschisis do not correlate with postnatal outcomes. *J Pediatr Surg.* 2008;43(4):647–653.
22. Long AM, Court J, Morabito A, et al. Antenatal diagnosis of bowel dilatation in gastroschisis is predictive of poor postnatal outcome. *J Pediatr Surg.* 2011;46(6):1070–1075.
23. Payne NR, Pfleghaar K, Assel B, et al. Predicting the outcome of newborns with gastroschisis. *J Pediatr Surg.* 2009;44(5):918–923.
24. Wilson MS, Carroll MA, Braun SA, et al. Is preterm delivery indicated in fetuses with gastroschisis and antenatally detected bowel dilation? *Fetal Diagn Ther.* 2012;32:262–266.
25. Vegunta RK, Wallace LJ, Leonardi MR, et al. Perinatal management of gastroschisis: analysis of a newly established clinical pathway. *J Pediatr Surg.* 2005;40(3):528–534.
26. Tawil A, Comstock CH, Chang CH. Prenatal closure of abdominal defect in gastroschisis: case report and review of the literature. *Pediatr Dev Pathol.* 2001;4(6):580–584.
27. Tonni G, Pattaccini P, Ventura A, et al. The role of ultrasound and antenatal single-shot fast spin-echo MRI in the evaluation of herniated bowel in case of first trimester ultrasound diagnosis of fetal gastroschisis. *Arch Gynecol Obstet.* 2011;283(4):903–908.
28. Bradnock TJ, Marven S, Owen A, et al. Gastroschisis: one year outcomes from national cohort study. *BMJ.* 2011;343:d6749.
29. Kalache KD, Bierlich A, Hammer H, et al. Is unexplained third trimester intrauterine death of fetuses with gastroschisis caused by umbilical cord compression due to acute extra-abdominal bowel dilatation? *Prenat Diagn.* 2002;22(8):715–717.
30. Christison-Lagay ER, Kelleher CM, Langer JC. Neonatal abdominal wall defects. *Semin Fetal Neonatal Med.* 2011;16(3):164–172.
31. Gorra AS, Needelman H, Azarow KS, et al. Long-term neurodevelopmental outcomes in children born with gastroschisis: the tiebreaker. *J Pediatr Surg.* 2012;47(1):125–129.
32. Needelman H, Jackson BJ, McMorris C. Referral for early intervention services in late preterm infants with a NICU experience. *J Neonatal Perinat Med.* 2008(1):169–174.
33. Luton D, de Lagausie P, Guibourdenche J, et al. Influence of amnioinfusion in a model of in utero created gastroschisis in the pregnant ewe. *Fetal Diagn Ther.* 2000;15(4):224–228.
34. Midrio P, Stefanutti G, Mussap M, et al. Amnioexchange for fetuses with gastroschisis: is it effective? *J Pediatr Surg.* 2007;42(5):777–782.
35. Logghe HL, Mason GC, Thornton JG, et al. A randomized controlled trial of elective preterm delivery of fetuses with gastroschisis. *J Pediatr Surg.* 2005;40(11):1726–1731.
36. Ergün O, Barksdale E, Ergün FS, et al. The timing of delivery of infants with gastroschisis influences outcome. *J Pediatr Surg.* 2005;40(2):424–428.
37. Henrich K, Huemmer HP, Reingruber B, et al. Gastroschisis and omphalocele: treatments and long-term outcomes. *Pediatr Surg Int.* 2008;24(2):167–173.
38. Weil BR, Leys CM, Rescorla FJ. The jury is still out: changes in gastroschisis management over the last decade are associated with both benefits and shortcomings. *J Pediatr Surg.* 2012;47(1):119–124.
39. Mortellaro VE, St Peter SD, Fike FB, et al. Review of the evidence on the closure of abdominal wall defects. *Pediatr Surg Int.* 2011;27(4):391–397.
40. Bonnard A, Zamakhshary M, de Silva N, et al. Non-operative management of gastroschisis: a case-matched study. *Pediatr Surg Int.* 2008;24(7):767–771.
41. Orion KC, Krein M, Liao J, et al. Outcomes of plastic closure in gastroschisis. *Surgery.* 2011;150(2):177–185.
42. Bucher BT, Mazotas IG, Warner BW, et al. Effect of time to surgical evaluation on the outcomes of infants with gastroschisis. *J Pediatr Surg.* 2012;47(6):1105–1110.
43. Kohl M, Wiesel A, Schier F. Familial recurrence of gastroschisis: literature review and data from the population-based birth registry "Mainz Model." *J Pediatr Surg.* 2010;45(9):1907–1912.
44. Islam S. Advances in surgery for abdominal wall defects: gastroschisis and omphalocele. *Clin Perinatol.* 2012;39(2):375–386.
45. Wilson RD, Johnson MP. Congenital abdominal wall defects: an update. *Fetal Diagn Ther.* 2004;19(5):385–398.
46. Port-Lis M, Leroy C, Manouvrier S, et al. A familial syndromal form of omphalocele. *Eur J Med Genet.* 2011;54(3):337–340.
47. Barisic I, Clementi M, Hausler M, et al. Evaluation of prenatal ultrasound diagnosis of fetal abdominal wall defects by 19 European registries. *Ultrasound Obstet Gynecol.* 2001;18(4):309–316.
48. Emanuel PG, Garcia GI, Angtuaco TL. Prenatal detection of anterior abdominal wall defects with US. *Radiographics.* 1995;15(3):517–530.
49. Bair JH, Russ PD, Pretorius DH, et al. Fetal omphalocele and gastroschisis: a review of 24 cases. *AJR Am J Roentgenol.* 1986;147(5):1047–1051.
50. Juhasz-Boss I, Goelz R, Solomayer EF, et al. Fetal and neonatal outcome in patients with anterior abdominal wall defects (gastroschisis and omphalocele). *J Perinat Med.* 2011;40(1):85–90.
51. Danzer E, Victoria T, Bebbington MW, et al. Fetal MRI-calculated total lung volumes in the prediction of short-term outcome in giant omphalocele: preliminary findings. *Fetal Diagn Ther.* 2012;31(4):248–253.
52. Hacivelioglu S, Tarim E. Limb body wall defect: three different presentations with abdominal wall defects. *J Obstet Gynaecol.* 2010;30(7):737–738.
53. Haas J, Achiron R, Barzilay E, et al. Umbilical cord hernias: prenatal diagnosis and natural history. *J Ultrasound Med.* 2011;30(12):1629–1632.
54. Salzman L, Kuligowska E, Semine A. Pseudoomphalocele: pitfall in fetal sonography. *AJR Am J Roentgenol.* 1986;146(6):1283–1285.
55. Hidaka N, Tsukimori K, Hojo S, et al. Correlation between the presence of liver herniation and perinatal outcome in prenatally diagnosed fetal omphalocele. *J Perinat Med.* 2009;37(1):66–71.
56. Kominiarek MA, Zork N, Pierce SM, et al. Perinatal outcome in the live-born infant with prenatally diagnosed omphalocele. *Am J Perinatol.* 2011;28(8):627–634.
57. Biard JM, Wilson RD, Johnson MP, et al. Prenatally diagnosed giant omphaloceles: short- and long-term outcomes. *Prenat Diagn.* 2004;24(6):434–439.
58. Cohen-Overbeek TE, Tong WH, Hatzmann TR, et al. Omphalocele: comparison of outcome following prenatal or postnatal diagnosis. *Ultrasound Obstet Gynecol.* 2010;36(6):687–692.

59. Montero FJ, Simpson LL, Brady PC, et al. Fetal omphalocele ratios predict outcomes in prenatally diagnosed omphalocele. *Am J Obstet Gynecol.* 2011;205(3):284.e1–284.e7.

60. Mann S, Blinman TA, Douglas Wilson R. Prenatal and postnatal management of omphalocele. *Prenat Diagn.* 2008;28(7):626–632.

61. Kilbride KE, Cooney DR, Custer MD. Vacuum-assisted closure: a new method for treating patients with giant omphalocele. *J Pediatr Surg.* 2006;41(1):212–215.

62. Martin AE, Khan A, Kim DS, et al. The use of intraabdominal tissue expanders as a primary strategy for closure of giant omphaloceles. *J Pediatr Surg.* 2009;44(1):178–182.

63. Ein SH, Langer JC. Delayed management of giant omphalocele using silver sulfadiazine cream: an 18-year experience. *J Pediatr Surg.* 2012;47(3):494–500.

64. Morales JM, Patel SG, Duff JA, et al. Ectopia cordis and other midline defects. *Ann Thorac Surg.* 2000;70(1):111–114.

65. Cantrell JR, Haller JA, Ravitch MM. A syndrome of congenital defects involving the abdominal wall, sternum, diaphragm, pericardium, and heart. *Surg Gynecol Obstet.* 1958;107(5):602–614.

66. Lampert JA, Harmaty M, Thompson EC, et al. Chest wall reconstruction in thoracoabdominal ectopia cordis: using the pedicled osteomuscular latissimus dorsi composite flap. *Ann Plast Surg.* 2010;65(5):485–489.

67. Carmi R, Boughman JA. Pentalogy of Cantrell and associated midline anomalies: a possible ventral midline developmental field. *Am J Med Genet.* 1992;42(1):90–95.

68. Engum SA. Embryology, sternal clefts, ectopia cordis, and Cantrell's pentalogy. *Semin Pediatr Surg.* 2008;17(3):154–160.

69. Martin RA, Cunniff C, Erickson L, et al. Pentalogy of Cantrell and ectopia cordis, a familial developmental field complex. *Am J Med Genet.* 1992;42(6):839–841.

70. Desselle C, Herve P, Toutain A, et al. Pentalogy of Cantrell: sonographic assessment. *J Clin Ultrasound.* 2007;35(4):216–220.

71. van Hoorn JH, Moonen RM, Huysentruyt CJ, et al. Pentalogy of Cantrell: two patients and a review to determine prognostic factors for optimal approach. *Eur J Pediatr.* 2008;167(1):29–35.

72. Peixoto-Filho FM, do Cima LC, Nakamura-Pereira M. Prenatal diagnosis of Pentalogy of Cantrell in the first trimester: is 3-dimensional sonography needed? *J Clin Ultrasound.* 2008;37(2):112–114.

73. Stein W, Haller F, Hawighorst T, et al. Pentalogy of Cantrell vs. limb body wall complex: differential diagnosis of a severe malformation in early pregnancy. *Ultraschall Med.* 2009;30(6):598–601.

74. Wheeler DS, St Louis JD. Pentalogy of Cantrell associated with hypoplastic left heart syndrome. *Pediatr Cardiol.* 2007;28(4):311–313.

75. Yuan SM, Shinfeld A, Mishaly D. An incomplete pentalogy of Cantrell. *Chang Gung Med J.* 2008;31(3):309–313.

76. Murphy A, Platt LD. First-trimester diagnosis of body stalk anomaly using 2- and 3-dimensional sonography. *J Ultrasound Med.* 2011;30(12):1739–1743.

77. Daskalakis G, Sebire NJ, Jurkovic D, et al. Body stalk anomaly at 10–14 weeks of gestation. *Ultrasound Obstet Gynecol.* 1997;10(6):416–418.

78. Hunter AG, Seaver LH, Stevenson RE. Limb-body wall defect. Is there a defensible hypothesis and can it explain all the associated anomalies? *Am J Med Genet A.* 2011;155A(9):2045–2059.

79. Pumberger W, Schaller A, Bernaschek G. Limb-body wall complex: a compound anomaly pattern in body-wall defects. *Pediatr Surg Int.* 2001;17(5–6):486–490.

80. Viscarello RR, Ferguson DD, Nores J, et al. Limb-body wall complex associated with cocaine abuse: further evidence of cocaine's teratogenicity. *Obstet Gynecol.* 1992;80(3, pt 2):523–526.

81. Litwin A, Fisch B, Tadir Y, et al. Limb-body wall complex with complete absence of external genitalia after in vitro fertilization. *Fertil Steril.* 1991;55(3):634–636.

82. Negishi H, Yaegashi M, Kato EH, et al. Prenatal diagnosis of limb-body wall complex. *J Reprod Med.* 1998;43(8):659–664.

83. Chen CP, Lin CJ, Chang TY, et al. Second-trimester diagnosis of limb-body wall complex with literature review of pathogenesis. *Genet Couns.* 2007;18(1):105–112.

84. Liu IF, Yu CH, Chang CH, et al. Prenatal diagnosis of limb-body wall complex in early pregnancy using three-dimensional ultrasound. *Prenat Diagn.* 2003;23(6):513–514.

85. Luehr B, Lipsett J, Quinlivan JA. Limb-body wall complex: a case series. *J Matern Fetal Neonatal Med.* 2002;12:132–137.

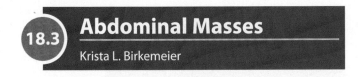

# Abdominal Masses

### Krista L. Birkemeier

## FETAL ABDOMINAL CYSTIC MASSES

Cystic abdominal masses in the fetus are common. Ozyuncu et al.[1] found a positive predictive value of 75% for identifying the body system of origin for prenatal cysts. Since the diagnosis rarely affects prenatal intervention or delivery, it is important to recognize the abnormality, give a differential diagnosis, and obtain postnatal follow-up to document resolution or make a definitive diagnosis for possible postnatal therapy.

## Ovarian Cyst

**Incidence:** Fetal ovarian cysts are the most common abdominal cysts reported prenatally. The incidence, however, is not documented. The presence of small ovarian cysts in the perinatal period is normal. Cohen et al.[2] evaluated postnatal ultrasounds (US) and found that 82% of normal infants in the first 3 months of life had ovarian cysts measuring 0.1 to 1.4 cm.

**Embryology and Pathology:** Neonatal cysts are of germinal or Graafian epithelial origin and consist of follicular, theca lutein,

corpus luteum, or simple cysts and result from enlargement of an otherwise normal follicle.[3]

A follicle may enlarge secondary to hormonal stimulation by follicle-stimulating hormone (FSH) the fetal pituitary, maternal estrogen, and placental human chorionic gonadotropin (HCG). There is increased incidence of fetal ovarian cysts in cases of maternal diabetes, rhesus sensitization, and preeclampsia, all of which are associated with increased serum chorionic gonadotropins. There is also a reported association with fetal hypothyroidism.[4]

After birth, HCG and estrogen drop, while FSH and luteinizing hormone (LH) increase until 3 months and then fall as the hypothalamic–pituitary axis matures. Cysts regress with time, likely because of hormonal changes.

### Diagnosis

*Ultrasound:* Fetal ovarian cysts are most often identified after 28 weeks' gestation, though they are also noted as early as 19 weeks.[4,5] They are typically unilateral, but may be bilateral.

Ovarian cysts may be simple (Fig. 18.3-1) or complicated (Fig. 18.3-2). Simple cysts are anechoic and smooth with thin or imperceptible walls on US. Complicated cysts demonstrate hemorrhage as a fluid–debris level, retracting clot, multiple internal septations, or a solid mass. The wall may be thick and echogenic from dystrophic calcification.[3]

*MRI:* Simple cysts are hyperintense on T2w and hypointense on T1w following fluid signal. On T2w, the blood products

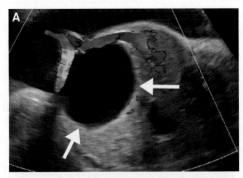

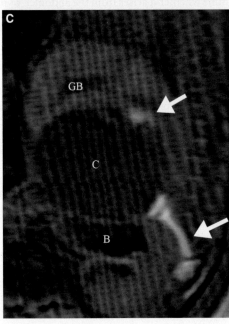

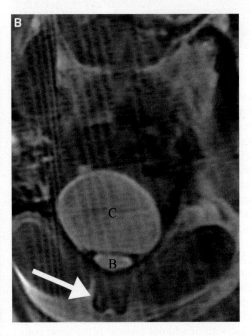

**FIGURE 18.3-1:** Simple ovarian cyst at 32 weeks' gestation. **A:** Axial color Doppler US demonstrates a large simple anechoic cyst *(arrows)* filling the pelvis and lower abdomen. **B:** Coronal fetal MRI demonstrates a large simple pelvic cyst *(C)* filling the pelvis and lower abdomen with hyperintense T2w signal. This cyst displaces the bladder *(B)* inferiorly. Gender is female *(arrow)*. **C:** Sagittal T1 fetal MR image demonstrates hypointense T1w fluid signal in this simple cyst *(C)* separate from the bladder *(B)* and gallbladder *(GB)*. Hyperintense signal posteriorly is from meconium in the rectum and colon *(arrows)*.

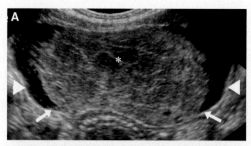

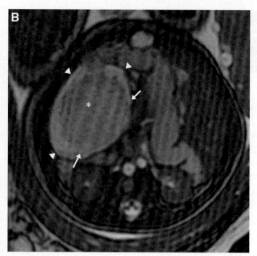

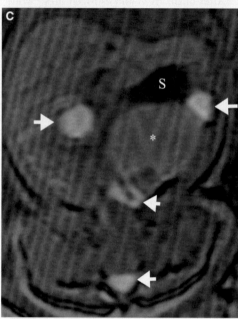

**FIGURE 18.3-2:** Complicated ovarian cyst secondary to ovarian torsion at 30 weeks' gestation. **A:** Axial US demonstrates peripheral anechoic fluid *(arrowheads)* and central lacelike echogenic mass *(asterisk)* representing retracting clot with acute margins *(arrows)* between the mass and the cyst wall. **B:** Axial fetal MRI demonstrates a complicated pelvic cyst with peripheral hyperintense T2w signal corresponding with fluid *(arrowheads)* and central intermediate signal *(asterisk)* with acute margins *(arrows)*, corresponding to retracting clot. **C:** Coronal MRI demonstrates mildly hyperintense T1w in this complicated cyst corresponding with clot *(asterisk)*. It is higher signal than the fluid-filled stomach *(S)*, but less intense than the bright meconium in the adjacent colon *(arrows)*.

in complicated cysts are lower signal than fluid. Hemorrhage causes hyperintense T1w. Marked hypointensity on gradient echo or echoplanar imaging indicates hemosiderin deposition. Nemac et al.[6] describes restricted diffusion and hyperintense FLAIR signal with intracystic hemorrhage. MRI can be useful to evaluate soft tissue components, but for the vast majority of cases, US diagnosis and follow-up is the imaging standard.[6]

Suggested criteria for fetal ovarian cyst include (1) female gender, (2) unilateral or bilateral pelvic or lower abdominal location, and (3) normal kidneys, bladder, and intestines. Cysts may be located anywhere in the abdomen or pelvis because of ligamentous laxity and a relatively long mesosalpynx, or because of torsion with autoamputation.[4,5] Cysts are considered pathologic if they measure 2 cm or greater. When very large, a cyst may fill the abdomen and pelvis, displacing normal structures and making it difficult or impossible to determine the source.

Cyst hemorrhage, with or without torsion, is the most common complication and is suspected when the cyst appears complicated. Ovarian cyst hemorrhage is highly associated with torsion. Ascites may occur with cyst rupture or torsion.[5] Anemia has been reported. Other complications are due to mass effect. Polyhydramnios occurs in up to 18% of cases,[7] and is likely secondary to extrinsic bowel obstruction by large cysts >6 cm.[8] Severe mass effect may rarely result in elevation of the diaphragm and pulmonary hypoplasia.[5]

**Differential Diagnosis:** The differential diagnosis for a fetal pelvic cyst includes lymphangioma, gastrointestinal (GI) duplication cyst, cystic teratoma, hydrocolpos, urachal cysts, and persistent cloaca. Identifying a normal urinary system excludes bladder outlet obstruction, megacystis microcolon intestinal hypoperistalsis syndrome, prune belly syndrome, and hydroureteronephrosis.

When a cyst is very large, it may not be possible to determine whether it arises from the abdomen or pelvis, and whether abdominal cysts should also be considered (Tables 18.3-1 and 18.3-2). Extremely rare fetal ovarian tumors such as benign cystic teratomas, mucinous and serous cystadenomas, and a single case of carcinoma have been reported.[5]

**Prognosis:** In a meta-analysis including 420 fetuses with ovarian cysts from 1984 to 2005, cysts spontaneously regress in 50%.[9] Spontaneous regression may occur either in utero or postnatally, and typically occurs within 1 to 12 months.[3,5] Both simple and complicated cysts may resolve, although there is a slightly lower regression rate of complicated cysts.[10]

Ovarian cysts are complicated by hemorrhage and/or torsion in 35%.[9] Regarding cyst size and prognosis, 98% of cysts <5 cm regressed spontaneously, whereas 93% of cysts greater than 5 cm resulted in complications.[9] However, there are studies indicating that size does not predict torsion and the complicated appearance, rate of growth, and length of the pedicle are more important.[3,7]

**Management:** Most authors recommended serial US follow-up for cysts less than 5 cm to document size and monitor for increasing complexity indicating hemorrhage/torsion. In utero needle

| Table 18.3-1 | Differential Diagnosis of Fetal Abdominal Cysts Based on Location |
|---|---|

Right upper quadrant
   Choledochal
   Hepatic cyst or cystic tumor
   Duodenal duplication
   Duodenal atresia
   Pancreatic (head)
Left upper quadrant
   Splenic
   Gastric duplication
   Pancreatic
Midabdomen
   Lymphatic (mesenteric, omental)
   Meconium pseudocyst
   Umbilical vein varix
Retroperitoneal
   Common
      Hydronephrosis
      Renal cystic disease
   Uncommon
      Urinoma
      Adrenal cyst
      Cystic neuroblastoma
      Lymphatic (retroperitoneal)
Lower abdomen and pelvis
   Common
      Hydrometrocolpos
      Ovarian
      Ureterocele
      Urachal
      Megacystis
   Uncommon
      Persistent cloaca
      Anterior sacral meningocele
      Sacrococcygeal teratoma
Any location
   Alimentary duplication
   Dilated bowel (obstruction, atresia)
   Cystic teratoma

aspiration appears to be safe and effective, but is used rarely, with an 89% regression rate after aspiration. Persistent complicated or persistent large simple cysts (>5 cm) can be treated surgically to decrease the possibility of torsion or exclude an alternative diagnosis.[9] Since torsion often occurs in utero, postnatal surgery is primarily for the purpose of preventing complications such as hemorrhage, rupture with peritonitis, and intestinal obstruction from adhesions, rather than for ovarian salvage.

**Recurrence Risk:** Since the hormonal stimulation is removed in the neonatal period, they are not expected to recur after they spontaneously resolve or are surgically treated.

## Hepatic Cyst

**Incidence:** Low but not precisely known.[11] There is a female predominance.

**Embryology and Pathology:** Simple hepatic cysts are presumed secondary to interruption of the intrahepatic biliary system with growth arrest and dilation, representing cysts of biliary origin.

Most antenatally diagnosed hepatic cysts are simple.[11] They most commonly have a cuboidal epithelial lining with positive CK-7 staining and a fibrous wall with occasional smooth muscle fibers, suggesting bile origin and supporting a biliary growth arrest etiology.[12] However, no epithelial lining[13] and simple squamous lining has also been reported.[11] Avni et al.[13] hypothesize that some hepatic cysts may represent areas of necrosis from an ischemic event, particularly those without an epithelial lining.

### Diagnosis
***Ultrasound:*** A hepatic cyst is most commonly seen in the second trimester (median gestational age 22 weeks), but has been reported in the third and first trimesters.[11,12] Hepatic cysts may be unilocular or multilocular. They may be clearly intrahepatic or subhepatic and attached to the liver capsule. Cysts as large as 20 cm have been reported.[14] Antenatally detected liver cysts are more often present in the left lobe.[11,14] On US, hepatic cysts are round, well defined, anechoic structures with posterior enhancement.

A large cyst may compress the umbilical vein, resulting in hydrops and fetal demise, may elevate the diaphragm and cause pulmonary hypoplasia, or may compress the bowel and cause polyhydramnios.[11,14]

***MRI:*** Hepatic cysts follow fluid signal on MRI with hyperintense T2-weighted signal and hypointense T1-weighted signal surrounded by higher signal liver parenchyma (Fig. 18.3-3).

**Differential Diagnosis:** Simple hepatic cysts, intrahepatic choledochal cysts (Caroli disease), and mesenchymal hamartomas may look identical on prenatal imaging,[11] although simple hepatic cysts are statistically more common.[11,12] Consider rare entities like cystic hepatoblastoma, cystic teratoma, and hemangioendothelioma, particularly if there is question of a solid component or multilocularity. If the cyst is large and/or subhepatic, it may be difficult to differentiate from extrahepatic fetal abdominal cysts (Tables 18.3-1 and 18.3-2).

**Prognosis:** Most simple hepatic cysts are asymptomatic and remain unchanged or regress over time.[11] Complications are rare and secondary to large size and mass effect. Infection, hemorrhage, and torsion of the cyst are theoretical complications.

**Management:** Hepatic cysts are typically managed with serial prenatal US examinations to document size and mass effect on adjacent structures. A very large cyst resulting in mass effect on the chest, umbilical cord, or bowel may require in utero aspiration to allow normal fetal development.[15]

Postnatally, cholangiography and/or hepatobiliary scan may help differentiate a choledochal cyst from a simple hepatic cyst, which is managed differently. Postnatal surgery for simple cysts, including aspiration, fenestration, cystectomy, or hepatic lobectomy, is typically reserved for patients with symptoms because of cyst size or uncertainty about the diagnosis.[11,12]

**Recurrence Risk:** Hepatic cysts tend to stay the same or regress on follow-up imaging.[11] Surgically resected cysts have not demonstrated recurrence.[11,12]

| Table 18.3-2 | **Comparison of Fetal Abdominal Cysts** | | | | |
|---|---|---|---|---|---|

| Cyst | Locularity | Trimester | Gender | Location |
|---|---|---|---|---|
| Ovarian | U > M | 3rd >> 2nd | F | Pelvis ± abdomen |
| Hepatic | U >> M | 2nd > 3rd > 1st | F >> M | RUQ |
| Choledochal | U | 2nd > 3rd | F >> M | RUQ |
| Gallbladder duplication | U | 2nd or 3rd | — | RUQ |
| Enteric | U >> M | 2nd or 3rd | M > F | Any |
| Lymphatic | M or U | 2nd > 3rd | M ≥ F | Any |
| Splenic | U | 3rd | — | LUQ |
| Pancreatic-isolated | M or U | 3rd > 2nd | F > M | Upper abdomen |
| Pancreatic-with anomalies | M or U | 2nd > 3rd | F ≥ M | Upper abdomen |

U, unilocular; M, multilocular; F, female; M, male; Trimester, trimester at diagnosis; RUQ, right upper quadrant; LUQ, left upper quadrant.

## Choledochal Cyst

**Incidence:** Variable depending on geography with two-thirds of reported cases involving the Japanese population. Females are affected more often than males by a ratio of 3:1 in the Japanese literature and 9:1 in the Western literature.[16,17]

**Embryology and Pathology:** The bile duct elongates and begins to recanalize at the end of the 5th week. By the 12th week, bile is secreted from the liver and transported to the duodenum by the extrahepatic biliary system.[18] The pancreas secretes enzymes in the 5th month.

The etiology is not proven. The most widely cited theory states that pancreaticobiliary reflux secondary to an anomalous long common pancreaticobiliary channel results in increased pressure, inflammation, and weakening resulting in cystic dilation. This does not explain cysts seen before pancreatic enzyme production. Alternatively, choledochal cysts may be due to distal obstruction by a web, stricture, biliary atresia, or sphincter of Oddi dysfunction.[19] Some hypothesize that prenatal infectious cholangitis causes biliary duct scarring resulting in a spectrum of obstructive cholangiopathy that includes choledochal cyst, biliary atresia, and neonatal hepatitis.[20] In utero accident has been suggested as well.

Choledochal cysts are classified by the Todani modified Alonso–Lej Classification (Fig. 18.3-4).[21–23]

There is evidence that 22% of patients in the United States with choledochal cysts have associated congenital cardiac anomalies including ASD, VSD, PDA, and persistent fetal circulation.[24] Choledochal cysts may also be associated with concurrent biliary atresia or be confused with the rare cystic biliary atresia.[25]

### Diagnosis

*Ultrasound:* A choledochal cyst is a cystic mass at the liver hilum, subhepatic, or in the liver parenchyma (Type V), that is separate from the gallbladder. Choledochal cysts have been detected during second-or-third trimester US. It can be differentiated from other cystic masses if one can demonstrate a fusiform shape with tapered ends in continuity with the biliary system. On US, it is typically anechoic with posterior enhancement, separate from the stomach, duodenum, and gallbladder, and

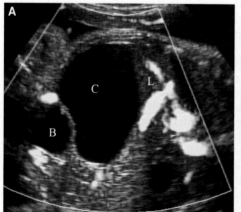
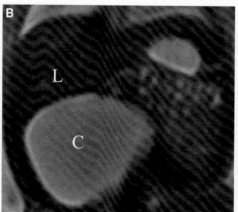
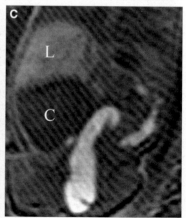

**FIGURE 18.3-3:** Hepatic cyst at 27 weeks' gestation. **A :** Coronal color Doppler US demonstrates a large anechoic cyst *(C)* along the inferior margin of the right lobe of the liver *(L)*, separate from the bladder *(B)*. There is no internal Doppler flow. **B:** Coronal MR image demonstrates hyperintense T2 fluid signal in the cyst *(C)* at the inferior margin of the right hepatic lobe *(L)*. **C:** Coronal T1w MR demonstrates hypointense fluid signal of the cyst *(C)* at the inferior margin of the right hepatic lobe *(L)*.

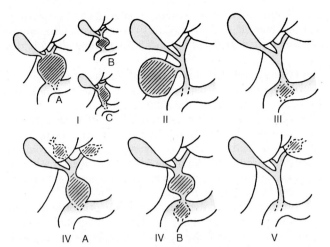

**FIGURE 18.3-4:** Classification of choledochal cysts as proposed by Alonso-Lej et al.[21] and modified by Todani et al.[22] Type IA, cystic extrahepatic biliary dilation; type IB, segmental extrahepatic biliary dilation; type IC, diffuse extrahepatic biliary dilation; type II, saccular diverticulum of extrahepatic bile duct; type III, choledochocele; IVA, multiple cysts of the intrahepatic and extrahepatic biliary tree; type IVB, multiple cysts of the extrahepatic biliary tree only; type V, intrahepatic cysts only (Caroli disease). (From Novak DA, Suchy FJ, Balistreri WF. Disorders of the liver and biliary system. In: McMillan JA, Feigin RD, DeAngelis C, et al, eds. *Oski's Solution*. Philadelphia, PA: Lippincott Williams & Wilkins; 2006:2035.)

without peristalsis (Fig. 18.3-5). Choledochal cysts with internal echoes have been reported.[26] Doppler US demonstrates lack of internal flow and intimate relationship with the portal vein and hepatic artery.[27]

*MRI:* Choledochal cysts follow fluid signal on MRI with hypointense T1w signal and hyperintense T2w signal. In some cases, MRI may be more useful than US in demonstrating the relationship to the biliary tree (Fig. 18.3-5).

**Differential Diagnosis:** If a cyst is in the porta hepatis and demonstrates intimate association with the portal vein and hepatic artery, the differential diagnosis includes choledochal

cyst, cystic biliary atresia, duodenal duplication cyst, and pancreatic head cyst. Biliary atresia with cystic dilation can look identical to a choledochal cyst on prenatal imaging. Amniotic fluid analysis for digestive enzymes may help differentiate these various cysts in utero; biliary atresia demonstrates decreased γ-glutamyl transferase.[19] Figure 18.3-6 schematically differentiates the types of prenatally diagnosed biliary anomalies. Some authors suggest that (1) choledochal cysts increase in size over time, whereas cystic biliary atresia does not, (2) cysts of biliary atresia tend to be <2.5 cm, whereas choledochal cysts tend to be >4 cm or have intrahepatic biliary dilation, or (3) anechoic cysts correspond to atresia whereas large, echoic, or enlarging cysts correspond with choledochal cysts; however, the number of cases is small and exceptions are reported, so these criteria should not be used for definitive prenatal diagnosis.[26,28]

Other abdominal or pelvic cysts, including hepatic cysts, mesenchymal hamartomas, ovarian cysts, and adrenal cysts, should be considered in the differential as well.

**Prognosis:** Untreated choledochal cysts may be complicated by rupture with peritonitis, biliary obstruction, recurrent cholangitis, pancreatitis, cirrhosis, portal hypertension, liver failure, and malignant degeneration. With modern early surgical treatment, symptoms resolve and prognosis is good, with increasing morbidity and mortality with delayed surgery.[28,29]

There is evidence that choledochal cysts are associated with congenital cardiac anomalies, so echocardiographic screening may be warranted before surgery.[24]

**Management:** Postnatal US, MRI and/or hepatobiliary scan confirm hepatobiliary origin and further differentiate a choledochal cyst from the rare cystic biliary atresia. Intraoperative cholangiography and/or pathology may be necessary to definitively exclude biliary atresia.[30]

Complete surgical excision of the choledochal cyst with bilioenteric reconstruction, typically Roux-en-Y hepaticojejunostomy, is the preferred treatment. Early surgery in the first month of life may be warranted since even asymptomatic (not jaundiced) patients tend to develop liver fibrosis immediately after birth.[29]

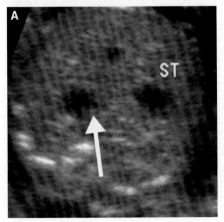
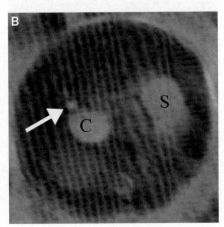
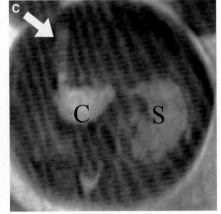

**FIGURE 18.3-5:** Choledochal cyst at 20 weeks' gestation. **A:** Transverse US through the fetal abdomen demonstrates a cyst in the liver hilum that tapers medially *(arrow)*. ST, stomach. **B:** Axial MRI demonstrates T2 hyperintense fluid signal of the cyst *(C)* at the hepatic hilum, separate from the stomach *(S)* and communicating with the bile duct *(arrow)* at the liver hilum. **C:** The next slice demonstrates the proximity of the cyst *(C)* to the gallbladder *(arrow)*, but separate from it. S, stomach.

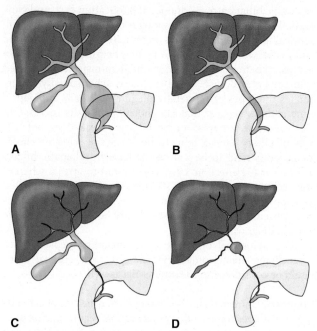

**FIGURE 18.3-6** Schematic diagram of congenital biliary anomalies diagnosed antenatally. **A:** Type I-c choledochal cyst. **B:** Type V choledochal cyst. **C:** Type 1 biliary atresia. **D:** Type 3 biliary atresia with segmental cystic dilation. (Reprinted from Redkar RM, Howard ER. Antenatal diagnosis of congenital anomalies of the biliary tract. *J Pediatr Surg.* 1998;33:700–704, copyright © 1998, with permission from Elsevier.)

**Recurrence Risk:** Postsurgical follow-up of antenatally diagnosed, postnatally resected choledochal cysts has not demonstrated recurrence with follow-up ranging from 10 months to 7 years.[25–29]

## Gallbladder Duplication

**Incidence:** One in 3,800 incidence is based on Boyden's 1926 work citing only 5 cases out of 19,000 autopsy and patient cases.[31] Bronshtein et al.[32] found 2 gallbladders described as septated, bilobed, or duplicated in 10,016 prenatal ultrasounds, for an estimated incidence of 1 in 5,008 screening ultrasounds.

**Embryology and Pathology:** The gallbladder arises from the caudal aspect of the hepatic diverticulum of the foregut in the 4th week and canalizes by the 12th week.[32]

In true duplication, there are two gallbladders, each with its own cystic duct.[33] It may result from continued growth, rather than the expected regression of diverticula that arise from the cystic or common bile duct in the 5th and 6th weeks.[31] Alternatively, two cystic primordia may arise separately from the common bile duct, resulting in an accessory gallbladder.[33]

A disturbance of cell division of the cystic primordium in the 5th or 6th week may result in splitting with two gallbladders in a septate, V-shaped, or Y-shaped duplication, but only one cystic duct entering the common duct.[33]

### Diagnosis

*Ultrasound:* A duplicated gallbladder appears as parallel elongated cysts in the gallbladder fossa. Duplicated gallbladder has been reported on prenatal imaging between 20 and 32 weeks gestation.[34–36] On US, fluid in the gallbladder is typically anechoic (Fig. 18.3-7).

*MRI:* On MRI, a duplicated gallbladder follows fluid signal with hyperintense T2-weighted signal and hypointense T1-weighted signal (Fig. 18.3-7C). In the third trimester, gallbladder content signal is more variable.

**Differential Diagnosis:** The primary differential consideration is a gallbladder fold, but this is oriented along the short axis of the gallbladder. Other considerations include choledochal cyst, hepatic cyst, enteric duplication cyst, or lymphatic cyst. Its parallel configuration in the gallbladder fossa is characteristic.[35]

**Prognosis:** Duplicated gallbladder is an incidental finding with a good prognosis. The greatest importance lies in knowledge of the anatomy prior to cholecystectomy for symptomatic disease

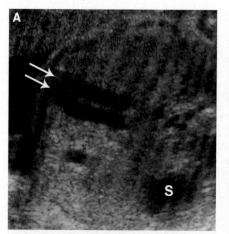
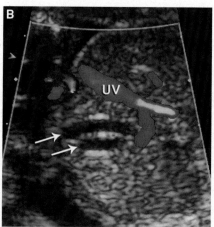
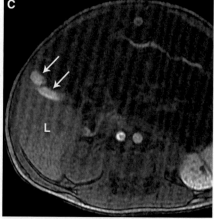

**FIGURE 18.3-7:** Gallbladder duplication at 30 weeks' gestation. **A:** Transverse US demonstrates two parallel elongated anechoic structures *(arrows)* in the gallbladder fossa. S, stomach. **B:** Color Doppler US demonstrates that the cystic structures *(arrows)* are to the right of the umbilical vein *(UV)* and lack internal flow. **C:** Postnatal MRI demonstrates hyperintense signal of bile in the parallel structures *(arrows)* in the gallbladder fossa of the liver *(L)*. (Reprinted from Gerscovich EO, Towner D, Sanchez T, et al. Fetal gallbladder duplication. *J Ultrasound Med.* 2011;30:1310–1312, with permission from American Institute of Ultrasound in Medicine.)

later in life, and for differentiating it from prenatal cysts that may require postnatal surgery.

**Management:** If the diagnosis is uncertain prenatally, postnatal US or MR may be useful for diagnosis. No intervention is required.

**Recurrence Risk:** None.

## Enteric Duplication Cyst

**Incidence:** Prenatal detection is reported to be 1 in 18,333 live births, compared to 1 in 4,500 detected by autopsy, suggesting that prenatal US detects approximately 25% of duplication cysts.[37] There is a 2:1 male predominance.[38]

**Embryology and Pathology:** Between the 6th and 8th weeks of gestation, the solid GI tract canalizes via coalescence of multiple vacuoles. Duplications of the esophagus and intestines may be related to an error of canalization according to the "aberrant recanalization theory." The split notochord theory states that an adhesion between the endoderm and the ectoderm during the fifth gestational week causes the notochord to split, resulting in vertebral abnormality and an intraspinal or extraspinal neurenteric cyst, mostly applying to foregut duplications. Other theories include incomplete twinning, persistent embryologic diverticula, and intrauterine vascular accident theories.[39]

Duplication cysts are spherical (74% to 82%) or tubular (18% to 26%), typically unilocular structures. They are often single but may be multiple in 5% to 7%[38,39] (Fig. 18.3-8). Duplication cysts occur anywhere along the alimentary tract from the mouth/tongue to the rectum, but most commonly involve the ileum. The spherical type usually does not communicate with the lumen, whereas the tubular type frequently communicates.[39] Intestinal duplications usually occur along the mesenteric border, and gastric duplications typically occur along the greater curvature. Rarely, a duplication cyst may have its own separate mesentery. By definition, they should be associated with the GI tract, but there are reports of cysts separate from the GI tract with the same histology as duplication cysts, often called isolated duplication cysts.

### Diagnosis

*Ultrasound:* On US, duplication cysts are typically anechoic. Intracystic hemorrhage results in internal echoes. Rarely, duplication cysts communicate with the bowel lumen, and enteric content/meconium is present in the cyst, causing internal echoes.[40] Enteric duplication cysts may demonstrate peristalsis and gut signature with echogenic mucosal and echolucent muscular layers. However, gut signature is easier to see on postnatal imaging and may not be detectable on prenatal US (Fig. 18.3-8).

Polyhydramnios may be present if the cyst results in GI obstruction or if there is concurrent bowel atresia, but this is uncommon. There is an association of bowel atresia with

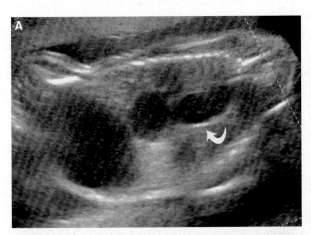
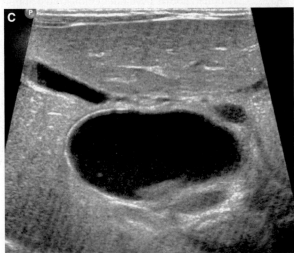
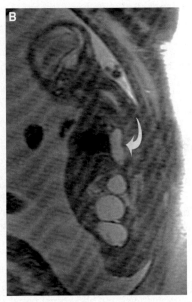

**FIGURE 18.3-8:** Multiple duplication cysts. **A:** Coronal prenatal US at 25 weeks demonstrates three cystic lesions in the chest and abdomen (*arrow* points to esophageal cyst). **B:** Sagittal MRI demonstrates hyperintense T2 fluid signal in multiple cysts (*arrow* points to esophageal cyst). **C:** Postnatal US documents gut signature sign with internal debris. Infant presented with vomiting at 2 weeks of age requiring surgery.

ileojejunal duplications in about 11%.[38] Half of foregut duplication cysts are associated with skeletal malformations and one-third of midgut and hindgut duplications are associated with GI or GU anomalies.[41]

**MRI:** On MRI, duplication cysts follow fluid signal, unless hemorrhage or meconium is present, resulting in hyperintense T1-weighted signal and hypointense T2-weighted signal (Fig. 18.3-8). Large field of view may help identify cyst origin and identify additional cysts. Associated GI or GU anomalies may be further assessed by MRI.

**Differential Diagnosis:** The differential diagnosis depends on location (Tables 18.3-1 and 18.3-2). Features that make a duplication cyst more likely include a thick wall with gut signature and peristalsis. Identification in the second trimester favors duplication cyst over ovarian cyst or bowel obstruction. Lymphatic cyst may be indistinguishable unless there is peristalsis.

**Prognosis:** Duplication cysts may be complicated by ulceration and hemorrhage if acid secreting gastric mucosa is present. Ectopic pancreatic tissue is most commonly found in gastric duplications and may cause pancreatitis. Duplications may result in mass effect on adjacent structures and intestinal obstruction. They may undergo torsion, become a lead point for intussusception or intestinal volvulus, or become infected or inflamed and perforate. Foley et al. found that of 12 prenatally detected duplications, 4 required surgery in the first 2 months for symptoms of bowel obstruction. Of the asymptomatic patients, 5/8 duplications demonstrated ulcerated acid secreting mucosa.[37] Prognosis is good with surgical resection.

**Management:** Since most enteric duplications become symptomatic in the first 2 years of life, they are typically completely excised, with or without segmental bowel resection.

**Recurrence Risk:** They do not recur after resection.

## Lymphatic Cyst

Lymphatic cysts (including mesenteric, omental, and retroperitoneal cysts) and lymphangiomas are often used as interchangeable terms, although some authors separate them based on histology and clinical course. Lymphangiomas tend to be more aggressive and infiltrative. For this discussion of prenatal imaging, both will be grouped together, with an emphasis on imaging follow-up to assess behavior.

**Incidence:** Lymphangioma of any location is common, occurring in 1 in 6,000 pregnancies, but abdominal lymphangiomas account for less than 5% of these.[42] Localized lymphatic cysts are often asymptomatic, and the incidence is not known.

**Embryology and Pathology:** Abdominal lymphatic cysts are hypothesized to arise from abnormal development of the lymphatic system in the 6th week of gestation with lack of lymphatic drainage resulting in cystic collections.[43]

Obstructed lymphatic drainage results in a benign cystic mass of lymphatic channels that most commonly occur in the small bowel mesentery, but may occur in the large bowel mesentery, omentum, or retroperitoneum.[44] Some authors describe them as obstructed lymphatics and others as hamartomatous lymphatic tumors.

## Diagnosis

*Ultrasound:* Review of case reports indicates that lymphatic cysts are commonly discovered on prenatal imaging in the second and early third trimesters (19 to 31 weeks), they increase in size over time, are more often left sided, and they may change from unilocular to multilocular over time. Small localized cysts are most often centrally located in the abdomen but may be anywhere in the abdomen or pelvis and may change position because of attachment to the mobile mesentery or omentum. Lymphangiomas may be isolated to the abdomen, or may infiltrate surrounding structures and may extend to the abdominal wall, chest, or legs.[43,45–47]

On US, lymphatic cysts are typically thin-walled anechoic unilocular or multilocular structures. Hemorrhage or chylous fluid may cause internal echoes. There may be associated skin edema, polyhydramnios, and hydrops.

**MRI:** MRI is useful for large field of view assessment. Lymphangiomas follow fluid signal with hypointense T1-weighted signal and hyperintense T2-weighted signal. If there is hemorrhage, T1 signal is hyperintense, T2 signal is more hypointense, and there may be marked hypointense signal on gradient echo imaging with hemosiderin deposition (Fig. 18.3-9).

**Differential Diagnosis:** Enteric duplication cysts and ovarian cysts may look identical to unilocular lymphatic cysts. Other cyst differential considerations depend on location (Tables 18.3-1 and 18.3-2). Pedunculated mesenchymal hamartoma and cystic teratoma are also considerations.

**Prognosis:** The prognosis depends on the location, rate of growth, extent, and effect on adjacent structures. The prognosis is good for small mesenteric cysts localized to the abdomen where there is often complete postnatal resection without recurrence. Poor prognosis is associated with early diagnosis, rapid growth, large size, hydrops/polyhydramnios, and extra-abdominal extension. Postnatally, localized cysts result in abdominal pain and/or distension from mass effect, torsion, hemorrhage, rupture, intussusception, or volvulus.

**Management:** Prenatally, follow-up USs are recommended to assess growth. Fetal karyotype is suggested because of the association with chromosomal abnormalities with lymphangiomas of the neck, but thus far the few reported cases of abdominal lymphangiomas have not demonstrated abnormal karyotype or other congenital abnormalities.

Cases have either been postnatally resected,[48–50] monitored clinically,[46] or, rarely, pregnancy was terminated because of the extent and fast growth of the lesion.[42,43,45,47]

Postnatally diagnosed symptomatic cysts have been treated surgically, preferably with complete enucleation, and bowel resection may be necessary. Marsupialization is the least preferable choice since incomplete resection may result in recurrence.[44]

**Recurrence Risk:** In children less than 10 years old, there is a 2% recurrence rate after resection. Recurrence is more likely for retroperitoneal cysts than mesenteric cysts.[44]

## Splenic Cyst

**Incidence:** Dankovcik et al.[51] found 3 fetal splenic cysts in 7,897 screening USs for an incidence of 1 in 2,632.

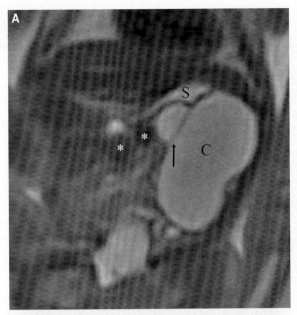

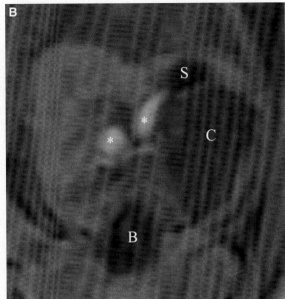

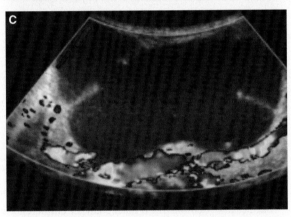

**FIGURE 18.3-9:** Mesenteric cyst. **A:** Coronal prenatal MRI at 30 weeks' gestation demonstrates a septated cyst *(C , arrow)* with hyperintense T2-weighted signal, slightly less bright than fluid in the stomach *(S)*, suggesting hemorrhage or debris. Adjacent hypointense meconium *(asterisks)* in the colon. **B:** Coronal T1 MRI demonstrates subtle hyperintense signal in the cyst *(C)* when compared with the stomach *(S)* and bladder *(B)*, representing hemorrhage or debris. There is hyperintense meconium *(asterisks)* in the adjacent colon. **C:** Postnatal color Doppler US demonstrates a large avascular, anechoic cyst containing septations.

**Embryology and Pathology:** The spleen begins development in the 6th to 7th week.

Prenatally diagnosed splenic cysts most likely represent lymphangiomas, epidermoids, or pseudocysts.[52] The pathogenesis is not proven, and theories include (1) pluripotent cell invasion of the spleen with subsequent metaplasia, (2) inclusion of coelomic mesothelial cells with squamous metaplasia, (3) invagination of peritoneal endothelial cells, and (4) lymphatic dilation.[51]

**Diagnosis**

***Ultrasound:*** A splenic cyst is unilocular with a thin or imperceptible smooth wall most often diagnosed in the third trimester. Published cases of splenic cysts in the English literature measure 6 to 31 mm.[51,53] On US, it is an anechoic left upper quadrant mass.

***MRI:*** On MRI, it follows fluid signal with hyperintense T2-weighted signal and hypointense T1-weighted signal.

**Differential Diagnosis:** Differential considerations include pancreatic cyst, hepatic cyst, lymphatic cyst, duplication cyst, renal cyst, urinoma, urinary collecting system dilation, and adrenal cyst.

**Prognosis:** Prenatally detected splenic cysts tend to be small and most often decrease in size or resolve in utero or in the first 2 years of life without symptoms.[51,52] Reports of splenic cyst complications of torsion, hemorrhage, rupture, and infection described in children and adults have not been described in the fetal/perinatal period.

**Management:** US monitoring in utero and postnatally is recommended to document cyst regression or stability and exclude growth, subsequent complications, or alternative diagnoses.

**Recurrence Risk:** Case reports of antenatally diagnosed splenic cysts indicate stability or regression without recurrence.

## Pancreatic Cyst

**Incidence:** Fetal pancreatic cysts are rare, with only seven reported cases of isolated congenital cysts[54–56] and rare cases associated with other congenital anomalies.[56–58]

**Embryology and Pathogenesis:** True pancreatic cysts are epithelium-lined cysts hypothesized to result from anomalous development of the pancreatic ducts.

It is suggested that they represent anomalous development of the pancreatic ductal system, where sequestered secretory cells give rise to cysts.[59] There is a predilection for female gender and body/tail location for isolated cysts. Prenatal pancreatic cysts have been prenatally associated with Beckwith–Weidemann syndrome, asphyxiating thoracic dysplasia, renal-hepatic-pancreatic dysplasia, and narrow thorax with short limb dwarfism.[56,58] Small cysts were reported with short rib polydactyly syndrome Type 1.[57] Postnatally, there is an association with polycystic renal disease, anorectal malformation, and Von Hippel Lindau disease.[59]

### Diagnosis

*Ultrasound:* Reported cases without congenital anomalies were diagnosed between 21 and 38 weeks' gestation, and cyst size at diagnosis was 21 to 58 mm. They may stay the same or increase in size.[54–56] Those with other congenital anomalies were diagnosed between 15 and 32 weeks with varied size, number, and appearance of cysts.[56–58]

Pancreatic cysts may be unilocular, multilocular, or transition from a unilocular to a septated cyst. They may be single or multiple. They are anechoic on US.

*MRI:* Pancreatic cysts follow fluid signal on MRI with hyperintense T2 signal and hypointense T1 signal.

**Differential Diagnosis:** Consider renal, liver, biliary, adrenal, or alimentary duplication cyst.

**Prognosis:** The prognosis is good for fetal pancreatic cysts without other congenital abnormalities where postnatal resection is successful (however, no long-term follow-up is documented in the literature). Potential serious postnatal complications of pancreatic cysts include infection, cholangitis, pancreatitis, cyst rupture, and peritonitis if not resected.

Prognosis is worse with concurrent congenital anomalies.

**Management:** Pancreatic cysts located in the body and tail are treated with surgical excision. Cysts in the pancreatic head are treated with internal drainage procedures.[56]

**Recurrence Risk:** There is one case report of recurrence in an incompletely resected antenatally diagnosed pancreatic cyst.[60]

## Hepatosplenomegaly

Fetal hepatosplenomegaly (HSM) may be secondary to immune or nonimmune hydrops, congenital infection, cardiac failure, hemolytic anemia, metabolic disease, overgrowth disorders, myeloproliferative disorders, or tumors (Table 18.3-3).[61–67] Detection of hepatic and/or splenic enlargement should prompt careful evaluation of the entire anatomy for other anomalies and clinical screening for congenital infection.

A myeloproliferative disorder may result in hepatomegaly or hepatosplenomegaly, with or without hydrops. It may represent either transient abnormal myelopoieses or acute leukemia; definitive diagnosis requires cordocentesis and analysis of blast forms. It has been mostly seen in infants with trisomy 21, but has also been described in infants with normal karyotype. Patients require intensive care after birth, so prenatal assessment of severity may be helpful. Ogawa et al.[68] suggest that the degree of HSM may correlate with severity of postnatal disease, but there are no large studies to prove it.

| Table 18.3-3 | Causes of Fetal Hepatosplenomegaly (HSM) |
| --- | --- |

Immune hydrops
Nonimmune hydrops
Cardiac failure
Congenital infection
   Toxoplasmosis
   CMV
   Syphilis
   Rubella
   Tuberculosis
Metabolic
   Hyperthyroidism
   Storage disease (Hunter, Gaucher, Niemann Pick, Wolman, Glycogen storage disease type IV have been described with prenatal HSM)
   Congenital disorders of glycosylation
   Mitochondrial hepatopathy
   Smith–Lemli–Opitz syndrome (defect in cholesterol synthesis)
   Enzyme deficiencies resulting in hemolytic anemia
      Congenital erythropoietic porphyria
      Pyruvate kinase deficiency
      Glucose–phosphate isomerase deficiency
      Transaldolase deficiency
Overgrowth disorders (Beckwith–Weidemann syndrome)
Zellweger syndrome
Myeloproliferative disorder/leukemia (usually associated with trisomy 21)
Primary tumor
Metastases

Studies have demonstrated that splenic circumference is an excellent predictor of severe fetal anemia secondary to Rh alloimmunization in nonhydropic fetuses not treated with transfusion, and is more useful late in pregnancy (after 30 weeks).[69] It was less sensitive and specific, but still useful, in the second-trimester evaluation of hemoglobin Bart (homozygous alpha thalassemia1).[63]

## SOLID LIVER MASSES

Solid hepatic masses of the fetus and neonate are rare and account for approximately 5% of total neoplasms in this age group. Primary hepatic tumors include infantile hemangioma/hemangioendothelioma, mesenchymal hamartoma, and hepatoblastoma. Liver metastases may be secondary to neuroblastoma, leukemia, or renal tumors. Less common liver metastases may be secondary to yolk sac tumor, rhabdomyosarcoma, or rhabdoid tumor.[70] Rare cases of fetal focal nodular hyperplasia and hepatic adenomas have been reported.[71,72]

### Hemangioendothelioma and Hepatic Vascular Lesions

**Incidence:** Hemangioendothelioma (HAE) accounts for 60% of perinatal liver tumors.[70]

**Embryology and Pathology:** North's placental theory suggests that placental mesodermal progenitor cells or placental angioblasts are responsible, as evidenced by the striking similarity of glucose transporter protein (GLUT)-1 positive infantile hemangioma tissue to placental tissue and supported by increased incidence after chorionic villous sampling. Alternatively, a vascular precursor cell may undergo somatic mutation or may be influenced by local inductive influences to proliferate.[73]

Hemangioendothelioma is a term applied to a benign vascular lesion of the liver. In the literature, several terms have been used, sometimes considered synonymous and sometimes discussed as separate entities (Table 18.3-4). These vascular liver lesions have more recently been grouped into solitary, multiple, and diffuse lesions, and into GLUT 1 reactive and nonreactive, which better describes their behavior.[74,75] *Focal lesions* are histologically GLUT-1 negative and behave similar to the rapidly involuting congenital hemangiomas (RICH) of the skin, which are fully grown at birth and regress over 12 to 14 months. These are more likely to be seen on prenatal imaging. *Multifocal lesions* are GLUT-1 positive and behave similar to infantile hemangiomas (IH) of the skin. They tend to present clinically in early infancy with a proliferative phase during infancy followed by an involutional phase over several years, and demonstrate female predominance. *Diffuse lesions* are multiple GLUT-1 positive lesions that are too numerous to count and may cause massive hepatomegaly with compartment syndrome, respiratory compromise, and impaired venous return.[74,75]

Multifocal and diffuse forms express type 3 iodothyronine-deiodinase, which degrades thyroid hormone and causes hypothyroidism. It is theorized that multifocal lesions may coalesce and become diffuse.[75] High-flow shunting may result in heart failure, more common in the diffuse form where more than half of patients are affected (Fig. 18.3-10F). Intralesional thrombosis may result in transient anemia and thrombocytopenia.[75]

**Diagnosis**

*Ultrasound:* On ultrasound, the *solitary* GLUT-1(−) lesions are typically large, well-circumscribed lesions with heterogeneous echogenicity from central necrosis and hemorrhage, and may have echogenic shadowing dystrophic calcification. They sometimes demonstrate high-flow arteriovenous or portovenous shunts with large tubular anechoic vessels (Fig. 18.3-10). *Multifocal* GLUT-1(+) lesions are homogeneous small round masses that are usually hypoechoic. There may be large vessels in or adjacent to the masses with shunting. *Diffuse* tumors may be difficult to discern because of near complete replacement of the liver parenchyma with hepatomegaly and heterogeneous echotexture.[74]

Doppler may demonstrate hypervascularity with high-velocity arterial waveforms and arterialized venous waveforms. Decreased aortic caliber below the celiac axis with hepatic artery, hepatic vein, and cardiac dilation suggest shunting.

| Table 18.3-4 | **Comparison of Infantile Hepatic Hemangioma Subtypes**[74,75] | | |
|---|---|---|---|
| *Subtype* | *Focal* | *Multifocal* | *Diffuse* |
| Synonyms | Hemangioendothelioma, cavernous hemangioma, arteriovenous malformation, solitary hemangioma, RICH of the liver, hepatic vascular malformation with associated capillary proliferation (HVMCP) | Hemangioendothelioma, capillary hemangioma, cellular hemangioma, infantile hepatic hemangioma | Hemangioendothelioma, capillary hemangioma, cellular hemangioma, infantile hepatic hemangioma, hemangiomatosis |
| GLUT 1 reactivity | GLUT 1 negative (−) | GLUT 1 positive (+) | GLUT 1 positive (+) |
| Time of clinical presentation | Prenatal imaging or first few weeks of life | First weeks–months of life | First weeks–months of life |
| Natural history | Fully grown at birth, involute in infancy | Proliferate in infancy, then involute | Proliferate in infancy, then involute |
| % Female | 48.5 | 66.2 | 70 |
| Prenatal appearance | Large, spherical, often heterogeneous with central necrosis/fibrosis, calcification | Multiple small spherical homogeneous masses, hepatomegaly | Innumerable masses or heterogeneous enlarged liver |
| Postnatal enhancement | Peripheral rim enhancement with no central enhancement of necrotic areas on delay | Centripetal enhancement with delayed homogeneous enhancement | Centripetal enhancement with delayed homogeneous enhancement |
| Cutaneous | 15.3% | 77.4% | 53.3% |
| Complications | High-flow shunts → CHF, mild anemia and thrombocytopenia | Occasional high-flow shunts → CHF, anemia, thrombocytopenia | Mass effect on IVC, renal and hepatic veins and chest with respiratory compromise, multiorgan failure |
| Hypothyroidism | 0% | 21.4% | 100%, profound hypothyroidism |
| Response to medical treatment | Unclear | Good | Poor |

*MRI:* All types are predominantly T2 hyperintense and T1 hypointense, but large solitary tumors may be heterogeneous secondary to necrosis, hemorrhage, thrombus, fibrosis, and calcification (Fig. 18.3-10). Dilated vessels are tubular flow voids on T2-weighted MRI. Shunting is suspected when there are large flow voids with aortic caliber change. Small nodules of the multifocal or diffuse subtypes may be more apparent on MRI rather than US because of the soft tissue contrast and tend to be homogeneous in signal.[74]

There is an association with cutaneous hemangiomas (Table 18.3-4). When HAE is diffuse, there may be extrahepatic involvement of many organs.[70] Hemangioendothelioma is rarely associated with other congenital anomalies.

**Differential Diagnosis:** Other hepatic tumors, including mesenchymal hamartoma, hepatoblastoma, and metastases, are the primary differential considerations. Urine catecholamines help differentiate neuroblastoma metastases in the case of multifocal disease. Alpha-fetoprotein (AFP) does not differentiate it from hepatoblastoma since AFP may be elevated in HAE and not elevated in half of congenital hepatoblastomas.

**Prognosis:** Asymptomatic patients have an excellent prognosis. Prognosis is poorer for patients with the diffuse form, hydrops, cardiac failure, jaundice, or thrombocytopenia.[75-77] Disseminated intravascular coagulation (DIC) rarely occurs.

**Management:** Prenatal fetal blood sampling to diagnose DIC with subsequent in utero platelet transfusion,[78] prenatal treatment with maternal oral steroids,[79] and intrauterine steroids via the umbilical vein and amniotic fluid[80] have been described. Rarely, tumor rupture during delivery may result in massive hemorrhage, so cesarean section should be considered.[70] Postnatally, asymptomatic patients are monitored with serial imaging. Symptomatic patients are treated medically. Corticosteroids are first-line treatment to hasten involution. Propranolol, vincristine, or interferon may be used in addition to steroids or separately. Medical therapy is often effective for GLUT-1(+) tumors, but effectiveness is unknown for GLUT-1(−) tumors.[75] Approximately one-third of patients with shunts fail pharmacologic therapy and require embolization. If medical management is ineffective, surgical options include hepatic artery ligation or embolization of shunts, rarely resection, and as

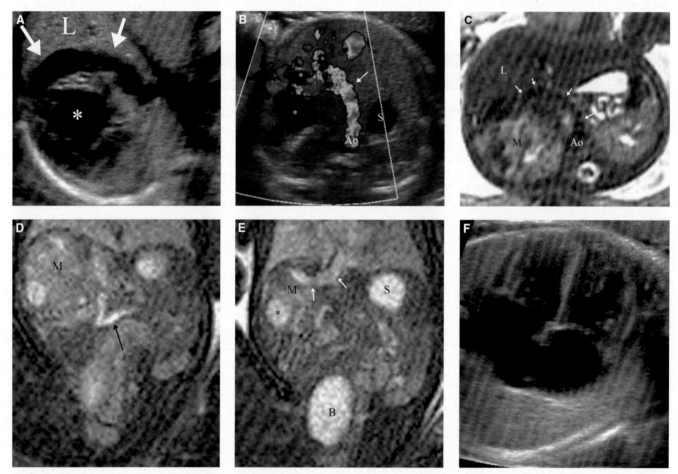

**FIGURE 18.3-10:** Hepatic hemangioma. **A:** Axial US image of the right lobe of the liver *(L)* demonstrates a heterogeneous, predominantly hypoechoic mass with a large round anechoic area centrally *(asterisk)* and a tubular anechoic structure anteriorly *(arrows)*. **B:** Doppler confirms that the tubular structure is a large celiac and hepatic artery *(arrow)* arising from the aorta *(Ao)*. There is no Doppler flow in anechoic cystic areas *(asterisks)* of degeneration. S, stomach. **C:** Axial MR T2w image demonstrates the heterogeneous, predominantly hyperintense mass *(M)*. The tubular hypointense flow void of the large artery *(arrows)* is displaced by the mass. Coronal SSFP images demonstrates **(D)** the large feeding artery *(arrow)* supplying the heterogeneous hepatic mass *(M)* and **(E)** large hepatic vein drains into the IVC *(arrows)*. S, stomach; B, bladder; asterisk, cystic degeneration. **F:** Four-chamber heart view demonstrates cardiomegaly secondary to high-flow shunt. (Courtesy of Chris Cassady, MD.)

a last resort, liver transplant. Symptomatic patients with diffuse disease should be quickly referred for transplant consideration while attempting medical therapy since their course is often short with high mortality. Thyroid function screening is recommended, since consumptive hypothyroidism associated with the multifocal and diffuse forms requires high-dose supplementation.[74]

**Recurrence Risk:** There are reports of hepatic IH regressing, and then recurring between 2½ and 5 years of age with malignant histology, and often metastatic disease, considered synonymous with angiosarcoma.[81]

## Mesenchymal Hamartoma

**Incidence:** Mesenchymal hamartomas (MH) account for 23% of liver tumors diagnosed in the perinatal period.[70]

**Embryology and Pathology:** Several chromosomal translocations have been described, favoring the hypothesis that MH may actually represent a neoplasia.[82]

There are four hypotheses (1) developmental, arising from a ductal plate malformation, (2) the result of a local vascular insult/ischemia, (3) a response to a toxic insult, or (4) a neoplasia rather than a hamartoma.[82]

MH is associated with placental mesenchymal stem villous hyperplasia (vascular malformation), and is not typically associated with other congenital anomalies.[82]

### Diagnosis

*Ultrasound:* MH is more common in the right lobe. Twenty percent are pedunculated and may not appear intrahepatic.[82] It has been diagnosed as early as 19 weeks gestation. Typically, it is a multilocular cystic structure with a variable soft tissue component (Fig. 18.3-11). There can be multiple thin mobile septations and hyperechoic intracystic nodules. Rare appearances include intracystic hemorrhage or debris, hypervascular angiomatous component or mixed MH-HAE, cysts so small that the mass appears solid on imaging, or echogenic calcifications.

Look for complications related to mass effect such as polyhydramnios, hydrops, and diaphragm elevation with pulmonary hypoplasia.

*MRI:* Large field of view is useful in assessing the origin of these masses by MRI. MH is T1-weighted hypointense, but variable signal intensity on T2-weighted imaging (Fig. 18.3-11).[82] Lung hypoplasia can be assessed.

**Differential Diagnosis:** The differential diagnosis for lesions in the liver includes hepatic cyst, hemangioendothelioma, and cystic hepatoblastoma. Pedunculated tumors may mimic intraabdominal cysts, particularly lymphatic cysts or cystic teratoma because of the septations.[82]

**Prognosis:** The prognosis is poorer for those diagnosed in utero than in childhood, with 29% mortality, predominantly because of mass effect.[83] There are reports of partial spontaneous regression, particularly in cases with a prominent angiomatous component. There are also rare reports of undifferentiated embryonal cell carcinoma of the liver arising within MH or after incomplete resection.[82]

**Management:** Prenatal follow-up with US is important to monitor size. They often enlarge quickly and can cause significant mass effect. Prenatal cyst decompression may alleviate mass effect and allow more normal fetal development, but fluid typically reaccumulates quickly. If the cyst is large, cesarean section may be performed for potential dystocia. Postnatally, symptomatic cysts are usually treated with surgical resection. Imaging and clinical follow-up is recommended for 5 years.[82]

**Recurrence Risk:** Recurrence rate is not documented, but recurrence of MH is reported after incomplete resection, and there are also cases of recurrence from small unrecognized satellite lesions.[82]

## Hepatoblastoma

**Incidence:** The incidence of hepatoblastoma in U.S. children under age 1 is 10.5/1,000,000, and has been increasing.[84] Less than

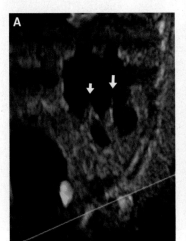
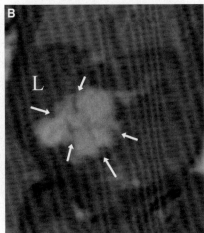
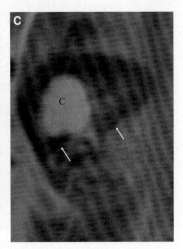

**FIGURE 18.3-11:** Mesenchymal hamartoma. **A:** Parasagittal US demonstrates an anechoic lobulated right upper quadrant abdominal mass with septations *(arrows)* and lack of internal Doppler signal. **B:** Coronal SSFP image demonstrates hyperintense signal in the lobulated mass in the liver *(L)* with several thin hypointense septations *(arrows)*. **C:** A sagittal T2w image best depicts its location within the liver (inferior margin of the liver is denoted by *arrows*). C, cyst.

10% of all hepatoblastomas occur in the perinatal period. It accounts for 17% of liver tumors diagnosed in the perinatal period.[70]

**Embryology and Pathology:** Multiple cytogenetic abnormalities have been described in association with childhood hepatoblastoma, including gain of chromosome 20, 2, or 8. There is also an association with trisomy 18.[84] An association with familial adenomatous polyposis has led to the discovery of adenomatous polyposis coli (APC)/β-catenin gene mutations found even in some sporadic hepatoblastoma cases. Changes in expression of *H19* and *IGF2* have been described, and are also commonly seen in Beckwith–Weidemann syndrome, with which hepatoblastoma is associated.[84,85]

It is hypothesized that oxygen free radicals may impede hepatocyte differentiation. There is also a high incidence of hepatoblastoma in very lowbirth weight infants, but whether the tumor is initiated or promoted by environmental factors of the NICU or owing to a common etiology is controversial and not proven.[84]

Hepatoblastoma is derived from undifferentiated embryonal tissue and may be classified as epithelial (subclassified as fetal, embryonal, or small cell undifferentiated) or mixed epithelial/mesenchymal subtypes. Congenital hepatoblastomas are more often the pure fetal histology. In childhood, metastases occur in the lung. In prenatal cases the lungs are spared, presumably because of fetal circulation, and metastases occur in the brain, bone, and placenta.[86]

### Diagnosis

*Ultrasound:* Review of the antenatally diagnosed case reports indicates that fetal hepatoblastomas are typically diagnosed by US late in the third trimester as a large mass measuring 6 to 10 cm, although it has been seen as early as 30 weeks, and as small as 2.5 cm.[87] They are typically single, but may be multiple, and are more common in the right lobe.[70] On US, it is usually hyperechoic but may be heterogeneous with areas of degeneration demonstrating necrosis, hemorrhage, and calcification. It is a vascular, predominantly solid tumor. It may appear polylobular with a "spoke-wheel appearance."[87]

Mass effect may result in compression of vessels (umbilical vein, portal vein, and IVC), hydrops and compression of the lungs resulting in respiratory distress.

*MRI:* Hepatoblastomas are typically T2-weighted hyperintense, and T1-weighted hypointense, but there may be heterogeneity in large tumors if there is associated degeneration (Fig. 18.3-12). MRI is useful for lung volume calculation and metastasis detection.

**Differential Diagnosis:** The differential diagnosis includes hemangioendothelioma, metastases, and mesenchymal hamartoma. The serum AFP is not a good discriminator. It is only elevated in half of congenital cases, and may rarely be elevated in hemangioendothelioma and mesenchymal hamartoma.[70]

**Prognosis:** The prognosis is poor. Mass effect may compress vessels, resulting in hydrops and stillbirth. Diaphragmatic elevation may compress the lungs, resulting in respiratory distress. Tumor hemorrhage, spontaneous or related to vaginal delivery, may result in anemia or death. Rarely, metastases contribute to mortality.[89] The survival rate for treated congenital hepatoblastoma patients is 40%, for untreated patients is 0%, and the overall survival is 25%. There is a difference in survival based on histology with 50% survival for pure fetal histology and 30% for fetal + embryonal.[70] There have been improved mortality rates with treatment of childhood hepatoblastomas, but it is not known whether modern treatment has improved mortality for those diagnosed in the perinatal period.

**Management:** Prenatally, hepatic masses are followed with imaging to assess growth, mass effect on adjacent structures, and to monitor for hydrops. Cesarean section should be considered since these tumors are known to bleed and rupture during delivery and are typically large and may cause dystocia.[70] Postnatally, they are treated with surgical resection. Chemotherapy may be used preoperatively to shrink the tumor, and/or postnatally to control microscopic disease.

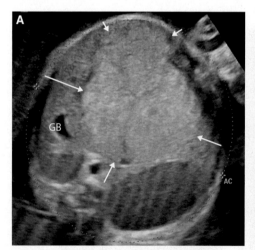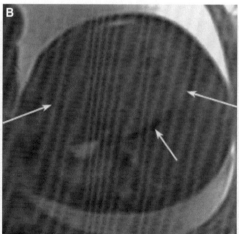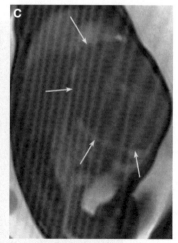

**FIGURE 18.3-12:** Hepatoblastoma. **A:** Transverse US demonstrates a large echogenic liver mass *(arrows)* displacing the gallbladder *(GB)*. There are subtle linear hypoechoic structures in a spoke-wheel orientation. **B:** Axial T2-weighted prenatal MR image demonstrates a large liver mass *(arrows)* with mild hyperintense T2-weighted signal relative to liver. **C:** Sagittal SSFP image demonstrates mild heterogeneous signal centrally within the mass *(arrows)*. (Reprinted from Al-Hussein H, Graham E, Tekes A, et al. Pre- and postnatal imaging of a congenital hepatoblastoma. *Fetal Diagn Ther*. 2011;30(2):157–159. Copyright © 2011, with permission from S. Karger AG, Basel, Switzerland.)[88]

**Recurrence Risk:** Hepatoblastoma diagnosed in childhood recurs, so presumably congenital hepatoblastoma may recur, but there are no data to cite a recurrence rate.

## OTHER ABDOMINAL MASSES

*Teratoma and fetus in fetu* both demonstrate heterogeneous appearance on US and MR, often with soft tissue, bone, and fat elements, and with varying degrees of organization. Fetus in fetu is a rare diagnosis in which a monochorionic, monozygotic twin is incorporated into the host twin. Some authors believe that presence of four limbs appropriately arranged relative to a vertebral column differentiates it from a teratoma, and others believe that a vertebral column is not required for the diagnosis.[90,91] Both fetus in fetu and teratoma are completely surgically excised with their surrounding membranes to reduce the risk of recurrence.[91]

*Gastric pseudomass* is a rounded echogenic area in the lumen of the stomach, possibly as a result of swallowed cells or hemorrhage in the amniotic fluid, which aggregates because of poor peristalsis in the second trimester. They resolve on follow-up imaging.[92]

*Meconium pseudocyst* is a well-defined hypoechoic mass with a hyperechoic-calcified wall and indicates bowel perforation[92] (see Chapter 18.1).

*Extralobar subdiaphragmatic pulmonary sequestration* occurs more commonly on the left (4:1) as an echogenic subdiaphragmatic mass, and the diagnosis is supported by identifying a thoracic aortic feeding vessel with Doppler. On MRI, it is homogeneously T2 hyperintense, and a feeding artery may be seen as a hypointense tubular flow void on T2-weighted imaging. They are typically seen in the second trimester and more often on the left, as opposed to neuroblastomas which are more hypoechoic and more often seen in the third trimester on the right[92] (see Chapter 17).

## The Gallbladder

The gallbladder is first visible by US at 13 to 14 weeks gestation as a fluid-filled, anechoic structure in the right upper quadrant, subhepatic or intrahepatic in location, and to the right of the umbilical vein. Size increases linearly with gestational age and plateaus at 32 to 35 weeks. It has a sinusoidal contractility pattern over a 3-hour interval that is independent of maternal meals. While the percent contractility increases through the third trimester, the minimum volume is relatively constant, so the gallbladder should be visible on imaging throughout the cycle.[93] The MRI signal of the gallbladder contents is variable and is age dependent. Before 27 weeks, gallbladder contents are T1 hypointense and T2 hyperintense. After 30 weeks, T1 and T2 signal are variable. This is likely due to sludge or accumulation of paramagnetic substances in the gallbladder mucous.[94]

### Nonvisualization of the Fetal Gallbladder

This is typically defined as not seeing the gallbladder on two USs within 7 to 15 days. With modern equipment and transvaginal technique at 14 to 16 weeks, the gallbladder is absent in only 0.1% of pregnancies.[95] The most recent data for transabdominal detection are from 1996 when nonvisualization was 68.6% at 12 to 16 weeks and decreased with gestational age to 7% at 20 to 24 weeks.[96] Blazer found that absent gallbladder was isolated in 59% (incidence 1 in 6,000 pregnancies) with normal outcome. Associated

structural malformations were present in 41%, and 36% of those also had abnormal karyotype. The gallbladder was detected later in pregnancy or postnatally in 4/5 structurally abnormal babies that were not terminated, and in 13/20 normal babies.[95] Nonvisualization of the gallbladder is associated with cystic fibrosis, biliary atresia, and aneuploidy, so amniocentesis with karyotype and evaluation of amniotic digestive enzymes may be useful.

### Cholecystomegaly

This is defined as gallbladder area more than 2 standard deviations above the mean for gestational age. Despite small retrospective studies suggesting an association with aneuploidy or biliary abnormalities, a large prospective study found cholecystomegaly in 43 of 775 (5.5%) fetuses and no such association.[97]

### Gallbladder Stones and Sludge

Echoes in the gallbladder with posterior acoustic shadowing suggest stones, and those without shadowing suggest sludge. There are few reported cases with an estimated incidence of 1% after 28 weeks' gestation.[98] They often resolve in utero or in the first year of life without symptoms. Management includes follow-up US and possibly postnatal ursodeoxycholic acid.[99]

## REFERENCES

1. Ozyuncu O, Canpolat FE, Ciftci AO, et al. Perinatal outcomes of fetal abdominal cysts and comparison of prenatal and postnatal diagnoses. *Fetal Diagn Ther.* 2010;28:153–159.
2. Cohen HL, Shapiro MA, Mandel FS, et al. Normal ovaries in neonates and infants: a sonographic study of 77 patients 1 day to 24 months old. *AJR Am J Roentgenol.* 1993;160:583–586.
3. Nussbaum AR, Sanders RS, Hartman DS, et al. Neonatal ovarian cysts: sonographic-pathologic correlation. *Radiology.* 1988;168:817–821.
4. Meizner I, Levy A, Katz M, et al. Fetal ovarian cysts: prenatal ultrasonographic detection and postnatal evaluation and treatment. *Am J Obstet Gynecol.* 1991;164(3):874–878.
5. Dimitraki M, Koutlaki N, Nikas I, et al. Fetal ovarian cysts: our clinical experience over 16 cases and review of the literature. *J Matern Fetal Neonatal Med.* 2012;25(3):222–225.
6. Nemac U, Nemac SF, Bettelheim D, et al. Ovarian cysts on prenatal MRI. *Eur J Radiol.* 2012;81:1937–1944.
7. Sakala E, Leon Z, Rouse GA. Management of antenatally diagnosed fetal ovarian cysts. *Obstet Gynecol Surv.* 1991;46(7):407–414.
8. Noia G, Riccardi M, Visconti D, et al. Invasive fetal therapies: approach and results in treating fetal ovarian cysts. *J Matern Fetal Neonatal Med.* 2012;25(3):299–303.
9. Słodki M, Respondek-Liberska M. Fetal ovarian cysts—420 cases from literature—metaanalysis 1984–2005. *Ginekol Pol.* 2007;78(4):324–328.
10. Shimada T, Miura K, Gotoh H, et al. Management of prenatal ovarian cysts. *Early Hum Dev.* 2008;84(6):417–420.
11. Charlesworth P, Ade-Ajayi N, Davenport M. Natural history and long-term follow-up of antenatally detected liver cysts. *J Pediatr Surg.* 2007;42(3):494–499.
12. Rogers T, Woodley H, Ramsden W, et al. Solitary liver cysts in children: not always so simple. *J Pediatr Surg.* 2007;42(2):333–339.
13. Avni EF, Rypens F, Donner C, et al. Hepatic cysts and hyperechogenicities: perinatal assessment and unifying theory on their origin. *Pediatr Radiol.* 1994;24(8):569–572.
14. Hackmon-Ram R, Wiznitzer A, Gohar J, et al. Prenatal diagnosis of a fetal abdominal cyst. *Eur J Obstet Gynecol Reprod Biol.* 2000;91(1):79–82.
15. Ito M, Yoshimura K, Toyoda N, et al. Aspiration of giant hepatic cyst in the fetus in utero. *Fetal Diagn Ther.* 1997;12(4):221–225.
16. Yamaguchi M. Congenital choledochal cyst: analysis of 1,433 patients in the Japanese literature. *Am J Surg.* 1980;140(5):653–657.
17. Edil BH, Cameron JL, Reddy S, et al. Choledochal cyst disease in children and adults: a 30 year single institution experience. *J Am Coll Surg.* 2008;206(5):1000–1005.
18. Ando H. Embryology of the biliary tract. *Dig Surg.* 2012;27:87–89.
19. Mackenzie TC, Howell LJ, Flake AW, et al. The management of prenatally diagnosed choledochal cysts. *J Pediatr Surg.* 2001;36(8):1241–1243.
20. Landing BH. Considerations of the pathogenesis of neonatal hepatitis, biliary atresia and choledochal cyst—the concept of infantile obstructive cholangiopathy. *Prog Pediatr Surg.* 1974;6:113–139.
21. Alonso-Lej F, Rever WB Jr, Pessagno DJ. Congenital choledochal cyst, with a report of 2, and an analysis of 94, cases. *Int Abstr Surg.* 1959;108(1):1–30.

22. Todani T, Watanabe Y, Narusue M, et al. Congenital bile duct cysts: classification, operative procedures, and review of thirty-seven cases including cancer arising from choledochal cyst. *Am J Surg.* 1977;134(2):263–269.

23. Lipsett PA, Pitt HA, Colombani PM, et al. Choledochal cyst: a changing pattern of presentation. *Ann Surg.* 1994;220(5):644–652.

24. Murphy A, Axt J, Lovvorn H. Associations between pediatric choledochal cysts, biliary atresia, and congenital cardiac anomalies. *J Surg Res.* 2012;177(2):e59–e63.

25. Lee HC, Yeung CY, Chang PY, et al. Dilatation of the biliary tree in children: sonographic diagnosis and its clinical significance. *J Ultrasound Med.* 2000;19(3):177–182.

26. Casaccia G, Bilancioni E, Nahom A, et al. Cystic anomalies of biliary tree in the fetus: is it possible to make a more specific prenatal diagnosis? *J Pediatr Surg.* 2002;37(8):1191–1194.

27. Gallivan EK, Crombleholme TM, D'Alton ME. Early prenatal diagnosis of choledochal cyst. *Prenat Diagn.* 1996;16(10):934–937.

28. Redkar R, Davenport M, Howard ER. Antenatal diagnosis of congenital anomalies of the biliary tract. *J Pediatr Surg.* 1998;33(5):700–704.

29. Diao M, Li L, Cheng W. Timing of surgery for prenatally diagnosed asymptomatic choledochal cysts: a prospective randomized study. *J Pediatr Surg.* 2012;47(3):506–512.

30. Tsuchida Y, Kawarasaki H, Iwanaka T, et al. Antenatal diagnosis of biliary atresia (type Icyst) at 19 weeks' gestation: differential diagnosis and etiologic implications. *J Pediatr Surg.* 1995;30(5):697–699.

31. Boyden EA. The accessory gall-bladder: an embryological and comparative study of aberrant biliary vesicles occurring in man and the domestic mammals. *Am J Anat.* 1926;38:177–231.

32. Bronshtein M, Weiner Z, Abramovici H, et al. Prenatal diagnosis of gall bladder anomalies—report of 17 cases. *Prenat Diagn.* 1993;13(9):851–861.

33. Harlaftis N, Gray SW, Skandalakis JE. Multiple gallbladders. *J Am Coll Surg.* 1977;145(6):928–934.

34. Gerscovich E, Towner D, Sanchez T, et al. Fetal gallbladder duplication. *J Ultrasound Med.* 2011;30(9):1310–1312.

35. Kinoshita L, Callen P, Filly R, et al. Sonographic detection of gallbladder duplication: two cases discovered in utero. *J Ultrasound Med.* 2002;21(12):1417–1421.

36. Sifakis S, Mantas N, Koumantakis G, et al. Prenatal diagnosis of gallbladder duplication. *Ultrasound Obstet Gynecol.* 2007;30(3):362–363.

37. Foley P, Sithasanan N, McEwing R, et al. Enteric duplications presenting as antenatally detected abdominal cysts: is delayed resection appropriate? *J Pediatr Surg.* 2003;38(12):1810–1813.

38. Holcomb GW III, Gheissari A, O'Neill JA, et al. Surgical management of alimentary tract duplications. *Ann Surg.* 1989;209(2):167–174.

39. Macpherson RI. Gastrointestinal tract duplications: clinical, pathologic, etiologic, and radiologic considerations. *Radiographics.* 1993;13(5):1063–1080.

40. Tseng JJ, Chou MM, Ho ES. In utero sonographic diagnosis of a communicating enteric duplication cyst in a giant omphalocele. *Prenat Diagn.* 2001;21(7):540–542.

41. Ildstad ST, Tollerud DJ, Weiss RG, et al. Duplications of the alimentary tract: clinical characteristics, preferred treatment, and associated malformations. *Ann Surg.* 1988;208(2):184–189.

42. Giacalone PL, Boulot P, Deschamps F, et al. Prenatal diagnosis of a multifocal lymphangioma. *Prenat Diagn.* 1993;13(12):1133–1137.

43. Deshpande P, Twining P, O'Neill D. Prenatal diagnosis of fetal abdominal lymphangioma by ultrasonography. *Ultrasound Obstet Gynecol.* 2001;17(5):445–448.

44. Kurtz RJ, Heimann TM, Holt J, et al. Mesenteric and retroperitoneal cysts. *Ann Surg.* 1986;203(1):109–112.

45. Kozlowski KJ, Frazier CN, Quirk JG. Prenatal diagnosis of abdominal cystic hygroma. *Prenat Diagn.* 1988;8(6):405–409.

46. Katz VL, Watson WJ, Thorp JM, et al. Prenatal sonographic findings of massive lower extremity lymphangioma. *Am J Perinatol.* 1992;9(2):127–129.

47. Kaminopetros P, Jauniaux E, Kane P, et al. Prenatal diagnosis of an extensive fetal lymphangioma using ultrasonography, magnetic resonance imaging and cytology. *Br J Radiol.* 1997;70(835):750–753.

48. Santo S, Marques J, Veca P, et al. Prenatal ultrasonographic diagnosis of abdominal cystic lymphangioma: a case report. *J Matern Fetal Neonatal Med.* 2008;21(8):565–566.

49. Devesa R, Muñoz A, Torrents M, et al. Prenatal ultrasonographic findings of intra-abdominal cystic lymphangioma: a case report. *J Clin Ultrasound.* 1997;25(6):330–332.

50. Salvador A, Rosenberg HK, Horrow MM, et al. Abdominal lymphangioma in a preterm infant. *J Perinatol.* 1996;16(4):305–308.

51. Dankovcik R, Urdzik P, Lazar I, et al. Conservative management in three cases of prenatally recognized splenic cyst using 2D, 3D, multi-slice and Doppler ultrasonography. *Fetal Diagn Ther.* 2009;26(3):177–180.

52. Garel C, Hassan M. Foetal and neonatal splenic cyst-like lesions: US follow-up of seven cases. *Pediatr Radiol.* 1995;25(5):360–362.

53. Lopes MA, Ruano R, Bunduki V, et al. Prenatal diagnosis and follow up of congenital splenic cyst: a case report. *Ultrasound Obstet Gynecol.* 2001;17(5):439–441.

54. Gerscovich EO, Fiels NT, Sanchez T, et al. Fetal true pancreatic cysts. *J Ultrasound Med.* 2012;31:811–813.

55. Choi SJ, Kang MC, Kim YH, et al. Prenatal detection of a congenital pancreatic cyst by ultrasound. *J Korean Med Sci.* 2007;22(1):156–158.

56. Liao Y, Chen H, Chou C, et al. Antenatal detection of a congenital pancreatic cyst. *J Formos Med Assoc.* 2003;102(4):273–276.

57. Balci S, Altinok G, Tekşen F, et al. A 34-week-old male fetus with short rib polydactyly syndrome (SRPS) type I (Saldino-Noonan) with pancreatic cysts. *Turk J Pediatr.* 2003;45(2):174–178.

58. Boopathy Vijayaraghavan S, Kamalam M, Raman ML. Prenatal sonographic appearance of congenital bile duct dilatation associated with renal-hepatic-pancreatic dysplasia. *Ultrasound Obstet Gynecol.* 2004;23(6):609–611.

59. Auringer ST, Ulmer JL, Sumner TE, et al. Congenital cyst of the pancreas. *J Pediatr Surg.* 1993;28(12):1570–1571.

60. Ishimaru T, Uchida H, Yotsumoto K, et al. Recurrence of a congenital pancreatic cyst mimicking omental cyst after laparoscopic cyst resection. *Eur J Pediatr Surg.* 2009;19(1):53–54.

61. Clayton P. Diagnosis of inherited disorders of liver metabolism. *J Inherit Metab Dis.* 2003;26(2–3):135–146.

62. Chen C, Lin S, Tzen C, et al. Prenatal diagnosis and genetic counseling of mucopolysaccharidosis type II (Hunter syndrome). *Genet Couns.* 2007;18(1):49–56.

63. Srisupundit K, Tongprasert F, Luewan S, et al. Splenic circumference at midpregnancy as a predictor of hemoglobin Bart's disease among fetuses at risk. *Gynecol Obstet Invest.* 2011;72:63–67.

64. Mignot C, Gelot A, Bessières B, et al. Perinatal-lethal Gaucher disease. *Am J Med Genet A.* 2003;120A(3):338–344.

65. Mochel F, Grébille AG, Benachi A, et al. Contribution of fetal MR imaging in the prenatal diagnosis of Zellweger syndrome. *AJNR Am J Neuroradiol.* 2006;27(2):333–336.

66. Patel S, DeSantis E. Treatment of congenital tuberculosis. *Am J Health Syst Pharm.* 2008;65(21):2027–2031.

67. Williams D, Gauthier D, Maizels M. Prenatal diagnosis of Beckwith-Wiedemann syndrome. *Prenat Diagn.* 2005;25(10):879–884.

68. Ogawa M, Hosoya N, Sato A, et al. Is the degree of fetal hepatosplenomegaly with transient abnormal myelopoiesis closely related to the postnatal severity of hematological abnormalities in Down syndrome? *Ultrasound Obstet Gynecol.* 2004;24(1):83–85.

69. Bahado-Singh R, Oz U, Mari G, et al. Fetal splenic size in anemia due to Rh-alloimmunization. *Obstet Gynecol.* 1998;92(5):828–832.

70. Isaacs H. Fetal and neonatal hepatic tumors. *J Pediatr Surg.* 2007;42(11):1797–1803.

71. Applegate KE, Ghei M, Perez-Atayde AR. Prenatal detection of a solitary liver adenoma. *Pediatr Radiol.* 1999;29(2):92–94.

72. Petrikovsky BM, Cohen HL, Scimeca P, et al. Prenatal diagnosis of focal nodular hyperplasia of the liver. *Prenat Diagn.* 1994;14(5):406–409.

73. North P, Waner M, Brodsky M. Are infantile hemangioma of placental origin? *Ophthalmology.* 2002;109(2):223–224.

74. Christison-Lagay ER, Burrows PE, Alomari A, et al. Hepatic hemangiomas: subtype classification and development of a clinical practice algorithm and registry. *J Pediatr Surg.* 2007;42(1):62–67; discussion 67-68.

75. Kulungowski A, Alomari A, Chawla A, et al. Lessons from a liver hemangioma registry: subtype classification. *J Pediatr Surg.* 2012;47(1):165–170.

76. Selby DM, Stocker JT, Waclawiw MA, et al. Infantile hemangioendothelioma of the liver. *Hepatology.* 1994;20(1, pt 1):39–45.

77. Kuroda T, Kumagai M, Nosaka S, et al. Critical infantile hepatic hemangioma: results of a nationwide survey by the Japanese Infantile Hepatic Hemangioma study group. *J Pediatr Surg.* 2011;46(12):2239–2243.

78. Gembruch U, Baschat AA, Gloeckner-Hoffmann K, et al. Prenatal diagnosis and management of fetuses with liver hemangiomata. *Ultrasound Obstet Gynecol.* 2002;19(5):454–460.

79. Morris J, Abbott J, Burrows P, et al. Antenatal diagnosis of fetal hepatic hemangioma treated with maternal corticosteroids. *Obstet Gynecol.* 1999;94(5, pt 2):813–815.

80. Mejides AA, Adra AM, O'Sullivan MJ, et al. Prenatal diagnosis and therapy for a fetal hepatic vascular malformation. *Obstet Gynecol.* 1995;85(5, pt 2):850–853.

81. Ackermann O, Fabre M, Franchi S, et al. Widening spectrum of liver angiosarcoma in children. *J Pediatr Gastroenterol Nutr.* 2011;53(6):615–619.

82. Stringer M, Alizai N. Mesenchymal hamartoma of the liver: a systematic review. *J Pediatr Surg.* 2005;40(11):1681–1690.

83. Cornette J, Festen S, van den Hoonaard T, et al. Mesenchymal hamartoma of the liver: a benign tumor with deceptive prognosis in the perinatal period. *Fetal Diagn Ther.* 2009;25(2):196–202.

84. Spector L, Birch J. The epidemiology of hepatoblastoma. *Pediatr Blood Cancer.* 2012;59(5):776–779.

85. Herzog CE, Andrassy RJ, Eftekhari F. Childhood cancers: hepatoblastoma. *Oncologist.* 2000;5(6):445–453.

86. Makin E, Davenport M. Fetal and neonatal liver tumours. *Early Hum Dev.* 2010;86(10):637–642.

87. Catanzarite V, Hilfiker M, Daneshmand S, et al. Prenatal diagnosis of fetal hepatoblastoma: case report and review of the literature. *J Ultrasound Med.* 2008;27(7):1095–1098.

88. Al-Hussein H, Graham E, Tekes A, et al. Pre- and postnatal imaging of a congenital hepatoblastoma. *Fetal Diagn Ther.* 2011;30(2):157–159.

89. Ammann RA, Plaschkes J, Leibundgut K. Congenital hepatoblastoma: a distinct entity? *Med Pediatr Oncol.* 1999;32(6):466–468.

90. Escobar M, Rossman J, Caty M. Fetus-in-fetu: report of a case and a review of the literature. *J Pediatr Surg.* 2008;43(5):943–946.

91. Basu A, Jagdish S, Iyengar K, et al. Fetus in fetu or differentiated teratomas? *Indian J Pathol Microbiol.* 2006;49(4):563–565.

92. McNamara A, Levine D. Intraabdominal fetal echogenic masses: a practical guide to diagnosis and management. *Radiographics.* 2005;25(3):633–645.

93. Tanaka Y, Senoh D, Hata T. Is there a human fetal gallbladder contractility during pregnancy? *Hum Reprod.* 2000;15(6):1400–1402.

94. Brugger P, Weber M, Prayer D. Magnetic resonance imaging of the fetal gallbladder and bile. *Eur Radiol.* 2010;20(12):2862–2869.

95. Blazer S, Zimmer EZ, Bronshtein M. Nonvisualization of the fetal gallbladder in early pregnancy: comparison with clinical outcome. *Radiology.* 2002;224(2):379–382.

96. Hertzberg BS, Kliewer MA, Maynor C, et al. Nonvisualization of the fetal gallbladder: frequency and prognostic importance. *Radiology.* 1996;199(3):679–682.

97. Hertzberg BS, Kliewer MA, Bowie JD, et al. Enlarged fetal gallbladder: prognostic importance for aneuploidy or biliary abnormality at antenatal US. *Radiology.* 1998;208(3):795–798.

98. Kiserud T, Gjelland K, Bognø H, et al. Echogenic material in the fetal gallbladder and fetal disease. *Ultrasound Obstet Gynecol.* 1997;10(2):103–106.

99. Iroh Tam P, Angelides A. Perinatal detection of gallstones in siblings. *Am J Perinatol.* 2010;27(10):771–774.

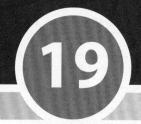

# 19 Genitourinary Abnormalities

## 19.1 Renal and Adrenal Abnormalities

Fred E. Avni

Congenital malformations of the urinary tract are among the most commonly identified abnormalities at antenatal ultrasound (US) with an incidence between 1 in 250 and 1 in 1,000 pregnancies. Abnormalities range from benign and simple conditions such as unilateral renal pelvic dilatation up to complex malformations or even life-threatening conditions, such as bilateral multicystic dysplasia. The kidney malformation can be an isolated finding or part of a polymalformative syndrome.[1–3]

US plays a central role in assessing the normal and abnormal fetal urinary tract. Fetal MR imaging has become a complementary examination in cases of complex malformations or when US is limited because of fetal or maternal limiting factors (e.g., oligohydramnios, fetal lie, maternal obesity). The findings of both techniques must be interpreted conjointly in order to provide the most accurate information to determine prognosis and appropriate management for delivery and postnatal care.[4–7]

Integrating imaging data along with familial, biological, and genetic data are of utmost importance as they can provide additional information for a proper diagnosis. Familial diseases clearly influence the course of the fetal development, as do maternofetal diseases. Advances in genetic research in isolated or polymalformative kidney diseases are obvious and increasing day after day; this has led to two important concepts: congenital anomalies of the kidney and urinary tract (CAKUT) (Table 19.1-1) and ciliopathies (Table 19.1-2). CAKUT account for the largest group of pediatric patients with end-stage renal diseases encompassing a broad phenotype spectrum. There is wide variability in genotype–phenotype correlation, indicating a complex process depending on many factors. Ciliopathies have brought a unifying concept in relation to hepatorenal fibrocystic diseases. In selected patients with urinary tract abnormalities,

| Table 19.1-1 | Principal Congenital Anomalies of the Kidney and Urinary Tract (CAKUT)[10,11] |
|---|---|

Duplex kidneys
Horseshoe kidneys
Multicystic dysplastic kidney
Polycystic kidneys
Posterior urethral valves
Renal agenesis
Renal dysplasia
Renal hypoplasia
Vesicoureteric reflux

| Table 19.1-2 | Principal Ciliary Disorders Associated with Congenital Hepatorenal Fibrocystic Diseases (Including Major Gene Mutations)[4] |
|---|---|

Autosomal dominant polycystic kidney disease (PKD1-PKD2)
Autosomal recessive polycystic kidney disease (PKHD-1)
Bardet–Biedl syndrome (BBSI → BBS10, MSK1)
Ellis van Creveld syndrome (EVC1-EVC2)
Glomerulocystic kidney disease (HNF-1β)
Jeune chondrodysplasia (IFT80)
Joubert syndrome (NHPH1)
Meckel–Gruber syndrome (MSK1, MSK3)
Nephronophithisis (NPH1, NPH3, NPH4, NPH8)
Orofaciodigital syndrome (OFD1)
Renal hepatic pancreatic dysplasia (NPHP3) (Zellweger syndrome)

chromosomal analysis needs to be performed and will provide information as well.[8–13]

## EMBRYOLOGY

The development of the human kidney starts when the primitive nephritic duct is formed on the embryonic day 22 from the intermediate mesoderm. The human urinary tract results from the progressive development and subsequent degeneration of three overlapping systems: the pronephros, the mesonephros, and the metanephros (Fig. 19.1-1). The *pronephros* forms a vestigial excretory unit that disappears by the end of the 4th week. The *mesonephros* development starts during the 4th week and results in primitive excretory tubules that eventually form primitive glomeruli at their medial extremity. These excretory tubules and primitive glomeruli form the renal corpuscle. These early structures degenerate rapidly, although some mesonephritic tubules remain and participate in the formation of the male reproductive system. The third system, the *metanephros* or permanent kidney, appears during the 5th week. On day 28, the definitive excretory units start to develop from the metanephric mesoderm; the definitive collecting ducts of the permanent kidney develop from the ureteric bud, an outgrowth of the vestigial mesonephritic duct. The ureteral bud invades the adjacent metanephric mesenchyme. Further development of the metanephros occurs via reciprocal inductive interactions between the ureteral bud and the mesenchyme. The ureteral bud end dilates progressively, forming the renal pelvis and subsequently, it splits into the future calyces. Each calyx forms new buds while penetrating the metanephritic tissue. At the periphery of the ureteral bud, initial generations of the ureteral bud are remodeled into the ureter, renal pelvis, and calyces; subsequent generations develop into collecting tubules (Fig. 19.1-2). The capillaries grow parallel to the collecting tubules and differentiate into the final

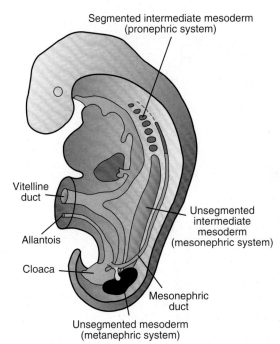

**FIGURE 19.1-1:** Relationship of the intermediate mesoderm of the pronephric, mesonephric, and metanephric systems. (From Sadler TW. The urogenital system. In: Sadler TW, ed. *Langman's Medical Embryology.* 9th ed. Philadelphia, PA: Lippincott Williams & Wilkins; 2004.321–362.)

glomeruli. The association of glomeruli and tubules represents a nephronic unit (Fig. 19.1-3). Nephrons are formed until the 36th week.

The embryo–fetal differentiation of the kidney involves epithelial/mesenchymal interactions under the regulation of many genes, the so-called renal developmental genes (RDG) that include transcription/growth factors and intracellular signaling molecules (e.g., RET, PAX2, HNF1Beta, UMOD, WT1); malfunction or mutation of these genes would induce urinary tract malformation.

The kidneys develop originally within the pelvis and ascend progressively to the lumbar areas (Fig. 19.1-4). The ureteral orifices move cranially into the bladder trigone, whereas the ejaculatory ducts, remains of the mesonephritic ducts, move

closer to the midline and enter the prostatic urethra where they open.

The bladder and urethra originate from the cloacal partition by the urorectal septum between the 7th and the 8th week. This partition separates the cloaca into the primitive urogenital sinus anteriorly and the anal canal posteriorly (Fig. 19.1-4). Subsequently, the urogenital sinus develops into three parts: *first*, the urinary bladder; *second*, the pelvic part of the urogenital sinus, which gives rise to the urethra (prostatic and membranous in the male, entire urethra in the female) and *third*, the phallic part that will correspond to the genital tubercle. The anterior urethra in the male develops as an ingrowth of the phallic ectoderm and closure of the urethral folds. Finally, the urogenital membrane breaks during the 7th week, establishing continuity between the developing urinary tract and the amniotic cavity. Chwalla membrane at the ureterovesical junction disappears during the 8th week. Intrinsic narrowings persist and can be discerned at the ureteropelvic and ureterovesical junction up to the 18th week.

If development is normal, urine production starts at the 9th week.[8–11,13,14]

## IMAGING OF THE NORMAL URINARY TRACT

### Ultrasound Imaging

The normal development of the urinary tract is well depicted by ultrasound. Bladder and ureter are clearly visible during the first trimester (Fig. 19.1-5). The fetal bladder is the first structure of the urinary tract to be visualized on US, appearing as an anechoic cystic structure within the fetal pelvis around 9 to 10 weeks' gestation. The kidneys themselves are visualized slightly later, appearing as two hyperechoic oval nodules, one at each side of the lumbar spine. During the first trimester, the kidneys appear globally hyperechoic, without corticomedullary differentiation (CMD). Throughout the rest of the pregnancy, the kidneys will grow and their echogenicity will evolve. The renal growth can be assessed by the measurement of the sagittal length compared with established nomograms (see Table 38 in Appendix A1). Renal length can be evaluated through the formula "renal length in cm = number of gestation weeks × 1.1 inches." This growth can also be assessed by the evaluation of renal parenchymal area or even volume calculation, although these types of measurements are not performed routinely. With evolving gestational

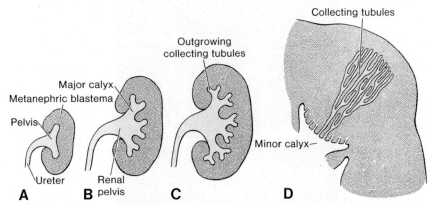

**FIGURE 19.1-2:** Development of the renal pelvis calyces and collecting tubules of the metanephros at 6 weeks **(A)**, at the end of 6 weeks **(B)**, at 7 weeks **(C)**, and in the newborn **(D)** . (From Sadler TW. The urogenital system. In: Sadler TW, ed. *Langman's Medical Embryology*. 9th ed. Philadelphia, PA: Lippincott Williams & Wilkins; 2004:321–362.)

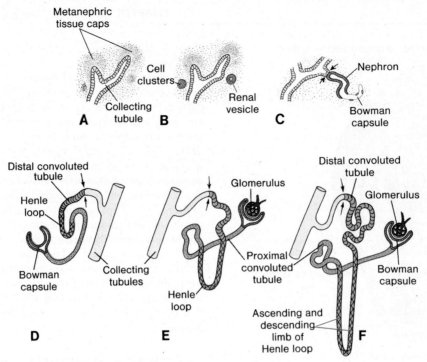

**FIGURE 19.1-3:** Stages in the development of a metanephric excretory unit (nephron) **(A)** Metanephric cap stage **(B)** Renal vesicle stage **(C)** S-shape tubule stage **(D)** Bowman's capsule stage **(E)** Glomerulus and proximal tubule stage **(F)** Distal convoluted tubule stage. The *arrows* point to the place where the excretory unit establishes an open communication that allows a flow of urine from the glomerulus into the collecting system. (From Sadler TW. The urogenital system. In: Sadler TW, ed. *Langman's Medical Embryology.* 9th ed. Philadelphia, PA: Lippincott Williams & Wilkins; 2004:321–362.)

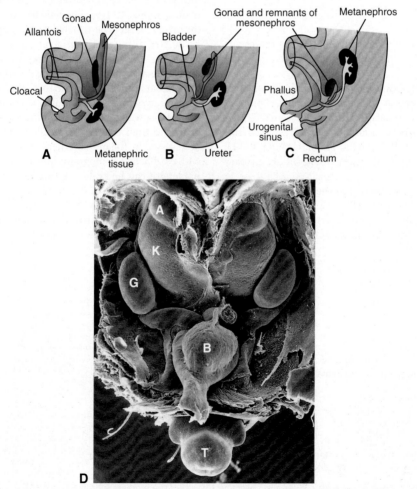

**FIGURE 19.1-4: A–C:** Cloacal partition into urogenital sinus and bladder anteriorly and rectum posteriorly. The ascent of the kidney is illustrated as well. **(D)** Scanning electron micrograph of a mouse embryo showing the kidneys in the pelvis. *B,* bladder; *K,* kidney; *A,* adrenal gland; *G,* gonad; *T,* tail. In: Sadler TW, ed. *Langman's Medical Embryology.* 9th ed. Philadelphia, PA: Lippincott Williams & Wilkins; 2004:321–362.)

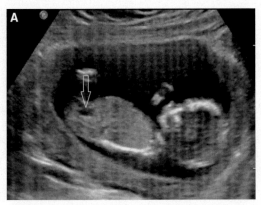
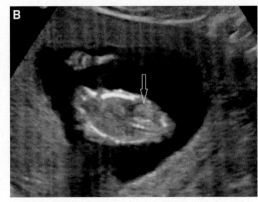

**FIGURE 19.1-5:** Fetal urinary tract at 13 weeks' gestation. **A:** The *arrow* points to the fluid-filled bladder. **B:** Coronal view. The *arrow* points to a hyperechoic normal kidney. Note the hypoechoic adrenal lying above the kidney.

age, the echogenicity of the renal cortex decreases with respect to the liver, and should be less echogenic than the liver by the third trimester. CMD should be progressively demonstrated—hypoechoic medulla compared to relatively hyperechoic cortex—starting at the 4th month of gestation (Figs. 19.1-6A and 19.1-7A). The renal vessels can easily be demonstrated with color or power Doppler (see Fig. 19.1-6B).[4,15–19]

The fetal bladder becomes larger, containing more urine (see Figs. 19.1-6C and 19.1-7B), and cycles of filling and emptying will be observed. These cycles slow at the end of the pregnancy especially in female fetuses. Even almost empty, it should be possible to identify the bladder using the umbilical arteries as

landmarks (see Fig. 19.1-6D). Filling of the bladder is influenced by maternal hydration. Normally, the fetal ureters are not visualized.[20,21]

Amniotic fluid volume should always be assessed. The kidney contributes by two-third to the amniotic fluid volume at the beginning of the 4th month of gestation.[22]

Information regarding the normal urinary tract can be obtained at each trimester of the pregnancy using US. In the first trimester, a fluid-filled bladder and hyperechoic kidneys should be identified. In the second and third trimesters, a systematic approach to evaluate the urinary tract includes identifying two kidneys, assessing size and echogenicity, including CMD,

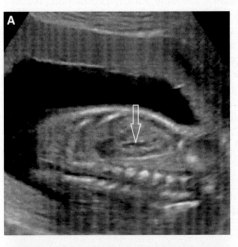
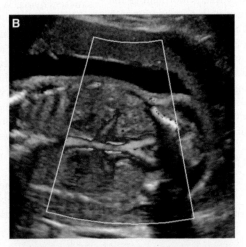
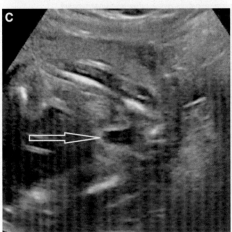
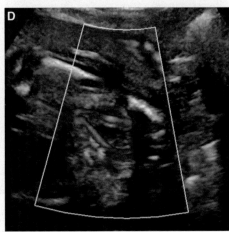

**FIGURE 19.1-6:** Fetal urinary tract. **A:** Sagittal ultrasound of a normal kidney in the second trimester. The renal cortical echogenicity has reduced as compared with Figure 19.1-5B. Some urine *(arrow)* distends the renal pelvis. A corticomedullary differentiation is beginning to appear (hyperechoic cortex/hypoechoic medulla). **B:** Coronal view of the fetal trunk with power Doppler displaying the aorta and renal vessels. **C:** Axial view of the lower pelvis and bladder *(arrow)*. **D:** Color Doppler demonstrates the two umbilical arteries along each side of the bladder.

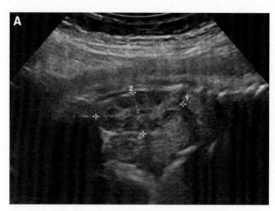
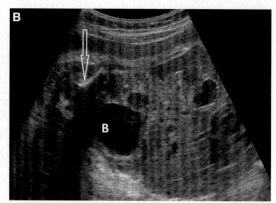

**FIGURE 19.1-7:** Fetal urinary tract. **A:** Sagittal view through the left kidney (limited by the *crosses*) in the third trimester. A corticomedullary differentiation is now obvious (hypoechoic medulla). The kidney measures 36 mm at 32 weeks, appropriate for the calculated length (number of weeks × 1.1 cm). **B:** Oblique view of the fetal abdomen; a round urine-filled bladder *(B)* is visible. The *arrow* points to the iliac wing.

identifying the bladder, including size and contour, and evaluating the amniotic fluid volume. If an anomaly is identified, it should be determined whether it is isolated or part of a polymalformative syndrome. MRI should be considered if assessment is incomplete.

## Magnetic Resonance Imaging

The advantages of MR imaging in the fetus with renal anomalies include a large field of view and multiplanar approach that can help to assess complex and large urinary tract abnormalities and also associated malformations. In cases with oligohydramnios, MR can provide better resolution of anomalies. T2w sequences are well adapted for the visualization of the kidneys, renal pelvis, and bladder. The fetal kidneys display a homogeneous intermediate hypersignal signal as compared with the liver. Urine in the renal pelvis and bladder is high in signal (Fig. 19.1-8). The use of T1w sequences is useful when a vesicourethral fistula is suspected.[5,23–28] Diffusion-weighted sequences can be helpful for locating renal parenchyma in cases of possible pelvic kidneys.

## URINARY TRACT ABNORMALITIES

### Bilateral Renal Agenesis

**Definition:** Congenital absence of both kidneys.

**Incidence:** Bilateral renal agenesis occurs in 1:4,000 births. The condition is threefold more common in male fetuses, with increased incidence in the offspring of diabetic mothers. It can be isolated or associated with other system malformations and part of syndromes (Table 19.1-3). Bilateral renal agenesis determines the so-called Potter syndrome or sequence (see later).[1,9,29–31]

**Embryology and Pathogenesis:** Renal agenesis can be explained from either failure of the ureteric bud to develop or from absent interaction between the ureteral bud and the metanephritic mesenchyma. Whatever the embryologic "explanation," it is obvious that mutations of the different genes that are involved in the normal renal development (RET, PAX2, WT1, HNFB1) are responsible for a wide range of anomalies that include uni- or bilateral renal agenesis, (multicystic) dysplasia, or hypoplasia. This explains the recurrence of the disease, sometimes under another phenotype; furthermore, these various genes are also involved in the development of the genital tract, and this explains why genital tract anomalies are associated in the case of their mutations.[2,9–11,14,32]

### Diagnosis
*Ultrasound:* The sonographic diagnosis of bilateral renal agenesis can be difficult during the first trimester since at this stage, the amniotic fluid volume is normal as it is mainly produced by

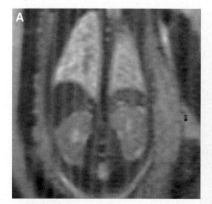
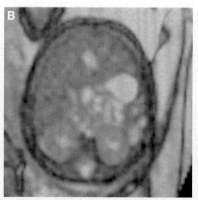
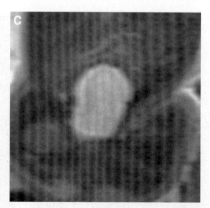

**FIGURE 19.1-8:** T2w MRI of the normal urinary tract. **A:** Coronal view through both kidneys, intermediate signal compared with the liver and spleen. **B:** Axial scan through the kidneys (and liver). **C:** Coronal view through the bladder.

| Table 19.1-3 | Syndromes Including Unilateral or Bilateral Renal Agenesis[3] |
| --- | --- |

**Autosomal Dominant**

Acro-renal-ocular syndrome
Branchio-oto-renal syndrome
Ectrodactyly–ectodermal dysplasia—cleft palate (EEC) syndrome
Pallister–Hall syndrome
Renal–Coloboma syndrome
Townes–Brocks syndrome
HNF1B (also sporadic)

**Autosomal Recessive**

Acro-renal-mandibular syndrome
Antley–Bixler syndrome
Fraser syndrome
Fryns syndrome
Rokitansky sequence
Smith–Lemli–Opitz syndrome

**X-linked**

Goltz–Gorlin syndrome
Kallmen syndrome
Lenz microphthalmia syndrome

**Sporadic**

Caudal regression syndrome
Goldenhar syndrome
MURCS association
Kabuki syndrome
Vater syndrome
HNF1beta

**Chromosomal**

Miller–Dieker syndrome
XXX
Deletion 22q

the placenta; the diagnosis is easier during the second and third trimesters, when it can be based on direct and indirect signs (Fig. 19.1-9). The main direct sign is the lack of visualization of kidneys in the lumbar fossae. Indirect signs include nonvisualization of the bladder (Fig. 19.1-9B), absent renal arteries on color Doppler, oligohydramnios, small chest, and club feet. In most cases, the urine-filled bladder is absent (still, a bladderlike structure can be filled backward through a patent urachus). The combination of renal agenesis, small chest, oligohydramnios, club feet, low-set ears, and facial deformation constitutes the so-called "Potter syndrome" or sequence. Other causes for bilateral nonfunctioning kidneys—e.g., bilateral multicystic dysplastic kidneys—are able to display the same sequence. With bilateral renal agenesis, the adrenals are present and appear elongated (Fig. 19.1-10).[32–35]

*MRI:* MR imaging is useful to confirm the absence of renal parenchyma and bladder on T2w sequences. Diffusion-weighted sequences may help identify residual renal parenchyma. Associated malformations may be better assessed by MR in the presence of oligohydramnios.[5,36]

**Differential Diagnosis:** The differential diagnosis of bilateral renal agenesis includes cases with poorly or nonfunctioning kidneys such as bilateral renal dysplasia or bilateral MCDK (Fig. 19.1-11). Other diagnoses to consider include bilateral pelvic kidneys or a solitary pelvic kidney (Fig. 19.1-12) (see later). Other causes of oligohydramnios such as intrauterine growth retardation or premature rupture of the membranes should also be considered.[36,37]

**Prognosis:** Bilateral renal agenesis is lethal.[2,36]

**Management:** Genetic counseling is important to evaluate the risk of recurrence.

Chromosomal analysis prenatally may be difficult because of the lack of amniotic fluid.

**Recurrence Risk:** The recurrence risk ranges between 3% and 6%. There are cases of autosomal dominant and recessive conditions with higher recurrence risks.[1–3]

## Unilateral Renal Agenesis

**Definition:** Congenital absence of one kidney.

**Incidence:** Unilateral renal agenesis occurs in about 1:500 to 1:1,000 births. There is a male predominance, and the left

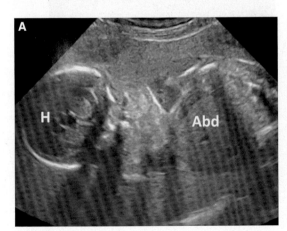
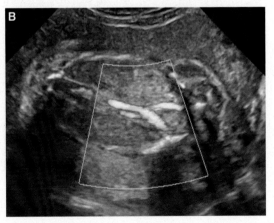

**FIGURE 19.1-9:** Bilateral renal agenesis. **A:** Ultrasound through the fetal head *(H)* and abdomen *(Abd)* through fetal head *(H)* and abdomen *(Abd)*. There is a striking anamnios; no renal structure could be demonstrated. **B:** Color Doppler enhancing the umbilical vessels. No urine-filled bladder is visible. (Courtesy of B. Broussin, MD.)

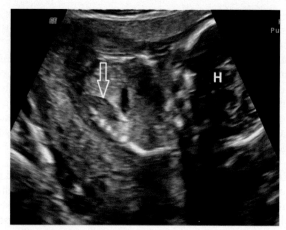

**FIGURE 19.1-10:** Bilateral renal agenesis. Sagittal ultrasound of the fetal body. A hypertrophied globular adrenal appears as an hypoechoic ovoid mass *(arrow)*. H, fetal head. (Courtesy of R. De Maubeuge, MD.)

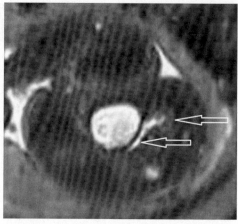

**FIGURE 19.1-12:** Hypoplastic solitary pelvic kidney. Axial T2w MRI through the fetal pelvis and bladder demonstrates a dilated ureter connected to a hypoplastic kidney *(arrows)* that was not visualized on simultaneous ultrasound.

kidney is more often the one missing. The condition can be isolated or part of polymalformative syndromes (see Table 19.1-3). The solitary kidney itself can display anomalies such as ureteropelvic junction (UPJ) or ureterovesical junction (UVJ) obstruction as well as vesicoureteric reflux (VUR). Associated genital tract anomalies are commonly encountered.[1,9,38]

**Embryology and Pathogenesis:** Renal agenesis can be explained from either failure of the ureteric bud to develop or from absent interaction between the ureteral bud and the metanephritic mesenchyma. Mutations of the different genes that are involved in the normal renal development (RET, PAX2, WT1, HNFB1) are responsible for a wide range of anomalies that include renal agenesis, multicystic dysplasia, and hypoplasia. This explains the recurrence of the disease, sometimes under another phenotype; furthermore, these mutations also explain why genital tract anomalies are associated as some of these genes are also involved in its development.

A pseudorenal agenesis can be the result of a complete involution of a multicystic dysplastic kidney (see later).[2,9–11,14,32]

**Diagnosis**

***Ultrasound:*** The sonographic diagnosis of a unilateral renal agenesis is based on the inability to visualize the kidney in one of the renal fossae. The corresponding renal artery tends to be absent on color Doppler (Fig. 19.1-13). The corresponding adrenal fills the empty space, as does the colon with left renal agenesis. Colonic loops should not be misinterpreted as a dilated ureter. Renal abnormalities such as UPJ, UVJ obstruction, or VUR can be associated findings within the solitary kidney. Often, the solitary kidney undergoes compensatory hypertrophy in utero.[33,34,38,39]

Whenever a renal fossa appears empty, one should look for an ectopic location. Renal agenesis can be the result of a complete involution of a multicystic dysplastic kidney (MCDK).[32]

***MRI:*** MR imaging is rarely performed for a diagnosis of solitary kidney. T2w and diffusion-weighted images can help search for a potential ectopic kidney. Assessment of other anomalies is useful in polymalformative syndromes (Fig. 19.1-14).[5]

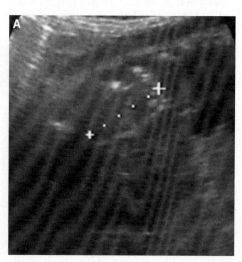

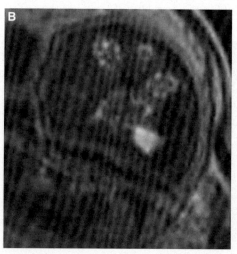

**FIGURE 19.1-11:** Bilateral multicystic dysplastic kidneys. **A:** Sagittal ultrasound through one kidney (between *crosses*), which appears small (20 mm at 30 weeks) and homogeneous, without corticomedullary differentiation. Oligohydramnios is striking. **B:** T2w MRI. The kidneys have multiple tiny cysts.

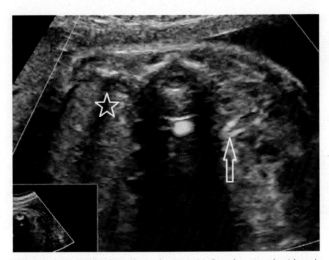

**FIGURE 19.1-13:** Unilateral renal agenesis. On ultrasound with color Doppler in the second trimester, neither renal parenchyma nor renal vessels can be visualized in the right renal fossa *(star)*, whereas both are visible present on the left side *(arrow)*. (Courtesy of R. De Maubeuge, MD.)

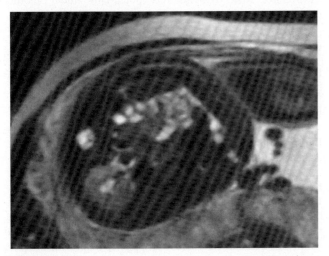

**FIGURE 19.1-14:** Unilateral renal agenesis. On this T2w MRI, only one kidney is visualized.

**Differential Diagnosis:** Unilateral renal hypoplasia, crossed fused ectopia, involuting MCDK, pelvic kidney.[40]

**Prognosis:** Excellent if isolated. Poor if the remaining kidney is dysplastic or obstructed and poorly functioning or unless the anomaly is part of a severe polymalformative syndrome. Solitary kidneys are at higher risk for developing cardiovascular diseases and renal failure.[41,42]

**Management:** Assessment of the remaining kidney is important to exclude UPJ, UVJ, and VUR.

**Recurrence Risk:** About 12%, possibly under other phenotypes.

## Renal Ectopia

**Definition:** Abnormal location of one or both kidneys. There are different types of ectopia: simple pelvic ectopia corresponds to a kidney that has not migrated from the pelvis, whereas complex ectopia with fusion that includes horseshoe kidneys (HSK) and crossed fused ectopia (CFE). HSK corresponds to kidneys

that fuse through an isthmus that connects (most usually) their lower poles. They are usually located lower than the normal kidneys. In CFE, both kidneys are fused on the same side. The ureters open within the bladder trigone in the normal location.[43,44]

**Incidence:** The incidence of pelvic kidneys is estimated at 1:2,500, HSK about 1:400 births and CFE around 1:7,500 births. All forms of renal ectopia are associated with a wide range of other renal anomalies, the commonest being UPJ and VUR. There is also a high prevalence of associated other system malformations, most commonly skeletal and genital (approximately 25%).[43,44]

**Embryology and Pathogenesis:** Ectopia results from an abnormal ascent of the kidney(s) during embryology. HSK may result from coalescence of the kidney poles during ascent, possibly in relation to abnormal caudal tilting. An abnormal tilting to a higher extent may explain the occurrence of CFE. Vascular and genetic factors are probably involved as well.[43,44]

**Diagnosis:** The discovery of an empty renal fossa (or bilateral fossae) may lead to the diagnosis of renal ectopia versus renal agenesis. An ectopic pelvic kidney tends to be small and malrotated. CMD in the renal parenchyma should be searched for (Fig. 19.1-15). The ectopic kidney may have a dilated collecting system, or it could be dysplastic or be multicystic dysplastic (Fig. 19.1-16A).

HSKs may be more difficult to diagnose prenatally since the isthmus can be thin. The axis of the fused kidneys may hint at the diagnosis as the lower poles are more oblique toward the midline than normal. The demonstration of CMD within the renal parenchyma, especially the isthmus, is confirmatory (Fig. 19.1-17). Each kidney can be affected by UPJ obstruction or MCDK.

Cross-fused ectopia is even more difficult to diagnose prenatally. It may be confused with a solitary kidney and/or unilateral renal duplication. The clue to the diagnosis is the axes of both kidneys that can be either parallel to each other or at right angles (L-ectopia). The CFE kidney is typically lower than the normally located one (Fig. 19.1-18).[43–46]

MR imaging may be useful in evaluating complicated ectopic kidneys, especially those presenting with a multicystic portion or with dilatation.[5]

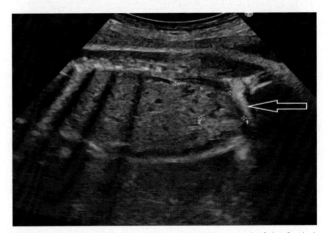

**FIGURE 19.1-15:** Pelvic kidney. Parasagittal ultrasound of the fetal abdomen shows the pelvic kidney is delineated by the crosses. The *arrow* points to the right iliac wing. No renal parenchyma could be demonstrated in the left lumbar fossa.

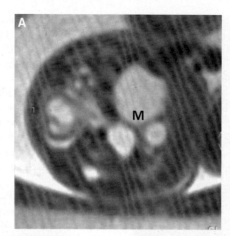
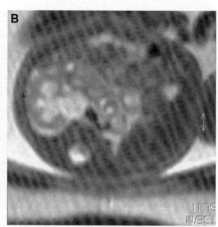

**FIGURE 19.1-16:** Pelvic MCDK and contralateral UPJ obstruction. **A:** Axial MRI through the fetal pelvis displays the MCDK *(M)*. **B:** Axial MRI through the left kidney shows UPJ obstruction.

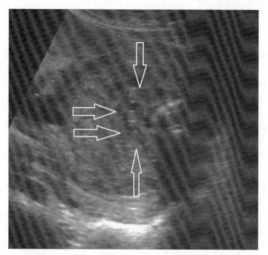

**FIGURE 19.1-17:** Horseshoe kidney. On axial ultrasound through fetal abdomen in the third trimester, the horseshoe kidney *(arrows)* can be identified by demonstration of the corticomedullary differentiation.

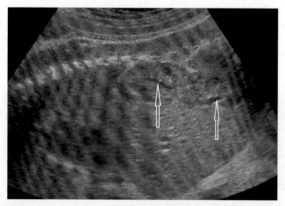

**FIGURE 19.1-18:** Crossed fused ectopia. On left parasagittal ultrasound in the third trimester, the kidney appears elongated owing to the fusion of both kidneys. Two renal pelves *(arrows)* are visualized. (Courtesy of C. Garel, MD.)

**Differential Diagnosis:** A pelvic kidney may be confused with a nonrenal pelvic mass, such as a pelvic teratoma. CFE can be confused with renal duplication or with solitary kidney.

**Prognosis:** Ectopic kidneys have a good prognosis unless associated with a significant renal malformation or part of a severe polymalformative syndrome.

**Management:** There is no specific in utero management. Chromosomal analysis should be considered in the case of polymalformative syndrome.

**Recurrence Risk:** Around 10% potentially under another phenotype.[47]

## Simple Renal Cyst

**Definition:** Unilateral, solitary, nongenetically transmitted cystic lesion within the renal parenchyma.[51,52,58]

**Incidence:** Rare, most resolving by 24 weeks' gestation.

**Embryology and Pathogenesis:** The origin of simple renal cysts is unclear; it may correspond to a sequel of localized ischemia.

### Diagnosis
***Ultrasound:*** A simple renal cyst appears as a single cystic structure without septa or calcifications; its size varies from a few millimeters to several centimeters (Fig. 19.1-19). It is localized within the renal cortex. Color Doppler is helpful in order to confirm the intrarenal location of the cyst (Fig. 19.1-19B).

***MRI:*** At MR imaging, on T2w, a renal cyst will appear as a cystic high-signal structure within the kidney.

**Differential Diagnosis:** The differential diagnosis includes a calyceal diverticulum, a hydrocalyx, and a cystic tumor. In the case of calyceal diverticulum and hydrocalyx, the diagnosis would be confirmed by the demonstration of a connection with the pyelocalyceal system. A tumor will usually appear as a cystic multiseptated mass. A hereditary renal cystic disease may start with a unilateral cyst; follow-up and familial history would help to reassess the diagnosis. Cysts in the upper pole of a kidney should be differentiated from a dilated upper pole moiety of a duplex kidney.

**Prognosis:** Excellent if isolated with no specific management in utero.

## Cystic Renal Diseases

**Definition:** Uni- or bilateral presence of multiple cystic lesions within the renal cortex or medulla or both. The cystic lesions may have a genetic (bilateral diseases) or nongenetic

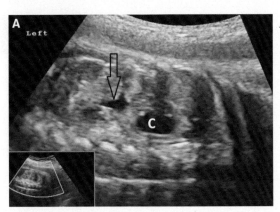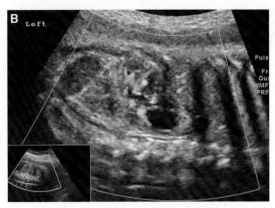

**FIGURE 19.1-19:** Simple renal cyst. **A:** On parasagittal ultrasound through the left kidney in the third trimester, a cystic structure *(C)* is visible within the upper pole of the kidney, and some urine distends the renal pelvis *(arrow)*. **B:** Color Doppler, same view as in **A**, confirms the intrarenal location of the cyst. (Courtesy of R. De Maubeuge, MD.)

transmission (uni- or bilateral diseases). Obstructive cystic dysplasia and multicystic dysplastic kidney (MCDK) are the commonest diseases without genetic transmission. Autosomal recessive (ARPKD) and dominant (ADPKD) polycystic kidney diseases are the commonest ones with genetic transmission. Cystic renal diseases can present as isolated renal anomalies or as part of a syndrome.[12,48–50]

**Embryology and Pathogenesis:** The Potter classification of renal cystic diseases has been replaced by a classification based on the genetic or nongenetic origin of the renal cystic diseases. Genetic renal cystic diseases include autosomal dominant and recessive polycystic kidney disease (ARPKD and ADPKD) as well as glomerulocystic kidney disease (GCKD), medullary cystic dysplasia associated with syndromes and nephronophthisis (NPHP)/medullary cystic dysplasia complex.[48,49] Among the nongenetic cystic diseases, obstructive cystic dysplasia and MCDK are the most common. Obstructive dysplasia is associated with urinary tract dilatation and various congenital uropathies. Noteworthy, some cases of MCDK are genetically transmitted.

A further step in the characterization and understanding of genetically transmitted cystic renal diseases has been achieved through their recognition as part of the group of *ciliopathies* (see Table 19.1-2). Primary cilia are microtubules, antennalike cellular organelles that extend outward from the surface of many cells of the renal tubule epithelium. These organelles are rich in receptors, ion channels, and signaling proteins activated by mechanical or chemical stimuli. Cilia regulate cell proliferation and differentiation in the developing and mature kidneys. Any defect in the structures or function of primary cilium may lead to various cystic phenotypes. Cilia are encountered in various sites and organs of the human body (i.e., liver, lungs), and this explains the potential association of cystic renal changes and other malformations encountered in various syndromes.[4,15,17] The cilia concept has induced a more global approach in renal cystic diseases combining renal and hepatic diseases. Hepatorenal fibrocystic diseases are characterized by developmental abnormalities of the porto-ciliary hepatic system in association with cystic degeneration of the kidney. They encompass various inherited diseases. The hepatic lesions are usually demonstrated by histology only and to a lesser extent by imaging. One or several genetic defects have been demonstrated (see Table 19.1-2). As some genetic loci mutations can be located close one to another, not surprisingly,

different diseases may have similar sonographic appearances (i.e., tuberous sclerosis and ADPKD).[49,50]

**Diagnosis**
***Ultrasound:*** Imaging plays an essential role in detecting and characterizing renal cystic diseases as well as follow-up.[51–54] Standard high-resolution sonographic images are essential. The knowledge of histologic changes that occur in cystic diseases helps one to understand their sonographic appearance (Table 19.1-4).[55] The exam includes measuring renal size, defining echogenicity of the cortex compared with liver and medulla (hypoechoic, absent, or hyperechoic), assessment of the CMD (present, absent, or reversed) and presence of cysts (number, size, and location), or calcifications as well as evaluation of the pelvicalyceal system.

Two main sonographic features lead to the suspicion of renal cystic diseases: the presence of renal cysts and the detection of hyperechoic kidneys (Fig. 19.1-20).[51,52,57] The "cysts" that are visualized on US result either from renal tubular dilatation, glomerular cysts, or from real cysts. They develop anywhere in the kidney and can be uni- or bilateral. Renal hyperechogenicity may involve the entire kidney, only the cortex, or only the medulla. The discovery of hyperechoic kidneys can be challenging as there are no objective US criteria defined up to 32 weeks' gestation; after 32 weeks, the hyperechogenicity is less subjective and should be considered abnormal whenever the renal cortex appears more echoic than the liver or spleen.[4] Once a suspicion of a renal cystic disease has arisen, the evaluation of the US findings should be standardized in a decision tree-type approach (Table 19.1-5).[51]

Color Doppler assessment is useful in selected cases.[9] Associated malformations should be searched for with particular assessment of the liver and genital tract. Family history is important, and whenever cystic kidneys are suspected, it is useful to perform a sonographic examination to the parents to check for "unknown" familial disease.

***MRI:*** In some patients, MR imaging provides additional information by demonstrating the renal cysts or associated brain malformation.[5,56]

**Management:** When bilateral renal cystic disease is identified, the evaluation of the US findings can be standardized in a decision tree-type approach. The first step is to rule out

| Table 19.1-4 | Main Histologic Changes in Renal Cystic Diseases[51] |
| --- | --- |
| **Disease** | **Histologic Changes** |
| Autosomal dominant polycystic kidney disease | Rounded cysts (from few millimeter to several centimeter) developing in the medulla and cortex anywhere on the renal tubules or collecting tubules. Glomerular cysts can be present |
| Autosomal recessive polycystic kidney disease | Fusiform dilatation (1–2 mm in diameter) of the collecting ducts mainly into the medulla but extending toward the cortex with normal glomeruli |
| Bardet–Biedl syndrome | Medullary cystic dysplasia with preservation of superficial cortex. Progressive tubulointerstitial nephropathy |
| Glomerulocystic kidney disease | Glomerular cysts without tubular dilatation anywhere in the renal cortex; most visible in the subcapsular areas |
| Nephronophthisis | Tubular distension. Cysts at the cortico-medullary junction with nonspecific tubulointerstitial nephritis and varying degrees of glomerulosclerosis |
| Medullary cystic dysplasia | Extensive dilatation of the medullary tubules extending toward the cortex, which is compressed and thinned |
| Obstructive dysplasia | Cystic dilatation of primitive ducts. Nodules of metaplastic cartilage and renal dysplasia may be present |
| Multicystic dysplastic kidney disease | Ductal dilatations, most marked peripherally. Paucity of nephrons. Diffuse renal dysplasia with occasional metaplastic cartilage |

| Table 19.1-5 | Differential Diagnosis of Fetal Hyperechoic and Cystic Kidneys |
| --- | --- |

**Hyperechoic Kidneys with Normal or Moderately Enlarged Kidneys**

Renal cystic diseases
   TCF2 gene mutation
   Autosomal recessive polycystic kidney disease
   Autosomal dominant polycystic kidney disease
Maternally induced diseases
   Diabetes
   Neutral endopeptidase autoimmune glomerulopathy
   Cytomegalovirus infection
   Antagonists
   Angiotensin II
Metabolic diseases
Nephrotic syndromes, Finnish type
Obstructive dysplasia
"Transient"

**Bilateral Multiple Cysts**

Autosomal recessive polycystic kidney disease
Autosomal dominant polycystic kidney disease
Bilateral multicystic dysplastic kidney disease (only in fetus)
Bilateral obstructive dysplasia
Syndromes (e.g., Bardet–Biedl, Zellweger)

**Fetal Macrocysts (>2 cm)**

Tuberous sclerosis
Simpson–Golabi–Behmel syndrome
TCF2-gene mutation
Joubert syndrome

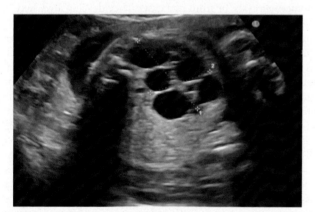

**FIGURE 19.1-20:** Left multicystic dysplastic kidney. Ultrasound in the second trimester shows typical multicystic patter, and no renal parenchyma or renal pelvis can be visualized.

dysplasia associated with an obstructive uropathy (with dilatation of the collecting system). Obstructive dysplasia is the commonest cause for a hyperechoic cortex with or without cysts. MCDK is the second diagnosis to consider. If these diagnoses are unlikely, inherited renal cystic diseases should be considered.

Knowledge of any familial history is essential. If *positive*, the finding of abnormal kidneys suggests recurrence (Fig. 19.1-21). If no familial history is present, cases can be further separated in patients where the renal findings are isolated and limited to the kidney and those where the renal anomalies are associated with malformations of other organs.

There are typical US patterns suggestive of specific diagnoses and nontypical US patterns. A "typical" pattern means typical

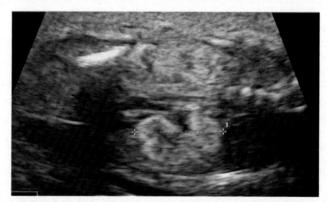

**FIGURE 19.1-21:** Glomerulocystic disease. Coronal ultrasound of both kidneys, which appear hyperechoic but normal sized. Family history was positive. (Reproduced from Avni FE, Garel C, Cassart M, et al. Imaging and classification of congenital cystic renal diseases. *AJR Am J Roentgenol.* 2012;198:1004–1013, with permission.)

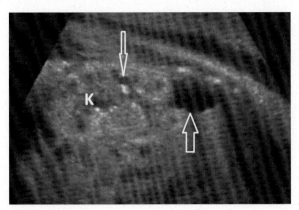

**FIGURE 19.1-22:** Simpson–Golarbi–Behmel syndrome with renal cysts. Sagittal ultrasound shows a kidney *(K)* that appears hyperechoic and contains one large and one tiny *(arrows)* cyst. Small cysts were visualized in the other kidney as well. Anomalies included signs of an overgrowth syndrome.

| Table 19.1.6 | Syndromes that Include Cystic Kidneys[3] |
|---|---|

Bardet–Biedl syndrome
COACH syndrome
Ellis–Van Creveld syndrome
Fryns syndrome
Glutaric acid II
Jeune syndrome
Marden–Walker syndrome
Joubert syndrome
Meckel–Gruber syndrome
Oro-facio-digital syndrome
Roberts syndrome
Smith–Lemli–Opitz syndrome
Zellweger syndrome
Tuberous sclerosis
Trisomy 13
Deletion 22q

pattern of all sonographic features that lead to a specific diagnosis (isolated or in association with other malformations). Nonspecific (or nontypical) means that there are no significant features that can lead to a specific diagnosis. For the latter, the diagnosis can be approached using tables of differential diagnosis (Fig. 19.1-22) (Table 19.1-6). In undetermined cases, supplementary examinations may help, such as genetic studies or MR to reach the most accurate diagnosis.

For example, in the fetus, bilateral, very large (>4 SD) hyperechoic kidneys with hyperechoic medulla (reversed CMD) is a typical pattern for fetal ARPKD (Fig. 19.1-23). The association of "renal cystic changes + malformations" can be characteristic for a specific syndrome (see Table 19.1-6). For example, GLMCK + Molar tooth sign in the CNS establishes the diagnosis of JOUBERT syndrome (Fig. 19.1-24).[57,51–53]

## Cystic Obstructive Dysplasia

See section on Urinary Tract Dilatation.

## Multicystic Dysplastic Kidney Disease

**Definition:** Multiple cysts of varying size that do not connect to a central pelvis. No functioning renal parenchyma.[39,40,59–63]

**Incidence:** Unilateral MCDK occurs in 1:2,500 births, bilateral MCDK occurs in 1:12,000 births.

**Embryology and Pathogenesis:** MCDK is classically considered to result from aberrant interactions between the ureteral bud and the metanephritic blastema. Most cases are sporadic, yet a genetic origin has been established in some cases. Mutations of PAX2, TCF2 (HNF1β), and uroplakin have been identified.

On histology, the kidney is highly dysplastic, displaying cysts, primitive abnormal tubules, few abnormal nephrons, and foci of cartilage. In rare instances, a few functioning normal nephrons are present, and the kidney would display some function. It can be uni- or bilateral (lethal form). It can develop in ectopic or duplex kidneys. Unilateral MCDK is associated with contralateral renal anomalies such as UPJ or VUR in 30% to 40% of cases. It can be associated with malformations of several other systems, especially of the genital tract.

*Ultrasound:* MCDK is usually detected during the second-trimester US examination. Its diagnosis is straightforward in typical cases: multiple cysts of varying sizes without normal renal parenchyma and without recognized renal pelvis (Fig. 19.1-20). The cysts may be tiny (microcystic form) (Fig. 19.1-25) or very large (giant form) (Fig. 19.1-26). The homolateral ureter may be enlarged. Furthermore, a MCDK may affect an ectopic kidney (see Fig. 19.1-16A) or any moiety of a duplex one (Fig. 19.1-27). Once a MCDK has been detected, associated anomalies should be searched at the level of the contralateral kidney (see Fig. 19.1-16B), the genital tract, or other systems. The contralateral kidney may undergo compensatory hypertrophy already in utero, which can be assessed through measurement of the contralateral kidney (see Fig. 19.1-25).[39] Furthermore, MCDK may undergo regression in utero or after birth, resulting eventually in a pseudorenal agenesis.[40,64]

*MRI:* MR imaging may be helpful to characterize very large or ectopic MCDK and unusual complications of the anomaly as well as complications of the contralateral kidney (see Figs. 19.1-16, 19.1-23, and 19.1-27). In the case of bilateral MCDK, cystic images are present in both kidneys, and oligohydramnios is the rule as both kidneys are nonfunctioning. MR imaging is helpful to differentiate bilateral hypoplasia from bilateral MCDK by showing the cystic lesions (see Fig. 19.1-11).[5]

**Differential Diagnosis:** The differential diagnosis of unilateral MCDK includes unusual UPJ obstruction, obstructive cystic dysplasia, cystic mesoblastic nephroma, and segmental dysplasia. The differential diagnosis of bilateral MCDK includes bilateral hypodysplasia, cystic dysplasia, and other inherited cystic renal diseases (see later).

**Prognosis:** The prognosis of unilateral MCDK is excellent as isolated anomaly. Bilateral MCDK is lethal, however.

**Management:** With unilateral MCDK, the other kidney should be evaluated for possible UPJ, UVJ, and VUR.

**Recurrence Rate:** About 12% in the case of genetic transmission.

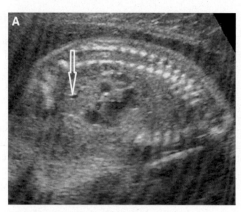
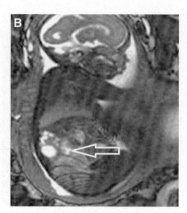

**FIGURE 19.1-23:** MCDK developing within the upper poles of a duplex kidney bilaterally. **A:** Parasagittal US of one kidney demonstrates multicystic appearance of the upper moiety. The lower pole pelvis is slightly dilated *(arrow)*. **B:** Parasagittal MRI confirms the lower moiety is displaced anteriorly and slightly distended *(arrow)*.

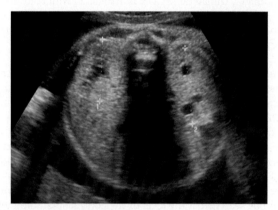

**FIGURE 19.1-24:** Joubert syndrome. Axial ultrasound shows both kidneys to be hyperechoic without CMD. There are scattered cysts within the parenchyma around the CM junction. The fetus displayed a molar tooth sign on fetal MR imaging (not shown). (Courtesy of M. Molho, MD.)

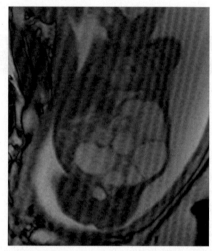

**FIGURE 19.1-26:** MCDK. T2w coronal MRI shows a large MCDK occupying a large part of the fetal abdomen. (Courtesy of K. Chaumoitre, MD.)

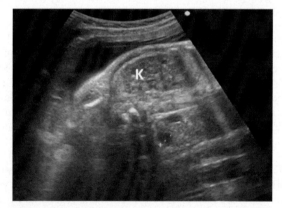

**FIGURE 19.1-25:** MCDK with contralateral hypertrophy. Oblique ultrasound in the third trimester shows the small MCDK (limited by the *crosses*), which is displaying small cysts. The contralateral kidney *(K)* measures 42 mm in length at 30 weeks, which confirms hypertrophy.

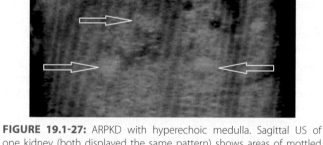

**FIGURE 19.1-27:** ARPKD with hyperechoic medulla. Sagittal US of one kidney (both displayed the same pattern) shows areas of mottled hyperechogenicities within the renal pyramids *(arrows)*. (Courtesy of C. Garel, MD.)

## Autosomal Recessive Polycystic Kidney Disease

**Definition:** Autosomal recessive polycystic kidney disease (ARPKD) is an autosomal recessively transmitted disease that causes fusiform dilatation of the renal collecting ducts and distal tubuli, resulting in large echogenic kidneys.[12,49,65–67]

**Incidence:** Estimated at 1:20,000 births.[65–67]

**Embryology and Pathogenesis:** ARPKD causes fusiform dilatation of the renal collecting ducts and distal tubuli to a variable extent, and that is invariably associated with congenital hepatic fibrosis. The variable involvement of the renal tubules leads to variable phenotypes and variable clinical expression. ARPKD results from mutation of the PKHD1 gene located on chromosome 6p12. Truncating mutations are associated with a higher perinatal mortality whereas missense mutations are associated with milder forms of the diseases. The disease has a variable expressivity even in the same family.[65–67]

### Diagnosis

*Ultrasound:* The diagnosis of ARPKD is usually achieved in the second and third trimesters, although there have been reports of cases detected in the 1st trimester.

Because of the histological variability, ARPKD displays a variety of US patterns; still, "markedly enlarged hyperechoic kidneys (4 to 8 SD above the mean) without CMD" is the most frequent pattern encountered on obstetrical US examination performed during the second and third trimesters (Figs. 19.1-18 and 19.1-28). Other possible appearances include hyperechoic very large kidneys with reversed CMD (very specific pattern; see Fig. 19.1-23), moderately enlarged hyperechoic kidneys, or even normal kidneys (at least at the start of the disease). Renal cysts may be observed already in utero; they tend to be located within the medulla (Fig. 19.1-29). The US patterns may evolve during pregnancy.

In cases with recurring disease, the US appearance may vary from one pregnancy to another.

Severely affected fetuses display a "Potter"-like phenotype as oligohydramnios and pulmonary hypoplasia are associated findings.

At the level of the liver, small hilar cysts can rarely be visualized. The hepatic fibrosis will not be detected in utero.

*MRI:* MR imaging may potentially display tiny cysts not visualized on US and help to characterize the diseases.[5,50–52,68,69]

**Differential Diagnosis:** The differential diagnosis of ARPKD includes the other causes of enlarged hyperechoic kidneys, including Bardet–Biedl syndrome, HNF1β mutation, other disorders with glomerulocystic kidneys, and rarely ADPKD.[50–52,57]

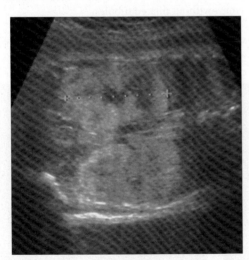

**FIGURE 19.1-28:** ARPKD. Coronal ultrasound through both kidneys demonstrates enlarged (8 cm), diffusely hyperechoic kidneys without CMD. (Reproduced from Avni FE, Garel C, Cassart M, et al. Imaging and classification of congenital cystic renal diseases. *AJR Am J Roentgenol.* 2012;198:1004–1013, with permission.)

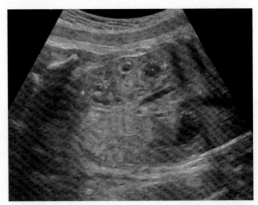

**FIGURE 19.1-29:** ARPKD with intramedullary cysts. Sagittal ultrasound through the enlarged right kidney shows cysts within several pyramids.

**Prognosis:** Of those affected, 50% will die in the perinatal period because of pulmonary hypoplasia and renal failure.

Survivors will display features of renal failure leading to renal transplantation in childhood. Furthermore, some patients with a mild form of the disease will be detected only later in childhood.[12,49,65–67]

Genetic counseling and evaluation of the postnatal prognosis at the light of US, genetic results, and degree of renal failure.

**Recurrence Risk:** ARPKD is transmitted as an autosomal recessive trait.

## Autosomal Dominant Polycystic Kidney Disease

**Definition:** Autosomal dominant polycystic kidney disease (ADPKD) is the most common genetically transmitted renal cystic disease in man and is characterized by the presence of multiple large cysts developing at any level of the nephron. The disease affects not only the kidneys but also the liver and the pancreas. There is also an increased risk of associated intracranial aneurisms.[12,49,55,70]

**Incidence:** One or 2 per 1,000 births.

**Embryology, Genetics, and Pathogenesis:** ADPKD includes at least three phenotypically similar but genetically different entities. Mutations of the gene PKD1, located on chromosome 6, and gene PKD2, located on chromosome 4, have been described. A 3D gene mutation PKD3 is suspected but not demonstrated. Ten percent de novo mutations occur as well. About 15% of cases may present asynchronously with the involvement of only one kidney first.[55]

**Diagnosis:** A typical pattern suggesting fetal ADPKD includes normal-sized kidneys with hyperechoic cortex leading to an increased CMD (Fig. 19.1-30). Some cortical renal cysts may be observed already in utero. In the case of US suspicion, US of the parents may reveal (even unrecognized) cystic disease as well. Normally appearing renal US in the fetus or in the parents does not exclude the disease. Associated urinary tract malformation such as duplex kidney or UPJ obstruction can be observed.

In rare cases, hyperechoic large kidneys with subcortical and/or diffuse parenchymal cysts may lead to a diagnosis of glomerulocystic type of ADPKD (see later) (Fig. 19.1-31).[55,71,72]

**Differential Diagnosis:** Hyperechoic kidneys with increased CMD can result from various anomalies, including consequences of infectious or vascular insults to the kidneys or fetuses affected by congenital nephrotic syndromes. It can also correspond to a normal variant[50–53] (Fig. 19.1-32).

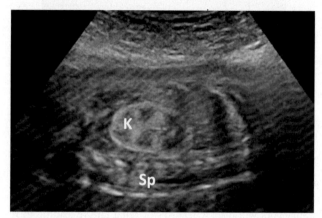

**FIGURE 19.1-30:** Autosomal dominant polycystic kidney disease (ADPKD). Sagittal ultrasound shows an enlarged kidney *(K)* with an echogenic cortex. The CMD is increased. Sp, fetal spine.

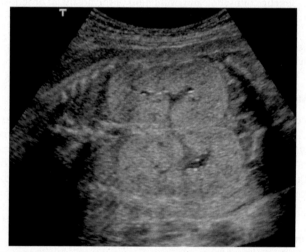

**FIGURE 19.1-31:** ADPKD, glomerulocystic type (GLMC). Coronal ultrasound in the third trimester shows both kidneys are markedly enlarged and hyperechoic and lack CMD. (Courtesy of C. Garel, MD.)

**Prognosis:** The disease becomes clinically obvious in the fourth and fifth decades, but because of US screening, fetal and neonatal cases are increasingly frequently detected. Patients with the GLMK type of ADPKD may develop neonatal hypertension and renal failure.

**Management:** Familial inquiry is mandatory and renal ultrasound should be performed to both parents (and if possible to grand-parents). One should keep in mind that absence of cysts in young parents does not exclude the disease as cysts may start to appear as late as 36 years old.

**Recurrence:** ADPKDs are transmitted as an autosomal dominant trait.

## Anomalies of the Gene TCF2 (or HNF1χ Mutations)

**Definition:** Anomalies of the gene TCF2 encompass a spectrum of diseases of the kidney that includes renal cystic disease, various renal malformations (uni- or bilateral agenesis, hypoplasia, dysplasia, MCDK) as well as pancreatic (diabetes type MODY V) and genital malformations. Histologically, the main feature is the demonstration of glomerular cysts—in over 5% of the surface of the renal parenchyma—without dilated tubules.[55,73–75]

**Incidence:** The incidence is unknown, but the condition is increasingly detected.

**Embryology, Genetics, and Pathogenesis:** Transcription gene factor 2 (TCF2) is localized on chromosome 17 and encodes the protein hepatocyte nuclear factor-1β (HNF1β). It is one of the principal genes involved in the development of the kidney, pancreas, and genital tract. HNF1β is also expressed in the neural tube, the biliary tract, the esophagus, and the lungs. HNF1β regulates various genes involved (in the mouse) in cilium formations (UMOD, PKHD1, PKD2). The genetic transmission is autosomal dominant but cases of sporadic occurrence are very common.[73–75]

Histologically, the main feature is the demonstration of glomerular cysts—in over 5% of the surface of the renal parenchyma—without dilated tubules.[55,73–75]

**Diagnosis:** The TCF2 mutation has become the most frequently recognized cause of hyperechoic kidneys in the fetus (usually

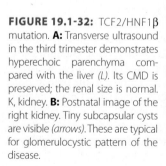

**FIGURE 19.1-32:** TCF2/HNF1β mutation. **A:** Transverse ultrasound in the third trimester demonstrates hyperechoic parenchyma compared with the liver *(L)*. Its CMD is preserved; the renal size is normal. K, kidney. **B:** Postnatal image of the right kidney. Tiny subcapsular cysts are visible *(arrows)*. These are typical for glomerulocystic pattern of the disease.

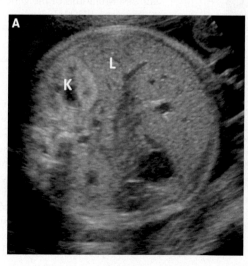

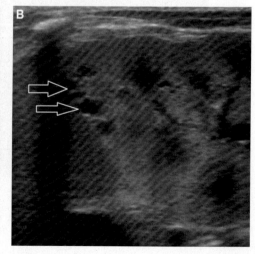

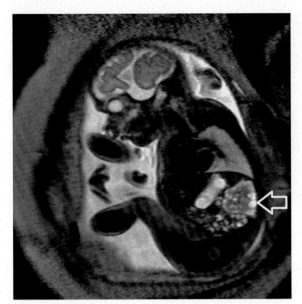

**FIGURE 19.1-33:** TCF2 mutation. Sagittal T2w MRI of the left kidney shows typical subcapsular cysts *(arrow)*. (Courtesy of L. Rausin, MD.)

normal-sized kidneys) (Fig. 19.1-32). Cysts may be either tiny and subcapsular or very large, resembling postnatal ADPKD (see later). The amniotic fluid volume is typically normal.

MR imaging may display the very characteristic subcapsular cysts (Fig. 19.1-33).[76,77]

**Differential Diagnosis:** Hyperechoic kidneys with increased CMD can result from various anomalies, including infectious or vascular insults to the kidneys, congenital nephrotic syndromes. It can also correspond to a normal variant[50–53,55,57] (see Table 19.1-5).

**Prognosis:** In utero, the prognosis is good and depends on the presence of associated malformation. Postnatally, the prognosis will depend upon the progression of renal disease and diabetes.

**Recurrence:** HNF1β is transmitted through a dominant trait, but a large number of sporadic mutations do occur.

## Other Renal Genetically Transmitted Renal Cystic Diseases

Renal cystic diseases can present as an isolated renal disease or can be a symptom of syndromes associating the renal cysts and other system anomalies. The kidney patterns can point to the diagnosis. See Figure 19.1-34 decision tree approach to renal cystic disease.

■ Bardet–Biedl syndrome (BBS): BBS associates hyperechoic large kidneys resembling ARPKD because of medullary cystic dysplasia. Associated postaxial polydactyly is the clue to the diagnosis (Fig. 19.1-35).[78]
■ Meckel–Gruber syndrome (MGS): MGS includes cystic kidneys, CNS anomalies, and polydactyly. Because of massive medullary cystic dysplasia, the renal pyramids will appear cystic and hypoechoic as early as the first trimester (Fig. 19.1-36).[79]
■ Nephronophtisis (NPHPH): NPHPH consists of a group of tubule–interstitial disorders that can be isolated or associated with other organs anomalies (e.g., Joubert or Jeune syndrome). The renal cysts develop mainly in the corticomedullary junction (see Fig. 19.1-24). Associated anomalies are the clue to the diagnosis.[80–83]
■ Glomerulocystic kidney diseases (GLMCK): GLMCK can be observed in ADPKD and HNF1B mutation as well as in Zellweger syndrome, trisomies, and with urinary tract dilatation (Fig. 19.1-37; see Fig. 19.1-21).[84]

## Urinary Tract Dilatation

**Definition:** Dilatation of the renal pelvis, calyces, and/or ureters. The urinary bladder may be dilated as well.

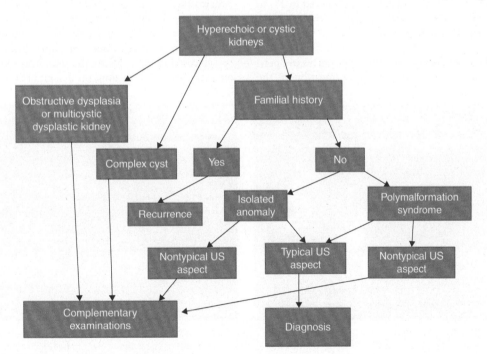

**FIGURE 19.1-34:** Decision-tree approach to renal cystic diseases.

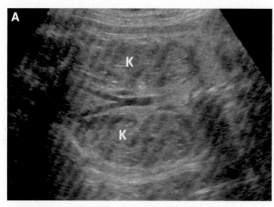
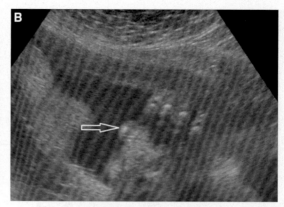

**FIGURE 19.1-35:** Bardet–Biedl syndrome. **A:** Coronal ultrasound in the third trimester shows kidneys *(K)* that are enlarged, hyperechoic, and without CMD. **B:** Postaxial polydactyly was present (the *arrow* points to a supernumerary digit). Both hands and feet were involved. (Courtesy of C. Garel, MD.)

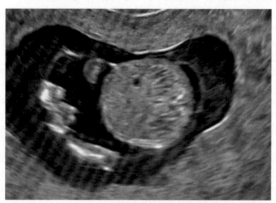

**FIGURE 19.1-36:** Meckel–Gruber syndrome. Transverse ultrasound in the first trimester shows cystic changes at the level of the renal pyramids. There was an associated CNS malformation. (Reproduced from Avni FE, Garel C, Cassart M, et al. Imaging and classification of congenital cystic renal diseases. *AJR Am J Roentgenol.* 2012;198:1004–1013, with permission.)

**Incidence:** Prenatal renal pelvis dilatation is observed in 1% to 5% of pregnancies; the male-to-female ratio is 2:1. Some 40% to 80% of cases will regress spontaneously.

**Embryology and Pathogenesis:** Ureteral kinks, delays in openings of the Chwalla membrane or of the permeation of the urethra can explain the occurrence of some of the dilatation. VUR has been identified in 50% of parents and siblings of affected individuals consistent with a genetic transmission.

**Diagnosis:** Various criteria are used to standardize urinary tract dilatation. The criterion usually used is the measurement of the A-P diameter of the renal pelvis on a transverse scan of the fetal abdomen. Many authors agree that the upper limit of the normal pelvic diameter should be 4 mm during the second and 7 mm during the third trimester of the pregnancy. These limits are set in order to detect not only patients that will need corrective surgery (in the case of obstructive dilatation) but also the majority of fetuses and neonates presenting vesicoureteric reflux. The latter are at risk for developing complications and eventually worsening their renal function.[4,6,85–88] Furthermore, there is a relation between higher degrees of dilatation and postnatal decreased renal function and need for corrective surgery; therefore, dilatation has been separated into groups of mild (7 to 9 mm), moderate (10 to 15 mm), and severe (>15 mm in the third trimester) dilatation (Fig. 19.1-38). Noteworthy, a pyelectasis (Fig. 19.1-39) refers to a visible renal pelvis below the significant threshold. During the second trimester, it is considered to be a minor sign of chromosomal anomaly.

Other sonographic evidence includes dilatation of the ureters or calyces (Fig. 19.1-40) or the demonstration of an enlarged bladder (over 12 mm long on a sagittal scan during the first,

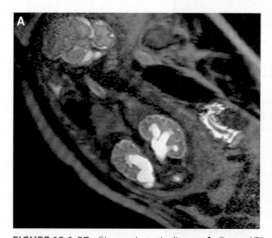
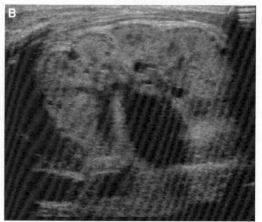

**FIGURE 19.1-37:** Glomerulocystic disease. **A:** Coronal T2w MRI of the fetal kidney shows bilateral urinary tract dilatation with multiple tiny cysts all around the kidney surfaces on both sides. **B:** Postnatal ultrasound of one kidney confirms the dilatation of the renal pelvis and the microscopic subcapsular tiny cysts. (Courtesy of L. Rausin, MD.)

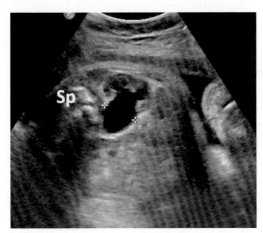

**FIGURE 19.1-38:** UPJ obstruction with marked dilatation. Transverse ultrasound in the second trimester shows the diameter of the dilatation (between the *crosses*) to be 21 mm. Sp, fetal spine.

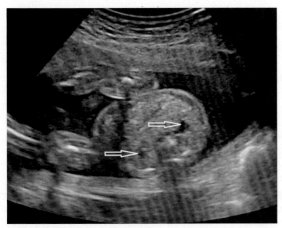

**FIGURE 19.1-39:** Bilateral mild pyelectasis (second trimester). Transverse ultrasound of the fetal abdomen reveals that some urine distends both renal pelves *(arrows)*.

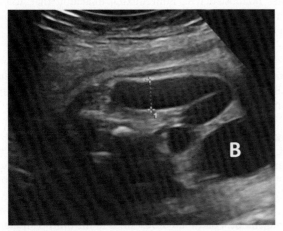

**FIGURE 19.1-40:** Primary megaureter (third trimester). Oblique ultrasound demonstrates a tortuous and dilated ureter (12 mm between *crosses*) above the bladder *(B)*.

3 cm during the second and 5 cm during the third trimester) (Fig. 19.1-41).

Once a dilatation has been detected in utero, usually through obstetrical US, the subsequent evaluation should answer three

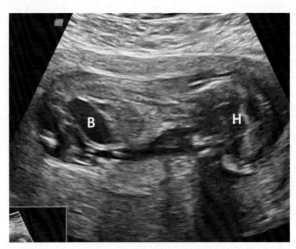

**FIGURE 19.1-41:** Megacystis (first trimester), prune belly sequence. Sagittal ultrasound demonstrates a distended bladder *(B)*. H, fetal head.

questions: the origin of the dilatation, the coexistence of associated anomalies, and, finally, the prognosis of the malformation. The most common cause for urinary tract dilatation is UPJ obstruction (around 30%). Other causes include nonobstructive and nonrefluxing dilatation (around 20%), UVJ obstruction (around 15%), VUR (around 25%), complicated duplex kidneys, and posterior urethral valves (PUVs).

In selected cases, fetal MR imaging can be useful, particularly when oligohydramnios is present. Assessment of ureteral dilatation and insertion may be better demonstrated by MR. MR provides additional information regarding associated malformations. T2-weighted sequences are useful for assessing the dilated collecting system. T1w sequence can demonstrate the relationship of the bladder to the rectum. Diffusion-weighted images can assess renal tissue.[5]

**Prognosis and Prenatal Management:** Whenever renal dilatation is detected, a complete survey of the fetal anatomy should be performed to detect associated malformations that would indicate the need for chromosomal analysis or the possibility of polymalformative syndromes. Bilateral renal dilatation and bladder outlet obstruction have an increased risk of associated chromosomal anomalies.

In the case of dilatation, the prognosis will depend upon the type and extent of anomalies; features of severity include early diagnosis, bilateral marked dilatation, obstructive dysplasia, persistently obstructed bladder, oligohydramnios, and secondary lung hypoplasia. The finding of associated echogenic and/or cystic renal parenchyma is frequently but only partially informative about renal function. Conversely, normal cortical echogenicity does not exclude dysplasia.

Still, for most uropathies, the prognosis is good, and the prenatal diagnosis will allow proper management after birth in order to apply best treatment and to prevent any further renal damage.[108–116]

**Postnatal Management:** After birth, any information relevant to the proper postnatal management should be transmitted to the postnatal team in charge of the newly born and, when necessary, delivery should occur in a tertiary care center. Some conditions require an immediate confirmation and treatment. For example, severe PUVs or prolapsed ectopic ureterocele into the urethra leading to oligoanuria necessitate immediate treatment.

Giant UPJ or MCDK—crossing the midline—may interfere with normal digestion with gastric compression, requiring close follow-up as well. Fetuses with oligohydramnios/renal failure may have pulmonary hypoplasia with pneumothoraxes requiring immediate support. In these cases, ultrasound and voiding cystourethrography may need to be performed immediately after birth in order to confirm the anomaly. In all other cases, the workup can be planned on an outpatient basis. Ultrasound should be performed after a few days of age to decrease false negative studies. Only patients with persistent ureteral dilatation should undergo a voiding cystourethrogram (VCUG).[4,6,7,116]

## UPJ Obstruction

**Definition:** Obstruction at the level of the ureteropelvic junction (see Figs. 19.1-38 and 19.1-42).

**Incidence:** The commonest cause for renal dilatation; approximately 1:2,000 births.

**Embryology and Pathogenesis:** The origin of the obstruction is unclear (ureteral kinking and/or vascular crossing). In most cases, the junction is patent, and the problem is likely functional.

### Diagnosis
*Ultrasound:* The classic appearance is dilation of the renal pelvis and calyces without hydroureter. UPJ obstruction is most commonly diagnosed in the second and/or third trimester. There might be an involution or a progression of the dilatation during pregnancy.[5,88–90]

With marked obstruction, the calyces may enlarge, and echogenic precipitates may be observed at the level of the precalyceal area. Obstruction may lead to rupture of renal calyces, and urinary extravasation collected as a perirenal urinoma (Fig. 19.1-43) or ascitis. In some instances, leakage may protect the renal parenchyma, while in others, renal growth is impaired.

*MRI:* MR imaging may be helpful in order to characterize the amount of leakage, as well as underlying renal parenchyma (Fig. 19.1-43B).

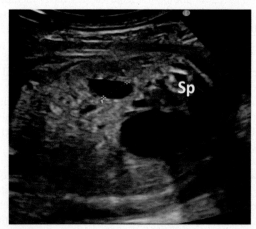

**FIGURE 19.1-42:** Bilateral UPJ obstruction (third trimester). Transverse ultrasound of the fetal abdomen shows bilateral asymmetrical dilatation. Sp, fetal spine.

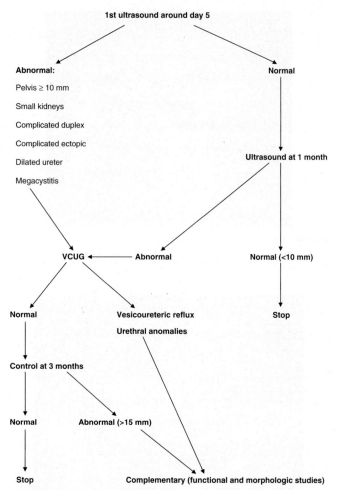

**FIGURE 19.1-42B:** Postnatal workup of antenatally diagnosed urinary tract dilatation.

**Differential Diagnosis:** The main differential diagnosis includes nonobstructive, nonrefluxing dilatation that accounts for a large proportion of urinary tract dilatation (approximately 20%) as well as MCDK, VUR, and UVJ obstruction.

**Associated Anomalies:** Renal anomalies in the contralateral kidney are common present in up to 25% of cases. This includes renal agenesis, MCDK, and vesicoureteral reflux. Extrarenal anomalies are noted in up to 12% of affected fetuses.

**Prognosis:** Outcome is usually good. There is poor correlation between prenatal pelvic dilatation and postnatal function. Thinned, echogenic cortex containing cortical cysts corresponds most likely to obstructive cystic dysplasia with potentially postnatal impaired renal function.

**Management:** Follow-up ultrasounds in the third trimester are useful to assess progression and amniotic fluid volume.

Following delivery, infants are usually begun on prophylactic antibiotics. Evaluation includes ultrasound, VCUG, and renal Lasix scans to assess severity of obstruction. Most cases are managed conservatively unless there is poor differential renal function and/or progressive obstruction. Pyeloplasty is performed in these cases to prevent further deterioration of renal function Figure 19.1-42.B.

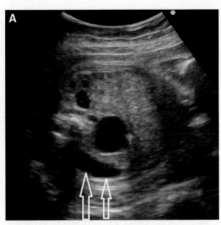 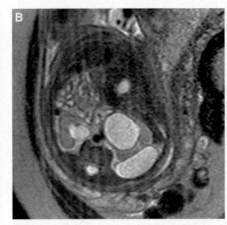

**FIGURE 19.1-43:** Urinoma associated with UPJ obstruction (third trimester). **A:** Transverse ultrasound displays asymmetrical dilatation in the right kidney, with perirenal fluid collection *(arrows)* corresponding to the urinoma. **B:** Axial T2w MR imaging of the fetal abdomen. The urinoma is well demarcated. The renal parenchyma has a homogeneous "normal" signal.

## UVJ Obstruction

**Definition:** Obstruction at the level of the uretero-vesicle junction (see Fig. 19.1-40).

**Incidence:** 1:6,500. Bilateral in up to 25% of cases. More common in males 2:1.

**Embryology and Pathogenesis:** Obstruction may be due to a localized region of dysfunction or secondary to an ectopic insertion, or ureterocele.

### Diagnosis
*Ultrasound:* The diagnosis of UVJ obstruction is suspected whenever the fetal ureter is visible and dilated (see Fig. 19.1-40). This can be differentiated from bowel as the urine is clear and the can be followed to the pelvis and/or bladder. The renal pelvic and calyces may be dilated as well. The dilatation may increase in utero but usually decreases progressively after birth.

*MRI:* MR imaging is helpful in the evaluation of ureteral insertion.

**Differential Diagnosis:** It can be difficult to differentiate UVJ obstruction from dilatation secondary to high-grade VUR.[88,89,91] Differential diagnosis includes nonobstructive, nonrefluxing dilatation as well as UPJ obstruction and PUVs.

**Prognosis and Management:** Follow-up scans are required to follow amniotic fluid stability. Prophylactic antibiotics is started until diagnosis is confirmed. Postnatal assessment includes US, VCUG, and renal Lasix scans. Reimplantation is performed on those with poor or deteriorating renal function. Patients with good renal function can be managed conservatively. Prognosis is generally good even when bilateral.

## Vesicoureteric Reflux

**Definition:** Retrograde flow of urine from the bladder into the ureter and pelvicalyceal system.

**Incidence:** Reflux is estimated to occur in up to 1% of all children. Up to 10% of neonates with antenatal diagnosis of dilatation likely have reflux.

**Embryology and Pathogenesis:** There are two types of reflux: low-grade VUR more commonly diagnosed in girls after a urinary tract infection, and high-grade VUR associated with dilated collecting systems, dysplastic kidneys that occur mainly in boys. The latter is more commonly detected in utero with damage occurring in utero prior to postnatal infections.

**Diagnosis:** The diagnosis can be suggested in patients where the dilatation varies at different moments of the same examination (Fig. 19.1-44) or in cases where renal dilatation is associated with impaired renal growth (Fig. 19.1-45).

**Differential Diagnosis:** Direct diagnosis of VUR in utero is difficult. Differential includes UPJ, UVJ obstruction, and PUVs. VUR should be included in the list of differential diagnosis of fetal megacystis, especially in female fetuses—in relation to the megacystis–microcolon intestinal hypoperistalsis syndrome (Fig. 19.1-46) (see later).[87,91–93]

**Associated Anomalies:** Associated with contralateral renal anomalies, including UPJ obstruction MCKD, Duplex kidney, and renal agenesis.

**Prognosis:** The majority of VUR resolve by age 2 years. In the rare cases of severe reflux nephropathy, the outcome can be poor.

## Renal Duplication

**Incidence:** Occurs in 1:500 births.

**Embryology and Pathology:** It results from a supernumerary ureteral bud budding from the primitive nephritic duct.

### Diagnosis
*Ultrasound:* Shows two collecting systems separated by a cortical band that can be visualized (Fig. 19.1-47); unless an associated urinary tract malformation is observed, it should be considered to be a normal variant. If dilatation is demonstrated in either upper or lower moiety, the condition should be considered abnormal and requires a complete workup postnatally (Figs. 19.1-48 and 19.1-49).

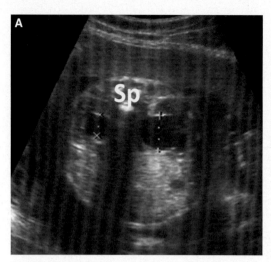
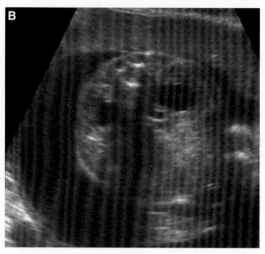

**FIGURE 19.1-44:** Vesicoureteric reflux (third trimester). **A:** Transverse ultrasound of the fetal abdomen through the kidneys. Bilateral dilatation 10 mm to the right and 16 mm to the left. Sp, fetal spine. **B:** Transverse scan at same level as in **A**, a few seconds later. The dilatation has modified.

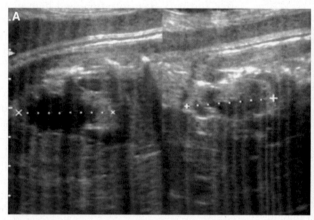
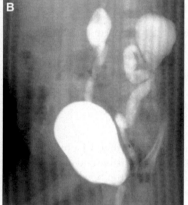

**FIGURE 19.1-45:** VUR associated with hypodysplastic kidneys (third trimester). **A:** Sagittal ultrasound through both kidneys (limited by *crosses*) shows that both are dilated and small, measuring 25 and 22 mm in length at 31 weeks. **B:** Postnatal voiding cystography shows bilateral grade IV VUR.

Obstruction (Fig. 19.1-48A), MCDK or reflux, may develop in either moiety of the duplication (Fig. 19.1-27). The upper pole may be completely dysplastic and large (Fig. 19.1-49A) or small. The upper pole may be associated with extravesical insertion of a ureter. An ectopic ureterocele is seen as a septum within the bladder (Fig. 19.1-49B). The ureterocele may collapse because of bladder filling or protrude into the bladder neck, inducing bladder outlet obstruction. "Disappearance" of a ureterocele has been described as urine production of the dysplastic upper pole may reduce. The renal parenchyma related to an obstructive moiety may display evidence for obstructive (cystic) dysplasia (Fig. 19.1-49A). Dysplastic parenchyma may also be associated with high-grade reflux.[94–96]

*MRI:* MR may better demonstrate an extravesical insertion of a ureter (see Fig. 19.1-48B,C).

**Differential Diagnosis:** VUR, UVJ obstruction, and upper pole renal cysts could be considered in the differential.

**Outcome/Management:** Prognosis is generally good. The function of the kidney depends on the degree of dysplasia affecting the upper pole moiety. The lower pole moiety may have severe vesico-ureteric reflux which may be associated with marked dysplasia. Large ureteroceles or bilateral ureteroceles can obstruct both kidneys, resulting in oligohydramnios, so follow-up sonograms are recommended.

Following delivery, infants are placed on prophylactic antibiotics. US, VCUG, and renal Lasix scans are performed postnatally at 2 to 3 weeks of age. Cystoscopy with puncture of the ureterocele may be performed to preserve function in the upper pole; still, rupture of the ureterocele predisposes to vesico-ureteric reflux. If the upper pole is nonfunctioning, heminephrectomy may be considered.

## Posterior Urethral Valves

**Definition:** Bladder outlet obstruction at the level of the posterior urethra.

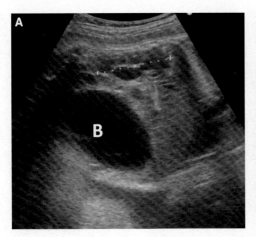

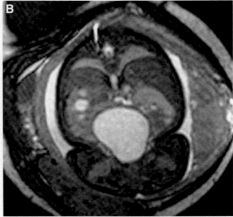

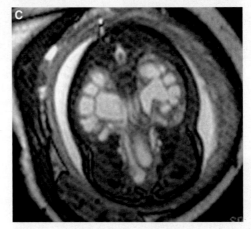

**FIGURE 19.1-46:** Megacystis associated with massive bilateral VUR. **A:** Sagittal ultrasound through one kidney (delineated by the *crosses*) and the enlarged bladder *(B)*. Amniotic fluid volume was normal. **B:** Coronal T2w MRI shows the enlarged bladder. **C:** Coronal T2w MRI through the dilated kidneys and ureters. T1w images demonstrated a normal colon, excluding megacystis, microcolon, and hypoperistalsis syndrome.

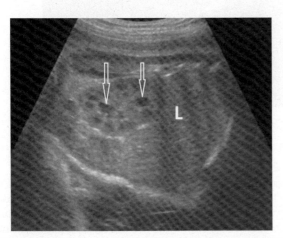

**FIGURE 19.1-47:** Uncomplicated duplex kidney (third trimester). Sagittal ultrasound through the kidney shows two separated collecting systems *(arrows)*. L, fetal liver.

**Incidence:** 1:5,000 males. The commonest cause of bladder outlet obstruction in male fetuses.

**Embryology and Pathology:** Incomplete regression of a urogenital membrane that develops during early embryological development.

**Diagnosis**
*Ultrasound:* The degree of obstruction and the timing of diagnosis vary greatly. Some cases are detected early during the first or early second trimester because of megacystis (Fig. 19.1-50; see Fig. 19.1-41) and/or oligohydramnios, while others will be detected during the third trimester or only after birth.

An enlarged bladder with thickened wall (above 3 mm) and a dilated posterior urethra are common findings.[47,58,59] Associated upper urinary tract dilatation is frequent but variable. Renal dilatation can be uni- or bilateral, related to obstruction and/or to VUR (Fig. 19.1-51A). The degree of associated renal dysplasia is variable as well. There seems to be a correlation between cortical echogenicity, cystic changes, and the degree of obstructive dysplasia (Fig. 19.1-51B). Unusual presentations include bladder rupture with ascitis and perirenal urinoma.

*MRI:* MR imaging may provide additional information, particularly when oligohydramnios is present.[5,97–101]

**Differential Diagnosis:** In the second and third trimesters, the differential diagnosis of enlarged bladder includes severe vesicoureteric reflux, megacystis–microcolon–hypoperistalsis syndrome and prune belly syndrome (Fig. 19.1-52; see Fig. 19.1-46). Medication-induced megabladder (e.g., cocaine) and a pseudoenlarged bladder in the female fetus should be considered. Anterior valves can very rarely be demonstrated in utero. A megalourethra (Fig. 19.1-53) is a particular abnormality of the urethra where in the corpus spongiosa are lacking and where the urethra is dilated.[102–106]

Bladder enlargement due to obstruction secondary to PUV must be differentiated from other causes of bladder outlet obstruction (BOO) (Table 19.1-7). During the first and early

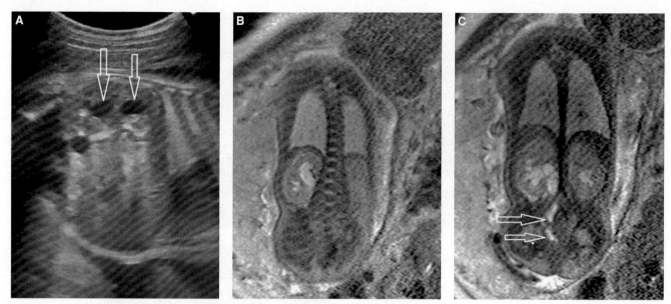

**FIGURE 19.1-48:** Duplex system with ectopic insertion of the upper pole ureter (third trimester). **A:** Sagittal ultrasound of the right kidney shows that the upper and lower moieties are dilated *(arrows).* **B:** Coronal T2w MRI of the fetal urinary tract shows a dilated upper pole. **C:** Coronal T2w MRI demonstrates the dilated lower pole as well as the distended upper pole ectopic ureter *(arrows)* that inserts below the bladder neck. (Courtesy of M. Cassart, MD.)

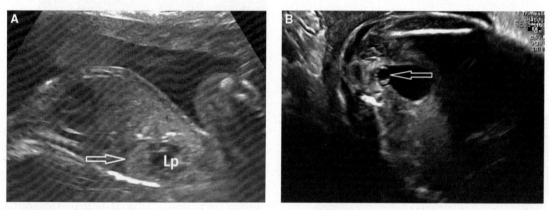

**FIGURE 19.1-49:** Duplex system. **A:** Sagittal ultrasound shows echogenic dysplastic upper pole *(arrow)* and dilated lower pole *(Lp).* **B:** Endovaginal ultrasound demonstrates a ureterocele within the bladder *(arrow).* (Courtesy of M. van Rysselberghe.)

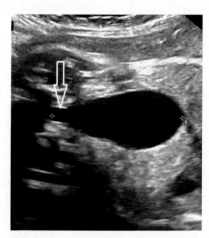

**FIGURE 19.1-50:** PUV (third trimester). Sagittal ultrasound shows a fetal megacystis (6 cm in length). The posterior urethra is dilated *(arrow).* (Courtesy of B. Broussin.)

second trimesters, BOO could result from urethral atresia (see Fig. 19.1-41). The kidneys will appear hyperechoic because of obstructive dysplasia. The prognosis is poor. Megabladder of the first trimester may be transitory or also associated with trisomies.

**Outcome:** The outcome is variable and depends on the severity of the obstruction. Postnatal mortality is around 8%, though prenatal mortality rates are higher—23% to 54%.

**Management:** The role of measuring urinary electrolytes in the fetal urine obtained through transabdominal puncture is controversial. Fetuses with renal damage show increased urinary concentration, especially of Na and Ca, without clear convincing confirmation. Measurements of B2-immunoglobulin on C cystatin in the fetal urine allow a better accuracy. Karyotyping can bring additional important information as chromosomal anomalies can be detected, especially in cases of lower urinary tract obstruction.

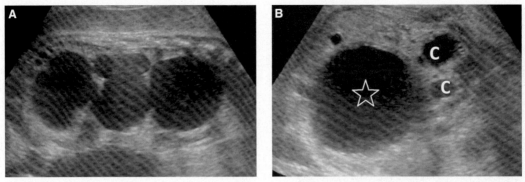

**FIGURE 19.1-51:** Obstructive cystic dysplasia in a case of PUV (third trimester). **A:** Sagittal ultrasound of one kidney shows a marked dilatation with cortical thinning and cortical cysts. **B:** Closeup of the dilated renal pelvis *(star)*. There are numerous cysts *(C)* within the renal cortex, consistent with obstructive cystic dysplasia. (Courtesy of C. Garel, MD.)

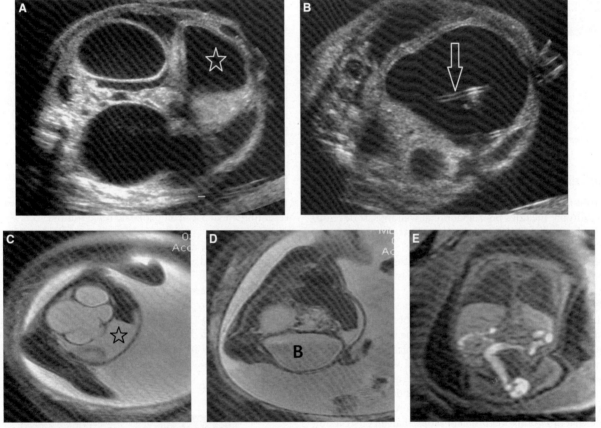

**FIGURE 19.1-52:** Megacystis–microcolon–hypoperistalsis syndrome (third trimester). **A:** Transverse ultrasound of the fetal abdomen at the level of the markedly dilated kidneys. Ascitis is also visible *(star)*. **B:** Transverse ultrasound through the fetal megacystis. A catheter had been inserted within the bladder *(arrow)*. **C:** Sagittal T2w MRI through one of the dilated kidneys. Star, ascites. **D:** Sagittal T2w MRI through the distended bladder *(B)* surrounded by ascitis. **E:** T1w MRI displays a short colon in the left upper quadrant. (Courtesy of L. Guibaud, MD.)

The role of vesicoamniotic shunting is controversial. Although technically easy, the long-term results of shunting have not been validated.[107–112]

In the poor prognosis group with severe oligohydramnios, bilateral hydroureteronephrosis, and echogenic dysplastic kidneys, termination may be offered because of the poor outcome in the neonatal period from pulmonary hypoplasia. Close follow-up with determination of optimal delivery coincides with the gestation age and timing of oligohydramnios. Before 32 weeks' gestation if oligohydramnios is developing, shunting may be useful. After 32 weeks' gestation if oligohydramnios develops, early delivery should be considered.

Postnatally, the patient should be placed on antibiotics, and emergency VCUG performed. If PUV is confirmed, urethral valve ablation or vesicostomy may be performed, depending on the size of the infant.

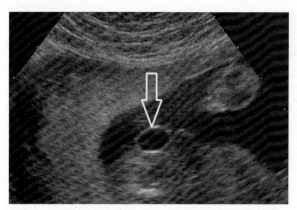

**FIGURE 19.1-53:** Megalourethra (second trimester). Ultrasound shows distension of the intrapenile urethra (arrow). (Courtesy of B. Broussin, MD.)

| Table 19.1-7 | Differential Diagnosis of Fetal Megabladder |
|---|---|

Posterior urethral valves
Prune belly sequence
Megacystis–megaureter syndrome (massive VUR)
Megacystis–microcolon–hypoperistalsis syndrome
Maternal sedative medication
Physiological (female, late third trimester)

## Prune Belly Syndrome

**Definition:** Also known as Eagle Barret or triad syndrome, prune belly syndrome includes poor abdominal wall muscle development, undescended testicles, and urinary tract abnormalities.

**Incidence:** Occurring in 1 in 40,000 live births, with 3% to 4% occurring in females. 4% are associated with twinning.[112A,112B]

**Embryology and Pathology:** Several theories have been suggested. One theory focuses on functional obstruction due to prostatic hypoplasia. The obstruction may be transient and result in reflux as well as an overdistended bladder that results in abnormal development of the abdominal wall musculature and prevents descent of testis. The mesodermal arrest theory is supported by histologic findings in the abdominal wall and urinary tract, where sparsely placed smooth muscle suggests a mesodermal differentiation problem rather than an obstruction problem.[112A,112B]

**Diagnosis:** Typically, megacystis is noted with a large protruberant abdomen. Obstruction can occur as high as the UPJ to as low as the prostatic membranous urethra with megalourethra at times observed. Dilated tortuous ureters are often present. Patent urachus is often associated with prune belly syndrome.

MRI can be useful in assessment of the ureters, bladder, and urachus, particularly if oligohydramnios develops.

**Differential Diagnosis:** PUVs, severe vesicoureteric reflux, megacystis–microcolon–hypoperistalsis syndrome should be considered (see Figs. 19.1-46 and 19.1-52). Isolated megalourethra (see Fig. 19.1-53) with absent corpus spongiosa is rare but should be included in the differential.[102–106]

**Associated Anomalies:** Patent urachus is commonly present. Anterior urethral abnormalities from atresia to megalourethra are common.

Orthopedic anomalies, including scoliosis and hip dislocation, can affect up to 50% of patients. Cardiac anomalies are noted in 10% of cases. Gastrointestinal abnormalities, including malrotation, atresia, and volvule, affect up to one-third of patients.[112B]

**Outcome:** Prognosis is variable. The spectrum extends from still birth due to severe pulmonary hypoplasia to undescended testis with minimal abdominal wall weakness. Long-term medial issues include renal failure, bladder incontinence, and infertility.[112B–112E]

**Management:** Vesicoamniotic shunting has had little effect in reducing the incidence of renal failure and need for transplantation.

In severe cases, immediate care is required because of pulmonary hypoplasia.

Prophylactic antibiotics should be initiated. US, VCUG, and renal Lasix scans should be performed to assess renal status. Urethral stenosis must be treated immediately. If there is no obstruction or reflux, management can be conservative. Abdominal wall reconstruction, vesicostomies, ureteral reimplantations, nephrostomies, and/or pyeloplasties may be required to help preserve renal function. Some individuals eventually require renal transplantation.[112B,112D,112E]

## Mesoblastic Nephroma

**Incidence:** The most common congenital renal neoplasm, representing 2% to 5% of all pediatric renal tumors.

**Pathology:** There are two main subtypes, a classical (resembling fibromatosis) and a cellular type (resembling fibrosarcoma).

**Diagnosis:** In the fetus, it appears as a solid tumor that is sometimes difficult to delineate from the adjacent renal normal parenchyma (Fig. 19.1-54). The tumor can display a partially cystic and septated pattern. In utero, polyhydramnios is typically present. MR imaging can provide better anatomical delineation of the mass from surrounding structures (Fig. 19.1-55).

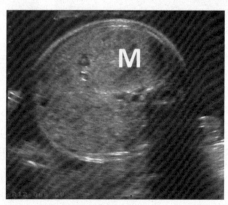

**FIGURE 19.1-54:** Mesoblastic nephroma (third trimester). Transverse ultrasound of the fetal abdomen shows a large solid-type mass (M) occupying the right renal fossa.

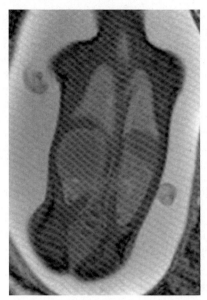

**FIGURE 19.1-55:** Mesoblastic nephroma (third trimester). Coronal T2w MRI of the kidneys shows a large mass, hyposignal compared with the rest of the kidney, occupying the upper pole of the right kidney. (Courtesy of K. Chaumoitre.)

**Differential Diagnosis:** Rare cases of fetal renal Wilms tumor have been reported (Fig. 19.1-56). Some syndromes, especially those associated with a mutation of WT1 gene, are at risk for developing Wilms tumor (e.g., Beckwith–Wiedemann, Wilms-Aniridia, or Drash Syndrome). Bilateral involvement suggests bilateral Wilms or nephroblastomatosis (see Fig. 19.1-56). The main differential diagnoses of cystic renal tumors include MCDK, cystic dysplasia, intrarenal lymphangiectasia, segmental dysplasia, and renal cysts.

**Prognosis and Management:** The prognosis is usually good. [117–122]Hypertension may develop after birth but resolves after nephrectomy. Survival rate is 95% after resection; a worse prognosis is reported with advanced stages of the cellular type and whenever excision is incomplete.

## Renal Hypodysplasia/Tubular Dysgenesis-Oligomeganephronia

**Definition:** A congenital small kidney is defined by a sagittal length below 2 SD compared to normal gestational age (see Table 38 in Appendix A1). The exact definitions of hypoplasia, dysplasia, tubular dysgenesis, or oligomeganephronia are histological ones.

**Embryology, Genetics, and Pathogenesis:** The origin of a congenital small kidney is multifactorial; it may be related to genetic mutations (e.g., HNF1β mutation, rennin angiotensin system mutation), associated with VUR or other uropathies, or acquired. Medications such as angiotensin-converting enzyme inhibitors and cocaine can cause hypodysplastic kidney. The condition can also be associated with chromosomal abnormalities.[3,8,10,11,14,123–126]

**Diagnosis:** Standard measures by gestation age are available (Table 38 and 39 renal measures in Appendix A1). Associated urinary tract dilatation should suggest VUR and renal dysplasia (see Fig. 19.1-45A).

Hyperechoic small kidneys with oligohydramnios is suggestive of tubular dysgenesis. The CMD is potentially preserved in these cases (Fig. 19.1-57).[126]

**Prognosis:** The prognosis depends on the degree of renal failure and oligohydramnios.

**Recurrence:** Recurrence depends upon the etiology. Cases that have genetic origin have a higher risk.

## Acquired Renal Pathologies

Renal anomalies can develop during pregnancy because of vascular impairment, maternal preexisting disease, maternofetal acquired disease, or toxic medications.[123–126] Fetal renal vein thrombosis may develop with maternal diabetes at any stage of the pregnancy. Sonographically, during the acute stage of the thrombosis, the kidney enlarges markedly and its

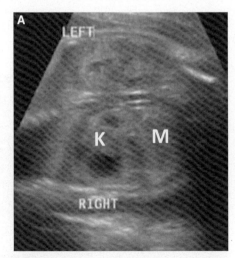
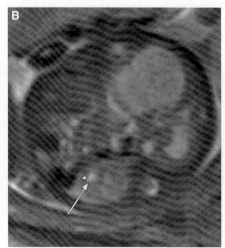

**FIGURE 19.1-56:** Bilateral Wilm tumor (third trimester). **A:** Coronal ultrasound of both kidneys shows solid-type mass *(M)* and the lower pole of the right kidney *(K)*. **B:** Axial T2w MRI demonstrates a large mass at the lower pole of the kidney. The *arrow* points to a contralateral Wilm tumor. (Courtesy of Beth Kline-Fath, MD.)

echogenicity becomes heterogeneous (Fig. 19.1-57). Doppler analysis may in some cases confirm the thrombosis. A thrombus within the inferior vena cava and adrenal hemorrhage may be associated findings (Figs. 19.1-58B and 19.1-59B). Rapidly, collateral vessels develop and the renal revascularization may resume. Vascular calcifications in the interlobar areas may remain as sequelae[127–130] (see Fig. 19.1-59). Kidney growth will be impaired in more severe cases with poorer prognosis.

Twin–twin transfusion syndrome, the death of one twin, may render the surviving one more vulnerable to ischemia. The ischemic kidneys might appear hyperechoic (Fig. 19.1-60).

Maternal deficit in neuropeptidase may induce an acute transient glomerulonephritis in the fetus, which will determine increased renal volume and cortical echogenicity. Transient renal failure may develop at birth. The renal appearance will return to normal progressively.[136]

Furthermore, maternofetal infection may involve the kidneys and determine increased echogenicity, as demonstrated in some cases with cytelomegalovirus (CMV).[132]

As mentioned above, some medications may result in impaired renal growth, neonatal renal failure, and intractable pneumothoraces.[123–126]

## Congenital Nephrotic Syndromes

Congenital nephrotic syndrome may start in fetal life. The kidneys appear diffusely hyperechoic (Fig. 19.1-61). The placenta is thick, and polyhydramnios is present. Affected fetuses are growth retarded, and birth is usually premature. The proteinuria

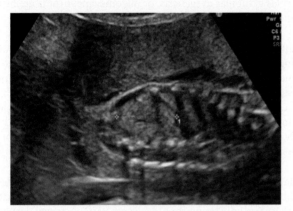

**FIGURE 19.1-57:** Tubular dysgenesis (third trimester). Sagittal ultrasound shows one kidney (limited by the *crosses*) that appears hyperechoic and small (the other kidney had similar findings). Oligohydramnios was present. The baby died at birth from pulmonary hypoplasia.

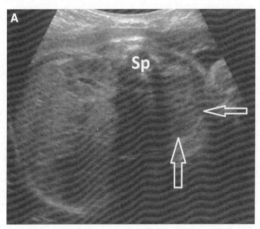
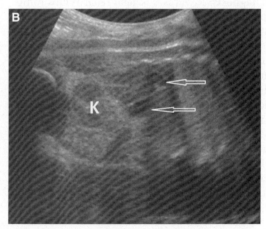

**FIGURE 19.1-58:** Renal vein thrombosis, acute phase. **A:** On transverse ultrasound of the kidneys on each side of the spine *(Sp)*, the left kidney *(arrows)* appears globular and lacks CMD. **B:** On sagittal ultrasound, the kidney *(K)* displays a heterogeneous pattern, and there is an associated acute adrenal hemorrhage *(arrows)*.

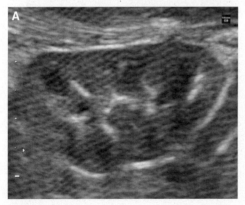
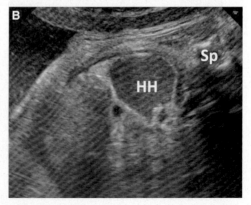

**FIGURE 19.1-59:** Renal vein thrombosis follow-up. **A:** Sagittal ultrasound in the third trimester reveals hyperechoic streaks in the interlobar areas, corresponding to calcifications. **B:** Transverse ultrasound of the corresponding adrenal gland shows an adrenal hemorrhage *(HH)*. Sp, fetal spine.

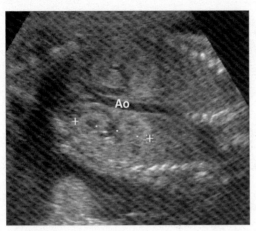

**FIGURE 19.1-60:** Ischemic kidney, twin-twin transfusion syndrome. On coronal ultrasound in the third trimester, both kidneys appear hyperechoic but normal in size. Ao, aorta.

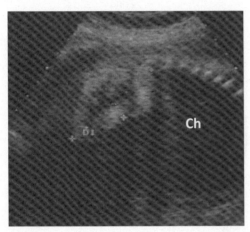

**FIGURE 19.1-61:** Congenital nephrotic syndrome. Sagittal ultrasound in the third trimester shows one kidney (limited by *crosses*) that is hyperechoic and heterogeneous. It corresponded to a mesangial sclerosis. Ch, fetal chest.

can be detected in the amniotic fluid. A particular association is the Drash syndrome that includes pseudohermaphrodism and a particular nephrotic syndrome (mesangial sclerosis). Patients affected by the syndrome carry an increased risk for Wilm tumor.[133]

## FETAL ADRENALS

### Embryology

The adrenal develops from two components: mesothelial cells and neural crest cells. During the 5th week of development, mesothelial cells close to the urogenital ridge proliferate and penetrate the underlying mesenchyme, where they differentiate into large acidophilic organs that will constitute the primitive fetal cortex. Thereafter, a second wave of cells surround the first ones and form the definitive cortex. Only the outermost layer will remain after birth. Simultaneously, neural crest cells invade the sympathetic system, where they are arranged in cords; they will form the adrenal medulla. These cells will migrate and penetrate the fetal cortex and coalesce within it. Both components,

cortex and medulla, will remain separated in the definitive adrenal (Fig. 19.1-62).[134]

### Normal Ultrasound Appearance

The fetal adrenals are easily visualized and measured during obstetrical ultrasound as early as 13 to 14 weeks. They appear as hypoechoic triangular-shaped structures above the kidneys (see Fig. 19.1-5B). During this period, the fetal adrenals are globular and large (their height is half of kidney height). Progressively, during the second and third trimesters a corticomedullary differentiation will become obvious (Fig. 19.1-63). The cortex appears hypoechoic, while the medulla is hyperechoic. The gland will display a Y or reverted V shape. The adrenal height should be one-third of that of the kidneys.[135,136]

### Tumors and Pseudotumors of the Adrenal Glands

**Differential Diagnosis:** The differential diagnosis of enlargement of the fetal adrenals includes tumoral and pseudotumoral enlargement. They must be differentiated from extra-adrenal tumors (Table 19.1-8).

*Tumoral enlargement* includes cysts and solid-type tumors. Simple adrenal cysts are detected during routine examinations. Their evolution is benign, and they may resolve spontaneously. Some syndromes (e.g., Beckwith–Wiedemann syndrome) include dysplastic, usually bilateral dysplastic cortical cysts. These cysts may become large and bleed (Fig. 19.1-64). Adrenal hemorrhage may develop in utero, associated or not with renal vein thrombosis (RVT) (see Figs. 19.1-57B and 19.1-58B).

*Neuroblastoma* is the main tumor affecting the fetal adrenals. Neuroblastomas represent 30% to 40% of fetal tumors and are the most common congenital malignancy (1:10,000 live births). The tumor is usually detected during the second trimester. The classic US appearance includes a suprarenal well-defined echogenic mass (Fig. 19.1-65A). Cystic changes may develop within the mass, and the tumor will become hypoechoic; at this stage, it becomes difficult to differentiate it from adrenal hemorrhage. The latter may develop isolated or in association with RVT. Color Doppler may demonstrate vascularization within the tumor helping the differentiation. Liver metastasis may develop already in utero in the case of neuroblastoma (Pepper syndrome). MR imaging may help to delineate the tumor or the metastasis (Figs. 19.1-65 and 19.1-66). Despite the malignant nature of neuroblastoma, the overall prognosis is excellent, even though metastasis has developed. Furthermore, cases of spontaneous regression have been described.[119–122,137–141]

### Congenital Adrenal Hyperplasia

CAH is the main cause of peusdotumoral enlargement. The clue to the prenatal diagnosis of CAH is usually the detection of a disorder of the sexual differentiation (DSD) (ambiguous genitalia) (see Chapter 19.3). Such a finding should prompt a detailed analysis of the fetal adrenals. In the case of CAH, the glands are markedly enlarged because of cortical hypertrophy; in typical cases, they would display the specific cerebriform pattern (Fig. 19.1-67). In the case of CAH, whenever a corticoid treatment is initiated in utero, sonography is helpful while demonstrating the progressive reduction in adrenal size. Enlargement of fetal adrenals due to CAH must be differentiated from the other causes of pseudotumoral enlargement.[142–145]

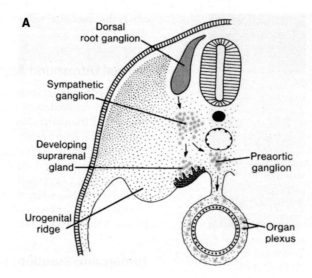

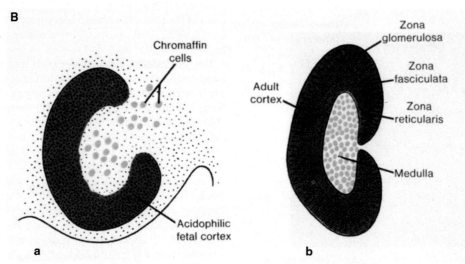

**FIGURE 19.1-62:** Embryology of the human adrenals. **A:** Formation of the sympathetic ganglia. A portion of neuroblasts migrates toward the mesothelium *(shaded area)* to form the medulla of the adrenal. **B:** The neuroblasts became the chromaffin cells; they penetrate the fetal cortex but remain separated from it in the definitive gland. (From Sadler TW. The urogenital system. In: Sadler TW, ed. *Langman's Medical Embryology.* 9th ed. Philadelphia, PA: Lippincott Williams & Wilkins; 2004:321–362.)

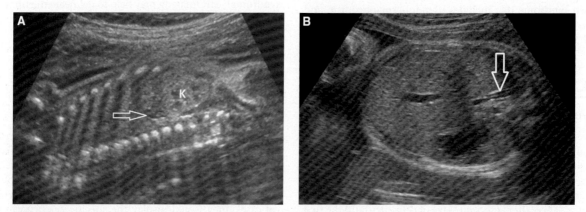

**FIGURE 19.1-63:** Normal adrenals. **A:** On parasagittal ultrasound in the second trimester, the adrenal *(arrow)* appears linear with an outer hypoechoic and central hyperechoic layer above the kidney *(K)*. **B:** On transverse ultrasound, the two-layered adrenal is visible *(arrow)*.

| Table 19.1-8 | Differential Diagnosis of Adrenal Masses |
|---|---|

Adrenal cortical cyst
Adrenal dysplastic cortical cyst
Adrenal hemorrhage
Neuroblastoma
Cortical adenoma
Congenital adrenal hyperplasia
Inflammatory hypertrophy
Upper pole of a duplex kidney
Intra-abdominal pulmonary sequestration
Hepatic and splenic cyst
Duplication cyst

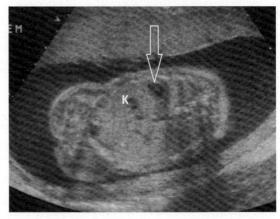

**FIGURE 19.1-64:** Adrenal dysplastic cyst, Beckwith–Wiedemann syndrome. Coronal ultrasound in the second trimester shows a hypoechoic mass *(arrow)* above the kidney *(K)*.

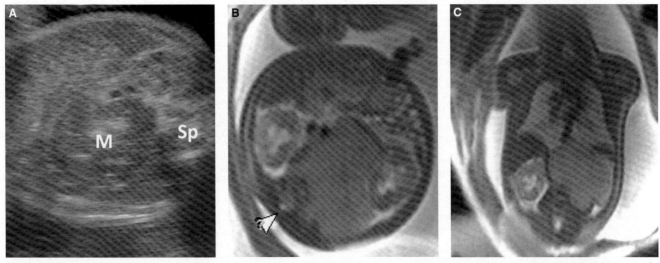

**FIGURE 19.1-65:** Neuroblastoma. **A:** Ultrasound in the third trimester demonstrates a heterogeneous solid-type mass *(M)* anterior to the fetal spine *(Sp)*. **B:** Axial MRI shows the mass displacing the left kidney anterioly. Fetal spine *(arrowhead)*. **C:** On coronal MRI, the neuroblastoma crosses the midline.

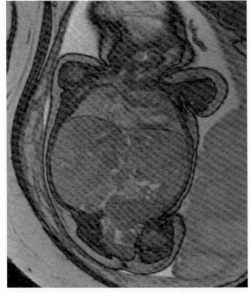

**FIGURE 19.1-66:** Neuroblastoma, Pepper syndrome. On coronal MRI, the liver is enlarged and heterogeneous pattern, related to the neuroblastoma metastasis. (Courtesy of O. Prodhomme, MD.)

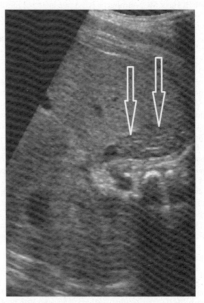

**FIGURE 19.1-67:** Congenital adrenal hyperplasia. On transverse ultrasound in the third trimester, the right adrenal appears multilayered *(arrows)* as compared with a normal adrenal as seen on Figure 19.1-63B.

# REFERENCES

1. Wiesel A, Queisser-Luft A, Clementi M, et al. Prenatal detection of congenital renal malformations by fetal ultrasonographic examination: an analysis of 709,030 births in 12 Europeans countries. *Eur J Med Genet.* 2005;48:131–144.
2. Carpenter MW, Corrado F, Sung J. Lethal fetal renal anomalies and obstetrics outcome. *Eur J Obstet Gynecol Reprod Biol.* 2000;89:149–153.
3. Desphande C, Hennekam RCM. Genetic syndromes and prenatally detected renal anomalies. *Semin Fetal Neonatal Med.* 2008;13:171–180.
4. Nguyen HT, Herndon CDA, Cooper C, et al. The Society for Fetal Urology consensus statement on the evaluation and management of antenatal hydronephrosis. *J Pediatr Urol.* 2010;6:212–231.
5. Cassart M, Massez A, Metens T, et al. Complementary role of MRI after sonography in assessing bilateral urinary tract anomalies in the fetus. *AJR Am J Roentgenol.* 2004;182:689–695.
6. Hubert KC, Palmer JS. Current diagnosis and management of fetal genitourinary abnormalities. *Urol Clin North Am.* 2007;34:89–101.
7. Riccabona M, Avni FE, Blickman JG, et al. Imaging recommendations in paediatric uroradiology: minutes of the ESPR workgroup session on urinary tract infection, fetal hydronephrosis, urinary tract US and voiding cystourethrography. *Pediatr Radiol.* 2008;38:138–145.
8. Wynyard P, Chitty LS. Dysplastic kidneys. *Semin Fetal Neonat al Med.* 2008;13:142–151.
9. Toka HR, Toka O, Hariri A, et al. Congenital anomalies of the urinary tract. *Semin Nephrol.* 2010;30:374–386.
10. Song R, Yosypiv IV. Genetics of congenital anomalies of the kidney and urinary tract. *Pediatr Nephrol.* 2011;26:353–364.
11. Woolf AS. A molecular and genetic view of human renal and urinary tract malformations. *Kidney Int.* 2000;58:500–512.
12. Deltas C, Papagregoriou G. Cystic diseases of the kidney. *Arch Pathol Lab Med.* 2010;134:569–582.
13. Sadler TW. The urogenital system. In: Sadler TW, ed. *Langman's Medical Embryology.* 9th ed. Baltimore, MD: Lippincott Williams & Wilkins; 2004:321–362.
14. Cuckow PM, Nyirady P, Winyard PJD. Normal and abnormal development of the urogenital tract. *Prenat Diagn.* 2001;21:908–916.
15. Zalel Y, Lotan D, Achiron R, et al. The early development of the fetal kidney—an in utero sonographic evaluation between 13 and 22 weeks' gestation. *Prenat Diagn.* 2002;22:962–965.
16. Brohnstein M, Kushnir O, Ben Zalel Z, et al. Transvaginal sonographic measurement of fetal kidneys in the first trimester of pregnancy. *J Clin Ultrasound.* 1990;18:299–301.
17. Chitty LS, Altman DG. Charts of fetal size: kidney and renal pelvis measurements. *Prenat Diagn.* 2003;23:891–897.
18. Kennedy WA II, Chitkara U, Abidari JM, et al. Fetal renal growth as assessed through renal parenchymal area derived from prenatal and perinatal US. *J Urol.* 2003;169:298–302.
19. Yu C, Chang C, Chang F, et al. Fetal renal volume in normal gestation: a three dimensional US study. *Ultrasound Med Biol.* 2000;26:1253–1256.
20. Stigler RH, Mulder EJH, Visser GHA. Hourly fetal urine production rate in the near term fetus: is it really increased during fetal quiet sleep? *Early Hum Dev.* 1998;50:263–272.
21. Oosterhof H, Haak MC, Aarnouche JG. Acute maternal rehydration increases the urine production rate in the near-term human fetus. *Am J Obstet Gynecol.* 2000;183:226–229.
22. Ross MG, Brace RA. Amniotic fluid biology: basic and clinical aspects. *J Matern Fetal Med.* 2001;10:2.
23. Hubbard AM. Ultrafast fetal MRI and prenatal diagnosis. *Semin Pediatr Surg.* 2003;12:143–153.
24. Farhataziz N, Engels JE, Ramus RM, et al. Fetal MRI of urine and meconium by gestational age for the diagnosis of genitourinary and gastrointestinal abnormalities. *AJR Am J Roentgenol.* 2005;184:1891–1897.
25. Abdelazim IA, Abdelrazak KM, Ramy RM, et al. Complementary roles of prenatal US and MR imaging in diagnosis of fetal renal anomalies. *Aust N Z J Obstet Gynaecol.* 2010;50:237–241.
26. Savelli S, Di Maurizio M, Perrone A, et al. MRI with diffusion weighted imaging (DWI) and apparent diffusion coefficient (ADC) assessment in the evaluation of normal and abnormal fetal kidneys: preliminary experience. *Prenat Diagn.* 2007;27:1104–1111.
27. Chaumoitre K, Colavolpe N, Shojah R, et al. DW MRI with ADC determination in normal and pathological fetal kidneys. *Ultrasound Med Gynecol.* 2007;29:22–31.
28. Lubusky M, Prochazka M, Dhaifalah I, et al. Fetal enterolithiasis: prenatal sonographic and MRI diagnosis in two cases of urorectal septum malformation (URSM) sequence. *Prenat Diagn.* 2006;26:345–349.
29. Schwarderer AL, Bates CM, McHugh KM. Renal anomalies in family members of infants with bilateral renal agenesis/adysplasia. *Pediatr Nephrol.* 2007;22:52–56.
30. Harewood L, Liu M, Keeling J, et al. Bilateral renal agenesis/hypoplasia/dysplasia (BRAHD): postmortem analysis of 45 cases with breakpoint mapping of two de novo translocations. *PLoS One.* 2010;5:e12375.
31. Nielsen BL, Norgard B, Puho E, et al. Risk of specific congenital anomalies in offspring of women with diabetes. *Diabet Med.* 2005;22:693–696.
32. Skinner MA, Safford SD, Reeves JG. Renal aplasia in humans is associated with RET mutations. *Am J Hum Genet.* 2008;82:344–351.
33. Hoffman CK, Filly RA, Callen PW. The lying down adrenal sign: a sonographic indicator of renal agenesis or ectopia in fetuses and neonates. *J Ultrasound Med.* 1992;11:533–536.
34. DeVore GR. The value of color Doppler US in the diagnosis of renal agenesis. *J Ultrasound Med.* 1995;14:443–449.
35. Bronshtein M, Amit A, Achiron R. The early prenatal US diagnosis of renal agenesis: technique and possible pitfalls. *Prenat Diagn.* 1994;14:291–297.
36. Hawkin JS, Dashe JS, Twickler DM. MRI diagnosis of severe fetal renal anomalies. *Am J Obstet Gynecol.* 2008;198:328.
37. Latini JM, Curtis MR, Cendron M, et al. Prenatal failure to visualize kidneys: a spectrum of diseases. *Urology.* 1998;52:306–311.
38. Ciasco S, Paran S, Puri P. Associated urological anomalies in children with unilateral renal agenesis. *Pediatr Nephrol.* 1992;6:412–416.
39. Cho JY, Moons MH, Lee YH, et al. Measurement of compensatory hyperplasia of the contralateral kidney: usefulness for differential diagnosis of fetal unilateral empty renal fossa. *Ultrasound Obstet Gynecol.* 2009;34:515–520.
40. Mesrobian HG, Rushton HG, Bulas D. Unilateral renal agenesis may result from in utero regression of multicystic renal dysplasia. *J Urol.* 1993;150:793–794.
41. Argueso LR, Ritchey ML, Boyle ET. Prognosis of patients with unilateral renal agenesis. *Pediatr Radiol.* 1992;6:412–416.
42. Sanna-Cherchi S, Ravani P, Corbani V, et al. Renal outcome in patients with congenital anomalies of the kidney and urinary tract. *Kidney Int.* 2009;76:528–533.
43. Glodny B, Peterson J, Hofmann KJ, et al. Kidney fusion anomalies revisited: clinical and radiological analysis of 209 cases of crossed fused ectopia and horseshoe kidney. *BJU Int.* 2009;103:224–235.
44. Decter RM. Renal duplication and fusion anomalies. *Pediatr Clin North Am.* 1997;44:1323–1341.
45. Hill LM, Grysbeck P, Mills A. Antenatal diagnosis of fetal pelvic kidneys. *Obstet Gynecol.* 1994;83:333–336.
46. Guarino N, Tadini B, Camardi P, et al. The incidence of associated urological abnormalities in children with renal ectopia. *J Urol.* 2004;172:1757–1759.
47. McPherson E. Renal anomalies in families of individuals with congenital solitary kidney. *Genet Med.* 2007;9:298–302.
48. Rizk D, Chapman AB. Cystic and inherited kidney diseases. *Am J Kidney Dis.* 2003;42:1305–1307.
49. Gunay-Aygun M. Liver and kidney disease in ciliopathies. *Am J Med Genet.* 2009;151C:269–306.
50. Hildebrandt F, Benzing T, Katsanis N. Ciliopathies. *N Engl J Med.* 2011;364:1533–1543.
51. Avni FE, Hall M. Renal cystic diseases in children: new concepts. *Pediatr Radiol.* 2010;40:939–946.
52. Avni FE, Garel L, Cassart M, et al. Perinatal assessment of hereditary cystic renal diseases: the contribution of sonography. *Pediatr Radiol.* 2006;36:405–414.
53. Avni FE, Garel C, Cassart M, et al. Imaging and classification of congenital cystic renal diseases. *AJR Am J Roentgenol.* 2012;198:1004–1013.
54. De Bruyn R, Gordon I. Imaging in cystic renal disease. *Arch Dis Child.* 2000;83:401–407.
55. Bisaglia M, Galliani CA, Senger C, et al. Renal cystic diseases: a review. *Adv Anat Pathol.* 2006;13:26–56.
56. Breysem L, Bosmans H, Dymarkowski S, et al. The value of fast MR imaging as an adjunct to ultrasound in prenatal diagnosis. *Eur Radiol.* 2003;13:1538–1548.
57. Chaumoitre K, Brun M, Cassart M, et al. Differential diagnosis of fetal hyperechogenic cystic kidneys unrelated to renal tract anomalies: a multicenter study. *Ultrasound Obstet Gynecol.* 2006;28:911–917.
58. Blazer S, Zimmer EZ, Blumenfels Z, et al. Natural history of fetal simple renal cysts detected in early pregnancy. *J Urol.* 1999;162:812–814.
59. Aubertin G, Cripps S, Coleman G, et al. Prenatal diagnosis of apparently isolated unilateral multicystic kidney: implications for counseling and management. *Prenat Diagn.* 2002;22:388–394.
60. Schreuder MF, Wesland R, van Wijk JAE. Unilateral MDK: a meta-analysis of observational studies on the incidence, associated urinary tract malformations and the contralateral kidney. *Nephrol Dial Transpl.* 2009;24:1810–1818.
61. Hains DS, Bates CM, Ingraham S, et al. Management and etiology of unilateral MDK: a review. *Pediatr Nephrol.* 2009;24:233–241.
62. Dahmen-Elias HAM, Stoutenbeek PH, Visser GHA, et al. Concomitant anomalies in 100 children with unilateral multicystic kidney. *Ultrasound Obstet Gynecol.* 2005;25:384–388.
63. Aslam M, Watson AR. Unilateral MDK: long term outcome. *Arch Dis Child.* 2006;91:820–823.
64. Siqueira Rabelo EA, Oliveira EA, Silva JMP, et al. US progression of prenatally detected MDK. *Urology.* 2006;68:1098–1102.
65. Bergman C, Senderek J, Windelen E, et al. Clinical consequences of PKHD1 mutations in 164 patients with ARPKD. *Kidney Int.* 2005;65:829–848.
66. Denamur E, Delezoide A, Alberti C, et al. Genotype-phenotype correlations in fetuses and neonates with ARPKD. *Kidney Int.* 2010;77:350–358.
67. Guay-Woodford LM, Desmond RA. Autosomal recessive polycystic kidney disease: the clinical experience in North America. *Pediatrics.* 2003;111:1072–1080.
68. Okumura M, Bunduki V, Shiang C, et al. Unusual sonographic features of ARPKD. *Prenat Diagn.* 2006;26:330–332.

69. Turkbey B, Ocak I, Daryanani K, et al. ARPKD and congenital hepatic fibrosis. *Pediatr Radiol*. 2009;39:100–111.

70. Wilson PO. Polycystic kidney disease. *N Engl J Med*. 2004;350:151–164.

71. Brun M, Maugey-Laulom B, Eurin D, et al. Prenatal sonographic patterns in autosomal dominant polycystic kidney disease: a multicenter study. *Ultrasound Obstet Gynecol*. 2004;24:55–61.

72. Mashiach R, Davidovits M, Einsenstein B, et al. Fetal hyperechogenic kidney with normal amniotic fluid volume: a diagnostic dilemma. *Prenat Diagn*. 2005;25:553–558.

73. Nakayama M, Nozu K, Goto Y, et al. HNF1B alterations with congenital anomalies of the kidney and urinary tract. *Pediatr Nephrol*. 2010;25:1073–1079.

74. Edghill EL, Bingham C, Ellard S, et al. Mutations in hepatocyte nuclear factor-1beta and their related phenotypes. *J Med Genet*. 2006;43:84–90.

75. Ulinski T, Lescure S, Beaufils S, et al. Renal phenotypes related to hepatocyte nuclear factor-1beta (TCF2) mutations in a pediatric cohort. *J Am Soc Nephrol*. 2006;17:497–503.

76. Decramer S, Parant O, Beaufils S, et al. Anomalies of the TCF2 gene are the main cause of fetal bilateral hyperechogenic kidneys. *J Am Soc Nephrol*. 2007;18:923–933.

77. Faguer S, Bouissou F, Dumazer P, et al. Massively enlarged polycystic kidneys in monozygotic twins with TCF2/HNF-1ß heterozygous whole gene deletion. *Am J Kidney Dis*. 2007;50:1023–1027.

78. Cassart M, Eurin D, Didier F, et al. Antenatal renal sonographic anomalies and postnatal follow-up of renal involvement in Bardet-Biedl syndrome. *Ultrasound Obstet Gynecol*. 2004;24:51–54.

79. Ickowicz V, Eurin D, Maugey-Laulom B, et al. Meckel-Grüber syndrome: sonography and pathology. *Ultrasound Obstet Gynecol*. 2006;27:296–300.

80. Hildebrandt F, Zhou W. Nephronophthisis-associated ciliopathies. *J Am Soc Nephrol*. 2007;18:1855–1871.

81. Salomon R, Saunier S, Niaudet P. Nephronophthisis. *Pediatr Nephrol*. 2009;24:2333–2344.

82. Blowey DL, Querfeld U, Geary D, et al. Ultrasound findings in juvenile nephronophthisis. *Pediatr Nephrol*. 1996;10:22–24.

83. Valente EM, Marsh SE, Castori M, et al. Distinguishing the four genetic causes of Jouberts syndrome-related disorders. *A nn Neurol*. 2005;57:513–519.

84. Woolf AS, Feather SA, Bringham C. Recent insights into kidney diseases associated with glomerular cysts. *Pediatr Nephrol*. 2005;17:229–235.

85. Ismaili K, Hall M, Donner C, et al. Results of systematic screening for minor degrees of fetal renal pelvis dilatation in an unselected population. *Am J Obstet Gynecol*. 2003;188:242–246.

86. John U, Kahler C, Schulz S, et al. The impact of fetal renal pelvic diameter on postnatal outcome. *Prenat Diagn*. 2004;24:591–595.

87. Lee RS, Kinnamon DD, Nguyen HT. Antenatal hydronephrosis as a predictor of postnatal outcome: a meta-analysis. *Pediatrics*. 2006;118:586–593.

88. Pates JA, Dashe JS. Prenatal diagnosis and management of hydronephrosis. *Early Hum Dev*. 2006;82:3–8.

89. Ismaili K, Hall M, Piepz A, et al. Insight into the pathogenesis and natural history of foetuses with renal pelvis dilatation. *Eur Urol*. 2005;48:207–214.

90. Thorup J, Jokela R, Cortes D, et al. The results of 15-years of consistent strategy in treating antenatally suspected PUJ obstruction. *BJU Int*. 2003;91:850–852.

91. Shukla AR, Cooper J, Paytel RK, et al. Prenatally detected primary megaureter: a role for extended follow-up. *J Urol*. 2005;173(4):1353–1356.

92. Van Eerde AM, Meutgeert MH, De Jong TPVM, et al. VUR in children with prenatally detected hydronephrosis: a systematic review. *Ultrasound Obstet Gynecol*. 2007;29:463–469.

93. Ismaili K, Hall M, Piepz A, et al. Primary VUR detected in neonates with a history of fetal pelvis dilatation: a prospective clinical and imaging study. *J Pediatr*. 2006;148:222–227.

94. Whitten SM, Wilcox DT. Duplex systems. *Prenat Diagn*. 2001;21:952–957.

95. Uphadhyay J, Bolduc S, Braga L, et al. Impact of prenatal diagnosis on the morbidity associated with ureterocele management. *J Urol*. 2002;167:2560–2565.

96. Austin PF, Cain MP, Casale AJ, et al. Prenatal bladder outlet obstruction secondary to ureterocele. *Urology*. 1998;52:1132–1135.

97. Harvie S, McLeod L, Acott P, et al. Abnormal antenatal sonogram: an indicator of disease severity in children with PUV. *Can Assoc Radiol J*. 2009;60:185–189.

98. Kousidis G, Thomas DFM, Morgan H, et al. The long term follow-up of prenatally detected PUV: a 10 to 23 year follow-up study. *BJU Int*. 2008;102:1020–1024.

99. Anumba DO, Scott JE, Plant ND, et al. Diagnosis and outcome of fetal lower urinary tract obstruction in the northern region of England. *Prenat Diagn*. 2005;25:7–13.

100. Morris RK, Malin GL, Khan KS, et al. Antenatal US to predict post natal renal function in congenital lower urinary tract obstruction: systematic review of test accuracy. *BJOG*. 2009;116:1290–1299.

101. Miller OF, Lashley DB, McAleer IM, et al. Diagnosis of urethral obstruction with prenatal MRI. *J Urol*. 2002;168:1158–1159.

102. Carlsson SA, Hokegard KH, Mattson LA. Megacystis-microcolon-hypoperistalsis syndrome: antenatal appearance in two cases. *Acta Obstet Gynecol Scand*. 1992;71:645–648.

103. McHugo J, Witthle M. Enlarged fetal bladders: aetiology, management and outcome. *Prenat Diagn*. 2001;21:958–963.

104. Osborne NG, Bonilla-Musoles F, Machado LE, et al. Fetal megacystis: differential diagnosis. *J Ultrasound Med*. 2011;30:833–841.

105. Gonzalez R, De Filippo R, Jednak R, et al. Urethral atresia: long term outcome in 6 children who survived the neonatal period. *J Urol*. 2001;165:2241–2244.

106. Stephens FD, Fortune DW. Pathogenesis of megalourethra. *J Urol*. 1993;149:1512–1516.

107. Klaassen I, Neuhaus TJ, Mueller-Wiefel DE, et al. Antenatal oligohydramnios of renal origin: long term outcome. *Nephrol Dial Transplant*. 2007;22:432–439.

108. Muller F, Dreux S, Audibert F, et al. Fetal serum B2-microglobulin and cystatin C in the prediction of post-natal renal function in bilateral hypoplasia and hyperechogenic enlarged kidneys. *Prenat Diagn*. 2004;24:327–332.

109. Morris RK, Quinlan-Jones E, Kilby MD, et al. Systematic review of accuracy of fetal urine analysis to predict poor postnatal renal function in cases of congenital urinary tract obstruction. *Prenat Diagn*. 2007;27:900–911.

110. Carr MC. Prenatal management of urogenital disorders. *Urol Clin North Am*. 2004;31:389–397.

111. Morris RK, Khan KS, Kilby MD. Vesico-amniotic shunting for lower urinary tract obstruction: an overview. *Arch Dis Child*. 2007;92:F166–F168.

112. Makino Y, Kobayashi H, Kyono K, et al. Clinical results of fetal obstructive uropathy treated by vesico-amniotic shunting. *Urology*. 2000;55:118–122.

112A. Terada S, Suzuki N, Uchide K, et al. Etiology of prune belly syndrome: evidence of megalocystic origin in an early fetus. *Obstet Gynecol*. 1994;83:865–868.

112B. Tonni G, Ida V, Alessandro V, et al. Prune-belly syndrome: case series and review of the literature regarding early prenatal diagnosis, epidemiology, genetic factors, treatment, and prognosis. *Fetal Pediatr Pathol*. 2013;31(1):13–24.

112C. Woods AG, Brandon DH. Prune belly syndrome: a focused physical assessment. *Adv Neonatal Care*. 2007;7:132–143.

112D. Biard JM, Johnson MP, Carr MC, et al. Long-term outcomes in children treated by prenatal vesicoamniotic shunting for lower urinary tract obstruction. *Obstet Gynecol*. 2005;106(3):503–508.

112E. Duckett J, Knutrud O, Hohenfellner R. Prune belly syndrome. *J Urol*. 1980;3:9.

113. Thomas DFM. Prenatal diagnosis: what do we know of long-term outcomes? *J Pediatr Urol*. 2010;6:204–211.

114. Valentin L, Marsal K. Does the prenatal diagnosis of fetal urinary tract anomalies affect perinatal outcome? *Ann N Y Acad Sci*. 1998;847:59–73.

115. Nakai H, Asanuma H, Shishido S, et al. Changing concepts in urological management of the congenital anomalies of kidney and urinary tract (CAKUT). *Pediatr Int*. 2003;45:634–641.

116. Riccabona M, Avni FE, Blickman JG, et al. Imaging recommendations in pediatric uroradiology: childhood obstructive uropathy, high grade fetal hydronephrosis, childhood haematuria, and urolithiasis in childhood. *Pediatr Radiol*. 2009;39:891–898.

117. Chan KL, Tang MHY, Tse HY, et al. Factors affecting outcomes of prenatally-diagnosed tumors. *Prenat Diagn*. 2002;22:437–444.

118. Woodward PJ, Sohaey R, Kennedy A, et al. A comprehensive review of fetal tumors with pathologic correlation. *Radiographics*. 2005;25:215–242.

119. Sebire NJ, Jauniaux E. Fetal and placental malignancies: prenatal diagnosis and management. *Ultrasound Obstet Gynecol*. 2009;33:235–244.

120. Avni FE, Massez A, Cassart M. Tumors of the fetal body: a review. *Pediatr Radiol*. 2009;39:1147–1157.

121. Linam LE, Yu X, Clvo-Garcia MA, et al. Contribution of MR imaging to prenatal differential diagnosis of renal tumors: report of two cases and review of the literature. *Fetal Diagn Ther*. 2010;28:100–108.

122. Ferguson MR, Chapman T, Dighe M. Fetal tumors: imaging features. *Pediatr Radiol*. 2010;40:1263–1273.

123. Celsi G, Kistner A, Aizman R, et al. Prenatal dexamethasone causes oligonephronia, sodium retention, and higher blood pressure in the offspring. *Pediatr Res*. 1998;44:317–322.

124. Peruzzi L, Gianoglio B, Porcellini MG, et al. Neonatal end-stage renal failure associated with maternal ingestion of COX-1 selective inhibitor nimesulide as tocolytic. *Lancet*. 1999;354:1615.

125. Saji H, Yamanaka M, Hagiwara A, et al. Losartan and fetal toxic effects. *Lancet*. 2001;357:363.

126. Lambot MA, Vermeylen D, Noel JC. Angiotensin II receptor inhibitors in pregnancy. *Lancet*. 2001;357:1619–1620.

127. Winyard PJD, Bharucha T, De Bruyn R, et al. Perinatal renal venous thrombosis: presenting renal length predicts outcome. *Arch Dis Child*. 2006;91:F273–F278.

128. Kraft JK, Brandao LR, Navarro OM. Sonography of renal venous thrombosis in neonates and infants: can we predict outcome? *Pediatr Radiol*. 2011;41:299–307.

129. Lau KK, Fernandez y Garcia E, Kwan WY, et al. Bilateral renal venous thrombosis and adrenal hemorrhage: sequential prenatal US with postnatal recovery. *Pediatr Radiol*. 2007;37:912–915.

130. Sohdi KS, Khandelwal S, Ray M, et al. Calcified neonatal renal vein and caval thrombosis. *Pediatr Radiol*. 2006;36:437–439.

131. Nortier JL, Debiec H, Tourney Y, et al. Neonatal disease in neutral endopeptidase alloimmunization: lessons for immunological monitoring. *Pediatr Nephrol*. 2006;10:1399–1405.

132. Chan M, Hecht JL, Boyd T, et al. Congenital CMV: a cause for renal dysplasia? *Pediatr Dev Pathol*. 2007;10:300–304.

133. Hofstaetter C, Neumann I, Lennert T, et al. Prenatal diagnosis of diffuse mesangial sclerosis by US: a longitudinal study of a case in an affected family. *Fetal Diagn Ther*. 1996;11:126–131.

134. Sadler TW. Central nervous system: sympathetic nervous system. In Sadler TW, ed. *Langman's Medical Embryology*. 9th ed. Lippincott Williams & Wilkins; 2004:474–477.

135. Van Vuuren SH, Dahmen-Elias HA, Stigter RH, et al. Size and volume of the fetal kidney, renal pelvis and adrenal gland. *Ultrasound Obstet Gynecol.* 2012;40(6):659–664.

136. Turan OM, Turan S, Funai EF, et al. US measurements of fetal adrenal gland enlargement on accurate predictor of preterm birth. *Am J Obstet Gynecol.* 2011;204; e1–e10.

137. Lin J, Lin G, Hung I, et al. Prenatally detected tumor mass in the adrenal gland. *J Pediatr Surg.* 1999;34:1620–1623.

138. Rubenstein SC, Benaceraff BR, Retik AB, et al. Fetal suprarenal masses: US appearance and differential diagnosis. *Ultrasound Obstet Gynecol.* 1995;5: 164–167.

139. Sherer DM, Dalloul M, Wagreich A, et al. Prenatal sonographic findings of congenital adrenal cortical adenoma. *J Ultrasound Med.* 2008;27(7): 1091–1093.

140. McCauley RGK, Beckwith JB, Elias ER, et al. Benign hemorrhagic adrenocortical macrocysts in Beckwith-Wiedemann syndrome. *AJR Am J Roentgenol.* 1991;157:549–552.

141. Niemec SF, Horcher E, Kasprian G, et al. Tumor disease and associated congenital abnormalities on prenatal MRI. *Eur J Radiol.* 2012;81:e15–e22.

142. Chambrier ED, Heinrichs C, Avni EF. US appearance of congenital adrenal hyperplasia in utero. *J Ultrasound Med.* 2002;21:97–100.

143. Saada J, Grebille A, Aubry MC, et al. Sonography in prenatal diagnosis of congenital adrenal hyperplasia. *Prenat Diagn.* 2004;24:627–630.

144. Cassart M, Massez A, Donner C, et al. Sonographic diagnosis of fetal adrenal hyperplasia: utility for prenatal corticotherapy. *Prenat Diagn.* 2005;25:1060–1061.

145. Buhimschi CS, Turan OM, Funai EF, et al. Fetal adrenal gland volume and cortisol/DHEA sulfate ratio in inflammation-associated preterm birth. *Obstet Gynecol.* 2008;111:715–722.

## PERSISTENT CLOACA

Cloacal malformations represent a spectrum of developmental defects in which the urinary tract, the vagina, and the rectum converge above the level of the perineum, creating a single perineal opening, the cloaca (Latin for "sewer") (Fig. 19.2-1).[1,2] Because of its prognostic and therapeutic implications, Peña[3] and Peña et al.[4] subdivided these anomalies into two major subgroups based on the length of the common channel. Cloacal malformations with a short common channel (less than 3 cm) have a lower incidence of associated defects and less difficult repair. Cloacal malformations with a long common channel (longer than 3 cm) have a high incidence of associated defects, complex anatomy, more difficult repair, and inferior functional results.

**Incidence:** The condition is seen typically in females with an incidence of 1 in 40,000 to 50,000 births.

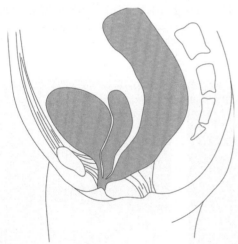

**FIGURE 19.2-1:** Diagram of a cloaca. Sagittal view of the pelvis. The rectum, vagina, and urethra are fused together, forming a single common channel opened to the perineum.

**Genetics and Embryology:** The most widely accepted theory is that cloacal malformations are related to failure in development of the urorectal septum. This is a structure that normally fuses with the cloacal membrane by the 6th week of gestation and subdivides the primitive cloaca into the urogenital sinus in front and the rectum posteriorly (Fig. 19.2-2). Development of these structures may be arrested at any stage, leading to a wide spectrum of defects unified under the term urorectal septum malformation sequence (URSM) (Fig. 19.2-3).[5,6] In this classification, persistent cloaca are termed partial URSM.

The aberrant drainage of urine can lead to bladder obstruction, hydrocolpos, and colonic dilatation. It is also thought that abnormalities in cloacal septation and urogenital sinus formation could interfere with normal mesonephric and paramesonephric duct development, explaining the high incidence of genital tract duplication or agenesis and increased anomalies of number and position of the kidneys in these patients. Associated lower spinal cord, lumbosacral spine, lower limbs, and bladder anomalies as well as ambiguous genitalia are also suggesting multiple disturbances during the embryonic development of the caudal pole.[2,7]

**Etiology:** The etiology is unknown. There are several case reports in monozygotic twins, in association with maternal drug abuse and one reported case of apparent genetic transmission.[8,9]

**Diagnosis:** Ultrasound diagnosis of cloacal malformations is challenging and usually considered when a pelvic cyst is seen in a female fetus (Fig. 19.2-4). In this situation, a differential diagnosis should include hydrocolpos or megacystis in the setting of cloaca, isolated hydrocolpos, urogenital sinus, obstructive uropathy, and other pelvic cystic lesions such as ovarian cyst, enteric duplication cyst, bowel atresia, cystic type IV sacrococcygeal teratoma, and anterior meningocele.[10,11] In addition, the sequence of findings on serial sonograms of transient ascites (from escape of urine via the fallopian tubes), progressive hydrocolpos, hydronephrosis, oligohydramnios with or without development of meconium peritonitis and peritoneal calcifications has been described as suggestive of this malformation, but is not clearly specific.[8,12–14]

The most specific sonographic signs supporting this diagnosis and the communication between the urinary system and the distal bowel in a female fetus are rectal fluid dilatation with intraluminal calcifications[8,13,15] and the detection of calcified meconium in the urinary system.[16] Unfortunately, these signs are not always present or easily detected.

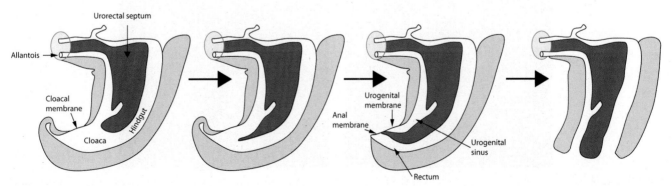

**FIGURE 19.2-2:** Normal development of the urorectal septum. The urorectal septum grows in a caudal direction to separate the cloaca into the dorsal rectum and the ventral urogenital sinus. The urorectal septum also divides the cloacal membrane into the urogenital and anal membranes. These structures will grow caudal, so they will be no longer be part of the ventral wall. Both membranes will subsequently rupture.

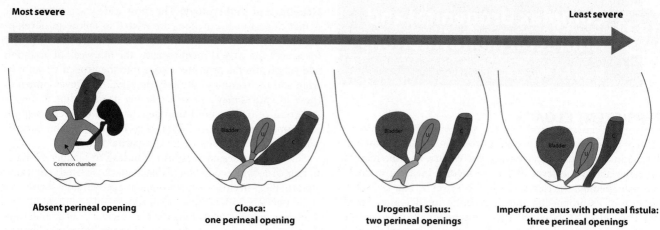

**Most severe**

**Least severe**

Common chamber

**Absent perineal opening**

**Cloaca:**
**one perineal opening**

**Urogenital Sinus:**
**two perineal openings**

**Imperforate anus with perineal fistula:**
**three perineal openings**

**FIGURE 19.2-3:** Spectrum of abnormalities related to the urorectal septum. Variations of these forms may also occur. C, colon; K, kidney; U, uterus.

In recent years, several authors have defined the normal appearance of the colon with fetal MRI. Starting around 20 to 21 weeks of gestation, meconium is expected to fill the rectum, and by 26 weeks, much of the colon is visualized with its characteristic bright T1 and dark T2 signal. The rectum is close to the bladder and its cul-de-sac at least 10 mm below the bladder neck.[11,17,18] MRI provides a resource to assess the rectum and its content and differentiate isolated hydrocolpos and urogenital sinus from cloacal malformation. Isolated hydrocolpos and urogenital sinus will present with a normal rectum.[19,20] Cloaca can have fluid signal instead of meconium in the rectum and/or rectal dilatation located high in the cul-de-sac, not extending below the bladder base. Content signal ranges from normal meconium to increased fluid signal in a series of long common channel cloacas. In addition, abnormal signal can be detected layering withing the bladder due to the presence of meconium.[21]

**Differential Diagnosis:** The differential diagnosis includes other etiologies presenting with megacystis and/or hydrocolpos. Megacystis can be seen in the setting of

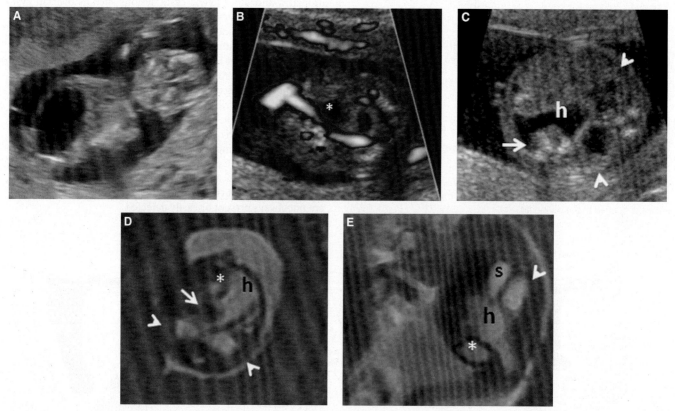

**FIGURE 19.2-4:** Cloacal malformation with hydrocolpos. **A:** Coronal US scan at 13 weeks GA shows a large abdominopelvic cyst. Axial US **(B)**, axial 2D SSFP and sagittal fetography **(C)** fetal MRI sequences on same fetus at 17w GA. There is bilateral hydronephrosis, large hydrocolpos *(h)* containing intraluminal echogenic foci with posterior shadowing *(arrow on **C**)* or dark T2 material as expected for meconium *(arrow on **D**)*. The bladder is anterior to the hydrocolpos *(asterisk)* and the stomach *(s)* anterior to the left kidney *(arrowhead on **E**)*.

mechanical obstruction such as urethral atresia, or in the setting of megacystis–microcolon intestinal hypoperistalsis syndrome and prune belly syndrome. Urethral atresia is typically associated with early development of oligo/anhydramnios, typically with normal rectal anatomy. Megacystis–microcolon intestinal hypoperistalsis syndrome, a process more frequently affecting females, is typically associated with polyhydramnios during the third trimester, and fetal MRI will be extremely helpful in defining the presence of microcolon.[11] Megacystis is also seen in prune belly syndrome, characterized by deficient abdominal musculature, urinary tract abnormalities, and cryptorchidism in males or major genital tract malformations in females including cloacal malformation.[21] Hydrocolpos due to underlying obstruction or urogenital sinus has a normal rectum and fetal MRI is helpful in differentiating it from cloacal malformation.[19]

It will be important to remember that transient ascites and meconium peritonitis (from urine and meconium scape through the tubes) can be seen with cloacal malformation in the absence of bowel perforation. Fetal MRI will help to define the appearance of the bowel and the pelvic structures to support one of the two possibilities.[11]

**Prognosis:** The prognosis is dictated by the presence of oligohydramnios and renal dysplasia, the type of cloaca, and the presence of other associated malformations. Amniotic fluid volume is easily tracked with ultrasound. Attempts to define the type of cloaca and potential additional malformations have been described with the use of fetal MRI during the third trimester in a series of six fetuses.[21] In this series, long common channel cloacas were linked to dilated and high rectums. Malformations consistent with VACTERL association were defined in one fetus.

With early diagnosis, management of associated anomalies, and efficient meticulous surgical repair, patients can have the best chance for a good anatomic outcome.[4] Functional results will depend as well on the degree of sacral development, nerve supply, and spinal cord anomalies. In cases with incontinence despite excellent anatomic repair, effective bowel and bladder management programs have been devised to improve the patient's quality of life.[22]

**Management:** Once the diagnosis is suspected with ultrasound, fetal MRI will help characterize the defect, assess renal parenchyma and help identify potential associated malformations. Fetal echocardiogram is recommended to rule out congenital heart defect as well. This approach will provide more accurate information, and a comprehensive multidisciplinary counseling session with the parents will be possible in the presence of pediatric and colorectal surgeons, pediatric urologist, neonatologist, and pediatric nephrologist.

Attempts to restore the amniotic fluid volume have been described in cases of bladder outlet obstruction with the use of vesicoamniotic shunts and serial amnioinfusions, and could be applied to cloacas with megacystis.[13] However, these options will not prevent renal dysfunction and vesicoamniotic shunts might lead to bladder dysfunction, in some cases severe enough to preclude kidney transplantation.[23] Open fetal vesicostomy would be a more effective way to decompress the bladder, preventing further renal damage but could precipitate preterm labor.[24]

Delivery is recommended at a tertiary center, and these infants need urgent clinical and radiological evaluation by experienced pediatric surgeons and radiologist with crucial decisions taken during the first 24 hours.[4,13,25]

**Recurrence Risk:** The condition is sporadic, with low recurrence risk.

## PERSISTENT UROGENITAL SINUS

Urogenital sinus is the persistence of an embryonic state in which there is a single-exit chamber for the bladder and the vagina in the presence of a normal rectum and anus. On physical exam, there are two perineal openings, one anterior for the urogenital sinus and the other for the anus.[1]

**Incidence:** The condition affects females and is rare.[1] The exact incidence is not well defined in the literature.

**Embryology:** The anomaly is the result of abnormal development of the lower vagina and failure of urethrovaginal septation. In this situation, urine flow can be impaired, leading to potential development of cystic dilatation of the vagina, also known as hydrocolpos (or hydrometrocolpos if the uterus is also involved). The hydrocolpos can compress the bladder forward, and can result in obstructive uropathy. Rarely, urine can reach the peritoneum through the fallopian tubes and present as urinary ascites.

**Etiology:** The most common etiology for persistent urogenital sinus is adrenogenital syndrome (congenital adrenal hyperplasia) or other in utero exposure to androgenic stimuli, with expected clitoral enlargement/ambiguous genitalia. It may also occur as pure urogenital sinus with normal external genitalia, or associated with gonadal dysgenesis and hermaphroditism.[1,26]

**Diagnosis:** Prenatal cystic dilatation of the vagina will compress and displace the bladder anteriorly. A pelvic cystic mass with fluid–fluid levels, representing thick, mucoid cervical or vaginal secretions, should be highly concerning for hydrocolpos.[27] Associated findings in the setting of urogenital sinus can include hydroureteronephrosis, urinary ascites, and in severe cases renal dysplasia and oligohydramnios (Fig. 19.2-5).[20,28]

Enlarged adrenal glands with a cerebriform pattern, typically seen in neonates with congenital adrenal hyperplasia, might not be detected in utero until the late third trimester.[29] Babies

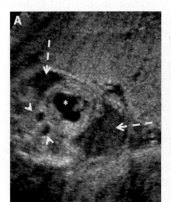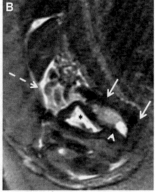

**FIGURE 19.2-5:** Fetus at 26 weeks gestation with urogenital sinus and severe oligohydramnios. **A:** Axial US image. **B:** Sagittal heavily T2w hydrography sequence (MR fetography). There is a septated hydrocolpos *(arrowheads)* posterior to a thick-walled bladder *(asterisk)*. There is ascites *(dashed arrow)* and normal meconium-filled (dark T2 signal) rectum *(arrows)* posterior to the hydrocolpos.

with urogenital sinus can present with normal or ambiguous genitalia.

Fetal MRI can detect the cervical imprint on the vagina confirming the diagnosis of hydrocolpos and will define the presence or absence of meconium in the rectum or potential abnormal content. With normal meconium in the rectum and hydrocolpos, urogenital sinus or vaginal obstruction should be suspected. If there is absence of meconium in the rectum or the rectum is identified but with fluid content, enteroliths, or dilatation, the underlying malformation is cloaca.[19,21,30]

**Differential Diagnosis:** One difficulty in diagnosing pelvic cystic masses in female fetuses is the potential confusion of the bladder with the hydrocolpos and an initial consideration of megacystis. However, the fetal bladder is outlined by the umbilical arteries, has an anterior midline position, and its volume is expected to change, allowing its correct identification.[19] In the setting of hydrocolpos, the possibility of cloaca, urogenital sinus, or obstructive vagina should be entertained. Other pelvic cystic lesions would be considered in the differential such as ovarian cyst, anterior meningocele, type IV sacrococcygeal teratoma, enteric duplication cyst, lymphatic malformations, and ectopic multicystic dysplastic kidney.[27]

**Prognosis:** The prognosis will be dictated by the degree of obstructive uropathy, and potential associated malformations. In survivors, the long-term outlook is reasonably good after reconstructive surgery. In the neonatal period, a correct prenatal diagnosis, absence of renal dysplasia, and coordinated work between the involved teams (obstetricians, neonatologists, radiologist, and pediatric surgeons) will significantly impact the clinical outcome.[28]

**Management:** Multidisciplinary counseling and delivery in a tertiary center is indicated. In the neonatal period, vaginal drainage will alleviate the abdominal distension and potential cardiorespiratory compromise and will improve any obstructive uropathy associated.[4] Metabolic assessment and treatment in cases of congenital adrenal hyperplasia and chromosomal studies will be indicated in cases of ambiguous genitalia.[1]

In families with known history of congenital adrenal hyperplasia, early medical treatment can start in utero with maternal glucocorticoid administration before the development of the urogenital sinus (6th to 7th week of gestation) and be maintained after confirmation of gene mutation and female karyotype (usually by the 13th week of gestation).[29]

**Recurrence Risk:** Persistent urogenital sinus, in the absence of congenital adrenal hyperplasia, is usually a sporadic condition with low recurrence risk. On the other hand, congenital adrenal hyperplasia is an autosomal recessive disorder with an incidence of approximately 1:14,000 live births.[31] When other malformations are associated including postaxial polydactyly, then an underlying genetic condition should be considered such as McKusick–Kaufman, Bardet–Biedl, Ellis van Creveld syndromes (with autosomal recessive inheritance), or Pallister–Hall syndrome (with autosomal dominant inheritance).[32]

# HYDROCOLPOS

Hydrocolpos is the cystic dilatation of the vagina. Hydrometrocolpos is distention of the uterus and vagina. We use the term hydrocolpos here to refer to both conditions.

**Incidence:** The condition is rare. The prevalence of congenital hydrocolpos is less than 1 per 30,000 births and represents 15% of the abdominal masses in female fetuses.[19]

**Embryology:** There are two types of hydrocolpos. The urinary type is related to a urogenital sinus or cloacal malformation. The secretory type is related to vaginal obstruction because of abnormal development of the lower vagina presenting as imperforate hymen, vaginal agenesis or hypoplasia, and transverse septum.

**Etiology:** Most cases of hydrocolpos are sporadic but can also be seen with genetic syndromes such as McKusick–Kaufman, Bander–Belt, Langer–Giedion (tricho–rhino–phalangeal syndrome), Pallister–Hall, and Mayer–Rokitansky–Küster–Hauser syndrome/MURCS (Müllerian duct, renal agenesis/ectopia, and cervical thoracic somite dysplasia) association (Fig. 19.2-6).[32]

**Diagnosis:** A pelvic cystic mass posterior to the bladder, with or without fluid–fluid levels, should be highly concerning for hydrocolpos in a female fetus. When there are Müllerian duct anomalies, it may appear as a septated cyst. Hydroureteronephrosis and ascites can be associated.[19,20,33] Fetal MRI can define the appearance of the rectum after 21 weeks of gestation.[17] With a normal rectal cul-de-sac filled with meconium, cloacal malformation is considered unlikely, and hydrocolpos could be related to urogenital sinus or vaginal obstruction. If there is absence of meconium in the distal rectum or the rectum is identified but with fluid content, enteroliths, or dilatation, the underlying malformation is a cloaca.[19]

At birth, they could present as a large abdominal mass with hydroureteronephrosis and possible respiratory distress from elevation of the diaphragm. If diagnosis and treatment are delayed, infection may follow, resulting in pyocolpos and sepsis.[4,33]

**Differential Diagnosis:** Differential diagnosis includes other cystic masses, such as ovarian cyst, enteric duplication cyst, megacystis, duplicated urinary bladder, anterior meningocele, and type IV sacrococcygeal teratoma.

In the setting of hydrocolpos, the possibility of cloaca, urogenital sinus, or obstructive vagina should be entertained. Complete assessment of the fetus will also help to define the defect as potentially isolated or in the setting of a syndromic association or genetic disease.

**Prognosis:** The prognosis will be dictated by the type of underlying defect (hydrocolpos versus urogenital sinus or cloacal malformation), the degree of obstructive uropathy present, and potential associated malformations or genetic syndromes. In isolated forms with preserved renal function, the outlook is excellent after final surgical reconstruction.[32,34]

**Management:** A complete assessment of the fetal anatomy is recommended to rule out other structural defects. Amniocentesis could be considered when there is concern for a major genetic anomaly. Multidisciplinary counseling and delivery in a tertiary center is indicated. In the immediate neonatal period, vaginal drainage will alleviate the abdominal distension and potential cardiorespiratory compromise and will improve urinary obstruction, if present.[4] In order to rule out syndromes, high-resolution chromosome studies as well as long-term clinical follow-up will be needed.[32]

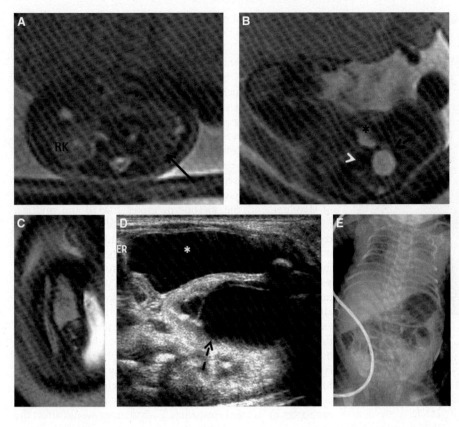

**FIGURE 19.2-6:** Hydrocolpos in the setting of MURCS association, also known as type II Mayer-Rokytansky-Küster-Hauser (MRKH) syndrome. Axial **(A,B)** and coronal **(C)** T2-weighted fetal MRI at 29 weeks GA. **A:** There is left kidney renal agenesis with bowel filling the left renal fossa *(arrow)*. A normal right kidney *(RK)* is present. **B:** Posterior to the bladder *(asterisk)*, normal rectum *(white arrowhead)*, and hydrocolpos *(black dashed arrow)* are noted. **C:** There is rightward thoracic scoliosis. Pelvic US **(D)** and chest-abdomen x-ray **(E)** on first day of life showing hydrocolpos *(black dashed arrow)* and focal segmentation vertebral anomaly at the lower thoracic spine accounting for thoracic scoliosis and short fourth ribs. There is also cardiomegaly and increased lung vascularity because of truncus arteriosus.

**Recurrence Risk:** Hydrocolpos is usually a sporadic condition with low recurrence risk. However, some syndromic forms are genetically transmitted.[32]

## CLOACAL EXSTROPHY

Cloacal exstrophy, also known as the OEIS complex (omphalocele, cloacal exstrophy, imperforate anus, spinal defects)[35] is one of the rarest and most complex anorectal and urogenital malformations. The entity represents an anterior wall defect that includes the persistence and exstrophy of a common cloaca that receives ureters, ileum, and a rudimentary blind-ending hindgut (Fig. 19.2-7). It is commonly associated with omphalocele, spinal dysraphism, and incompletely formed external genitalia and is always associated with imperforate anus.[36] Typically in females, there are usually two vaginal openings, widely separated and entering the lower aspect of each hemibladder and bilateral hemiuteri as well as two widely separated clitoral halves, while in males there is usually a rudimentary hemipenis on each side caudal to the exstrophy.[1] The terminal ileum could prolapse, giving the appearance of an elephant's trunk (Fig. 19.2-8).[37]

**Incidence:** The reported incidence is 1 in 200,000 to 400,000 live births.[1] The condition can affect both genders, with most recent studies suggesting no predilection toward either gender[38] or female preponderance.[39] It has also been described as increased

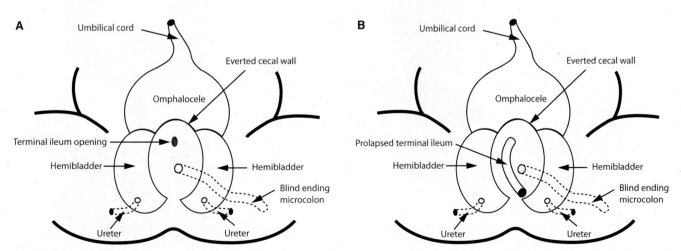

**FIGURE 19.2-7:** Diagrams of typical anatomical appearances of cloacal exstrophy without **(A)** and with **(B)** prolapse terminal ileum. (Reproduced with permission from Calvo-Garcia MA, Kline-Fath BM, Rubio EI, et al. Fetal MRI of cloacal exstrophy. *Pediatr Radiol.* 2013;43:593–604.)

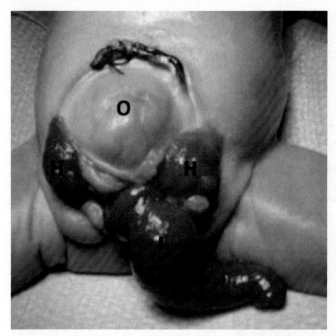

**FIGURE 19.2-8:** Cloacal exstrophy with prolapsed terminal ileum photograph. There is a low-lying omphalocele *(O)*. Extending from the back of the cecal plate is a prolapsed terminal ileum *(I)*. The exstrophied hemibladders *(H)* are seen on each side. (Reproduced with permission from Bischoff A, Calvo-Garcia MA, Baregamian N, et al. Prenatal counseling for cloaca and cloacal exstrophy: challenges faced by the pediatric surgeons. *Pediatr Surg Int.* 2012;28:781–788.)

incidence of cloacal exstrophy in multiple gestations, especially monozygotic twins.[39,40]

**Embryology:** Cloacal exstrophy is a severe and rare malformation thought to be a developmental field defect affecting the mesoderm, which later contributes to infraumbilical mesenchyme, urorectal septum, and caudal vertebrae during early embryogenesis (Figs. 19.2-2 and 19.2-9).[39]

Before the 5th week of embryonic development, the urinary, genital, and gastrointestinal tracts empty into a common chamber, the cloaca. At the caudal end of the cloaca, ectoderm lies directly over endoderm, forming the cloacal membrane, which at this stage forms part of the ventral wall. During the 6th week of development, the mesoderm grows toward the midline, forming the infraumbilical abdominal wall. Simultaneously, the urorectal septum extends caudally toward the cloacal membrane, and by the 8th week of gestation, the cloaca is divided into an anterior chamber, the primitive urogenital sinus, and a posterior chamber, the rectum. There is also caudal retraction of the cloacal membrane, so it is no longer a part of the abdominal wall and eventually ruptures at the end of the 10th week of gestation. Abnormal mesodermal migration between the ectodermal and the endodermal layers of the cloacal membrane or failure of the mesoderm to grow between those two layers is thought to cause its premature rupture. Some authors think that the stage of development when the abnormality occurs determines the type of defect: cloacal exstrophy, bladder exstrophy, or isolated epispadias. Early damage would affect the

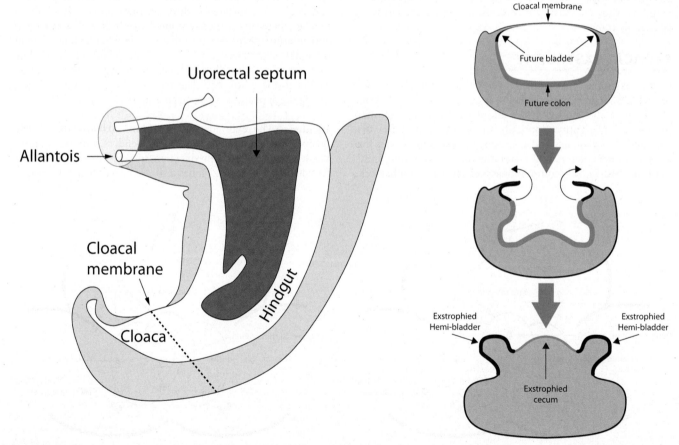

**FIGURE 19.2-9:** Diagram of events leading to cloacal exstrophy. The urorectal septum fails to grow caudal. Subsequently, there is premature rupture of the cloacal membrane while it is still part of the infraumbilical ventral wall. There is a resultant infraumbilical abdominal wall defect with everted bladder plates and cecal wall.

mesenchyme that contributes to the infraumbilical mesoderm, the urorectal septum, and the lumbosacral somites. This results in failure of cloacal septation. This leads to persistent cloaca and rudimentary hindgut with imperforate anus. A breakdown of the cloacal membrane, causes exstrophy of the cloaca, failure of fusion of the genital tubercles, and diastasis of the pubic rami. Occasionally there is also an omphalocele, and incomplete development of the lumbosacral vertebrae with commonly a closed neural tube defect. This constitutes what has been classically recognized as cloacal exstrophy. A later failure in migration of the infraumbilical mesoderm, after the caudal movement of the urorectal septum has been completed will result in bladder exstrophy.[41]

### Etiology:
The underlying cause remains unknown, but genetic and environmental factors are thought to play a role.[42] However, no single environmental exposure or consistent genetic defect has yet been identified.[38]

### Diagnosis:
Prenatal diagnosis with ultrasound has been suggested with the following criteria: failure to visualize the bladder in the presence of normal amniotic fluid volume, large midline infraumbilical anterior wall defect, omphalocele, cystic anterior wall structure, and/or neural tube defect.[43] In 1999, Hamada et al.[37] reported the "elephant trunk-like" image as a new criterion for the diagnosis. This sign represents the prolapse of the terminal ileum through the exstrophy, and it is the most specific sonographic sign supporting this diagnosis (Fig. 19.2-10). However, it is inconsistently found as the prolapse can be intermittent or potentially obscured by an adjacent omphalocele or umbilical cord.[44]

In the case of delayed rupture of the cloacal membrane, a protruding infraumbilical cyst will be seen outlined by the umbilical arteries.[45] Later in the pregnancy, usually it breaks down, and by the time of delivery, a classic cloacal exstrophy is observed.

When a classic elephant trunk-like sign is not seen, fetal MRI will be able to define the infraumbilical anterior wall defect with or without associated omphalocele. It will provide improved renal and spine assessment, and helps confirm a primitive hindgut with imperforate anus in the absence of meconium signal in the expected distribution of the colon and rectum.[46]

### Differential Diagnosis:
In the absence of an elephant trunk-like sign, a prenatal diagnosis with ultrasound can be challenging, and several cases have been misdiagnosed as omphalocele, gastroschisis, or sacrococcygeal teratoma.[43,47] In other cases, a differential diagnosis with bladder exstrophy is considered.[48] The first clues for the correct diagnosis would be the absence of the bladder despite normal amniotic fluid and a protuberant anterior pelvic contour with or without associated omphalocele. In that situation, cloacal or bladder exstrophy should be considered, and fetal MRI performed after 21 weeks, when meconium is expected to fill the rectum, could provide a definitive diagnosis.

### Prognosis:
With modern surgical and medical treatment and in the absence of other severe malformations, the long-term survival rate is 83% to 100%. However, the challenge remains in how to improve the quality of life of these children, and in order to optimize functional results, it is paramount that a correct unified surgical management plan be instituted from birth.[49] Lifelong colostomy could be necessary, but pull-through procedures of the distal colon to the perineum might be successful together with the use of daily enemas. The majority of the patients achieve urinary continence with modern surgical reconstructive techniques, but most of them require intermittent bladder catheterization. Renal function has also a great impact on long-term outcome. Sexual function might be impaired, and reproduction is unlikely.[40]

### Management:
Once a confident diagnosis is established, parental counseling with a multidisciplinary team, including colorectal surgeons, pediatric urologists, pediatric neurosurgeons, and neonatologists, must be provided. After thorough patient education and counseling, parents can make an informed decision about available options. If parents choose postnatal treatment, referral to centers with experience in treating cloacal exstrophy is recommended.[40,42]

### Recurrence Risk:
The vast majority of cases are sporadic without a recognized associated chromosomal abnormality. There is, however, a higher reported incidence of cloacal exstrophy in monozygotic twins and in families in which one member is affected.[50]

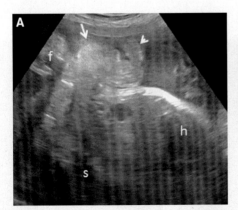
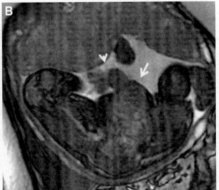
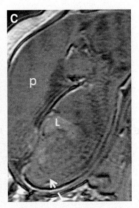

**FIGURE 19.2-10:** US and fetal MRI at 33 weeks of gestation. **A:** Sagittal oblique US image shows a protruding "mass" *(arrow)* in the infraumbilical abdominal wall with a tubular extension *(arrowhead)* representing the "elephant trunk-like" image. Spine *(s)*, femur *(f)*, and heart *(h)* are labeled. **B:** Axial 2D FIESTA. There is absent bladder despite normal amniotic fluid volume and protruding anterior pelvic contour *(arrow)* with a tubular extension *(arrowhead)*, the prolapsed terminal ileum. **C:** Sagittal midline T1-weighted MRI shows lack of bright meconium signal in the rectum *(dashed arrow)*. Liver *(L)* and placenta *(p)* are labeled.

# BLADDER EXSTROPHY

Bladder exstrophy is characterized by a defect involving the infraumbilical abdominal wall and anterior wall of the urinary bladder. As a result, the open bladder mucosa becomes exposed and everted through the wall defect (Fig. 19.2-11). The umbilical cord is low set and the pubic symphysis is always widened. In males, there is complete epispadias with the urethral plate open to the tip of the phallus, resulting in a short, wide, anteriorly displaced penis. In females, there is an open urethral plate, a bifid clitoris, and wide separation of the labia.[42,51] In the most severe form, it may be accompanied by omphalocele, inguinal hernia, undescended testis, ventrally located anal orifice, relaxed anal sphincter, and intermittent rectal prolapse.[52] Imperforate anus, spine defects, and spina bifida, more typical in cloacal exstrophy, have been found only in a low number of cases.[39]

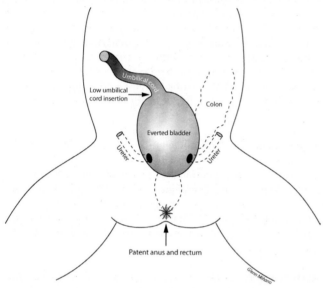

**FIGURE 19.2-11:** Diagram of typical anatomical appearance of bladder exstrophy. The everted and opened bladder is exposed through an infraumbilical wall defect. There is a patent anus with normal rectum. (Reproduced with permission from Calvo-Garcia MA, Kline-Fath BM, Rubio EI, et al. Fetal MRI of cloacal exstrophy. *Pediatr Radiol.* 2013;43:593–604.)

**Incidence:** It occurs in 1 per 30,000 live births and is more common in males, with a 2:1 male-to-female ratio.[42]

**Embryology:** Bladder exstrophy represents a slightly later abnormality in embryogenesis than does cloacal exstrophy. Both processes start in the 4th week of gestation because of failure of mesenchymal cells to migrate between the ectoderm of the abdominal wall and the endoderm of the cloacal membrane. As a result, the cloacal membrane ruptures prematurely. If the defect occurs after the urorectal septation of the cloaca, it will result in bladder exstrophy.

**Etiology:** The etiology remains unclear, but is thought to represent a multifactorial disorder in which environmental and genetic factors are likely to play a role.[53]

**Diagnosis:** Usual sonographic findings include persistent nonvisualization of the fetal bladder despite a normal amniotic fluid volume with a lower abdominal bulge, low umbilical insertion, small penis with anteriorly displaced scrotum, and widening of the iliac crests (Fig. 19.2-12).[51] Color Doppler can help identify the umbilical arteries running alongside the bulging mass, also noted in the case of cloacal exstrophy and linking the bulging mass with the bladder.[47,54] Three-dimensional (3D) ultrasound has also been reported to help in the diagnosis of bladder and cloacal exstrophy.[55]

Similar findings will be noted with fetal MRI.[56] In addition, normal appearance of the rectum and colon will allow a more definitive diagnosis, excluding cloacal exstrophy, especially in cases where omphalocele or other malformations are noted.

**Differential Diagnosis:** The main differential diagnosis is cloacal exstrophy. The absence of associated malformations such as omphalocele or spinal defects would make cloacal exstrophy less likely. However, bladder exstrophy has been reported in a low number of cases with those same associated defects, and cases of cloacal exstrophy might not show obvious spinal defects. Fetal MRI will be able to differentiate between the two in those situations.

Other abdominal wall defects, such as omphalocele and gastroschisis, need to be considered, but they are easily differentiated, and there should be a normally filled bladder.

**FIGURE 19.2-12:** Bladder exstrophy. **A:** Axial US image at 24 weeks of gestation shows a protruding anterior pelvic wall "mass" *(arrowheads)* and lack of visualization of fluid-filled bladder in the presence of normal amniotic fluid volume. The spine *(SP)* and thighs *(white asterisks)* are denoted for orientation. Umbilical cord *(UC)*. **B:** Postnatal frontal abdomen x-ray on the first day of life. Note also the pubic symphysis diastasis *(black asterisks)*.

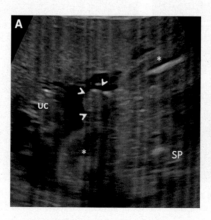
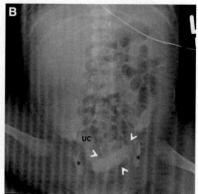

**Prognosis:** The prognosis for bladder exstrophy has improved quite significantly in recent years, and the overall outcome is relatively good with expected urinary continence and normal sexual function in many patients.[57]

**Management:** Prenatal diagnosis will allow appropriate parental counseling,[57] as well as optimal perinatal management and prompt postnatal surgical intervention. Early intervention, in the first 48 hours of life, minimizes damage to the exposed bladder and permits early closure and possibly avoids the need for pelvic osteotomy.[51]

**Recurrence Risk:** The recurrence risk for offspring of affected individuals is 1 in 70. Among siblings, the estimated recurrence risk has been reported to be between 0.3% and 1%.[58–60]

## PATENT URACHUS

The urachus is a vestigial remnant of the allantois, extending from the anterosuperior aspect of the bladder toward the umbilicus. Complete or partial persistence of its lumen gives rise to urachal disorders. The anomalies of the urachus are classified according to the persisting patent segment and include congenital patent urachus, urachal cyst, umbilico-urachal sinus, and vesico-urachal diverticulum (Fig. 19.2-13).[61]

**Incidence:** Urachal anomalies are uncommon, with a male-to-female ratio of 2 to 1.[62] Patent urachus accounts for about 50% of all cases, urachal cyst 30%, umbilical-urachal sinus about 15%, and vesico-urachal diverticulum 3% to 5%.[63]

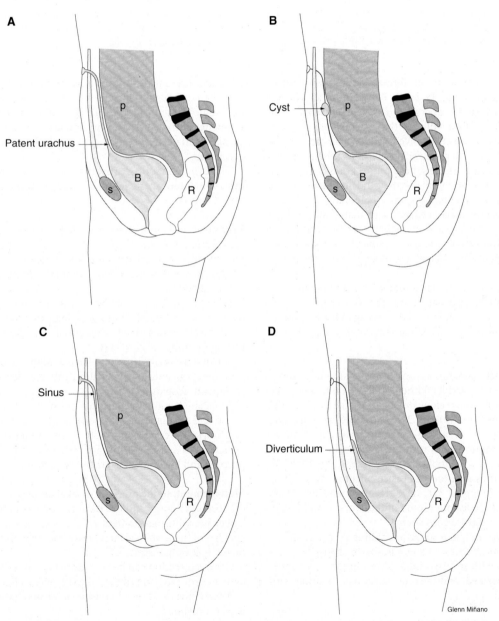

Glenn Miñano

**FIGURE 19.2-13:** Types of congenital urachal anomalies. **A:** Patent urachus. **B:** Urachal cyst. **C:** Urachal sinus. **D:** Urachal diverticulum. B, bladder; p, peritoneal cavity; r, rectum; s, symphysis pubis.

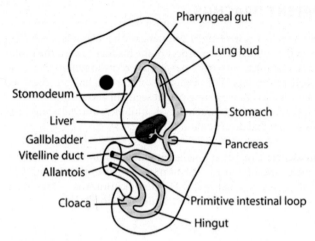

**FIGURE 19.2-14:** Embryo with primitive umbilical cord. (Reproduced with permission from Bunch PT, Kline-Fath BM, Imhoff SC, et al. Allantoic cyst: a prenatal clue to patent urachus. *Pediatr Radiol.* 2006;36:1090–1095.)

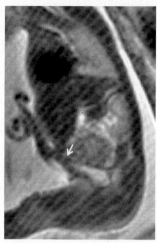

**FIGURE 19.2-15:** 25-Week-old fetus with patent urachus. T2w sagittal MR image demonstrates elongation of the bladder dome toward the abdominal cord insertion (*white arrow*).

**Embryology:** The urachus is the intraabdominal remnant of the embryonic allantois (Fig. 19.2-14). The allantois appears on approximately the 16th day of gestation as a small diverticulum from the caudal wall of the yolk sac that extends into the connecting stalk. The allantois is involved with development of the dome of the urinary bladder and the umbilical vessels, and forms a hollow tube that connects the superior aspect of the urogenital sinus with the anterior abdominal wall at the umbilicus. As the bladder enlarges, the allantois becomes obliterated to form a thick tube, the urachus, also known as the median umbilical ligament, situated in the prevesical space, between the peritoneum behind and the transversalis fascia in front. Defective closure may happen and leads to congenital pathology of the urachus.[62]

**Etiology:** The etiology of urachal anomalies is unknown. Urachal anomalies, particularly patent urachus, have been reported, in up to one-third of these cases, in the setting of bladder outlet obstruction as a "pop-off" mechanism to protect the upper urinary tract.[61]

**Diagnosis:** A patent urachus results from persistent communication between the bladder lumen and the umbilicus. The bladder dome will show elongated appearance toward the abdominal cord insertion (Fig. 19.2-15). In some cases, it could lead to the development of a true cyst at the base of the umbilical cord, which communicates with the bladder dome and will lead to separation of the umbilical cord vessels (Fig. 19.2-16). The cyst is known as allantoic, or vesico-allantoic cyst. Ultrasound with color Doppler, 3D, 4D ultrasound, and fetal MRI can characterize these lesions. Some of these cysts can be very large or progress to diffuse cord edema.[64]

Urachal cysts are noted as anterior midline cysts, cranial to the bladder without dynamic changes in size or shape.[65]

Patent urachus with in utero interval resolution of allantoic cyst has been described, and in some cases in association with subsequent bladder prolapse.[66,67]

**Differential Diagnosis:** Allantoic cysts in the setting of patent urachus will present as a cyst near the fetal anterior abdominal wall. Omphalomesenteric cysts are also true umbilical cord

cysts and present in this same location, but they do not separate the cord vessels and do not communicate with the bladder dome. Umbilical cord pseudocysts will affect more distal segments of the cord.[64] Color Doppler ultrasound will be able to differentiate from umbilical vein varix or umbilical artery aneurysm.[62,68]

The differential diagnosis of a urachal cyst includes ovarian cyst, mesenteric cyst, omphalomesenteric duct remnant, and bowel atresia.

**Prognosis:** Allantoic cysts have no increased risk for chromosomal anomaly. One-third of these cases occur in association with bladder outlet obstruction, and its presence supports a patent urachus with urine leakage from the umbilicus noted in the neonatal period.[64]

Potential umbilical cord vessel compression, umbilical cord hematoma or torsion leading to fetal distress and even fetal death has been described as potential rare complications in the setting of umbilical cord cysts.[69]

All urachal malformations have a high incidence of recurrent infection and stone formation and may develop benign and malignant neoplasms.[61,63]

Associated anomalies are uncommon but include omphalocele and omphalomesenteric remnants[64,66,70] as well as other genitourinary conditions such as hypospadias, undescended testicles, crossed renal ectopia, vesicoureteral reflux, hydronephrosis, and lower urinary tract obstruction.[61,66]

**Management:** In the presence of an allantoic cyst or any umbilical cord cyst, some authors recommend close prenatal surveillance, including assessment of the size of the cyst, Doppler analysis of the umbilical circulation and delivery as soon as fetal maturity is demonstrated.[69]

Cesarean section can be considered in cases of large allantoic cysts in order to better define the site of cord ligation.[64]

After delivery, surgical consult of all urachal malformations is recommended.[63]

**Recurrence Risk:** These conditions are sporadic with a low recurrence risk.[64]

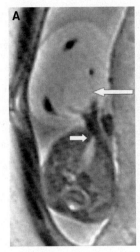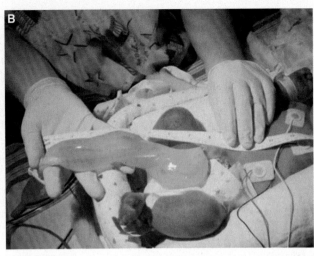

**FIGURE 19.2-16:** Patent urachus with allantoic cyst. **A:** Fetal MRI axial T2-weighted image shows elongation of the bladder dome toward the abdominal cord insertion *(short arrow)* with a cyst *(long arrow)* at the base of the cord. Note the splaying of the umbilical vessels *(dark structures)*. **B:** First day of life photograph. There is a large edematous mass in the umbilical cord. (Reproduced with permission from Bunch PT, Kline-Fath BM, Imhoff SC, et al. Allantoic cyst: a prenatal clue to patent urachus. *Pediatr Radiol.* 2006;36:1090–1095.)

# REFERENCES

1. Hendren WH. Urogenital sinus and cloacal malformations. *Semin Pediatr Surg.* 1996;5(1):72–79.
2. Jaramillo D, Lebowitz RL, Hendren WH. The cloacal malformation: radiologic findings and imaging recommendations. *Radiology.* 1990;177(2):441–448.
3. Peña A. Anorectal malformations. *Semin Pediatr Surg.* 1995;4(1):35–47.
4. Peña A, Levitt MA, Hong A, et al. Surgical management of cloacal malformations: a review of 339 patients. *J Pediatr Surg.* 2004;39(3):470–479; discussion 470–479.
5. Escobar LF, Weaver DD, Bixler D, et al. Urorectal septum malformation sequence: report of six cases and embryological analysis. *Am J Dis Child.* 1987; 141(9):1021–1024.
6. Wheeler PG, Weaver DD. Partial urorectal septum malformation sequence: a report of 25 cases. *Am J Med Genet.* 2001;103(2):99–105.
7. Stephens FD. Embryology of the cloaca and embryogenesis of anorectal malformations. *Birth Defects Orig Artic Ser.* 1988;24(4):177–209.
8. Cilento BG Jr, Benacerraf BR, Mandell J. Prenatal diagnosis of cloacal malformation. *Urology.* 1994;43(3):386–388.
9. Lubusky M, Prochazka M, Dhaifalah I, et al. Concordant partial urorectal septum malformation sequence in monozygotic twins. *Am J Med Genet A.* 2006;140(24):2828–2831.
10. Zaccara A, Gatti C, Silveri M, et al. Persistent cloaca: are we ready for a correct prenatal diagnosis? *Urology.* 1999;54(2):367.
11. Veyrac C, Couture A, Saguintaah M, et al. MRI of fetal GI tract abnormalities. *Abdom Imaging.* 2004;29(4):411–420.
12. Petrikovsky BM, Walzak MP Jr, D'Addario PF. Fetal cloacal anomalies: prenatal sonographic findings and differential diagnosis. *Obstet Gynecol.* 1988; 72(3, pt 2):464–469.
13. Warne S, Chitty LS, Wilcox DT. Prenatal diagnosis of cloacal anomalies. *BJU Int.* 2002;89(1):78–81.
14. Shono T, Taguchi T, Suita S, et al. Prenatal ultrasonographic and magnetic resonance imaging findings of congenital cloacal anomalies associated with meconium peritonitis. *J Pediatr Surg.* 2007;42(4):681–684.
15. Mandell J, Lillehei CW, Greene M, et al. The prenatal diagnosis of imperforate anus with rectourinary fistula: dilated fetal colon with enterolithiasis. *J Pediatr Surg.* 1992;27(1):82–84.
16. Chaubal N, Dighe M, Shah M, et al. Calcified meconium: an important sign in the prenatal sonographic diagnosis of cloacal malformation. *J Ultrasound Med.* 2003;22(7):727–730.
17. Saguintaah M, Couture A, Veyrac C, et al. MRI of the fetal gastrointestinal tract. *Pediatr Radiol.* 2002;32(6):395–404.
18. Brugger PC, Prayer D. Fetal abdominal magnetic resonance imaging. *Eur J Radiol.* 2006;57(2):278–293.
19. Picone O, Laperelle J, Sonigo P, et al. Fetal magnetic resonance imaging in the antenatal diagnosis and management of hydrocolpos. *Ultrasound Obstet Gynecol.* 2007;30(1):105–109.
20. Dhombres F, Jouannic J-M, Brodaty G, et al. Contribution of prenatal imaging to the anatomical assessment of fetal hydrocolpos. *Ultrasound Obstet Gynecol.* 2007;30(1):101–104.
21. Calvo-Garcia MA, Kline-Fath BM, Levitt MA, et al. Fetal MRI clues to diagnose cloacal malformations. *Pediatr Radiol.* 2011;41(9):1117–1128.
22. Levitt MA, Pena A. Anorectal malformations. *Orphanet J Rare Dis.* 2007;2:33.
23. Biard JM, Johnson MP, Carr MC, et al. Long-term outcomes in children treated by prenatal vesicoamniotic shunting for lower urinary tract obstruction. *Obstet Gynecol.* 2005;106(3):503–508.
24. Lissauer D, Morris RK, Kilby MD. Fetal lower urinary tract obstruction. *Semin Fetal Neonatal Med.* 2007;12(6):464–470.
25. Levitt MA, Pena A. Pitfalls in the management of newborn cloacas. *Pediatr Surg Int.* 2005;21(4):264–269.
26. Jenak R, Ludwikowski B, Gonzalez R. Total urogenital sinus mobilization: a modified perineal approach for feminizing genitoplasty and urogenital sinus repair. *J Urol.* 2001;165(6, pt 2):2347–2349.
27. Taori K, Krishnan V, Sharbidre KG, et al. Prenatal sonographic diagnosis of fetal persistent urogenital sinus with congenital hydrocolpos. *Ultrasound Obstet Gynecol.* 2010;36(5):641–643.
28. Pauleta J, Melo MA, Borges G, et al. Prenatal diagnosis of persistent urogenital sinus with duplicated hydrometrocolpos and ascites—a case report. *Fetal Diagn Ther.* 2010;28(4):229–232.
29. Chambrier ED, Heinrichs C, Avni FE. Sonographic appearance of congenital adrenal hyperplasia in utero. *J Ultrasound Med.* 2002;21(1):97–100.
30. Subramanian S, Sharma R, Gamanagatti S, et al. Antenatal MR diagnosis of urinary hydrometrocolpos due to urogenital sinus. *Pediatr Radiol.* 2006;36(10):1086–1089.
31. Farkas A, Chertin B. Feminizing genitoplasty in patients with 46XX congenital adrenal hyperplasia. *J Pediatr Endocrinol Metab.* 2001;14(6):713–722.
32. Puhl AG, Steiner E, Krämer WW, et al. Fetal urogenital sinus with consecutive hydrometrocolpos because of labial fusion: prenatal diagnostic difficulties and postpartal therapeutic management. *Fetal Diagn Ther.* 2008;23(4):287–292.
33. Hahn-Pedersen J, Kvist N, Nielsen OH. Hydrometrocolpos: current views on pathogenesis and management. *J Urol.* 1984;132(3):537–540.
34. Parlakgumus A, Yalcinkaya C, Kilicdag E. Prenatal diagnosis of McKusick-Kaufman/Bardet-Biedl syndrome. *BMJ Case Rep.* 2011. doi:10.1136/bcr.02.2011.3808.
35. Carey JC. Exstrophy of the cloaca and the OEIS complex: one and the same. *Am J Med Genet.* 2001;99(4):270.
36. Carey JC, Greenbaum B, Hall BD. The OEIS complex (omphalocele, exstrophy, imperforate anus, spinal defects). *Birth Defects Orig Artic Ser.* 1978;14(6B):253–263.
37. Hamada H, Takano K, Shiina H, et al. New ultrasonographic criterion for the prenatal diagnosis of cloacal exstrophy: elephant trunk-like image. *J Urol.* 1999;162(6):2123–2124.
38. Boyadjiev SA, Dodson JL, Radford CL, et al. Clinical and molecular characterization of the bladder exstrophy-epispadias complex: analysis of 232 families. *BJU Int.* 2004;94(9):1337–1343.
39. Martinez-Frias ML, Bermejo E, Rodríguez-Pinilla E, et al. Exstrophy of the cloaca and exstrophy of the bladder: two different expressions of a primary developmental field defect. *Am J Med Genet.* 2001;99(4):261–269.
40. Tiblad E, Wilson RD, Carr M, et al. OEIS sequence—a rare congenital anomaly with prenatal evaluation and postnatal outcome in six cases. *Prenat Diagn.* 2008;28(2):141–147.

41. Purves JT, Gearhart JP. The bladder exstrophy-epispadia-cloacal exstrophy complex. In: Gearhart JP, Rink RC, Mouriquand P, eds. *Pediatric Urology.* Philadelphia, PA: WB Saunders; 2010:410–415.

42. Ebert AK, Reutter H, Ludwig M, et al. The exstrophy-epispadias complex. *Orphanet J Rare Dis.* 2009;4:23.

43. Austin PF, Homsy YL, Gearhart JP, et al. The prenatal diagnosis of cloacal exstrophy. *J Urol.* 1998;160(3, pt 2):1179–1181.

44. Richards DS, Langham MR Jr, Mahaffey SM. The prenatal ultrasonographic diagnosis of cloacal exstrophy. *J Ultrasound Med.* 1992;11(9):507–510.

45. Langer JC, Brennan B, Lappalainen RE, et al. Cloacal exstrophy: prenatal diagnosis before rupture of the cloacal membrane. *J Pediatr Surg.* 1992; 27(10):1352–1355.

46. Calvo-Garcia MA, Kline-Fath BM, Rubio EI, et al. Fetal MRI of cloacal exstrophy. *Pediatr Radiol.* 2013;43:593–604.

47. Wu JL, Fang KH, Yeh GP, et al. Using color Doppler sonography to identify the perivesical umbilical arteries: a useful method in the prenatal diagnosis of omphalocele-exstrophy-imperforate anus-spinal defects complex. *J Ultrasound Med.* 2004;23(9):1211–1215.

48. Gobbi D, Fascetti Leon F, Tregnaghi A, et al. Early prenatal diagnosis of cloacal exstrophy with fetal magnetic resonance imaging. *Fetal Diagn Ther.* 2008;24(4):437–439.

49. Soffer SZ, Rosen NG, Hong AR, et al. Cloacal exstrophy: a unified management plan. *J Pediatr Surg.* 2000;35(6):932–937.

50. Siebert JR, Rutledge JC, Kapur RP. Association of cloacal anomalies, caudal duplication, and twinning. *Pediatr Dev Pathol.* 2005;8(3):339–354.

51. Gearhart JP, Ben-Chaim J, Jeffs RD, et al. Criteria for the prenatal diagnosis of classic bladder exstrophy. *Obstet Gynecol.* 1995;85(6):961–964.

52. Pinette MG, Pan YQ, Pinette SG, et al. Prenatal diagnosis of fetal bladder and cloacal exstrophy by ultrasound: a report of three cases. *J Reprod Med.* 1996;41(2):132–134.

53. Reutter H, Qi L, Gearhart JP, et al. Concordance analyses of twins with bladder exstrophy-epispadias complex suggest genetic etiology. *Am J Med Genet A.* 2007;143A(22):2751–2756.

54. Lee EH, Shim JY. New sonographic finding for the prenatal diagnosis of bladder exstrophy: a case report. *Ultrasound Obstet Gynecol.* 2003;21(5):498–500.

55. Evangelidis A, Murphy JP, Gatti JM. Prenatal diagnosis of bladder exstrophy by 3-dimensional ultrasound. *J Urol.* 2004;172(3):1111.

56. Hsieh K, O'Loughlin MT, Ferrer FA. Bladder exstrophy and phenotypic gender determination on fetal magnetic resonance imaging. *Urology.* 2005; 65(5):998–999.

57. Cacciari A, Pilu GL, Mordenti M, et al. Prenatal diagnosis of bladder exstrophy: what counseling? *J Urol.* 1999;161(1):259–261; discussion 262.

58. Shapiro E, Lepor H, Jeffs RD. The inheritance of the exstrophy-epispadias complex. *J Urol.* 1984;132(2):308–310.

59. Messelink EJ, Aronson DC, Knuist M, et al. Four cases of bladder exstrophy in two families. *J Med Genet.* 1994;31(6):490–492.

60. Reutter H, Shapiro E, Gruen JR. Seven new cases of familial isolated bladder exstrophy and epispadias complex (BEEC) and review of the literature. *Am J Med Genet A.* 2003;120A(2):215–221.

61. Cilento BG Jr, Bauer SB, Retik AB, et al. Urachal anomalies: defining the best diagnostic modality. *Urology.* 1998;52(1):120–122.

62. Sepulveda W, Bower S, Dhillon HK, et al. Prenatal diagnosis of congenital patent urachus and allantoic cyst: the value of color flow imaging. *J Ultrasound Med.* 1995;14(1):47–51.

63. Yu JS, Kim KW, Lee HJ, et al. Urachal remnant diseases: spectrum of CT and US findings. *Radiographics.* 2001;21(2):451–461.

64. Bunch PT, Kline-Fath BM, Imhoff SC, et al. Allantoic cyst: a prenatal clue to patent urachus. *Pediatr Radiol.* 2006;36(10):1090–1095.

65. Goldstein I, Shalev E, Nisman D. The dilemma of prenatal diagnosis of bladder exstrophy: a case report and a review of the literature. *Ultrasound Obstet Gynecol.* 2001;17(4):357–359.

66. Matsui F, Matsumoto F, Shimada K. Prenatally diagnosed patent urachus with bladder prolapse. *J Pediatr Surg.* 2007;42(12):e7–e10.

67. Sepulveda W, Rompel SM, Cafici D, et al. Megacystis associated with an umbilical cord cyst: a sonographic feature of a patent urachus in the first trimester. *J Ultrasound Med.* 2010;29(2):295–300.

68. Sepulveda W. Beware of the umbilical cord "cyst." *Ultrasound Obstet Gynecol.* 2003;21(3):213–214.

69. Sepulveda W, Wong AE, Gonzalez R, et al. Fetal death due to umbilical cord hematoma: a rare complication of umbilical cord cyst. *J Matern Fetal Neonatal Med.* 2005;18(6):387–390.

70. Kita M, Kikuchi A, Miyashita S, et al. Umbilical cord cysts of allantoic and omphalomesenteric remnants with progressive umbilical cord edema: a case report. *Fetal Diagn Ther.* 2009;25(2):250–254.

## 19.3 Fetal Gender and Ambiguous Genitalia

### Christopher Cassady

Genetic, or chromosomal, sex is determined at conception by the absence or presence of a Y chromosome. The complex process of sexual differentiation then unfolds with the expression of a gonadal (or internal) sex, and a phenotypic (or external, anatomic) sex. When these three facets of sex expression are inconsistent, there is sexual ambiguity, or what is now preferentially termed a *disorder of sex development (DSD)*.

## INCIDENCE

Nearly all of the time, an XY genotype results in a baby with a typical male phenotype of penis and scrotum with median raphe, testes, vas deferens, and a prostate gland; likewise, an XX genotype has labia majora and minora, a clitoris, and a uterus with fallopian tubes and ovaries. However, approximately 1/5,000 liveborn infants has a disorder of sexual development in which the genotype and classic phenotype are not consistently aligned.[1,2] This may occur for any number of complex reasons, including both in isolated instances and with other manifestations of syndromic or chromosomal anomalies (Table 19.3-1).

| **Table 19.3-1** | **Conditions Associated with Nonisolated Ambiguous Genitalia** |
|---|---|

Chromosomal abnormalities
   Trisomies 13 and 18
   Triploidy
   Abnormal sex chromosome complements
   del(4)(p16.3)
   del(11)(q23.3)
   del(13)(q33.2)
Single-gene disorder syndromes
   Aarskog (X-linked)
   ATRX (X-linked)
   Carpenter (AR)
   Cornelia de Lange (AD)
   Fraser (AR)
   Frasier (AD)
   Fryns (AR)
   McKusick–Kaufman (AR)
   Noonan (AD)
   Robinow (AR and AD)
   Russell–Silver (AR and AD)
   Smith–Lemli–Opitz (AR)
Imprinting disorders
   Prader–Willi
Associations
   CHARGE (AD)
   EEC (epispadius, exstrophy, OEIS)
   MURCS (Mullerian duct, renal and cervicothoracic somite a/dysplasia)

Adapted from Chitayat D, Glanc P. Diagnostic approach in prenatally detected genital abnormalities. *Ultrasound Obstet Gynecol.* 2010;35:637–646.

## EMBRYOLOGY

While it is true that without the protein encoded by the sex-determining region Y (SRY) gene on the short arm of the Y chromosome there can be no male gonadal or phenotypic sexual expression, it would be incorrect to believe that the absence of SRY alone produces a normal female; genes on the X and other chromosomes, including WNT4 on chromosome 1, are necessary for ovarian development.[3] Internal differentiation begins in the 4th gestational week with the migration of primitive germ cells from the yolk sac to form genital ridges medial to both the lateral paramesonephric (Mullerian) ducts and the mesonephric (Wolffian) ducts that will end caudally in the cloaca. In week 8, gonadal differentiation is thought to begin in the fetus. The SRY protein differentiates Sertoli cells in the testes to secrete Mullerian inhibitory factor or substance (also called anti-Mullerian hormone, AMH), inducing degeneration of paramesonephric ducts. The gonadal ridges form testes, and the mesonephric ducts form the rete testis, efferent ducts, and vas deferens under the influence of testosterone secreted by testicular Leydig cells beginning in week 9. Over weeks 9 to 20 in the female, the gonad becomes the ovary, and, under the influence of ovarian follicular estrogen, the paramesonephric ducts form the fallopian tubes, uterus, and upper vagina; the mesonephric duct regresses because of a lack of MIF and testosterone. Ovarian follicles appear after week 14.

Externally, fetuses are identical early. In week 5, cloacal folds form on either side of the cloacal membrane, then join to make a genital tubercle and the urogenital (UG) folds on each side of the UG membrane that has been subdivided separate from the anal orifice out of the cloacal membrane in week 7. Two additional labioscrotal folds form alongside the UG folds. After 7 (generally by 9 to 12) weeks, in a female phenotype, the genital tubercle becomes the clitoris and the UG sinus becomes the lower vagina and the urethra. The UG folds make the labia minora, and the labioscrotal folds make the labia majora. For a male phenotype, the genital tubercle becomes the penis and the UG folds the penile urethra, while the UG sinus becomes the proximal urethra and the prostate. The labioscrotal folds form the scrotum.[3–5] Initially, the phallus created by the genital tubercles is identical in length in both males and females, and it is not until 11 weeks that the external genitalia begin to become more distinct.[6]

Testicular descent begins from a gonadal position in the abdomen and continues to the inguinal canals and then to the scrotum. Between 10 and 23 weeks, nearly 10% of testes have migrated from the abdomen and are situated in the inguinal canal. At 24 to 26 weeks, 58% have migrated from the abdomen and descent of the testes from the inguinal canal to the scrotum begins. By 29 weeks, less than 20% have not descended to the scrotum, and by 32 weeks, 90% to 95% of testes are intrascrotal.[7,8]

## PATHOGENESIS

When there is a disruption in the coordination among all the processes involved from genotypic sex establishment through phenotypic expression, a disorder of sex development occurs. DSDs have been categorized by the International Intersex Consensus Conference, which in 2006 published a revised nomenclature incorporating genetic assignment and description, and removing

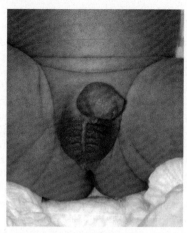

**FIGURE 19.3-1:** Congenital adrenal hyperplasia. Newborn with XX genotype and male phenotype.

reference to gender.[9] Classification systems vary because some diagnoses overlap categories but, in general, pathologies can be assigned to one of six groups,[10] as described below.

## 46, XX Disorder of Sex Development (Female Pseudohermaphroditism)

This is the most common DSD. Ovaries and Mullerian structures are normal, but external genitalia are masculinized secondary to androgen exposure. Though the exposure could be exogenous, the most common cause is congenital adrenal hyperplasia (CAH), a collection of autosomal recessive disorders from five genes that code for enzymes involved in cortisol synthesis. CAH can affect either genetic sex, but only when there is masculinization of a genetic female is it considered a cause of 46, XX DSD. Depending on the enzyme deficiency, there may be an overproduction of adrenal androgens (masculinized female genitalia, normal male genitalia) or a lack of gonadal steroid production (normal female genitalia, and undermasculinized male genitalia) (Fig. 19.3-1).

## 46, XY Disorder of Sex Development (Male Pseudohermaphroditism)

Testes are at least initially present, but internal or external genitalia are not at all or incompletely masculinized. There are eight categories, and these are generally assigned after birth (Table 19.3-2).

| Table 19.3-2 | Etiology of Male Pseudohermaphroditism |
| --- | --- |

Leydig cell failure
Testosterone biosynthesis enzyme defects
Androgen insensitivity syndrome (testicular feminization syndrome), complete or partial
5 Alpha reductase deficiency
Persistent Mullerian duct syndrome
Congenital anorchia (vanishing testes syndrome)
Exogenous progesterone exposure
Smith-Lemli-Opitz syndrome

## Ovotesticular Disorder of Sex Development (True Hermaphroditism)

Both testicular and ovarian tissues are present. There are three types: lateral, with a testis on one side and ovary on the other (typically left); bilateral ovotestis; or ovotesis on one side and either testis or ovary on the other, which is most common. External genitalia are ambiguous: there may be hypospadius, cryptorchidism, and incomplete labioscrotal fold fusion. Internal genitalia generally follow the gonad per side.

## Gonadal Dysgenesis

There is ambiguous development of internal genitalia, the genitourinary sinus, and external genitalia with dysgenetic gonads from lack of development or loss of primordial germ cells. Phenotypic variability occurs from mixed or partial to pure gonadal dysgenesis, a term that describes conditions with normal sets of sex chromosomes (e.g., 46, XX or 46, XY) but with no gonads, for example, Swyer syndrome (46, XY with female external genitalia because of a lack of testicular development), and Perrault syndrome (46, XX without ovaries). Partial GD has a streak gonad on one side and a typically dysgenetic testis on the other; these patients are at risk for development of gonadal tumors, including dysgerminoma.[11] This category includes patients with Denys-Drash syndrome, WAGR and Frasier syndrome, each of which can express "sex reversal", in which the phenotypic sex appears normal but is discordant with the chromosomal sex (Table 19.3-3).

## Sex Chromosome Disorder of Sex Development

There is an abnormal number or complement of sex chromosomes. Examples include Klinefelter syndrome (XXY/XXXY), Triple X (47XXX), or Turner Syndrome (45XO or 45XO/46XX). This would include individuals with four or more sex chromosomes. These will not be diagnosed in utero other than by karyotype as there is typically no genital abnormality appreciated.

| Table 19.3-3 | Sex Reversal ("Chromosome–Phenotype Discordance") |
| --- | --- |

Campomelic dysplasia
Gonadal dysgenesis DSD
  Swyer syndrome (XY female)
  WT1 gene alterations (chromosome 11)
    WAGR (Wilm tumor, aniridia, genitourinary abnormalities, mental retardation)
    Frasier syndrome
    Denys–Drash syndrome
Sex chromosome DSD
  Mosaicism (e.g. 45XO/46XY)
46, XX DSD
  Congenital adrenal hyperplasia
46, XY DSD
  Complete androgen insensitivity syndrome (testicular feminization syndrome)
46, XX testicular DSD
  De la Chappelle syndrome
Smith–Lemli–Opitz syndrome

## 46, XX Testicular/Ovotesticular Disorder of Sex Development

The genotype is 46, XX with male external genitalia. Nearly all (80% to 90%) are from anomalous Y-X translocation involving the SRY gene in meiosis; the greater the amount of Y DNA, the more virilized the phenotype. Therefore, there is wide variability in appearance, including what looks like "sex reversal" (de la Chappelle syndrome, or XX male syndrome). Differentiation between testicular and ovotesticular varieties is made by histology. These are mostly SRY +, in comparison with 46, XX DSD (female pseudohermaphroditism), which is SRY −; note, however, that the phenotypes overlap.

## IMAGING

Although parental curiosity often drives the initial imaging investigation of fetal gender, there are medical reasons for understanding gender assignment, as with fetuses at risk for x-linked and gender-specific conditions. It can be important in the determination of zygosity in multiple gestations. Additionally, abnormal genitalia may be among the clues to a potentially antenatally diagnosable syndrome or chromosomal defect.[7]

Given the embryology, it is unsurprising that distinguishing male from female external genitalia is not reliably possible before 12 weeks. However, using the "sagittal sign" and transabdominal scanning, many report extremely high levels of accuracy from 12 weeks onwards in fetal gender assignment. Male gender is assigned if the angle of the phallus at the genital tubercle is >30° from parallel to the fetal lumbosacral skin, and female if the angle is <10°. Angles between 10° and 30° are labelled "indeterminate," and this small number of fetuses (3-4%) is scanned again at later gestational ages[12,13] (Figs. 19.3-2 and 19.3-3). It has been suggested that the ultrasonographer also verify a male phenotype by recognizing the "dome sign," which is the rounded scrotum and its midline echogenic median raphe, both at the penile base, as differentiated from the parallel and separate echogenic lines of the labia in a female phenotype.[14,15] Knowing that there is a normally larger anogenital distance in males starting at 12 weeks' gestation also can prove to be useful in certain cases.[16]

From the early second trimester on both ultrasound (US) and MRI, female external genitalia in the axial plane can be seen as a series of parallel lines and three to five protruberances, with

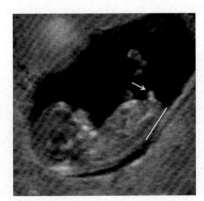

**FIGURE 19.3-2:** Male fetus first trimester. Sagittal US demonstrating the oblique angulation of the phallus *(arrow)* from a line parallel to the lumbosacral skin.

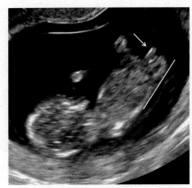

**FIGURE 19.3-3:** Female fetus first trimester. Sagittal US demonstrates the parallel configuration of the phallus *(arrow)* with the lumbosacral line.

the labia majora on the periphery, and the clitoris ± the labia minora more centrally[17] (Fig. 19.3-4). Data on normal bilabial diameter are available for both US and MRI.[18,19] In males, the scrotum has a midline raphe, and the penis is tapered distally because of the foreskin; aposthia, or foreskin aplasia, is exceedingly uncommon.[20] Testicular descent is first observed on MRI at 25 + 4 weeks. Starting at 27 weeks, approximately 50% of testicles are bilaterally descended; at 28 weeks, about two-thirds are intrascrotal; and from 30 weeks <5% are nondescended. The testes do not necessarily descend simultaneously. Testes are hypointense on T2-weighted imaging[21] (Fig. 19.3-5). In US studies, bilateral testicular descent has been documented in 97% of males by 32 weeks.[22]

General consensus would suggest that surface-rendered 3D US does not provide an advantage over two dimensional US in the routine assignment of fetal gender, and, while occasionally useful, is potentially misleading in cases of sexual ambiguity.[1,23–26] There is potential for using virtual reality techniques to effect.[27]

Because a gender assignment may need to rely on more than an assessment of the external genitalia, pelvic content evaluation can be important. Measurements of the distance between the bladder and the rectum are useful to distinguish the presence of a uterus between them. Males lie below the line determined by *distance (mm) = (0.26 × weeks' GA) − 2.17*, and 99% of females lie above.[28] A convex uterine impression on the dorsum of the bladder may also be detectable. Using 3D Volume Contrast Imaging (VCI), approximately 85% of fetal uteri may be confirmed after 20 weeks, increasing to nearly 100% after 32 weeks' gestational age (GA).[29]

Occasionally, findings other than those associated with ambiguous genitalia can affect the fetal genital system, and this pertains in particular to the scrotum. A small amount of simple fluid (hydrocele) is often seen and is normal (see Fig. 19.3-5). Complex fluid, or debris, is characteristic of contamination that has flowed through the patent processus vaginalis into the scrotum from the peritoneal space, and meconium peritonitis from a gastrointestinal tract perforation, or blood product, should be considered first.[30–32] Solid-appearing masses other than the testis in the scrotum are extremely rare prenatally; inguinal hernia has been reported.[33] Also, testes can undergo in utero torsion and enlarge the scrotum, just as ovarian torsion can present as a fetal abdominal mass. Color or pulsed wave Doppler is very useful in this circumstance to show a lack of internal vascularity to the mass.[34–36] The prostatic utricle can persist in the midline just caudal to the bladder as a Mullerian derivative in a male fetus,

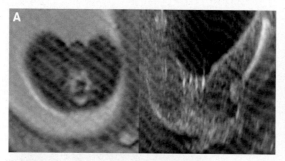
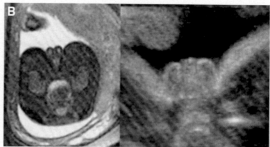

**FIGURE 19.3-4:** Female fetus. T2W MRI **(left)** and US images in axial plane at 20 weeks, **(A)** and 32 weeks, **(B)** GA. Note the parallel lines on ultrasound representing the interfaces between labia and clitoris. It is neither unusual nor abnormal to see a small amount of high signal in the labia on MRI.

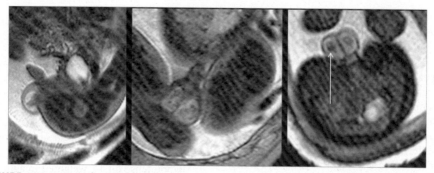

**FIGURE 19.3-5:** Male fetus. Sagittal, coronal, and axial T2W MRIs of the male external genitalia. Testes *(arrow)* are intermediate to low signal and typically surrounded by a small volume of high-signal fluid. The median raphe is equal to or of lesser thickness than the scrotal wall. The normal penis is tapered and central.

and is typically incidental, though may be secondary to bladder outlet obstruction, as with posterior urethral valves (Fig. 19.3-6).

## DIFFERENTIAL DIAGNOSIS

When the external genitalia do not appear as expected, further investigation is initiated. The anatomy should be characterized as precisely as the imaging allows:

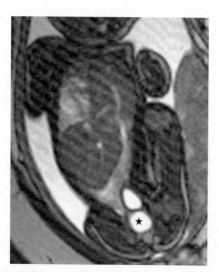

**FIGURE 19.3-6:** Prostatic utricle. Coronal T2W MRI in a patient with left congenital diaphragmatic hernia and an incidental cyst *(star)* in the midline caudal to the bladder.

- *Aphallia*—A failure of the fetal genital tubercle to form. The urethra opens directly onto the perineum.[37]
- *Micropenis*—A stretched penile length of <2 cm in a term neonate. There are penile length charts for the fetus on both US and MRI, although norms vary among investigators[38–41] (Fig. 19.3-7).
- *Hypospadius*—The penis is short and broad, and the urination stream (with color Doppler) is directed caudally and comes not from the penile tip but from the midshaft or base.
- *Chordee*—Atresia of the corpus spongiosum distal to the abnormally placed urethral meatus in hypospadius, causing an angulation to the penis (Fig. 19.3-8).
- *Penoscrotal transposition*—A ventrally bent penis between scrotal folds owing to severe hypospadius and a bifid (or

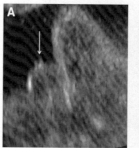
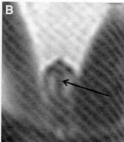

**FIGURE 19.3-7:** Micropenis. Axial US **(A)** and T2W MRI **(B)** in this XY fetus demonstrate both a micropenis *(white arrow)* and a thickened median raphe *(black arrow)*.

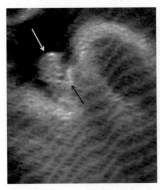
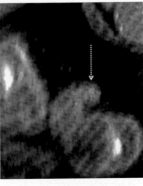

**FIGURE 19.3-8:** Hypospadius on axial US. On the left, the penile tip is clubbed and rounded *(white arrow)*, and there is a bifid *(shawl)* scrotum *(black arrow)*. The *dotted arrow* on the right indicates the lateral angulation of the penis that results from the chordee often associated with hypospadius.

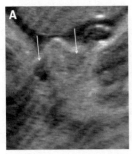
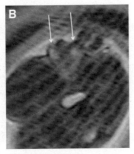

**FIGURE 19.3-9:** Penoscrotal hypospadias—the "tulip sign." The shortened penis is interposed between the hemiscrota *(arrows)*, resembling a flower in axial ultrasound **(A)** and MRI **(B)**.

shawl) scrotum. On imaging, this has been dubbed the "tulip sign"[42] (Fig. 19.3-9).

- *Epispadius*—The meatal orifice is on the dorsal side of the penis. In severe cases, the penis is split; this condition is associated with bladder or cloacal (OEIS) exstrophy.
- *Concealed penis*—A syndrome consisting of a paucity of penile shaft skin and a short penile shaft, not associated typically with a DSD.[43]
- *Clitoromegaly*—A clitoris 5 mm or more beyond the labia majora. Serial US is generally indicated, as clitoromegaly may resolve over time; however, it would be prudent to examine the fetal adrenal glands for enlargement and/or a cerebriform configuration if considering CAH.[44] Should there be fused labia, the imaging can be indistinguishable from an early stage or hypospadic male. Several sonographic examinations and karyotyping may be needed to assign gender correctly.
- *Split labia and clitoris, or scrotum and penis* (in conjunction with lack of a normal bladder)—cloacal or bladder exstrophy[45] (Fig. 19.3-10).

In terms of the revised DSD classifications,[46] *46 XX DSD* is not very accurately recognized prenatally. Clitoromegaly is the sign, but as a single finding overestimates an abnormality, resulting in false positives. Vulvar or vaginal abnormalities may be more specific. *46 XY DSD* is the most reliably identified by an experienced ultrasonographer, and the imaging findings include hypospadius with chordee and scrotal anomaly ± cryptorchidism.[46] However, none of the imaging findings is diagnostic of a particular category of DSD, and each case needs a complete

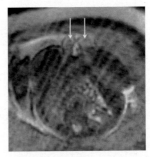

**FIGURE 19.3-10:** XY fetus with cloacal exstrophy. Axial T2W MRI at the expected level of the scrotum showing complete division of the hemiscrota containing the testes *(arrows)*. (Courtesy of Maria Calvo-Garcia, MD, Cincinnati Children's Hospital, Cincinnati, OH.)

evaluation to arrive at an appropriate diagnosis. Even then, it will not be possible to determine many etiologies prenatally since only about half of children ultimately diagnosed with 46, XY DSD, for example, will reach a definitive clinical diagnosis.[47] A specific molecular diagnosis for chromosomal gonadal differentiation defects is identified postnatally in only about 20% of cases.[10] Additionally, for ultimate differential diagnosis and treatment purposes, the identification of 0, 1, or 2 gonads and the determination about the presence of a uterus are critical, and some of these findings are not reliably made antenatally. Finally, some disorders typically present past infancy because they are phenotypically unremarkable, and therefore will have a very low prenatal detection rate unless there is a specific history to prompt investigation.

A differential diagnostic algorithm for the fetus with ambiguous genitalia (Fig. 19.3-11) should include both phenotypic (external) and gonadal (internal) genitourinary tract evaluation by imaging, and chromosomal evaluation with microarray analysis if at all possible. In the absence of other fetal anomalies or intrauterine growth retardation (IUGR), a prenatal karyotype with in situ hybridization (FISH) for SRY is the most useful test to work up ambiguous genitalia.[48] A maternal and family history should be taken, assessing ingestion of exogenous maternal hormones (as in ART), oral contraceptives during pregnancy, neonatal deaths, urologic abnormalities, precocious puberty, amenorrhea, infertility, and consanguinity; a maternal physical examination for virilization or cushingoid appearance may be appropriate. Once chromosomal, urinary tract, and syndromic etiologies are excluded, consideration should turn to steroid profiling or sequencing of the androgen receptor gene.[49]

## PROGNOSIS AND MANAGEMENT

The prognosis in these cases is highly variable, depending first on whether there is a chromosomal anomaly with systemic expression of abnormalities or whether anomalies are isolated to the genitourinary system. Isolated disorders of sexual differentiation have no impact on mode of delivery, and are not life threatening with the exception of congenital adrenal hyperplasia, the most common cause for the most common category of DSD at approximately 1/16,000 live births.[50] These children need to be medically managed carefully immediately at birth.[10] If a prenatal diagnosis is made early enough, steroid administered antenatally has been used to prevent virilization; however, the use of prenatal dexamethasone for CAH has been challenged on an ethical basis.[51] Even if there is no immediate concern for the

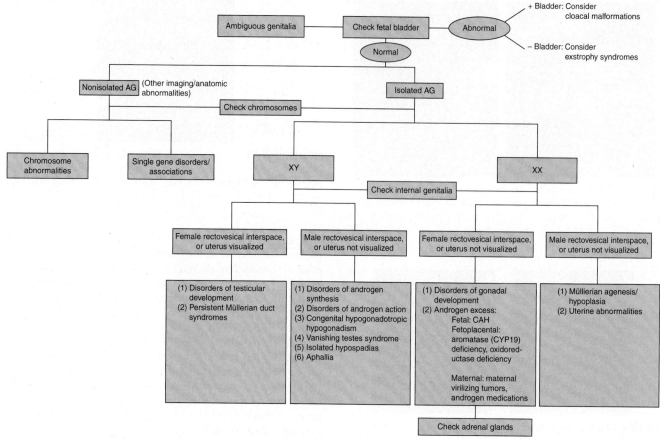

**FIGURE 19.3-11:** An algorithm for the workup of genital abnormalities in the fetus. (Adapted from Chitayat D, Glanc P. Diagnostic approach in prenatally detected genital abnormalities. *Ultrasound Obstet Gynecol.* 2010;35:637–646.)

infant's stability, most clinicians involved with caring for a child diagnosed with any DSD consider the evaluation psychosocially urgent for the family, requiring a high degree of sensitivity. Additionally, some disorders, particularly those with gonadal dysgenesis, are at high risk for gonadal malignancies in childhood.

## RECURRENCE RISK

Isolated DSD is not thought to have significant recurrence risk, but multiple chromosomal disorders have been identified that carry a certain risk for subsequent pregnancies, depending on the type of transmission (Table 19.3-1).

## REFERENCES

1. Naylor CS, Carlson DE, Santulli T Jr, et al. Use of three-dimensional ultrasonography for prenatal diagnosis of ambiguous genitalia. *J Ultrasound Med.* 2001;20:1365–1367.
2. Hamerton JL, Canning N, Ray M, et al. A cytogenetic survey of 14,068 newborn infants, I: incidence of chromosome abnormalities. *Clin Genet.* 1975;4:223–243.
3. Parker KL, Schimmer BP. Embryology and genetics of the mammalian gonads and ducts. In: Neill JD, ed. *Knobil and Neill's Physiology of Reproduction.* 3rd ed. St Louis, MO: Elsevier; 2006.
4. Carlson BM. *Human Embryology and Developmental Biology.* 4th ed. Philadelphia, PA: Mosby Elsevier; 2009.
5. Schoenwolf GC, Bleyl SB, Brauer PR, et al, eds. *Larsen's Human Embryology.* 4th ed. Philadelphia, PA: Churchill Livingstone.Elsevier; 2009.
6. Ammini AC, Pandey J, Vijyaraghavan M, et al. Human female phenotypic development: role of fetal ovaries. *J Clin Endocrinol Metab.* 1994;79(2):604–608.
7. Smith DP, Felker RE, Noe HN, et al. Prenatal diagnosis of genital anomalies. *Urology.* 1996;47(1):114–117.
8. Sampaio FJ, Favorito LA. Analysis of testicular migration during the fetal period in humans. *J Urol.* 1998;159(2):540–542.
9. Houk CP, Hughes IA, Ahmed SF, et al. Summary of concensus statement on intersex disorders and their management. International Intersex Consensus Conference. *Pediatrics.* 2006;118:753–757.
10. Lambert SM, Vilain EJN, Kolon TF. A practical approach to ambiguous genitalia in the newborn period. *Urol Clin North Am.* 2010;37:195–205.
11. Casey AC, Bhodauria S, Shapter A, et al. Dysgerminoma: the role of conservative surgery. *Gynecol Oncol.* 1996;63:352–357.
12. Efrat Z, Perri T, Ramati E, et al. Fetal gender assignment by first-trimester ultrasound. *Ultrasound Obstet Gynecol.* 2006;27:619–621.
13. Emerson DS, Felker RE, Brown DL. The sagittal sign: an early second trimester sonographic indicator of fetal gender. *J Ultrasound Med.* 1989;8:293–297.
14. Odeh M, Ophir E, Bornstein J. Hypospadius mimicking female genitalia on early second trimester sonographic examination. *J Clin Ultrasound.* 2008;36(9):581–583.
15. Bronshtein M, Rottem S, Yoffe N, et al. Early determination of fetal sex using transvaginal sonography: technique and pitfalls. *J Clin Ultrasound.* 1990;18(4):302–306.
16. Natsuyama E. Sonographic determination of fetal sex from 12 weeks of gestation. *Am J Obstet Gynecol.* 1984;149:748–757.
17. Martin C, Darnell A, Duran C, et al. Magnetic resonance imaging of the intrauterine fetal genitourinary tract: normal anatomy and pathology. *Abdom Imaging.* 2004;29:286–302.
18. Pinette MG, Wax JR, Blackstone J, et al. Normal growth and development of fetal external genitalia demonstrated by sonography. *J Clin Ultrasound.* 2003;31:465–472.
19. Nemec SF, Nemec U, Weber M, et al. Female external genitalia on fetal magnetic resonance imaging. *Ultrasound Obstet Gynecol.* 2011;38:695–700.
20. James T. Aplasia of the male prepuce with evidence of hereditary transmission. *J Anat.* 1951;85(4):370–372.
21. Nemec SF, Nemec U, Weber M, et al. Male sexual development *in utero*: testicular descent on prenatal magnetic resonance imaging. *Ultrasound Obstet Gynecol.* 2011;38:688–694.
22. Achiron R, Pinhas-Hamiel O, Zalel Y, et al. Development of male fetal gender: prenatal sonographic measurement of the scrotum and evaluation of testicular descent. *Ultrasound Obstet Gynecol.* 1998;11:242–245.

23. Cafici D, Iglesius A. Prenatal diagnosis of severe hypospadias with 2- and 3-dimensional sonography. *J Ultrasound Med.* 2002;21:1423–1426.

24. Hackett LK, Tarsa M, Wolfson TJ, et al. Use of multiplanar 3-dimensional ultrasonography for prenatal sex identification. *J Ultrasound Med.* 2010;29:195–202.

25. Abu-Rustum R, Chaaban M. Is 3-dimensional sonography useful in the diagnosis of ambiguous genitalia? *J Ultrasound Med.* 2009;28:95–97.

26. Wang Y, Cai A, Sun J, et al. Prenatal diagnosis of penoscrotal transposition with 2- and 3-dimensional ultrasonography. *J Ultrasound Med.* 2011;30:1397–1401.

27. Verwoerd-Dikkeboom CM, Koning AHJ, Groenenberg IAL, et al. Using virtual reality for evaluation of fetal ambiguous genitalia. *Ultrasound Obstet Gynecol.* 2008;32:510–514.

28. Glanc P, Umranikar S, Koff D, et al. Fetal sex assignment by sonographic evaluation of the pelvic organs in the second and third trimesters of pregnancy. *J Ultrasound Med.* 2007;26:563–569.

29. Jouannic J-M, Rosenblatt J, Demaria F, et al. Contribution of three-dimensional volume contrast imaging to the sonographic assessment of the fetal uterus. *Ultrasound Obstet Gynecol.* 2005;26:567–570.

30. Cesca E, Midrio P, Tregnaghi A, et al. Meconium periorchitis: a rare cause of fetal scrotal cyst—MRI and pathologic appearance. *Fetal Diagn Ther.* 2009;26:38–40.

31. Gililland A, Carlan SJ, Greenbaum LD, et al. Undescended testicle and a meconium-filled hemiscrotum: prenatal ultrasound appearance. *Ultrasound Obstet Gynecol.* 2002;20(2):200–202.

32. Regev RH, Markovich O, Arnon S, et al. Meconium periorchitis: intrauterine diagnosis and neonatal outcome: case reports and review of the literature. *J Perinatol.* 2009;29(8):585–587.

33. Frati A, Ducarme G, Vuillard E, et al. Prenatal evaluation of a scrotal mass using a high-frequency probe in the diagnosis of inguinoscrotal hernia. *Ultrasound Obstet Gynecol.* 2008;32(7):949–950.

34. Herman A, Schvimer M, Tovbin J, et al. Antenatal sonographic diagnosis of testicular torsion. *Ultrasound Obstet Gynecol.* 2002;20(5):522–524.

35. Devesa R, Muñoz A, Torrents M, et al. Prenatal diagnosis of testicular torsion. *Ultrasound Obstet Gynecol.* 1998;11(4):286–288.

36. Youssef BA, Sammak BM, Al Shahed M. Pre-natally diagnosed testicular torsion ultrasonographic features. *Clin Radiol.* 2000;55(2):150–151.

37. Skoog SJ, Belman AB. Aphallia: its classification and management. *J Urol.* 1989;41(3):589–592.

38. Perlitz Y, Keselman L, Haddad S, et al. Prenatal sonographic evaluation of the penile length. *Prenat Diagn.* 2011;31(13):283–285.

39. Danon D, Ben-Shitrit G, Bardin R, et al. Reference values for fetal penile length and width from 22 to 36 gestational weeks. *Prenat Diagn.* 2012;32(9):829–832.

40. Johnson P, Maxwell D. Fetal penile length. *Ultrasound Obstet Gynecol.* 2000;15(4):308–310.

41. Nemec SF, Nemec U, Weber M, et al. Penile biometry on prenatal magnetic resonance imaging. *Ultrasound Obstet Gynecol.* 2012;39(3):330–335.

42. Meizner I, Mashiach R, Shalev J, et al. The "tulip sign": a sonographic clue for in-utero diagnosis of severe hypospadius. *Ultrasound Obstet Gynecol.* 2002;19:250–253.

43. Redman JF. Buried penis: congenital syndrome of a short penile shaft and a paucity of penile shaft skin. *J Urol.* 2005;173(5):1714–1717.

44. Chambrier ED, Heinrichs C, Avni FE. Sonographic appearance of congenital adrenal hyperplasia in utero. *J Ultrasound Med.* 2002;21(1):97–100.

45. Calvo-Garcia MA, Kline-Fath BM, Rubio EI, et al. Fetal MRI of cloacal exstrophy. *Pediatr Radiol.* 2013;43(5):593–604.

46. Cheikhelard A, Luton D, Philipp-Chomette P, et al. How accurate is the prenatal diagnosis of abnormal genitalia? *J Urol.* 2000;164:984–987.

47. Morel Y, Rey R, Teinturier C, et al. Aetiological diagnosis of male sex ambiguity: a collaborative study. *Eur J Pediatr.* 2002;161:49.

48. Adam MP, Fechner PY, Ramsdell LA, et al. Ambiguous genitalia: what prenatal genetic testing is practical? *Am J Med Genet A.* 2012;158A:1337–1343.

49. Katorza E, Pinhas-Hamiel O, Mazkereth R, et al. Sex differentiation disorders (SDD): prenatal sonographic diagnosis, genetic and hormonal work-up. *Pediatr Endocrinol Rev.* 2009;7:12–21.

50. Speiser PW, White PC. Congenital adrenal hyperplasia. *N Engl J Med.* 2003;349:776.

51. Dreger A, Feder EK, Tamar-Mattis A. Prenatal dexamethasone for congenital adrenal hyperplasia: an ethics canary in the modern medical mine. *J Bioeth Inq.* 2012;9(3):277–294.

# 20  Genetic Abnormalities and Syndromes*

Teresa Chapman • Stephanie L. Santoro • Robert J. Hopkin

Advances in prenatal imaging using ultrasound (US) and magnetic resonance imaging (MRI) have enabled earlier and more accurate identification of developmental features that point to various chromosomal abnormalities and syndromes. Because of the high perinatal death rate and childhood disability rates associated with these abnormalities, invasive prenatal testing by chorionic villous sampling, amniocentesis, or cordocentesis may be legitimately pursued. The body of identified genes attributed causally to a wide array of developmental anomalies and syndromes continues to expand, enabling families and physicians to make steadily more informed decisions about pregnancy management and future family planning.

In this chapter, the pathogenesis, imaging characteristics, and management issues are described for several common and/or well-described conditions, including the most important chromosomal anomalies, heritable and sporadic syndromes, craniofacial abnormalities, and nongenetic associations leading to multisystem anomalies.

*Editors' note: An overwhelming number of genetic and nongenetic associations can be encountered in the fetus. Determining which entities to include in this chapter was difficult, but the synopsis is a review of disorders that may be imaged more commonly in a perinatal practice. The section is separated into chromosomal, genetic, craniosynostosis syndromes, syndromes affecting mandible and auricle and nongenetic associations. The review of each of these disorders focuses on the most common organ systems affected but cannot include every anomaly cited in the literature. For tables or lists of all abnormalities possible in the syndromes discussed below and for others not reviewed, dedicated genetic texts or internet resources, especially OMIM (Online Mendelian Inheritance in Man www.omim.org) or Genereviews (http://www.ncbi.nlm.nih.gov/books/NBK1116/), may be helpful.

## CHROMOSOMAL ANOMALIES

Any individual pregnant woman's background risk of having a baby affected by a chromosomal abnormality is influenced by her age (the higher the age of the mother, the higher the risk), the gestational age (the earlier the gestation, the higher the risk), and a history of having had a previous fetus or infant with a chromosomal defect. Specifically, the risk for trisomies in women who have had a prior fetus or child with a trisomy is 0.75% higher than the risk would be otherwise.[1] Maternal age positively correlates with various chromosomal abnormalities, including trisomies 13, 18, and 21, XXX and XXY, but not with 45X.[2] Further noninvasive tests can contribute to the calculation of a risk for a trisomy or chromosomal defect. First-trimester tests performed at 11 to 14 weeks include nuchal translucency (NT) screening and maternal serum biochemistry assessment of human chorionic gonadotropin (hCG) and pregnancy-associated plasma protein A (PAPP-A). In the second trimester, a fetal anatomy screening ultrasound typically between 18 and 22 weeks and maternal serum biochemistry assessment at 15 to 20 weeks known as the quad or tetra screen includes measurements of alpha-fetoprotein (AFP), hCG, estriol, and inhibin-A. Any time a screening test is performed, the background risk, based on maternal age,

gestational age, and prior history of a trisomy, is factored into a complex calculation that includes all variables measured, and this product becomes the updated background risk for the pregnancy.

### Trisomy 21

Down syndrome (DS) is also known as trisomy 21, as it is caused by the presence of additional genetic material from chromosome 21. DS is the most common autosomal trisomy and is also the most common genetic cause of developmental delay. There is an increased risk of trisomy 21 with increasing maternal age (Table 20.1). DS is associated with a number of congenital anomalies and medical issues.[3]

| Table 20.1 | Risk Table for Chromosomal Anomalies | |
|---|---|---|
| **Maternal Age (y)** | | **Odds (1 in_)** |
| 20 | | 1,176 |
| 21 | | 1,160 |
| 22 | | 1,136 |
| 23 | | 1,114 |
| 24 | | 1,087 |
| 25 | | 1,040 |
| 26 | | 990 |
| 27 | | 928 |
| 28 | | 855 |
| 29 | | 760 |
| 30 | | 690 |
| 31 | | 597 |
| 32 | | 508 |
| 33 | | 421 |
| 34 | | 342 |
| 35 | | 274 |
| 36 | | 216 |
| 37 | | 168 |
| 38 | | 129 |
| 39 | | 98 |
| 40 | | 74 |
| 41 | | 56 |
| 42 | | 42 |
| 43 | | 31 |
| 44 | | 23 |

Data from Snijders RJ, Sundberg K, Holzgreve W, et al. Maternal age- and gestation-specific risk for trisomy 21. *Ultrasound Obstet Gynecol.* 1999;13(3):167–170.

**Incidence:** The incidence of DS is approximately 1.3 in 1,000 live births, with a similar prevalence across ethnicities.[3]

**Pathogenesis/Etiology:** The additional chromosomal material can be identified as an entire additional copy of chromosome 21, which is known as full trisomy 21 and is present in 90% to 95% of individuals with DS, an unbalanced Robertsonian translocation noted in 3% to 4% of individuals wherein a portion of chromosome 21 translocates to another acrocentric chromosome, usually to chromosome 14, or from mosaicism for chromosome 21 in 1% of cases.[4] In a Robertsonian translocation, all the genes on each chromosome are included since the p arms of the acrocentric chromosomes contain only repeat elements. Translocations of part of the q arm are also possible but are much less common. The additional chromosomal material is due to either nondisjunction, in the case of full trisomy, or from random inheritance of a derivative chromosome in the case of an unbalanced translocation. A known relationship between increasing maternal age and prevalence of DS is theorized to be due to prolonged time in meiotic arrest and increased likelihood of meiotic nondisjunction during egg formation.[5] In the subset of cases attributable to translocation, however, the age of the mother does not seem to be relevant.

**Diagnosis:** Diagnosis cannot be made from ultrasound findings or first-trimester screening alone. Measurement of the NT, combined with the maternal age and maternal serum markers, including hCG and PAPP-A, can increase the detection of chromosomal defects substantially.[6] Further diagnostic testing via amniocentesis or chorionic villus sampling (CVS) should be offered. New laboratory techniques have allowed for isolation of cell-free fetal DNA from maternal serum and for detection of increased ratios of the presence of chromosome 21 suggestive of DS.[7] This testing is considered by the National Society of Genetic Counselors (NSGC) to be a form of screening and not diagnostic at this time.[8] If diagnosis of DS is made by chromosome analysis, parents should be offered referral to a geneticist to discuss outcomes and options.

*Imaging:* First-trimester ultrasound between 11 and 14 weeks for measurement of the fetal NT, when combined with maternal serum biochemical evaluation, can detect 90% of trisomy 21 cases with a false-positive rate of 5%.[6] At the same time that the NT is measured, the nasal bone should be evaluated. Either

an absent or short nasal bone is an important imaging feature associated with trisomy 21 and other chromosomal defects. At the 11- to 14-week scan, absence of the nasal bone may be seen in as high as 70% of fetuses affected by trisomy 21 (Fig. 20.1A). In contrast, a normal nasal bone is visualized in 97.3% to 99.5% of chromosomally normal fetuses.[9] As with measurement of the NT, assessment of the fetal nasal bone is technically difficult, and the Fetal Medicine Foundation UK has established standards for this technique. A midline sagittal view of the fetal profile is captured, and the image is magnified such that only the fetal head and thorax fill the screen. The angle between the ultrasound transducer and the midline of the face should be about 45°. The observer should look for three echogenic lines, representing the skin of the nose, the nasal bone, and the nasal tip (Fig. 20.1B).

The fetal anatomic assessment by ultrasound in the second trimester serves to identify both minor and major defects (Table 20.2 and Fig. 20.2). Minor defects include increased nuchal fold thickness, echogenic bowel, echogenic intracardiac focus, mild hydronephrosis, short humerus, and short femur (Fig. 20.3). Major defects include cardiac anomalies (most commonly endocardial cushion defects), duodenal atresia, cervical lymphatic malformation, and hydrops. The risk for a chromosomal abnormality increases with the number of defects identified.[10]

A second-trimester ultrasound examination to screen for abnormal fetal anomalies may show few or extensive systems affected by trisomy 21. The "genetic sonogram" refers to evaluation for anatomic abnormalities, or markers, seen in the second-trimester fetal anatomic assessment. Detection of even minor markers increases the risk of an abnormal karyotype (Table 20.3). A recent meta-analysis of 48 studies summarizing prenatal ultrasounds from gestational ages 14 to 24 weeks found that the combined negative likelihood ratio of all markers, including short femur, but not short humerus, was 0.13, implying that if a systematic ultrasound examination excludes all markers, there is a 7.7-fold reduction in risk.[11]

Skull and facial imaging should evaluate for acrobrachycephaly, mild ventriculomegaly, nasal bone hypoplasia, and nuchal thickening. Cardiac defects might include ventricular septal defect, atrioventricular canal defect, tetralogy of Fallot, or the finding of an echogenic intracardiac focus. Intra-abdominal abnormalities to consider are duodenal atresia, echogenic bowel, and pyelectasis. Duodenal atresia would be inferred

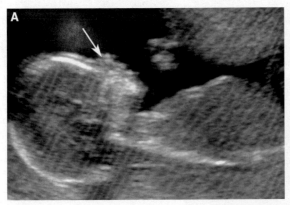 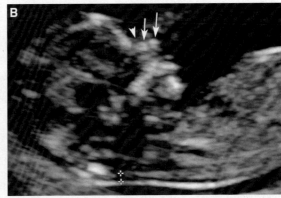

**FIGURE 20.1:** Absent and normal nasal bone. **A:** First-trimester fetal ultrasound shows absence of a nasal bone (*arrow* indicates nasal soft tissue) in a fetus at gestational age 16 weeks with trisomy 21. **B:** First-trimester ultrasound in a different fetus at gestational age 13 weeks shows the expected echogenicity of the skin (*arrowhead*) and nasal bone and tip (*arrows*).

| Table 20.2 | Common Features of Major Trisomies | | |
| --- | --- | --- | --- |
| | **Trisomy 21** | **Trisomy 18** | **Trisomy 13** |
| Major features | Cardiac defects, duodenal atresia, cystic hygroma, hydrops | Cardiac defects, spina bifida, cerebellar dysgenesis, micrognathia, diaphragmatic hernia, omphalocele, clenched hands/wrists, radial aplasia, clubfeet, cystic hygroma | Cardiac defects, central nervous system abnormalities, facial anomalies, cleft lip/palate, urogenital anomalies/echogenic kidneys, omphalocele, polydactyly, rocker-bottom feet, cystic hygroma |
| Makers or subtle finding | Nuchal thickening, hyperechoic bowel, EIF, shortened limbs, pyelectasis, mild ventriculomegaly, widened pelvic angle, shortened frontal lobe, clinodactyly, widened sandal gap, hypoplastic or absent nasal bone | Choroid cysts, brachycephaly, shortened limbs, IUGR, single umbilical artery | EIF, mild ventriculomegaly, pyelectasis, IUGR, single umbilical artery |

EIF, echogenic intracardiac focus; IUGR, intrauterine growth restriction.
From Nyberg DA, Souter VL. Chromosomal abnormalities. In: Nyberg DA, McGahan JP, Pretorius DH, et al, eds. *Diagnostic Imaging of Fetal Anomalies*. Philadelphia, PA: Lippincott Williams & Wilkins; 2003:861–906.

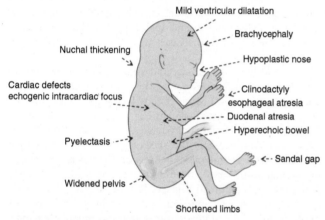

**FIGURE 20.2:** Common features of trisomy 21.

by duodenal bulb distension proximal to the atretic segment. This pathology results in the "double-bubble" sign (Fig. 20.4A), reflecting the fluid-filled stomach adjacent to the distended duodenal bulb. Trisomy 21 may affect musculoskeletal development and manifest with short humerus and femur, clinodactyly, hypoplasia of the fifth digit middle phalanx, and sandal-foot deformity (Fig. 20.4B).

Fetal MR imaging is not commonly required for the diagnosis of trisomy 21, given the number of identifiable abnormalities evident sonographically and the biochemical and genetic testing available for diagnosis. There is no published literature showing improved diagnosis of trisomy 21 by fetal MR. However, brain abnormalities, including mild ventriculomegaly (Fig. 20.5), are common indications for fetal MRI. When imaging a fetus for ventriculomegaly, it is important to focus not only on the fetal brain, but on the entire fetal body to exclude other associated

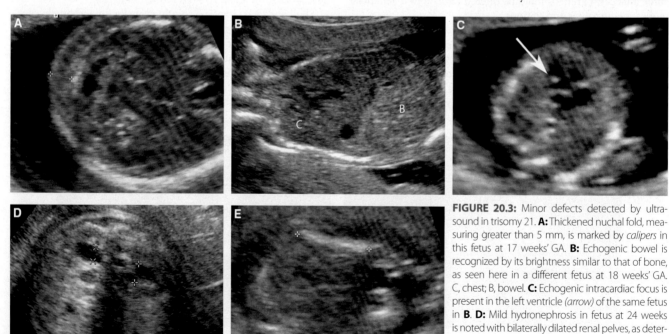

**FIGURE 20.3:** Minor defects detected by ultrasound in trisomy 21. **A:** Thickened nuchal fold, measuring greater than 5 mm, is marked by *calipers* in this fetus at 17 weeks' GA. **B:** Echogenic bowel is recognized by its brightness similar to that of bone, as seen here in a different fetus at 18 weeks' GA. C, chest; B, bowel. **C:** Echogenic intracardiac focus is present in the left ventricle (*arrow*) of the same fetus in **B**. **D:** Mild hydronephrosis in fetus at 24 weeks is noted with bilaterally dilated renal pelves, as determined by measuring the anterior–posterior renal pelvis diameter. **E:** Short long bones (<5th percentile; femur length is 21 mm = 16 and 2/7 weeks ± 1.38 weeks) present in the same fetus as in **A**.

| Table 20.3 | Pooled Estimates of Detection Rate (DR), False-Positive Rate (FPR), and Positive and Negative Likelihood Ratios (LR+ and LR−) of Sonographic Markers for Trisomy 21 and Estimated Likelihood Ratio (LR) of Individual Isolated Markers | | | | |
|---|---|---|---|---|---|
| *Marker* | *DR (95% CI) (%)* | *FPR (95% CI) (%)* | *LR+ (95% CI) (%)* | *LR− (95% CI) (%)* | *LR Isolated Marker[a]* |
| Intracardiac echogenic focus | 24.4 (20.9–28.2) | 3.9 (3.4–4.5) | 5.83 (5.02–6.77) | 0.80 (0.75–0.86) | 0.95 |
| Ventriculomegaly | 7.5 (4.2–12.9) | 0.2 (0.1–0.4) | 27.52 (13.61–55.68) | 0.94 (0.91–0.98) | 3.81 |
| Increased nuchal fold | 26.0 (20.3–32.9) | 1.0 (0.5–1.9) | 23.30 (14.35–37.83) | 0.80 (0.74–0.85) | 3.79 |
| Echogenic bowel | 16.7 (13.4–20.7) | 1.1 (0.8–1.5) | 11.44 (9.05–14.47) | 0.90 (0.86–0.94) | 1.65 |
| Mild hydronephrosis | 13.9 (11.2–17.2) | 1.7 (1.4–2.0) | 7.63 (6.11–9.51) | 0.92 (0.89–0.96) | 1.08 |
| Short humerus | 30.3 (17.1–47.9) | 4.6 (2.8–7.4) | 4.81 (3.49–6.62) | 0.74 (0.63–0.88) | 0.78 |
| Short femur | 27.7 (19.3–38.1) | 6.4 (4.7–8.8) | 3.72 (2.79–4.97) | 0.80 (0.73–0.88) | 0.61 |
| Absent or hypoplastic NB | 59.8 (48.9–69.9) | 2.8 (1.9–4.0) | 23.27 (14.23–38.06) | 0.46 (0.36–0.58) | 6.58 |

[a]Derived by multiplying the positive LR for the given marker by the negative LR of each of all other markers; NB, nasal bone.
Adapted from Agathokleous M, Chaveeva P, Poon LC, et al. Meta-analysis of second-trimester markers for trisomy 21. *Ultrasound Obstet Gynecol.* 2013;41:247–261.

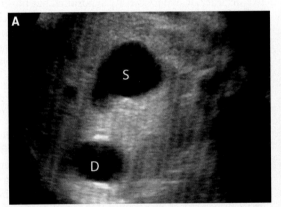

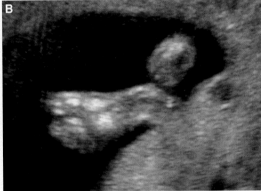

**FIGURE 20.4:** Additional anomalies in fetus affected by trisomy 21. **A:** Duodenal atresia is evident by a fluid-distended stomach *(S)* and proximal duodenum *(D)* in this 30-week-GA fetus with trisomy 21. Polyhydramnios was also found in this pregnancy (not shown here). **B:** Sandal-foot deformity in a 20-week-GA fetus with trisomy 21. There is a gap between the first and second toes. Considerations for a gap between the second and third toes include syndactyly, ectrodactyly spectrum, and amniotic band syndrome.

anomalies. In the presence of DS, mild ventriculomegaly is often present without associated CNS anomalies. Gastrointestinal anomalies, such as Hirschsprung disease or anal atresia, may also be detected on second- or third-trimester MR imaging.

**Differential Diagnosis:** In the first trimester, an abnormally thick NT (>3.0 mm) can offer useful information, even with a normal chromosomal evaluation, as a thick NT is also associated with other developmental anomalies, including cardiac defects, diaphragmatic hernia, abdominal wall defects, and renal abnormalities. The NT is also useful in multiple gestation pregnancies, where maternal serum evaluation is not applicable. Discordant NT measurements in a dichorionic pregnancy would be concerning for genetic abnormalities, and in a monochorionic pregnancy would be concerning for twin-twin transfusion.[12]

In the second trimester, multisystem developmental anomalies may be identified, and, taken separately, each of these developmental anomalies has its own set of differential considerations. Thickening of the nuchal soft tissues could indicate a cervical lymphatic malformation, which may be present in isolation or as part of other trisomies (13 and 18), Turner

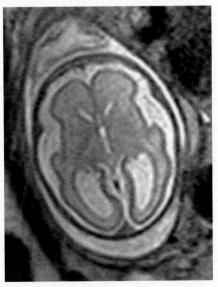

**FIGURE 20.5:** Axial SSFSE T2 MRI of a 24-week fetus with mild ventriculomegaly measuring 12 mm at atrium but no other associated CNS abnormalities.

syndrome, microdeletion syndromes (13q-, 18p-) and triploidy. Nonimmune hydrops fetalis, characterized by generalized skin edema, ascites, pericardial and pleural effusions, is a nonspecific condition resulting from a wide variety of maternal and fetal disorders.[13]

Echogenic bowel is also a nonspecific finding and is most often seen in normal fetuses. However, in addition to its increased frequency among fetuses with aneuploidy, and particularly trisomy 21, it is also associated with bowel atresia, congenital infection, and, uncommonly, with meconium ileus secondary to cystic fibrosis. Further, an increased risk of intrauterine growth retardation, fetal demise, and placenta-related complications has been associated with echogenic bowel.[14]

Duodenal atresia, manifested by the "double-bubble" sign and polyhydramnios (see Fig. 20.4A), may not be apparent until well into the second trimester, after 20 weeks' gestational age. It is important to keep in mind that this sign may be seen in the normal fetus, and it is not specific for trisomy 21. Approximately 40% of prenatally detected duodenal atresia cases are not associated with a genetic defect.[15] In one-third of these cases, the fetus will be affected by trisomy 21. Other conditions leading to distension of the descending duodenum would include nonsyndromic duodenal atresia, pyloric atresia, extrinsic compression by a mass or by annular pancreas (a diagnosis further supported by the presence of echogenic bands around the descending duodenum), midgut volvulus secondary to malrotation, diaphragmatic hernia, or colonic duplication.[16]

Mild pyelectasis is defined differently among various imaging centers, but is roughly defined as an anterior–posterior renal pelvis diameter of 4 to 7 mm in the second trimester and as 7 to 10 mm in the third trimester.[17] Although this finding has been shown to be associated with aneuploidy (and specifically trisomy 21), the abnormality is commonly seen in screening ultrasound, with an incidence of approximately 2% of all pregnancies.[17] The main etiologic considerations include an obstructive lesion, such as ureteropelvic junction, and vesicoureteral reflux. The anomaly may be isolated or may be seen as part of a number of multisystemic syndromes.

Short long bones (femur and humerus) and other limb reduction anomalies are seen in many syndromes. Trisomy 21 should be considered if the measured-to-expected femur length ratio is less than 0.91. It would then be relevant to measure the humerus, which is confirmed abnormal if the measured:expected humerus length ratio <0.90.[18] Primary differential considerations include constitutional shortening of the limbs or of the femurs, the latter being more common in Hispanic and Asian populations,[18] and skeletal dysplasias with either rhizomelic or micromelic shortening.

**Prognosis:** The prognosis for infants and children with trisomy 21 varies greatly and depends on the combination of the congenital malformations. Approximately 75% of fetuses known to have trisomy 21 will spontaneously abort or are stillborn.[19] The median age at death of individuals with DS has risen significantly in the US, from 25 years in the early 1980s to 60 years today (http://www.ndss.org). Congenital heart disease and respiratory infections are the most frequently reported medical cause of death.[20] Trisomy 21 is the most common genetic cause of intellectual disability, and affected individuals have intelligent quotients typically ranging from 40 to 70.[21] By 40 years of age, approximately 22% to 25% of individuals with DS develop Alzheimer dementia.[22]

**Management:** With early prenatal diagnosis, education regarding trisomy 21 should be offered to the family to help them evaluate options and identify needed resources. Decisions regarding pregnancy termination or planning for delivery and care may be influenced by detailed imaging to identify malformations that require immediate postnatal attention or impact long-term prognosis. Following delivery, the infant should have a complete physical exam, chromosome analysis, and evaluation by a geneticist shortly after delivery. Common issues immediately after birth can include hypotonia and feeding difficulties.[3] GI anomalies (duodenal atresia, imperforate anus, Hirschsprung disease, celiac disease, and pancreas abnormalities) are seen in up to 12% of DS patients.[3] Congenital heart disease (CHD) is also common, affecting up to 50% of children with DS. The CHD can range from AV canal defects (40% to 60%) to tetralogy of Fallot to atrial or ventricular septal defects.[3] For this reason, echocardiography should be performed in the first month of life or sooner if symptomatic. Pulmonary hypoplasia is common in patients with DS and can result in respiratory difficulty.[3] Blood abnormalities commonly seen include transient myeloproliferative disorder or hyperviscosity syndrome, but thrombocytopenia, polycythemia, and leukemias are also possible; therefore, a screening complete blood count at the time of birth is necessary.[23] Hypothyroidism is common and is diagnosed through newborn screen.[3] Referral to early intervention services should be made in the first few months after birth.[3]

**Recurrence Risk:** Genetic counseling should be offered to all parents of a child with DS for review of their specific recurrence risks based on the chromosomal pathogenesis. If a translocation is present (3% to 4% of cases), parents should be offered chromosome analysis to determine whether one of them is a carrier of a balanced translocation. If the translocation is de novo and neither parent has a balanced translocation, then there is no increased risk of recurrence. If the mother carries a balanced translocation, then the risk for future pregnancies is about 10% to 15%, whereas if the father carries the balanced translocation, the risk is about 3% to 5%.[4] Rarely, the translocation involves both of the chromosomes 21. In this circumstance, the carrier parent of the 21/21 translocation would have a 100% risk of recurrence. There is not an increased rate of trisomy 21 in second-degree relatives.[24]

## Trisomy 18

Trisomy 18 is the second most common autosomal trisomy in live born infants. It was described by Edwards in 1960 and is also known as Edwards Syndrome. It is associated with multiple congenital anomalies, including cardiac defects, neural tube defects, diaphragmatic hernia, omphalocele, cervical lymphatic malformation, limb anomalies, as well as profound developmental delay and short life expectancy.

**Incidence:** Trisomy 18 affects 1 in 3,000 live births.[25]

**Pathogenesis/Etiology:** Trisomy 18 is caused by additional genetic material from chromosome 18. Eighty percent to 85% of cases are the result of a full trisomy, 5% are due to unbalanced translocation, and 10% are mosaic. The additional chromosomal material is due to either nondisjunction in the case of full trisomy or from random inheritance of a derivative chromosome in the case of an unbalanced translocation. Trisomy

18 from a translocation is always partial trisomy since chromosome 18 is not an acrocentric chromosome and some genes will be lost at the break point. The phenotype is often different for partial trisomy 18 due to a translocation than for classical trisomy 18 secondary to nondisjunction. Trisomy 18 and 21 differ in that the majority of meiotic errors in trisomy 18 occur in meiosis II, while trisomy 21 is typically due to meiosis I errors.[26]

**Diagnosis:** First-trimester screening shows low PAPP-A and low hCG. The second-trimester serum screening shows low estriol and AFP.[27] Maternal serum derived cell-free fetal DNA testing can also detect most cases of trisomy 18 with a sensitivity and specificity similar to that found in trisomy 21. The suspected diagnosis should be confirmed with chromosomal analysis on CVS or amniocentesis regardless of the screening method used.

*Imaging:* Concern for aneuploidy may arise in the first trimester if the NT is thickened. In the second trimester, suspicion for trisomy 18 is typically due to multiple anomalies seen on ultrasound.[28,29] Sonographic markers seen with trisomy 18 are summarized in Table 20.2 and Figure 20.6 and include the following: a strawberry-shaped cranium (narrow frontal diameter and wide occipitoparietal diameter), choroid plexus cysts, clenched hands with overlapping fingers, a small omphalocele, single umbilical artery, shortened limbs, and cavovarus/clubfoot and rockerbottom foot deformities (Fig. 20.7). Major abnormalities include early-onset intrauterine growth restriction (IUGR), cardiac defects, cervical lymphatic malformation, radial aplasia, spina bifida, esophageal atresia, and cerebellar anomalies (Fig. 20.8).

IUGR is seen in 51% of fetuses with trisomy 18 before 24 weeks and in 89% of fetuses after 24 weeks of gestation.[29] CHD is seen

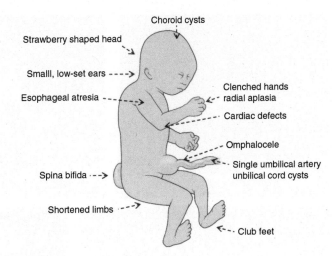

**FIGURE 20.6:** Common features of trisomy 18.

in 73% to 90% of fetuses and can include atrioventricular canal defect, tetralogy of Fallot and left heart disease.[30] Cervical lymphatic malformations can be evident both sonographically and by fetal MR imaging, and may range in appearance from mere nuchal thickening to a large cystic neck mass.

Neural tube defects suspected on ultrasound may be better seen by fetal MR imaging. Fetal karyotyping is recommended after the diagnosis of spina bifida, as approximately 17% of prenatally diagnosed cases of spina bifida are later recognized as having aneuploidy, including trisomy 18, trisomy 13, triploidy, and translocation.[31]

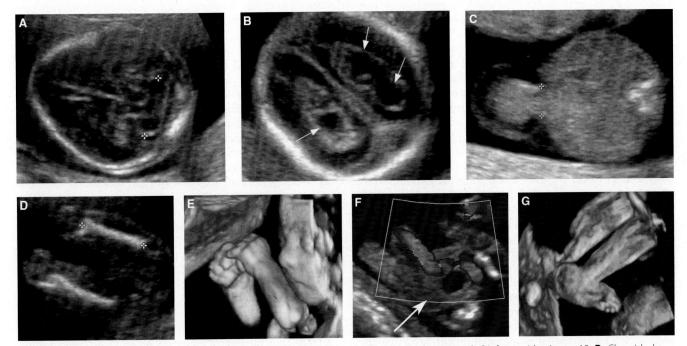

**FIGURE 20.7:** Sonographic markers of trisomy 18. **A:** A strawberry-shaped calvarium in this 19-week-GA fetus with trisomy 18. **B:** Choroid plexus cysts are noted as well-demarcated anechoic spaces within the bulk *(arrows)* of the echogenic choroid. **C:** Small omphaloceles are additional features of this disorder. **D:** Bilateral femurs and remaining long bones are abnormally short (<5th percentile; femur length of 22 mm = 16 and 4/7 weeks = ±1.38 weeks). **E:** Clenched hands may be observed by two-dimensional ultrasound and easily seen with three-dimensional ultrasound. **F:** A single umbilical artery in isolation is usually of no clinical significance, but, with other malformations, contributes to the likelihood of a chromosomal anomaly. Here, an *arrow* indicates the expected location of a nonvisualized umbilical artery. **G:** Foot abnormalities include rockerbottom foot, as seen in a different 23-week fetus on three-dimensional ultrasound.

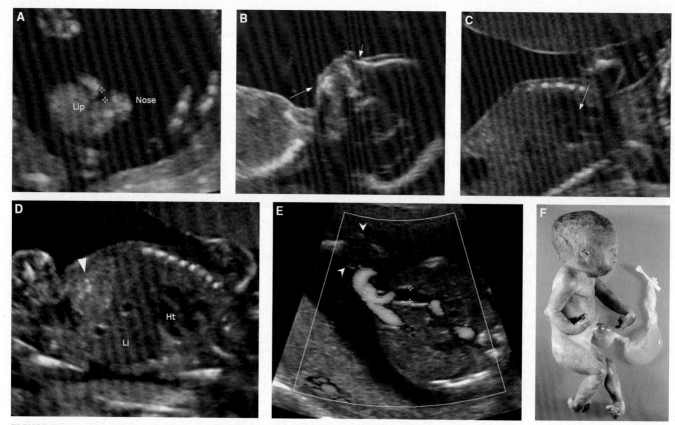

**FIGURE 20.8:** Additional sonographic findings in a different fetus with trisomy 18 at gestational age 20 weeks and 5 days. Facial developmental anomalies include **(A)** a unilateral cleft lip, marked by *calipers*, and **(B)** micrognathia seen on the sagittal view of the facial profile (*short arrow* indicates the nasal bone and *long arrow* points to the chin). **C:** Atrioventricular canal defect (*arrow*) is apparent. Axial views of the abdomen and pelvis are notable for **(D)** echogenic bowel (*arrowhead*; Ht, heart; Li, liver) and an umbilical cord cyst (*arrowheads*) **(E).** Calipers are measuring the umbilical vein. **F:** A postmortem photograph of a different fetus with trisomy 18 shows multiple anomalies, including flexed hands and wrists, clubfeet, brachycephaly, omphalocele, and umbilical cord pseudocyst. (Courtesy of Raj Kapur, Pathology Department, Seattle Children's Hospital, Washington, DC.)

A mild marker for trisomy 18 and 21 are choroid plexus cysts. These are visualized commonly in the second trimester by ultrasound and bear no implication on prognosis when the karyotype is normal. The finding, when isolated, can be considered a transient, benign observation. A meta-analysis by Yoder et al.[32] reports a likelihood ratio of 13.8 (CI, 7.7 to 25.0) for trisomy 18 and 1.87 (CI, 0.78 to 4.46) for trisomy 21. In this study, including 1,346 fetuses with isolated choroid plexus cysts, 7 had trisomy 18, and 5 had trisomy 21. Two important variables that further increase the risk of trisomy 18 are a size greater than 10 mm and advanced maternal age.[33] Brain malformations that are recognized in fetuses affected by trisomy 18 may include cerebellar hypoplasia, cerebellar vermian hypoplasia, agenesis of the corpus callosum, and holoprosencephaly, which can be recognized sonographically. Fetal MR is ideal for further evaluation of the cerebellar vermis and hemispheres. The degree of incomplete fusion of the hemispheres in holoprosencephaly is also readily detected by fetal MRI. Facial abnormalities that may be found in trisomy 18 fetuses include cleft lip, cleft palate, ocular abnormalities (particularly in the context of severe midline brain anomalies), and micrognathia. Cleft defects, ocular anomalies, and micrognathia are well seen by ultrasound (Fig. 20.8). However, brain anomalies not detected by ultrasound may accompany these facial anomalies and could be elucidated by the adjunctive use of MR imaging.

Intrathoracic and abdominal malformations, including diaphragmatic hernia and omphalocele, are typically recognized in the second trimester. Fetal MRI can clarify location of intrathoracic and intra-abdominal structures and assess compromise of pulmonary development by calculation of fetal lung volumes. Skeletal anomalies can be evaluated in real time with ultrasound, and it is uncommon that fetal MR is required for clarification of clubfoot and rockerbottom deformities or radial ray anomalies. When performing fetal MR for other reasons, however, it is important to attempt to visualize the extremities, and thick-slab T2-weighted images and cine sequences can allow for a global assessment of skeletal position and movement.

**Differential Diagnosis:** First-trimester findings of increased nuchal thickness and early IUGR may be seen with other major chromosomal abnormalities. It has been reported that the risk for aneuploidy is substantially increased (odds ratio of 9.04) when the crown-rump length is shortened by 14 mm or more from that expected for the menstrual age.[34]

There are a number of prenatally detected anatomic features of trisomy 18 that each independently has other differential considerations. A single umbilical artery is a frequent association of congenital anomalies and chromosomal abnormalities.[35] Over 50% of fetuses with trisomy 18 have a single umbilical artery. Other entities with a high incidence of single umbilical artery include trisomy 13, Turner syndrome, and triploidy.

Central nervous system abnormalities may be seen in trisomy 18, and there is wide overlap with other syndromes and disease processes in this category. Cerebellar hemispheric and vermian hypoplasia may also be seen with various chromosomal abnormalities, including trisomy 13, and may be seen in the context of other more complex hindbrain malformations such as Dandy–Walker malformations, rhombencephalosynapsis, and Joubert syndrome. Holoprosencephaly has a high association with chromosomal anomalies, most often trisomy 13, but is also seen with trisomy 18, triploidy, and many chromosomal deletions (see Table 12.1-4 in chapter 12.1). Congenital diaphragmatic hernia and omphalocele are each observed in a wide number of fetuses affected by chromosomal abnormalities. CDH is most often associated with trisomies 18, 13, and 21, and Turner syndrome.[36] Omphalocele carries an even higher risk of aneuploidy than does CDH, particularly if the omphalocele contains liver. Trisomies 18 and 13 are reported most often, followed by Trisomy 21, Turner syndrome and triploidy. A syndrome that often presents with an omphalocele is Beckwith-Wiedemann.

**Prognosis:** Trisomy 18 is highly lethal in utero. Without elective termination, 64% of fetuses die. Interestingly, there is a gender selection in fetuses with trisomy 18. Females with trisomy 18 are more likely to be born alive and survive longer than males with trisomy 18.[37]

A review of outcomes of patients with trisomy 18 has shown that the average survival is 7 to 14 days. For infants discharged home, median survival is 1 to 2 months for males and 9 to 10 months for females.[38] Five percent to 10% of infants with trisomy 18 survive to 1 year.[37] The most common causes of death include apnea, cardiopulmonary arrest, CHD, and pneumonia.[38] Of patients who survive beyond 1 year of age, major medical problems include scoliosis, hearing loss, and Wilms tumor.[39] Developmental delays are severe to profound.

**Management:** If not obtained prenatally, chromosome analysis should be performed to confirm the diagnosis. If the pregnancy is not terminated electively, infants that survive to delivery can have multiple complications. A complete physical exam should evaluate for growth restriction, abnormal head shape, and an abnormal thorax due to a short sternum and narrow transverse chest diameter. Other typical findings include hypertonia, hypoplastic toenails, micrognathia, and low-arch dermal ridges.[25] Because of the high likelihood of CHD, echocardiography should be performed after birth.[39] Very few infants with trisomy 18 are able to feed orally, so nasogastric or gastrostomy tube feedings is often necessary.

**Recurrence Risk:** Families should receive genetic counseling when a diagnosis is made or suspected. The recurrence risk for full trisomy 18 is 1% or maternal age–associated risk or whichever is greater. The recurrence risk for parents with a balanced translocation may be as high as 50%.[38]

## Trisomy 13

Trisomy 13 is the third most common autosomal aneuploidy in live-born infants. It was described by Patau in 1960 and is also known as Patau Syndrome. It is associated with multiple congenital anomalies, including cardiac defects, CNS and facial anomalies, urogenital defects, omphalocele, cervical lymphatic malformation, and limb anomalies, as well as profound developmental delay and short life expectancy.[38]

**Incidence:** Trisomy 13 affects 1 in 5,000 live births.[38]

**Pathogenesis/Etiology:** Trisomy 13 is caused by additional genetic material from chromosome 13. Eighty percent of cases are the result of a full trisomy, and 20% are due to unbalanced translocation or mosaicism. The additional chromosomal material is due to either nondisjunction usually during maternal meiosis I in the case of full trisomy, or random inheritance of a derivative chromosome in the presence of an unbalanced translocation.[40] Both Robertsonian and non-Robertsonian translocations are associated with trisomy 13. Non-Robertsonian translocations are more likely to be associated with long-term survival. The phenotype of trisomy 13 with Robertsonian translocation is similar to that associated with nondisjunction.

**Diagnosis:** The standard tetra biochemistry serum screen does not detect fetuses with trisomy 13; however, screening for PAPP-A in the first trimester can identify trisomy 13.[41] Maternal serum cell-free fetal DNA testing can detect trisomy 13 but is not as sensitive for chromosome 13 as for chromosomes 18 or 21. This may lead to false negative results. Amniocentesis or CVS should be offered to confirm an abnormal screen or in case of high suspicion based on the pattern of malformations identified. Fluorescence in situ hybridization (FISH) may be performed to obtain a more rapid diagnosis.

*Imaging:* Abnormal ultrasound findings are a common cause for suspicion of the diagnosis of trisomy 13. In the first trimester, the only discernible abnormality might be a thickened NT.[42] There are minor and major markers that should be excluded on the second-trimester fetal anatomy ultrasound (summarized in Table 20.2 and in Fig. 20.9). The more subtle sonographic abnormalities that might raise suspicion for trisomy 13 include low-set ears, cleft lip or palate, mild ventriculomegaly, polydactyly, echogenic intracardiac focus, small omphalocele, single umbilical artery, and cavovarus deformity (Fig. 20.10A–D).[43] Severe abnormalities include holoprosencephaly, cardiac defects, and renal anomalies (Fig. 20.10E,F). The most common ultrasound finding is holoprosencephaly and can be seen as early as 12 weeks of gestation.[42] Cardiac defects are often seen (in 80% to 100% of cases), and lesions include atrioventricular septal defect, hypoplastic left ventricle, or double outlet right ventricle.[43]

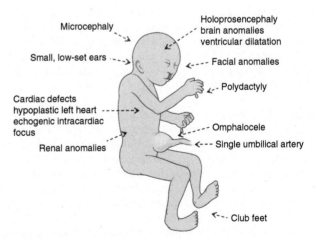

**FIGURE 20.9:** Common features of trisomy 13.

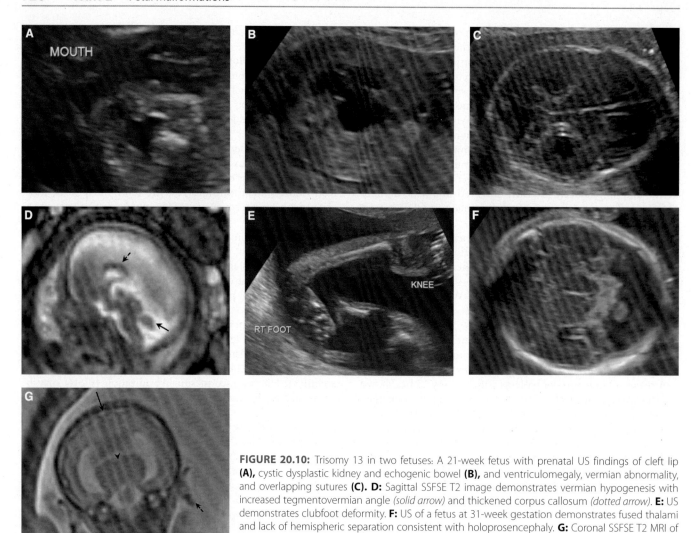

**FIGURE 20.10:** Trisomy 13 in two fetuses: A 21-week fetus with prenatal US findings of cleft lip **(A),** cystic dysplastic kidney and echogenic bowel **(B),** and ventriculomegaly, vermian abnormality, and overlapping sutures **(C). D:** Sagittal SSFSE T2 image demonstrates vermian hypogenesis with increased tegmentovermian angle *(solid arrow)* and thickened corpus callosum *(dotted arrow).* **E:** US demonstrates clubfoot deformity. **F:** US of a fetus at 31-week gestation demonstrates fused thalami and lack of hemispheric separation consistent with holoprosencephaly. **G:** Coronal SSFSE T2 MRI of the same fetus in **F** confirms fusion of the thalami *(arrowhead)* and hemispheres *(solid arrow).* The ears are prominent and low in position *(dashed arrows).*

Fetal MR imaging may clarify findings of the fetal brain, specifically features of holoprosencephaly. Delineation of anatomic structures using fetal MR may be required for further evaluation of CDH, omphalocele, and renal and genitourinary abnormalities.

**Differential Diagnosis:** The observation of multisystem anomalies strongly supports a chromosomal abnormality or a severe manifestation of a syndrome. Many of the abnormalities overlap with trisomy 21 and 18, which would be differential consideration. Additional considerations could include Smith–Lemli–Opitz syndrome and Meckel–Gruber syndrome.

**Prognosis:** Trisomy 13 is highly lethal in utero. In a study evaluating the timing of miscarriage in fetuses with trisomy 13, it has been noted that the mean gestation is approximately 80 days and that only 5 of 62 fetuses carried beyond 100 days will survive beyond gestation.[44] This suggests that there are specific times during development when fetuses with trisomy 13 are more likely to die. Median postnatal survival is 7 to 10 days, and only 5% to 10% of infants with trisomy 13 survive 1 year.[37] Those who live beyond the perinatal period have severe developmental disabilities, feeding difficulties, apnea, poor growth, seizures,

and hypertension.[39] A case report of a female with trisomy 13 at age 12 years has been described.

**Management:** Once diagnosed, implications exist for both the fetus and the mother. Mothers of infants with trisomy 13 have an increased risk of developing severe preeclampsia.[45] This is theorized to be due to an increase in soluble fms-like tyrosine kinase (sFlt-1), an antiangiogenic protein whose gene is on chromosome 13. The protein can be released from the placenta into the maternal circulation and lead to endothelial dysfunction that may result in hypertension, proteinuria, and edema.[46]

Infants that survive to delivery should have chromosomal confirmation if not performed prenatally. Complete physical exam may show scalp defects, microcephaly, microphthalmia, cleft lip and palate, omphalocele, genital abnormalities, and polydactyly. Supportive care may be necessary for feeding difficulties and seizures.

**Recurrence Risk:** The recurrence risk for full trisomy 13 is 1% or the maternal age–associated risk or whichever is greater. The recurrence risk for parents with a balanced translocation is highly variable. The risk is estimated to be 20% for spontaneous abortion.[47] Recurrence risk for trisomy 13 can range from less than 1% for cases that involve mosaicism to 100% for rare cases of a parental balanced 13–13 Robertsonian translocation.

## Triploidy and Tetraploidy

Triploidy and tetraploidy are two forms of polyploidy syndromes. Unlike the aneuploidy syndromes described with one extra chromosome, the polyploidy syndromes consist of entire additional sets of genetic material. A haploid cell has 23 chromosomes; therefore, a triploid cell has 69 chromosomes and a tetraploid cell 92 chromosomes.

**Incidence:** Polyploidies can occur in up to 1% to 2% of conceptions, but are only seen in 1/10,000 live births.[48]

**Pathogenesis/Etiology:** In triploidy, the additional set of chromosomal material is due to failure of division in meiosis I or II in the spermatocyte (diandry) or oocyte (digyny), or, alternatively, the additional chromosomal material may arise from double fertilization of a normal ovum (dispermy). The source is most often paternal (75%), with the most common karyotype being 69 XXY (60%), and less frequent 69 XXX (37%) or 69 XYY (3%).[48] There is no association between triploidy and advanced maternal age, but there have been associations made between triploidy and delayed fertilization, for example in the presence of prolonged menstrual cycles or with oral contraceptive discontinuation.[49]

Triploid fetuses can have variable features that range from nearly normal-appearing to multiple anomalies (Fig. 20.11). Interestingly, the underlying meiotic error has been associated with the features of the fetus.[50] In one type, typically due to diandry, the fetus is well developed, but the placenta is large and cystic. The second type is associated with a growth-restricted fetus having a relatively large head, but a small and noncystic placenta.

**Diagnosis:** An increased AFP level on quad screen may suggest triploidy. A low PAPP-A can also be seen with triploidy.[51] It is possible to diagnose fetal tetraploidy from amniocentesis or CVS, although it is important to consider false-positive results on CVS due to confined placental mosaicism and placental artifact.[52] Maternal serum cell-free fetal DNA testing does not detect triploidy or tetraploidy. Chromosomal analysis should be offered to confirm the suspected diagnosis based on screening or imaging studies.

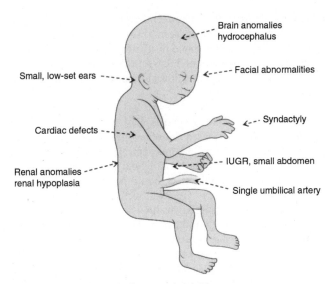

**FIGURE 20.11:** Common features of triploidy.

*Imaging:* Suspicion for triploidy should be raised when cystic placental changes or fetal anomalies, especially IUGR or disproportionately large head, are seen[53] (Fig. 20.12). Other features that can be seen on ultrasound include oligohydramnios, hydrocephalus, micrognathia, microphthalmia, omphalocele, neural tube defects, and 3–4 digital syndactyly.[53]

Tetraploidy is even more rare than triploidy. Only 24 fetuses with tetraploidy have been reported to date. Tetraploid fetuses can also have variable features, which include growth retardation, limb anomalies, abnormal positioning, low-set ears, increased nuchal thickness, and internal abnormalities.[54]

**Differential Diagnosis:** The differential diagnosis may include IUGR-related causes or other aneuploidy. A complete molar pregnancy (complete mole or hyatidiform mole) should also be considered. A complete mole occurs when a single sperm or two sperm fertilize an egg that has lost its DNA. If two sperm fertilize the egg, a diploid karyotype of either 46 XX or 46 XY could be seen. If a single sperm fertilizes such an egg, mitosis leads to replication of its genetic material, the genotype is diploid (46 XX—46 YY is not seen). The result is gestational trophoblastic disease, wherein a mass of trophoblastic tissue with dilated chorionic villi, grossly appearing as a cluster of grapes, grows within the uterus.[55]

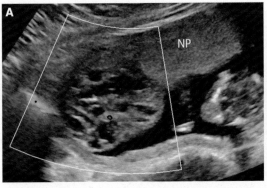 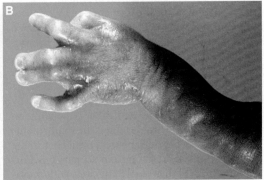

**FIGURE 20.12:** Cystic placental changes in triploidy. **A:** Ultrasound of a twin pregnancy at 17 weeks' GA shows the normal placenta *(NP)* of a healthy twin adjacent to an abnormally cystic placenta of the twin affected by triploidy. **B:** A pathologic photograph shows characteristic syndactyly of the third and fourth fingers. (Courtesy of Joe Siebert, Pathology Department, Seattle Children's Hospital, Washington, DC.)

**Prognosis:** Most triploid fetuses miscarry. Triploidy is one of the most common diagnoses seen in first-trimester products of conception.[56] For each triploid born alive, approximately 1,200 are miscarried. There are no known triploidy survivals beyond 10.5 months.[57] There are no known tetraploidy survivals beyond 2 years.[54]

**Management:** Triploid diagnosis has implications for the mother as there is increased risk of vaginal bleeding and severe preeclampsia. The large placenta can also cause postpartum hemorrhage.[58] Maternal risks and fetal prognosis should be discussed. Elective termination should be offered, if before 24 weeks in the United States. Cesarean section is indicated only to assist in delivery for maternal health.

In all cases of triploidy and tetraploidy, chromosomal analysis should be performed to confirm the diagnosis. Supportive comfort care is recommended as both typically present with multiple complications. Infants with triploidy that survive to delivery often have growth restriction, macrocephaly, colobomas, cleft palate, micrognathia, and hypotonicity. Infants with tetraploidy have growth restriction, developmental delay and dysmorphic features, such as microcephaly, a prominent narrow forehead, microphthalmia or anophthalmia, and cleft palate.[54] It is important to keep in mind that exam findings can be subtle, so the diagnosis can be unsuspected for both disorders.

**Recurrence Risk:** The cause of triploidy and tetraploidy is unclear. Parents with a fetus with triploidy or tetraploidy are thought to be at slightly increased risk for chromosomal abnormalities, not solely triploidy or tetraploidy.[54]

## Turner Syndrome

Turner syndrome (TS), also known as XO syndrome and monosomy X owing to loss of the second sex chromosome, is the most common chromosomal abnormality in females.[59] The syndrome was first described in 1938 by Henry Turner.

**Incidence:** TS is present in 1 in 2,500 female live births.[59] However, it is highly lethal in utero.[60] There is no relationship between increasing maternal age and prevalence of TS.[61]

**Pathogenesis/Etiology:** The loss of chromosomal material is variable and can be seen as an entirely lost chromosome, full 45X, in 50% of individuals, a structural abnormality of one X chromosome in 10% to 20%, or a mosaicism in 30% to 40%.[61] A common structural abnormality is the formation of an isochromosome, wherein one arm of the chromosome is duplicated and the other portion of the arm is lost. The lost sex chromosome can be due to either nondisjunction in the case of full 45X or from random inheritance of a derivative chromosome, as in the case of a structural chromosome abnormality.

The severity of clinical phenotype cannot be predicted by type of karyotype, but the phenotype may differ depending on parental origin of remaining X chromosome.[62] In some infants with TS, the disease may not become apparent until later in life when a female presents with short stature and primary amenorrhea.[60] Mosaicism is quite common in TS. In cases with mosaicism, the unaffected cells may contain a Y chromosome.

**Diagnosis:** Serum screening findings include reduced AFP, reduced estriol, and elevated β-hCG.[63] Detection of abnormal X chromosome ratios in cell-free fetal DNA is now available as a clinical screening test. Amniocentesis or CVS should be offered.

**Imaging:** Multiple anomalies may be present on ultrasound (Fig. 20.13), though biochemical markers and chromosomal analysis are more accurate at diagnosis. MRI typically is not necessary to aid in diagnosis.

TS results in lymphangiectasia and lymphatic malformations, manifesting in early pregnancy by fetal hydrops and large, septated cervical anechoic masses. The first-trimester manifestation of TS is typically an increased NT. A large yolk sac greater than 6 mm has also been reported.[64] Fetal hydrops may develop in either the first or the second trimester and is evident by pronounced skin thickening, pleural effusions, and ascites (Fig. 20.14A,B). Additional systems affected include the heart, kidneys, and the skeletal system. A full anatomy assessment in the second trimester may reveal left-heart congenital anomalies, such as coarctation or hypoplastic left heart syndrome. These cardiac lesions are the most common prenatal finding, whereas bifid aortic valve followed by mitral valve disease is the most common postnatally.[65] Findings of coarctation on grayscale and Doppler imaging are poststenotic dilatation distal to the level of narrowing in the descending thoracic aorta and an abrupt velocity increase at the site of stenosis. Renal abnormalities in affected fetuses are usually not evident until the second trimester. Malformations of the urinary system are present in 30% to 40% of patients with TS, with collecting-system anomalies most common, followed by horseshoe kidneys (Fig. 20.14C), malrotation, and ectopia.[66]

Short stature is a common clinical feature of TS, and the earliest prenatal manifestation of this is intrauterine growth retardation and short femur. Other skeletal abnormalities manifest postnatally and may include hip dislocation in infancy, scoliosis, and kyphosis. Short neck, broad chest, cubitus valgus, genu valgum, and short fourth metacarpals are also seen in TS.[67] Edema of the hands and feet in female fetuses is also potentially suggestive of TS. This may be seen both prenatally and postnatally.

**Differential Diagnosis:** In the first trimester of a monosomy X fetus, a thick NT reflects the development of a lymphatic malformation. The differential diagnosis for a thick NT is extensive and includes aneuploidy and multiple syndromes (Table 20.4).

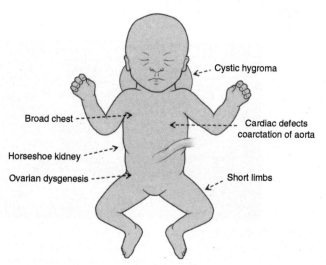

**FIGURE 20.13:** Common features of Turner syndrome (45,X).

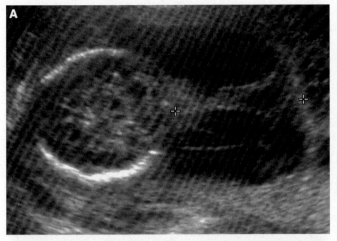
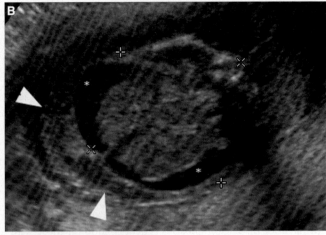
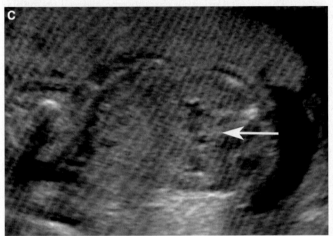
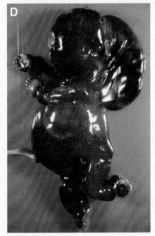

**FIGURE 20.14:** Turner syndrome in a 17-week fetus. **A:** A complex predominantly anechoic structure containing multiple septations along the posterior subcutaneous tissues of the neck *(calipers demarcating)*, consistent with a lymphatic malformation. **B:** Fetal hydrops was also observed, with ascites *(asterisks)* and extensive skin thickening *(arrowheads)*. **C:** The kidneys of this fetus are fused across the midline consistent with horseshoe kidney *(arrow)*. **D:** A postmortem photograph of another fetus with Turner syndrome shows a large nuchal lymphatic malformation.

---

| Table 20.4 | Differential Diagnosis for Abnormally Thick Nuchal Translucency (≥3 mm)[a,12,289,290] |
|---|---|

| *Chromosomal Anomalies* | *Skeletal Abnormalities* | *Other Syndromes and Sequences* | *Other Causes* |
|---|---|---|---|
| Trisomies: | Limb deletions syndromes: | Noonan syndrome | Congenital cardiac disease. |
| ■ Trisomy 21 (Down syndrome) | ■ Fanconi anemia | CHARGE syndrome | Chance of CHD increases |
| ■ Trisomy 18 (Edwards syndrome) | ■ Holt–Oram syndrome | Limb-body-wall complex | exponentially with increasing NT: 0.6%–5% with NT |
| ■ Trisomy 13 (Patau syndrome) | ■ Roberts syndrome | Arthrogryposis | between 2.5 and 3.5 mm; |
| ■ Other trisomies (9, 10, 22) | ■ Cornelia de Lange syndrome | | 64% with NT > 8.5 mm |
| | ■ Smith–Lemli–Opitz syndrome | | |
| Triploidy | ■ Ectrodactyly–ectodermal dysplasia–clefting (EEC) syndrome | Caudal regression syndrome | |
| Tetraploidy | ■ Thrombocytopenia-absent radius (TAR) syndrome | Congenital adrenal hyperplasia | |
| | ■ Orofaciodigital syndrome type IV | Congenital high airway obstruction syndrome | |
| Turner syndrome (XO syndrome) | Skeletal dysplasias: | Fryns syndrome | |
| Deletion syndromes: | ■ Achondrogenesis | Cerebro-fronto-facial syndrome | |
| ■ DiGeorge syndrome (22q11.2) | ■ Achondroplasia | Multiple pterygium syndrome | |
| ■ Deletion 5p (Cri du Chat syndrome) | ■ Camptomelic dysplasia | | |
| ■ Deletion 11q (Jacobsen syndrome) | ■ Ellis–van Creveld syndrome | | |
| | ■ Jeune thoracic dystrophy | | |
| | ■ Thanatophoric dysplasia | | |
| | ■ Spondylothoracic dysplasia | | |
| | ■ Diastrophic dysplasia | | |
| | ■ Spondyloepiphyseal dysplasia congenita (SEDC) | | |
| | Split-hand/foot malformation | | |
| | Spinal muscular atrophy | | |

[a]Over 100 chromosomal aberrations and syndromes have been described in association with a thickened NT, and this table only includes the more commonly seen entities.

Observed chromosomal syndromes other than TS include trisomy 13, trisomy 18, trisomy 21, and triploidy with mosaicism. In one series, the most frequently observed abnormality in non-septated cervical lymphatic malformation was trisomy 21, and that in septated malformations was TS.[68]

**Prognosis:** A small minority of conceptions with TS will survive to delivery. Girls with mosaicism for TS may have cells with all or a portion of the Y chromosome and are at risk for gonadoblastoma.[69] Intelligence is typically normal, but girls with TS may have learning disabilities.[60] Infants with TS may have a wide variety of clinical manifestations, but some are clinically normal at birth. The prognosis is generally good for those with only mild manifestations on prenatal imaging.

**Management:** The presence of a cervical lymphatic malformation, particularly in the setting of an abnormal karyotype, merits offering the option of termination of pregnancy. The newborn infant should have a complete physical exam with confirmed chromosome analysis. The typical phenotype includes short stature and a webbed appearance of the neck soft tissues, attributable to regression of the lymphatic malformation. Common issues immediately after birth include small for gestational age (SGA), lymphedema and feeding difficulty due to inefficient sucking and swallowing.[60]

Increasing recognition of silent CHD leading to shorter life span has led to an increased referral to pediatric cardiologist with echocardiography and cardiac MRI as needed. Cardiac lesions, such as coarctation, will most commonly require intervention. Renal anomalies may require renal ultrasound with routine follow-up to ensure continued normal renal function and to evaluate for complications, such as recurrent urinary tract infection and nephrolithiasis. Evaluation for congenital hip dysplasia is indicated.[60]

Long-term management of TS includes hormone treatment, especially growth hormone for short stature and estrogen for feminization and bone health. Close monitoring for other medical complications such as cardiovascular and autoimmune disease are warranted.[60–66]

**Recurrence Risk:** The recurrence risk for TS is very low as inheritance is sporadic. However, when women with TS conceive, amniocentesis should be offered as there is up to 30% risk of chromosome or congenital abnormalities.[69]

# GENETIC SYNDROMES

## Beckwith–Wiedemann Syndrome

Beckwith–Wiedemann Syndrome (BWS) is one in a group of syndromes known as the overgrowth syndromes.[70] Affected individuals may have asymmetric growth of the body, including hemihypertrophy of solid organs, and patients with BWS have an increased risk of Wilms tumor, hepatoblastoma, neuroblastoma, rhabdomyosarcoma, and adrenocortical carcinoma.[70]

**Incidence:** BWS affects 1 in 13,700 live births.[70] BWS is more common in women who have undergone in vitro fertilization (IVF) treatment. It is seen in 1 in 4,000 deliveries that have used assisted reproductive technology.

**Pathogenesis/Etiology:** Abnormal imprinting on chromosome 11p15.5 is the underlying genetic cause of this syndrome.[71] Imprinting refers to the phenomenon whereby addition of methyl groups to the genetic material from one parent determines its expression. In general, children of parents with impaired fertility who are conceived by assisted reproductive technology may have an increased risk for all imprinting disorders.[71]

Most individuals with BWS are reported to have normal chromosome studies or karyotypes, and approximately 85% of individuals with BWS have no family history.[72] Up to 20% of BWS is due to paternal uniparental disomy. In this scenario, both copies of 11p15.5 come from the father, and the maternal copy is lost. The parental origin of chromosome material on routine chromosome analysis is not discernible; therefore, this genetic abnormality is undetectable on karyotype. Methylation studies for the critical region on chromosome 11 are the most sensitive initial study. A minority of cases are due to mutation in the *CDKN1C* gene. This accounts for up to 15% of cases but is the most common cause of cases with apparent autosomal dominant inheritance.[73] Only 1% to 2% of cases have a recognizable cytogenetic abnormality, with duplication, inversion, or deletion as the cause.[70]

**Diagnosis:** Consideration of chromosome analysis and/or molecular genetic testing should be based on ultrasound findings (e.g., omphalocele, macrosomia, and macroglossia). Molecular studies for BWS are clinically available but must be specifically requested (Table 20.5). In cases with a known genetic mechanism in the family, testing could be performed on an amniocentesis sample. Without a known genetic mechanism, testing may be negative, but this does not exclude BWS due to the complex genetics of this syndrome. Regardless, diagnostic testing should be offered to evaluate for chromosomal abnormalities by amniocentesis or CVS.

*Imaging:* Abdominal wall defects are common in BWS.[72] The diagnosis may be suspected as early as 12 weeks' gestational age if an omphalocele is observed. Between 10% and 43% of fetuses with apparently isolated omphalocele have BWS.[74]

Second-trimester fetal anatomic ultrasound may detect the classic features of BWS, which include global macrosomia, macroglossia, omphalocele, enlargement and echogenicity of the kidneys, and polyhydramnios (Fig. 20.15A). Beckwith–Wiedemann should always be considered when macrosomia and an omphalocele are both observed either via US or MRI (Fig. 20.15B,C). However, the development of macrosomia is not usually seen until the late second trimester or third trimester. Routine ultrasound may also detect placentomegaly, with placental abnormalities suggesting a partial mole.[75] A higher-level focused ultrasound can reveal cardiomyopathy with cardiomegaly.

Additional occasional findings that standard ultrasound screening is unlikely to detect include cryptorchidism, hypospadias, embryonal tumors, pancreas enlargement, and renal cystic dysplasia. Although fetal MR imaging is not generally indicated to make this diagnosis, more detailed evaluation of the anatomy by MRI may be pursued for suboptimal imaging by ultrasound. On MRI, renal enlargement, a suspected neoplasm, and more subtle findings of BWS might be discernible (Fig. 20.15D).[76] Not only will MR imaging allow for evaluation of the extent of newly recognized fetal tumors in fetuses with BWS, but the technique

| Cause of BWS by Molecular Mechanism | Test Method | Mutations/Alterations Detected | Proportion of BWS Alterations Detected[1] |
|---|---|---|---|
| Loss of methylation at IC2 on the maternal chromosome | Methylation analysis | Methylation abnormalities at IC2 on the maternal chromosome | 50% |
| Gain of methylation at IC1 on the maternal chromosome | | Methylation abnormalities at IC1 on the maternal chromosome | 5% |
| Mutation of the maternal *CDKN1C* allele | Sequence analysis | *CDKN1C* mutations | 5% in persons with no family history of BWS ~40% in persons with a positive family history of BWS |
| Paternal uniparental disomy of 11p15.5 | UPD analysis | 11p15.5 paternal uniparental disomy | 20% |
| Duplication, inversion, or translocation of 11p15.5 | Cytogenetic analysis (karyotype) FISH | Cytogenetic duplication, inversion, or translocation Primarily used to clarify the relative positions of a chromosome 11 inversion or translocation and to confirm duplication of chromosome 11 | 1% |
| Submicroscopic genomic alteration within chromosome 11p15.5 | Microdeletion/ microduplication analysis | Genomic alterations involving IC1 and/or IC2 | Not yet accurately determined |

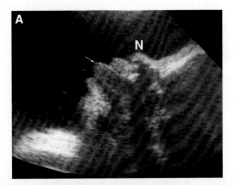

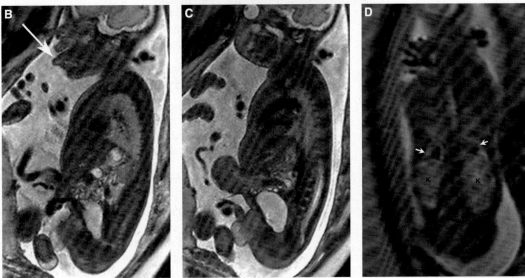

**FIGURE 20.15:** Beckwith–Weidemann syndrome ultrasound and MR images in three separate fetuses. **A:** Third-trimester sagittal view of the face shows macroglossia *(arrow)*; N, nose. **B:** Sagittal SSFSE T2 Fetal MR in a 30-week fetus with enlargement of the tongue *(arrow)* persistently protruding beyond the lips. **C:** Sagittal T2 image of same fetus demonstrates a small omphalocele containing loops of bowel. (Courtesy of Dr. Chris Cassady, Houston, TX.) **D:** Coronal SSFSE T2 image of a third fetus diagnosed with BWS after birth. Fetus has enlarged adrenal glands *(arrow)* and kidneys (K) bilaterally.

has been shown to be useful in the distinction of adrenal cystic changes from neuroblastoma.[77]

**Differential Diagnosis:** Other causes of macrosomia include incorrect dates, maternal diabetes, genetic anomalies, and chromosomal defects (Table 20.6). Genetic syndromes, including Perlman (small mouth, small upturned nose, bilateral renal enlargement, macrosomia, renal hamartomas, hydronephrosis, hydroureter, developmental delay, and cryptorchidism), Sotos (pre- and postnatal overgrowth, developmental delay, macrocephaly, dolichocephaly, a prominent forehead, large hands and feet, advanced bone age, prominent jaw, and variable psychomotor developmental delay), Weaver (prenatal overgrowth, developmental delay, macrocephaly, and camptodactyly), and Simpson–Golabi–Behmel (pre- and postnatal overgrowth, macrocephaly, congenital diaphragmatic hernia, coarse facies, palatal abnormalities, congenital heart defects, generalized hypotonia, and ventriculomegaly).[75] Chromosomal abnormalities associated with fetal overgrowth as noted in Table 20.6 include mosaic tetrasomy 12p, also known as Pallister–Killian syndrome, which is characterized by normal growth or overgrowth, congenital diaphragmatic hernia, CHD, and postaxial polydactyly.[78]

Confirmation of gestational dates and evaluation for maternal diabetes should be done first. Next, a detailed ultrasound

| Table 20.6 | Differential Diagnosis of Fetal Overgrowth | | |
|---|---|---|---|
| | | Gene Involved | Inheritance Pattern |
| **Incorrect gestational dating** | | N/A | N/A |
| **Maternal diabetes** | | N/A | N/A |
| **Genetic** | | | |
| Sotos syndrome | | NSD1 | Sporadic/AD |
| Weaver syndrome | | NSD1 | Sporadic/AD |
| Beckwith–Wiedemann syndrome | | Imprinted gene on 11p15 | 85% sporadic/ 15% AD |
| Simpson–Golabi–Behmel syndrome | | GPC3 | X-linked |
| Bannayan–Riley– Ruvalcaba syndrome | | PTEN | AD |
| **Chromosome** | | | |
| Trisomy 4p16.3 | | N/A | N/A |
| Trisomy 5p | | N/A | N/A |
| Trisomy 12p | | N/A | N/A |
| Pallister–Killian syndrome (mosaic tetrasomy 12p) | | N/A | N/A |
| Trisomy 15q25 | | N/A | N/A |
| Deletion (monosomy) 22q13 | | N/A | N/A |
| Mosaic trisomy 8 | | N/A | N/A |

AD means autosomal dominant.

should be performed to evaluate for renal and cardiac anomalies. BWS is rarely associated with cardiac anomalies, but other overgrowth syndromes (e.g., Simpson–Golabi–Behmel syndrome) have a high incidence of cardiac defects (up to 50%).[71]

**Prognosis:** The reported perinatal mortality rate in BWS from prematurity, macroglossia, and cardiomyopathy is as high as 20%.[79] Patients with BWS have a higher risk of developing tumors in their first decade of life, after which the risk approaches the baseline risk of the general population. The most frequently observed tumors in BWS are Wilms tumor and hepatoblastoma, which comprise 43% and 12% of reported cancers, respectively.[80] Less common tumors include adrenocortical carcinoma, neuroblastoma, and rhabdomyosarcoma, as well as other benign or malignant neoplasms.[81] Intelligence and development are often normal.[82]

**Management:** The degree of macrosomia may influence the mode of delivery. An antenatal diagnosis can prepare the neonatology team for management of airway obstruction by macroglossia and for the severe hypoglycemia that can affect these patients.[79] Conservative postnatal surveillance for intra-abdominal tumors is performed with renal ultrasound examinations every 3 months until the age of 8 years; liver ultrasound examinations every 3 months until the age of 4 years; and measurements of serum AFP levels every 6 weeks until the age of 4 years.[80] Alpha-fetoprotein is normally very high in neonates, and it is not until 6 to 8 months of age that the AFP in a normal patient decreases to adult levels. AFP levels in BWS patients are less abnormal than previously expected; however, an increase in the AFP level in these patients, even if the levels remain relatively low, could indicate the growth of a hepatoblastoma.[80]

**Recurrence Risk:** Identification of the underlying genetic mechanism causing BWS permits better estimation of recurrence risk. In families with suspected autosomal dominant inheritance (15%), the recurrence risk is up to 50%, but in other forms of inheritance (e.g., methylation abnormalities), the recurrence risk would be expected to be very low.[83]

## Holt–Oram Syndrome

Holt–Oram syndrome (HOS), also known as Heart and Hand syndrome, was first described in 1960 as a disease affecting cardiac and skeletal development.[84] The syndrome is characterized by asymmetric abnormalities of the limbs (usually the left upper extremity) and cardiac defects (most commonly secundum atrial septal defects).

**Incidence:** HOS affects approximately 1 in 100,000 live births.[85]

**Pathogenesis/Etiology:** HOS is caused by mutations in the T-box transcription factor 5 (TBX5) gene (at 12q24.1).[86,87] Point mutations and other sequence variants account for more than 70% of cases, while deletions and duplications are seen in less than 1%.[87] Interestingly, the sal-like 4 (Drosophila) SALL4 gene (at 20q13) has also been associated with a phenotype clinically indistinguishable from HOS and accounts for a small portion of the identified mutations, but mutations in this syndrome may be associated with additional congenital anomalies, especially renal, tympanic, and ocular.[88]

**Diagnosis:** There is no recognized serum screening abnormality that would alert the clinician to a diagnosis of HOS prenatally. If HOS is suspected, amniocentesis could be offered, though genetic testing is not required for diagnosis and could be falsely negative. Karyotype alone would not be expected to detect the vast majority of molecular genetic causes of HOS; *TBX5* gene testing would be required.

*Imaging:* The only first-trimester abnormality that may be evident with this syndrome is an abnormal nuchal translucency. The diagnosis is typically made in the mid-to-late second trimester by ultrasound, although the findings may be overlooked depending on ability to view the extremities carefully. Three-dimensional ultrasound offers significant detail of the bones and soft tissues of the fetus, enabling the diagnosis to be made more accurately in the second trimester.[89] It has been suggested that the ideal time to sonographically evaluate the upper extremity is between 13 and 16 weeks of gestation when the amniotic fluid volume enables free movement of the fetus, thereby permitting rotation of the forearm such that the radius and ulna can be viewed in a single plane. Outside of this gestational period, hypoplasia of the ulna or radius can be more easily missed.[89]

HOS may present in a highly variable way, with limb anomalies identified from the shoulder through the hand, summarized in Table 20.7 (Fig. 20.16).[90] Deformity of the sternum has also been described.[91]

Cardiac defects affect approximately 85% of fetuses with this disorder. The most common cardiac defect is an ostium secundum atrial septal defect (ASD).[84] The cardiac abnormalities span a spectrum from normal cardiac development to combined severe ASD, ventricular septal defect (VSD), and pulmonic stenosis.[92] Other reported cardiac anomalies include Ebstein anomaly, mitral valve prolapse, transposition of the great vessels, tetralogy of Fallot, and anomalous pulmonary venous return.[91]

**Differential Diagnosis:** Numerous conditions may lead to an abnormal NT (see Table 20.4). Other conditions that manifest

| Table 20.7 | Extremity Findings That May Be Seen in Holt–Oram Syndrome |
|---|---|
| Shoulder | Clavicle hypoplasia |
| | Deformity of scapula |
| | Deformed head of humerus |
| | Accessory bones at shoulder joint |
| Forearm | Synostosis of radius and ulna |
| | Partial or complete radial hypoplasia |
| Carpus | Deformed carpal bones |
| | Supernumary carpal bones |
| Thumb and digits | Hypoplastic thenar eminences |
| | Triphalangia |
| | Absent thumbs |
| | Clinodactyly of thumb |
| | Syndactyly |
| | Absent first metacarpal |
| | Short middle phalanx of fifth digit |
| | Clinodactyly of fifth digit |
| Whole limb | Phocomelia |

with limb anomalies include the VACTERL/VATER association, thrombocytopenia-absent radius (TAR) syndrome, Goldenhar syndrome, trisomy 13, and trisomy 18. Rare conditions such as Fanconi syndrome, Nager syndrome, Townes–Brocks syndrome, and Roberts syndrome should be considered in the differential diagnosis, but additional findings, such as micrognathia or in utero growth restriction, microcephaly, and radial ray deficiencies, would be apparent. Poorly controlled diabetes may also lead to overlapping findings, including heart disease and radial malformations.

**Prognosis:** This syndrome is not associated with an increased rate of fetal demise. The prognosis will depend on the severity of cardiac disease.

**Management:** When an infant with suspected HOS is born, complete physical exam should be performed. Postnatal diagnostic criteria include: (1) upper limb malformation involving carpal bone, (2) personal or family history of congenital heart malformation, and (3) personal history of cardiac conduction

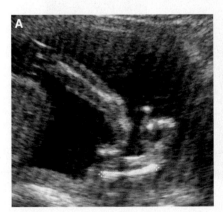 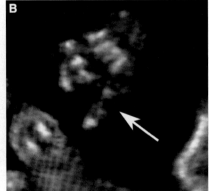 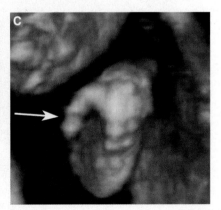

**FIGURE 20.16:** Radial deficiencies and suspected Holt-Oram syndrome. **A:** Ultrasound of the left upper extremity in this 17-week-GA fetus shows a single forearm bone and radial angulation of the wrist. **B,C:** In a different fetus evaluated at 20-week-GA with suspected Holt–Oram syndrome, there is absence of the thumb and pollicization of the index finger *(arrows)* of the right hand seen by 2D **(B)** and 3D **(C)** ultrasound. Findings were symmetric (left upper extremity not shown). Anatomic assessment was also notable for a two-vessel cord and an atrial septal defect (not shown).

disease.[67] Exclusion criteria for HOS include other specific congenital anomalies such as ulnar ray anomalies only, lower limb anomalies, the presence of renal, vertebral, craniofacial, or anal anomalies, or abnormalities in auditory or visual systems.[67] Because of the varied clinical presentations, hand x-rays should be taken to evaluate for carpal bone anomalies.[90] If an infant meets the clinical diagnosis of HOS, *TBX5* gene testing should be sent. Cardiology consultation, electrocardiography (ECG), and echocardiography should be performed in view of the high incidence of cardiac disease.[87]

**Recurrence Risk:** The recurrence risk depends on the underlying genetic mechanism. If one parent carries the same mutation, the recurrence risk would be expected to be up to 50%; if neither parent carries the mutation, the syndrome is isolated with a very low recurrence risk.

## Meckel–Gruber Syndrome

Meckel–Gruber syndrome (MKS) is also referred to as dysencephalia splanchnocystica and is invariably lethal. The syndrome was first described by Meckel in 1822 and later by Gruber in 1934,[93] and is most frequently characterized by an occipital encephalocele in 80% of cases, nephromegaly with microcystic dysplasia, and postaxial polydactyly.[93,94]

**Incidence:** The incidence of MKS ranges from 1 in 13,250 to 1 in 140,000 live births worldwide with a predilection for the Finnish population (up to 1 in 9,000).[85,95]

**Pathogenesis/Etiology:** MKS is inherited autosomal recessive and has some variability to its expression, even among affected siblings.[93] The disease is now recognized to be secondary to a ciliary dysfunction and is categorized with other primary ciliopathies such as Bardet–Biedl and Joubert syndromes.

MKS demonstrates locus heterogeneity. There are a number of genes associated with MKS, including *TMEM216, TMEM67, CEP290, RPGRIP1L,* and *CC2D2A,* which are located on a number of different chromosomes.[96,97] Regardless of the specific

gene change, the result in embryogenesis is dysfunction of primary cilia.[98] The diagnosis is made clinically, though there is controversy over the specific criteria that should be used.[85,99]

**Diagnosis:** There is no recognized serum screening abnormality that would alert the clinician to a diagnosis of MKS prenatally.

**Imaging:** The diagnosis may be made as early as the first trimester at 10 to 11 weeks, with visualization of the posterior encephalocele and polydactyly.[100,101] Anomalies of the central nervous system may be detected by screening ultrasound, and further evaluated with fetal MR imaging.

Malformations of the brain and face, in addition to an occipital encephalocele noted in 80% of cases, might include a Dandy–Walker malformation (approximately one-third of cases), cerebellar hypoplasia, ventriculomegaly, microcephaly, brainstem dysplasia, cleft palate, and micrognathia (Fig. 20.17A,B).[93,99]

Renal disease may be evident sonographically by abnormal renal enlargement, microcystic changes, heterogeneous corticomedullary differentiation, and large hypoechoic medullary regions. When present, hyperechogenicity of affected kidneys is appreciable as early as 17 weeks' gestational age, when the renal cortex appears brighter than that of the fetal liver and spleen.[17] Nephromegaly and abnormally increased T2 signal is appreciable on fetal MR (Fig. 20.17C). The renal disease may manifest with oligohydramnios, although the amniotic fluid volume may remain normal. In the setting of oligohydramnios, fetal MR imaging is particularly helpful, given the limitations of evaluation by ultrasound without sufficient amniotic fluid.[102] Hepatic fibrosis may also be evident on necropsy, although this is not discernible on prenatal imaging.

Other features that could be detected prenatally include sloping forehead and bowing of the long bones of extremities. Cleft lip and palate, micrognathia, microphthalmia, and genital ambiguity are also reported.

**Differential Diagnosis:** Other syndromes that manifest with both brain and renal anomalies and polydactyly include trisomy 13, Joubert syndrome, oral-facial-digital (OFD) syndromes

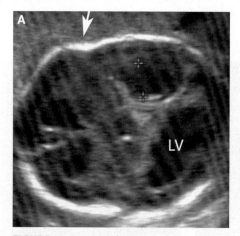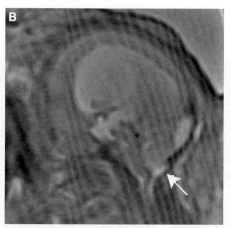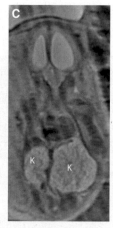

**FIGURE 20.17:** Meckel–Gruber syndrome in a 23-week-GA fetus. **A:** Axial US through the brain shows abnormally dilated ventricles (*LV,* lateral ventricle and calipers), as well as abnormal shape of the skull, with a buckled appearance in the region of the coronal suture (*arrow*), possibly related to hydrocephalus or to an abnormal suture. **B:** Subsequent fetal MR T2 SSFSE image in sagittal plane shows aqueductal stenosis (*asterisk* marks the tectum, dorsal to the expected aqueduct), kinked deformity of the brainstem, and a small occipital cephalocele (*arrow*). **C:** Coronal MR SSFSE T2 image shows marked enlargement and abnormal widespread cystic change of the bilateral renal parenchyma (denoted by *K*).

types I and II, short rib polydactyly syndrome, and Smith–Lemli–Opitz syndrome. Another closely related ciliopathy to MKS is Joubert syndrome, a nonlethal condition characterized by vermian hypoplasia, thick horizontal superior cerebellar peduncles, and a deep interpeduncular cistern, creating a molar tooth sign.[103] Distinguishing the two syndromes from one another is important given the fatality of MKS.[104]

The primary differential for cystic renal disease in the absence of other associated anomalies are autosomal recessive and autosomal dominant polycystic kidney disease. The increased renal echogenicity seen with MKS can be similar in other renal conditions that have innumerable microscopic cysts, tubular dilatation, or parenchymal dysplasia. Other syndromes to consider in the differential diagnosis of large and echogenic kidneys include Bardet–Biedl (also features ventriculomegaly and polydactyly), Ivermark II, and Jarcho–Levin syndromes (also features platyspondyly and spondylocostal dysplasia).[17,105]

**Prognosis:** This syndrome is lethal, and infants that survive gestation die within a few days after birth.[85]

**Management:** Families should receive genetic counseling if the diagnosis is suspected. Amniocentesis should be offered to exclude a chromosomal abnormality, though MKS has complex genetics and cannot be diagnosed by karyotype alone. Termination can be offered in the United States if diagnosis is made before 24 weeks. If an infant with suspected MKS is carried to delivery, supportive comfort care should be suggested at the time of birth. An autopsy should be performed and genetic testing to provide counseling for future pregnancies.

**Recurrence Risk:** As MKS is autosomal recessive, the recurrence risk is 25%.[85]

## Cornelia de Lange Syndrome

Cornelia de Lange syndrome (CdLS) is also known as Brachmann-de Lange syndrome, as Brachmann first described it in the early 1900s, and later, de Lange contributed to the description. Features of this syndrome (summarized in Table 20.8)

| Table 20.8 | Features of Cornelia de Lange Syndrome and Their Respective Frequencies | |
|---|---|---|
| | | **Frequency (%)** |
| Growth failure | | >95 |
| Intellectual disability | | >95 |
| Limb abnormalities | | >95 |
| Hirsutism | | >80 |
| Micrognathia | | 80 |
| High and arched palate with clefts | | 30 |
| Mandibular spurs | | 42 |
| Seizures | | 25 |
| GI abnormalities | | 1–4 |
| Sensorineural hearing loss | | >80 |
| Ptosis or other ocular problems | | 50 |
| Cryptorchidism | | 73 |
| Congenital heart disease | | 25 |

include pre- and postnatal growth restriction, limb anomalies, distinctive facial features, cardiac defects, and congenital diaphragmatic hernia.[106] The facial features include hypertrophy and fusion of the eyebrows, arched eyebrows, long eyelashes, small upturned nose, and microcephaly.[107]

**Incidence:** Estimates of the incidence of CdLS vary from 1 in 10,000 to 1 in 100,000.[106,107]

**Pathogenesis/Etiology:** Several genes are known to cause CdLS.[108,109] The gene responsible determines the inheritance pattern; *NIPBL* and *SMC3* are inherited in an autosomal dominant manner, while *SMC1A* and *HDAC8* show X-linked inheritance. Both point mutations and deletions/duplications are known to cause CdLS.

**Diagnosis:** A helpful adjunct to first- and second-trimester imaging may be measurement of pregnancy-associated plasma protein (PAPP-A), which is abnormally low in this syndrome.[110] Diagnostic testing with amniocentesis or CVS can be offered to families in which a diagnosis of CdLS is suspected, but typically karyotype does not demonstrate abnormality. Further, even if the three genes known to cause CdLS are tested, a negative result does not exclude the diagnosis of CdLS. Amniocentesis can evaluate for other chromosomal anomalies in the differential diagnosis.

**Imaging:** US is the primary mode of detection, with fetal MRI less helpful given the anatomic areas affected. The syndrome may be among many suspected as early as the first trimester on the basis of sonographic detection of a thickened nuchal translucency and generalized skin edema (Fig. 20.18A,B). The diagnosis of CdLS can be suspected on the basis of ultrasound features of limb reduction defects, cardiac defects, and IUGR, although the in utero growth restriction is not usually recognized until 20 to 25 gestational weeks (Fig. 20.18C,D). Growth retardation typically occurs prenatally and is symmetric.[111]

Head and facial abnormalities that may be detected prenatally include brachycephaly, microcephaly, micrognathia, short broad nose with anteverted nares, fusion of eyebrows, low-set ears, hypertrichosis, and long eyelashes (Fig. 20.19A,B).[112] Recognition of the facial features seen in CdLS is enhanced by three-dimensional US in the second and third trimesters.

The limb malformations, if present, are quite variable, although most commonly affect the ulnar aspect of the upper extremities and also include syndactyly, micromelia, contractures at the elbows and oligodactyly (Fig. 20.18C,D). Lower extremities are less likely to show abnormalities.

Cardiac abnormalities frequently identified are atrial and ventricular septal defects, but there have also been descriptions of hypoplastic left ventricle and coarctation of the aorta.[113] Genitourinary tract anomalies include polycystic kidneys, renal ectopia, pyelectasis, cryptorchidism, and ambiguous genitalia.[114] Bilateral diaphragmatic hernia is a rarer finding, but confirmation with fetal MRI can be helpful (Fig. 20.19C).

Interestingly, despite the number of systems that are maldeveloped in this syndrome, prenatal diagnosis can be elusive, with one report showing nearly 70% of postnatally diagnosed cases of de Lange syndrome missed by routine prenatal imaging.[115] The disease should be suspected with the observations of IUGR, ulnar deficiencies of the upper extremities, and cardiac defects and/or congenital diaphragmatic hernia.[106]

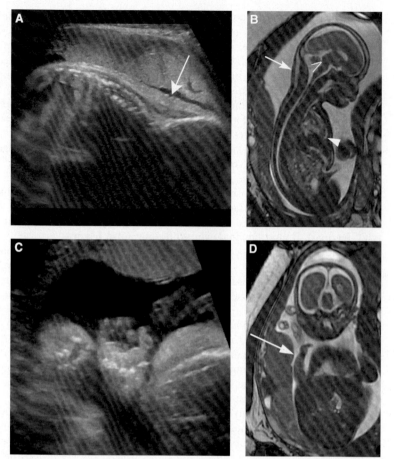

**FIGURE 20.18:** Cornelia de Lange syndrome in a 29-week fetus. **A:** Progressive hydrops had been monitored in this fetus, with worsening pleural effusions, a small pericardial effusion, minimal ascites, diffuse skin thickening *(arrow)*, and increasing amniotic fluid index. **B:** Sagittal SSFP T2 MR image shows skin thickening *(arrow)*, pericardial effusion *(arrowhead)*, and cerebellar vermian hypoplasia, with an increased tegmentovermian angle (marked by *white lines*). **C:** Ultrasound of the extremities was notable for abnormally short right upper extremity containing a single forearm bone and an abnormal number of digits. The left hand was in a fixed flexed position (not shown here). **D:** Coronal MR image again depicts the abnormal shortened right upper extremity *(arrow)*.

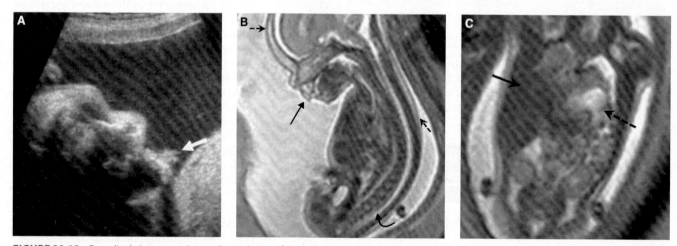

**FIGURE 20.19:** Cornelia de Lange syndrome. **A:** Axial view of the orbits shows the characteristic long eyelashes *(arrow)* seen in this syndrome. **B:** Fetal MRI at 23 weeks. Sagittal SSFSE T2 MR demonstrates prominent philtrum *(arrow)*, diffuse soft tissue edema *(dashed arrows)* and low conus *(curved arrow)*. **C:** Cor SSFSE T2 in same fetus shows bilateral congenital diaphragmatic hernia with liver in the right chest *(arrow)* and stomach in the left *(dashed arrow)*.

**Differential Diagnosis:** CdLS overlaps with a number of other syndromes. Abnormal nuchal translucency and limb anomalies may be seen with Apert syndrome, chromosomal abnormalities, multiple pterygium syndrome, Roberts syndrome, and Smith–Lemli–Opitz syndrome. The facial appearance in CdLS is similar to that seen in Roberts syndrome, but the limb anomalies will distinguish the two. Short radial ray may be observed in Fanconi anemia, TAR and in HOS.

**Prognosis:** Developmental delay is nearly universal (up to 95%), but varies in severity. Mean IQ is 53 but can range from below 30 to 100.[116] Behavioral problems are also seen and include autistic features and self-mutilating behaviors. Life expectancy can be normal, as patients with CdLS have been reported to live into their 60s. Causes of death are varied but can include aspiration pneumonia, apnea, CHD, intestinal obstruction, and postsurgical complications.[117]

**Management:** Prenatal surveillance of the IUGR is routine. Genetic evaluation should be sought shortly after birth to discuss diagnosis and options for testing. Postnatal difficulties are numerous and require multidisciplinary attention. Children affected by this syndrome have severe developmental delay and behavioral difficulties, failure to thrive, feeding difficulties, swallowing difficulties, and postnatal growth restriction. Early intervention should be initiated to optimize psychomotor development and communication skills.

After an infant with suspected CdLS is born, complete physical exam should be performed. Common issues after birth include gastroesophageal reflux disease (GERD) and feeding difficulties. Many patients with CdLS require gastrostomy tube or supplemental formula. Gastrointestinal evaluation should be completed and include upper GI series, endoscopy, and possibly pH probe.[106] Growth parameters should be plotted on CdLS-specific growth charts.[118] With increased risk of cardiac defects, echocardiography should be performed. Upper extremity radiographs should be considered to evaluate any upper extremity anomalies.[106] Ophthalmology evaluation including dilated exam and evaluation for blocked tear ducts should be performed.[119] Renal ultrasound should be obtained to evaluate for renal anomalies, physical exam for cryptorchidism, and hearing tests to exclude hearing loss.[106]

**Recurrence Risk:** With a negative family history, recurrence risk is estimated at 1.5% because of the potential for germline mosaicism. With family history of CdLS, recurrence risk is based on genetic transmission, but may be as high as 50%.[108]

## Smith–Lemli–Opitz Syndrome

Smith–Lemli–Opitz syndrome (SLOS) was first recognized in 1964 as a constellation of clinical findings, including microcephaly, broad alveolar ridge, severe feeding disorder, hypospadias, and global developmental delay.[120]

**Incidence:** Incidence is 1 in 20,000 to 1 in 40,000 live births.[121]

**Pathogenesis/Etiology:** This syndrome arises from a genetic abnormality causing absent or deficient levels of 7-dehydrocholesterol reductase (DHCR7), an enzyme required in the cholesterol formation pathway.[121] The resulting overproduction of 7-dehydrocholesterol (a cholesterol precursor) is thought to affect several systems during fetal development, and the phenotypic manifestations cover a spectrum from mild developmental delay and syndactyly to lethality.[122] The wide variability of malformations is reflected in a scoring system (Table 20.9) used by Bialer et al.[123] to analyze phenotypic correlations between individuals and siblings. The study assigned a numeric value of 0, 1, or 2 to the relative severity of various anomalies across all systems. This evaluation determined that males with complete feminization, tending to have polydactyly and cleft palate, are among the more severely affected patients. Other findings in SLOS include cleft palate and cardiac defects.[124]

Mutations in *DHCR7* are detected by sequence analysis in 96% of SLOS cases.[125]

**Diagnosis:** Detection of elevated levels of 7-dehydrocholesterol in the amniotic fluid, as well as absence of unconjugated estriol, confirms the diagnosis.[126] However, up to 10% of affected

| | | Possible Features Seen in Smith–Lemli–Opitz Syndrome Are Summarized in a Scoring System Established to Evaluate Phenotypic Correlations between Individuals and Siblings |
|---|---|---|
| **Table 20.9** | | |

| Organ | Score | Criteria |
|---|---|---|
| Brain | 1 | Seizures; qualitative MR abnormality |
| | 2 | Major CNS malformations; gyral abnormalities |
| Oral | 1 | Bifid uvula or submucous cleft |
| | 2 | Cleft hard palate or median cleft lip |
| Acral | 0 | Non–Y-shaped minimal toe syndactyly |
| | 1 | Y-shaped 2/3 toe syndactyly; club foot; upper or lower polydactyly; other syndactyly |
| Eye | 2 | Cataract; frank microphthalmia |
| Heart | 0 | Functional defects |
| | 1 | Single-chamber or vessel defect |
| | 2 | Complex cardiac malformation |
| Kidney | 0 | Functional defect |
| | 1 | Simple cystic kidney disease |
| | 2 | Renal agenesis; clinically important cystic disease |
| Liver | 0 | Induced hepatic abnormality |
| | 1 | Simple structural abnormality |
| | 2 | Progressive liver disease |
| Lung | 0 | Functional pulmonary disease |
| | 1 | Abnormal lobation; hypoplasia |
| | 2 | Pulmonary cysts; other major malformations |
| Bowel | 0 | Functional GI disease |
| | 1 | Pyloric stenosis |
| | 2 | Hirschsprung disease |
| Genitalia | 1 | Simple hypospadias |
| | 2 | Ambiguous for female genitalia in 46,XY; frank genital malformation in 46,XX |

Adapted from Bialer MG, Penchaszadeh VB, Kahn E, et al. Female external genitalia and mullerian duct derivatives in a 46,XY infant with the Smith-Lemli-Opitz syndrome. *Am J Med Genet.* 1987;28:723–731.

patients may have estriol and cholesterol levels in the normal range.[127] Gene sequencing can also be done.[125]

Prenatal diagnostic testing options for ambiguous genitalia include multiple molecular tests and amniotic fluid hormone concentrations. In the absence of other fetal anomalies or growth retardation on ultrasound, prenatal karyotype with testing for the sex-determining region Y gene (SRY gene) on the Y chromosome is the most useful test when ambiguous genitalia is suspected.

**Imaging:** Ultrasound findings that may raise suspicion for SLOS include growth restriction, limb anomalies, holoprosencephaly and cardiac defects. The primary features present in SLOS include microcephaly, limb malformations, and genital abnormalities, and variable features include brain malformations, cardiac defects, renal anomalies, and late-onset intrauterine growth retardation. Syndactyly of the second and third toes is clinically present in 97% of cases.[127]

The prenatal detection of this disorder might be seen in the late first trimester by recognition of a thick NT.[128] Abnormalities of the limbs, such as polydactyly, might be apparent as early as 12 weeks' GA. At this stage, karyotyping is helpful to rule out chromosomal causes.

Second-trimester ultrasound and fetal MR may show findings that range from normal to multisystem anomalies. The most frequent detectable trait prenatally is IUGR.[122,129] Previously described brain anomalies in SLOS fetuses include ventriculomegaly, agenesis of the corpus callosum, cerebellar hypoplasia, and holoprosencephaly, which may be better elucidated on fetal MRI (Fig. 20.20A,B). Facial abnormalities that may be detected prenatally include hypertelorism, micrognathia, and cleft palate (Fig. 20.20C).

Limb abnormalities may involve the upper or lower extremities. Postaxial polydactyly of the hands, clenched hands, and valgus deformity of the feet are additional findings described in this syndrome (Fig. 20.20D). Soft tissue syndactyly of the second and third toes is the most common anomaly of the skeletal system (Fig. 20.20E). Renal abnormalities seen in SLOS include hypoplasia, hydronephrosis, or cystic change.[129] Although the fetal genitalia can usually be assessed by 20 weeks' gestational age, the prenatal recognition of ambiguous genitalia is difficult, with studies showing prenatal identification in only approximately 25% of postnatal diagnosed cases.[130] Fetal MRI may be helpful in genitalia evaluation.

**Differential Diagnosis:** The differential considerations for a thickened NT are extensive (see Table 20.4). In the presence of postaxial polydactyly and genital anomalies, two main categories of syndromes should be considered in the differential of SLOS. Polydactyly syndromes include Meckel–Gruber, Joubert, OFD syndrome, trisomy 13, Ellis-van Creveld, and short rib polydactyly syndromes. Many of these syndromes have associated limb anomalies, but they do not include the 2–3 syndactyly classically associated with SLOS. Syndromes manifesting with genital abnormalities include Carpenter syndrome, which also shares abnormal head shape and polydactyly in common with SLOS, congenital adrenal hyperplasia, CdLS, Opitz G/BBB syndrome, and the MURCS association (müllerian duct aplasia, renal aplasia, cervicothoracic somite dysplasia).

**Prognosis:** The severity of disease depends on the amount of DHCR7 activity. Two types of Smith–Lemli–Optiz syndrome have been described: type I and type II. Type II is associated with absent DHCR7 activity altogether, whereas in type I, some amount of activity is present. In type II, neonatal death occurs. In less severe cases (type I), the children exhibit growth retardation, intellectual disability, behavior abnormalities, and failure to thrive. Life expectancy depends on the degree of internal malformations and on the amount of supportive care during childhood and adulthood.[122]

**Management:** Infants with suspicion for SLOS should have complete physical exam. During the newborn period, feeding difficulty is the most likely complication, and gastrostomy is frequently required. Airway management may be necessary.

Other medical issues include GI problems (pyloric stenosis, GERD, Hirschsprung disease or constipation), recurrent acute otitis media, and eye problems (cataracts, ptosis, or strabismus).

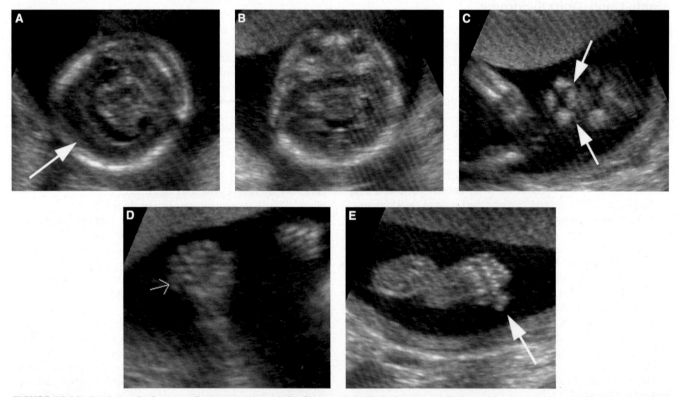

**FIGURE 20.20:** Smith–Lemli–Opitz syndrome in a 21-week-GA fetus, with IUGR, holoprosencephaly, and limb anomalies. **A:** Ultrasound images through the fetal head show characteristic features of alobar holoprosencephaly, with fusion of the cerebral hemispheres *(arrow)*. **B:** Hypotelorism and fusion of the thalami are noted. **C:** Coronal image through the fetal face shows bilateral cleft palate defects *(arrows)*. **D:** Both the upper extremities and lower extremities were notable for postaxial polydactyly *(arrow* marks the supernumary digits). **E:** Soft tissue fusion of the second and third toes is observed *(arrow)*.

Ophthalmology evaluation should be obtained to evaluate for associated eye findings, as up to 20% of patients with SLOS have congenital cataracts.[131] Hearing screening should be completed to evaluate for conductive or sensorineural hearing loss.

CNS malformations are seen in SLOS (including Dandy–Walker malformation, holoprosencephaly); therefore, postnatal brain MRI is often helpful for accurate diagnosis.[132] Renal malformations (hypoplastic or cystic kidneys) have been reported, and renal ultrasound is typically performed.[133]

Cholesterol supplementation has been reported to result in improved growth, reduced photosensitivity, and increased nerve conduction velocity.[134,135] However, improvement in cognitive outcomes has not been documented. Cholesterol supplementation in young patients can be given with dried or pasteurized egg yolk and has minimal side effects.[136] Patients with SLOS may require stress-dosed steroid treatment during acute illness.[137]

Developmental delay ranges from near-normal intelligence to severe cognitive disability, but is generally severe. Long-term issues include failure to thrive, risk of behavioral problems, and psychiatric disorders.[138]

**Recurrence Risk:** Gene testing can be performed to allow for prenatal testing in future at-risk pregnancies.[139] SLOS demonstrates autosomal recessive inheritance; thus, recurrence risk is 25%.[125]

## Klippel–Trenaunay Syndrome

Klippel–Trenaunay syndrome (KTS) is characterized by asymmetric limb or trunk enlargement coupled with deep and superficial lymphatic malformations, venous malformations, and cutaneous hemangiomata of the affected limb or body part. The entity was first described by Klippel and Trenaunay in 1900 as a syndrome with cutaneous hemangiomas, asymmetric limb overgrowth, and varicosities, and later in 1907, Weber contributed the observation of occasional arteriovenous malformations in affected individuals.[140] The first prenatal recognition of this syndrome was described in 1988 as limb hypertrophy and numerous subcutaneous cysts.[141]

**Incidence:** The incidence of KTS is less than 1:10,000.[140]

**Pathogenesis/Etiology:** The genetic basis for KTS is thought to be a somatic mutation resulting in vascular malformations. Inheritance is sporadic with all cases thought to involve mosaicism.[140] Multiple candidate genes have been identified, but currently, no clinical genetic testing is available. Diagnosis is clinical and is documented with two of three criteria: (1) capillary malformation, (2) venous malformation or atypical varicose veins, and (3) hypertrophy of soft tissues and/or bone.[142] Most patients (63%) have all three clinical criteria.[143]

**Diagnosis:** There is no recognized serum screening abnormality that would alert the clinician to a diagnosis of KTW prenatally.

*Imaging:* The diagnosis may be made as early as middle second trimester, based on marked enlargement of the soft tissues of the involved limb or body part (Fig. 20.21A). The soft tissue abnormalities may appear as masslike tumors. Ultrasound may be insufficient to completely evaluate the extent of abnormalities, in which case fetal MR imaging may offer additional information (Fig. 20.21B,C).[144]

The vascular malformations may enlarge rapidly, leading to life-threatening complications, including high-output cardiac failure and platelet trapping with a consumptive coagulopathy.[141] Overgrowth of the long bones in the affected limb will be apparent by prenatal ultrasound. Occasionally, the syndrome can affect the face and manifest with asymmetric facial hypertrophy. Intrapelvic and intra-abdominal involvement is also possible, evidenced by either distinct masses or visceromegaly. There has also been description of a case diagnosed by hemihypertrophy and subcutaneous cysts coupled with ascites and an abnormal maternal serum panel, and it is theorized that the ascites was secondary to cardiac failure or lymphatic abnormalities.[145]

**Differential Diagnosis:** Other syndromes that might present prenatally with lymphatic malformations, lymphedema, and limb hypertrophy include Beckwith–Wiedemann, disseminated hemangiomatosis syndrome, Maffuci syndrome, Banyan–Riley–Ruvalcaba, Proteus syndrome, Russell–Silver syndrome, and TS. Soft tissue masses in the sacrococcygeal region should prompt consideration of a sacrococcygeal teratoma in the

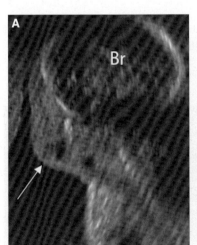
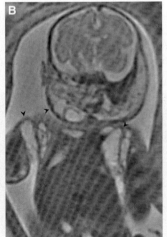
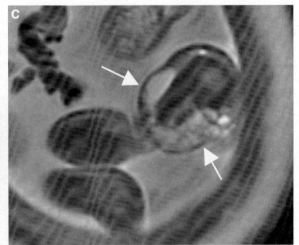

**FIGURE 20.21:** Klippel–Trenaunay syndrome. **A:** Sagittal view of the fetal head and neck at 17 weeks' GA shows abnormal subcutaneous soft tissue thickening (*arrow; Br, brain*) containing cystic spaces. **B:** Coronal fetal MR imaging using SSFSE T2 imaging shows the extent of the superficial soft tissue abnormality (*arrowheads*), involving the bilateral neck and chest. **C:** Extension along an upper extremity (marked by *arrows*) was also observed.

differential diagnosis, and fetal MR would be advantageous for evaluating the intrapelvic extent of disease in this situation.

**Prognosis:** Prognosis of KTW depends on the location, size, and type of malformations seen. In severe fetal cases, hydrops may develop, and this is likely to lead to in utero demise. Routine monitoring for signs of cardiac failure is important, and if detected, delivery should be promptly performed in a medical setting where intensive neonatal care is available. Intelligence is normal. Life expectancy can be in the normal range.[143]

**Management:** Fetal congestive heart failure associated with KTW has been observed, so close monitoring during the pregnancy is warranted.[141] An infant with suspected KTW should have a screening complete blood count after birth to evaluate for thrombocytopenia that can develop from platelet consumption in the hemangioma.[140] Because some of the diagnoses in the differential have associated cardiac defects and the risk of heart failure, echocardiography is typically performed.

Depending on the severity of the hemangioma and hypertrophy, limb amputations in the neonatal period have been required.[144] In those infants that are stable postnatal, the disorder is treated symptomatically. Options for therapy include observation only, compressive stockings, anticoagulation, steroid therapy, laser ablation, sclerotherapy, and surgical resection.[144]

**Recurrence Risk:** Recurrence risk is expected to be very low owing to sporadic nature, though some reports of familial recurrence suggest the possibility of higher recurrence risk.[140]

## Roberts Syndrome

Roberts syndrome (RBS), also called pseudothalidomide syndrome or SC syndrome, was first described in 1919 as a combination of cleft lip, cleft palate, and maldevelopment of all four extremities. Numerous cases have since been described, sharing the primary features of intrauterine growth retardation, severe shortening of the limbs, cleft lip and palate, hypertelorism, microcephaly, and micrognathia.[146]

**Incidence:** RBS is rare; around 150 cases have been reported to date.[147]

**Pathogenesis/Etiology:** RBS is an autosomal recessive inherited disorder.[146] Clinical variability is even seen among affected individuals in families.[147] There is one gene known to cause RBS (*ESCO2*), and diagnosis is based on genetic testing.[148] A mutation

in the *ESCO2* gene has been found in all patients with RBS. A negative result from amniocentesis nearly excludes RBS.[148]

**Diagnosis:** Karyotyping will show premature centromere separation of some chromosomes, and, therefore, if a genetic workup is time-sensitive, a search for these chromosome abnormalities can provide information about the diagnosis.[148] Similar, but distinct, metaphase abnormalities can be seen in other syndromes (aneuploidies and CdLS).[149] Typically, if these findings are not seen, the diagnosis of RBS is unlikely but not definitively excluded.

*Imaging:* Fetuses with growth delay and limb anomalies on ultrasound may be suspected to have RBS. This disorder may be recognized as early as 12 weeks, on the basis of limb shortening, cervical lymphatic malformation, and polyhydramnios (Fig. 20.22). The degree of limb reduction in the upper and lower extremities is variable, and the bones may be absent or hypoplastic. Tetraphocomelia is classically observed. Flexion contractures are typically seen. Oligo- and syndactyly are also common features, which are more readily detected by 3D ultrasound than by 2D ultrasound.[150]

Additional less common findings in RBS are numerous: cryptorchidism, CNS malformations, cardiac lesions, renal anomalies, abnormal genitalia, and cervical lymphatic malformations.[146] Confusing findings on ultrasound may be elaborated with fetal MR, although there is no published case of a prenatal diagnosis of Robert syndrome by fetal MR imaging.

**Differential Diagnosis:** Other syndromes that can cause these severe limb abnormalities include amniotic band syndrome, Fanconi anemia (in utero growth restriction, microcephaly, and radial ray deficiencies), HOS, autosomal recessive tetra-amelia associated with *WNT3* gene, thalidomide embryopathy, Nager syndrome, OFD syndrome, and TAR. Table 20.10 lists the recognized disorders that manifest with limb reduction abnormalities.[151]

**Prognosis:** The prognosis is poor. Rates of pregnancy loss and postnatal mortality are high.[147] Affected children that survive generally die after a few years, owing to associated malformations.

**Management:** An infant born with features of RBS should receive genetic counseling and confirmatory gene testing. A complete physical exam and extremity radiographs are typically performed to evaluate for limb reduction malformations.

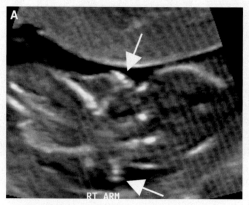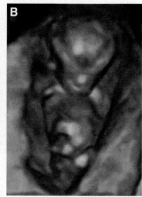

**FIGURE 20.22:** Tetraphocomelia in a 14-week fetus, raising suspicion for Roberts syndrome. **A:** Two-dimensional coronal ultrasound shows absence of the bilateral arms and forearms, with discernible bilateral hands *(arrows)* arising directly from the shoulder regions. **B:** Three-dimensional ultrasound shows four diminutive limbs.

| Table 20.10 | Expected Limb Reduction Anomalies in Recognized Chromosomal and Syndromic Conditions |
|---|---|
| **Diagnosis** | **Malformations** |
| Trisomy 18 | Hypoplasia of phalanges and/or short hallux |
| Poland anomaly | Hypoplasia of hands; hypoplasia of entire arm |
| Ectrodactyly–ectodermal dysplasia–clefting (EEC) | Ectrodactyly of hands and/or feet |
| Thrombocytopenia-absent radius (TAR) syndrome | Bilateral absence of the radius, mild shortening and bending of the ulna |
| Smith–Lemli–Opitz syndrome | Terminal transverse limb deficiencies |
| Oral-facial-digital syndrome | Asymmetric shortening of digits |
| Townes–Brocks | Hypoplasia of the thumb and of the third toe |
| Moebius | Terminal transverse limb deficiencies |
| Du Pan | Bilateral absence of the fibula, short metacarpals |
| Hypoglossia/hypodactyly | Absence of digits |
| Cornelia de Lange | Oligodactyly |
| Fanconi anemia | Hypoplasia of the thumb |
| Roberts | Phocomelia |
| Holt–Oram | Radial hypoplasia |
| VACTERL association | Hypoplasia of the thumb and/or radius |
| Oculo-auriculo-vertebral defect spectrum | Bilateral or unilateral hypoplasia of fingers |
| Amniotic bands | Terminal transverse limb deficiencies |

Adapted from Stoll C, Alembik Y, Dott B, et al. Associated malformations in patients with limb reduction deficiencies. *Eur J Med Genet*. 2010;53:286–290.

Prostheses may be indicated.[152] In the neonatal period, feeding is often an issue, especially if cleft lip or palate is present.[153] Additionally, echocardiography and cardiology evaluation are recommended because of the association with congenital heart defects.[146] Renal ultrasound is performed to evaluate for renal cysts.[152] Ophthalmology evaluation should be completed as corneal clouding and visual impairment are often seen.[146] Intellectual disability is nearly universal. However, patients with mild disease can have had normal intelligence and survive into adulthood.[154]

**Recurrence Risk:** Recurrence risk in future pregnancies is 25%.[140]

## Noonan Syndrome

Noonan syndrome (NS) is similar to TS, but with a normal karyotype. The syndrome is characterized by postnatal short stature, identified in 50% to 70% of cases, a broad and webbed neck, and anterior chest wall deformity due to superior pectus carinatum and inferior pectus excavatum.[155] Characteristic facies are low-set and posteriorly rotated ears, hypertelorism, epicanthal folds, and thick eyelids. Coagulation defects, lymphatic dysplasias, renal anomalies, and ocular abnormalities are also associations.[156,157]

**Incidence:** The incidence of NS is estimated to be between 1 in 1,000 and 1 in 2,500 live births.[156]

**Pathogenesis/Etiology:** NS is inherited autosomal dominant but with a normal karyotype. The genetic basis of NS is complex with numerous genes identified.[158] All of the genes identified are in the RAS pathway (group of proteins in human cells) which lead to overactivation of the RAS, turning on genes responsible for cell growth, proliferation, and survival. A *PTPN11* gene mutation is found in approximately 50% of patients.[159]

**Diagnosis:** When this syndrome is suspected, an NS gene panel could be considered. A positive result would have prognostic implications, but a negative result would not exclude NS.

*Imaging:* The diagnosis may be considered in the late first trimester based on a thickened NT. The primary prenatal feature is cervical lymphatic malformation, particularly in the lateral aspects of the neck. In the presence of a normal karyotype and cervical lymphatic lesion, NS should be suspected. In a minority of cases, the lymphatic abnormalities will lead to overt development of fetal hydrops, which portends a poor prognosis (Fig. 20.23A).

Whereas intrauterine growth retardation is a feature of TS, prenatal growth restriction is not a feature of NS. Body length is usually normal in affected infants, and subsequently, short stature becomes apparent in 50% to 70% of children.[155]

Cardiac defects are seen in 50% to 80% of individuals with this syndrome. While left-heart lesions are more common in TS, right-heart lesions, especially pulmonic stenosis and septal defects, are typically seen in NS (Fig. 20.23B). Pulmonary valve stenosis should raise suspicion for NS. Other types of cardiac diseases that might be prenatally diagnosed include atrioventricular canal defect, pulmonary artery stenosis, and tetralogy of Fallot.[160]

Additional findings that may be seen with NS include hypertelorism, low-set ears, cryptorchidism, micropenis, renal anomalies, including solitary kidney and collecting system anomalies, and scoliosis secondary to hemivertebrae.[155,161]

These features are typically detected by prenatal ultrasound. There is no published description of fetal MR imaging offering further advantage in the prenatal diagnosis of NS, but when imaging for further definition in a fetus with anomalies, diffuse edema with normal karyotype should raise suspicion for NS (Fig. 20.23C).

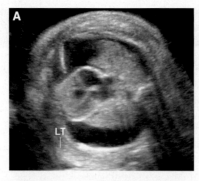
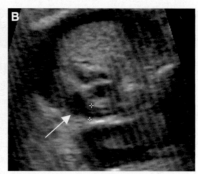
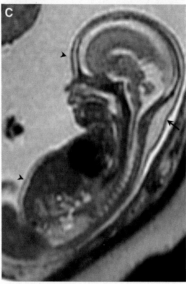

**FIGURE 20.23:** Noonan syndrome. **A,B:** Fetus at 35-week-GA. **A:** Axial ultrasound of the chest shows large bilateral anechoic pleural effusions (*Lt*, left). **B:** Focused image of the right ventricular outflow tract shows the pulmonary artery (marked by *calipers*) and poststenotic dilatation (*arrow*). Pulmonic stenosis and evidence of hydrops portend a poor prognosis. **C:** Fetus at 23 weeks with significant nuchal soft tissue thickening (*arrow*) and diffuse soft tissue edema (*arrowheads*). AV canal was also present in this patient with confirmed Noonan syndrome.

**Differential Diagnosis:** There are several rare syndromes caused by mutations in RAS pathway genes. These include LEOPARD syndrome, Costello syndrome, and cardio-facio-cutaneous syndrome. As with many of the syndromes and genetic abnormalities discussed in this chapter (see Table 20.4), the NT is abnormal in fetuses affected by NS. Cervical lymphatic malformations may be seen with a number of genetic abnormalities and have a high association with other major congenital anomalies.[162] This finding, combined with detection of cardiac defects, might also be seen with DiGeorge syndrome, Pallister–Killian syndrome, trisomy 10, trisomy 13, trisomy 18, trisomy 21, and TS.

**Prognosis:** Survival through gestation and in the first year of life typically depends on the severity of cardiac disease. Twenty percent to 30% of NS patients are affected by hypertrophic cardiomyopathy. The leading genetic cause of infantile hypertrophic cardiomyopathy is NS.[160] The combination of hypertrophic cardiomyopathy and NS carries a significant mortality, 22% at 1 year.[163]

Interestingly, some cases of NS are mild and may not be diagnosed until adulthood when the affected person has an affected child. Diagnosis of an affected fetus or neonate should prompt evaluation of family members.

**Management:** Prenatally, fetuses should be routinely assessed by ultrasound to monitor for the development of diffuse lymphedema, which places the fetus at risk for intrauterine death. Children born with this syndrome can develop peripheral edema,

and like children affected by TS, the neck appears webbed owing to regression of the lymphatic malformations.

Feeding difficulties are common in the newborn period but are typically self-limited.[164] Newborns should have screening echocardiography, renal ultrasound, and an ophthalmology exam.[165] Growth parameters should be plotted on NS-specific growth charts.[164] Approximately 80% of affected males will have cryptorchidism.[161] Management of scoliosis secondary to vertebral segmentation anomalies may require orthopedic intervention.

Approximately 25% of children with NS have some degree of intellectual disability, but it is often mild.[166] Early referral for intervention should be obtained to limit developmental delay. Individuals with NS have a genetic predisposition to leukemia and certain solid tumors, including neuroblastoma and embryonal rhabdomyosarcoma.[167] Additionally, a variety of coagulation defects have been seen in patients with NS; thus, biochemical tests to evaluate for coagulation defects should be performed.[165]

**Recurrence Risk:** Recurrence risk is up to 50% if the parents are found to carry a mutation.[158]

## Velocardiofacial Syndrome

Velocardiofacial syndrome (VCFS), also referred to as DiGeorge syndrome, is characterized by palate anomalies, characteristic facial features, and developmental delay. Conotruncal heart defects, such as tetralogy of Fallot, interrupted aorta, VSD, and truncus arteriosus, are seen in up to 74% of patients.[168] Immune problems are less common but may be severe.[168] Other features include hypocalcemia, seizures, hearing loss, feeding difficulty, renal anomalies, and growth hormone deficiency.[168] Marked variability is seen both within and among families with VCFS.[169]

**Incidence:** Incidence estimates range from 1 in 4,000 to 1 in 6,395 live births.[168]

**Pathogenesis/Etiology:** The syndrome arises from a deletion on chromosome 22q11.2.[169] Ninety percent of cases are due to new mutations, but the remaining 10% are autosomal dominant.

**Diagnosis:** Fluorescence in situ hybridization specific for VCFS can detect the submicroscopic deletion on chromosome 22.[170] The deletion can also be identified on microarray. Microarray will also detect smaller or atypical deletions in this region. Karyotype from amniocentesis alone would not be expected to detect the deletion associated with most cases of VCFS.

*Imaging:* Sonographic findings of CHD (Fig. 20.24) or cleft palate may raise suspicion for VCFS. Amniocentesis should be offered for all pregnancies with a conotruncal heart defect since 10% to 20% will have abnormal FISH for VCFS. Three-dimensional ultrasound may assist further in the diagnosis by demonstrating hypotelorism, small low-set ears with abnormal helices, downturned oral commissures, small mouth and jaw, and a straight facial profile (Fig. 20.25).[171]

Severe central nervous system malformations have also been described in fetuses affected by 22q11.2 microdeletion syndromes and include posterior encephalocele, myelomeningocele, and holoprosencephaly.[171] Fetal MR imaging would be ideal for evaluating brain and spine anomalies.

**Differential Diagnosis:** Other syndromes to consider in the differential diagnosis include CHARGE, diabetic embryopathy, SLOS, Alagille syndrome, VATER or Goldenhar.

**Prognosis:** The heart defects associated with deletion 22q11.2 are generally repairable, but feeding problems are very common, and cognitive impairment is essentially universal. Mental health problems, especially schizophrenia, may be seen in up to 30% of affected adults and adolescents. Combinations of heart disease, kidney disease, and/or other malformations may complicate management. Severe T-cell deficiency with congenital heart has a mortality rate of approximately 65% to 70%.[168]

**Management:** Infants with suspicion for VCFS or DiGeorge syndrome should receive a number of evaluations at the time of birth. A complete physical exam should be performed. Feeding evaluation may be necessary as many infants have difficulty with suck and swallow (30%) and often require nasogastric tube feedings or gastrostomy tube.[172] Serum ionized calcium level should be checked as hypocalcemia is common and is most severe in neonatal period. A lymphocyte count screens for immune defects; an abnormal value should prompt further testing and referral to an immunologist or hematologist. Ophthalmology evaluation is performed on the basis of the wide variety of eye findings associated with VCFS, including cataracts, colobomas, ptosis, and small optic nerves.[170] Hearing loss has been reported and should be screened.

Postnatal imaging is important to evaluate the extent of anomalies. Renal anomalies are seen in approximately 20% of affected patients and are evaluated with renal ultrasound. Radiography is performed to evaluate for vertebral anomalies.[173] Echocardiography and referral to a cardiologist should be obtained.[168] CNS malformations include cerebellar atrophy, polymicrogyria, cystic white matter lesions, and pituitary gland defects. MRI could be considered, especially with seizure activity.[174]

Many long-term issues are present in VCFS. Developmental delays, behavioral problems, and psychiatric disorders are nearly universal, but have varying significance. Delays can range from mild, isolated language delay to significant global delay.[175] Speech assessment by age 1 year is recommended in view of the high incidence of velopalatine insufficiency and speech disorders, even without clefts.[176]

**Recurrence Risk:** Since 90% of cases are due to new mutations, recurrence risks are generally low. However, if a parent is affected, recurrence risk is 50%. Because of the variability in presentation, a mildly affected parent could have the 22q11.2 deletion and have gone undiagnosed.[176]

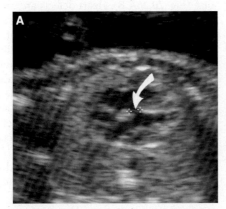
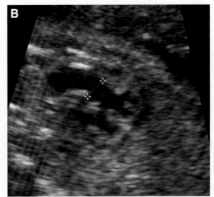

**FIGURE 20.24:** Velocardiofacial syndrome. **A:** A transverse view of the heart shows a ventricular septal defect *(arrow)* measuring 3 mm. **B:** A single great vessel (marked by calipers) arises from the heart. Single umbilical artery was also present. Fluorescent in situ hybridization analysis revealed a 22q deletion consistent with velocardiofacial syndrome.

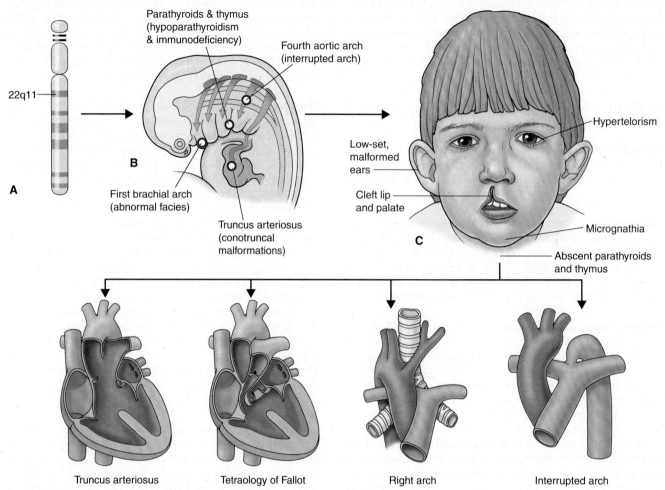

**FIGURE 20.25:** Characteristic features of velocardiofacial syndrome. (Adapted from Sze RW, Yutzey KE. The molecular genetic revolution in congenital heart disease. *AJR Am J Roentgenol.* 2001;176:575–581.)

## CRANIOFACIAL SYNDROMES

### CHARGE Syndrome

CHARGE syndrome is a rare set of associations consisting of *c*olobomas, *h*eart defects, choanal *a*tresia, *r*etarded growth and development, *g*enital abnormalities, and *e*ar anomalies.[177]

**Incidence:** The incidence of CHARGE syndrome is 1 in 8,500 to 1 in 10,000 live births.[177]

**Pathogenesis/Etiology:** The majority of CHARGE cases are sporadic because of new mutations. Rare recurrence has been attributed to germline mosaicism in a parent.[178] The chromodomain helicase DNA-binding protein 7 (*CHD7*) is the only gene known to be associated with CHARGE syndrome. An abnormality in CHD7 is seen in 65% to 70% of patients, but is not necessary for diagnosis.[178] Truncating mutations (those that induce a premature translational "stop" signal) may cause haploinsufficiency of CHD7 in some cases. Missense mutations (resulting in a single nucleotide change rendering its encoded protein nonfunctional) seem to be related to a less severe, less specific phenotype.[179]

**Diagnosis:** An amniocentesis with gene testing for *CHD7* could be offered and has been described in confirming a prenatally suspected case of CHARGE syndrome.[180] Karyotype from amniocentesis is expected to be normal.

*Imaging:* Postnatal diagnosis is based on clinical findings and temporal bone imaging.[177,181] Colobomas, which are seen in 80% to 90% of patients with CHARGE syndrome, can be unilateral or bilateral and can involve the iris, retina-choroid or disc (Fig. 20.26A,B). Heart defects are variable but common in 75% to 85% of cases. Choanal atresia or stenosis can be unilateral or bilateral in 50% to 60% of patients (Fig. 20.26C,D). Growth deficiency is noted in 70% to 80%.[182] Genital anomalies seen in CHARGE include cryptorchidism or hypogonadotrophic hypogonadism.[183] Ear abnormalities, seen in greater than 90% of affected individuals, include abnormal outer ears, malformed ossicles, cochlear defects, or abnormal semicircular canals (Fig. 20.26E,F).[184] Other features of CHARGE syndrome include cranial nerve dysfunction, orofacial clefts, and tracheoesophageal fistula.[178]

Prenatal suspicion for CHARGE syndrome could be raised owing to abnormal prenatal ultrasound and MRI findings. Sanlaville et al.[185] summarize a series of 10 fetuses affected by a *CDH7* gene mutation. The most commonly seen findings included bilateral and asymmetric external ear abnormalities manifesting as low-set, posteriorly rotated, and triangular or square-shaped auricle, semicircular canal hypoplasia or

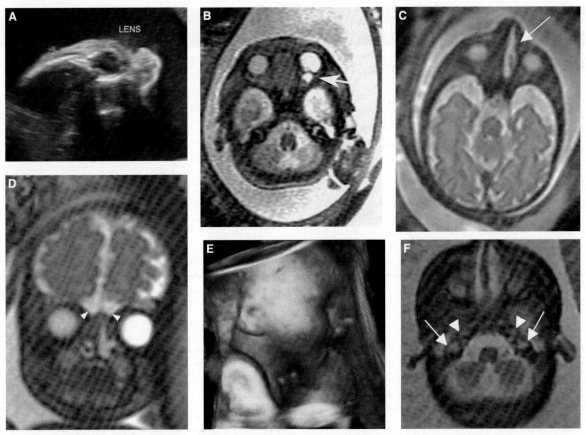

**FIGURE 20.26:** Prenatal imaging findings seen in CHARGE syndrome. **A:** Axial ultrasound demonstrates globe with eccentric posterior cyst protrusion consistent with coloboma. **B:** Axial MR image in a 33-week fetus shows a small well-demarcated T2-hyperintense structure posterior to the globe *(arrow)*, consistent with a small coloboma. **C,D:** 34-Week fetus diagnosed with CHARGE. Axial SSFSE T2 **(C)** and coronal SSFP **(D)** demonstrates fluid-distended nasal cavity *(arrow)*, proven to represent choanal atresia. On the coronal imaging, there is also absence of the olfactory bulbs *(arrowheads)*. **E,F:** Fetus at 31 weeks confirmed postnatal with CHARGE. **E:** 3D ultrasound demonstrates malformed ear. **F:** Axial SSFP demonstrates misshapen ears and dysplasia of the lateral semicircular canals *(arrows)*, which should be distinct from the vestibule at this gestational age *(arrowheads mark the cochlea).*

agenesis, and arhinencephaly. Seven out of 10 fetuses also had a coloboma, always affecting the retina or choroid segment. Nine out of 10 fetuses had a congenital heart defect, usually complex lesions and often involving the conotruncal region with septal defects. Six of the fetuses had choanal atresia. Less common findings included polyhydramnios, microphthalmia, and cleft lip and/or palate. Interestingly, although postnatal growth retardation is a feature of CHARGE syndrome, intrauterine growth retardation is not observed.

On the basis of their observation that four of six major criteria of CHARGE (coloboma, choanal atresia and/or cleft lip/palate, heart defect, arhinencephaly, semicircular canal agenesis, and external ear anomalies) were sufficient for the diagnosis of CHARGE, it has been proposed that the presence of four of these major findings are necessary for the prenatal diagnosis of CHARGE syndrome. Major and minor diagnostic criteria are summarized in Tables 20.11 and 20.12.

Two-dimensional and three-dimensional ultrasound can readily evaluate the pinna; however, sonographic evaluation of the temporal bone is limited. Identification of the fetal cochlea caudal to the temporal lobes can be obtained in approximately 50% of cases in the second trimester by using the fetal anterior fontanelle and coronal plane insonation.[186] The semicircular canals may be identified by second-trimester ultrasound as well, although with limited resolution. Fetal MR imaging has been

shown to distinguish the cochlea from the semicircular canals, and it also permits the identification of the external auditory canals, with improved resolution as gestational age advances.[187] The fetal ear anomalies seen in CHARGE syndrome may be found by prenatal MR imaging, but it is important to keep in mind that evaluation of the cochlea, semicircular canals, and vestibule in the fetus by T2-weighted MR imaging (Fig. 20.27) is usually possible only after 25 weeks' gestational age, and the external auditory canals are not well seen before 29 weeks' gestational age. Of note, the vestibule is more readily discernible than the cochlea and the ossicles earlier in gestation. Fetal MRI can also define subtle anomalies like coloboma (see Fig. 20.26B), absence of the olfactory tracts after 30 weeks' gestational age (Fig. 20.26D), choanal atresia (see Fig. 20.26C), cleft palate, or genital anomalies.[187]

**Differential Diagnosis:** The differential diagnosis includes mosaic trisomy 9, diabetic embryopathy, Carpenter syndrome, VCFS, VACTERL association, Kabuki syndrome, and Joubert syndrome. These could be differentiated on the basis of physical findings, but some may be subtle and might not be identified until the child is born.

**Prognosis:** Survival depends on the severity of an individual's phenotype. Cyanotic heart disease, tracheoesophageal fistula,

---

| Table 20.11 | Major Diagnostic Characteristics of CHARGE Syndrome | |
| --- | --- | --- |
| **Characteristics** | **Manifestations** | **Frequency** |
| Ocular coloboma | Coloboma of the iris, retina, choroid, disc; microphthalmos | 80%–90% |
| Choanal atresia or stenosis | Unilateral/bilateral: bony or membranous atresia/stenosis | 50%–60% |
| Cranial nerve dysfunction or anomaly | I: hyposmia or anosmia | Frequent |
| | VII: facial palsy (unilateral or bilateral) | >40% |
| | VIII: hypoplasia of auditory nerve | Frequent |
| | IX/X: swallowing problems with aspiration | 70%–90% |
| Characteristic CHARGE syndrome ear | Outer ear: short, wide ear with little or no lobe, "snipped off" helix, prominent antihelix that is often discontinuous with tragus, triangular concha, decreased cartilage; often protruding and usually asymmetric | 80%–100% |
| | Middle ear: ossicular malformations | |
| | Mondini defect of the cochlea | |
| | Temporal bone abnormalities; absent or hypoplastic semicircular canals | |

Data from Sanlaville D, Etchevers HC, Gonzales M, et al. Phenotypic spectrum of CHARGE syndrome in fetuses with CHD7 truncating mutations correlates with expression during human development. *J Med Genet*. 2006;43:211–217.

and bilateral choanal atresia have the lowest survival.[188] It is highly recommended that affected infants be delivered at a tertiary care center. Observed intelligent quotients tend to be below average, and cognitive impairments may be partially explained by sensory deficits and by dysfunction in integrating regions of the brain.[182]

**Management:** An infant born with suspected CHARGE syndrome should have a full physical exam. In the newborn period, associated medical conditions can be life-threatening.[188] Airway management typically requires tracheostomy and surgical correction of choanal atresia.[189] Feeding difficulties are common, and evaluation by a speech pathologist should be performed. Need for gastrostomy is not uncommon.[190] Echocardiography as well as cardiology consultation, renal ultrasound, and hearing screening should be included in management shortly after birth.

Long-term needs include hearing and vision evaluations, assessment for hypogonadism as puberty onset can be delayed, and consideration of airway anomalies if anesthesia is required.[188]

**Recurrence Risk:** If parents are unaffected, risk is approximately 1% to 2% due to germline mosaicism.[191]

## Oral-Facial-Digital Syndrome Type 1

The OFD syndrome is a group of at least nine disorders all consistently characterized by abnormalities of mouth, face, and digits.[192] Type 1 OFD is the most common and will be the focus of the following discussion. Additional frequent anomalies in OFD include those of the central nervous system and genitourinary tract.

---

| Table 20.12 | Minor Diagnostic Characteristics of CHARGE Syndrome | |
| --- | --- | --- |
| **Characteristics** | **Manifestations** | **Frequency** |
| Genital hypoplasia | Males: micropenis, cryptorchidism | 50%–60% |
| | Females: hypoplastic labia | |
| | Males and females: delayed puberty secondary to hypogonadotropic hypogonadism | Frequent |
| Developmental delay | Delayed milestones, hypotonia | ≤100% |
| Cardiovascular malformation | Including conotruncal defects (e.g., tetralogy of Fallot), AV canal defects, and aortic arch anomalies | 75%–85% |
| Growth deficiency | Short stature, usually postnatal with or without growth hormone deficiency | 70%–80% |
| Orofacial cleft | Cleft lip and/or palate | 15%–20% |
| Tracheoesophageal (TE) fistula | TE defects of all types | 15%–20% |
| Distinctive facial features | Square face with broad prominent forehead, prominent nasal bridge and columella, flat midface | |

Data from Sanlaville D, Etchevers HC, Gonzales M, et al. Phenotypic spectrum of CHARGE syndrome in fetuses with CHD7 truncating mutations correlates with expression during human development. *J Med Genet*. 2006;43:211–217.

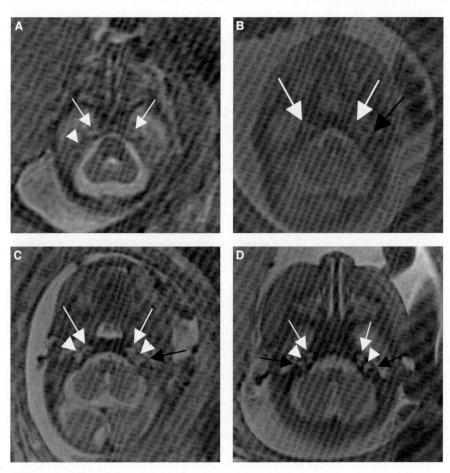

**FIGURE 20.27:** Normal temporal bone anatomy with fetal MRI in fetuses from gestation ages 21 to 30 weeks. The first structure most readily identified is the vestibule. This gradually becomes distinct from the cochlea. Identification of the lateral semicircular canals may be possible after 27 weeks'. Distinct turns in the cochlea may be identified in the late second and early third trimesters. Axial images are shown in **(A)** a 21-week fetus, **(B)** 26-week fetus, **(C)** 29-week fetus, and **(D)** 36-week fetus. When structures are distinguishable, the *white arrows* indicate the cochlea, *white arrowheads* indicate the vestibule, and *black arrows* indicate the lateral semicircular canal.

**Incidence:** The incidence of type 1 OFD syndrome is 1 in 50,000 to 1 in 250,000 live births.[192]

**Pathogenesis/Etiology:** The *OFD1* gene is the only gene known to be associated with OFD1 syndrome. On clinical testing of *OFD1*, a mutation is found in approximately 80% of patients with the syndrome.[193] The gene mutation leads to dysfunction of primary cilia mechanosensation. The location of the mutation likely influences the severity of the phenotype. The underlying genetics and the effect upon ciliary function overlap with other ciliopathies, including Joubert syndrome and polycystic kidney disease.[194] OFD1 is on the short (p) arm of the X chromosome, exhibiting an X-linked dominant inheritance. The genetic disorder is lethal in males, with intrauterine demise usually in the first or second trimester.[194]

**Diagnosis:** Gene sequencing of *OFD1* should be offered but is not required for diagnosis. The *OFD1* gene demonstrates X-linked inheritance. There is a high de novo mutation rate.[195]

***Imaging:*** It is helpful to understand the breadth of clinical findings of OFD syndrome. In type 1 OFD, oral findings can include lobed tongue, hamartomas or lipomas of the tongue, cleft of the hard or soft palate, accessory frenulae with tethering of the tongue, and hypodontia or other dental abnormalities.[195] Facial features include hypertelorism, telecanthus, hypoplastic alae nasi, clefts of upper lip, and micrognathia (Fig. 20.28A). Digital anomalies consist of brachydactyly, syndactyly, clinodactyly, duplicated digits, or polydactyly (Fig. 20.28B).[192] As is seen with other ciliopathies, some mild cases may present with isolated polycystic kidney disease in adulthood.[196] Brain malformations

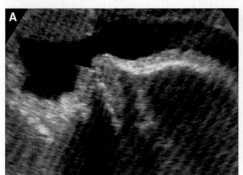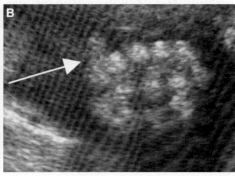

**FIGURE 20.28:** Imaging findings seen in oro-facial-digital syndrome. **A:** Ultrasound of the midline face in sagittal projection shows micrognathia in this 23-week fetus. No cleft palate was found. **B:** Evaluation of the hand shows polydactyly (*arrow* indicate supernumary digit). Abnormality was bilateral.

are relatively common, noted in 65% of cases, and include intracerebral cysts, agenesis of corpus callosum, cerebellar agenesis, and Dandy–Walker malformation.[195]

Prenatal diagnosis of OFD syndrome has been described for types I, II, IV, and VI.[197] Because of the X-linked nature of OFD1 and its lethality in male fetuses, type 1 OFD will only be diagnosed in female fetuses. Prenatal ultrasound and fetal MR imaging are capable of detecting cleft lip, cleft palate, hypertelorism, micrognathia, facial asymmetry, ear anomalies, brain malformations, echogenic or cystic kidneys, and anomalies of the extremities. However, diagnosis is typically made after birth when subtle characteristic features are more obvious. In the mildest cases, diagnosis is not made until polycystic kidney disease develops later in life.[196]

**Differential Diagnosis:** The differential diagnosis for OFD includes syndromes that affect the face and extremities. Meckel–Gruber syndrome exhibits central nervous system abnormalities and polydactyly as well as cystic kidneys. SLOS is associated with facial, digital, and renal anomalies. Other syndromes not discussed in this chapter but that overlap with OFD findings include Carpenter syndrome, which features a bifid hallux and hydrolethalus syndrome, which has both central nervous abnormalities and preaxial polydactyly.[198] Majewski syndrome is a skeletal dysplasia featuring a midline facial cleft, polydactyly, and short limbs. The differential diagnosis includes other OFD syndromes, all of which have polydactyly and associated characteristic oral-facial findings.

**Prognosis:** The prognosis of any individual with OFD syndrome depends on the phenotypic severity.

**Management:** Oral-facial issues typically cause feeding difficulty at birth. Management includes surgery for defects such as cleft lip/palate, tongue nodules, and accessory frenulae. Nutrition consultation and speech therapy are typically necessary.[192] Postnatal brain imaging should be performed to evaluate for structural brain abnormalities.[195] Although polycystic kidney disease is common, seen in up to 50% of cases, it typically does not develop until adulthood. A screening renal ultrasound could be performed but would be expected to be negative and does not exclude the potential to develop cystic disease later in life.[196]

Long-term issues include orthodontia for malocclusion, surgical management of syndactyly, and special education for developmental delay.[192] Developmental delay is typically mild and is seen in up to 50% of patients.[195]

**Recurrence Risk:** If the mother does not have the mutation found in the child, recurrence risk is very low. However, the recurrence risk increases by one-third in a live born if the mother carries the same mutation.[192]

## CRANIOSYNOSTOSIS

There are a number of craniosynostosis syndromes; however, only the most common types will be described. Apert, Pfeiffer, and Crouzon syndromes are related syndromes as all are characterized by craniosynostosis resulting from abnormalities of fibroblast growth factor receptor (*FGFR*) genes.[199] Whereas the skull base develops from enchondral ossification, the calvarial ossification occurs within membrane-derived mesodermal tissue. The gradually apposing calvarial ossification centers meet at fibrous sutures. Complete, solid fusion of these sutures in a normal individual does not occur until well into adulthood, with the exception of the metopic and mendosal suture, which typically fuse within the first year of life.

Clinically, the most important growth occurs along the sagittal and coronal sutures. The growth of the cranium is perpendicular to the suture, so that the skull increases in width through the sagittal suture and in anteroposterior diameter through the coronal sutures.[199] Premature fusion of the sutures leads to abnormal head shape, summarized in Table 20.13 (Fig. 20.29).

Characteristic facial features include hypertelorism, downslanting palpebral fissures, proptosis, midface hypoplasia, small beaked nose, and prognathism. Other common features include high arch or cleft palate abnormalities, hearing loss, visual problems, and choanal stenosis or atresia. Developmental delay is also common.[200]

In this section, global features of the main craniosynostosis syndromes will be provided, followed by more specific details about the clinical features, genetics, imaging, and management of Apert, Pfeiffer, Crouzon, and Antley–Bixler syndromes.

**Incidence:** The incidence of craniosynostosis is approximately 1 in 2,000 live births. Interestingly, advanced paternal age has been shown to be associated with de novo mutations in Apert, Pfeiffer, and Crouzon syndromes.[201]

**Pathogenesis/Etiology:** The specific genetics of each syndrome will be discussed separately, below. Genetic testing for all three of the *FGFR* genes is clinically available. Karyotype from amniocentesis would be expected to be normal.

| Table 20.13 | Summary of Resulting Head Shapes with Various Calvarial Suture Synostoses and the Syndromes Featuring Each | | |
|---|---|---|---|
| **Fused Suture** | **Head Shape** | **Description of Condition** | **Syndrome** |
| Sagittal | Scaphocephaly | Long, narrow skull | Crouzon, Philadelphia type |
| Coronal, bilateral | Acrobrachycephaly | Broad, short skull | Apert, Crouzon, Pfeiffer, Saethre–Chotzen, Muenke, Antley–Bixler |
| Unilateral lambdoid or unilateral coronal | Plagiocephaly | Asymmetric, trapezoid | |
| Metopic | Trigonocephaly | Keel forehead | Baller–Gerold |
| All sutures | Oxycephaly Kleeblattschadel | Cloverleaf skull | Carpenter, Pfeiffer |

Adapted from Flores-Sarnat L. New insights into craniosynostosis. *Semin Pediatr Neurol.* 2002;9:274–291.

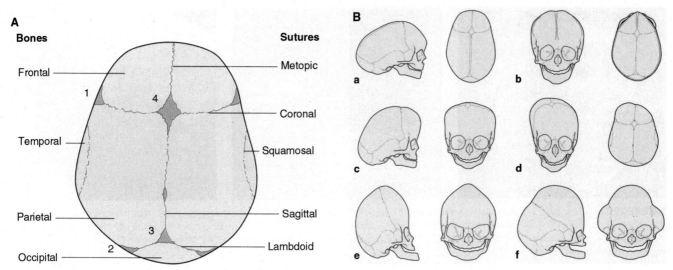

**FIGURE 20.29:** Craniosynostosis. **A:** Normal bones and sutures of fetal calvaria *(top view)* and anterolateral *(1)*, posterolateral *(2)*, posterior *(3)*, and anterior *(4)* fontanelles. **B:** Forms of craniosynostosis resulting from premature closure of the sagittal suture *(a)*, metopic suture *(b)*, coronal sutures *(c)*, unilateral coronal suture *(d)*, coronal and sagittal sutures *(e)*, and cloverleaf skull deformity with fusion of all sutures *(f)*.

**Diagnosis:** First-trimester diagnosis may be made with chorionic villus sampling and genetic analysis in patients with a known family history.

*Imaging:* It is possible to detect the presence of craniosynostosis prenatally by US. The biparietal distance (BPD) measures the transverse plane where the skull is widest. The occipitofrontal diameter represents the anteroposterior direction with the measurement obtained from outer skull to outer skull. The cephalic index is the ratio of the biparietal to occipitofrontal diameters, calculated as a percentage. Eighty percent is the normal intrauterine cephalic index (Fig. 20.30A). Brachycephaly, correctly known as acrobrachycephaly, is diagnosed if the cephalic index is more than 85% (Fig. 20.30B). Scaphocephaly, also previously called dolicocephaly, is defined if the index is less than 75% (Fig. 20.30C). Head measurements may be correlated with abdominal circumference or femur length. The normal head circumference/abdominal circumference (HC/AC) is 1.07% to 1.26%. An abnormal ratio should raise suspicion of a cranial anomaly.[202]

Fetal MR imaging may also show findings that suggest craniosynostosis.[203] Abnormal skull shape is readily apparent. Bone thickening and slight temporal indentations suggest bilateral coronal synostosis (Fig. 20.31A), whereas an indentation in the midline with scaphocephaly is suggestive of sagittal synostosis (Fig. 20.32A).

In general, prenatal diagnosis of craniosynostosis is very challenging and often missed.[203] The diagnosis of syndromic synostosis relies mainly on cranial deformity and associated abnormalities, in particular, limb malformations.

**Differential Diagnosis:** Differentiating between Apert, Crouzon, and Pfeiffer is based on characteristic features (see Tables 20.13 and 20.14). However, accurate diagnosis is often difficult prenatally and may be dependent upon postnatal clinical findings and genetic testing.[200] The differential diagnosis includes other craniosynostosis syndromes (Muenke syndrome, Saethre–Chotzen syndrome, Antley–Bixler syndrome, Carpenter syndrome, or Baller–Gerold syndrome) or isolated, nonsyndromic craniosynostosis. Muenke syndrome has variable findings that may include unilateral coronal synostosis or megalencephaly without craniosynostosis.[204] Saethre–Chotzen syndrome is typically diagnosed via characteristic ear findings.[205] Baller–Gerold syndrome typically has radial ray defects. Carpenter syndrome has preaxial polydactyly of the feet.[199]

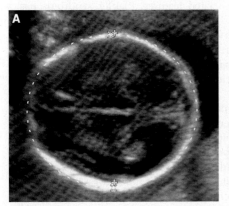
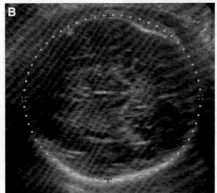
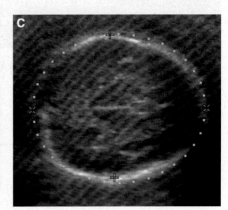

**FIGURE 20.30:** Assessment of the skull shape by ultrasound. **A:** The cephalic index is the ratio of the biparietal diameter to the occipitofrontal diameter, and this is typically near 80% (19 weeks' GA). **B:** An abnormally high index is diagnostic of acrobrachycephaly (19 weeks' GA). **C**. An abnormally low index is diagnostic of scaphocephaly (27 weeks' GA) + calipers represent biparietal and X calipers represent occipitofrontal diameters.

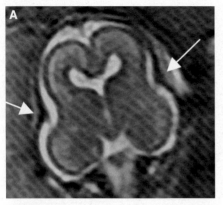
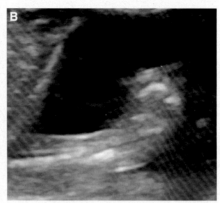
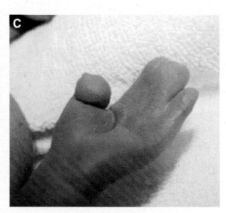

**FIGURE 20.31:** Apert syndrome diagnosed prenatally in a 21-week fetus. **A:** Coronal SSFSE T2-weighted image through the fetal head shows abnormal indentations *(arrows)* in the bilateral frontotemporal regions, indicating early coronal synostosis. **B:** Ultrasound of the right hand shows abnormal clenching of the hand and fingers, with indistinct digits, indicating complete syndactyly, called the "mitten" hand deformity. **C:** Photograph of hand of a newborn infant with Apert syndrome showing syndactyly deformity.

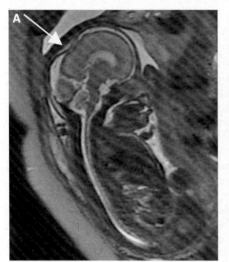
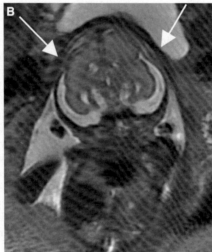
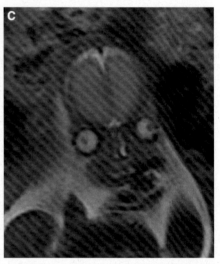

**FIGURE 20.32:** Pfeiffer syndrome diagnosed prenatally in a 27-week fetus. Sagittal **(A)** and coronal **(B)** T2-weighted SSFSE images through the fetal head show abnormal concave contours of the skull in the midline *(arrow in A)* at the vertex and along the frontotemporal regions *(arrows in B)*, creating a cloverleaf-shaped skull. Midface hypoplasia is also appreciable. **C:** Coronal SSFSE T2 image through the fetal face demonstrates hypertelorism. No polydactyly or syndactyly was appreciable.

| Table 20.14 | Classic Extremity Abnormalities Commonly Observed in Each Craniosynostosis Syndromes | |
| --- | --- | --- |
| *Craniosynostosis Syndrome* | *Extremity Anomaly* | |
| Apert | Mitten syndactyly | |
| Pfeiffer | Broad toes and thumbs | |
| Antley–Bixler | Arachnodactyly | |
| Crouzon | Normal extremities | |

Isolated craniosynostosis will present without other extremity or craniofacial anomalies, other than hyper- or hypotelorism due to abnormal skull shape. There are a number of other syndromes that can present with craniosynostosis as a minor feature. Evaluation by a geneticist is warranted.

**Prognosis:** The prognosis will vary with each syndrome and depends on the associated features. Pfeiffer syndrome has a higher morbidity and mortality than the other syndromes owing to the severity of airway abnormalities, which include midface hypoplasia, nasopharyngeal stenosis, and tracheal anomalies.[206] Obstruction to the airway can cause failure to thrive, suboptimal neurologic development, and developmental delay.

**Management:** An infant with syndromic craniosynostosis often has breathing problems in the first few months of life.[200] Respiratory issues are typically due to upper airway obstruction as a result of midface hypoplasia or choanal atresia/stenosis. Tracheostomy is often needed. Feeding difficulties are also common and can result in failure to thrive, if not addressed.[199] Management of syndromic craniosynostosis involves care at a multidisciplinary craniofacial clinic. Head imaging with cat scan (CT) using three-dimensional surface reconstructions of the face and skull are typically obtained in preparation for possible surgical management. Brain MR imaging may be added to evaluate for hydrocephalus.[207] Craniosynostosis typically requires serial surgical procedures. Earlier surgical treatment, including craniotomy and fronto-orbital advancement, can reduce the risk of complications such as hydrocephalus and cognitive impairment. Ophthalmology evaluation and treatment may be necessary, especially if proptosis is present, as this can lead to exposure keratopathy.[208] Spinal radiographs are performed to evaluate for vertebral anomalies.[209]

**Recurrence Risk:** Inheritance of the *FGFR* gene is autosomal dominant; therefore, recurrence risk is 50% for affected individuals.[210]

## Apert Syndrome

Apert syndrome, also known as acrocephalosyndactyly, was first described in the early 20th century and is one of the most severe craniosynostosis syndromes.[207,208] Patients with this disorder have a short AP skull diameter owing to bilateral coronal synostosis, a high forehead, a flat occiput, shallow orbits, hypertelorism, a flat face, midface hypoplasia, and a small nose.[199] Apert syndrome classically presents with fused fingers or toes and soft tissue or bony syndactyly in hands or feet. Occasionally, rhizomelic shortening or elbow ankylosis can be seen. During infancy, there is a large midline calvarial defect replacing the sagittal and metopic suture. This defect gradually closes by the age of 3 to 4 years.[211] Other features of Apert syndrome include fused cervical vertebrae, hydrocephalus, cardiac, and gastrointestinal abnormalities.[212]

**Incidence:** The incidence of Apert is approximately 1 in 100,000.[213]

**Pathogenesis/Etiology:** Apert syndrome results from *FGFR*-2 mutations, which map to chromosome 10q25–q16 and apparently arise exclusively from the paternally derived chromosome. The disorder has been associated with older paternal age.[212] Two specific mutations, p.Ser252Trp and p.Pro253Arg, are most common.

**Diagnosis:** Targeted testing for the two mutations, p.Ser252Trp and p.Pro253Arg, can be performed. If negative, sequencing of the *FGFR2* gene is done.[214]

*Imaging:* Prenatal recognition of Apert syndrome is difficult because the characteristic features of craniosynostosis do not usually present until the third trimester. Affected fetuses are usually identified by US between gestational weeks 20 and 27 when there is notation of either a brain abnormality, an abnormal skull shape, or syndactyly.[215] Ultrasound and MR imaging may show the abnormal head shape (see Fig. 20.31A). The most common brain abnormality is ventriculomegaly, which may be assessed by MRI. Three-dimensional ultrasound can illustrate the craniofacial abnormalities more readily than two-dimensional ultrasound. This technique may not only decisively influence diagnosis, it may assist the parents in understanding the anomalies when being counseled.[215] Ultrasound is ideal for evaluating the feet and hands, which are characteristically affected by bilateral syndactyly. A clenched "mitten" type appearance of the hand is typical and reflects near complete syndactyly (Fig. 20.31B,C). The feet may appear small and unusually arched. Other associated abnormalities such as congenital cardiac lesions may be directly visualized on prenatal sonography.

**Prognosis and Management:** Neonates may require management of their airway. Surgery, such as craniofacial expansion or ventricular shunting, is often performed in early childhood to reduce intracranial pressure as it has been shown to diminish the incidence of developmental delay. Affected individuals are at risk for developmental delay, although the degree of developmental delay is variable.[200] Management of a patient with Apert syndrome should include management of hydrocephalus, screening echocardiography for cardiac defects, and gastrointestinal imaging to evaluate for intestinal malrotation or esophageal atresia.

## Pfeiffer Syndrome

Pfeiffer syndrome, also called Pfeiffer-type acrocephalosyndactyly, was initially described in 1964 and is characterized by acrobrachycephaly, hypertelorism, depressed nasal bridge, broad-appearing and medially deviated thumb and great toe as well as partial syndactyly in the hands and feet.[216] Pfeiffer syndrome can be subdivided into three types with all having extremity findings but varying on other features. Pfeiffer syndrome type I typically has normal cognition, characteristic moderate to severe midface hypoplasia, hearing loss, and hydrocephalus. Type I is less common and less severe than types II and III. Pfeiffer syndrome types II and III commonly present with developmental delay, characteristic extreme proptosis, choanal and palatal abnormalities, hydrocephalus, and seizures.[217] Proptosis is often so severe that patients are unable to close their eyelids.[216] Visceral anomalies, including CHD and genitourinary anomalies, also occur. Type II is more likely to include a broad thumb and great toe than type III. Skull shape is also a distinguishing feature in Pfeiffer syndrome types II and III. Type II typically has a cloverleaf skull shape, while type III presents with an oxycephalic skull shape, which is a conical shape secondary to coronal and lambdoid synostosis.[218]

**Incidence:** The incidence of Pfeiffer syndrome is approximately 1–1.6:100,000.[213] Nearly all cases of Pfeiffer syndrome result from de novo mutation.[201]

**Pathogenesis/Etiology:** Regardless of subtype, nearly all mutations in Pfeiffer syndrome are related to the *FGFR2* gene, which map at chromosome 10q25–q26. However, it should be noted that 5% of mutations in Pfeiffer syndrome type 1 are associated with the *FGFR1* gene, which map at chromosome 8p11.22–p1.[219] Approximately 80% of mutations are in exons 8 and 10.

**Diagnosis:** In a stepwise gene analysis for this suspected disorder, exons 8 and 10 are sequenced first, then other exons are sequenced if negative.[219]

*Imaging:* Sonographic findings of Pfeiffer syndrome type I in the second trimester include acrobrachycephaly, hypertelorism, a small nose, syndactyly, a broad thumb, and large toes.[220] MR imaging may also show these findings, as well as better detailing abnormal brain development (Fig. 20.32).[203,218] Although ultrasound is superior for evaluation of the bones, MR imaging may improve assessment of the hands in certain cases using a thick-slab imaging technique that provides detail about the surface of the extremities. This has been shown to be useful in demonstrating the broad thumb of a fetus affected by Pfeiffer syndrome Type II, thereby differentiating it from a fetus affected by the other craniosynostoses.[218]

**Prognosis and Management:** Prognosis depends on the severity of associated anomalies and primarily on the severity of the central nervous system compromise. Type I is compatible with life, and the individual is expected to have normal intelligence. Postnatal evaluation includes management of the craniosynostosis and surgical correction of the extremity anomalies. Types II and III usually result in early death.

## Crouzon Syndrome

Crouzon syndrome, also known as craniofacial dysostosis, was initially described in 1912. This craniosynostosis syndrome does not have clinically apparent abnormalities of hands and feet, although radiographs may show shortening of metacarpals and phalanges. Facial features that are more distinct in Crouzon syndrome include significant proptosis, external strabismus, and mandibular prognathism.[217] Progressive hydrocephalus occurs in approximately 30% of individuals affected by Crouzon syndrome. Development and cognition are typically normal in Crouzon syndrome.[221]

**Incidence:** Crouzon syndrome is the most common autosomal dominant craniosynostosis and occurs in 1 in 25,000 live births.[213]

**Pathogenesis/Etiology:** The most common gene known to be associated with Crouzon syndrome is the *FGFR2* gene, which maps to chromosome 10q25–q26.[199] A variant of this syndrome is Crouzon syndrome with acanthosis nigricans, which is associated with the *FGFR3* gene.[209]

**Diagnosis:** Gene sequencing should be approached as in Pfeiffer syndrome with sequencing exons 8 and 10 first, then sequencing others if negative. If a young child presents with acanthosis nigricans or other characteristic findings including choanal atresia, hydrocephalus, or skeletal abnormalities, testing for the most common mutation in the *FGFR3* gene could be considered.[222]

*Imaging:* Imaging does not play a diagnostic role until the second or third trimesters.[223] Both second and third trimester ultrasound and fetal MRI are capable of demonstrating the abnormal skull shape and striking ocular features of Crouzon syndrome. However, these findings may be apparent only late in pregnancy and may escape diagnosis.

**Prognosis and Management:** The severe proptosis frequently associated with Crouzon syndrome leads to exposure conjunctivitis and keratitis. Visual abnormalities include poor acuity and nystagmus. Scaphocephaly and acrobrachycephaly are the most common calvarial manifestations that are approached surgically with cranial osteotomies and orbitofacial advancement. Conductive hearing loss is also a prominent feature and will require postnatal management. Crouzon syndrome individuals uncommonly have intracranial hypertension or hydrocephalus. There are no associated extremity malformations. Development and cognition are typically normal.[221]

## Antley–Bixler Syndrome

Antley–Bixler syndrome, also known as trapezoidocephaly or multiple synostosis syndrome, involves premature closure of the coronal and lambdoidal sutures, resulting in brachycephaly with frontal bossing.[224] Characteristic facial features include proptosis, downslanting palpebral fissures, depressed nasal bridge, low-set, and protruding ears. Choanal stenosis and atresia are frequent. Limb defects include radiohumeral synostosis, ulnar and femoral bowing, slender hands and feet, contractures, fractures, and advanced bone age. Other congenital abnormalities include congenital heart disease, renal anomalies, and genital abnormalities. Renal anomalies that can be associated include ectopic kidney, duplication, horseshoe kidney, hypoplasia, or hydronephrosis. Congenital adrenal hyperplasia may be seen.[224]

**Incidence:** The incidence is unknown because of diagnostic controversies in the reporting of *FGFRS*-related craniosynostosis as Antley–Bixler syndrome. More than 60 cases have been reported.

**Pathogenesis/Etiology:** The underlying etiology is a defect in sterol biosynthesis caused by mutation in a gene for cytochrome p450 reductase. The only gene known to be associated with Antley–Bixler syndrome is the cytochrome P450 oxidoreductase (*POR*) gene.

**Diagnosis:** Diagnosis is based on clinical findings, but gene sequencing of the *POR* gene is available to confirm the diagnosis.[225] Amniocentesis with Cytochrome P450 reductase (*POR*) gene sequencing can be offered, though not required for diagnosis and not routinely performed. During pregnancy, some mothers of fetuses with Antley–Bixler syndrome will have abnormal virilization that does not require intervention and resolves after delivery. Low maternal serum unconjugated estriol or lack of increase in urinary unconjugated estriol may be noted. There are reports of abnormal sterol profiles, particularly di- and trimethylated sterols, in the amniotic fluid, although the finding is not specific for this syndrome.[226] Some infants are not diagnosed until the newborn screen is abnormal for 21-hydroxylase deficiency.[225]

*Imaging:* Ultrasound findings of brachycephaly with frontal bossing and limb anomalies, especially radiohumeral synostosis, ulnar and femoral bowing, contractures, and fractures, may be evident with two-dimensional ultrasound. Dedicated fetal echocardiography is recommended to assess for congenital cardiac lesions. Three-dimensional ultrasound will increase the ability to detect characteristic facial features such as depressed nasal bridge and low-set ears. Renal anomalies and genital abnormalities may be more readily detected by fetal MR than by fetal ultrasound if sonography is limited owing to maternal factors, fetal positioning, or oligohydramnios. Prenatally discernible features of congenital adrenal hyperplasia, including adrenal gland enlargement and ambiguous genitalia, may be seen.[227]

**Differential Diagnosis:** The differential diagnosis includes other craniosynostosis syndromes, thanatophoric dysplasia, and Shprintzen-Goldberg syndrome. Shprintzen–Goldberg syndrome lacks the characteristic facial features and ambiguous genitalia seen in Antley–Bixler syndrome.[228]

**Prognosis and Management:** Prognosis is guarded. Respiratory complications, typically due to choanal stenosis and atresia, can result in early death, but if respiratory issues are addressed, outcomes can be reasonably good. Interventions that have been utilized include endotracheal intubation, nasal stents, tracheotomy, and tracheostomy. Evaluation by an endocrinologist and assessment of adrenal axis should be performed even without ambiguous genitalia.[225] Identification of ambiguous genitalia requires a multidisciplinary team working with the family, ideally prenatally.[130] Imaging with CT or MRI should be done to describe location and extent of craniosynostosis, the presence of choanal stenosis, and the evaluation of orbital depth, to assist with surgical planning. Radiographs of long bone should be performed to evaluate for fractures, bowing, synostoses or joint contractures.[229] Congenital heart defects, such as transposition of the great vessels, atrioventricular septal defects, patent foramen ovale, and hypoplastic right atrium should be excluded by screening echocardiography. Gastrointestinal malformations are rare, but screening for malrotation and imperforate anus should be considered.[224] Hydrocortisone replacement therapy is often needed for cortisol deficiency with stress-dose steroids.[225] Joint contractures are common, requiring physical therapy referral.[229]

**Recurrence Risk:** Inheritance is autosomal recessive; thus, recurrence risk is 25%.

## SYNDROMES CHARACTERIZED BY MANDIBULAR/AURICULAR ANOMALIES

Mandible anomalies are commonly encountered prenatally, and are a feature of numerous genetic syndromes and various chromosomal anomalies such as trisomies 18 and 13, triploidy, and those involving gene deletions or translocations. Fetuses with mandible anomalies are at risk of acute neonatal respiratory distress due to mechanical airway obstruction by the tongue in the presence of an abnormally formed mandible or due to an associated defect of the central nervous system.[230] At birth, an airway emergency may necessitate the presence of a neonatologist in the delivery room to provide immediate care for the infant. Prenatal assessment between 20 and 25 weeks' gestational age by two-dimensional ultrasound may identify mandibular hypoplasia/micrognathia and posterior displacement of the mandible/retrognathia, both by subjective perception and by measurements of the mandible width/maxilla width with a ratio of <0.785 defining micrognathia. The inferior facial angle, which is the angle between two lines on the sagittal midline profile view, one line drawn orthogonal to the forehead at the nasal bone synostosis and the other line drawn along the connection between the more prominent lip and the chin, may confirm retrognathism when the angle is <49.2° (Fig. 20.33).[231] Another manner of diagnosing micrognathia is using the jaw index, which can be measured sonographically and by MR imaging. This measurement of the mandible is assessed in the axial plane at the base of the cranium just caudad to the lower dental arch, where the whole horseshoe mandible is imaged (Fig. 20.34). Anteroposterior and laterolateral diameters are measured as follows: the laterolateral diameter is traced joining the bases of the two rami; the anteroposterior diameter is from the symphysis to the middle of the laterolateral diameter. The jaw index is then calculated as follows: anteroposterior mandibular diameter/BPD. A jaw index less than 23 indicates micrognathia with a sensitivity and specificity of 100% and 98.1%, respectively.[232]

## Goldenhar Syndrome

Goldenhar syndrome is one of the craniofacial microsomia syndromes, which are caused by malformations involving the first and second branchial apparatus derivatives. Goldenhar syndrome, also known as oculoauriculovertebral spectrum, consists of hemifacial microsomia as well as auricular malformations and specific eye malformations. Facial features include lip and palate clefting, temporomandibular joint ankylosis, asymmetric mandible, palpebral fissures, and midface hypoplasia.[233] Eye findings include possible coloboma or microphthalmia/anophthalmia, in addition to the presence of the characteristic epibulbar dermoid.[234] Hearing loss is common and may be sensorineural or conductive, surprisingly not associated with severity of dysmorphic features.[233] Other anomalies include vertebral abnormalities, such as malformed or hemivertebrae, pulmonary agenesis, absent thyroid gland, and cranial nerve findings, including facial palsy, sensorineural hearing loss, impaired eye movements, or trigeminal palsy.[235]

**Incidence:** The incidence of Goldenhar syndrome is unknown. The incidence of hemifacial microsomia ranges from 1 in 3,000 to 1 in 45,000 live births.[236]

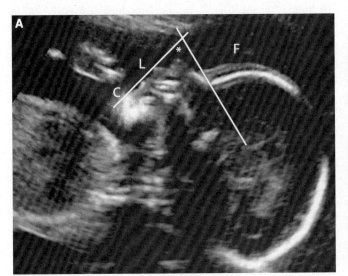
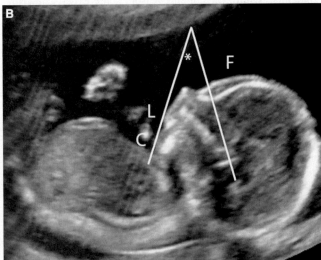

**FIGURE 20.33:** Inferior facial angle used to diagnose retro-micrognathia. **A:** Normal profile of a 22-week-GA fetus in which the angle (*asterisk*) between two lines (*one line* along the chin-lip anterior surface and the *other line* orthogonal to the forehead) should be greater than 50°. **B:** A different fetus at 19 weeks has an abnormally low inferior facial angle, signifying an abnormally posteriorly positioned mandible. F, forehead; L, lip; C, chin.

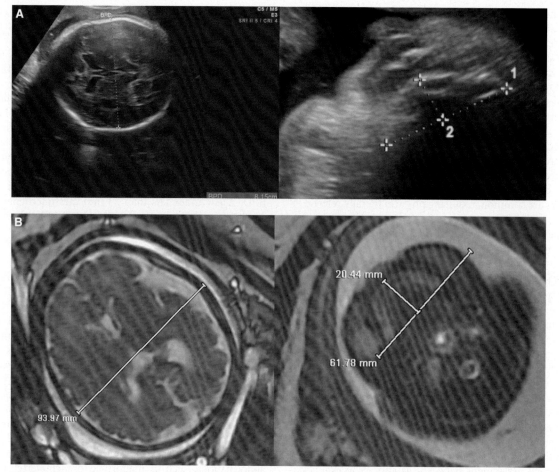

**FIGURE 20.34:** Mandibular index showing micrognathia. Anteroposterior and laterolateral diameters are measured, and the jaw index is then calculated as follows: anteroposterior mandibular diameter/BPD. A jaw index less than 23 indicates micrognathia. **A:** Measurement of the mandible by ultrasound. First image is standard BPD.  On second image, calipers designated 1 indicate laterolateral diameters and that marked 2 represent anterior to posterior dimension of the mandible. Jaw index was low at 17. **B:** Jaw index on MRI measured 21, which is low. Image to the left is BPD obtained as a standard US measurement.  On image to the right, calipers measuring 61.78 mm represent laterolateral dimension and 20.44 anteroposterior measurement of mandible.

**Pathogenesis/Etiology:** There is no known gene associated with Goldenhar syndrome. For this reason, some experts describe this grouping of abnormalities as an association rather than a syndrome. Few reports support a hypothesis that Goldenhar syndrome may be part of a mesodermal dysplasia complex involving maldevelopment of asymmetric structures, such as interrupted inferior vena cava with azygous continuation and persistent left superior vena cava.[235]

**Diagnosis:** No genetic testing is available. Amniocentesis has been noted to show inconsistent chromosome abnormalities; however, in the majority of cases, karyotype is normal in Goldenhar syndrome.[237] Diagnosis is made clinically, but debate on the specific diagnostic criteria continues.[236]

*Imaging:* Asymmetric facial appearance may rarely be visible on ultrasound. Other congenital anomalies may be seen and prompt further imaging with fetal MRI, which can improve detection of the asymmetry and raise concern for a hemifacial microsomia syndrome. Most often, characteristic facial features are obvious after delivery, leading to diagnosis.[233] Nevertheless, Goldenhar syndrome has been described as being suspected on the basis of ultrasound as early as 15 weeks' gestational age,

with observations of cleft palate and unilateral severe microphthalmia (Fig. 20.35A).[238] In the late third trimester, subtle abnormalities such as preauricular skin tags and colobomas can be recognized.[239] Additional anomalies such as pulmonary agenesis may be suggested by displacement of the fetal heart (Fig. 20.35B,C). Fetal MR has also been shown to be helpful in identifying abnormalities in development of the outer and middle ear, with absence of the expected T2 hyperintensity within the external auditory canal and tympanic cavity from the mid-second trimester through gestation (Fig. 20.35D).[240]

**Differential Diagnosis:** The differential diagnosis includes other craniofacial conditions, associations, or syndromes with spine anomalies: Emmanuel syndrome (due to an unbalanced 11/22 translocation that results in partial trisomy 11q and partial trisomy 22q), Treacher Collins, Townes–Brocks, in which there may be asymmetry of the ear size and cupping of one ear, CHARGE, branchio-oto-renal (BOR), or chromosomal deletions/duplications. Table 20.15 summarizes entities that may feature facial clefts.

**Prognosis:** Postnatal mortality primarily depends on the severity of congenital cardiac disease or airway malformations. If severe defects are not present, the long-term prognosis is good.[235]

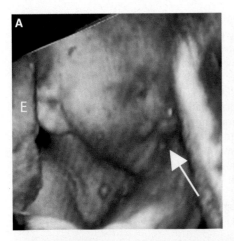
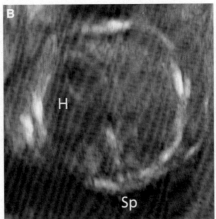
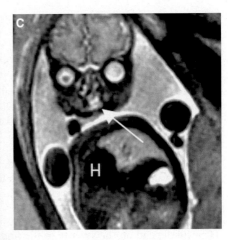

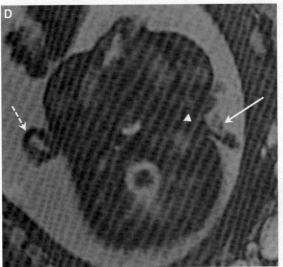
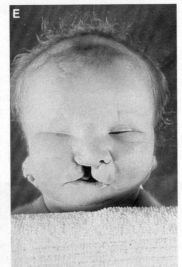

**FIGURE 20.35:** Goldenhar syndrome diagnosed prenatally in a 34-week-GA fetus. **A:** Three-dimensional ultrasound of the fetal face shows a low-set ear *(E)* and a cleft palate *(arrow)*. **B:** Axial ultrasound image through the chest demonstrates agenesis of one lung, with lateral displacement the fetal heart (H, heart; Sp, spine). **C:** Subsequent evaluation with fetal MRI of same fetus readily shows aplasia of the right lung with normal left lung and cleft palate *(arrow)* on coronal SSFSE T2 image. **D:** Axial SSFP sequence through the temporal bones shows asymmetry of earlobes with the left *(solid arrow)* normal and the right malformed *(dotted arrow)*. Normal external auditory canal is present on the left *(arrowhead)* but absent on the right. **E:** A postmortem photograph of a different patient with Goldenhar syndrome shows these similar facial features.

| Table 20.15 | Syndromes Associated with Facial Clefts |
| --- | --- |
| **Syndrome** | **Other Features** |
| Goldenhar syndrome | Asymmetric facial hypoplasia, microtia, preauricular skin tags, hemivertebrae, cardiac defects |
| Pierre-Robin sequence | Micrognathia, cleft of soft palate |
| Velocardiofacial syndrome | Cardiac defects, hypotonia, growth restriction, chromosome 22q microdeletion, autosomal dominant |
| Stickler syndrome | Flat facies, micrognathia, hypotonia, myopia, scoliosis, autosomal dominant |
| Treacher Collins syndrome | Malar and mandibular hypoplasia, downslanting palpebral fissures, ear malformations, absent lower eyelashes, autosomal dominant |
| Trisomy 13 | Polydactyly, congenital heart disease, CNS abnormalities |
| Trisomy 18 | IUGR, congenital heart disease |
| Van der Woude syndrome | Lower lip pits, missing teeth, autosomal dominant |

**Management:** Infants suspected of having a craniofacial microsomia syndrome should have a neonatology support at the time of delivery. Full physical exam should be performed to exclude other congenital anomalies. Referral to ophthalmology and audiology evaluations, screening echocardiography, and renal ultrasound should be obtained.[241] Echocardiography is especially important because of the possibility of severe conotruncal defects that result in high postnatal mortality. Postnatal spine radiographs are also recommended to evaluate for vertebral malformations.[233] Most affected individuals (>90%) have normal intelligence. Long-term management should focus on hearing abnormalities and possible facial nerve weakness.[242] Reconstructive surgery to address the facial asymmetry is often helpful.

**Recurrence Risk:** Most cases are de novo. Recurrence risk is 2% to 3%.[242]

## Treacher Collins Syndrome

Treacher Collins syndrome (TCS), also referred to as Treacher Collins–Fransceschetti syndrome and mandibulofacial dysostosis, consists of hypoplastic zygomatic bones and mandible, ear anomalies, coloboma of the eyelid rather than of the globe, absent lower eyelashes, and displaced hair growth onto cheeks.[243]

**Incidence:** The incidence of TCS ranges from 1:10,000 to 1:50,000.[244]

**Pathogenesis/Etiology:** Inheritance of TCS is autosomal dominant with most mutations being de novo.[244] Karyotype would be expected to be normal. There are several genes known to be associated with TCS, including *TCOF1, POLR1C,* and *POLR1D.* The *TCOF1* gene is the most common and accounts for 71% to 93% of mutations.[245]

**Diagnosis:** If genetic testing is performed, the *TCOF1* gene is typically evaluated first. If no mutation is found, the *POLR1D* and then the *POLR1C* genes are evaluated.

**Imaging:** The reliability of prenatal ultrasound in diagnosing TCS will depend on the severity of the findings. The principal findings in TCS are polyhydramnios, micrognathia, low-set ears, slanting palpebral fissures, and cleft palate (Fig. 20.36A). Typical facial features are better illustrated with three-dimensional ultrasound (Fig. 20.36B) than with standard two-dimensional imaging.[246] MRI may be helpful to evaluate airway and temporal bone anatomy (Fig. 20.36C,D).[246]

**Differential Diagnosis:** The differential diagnosis may include Goldenhar syndrome, though abnormalities in Goldenhar syndrome are almost always unilateral and involve notching of the upper rather than the lower lid, as well as epibulbar dermoids.

Fetuses with Goldenhar may also have vertebral anomalies and cardiac defects. Nager syndrome is also possible, but would have preaxial reduction defects of the upper extremities ranging from hypoplasia to aplasia of the thumb with or without involvement of the radius. Miller syndrome, also known as postaxial acrofacial dysostosis (POADS), may have similar findings, but is characterized by micrognathia, cleft palate, postaxial reduction defects, and vertebral anomalies.[247] Pierre-Robin sequence or nonsyndromic mandibular hypoplasia is characterized by early mandibular hypoplasia alone. It should be emphasized that limb anomalies are not a feature of TCS, and if present, Miller and Nager syndromes should be considered.

**Prognosis:** The prognosis depends on the severity of the phenotype expressed.

**Management:** Craniofacial abnormalities seen in this syndrome can lead to respiratory distress, requiring special positioning or tracheostomy,[248] and an ex utero intrapartum therapy (EXIT) procedure may be discussed for delivery planning if micrognathia is severe and airway access is questionable. In this instance, the child will remain on placental support until the airway is secured.

Management should involve a multidisciplinary craniofacial team. Surgical management is often needed for craniofacial reconstruction and cleft repair.[249] Diagnostic imaging with postnatal CT of the head and face to delineate abnormalities of the zygomatic arch, malar bones, and mandible is often

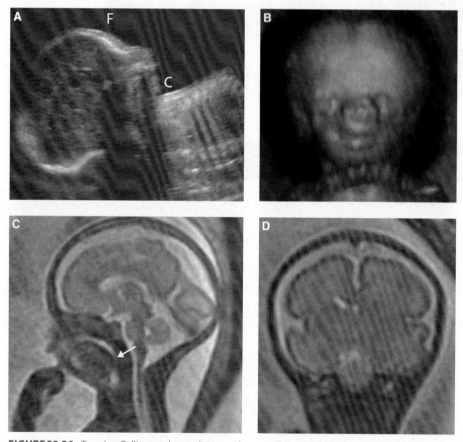

**FIGURE 20.36:** Treacher Collins syndrome diagnosed prenatally in a 29-week fetus. **A:** Two-dimensional sagittal ultrasound of the face shows retrognathia. F, face; C, chin. **B:** Three-dimensional view of the fetal face demonstrates abnormal flattening of the fetal nose and lack of visualization of the pinna bilaterally. **C:** Further evaluation with fetal MRI in sagittal plane with SSFSE T2 imaging also depicts the small mandible and the flattened nose. The tongue partly occludes the oropharyngeal airway *(arrow).* **D:** Coronal MR image shows absence of the bilateral ears.

pursued. An ophthalmology examination is important to evaluate for vision loss, amblyopia, refractive errors, and strabismus.[250] Auricular malformations of ossicles and the tympanic cavity can lead to conductive hearing loss in 40% to 50% of cases.[245] Speech therapy evaluations to assess for swallowing and feeding difficulty may determine the need for gastrostomy tube.[246] Rarely, palatal clefting and abnormalities of choanae can be seen.[251] Dental anomalies are present in 60% of TCS cases and can include dental agenesis, enamel abnormalities, and ectopic molars.[252]

**Recurrence Risk:** The inheritance of TCS is autosomal dominant, and most mutations are de novo.[244] Intrafamilial variability is marked. It is not uncommon for a parent to be mildly affected and undetected, so parental testing should be considered to guide recurrence risk counseling.

## Nager Syndrome

Nager syndrome was first described in 1948 and is one of a group of disorders referred to as the acrofacial dysostoses, a group of syndromes associated with craniofacial and skeletal malformations. Of the acrofacial dysostoses, Nager can be distinguished by characteristic facial features, including downslanting palpebral fissures, external ear malformations, midface/malar hypoplasia, and micrognathia.[253] Cleft lip and palate are also seen.[254] Limb malformations involve the radial distribution and include small or absent thumbs, triphalangeal thumbs, radial hypoplasia/aplasia and radioulnar synostosis. Reports of patients with typical features of Nager syndrome and other congenital anomalies, including

Hirschsprung disease, CNS anomalies, congenital heart defects, and cardiac conduction abnormalities, have been described.[255]

**Incidence:** Nager syndrome is rare, with fewer than 100 reported cases.[256]

**Pathogenesis/Etiology:** Nager syndrome is associated with mutation of the acrofacial dysostosis 1 gene (*AFD1*) on chromosome 9q32, but numerous other genetic etiologies have been reported in patients with clinical features of Nager syndrome.[253] Families with both autosomal dominant and autosomal recessive inheritance have been reported.[257]

**Diagnosis:** *AFD1* gene testing could be offered if Nager syndrome is suspected. Postnatal assessment of clinical features is more definitive than genetic testing.

*Imaging:* Suspicion for Nager syndrome may be raised on prenatal ultrasound, although craniofacial and extremity findings can be subtle and are often not well delineated. As with Goldenhar and Treacher Collins syndromes, prenatal diagnosis depends on the severity of the disorder. The vast majority of these rare cases have been described in the pediatric literature, and very few fetuses with Nager have been described prenatally.[258] Prenatal diagnosis has been suspected as early as 22 weeks' gestational age based on ultrasound.[259] The most readily recognized features by prenatal two-dimensional ultrasound are micrognathia and radial hypoplasia (Fig. 20.37A,B). Adding three-dimensional technique will enable further detail of the external

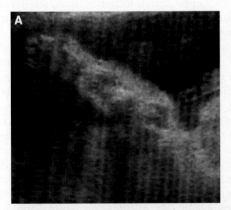
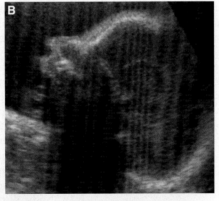
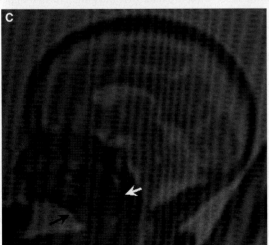
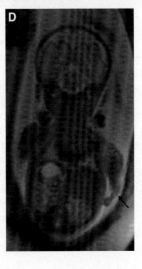

**FIGURE 20.37:** A 28-week fetus with confirmed Nager syndrome. **A:** US of the arm demonstrates lack of visualization of bones of the forearm. **B:** Severe micrognathia was present on US. **C:** Sagittal SSFSE T2 of the same fetus shows severe micrognathia *(black arrow)* with obstruction of the oropharyngeal airway *(white arrow)*. **D:** Coronal SSFSE T2 depicts significant shortening of the arm *(arrow)*. The lower extremities were normal.

ears, which are typically small, low-set, and posteriorly rotated. Sometimes, it is possible to identify down-sloping palpebral fissures. Unilateral limb involvement has also been described in a prenatally diagnosed case without any family history of acrofacial dysostosis.[260] MRI is often performed in the presence of severe micrognathia to evaluate severity of airway obstruction (Fig. 20.37C,D).

**Differential Diagnosis:** The differential diagnosis depends on severity of associated anomalies. Other facial dysostoses in the differential would include Treacher Collins, which is distinguished by lack of limb anomalies. Orofacial digital syndromes typically have polydactyly or bifid hallux, while reduction defects are noted in Nager syndrome. Other syndromes associated with radial ray anomalies include Fanconi anemia and trisomy 18. Lower extremity malformations are rarely seen in Nager syndrome. This finding may help distinguish Nager from Miller syndrome, which is another disorder within the acrofacial dysostoses group and is characterized by postaxial reduction defects, vertebral anomalies, and cardiac defects.[253]

**Prognosis:** Prognosis depends upon the severity and medical management of the conductive hearing loss and upper airway obstruction that is responsible for early feeding and respiratory difficulties. Intelligence is expected to be normal, unless impacted by delayed diagnosis of these anomalies.[258]

**Management:** Infants born with suspected Nager syndrome often have respiratory issues related to micrognathia. In the presence of severe micrognathia, an EXIT procedure to airway may be necessary. Tracheostomy is sometimes required.[261] Feeding issues are common. Orthopedic management of extremity anomalies may be necessary, and a radiographic survey of the infant will be important to define skeletal malformations. Nearly all affected fetuses have some degree of hearing loss, and postnatal imaging with CT or MR of the temporal bones may be indicated. Because of the associated incidence of CHD and conduction abnormalities, echocardiography should be performed to screen for structural heart disease.[261]

**Recurrence Risk:** Recurrence risk varies according to inheritance pattern. Both autosomal dominant and recessive inheritance have been reported. In sporadic cases, recurrence risk is cited at 3% to 5%.[261]

# NONHERITABLE SYNDROMES AND ASSOCIATIONS

The following section includes multisystemic disorders arising from sporadic mutations or nongenetic processes.

## VATER/VACTERL

The VATER association refers to a nonrandom association of the following anomalies: *v*ertebral defects, *a*nal atresia, *tr*acheoesophageal fistula with *e*sophageal atresia, and *r*enal dysplasia. The association, originally described in 1973, was later expanded to include *c*ardiac anomalies and *l*imb anomalies in the VACTE*RL* association. The entity is not considered syndromic, as there is no known common underlying etiology. Of the cardiac defects in patients with VACTERL, the most

common type is ventricular septal defect.[262] The most common type of renal anomaly is renal agenesis, and the most common limb defects are reduction deformities and polydactyly. Three of the core findings are required to make the diagnosis of VATER.[262]

**Incidence:** The incidence ranges from 1 in 10,000 to 1 in 40,000.[263]

**Pathogenesis/Etiology:** It is postulated that the grouping of disorders arise from abnormal mesodermal organization before 35 weeks' gestational age.[264] Interestingly, nearly all cases are sporadic, and no established gene has been found, although one patient with features was found to have a mutation in the Homeobox protein Hox-D13 (*HOXD13*) gene.[265] There are a few reports of families with inherited VACTERL features.[266] There is also a published report of both dichorionic, diamniotic twin fetuses affected by the VATER association. However, this twin pregnancy was conceived with intracytoplasmic sperm injection (ICSI) and embryo transfer, and the incidence of anomalies in pregnancies arising from ICSI is higher than seen with spontaneous conceptions.[267]

### Diagnosis

*Imaging:* Prenatal imaging can detect anomalies that may lead to suspicion of the VACTERL association (Fig. 20.38). Diagnosis of VACTERL by ultrasound has been described as early as 17 weeks.[268] The most commonly recognized findings include radial ray anomalies, vertebral anomalies, and renal agenesis. Other less commonly identified findings include absent stomach, ventricular septal defect, hydronephrosis, and lower extremity reduction defects. The minority of diagnosed cases exhibit more than three of the classic findings.[269]

Esophageal atresia may be difficult to diagnose by ultrasound, inferred either by an absent stomach or by polyhydramnios, and fluid may still be present in the stomach owing to an esophageal fistula. The diagnosis of esophageal atresia can be made by fetal MR imaging, which may show fluid distension of the hypopharynx and upper esophagus, and absence of the intrathoracic esophagus (Fig. 20.38E).[270] Fetal MR imaging may be useful for further evaluation of the abdomen, elucidating details of renal development, and allowing for problem-solving in cases of urogenital sinus formation and obstructive tract lesions, which may be confusing due to cyst formation. Spine and limb anomalies may also be discernible by fetal MR imaging. Normal appearance of the fetal brain is expected.

Secondary findings of VACTERL include single umbilical artery, abnormal fetal respirations, and intrauterine growth retardation.[268]

**Differential Diagnosis:** Findings present determine the differential diagnosis, but could include CHARGE syndrome, diabetic embryopathy, and Townes–Brocks syndrome, which share features including anorectal malformation, ear anomalies, vertebral anomalies, renal hypoplasia or dysplasia, cardiac anomalies, and limb anomalies. Fanconi anemia, chromosomal abnormalities, or MURCS association, which includes Mullerian hypoplasia/aplasia, renal agenesis, and cervicothoracic somite dysplasia, may be considered. There is also a genetically distinct condition referred to as VATER with hydrocephaly that has overlapping features but may be X-linked, and with hydrocephaly as a feature, is often associated with intellectual disability.

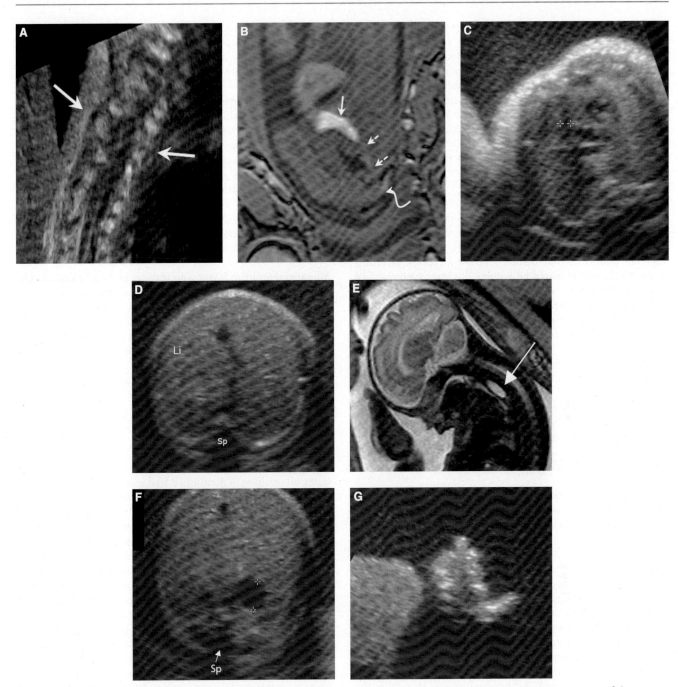

**FIGURE 20.38:** VACTERL association in multiple fetuses. **A: V**ertebral defects. Coronal ultrasound demonstrating curvature of the spine and multiple segmentation errors *(arrows)*. **B: A**nal atresia. Sagittal T1 image demonstrates dilated meconium *(solid arrow)* proximal to diminutive meconium in rectosigmoid *(dotted arrows)*, and complete absence in the rectum *(curved arrow)* in fetus at 28 weeks with VACTERL and anal atresia. **C: C**ardiac. Ultrasound shows a ventricular septal defect. **D: T**racheoesophageal fistula. Initial survey demonstrates an abnormally high amniotic fluid index (30 mm) and absence of the stomach (Li, liver; Sp, spine). **E: E**sophageal atresia. Sagittal SSFSE T2 image depicts a fluid-distended esophageal pouch above the atresia, which was noted transiently during imaging. (Courtesy of Dr. Chris Cassady, Houston, TX.) **F: R**enal anomalies. Axial view through the fetal abdomen at the level of the kidneys shows abnormally dilated renal pelves with an AP diameter of 15 mm on the right (calipers) and 8 mm on the left (not shown). Sp, spine. **G: L**imb defects. Polydactyly was observed in the left hand.

**Prognosis:** Neonatal survival is high with the VACTERL association; however, affected infants require considerable medical and surgical attention.[268]

**Management:** An infant born with features of VACTERL should have full physical exam and imaging to identify all anomalies. Examination should focus on detecting malformations that could exclude or verify diagnoses. Screening should include spine and extremity radiographs, echocardiography, and renal ultrasound. If there is difficulty or hypoxia with feeding, airway and esophageal evaluation should be performed to exclude tracheoesophageal fistula. Postnatal management of patients with VACTERL/VATER association focuses on surgical correction of the specific congenital anomalies. Long-term medical management is aimed at addressing the sequela of congenital malformations. If optimal surgical correction is achievable, the prognosis can be relatively positive. However, some patients will continue to be affected by their congenital malformations throughout life. Importantly, patients with VACTERL association do not tend to have neurocognitive impairment.

**Recurrence Risk:** VACTERL association is typically sporadic.

## Amniotic Band Syndrome

Amniotic band syndrome (ABS) refers to fetal anomalies resulting from fibrous bands adhering to and entrapping fetal parts, leading potentially to structural deformity and even amputation. The anomalies may involve multiple locations, including limbs, trunk, and craniofacial regions.[271] Other synonyms for this disorder include constriction band syndrome, amniotic band disruption complex, amniotic deformity, adhesion and mutilation (ADAM) complex, amniotic adhesion malformation syndrome, and limb and body wall defect complex.[272]

**Incidence:** Depending on how ABS is defined, incidence ranges from 1 in 1,200 to 1 in 15,000 live births.[273]

**Pathogenesis/Etiology:** Numerous theories for the underlying mechanism of ABS exist. Common considerations include a disruption in embryogenesis and primary rupture of amnion early in gestation.[272] Most cases of ABS are sporadic. No genes have been found to predispose to ABS.

**Diagnosis:** Amniocentesis is not necessary in situations in which diagnosis of ABS is clear. If diagnosis is unclear owing to the appearance of associated anomalies, amniocentesis should be offered.

*Imaging:* Amniotic bands can be identified both by two-dimensional ultrasound and by fetal MRI with a similar sensitivity, although the two modalities used in conjunction may aid the diagnosis in a small percentage of cases. The bands usually appear as thin, wispy strands that are freely floating within the amniotic fluid (Fig. 20.39A). In approximately one-third of focal or regional cases, an amniotic band will be identified in close approximation to the involved fetal part (Fig. 20.39B). Three-dimensional ultrasound has been shown to solidify the diagnosis by visualizing the physical relationship of a band with the affected fetal part.[274]

Limb involvement is appreciable as focal constriction of the soft tissues, possibly with edema distal to the site of constriction (Fig. 20.39C). This edema appears as hypoechoic subcutaneous skin thickening on US, and as fluid signal thickening the subcutaneous space on MR imaging (Fig. 20.39D,E). On MRI, SSFP or heavy T2-weighted images can improve visualization of the amniotic bands (Fig. 20.39F). Real-time imaging by US or cine imaging with MR may show synchronous movement of separate fetal parts bound by a single band. Circumferential involvement by a band or bands may cause constriction of growth and deformity of the chest, abdomen, and skull or may also cause amputation of a limb.[274]

Involvement of the umbilical cord by amniotic bands is also a potential complication of this disorder. The bands may envelop several loops of cord or may constrict a focal segment, leading to congestion of flow. Doppler spectral wave analysis may show pulsatility of the umbilical vein, absent end-diastolic flow in the umbilical artery, and elevation of the middle cerebral artery peak systolic velocity (Fig. 20.39G).[274]

**Differential Diagnosis:** The differential diagnosis is based on the findings and could include lymphatic or vascular malformations in the setting of a focal limb soft tissue swelling. More severe limb involvement with distortion of normal bone development may raise the question of limb reduction defects in other syndromes such as Fanconi anemia or Adams–Oliver syndrome. Constriction and deformity of the skull may mimic a craniosynostosis.

**Prognosis:** The long-term outcome depends on the location and severity of deformations.

**Management:** In an infant with features of ABS, umbilical cord involvement may necessitate intrauterine lysis or early delivery if fetal compromise develops.[275] After birth, care is focused on management of deformities present, many requiring surgical therapy.[271] Reconstructive surgery for craniofacial clefts, anophthalmia, and encephalocele may be required.

**Recurrence Risk:** Most cases of ABS are sporadic with low recurrence.[271] A small number of families have reported recurrent pregnancies with amniotic bands.

## Arthrogryposis

Arthrogryposis describes joint contractures in many different states, all resulting in diminished fetal movement. Arthrogyposis was first described in 1841.[276] There is a debate on the use of the phrase "multiple congenital contractures" versus the term arthrogryposis. Although both names may be used interchangeably, it should be emphasized that the term arthrogryposis is a descriptive rather than a definitive diagnosis. Any disease process that reduces fetal movement after 8 weeks' gestational age will impact fetal growth. The etiologies are extensive and include neurologic disease that may be either congenital or acquired and may affect the central or peripheral nervous system sometimes occurring due to a vascular insult, infection, or drugs. Connective tissue defects and muscle abnormalities, including muscular dystrophies and mitochondrial abnormalities, in utero space limitations from oligohydramnios, multiple gestation pregnancy or uterine fibroids, or maternal diseases such as diabetes mellitus, myasthenia gravis, and toxic effect from drugs, are also potential causes. All may impact fetal movement and lead to joint contractures.[276]

**Incidence:** The incidence is approximately 1 in 2,000 to 3,000 live births.[277]

**Pathogenesis/Etiology:** Arthrogryposis multiplex congenital (AMC) refers to categorized types of arthrogryposis, some associated with a genetic defect. There are many subgroups of AMC, all differing in signs and causes. The most commonly seen form of AMC is a sporadic, symmetric disorder known as amyoplasia.[278] This type of AMC is characterized by symmetric replacement of extremity muscles by fat and connective tissue. Midline hemangiomas are also described in these patients, and, importantly, affected patients have normal cognitive function. Another subtype of AMC is called distal arthrogryposis,

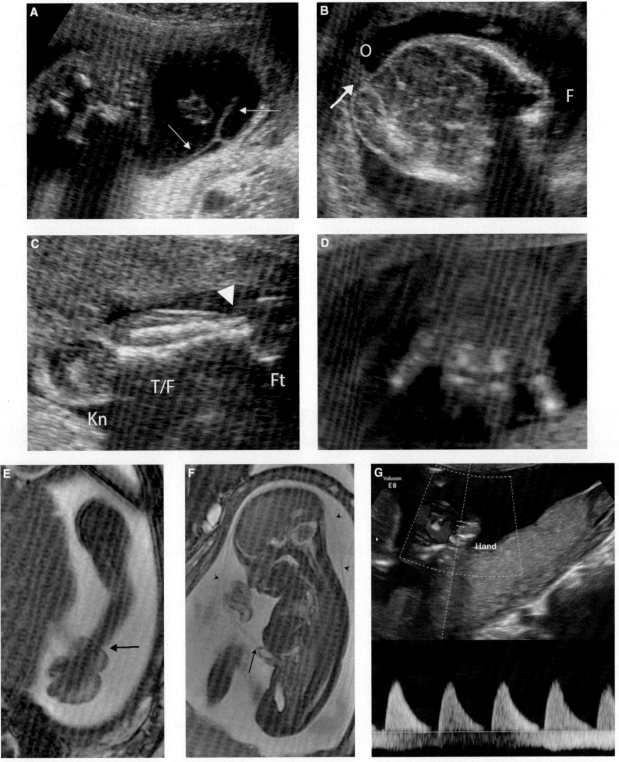

**FIGURE 20.39:** Amniotic band syndrome. **A–C:** A 19-week-GA fetus. **A:** Images through the lower left quadrant of the amniotic cavity show abnormal septations consistent with amniotic bands *(arrows)*. **B:** Axial image through the fetal head shows apparent herniation of the occipital lobes through the posterior skull, consistent with encephalocele caused by amniotic bands next to defect, *arrow* (O, occiput; F, face). **C:** The left lower extremity is abnormal, with constriction of the soft tissues around the ankle *(arrowhead)*, and swelling of the subcutaneous tissues in the foot, distal to the constriction (Kn, knee; T/F, tibia/fibula; Ft, foot). **D,E:** 23-week fetus, **(D)** there is amputation of the distal second and third digits. **E:** Sagittal SSFP through the hand demonstrates constriction *(arrow)* from the band and distal T2 hyperintense swelling. **F:** SSFP imaging best depicts bands on this sagittal image of a fetus in which the band is identified as a thin membrane attaching to the umbilical cord *(arrow)*, deforming abdominal wall, and encircling fetus *(arrowheads)*. **G:** 18-week fetus with bands encircling umbilical cord. Spectral Doppler of the tangled compromised cord demonstrates loss of diastolic flow in the umbilical artery and pulsatile umbilical vein.

which is transmitted autosomal dominant but can have variable expression. In this disorder, there is characteristic involvement of distal joints with talipes equinovarus, calcaneovalgus, vertical talus, and metatarsus varus. The upper limbs can also be affected and may show ulnar deviation, camptodactyly, hypoplastic, or absent flexed overriding fingers. The large joints are spared. A number of distal arthrogryposis syndromes have been described.[279] Several genes, *TPM2, TTNI2, TNNT3,* and *MYH3,* have been found responsible for the distal arthrogryposis syndromes and are available for clinical testing. The testing, however, is not required for diagnosis and may be falsely negative because of the number of subtypes of arthrogryposis and locus heterogeneity.[280,281]

Another subtype of AMC, multiple pterygium syndrome, is a group of autosomal dominant, recessive, or X-linked inherited syndromes that manifests with multiple contractures associated with webbing ("pterygia") of the joints, micrognathia, low-set ears, cardiac abnormaltiies, lung hypoplasia, cystic hygroma, and hydrops.[276] As opposed to the above-described entities, abnormal neurologic function is common in this group of disorders. Also worthy of mention is Pena-Shokeir syndrome,[282,283] which is a recessive disorder characterized by arthrogryposis and pulmonary hypoplasia. The pathophysiology in this disorder may reflect a primary motor neuropathy with a paucity of anterior horn cells in the spinal cord, although it has also

been postulated that the phenotype results from fetal akinesia.[248] Table 20.16 summarizes disorders exhibiting evidence of arthrogryposis.

**Diagnosis:** Amniocentesis should be offered to exclude chromosomal abnormalities. Families of infants with arthrogryposis should be evaluated by a geneticist to assist with diagnosis of the underlying mechanism for the features seen, to discuss potential for genetic testing, and to receive counseling on recurrence risk.

*Imaging:* First-trimester ultrasound may show increased nuchal translucency between weeks 10 and 14, and scoliosis has been reported as early as 15 weeks' gestational age.[284] Arthrogryposis should be suspected when decreased or lack of fetal movement is observed along with an abnormal fetal position. These observations should prompt a careful inspection of the joints, bone for fractures, spine, and thoracic circumference (Fig. 20.40A–C). Features seen by prenatal ultrasound are summarized in Table 20.17. Fetal MRI may be helpful in identifying CNS malformations; for example, polymicrogyria can be present in some types (Fig. 20.40D,E).

**Differential Diagnosis:** Arthrogryposis is not a diagnosis; it is a physical finding that simply refers to contractures of multiple joints regardless of etiology. Therefore, any condition that may

| **Table 20.16** | **Major Features of Disorders Exhibiting Evidence of Arthrogryposis** | | |
|---|---|---|---|
| **Disorder** | **Major Features** | **Inheritance** | **Prognosis** |
| Pena-Shokeir syndrome | Growth retardation, multiple joint contractures, facial anomalies, pulmonary hypoplasia, hypertelorism, abnormal bone morphology with decreased calcification, short umbilical cord | Autosomal recessive or sporadic | Usually lethal |
| Lethal multiple pterygium syndrome | Soft tissue webbing and flexion contractures of neck, axilla, antecubital, and popliteal regions; hypoplastic lungs; intrauterine growth restriction; cystic hygroma; hydrops | Usually autosomal recessive | Uniformly lethal |
| Arthrogryposis multiplex congenital | Fixed contractures, clubfeet, involvement of all four extremities in two-thirds of cases, normal intelligence | Sporadic | Variable, usually lethal when severe |
| Congenital myotonic dystrophy | Clubfoot (50%), hypotonia, facial muscle weakness, swallowing and speech difficulties, respiratory distress, occasional joint contractures, mental retardation | Autosomal dominant; affected infants are born only to mothers with myotonic dystrophy | Mental retardation and motor delay common |
| Restrictive dermopathy | Hyperkeratosis; flexion of knees, elbows, wrists, and ankles; camptodactyly; short umbilical cord; prematurity; hypertelorism; tight, rigid, shiny skin | Autosomal recessive | Lethal after birth |
| Cerebro-oculo-facial-skeletal syndrome | Microcephaly, microphthalmos, cataract, scoliosis, hip and pelvic defects, flexion contractures, sloping forehead, rockerbottom feet | Autosomal recessive | Survival typically <3 y |
| Alpers disease (progressive infantile poliodystrophy) | Intrauterine growth restriction, microcephaly, retrognathia, joint contractures, seizures | Autosomal recessive | Survival typically <3 y |
| Gaucher disease type 2 | Multiple contractures, visceromegaly, pulmonary hypoplasis, ichthyosis | Autosomal recessive | Survival typically <1 y |

Adapted from Hammond E, Donnenfield AE. Fetal akinesia. *Obstet Gynecol Surv.* 1995;50:140–149.

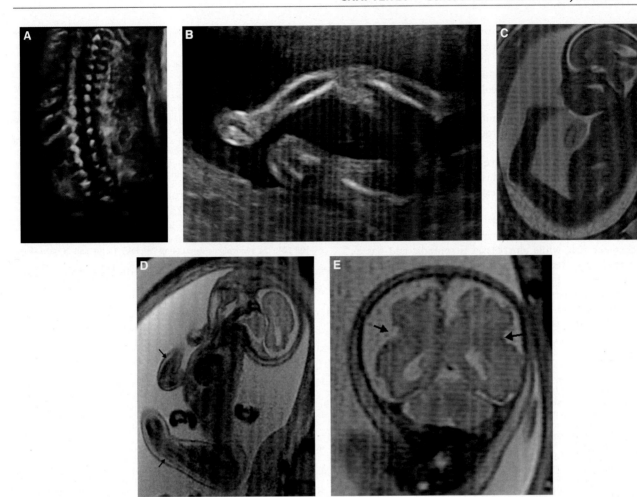

**FIGURE 20.40:** Arthrogryposis in two fetuses. **A–C:** Fetus at 22 weeks. **A:** Fixed curvature of the spine was noted on 3D ultrasound. **B:** Unusual fixed positioning of the lower extremities was noted with persistent hyperextension and rotation at the knee. **C:** Sagittal SSFP image shows similar findings. **D,E:** Fetus at 27 weeks. **D:** Sagittal SSFSE T2 demonstrates fixed flexion deformities at the elbow and knee. The subcutaneous fat *(arrows)* is prominent, and the muscles *(dark signal)* are thin. **E:** Coronal SSFSE T2 image of the brain demonstrates irregular appearance of the Sylvian fissures *(arrows)* consistent with polymicrogyria. Patient expired with postmortem diagnosis of arthrogryposis, Pena-Shokeir phenotype.

lead to multiple congenital contractures can be included in the differential. There are over 100 such conditions. The major categories can be divided into central nervous system anomalies or dysfunction, peripheral nervous system problems, muscle

| Table 20.17 | **List of Features of Arthrogryposis Seen by Prenatal Ultrasound** |
|---|---|

Diminished or absent mobility
Abnormal fetal position
Fixed flexion deformities
Growth retardation
Small chest
Thin ribs
Multiple diaphyseal fractures
Increased NT/lymphatic malformation
Scoliosis
Fetal seizures
Ventriculomegaly

Adapted from Bilardo CM, Timmerman E, Pajkrt E, et al. Increased nuchal translucency in euploid fetuses—what should we be telling the parents? *Prenat Diagn.* 2010;30:93–102.

pathology, and constraint. In addition to those described above, neonatal myasthenia, spinal muscular atrophy, or chromosomal abnormalities may be identified.

**Prognosis:** Short-term and long-term prognosis depends on the extent of abnormalities and number of systems impacted. Some patients with arthrogryposis multiplex congenita (AMC) may require intubation. Those patients with AMC who require ventilator support have much worse long-term outcomes[285]

**Management:** An infant with arthrogryposis should have a complete physical exam with attention to joints. Characteristic features include rigidity of joints from contractures, dislocations, absence of normal skin creases, increase in subcutaneous fat, deep skin dimples, and decreased muscle mass.[286]

Respiratory distress may be seen in patients with arthrogryposis shortly after birth owing to pulmonary hypoplasia. Feeding issues may also occur. Management of joint abnormalities includes physical therapy, which should be initiated in the newborn period to maintain and develop joint mobility.[286] It is important to exclude central nervous system abnormalities; therefore, MR imaging of the brain and spine is recommended.[286] Renal dysfunction and cholestasis can be associated with some subtypes of the distal arthrogryposis syndromes and should be screened with ultrasound and biochemical testing.[287]

Long-term management issues focus on joint disorders, including potential for knee contractures. There is an increased incidence of hip dislocation and scoliosis.[288] A study of teens and adults with arthrogryposis showed that they had limited shoulder motion and elbow deformities, but no other significant handicaps. Half of the study group walked independently, and most had normal intelligence.[287] However, complex cases of arthrogryposis that did not survive were not included in this study, and therefore the information is limited to cases of amyoplasia, which, in general, have the best long-term outcomes.

**Recurrence Risk:** Recurrence risk varies according to the underlying cause. Distal arthrogryposis syndromes have a 50% recurrence risk, while amyoplasia is sporadic and has a low recurrence risk. Recurrence risk is 25% for the forms with autosomal recessive inheritance. In one study of nonsyndromic forms of arthrogryposis for which no cause was found, recurrence risk ranged from 1.4% to 7%, depending on the location of contractures and organ systems involved.[277]

# REFERENCES

1. Snijders RJ, Sundberg K, Holzgreve W, et al. Maternal age- and gestation-specific risk for trisomy 21. *Ultrasound Obstet Gynecol.* 1999;13:167–170.
2. Munne S, Sultan KM, Weier HU, et al. Assessment of numeric abnormalities of X, Y, 18, and 16 chromosomes in preimplantation human embryos before transfer. *Am J Obstet Gynecol.* 1995;172:1191–1199.
3. Bull MJ. Health supervision for children with Down syndrome. *Pediatrics.* 2011;128:393–406.
4. Antonarakis SE. Parental origin of the extra chromosome in trisomy 21 as indicated by analysis of DNA polymorphisms: Down Syndrome Collaborative Group. *N Engl J Med.* 1991;324:872–876.
5. Huether CA, Ivanovich J, Goodwin BS, et al. Maternal age specific risk rate estimates for Down syndrome among live births in whites and other races from Ohio and metropolitan Atlanta, 1970–1989. *J Med Genet.* 1998;35:482–490.
6. Cicero S, Bindra R, Rembouskos G, et al. Integrated ultrasound and biochemical screening for trisomy 21 using fetal nuchal translucency, absent fetal nasal bone, free beta-hCG and PAPP-A at 11 to 14 weeks. *Prenat Diagn.* 2003;23:306–310.
7. Canick JA, Kloza EM, Lambert-Messerlian GM, et al. DNA sequencing of maternal plasma to identify Down syndrome and other trisomies in multiple gestations. *Prenat Diagn.* 2012;32:730–734.
8. Devers PL, Cronister A, Ormond KE, et al. Noninvasive prenatal testing/noninvasive prenatal diagnosis: the position of the National Society of Genetic Counselors. *J Genet Couns.* 2013;22(3):291–295.
9. Vintzileos A, Walters C, Yeo L. Absent nasal bone in the prenatal detection of fetuses with trisomy 21 in a high-risk population. *Obstet Gynecol.* 2003;101:905–908.
10. Canick J. Prenatal screening for trisomy 21: recent advances and guidelines. *Clin Chem Lab Med.* 2012;50:1003–1008.
11. Agathokleous M, Chaveeva P, Poon LC, et al. Meta-analysis of second-trimester markers for trisomy 21. *Ultrasound Obstet Gynecol.* 2013;41:247–261.
12. Nicolaides KH, Heath V, Cicero S. Increased fetal nuchal translucency at 11–14 weeks. *Prenat Diagn.* 2002;22:308–315.
13. Holzgreve W, Curry CJ, Golbus MS, et al. Investigation of nonimmune hydrops fetalis. *Am J Obstet Gynecol.* 1984;150:805–812.
14. Sepulveda W, Reid R, Nicolaidis P, et al. Second-trimester echogenic bowel and intraamniotic bleeding: association between fetal bowel echogenicity and amniotic fluid spectrophotometry at 410 nm. *Am J Obstet Gynecol.* 1996;174:839–842.
15. Choudhry MS, Rahman N, Boyd P, et al. Duodenal atresia: associated anomalies, prenatal diagnosis and outcome. *Pediatr Surg Int.* 2009;25:727–730.
16. Dankovcik R, Jirasek JE, Kucera E, et al. Prenatal diagnosis of annular pancreas: reliability of the double bubble sign with periduodenal hyperechogenic band. *Fetal Diagn Ther.* 2008;24:483–490.
17. Chapman T. Fetal genitourinary imaging. *Pediatr Radiol.* 2012;42(suppl 1):S115–S123.
18. Kovac CM, Brown JA, Apodaca CC, et al. Maternal ethnicity and variation of fetal femur length calculations when screening for Down syndrome. *J Ultrasound Med.* 2002;21:719–722.
19. Ranweiler R. Assessment and care of the newborn with Down syndrome. *Adv Neonatal Care.* 2009;9:17–24; quiz 25–16.
20. Yang Q, Rasmussen SA, Friedman JM. Mortality associated with Down's syndrome in the USA from 1983 to 1997: a population-based study. *Lancet.* 2002;359:1019–1025.
21. Roberts JE, Price J, Malkin C. Language and communication development in Down syndrome. *Ment Retard Dev Disabil Res Rev.* 2007;13:26–35.
22. Holland AJ, Hon J, Huppert FA, et al. Incidence and course of dementia in people with Down's syndrome: findings from a population-based study. *J Intellect Disabil Res.* 2000;44(pt 2):138–146.
23. Henry E, Walker D, Wiedmeier SE, et al. Hematological abnormalities during the first week of life among neonates with Down syndrome: data from a multi-hospital healthcare system. *Am J Med Genet A.* 2007;143:42–50.
24. Eunpu DL, McDonald DM, Zackai EH. Trisomy 21: rate in second-degree relatives. *Am J Med Genet.* 1986;25:361–363.
25. Lin HY, Lin SP, Chen YJ, et al. Clinical characteristics and survival of trisomy 18 in a medical center in Taipei, 1988–2004. *Am J Med Genet A.* 2006;140:945–951.
26. Eggermann T, Nothen MM, Eiben B, et al. Trisomy of human chromosome 18: molecular studies on parental origin and cell stage of nondisjunction. *Hum Genet.* 1996;97:218–223.
27. Palomaki GE, Neveux LM, Knight GJ, et al. Maternal serum-integrated screening for trisomy 18 using both first- and second-trimester markers. *Prenat Diagn.* 2003;23:243–247.
28. Nyberg DA, Kramer D, Resta RG, et al. Prenatal sonographic findings of trisomy 18: review of 47 cases. *J Ultrasound Med.* 1993;12:103–113.
29. Hill LM. The sonographic detection of trisomies 13, 18, and 21. *Clin Obstet Gynecol.* 1996;39:831–850.
30. Moyano D, Huggon IC, Allan LD. Fetal echocardiography in trisomy 18. *Arch Dis Child.* 2005;90:F520–F522.
31. Babcock CJ, Goldstein RB, Filly RA. Prenatally detected fetal myelomeningocele: is karyotype analysis warranted? *Radiology.* 1995;194:491–494.
32. Yoder PR, Sabbagha RE, Gross SJ, et al. The second-trimester fetus with isolated choroid plexus cysts: a meta-analysis of risk of trisomies 18 and 21. *Obstet Gynecol.* 1999;93:869–872.
33. Snijders RJ, Shawa L, Nicolaides KH. Fetal choroid plexus cysts and trisomy 18: assessment of risk based on ultrasound findings and maternal age. *Prenat Diagn.* 1994;14:1119–1127.
34. Bahado-Singh RO, Lynch L, Deren O, et al. First-trimester growth restriction and fetal aneuploidy: the effect of type of aneuploidy and gestational age. *Am J Obstet Gynecol.* 1997;176:976–980.
35. Byrne J, Blanc WA. Malformations and chromosome anomalies in spontaneously aborted fetuses with single umbilical artery. *Am J Obstet Gynecol.* 1985;151:340–342.
36. Benjamin DR, Juul S, Siebert JR. Congenital posterolateral diaphragmatic hernia: associated malformations. *J Pediatr Surg.* 1988;23:899–903.
37. Rasmussen SA, Wong LY, Yang Q, et al. Population-based analyses of mortality in trisomy 13 and trisomy 18. *Pediatrics.* 2003;111:777–784.
38. Baty BJ, Blackburn BL, Carey JC. Natural history of trisomy 18 and trisomy 13, I: growth, physical assessment, medical histories, survival, and recurrence risk. *Am J Med Genet.* 1994;49:175–188.
39. Carey JC. Health supervision and anticipatory guidance for children with genetic disorders (including specific recommendations for trisomy 21, trisomy 18, and neurofibromatosis I). *Pediatr Clin North Am.* 1992;39:25–53.
40. Hassold T, Jacobs PA, Leppert M, et al. Cytogenetic and molecular studies of trisomy 13. *J Med Genet.* 1987;24:725–732.
41. Brizot ML, Snijders RJ, Bersinger NA, et al. Maternal serum pregnancy-associated plasma protein A and fetal nuchal translucency thickness for the prediction of fetal trisomies in early pregnancy. *Obstet Gynecol.* 1994;84:918–922.
42. Lehman CD, Nyberg DA, Winter TC III, et al. Trisomy 13 syndrome: prenatal US findings in a review of 33 cases. *Radiology.* 1995;194:217–222.
43. Wladimiroff JW, Bhaggoe WR, Kristelijn M, et al. Sonographically determined anomalies and outcome in 170 chromosomally abnormal fetuses. *Prenat Diagn.* 1995;15:431–438.
44. Jacobs PA, Hassold TJ, Henry A, et al. Trisomy 13 ascertained in a survey of spontaneous abortions. *J Med Genet.* 1987;24:721–724.
45. Tuohy JF, James DK. Pre-eclampsia and trisomy 13. *BJOG.* 1992;99:891–894.
46. Bdolah Y, Palomaki GE, Yaron Y, et al. Circulating angiogenic proteins in trisomy 13. *Am J Obstet Gynecol.* 2006;194:239–245.
47. Schreinemachers DM, Cross PK, Hook EB. Rates of trisomies 21, 18, 13 and other chromosome abnormalities in about 20 000 prenatal studies compared with estimated rates in live births. *Hum Genet.* 1982;61:318–324.
48. Hassold T, Chen N, Funkhouser J, et al. A cytogenetic study of 1000 spontaneous abortions. *Ann Hum Genet.* 1980;44:151–178.
49. Rochon L, Vekemans MJ. Triploidy arising from a first meiotic nondisjunction in a mother carrying a reciprocal translocation. *J Med Genet.* 1990;27(11):724–726.
50. McFadden DE, Kalousek DK. Two different phenotypes of fetuses with chromosomal triploidy: correlation with parental origin of the extra haploid set. *Am J Med Genet.* 1991;38:535–538.
51. de Graaf IM, van Bezouw SM, Jakobs ME, et al. First-trimester non-invasive prenatal diagnosis of triploidy. *Prenat Diagn.* 1999;19:175–177.
52. Schluth C, Doray B, Girard-Lemaire F, et al. Prenatal diagnosis of a true fetal tetraploidy in direct and cultured chorionic villi. *Genet Couns.* 2004;15:429–436.
53. Pircon RA, Porto M, Towers CV, et al. Ultrasound findings in pregnancies complicated by fetal triploidy. *J Ultrasound Med.* 1989;8:507–511.
54. Stefanova I, Jenderny J, Kaminsky E, et al. Mosaic and complete tetraploidy in live-born infants: two new patients and review of the literature. *Clin Dysmorphol.* 2010;19:123–127.

55. Di Cintio E, Parazzini F, Rosa C, et al. The epidemiology of gestational trophoblastic disease. *Gen Diagn Pathol.* 1997;143:103–108.

56. Lindor NM, Ney JA, Gaffey TA, et al. A genetic review of complete and partial hydatidiform moles and nonmolar triploidy. *Mayo Clin Proc.* 1992;67:791–799.

57. Sherard J, Bean C, Bove B, et al. Long survival in a 69,XXY triploid male. *Am J Med Genet.* 1986;25:307–312.

58. Jauniaux E. Partial moles: from postnatal to prenatal diagnosis. *Placenta.* 1999;20:379–388.

59. Gravholt CH, Juul S, Naeraa RW, et al. Prenatal and postnatal prevalence of Turner's syndrome: a registry study. *BMJ.* 1996;312:16–21.

60. Frias JL, Davenport ML. Health supervision for children with Turner syndrome. *Pediatrics.* 2003;111:692–702.

61. Jacobs P, Dalton P, James R, et al. Turner syndrome: a cytogenetic and molecular study. *Ann Hum Genet.* 1997;61:471–483.

62. Sagi L, Zuckerman-Levin N, Gawlik A, et al. Clinical significance of the parental origin of the X chromosome in turner syndrome. *J Clin Endocrinol Metab.* 2007;92:846–852.

63. Ruiz C, Lamm F, Hart PS. Turner syndrome and multiple-marker screening. *Clin Chem.* 1999;45:2259–2261.

64. Gersak K, Veble A, Mulla ZD, et al. Association between increased yolk sac diameter and abnormal karyotypes. *J Perinat Med.* 2012;40:251–254.

65. Carvalho AB, Guerra Junior G, Baptista MT, et al. Cardiovascular and renal anomalies in Turner syndrome. *Rev Assoc Med Bras.* 2010;56:655–659.

66. Bondy CA. Care of girls and women with Turner syndrome: a guideline of the Turner Syndrome Study Group. *J Clin Endocrinol Metab.* 2007;92:10–25.

67. McDermott DA, Bressan MC, He J, et al. TBX5 genetic testing validates strict clinical criteria for Holt-Oram syndrome. *Pediatr Res.* 2005;58:981–986.

68. Gedikbasi A, Oztarhan K, Aslan G, et al. Multidisciplinary approach in cystic hygroma: prenatal diagnosis, outcome, and postnatal follow up. *Pediatr Int.* 2009;51:670–677.

69. Bianco B, Lipay MV, Melaragno MI, et al. Detection of hidden Y mosaicism in Turner's syndrome: importance in the prevention of gonadoblastoma. *J Pediatr Endocrinol Metab.* 2006;19:1113–1117.

70. Baujat G, Rio M, Rossignol S, et al. Clinical and molecular overlap in overgrowth syndromes. *Am J Med Genet C Semin Med Genet.* 2005;137C:4–11.

71. Cytrynbaum CS, Smith AC, Rubin T, et al. Advances in overgrowth syndromes: clinical classification to molecular delineation in Sotos syndrome and Beckwith-Wiedemann syndrome. *Curr Opin Pediatr.* 2005;17:740–746.

72. Reish O, Lerer I, Amiel A, et al. Wiedemann-Beckwith syndrome: further prenatal characterization of the condition. *Am J Med Genet.* 2002;107:209–213.

73. Shuman C, Beckwith JB, Smith AC, et al. Beckwith-Wiedemann syndrome. In: Pagon RA, Adam MP, Bird TD, et al, eds. *GeneReviews™* [Internet]. Seattle, WA: University of Washington; 1993–2014. Available from http://www.ncbi.nlm.nih.gov/books/NBK1394/. Intially posted on March 3, 2000. Updated December 14, 2010.

74. Porter A, Benson CB, Hawley P, et al. Outcome of fetuses with a prenatal ultrasound diagnosis of isolated omphalocele. *Prenat Diagn.* 2009;29:668–673.

75. Elliott M, Bayly R, Cole T, et al. Clinical features and natural history of Beckwith-Wiedemann syndrome: presentation of 74 new cases. *Clin Genet.* 1994;46:168–174.

76. Storm DW, Hirselj DA, Rink B, et al. The prenatal diagnosis of Beckwith-Wiedemann syndrome using ultrasound and magnetic resonance imaging. *Urology.* 2011;77:208–210.

77. Gocmen R, Basaran C, Karcaaltincaba M, et al. Bilateral hemorrhagic adrenal cysts in an incomplete form of Beckwith-Wiedemann syndrome: MRI and prenatal US findings. *Abdom Imaging.* 2005;30:786–789.

78. Vora N, Bianchi DW. Genetic considerations in the prenatal diagnosis of overgrowth syndromes. *Prenat Diagn.* 2009;29:923–929.

79. Williams DH, Gauthier DW, Maizels M. Prenatal diagnosis of Beckwith-Wiedemann syndrome. *Prenat Diagn.* 2005;25:879–884.

80. Zarate YA, Mena R, Martin LJ, et al. Experience with hemihyperplasia and Beckwith-Wiedemann syndrome surveillance protocol. *Am J Med Genet Part A.* 2009;149A:1691–1697.

81. Lapunzina P. Risk of tumorigenesis in overgrowth syndromes: a comprehensive review. *Am J Med Genet C Semin Med Genet.* 2005;137C:53–71.

82. Slavotinek A, Gaunt L, Donnai D. Paternally inherited duplications of 11p15.5 and Beckwith-Wiedemann syndrome. *J Med Genet.* 1997;34:819–826.

83. Sparago A, Cerrato F, Vernucci M, et al. Microdeletions in the human H19 DMR result in loss of IGF2 imprinting and Beckwith-Wiedemann syndrome. *Nat Genet.* 2004;36:958–960.

84. Majeed SM, Khan A, ul Haq M, et al. Holt-Oram syndrome. *J Pak Med Assoc.* 1991;41:139–140.

85. Salonen R, Norio R. The Meckel syndrome in Finland: epidemiologic and genetic aspects. *Am J Med Genet.* 1984;18:691–698.

86. Terrett JA, Newbury-Ecob R, Smith NM, et al. A translocation at 12q2 refines the interval containing the Holt-Oram syndrome 1 gene. *Am J Hum Genet.* 1996;59:1337–1341.

87. Basson CT, Bachinsky DR, Lin RC, et al. Mutations in human TBX5 [corrected] cause limb and cardiac malformation in Holt-Oram syndrome. *Nat Genet.* 1997;15:30–35.

88. Borozdin W, Wright MJ, Hennekam RC, et al. Novel mutations in the gene SALL4 provide further evidence for acro-renal-ocular and Okihiro syndromes being allelic entities, and extend the phenotypic spectrum. *J Med Genet.* 2004;41:e102.

89. Sunagawa S, Kikuchi A, Sano Y, et al. Prenatal diagnosis of Holt-Oram syndrome: role of 3-D ultrasonography. *Congenit Anom.* 2009;49:38–41.

90. Poznanski AK, Gall JC Jr, Stern AM. Skeletal manifestations of the Holt-Oram syndrome. *Radiology.* 1970;94:45–53.

91. Tongsong T, Chanprapaph P. Prenatal sonographic diagnosis of Holt-Oram syndrome. *J Clin Ultrasound.* 2000;28:98–100.

92. Hurst JA, Hall CM, Baraitser M. The Holt-Oram syndrome. *J Med Genet.* 1991;28:406–410.

93. Ickowicz V, Eurin D, Maugey-Laulom·B, et al. Meckel-Gruber syndrome: sonography and pathology. *Ultrasound Obstet Gynecol.* 2006;27:296–300.

94. Eckmann-Scholz C, Jonat W, Zerres K, et al. Earliest ultrasound findings and description of splicing mutations in Meckel-Gruber syndrome. *Arch Gynecol Obstet.* 2012;286:917–921.

95. Auber B, Burfeind P, Herold S, et al. A disease causing deletion of 29 base pairs in intron 15 in the MKS1 gene is highly associated with the campomelic variant of the Meckel-Gruber syndrome. *Clin Genet.* 2007;72:454–459.

96. Valente EM, Logan CV, Mougou-Zerelli S, et al. Mutations in TMEM216 perturb ciliogenesis and cause Joubert, Meckel and related syndromes. *Nat Genet.* 2010;42:619–625.

97. Tallila J, Jakkula E, Peltonen L, et al. Identification of CC2D2A as a Meckel syndrome gene adds an important piece to the ciliopathy puzzle. *Am J Hum Genet.* 2008;82:1361–1367.

98. Kyttala M, Tallila J, Salonen R, et al. MKS1, encoding a component of the flagellar apparatus basal body proteome, is mutated in Meckel syndrome. *Nat Genet.* 2006;38:155–157.

99. Wright C, Healicon R, English C, et al. Meckel syndrome: what are the minimum diagnostic criteria? *J Med Genet.* 1994;31:482–485.

100. Celentano C, Prefumo F, Liberati M, et al. Prenatal diagnosis of Meckel-Gruber syndrome in a pregnancy obtained with ICSI. *J Assist Reprod Genet.* 2006;23:281–283.

101. Liu SS, Cheong ML, She BQ, et al. First-trimester ultrasound diagnosis of Meckel-Gruber syndrome. *Acta Obstet Gynecol Scand.* 2006;85:757–759.

102. Hosny IA, Elghawabi HS. Ultrafast MRI of the fetus: an increasingly important tool in prenatal diagnosis of congenital anomalies. *Magn Reson Imaging.* 2010;28:1431–1439.

103. Maria BL, Quisling RG, Rosainz LC, et al. Molar tooth sign in Joubert syndrome: clinical, radiologic, and pathologic significance. *J Child Neurol.* 1999;14:368–376.

104. Mougou-Zerelli S, Thomas S, Szenker E, et al. CC2D2A mutations in Meckel and Joubert syndromes indicate a genotype-phenotype correlation. *Hum Mutat.* 2009;30:1574–1582.

105. Chaumoitre K, Brun M, Cassart M, et al. Differential diagnosis of fetal hyperechogenic cystic kidneys unrelated to renal tract anomalies: a multicenter study. *Ultrasound Obstet Gynecol.* 2006;28:911–917.

106. Kline AD, Krantz ID, Sommer A, et al. Cornelia de Lange syndrome: clinical review, diagnostic and scoring systems, and anticipatory guidance. *Am J Med Genet A.* 2007;143A:1287–1296.

107. Jackson L, Kline AD, Barr MA, et al. de Lange syndrome: a clinical review of 310 individuals. *Am J Med Genet.* 1993;47:940–946.

108. Borck G, Redon R, Sanlaville D, et al. NIPBL mutations and genetic heterogeneity in Cornelia de Lange syndrome. *J Med Genet.* 2004;41:e128.

109. Deardorff MA, Kaur M, Yaeger D, et al. Mutations in cohesin complex members SMC3 and SMC1A cause a mild variant of cornelia de Lange syndrome with predominant mental retardation. *Am J Hum Genet.* 2007;80:485–494.

110. Arbuzova S, Nikolenko M, Krantz D, et al. Low first-trimester pregnancy-associated plasma protein-A and Cornelia de Lange syndrome. *Prenat Diagn.* 2003;23:864.

111. Bruner JP, Hsia YE. Prenatal findings in Brachmann-de Lange syndrome. *Obstet Gynecol.* 1990;76:966–968.

112. Spaggiari E, Vuillard E, Khung-Savatovsky S, et al. Ultrasound detection of eyelashes: a clue for prenatal diagnosis of Cornelia de Lange syndrome. *Ultrasound Obstet Gynecol.* 2013;41:341–342.

113. Ranzini AC, Day-Salvatore D, Farren-Chavez D, et al. Prenatal diagnosis of de Lange syndrome. *J Ultrasound Med.* 1997;16:755–758.

114. Charles AK, Porter HJ, Sams V, et al. Nephrogenic rests and renal abnormalities in Brachmann-de Lange syndrome. *Pediatr Pathol Lab Med.* 1997;17:209–219.

115. Barisic I, Tokic V, Loane M, et al. Descriptive epidemiology of Cornelia de Lange syndrome in Europe. *Am J Med Genet A.* 2008;146A:51–59.

116. Kline AD, Stanley C, Belevich J, et al. Developmental data on individuals with the Brachmann-de Lange syndrome. *Am J Med Genet.* 1993;47:1053–1058.

117. Beck B, Fenger K. Mortality, pathological findings and causes of death in the de Lange syndrome. *Acta Paediatr.* 1985;74:765–769.

118. Kline AD, Barr M, Jackson LG. Growth manifestations in the Brachmann-de Lange syndrome. *Am J Med Genet.* 1993;47:1042–1049.

119. Levin AV, Seidman DJ, Nelson LB, et al. Ophthalmologic findings in the Cornelia de Lange syndrome. *J Pediatr Ophthalmol Strabismus.* 1990;27:94–102.

120. Kelley RI, Hennekam RC. The Smith-Lemli-Opitz syndrome. *J Med Genet.* 2000;37:321–335.

121. Tint GS, Irons M, Elias ER, et al. Defective cholesterol biosynthesis associated with the Smith-Lemli-Opitz syndrome. *N Engl J Med.* 1994;330:107–113.

122. Porter FD. Smith-Lemli-Opitz syndrome: pathogenesis, diagnosis and management. *Eur J Hum Genet.* 2008;16:535–541.

123. Bialer MG, Penchaszadeh VB, Kahn E, et al. Female external genitalia and mullerian duct derivatives in a 46,XY infant with the Smith-Lemli-Opitz syndrome. *Am J Med Genet.* 1987;28:723–731.

124. Lin AE, Ardinger HH, Ardinger RH Jr, et al. Cardiovascular malformations in Smith-Lemli-Opitz syndrome. *Am J Med Genet.* 1997;68:270–278.

125. Witsch-Baumgartner M, Loffler J, Utermann G. Mutations in the human DHCR7 gene. *Hum Mutat.* 2001;17:172–182.

126. Bradley LA, Palomaki GE, Knight GJ, et al. Levels of unconjugated estriol and other maternal serum markers in pregnancies with Smith-Lemli-Opitz (RSH) syndrome fetuses. *Am J Med Genet.* 1999;82:355–358.

127. Cunniff C, Kratz LE, Moser A, et al. Clinical and biochemical spectrum of patients with RSH/Smith-Lemli-Opitz syndrome and abnormal cholesterol metabolism. *Am J Med Genet.* 1997;68:263–269.

128. Hyett JA, Clayton PT, Moscoso G, et al. Increased first trimester nuchal translucency as a prenatal manifestation of Smith-Lemli-Opitz syndrome. *Am J Med Genet.* 1995;58:374–376.

129. Goldenberg A, Wolf C, Chevy F, et al. Antenatal manifestations of Smith-Lemli-Opitz (RSH) syndrome: a retrospective survey of 30 cases. *Am J Med Genet A.* 2004;124A:423–426.

130. Moshiri M, Chapman T, Fechner PY, et al. Evaluation and management of disorders of sex development: multidisciplinary approach to a complex diagnosis. *Radiographics.* 2012;32:1599–1618.

131. Finley SC, Finley FW, Monsky DB. Cataracts in a girl with features of the Smith-Lemli-Opitz syndrome. *J Pediatr.* 1969;75:706–707.

132. Caruso PA, Poussaint TY, Tzika AA, et al. MRI and 1H MRS findings in Smith-Lemli-Opitz syndrome. *Neuroradiology.* 2004;46:3–14.

133. Thompson E, Baraitser M. An autosomal recessive mental retardation syndrome with hepatic fibrosis and renal cysts. *Am J Med Genet.* 1986;24:151–158.

134. Starck L, Lovgren-Sandblom A, Bjorkhem I. Cholesterol treatment forever? The first Scandinavian trial of cholesterol supplementation in the cholesterol-synthesis defect Smith-Lemli-Opitz syndrome. *J Intern Med.* 2002;252:314–321.

135. Azurdia RM, Anstey AV, Rhodes LE. Cholesterol supplementation objectively reduces photosensitivity in the Smith-Lemli-Opitz syndrome. *Br J Dermatol.* 2001;144:143–145.

136. Nwokoro NA, Mulvihill JJ. Cholesterol and bile acid replacement therapy in children and adults with Smith-Lemli-Opitz (SLO/RSH) syndrome. *Am J Med Genet.* 1997;68:315–321.

137. Chemaitilly W, Goldenberg A, Baujat G, et al. Adrenal insufficiency and abnormal genitalia in a 46XX female with Smith-Lemli-Opitz syndrome. *Horm Res.* 2003;59:254–256.

138. Tierney E, Nwokoro NA, Porter FD, et al. Behavior phenotype in the RSH/Smith-Lemli-Opitz syndrome. *Am J Med Genet.* 2001;98:191–200.

139. Abuelo DN, Tint GS, Kelley R, et al. Prenatal detection of the cholesterol biosynthetic defect in the Smith-Lemli-Opitz syndrome by the analysis of amniotic fluid sterols. *Am J Med Genet.* 1995;56:281–285.

140. Berry SA, Peterson C, Mize W, et al. Klippel-Trenaunay syndrome. *Am J Med Genet.* 1998;79:319–326.

141. Zoppi MA, Ibba RM, Floris M, et al. Prenatal sonographic diagnosis of Klippel-Trenaunay-Weber syndrome with cardiac failure. *J Clin Ultrasound.* 2001;29:422–426.

142. Aelvoet GE, Jorens PG, Roelen LM. Genetic aspects of the Klippel-Trenaunay syndrome. *Br J Dermatol.* 1992;126:603–607.

143. Samuel M, Spitz L. Klippel-Trenaunay syndrome: clinical features, complications and management in children. *Br J Surg.* 1995;82:757–761.

144. Peng HH, Wang TH, Chao AS, et al. Klippel-Trenaunay-Weber syndrome involving fetal thigh: prenatal presentations and outcomes. *Prenat Diagn.* 2006;26:825–830.

145. Chen CP, Lin SP, Chang TY, et al. Prenatal sonographic findings of Klippel-Trenaunay-Weber syndrome. *J Clin Ultrasound.* 2007;35:409–412.

146. Van Den Berg DJ, Francke U. Roberts syndrome: a review of 100 cases and a new rating system for severity. *Am J Med Genet.* 1993;47:1104–1123.

147. Maheshwari A, Kumar P, Dutta S, et al. Roberts-SC phocomelia syndrome. *Indian J Pediatr.* 2001;68:557–559.

148. Shule B, Oviedo A, Johnston K, et al. Inactivatiing mutations in ESCO2 cause SC phocomelia and Roberts syndrome: no phenotype-genotype correlation. *Am J Hum Genet.* 2005;77:1117–1128.

149. Kaur M, DeScipio C, McCallum J, et al. Precocious sister chromatid separation (PSCS) in Cornelia de Lange syndrome. *Am J Med Genet A.* 2005;138:27–31.

150. Rios LT, Araujo Junior E, Caetano AC, et al. Prenatal Diagnosis of EEC syndrome with "lobster claw" anomaly by 3D ultrasound. *J Clin Imaging Sci.* 2012;2:40.

151. Stoll C, Alembik Y, Dott B, et al. Associated malformations in patients with limb reduction deficiencies. *Eur J Med Genet.* 2010;53:286–290.

152. Holden KR, Jabs EW, Sponseller PD. Roberts/pseudothalidomide syndrome and normal intelligence: approaches to diagnosis and management. *Dev Med Child Neurol.* 1992;34:534–539.

153. Karabulut AB, Aydin H, Erer M, et al. Roberts syndrome from the plastic surgeon's viewpoint. *Plast Reconstr Surg.* 2001;108:1443–1445.

154. Goh ES, Li C, Horsburgh S, et al. The Roberts syndrome/SC phocomelia spectrum—a case report of an adult with review of the literature. *Am J Med Genet A.* 2010;152A:472–478.

155. Chacko E, Graber E, Regelmann MO, et al. Update on Turner and Noonan syndromes. *Endocrinol Metab Clin North Am.* 2012;41:713–734.

156. van der Burgt I. Noonan syndrome. *Orphanet J Rare Dis.* 2007;2:4.

157. Burch M, Sharland M, Shinebourne E, et al. Cardiologic abnormalities in Noonan syndrome: phenotypic diagnosis and echocardiographic assessment of 118 patients. *J Am Coll Cardiol.* 1993;22:1189–1192.

158. Jongmans M, Otten B, Noordam K, et al. Genetics and variation in phenotype in Noonan syndrome. *Horm Res.* 2004;62(suppl 3):56–59.

159. Beneteau C, Cave H, Moncla A, et al. SOS1 and PTPN11 mutations in five cases of Noonan syndrome with multiple giant cell lesions. *Eur J Hum Genet.* 2009;17:1216–1221.

160. Marino B, Digilio MC, Toscano A, et al. Congenital heart diseases in children with Noonan syndrome: an expanded cardiac spectrum with high prevalence of atrioventricular canal. *J Pediatr.* 1999;135:703–706.

161. Romano AA, Allanson JE, Dahlgren J, et al. Noonan syndrome: clinical features, diagnosis, and management guidelines. *Pediatrics.* 2010;126:746–759.

162. Descamps P, Jourdain O, Paillet C, et al. Etiology, prognosis and management of nuchal cystic hygroma: 25 new cases and literature review. *Eur J Obstet Gynecol Reprod Biol.* 1997;71:3–10.

163. Wilkinson JD, Lowe AM, Salbert BA, et al. Outcomes in children with Noonan syndrome and hypertrophic cardiomyopathy: a study from the Pediatric Cardiomyopathy Registry. *Am Heart J.* 2012;164:442–448.

164. Otten BJ, Noordam C. Growth in Noonan syndrome. *Horm Res.* 2009;72(suppl 2):31–35.

165. Romano AA, Allanson JE, Dahlgren J, et al. Noonan syndrome: clinical features, diagnosis, and management guidelines. *Pediatrics.* 2010;126:746–759.

166. van der Burgt I, Thoonen G, Roosenboom N, et al. Patterns of cognitive functioning in school-aged children with Noonan syndrome associated with variability in phenotypic expression. *J Pediatr.* 1999;135:707–713.

167. Jongmans MC, van der Burgt I, Hoogerbrugge PM, et al. Cancer risk in patients with Noonan syndrome carrying a PTPN11 mutation. *Eur J Hum Genet.* 2011;19:870–874.

168. Shprintzen RJ, Higgins AM, Antshel K, et al. Velo-cardio-facial syndrome. *Curr Opin Pediatr.* 2005;17:725–730.

169. Yamagishi H, Srivastava D. Unraveling the genetic and developmental mysteries of 22q11 deletion syndrome. *Trends Mol Med.* 2003;9:383–389.

170. Emanuel BS, McDonald-McGinn D, Saitta SC, et al. The 22q11.2 deletion syndrome. *Adv Pediatr.* 2001;48:39–73.

171. Basgul A, Kavak ZN, Kotiloglu E, et al. Antenatal diagnosis of velocardiofacial syndrome by 3D ultrasonography. *J Perinat Med.* 2006;34:177–178.

172. Eicher PS, McDonald-Mcginn DM, Fox CA, et al. Dysphagia in children with a 22q11.2 deletion: unusual pattern found on modified barium swallow. *J Pediatr.* 2000;137:158–164.

173. Ming JE, McDonald-McGinn DM, Megerian TE, et al. Skeletal anomalies and deformities in patients with deletions of 22q11. *Am J Med Genet.* 1997;72:210–215.

174. Kates WR, Burnette CP, Bessette BA, et al. Frontal and caudate alterations in velocardiofacial syndrome (deletion at chromosome 22q11.2). *J Child Neurol.* 2004;19:337–342.

175. McDonald-McGinn DM, Tonnesen MK, Laufer-Cahana A, et al. Phenotype of the 22q11.2 deletion in individuals identified through an affected relative: cast a wide FISHing net! *Genet Med.* 2001;3:23–29.

176. Bassett AS, Chow EW, Husted J, et al. Clinical features of 78 adults with 22q11 deletion syndrome. *Am J Med Genet A.* 2005;138:307–313.

177. Issekutz KA, Graham JM Jr, Prasad C, et al. An epidemiological analysis of CHARGE syndrome: preliminary results from a Canadian study. *Am J Med Genet A.* 2005;133A:309–317.

178. Bergman JE, Janssen N, Hoefsloot LH, et al. CHD7 mutations and CHARGE syndrome: the clinical implications of an expanding phenotype. *J Med Genet.* 2011;48:334–342.

179. Pampal A. CHARGE: an association or a syndrome? *Int J Pediatr Otorhinolaryngol.* 2010;74:719–722.

180. Colin E, Bonneau D, Boussion F, et al. Prenatal diagnosis of CHARGE syndrome by identification of a novel CHD7 mutation in a previously unaffected family. *Prenat Diagn.* 2012;32:692–694.

181. Amiel J, Attiee-Bitach T, Marianowski R, et al. Temporal bone anomaly proposed as a major criteria for diagnosis of CHARGE syndrome. *Am J Med Genet.* 2001;99:124–127.

182. Davenport SL, Hefner MA, Mitchell JA. The spectrum of clinical features in CHARGE syndrome. *Clin Genet.* 1986;29:298–310.

183. Ragan DC, Casale AJ, Rink RC, et al. Genitourinary anomalies in the CHARGE association. *J Urol.* 1999;161:622–625.

184. Davenport SL, Hefner MA, Thelin JW. CHARGE syndrome, part I: external ear anomalies. *Int J Pediatr Otorhinolaryngol.* 1986;12:137–143.

185. Sanlaville D, Etchevers HC, Gonzales M, et al. Phenotypic spectrum of CHARGE syndrome in fetuses with CHD7 truncating mutations correlates with expression during human development. *J Med Genet.* 2006;43:211–217.

186. Leibovitz Z, Egenburg S, Arad A, et al. Sonography of the fetal cochlea in the early second trimester of pregnancy. *J Ultrasound Med.* 2013;32:53–59.

187. Moreira NC, Teixeira J, Raininko R, et al. The ear in fetal MRI: what can we really see? *Neuroradiology.* 2011;53:1001–1008.

188. Blake KD, Davenport SL, Hall BD, et al. CHARGE association: an update and review for the primary pediatrician. *Clin Pediatr.* 1998;37:159–173.

189. Roger G, Morisseau-Durand MP, Van Den Abbeele T, et al. The CHARGE association: the role of tracheotomy. *Arch Otolaryngol Head Neck Surg.* 1999;125:33–38.

190. Dobbelsteyn C, Marche DM, Blake K, et al. Early oral sensory experiences and feeding development in children with CHARGE syndrome: a report of five cases. *Dysphagia.* 2005;20:89–100.

191. Jongmans MC, Hoefsloot LH, van der Donk KP, et al. Familial CHARGE syndrome and the CHD7 gene: a recurrent missense mutation, intrafamilial recurrence and variability. *Am J Med Genet A.* 2008;146A:43–50.

192. Gurrieri F, Franco B, Toriello H, et al. Oral-facial-digital syndromes: review and diagnostic guidelines. *Am J Med Genet A.* 2007;143A:3314–3323.

193. Ferrante MI, Giorgio G, Feather SA, et al. Identification of the gene for oral-facial-digital type I syndrome. *Am J Hum Genet.* 2001;68:569–576.

194. Field M, Scheffer IE, Gill D, et al. Expanding the molecular basis and phenotypic spectrum of X-linked Joubert syndrome associated with OFD1 mutations. *Eur J Hum Genet.* 2012;20:806–809.

195. Thauvin-Robinet C, Cossee M, Cormier-Daire V, et al. Clinical, molecular, and genotype-phenotype correlation studies from 25 cases of oral-facial-digital syndrome type 1: a French and Belgian collaborative study. *J Med Genet.* 2006;43:54–61.

196. Coll E, Torra R, Pascual J, et al. Sporadic orofaciodigital syndrome type I presenting as end-stage renal disease. *Nephrol Dial Transplant.* 1997;12:1040–1042.

197. Shipp TD, Chu GC, Benacerraf B. Prenatal diagnosis of oral-facial-digital syndrome, type I. *J Ultrasound Med.* 2000;19:491–494.

198. Muenke M, Ruchelli ED, Rorke LB, et al. On lumping and splitting: a fetus with clinical findings of the oral-facial-digital syndrome type VI, the hydrolethalus syndrome, and the Pallister-Hall syndrome. *Am J Med Genet.* 1991;41:548–556.

199. Flores-Sarnat L. New insights into craniosynostosis. *Semin Pediatr Neurol.* 2002;9:274–291.

200. Passos-Bueno MR, Serti Eacute AE, Jehee FS, et al. Genetics of craniosynostosis: genes, syndromes, mutations and genotype-phenotype correlations. *Front Oral Biol.* 2008;12:107–143.

201. Glaser RL, Jiang W, Boyadjiev SA, et al. Paternal origin of FGFR2 mutations in sporadic cases of Crouzon syndrome and Pfeiffer syndrome. *Am J Hum Genet.* 2000;66:768–777.

202. Miller C, Losken HW, Towbin R, et al. Ultrasound diagnosis of craniosynostosis. *Cleft Palate Craniofac J.* 2002;39:73–80.

203. Fjortoft MI, Sevely A, Boetto S, et al. Prenatal diagnosis of craniosynostosis: value of MR imaging. *Neuroradiology.* 2007;49:515–521.

204. Muenke M, Gripp KW, McDonald-McGinn DM, et al. A unique point mutation in the fibroblast growth factor receptor 3 gene (FGFR3) defines a new craniosynostosis syndrome. *Am J Hum Genet.* 1997;60:555–564.

205. Gebb J, Demasio K, Dar P. Prenatal sonographic diagnosis of familial Saethre-Chotzen syndrome. *J Ultrasound Med.* 2011;30:420–422.

206. Greig AV, Wagner J, Warren SM, et al. Pfeiffer syndrome: analysis of a clinical series and development of a classification system. *J Craniofac Surg.* 2013;24:204–215.

207. Renier D, Lajeunie E, Arnaud E, et al. Management of craniosynostoses. *Childs Nerv Syst.* 2000;16:645–658.

208. Wong GB, Kakulis EG, Mulliken JB. Analysis of fronto-orbital advancement for Apert, Crouzon, Pfeiffer, and Saethre-Chotzen syndromes. *Plast Reconstr Surg.* 2000;105:2314–2323.

209. Schweitzer DN, Graham JM Jr, Lachman RS, et al. Subtle radiographic findings of achondroplasia in patients with Crouzon syndrome with acanthosis nigricans due to an Ala391Glu substitution in FGFR3. *Am J Med Genet.* 2001;98:75–91.

210. Ferreira JC, Carter SM, Bernstein PS, et al. Second-trimester molecular prenatal diagnosis of sporadic Apert syndrome following suspicious ultrasound findings. *Ultrasound Obstet Gynecol.* 1999;14:426–430.

211. Kanauchi Y, Muragaki Y, Ogino T, et al. FGFR2 mutation in a patient with Apert syndrome associated with humeroradial synostosis. *Congenit Anom.* 2003;43:302–305.

212. Lajeunie E, Cameron R, El Ghouzzi V, et al. Clinical variability in patients with Apert's syndrome. *J Neurosurg.* 1999;90:443–447.

213. Wilkie AO, Byren JC, Hurst JA, et al. Prevalence and complications of single-gene and chromosomal disorders in craniosynostosis. *Pediatrics.* 2010;126:e391–e400.

214. Moloney DM, Slaney SF, Oldridge M, et al. Exclusive paternal origin of new mutations in Apert syndrome. *Nat Genet.* 1996;13:48–53.

215. Mahieu-Caputo D, Sonigo P, Amiel J, et al. Prenatal diagnosis of sporadic Apert syndrome: a sequential diagnostic approach combining three-dimensional computed tomography and molecular biology. *Fetal Diagn Ther.* 2001;16:10–12.

216. Cohen MM Jr. Pfeiffer syndrome update, clinical subtypes, and guidelines for differential diagnosis. *Am J Med Genet.* 1993;45:300–307.

217. Stoler JM, Rosen H, Desai U, et al. Cleft palate in Pfeiffer syndrome. *J Craniofac Surg.* 2009;20:1375–1377.

218. Itoh S, Nojima M, Yoshida K. Usefulness of magnetic resonance imaging for accurate diagnosis of Pfeiffer syndrome type II in utero. *Fetal Diagn Ther.* 2006;21:168–171.

219. Cornejo-Roldan LR, Roessler E, Muenke M. Analysis of the mutational spectrum of the FGFR2 gene in Pfeiffer syndrome. *Hum Genet.* 1999;104:425–431.

220. Medina M, Cortes E, Eguiluz I, et al. Three-dimensional features of Pfeiffer syndrome. *Int J Gynaecol Obstet.* 2009;105:266–267.

221. Dodge HW Jr, Wood MW, Kennedy RL. Craniofacial dysostosis: Crouzon's disease. *Pediatrics.* 1959;23:98–106.

222. Reardon W, Winter RM, Rutland P, et al. Mutations in the fibroblast growth factor receptor 2 gene cause Crouzon syndrome. *Nat Genet.* 1994;8:98–103.

223. Gollin YG, Abuhamad AZ, Inati MN, et al. Sonographic appearance of craniofacial dysostosis (Crouzon syndrome) in the second trimester. *J Ultrasound Med.* 1993;12:625–628.

224. McGlaughlin KL, Witherow H, Dunaway DJ, et al. Spectrum of Antley-Bixler syndrome. *J Craniofac Surg.* 2010;21:1560–1564.

225. Huang N, Pandey AV, Agrawal V, et al. Diversity and function of mutations in p450 oxidoreductase in patients with Antley-Bixler syndrome and disordered steroidogenesis. *Am J Hum Genet.* 2005;76:729–749.

226. Shackleton C, Marcos J, Arlt W, et al. Prenatal diagnosis of P450 oxidoreductase deficiency (ORD): a disorder causing low pregnancy estriol, maternal and fetal virilization, and the Antley-Bixler syndrome phenotype. *Am J Med Genet A.* 2004;129A:105–112.

227. New MI, Abraham M, Yuen T, et al. An update on prenatal diagnosis and treatment of congenital adrenal hyperplasia. *Semin Reprod Med.* 2012;30:396–399.

228. Robinson PN, Neumann LM, Demuth S, et al. Shprintzen-Goldberg syndrome: fourteen new patients and a clinical analysis. *Am J Med Genet A.* 2005;135:251–262.

229. Rumball KM, Pang E, Letts RM. Musculoskeletal manifestations of the Antley-Bixler syndrome. *J Pediatr Orthop B.* 1999;8:139–143.

230. Nicolaides KH, Salvesen DR, Snijders RJ, et al. Fetal facial defects: associated malformations and chromosomal abnormalities. *Fetal Diagn Ther.* 1993;8:1–9.

231. Rotten D, Levaillant JM, Martinez H, et al. The fetal mandible: a 2D and 3D sonographic approach to the diagnosis of retrognathia and micrognathia. *Ultrasound Obstet Gynecol.* 2002;19:122–130.

232. Paladini D, Morra T, Teodoro A, et al. Objective diagnosis of micrognathia in the fetus: the jaw index. *Obstet Gynecol.* 1999;93(3):382–386.

233. Cohen MM Jr, Rollnick BR, Kaye CI. Oculoauriculovertebral spectrum: an updated critique. *Cleft Palate Craniofac J.* 1989;26:276–286.

234. Harris J, Kallen B, Robert E. The epidemiology of anotia and microtia. *J Med Genet.* 1996;33:809–813.

235. Volpe P, Gentile M. Three-dimensional diagnosis of Goldenhar syndrome. *Ultrasound Obstet Gynecol.* 2004;24:798–800.

236. Gougoutas AJ, Singh DJ, Low DW, et al. Hemifacial microsomia: clinical features and pictographic representations of the OMENS classification system. *Plast Reconstr Surg.* 2007;120:112e–120e.

237. Aouchiche M, Boyer R, Nouar A. Karyotype results in Goldenhar's syndrome. *Bull Mem Soc Fr Ophtalmol.* 1972;85:57–69.

238. De Catte L, Laubach M, Legein J, et al. Early prenatal diagnosis of oculoauriculovertebral dysplasia or the Goldenhar syndrome. *Ultrasound Obstet Gynecol.* 1996;8:422–424.

239. Ghi T, Contro E, Carletti A, et al. Prenatal sonographic imaging of Goldenhar syndrome associated with cystic eye. *Prenat Diagn.* 2008;28:362–363.

240. Hattori Y, Tanaka M, Matsumoto T, et al. Prenatal diagnosis of hemifacial microsomia by magnetic resonance imaging. *J Perinat Med.* 2005;33:69–71.

241. Gorlin RJ, Cohen MM, Hennekam RCM. *Syndromes of the Head and Neck.* Oxford, England: Oxford University Press; 2001.

242. Ala-Mello S, Siggberg L, Knuutila S, et al. Further evidence for a relationship between the 5p15 chromosome region and the oculoauriculovertebral anomaly. *Am J Med Genet A.* 2008;146A:2490–2494.

243. Dixon MJ. Treacher Collins syndrome. *Hum Mol Genet.* 1996;5 Spec No:1391–1396.

244. Trainor PA, Dixon J, Dixon MJ. Treacher Collins syndrome: etiology, pathogenesis and prevention. *Eur J Hum Genet.* 2009;17:275–283.

245. Teber OA, Gillessen-Kaesbach G, Fischer S, et al. Genotyping in 46 patients with tentative diagnosis of Treacher Collins syndrome revealed unexpected phenotypic variation. *Eur J Hum Genet.* 2004;12:879–890.

246. Tanaka Y, Kanenishi K, Tanaka H, et al. Antenatal three-dimensional sonographic features of Treacher Collins syndrome. *Ultrasound Obstet Gynecol.* 2002;19:414–415.

247. Miller M, Fineman R, Smith DW. Postaxial acrofacial dysostosis syndrome. *J Pediatr.* 1979;95:970–975.

248. Moessinger AC. Fetal akinesia deformation sequence: an animal model. *Pediatrics.* 1983;72:857–863.

249. Thompson JT, Anderson PJ, David DJ. Treacher Collins syndrome: protocol management from birth to maturity. *J Craniofac Surg.* 2009;20:2028–2035.

250. Posnick JC. Treacher Collins syndrome: perspectives in evaluation and treatment. *J Oral Maxillofac Surg.* 1997;55:1120–1133.

251. Hayashi T, Sasaki S, Oyama A, et al. New grading system for patients with Treacher Collins syndrome. *J Craniofac Surg.* 2007;18:113–119.

252. da Silva Dalben G, Costa B, Gomide MR. Prevalence of dental anomalies, ectopic eruption and associated oral malformations in subjects with Treacher Collins syndrome. *Oral Surg Oral Med Oral Pathol Oral Radiol Endod.* 2006;101:588–592.

253. Bernier FP, Caluseriu O, Ng S, et al. Haploinsufficiency of SF3B4, a component of the pre-mRNA spliceosomal complex, causes Nager syndrome. *Am J Hum Genet.* 2012;90:925–933.

254. Richieri-Costa A, Gollop TR, Colletto GM. Brief clinical report: syndrome of acrofacial dysostosis, cleft lip/palate, and triphalangeal thumb in a Brazilian family. *Am J Med Genet.* 1983;14:225–229.

255. Aylsworth AS, Lin AE, Friedman PA. Nager acrofacial dysostosis: male-to-male transmission in 2 families. *Am J Med Genet.* 1991;41:83–88.

256. Schlieve T, Almusa M, Miloro M, et al. Temporomandibular joint replacement for ankylosis correction in Nager syndrome: case report and review of the literature. *J Oral Maxillofac Surg.* 2012;70:616–625.

257. McDonald MT, Gorski JL. Nager acrofacial dysostosis. *J Med Genet.* 1993;30:779–782.

258. Paladini D, Tartaglione A, Lamberti A, et al. Prenatal ultrasound diagnosis of Nager syndrome. *Ultrasound Obstet Gynecol.* 2003;21:195–197.

259. Ansart-Franquet H, Houfflin-Debarge V, Ghoumid J, et al. Prenatal diagnosis of Nager syndrome in a monochorionic-diamniotic twin pregnancy. *Prenat Diagn.* 2009;29:187–189.

260. Couyoumjian CA, Treadwell MC, Barr M. Prenatal sonographic diagnosis of Nager acrofacial dysostosis with unilateral upper limb involvement. *Prenat Diagn.* 2008;28:964–966.

261. Palomeque A, Pastor X, Ballesta F. Nager anomaly with severe facial involvement, microcephaly, and mental retardation. *Am J Med Genet.* 1990;36:356–357.

262. Khoury MJ, Cordero JF, Greenberg F, et al. A population study of the VACTERL association: evidence for its etiologic heterogeneity. *Pediatrics.* 1983;71:815–820.

263. Solomon BD. VACTERL/VATER association. *Orphanet J Rare Dis.* 2011;6:56.

264. Weaver DD, Mapstone CL, Yu PL. The VATER association: analysis of 46 patients. *Am J Dis Child.* 1986;140:225–229.

265. Garcia-Barcelo MM, Wong KK, Lui VC, et al. Identification of a HOXD13 mutation in a VACTERL patient. *Am J Med Genet A.* 2008;146A:3181–3185.

266. Solomon BD, Pineda-Alvarez DE, Raam MS, et al. Analysis of component findings in 79 patients diagnosed with VACTERL association. *Am J Med Genet A.* 2010;152A:2236–2244.

267. Sunagawa S, Kikuchi A, Yoshida S, et al. Dichorionic twin fetuses with VACTERL association. *J Obstet Gynaecol Res.* 2007;33:570–573.

268. Miller OF, Kolon TF. Prenatal diagnosis of VACTERL association. *J Urol.* 2001;166:2389–2391.

269. Tongsong T, Wanapirak C, Piyamongkol W, et al. Prenatal sonographic diagnosis of VATER association. *J Clin Ultrasound.* 1999;27:378–384.

270. Langer JC, Hussain H, Khan A, et al. Prenatal diagnosis of esophageal atresia using sonography and magnetic resonance imaging. *J Pediatr Surg.* 2001;36:804–807.

271. Seeds JW, Cefalo RC, Herbert WN. Amniotic band syndrome. *Am J Obstet Gynecol.* 1982;144:243–248.

272. Orioli IM, Ribeiro MG, Castilla EE. Clinical and epidemiological studies of amniotic deformity, adhesion, and mutilation (ADAM) sequence in a South American (ECLAMC) population. *Am J Med Genet A.* 2003;118A:135–145.

273. Ray M, Hendrick SJ, Raimer SS, et al. Amniotic band syndrome. *Int J Dermatol.* 1988;27:312–314.

274. Neuman J, Calvo-Garcia MA, Kline-Fath BM, et al. Prenatal imaging of amniotic band sequence: utility and role of fetal MRI as an adjunct to prenatal US. *Pediatr Radiol.* 2012;42:544–551.

275. Kanayama MD, Gaffey TA, Ogburn PL Jr. Constriction of the umbilical cord by an amniotic band, with fetal compromise illustrated by reverse diastolic flow in the umbilical artery: a case report. *J Reprod Med.* 1995;40:71–73.

276. Kalampokas E, Kalampokas T, Sofoudis C, et al. Diagnosing arthrogryposis multiplex congenita: a review. *ISRN Obstet Gynecol.* 2012;2012:264918.

277. Hall JG. Genetic aspects of arthrogryposis. *Clin Orthop Relat Res.* 1985;(194):44–53.

278. Bevan WP, Hall JG, Bamshad M, et al. Arthrogryposis multiplex congenita (amyoplasia): an orthopaedic perspective. *J Pediatr Orthop.* 2007;27:594–600.

279. Beals RK. The distal arthrogryposes: a new classification of peripheral contractures. *Clin Orthop Relat Res.* 2005;(435):203–210.

280. Zhao N, Jiang M, Han W, et al. A novel mutation in TNNT3 associated with Sheldon-Hall syndrome in a Chinese family with vertical talus. *Eur J Med Genet.* 2011;54:351–353.

281. Toydemir RM, Rutherford A, Whitby FG, et al. Mutations in embryonic myosin heavy chain (MYH3) cause Freeman-Sheldon syndrome and Sheldon-Hall syndrome. *Nat Genet.* 2006;38:561–565.

282. Pena SDJ, Shokeir MHK. Syndrome of camptodactyly, multiple ankyloses facial anomalies and pulmonary hypoplasia: a lethal condition. *J Pediatr.* 1974;85:373–375.

283. Moerman P, Fryns JP, Goddeeris P, et al. Multiple ankyloses, facial anomalies, and pulmonary hypoplasia associated with severe antenatal spinal muscular atrophy. *J Pediatr.* 1983;103:238–241.

284. Madazli R, Tuysuz B, Aksoy F, et al. Prenatal diagnosis of arthrogryposis multiplex congenita with increased nuchal translucency but without any underlying fetal neurogenic or myogenic pathology. *Fetal Diagn Ther.* 2002;17:29–33.

285. Bianchi DW, Van Marter LJ. An approach to ventilator-dependent neonates with arthrogryposis. *Pediatrics.* 1994;94:682–686.

286. Hageman G, Ippel EP, Beemer FA, et al. The diagnostic management of newborns with congenital contractures: a nosologic study of 75 cases. *Am J Med Genet.* 1988;30:883–904.

287. Carlson WO, Speck GJ, Vicari V, et al. Arthrogryposis multiplex congenita: a long-term follow-up study. *Clin Orthop Relat Res.* 1985;(194):115–123.

288. Thomas B, Schopler S, Wood W, et al. The knee in arthrogryposis. *Clin Orthop Relat Res.* 1985;(194):87–92.

289. Bilardo CM, Timmerman E, Pajkrt E, et al. Increased nuchal translucency in euploid fetuses—what should we be telling the parents? *Prenat Diagn.* 2010;30:93–102.

290. Pergament E, Alamillo C, Sak K, et al. Genetic assessment following increased nuchal translucency and normal karyotype. *Prenat Diagn.* 2011;31:307–310.

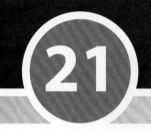

# 21 Skeletal Dysplasia

Teresa Victoria • Beverly Coleman • Christopher Cassady

Skeletal dysplasias (SDs) are a heterogeneous group of disorders resulting from a generalized abnormality of the skeleton. Individually rare, collectively they occur in approximately 1 per 5,000 live births.[1] Clinically, these disorders may manifest as short stature, with malformation and deformation of the skeleton. Severity ranges among individuals, from minor handicaps to death in the perinatal period.

A group of experts have developed an approach to classify dysplasias. Their work, which has been revised on several occasions, is presented under the umbrella name of the Nosology and Classification of Genetic Skeletal Disorders. In their 2010 revision, it included 456 conditions placed in 40 groups according to their molecular, biochemical, and/or radiographic criteria.[2] Of these, 316 were associated with mutations in one or more of 226 different genes. A hundred or so dysplasias have prenatal onset, while others may present during the newborn period or beyond 2 or 3 years of age.[3]

Broadly, SDs can be classified as osteodysplasias, chondrodysplasias, and dysostosis.[4,5] *Osteodysplasias* refer to abnormalities of the bone leading to altered bone density and mineralization. The *chondrodysplasias* result from genetic abnormalities affecting the cartilage. These usually affect the entire appendicular skeleton, with progressive abnormalities that may lead to changes in size and shape of limbs, trunk, and/or skull, and frequently result in short stature. Often, the osteodysplasias and chondrodysplasias are grouped together into the more encompassing heading of osteochondrodysplasia, or SDs, overall describing entities that may affect bone and cartilage. As a result of varied gene expression through fetal and postnatal life, the phenotype of an osteochondrodysplasia may change throughout life, such that previously unaffected bones may eventually become involved. This is in contraposition with the *dysostosis*, which are malformations of individual bones or group of bones, the result of abnormal blastogenesis during the first 6 weeks of fetal life. In contrast to the osteochondrodysplasias, the phenotype in the dysostosis is static, such that the malformations do not spread or progress.

SDs can be difficult entities to diagnose both pre- and postnatally. The large phenotypic variability among different patients with the same disease, or just within the same patient at different times of life, the overlapping features of some syndromes, and the lack of precise molecular diagnosis in certain entities, present considerable diagnostic challenges. In this chapter, we will review the different imaging modalities utilized prenatally to help evaluate and diagnose the fetus with suspected SD and will discuss the most commonly encountered dysplasias prenatally. Some of the entities discussed below, including arthrogryposis and craniosynostosis, are not strictly SDs, but are included in this chapter because they are severe osseous abnormalities that may be included in the differential diagnosis of the fetus with marked abnormalities of the skeleton.

## EMBRYOLOGY

The fetal skeleton develops relatively early during gestation. The appendicular and axial skeletons undergo a programmed pattern of endochondral ossification during which a cartilage template is replaced by bone. In contrast, the calvarium and portions of the clavicle and pubis ossify via membranous ossification, whereby mesenchymal cells differentiate directly into osteoblasts.[6] Limb buds begin to develop during the 4th week of embryonic life as clusters of mesenchymal cells covered by a layer of ectoderm. Mesenchymal models of bone or anlages form during the 5th week of gestation. Development of the upper limb antecedes that of the lower limbs in bud appearance, differentiation, and final size. The limbs develop in a proximodistal sequence, with the humerus and femur forming first, followed by radius and ulna, tibia and fibula, metacarpals and metatarsals, and, finally, phalanges. Clavicles and mandibles ossify at 8 weeks of gestation; appendicular skeleton, ileum, and scapula by 12 weeks; metacarpals and metatarsals are ossified by 12 to 16 weeks.[7]

The skeleton is composed of 2 tissues (bone and cartilage), 3 cell types (osteoblasts, osteoclasts, and chondrocytes), and more than 200 skeletal elements. This intricate interplay among the different components allows for inborn errors of metabolism to occur along the path, giving rise to the SDs. These genetic "errors" may be inherited as autosomal dominant, autosomal recessive, or X-linked disorders; while other SDs are due to imprinting errors, somatic mosaicism, or teratogen exposure.[8] Within the last few decades, there has been marked progress in the field of molecular genetics, advancing the knowledge and genetic cause of many of these disorders. Yet, in order to fully evaluate the fetus with a suspected SD, highly detailed prenatal imaging is crucial, so that tailored genetic testing can be done.

## PRENATAL IMAGING OF SKELETAL DYSPLASIAS

### Ultrasound

Ultrasound (US) is the primary imaging modality in the evaluation of the affected fetus. By US, the fetal skeleton is readily visualized by 14 weeks of gestation. Suspicion of a possible fetal SD is usually first suggested when the measurement of the long bones is more than 3 standard deviations from the mean for gestational age, or when focal abnormalities, such as bone bowing, fractures, or demineralization, are detected. The presence of an increased nuchal translucency may be the first sign of a dysplasia in the first trimester (Fig. 21.1). When evaluating a fetus for SD, a systematic and meticulous evaluation of the fetal skeleton must be undertaken of the long bones, skull, profile, and chest. Detailed evaluation of the internal structures for additional abnormalities may provide additional clues in reaching a diagnosis. A proposed systematic approach of the fetal skeleton follows.

1. *Skull.* Examination of the acoustic shadow behind the calvarium and the echogenicity of the bone itself allow evaluation for possible demineralization. Frontal bossing, craniosynostosis, cleft palate, micrognathia, or hypertelorism are features

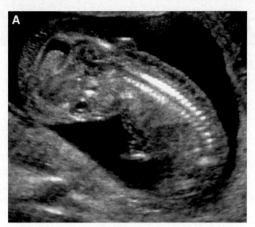
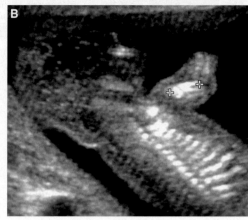

**FIGURE 21.1:** Cystic hygroma. Osteogenesis imperfecta type II at 14 weeks' gestation. **A:** Sagittal US demonstrates subcutaneous edema along the cranium and spine. **B:** Coronal view demonstrates markedly short bowed humerus *(cursers)* and irregular beaded appearance of the ribs consistent with fractures.

that may be seen in different SDs, and should be assessed when evaluating the fetus with a possible dysplasia.

2. *Clavicle, scapula.* A hypoplastic scapula may be seen in campomelic dysplasia (CD) or cleidocranial dysplasia; total or partial aplasia of the clavicles may occur in cleidocranial dysplasia.

3. *Spine.* The presence of segmentation anomalies, platyspondyly, abnormal curvature of the spine, and possible nonossification of the spine must be carefully evaluated.

4. *Thorax.* Detailed examination of the thorax is crucial, as chest restriction leads to pulmonary hypoplasia, a frequent cause of death in the neonate with SD (see below). A chest circumference measured at the level of the four-chamber heart of less than the 5th percentile for GA is a strong indicator of pulmonary hypoplasia. Other parameters indicative of pulmonary hypoplasia and/or lethality include chest circumference–abdominal circumference ratio less than the 5th percentile, chest–trunk length ratio less than 0.32, and a femur length–abdominal circumference ratio less than 0.16.[9] Evaluation of the thorax should include a full analysis of the ribs, including number, shape, mineralization, and overall configuration.

5. *Long bones.* Evaluation of the long bones includes analysis of the degree of mineralization, presence of fractures or abnormal curvature of the long bones, as well as absence, hypoplasia, and malformation of the bone. Comparison among segments for shortening establishes whether the entity is a rhizomelic, mesomelic, or acromelic dysplasia, or if it involves all the segments of the extremities (micromelia) (Fig. 21.2).

6. *Pelvis.* Abnormalities in the shape of the pelvis can provide clues as to the diagnosis of the SD at hand. A flared iliac wing may be found in entities such as Kniest dysplasia, a small pelvis may be seen in achondrogenesis or CD, and delayed ossification of the pubic bones may occur in ischiopatellar dysplasia.

7. *Hands and feet.* Polydactyly (more than 5 digits per hand) is classified as pre- or postaxial when the extra digits are located on the radial or ulnar side of the hand, respectively (Fig. 21.3). Other abnormalities, such as syndactyly (soft-tissue or bone fusion of adjacent digits), clinodactyly (deviation of the finger), postural deformities ("hitchhiker's thumb," "sandal toe deformity," clinched hands), or abnormal extremities (broad tubular phalanges) must be evaluated (Fig. 21.4).

One of the most important determinations when evaluating the fetus with presumed dysplasia by US is the assessment and prediction of postnatal lethality. Lethality is mainly determined by the presence of pulmonary hypoplasia, whereby the small lungs are unable to maintain adequate oxygen exchange postnatally. Sonographic indicators of pulmonary hypoplasia are discussed.

Despite being the main imaging modality in the prenatal evaluation of the fetus, US has limited sensitivity in diagnosing SD

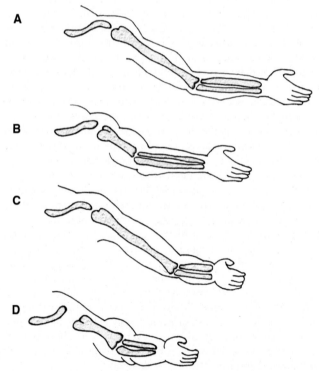

**FIGURE 21.2:** Nomenclature for long bone shortening. **A:** Normal. **B:** Rhizomelia—shortening of the proximal segment. **C:** Mesomelia—shortening of the midsegments (radius and ulna/tibia and fibula). **D:** Micromelia—overall extremity length is small. Not depicted is *acromelia*, where the distal segments are short in length.

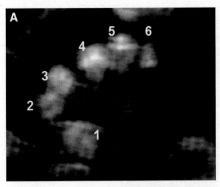
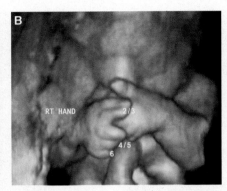
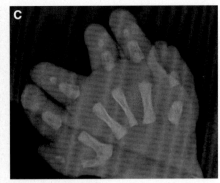

**FIGURE 21.3:** Polydactyly. Pallister–Hall syndrome at 28-week gestation. 2D **(A)** and 3D **(B)** US of the right hand demonstrate postaxial polydactyly and syndactyly of the 2nd and 3rd, as well as 4th and 5th digits. **C:** Postnatal radiograph of the hand confirmed the prenatal findings.

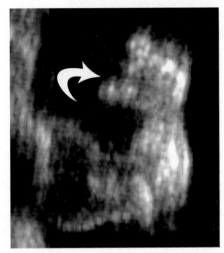

**FIGURE 21.4:** Diastrophic dysplasia. An 18-week fetus with short limbs. US of the hand demonstrates a classic "hitchhiker thumb" (arrow) with thumb abducted, helping confirm the diagnosis.

prenatally. Diagnosis remains inaccurate with both false positive and false negative results. Published accuracy values range between 40% and 60%,[10,11] opening the door to other imaging modalities to help confirm a diagnosis.

## Magnetic Resonance Imaging

The use of magnetic resonance imaging (MRI) in the assessment of the fetal skeleton has advanced as technology improves.[12,13] The development of fast echoplanar imaging (repetition time/echo time 3,000/45–60) has been particularly valuable in the evaluation of fetal cartilage and bone (Figs. 21.5 and 21.6). Connolly et al. documented the ability of MR to delineate cartilage transformation and development of secondary ossification centers in the fetal pig.[14,15] Nemec et al.[12] reviewed the long bone development of 253 fetuses from 19 to 36 weeks' gestations by MR. In their series, the epiphysis changed in shape from spherical to hemispherical with a notch. The metaphysis was flat early in the second trimester and became undulated, while the perichondrium decreased in thickness with advancing gestational age. The range of diaphyseal lengths was wider than corresponding US values likely related to variability in fetal positioning.

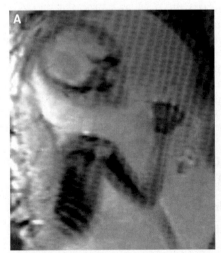
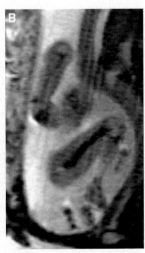
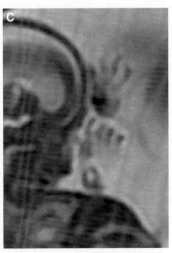

**FIGURE 21.5:** MRI of the fetal skeleton. Echoplanar image (EPI) of a 22-week fetus demonstrates low-signal skeleton and high-signal cartilage of the humerus, ribs, and hand **(A)** and humerus, femur, and portion of the tibia **(B)**. **C:** SSFSE T2w MR image of a 17-week fetus demonstrates hands and fingers.

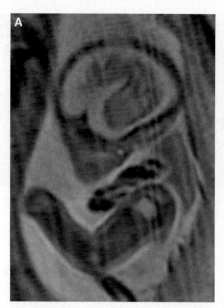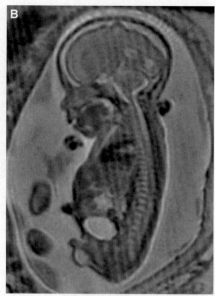

**FIGURE 21.6:** Kneist dysplasia. SSFSE T2w MR demonstrates unusually prominent high-signal epiphysis **(A)** and bright discs **(B)** in this fetus with moderate micromelia and platyspondyly. This nonlethal dysplasia is caused by mutations in COL2A1 with resultant joint contractures, scoliosis, and premature arthropathy.

Anecdotal cases of fetal MRI in the evaluation of specific SDs have been published.[16–21] MR is particularly helpful when other anomalies are present such as cranial (craniosynostosis) or when oligohydramnios is present.[20,21]

## Computed Tomography

The use of low-dose fetal CT in the evaluation of the fetal skeleton has developed as well.[22–25] Given the obvious radiation dose to the fetus, this type of study is relegated exclusively to the fetus with *severe* osseous abnormalities, when the diagnosis is still in question and will impact outcome. Fetal CT should only be performed in the second or third trimester, when fetal organogenesis has already taken place.

When the decision is made to undergo this test, the patient is placed supine on the CT table. The top and bottom of the uterus are marked by US, providing the strict borders for CT scanning. The study is done without contrast and at such a low radiation dose that only the fetal bones (and not the solid organs) are visualized. Images are reviewed in the 3D console, following sectioning of the maternal structures, and rendering exquisite detail of the fetal skeleton (Figs. 21.7 to 21.9). By CT, the skull, clavicles, scapula, ribs, vertebral bodies, and long bones should be visualized in a normal fetus in the second and third trimester, and their absence implies pathology. Because of the low radiation used, the fetal hands and feet may not be seen, particularly in the second trimester; however, these are usually seen by US, obviating the need to increase the radiation dose to the fetus.

The analysis of a fetal CT should follow a systematic approach, as with US. It can demonstrate additional findings demonstrating bones in exquisite detail.[25] Because of the radiation dose, however, fetal CT should be done only if the osseous findings are severe, and if the diagnosis in question is still uncertain by US.

There are some limitations in the evaluation of the fetus with SD when utilizing this imaging technique. First, the length of long bones in normal fetuses by CT has not yet been established. Secondly, assessment of mineralization currently is subjective. Using a fetal radiology atlas such as Schumacher et al.,[26] which has postmortem radiographs of the normal fetus up to 23 weeks' gestational age is useful as a reference. For older fetuses, mineralization can be assessed by comparing the skull with other cases of similar gestational age.

When performing a fetal CT, the goal is to use the lowest radiation dose possible while still having a diagnostically adequate study. We aim at a radiation dose of approximately 5 mSv. To put this in context, a study by McCollough et al.[27] postulates that the absolute risk of fetal effects (including cancer induction) is small at a conceptus dose of 100 mSv, and negligible at a dose of less than 50 mSv. Assuming a normal incidence of 0.07% incidence of childhood cancer and a natural incidence of malformation risk in the order of 4% in the normal population, the risk to the conceptus given a fetal dose of about 50 mSv results in a 96% probability of birthing a child with no malformation, or a 99.9% chance that the child will not develop cancer, or 95.9% chance that the child will have no malformation nor cancer.[22–28] The radiation risk to the fetus from a low-dose fetal CT is small, but real. Great care must be placed in proceeding with this type of study, and the decision should be taken by consensus by a group of radiologists, maternal fetal medicine specialists, and geneticists as well as the parents.

## COMMONLY ENCOUNTERED PRENATAL SKELETAL DYSPLASIAS

### Achondrogenesis

**Differential Diagnosis:** The term "achondrogenesis" (Greek for "not producing cartilage") was coined by Marco Fraccaro, an Italian pathologist who observed a stillborn female with severe micromelia and marked histological changes of the cartilage.[29] This is a lethal entity characterized by a relatively large head, short

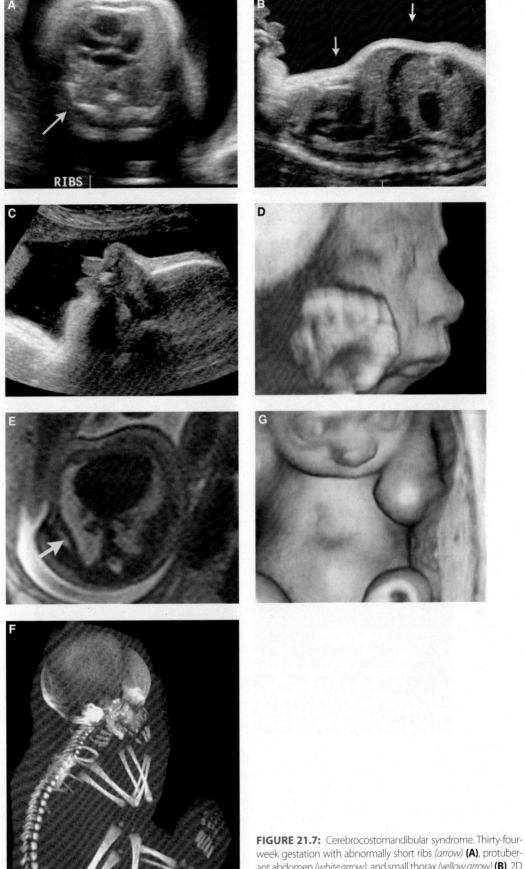

**FIGURE 21.7:** Cerebrocostomandibular syndrome. Thirty-four-week gestation with abnormally short ribs *(arrow)* **(A)**, protuberant abdomen *(white arrow)*, and small thorax *(yellow arrow)* **(B)**. 2D **(C)** and 3D **(D)** US showed pronounced micrognathia. SSFSE T2 MR confirms short ribs *(arrow)* **(E)**. Low-dose fetal CT demonstrates hypoplastic ribs with rib defects and gaps **(F)**. 3D US reconstruction of the chest in the coronal plane depicts a pectus excavatum deformity **(G)**.

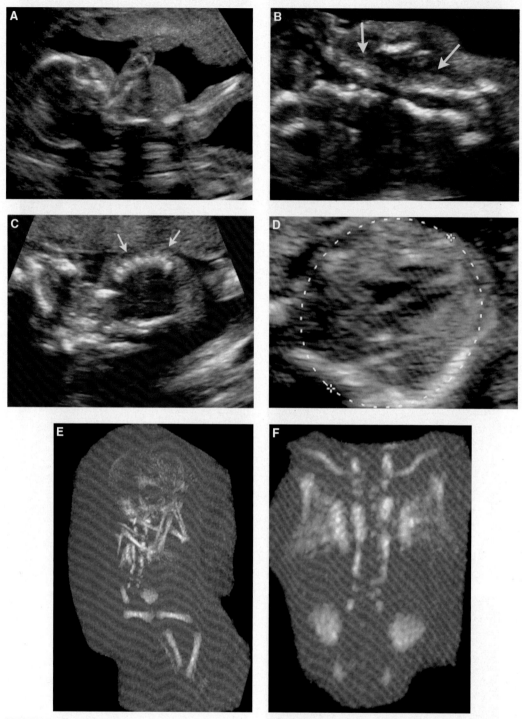

**FIGURE 21.8:** Spondylothoracic dysostosis. Twenty-one-week gestation with an overall short trunk and small chest/abdomen, on sagittal US **(A)**. The vertebral bodies were disorganized (*arrows* in **B**). The ribs appeared close together (*arrows*) **(C)**. In the axial plane, calipers are measuring the chest circumference, the ribs were short **(D)**. the ribs were short **(D)**. **E:** Low-dose fetal CT showed an overall short spine with normal-size long bones and head. The ribs were fused posteriorly and appeared to separate anteriorly, resembling a crab-like configuration. Magnified view of the thorax showed the ribs to better advantage **(F)**. Also seen is a disorganized spine with multiple segmentation anomalies.

neck, extreme micromelia, and a defect in vertebral ossification. Achondrogenesis usually results in stillbirth or neonatal demise.

**Incidence and Molecular Pathology:** Birth prevalence is about 0.2 in 10,000 live births. It is inherited as autosomal recessive (type IA and IB) and autosomal dominant (type II). The locus for type IA is not yet known; the gene for type IB is responsible for a sulfate transporter, DTDST, located on chromosome 5q,[29] also responsible for other forms of SDs including diastrophic dysplasia, atelogenesis type II, and multiple epiphyseal dysplasia. Type II achondrogenesis belongs to the type II collagenopathies and has a defect in the COL2A1 gene located in chromosome 12.

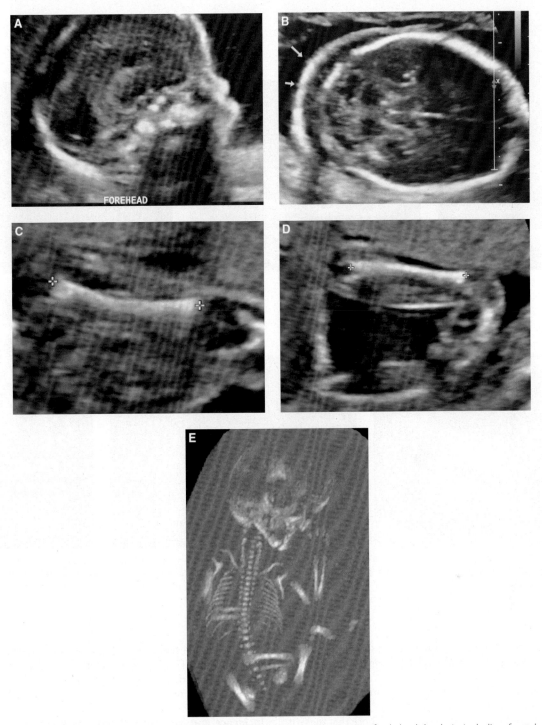

**FIGURE 21.9:** Pallister–Killian syndrome. Twenty-two-week fetus with non specific skeletal dysplasia, including: frontal bossing **(A)**, nuchal thickening (*arrows* in **B**), short long bones without bowing or fractures **(C)**, Flexion deformities at the wrist and ankles **(D)** were present by US. A normal-size rib cage was confirmed by low-dose fetal CT **(E)**. Diagnosis of Pallister–Killian syndrome was confirmed molecularly with identification of isochromosome at 12p.

**Radiologic Manifestations:** Type I manifests with poorly mineralized skull, absent or minimal ossification of the vertebral bodies, pubis and sacrum, as well as short and thin ribs (with fractures, in the case of the fetus with type IA), short and deformed iliac wings, and marked shortness and bowing of the tubular bones. Type II has variable degrees of shortness of the long bones (from near normal to very short), lack of mineralization of many vertebral bodies, nonossified sacrum and ischium,

small iliac wings with concave inferior and medial margins, and shortening of the ribs. Unlike type I, the calvaria demonstrates normal mineralization in type II achondrogenesis.

**Diagnosis:** Achondrogenesis can be diagnosed in the second trimester by US (Fig. 21.10). Limbs are abnormally short with small chest circumference. Unossified vertebrae may be missed sonographically if not carefully evaluated. At times, the fetus can

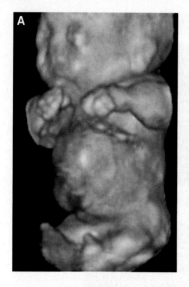
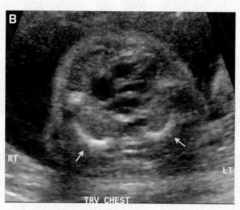
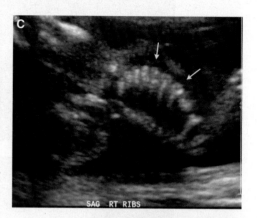
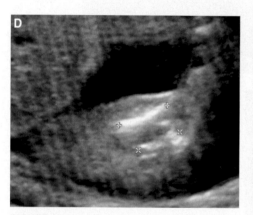
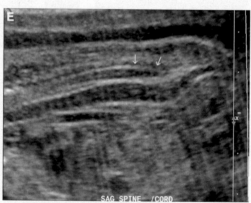
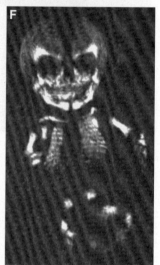

**FIGURE 21.10:** Achondrogenesis. 3D-US rendering of this 21-week fetus demonstrates shortening of the upper and lower extremities and a protuberant stomach **(A)**. Axial sonographic image at the level of the heart shows markedly foreshortened ribs, denoted by *arrows* **(B)**, which appear rather crowded and stacked (*arrows*) **(C)**. The long bones are short **(D)**. The spine is nonossified (*arrows* in **E**). Coronal 3D CT shows complete nonossification of the spine **(F)** with a "floating skull" appearance. The ribs and long bones are short. The iliac bones are small, and acetabula are flat.

present with hydrops (Fig. 21.11). Fetal CT can be helpful in confirming the unossified spine and short–long bones (see Fig. 21.10).

**Course and Prognosis:** Achondrogenesis is uniformly lethal. If hydrops develops, in utero demise may occur. Polyhydramnios may be present and may accelerate delivery. Those that make it to term die in the neonatal period.

**Differential Diagnosis:** In achondrogenesis IB, there are no rib fractures, and the vertebral pedicles may be ossified, whereas type IA may have rib fractures. In achondrogenesis type II, the ribs are not as thin and show no fractures. Differential includes osteogenesis imperfecta (OI) and hypophosphatesia, which have absent or delayed ossification of the calvaria that is compressible.

## Achondroplasia

**Description:** The term "achondroplasia" was used in the past to define all short-limb dysplasias. With recognition of the

heterogeneity of these disorders, this term is currently used to describe a specific disease characterized by predominantly rhizomelic dwarfism, limb bowing, lordotic spine, bulky head, and depressed nasal bridge.

**Incidence and Molecular Pathology:** It is the most common nonlethal SD (approximately 1 in 25,000 births) that may be transmitted as an autosomal dominant pattern or, in 80% to 90% of cases, a spontaneous mutation. It is caused by a gain-of-function mutation in the fibroblast growth receptor 3 gene (FGFR3), a transmembrane tyrosine kinase receptor that binds fibroblast growth factors. The gene is located in the short arm of chromosome 4 and codifies a highly conserved protein. The most common mutation, a G>A transition at nucleotide 1,138 (Gly380Arg), is observed in 95% of affected patients. The gain-of-function mutation causes ligand-independent activation of FDFR3, resulting in inappropriate cartilage growth plate differentiation and deficient endochondral growth and ossification.[30] Targeted molecular confirmation can be carried out using cell-free fetal DNA.[31]

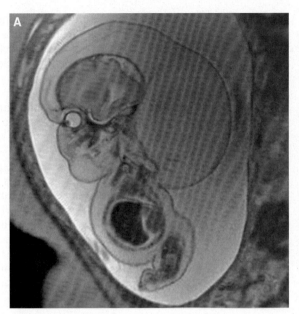
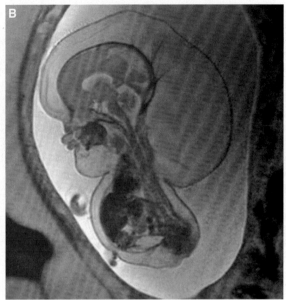

**FIGURE 21.11:** Achondrogenesis. **A:** SSFSE T2w MR demonstrates severe hydrops, hygroma, and ascites. The long bones are markedly short and bowed, the ribs short. **B:** The vertebrae are small and unossified.

The homozygous form is more severe, resembling thanatophoric dysplasia and is lethal.

**Radiologic Manifestations:** Achondroplasia is a rhizomelic micromelia with mild bowing of the long bones and disproportionately large head. The nasal bridge is depressed, there is frontal bossing and decreased size of the skull base and foramen magnum. Hydrocephalus may develop. Short, flat vertebral bodies that may be bullet-shaped, progressive narrowing of the interpediculate distance in the lumbar spine, square iliac wings, short narrow sciatic notch, and flat acetabular roofs are findings encountered in achondroplasia. A trident hand with fingers of equal length and separation of the third and fourth fingers may be present.

**Diagnosis:** Heterozygous achondroplasia is typically not diagnosed in the first and early second trimester. Femoral length crosses below the 3rd percental only after 18 to 26 weeks gestation with the affected fetus having relatively normal long bone growth before then.[32] Establishment of a femoral growth curve in the second trimester helps to distinguish between homozygous, heterozygous, and unaffected fetuses. Fetal size charts show femoral length on or below the 3rd percentile by 25 weeks' gestation and always below the 3rd percentile by 30 weeks.[31] The head circumference increases to above the 95th percentile in a majority of cases, with a slight increase in abdominal circumference as well. Additional US findings include frontal bossing, slightly bowed femora, short fingers, small chest, and polyhydramnios (Fig. 21.12).

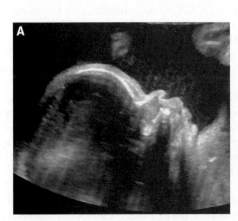
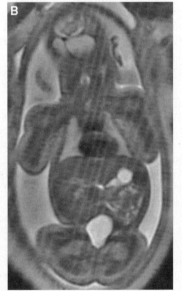
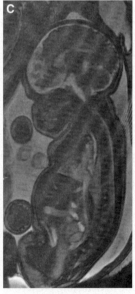

**FIGURE 21.12:** Achondroplasia. **A:** Sagittal US demonstrates frontal bossing at 32 weeks' gestation. **B:** Coronal SSFSE T2w MR demonstrates short humeri but normal lung volume. **C:** Sagittal SSFP MR confirms frontal bossing and documents narrowing of the foramen magnum.

Fetal MRI can help confirm the diagnosis documenting narrowing of the foramen magnum (Fig. 21.12C).

Homozygous achondroplasia can be diagnosed much earlier due to the presence of severe micromelia. Femoral length will fall below the 3rd percentile by 14 to 16.5 weeks' gestation.[33,34]

**Course and Prognosis:** Intelligence and life span are usually normal. Postnatal complications are mainly neurologic and are related to the degree of foramen magnum narrowing and spinal cord compression.

Homozygous achondroplasia (when both parents are affected) is lethal, with either stillbirth or early neonatal death from respiratory failure.

**Differential Diagnosis:** Differential diagnosis includes asymmetric IUGR and familial short stature. Assessment for fetal health and family history is important in distinguishing between these entities. Hypochondroplasia is a relatively common milder form that varies within and between families and lacks the cranial complications with lack of frontal bossing.[35]

Fetuses with the severe form of homozygous achondroplasia present early in the second trimester with severe micromelia. In these cases, other lethal SDs such as thanatophoric should be included in the differential and correlated with family history.[33,34]

## Arthrogryposis

**Description:** Arthrogryposis multiplex congenital (AMC) is a descriptive term that refers to multiple joint contractures present at birth. This term is often misused as a specific diagnosis instead of a descriptor or clinical finding. Arthrogryposis is not a specific disorder nor a SD, but the consequence of neurological, muscular, connective tissue, and skeletal abnormalities or intrauterine crowding, which may lead to limitation of fetal joint mobility and subsequent development of contractures. Potential etiologies include neuropathic abnormalities (brain, spine, or peripheral nerve), abnormalities of muscle structure or function (muscular dystrophies, mitochondrial abnormalities), abnormalities of connective tissue (diastrophic dysplasia), space limitation (multiple gestations, oligohydramnios), maternal diseases (multiple sclerosis, myasthenia gravis), and impaired intrauterine or fetal vascularity.[36] The common outcome is the decrease or lack of fetal movement leading to collagen proliferation, fibrotic replacement of the muscle, and marked thickening of the joint capsules.

**Incidence and Molecular Pathology:** Approximately 1% of all live births demonstrate some type of contracture involving one or more joints. The overall incidence of arthrogryposis, with multiple joint involvements, is 1 in 3,000 live births.[37] Arthrogryposis may be caused by genetic and environmental factors. Among the genetic factors, more than 35 specific genes have been associated with this condition. Since the evaluation of every single one is beyond the scope of this article, the reader is directed to a comprehensive review of the genetic etiologies.[38]

### Diagnosis
*Ultrasound:* Decreased fetal motion as detected by US during the second or third trimester or by maternal perception may be the first clue in detecting prenatal arthrogryposis. Real-time sonographic evaluation may show contractures with decreased fetal motion or severe flexion/extension deformities, unchanged in appearance during the time of scanning (Fig. 21.13).

*MRI:* MR cine sequences may be helpful in evaluating fetal movement as well. Fetal MR can help delineate intracranial and/or spine pathology that may be directly responsible for decreased fetal movement. Subjective evaluation of muscle mass can be provided by both US and MR.

*CT:* Fetal CT may provide 3D rendering of the bones that may be more easy to visually relate to for parents, obstetricians, and orthopedic surgeons (Fig. 21.13E).

**Course and Prognosis:** The prognosis is related to the specific etiology. In some severe cases, the underlying disease is lethal, with death occurring shortly after birth. In other cases, musculoskeletal impairment is minimal, and intelligence is normal. In between these two extremes, infants may have different degrees of disabilities. It is estimated that up to 50% of children born with arthrogryposis and CNS involvement will die in the neonatal period.[36] For those with contractures, treatment is directed toward achieving stable functional weight-bearing and manual dexterity.

## Asphyxiating Thoracic Dysplasia

**Synonym:** Jeune syndrome

**Description:** This autosomal recessive osteochondrodysplasia is grouped among the short-rib dysplasias including the lethal short-rib polydactyly syndromes (SRPS I–V) and less severe Ellis–van Creveld syndrome. These short-rib dysplasias (with or without polydactyly) appear to share a common primary cilium function defect and form a subset of ciliopathy disease. Jeune and Ellis–van Creveld have overlapping but milder phenotype as compared with the SRPS 1–V.[39]

Characteristic skeletal abnormalities include small, narrow thorax, short ribs, short squared iliac wings, and limb shortening. The spectrum of clinical manifestations is wide, ranging from lethal pulmonary hypoplasia to mild forms without respiratory compromise. Renal, hepatic, pancreatic, and retinal complications may also occur. Renal hypertension and failure have been reported findings. Hepatic involvement may include prolonged neonatal jaundice, polycystic liver disease, and hepatic cirrhosis. Pancreatic cystic disease may be present. Retinal abnormalities include retinal dystrophy and abnormalities in pigmentation. Other pathologic findings, including agenesis of the corpus callosum or Dandy Walker malformation, may be present.

**Incidence and Molecular Pathology:** The estimated prevalence is 0.14 per 10,000 births. Most mild and severe forms map to chromosome 15q13.[40] The causative gene has not yet been found.

**Radiologic Manifestations:** Short, horizontally directed ribs with bulbous anterior ends, narrow, bell-shaped thorax, horizontal or handlebar configuration of the clavicles, small pelvis, trident acetabulum, and normal vertebrae are some of the findings.[41] The extremities, including hand and feet, may be short with possible polydactyly.

**Diagnosis:** The diagnosis may be detected by US early in the second trimester if the findings are severe.[41–43] Chest circumference is small. Polyhydramnios may develop. Polydactyly may be present. MR can be helpful to confirm small rib cage and low lung volumes[43] (Fig. 21.14).

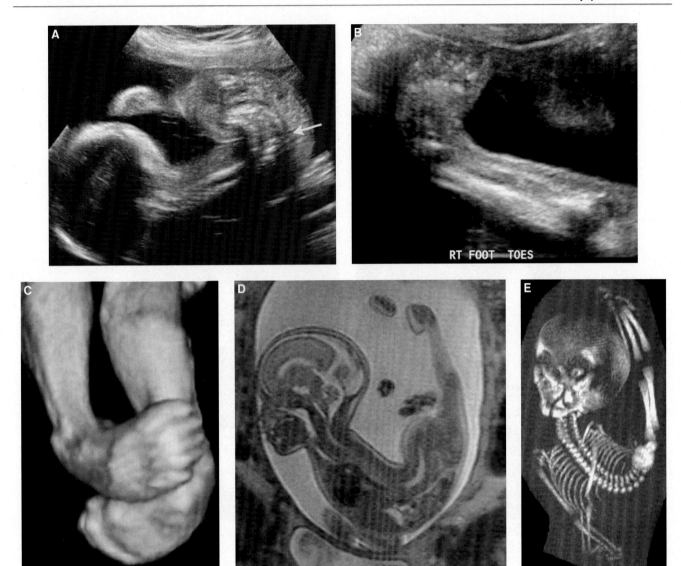

**FIGURE 21.13:** Arthrogryposis. 2D sonographic view of this 23-week fetus demonstrates a severe lumbosacral lordosis (*arrow* in **A**). Bilateral clubfeet are shown in this 2D image **(B)** and 3D US rendering **(C)**. SSFSE T2w sagittal MR image of the fetus demonstrates the scoliosis with marked extension contractures of the lower extremities and partial visualization of the clubfoot deformity **(D)**. Low-dose fetal CT shows abnormal spinal curvature and the abnormal posturing of the extremities **(E)**.

**Course and Prognosis:** Outcome is variable depending on the severity of symptoms. In severe cases, thoracic narrowing is responsible for pulmonary hypoplasia, respiratory failure, and death. In the milder forms, it is the degree of renal involvement that constitutes the main prognostic indicator. Indeed, progressive renal disease appears to be the norm rather than the exception.

**Differential Diagnosis:** Absence of mesomelic shortness and smooth metaphyseal margins differentiate asphyxiating thoracic dysplasia from other short-rib (minus polydactyly) syndromes. The pelvic configuration is indistinguishable from chondroectodermal dysplasia (Ellis–van Crevald), but polydactyly is a constant feature in this syndrome that may not necessarily be present in asphyxiating thoracic dysplasia. Ellis–van Crevald typically has cardiac anomalies as well.

## Campomelic Dysplasia

*Campomelic dysplasia* (CMD) is derived from the Greek "bent bones," a condition characterized by bowing of the long bones,

particularly lower extremities, hypoplastic scapulae, and other associated abnormalities, including hydrocephalus, congenital heart disease, and hydronephrosis. Craniofacial abnormalities (macrocephaly, cleft palate, micrognathia) have been reported in 90% to 99% of cases.[44] Approximately 75% with a 46, XY karyotype have ambiguous or normally appearing female external genitalia. The internal genitalia are variable, often with a mixture of Müllerian and Wolffian duct structures. Pretibial skin dimples may be seen in the neonate.

**Incidence and Molecular Pathology:** 0.05 per 10,000 births. Inherited as an autosomal dominant manner as a de novo mutation in the SOX9 gene mapped to chromosome 17 (17q24.3–q25.1). The SOX9 gene is a transcription factor involved in chondrogenesis and sex determination.

**Radiologic Manifestations:** Enlarged, elongated skull, hypoplasia, and poor ossification of the cervical vertebrae, small bell-shaped thorax with 11 pairs of ribs, hypoplastic scapula, short and angulated long bones, narrow and tall iliac wings, poor or

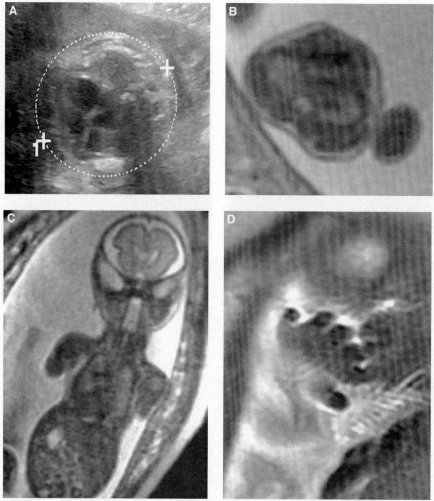

**FIGURE 21.14:** Asphyxiating thoracic dystrophy. **A:** Axial US demonstrates a small chest circumference (calipers). SSFSE T2 MR axial **(B)** and coronal **(C)** images confirm the short ribs and small lung volume. **D:** Postaxial polydactyly is also present.

absent ossification of the pubis, angulated proximal femoral shaft with apex located anterolaterally, hypoplasia, and angulation of tibia and hypoplastic fibula may be present.

**Diagnosis:** US can demonstrate marked anterior bowing of the long bones, particularly the tibia and femora. Bowing may be unilateral and mimic fractures. Other findings include hypoplastic scapulae, small thorax and vertically narrowed iliac bones. Flat face, micrognathia, hypertelorism, hydrocephalus, and ambiguous genitalia have also been described. 3D is useful in further assessment of hypoplastic scapula. As with other SDs, nuchal thickening may be noted early in gestation. Polyhydramnios, CNS, cardiac, and renal anomalies can be present (Fig. 21.15).

When CMD is being considered, genetic analysis of the *SOX9* gene is recommended.

**Course and Prognosis:** Many newborns with CMD die shortly after birth secondary to respiratory insufficiency. However, unlike other SDs, the cause of death may not be related to thoracic cage hypoplasia, but rather airway instability (tracheobronchomalacia) or cervical instability.

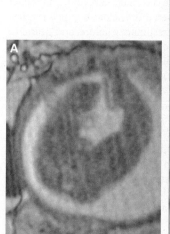
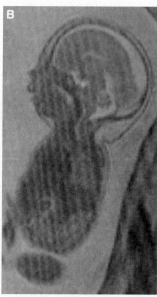

**FIGURE 21.15:** Campomelic dysplasia. **A:** SSFSE T2 MR axial image demonstrates short bowed tibia and equinovarus deformity. **B:** Sagittal image demonstrates micrognathia and cystic hygroma.

**Differential Diagnosis:** The most common error is to confuse CMD with OI. CMD is characterized by hypoplastic scapula and may have renal anomalies. Facial features of CMD are not present in OI. Irregularbeaded ribs representing fractures in OI are not present in CMD. Bowing of long bones in the fetus with OI may be more asymmetric secondary to healing fractures. Other differentials include hypophosphatasia, thanatophoric dysplasia, mesomelic dysplasia, and diastrophic dysplasia.

## Chondroectodermal Dysplasia

**Synonym:** Ellis–van Creveld syndrome.

**Description:** An autosomal recessive SD in the short-rib polydactyly group characterized by disproportionate short-limb dwarfism with centrifugal shortening, short ribs, postaxial polydactyly (generally involving the fingers, less commonly the toes), and dysplasia of ectodermal derivatives (hypoplastic or absent nails, partial anodontia, scant or fine hair). Approximately 60% of patients have congenital heart malformations, especially atrial septal defects.

**Incidence and Molecular Pathology:** 0.9 per 10,000 births, with a high incidence among the Amish community of Lancaster, Pennsylvania. Two EVC genes, linked to the 4p16 chromosome, are thought to be causative of the disease, although these may not be the only genes involved in this phenotype.

**Radiologic Manifestations:** Disproportionate short-limb dwarfism with progressive distal shortening of the extremities, bony spike in the medial side of distal metaphysis of humerus in newborns, polydactyly of hands (almost 100%) and feet (about 25%), short ribs, narrow thorax, dysplasia of the pelvis with low iliac wings and hook-like protrusion of the medial and/or lateral aspect of the acetabulum (trident pelvis), often premature ossification of the capital femoral epiphysis, slanting of the proximal medial tibial metaphysis, and cone-shaped epiphysis of the middle phalanges.

**Diagnosis:** Abnormal osseous findings may be detected during the second or third trimester of pregnancy, although distinction with other short ribs dysplasia is challenging by US. The presence of mesomelic shortened long bones, polydactyly, small chest with small ribs, and cardiac defects are clues suggestive of this entity.

**Course and Prognosis:** One-third of the infants die in the first month of life because of cardiopulmonary problems. Survivors may reach adulthood, usually with normal intellectual development but short stature.

**Differential Diagnosis:** Differentiating between chondroectodermal dysplasia and asphyxiating thoracic dysplasia (Jeune syndrome) is challenging because of the significant overlap: polydactyly, narrow thorax, and similar but less severe pelvic dysplasia occur in asphyxiating thoracic dysplasia as well. Hexadactyly of the fingers is a constant finding in chondroectodermal dysplasia but rare in asphyxiating thoracic dysplasia.

## Chondrodysplasia Punctata

**Synonyms:** Conradi–Hunermann syndrome, chondrodystrophia calcificans congenita.

**Description:** Chondrodysplasia punctata (CDP) describes the radiographic appearance of abnormal cartilaginous stippling, the result of abnormal deposition of calcium during endochondral bone formation. Stippling may arise secondary to premature calcification of the cartilage in the epiphyseal growth plate, later resolving during the first year of life, or may also be found in cartilaginous sites not expected to calcify, like the trachea.[45,46] These findings may be seen in a number of different entities, including errors of metabolism, chromosomal abnormalities, and abnormal vitamin K metabolism. Irving et al.[45] proposed the following classification of disorders with cartilage stippling: (1) metabolic abnormalities, including errors of peroxisomal function, cholesterol biosynthesis, and other inborn errors of metabolism; (2) disorders resulting in disruption of vitamin K metabolism; and (3) various chromosomal abnormalities, including trisomy 13, 21 and Turner syndrome. It is important to note that CDP does not constitute a diagnosis, and that, as such, an appropriate investigation must be done in order to find the underlying diagnosis.

Prenatally, a classification of rhizomelic (potentially lethal) and nonrhizomelic (Conradi–Hünermann syndrome, more common and generally benign) is made.

**Incidence and Molecular Pathology:** Incidence is 0.09 per 10,000 births. CDP is seen in a number of different conditions, as above.[35,45] The rhizomelic type is inherited as autosomal recessive pattern and is usually lethal. The nonrhizomelic Conradi–Hünermann type may be inherited as autosomal dominant or recessive and X-linked pattern. It can present with asymmetric short stature, scoliosis, cataracts, and/or flat facies with nasal hypoplasia.

**Radiologic Manifestations:** The rhizomelic type is characterized by marked limb shortening. Contractions, flexed fingers, and hypertelorism are commonly seen. There is calcific stippling of the epiphyses. Metaphyseal splaying and coronal clefts of the spine may be seen.

The nonrhizomelic Conradi–Hünermann type is a milder, with minimal or no limb shortening. The metaphyses are not splayed. Stippling is very fine and may be limited to the tarsal or carpal bones.[44]

**Diagnosis:** Prenatal findings are variable. One case describes a normal first trimester scan that on follow-up at week 19 showed profound shortening of the humeri with hypomineralization, and epiphyseal fractures and stippled hyperechoic foci in the epiphyseal cartilage.[47] By 21 weeks, humeri became bowed, and femora became short with abnormalities of the epiphyseal cartilage. Another report describes a 23-week fetus with rhizomelic limb shortening and epiphyseal calcifications. A fetal CT demonstrated the epiphyseal calcifications as well as bowed long bones, scoliosis, and distal phalangeal hypoplasia.[48]

With milder forms, isolated midface hypoplasia may be the only finding (Fig. 21.16).

**Course and Prognosis:** The rhizomelic type of CDP is often fatal within the first year of life secondary to respiratory failure. Severe mental deficiency and psychomotor delay is present in survivors.

With the nonrhizomelic-type bone changes can actually improve with a normal life span and intelligence. The only marker in adults may be the nasal anomaly.[30]

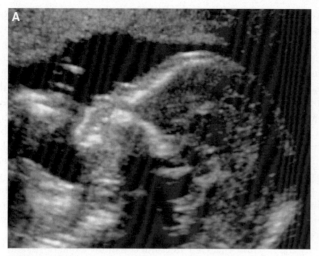
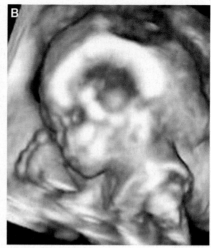

**FIGURE 21.16:** Chondrodysplasia punctata. Family history of chondrodysplasia punctata X-linked. In this 20-week fetus, isolated midface hypoplasia with a small nose was identified by 2D **(A)** and 3D **(B)** US consistent with Conradi–Hünermann syndrome.

**Differential Diagnosis:** Other forms of chondrodysplasia punctata such as Warfarin embryopathy, aneuploidy, phenytoin and alcohol exposure, Smith–Lemli–Opitz syndrome, and GM1 gangliosidosis.

## Craniosynostosis

**Description:** Abnormal development or premature closure of one or more cranial sutures resulting in abnormal head shape. It may occur in isolation or in the presence of a syndrome. The syndromic form tends to be associated with multiple sutures, whereas the isolated form tends to involve a single suture, most commonly the sagittal followed by the coronal, metopic, and lambdoid sutures. In severe cases, craniosynostosis can cause compression of cranial nerves and increased pressure on the growing brain.

**Incidence and Molecular Pathology:** Isolated craniosynostosis occurs in about 3.4 per 1,000 live births. When associated with a syndrome, it is a rare occurrence (<1 in 50,000 to 100,000). Most isolated cases have multifactorial or sporadic inheritance; as part of a syndrome, inheritance is usually autosomal dominant, depending on the specific syndrome. The causes of craniosynostosis are numerous and include chromosomal, metabolic, teratogenic (aminopterin, sodium valproate), and infection as possible culprits. For a more extensive list, the reader is referred to the excellent review by Dr. Lachman.[49]

**Radiologic Manifestations:** The findings seen in a fetus with craniosynostosis depend on the underlying syndrome. In Crouzon syndrome, findings may include premature fusion of the coronal sutures leading to brachycephaly and in severe cases, a cloverleaf skull. In Apert syndrome, cloverleaf deformity of the skull may also be found, along with hypertelorism, ventriculomegaly, and "mitten hands" or osseous/cutaneous syndactyly of the second, third, and fourth fingers (Fig. 21.17). In Pfeiffer syndrome, brachycephaly and acrocephaly relate to fusion of the coronal and sometimes sagittal sutures.

**Diagnosis:** Cranial sutures can be visualized by three-dimensional sonography as early as the 13 weeks' gestation. However, the

prenatal diagnosis of craniosynostosis is usually made on the basis of secondary features such as cranial deformation and hyper- or hypotelorism later in gestation.[50]

MRI has been shown to be a helpful imaging adjunct,[33] providing additional detail about the brain and possible cranial dysmorphism[51] (Figs. 21.17 to 21.19).

Expected findings if there is premature fusion of a single coronal suture include ipsilateral cranial flattening or plagiocephaly with elevation and posterior displacement of the ipsilateral orbit and anterior displacement of the ipsilateral ear canal. If two coronal sutures are fused, the result is brachycephaly or turribrachycephaly, with decreased anteroposterior dimension of the skull (Fig. 21.20). Premature fusion of the metopic suture leads to a triangular shape of the anterior skull (trigonocephaly), resulting in bitemporal narrowing and hypotelorism as seen in

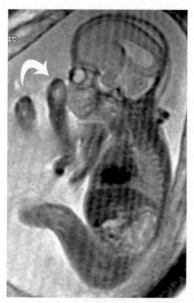

**FIGURE 21.17:** Apert syndrome. Sagittal SSFSE T2w MR demonstrates mitten hands *(arrow)* as well as brachycephaly in this fetus with evolving craniosynostosis.

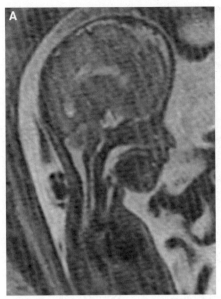
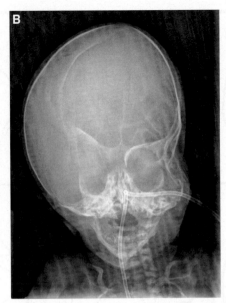
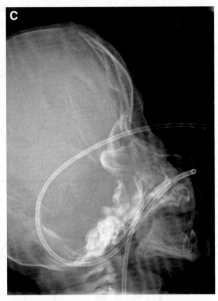

**FIGURE 21.18:** Craniosynostosis. Twenty-eight-week gestation with turricephaly (increased craniocaudal and decreased anteroposterior diameter of skull), flattened facial profile by sagittal SSFSE T2w MR image **(A)**. Postnatal radiographs of the skull AP **(B)** and lateral **(C)** confirm prenatal findings with bicoronal craniosynostosis, resulting in brachycephaly and partial closure of the lambdoid suture with pronounced left plagiocephaly.

prenatal US and MR. Synostosis of the sagittal suture results in a decreased biparietal dimension of the cranium (scaphocephaly or dolichocephaly). Premature closure of the coronal and lambdoid sutures may result in the cloverleaf deformity of the skull or Kleeblattschädel, with bitemporal and bifrontal bulging, findings that may be seen in entities such as thanatophoric dysplasia. Early fusion of the lambdoid suture may produce parieto-occipital plagiocephaly.

**Course and Prognosis:** A prenatal diagnosis of craniosynostosis carries significant cosmetic and surgical implications. The prognosis for isolated craniosynostosis is very good with reconstructive surgery. Prognosis for individuals with a genetic syndrome with craniosynostosis ranges from very good (Crouzon, Jackson–Weiss syndrome) to developmental delay and mental retardation (Apert and Pfeiffer syndromes) or lethality (thanatophoric dysplasia type II).

## Hypophosphatasia

**Description:** Congenital disease characterized by demineralization of bones and low alkaline phosphatase (ALP) in the tissue and serum. ALP acts on pyrophosphate and other phosphate esters, leading to the accumulation of inorganic phosphates that are crucial for the formation of bone crystals. Bone fragility is thought to be the result of deficient generation of bone crystals. The severity of the disease is inversely related to the serum levels of ALP activity. Hypophosphatasia has been subdivided into four clinical types according to the age of onset: (1) perinatal, (2) infantile, (3) childhood, and (4) adult.

**Incidence and Molecular Pathology:** Incidence is 1 per 100,000 live births. It is inherited as autosomal recessive in the infantile/childhood type and autosomal dominant for the adult form of the disease. Loss of function of the ALP liver gene,

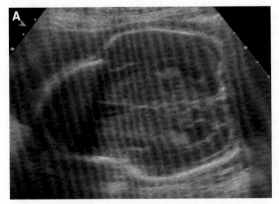
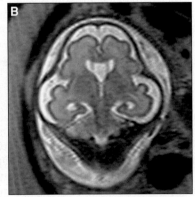

**FIGURE 21.19:** Craniosynostosis. US **(A)** and SSFSE T2w MR sequence **(B)** in this 29-week fetus with a cloverleaf deformity of the skull (Kleeblattschädel), characterized by a trilobar skull with bossing of the forehead, temporal bulging, and a flat posterior skull.

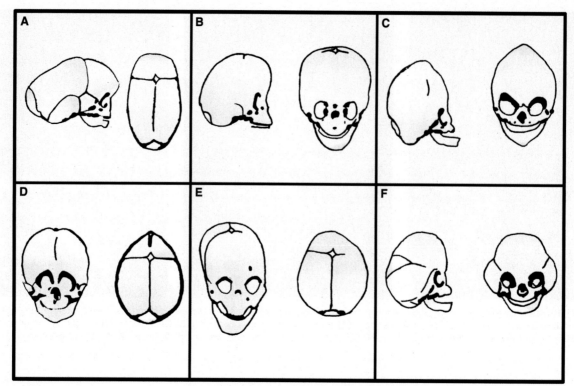

**FIGURE 21.20:** Common forms of craniosynostosis. **A:** *Scaphocephaly*: elongated and narrow cranial vault secondary to the premature closure of sagittal suture. **B:** *Turricephaly* or *oxycephaly*: tall head. **C:** *Oxycephaly* with prominent bregmatic junction. **D:** *Trigonocephaly*: premature fusion of the metopic suture resulting in a triangular-shaped anterior skull. **E:** *Plagiocephaly*: asymmetric distortion and flattening of one side of the head. **F:** *Cloverleaf skull* or *kleblattschädel*: deformity of the skull resulting in a trilobed cranium.

also called tissue nonspecific alkaline phosphatase (TNSALP), located on chromosome 1p36.1–p34, is responsible for the genotype in hypophosphatasia. A large spectrum of mutations have been observed, resulting in different ranges of enzymatic activity, leading to the wide phenotypic variability seen in hypophosphatasia.

**Radiologic Manifestations:** The congenital form is characterized by marked demineralization of the calvarium. The skull appears soft ("caput membranaceum"). Tubular bones are short and may have numerous fractures. The skeleton may be poorly and irregularly ossified.

**Diagnosis:** By US, demineralization of the skull is seen with increased echogenicity of the falx cerebri, attributed to enhanced sound transmission in a poorly mineralized skull. Deformation of the skull from external compression with the US transducer is consistent with skull demineralization (see "Osteogenesis Imperfecta"). Demineralization and fractures of the long bones may also be noted. Amniotic fluid is increased.

**Course and Prognosis:** The perinatal form is lethal because of intracranial hemorrhage or respiratory insufficiency secondary to the poorly developed ribs and reduced thoracic cavity volume. In the infantile or juvenile form, symptoms may appear shortly after birth (failure to thrive, irritability, convulsion, cyanotic episodes, angulated limbs, and other signs of hypercalcemia) or early in childhood (delayed onset of walking, myopathy, weakness). In the adult form, bone pain, tendency to fracture, and abnormal teeth may be presenting symptoms.

**Differential Diagnosis:** In achondrogenesis, there is lack of ossification of the spine; however, it is the vertebral bodies that are not ossified as opposed to the neural arches in hypophosphatasia. In addition, the calvarium will be ossified in achondrogenesis, as opposed to hypophosphatasia.

Fractures and bowed and short bones may be found in osteogenesis imperfect as well, but the calvarium may be partially ossified in OI.

## Mesomelic Dysplasia

**Description:** Group of disorders with disproportionate limb shortening of the middle segments of the extremities. It includes dyschondrosteosis, Nievergelt mesomelic dysplasia, Langer mesomelic dysplasia, Reinhardt mesomelic dysplasia, Robinow (fetal face syndrome) mesomelic dysplasia, and Werner mesomelic dysplasia. The tibia/fibula and/or radius/ulna are hypoplastic, but the bones can also be malformed or fused. Associated anomalies include ulnar deviation of the hands, talipese equinovarus, bony spurs, and carpal and/or tarsal synostosis.

**Incidence and Molecular Pathology:** These are rare entities, with no known incidence defined.

Many, but not all, of the mesomelic dysplasias are autosomal dominant. For a detailed listing of known genes involved in these disorders, the reader is directed to Dr. Spranger's review in his book on SDs.[35]

**Radiologic Manifestations:** Variable. *Langer mesomelic dysplasia* is characterized by a hypoplastic ulna, fibula, and mandible, with the ulna being shorter than the radius. The lower extremities are more affected than the upper extremities. Some people consider the Langer type as the homozygous state of *dyschondrosteosis*, a mesomelic dysplasia recognized in late childhood and characterized by mesomelic shortening with Madelung deformity.

In *Nievergelt mesomelic dysplasia*, there is mesomelia in the presence of clubfoot deformity. *Robinow mesomelic dysplasia* has acromelic brachymelia with short hands and feet and stubby fingers and toes. There is macrocephaly with a prominent forehead, hypertelorism, and hypoplastic mandible.

*Werner mesomelic dysplasia* is characterized by extreme bilateral hypoplasia of the tibia, polydactyly, absence of the thumbs, and, frequently, webbing of the fingers.

**Diagnosis:** Few prenatal diagnoses of mesomelic cases have been reported.[52,53] By US, shortening of the midsegments of the limbs is identified. Ribs, scapula, and clavicles are typically normal. Increased nuchal translucency has been described in the first trimester.[52]

**Course and Prognosis:** These disorders are associated with normal intelligence, with the exception of the Robinow type. Orthopedic problems are expected.

**Differential Diagnosis:** Other mesomelic dysplasias. VACTERL sequence, TAR, chondroectodermal dysplasia.

## Osteogenesis Imperfecta

**Description:** Heritable disorder of connective tissue whose cardinal manifestation is bone fragility caused by abnormal collagen microfibril assembly. About 90% of cases of OI are caused by mutations in genes that encode the proα1 and proα2 polypeptide chains that comprise the type I collagen molecule. Type I collagen is the most abundant type of collagen and is widely distributed in almost all connective tissues with the exception of hyaline cartilage. It is the major protein in bone, skin, tendon, ligament, sclera, cornea, and blood vessels. It comprises approximately 95% of the entire collagen content of bone and about 80% of the total protein content in bone.[54] Type I collagen is composed of two identical α1 polypeptide chains and one α2 chain, with the three strands twisted in a triple helix. Each polypeptide chain is composed of about 1,000 amino acids arranged in uninterrupted repeats of Gly-X-Y triplets. A complex pathway of postprocessing occurs with the triple helix as its final form. A mutation in one of the two genes that comprise the proα1 and proα2 polypeptide chains may induce a change either in the structure of the protein or in the number of collagen molecules made, resulting in OI. Both severe and mild forms of the disease have in common the presence of bone fractures after no or little trauma, and low bone mass.

Classification: The classification of OI is disputed. In its original form, it is divided into four subtypes, as proposed by Sillence et al.[55] in 1979, on the basis of clinical, genetic, and radiographic findings.

- Type I OI is the most common and the mildest form, characterized by relatively mild bone fragility, blue sclera, and conductive hearing loss.
- Type II OI is the most severe form, with findings seen prenatally expressed as intrauterine fractures, and is essentially fatal.

- Type III is the most severe form that is compatible with survival into adulthood with findings that may range between mild and severe.
- Type IV may present with dentinogenesis imperfecta and fractures.

There are other subtypes of OI that escape the Sillence classification, prompting investigators to add the additional types V–VII OI.[56] These are thought not to be associated with type I collagen mutations.

**Incidence and Molecular Pathology:** The precise incidence depends on the criterion used to define this entity, with reports ranging between 1 in 25,000 and 1 in 100,000.[56] The genes that encode the α1 and α2 polypeptide chains of type 1 collagen are referred to as COL1A1 and COL1A2 respectively, located on chromosome17q21.31–q22 and chromosome 7q22.1. Type I OI, the relatively mild form, is inherited as an autosomal dominant pattern, caused by a mutation in the type I collagen gene that results in normal type I collagen, but in reduced amounts. Type II OI is predominantly autosomal dominant (fewer than 5% are autosomal recessive), inherited as a de novo mutation in the type I collagen gene. Type III OI is a predominantly autosomal dominant mutation, also called progressively deforming OI, as the incidence of fractures usually increases with age. Finally, the autosomal dominant Type IV OI has marked intra- and interfamilial expression with clinical and radiographic manifestations that may overlap with type I in mild cases, and with type II/III in severe cases.

**Radiologic Manifestations:** Types I and IV demonstrate one or more fractures with normal or mildly shortened long bones that may appear angulated, with irregular contour of the bone and evidence of callus formation. Type I and IV may not demonstrate abnormalities until the postnatal period.

Type II is the most common type seen in utero, demonstrated by generalized bone deossification, a crumpled and coarsened appearance of the long bones, and irregularity and beading of the ribs (Figs. 21.21 to 21.23).

In type III, fractures may be present in the second trimester, although not as severe as in type II.

**Diagnosis:** Type I and IV may not demonstrate prenatal deformities, with the diagnosis often made after birth when fractures later develop.

Type II presents with wrinkling of the surface of the bones because of multiple fractures. The bones are typically <3% by the second trimester, and nuchal thickening can be present in the first trimester (Fig. 21.1). The ribs are beaded from multiple rib fractures with the chest bell-shaped. There is significant demineralization of the skull. The head may be compressible and the intracranial structures easily seen (see Fig. 21.21). Because of the degree of demineralization, both cortices of the bone may be visualized by US. Polyhydramnios may be present.

Type III may present as isolated fracture or multiple short-bowed bones. Findings may be similar to type II, but less severe, with long bones not severely micromelic in the early second trimester unlike type II OI.

While the diagnosis can be made by US, MR and CT have been used as an adjunct to confirm findings and help differentiate from other dysplasias (Figs. 21.22 and 21.23).

**Course and Prognosis:** Prognosis depends on the severity and type of the disease. Infants with type II are born with multiple

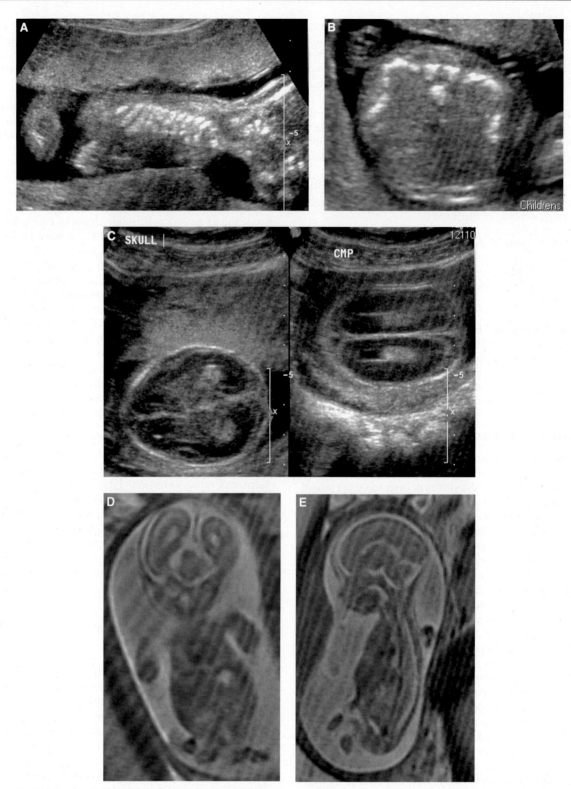

**FIGURE 21.21:** Osteogenesis imperfecta type II. Sagittal **(A)** and axial **(B)** US images of the chest at 18 weeks' gestation demonstrate multiple irregular rib fractures. **C:** Axial image of the skull without and with compression demonstrate decreased skull echogenicity with compressibility (*right*). SSFSE T2w MR Coronal image **(D)** demonstrates unossified calvarium, small chest, accordion appearance to the humerus. **E :** Sagittal image demonstrates lack of vertebral ossification.

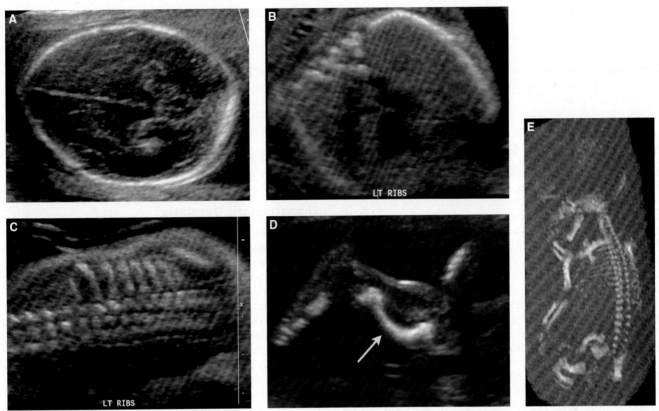

**FIGURE 21.22:** Osteogenesis imperfecta. **A:** 2D US in this 21-week fetus shows a pointed anterior skull. The ribs appear to be normal in length and morphology **(B ,C )**, with no definite fractures. The long bones of the lower extremity appear bowed and irregular *(arrow)* **(D)**. **E:** Low-dose fetal CT shows with irregularity of the long bones, consistent with fractures.

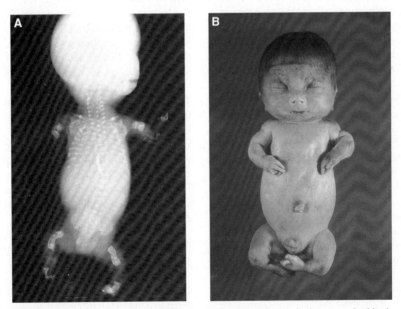

**FIGURE 21.23:** Osteogenesis imperfecta. **A:** Frontal radiograph shows marked limb shortening with numerous fractures. **B:** Postmortem photograph of a case of osteogenesis imperfecta. (From Jeanty P, Valero G, Bircher ME, et al. Skeletal dysplasias. In: Nyberg DA, McGahan JP, Pretorius DH, et al, eds. *Diagnostic Imaging of Fetal Anomalies*. Philadelphia, PA: Lippincott Williams & Wilkins; 2003:661–712.)

fractures and most often die in the neonatal period from respiratory compromise. In the milder types, fractures may not occur until later in life.

**Differential Diagnosis:** Differential diagnosis includes thanatophoric dysplasia, hypophosphatasia, achondrogenesis and campomelic dysplasia. The key in differentiation includes asymmetric fractures in various stages of healing and beaded ribs.

## Short-Rib Polydactyly Syndrome

**Description:** Short-rib polydactyly syndromes (SRPS I–V) are a group of lethal congenital disorders characterized by shortening of the ribs and long bones, polydactyly, and a range of extraskeletal anomalies (heart, intestine, genitalia, kidney, liver, and pancreas).[57] Other disorders in this grouping, including Jeune and Ellis–van Creveld syndromes, have overlapping but typically milder phenotype. These short-rib dysplasias (with or without polydactyly) appear to share a common primary cilium function defect and form a subset of ciliopathy disease.[39]

Four types of SRP syndromes have been described, but overlap in the clinical and radiological features of the four types has led to difficulty in distinguishing between them. Polydactyly occurs frequently, but is not obligatory.

**Incidence and Molecular Pathology:** Because of the rarity of the syndrome, its true incidence is not known. The candidate genes for the different SRPS are delineated in the excellent revision of the Nosology and Classification of Genetic Skeletal Disorders from 2012.

**Radiologic Manifestations**
*SRP Type I or Saldino-Noonan Syndrome:* Findings include dolichocephaly, poor mineralization of the frontal bones, metacarpals, metatarsal and phalanges, severe micromelia, hypoplastic tubular bones, narrow thorax, extremely short and horizontally oriented ribs, pointed femurs, and absent fibula. Cardiac, gastrointestinal, and urogenital malformations can be found. Polydactyly can be pre- or postaxial.

*SRP Type II or Majewski Syndrome:* Findings include extremely short and horizontally located ribs, mesomelia with marked shortening of the tubular bones, extremely short tibia with an ovoid configuration, rounded metaphyseal ends of the long tubular bones, pre- and postaxial polysyndactyly, and distal phalangeal hypoplasia. Genitalia may be ambiguous. Hydrops and polyhydramnios have been described.

*SRP Type III or Verma-Naumorff Syndrome:* Similar to type I, but with milder findings, including vertebral hypoplasia, short ribs, short base of skull, shortening of all short tubular bones, and long bones with widened metaphyseal ends that contain lateral spikes.

*SRP Type IV or Beemer-Langer Syndrome:* Same as SRP type II but without polydactyly.

**Diagnosis:** The triad of micromelia, short ribs, and polydactyly is suggestive of SRP syndrome. By US, these findings may be detected in the early second trimester.

**Course and Prognosis:** All of these four types are uniformly fatal and need to be differentiated from the potentially surviving SRPS conditions of asphyxiating thoracic dystrophy (Jeune syndrome) and chondroectodermal dysplasia (Ellis–van Creveld syndrome).

**Differential Diagnosis:** Included in the differential diagnoses are Jeune and Ellis–van Creveld syndromes. Thanatophoric dysplasia chondrodysplasia punctata, osteogenesis imperfecta, a CMD and orofaciodigital syndrome type II should also be considered. Often diagnosis can only be confirmed after birth.

Recurrence Risk: SRPS is autosomal recessive (25% recurrence).

## Thanatophoric Dysplasia

**Description:** The term thanatophoric is derived from the Greek word thanatophorus, which means "death bringing" or "death bearing." Salient features of thanatophoric dysplasia (TD) include macrocephaly, narrow bell-shaped thorax, normal trunk length, and severe shortening of all the limbs (micromelia).

**Incidence and Molecular Pathology:** Most common form of lethal SD with an incidence of about 0.5 in 10,000 births. Two forms have been described: TD type I, which originates from several described mutations in the FGFR3gene46, and TD type II, accounted for by a single described mutation in the same FGFR3gene (Lys650Glu).[58]

**Radiologic Manifestations:** Prenatally, the findings of TD are characteristic: a relatively large head, marked shortening of the long bones, normal trunk length, small thoracic cage with very short ribs, platyspondyly, U- or H-shaped vertebral bodies seen in AP view, small iliac bones, flat acetabular roofs, and trident hands. In TD type I, the affected fetus has bowing of the long bones and a characteristic "telephone receiver" appearance of the femora. In TD type II, the long bones are short, but straight. The morphology of the skull also differs and is typically described as cloverleaf deformity in TD type I, but normal in shape in TD type II (Figs. 21.24 to 21.27).

**Diagnosis:** By US, the diagnosis can be made early in the second trimester with severe micromelia (long bones <3% for GA). Chest circumference is small with a bell-shaped thorax. The ribs are short but not beaded. No discreet fractures are present, although the short bones may appear bowed, which can be confused with fractures. Symmetrical findings and lack of callous formation can help to differentiate these findings from OI. In addition, the skull should be normally mineralized and not compressible (see Fig. 21.24).[59,60]

MR and CT may increase diagnostic accuracy and confidence if the sonographic findings are still in question (see Figs. 21.24 to 21.26).

**Course and Prognosis:** TD is fatal in the prenatal period. With intensive medical intervention, a few patients have survived relatively longer periods.

**Differential Diagnosis:** Type II OI is often confused with TD prenatally by US due to the severe micromelia and short ribs present in both. Key differentiating features include asymmetric beading and irregular bowing of the long bones and ribs in OI. Homozygous achondroplasia may be similar to TD; the

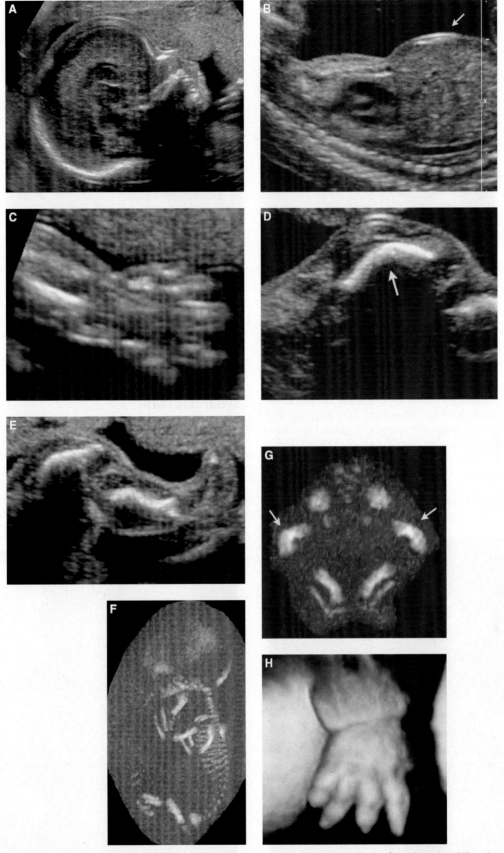

**FIGURE 21.24:** Thanatophoric dysplasia. Twenty-week gestation. Sagittal US shows frontal bossing **(A)** and a protuberant abdomen (*arrow* in **B**). The hand shows short tubular bones **(C)**. Short bowed femur (*arrow*), with normal mineralization **(D)** and short tibia **(E)**. Low-dose fetal CT reveals short ribs and extremities, subjective demineralization of the skull, and platyspondyly **(F)**. Coned view of the pelvis demonstrates bowed femora (*arrows*), decreased vertical diameter of the ischial bones, and flattened acetabula **(G)**. **H:** 3D US demonstrating brachydactyly with equal length of the digits in a different fetus with thanatophoric dysplasia at 34 weeks' gestation.

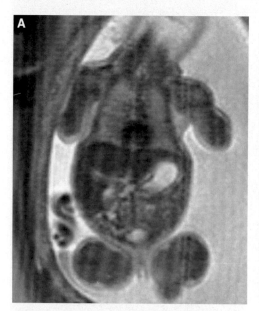

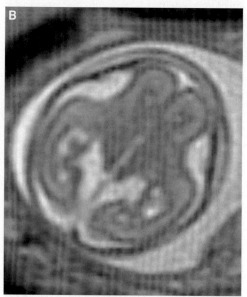

**FIGURE 21.25:** Thanatophoric dysplasia 22-week gestation. **A:** SSFSE T2w MR confirms the presence of short ribs with small lung volume. **B:** Axial image of the brain demonstrates mild changes of craniosynostosis. Deep sulci at the medial temporal lobes are present consistent with temporal lobe dysplasia of TD

final verdict is genetic analysis of the FGFR3 gene. Interestingly, several SDs are caused by different mutations in one single gene, FGFR3. Although all FGFR3-related SDs manifest with shortening of the long bones, they display a graded spectrum of phenotypic severity, ranging from the relatively mild (hypochondroplasia) to the more severe (achondroplasia), to lethal type (TD).[61] In all cases, this is the result of gain-of-function mutations that deregulate the receptor gene, leading to inhibition of chondrocyte growth and proliferation.[58]

## Thrombocytopenia Absent Radius Syndrome (TAR)

**Description:** Thrombocytopenia that is generally transient (platelet count of less than $100,000/mm^3$) and bilateral absence of radii are keys to the diagnosis. Other anomalies of the skeleton (upper and lower limbs, ribs, and vertebrae), heart, and genitourinary system (renal anomalies and agenesis of the uterus, cervix, and upper part of the vagina) may occur.

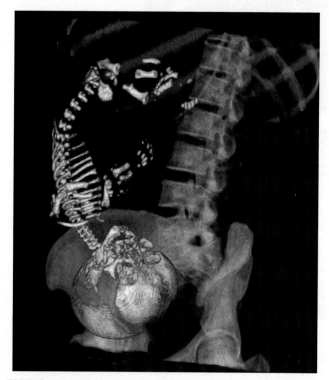

**FIGURE 21.26:** Thanatophoric dysplasia. Low-dose fetal CT 3D rendering of a 34-week fetus with TD. (Image courtesy of Monica Epelman, MD.)

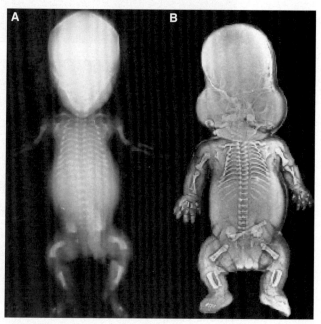

**FIGURE 21.27:** Two types of thanatophoric dysplasia. Type 1 **(A)** shows bowed femurs, and type II **(B)** shows straight femurs with cloverleaf skull deformity. (From Jeanty P, Valero G, Bircher ME, et al. Skeletal dysplasias. In: Nyberg DA, McGahan JP, Pretorius DH, et al, eds. *Diagnostic Imaging of Fetal Anomalies*. Philadelphia, PA: Lippincott Williams & Wilkins; 2003:661–712.)

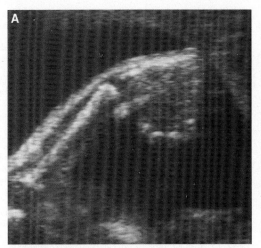 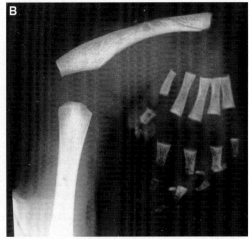

**FIGURE 21.28:** Radial aplasia. **A:** Radial aplasia with medial deviation of the wrist and hand. **B:** Radiograph after birth. (From Jeanty P, Valero G, Bircher ME, et al. Skeletal dysplasias. In: Nyberg DA, McGahan JP, Pretorius DH, et al, eds. *Diagnostic Imaging of Fetal Anomalies*. Philadelphia, PA: Lippincott Williams & Wilkins; 2003:661–712.)

**Incidence and Molecular Pathology:** Thought to be inherited as an autosomal recessive pattern. Although a microdeletion at chromosome band 1q21.1 has been involved, deletion of this segment is not sufficient to cause the phenotype and suggests an additional modifier gene.[62]

**Radiologic Manifestations:** Bilateral absent radii. The lower limbs may be short or absent. The ulna and humerus may be unilaterally or bilaterally absent. Thumbs and metacarpals are always present. Clubfoot deformity may occur.

**Diagnosis:** Highly suggested when there is bilateral absence of the radii in the presence of both thumbs, findings that can be seen by US (Fig. 21.28).

**Course and Prognosis:** Delivery by Cesarian section is recommended because these fetuses are at risk for intracranical hemorrhage. There is a high fatality rate within the first few months of life, but prognosis improves considerably after the first year.[44] Mental retardation may be present in 8% of patients, thought to be related to intracranial bleeding. Long-term disability is related to skeletal deformity with orthopedic intervention as needed to maximize function of limbs.

**Differential Diagnosis:** Holt–Oram syndrome: the thumb is often absent or hypoplastic in this condition; Roberts syndrome: thumb may be present sometimes, thrombocytopenia not reported; Fanconi anemia: absent thumbs, marrow failure.

## CONCLUSION

The evaluation of a fetus carrying a presumed diagnosis of SD is very challenging. Different phenotypes for a single disorder, evolving manifestations of the disease through gestation and the postnatal period, lack of specific genetic testing of certain entities, and overlapping features make this a complex group of disorders to diagnose accurately prenatally.

US is always the initial screening tool for evaluating the fetus with abnormal bones. MRI is becoming a useful adjunct particularly in the evaluation of anomalies associated with these dysplasias. Low-dose fetal CT has emerged as a method of delineating bony anomalies, but is limited to a small subset of cases with *severe* osseous abnormalities in which accurate diagnosis will impact management due to the low, but real, risk of radiation exposure to the fetus.

Once all of the fetal imaging is obtained, it is helpful to discuss the observed findings with consultants in radiology, genetics, and maternal fetal medicine,[35,49] so that appropriate additional genetic testing, if available, should be planned for.

## REFERENCES

1. Orioli IM, Castilla EE, Barbosa-Neto JG. The birth prevalence rates for the skeletal dysplasias. *J Med Genet*. 1986;23:328–332.
2. Warman ML, Cormier-Daire V, Hall C, et al. Nosology and classification of genetic skeletal disorders: 2010 revision. *Am J Med Genet A*. 2011;155A:943–968.
3. Alanay Y, Lachman RS. A review of the principles of radiological assessment of skeletal dysplasias. *J Clin Res Pediatr Endocrinol*. 2011;3:163–178.
4. Hall CM. International nosology and classification of constitutional disorders of bone (2001). *Am J Med Genet*. 2002;113:65–77.
5. Offiah AC, Hall CM. Radiological diagnosis of the constitutional disorders of bone: as easy as A, B, C? *Pediatr Radiol*. 2003;33:153–161.
6. Eames BF, de la Fuente L, Helms JA. Molecular ontogeny of the skeleton. *Birth Defects Res C Embryo Today*. 2003;69:93–101.
7. Schoenwolf GC, Larsen WJ. *Larsen's Human Embryology*. 4th ed. Philadelphia, PA: Elsevier Churchill Livingstone; 2009.
8. Krakow D, Lachman RS, Rimoin DL. Guidelines for the prenatal diagnosis of fetal skeletal dysplasias. *Genet Med*. 2009;11:127–133.
9. Dighe M, Fligner C, Cheng E, et al. Fetal skeletal dysplasia: an approach to diagnosis with illustrative cases. *Radiographics*. 2008;28:1061–1077.
10. Doray B, Favre R, Viville B, et al. Prenatal sonographic diagnosis of skeletal dysplasias: a report of 47 cases. *Ann Genet*. 2000;43:163–169.
11. Parilla BV, Leeth EA, Kambich MP, et al. Antenatal detection of skeletal dysplasias. *J Ultrasound Med*. 2003;22:255–258.
12. Nemec U, Nemec SF, Weber M, et al. Human long bone development in vivo: analysis of the distal femoral epimetaphysis on MR images of fetuses. *Radiology*. 2013;267(2):570–580.
13. Nemec SF, Nemec U, Brugger PC, et al. MR imaging of the fetal musculoskeletal system. *Prenat Diagn*. 2012;32(3):205–213.
14. Connolly SA, Jaramillo D, Hong JK, et al. Skeletal development in fetal pig specimens: MR imaging of femur with histologic comparison. *Radiology*. 2004;233(2):505–514.
15. Applegate KE. Can MR imaging be used to characterize fetal musculoskeletal development? *Radiology*. 2004;233(2):305–306.
16. Servaes S, Hernandez A, Gonzalez L, et al. Fetal MRI of clubfoot associated with myelomeningocele. *Pediatr Radiol*. 2010;40(12):1874–1879.
17. Nemec SF, Kasprian G, Brugger PC, et al. Abnormalities of the upper extremities on fetal magnetic resonance imaging. *Ultrasound Obstet Gynecol*. 2011;38(5):559–567.

18. Yazici Z, Kline-Fath BM, Laor T, et al. Fetal MR imaging of Kniest dysplasia. *Pediatr Radiol.* 2010;40:348–352.
19. Suzumura H, Kohno T, Nishimura G, et al. Prenatal diagnosis of hypochondrogenesis using fetal MRI: a case report. *Pediatr Radiol.* 2002;32:373–375.
20. Miller E, Blaser S, Miller S, et al. Fetal MR imaging of atelosteogenesis type II (AO-II). *Pediatr Radiol.* 2008;38(12):1345–1349.
21. Fink AM, Hingston T, Sampson A, et al. Malformation of the fetal brain in thanatophoricdysplasia: US and MRI findings. *Pediatr Radiol.* 2010;40(suppl 1):S134–S137.
22. Victoria T, Epelman M, Bebbington M, et al. Low-dose fetal CT for evaluation of severe congenital skeletal anomalies: preliminary experience. *Pediatr Radiol.* 2012;42(suppl 1):S142–S149.
23. Cassart M, Massez A, Cos T, et al. Contribution of three-dimensional computed tomography in the assessment of fetal skeletal dysplasia. *Ultrasound Obstet Gynecol.* 2007;29:537–543.
24. Miyazaki O, Nishimura G, Sago H, et al. Prenatal diagnosis of fetal skeletal dysplasia with 3D CT. *Pediatr Radiol.* 2012;42:842–852.
25. Victoria T, Epelman M, Coleman BG, et al. Low-dose fetal CT in the prenatal evaluation of skeletal dysplasias and other severe skeletal abnormalities. *AJR Am J Roentgenol.* 2013;200(5):989–1000.
26. Schumacher R, Seaver LH, Spranger J. *Fetal Radiology: A Diagnostic Atlas.* Berlin, Germany: Springer; 2004.
27. McCollough CH, Schueler BA, Atwell TD, et al. Radiation exposure and pregnancy: when should we be concerned? *Radiographics.* 2007;27:909–917; discussion 917–918.
28. Wagner LK, Hayman LA. Pregnancy and women radiologists. *Radiology.* 1982;145:559–562.
29. Superti-Furga A. Achondrogenesis type 1B. *J Med Genet.* 1996;33:957–961.
30. Trujillo-Tiebas MJ, Fenollar-Cortes M, Lorda-Sanchez I, et al. Prenatal diagnosis of skeletal dysplasia due to FGFR3 gene mutations: a 9-year experience: prenatal diagnosis in FGFR3 gene. *J Assist Reprod Genet.* 2009;26:455–460.
31. Chitty LS, Griffin DR, Meaney C, et al. New aids for the non-invasive prenatal diagnosis of achondroplasia: dysmorphic features, charts of fetal size and molecular confirmation using cell-free fetal DNA in maternal plasma. *Ultrasound Obstet Gynecol.* 2011;37(3):283–289.
32. Modaff P, Horton VK, Pauli RM. Errors in the prenatal diagnosis of children with achondroplasia. *Prenat Diagn.* 1996;16:525–530.
33. Lemyre E, Azouz EM, Teebi AS, et al. Bone dysplasia series: achondroplasia, hypochondroplasia and thanatophoric dysplasia: review and update. *Can Assoc Radiol J.* 1999;50(3):185–197.
34. Patel MD, Filly RA. Homozygous achondroplasia: US distinction between homozygous, heterozygous, and unaffected fetuses in the second trimester. *Radiology.* 1995;196(2):541–545.
35. Spranger JW, Brill PW, Poznanski AK. *Bone Dysplasias: An Atlas of Genetic Disorders of Skeletal Development.* 2nd ed. Oxford, UK: Oxford University Press; 2002.
36. Bevan WP, Hall JG, Bamshad M, et al. Arthrogryposis multiplex congenita (amyoplasia): an orthopaedic perspective. *J Pediatr Orthop.* 2007;27:594–600.
37. Rink BD. Arthrogryposis: a review and approach to prenatal diagnosis. *Obstet Gynecol Surv.* 2011;66:369–377.
38. Hall JG. Genetic aspects of arthrogryposis. *Clin Orthop Relat Res.* 1985;(194):44–53.
39. McInerney-Leo AM, Schmidts M, Cortés CR, et al. Short-rib polydactyly and Jeune syndromes are caused by mutations in *WDR60. Am J Hum Genet.* 2013;93(3):515–523.
40. Keppler-Noreuil KM, Adam MP, Welch J, et al. Clinical insights gained from eight new cases and review of reported cases with Jeune syndrome (asphyxiating thoracic dystrophy). *Am J Med Genet A.* 2011;155A:1021–1032.
41. den Hollander NS, Robben SG, Hoogeboom AJ, et al. Early prenatal sonographic diagnosis and follow-up of Jeune syndrome. *Ultrasound Obstet Gynecol.* 2001;18:378–383.
42. Rahmani R, Sterling CL, Bedford HM. Prenatal diagnosis of Jeune-like syndromes with two-dimensional and three-dimensional sonography. *J Clin Ultrasound.* 2012;40:222–226.
43. Tonni G, Panteghini M, Bonasoni M, et al. Prenatal ultrasound and MRI diagnosis of Jeune syndrome type I with histology and post-mortem three-dimensional CT confirmation. *Fetal Pediatr Pathol.* 2013;32(2):123–132.
44. Romero R. *Prenatal Diagnosis of Congenital Anomalies.* Norwalk, CT: Appleton & Lange; 1988.
45. Irving MD, Chitty LS, Mansour S, et al. Chondrodysplasia punctata: a clinical diagnostic and radiological review. *Clin Dysmorphol.* 2008;17:229–241.
46. Kaufmann HJ, Mahboubi S, Spackman TJ, et al. Tracheal stenosis as a complication of chondrodysplasia punctata [in French]. *Ann Radiol.* 1976;19:203–209.
47. Zwijnenburg PJ, Deurloo KL, Waterham HR, et al. Second trimester prenatal diagnosis of rhizomelic chondrodysplasia punctata type 1 on ultrasound findings. *Prenat Diagn.* 2010;30:162–164.
48. Ulla M, Aiello H, Cobos MP, et al. Prenatal diagnosis of skeletal dysplasias: contribution of three-dimensional computed tomography. *Fetal Diagn Ther.* 2011;29:238–247.
49. Lachman RS, Taybi H. *Taybi and Lachman's Radiology of Syndromes, Metabolic Disorders, and Skeletal Dysplasias.* 5th ed. Philadelphia, PA: Mosby Elsevier; 2007.
50. Robson CD, Barnewolt CE. MR imaging of fetal head and neck anomalies. *Neuroimaging Clin N Am.* 2004;14:273–291, viii.
51. Fjortoft MI, Sevely A, Boetto S, et al. Prenatal diagnosis of craniosynostosis: value of MR imaging. *Neuroradiology.* 2007;49:515–521.
52. Vseticka J, Gattnarova Z, Marik I, et al. Ultrasound diagnosis of severe mesomelic dysplasia in two fetuses, associated with increased neck translucency and tetralogy of Fallot in one and cystic hygroma in the other. *Am J Med Genet A.* 2010;152A:815–818.
53. Thomas NS, Maloney V, Bass P, et al. SHOX mutations in a family and a fetus with Langer mesomelic dwarfism. *Am J Med Genet A.* 2004;128A:179–184.
54. Niyibizi C, Wang S, Mi Z, et al. Gene therapy approaches for osteogenesis imperfecta. *Gene Ther.* 2004;11:408–416.
55. Sillence DO, Senn A, Danks DM. Genetic heterogeneity in osteogenesis imperfecta. *J Med Genet.* 1979;16:101–116.
56. Basel D, Steiner RD. Osteogenesis imperfecta: recent findings shed new light on this once well-understood condition. *Genet Med.* 2009;11:375–385.
57. Elcioglu NH, Hall CM. Diagnostic dilemmas in the short rib-polydactyly syndrome group. *Am J Med Genet.* 2002;111:392–400.
58. Chitty LS, Khalil A, Barrett AN, et al. Safe, accurate, prenatal diagnosis of thanatophoric dysplasia using ultrasound and free fetal DNA. *Prenat Diagn.* 2013;33(5):416–423.
59. Vasilj O, Miškoviæ B. Diagnosis and counseling of thanatophoric dysplasia with four-dimensional ultrasound. *J Matern Fetal Neonatal Med.* 2012;25(12):2786–2788.
60. Giancotti A, Castori M, Spagnuolo A, et al. Early ultrasound suspect of thanatophoric dysplasia followed by first trimester molecular diagnosis. *Am J Med Genet A.* 2011;155A(7):1756–1758.
61. Foldynova-Trantirkova S, Wilcox WR, Krejci P. Sixteen years and counting: the current understanding of fibroblast growth factor receptor 3 (FGFR3) signaling in skeletal dysplasias. *Hum Mutat.* 2012;33:29–41.
62. Toriello HV. Thrombocytopenia-absent radius syndrome. *Semin Thromb Hemost.* 2011;37:707–712.

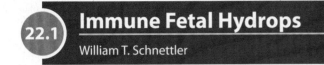

## Immune Fetal Hydrops

**22.1** William T. Schnettler

Immune hydrops represents the visible manifestation of complex pathophysiologic processes initiated by red blood cell alloimmunization (also known as hemolytic disease of the fetus and newborn, or HDFN)—the maternal immunologic response to "nonself" fetal red blood cell antigens. Historians theorize that Catherine of Aragon's recurrent fetal and neonatal demises were attributable to red cell alloimmunization and ultimately led to Henry VIII's decision to divorce her without a papal annulment.[1] This led to England's split from the Roman Catholic Church and the subsequent creation of the Church of England—highlighting the morbid and historic impact of HDFN. Advances in the understanding, detection, management, and prevention of pregnancies complicated by red cell alloimmunization stand among quintessential achievements of the 20th century. However, perinatal morbidity and mortality attributable to red cell alloimmunization continue to plague the developing world at rates comparable to those of prior centuries.[2] In the absence of effective identification and preventative strategies, alloimmunization claims hundreds of thousands of fetuses and neonates every year.[2]

### INCIDENCE

Fetal and neonatal effects of red cell alloimmunization range from mild hyperbilirubinemia to hydrops and death. The frequency of these effects depends upon the prevalence of specific antigens among the population and whether an effective prevention program utilizing antepartum and postpartum Rhesus immunoglobulin (RhIg) is in place. The prevalence of Rh(D) negativity varies considerably by ethnicity from less than 5% among Southeast Asian and individuals of African descent to 30% among the Basque population of Spain.[3] In the United States, 14.6% of the total population demonstrates Rh(D) negativity, with rates ranging from 1.7% among those of Asian ethnicity to 17.6% among non-Hispanic Whites.[4] The rates of immune hydrops and stillbirth due to Rh-alloimmunization are highest in South Asia and Africa, where little prevention or treatment with RhIg occurs.[3] The percentage of Rh(D)-negative women who become alloimmunized after giving birth to a Rh(D)-positive baby in those countries approximates 15% compared with 1% to 2% in the industrialized world.[3] Alloimmunized pregnancies have a 14% risk for stillbirth, and up to 50% of the surviving newborns will die or experience brain injury due to severe hyperbilirubinemia.[2] In the year 2010, rates for stillbirth and kernicterus attributable to Rh disease are an estimated 20- to 40-fold greater in South Asia and Sub-Saharan Africa than in high-income countries.[3] Data from the 2008 U.S. National Vital Statistics Report revealed that 540 out of 100,000 live births with HDFN resulted in neonatal death.[5]

Alloantibodies other than the anti-Rh(D) antibody have begun to contribute to a larger proportion of the responsibility for HDFN and immune hydrops.[6] Dutch scientists published a large prospective cohort study in 2008 that yielded a prevalence of 400 per 100,000 (0.4%) first trimester pregnancies with a positive screen for alloantibodies capable of causing hemolytic disease.[6] Of these, 79% were antibodies other than anti-D, and the most common were anti-E, anti-c, and anti-K (Kell). Among at-risk pregnancies, the incidence of severe HDFN was 26.3% of those who screened positive for anti-K, 10.2% for anti-c, 2.1% for anti-E, and 5% for those positive for anti-Rh antibodies other than c, D, and E.[6]

### GENETICS

The Rhesus blood antigen group was discovered nearly 75 years ago and includes the D, C, c, E, and e antigens.[7,8] Two linked genes on chromosome 1 encode for the red cell transmembrane proteins RhD and RhCcEe such that an individual's red blood cells display either the C or c antigen, E or e antigen, and D or no "D" antigen.[9] Whereas all Rhesus antigens have the potential to cause immune hydrops, the D antigen is the most immunogenic and historically responsible for more than 50% of cases of maternal alloimmunization.[6,9] Common nomenclature denotes individuals lacking the D antigen as Rh negative without regard to the genotypic presence of the other antigens. Most Caucasian, Rh(D)-negative individuals lack the RHD gene altogether. In other populations, certain individuals possess a normal RHD gene, but display the Rh(D)-negative phenotype owing to an error at the level of transcription or pre-mRNA processing (known as "partial D").[9] This regional genetic heterogeneity suggests a possible "founder-effect" within the Spanish population of the RHD gene deletion. Figure 22.1-1 depicts the RHD and RHCE genes with their possible phenotypic outcomes. The risk for HDFN is determined by whether the fetus is suspected or confirmed to carry the red cell antigen against which maternal alloantibodies are directed. Paternal zygosity denotes whether the risk is 50% (father is heterozygous for the gene) or 100% (father is homozygous).

### PATHOGENESIS

As Levine and Stetson[7] first reported in 1939, a breech in the fetal-maternal interface may expose the mother to various fetal red cell antigens, inciting an immunologic response. The antigen is presented to B lymphocytes of the maternal reticuloendothelial system (RES), activating a primary immune response characterized by large-scale immunoglobulin M (IgM) antibody production over the first several weeks. These antibodies are large and do not cross the placenta, posing no risk to the fetus. Following the initial phase, the maternal response shifts to clonal expansion of immunoglobulin G (IgG)-type antibodies and maturation of small resting lymphocytes into memory B lymphocytes targeted against the specific antigen. Memory B lymphocytes can persist in the mother for decades

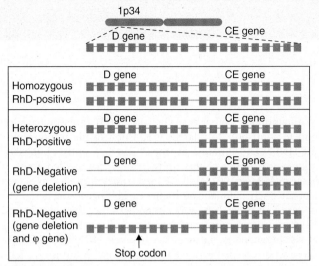

**FIGURE 22.1-1:** Schematic diagram of the RH gene locus on chromosome 1 with the four possible genotypes, including the "partial D" genotype phenotypically mimicking RhD-negative. (From Moise KJ Jr. Hemolytic disease of the fetus and newborn. In: Creasy RK, Resnick R, Iams JD, et al, eds. *Creasy and Resnik's Maternal-Fetal Medicine: Principles and Practice.* 6th ed. Philadelphia, PA: Saunders; 2009:479.)

awaiting reappearance of the relevant antigen to differentiate into plasma cells. If the antigen is presented in a subsequent pregnancy, plasma cells can rapidly proliferate and produce large quantities of IgG antibodies that can cross the placenta and bind to fetal red cells. Factors that increase the likelihood of alloimmunization include the volume of fetal-maternal transplacental hemorrhage (0.2 mL or greater), antigen density, gestational age, and ABO-compatibility. Maternal destruction of ABO-incompatible fetal red cells often occurs prior to presentation of other antigens such that the risk of Rh-alloimmunization is reduced from 16% to 2%.[10]

Once maternal alloantibodies bind fetal red cells, macrophages within the fetal circulation and spleen adhere and lyse the cells. To counter this destruction, the fetus increases plasma erythropoietin, prompting extramedullary erythropoiesis (primarily in the liver) and release of immature erythroblasts.[11] The resultant hepatosplenomegaly may alter the portal and venous architecture leading to portal hypertension and decreased hepatic albumin production. Increased umbilical venous pressure and decreased colloid oncotic pressure trigger extravasation of fluid from the fetal vasculature into the fetal and placental interstitial spaces.[12] The fetus attempts to compensate and maintain intravascular volume by increasing plasma aldosterone concentration, but this further decreases the fetal osmolality and hematocrit in a feed-forward cycle, ultimately resulting in the visible fetal and placental edema seen with immune hydrops.[13]

The mechanism underlying fetal anemia and the development of immune hydrops in fetuses affected by Kell-alloimmunization differs from the processes taking place in the Rh-alloimmunized fetus. In vitro studies of hematopoietic progenitor cells from cord blood reveal suppressed growth of the erythroid progenitor cells in the presence of monoclonal anti-Kell antibodies but not anti-Rh(D) antibodies.[14] Anti-Kell antibodies cause fetal anemia by inhibiting erythropoiesis at the progenitor-cell level rather than by RES-mediated hemolysis, as seen in Rh-alloimmunization. This finding becomes important in differentiating the diagnostic workup of Kell-mediated alloimmunization from that caused by most of the other blood-group allo-antigens.

## DIAGNOSIS

**Imaging:** Immune hydrops is generally defined by the sonographic detection of excess fluid accumulation within two separate fetal body compartments in conjunction with a positive maternal indirect Coombs test for an antibody known to cause HDFN. Excess fluid accumulation may manifest as ascites, pleural effusion, pericardial effusion, polyhydramnios, skin edema, and placental enlargement. True ascites appears as an echolucent rim of fluid encircling the entire contents of the fetal abdomen such that bowel, liver, and spleen are more easily identified (Fig. 22.1-2). Pleural effusions are often seen bilaterally compressing the lungs and mediastum, potentially leading to pulmonary hypoplasia (Fig. 22.1-3). The diagnosis of pericardial effusion requires visualization of at least 3 mm of fluid surrounding both cardiac ventricles (Fig. 22.1-4). Skin edema must measure 5 mm or greater in thickness (Fig. 22.1-5), and placentomegaly must measure 5 cm or greater in thickness (Fig. 22.1-6). If one such finding is seen in isolation, it should simply be described in terms of its location and not as hydrops fetalis. Although fluid accumulation in two separate fetal compartments denotes hydrops, no sonographic pattern specifies the etiology or severity of anemia.[15,16]

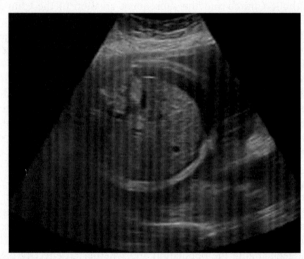

**FIGURE 22.1-2:** Ascites. Axial image of the fetal abdomen demonstrating ascites.

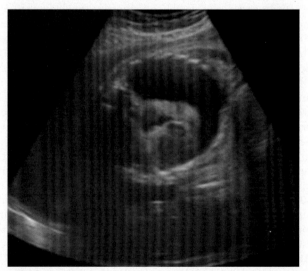

**FIGURE 22.1-3:** Pleural effusions. Axial image of the fetal thorax demonstrating bilateral pleural effusion with lung compression and mediastinal displacement.

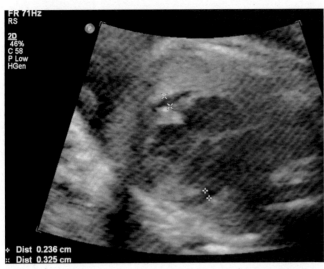

FR 71Hz
RS
2D
46%
C 58
P Low
HGen

Dist 0.236 cm
Dist 0.325 cm

**FIGURE 22.1-4:** Pericardial effusion. Axial view of the fetal thorax at the level of the four-chamber cardiac view demonstrating more than 3 mm of fluid surrounding both cardiac ventricles.

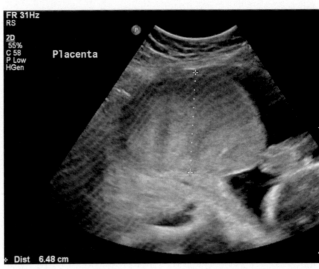

FR 31Hz
RS
2D
55%
C 58
P Low
HGen

Placenta

Dist 6.48 cm

**FIGURE 22.1-6:** Placental edema greater than 5 cm in thickness.

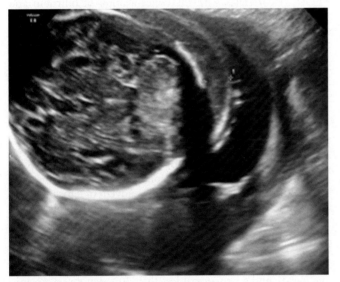

**FIGURE 22.1-5:** Skin edema of more than 5 mm.

A variety of fetal sonographic measures have been investigated in attempts at identifying methods for noninvasive quantification of fetal anemia. Measurement of the axial splenic circumference (Fig. 22.1-7) demonstrated 100% sensitivity and 94.7% specificity for severe anemia in cases without prior intrauterine transfusion in one prospective study.[17] The pathophysiologic association of splenomegaly with hemolytic anemia is easily understood, and this finding was promising. Unfortunately, enlargement of the splenic circumference was not predictive of mild anemia or the decrease in hematocrit following intrauterine transfusion (IUT). To achieve earlier detection and follow-up, investigators have employed Doppler assessment of the fetal blood velocity in the umbilical artery, umbilical vein, descending aorta, ductus venosus, splenic artery, and middle cerebral artery.

In 2000, Mari and coauthors[18] presented convincing evidence supporting the hypothesis that the decreased blood viscosity associated with fetal anemia manifests as an elevation in peak systolic velocity of blood flow within the middle cerebral artery. They prospectively compared cordocentesis-derived hemoglobin concentrations with middle cerebral artery peak systolic velocity measurements in 111 fetuses deemed at-risk for anemia and 265 nonanemic "normal" fetuses. Their findings provided essential normative data and threshold values representing mild, moderate, and severe anemia (see Table 53 in Appendix A1). With appropriate technique (Fig. 22.1-8), this measurement can noninvasively diagnose early anemia prior to the development of hydrops and provide surveillance following IUT to guide timing of repeat percutaneous umbilical cord blood sampling (PUBS) and transfusion. The measurements can be initiated at 18 weeks' gestation, and the fetal middle cerebral artery closest to the transducer should be evaluated with the Doppler gate placed immediately distal to the bifurcation of the carotid siphon. The angle of insonation should be as close to zero degrees (parallel) to the vessel direction as possible, and the baseline should be adjusted close to zero. Values greater than 1.50 multiples of the median (MoM) for gestational age denote moderate or severe anemia with 100% sensitivity and 88% specificity. The test's validity is preserved in the cases of Kell-mediated fetal anemia and hydrops.

Additional diagnostic tools may be employed for situations where the cause of hydrops fetalis is less clear. Fetal echocardiography may be reserved for nonimmune causes of hydrops. Magnetic resonance imaging may prove useful for investigating brain abnormalities resulting from infectious causes such as congenital parvovirus B19 infection, but its use has been limited to cases of nonimmune hydrops.[19]

**Laboratory Testing:** Maternal Rh typing and antibody screening are typically performed in the first trimester, but should be repeated if sonographic evidence of hydrops develops. Although a woman may demonstrate Rh(D) positivity and have a negative first trimester antibody screen, she may acquire atypical blood-group antibodies or become alloimmunized during gestation (following packed red blood cell or platelet transfusion, for example).[20] Antibody titers may vary slightly among different laboratories, but most consider titers greater than 1:16 potentially causative of severe fetal anemia. When a maternal antibody screen is positive for non-Kell antibodies and the titer

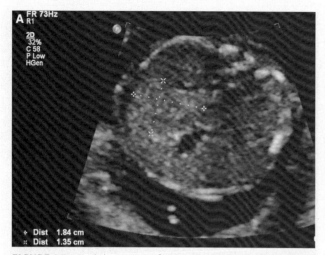
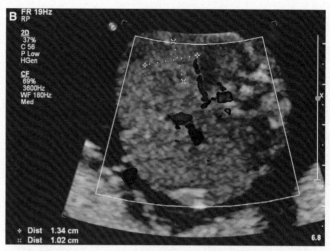

**FIGURE 22.1-7:** Splenic circumference. **A:** Axial view of the fetal abdomen at the standard level for abdominal circumference measurement. Splenic circumference (millimeters) = (length + width) × 1.57. **B:** Color Doppler identifying the splenic artery can aid in location of the spleen.

is at or below 1:16, titers are repeated monthly. Maternal Kell antibody titers are not correlative with risk for fetal anemia.[14]

To determine the likelihood of fetal expression of the suspected antigen, paternal zygosity may be accurately determined by quantitative polymerase chain reaction for the RHD gene or by serology for the other blood-group antigens with a nondominant allele such as the "k" of the (K1) Kell gene.[21] Paternal homozygosity essentially confers a 100% likelihood that the fetus is a carrier of the putative blood-group antigen. However, paternal heterozygosity equates to a 50% risk, and determination of fetal antigen status is required. Cell-free fetal DNA testing is now available in the United States such that the exons of the RHD gene are detected with a sensitivity of 97.2% and a specificity of 96.8%.[22] This technology has proven reliable for predicting fetal K, C, c, and E phenotypes as well, and these methods are now being used routinely in the United Kingdom but not in the United States.[23]

Invasive techniques have historically been required to confirm fetal antigen status and quantify anemia as the cause of hydrops fetalis. Amniocentesis accurately determines fetal Rh(D) status with a sensitivity of 98.7% and a specificity of 100%, and it is equally reliable for identifying dominant and nondominant alleles of the other blood-group antigens.[24] Amniocentesis for spectrophotometric analysis of amniotic fluid bilirubin levels was first described by Bevis[25] and then

further characterized by Liley[26] and Queenan et al.[27] The shift in optical density of amniotic fluid at a wavelength of 450 nm ($\Delta OD_{450}$) correlates with the concentration of bilirubin and provides an indirect measure of fetal hemolysis. Liley was first to plot $\Delta OD_{450}$ values as three "zones" of anemia severity according to gestational age (weeks 27 through 42). Queenan and colleagues[27] extrapolated this concept to earlier gestational ages and additional zones in a study of 789 amniotic fluid samples with improved sensitivity and specificity (Fig. 22.1-9). Serial amniotic fluid assessments demonstrating elevation to the IUT zone on the Queenan curve or the 80th percentile of Zone 2 on the Liley curve suggest severe anemia and warranted premature delivery or attempts at fetal intraperitoneal transfusion. Unfortunately, nonhemolytic anemia, as in Kell-mediated erythropoiesis inhibition, was not identifiable with this method. The 1980s witnessed the advent of fetoscopic and ultrasound-guided umbilical vein needle sampling (also called PUBS—percutaneous umbilical blood sampling, cordocentesis, or funipuncture), which allowed for direct measurement of the fetal serum bilirubin concentration and hematocrit.[28] An umbilical venous total bilirubin concentration greater than 3 mg per dL and a hematocrit less than 30% denote severe anemia, warranting potential IUT. This procedure is successful in more than 95% of cases and applicable to all causes of anemia, but is not employed on a routine basis owing to the associated

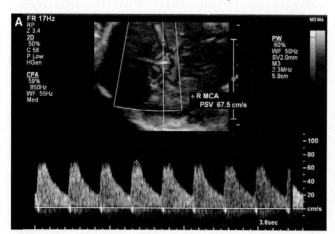
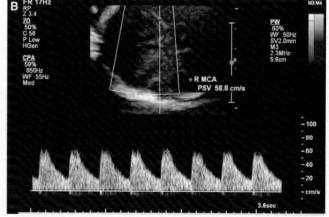

**FIGURE 22.1-8:** Doppler imaging of the middle cerebral artery. **A:** Transverse view of the fetal head shows Doppler sampling and peak systolic velocity measurement of the middle cerebral artery with the correct angle of insonation. **B:** Note the change in the measured value with too large an angle of insonation.

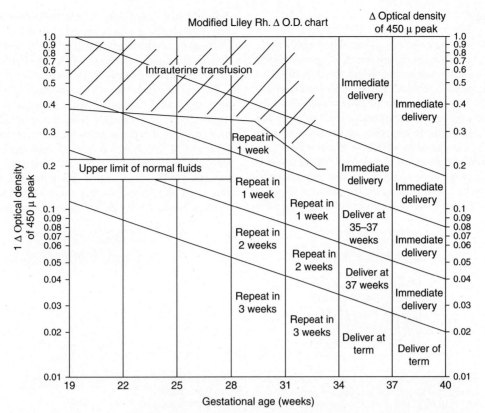

**FIGURE 22.1-9:** Normal Liley curves. Modification of Liley $\Delta OD_{450}$ reading zone boundaries before 24 weeks' gestation is the same as the zone boundary angle of inclination after 24 weeks' gestation. (From Ulreich S, Gruslin A, Nodell CG, et al. Fetal hydrops and ascites. In: Nyberg DA, McGahan JP, Pretorius DH, et al, eds. *Diagnostic Imaging of Fetal Anomalies*. Philadelphia, PA: Lippincott Williams & Wilkins; 2003:713–744.)

1% to 2% fetal loss rate and potential for worsened fetomaternal hemorrhage.[29]

Additional diagnostic tools may be employed for situations where the cause of hydrops fetalis is less clear. Fetal karyotype and microarray analysis are generally not required for cases of hydrops in the setting of a positive maternal indirect Coombs test unless concern exists for additional fetal abnormalities. Maternal and paternal serologies in combination with two-dimensional and Doppler sonography comprise the standard tools for diagnosis of immune hydrops.

## DIFFERENTIAL DIAGNOSIS

If excess fluid is identified in only one fetal compartment, organ-specific causes of fluid accumulation such as cardiomyopathy or thoracic duct abnormalities should be considered. Aneuploidies, skeletal dysplasias, and certain fetal structural anomalies may result in true fetal hydrops, and these should be considered even in the presence of a maternal antibody known to cause HDFN. Initial assessment should also include Doppler evaluation of the middle cerebral artery peak systolic velocity. If this velocity is found to be normal, additional anatomic abnormalities are identified, or maternal indirect Coombs testing is negative, one should consider nonimmune causes of hydrops as described later in this chapter.

## PROGNOSIS

The finding of immune hydrops signifies progression of the pathophysiologic processes involved in fetal alloimmune anemia toward the near-fatal stages. If left uncorrected, the prognosis is invariably fatal for the fetus or neonate. Intrauterine fetal transfusion provides an effective therapy temporarily correcting the anemia and potentially reversing the hydrops. This benefit was demonstrated in a large retrospective cohort study from the national referral center for management of fetal anemia in the Netherlands.[30] Of 210 fetuses with alloimmune anemia, 80 (36%) were hydropic and underwent intrauterine fetal transfusion with a survival rate of 78%. Logistic regression revealed that survival was decreased among cases where the first transfusion occurred prior to 20 weeks (55%), among cases in which the hydrops was not reversed (55%), and among cases of Kell-alloimmunization (60%). A meta-analysis of 19 publications demonstrated a similar rate of survival (74%) among hydropic fetuses following IUT.[31]

Concern exists for the long-term neurodevelopmental outcomes of fetuses that have successfully undergone treatment for immune hydrops. Anemia may lead to hypoxemia and hyperbilirubinemia that potentially impairs critical brain development. However, a report on 18 consecutively treated hydropic fetuses revealed that physical and neurologic outcomes were similar in comparison with their unaffected siblings for most immune hydrops survivors (13 of 16 children; 81%) at a mean age of 10 years.[32] A large national cohort study of 291 survivors of immune hydrops evaluated at a median age of 8.2 years revealed rates of cerebral palsy of 2.1%, severe developmental delay of 3.1%, bilateral deafness of 1.0%, and overall neurodevelopmental impairment of 4.8%.[33] Thus, the risk of neurodevelopmental impairment among survivors of intrauterine transfusion IUT for fetal alloimmune anemia appears low.

## MANAGEMENT

Management begins with prevention against alloimmunization. Although the exact mechanism is unknown, exogenous RhIg reduces the risk of alloimmunization to the Rh(D) antigen to 0.1% to 0.2% when given at 28 weeks' gestation and again within 72 hours of delivery.[34] Once bound to the RhD sites on red cells, the RhIg can bind to the IgG Fc receptors on macrophages and natural killer cells, resulting in clearance of the RhD-positive red cells from circulation prior to activation of memory B lymphocytes.[35] The standard intramuscular dose of 300 μg protects against 30 mL of fetal blood or 15 mL of packed fetal red cells, but a Kleihauer-Betke test can quantify the amount of fetal-maternal hemorrhage to further guide dosing of RhIg. Since it is

derived from pooled donors' sera, the potential to transmit hepatitis C infection has been reported in a case report.[36] The cold alcohol fractionation used in isolating the antibodies appears to destroy the human immunodeficiency virus such that the possibility for transmission of HIV is considered nonexistent.

Differentiation between immune hydrops and other nonimmunologic fetal conditions relies on an algorithmic approach beginning with a detailed fetal sonographic assessment and maternal blood type assessment and indirect Coombs testing (Fig. 22.1-10). Confirmed cases of immune hydrops should be assessed for maternal transport to a tertiary care center with expertise in management of this potentially critical situation. The team should include experienced perinatologists, sonographers, blood bank personnel, neonatologists, and anesthesia

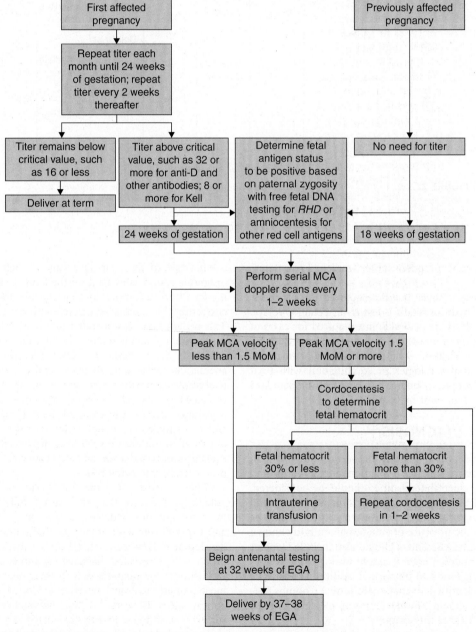

**FIGURE 22.1-10:** Algorithm for clinical management of red cell alloimmunization. MCA, middle cerebral artery; MoM, multiples of the median; EGA, estimated gestational age. (From Moise KJ Jr, Argoti PS. Management and prevention of red cell alloimmunization in pregnancy: a systematic review. *Obstet Gynecol.* 2012;120:1132–1139.)

and nursing staff. If the gestational age lies between 24 and 34 weeks, maternal administration of an antenatal course of corticosteroids is advised. Preparations for PUBS are undertaken, including the early notification of the blood bank and collection of a maternal blood sample for typing, antibody determination, and preparation of appropriate blood for fetal transfusion. This blood should be irradiated group O negative red cells packed to a hematocrit of at least 75% and negative for Kell, CMV, and the putative antigen. If the fetal blood type is known from a prior PUBS and there is no maternal ABO incompatibility, red cells of the same ABO status of the fetus may be used for transfusion. A detailed ultrasound should be performed to evaluate the severity of the hydrops, the estimated fetal weight, and the target for fetal intravascular sampling and transfusion.

In 1963, prior to the technologic advancement of sonography, Liley[37] introduced the concept of intrauterine transfusion and ushered in the age of fetal therapeutics. The technique involved intraperitoneal transfusion (IPT) of packed red cells to allow for lymphatic and venous absorption into the anemic fetus, and this remained the standard approach until the method of direct intravascular access (IVT) under fetoscopic and sonographic guidance was introduced in the mid-1980s.[28] Direct comparison of these two techniques revealed a 13% increased survival rate for nonhydropic fetuses undergoing IVT in comparison with those undergoing IPT; the survival advantage was nearly 2-fold among hydropic fetuses.[38] The lymphovascular congestion and distortion of the portal and hepatic venous architecture associated with fetal hydrops likely prohibit timely absorption of transfused packed red cells from the peritoneal cavity. Thus, the intravascular approach is preferred, and the placental insertion of the umbilical vein often offers the most reliable intravascular access with minimal risk for fetal bradycardia (approximately 3%).[29] Free floating and periumbilical portions of the cord can be more challenging to puncture (often requiring fetal paralysis), and have demonstrated higher rates of fetal bradycardia.[29] If the placental insertion site is not accessible, one may safely attempt to access the intrahepatic portion of the umbilical vein with similar low likelihood of fetal bradycardia.[39]

Once the access site has been determined, a sedative or regional neuraxial anesthesia is administered to the mother. A neuromuscular blocker may also be directly injected into the fetal circulation. An operating room is prepared for both the procedure and for possible emergent cesarean delivery of the viable fetus should severe complications arise. The appropriate blood for transfusion should be available in the operating room, and the hematology laboratory should be immediately available to quickly analyze and report results of the fetal blood samples. A broad-spectrum cephalosporin with coverage against gram-positive skin flora can be given as prophylaxis. The patient's abdomen is then prepared for surgery, and sterile technique is used while a 20- or 22-gauge spinal needle is advanced through the maternal abdomen into the fetal umbilical vein under direct ultrasound guidance (Fig. 22.1-11). Free return of blood confirms venous entry, and a 1- or 2-mL sample should be drawn into a heparinized tuberculin syringe for immediate analysis of hematocrit, hemoglobin, and mean corpuscular volume (values greater than 110 $\mu m^3$ confirm the source as fetal). Fetal blood should also be measured for platelet count, total bilirubin concentration, blood type, antibody screen, and reticulocyte count. Given that the hematocrit is less than 30% in most cases of immune hydrops, the fetal transfusion can be started while awaiting results from the laboratory.

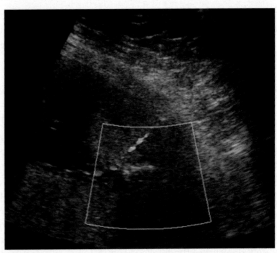

**FIGURE 22.1-11:** Percutaneous umbilical blood sampling. Color Doppler scan demonstrating aspiration of fetal blood from the umbilical vein at the placental cord insertion site with a 20-gauge spinal needle.

Calculation of the total volume to transfuse relies on determination of the estimated fetal weight, the correction factor for the volume of blood in the fetoplacental circulation, the initial fetal hematocrit, the hematocrit of the transfused blood, and the target hematocrit. The following formula is commonly used for determining the total milliliters of transfusion volume ($V_T$):

$$V_T = \frac{V_{(fetoplacental)} \times (\text{Target fetal hematocrit} - \text{Initial fetal hematocrit})}{\text{Hematocrit of transfused blood}}$$

where $V_{(fetoplacental)}$ (mL) is calculated by multiplying the estimated fetal weight in grams by 0.14. The target fetal hematocrit should approximate the physiologic fetal value (45% to 50%), but should not increase 25% above the initial fetal hematocrit, owing to concerns for fluid overload and intrauterine fetal demise.[40] In general, initial fetal hematocrit values less than 30% warrant IVT. Severely anemic fetuses with hematocrits below 10% should potentially undergo a two-step IVT with the initial goal of achieving a hematocrit of 25% to 30% followed by a second transfusion 48 to 72 hours later to achieve a final hematocrit of 45% to 50%. Another option for severe anemia is to perform a combined intravascular and intraperitoneal transfusion, where the IVT is performed to reach a hematocrit of 35% to 40%.[41] The needle is then inserted into the fetal peritoneal cavity, where a portion of the ascites can be aspirated and replaced with a volume (mL) of packed red cells determined by Bowman's formula, subtracting 20 from the gestational age in weeks and multiplying the result by 10.[42] This method has been shown to provide a more stable fetal hematocrit declining only 0.01% per day rather than the 1% per day with IVT alone.[43]

Timing of subsequent transfusions depends on the final hematocrit achieved and whether a combined approach or IVT alone was performed. Additionally, weekly measurement of the peak systolic velocity of the middle cerebral artery can help time subsequent transfusions. Values greater than 1.32 MoM demonstrate 100% sensitivity and 63% specificity in predicting reoccurrence of moderate anemia and warrant repeat IUT.[44] Fetal surveillance with twice weekly biophysical profiles, including non stress test, should be instituted until delivery. The last transfusion is typically performed around 35 weeks' gestation with planned delivery near 37 weeks. The false positive rate of middle cerebral artery peak systolic velocity measurement increases after 35 weeks, but its sensitivity remains excellent and may convey reassurance against moderate to severe anemia until delivery.[45]

## RECURRENCE RISK

The recurrence risk for immune hydrops is substantial and dependent upon the gestational age and severity of the first alloimmunized pregnancy. Among women with a history of a prior perinatal loss attributable to HDFN, prior need for IUT, or delivery of an infant requiring neonatal exchange transfusion, maternal titers are not reliable in predicting HDFN in subsequent pregnancies. Paternal homozygosity for the responsible antigen confers a 100% risk for recurrence, whereas heterozygosity equates to a 50% risk. Preimplantation genetic diagnosis can accurately determine the fetal antigen status in situations of paternal heterozygosity, but this is costly and requires in vitro fertilization.[46] Cell-free fetal DNA analysis can accurately determine the fetal antigen status beginning around 10 weeks of gestation, and can determine the need to initiate surveillance at 18 weeks with serial Doppler evaluation of the middle cerebral artery.

## REFERENCES

1. Moise KJ Jr. Hemolytic disease of the fetus and newborn. In: Creasy RK, Resnik R, eds. *Maternal-Fetal Medicine.* 6th ed. Philadelphia, PA: Saunders Elsevier; 2009:191–207.
2. Zipursky A, Paul VK. The global burden of Rh disease. *Arch Dis Child Fetal Neonatal Ed.* 2011;96(2):F84–F85.
3. Bhutani VK, Zipursky A, Blencowe H, et al. Neonatal hyperbilirubinemia and Rhesus disease of the newborn: incidence and impairment estimates for 2010 at regional and global levels. *Pediatr Res.* 2013;74(suppl 1):86–100.
4. Garratty G, Glynn SA, McEntire R. ABO and Rh(D) phenotype frequencies of different racial/ethnic groups in the United States. *Transfusion.* 2004;44(5):703–706.
5. Martin JA, Hamilton BE, Sutton PD, et al. Births: final data for 2008. *Natl Vital Stat Rep.* 2010;59(1):1–71.
6. Koelewijn JM, Vrijkotte TG, van der Schoot CE, et al. Effect of screening for red cell antibodies, other than anti-D, to detect hemolytic disease of the fetus and newborn: a population study in the Netherlands. *Transfusion.* 2008;48(5):941–952.
7. Levine P, Stetson RE. An unusual case of intragroup agglutination. *JAMA.* 1939;113:126–127.
8. Fisher RA, Race RR. Rh gene frequencies in Britain. *Nature.* 1946;157:48.
9. Avent ND, Reid ME. The Rh blood group system: a review. *Blood.* 2000;95(2):375–387.
10. Nevanlinna HR. ABO protection in Rh immunization. *Ann Med Exp Biol Fenn.* 1966;44(2):318–321.
11. Moya FR, Grannum PA, Widness JA, et al. Erythropoietin in human fetuses with immune hemolytic anemia and hydrops fetalis. *Obstet Gynecol.* 1993;82(3):353–358.
12. Ville Y, Sideris I, Hecher K, et al. Umbilical venous pressure in normal, growth-retarded, and anemic fetuses. *Am J Obstet Gynecol.* 1994;170(2):487–494.
13. Ville Y, Proudler A, Kuhn P, et al. Aldosterone concentration in normal, growth-retarded, anemic, and hydropic fetuses. *Obstet Gynecol.* 1994;84(4):511–514.
14. Vaughan JI, Manning M, Warwick RM, et al. Inhibition of erythroid progenitor cells by anti-Kell antibodies in fetal alloimmune anemia. *N Engl J Med.* 1998;338(12):798–803.
15. Chitkara U, Wilkins I, Lynch L, et al. The role of sonography in assessing severity of fetal anemia in Rh- and Kell-isoimmunized pregnancies. *Obstet Gynecol.* 1988;71(3, pt 1):393–398.
16. Nicolaides KH, Fontanarosa M, Gabbe SG, et al. Failure of ultrasonographic parameters to predict the severity of fetal anemia in rhesus isoimmunization. *Am J Obstet Gynecol.* 1988;158(4):920–926.
17. Bahado-Singh R, Oz U, Mari G, et al. Fetal splenic size in anemia due to Rh-alloimmunization. *Obstet Gynecol.* 1998;92(5):828–832.
18. Mari G, Deter RL, Carpenter RL, et al. Noninvasive diagnosis by Doppler ultrasonography of fetal anemia due to maternal red-cell alloimmunization. *N Engl J Med.* 2000;342(1):9–14.
19. Courtier J, Schauer GM, Parer JT, et al. Polymicrogyria in a fetus with human parvovirus B19 infection: a case with radiologic-pathologic correlation. *Ultrasound Obstet Gynecol.* 2012;40(5):604–606.
20. Yun JW, Kang ES, Ki CS, et al. Sensitization to multiple rh antigens by transfusion of random donor platelet concentrates in a -D- phenotype patient. *Ann Lab Med.* 2012;32(6):429–432.
21. Pirelli KJ, Pietz BC, Johnson ST, et al. Molecular determination of RHD zygosity: predicting risk of hemolytic disease of the fetus and newborn related to anti-D. *Prenat Diagn.* 2010;30(12–13):1207–1212.
22. Bombard AT, Akolekar R, Farkas DH, et al. Fetal RHD genotype detection from circulating cell-free fetal DNA in maternal plasma in non-sensitized RhD negative women. *Prenat Diagn.* 2011;31(8):802–808.
23. Finning K, Martin P, Summers J, et al. Fetal genotyping for the K (Kell) and Rh C, c, and E blood groups on cell-free fetal DNA in maternal plasma. *Transfusion.* 2007;47(11):2126–2133.
24. Van den Veyver IB, Moise KJ Jr. Fetal RhD typing by polymerase chain reaction in pregnancies complicated by rhesus alloimmunization. *Obstet Gynecol.* 1996;88:1061–1067.
25. Bevis DC. Blood pigments in haemolytic disease of the newborn. *J Obstet Gynaecol Br Emp.* 1956;63(1):68–75.
26. Liley AW. Liquor amnii analysis in the management of the pregnancy complicated by rhesus sensitization. *Am J Obstet Gynecol.* 1961;82:1359–1370.
27. Queenan JT, Tomai TP, Ural SH, et al. Deviation in amniotic fluid optical density at a wavelength of 450 nm in Rh immunized pregnancies from 14 to 40 weeks' gestation: a proposal for clinical management. *Am J Obstet Gynecol.* 1993;168(5):1370–1376.
28. Rodeck CH, Holman CA, Karnicki J, et al. Direct intravascular fetal blood transfusion by fetoscopy in severe rhesus isoimmunization. *Lancet.* 1981;1(8221):625–627.
29. Weiner CP, Wenstrom KD, Sipes SL, et al. Risk factors for cordocentesis and fetal intravascular transfusion. *Am J Obstet Gynecol.* 1991;165:1020–1025.
30. van Kamp IL, Klumper FJ, Meerman RH, et al. Treatment of fetal anemia due to red-cell alloimmunization with intrauterine transfusions in the Netherlands, 1988–1999. *Acta Obstet Gynecol Scand.* 2004;83(8):731–737.
31. Schumacher B, Moise KJ Jr. Fetal transfusion for red blood cell alloimmunization in pregnancy. *Obstet Gynecol.* 1996;88(1):137–150.
32. Harper DC, Swingle HM, Weiner CP, et al. Long-term neurodevelopmental outcome and brain volume after treatment for hydrops fetalis by in utero intravascular transfusion. *Am J Obstet Gynecol.* 2006;195(1):192–200.
33. Lindenburg IT, Smits-Wintjens VE, van Klink JM, et al; for the LOTUS Study Group. Long-term neurodevelopmental outcome after intrauterine transfusion for hemolytic disease of the fetus/newborn: the LOTUS study. *Am J Obstet Gynecol.* 2012;206(2):141.e1–141.e8.
34. Bowman JM. The prevention of Rh immunization. *Transfus Med Rev.* 1988;2(3):129.
35. Siberil S, de Romeuf C, Bihoreau N, et al. Selection of human anti-RhD monoclonal antibody for therapeutic use: impact of IgG glycosylation on activating and inhibitory Fc gamma R functions. *Clin Immunol.* 2006;118(2–3):170–179.
36. Power JP, Lawlor E, Davidson F, et al. Molecular epidemiology of an outbreak of infection with hepatitis C virus in recipients of anti-D immunoglobulin. *Lancet.* 1995;345(8959):1211–1213.
37. Liley AW. Intrauterine transfusion of foetus in haemolytic disease. *Br Med J.* 1963;2(5365):1107–1109.
38. Harman CR, Bowman JM, Manning FA, et al. Intrauterine transfusion—intraperitoneal versus intravascular approach: a case-control comparison. *Am J Obstet Gynecol.* 1990;162(4):1053–1059.
39. Nicolini U, Santolaya J, Ojo OE, et al. The fetal intrahepatic umbilical vein as an alternative to cord needling for prenatal diagnosis and therapy. *Prenat Diagn.* 1988;8(9):665–671.
40. Radunovic N, Lockwood CJ, Alvarez M, et al. The severely anemic and hydropic isoimmune fetus: changes in fetal hematocrit associated with intrauterine death. *Obstet Gynecol.* 1992;79(3):390–393.
41. Moise KJ Jr, Carpenter RJ Jr, Kirshon B, et al. Comparison of four types of intrauterine transfusion: effect on fetal hematocrit. *Fetal Ther.* 1989;4(2–3):126–137.
42. Bowman JM. The management of Rh-isoimmunization. *Obstet Gynecol.* 1978;52:1–16.
43. Moise KJ Jr, Argoti PS. Management and prevention of red cell alloimmunization in pregnancy: a systematic review. *Obstet Gynecol.* 2012;120(5):1132–1139.
44. Detti L, Oz U, Guney I, et al; for the Collaborative Group for Doppler Assessment of Blood Velocity in Anemic Fetuses. Doppler ultrasound velocimetry for timing the second intrauterine transfusion in fetuses with anemia from red cell alloimmunization. *Am J Obstet Gynecol.* 2001;185(5):1048–1051.
45. Zimmerman R, Carpenter RJ Jr, Durig P, et al. Longitudinal measurement of peak systolic velocity in the fetal middle cerebral artery for monitoring pregnancies complicated by red cell alloimmunisation: a prospective multicentre trial with intention-to-treat. *BJOG.* 2002;109(7):746–752.
46. Van den Veyver IB, Chong SS, Cota J, et al. Single-cell analysis of the RhD blood type for use in preimplantation diagnosis in the prevention of severe hemolytic disease of the newborn. *Am J Obstet Gynecol.* 1995;172:533–540.

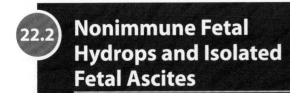

# 22.2 Nonimmune Fetal Hydrops and Isolated Fetal Ascites

Eva I. Rubio

Fetal hydrops refers to abnormal fluid accumulation in two or more spaces in the developing fetus. The finding occurs when there is an imbalance between the production and resorption of interstitial fluid, with the excess fluid filling interstitial spaces of the fetal skin, pleural or pericardial spaces, or peritoneal cavity. The individual entities of pleural and pericardial effusions, and in particular ascites, seen in isolation without progression to frank hydrops often indicate specific disease processes and warrant a more targeted evaluation. The fetus with true hydrops is at high risk for intrauterine demise or significant postnatal morbidity and mortality, and a thorough search for an underlying etiology should be sought, with appropriate maternal counseling. Detailed prenatal ultrasound with Doppler evaluation is a fundamental tool in the evaluation of the hydropic fetus, with fetal MRI employed for specific investigations.

The distinction between nonimmune hydrops and immune hydrops was first made in 1943 by Edith Potter.[1] At that time in the mid-20th century, nonimmune hydrops was comparatively uncommon, representing less than a quarter of all infants born with fetal hydrops. Today, in developed countries, owing to successful prophylactic Rh immunization, nonimmune hydrops represents approximately 90% of all cases of fetal hydrops.[2,3]

The underlying causes of nonimmune hydrops are myriad, and include cardiac disease, infection, abdominal or thoracic lesions, chromosomal abnormalities, metabolic disorders, neurologic disorders, urinary tract anomalies, and placental tumors.[3]

## NONIMMUNE FETAL HYDROPS

### Incidence

The prevalence of nonimmune hydrops remains at approximately 1 in 2,000 to 3,000 pregnancies.[3,4]

### Pathogenesis

Nonimmune hydrops fetalis (NIHF) may be considered an end-stage manifestation of any one of a growing list of fetal etiologies.[5,6] Despite the increasing availability of diagnostic tests for specific causes, approximately 18% remain categorized as idiopathic.[6] Even in cases where a compelling primary diagnosis is identified, the exact mechanism causing hydrops may not be clear.[5]

In normal physiology, fluid is released into the interstitial space by the capillary circulation and is returned to the vascular space by lymphatic vessels and reabsorbed via capillaries. The pathophysiologic mechanisms leading to hydrops result in either increase in fluid production or obstruction to normal return. The fetus is at high risk for hydrops, given that the body has higher water content (90% to 95% at 8 weeks decreasing to 70% at term) and also a highly compliant interstitial compartment, great capillary permeability, and a lymphatic return that is strongly influenced by central venous pressure.[2] Underlying pathophysiology may be organized into the following categories. However, in reality, these mechanisms often occur together in a cascade of systemic failure (Fig. 22.2-1).[3,5,6]

**Increase in Capillary Pressure** is among the most common mechanisms. Pressure can rise in the capillary bed when there is increased central venous pressure, increased arterial pressure, or obstruction in venous drainage.[3] Increased fetal central venous pressure may result from cardiac failure or thoracic mass effect. Cardiac failure may be primary (arrhythmias, structural defects, viral or autoimmune myocarditis) or secondary, resulting from high-output conditions (twin-twin transfusion syndrome, anemia, vascular malformations, and high-flow tumors). The subsequent impedance of lymphatic flow occurring with venous hypertension also results in accumulation of fluid in the highly compliant fetal interstitial space.[6]

**Increased Capillary Membrane Permeability** is the result of injury to the capillary endothelium, allowing efflux of plasma proteins from the vascular space into the interstitial tissues. The fluid follows the proteins into the interstitium because of a reverse in the osmotic pressure gradient, being higher in the protein-filled interstitium than vasculature. The injury may result from hypoxia or inflammatory mediators and endotoxins in the setting of infection.[3]

**Diminished Plasma Oncotic Pressure** occurs when large intravascular molecules, such as albumin, are decreased. In their absence in the plasma, the intravascular osmotic pressure is decreased, causing loss of fluid to the interstitial space. Most hypoproteinemic states indicate a degree of liver impairment or, less commonly, renal disease that results in loss of protein in the urine. Organ damage resulting from infection, hepatic congestion, or hypoxic injury leads to an overall reduction in plasma albumin levels.[3,6]

**Impedance of Lymphatic Flow** may occur via several mechanisms. Lymph vessels are made of smooth muscle with one-way valves which contract when filled. However, other important factors for lymph flow include body and limb movement, skeletal muscle contraction, arterial pulsations, and tissue compression. The lymph flow may be impaired due to intrinsic lymphatic aberrations, decreased activity in a fetus with severe musculoskeletal or central nervous system abnormalities, or intrathoracic/cardiac abnormalities characterized by increased central venous pressure.[3]

### Diagnosis

In many cases, the cause of NIHF is not readily apparent. A thorough assessment of family history and ethnic background in conjunction with detailed imaging and, often, more invasive diagnostic testing will be necessary to explore all possible diagnostic entities.

Stepwise evaluation of a pregnancy affected by hydrops fetalis begins with exclusion of Rh incompatibility. Once this has been ruled out, the degree of invasiveness of further maternal and fetal testing is at the discretion of the mother. A complete anatomic survey is warranted to identify any structural abnormalities. Maternal minimally invasive investigations include serum testing for viral exposures, metabolic disorders, and anemia, as well as for the presence of fetal genetic material consistent with aneuploidies. Other conditions, including fetal thalassemia, metabolic and single gene disorders, and aneuploidy will require amniocentesis or fetal blood sampling for diagnosis.

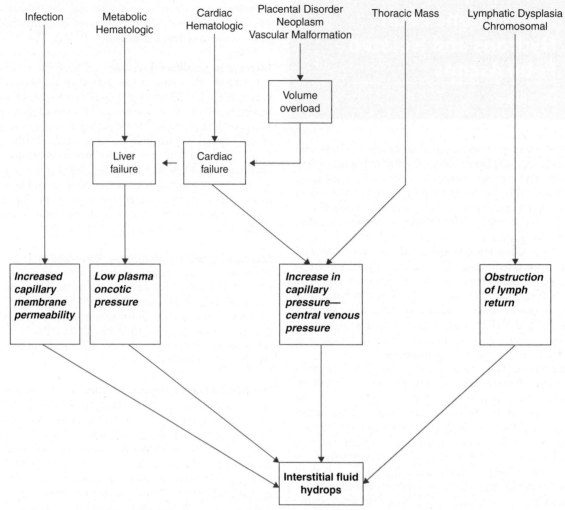

**FIGURE 22.2-1:** Etiologies and mechanisms for hydrops. (Adapted from Bellini C, Hennekam RC. Etiology of nonimmune hydrops fetalis: a systematic review. *Am J Med Genet A.* 2009;149A:844–851.)

**Imaging:** Initial presentation in a pregnancy with hydrops may include decreased fetal movements, polyhydramnios, and maternal preeclampsia. Confirmation of hydrops is generally accepted as the presence of excess fluid in two or more compartments of the fetal body, with the skin counted as one of the compartments. On US or MRI, there may be skin thickening of more than 5 mm, more than 3 mm of pericardial fluid, pleural fluid, ascites, and often placental enlargement of greater than 5 or 6 cm (Fig. 22.2-2). In most cases, the pattern of the hydropic findings offers few, if any, clues to the diagnosis. A detailed and systematic approach to the fetal anatomic survey is helpful and may reveal an etiology. In complex cases, especially when there is concern for a mass, syndrome, or intracranial abnormality, fetal MRI may be helpful.

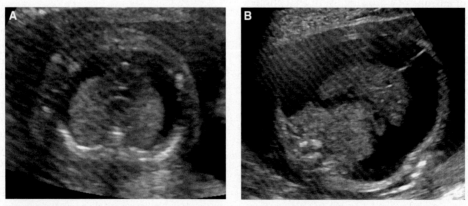

**FIGURE 22.2-2:** A 21-week fetus with hydrops of unknown etiology. **A:** Axial view of the lower chest demonstrates collapsed echogenic lungs, pleural effusions, and skin edema. **B:** Axial view of the abdomen demonstrates large ascites surrounding the liver and collapsed, centralized bowel.

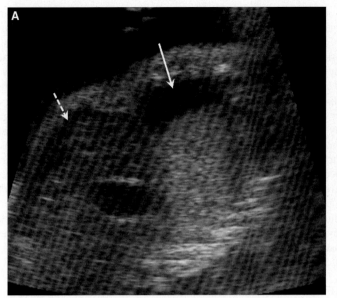
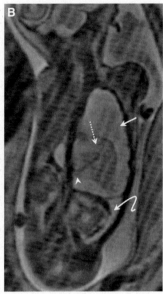

**FIGURE 22.2-3:** Hybrid sequestration and hydrops in a fetus at 31 weeks. **A:** Sagittal ultrasound of chest and abdomen shows large pleural effusion *(solid arrow)* and small ascites *(dotted arrow)*. The fetus also had skin edema and presented with polyhydramnios. **B:** Coronal MRI of the fetal chest demonstrates a complex lung lesion *(dotted arrow)* with feeding vessel *(arrowhead)*. Note large pleural effusion *(solid arrow)* and small ascites *(curved arrow)*.

Pleural effusions may be small or large, and the mass effect of large pleural effusions may place the fetus at risk for pulmonary hypoplasia. Thoracic lesions such as sequestrations and congenital pulmonary airway malformations should be considered. Fetal MRI can be helpful in excluding underlying thoracic lesions as the inciting cause (Fig. 22.2-3). Occasionally, a congenital diaphragmatic hernia will be associated with a pleural effusion. Chylothorax may be unilateral or bilateral.

Ascites may be subtle and in early stages only well seen around the liver. Massive ascites may likewise contribute to impaired lung development owing to upward mass effect on the diaphragm. Fluid complexity and the presence of calcifications may offer clues to the diagnosis. Genitourinary tract obstructive processes with rupture may yield massive urinary ascites; attention to the kidneys and bladder wall thickness is imperative.

Skin thickening will often be present in the nuchal and scalp area prior to visualization of thoracic or abdominal wall edema. Anasarca is best reserved for diffuse skin thickening without septations, and often progresses in a cephalocaudal direction. It may herald impending hydrops and should be followed closely once identified.

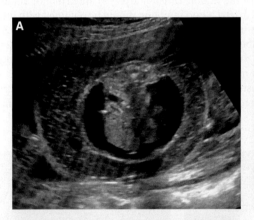
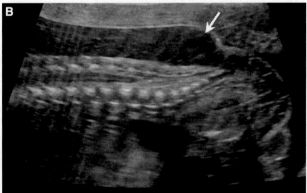
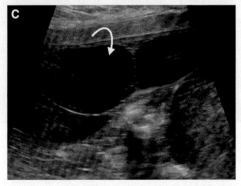

**FIGURE 22.2-4:** Turner syndrome, 23-week fetus. **A:** Axial view, thorax. Skin edema and large bilateral effusions. **B:** Sagittal image shows skin edema *(solid arrow)* filling the amniotic cavity. **C:** Cystic hygroma may easily be mistaken for amniotic fluid *(curved arrow)*.

Severe hydrops and large cystic hygromas may be mistaken for amniotic fluid (Fig. 22.2-4). Obliquity in the plane of imaging can create a spuriously thickened appearance of normal fetal skin. In cases of arthrogryposis and other musculoskeletal disorders, fatty replacement of the fetal musculature may create a featureless and redundant appearance of the skin and soft tissues.

The findings of polyhydramnios, oligohydramnios, and placental edema are also worth noting. Although they are not considered among the criteria defining hydrops, they may have a clear correlation with the underlying disease process. Polyhydramnios is associated with maternal morbidity, including postpartum hemorrhage and retained products of conception.[5]

Doppler is essential in a fetus with NIHF. Careful interrogation of the middle cerebral artery for elevated peak systolic velocity may indicate fetal anemia. Abnormal ductus venous or umbilical venous waveforms often suggest elevated venous pressure and/or cardiac dysfunction. Loss of diastolic flow in the umbilical artery reflects high placental resistance and/or increased cardiac afterload.

Because a significant percentage of cases of NIHF stem from a cardiac cause, a fetal echocardiogram with complete assessment of cardiac structure, contractility, and rhythm is imperative. Attention to M-mode is essential to evaluate for subtle arrhythmias. The presence of a pericardial effusion may suggest an underlying cardiac abnormality.[5]

## Prognosis

While it is true that fetal prognosis in the setting of hydrops fetalis remains poor, one should bear in mind that this generalization may not apply to certain specific etiologies (Fig. 22.2-5). The overall mortality of NIHF is variably reported between 70% and 90%.[7] Approximately 50% of cases diagnosed in utero will end in fetal demise, and of those live-born, 50% will not survive the neonatal period.[3,8] Fetuses presenting earlier in pregnancy (<20 weeks) are much more likely to have an underlying chromosomal disorder, and these cases are uniformly fatal.[7] In contrast, fetuses with conditions amenable to intrauterine therapy may have a much better prognosis. These include anemia resulting from alpha thalassemia, infection (especially parvovirus), drainable cystic lesions or fluid collections, and cardiac arrhythmias correctable via intravascular or intraperitoneal therapy.[7,8] These observations are supported by postnatal studies that also

describe a much higher mortality rate (57.7%) among hydropic newborns with congenital anomalies as compared with a mortality rate of 5.9% among newborns presenting with isolated, treatable abnormalities such as congenital chylothorax.[9]

Allowing for maternal preferences, discovery of NIHF mandates a thorough search for an etiology. Currently available testing strategies may be successful in identifying a cause in 80% to 90% of cases with the most common etiologies for NIHF in the literature being aneuploidies, infection, cardiovascular and thoracic disorders.[7,8,10] The etiology of hydrops is an essential consideration in determining the prognosis in an individual case and can provide meaningful guidance to the family for current and future pregnancies. It is interesting, though, that despite postnatal workup, as high as 68% of prenatal idiopathic NIHF cases remain undiagnosed.[8] Of those surviving NIFH, approximately 61% will have normal development.[8]

## Management

Decisions about management of a pregnancy complicated by NIHF depend directly upon determination of the underlying cause, which should ultimately be defined in 80% to 90% of cases.[7,10] Therefore, prompt initiation of an organized search for a diagnosis is crucial. A detailed maternal history and physical exam are indicated. Investigations often proceed from noninvasive to increasingly invasive to minimize risk. Much information can be gathered via noninvasive methods, which include comprehensive US with Doppler, maternal serum testing for an ever-increasing array of disorders, fetal echocardiogram, and fetal MRI as indicated. Further investigation with amniocentesis for karyotype and possible genetic microarray molecular testing may be necessary. Referral to a geneticist may help guide management and therapy and direct further enzymatic testing for metabolic abnormalities. In women at risk for infection or blood dyscrasias, other directed laboratory testing may be performed. If the Doppler of the middle cerebral artery is abnormal or anemia is suspected, fetal blood sampling should be obtained with intrauterine transfusion as indicated.[11] Some entities, such as thoracic lesions, may be candidates for surgical intervention (Table 22.2-1). However, many cases of NIHF are not amenable to interventions, and close monitoring may be all that can be offered.

Postnatally, infants born with hydrops are typically critically ill and require intensive therapy, including assisted ventilation and

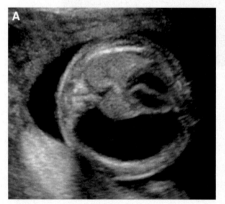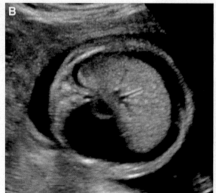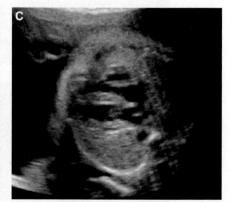

**FIGURE 22.2-5:** A 20-week pregnancy complicated by hydrops of unknown etiology. **A:** Axial view of the lower thorax demonstrates large effusion and compressed echogenic lungs. **B:** Axial view of the abdomen demonstrates large volume anechoic ascites. **C:** Same patient, 7 weeks later. There was spontaneous interval resolution of pleural effusions; only trace ascites (not shown) remained.

| Table 22.2-1 | Intrauterine Therapies to Treat NIFH |
|---|---|
| **Fetal Conditions with NIHF** | **Intrauterine Intervention** |
| Anemia | Fetal intravascular blood transfusion |
| Fetal cardiac arrhythmias | Transplacental or direct administration antiarrhythmic, fetal ventricular pacing |
| Cardiac defects | Intrauterine heart surgery |
| Infection | Transplacental antiviral or antibiotic therapy |
| Obstructive uropathy | Fetal bladder decompression with vesicoamniotic shunt or open fetal surgery |
| Pleural effusion/cystic mass | Fetal thoracoamniotic drainage or fetal surgery |
| Thoracic congenital anomaly | Open fetal surgery or ex-utero intrapartum treatment (EXIT) procedure |
| Tumor | Surgical resection |
| Twin-twin transfusion syndrome | Fetoscopic laser photocoagulation, amnioreduction, septostomy |

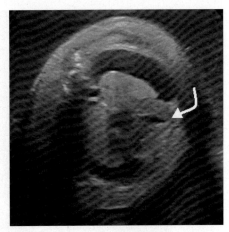

**FIGURE 22.2-6:** A 31-week fetus with critical aortic stenosis. Axial ultrasound of the thorax. The myocardium is conspicuously thickened (*curved arrow*). Note large pleural effusions and skin thickening.

fluid resuscitation due to low intravascular volume.[6] Postnatal evaluation by a comprehensive medical team including genetics is warranted. If demise occurs without known cause for NIFH, autopsy may be considered.

## Conditions Associated with NIFH

**Cardiac Anomalies:** Cardiac abnormalities are the most common underlying etiology for nonimmune fetal hydrops, especially after 22 to 24 weeks, representing approximately 18% to 22% of all cases.[2,5,12,13] The mechanisms by which congestive heart failure causes hydrops include one or more of the following: elevated central venous pressures or decreased ventricular output affecting fluid balance at the capillary level, fetal capillary damage due to hypoxia, insufficient oncotic pressure due to hepatic dysfunction and protein loss, and decreased lymphatic drainage.[3] For reasons not readily apparent, fetal hydrops will manifest in some cases of cardiac anomalies, while other fetuses remain unaffected. However, the prognosis is often questionable, with a live-born rate of 48% and a combined fetal and infant mortality rate of approximately 70% in cases of NIFH with an underlying cardiogenic cause.[12]

Categories of cardiovascular conditions implicated in fetal hydrops include *structural defects, rhythm disturbances, cardiomyopathy, and tumors.*[3,5]

*Structural cardiac defects* known to be associated with nonimmune fetal hydrops tend to be anomalies of the right heart as an increase in right atrial pressure will increase venous pressure.[3] However, left heart defects with obstructive outflow can be transmitted to the right heart via the foramen ovale, thus also increasing pressures. Types of heart lesions include mitral and tricuspid valve abnormalities, atrial and ventricular septal defects, hypoplastic right and left heart syndromes, and great vessel derangements (Fig. 22.2-6).[3,5] Hydrops occurring in the setting of a structural defect indicates an especially poor prognosis, with a combined fetal and infant mortality of 92% in one

meta-analysis.[12] A significant percentage will also have a chromosomal anomaly.

*Fetal cardiac arrhythmias* include tachycardia, bradycardia, and heart block, all which may result in hydrops due to impaired tissue perfusion, elevated central venous pressures, and hepatic congestion.[3] Fetal supraventricular tachycardia (SVT) is the most common tachyarrhythmia causing hydrops.[6] Congenital heart block with heart rates of <90 bpm frequently have NIFH, with the most common etiology being a maternal autoimmune disorder.[6] The M-mode tracing should be carefully inspected for irregularities or an abnormal heart rate. The fetus is more vulnerable to sequelae of tachyarrhythmias earlier in gestation,[3] although, fortunately, this is a treatable cause of fetal hydrops with available pharmacologic agents.[14]

*Fetal cardiomyopathy* may arise from one of many pathologic entities, including autoimmune disorders such as lupus, infectious agents (in particular, Parvovirus B19), lysosomal storage disorders, Noonan syndrome, maternal insulin-dependent diabetes, and a variety of high-output conditions including vascular lesions and twin-twin transfusion syndrome.[3] In a pregnancy with maternal systemic lupus erythematosus, anticardiolipin crosses the placenta, causing fetal heart dysfunction. Fetal/neonatal lupus complicated by hydrops carries a significantly higher risk of demise with typical manifestations, including fetal heart block, dilated cardiomyopathy, and endocardial fibroelastosis.[15] Parvovirus B19 cardiac sequelae include high-output failure related to anemia and fetal viral myocarditis.[16,17] High-output failure may also result from any condition demanding abnormally increased blood flow, a list including, but not limited to, twin-twin transfusion syndrome,[18] twin reversal arterial perfusion sequence,[19] vein of Galen aneurysm,[20] and large neck or abdominopelvic tumors (often teratomas). Vein of Galen aneurysms are readily identified by ultrasound as a large, hypoechoic, central intracranial, tubular structure with robust flow on Doppler imaging. While commonly associated with cardiomegaly and congestive heart failure, hydrops may also follow.[5] MRI can be useful to evaluate brain parenchymal injury (Fig. 22.2-7).[21]

*Cardiomediastinal tumors* are uncommon, but carry a significant risk of precipitating hydrops. The mass effect and obstruction observed in cases of atrial rhabdomyomas (typically seen in fetuses with tuberous sclerosis) and pericardial/mediastinal teratomas induce hydropic changes primarily via impedance of

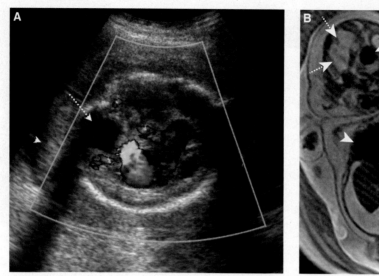

**FIGURE 22.2-7:** A 27-week fetus with vein of Galen malformation. **A:** Axial Color Doppler US shows massive cardiomegaly, soft tissue edema *(arrowhead),* and pleural effusions *(dotted arrow).* **B:** Coronal MRI demonstrates large vein of Galen aneurysm *(solid arrow),* massive cardiomegaly *(arrowheads),* ascites, and soft tissue edema. Notice that there is absence of normal right hemispheric tissue *(dotted arrows)* consistent with brain injury.

venous return to the heart.[3] Atrial hemangiomas have also been reported as a cause of fetal hydrops.[22]

**Chromosome Abnormalities:** Following cardiac disease, chromosomal anomalies have one of the highest associations with nonimmune hydrops. Although estimates vary, and a causal relationship is not always clear, approximately 18% of combined fetal and infant cases of nonimmune hydrops are affected by chromosomal defects.[12] The cause of hydrops is favored to be incomplete formation of the lymphatics and hypoabluminemia, with less likely contributing factors being hypotonia and hematologic disturbances.[6] The mortality rate with NIFH is 58% for live-born, but increases to 98% with combined fetal and infant data.[12]

The likelihood of an underlying chromosomal abnormality is increased with presentation of hydrops earlier in gestation.[10] The most common chromosomal abnormalities associated with

hydrops are Turner syndrome and trisomy 21, although other culprits include trisomies 13, 18, 15, 16 and various chromosomal rearrangements (Fig. 22.2-8; see Fig. 22.2-4).[3,5,23] In pregnancies complicated by nonimmune hydrops without a clear etiology, diagnostic interventions including maternal serum testing (mateniT21), amniocentesis, cordocentesis, and placental sampling should be presented and considered in accordance with maternal preference.

**Lymphatic Dysplasias:** Lymphatic lesions, which include lymphatic malformations, lymphangiectasia, and chylothorax, typically result in reduced lymphatic clearance. Mortality rate for lymphatic abnormalities in the presence of NIFH is 24% for live-born, and 66% for fetal and infant data.[12]

Lymphatic malformations contain dysplastic lymph channels. Terminology for these lesions, including cystic hygroma,

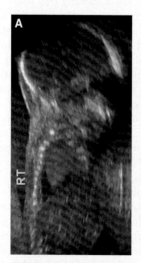
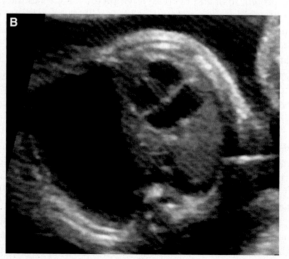

**FIGURE 22.2-8:** Hydropic changes in a 23-week fetus with Down syndrome. **A:** Sagittal view demonstrates nuchal thickening. **B:** Axial view of the thorax shows bilateral effusions, right greater than left, with compressed lung.

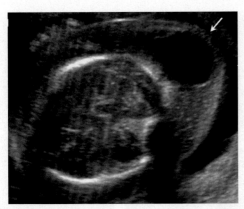

**FIGURE 22.2-9:** Axial view of the posterior neck of a 25-week fetus with a large, septated lymphatic malformation *(arrow)*, in the setting of multiple additional anomalies.

lymphangioma, and venolymphatic malformation, was confusing, until recently when it was replaced by the nomenclature lymphatic malformation. Lymphatic malformations commonly known as cystic hygromas are complex, usually septated, anomalous malformations of the lymphatic system located in the posterior neck. These posterior-neck malformations may be identified earlier or later in pregnancy and have a high association with chromosomal and genetic disorders (particularly Turner syndrome) and hydrops.[3,5,20] (Fig. 22.2-9; see Fig. 22.2-4). Lymphatic malformations localized in the anterolateral soft tissues of the fetal neck are often isolated entities. These lesions, which may appear somewhat later in pregnancy, are not typically associated with chromosomal abnormalities or complicated by hydrops.

*Lymphangiectasia* is a pathologic dilatation of lymph vessels, and when primary or congenital is a severe and extensive lymphatic aberration throughout the subcutaneous tissues, lung, and intestines, often with manifestations of hydrops. It is associated with a high likelihood of an underlying chromosomal abnormality, and is generally considered incompatible with survival[20,23] (Fig. 22.2-10A). Secondary lymphangiectasia is usually due to cardiac or thoracic duct anomalies and typically presents as pulmonary interstitial findings in the lung (Fig. 22.2-10B).

*Chylothorax* is a common primary cause for fetal hydrothorax; however, pleural fluid accumulation can be due to multiple secondary etiologies, including pulmonary sequestrations.[20] Large unilateral or bilateral effusions may precipitate frank hydrops due to cardiomediastinal compression and impaired venous return. In the presence of chylothorax, loss of albumin in the chyle of the pleural space may also aggravate interstitial fluid accumulation.[6] Management options include thoracentesis, thoracoamniotic shunting, and expectant management/counseling, were appropriate. Timely shunting may successfully reverse fetal deterioration, particularly in cases of primary fetal chylothorax (Fig. 22.2-11).

**Infection:** Intrauterine infection is a cause of nonimmune hydrops in 7% of cases.[12] Infection primarily targets the fetal bone marrow, myocardium, and vascular endothelium. Heart failure, anemia, fetal sepsis leading to anoxia and endothelial cell damage may result in hepatic dysfunction and increased capillary permeability, which are likely mechanisms for interstitial fluid accumulation. Mortality rates are 37% in live-born and 72% in fetal and neonatal groups.[3]

Common culprits include parvovirus B19, toxoplasma, *Treponema pallidum*, cytomegalovirus, herpes simplex virus, congenital hepatitis, coxsackievirus, hepatitis B, adenovirus, human immunodeficiency virus, and *Listeria monocytogenes*.[3,5] Pregnancies affected by infection with subsequent hydrops have variable outcomes, and additional characteristic sonographic features may help in elucidating the diagnosis (see Chapter 23).

The most common organism known to cause fetal hydrops is parvovirus B19, which in some reports is stated as the etiology of 8% to 30% of all cases of nonimmune hydrops (Fig. 22.2-12).[3,17] The mechanisms for development of fetal hydrops in the setting of parvovirus infection can be characterized as both direct and indirect and includes: destruction of fetal red blood cell progenitor cells resulting in both anemia and hypoxia, fetal viral myocarditis as well as output failure associated with anemia, liver failure due to hepatocyte damage and hemosiderin deposits, and placentitis.[5,16,17] The fetus is at highest risk for adverse outcome in the first and second trimesters because of increased vulnerability and red blood cell requirements earlier in gestation, as well as changes in placental receptors over the course of the pregnancy.[17] Establishment of the diagnosis of acute parvovirus B19 infection

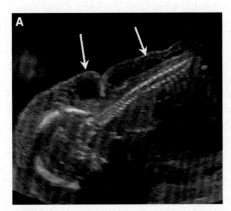
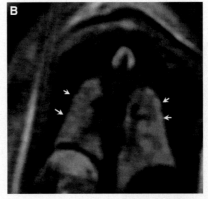

**FIGURE 22.2-10:** Lymphangiectasia. **A:** Sagittal US image of a 19-week fetus demonstrating lymphangiectasia: profound, extensive skin edema with scattered macrocysts *(arrows)*, enveloping the entire fetus, without known etiology. Other manifestations of hydrops were not present. **B:** Coronal T2 MRI showing linear and rounded areas of inhomogeneous hyperintensity in the lung *(arrows)* of a fetus at 30 weeks with myocarditis and secondary lymphangiectasia.

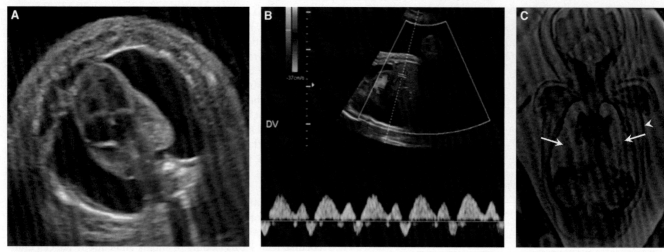

**FIGURE 22.2-11:** Primary chylothorax in a 31-week fetus. **A:** Axial US of the thorax demonstrates large bilateral effusions with collapsed lungs and central compression of the heart. Note skin edema. **B:** A-wave reversal of the ductus venosus. **C:** Coronal MRI: large effusions (*solid arrows*) and skin edema (*arrowhead*). No mass was identified. The pleural effusions were successfully treated with thoracoamniotic shunts.

begins with maternal immunoglobulin M (IgM) and immunoglobulin G (IgG) serologic testing and may proceed to amniotic fluid or fetal cord blood PCR testing for viral RNA or DNA.[17] Although most (>80%) pregnancies affected by parvovirus have no fetal sequelae, overall fetal mortality is approximately 5% to 10% of cases.[5,16,17] The infection may affect fetuses of a twin pregnancy with asymmetric severity,[17] and can even mimic other conditions such as twin-twin transfusion syndrome and intrauterine growth restriction. When fetal hydrops develops in the setting of parvovirus B19, fetal blood transfusion has been shown to decrease the likelihood of fetal demise by 5- to 7-fold.[16,17]

**Anemia and Hematologic Disorders:** Nonimmune hydrops is the result of hematologic abnormalities in approximately 10% of cases.[2,5] The primary pathophysiologic mechanism precipitating hydrops is often anemia,[5] but other contributing factors include high-output cardiomyopathy[16,17] and liver failure with associated fetal hypoalbuminemia.[24] Differential diagnostic considerations should include alpha thalassemia, parvovirus B19, and transient abnormal myelopoiesis. The mortality rate is 57% in live-born and 88% in fetal and infant data.[12]

Alpha thalassemia is commonly found among southeastern Asian populations.[5] The two severe forms at risk of developing

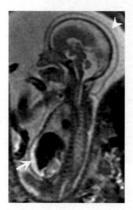

**FIGURE 22.2-12:** Sagittal MR image of a 20-week fetus with parvovirus B19. Note diffuse skin thickening (*arrowhead*) and ascites (*arrow*).

fetal hydrops include Hb Bart, characterized by total absence of hemoglobin alpha chains, and Hb H, in which three of four alpha chain genes are absent.[25] These conditions result in fetal hydrops with anemia, hypoxemia, and marked hepatosplenomegaly, which is explained by both congestive heart failure and extramedullary hematopoiesis.[25] Hb Bart is considered essentially incompatible with survival of the fetus. Significant maternal morbidity in the form of mirror syndrome may occur and should be recognized promptly. Beta thalassemia is not associated with fetal hydrops.

Transient abnormal myelopoiesis is usually seen in fetuses with trisomy 21. Well known postnatally, the condition affects 10% of newborns with trisomy 21.[24] It has also been documented prenatally via percutaneous umbilical cord sampling.[25,26] Imaging findings in the hydropic fetus with trisomy 21 that may raise suspicion for this entity include hepatosplenomegaly and declining cardiac function.[24,26]

**Genetic and Metabolic Disorders:** Genetic and metabolic disorders may cause hydrops; identification of these entities is important, as some are inherited with a recurrence risk of 25%. Mortality with these disorders in the presence of NIHF is high at 67% in live-born and 93% in studies with combined fetal and infant data.[12]

In genetic disorders, many mechanisms are suggested to cause NIHF, including increased venous pressure due to low thoracic volume, hypomobility, lymphatic abnormalities, and hemolytic anemias. X-linked and autosomal dominant genetic disorders include achondrogenesis, chondrodysplasia, G6PD, Noonan syndrome, and myotonic dystrophy. Autosomal recessive disorders include arthrogryposis multiplex congenita and thalassemia. Skeletal dysplasias and other assorted autosomal recessive and autosomal dominant single gene disorders have been cited.[3,5,27,28] Among the skeletal dysplasias are achondrogenesis, thoracic asphyxiating dysplasia (Jeune syndrome), osteogenesis imperfecta, and the short-rib polydactyly syndromes[5,27] (Fig. 22.2-13).

The percentage of cases of NIHF caused by inborn errors of metabolism was previously estimated at approximately 1%.[6,29] However, more recent studies indicate that inborn errors

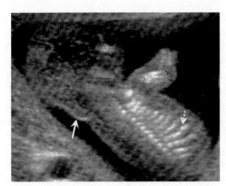

**FIGURE 22.2-13:** 14-week fetus with osteogenesis imperfecta. Coronal oblique image demonstrates extensive lymphedema *(solid arrow)*, beaded ribs *(dashed arrow)*. *Calipers* indicate abnormally shortened humerus.

of metabolism may be more common than once assumed, accounting for 5.7% of NIHF cases in one series.[10] Proposed mechanisms for precipitating hydrops include organomegaly causing impedance of venous return, lymph dysplasia, anemia, hypoproteinemia, and congestive heart failure.[29] Most genetic and metabolic disorders are autosomal recessive in their inheritance pattern. A variety of lysosomal storage disorders may present in the prenatal period with hydrops, including Gaucher disease, sialidosis, I-cell disease, Niemann-Pick, GM1 gangliosidosis, infantile sialic acid storage disease, mucopolysaccharidoses, Wolman disease, and Farber disease.[29] Hydrops fetalis affecting multiple pregnancies in a family, in ethnic groups with higher risk or with consanguinuity should prompt further investigation.[29]

**Thoracic Abnormalities:** Intrathoracic structural abnormalities are a recognized cause of fetal nonimmune hydrops, estimated to be the underlying cause in approximately 6% of cases.[2,5] The mechanism for development of fetal hydrops is generally accepted as a combination of impaired venous return, obstructed lymphatics, and direct impingement upon the cardiac chambers negatively affecting contractility.[3,21] Mortality is high in the setting of hydrops, 73% for fetal and 85% for combined fetal and neonatal data.[12]

Thoracic lesions that are most likely to result in fetal hydrops are large congenital pulmonary airway malformations (CPAM), mediastinal/pericardial teratomas, and fetal chylothorax (Fig. 22.2-14). Other lesions such as congenital diaphragmatic hernias, lymphatic malformations, pulmonary sequestrations, and bronchogenic cysts are also candidates, but less likely to be complicated by hydrops. Fetuses with hydrops in the setting of a thoracic lesion carry a relatively dire prognosis.[5] CPAMs range in size from sub centimeter to massive lesions that occupy a majority of the fetal thorax. Although the vast majority of these lesions carry a favorable prognosis, the larger masses carry a risk of hydrops and fetal demise. A CPAM volume ratio (CVR) is calculated by obtaining three orthogonal lesional measurements, multiplying by 0.52, and dividing this value by the head circumference. A CVR of greater than 1.6 indicates a high risk of development of hydrops. A CVR of less than 1.6 without a dominant intralesional cyst indicates a low risk of hydrops, below 3%.[30]

Fetal mediastinal and pericardial teratomas are exceedingly rare lesions with a poor prognosis. They are typically complicated by hydrops and cardiovascular compromise due to compression. The imaging appearance reflects their complex composition of fat, cysts, calcifications and various soft tissues. Not infrequently mistaken for other diagnoses (in particular CPAMs), mediastinal/pericardial teratomas often displace the heart inferiorly, a feature not demonstrated by masses arising from the lung. Pericardial/mediastinal teratomas portend a grim prognosis unless intervention is carried out in a timely fashion, either during fetal life or soon after delivery (Fig. 22.2-15). The large pericardial effusions commonly associated with these lesions may precipitate the development of hydrops due to cardiovascular compromise; pericardiocentesis has been utilized as temporizing measure to stabilize the fetus in these cases.[31]

A distinct entity in which hydrops is commonly seen is congenital high airway obstruction syndrome (CHAOS). Its typical imaging appearance results from upper airway (often laryngeal) atresia or occlusion and is characterized by severely hyperexpanded, echogenic lungs which compress central cardiomediastinal structures, dilated central airways, everted diaphragms, anasarca and ascites. The hydropic changes presumably reflect obstructed venous and lymphatic return due to central cardiomediastinal compression by the lungs[32] (Fig. 22.2-16).

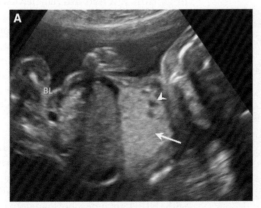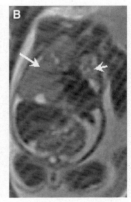

**FIGURE 22.2-14:** Hydrops complicating a large congenital pulmonary airway malformation in a 21-week fetus. **A:** Coronal US image demonstrates an echogenic lesion *(arrow)* containing cystic areas *(arrowhead)*. Ascites was present. BL represents bladder. **B:** Coronal MRI depicts heterogeneous lung mass *(arrows)* occupying the right and part of the left thoracic cavity. MRI also depicts ascites. Open fetal surgery was attempted, but the fetus did not survive.

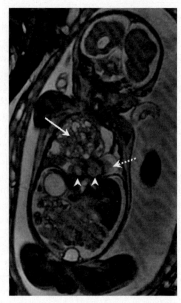

**FIGURE 22.2-15:** Mediastinal teratoma. Coronal SSFP image of a complex fetal mediastinal mass *(solid arrow)* displacing the heart *(arrowheads)* inferiorly. Note effusion *(dotted arrow)* and ascites. Mild skin thickening is also present. The fetus died shortly after the study.

**Neoplasms and Vascular Malformations:** Tumors and vascular anomalies are a well-known cause of fetal nonimmune hydrops, accounting for 6% to 7% of all cases.[6] Neoplasms and vascular lesions precipitate high-output cardiac failure owing to demands of increased flow volume.[31]

Intrathoracic tumors lead the list and are described under thoracic masses. Other culprits include cervical and sacrococcygeal teratomas and liver lesions. Sacrococcygeal teratomas, in particular, may grow rapidly, which places the fetus at risk for hydrops (Fig. 22.2-17).[21] The development of hydrops indicates a high likelihood of intrauterine demise.[20] Other specific indicators of high-risk lesions include elevated aortic velocity, increased inferior vena cava (IVC) diameter, high cardiac output, and umbilical arterial diastolic flow reversal.[20]

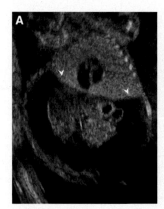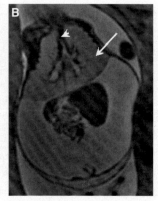

**FIGURE 22.2-16:** A 19-week fetus with congenital high airway obstruction syndrome (CHAOS). **A:** Coronal US depicts echogenic, hyperexpanded lungs and ascites. Note everted diaphragms *(arrowheads)*. **B:** Coronal T2 MRI demonstrates hyperexpanded increased signal lungs *(solid arrow)* and large ascites. *Arrowhead* indicates area of airway obstruction. Fluid-dilated trachea and bronchi are noted below the obstruction.

Fetal intracardiac tumors include rhabdomyomas, myxomas, and hemangiomas, although rhabdomyomas are by far the most common in this category, representing up to 80% to 90% of prenatally diagnosed cardiac tumors.[33] Typically echogenic and homogeneous by ultrasound, they may be single or multiple.[33] They are of low signal intensity on T2-weighted MR imaging. Rhabdomyomas are commonly associated with tuberous sclerosis, which may be familial or represent a de novo mutation. While hydrops resulting from rhabdomyomas is unusual, it has been reported.[33]

Liver tumors diagnosed in the prenatal period are an uncommon cause of hydrops. Hepatic hemangiomas/hemangioendotheliomas may precipitate hydrops via high cardiac output physiology, while mesenchymal hamartomas may cause hydrops via umbilical vein or IVC compression if they grow to a very large size.[34]

**Placental Abnormalities:** Nonimmune fetal hydrops may occur in the setting of placental or umbilical cord abnormalities. These disorders account for approximately 10% of cases of NIHF with a mortality rate of 51% in live-born and 71% among combined fetal and neonatal deaths.[12]

***Monozygotic Twin Pregnancies:*** Monozygotic pregnancies have a higher risk for fetal hydrops due to the presence of vascular anastomoses across the single placenta. In twin-twin transfusion syndrome (TTTS), the occurrence of hydrops in either twin is approximately 8%.[5,18] The donor twin is characterized by oligohydramnios, nonfilling of the urinary bladder, and smaller size. In the recipient, expected findings include polyhydramnios, urinary tract distension, cardiomegaly, and venous sinus enlargement.[18] The recipient twin tends to develop hydrops due to a hypertensive cardiomyopathy (Fig. 22.2-18). The donor is less likely to manifest hydrops, which when present is typically the consequence of severe anemia resulting in hypoxia and increased cardiac output, eventually precipitating cardiac failure.[6] Pregnancies affected by TTTS are organized according to imaging signs into stages established by Quintero, and subsequently revised by the Cincinnati Staging System.[20] Development of hydrops indicates Stage IV which is uniformly fatal without therapeutic intervention.

In the infrequent scenario of acardiac twinning, also referred to as twin reversed arterial perfusion sequence (TRAP), the acardiac twin is typically hydropic due to lymphatic abnormalities (Fig. 22.2-19).[19] However, the pump twin is at risk to develop myocardial failure, subsequent hydrops, and fetal demise. Volume calculations of the acardiac twin are assessed as a ratio to the pump twin to predict the risk of morbidity and mortality for the pump twin. The pump twin is at increased risk for demise when the acardiac twin's calculated weight is greater than 70% of the pump twin.[35]

***Primary Placental/Cord Anomalies:*** NIHF may occur due to fetal anemia secondary to fetomaternal hemorrhage from malformation of the placenta, umbilical cord accident or obstetric accident. Other placental abnormalities which are associated with NIFH include chorioangioma,[3,5,20,36] choriocarcinoma,[37] chorionic vein thrombosis,[20] and hemorrhagic endovasculitis.[5,20] Chorioangioma of the placenta is a benign but vascular lesion (Fig. 22.2-20). Hydrops may result from one or more of the following mechanisms: high-output failure from arteriovenous shunting[3,5,36]; hemolytic anemia due to intralesional

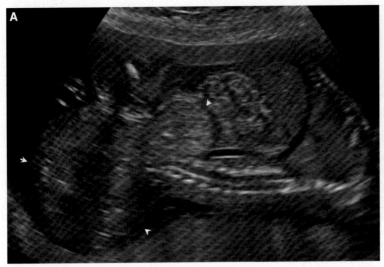
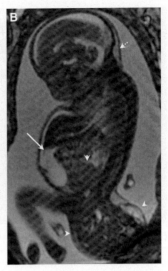

**FIGURE 22.2-17:** Hydrops in a fetus at 20 weeks with large sacrococcygeal teratoma. **A:** Sagittal ultrasound demonstrates large exophytic mass with extension into the pelvis and lower abdomen *(arrowheads)*. There is small ascites and pleural fluid. **B:** Sagittal SSFP image from same fetus shows complex mass *(arrowheads)*, ascites *(solid arrow)*, and nuchal thickening *(dotted arrow)*.

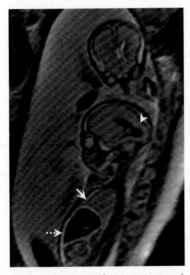

**FIGURE 22.2-18:** Complications of twin-twin transfusion syndrome at 21 weeks. Sagittal MRI demonstrates recipient twin ascites *(dotted arrow)*, pleural effusions *(solid arrow)*, and germinal matrix hemorrhage *(arrowhead)*.

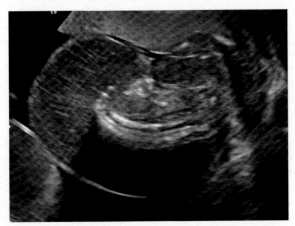

**FIGURE 22.2-19:** TRAP sequence. Dysmorphic and diffusely edematous appearance of the acardiac twin.

trapping of fetal erythrocytes[3,5,36]; or fetal hypoxia with subsequent organ and tissue damage due to both abnormal shunting of unoxygenated blood[4] and concomitant anemia.

Cord abnormalities that may be associated with fetal hydrops include umbilical vein thrombosis,[5,20] umbilical cord knot,[5,20] and umbilical cord tumors such as angiomyxoma.[20] Monochorionic monoamniotic twins are at particularly high risk of developing true knots of the umbilical cord(s).

**Miscellaneous Conditions:** In addition to the disease entities reviewed in the foregoing sections, a growing number of other disorders are reported to be associated with nonimmune fetal hydrops. These include neurologic abnormalities, multiple pterygium syndrome, and arthrogryposis multiplex syndromes, which may cause hypomobility with secondary decreased respiratory movements and increased intrathoracic and venous pressure.[3,28] Urinary obstructive abnormalities may result in increase in venous pressure and lymphatic overload, while congenital nephrotic diseases, such as polycystic disease, can cause hypoalbuminemia. Gastrointestinal disorders, such as bowel perforation, bowel obstruction or mass, may increase venous pressure, prevent normal lymphatics drainage, or injure capillaries due to infection or inflammation.[3] These are only representative samples in their respective categories. The complete lists are exhaustive including many rare etiologies.

## Summary

The findings of hydrops fetalis are readily identified and confirmed by ultrasound and fetal MRI. Nonimmune hydrops accounts for most cases, approximately 90% in various studies.[2,3] A systematic approach using a combination of medical history, thorough imaging, maternal serum testing, and more invasive investigations such as amniocentesis and fetal blood sampling as needed or desired by the family should be employed. In spite of extensive workup, approximately 18% will remain categorized as idiopathic.[6,8] Sonography plays an important role in monitoring the pregnancy for signs of deteriorating fetal status. Fetal mortality remains a significant risk once hydrops has developed.

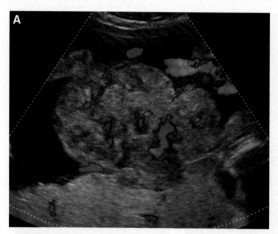
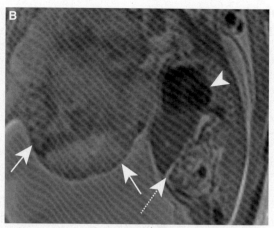

**FIGURE 22.2-20:** 26-week gestation pregnancy with large chorioangioma. **A:** Color Doppler shows large vascular placental mass. **B:** Sagittal T2 MR through the fetus shows large inhomogeneous placental mass *(solid arrows)*. The fetus has cardio-megaly *(arrowhead)* and hydrops–skin edema and ascites *(dotted arrow)*.

## ISOLATED FETAL ASCITES

When fetal ascites is identified, it may be considered as an iso-lated finding, or it may be the first manifestation of impending frank nonimmune fetal hydrops. In either case, for optimal man-agement and to avoid fetal demise, the pregnancy deserves both close monitoring and a thorough investigation to determine the cause, when possible. A number of studies in the literature have examined the prevalence and prognosis for isolated ascites, but the variability among the studies in inclusion criteria and ter-minology contribute to a lack of clarity in predicting outcomes. For the purposes of this discussion, isolated ascites is defined as intra-abdominal fluid without other manifestations of hydrops such as pleural or pericardial effusions or skin thickening.

### Diagnosis

On ultrasound, fetal ascites appears as fluid around the liver or spleen, among bowel loops, or outlining the umbilical vein or falciform ligament.[5] The smallest volume of ascites is most eas-ily identified around the liver (Fig. 22.2-21). Specific features which deserve particular attention include location of the fluid, the presence of calcifications, the echogenicity, and the sono-graphic appearance of the fetal kidneys and liver, all of which may offer clues to the diagnosis. Massive fluid collections which displace bowel loops posteriorly or laterally may rep-resent meconium pseudocyst formation. Echogenic or cystic dysplastic kidneys suggest an underlying urinary tract obstruc-tion. Large perinephric urinomas should not be mistaken for ascites. Calcifications intraperitoneal suggest meconium peri-tonitis, whereas hepatic calcifications may be seen in infection or aneuploidy.

The thin hypoechoic rim of abdominal wall musculature seen on transverse views of the abdomen should not be mistaken for small free fluid. This has been described as pseudoascites.[5] Sag-ittal or coronal views of the abdomen should help clarify this observation.

### Pathogenesis and Management

Isolated fetal ascites that does not progress to fetal hydrops is more likely to result from an intra-abdominal disturbance, and less likely to indicate an underlying systemic hydropic failure mechanism, as described earlier in the chapter.[5] Newly identi-fied fetal ascites deserves repeat ultrasound evaluation in 5 to 7 days,[5] with biophysical profile to document stability or pro-gression in ascites as well as fetal well-being. Increasing ascites or deterioration of the biophysical profile score should prompt consideration for early delivery. Potential etiologies of isolated fetal ascites are many, and include genitourinary structural ab-normalities, bowel obstruction, infection, lymphatic malfor-mations, liver disease, cardiac abnormalities, and pulmonary abnormalities.[38] Some cases remain classified as idiopathic, and among those, many resolve spontaneously.[38,39]

*Genitourinary tract* abnormalities are frequently cited as the most common cause of isolated ascites, with the most frequent culprit being posterior urethral valves.[38] Urinary ascites may result from rupture of the bladder, ureters, or a perinephric uri-noma. Less common genitourinary sources of ascites include cloacal anomalies, ruptured ovarian cysts, polycystic kidneys, and nephrotic syndrome.[5] Cases of genitourinary tract obstruction are often obvious on imaging due the presence of abnormal kidneys, oligohydramnios, and thick-walled bladder or cloaca. Karyotyping

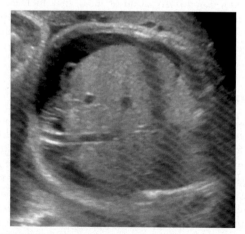

**FIGURE 22.2-21:** Unexplained progressive isolated ascites in a 34-week fetus being followed for a low-risk lung lesion; note the outlines of the umbilical vein. The fetus was delivered early and the ascites resolved spontaneously.

may provide additional information. Although options include monitoring, serial beta-microglobulin levels and placement of vesicoamniotic shunts, in general, the prognosis is poor.

*Intestinal abnormalities* are another important source for isolated fetal ascites. Not uncommonly, jejunal or ileal atresia account for unexplained fetal ascites. The prenatal imaging manifestations are variable and range from no detectable abnormalities to dilated bowel loops and meconium pseudocyst.[40] Additional intestinal abnormalities may also be present, including malrotation, intussusception, and bands.[5,40] A search for other fetal abnormalities is warranted, including fetal echocardiogram, as associated cardiac and renal structural defects have been described.[40]

An *infectious origin* should be considered a potential cause for isolated fetal ascites. Well-known agents include parvovirus B19, cytomegalovirus (CMV), toxoplasmosis, hepatitis A, and *E. coli*.[38] Varicella and congenital syphilis have also been implicated. Investigation may include maternal serum titers of antigen-specific IgM/IgG antibodies or amniotic fluid sampling for PCR analysis. Sequelae of parvovirus B19 may be ameliorated by fetal blood transfusion.[16,17] Timely initiation of postnatal therapies for CMV may lessen the long-term sequelae related to hearing loss.

*Isolated primary fetal chylous ascites* may result from congenital lymphatic dysplasia, lymphatic vessel obstruction, or lymphatic duct leakage. These cases may be amenable to dietary regimens or may require surgical intervention.[41] The diagnosis may be considered a diagnosis of exclusion in the prenatal period. Mirroring a trend of general fetal hydrops, gestational age of onset has an inverse relationship to prognosis. Later onset after 30 weeks is generally associated with a significantly more favorable outcome.[41]

Although uncommon, *inborn errors of metabolism and lysosomal storage disorders* are an established cause of nonimmune fetal hydrops or ascites. Thirteen of these disorders have been implicated, including type 2 Gaucher disease, sialidosis type II, galactosialidosis, infantile sialic acid storage disease (ISSD), Salla disease, MPS types IV and VII, GM gangliosidosis, I-cell disease, Niemann-Pick types A and C, Wolman disease, and Farber disease.[29] Proposed mechanisms include obstruction stemming from hepatomegaly, hypoproteinemia resulting from hepatic dysfunction, anemia, and congestive heart failure. Any of these mechanisms may incite the pathophysiologic cascade of fetal hydrops.[29]

The classic imaging presentation of *congenital high airway obstruction* sequence includes ascites, in addition to massively hyperexpanded lungs, laryngeal obstruction, and dilated central airways. Presumably, the ascites results from profound mass effect on the heart and inferior vena cava by the tense, fluid-filled lungs, causing obstruction of venous return.[32] These may be complicated by eventual hydrops and polyhydramnios. Delivery in these cases is often via ex-utero intrapartum treatment (EXIT) procedure.[32]

Ascites may also be the initial presentation of *fetal hydrops resulting from cardiac abnormalities, either structural or arrhythmias*.[5] Considerations include fibroelastosis, tachyarrhythmias, critical pulmonary stenosis, restrictive foramen ovale, restrictive ductus arteriosus, Ebstein anomaly, AV canal defect, and other lesions affecting the right side of the heart.[5,38] Fetal echocardiography should be included in the initial workup of a new diagnosis of isolated ascites.

In spite of combined antenatal and postnatal investigation, some case of isolated fetal ascites will ultimately remain categorized as *idiopathic*. Many of these will resolve spontaneously either prenatally or postnatally without further intervention.[38,39]

## Summary

There is significant overlap in diagnostic considerations between isolated ascites and NIFH. Fetuses with isolated ascites who do not go on to develop NIHF tend to have a better prognosis, although the long-term prognosis will depend on the underlying etiology. A complete anatomic survey and search for a diagnosis is still warranted in these cases, to allow for optimal counseling and therapeutic guidance.

## REFERENCES

1. Potter EL. Universal edema of fetus unassociated with erythroblastosis. *Am J Obstet Gynecol.* 1943;46:130–134.
2. Bellini C, Hennekam RC. Non-immune hydrops fetalis: a short review of etiology and pathophysiology. *Am J Med Genet A.* 2012;158A(3):597–605.
3. Randenberg AL. Nonimmune hydrops fetalis, part I: etiology and pathophysiology. *Neonatal Netw.* 2010;29(5):281–295.
4. Carlson DE, Platt LD, Medearis AL, et al. Prognostic indicators of the resolution of nonimmune hydrops fetalis and survival of the fetus. *Am J Obstet Gynecol.* 1990;163(6, pt 1):1785–1787.
5. Ulreich S, Gruslin A, Nodell G, et al. Fetal hydrops and ascites. In: Nyberg DA, McGahan JP, Pretorius DH, et al., eds. *Diagnostic Imaging of Fetal Anomalies.* Philadelphia, PA: Lippincott Williams & Wilkins; 2003;713–743.
6. Bellini C, Hennekam RC. Etiology of nonimmune hydrops fetalis: a systematic review. *Am J Med Genet A.* 2009;149A:844–851.
7. Anandakumar C, Biswas A, Wong YC, et al. Management of non-immune hydrops: 8 years' experience. *Ultrasound Obstet Gynecol.* 1996;8(3):196–200.
8. Santo S, Mansour S, Thilaganathan B, et al. Prenatal diagnosis of non-immune hydrops fetalis: what do we tell the parents? *Prenat Diagn.* 2011;31:186–195.
9. Abrams ME, Meredith KS, Kinnard P, et al. Hydrops fetalis: a retrospective review of cases reported to a large national database and identification of risk factors associated with death. *Pediatrics.* 2007;120(1):84–89.
10. Moreno CA, Kanazawa T, Barini R, et al. Non-immune hydrops fetalis: a prospective study of 53 cases. *Am J Med Genet A.* 2013;161A(12):3078–3086.
11. Dijkmans AC, de Jong EP, Dijkmans BA, et al. Parvovirus B19 in pregnancy: prenatal diagnosis and management of fetal complications. *Curr Opin Obstet Gynecol.* 2012;24(2):95–101.
12. Randenberg AL. Nonimmune hydrops fetalis, part II: does etiology influence mortality? *Neonatal Netw.* 2010;29(6):367–380.
13. Fukushima K, Morokuma S, Fujita Y, et al. Short-term and long-term outcomes of 214 cases of non-immune hydrops fetalis. *Early Hum Dev.* 2011;87(8):571–575.
14. Simpson JM, Sharland GK. Fetal tachycardias: management and outcome of 127 consecutive cases. *Heart.* 1998;79(6):576–581.
15. Izmirly PM, Saxena A, Kim MY, et al. Maternal and fetal factors associated with mortality and morbidity in a multi-racial/ethnic registry of anti-SSA/Ro-associated cardiac neonatal lupus. *Circulation.* 2011;124(18):1927–1935.
16. Giorgio E, De Oronzo MA, Iozza I, et al. Parvovirus B19 during pregnancy: a review. *J Prenat Med.* 2010;4(4):63–66.
17. Lamont R, Sobel J, Vaisbuch E, et al. Parvovirus B19 in human pregnancy. *BJOG.* 2011;118:175–186.
18. Kline-Fath BM, Calvo-Garcia MA, O'Hara SM, et al. Twin-twin transfusion syndrome: cerebral ischemia is not the only fetal MR imaging finding. *Pediatr Radiol.* 2007;37:47–56.
19. Guimaraes CV, Kline-Fath BM, Linam LE, et al. MRI findings in multifetal pregnancies complicated by twin reversed arterial perfusion sequence (TRAP). *Pediatr Radiol.* 2011;41(6):694–701.
20. Bianchi D, Crombleholme T, D'Alton M, et al. *Fetology: Diagnosis and Management of the Fetal Patient.* 2nd ed. New York, NY: McGraw Hill; 2010.
21. Cass DL, Olutoye OO, Ayres NA, et al. Defining hydrops and indications for open fetal surgery for fetuses with lung masses and vascular tumors. *J Pediatr Surg.* 2012;47:40–45.
22. Platt LD, Geierman CA, Turkel SD, et al. Atrial hemangioma and hydrops fetalis. *Am J Obstet Gynecol.* 1981;141(1):107–109.
23. Weingst GR, Hopper KD, Gottesfeld SA, et al. Congenital lymphangiectasia with fetal cystic hygroma: report of two cases with coexistent Down's syndrome. *J Clin Ultrasound.* 1988;16:663–668.
24. Kim GJ, Lee ES. Prenatal diagnosis of transient abnormal myelopoiesis in a Down syndrome fetus. *Korean J Radiol.* 2009;10(2):190–193.
25. Taweevisit M, Thorner PS. The contribution of extramedullary hematopoiesis to hepatomegaly in anemic hydrops fetalis: a study in alpha-thalassemia hydrops fetalis. *Pediatr Dev Pathol.* 2012;15(3):206–212.
26. Baschat AA, Wagner T, Malisius R, et al. Prenatal diagnosis of a transient myeloproliferative disorder in trisomy 21. *Prenat Diagn.* 1998;18:731–736.

27. Van Maldergem L, Jauniaux E, Fourneau C, et al. Genetic causes of hydrops fetalis. *Pediatrics.* 1992;89(1):81–86.

28. Jauniaux E, Van Maldergem L, De Munter C, et al. Nonimmune hydrops fetalis associated with genetic abnormalities. *Obstet Gynecol.* 1990;75(3, pt 2):568–572.

29. Staretz-Chacham O, Lang TC, LaMarca ME, et al. Lysosomal storage disorders in the newborn. *Pediatrics.* 2009;123(4):1191–1207.

30. Crombleholme TM, Coleman B, Hedrick H, et al. Cystic adenomatoid malformation volume ratio predicts outcome in prenatally diagnosed cystic adenomatoid malformation of the lung. *J Pediatr Surg.* 2002;37(3):331–338.

31. Woodward PJ, Sohaey R, Kennedy A, Koeller KK. A Comprehensive Review of Fetal Tumors with Pathologic Correlation. *Radiographics.* 2005; 25:215–242.

32. Guimaraes CVA, Linam LE, Kline-Fath BM, et al. Prenatal MRI findings of fetuses with congenital high airway obstruction sequence. *Korean J Radiol.* 2009;10(2):129–134.

33. Pruksanusak N, Suntharasaj T, Suwanrath C, et al. Fetal cardiac rhabdomyoma with hydrops fetalis: report of 2 cases and literature review. *J Ultrasound Med.* 2012;31(11):1821–1824.

34. Makin E, Davenport M. Fetal and neonatal liver tumours. *Early Hum Dev.* 2010;86(10):637–642.

35. Moore TR, Gale S, Benirschke K. Perinatal outcome of 49 pregnancies complicated by acardiac twinning. *Am J Obstet Gynecol.* 1990;163:907–912.

36. D'Ercole C, Cravello L, Boubli L, et al. Large chorioangioma associated with hydrops fetalis: prenatal diagnosis and management. *Fetal Diagn Ther.* 1996; 11(5):357–360.

37. Santamaria M, Benirschke K, Carpenter PM, et al. Transplacental hemorrhage associated with placental neoplasms. *Pediatr Pathol.* 1987;7(5–6):601–615.

38. Favre R, Dreux S, Dommergues M, et al. Nonimmune fetal ascites: a series of 79 cases. *Am J Obstet Gynecol.* 2004;190(2):407–412.

39. El Bishry G. The outcome of isolated fetal ascites. *Eur J Obstet Gynecol Reprod Biol.* 2008;137(1):43–46.

40. Jo YS, Jang DG, Nam SY, et al. Antenatal sonographic features of ileal atresia. *J Obstet Gynaecol Res.* 2012;38(1):215–219.

41. Nose S, Usui N, Soh H, et al. The prognostic factors and the outcome of primary isolated fetal ascites. *Pediatr Surg Int.* 2011;27(8):799–804.

# 23 Congenital Infections

Cristiano Jodicke • Paul Singh • Dev Maulik

Fetal infections account for 2% to 3% of all congenital anomalies.[1] Infections acquired during pregnancy may be associated with significant maternal–fetal morbidity and mortality. Pregnant women are commonly exposed to young children who may be a potential source of infectious disease. Maternal infections may be transmitted to the fetus, leading to poor perinatal and neonatal outcomes. Congenital infections pose many difficult issues for physicians and parents because of the obscure short and potential long-term sequelae that may adversely affect a variety of organ systems. Over the last few decades the prevention, detection, and treatment of congenital infections have improved dramatically. Despite being more common in underdeveloped countries, perinatal infections remain a concern worldwide. Thus, a sound knowledge of congenital infection is important for the clinician involved in maternal–child health. It is estimated that congenital infections account for nearly 20% of fetal and neonatal diseases.

Several organisms, such as cytomegalovirus (CMV), parvovirus, herpes simplex virus (HSV), human immunodeficiency virus (HIV), *Toxoplasma gondii*, varicella zoster virus (VZV), rubella, and *Treponema pallidum* are known to cause fetal infections. Less commonly considered pathogens include enteroviruses, *Listeria monocytogenes*, *Plasmodium*, and *Mycobacterium tuberculosis*. Efforts such as universal immunizations, preconceptional screening, and good hygienic practices have been instrumental in the reduction of incidence of these diseases.

Concern for exposure to infectious agents during pregnancy should prompt the workup of both the mother and fetus. Sonographic findings may assist in fetal prognostication, aid in patient counseling, and influence perinatal management. Apart from ultrasound, other commonly employed methods for prenatal diagnosis of congenital infection include magnetic resonance imaging (MRI) and amniotic fluid and fetal blood sampling.

Improvement in ultrasound technology has enhanced our understanding of fetal diagnosis and management. However, ultrasound is not a sensitive test for fetal infection and a normal targeted sonogram cannot reliably predict a favorable outcome. Although, most affected fetuses appear sonographically normal, serial imaging may reveal evolving findings. Crino[2] reported that the initial screening ultrasound may not demonstrate any abnormalities; however, the fetus may show signs of undetected clinical infection only during the latter part of pregnancy. Various sonographic abnormalities have been associated with congenital infections, such as ascites, hydrops, ventriculomegaly, intracranial calcifications, hydrocephaly, microcephaly, cardiac anomalies, hepatosplenomegaly, echogenic bowel, and placentomegaly. Multiple organ systems are affected in approximately 50% of cases. Different intrauterine infections may have similar sonographic findings, but certain patterns of images in high-risk patients may lead to a specific diagnosis. Thus, practitioners should understand the limitations of ultrasound for the detection of congenital infection.

Since the central nervous system (CNS) is often affected by infectious exposures, fetal MRI may be utilized as an adjunct to ultrasound to provide further definition of brain injury. MRI will not be emphasized in this chapter, but findings with regard to CNS infection can be found in Chapter 12.2 (Fetal CNS

Infection). Sometimes, MRI may also be helpful in evaluation of the gastrointestinal tract and hydropic fetus when the etiology of abnormality is unknown. Discussion of ultrasound and MRI in the evaluation of the GI tract and nonimmune hydrops can be found in Chapters 18.1 and 22.2, respectively.

This chapter reviews the agents most commonly associated with congenital infection and their respective ultrasound findings. In addition, a discussion about pathogenesis and other maternal–fetal diagnostic modalities and management is provided.

## VIRAL INFECTIONS

### Cytomegalovirus

**Definition and Incidence:** Cytomegalovirus (CMV) occurs in 0.2% to 2.2% of all live births and is the most common cause of intrauterine infection and the leading infectious cause of sensorineural hearing loss and mental retardation.[3–5]

**Pathogenesis:** CMV is the largest known member of the human herpes virus family. These viruses are large, enveloped, DNA viruses sharing the biologic properties of latency and reactivation. Endogenous latent virus reactivation may occur regularly. Although CMV is found throughout all geographic locations, it is more widespread in developing countries and in areas of lower-socioeconomic conditions. The seroprevalence increases with age and is due to many other factors such as poor hygiene, underdeveloped infrastructure, and high-risk sexual behavior.[6] Transmission of CMV occurs from person to person and requires intimate contact with infected excretions, such as saliva, urine, breast milk, or other body fluids.[7,8]

Vertical transmission can occur through the placenta from maternal–fetal hematogenous exchange. In addition, fetal infection can also occur as a result of exposure to infected cervical secretions and blood during delivery. The risk for transmission of the virus to the fetus is higher in primary-infected mothers than in those with reactivated disease. Although, primary CMV infections are reported in 1% to 4% of seronegative women during pregnancy, the risk for viral transmission to the fetus is 30% to 40%.[5] Pregnant women who experience recurrent or reactivated CMV infection are much less likely to transmit infection to their fetus. While reactivation of CMV infection during pregnancy is reported to occur in 10% to 30% of seropositive women, the risk of transmitting the virus is only 1% to 3%.

The overall risk of congenital infection is highest when maternal CMV occurs during the third trimester; however, the probability of severe fetal injury is greatest when fetal infection takes place during the first trimester. During early pregnancy, CMV infection may cause disturbances during early brain development. CMV infections acquired during delivery or via breast milk have no effect on future, neurodevelopmental outcome in full-term infants. In contrast, in premature infants (<32 weeks), sepsis-like symptoms have been reported after exposure to contaminated secretions.[6]

**Diagnosis:** During diagnosis, two important steps must be followed. Initially, maternal infection must be investigated, and differentiation should be made between maternal primary and secondary infection based on serologic testing. Next, after maternal infection has been demonstrated, congenital infection should be investigated using both noninvasive (ultrasound examination) and invasive (amniocentesis) prenatal testing.

The best method for the diagnosis of asymptomatic maternal primary infection is seroconversion; however, this is clinically problematic due to the lack of universal screening. The detection of IgM antibodies in maternal sera can be helpful, but interpretation is somewhat complicated. Although CMV-IgM antibodies occur in all primary infections, they may also be detected after reactivation or reinfection and remain present for months. Hence, finding CMV-IgM antibodies in a single serum sample is not definitive for the diagnosis of a primary CMV infection and may indicate either remote primary infection acquired before pregnancy or recurrent disease.[5,9]

Apart from seroconversion, the combination of anti-CMV-IgM and low-avidity anti-CMV IgG testing is the best way to diagnose a primary maternal infection. Antibody avidity is an indirect measure of the tightness of antibody binding to its target antigen and increases during the first months after a primary infection. The IgG avidity assay can be a useful tool to assist in distinguishing primary infection from past or recurrent infection as well as to determine when the primary infection occurred. An avidity index <30% strongly suggests a primary infection of less than 12 weeks.[10,11]

The clinical spectrum of congenital CMV infection is wide, ranging from a complete lack of symptoms to severe disease with multi-organ involvement and postnatal complications. The most sensitive and specific test for diagnosing congenital CMV infection is the identification of CMV in amniotic fluid using virus culture or CMV-DNA analysis by polymerase chain reaction (PCR). CMV-DNA and CMV-IgM antibody activity may also be demonstrable in cord blood. Amniocentesis is generally the procedure of choice because it is safer and has a higher diagnostic sensitivity compared to cordocentesis. The amniotic fluid should be sampled after the 21st week of pregnancy and at least 5 to 6 weeks after the estimated onset of infection.[6]

Approximately 5% to 15% of infants who develop congenital CMV infection as a result of primary maternal infection are symptomatic at birth. The most common clinical manifestations of severe neonatal infection are hepatosplenomegaly, intracranial calcifications, jaundice, growth restriction, microcephaly, chorioretinitis, hearing loss, thrombocytopenia, hyperbilirubinemia, and hepatitis.[6] Approximately 30% of severely infected infants die, and 80% of survivors have major morbidity. Among the 85% to 90% of infants with congenital CMV infection who are asymptomatic at birth, 10% to 15% subsequently develop hearing loss, chorioretinitis, or dental defects within the first 2 years of life.[12,13]

***Ultrasound:*** Ultrasound evaluation is invaluable in providing information about the condition of the fetus. The presence of characteristic ultrasound findings has a high predictive value for fetal infection and also may have prognostic significance. Because routine maternal CMV screening is not recommended, congenital CMV infection is underdiagnosed, and detection during pregnancy is often noted when suspicious sonographic abnormalities are found during routine screening examinations.

The main sonographic findings suggestive of congenital CMV infection are echogenic bowel (Fig. 23.1), ventriculomegaly (Fig. 23.2), microcephaly, periventricular calcifications

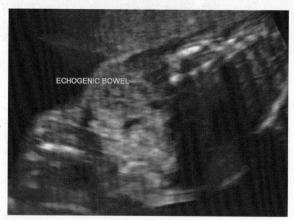

**FIGURE 23.1:** Sagittal-oblique ultrasound view demonstrating echogenic bowel at 26 gestational weeks in a fetus with known congenital CMV.

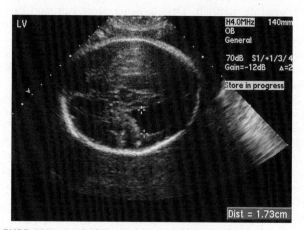

**FIGURE 23.2:** Axial ultrasound view showing ventriculomegaly in a patient with known congenital CMV at 27 weeks' gestation.

(Fig. 23.3), fetal hydrops, intrauterine growth restriction (IUGR), placentomegaly (Fig. 23.4), and oligohydramnios. Less common findings include supraventricular tachycardia, meconium peritonitis, renal dysplasia, ascites, and pleural effusions.

Ventriculomegaly is frequently diagnosed during fetal life and has multiple etiologies, including CMV infection. Around 5% of all cases of ventriculomegaly are caused by fetal infection. De Vries et al.[14] found periventricular calcifications associated with mild-to-moderate ventriculomegaly in 10 out of 11 children with symptomatic congenital CMV infection. Malinger et al. demonstrated similar findings in five of eight affected fetuses with congenital CMV. In addition, fetuses with ventriculomegaly were identified at a more advanced gestational age (28.6 weeks) and had other associated sonographic findings than those without ventriculomegaly.[15]

Microcephaly is associated with a poor prognosis in cases of congenital CMV, usually due to mental retardation. Noyola et al.[16] reported that microcephaly is the most specific predictor for mental retardation (100%; 95% CI, 84.5–100) and major motor disability (92.3%; 95% CI, 74.8–90) in children with symptomatic congenital CMV infection. Of note, microcephaly may not be apparent during the second-trimester ultrasound examination and generally is not an isolated finding. More common associated findings include intracranial calcifications, increased echogenicity of the lining of the ventricles, and ventriculomegaly.

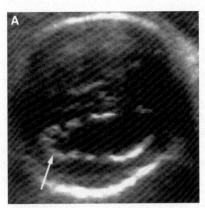
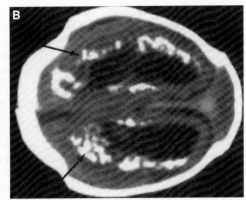

**FIGURE 23.3:** Cytomegalovirus. **A:** Transverse view of fetal brain shows ventricular dilatation and periventricular echogenic nodules *(arrow)*. **B:** Computed tomography scan (oriented to correspond with ultrasound image) after birth confirms hydrocephalus and marked periventricular calcifications *(arrows)*. (Courtesy of Luis Izquierdo, MD, Miami, FL.)

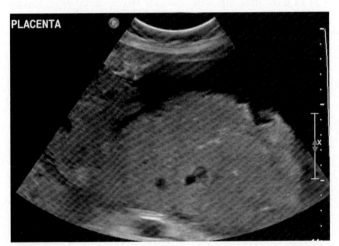

**FIGURE 23.4:** Thickened placenta in a pregnancy diagnosed with congenital CMV at 30 weeks' gestation.

Ventriculitis, which manifests as an increased echogenicity surrounding the lateral ventricles, is an ultrasound finding that may be present in CMV infection, although it also may be a normal variant. As with ventriculomegaly, it will rarely be an isolated ultrasound finding. Periventricular pseudocysts and intraventricular synechiae (IVS) have also been described in association with CMV infection.

Brain calcifications are considered a strong and common ultrasound marker of intrauterine infections. It is not an exclusive ultrasound finding in CMV infection and has been described in fetuses with other infections such as congenital toxoplasmosis, rubella, herpes simplex, and varicella. The calcifications do not usually have an acoustic shadowing, and although they may be found in any portion of the brain, they have particular predilection for the periventricular zone.

Congenital CMV infection during the late first or early second trimester may interfere with neuronal proliferation and migration, and result in abnormal cortical development, including lissencephaly and schizencephaly. Microcephaly, ventriculomegaly, callosal dysgenesis, and abnormally developed sulci and gyration are the most common initial ultrasound findings in fetuses with congenital CMV infection and malformations

of cortical development. A detailed ultrasound, including dedicated neurosonography, and perinatal MRI are indicated when the above-mentioned intracranial ultrasound findings are detected during the initial routine screening examination.

Hyperechogenic bowel and ventriculomegaly are the most common abnormal ultrasound findings in CMV infection, although they may also be seen in uninfected fetuses. Guerra et al.[17] reported the following sonographic abnormalities in 23 cases of CMV-infected fetuses/infants: hyperechogenic bowel ($n = 7$), cerebral ventriculomegaly ($n = 7$), IUGR ($n = 3$), hydronephrosis ($n = 1$), hydrops ($n = 1$), cerebral periventricular echogenicity ($n = 1$), and the association of two or more fetal abnormalities (hyperechogenic bowel and cerebral ventriculomegaly, $n = 3$).

Hepatomegaly and hepatic calcifications may be also found in cases of fetal infection. Hydrops and ascites have been documented and may be related to hepatic dysfunction and portal hypertension from liver congestion. Supraventricular tachycardia and pericardial effusion have also been reported in association with CMV infection. During a 6-year study period, Gonce et al.[18] diagnosed 19 fetuses with CMV infection. The main sonographic findings were the following: brain abnormalities ($n = 14$), fetal hydrops ($n = 4$), hyperechogenic bowel ($n = 4$), pericardial effusion ($n = 1$), cardiomegaly ($n = 1$), oligohydramnios ($n = 4$), and placentomegaly ($n = 2$).

Although ultrasound is a valuable tool in evaluating a fetus with CMV infection, its limitations should be discussed when counseling patients. Guerra et al.[17] studied the effectiveness of ultrasound in the antenatal detection of symptomatic congenital CMV infection. Six hundred and fifty ultrasound examinations of fetuses from mothers with primary CMV infection were correlated to fetal or neonatal outcome. Ultrasound abnormalities were found in 51 of 600 mothers with primary infection (8.5%) and 23 of 154 congenitally infected fetuses (14.9%). They concluded that ultrasound abnormalities predict symptomatic congenital infection in only a third of cases. Liesnard et al.[9] reported characteristic sonographic findings in 9 of 55 infected fetuses (16.4%), but the majority of infected newborns were asymptomatic. Another issue is that abnormal sonographic findings may be only detected for the first time during the third trimester after a normal ultrasound examination earlier in the pregnancy. Although repeat ultrasound examination during the third-trimester scan may lead to a more accurate diagnosis and help with counseling, pregnancy termination would not be an option due to advanced gestational age.

**Management:** The best prevention for congenital CMV infection is primary prevention with personal hygiene practices, such as hand-washing and avoiding intimate contact with salivary secretions and urine from young children. Vaccination to CMV is currently under investigation and is not available for clinical use yet.

Although there are several methods for the prenatal diagnosis of congenital CMV infection, there is no effective treatment to offer once a diagnosis has been made. The use of CMV-specific hyperimmune globulin for treatment was evaluated by Nigro et al.[19] in 157 pregnant women with primary CMV infection. Forty-five women who had a primary infection longer than 6 weeks and congenital infection confirmed by amniocentesis were enrolled. Thirty-one of these women received intravenous treatment with CMV-specific hyperimmune globulin (200 U per kg of maternal body weight), and only one had an infant with clinical CMV disease at birth. In comparison, of the 14 women who declined treatment, 7 had infants who were symptomatic at delivery (adjusted OR, 0.02, $P < .001$). The maternal administration of valaciclovir and ganciclovir to treat intrauterine CMV infection has also been reported.[20,21] Although these studies were not randomized, they are promising and offer a possible treatment option for congenital CMV infection.

Intrauterine therapy with cytomegalovirus hyperimmunoglobulin has also been attempted. Negishi et al.[22] was the first to report intraperitoneal CMV hyperimmunoglobulin administration in a fetus at 28 and 29 weeks of pregnancy. Since then, other investigators have reported the use of intraperitoneal CMV hyperimmunoglobulin as a possible treatment alternative for congenital CMV.[23-25] In addition, both the intraumbilical and intra-amniotic fluid administration of CMV-specific hyperimmune globulin has been performed.[26]

## Parvovirus

**Definition and Incidence:** Human parvovirus B19 is a small single-stranded DNA virus from the Parvoviridae family that is responsible for erythema infectiosum, also known as fifth disease, and is a common childhood illness. It is a worldwide infection that affects individuals from infancy through adulthood. Infection can occur at any age but most commonly affects children from 6 to 10 years of age. The prevalence of parvovirus IgG antibodies steadily rises throughout life. In children aged from 1 to 5 years and from 6 to 19 years, the prevalence of IgG antibodies is 2% to 15% and 15% to 60%, respectively. In the geriatric population, the prevalence is more than 85%.[27,28]

More than half of reproductive-age women have developed immunity to parvovirus B19. About 35% to 45% of women of childbearing age, however, do not have protective IgG antibodies against parvovirus. During pregnancy, the risk of acquiring parvovirus infection is low. The incidence of acute infection in pregnancy is approximately 1% to 2% during endemic periods.[29] Women at increased risk include mothers of preschool and school-age children, workers at day-care centers, and school teachers. Vertical transmission occurs in about 30% to 50% of mothers infected with parvovirus during pregnancy.[30] Congenital infection can cause severe fetal consequences, such as anemia, nonimmune hydrops fetalis (NIHF), and fetal death. The risk of adverse fetal outcome is increased if maternal infection occurs during the first two trimesters of pregnancy; however, fetal infection can still occur during the third trimester.[31-33] It is highly unlikely that fetal infection will occur if the mother has IgG antibodies, since prior infection with parvovirus B19 confers lifelong immunity.[34]

**Pathogenesis:** The risk of fetal complications depends upon the gestational age at the time of maternal infection. The incidence of fetal morbidity and mortality decreases with gestational age. The highest risk for fetal loss happens when maternal infection develops during the 9th through the 16th weeks of pregnancy.[35,36] The risk of vertical transmission is maximal at the time IgM antibodies appear. This coincides with maternal peak viral load which occurs generally 7 days after maternal inoculation.[37]

The virus is spread by respiratory droplets, hand-to-mouth contact and by blood products containing factor XIII and IX concentrates.[31-33,38,39] Outbreaks usually occur during the spring every 4 to 5 years and may last up to 6 months. Viremia occurs 4 to 14 days after exposure and may last up to 20 days. Serum and respiratory secretions become positive for parvovirus DNA 5 to 10 days after intranasal inoculation. Symptoms such as erythema infectiosum, mild fever, arthralgias, and headaches start approximately 10 to 14 days after infection; however, many people remain asymptomatic. By the time erythema infectiosum develops, the person is usually no longer infectious.

The fetal liver, the main site of erythrocyte production, is the virus's main target of infection.[31] The fetus is more vulnerable during the second trimester when the liver is the main source of hematopoietic activity, and the half-life of red blood cells is short. Parvovirus is a potent inhibitor of hematopoiesis because it infects erythroid precursor cells such as erythroblasts and megakaryocytes. Resultant severe anemia may occur, leading to congestive heart failure and the development of hydrops fetalis. Parvovirus may infect fetal cardiac myocytes and hepatocytes, resulting in myocarditis and impaired hepatic function, respectively.[40] Subsequent development of fetal high-output cardiac failure, generalized edema, and death may occur.[40] Thus, the development of hydrops may not correlate with the severity of fetal anemia. Placental trophoblastic cells also express the P antigen, the main cellular receptor for the virus, and are thus susceptible to infection by parvovirus. Poor fetal outcomes have been associated with placental villous trophoblast apoptosis in patients with congenital infection.[41] Such observations suggest that parvovirus infection may be associated with placental insufficiency. Stillbirth in nonhydropic fetuses may result from placental damage and occurs in 0.9% to 23% of pregnancies with documented maternal infection.[42,43]

**Diagnosis:** Serologic examination of maternal blood is the initial and most useful diagnostic tool for parvovirus. Specific IgM and IgG testing should be performed as soon as possible once maternal infection is suspected during pregnancy.[44] IgM antibodies become detectable in maternal serum within 7 to 10 days after infection, sharply peak at 10 to 14 days, and can persist in the circulation for 3 to 4 months or longer.[45] IgG antibodies will rise considerably more slowly and reach a plateau at 4 weeks after infection. Of note, after a recent contact, there will be a serologic window of 7 days, during which both IgG and IgM remain undetectable.[44] Women who are IgG-positive and IgM-negative can be reassured that there is no evidence of recent infection. Patients with IgG- and IgM-negative–specific antibody should be considered susceptible, and further serological testing should be carried out 4 weeks after the last contact or if signs of the disease develop.[35] IgM-positive patients, irrespective of IgG status, should receive serial fetal evaluation to rule out congenital infection.

Since most infected pregnancies have a favorable outcome, invasive prenatal diagnostic testing should only be used if there are definitive signs of fetal anemia or hydrops fetalis.[35] Ultrasound must be used for diagnosis and surveillance. Fetal infection may be identified by using PCR of parvovirus viral DNA in amniotic fluid or fetal cord blood. Amniocentesis is the preferred method of choice due to less complications and increased availability. Serologic examination of fetal blood samples is highly unreliable since the IgG and IgM response to parvovirus is not produced during intrauterine life. Detection of parvovirus using specific IgM in fetal blood has a sensitivity of 29% compared to almost 100% for PCR.[35,44,46]

***Ultrasound:*** As soon as a recent parvovirus maternal infection is suspected during pregnancy, ultrasound examination should be performed to exclude the presence of fetal anemia and hydrops. The virus infects the liver which is the main site of erythrocyte production in the fetus leading to anemia, most often occurring during the second trimester. Increased cardiac output and decreased viscosity of fetal blood caused by anemia are responsible for the changes in fetal blood during congenital infection. An increase in the middle cerebral artery peak systolic velocity (MCA-PSV) (Fig. 23.5) is a very sensitive measure to identify fetal anemia caused by parvovirus infection.[47] Weekly measurements of MCA-PSV are recommended after maternal infection is documented. Timing of intrauterine transfusion for treatment of fetal anemia and prevention of fetal hydrops can be based on these MCA-PSV measurements. The infection causes anemia and possible myocarditis, leading to high-output cardiac failure and subsequent development of generalized edema. Fetal hydrops, an accumulation of excess fluid in at least two body compartments of the fetus, can be easily seen with ultrasound. The median interval between maternal parvovirus infection and diagnosis of hydrops fetalis is about 3 weeks, but may vary between 1 and 20 weeks.[48] The ultrasonographic findings include fetal ascites, skin edema, pericardial effusion, pleural effusions, and placental edema (Figs. 23.6 to 23.11). Enlargement and thickening of the fetal heart also may be documented during

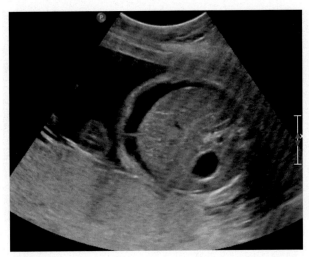

**FIGURE 23.6:** Cross-sectional ultrasound view of the abdomen showing marked ascites in a fetus with congenital parvovirus.

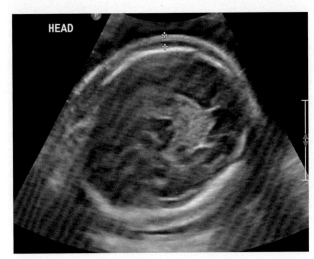

**FIGURE 23.7:** Axial ultrasound image of the fetal head showing scalp edema in a pregnancy exposed to parvovirus and positive IgM titers.

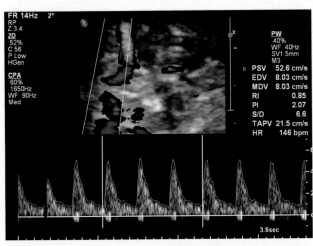

**FIGURE 23.5:** Duplex Doppler of the middle cerebral artery at 24 gestational weeks demonstrating increased peak systolic velocity in a fetus exposed to parvovirus.

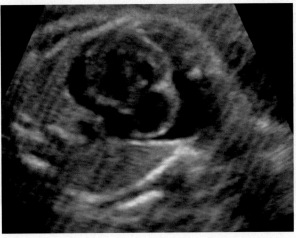

**FIGURE 23.8:** Cross-sectional ultrasound view of the fetal chest demonstrating marked pericardial effusion in a pregnancy with confirmed parvovirus infection by amniotic fluid PCR.

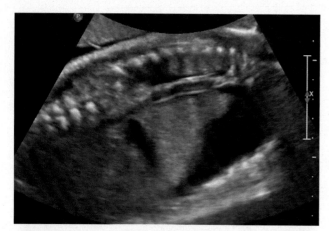

**FIGURE 23.9:** Sagittal view of chest demonstrating pleural effusion at 20 gestational weeks in a fetus with congenital parvovirus.

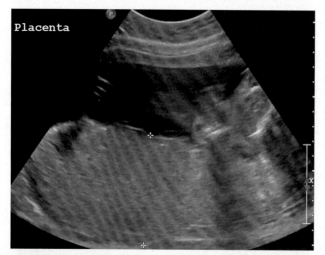

**FIGURE 23.10:** Placentomegaly demonstrated by ultrasound in a pregnancy complicated by fetal parvovirus infection.

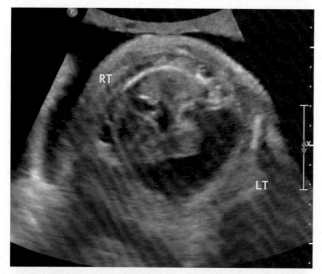

**FIGURE 23.11:** Cross-sectional view of the chest in a fetus with congenital parvovirus showing bilateral pleural effusions, more prominent in the left hemithorax. The fetal heart is displaced to the right side of the chest.

the examination. Fetal structural anomalies associated with parvovirus are uncommon; however, ultrasound findings such as hydrocephalus, hyperechogenic bowel, meconium peritonitis, fetal liver calcifications, cleft lip and palate, and increased fetal nuchal translucency have been reported.[48–52]

**Management:** Maternal infection with parvovirus is self-limited and is treated symptomatically. Acute red cell aplasia may rarely occur and requires serial measurements of hemoglobin and possible blood transfusions to prevent maternal complications due to severe anemia. The confirmation of fetal infection is not required for suspected maternal infection.

If serologic evidence suggests possible maternal infection, weekly measurements of fetal MCA-PSV and US assessment for hydrops should be performed. The MCA-PSV may diagnose significant fetal anemia with a sensitivity of as high as 100%.[53] In parvovirus infection, the MCA-PSV was reported to have a sensitivity of 94.1% for the diagnosis of fetal anemia.[47] Percutaneous umbilical blood sampling (PUBS) should be considered once the MCA-PSV reaches 1.5 multiples of the median (MOM) for gestational age. If fetal anemia is confirmed, fetal blood transfusion is indicated. Intrauterine transfusion with packed red blood cells for cases of severe fetal anemia has been shown to reduce perinatal morbidity and mortality. Fetal survival may be as high as 60% to 80% when intrauterine transfusion is attempted, compared to only 15% to 30% with hydrops and no intervention. Fairley et al.[54] compared outcomes of expectant management with intrauterine transfusion in cases of maternal parvovirus infection, and found a greater than 7-fold reduction in fetal death with the use of intrauterine transfusion.

In addition, a targeted fetal ultrasound and echocardiography should be performed, especially in cases complicated by hydrops fetalis. Delivery is recommended at 34 gestational weeks in pregnancies affected with hydrops fetalis. An attempt to correct fetal anemia should be considered before delivery to improve neonatal outcome.

**Prognosis:** The long-term prognosis for children who received intrauterine transfusion (IUT) for congenital parvovirus infection is controversial. Some studies have shown that children who underwent a successful intrauterine transfusion have good neurodevelopmental outcomes.[36,55] Miller et al.[36] described seven cases of fetal hydrops, two of which received IUT. They were unable to find any long-term developmental problems in the patients who received fetal blood transfusion. Similarly, Dembinski et al.[55] followed up 20 children with parvovirus infection treated with IUT and found no evidence of developmental delay. On the other hand, de Jong et al.[44] described an increased risk of both neurodevelopmental delay and cerebral palsy in children treated with intrauterine transfusions for congenital parvovirus infection. Parvovirus DNA has been detected within white matter multinucleated, reactive microglial cells, suggesting that the virus itself may play a direct role in perivascular changes and white matter damage.[56] Alternatively, severe fetal anemia and hydrops may cause hypoxic-ischemic cerebral injury, thereby, contributing to the increased rate of neurodevelopmental complications. Lindenburg et al.[57] demonstrated similar findings of developmental delay and cerebral palsy in neonates that underwent IUT for severe fetal anemia. However, for a number of reasons, these fetuses are likely to be delivered prematurely, which is itself a significant risk factor for pediatric developmental disorders.

## Rubella Virus

**Definition and Incidence:** Rubella, also known as German measles and "third" disease, is caused by a lipid-enveloped, single-stranded RNA togavirus.[58] Congenital rubella syndrome (CRS) was one of the earliest-described vertically transmitted infections in the newborn infant.[59] The last major epidemic of rubella in the United States occurred between 1964 and 1965, during which time 20,000 cases of infants were born with CRS. Cases of infection during pregnancy have been significantly reduced following vaccine development in 1969. From 1995 to 2000, an average of five cases of CRS has been reported annually in the United States. Newborns affected by CRS are most commonly born in countries where routine rubella vaccination programs are not used.

**Pathogenesis:** Rubella is an airborne transmitted infection spread by small respiratory droplets which becomes infectious 7 days prior to the appearance of the initial symptoms. Vertical transmission is hypothesized to occur 5 to 7 days following maternal inoculation.[60] The clinical features of rubella are a rash, fever, arthralgias, and lymphadenopathy. The rash generally manifests initially on the face and then gradually migrates toward the trunk and then to the lower extremities.[60] Generally self-limited complications such as encephalitis, thrombocytopenia, neuritis, conjunctivitis, and orchitis have rarely been reported to occur as a result of rubella.[60-62] Importantly, encephalitis from rubella infection has been associated with a 50% mortality. Subclinical infection can occur in up to 50% of patients; however, in these patients, fetal anomalies as a result of congenital infection rarely occur. Reinfection with rubella after prior documented infection or immunization is extremely rare during pregnancy.[63,64] Antibody titers lower than 1/64 has been associated with reinfection.[65] The risk of vertical transmission depends upon gestational age and is 90%, 25%, and 95% during the first, second, and third trimesters, respectively. During the first trimester, CRS is extremely rare if the maternal rash occurs within the first 2 gestational weeks. If the rash appears during the 3rd gestational week, the infection rate is 31%, and nearly 100% afterwards.[66] Congenital heart defects and deafness most commonly occur in infected fetuses during the first trimester, but are rare afterwards.

**Laboratory Studies:** Serological analysis is based on the detection of IgG, IgM, and also IgG avidity antibodies.[60,67] The enzyme-linked immunosorbent assays (ELISA), hemoagglutination inhibition test (HI), and the immunofluorescent antibody assay (IFA) are the most common methods of antibody detection.[59,60,67-69] Acute rubella infection is characterized by the appearance of rubella IgM about 5 days after the onset of the maternal rash and persists for 6 weeks.[70] The presence of IgM antibodies does not always correspond to an acute infection. A false-positive IgM for rubella can result in patients with parvovirus, mononucleosis, or a positive rheumatoid factor.[71] In addition, IgM antibodies may persist for 1 year or more in a chronic rubella carrier. Thus, in order to properly establish a timeline of infection, it is important to measure the Rubella IgG avidity. A high IgG avidity indicates chronic carrier status, while a lower IgG avidity indicates a more recent infection. The evaluation of IgG, IgM, or the RNA virus in the saliva instead of in the blood has been proposed to diagnose rubella.[72-75] Ramsay et al.[75] found a sensitivity of 98% and a specificity of 100% for IgG, and a specificity of 99% for IgM detected in the saliva.

Amniotic fluid sampling for fetal diagnosis of CRS should be performed 6 to 8 weeks after maternal infection to avoid false-negative results. Samples of amniotic fluid may be sent for viral cultures; however, this method lacks sensitivity and final results may take up to 6 weeks. PCR technology may be used to diagnose CRS, having the advantage of increased detection rates and faster result times.[69] The diagnosis of CRS via chorionic villus sampling has been described.[76]

*Ultrasound:* Ultrasound has an important role in the prenatal diagnosis of CRS. Migliucci et al.[77] performed a retrospective study on 175 women referred for rubella infection. Sonographic findings of IUGR, polyhydramnios, cardiomegaly, atrial septal defect, hepatosplenomegaly, ascites, echogenic bowel, and placentomegaly were detected. Ugurbas et al.[78] reported an association between microphthalmos and CRS. Ventricular septal defect and pulmonary stenosis have also been reported in cases of CRS.[79] Exencephaly was diagnosed in one case.[80]

**Management:** Maternal rubella is a self-limited disease requiring only symptomatologic care. Severe complications of rubella infection such as encephalitis, thrombocytopenia, neuritis, conjunctivitis, and orchitis should be aggressively managed. Termination of pregnancy may be offered in cases of maternal infection. The maternal administration of immune globulin in large doses (20 mL in adults) in cases of susceptible women exposed to rubella during gestation has been proposed.[67] This treatment, however, has not produced encouraging results because it does not seem to prevent fetal infection. Post exposure prophylaxis for rubella in early pregnancy is not recommended due to unproven clinical efficacy. The rubella vaccine is contraindicated during pregnancy; therefore, susceptible women should be immunized postpartum.

**Prognosis:** Up to two-thirds of children with congenital rubella may be asymptomatic at birth, but will develop sequelae within the first 5 years of life.[74] Classic findings associated with neonatal rubella are low birth weight with a cluster of abnormalities, including cataracts, sensorineural deafness, and cardiac defects such as patent ductus arteriosus, pulmonary artery stenosis, and coarctation of aorta. Less common neonatal heart defects that have been reported are aortic stenosis and Ebstein anomaly.[81-84] Purpura (blueberry muffin spots), microphthalmia, corneal opacity, glaucoma, hepatosplenomegaly, thrombocytopenia, and radiolucent bone lesions may also be found.[85] Late manifestations of congenital rubella include hearing loss, pancreatic insufficiency, and behavioral disorders.[74,85] Diagnosis is made by serum detection of rubella IgM before 3 months of age or persistent IgG between 6 and 12 months of age.

## Herpes Simplex Virus

**Definition and Incidence:** Genital HSV type 1 (HSV-1) or HSV type 2 (HSV-2) is a common infection in United States, affecting 16.2% or 1 in 6 people between the ages of 14 and 49 years.[86] Approximately 25% to 65% of pregnant patients in the United States have genital infection with HSV. The frequency of neonatal HSV infection in the United States varies according to the patient population, with the rate of infection ranging from 1 case per 12,500 to 1 case per 1,700 live births. Whitley et al.[87] analyzed the data from 30 U.S. health plans and showed a rate of 60 cases per 100,000 live births. This incidence is higher than that of congenital syphilis, toxoplasmosis, and congenital rubella.

**Pathogenesis:** HSV belongs to the family of double-stranded DNA viruses known as Alphaherpesvirinae, a subfamily of the Herpesviridae. HSV type 1 (HSV-1) and type 2 (HSV-2) are differentiated based on the glycoproteins within the lipid envelope. Glycoproteins G1 and G2 are associated with HSV-1 and HSV-2, respectively. The hallmark of herpes infection is the ability to infect epithelial mucosal cells where replication occurs. The virus, then, gains access to sensory neurons and stay latent in the sensory ganglia for years, followed by reactivation.

HSV is transmitted from person to person through direct contact. HSV-1 is usually acquired orally, but may also be sexually transmitted. HSV-2 is primarily a sexually transmitted infection. Most neonatal infections result from exposure to HSV in the genital tract during delivery, although both viruses may also be transmitted vertically during pregnancy. Traditionally, HSV-1 was typically associated with orofacial lesions while HSV-2 was felt to cause genital herpes. Although HSV-2 still predominates as the major etiology for genital herpes, an increasing proportion has been ascribed to HSV-1 recently, especially in younger women. According to the Centers for Disease Control and Prevention (CDC), the rate of HSV-2 seroprevalence in the United States has remained stable since the mid-1990s at 16.2%.[86]

The three categories of genital herpes infections are primary, nonprimary, and recurrent. A primary HSV infection is a newly acquired infection in the absence of preexisting antibodies to either HSV-1 or HSV-2. Primary symptomatic genital herpes have an incubation of a period of 2 to 20 days and cause ulceration of the external genitalia and cervix as well as blistering lesions on the internal thigh, buttocks, and perineal skin. Primary HSV infections can also be associated with a number of systemic symptoms such as fever, malaise, and headache.

Nonprimary episode infection refers to newly acquired antibodies to HSV-1 or 2 in the presence of preexisting antibodies to the other type. Nonprimary infections tend to be less severe than primary HSV infections and to have less systemic symptoms and quicker recovery times. HSV-2 antibodies are highly protective against new HSV-1 infection, thus, nonprimary HSV-1 infections are much less common.

Recurrent genital HSV infections refer to the reactivation of a latent genital HSV. The HSV type obtained from the lesion matches the HSV type obtained from the serum. Recurrent infections are typically less severe, unilateral, and have fewer lesions than either primary or nonprimary infections.[88] As in nonprimary HSV, recurrent genital HSV infections are more common with HSV-2 as opposed to HSV-1. Asymptomatic viral shedding may occur during phases in between clinical outbreaks of genital herpes, where HSV reactivates within the sensory neurons of the genital mucosa. Most sexual transmission of HSV occurs during periods of asymptomatic viral shedding because patients are unaware that they are infectious.[89] Most cases of genital HSV infection in women occur without signs or symptoms of disease and are associated with cervical viral shedding.

**Diagnosis:** There are a variety of methodologies for the diagnosis of HSV infection, including viral culture, PCR, direct fluorescent antibodies, Tzanck smears, and serologic identification of IgG and IgM. Pregnant women who present with symptoms

suggestive of genital herpes should undergo both type-specific assay and viral identification testing. Routine antepartum screening in asymptomatic patients is not recommended.

*Ultrasound:* Since intrauterine HSV infection is very uncommon, limited experience exists regarding the sonographic prenatal diagnosis. Various fetal malformations have been associated with congenital herpes, including microcephaly, cerebral atrophy, hydranencephaly, intracranial calcifications, ventriculomegaly, microphthalmia, chorioretinitis, cataracts, congenital herpetic keratitis, congenital heart disease, hepatic calcifications, nonimmune hydrops, bullous skin lesions and scars, lower-limb hypoplasia, and abnormal digits. Fetal cerebral malformation, echogenic bowel (Fig. 23.12), and skin lesions seem to be more common ultrasound findings in fetuses with congenital herpes. Brain lesions are considered as secondary to the cytotoxic virus effects, or subsequent ischemia caused by vascular occlusion of cerebral vessels. Lanouette et al.[90] reported a 14-fold increase in $\alpha$-fetoprotein (AFP) noted during second trimester screening in a patient with multiple fetal congenital anomalies. At 19 weeks' gestation, the patient underwent an amniocentesis and cordocentesis with results consistent with HSV infection.

Jayaram and Wake[91] reported a case with confirmed maternal HSV-2 infection in which a screening ultrasound at 20 weeks did not show any abnormalities. During the third trimester, the patient was admitted with reduced fetal movements. An ultrasound examination then noted absent corpus callosum and gross ventriculomegaly associated with absent end-diastolic flow of umbilical artery Doppler. Interestingly, an irregular heart rate with fluctuating baseline between 60 and 160 beats per minute was also documented.

In a case report by Diguet et al.,[92] during a screening ultrasound at 23 weeks of gestation, IUGR, absence of limb movements, thickened skin, hyperechogenic bowel, placental micronodular alterations, moderate pericardial effusion, and a reverse flow of the ductus venosus were noted. Because of a previous clinical episode of HSV at the beginning of pregnancy, amniocentesis was performed, revealing a positive PCR for HSV-1. On follow-up sonographic examination at 27 weeks of gestation, oligohydramnios associated with fetal abdominal and lower-limb skin irregular thickness, esophageal hyperechogenicity, and persistence of IUGR were found. The pregnancy was terminated, and fetal examination revealed extensive skin ulceration on the trunk and limbs, splenomegaly, and cardiomegaly.

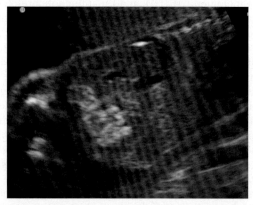

**FIGURE 23.12:** Sagittal-oblique ultrasound view demonstrating echogenic bowel at 26 gestational weeks in a fetus with congenital herpes simplex virus.

Duin et al.[93] reported a case in a patient with confirmed HSV in which a normal ultrasound at 20 weeks' gestation with symmetric fetal growth was obtained; however, during a third-trimester examination, marked cerebral ventriculomegaly, third ventricle enlargement, frontal thinning of the cerebral cortex, and microcephaly were noted. A follow-up ultrasound demonstrated a slight dissolution of the cortical mantle. Severe parenchymal destruction, particularly in the temporal and parietal lobes, was confirmed by a prenatal MRI. The occipital cerebral cortex was also globally thinned with microgyria. Postmortem examination confirmed the prenatal diagnosis of hydranencephaly. This report suggests that fetal MRI may provide significant additional information in assessing the extensiveness of the fetal HSV infection. Interestingly, fetal malformation caused by congenital herpes infection may be only evident during the late part of pregnancy despite an initial normal screening ultrasound. Thus, third-trimester ultrasound evaluation for an anatomy follow-up and biometry should be considered in pregnancies with known herpes virus infection.

**Management:** Although considerable effort is made for the viral identification of genital HSV, treatment regiments do not vary by virus type. During a primary outbreak in pregnancy, oral antibiotic therapy is indicated to reduce the duration and severity of symptoms. Viral shedding is also decreased with proper therapy. No data indicates that maternal treatment reduces the risk of neonatal herpes. Acyclovir is not teratogenic and may be administered either orally in pregnant women with a first episode of genital herpes or intravenously in pregnant women with severe genital or disseminated herpetic disease.

Transabdominal invasive procedures, such as chorionic villus sampling, amniocentesis, and percutaneous umbilical sampling, may be performed even when genital lesions are present. Transcervical procedures should not be performed during the presence of active lesions.

**Prognosis:** Neonatal HSV infection is defined as infection in a newborn within 28 days after birth. There are three categories of neonatal infections: cutaneous disease, CNS disease, and disseminated disease. Cutaneous disease is a HSV disease localized to the skin, eye, and/or mouth. Although cutaneous disease has a low mortality, it may progress to CNS or disseminated disease. CNS disease manifests with neurologic symptoms as well as positive CSF PCR findings and carries a mortality of approximately 15%. Disseminated disease has the worst prognosis with the highest fatality rate. Involvement of multiple organs (e.g., hepatitis, pneumonitis, or disseminated intravascular coagulation) is common and has a mortality rate of 31% and 85%, with and without therapy, respectively.

## Human Immunodeficiency Virus

**Definition and Incidence:** Acquired immune deficiency syndrome (AIDS) is a severe immunological disorder caused by the HIV RNA retrovirus, resulting in a defect in cell-mediated immune response leading to an increased susceptibility to opportunistic infections. Despite aggressive efforts by the health community to reduce vertical transmission, HIV remains a significant perinatal risk globally. Almost 33.3 million people worldwide are infected, with 88% of infected infants born to mothers who did not receive any antiretroviral treatment.[94,95] In the United States, approximately 21% of patients with HIV are unaware of their infection[96]; so the CDC recommends routine preconceptional HIV-testing for all women.[97]

**Pathogenesis:** HIV attaches to the CD4 molecule on T lymphocytes via the external glycoprotein (gp120) and the transmembrane protein (gp41) located on the HIV envelope.[98] Following release into the cell cytoplasm, the viral RNA is reverse transcribed into DNA by the virus' own reverse transcriptase enzyme. After host-cell synthesis of HIV viral proteins, they are transported in close proximity to the cell membrane for assembly and egress. Destruction of the host's immune system ensues as CD4 T-cells are consumed by the HIV virus. HIV is transmitted primarily by exposure to contaminated body fluids, especially blood and semen. During pregnancy, HIV may be transmitted to the fetus either transplacentally, at the time of vaginal delivery, or through breast milk.

**Diagnosis:** The enzyme-linked immunosorbent assay performed on a blood sample or the rapid HIV test performed on blood or oral mucosa is the screening test of choice. Any positive HIV-screening test should be followed by a confirmatory western blot assay. Patients with a positive confirmatory testing result are considered to be infected with HIV and should be referred for consultation to an HIV specialist. A thorough laboratory evaluation, including CD4+ T-cell count, and plasma HIV RNA PCR is recommended.

***Ultrasound:*** HIV infection has not been associated with any specific fetal anomalies. Joao et al.[99] followed 995 HIV-infected pregnant patients undergoing antiretroviral therapy (ART). No significant increase in the rate of congenital anomalies was found compared to the overall population. In addition, they found that the prevalence of congenital anomalies was not affected by the timing of ART exposure during pregnancy.[99] However, the increasing complexity of antiretroviral (ARV) regimens used antenatally for HIV treatment may result in potential drug-related adverse events such as low birth weight and preterm birth.[100-103] Late IUGR has been demonstrated in HIV-infected pregnant women.[104] Similarly, in a prospective cohort study, Aaron et al.[105] found an increase in small for gestational age (SGA) births in HIV patients compared to an HIV-negative population. Therefore it is suggested to follow up HIV patients with serial growth ultrasounds. Ultrasound has been used to investigate abnormal placental implantation in HIV-positive women. Savvidou et al. investigated the effect of maternal HIV infection on the degree of placental invasion through pulsatility index measurements of the uterine arteries during the first trimester. No significant differences, however, were found in placental perfusion of HIV patients compared to non-HIV patients.[106]

**Management:** All women should be tested immediately upon diagnosis of pregnancy. Repeat testing should be done during the third trimester for patients at high risk of acquiring HIV antenatally. Instrumentation and invasive procedures, such as fetal scalp electrodes, forceps, vacuum suction devices, amniocentesis, cordocentesis, and chorionic villus sampling, may increase the risk of vertical transmission and should be avoided. Davies et al.[107] reviewed the risk of fetal infection with amniocentesis in women with HIV. They concluded that in HIV-positive women noninvasive screening tools, such as maternal serum and fetal ultrasound screening, be preferentially performed prior to the consideration of amniocentesis.[107] Furthermore, artificial rupture of membranes should be avoided in the absence of obstetrical indications.

Plasma viral load prior to delivery is the strongest predictor of vertical transmission and also will determine the mode of delivery. The American College of Obstetricians and Gynecologists recommend a scheduled cesarean delivery at 38 weeks of gestation for HIV-infected women with viral loads >1,000 copies per mL regardless of the ART regimen.[108] The combination of ART antenatally and intrapartum Zidovudine (AZT) has led to a significant decrease in the rate of vertical transmission of HIV. Prior to vaginal delivery, patients should receive a 2 mg per kg intravenous loading dose of AZT over 1 hour, followed by 1 mg per kg of intravenous AZT until cord clamp.[109] For HIV patients undergoing cesarean delivery, AZT should begin 3 hours before the surgery. Aside from AZT, all other ART drugs should be continued intrapartum.[109] Lastly, antibiotic prophylaxis for Pneumocystis and *Mycobacterium avium* complex may be required according to the CD4 count.

**Prognosis:** Pregnant patients affected with HIV should be counseled that in the absence of ART, the risk of vertical transmission is approximately 25%. With AZT, the risk is reduced to 5% to 8%. When care includes both AZT and scheduled cesarean delivery, the risk is decreased to 2% or less. A similar risk is seen among women with viral loads of less than 1,000 copies per mL despite the mode of delivery. Neonatal administration of ART has been shown to decrease the rate of seroconversion in a newborn of an HIV-infected mother.[110]

## Varicella Zoster Virus

**Definition and Incidence:** Varicella infection, also known as chickenpox, is uncommon during pregnancy though an important cause of maternal and fetal complications. An incidence of 1.6 to 4.6 per 1,000 has been reported among individuals between 15 and 45 years of age in the United States of America (USA).[111,112] Approximately 90% of adults born in the United States and Europe are immune to VZV. The introduction of universal varicella vaccination has reduced the rate of VZV transmission in some countries.

Serious fetal complications have been associated with varicella acquired during pregnancy. Congenital varicella syndrome (CVS) is more common with maternal infection during the first half of pregnancy and may lead to multiple fetal anomalies. Since the first description of CVS in 1947 by Laforet et al.,[113] several other cases have been reported. Primary VZV during pregnancy may result in congenital infection 25% of the time.[114] Fetal outcomes depend on the time when the infection occurs. If maternal infection takes place during the first 20 weeks of gestation, the incidence of CVS is approximately 1% to 2%. The risk for spontaneous abortion is also increased during this period.[115]

**Pathogenesis:** Varicella zoster virus (VZV) is a DNA virus of the herpes family and is highly contagious. The primary infection, also referred to as chickenpox, is self-limited. It is transmitted from person to person by direct contact, via respiratory droplets or secretions, or via aerosolization of vesicular fluid from skin lesions. The virus enters the host through the upper respiratory tract.[116] The incubation period usually lasts between 14 and 16 days but can vary from as few as 10 or as many as 21 days after contact.[115] Initially, nonspecific prodromal symptoms, such as fever, chills, headache, malaise, and sore throat, occur,

followed by pruritus and a maculopapular rash that becomes vesicular. The rash will crust over in approximately 5 days. The period of contagiousness is 1 to 2 days before the onset of the rash and continues until all lesions are crusted.

Intrauterine infection occurs via transplacental transmission following maternal viremia. The vertical transmission rate increases with advancing gestation age. In a large prospective study, Enders et al.[117] demonstrated that IgM was detected in 5%, 10%, and 25% of infants at birth, following maternal varicella infection during the first, second, and third trimester, respectively. The type of fetal infection depends on the gestational age when the disease takes place. Infection during the first half of pregnancy may be complicated by CVS, while maternal disease around the time of delivery results in neonatal varicella.[118,119]

**Diagnosis:** The diagnosis of varicella generally is based on its classic clinical manifestations, and laboratory testing is unnecessary. Cases in which clinical manifestations are ambiguous but infection is suspected, culture, fluorescent antigen staining, or PCR testing for VZV DNA can be performed on vesicular fluid or scrapings from the lesions. Serologic tests are generally not of use for diagnosis, because specific antibodies only become detectable after the rash has occurred. At present, there are no reliable prenatal markers to predict fetal disease or severity. Serial ultrasound examinations of the fetus may be useful since some anomalies are not detected sonographically during the first examination.[120] PCR testing has been used to detect VZV infection in amniotic fluid with a high sensitivity and specificity.[121,122] Amniocentesis should not be performed until 1 month after maternal infection to avoid false-negative results.[120,123] VZV cultures from amniotic fluid have a poor sensitivity.[124] Disruptions in the fetal skin may cause an elevation of $\alpha$-fetoprotein (AFP) in maternal blood and amniotic fluid as well as an increase in acetylcholinesterase within the amniotic fluid.[120]

**Ultrasound:** Targeted ultrasound is recommended for all patients with documented infection to identify fetal anomalies associated with congenital varicella. Possible findings include IUGR, microcephaly, ventriculomegaly, cerebellar dysplasia, polyhydramnios, oligohydramnios, hydrops, and calcifications in the liver (Fig. 23.13), abdomen, and lungs.[120,125,126]

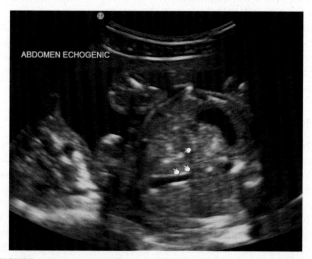

**FIGURE 23.13:** Liver calcifications seen on cross-sectional ultrasound view of abdomen in a fetus with suspected congenital varicella syndrome.

Limb anomalies, including hypoplasia and contractures, are commonly found in cases of congenital varicella. Free-floating echogenic material and spicular echo reflections surrounding the skin may be indicative of cutaneous lesions.[126] Fetal ocular defects such as cataracts and microphthalmia may be visualized, as well. Interestingly, during a second-trimester ultrasound in a patient with documented varicella infection, a case of congenital pulmonary airway malformation (CPAM) was documented.[127] Multiple bilateral, diffuse hyperechogenic lesions in the lungs as well as multiple sonolucent areas in the liver were the only other noted abnormal images. Of note, sonographic findings associated with varicella fetopathy are nonspecific and may be associated with several other congenital infections, creating a difficulty in obtaining a clear diagnosis.

Fetal MRI may be a valuable adjunct to prenatal ultrasound. Verstraelen et al.[126] reported a case of congenital varicella infection in which additional information was obtained using MRI. During a routine prenatal ultrasound at 26 weeks' gestation, diminished gross fetal body movements, left lower-limb hypoplasia with club-foot deformity, right-kidney pyelectasis, echogenic bowels, and multiple calcifications in the liver and thorax were visualized. CNS lesions including cerebellar hypoplasia, pachygyria, and incomplete opercularization of the Sylvian fissure were missed by ultrasound, but were clearly demonstrated by MRI at 32 weeks. Prenatal MRI may, therefore, contribute to initial sonographic findings which may help enhance patient counseling.[126]

**Management:** Among adults who do not recall having varicella, the majority of patients are actually immune.[128] A history of varicella or two-dose vaccination is sufficient to reassure a pregnant patient that she is not susceptible to varicella infection. If maternal serology is negative, secondary prevention during pregnancy must be considered. Susceptible pregnant seronegative women exposed to varicella should be offered varicella zoster immunoglobulin (VZIG) to limit maternal disease. Although, optimum protection is obtained when the dose is administered within 96 hours of exposure, some experts suggest that VZIG may be administered with benefit up to 10 days after exposure.[129] VZIG should not be given once active disease has begun.[116] The recommended dose of VZIG is 125 units per 10 kg of body weight, up to a maximum of 625 units. Intravenous immune globulin (IVIG) can be substituted if necessary at a dose of 400 mg per kg if VZIG is not available. If VZIG is not administered within 4 to 10 days of exposure, antiviral therapy may be considered for postexposure prophylaxis; however, some authorities question its safety or efficacy compared to VZIG.

Even though VZIG has been shown to reduce the incidence of symptomatic disease in pregnant women, it does not influence the risk of development of CVS. Since serial ultrasound may lack sensitivity or specificity as a diagnostic tool for fetal varicella syndrome (FVS), invasive prenatal diagnosis to confirm congenital infection should be considered. Although, there is no validated in utero treatment for FVS, a negative amniocentesis result can reassure parents that their child has no risk of FVS or of any long-term impairment.

**Prognosis:** Maternal infection during the second trimester and early third trimester most often does not result in CVS and is associated with a good prognosis.[130–133] Generally neonates born with CVS have poor outcomes. Isolated cases of more favorable scenarios have been reported.[134,135] Neonatal death

usually occurs from intractable gastroesophageal reflux, severe recurrent aspiration pneumonia, or respiratory failure. Structural anomalies are usually not seen with neonatal varicella syndrome. Before VZIG was available, the mortality rate from neonatal varicella syndrome was 31%.[136] Since the introduction of VZIG, the mortality rate has dropped to 7%.[118]

## Other Viral Infections

Congenital viral infection with Coxsackie B1 and B5 during the first trimester has been associated with fetal myocarditis resulting in severe heart failure.[79] (pp762–763) Intrauterine infection with enterovirus has been postulated as a possible cause of future development of type 1 diabetes during adolescence.[137]

## PARASITIC INFECTIONS

### Toxoplasmosis

**Definition and Incidence:** Toxoplasmosis is a parasitic infection caused by *Toxoplasma gondii*. It is estimated that 400 to 4,000 cases occur in the United States each year.[138–140] Furthermore, recent data suggests that congenital toxoplasmosis occurs in approximately 1 in 10,000 live births.[139] Treatment has been shown to decrease fetal infection rate, thus underscoring the importance of prenatal diagnosis.

**Pathogenesis:** *T. gondii* undergoes a complex life cycle comprised of three stages known as the tachyzoite, bradyzoite, and sporozoite phases. The tachyzoite phase represents the acute stage of infection where the protozoan invades and replicates within host cells. The bradyzoite phase represents the latent stage of infection where the protozoan exists as a tissue cyst. During the sporozoite phase, the protozoan exists as an environmentally resistant cyst. It is the tachyzoite form of the organism that is responsible for congenital infection. Members of the family Felidae are the definitive reservoir of *T. gondii* while humans are temporary hosts only. During acute infections, cats excrete *T. gondii* oocysts in their feces, and humans are then infected by fecal–oral contact. Other routes of transmission to humans include ingestion of raw or inadequately cooked infected meat or unwashed fruits or vegetables and exposure to contaminated soil from gardening.[141] Sporozoites penetrate the human host's gastrointestinal mucosa and are released in the tachyzoite phase into the systemic circulation. A woman can then transmit the infection to her fetus transplacentally. The incubation period may range from 10 to 23 days after ingestion of undercooked meat, and from 5 to 20 days after ingestion of oocysts from cat feces.[142]

Maternal infection with *T. gondii* prior to conception rarely results in congenital infection.[143] The prevalence of maternal infection is 0.4%, and out of those patients, 40% will develop congenital toxoplasmosis. The risk of congenital infection is directly related to the fetal gestational age. While acute maternal infection occurs between 10% and 25% of the time during the first trimester, it will occur between 60% and 90% of the time during the third trimester.[144,145] The severity of congenital toxoplasmosis, however, is inversely related to fetal gestational age with the most devastating fetal infections occurring during the first half of pregnancy. Significant fetal morbidity and mortality decreases from 75% during the first trimester to almost 0% toward the end of the pregnancy.[79] (763)

**Diagnosis:** In adults the severity of *T. gondii* infection is correlated with the immune status of the host.[142] Generally, for immunocompetent adults, toxoplasmosis infections result in mild symptoms of lymphadenopathy, fever, fatigue, and malaise that are self-limited and resolve in weeks to months without any specific treatments. In contrast, however, patients who are immunocompromised as a result of AIDS, organ transplants, malignancies, or chronic steroid administration demonstrate severe neurologic manifestations such as meningoencephalitis.

The most common method of diagnosis for acute toxoplasmosis is maternal serum antibody detection; however, individual variation in titers may confound the serologic results. Also, IgM antibodies have been reported to persist for up to 18 months post infection.[146] A negative IgM with a positive IgG result indicates chronic infection. A positive IgM result, on the other hand, may indicate more recent infection or a false-positive reaction. Commercially available test kits for *Toxoplasma* IgG and IgM antibodies have significant variation in sensitivities and specificities.[147] In response to this problem, the FDA in 1997 issued a guide for the interpretation of toxoplasmosis serologic results.[148] Determining when *T. gondii* infection occurred in a pregnant woman is important since infection before conception poses little risk for transmission to the fetus. IgG avidity testing measures the strength with which IgG binds to *T. gondii* and may help to determine when the infection occurred. High IgG avidity indicates that the infection occurred at least 5 months ago; while low IgG avidity reflects a more recent infection.[149] Women with positive serum IgM antibodies should undergo IgG avidity testing by an experienced toxoplasmosis reference laboratory.[149]

After maternal infection is confirmed, congenital toxoplasmosis must be investigated. The identification of *T. gondii* intrauterine infection by amniocentesis using PCR testing has been found to have both high sensitivities and specificities.[150] Foulon et al.[151] reported that a combination of PCR and mouse inoculation of amniotic fluid may improve sensitivities even further. Given the advances in PCR testing of amniotic fluid as well as the risk associated with cordocentesis, amniocentesis is the procedure of choice for the diagnosis of congenital toxoplasmosis infection.

*Ultrasound:* Ultrasound findings of congenital toxoplasmosis include hydrocephalus, intracranial calcifications, fetal growth restriction, ascites (Fig. 23.14), and hepatosplenomegaly. In a case series published by Hohlfeld et al.,[152] 32 of 89 fetuses with proven congenital toxoplasmosis developed sonographic signs of infection. Ventriculomegaly was found in 25 fetuses, while intracranial calcifications (Fig. 23.15) were found in only 6 fetuses.[152] Furthermore, a number of false negatives were found, with postnatal brain examinations revealing multiple areas of brain necrosis and abscesses in normally reported prenatal studies.[152] With the improvement of ultrasound resolution, the advent of neurosonography, and the addition of fetal MRI, recent studies have been able to better delineate fetal neurologic signs of congenital toxoplasmosis. Malinger et al.[153] in a recent review of eight patients with congenital toxoplasmosis described ventriculomegaly ($n = 7$) and multiple echogenic nodular foci consistent with calcifications in the brain parenchyma ($n = 7$), in the periventricular zone ($n = 3$), and in the caudothalamic zone 9 ($n = 3$). Good correlation has been demonstrated between ultrasound and fetal MRI for diagnosing brain abnormalities in fetal toxoplasmosis.[154,155] Interestingly,

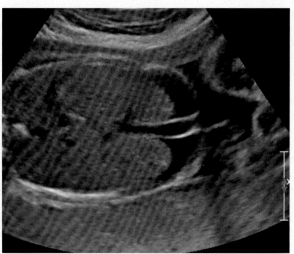

**FIGURE 23.14:** Cross-sectional ultrasound view of the abdomen at the level of the cord insertion demonstrating ascites in a fetus with congenital toxoplasmosis.

while ultrasound signs of fetal toxoplasmosis are not identified during the routine second trimester ultrasound examination, they may be more commonly detected during the third trimester. It has been speculated that this occurs because of the prolonged time for the fetal insult to develop.[156] Unlike in CMV infection where intracranial echogenic nodules occur most often in the periventricular zone,[157] in toxoplasmosis they may be found dispersed in multiple areas of the fetal brain. Furthermore, periventricular cysts and microcephaly which are characteristic of CMV infections are not common in fetal toxoplasmosis.[153,158] Other non-CNS ultrasound findings such as thickened placenta with hypoechoic areas, liver echogenicities (Fig. 23.16), and hepatomegaly may be visualized, but are not specific for fetal toxoplasmosis.[153]

**Management:** Since the prevalence of congenital toxoplasmosis is so rare, routine screening during pregnancy for acute toxoplasmosis is not advocated by the American College of Obstetrics and Gynecology[159] and the Royal College of Obstetrics and Gynecology.[160] Routine screening may not be cost effective, but more importantly may result in equivocal or false-positive values, leading to unnecessary treatment and fetal interventions. Interestingly, other countries such as Austria and France have implemented screening programs for toxoplasmosis, demonstrating a decline in the incidence of congenital infection.[161,162] It is difficult to determine whether the proportion of the decline is directly attributable to the program or to the overall general decline in European toxoplasmosis rate.

Treatment for toxoplasmosis infection is available and should be instituted as soon as maternal infection is confirmed. Spiramycin should be started at a maximum dose of 3 g per day in all pregnant women found to have serologic evidence of toxoplasmosis. In the United States, however, spiramycin is not available, but may be obtained from Europe with special approval from the United States Food and Drug Administration. Spiramycin is a macrolide antibiotic that itself does not cross the placenta, but is thought to prevent passage of toxoplasmosis to the fetus.[79] (p165) A combination of pyrimethamine and sulfadiazine has been recommended when congenital infection is confirmed by amniocentesis.[163] Both drugs, however, are contraindicated during the first trimester due to their

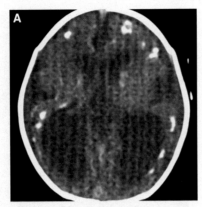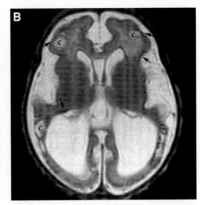

**FIGURE 23.15:** Congenital toxoplasmosis. **A:** Axial noncontrast CT image in a newborn shows extensive parenchymal calcifications that are predominantly cortical and subcortical in location. Also note moderate ventriculomegaly. Hydrocephalus is more common in toxoplasmosis than in CMV infection. **B:** Axial T2-weighted image shows multiple foci of T2 hypointensity corresponding to CT-confirmed calcification (*black arrows*). Also note the subcortical cysts (*c*). Ventriculomegaly is moderate. (From Hedlund G, Bale JF, Barkovich AJ. Infections of the developing and mature nervous system. In: Barkovich AJ, Raybaud C, eds. *Pediatric Neuroimaging*. 5th ed. Philadelphia, PA: Lippincott Williams & Wilkins; 2012:954–1050.)

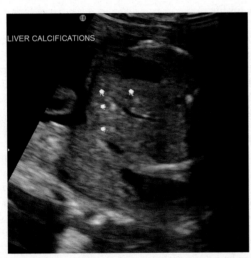

**FIGURE 23.16:** Axial cross-sectional ultrasound view of multiple nonshadowing hepatic calcifications at 28 weeks' gestation.

teratogenicity. Pyrimethamine is a folic acid antagonist; thus, increasing the risk of neural tube defects if used early in pregnancy. Also, pyrimethamine has been associated with fetal heart and kidney malformations as well as maternal and fetal bone marrow suppression.[164] Sulfadiazine has been associated with an increased incidence of oral clefting. Thus, spiramycin is generally prescribed initially and changed to a pyrimethamine and sulfonamide combination if fetal infection is diagnosed after 15 weeks.[165]

In 2000, the CDC published primary prevention recommendations for pregnant women to avoid toxoplasmosis infection. These guidelines centered around patient and provider education as well as specific hygienic and dietary precautions.[162] Foulon et al.[166] examined the impact of primary prevention on the incidence of toxoplasmosis in pregnancy. Periconceptional education and antenatal education are fundamental in the prevention of maternal and fetal infections. It has been demonstrated that pregnant women who received education sessions were associated with a 63% decrease in toxoplasmosis seroconversion rates compared to women who did not.[166]

**Prognosis:** The likelihood of long-term sequelae as a result of congenital toxoplasmosis decreases as gestational age increases. Toxoplasmosis acquired during the first trimester may result in a spontaneous abortion while infection incurred during third trimester may be asymptomatic. Although the classic neonatal triad of chorioretinitis, intracranial calcifications, and hydrocephalus is suggestive of congenital toxoplasmosis, up to 90% of neonates affected with congenital toxoplasmosis do not demonstrate obvious signs on routine examination.[152,167] Other findings often seen in congenital toxoplasmosis include lymphadenopathy, hepatosplenomegaly, mental retardation, seizures, encephalitis, malaise, arthralgia, low-grade fever, and occipital and cervical lymphadenopathy. Indeed, disease sequelae may only become apparent when visual impairment, mental and cognitive abnormalities of variable severity, seizures, or learning disabilities present after several months or years.

## Other Parasitic Infections

Apart from congenital toxoplasmosis, other sources of congenital parasitic infections include malaria, schistosomiasis, and trypanosomiasis. Malaria infection during pregnancy can have a huge impact on both the mother and the fetus, leading to still birth, premature delivery, or fetal growth restriction. Fetal anemia and splenomegaly have also been described in cases of congenital malaria.[168] Considering the poor outcomes associated with congenital malaria,[169,170] fetal ultrasound surveillance in endemic areas to detect and treat cases during pregnancy needs to be actively implemented.

*Schistosomiasis mansoni* has also been demonstrated to cause placental insufficiency, leading to fetal growth restriction.[171] *Trypanosoma cruzi* can cause congenital Chagas disease. Fetal organs, including the heart, brain, integumentary and gastrointestinal systems, may be affected, leading to hepatosplenomegaly, anemia, jaundice, and encephalitis.

## BACTERIAL INFECTIONS

### Syphilis

**Definition and Incidence:** Syphilis is a sexually transmitted disease caused by the bacterium *Treponema pallidum.* According to World Health Organization (WHO), 12 million people are infected with syphilis each year.[172] In the Unites States, the rate of syphilis among women was 1.1 cases per 100,000 women in 2010, while the rate of congenital syphilis was 8.7 cases per 100,000 live births.[173] In 2008, the WHO reported that approximately 1.9 million pregnant women had active syphilis.[174] The importance of accurate prenatal diagnosis of syphilis was emphasized by Hawkes et al.[175] in a recent meta-analysis, who stated that approximately 70% of pregnant women infected with syphilis will have an adverse pregnancy outcome. Both the American College of Obstetricians and Gynecologists and the American Academy of Pediatrics recommend screening for syphilis at the first prenatal visit and again at 32 to 36 weeks, in high-risk women. Furthermore, CDC recommends screening at delivery.[176]

**Pathogenesis:** Syphilis is horizontally transmitted via vaginal, anal, or oral sex. Approximately 3 weeks after infection, a round, small, and painless syphilitic chancre may appear on the vulva, vagina, cervix, anus, or rectum indicating primary infection. This lesion may last for 3 to 6 weeks and often goes unrecognized by the host. Eventually *Treponema spirochetes* disseminate systemically, resulting in the cutaneous and mucosal manifestations of secondary infection, lasting for up to a year. During this time the disease can be especially contagious. After primary or secondary syphilis, the infection may enter a latent phase, causing no symptoms to the host. This phase of the disease is divided into early and late depending on the duration of the infection. Initial infection occurring within the previous 12 months and beyond 12 months is characterized as early latent and late latent syphilis respectively. Importantly, during the latent phase, transmission to the fetus may still occur.[177] In approximately one-third of the people who go untreated, tertiary syphilis may develop. Skin, bone, or liver gumma, CNS abnormalities, and cardiovascular disorders are associated with tertiary syphilis. During this stage, individuals are not considered infectious.[178]

**Diagnosis:** The most specific test for the diagnosis of syphilis when an active chancre or condyloma latum is present is dark field microscopy. In the absence of active lesions, serologic testing for syphilis is performed. Serologic testing includes nontreponemal tests (NTTs) and treponemal tests (TTs). Generally, NTTs are used for screening and monitoring therapy, while TTs are for diagnostic confirmation. The Venereal Disease Research Laboratory (VDRL) test and the rapid plasma reagin (RPR) test are the most commonly used NTTs. Since NTTs detect antibodies to cardiolipin, a compound commonly found in human tissue, false-positive reactions can occur. TTs detect an interaction between serum immunoglobulins and surface antigens of *T. pallidum.* They include the fluorescent treponemal antibody absorption (FTA-ABS) test, the treponemal-specific, microhemagglutination assay for *T. pallidium* (MHA-TP), and

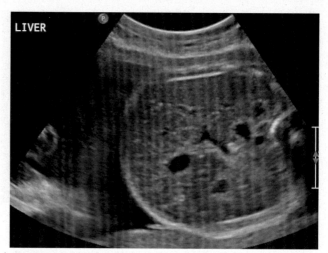

**FIGURE 23.17:** Axial ultrasound view of the abdomen demonstrating hepatomegaly in a fetus with congenital syphilis.

*T. pallidum* particle agglutination test (TP-PA). Although far less common than in NTTs, false-positive reactions may still occur in diseases such as Lyme disease and leptospirosis.[177] Unlike NTTs which may become negative, TTs usually remain positive for life.

***Ultrasound:*** In the presence of maternal syphilis, ultrasound findings of fetal hydrops, hepatosplenomegaly (Fig. 23.17), polyhydramnios, and thick placenta strongly suggest congenital syphilis. Other sonographic features include intrahepatic calcifications, ascites, hyperechogenic bowel, and even fetal death. Amniotic fluid dark field testing or PCR may be performed for confirmatory diagnosis. Hematologic sampling for fetal IgM anti-treponemal antibodies has been reported.[179] The degree of fetal hepatomegaly in pregnancies with syphilis has been correlated with amniotic fluid infection.[180] Dilatation of fetal bowel segments has been reported in case of congenital syphilis.[181] Hill and Maloney[182] reported fetal GI tract obstruction involving the stomach and small bowel in a case of congenital syphilis. Treponemal involvement of the intestine causing syphilitic enterocolitis has been described previously in stillbirths.[183] Wendel and Gilstrap[184] reported an association between hyperechogenicity of the vasculature in the basal ganglia and congenital syphilis. It has been demonstrated that congenital infection can result in placental villitis and obliterative arteritis; therefore, resulting in placentomegaly and increased placental vascular resistance.[182] Lucas et al.[185] showed that mean S/D ratios of both the uterine and umbilical arteries were significantly increased in pregnancies affected by syphilis. Interestingly, in a case described by Schulman et al.[186] where decreased fetal movement was the initial complaint, fetal cardiac failure followed by bradycardia was noted. The pathologic examination revealed acute syphilitic funisitis. Using 3D ultrasound, Araujo et al.[187] demonstrated oligodactyly and twisting of the toes in a case of congenital syphilis.

**Management:** Treatment of maternal infection is effective for both the prevention and the treatment of congenital syphilis. Penicillin G, parenterally administered, is the recommended treatment. In a randomized controlled trial performed by Radcliffe et al.,[188] penicillin G was found to be the most effective treatment for syphilis. The appropriate penicillin regimen varies according to the stage of infection.[189] A single dose of 2.4 million units of benzathine penicillin G is recommended for the treatment of primary syphilis, secondary syphilis, and early latent syphilis.[189] In cases of late latent syphilis or latent syphilis of unknown duration, the same dosage should be given and repeated twice at weekly intervals.[189] Because penicillin G does not cross the blood–brain barrier, aqueous crystalline penicillin G of 3 to 4 million units parenterally every 4 hours for 10 to 14 days is the treatment of choice for neurosyphilis.[189] Pregnant women who have a history of a penicillin allergy should be desensitized and treated. The titer of NTT antibodies reflects disease activity, with a 4-fold decrease suggesting adequate therapy and a 4-fold increase indicating active disease.

**Prognosis:** Congenital syphilis is classified as either early congenital syphilis (ECS) or late congenital syphilis (LCS). ECS appears in the first 2 years of life while LCS appears afterwards. Both ECS and LCS affect a variety of organ systems. Findings of ECS include hepatomegaly, splenomegaly, anemia, thrombocytopenia, leukopenia, macular–papular lesions over the hands and feet, ulceration of the nasal mucosa and cartilage (saddle nose deformity), periostitis, osteochondritis, nephrosis, neurosyphilis, and ocular malformations. Findings of LCS include peg-shaped, notched central incisors (Hutchinson teeth), multicuspid first molars (mulberry molars), interstitial keratitis, palsy of cranial nerve 8, rhinitis, impaired maxillary growth, saddle nose deformity, mental retardation, hydrocephalus, seizure disorders, periostitis of the skull, tibia (saber shin), and the clavicle (Higouménakis sign), and symmetric, tender joints (Clutton joints). The prognosis of congenital syphilis is dependent upon a number of factors, including the gestational age when vertical transmission occurred, stage of maternal syphilis, maternal treatment, and immunological response of the fetus.[190]

## Other Bacterial Infections

Other bacteria that may cause congenital infections include *Listeria, Chlamydia, Mycoplasma, Mycobacterium,* and *Coxiella.* Q fever infection in pregnancy, caused by *Coxiella burnetii,* is associated with various maternal and neonatal adverse outcomes, including IUGR, stillbirth, preterm delivery, and oligohydramnios.[191,192] Shinar et al.[192] described two pregnancies complicated by Q fever, that resulted in placental infection and abruption remote from term.

Although congenital tuberculosis is rare, a perinatal mortality of nearly 50% has been reported.[193] Clinical presentation of tuberculosis during pregnancy and infancy is often nonspecific, making recognition difficult. Tuberculosis has been associated with increased antenatal admission, premature delivery, IUGR, and maternal–fetal mortality.[194–196] Abramowsky et al.[197] described two cases of placental involvement with *Mycobacterium tuberculosis* causing acute villitis and intervillitis. Principal neonatal sites of involvement include the liver and lungs; however, the bones, kidneys, spleen, GI tract, skin, and lymph nodes may also be affected. Generally, the diagnosis of congenital infection only occurs during the early neonatal period when clinical manifestations present. Common nonspecific clinical symptoms such as fever, respiratory distress, and hepatosplenomegaly most commonly appear within 2 to 3 weeks of delivery.[198] A high index of suspicion by health professionals is paramount in order to detect and manage tuberculosis in pregnancy and the early newborn period.

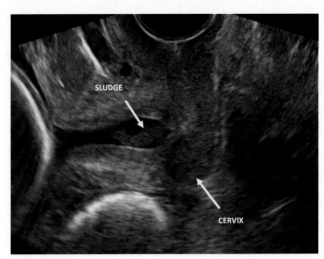

**FIGURE 23.18:** Transvaginal ultrasound demonstrating intra-amniotic sludge associated with cervical funneling at 24 gestational weeks.

*Listeria monocytogenes* infection is a rare complication of pregnancy.[199] Intrauterine infection by *L. monocytogenes* has been associated with preterm delivery, meconium-stained amniotic fluid, hydrocephalus, chorioamnionitis, stillbirth, and neonatal death.[200,201] Prompt treatment with antibiotics is paramount in improving maternal and neonatal outcome.[202]

Mycoplasma and ureaplasma have been associated with chorioamnionitis, preterm delivery, and pregnancy loss.[203,204] Intrauterine infection with ureaplasma has also been associated with congenital pneumonia.[205]

### Intra-amniotic Sludge

Intra-amniotic sludge is represented by the sonographic appearance of free-floating hyperechoic matter close to the internal cervical os (Fig. 23.18). It has been associated with an increased risk for preterm delivery and other adverse pregnancy outcomes. The precise nature of this material is unclear; however, it has been attributed to bleeding, meconium, vernix, and intrauterine infection.[206–209] For a more comprehensive review, please refer to chapters 7 and 10.

## SUMMARY

In summary, the global impact of congenital infections is significant. Although sonography by itself is not a sensitive test for fetal infection, the utilization of ultrasound technology assited by fetal MRI along with other markers for congenital infection may influence clinical management, assist in prognostication, and aid in patient counseling. Indeed, particular findings such as an elevated MCA-PSV in the setting of congenital parvovirus may indicate the need for in utero fetal treatment. As diagnostic fetal imaging continues to advance, sonography will remain an invaluable tool for clinicians involved in the prenatal diagnosis of congenital infections.

## REFERENCES

1. Stegmann BJ, Carey JC. TORCH infections: toxoplasmosis, other (syphilis, varicella-zoster, parvovirus B19), rubella, cytomegalovirus (CMV), and herpes infections. *Curr Womens Health Rep.* 2002;2(4):253–258.
2. Crino JP. Ultrasound and fetal diagnosis of perinatal infection. *Clin Obstet Gynecol.* 1999;42(1):71–80.

3. Pultoo A, et al. Detection of cytomegalovirus in urine of hearing-impaired and mentally retarded children by PCR and cell culture. *J Commun Dis.* 2000;32(2):101–108.

4. Stagno S, et al. Primary cytomegalovirus infection in pregnancy: incidence, transmission to fetus, and clinical outcome. *JAMA.* 1986;256(14):1904–1908.

5. Yinon Y, Farine D, Yudin MH. Screening, diagnosis, and management of cytomegalovirus infection in pregnancy. *Obstet Gynecol Surv.* 2010;65(11):736–743.

6. Malm G, Engman ML. Congenital cytomegalovirus infections. *Semin Fetal Neonatal Med.* 2007;12(3):154–159.

7. Hanshaw JB. Cytomegalovirus infections. *Pediatr Rev.* 1995;16(2):43–48.

8. Stagno S, et al. Maternal cytomegalovirus infection and perinatal transmission. *Clin Obstet Gynecol.* 1982;25(3):563–576.

9. Liesnard C, et al. Prenatal diagnosis of congenital cytomegalovirus infection: prospective study of 237 pregnancies at risk. *Obstet Gynecol.* 2000;95(6, pt 1): 881–888.

10. Adler SP, Nigro G, Pereira L. Recent advances in the prevention and treatment of congenital cytomegalovirus infections. *Semin Perinatol.* 2007;31(1):10–18.

11. Grangeot-Keros L, et al. Value of cytomegalovirus (CMV) IgG avidity index for the diagnosis of primary CMV infection in pregnant women. *J Infect Dis.* 1997;175(4):944–946.

12. Boppana SB, et al. Symptomatic congenital cytomegalovirus infection: neonatal morbidity and mortality. *Pediatr Infect Dis J.* 1992;11(2):93–99.

13. Jones CA. Congenital cytomegalovirus infection. *Curr Probl Pediatr Adolesc Health Care.* 2003;33(3):70–93.

14. de Vries LS, et al. The spectrum of cranial ultrasound and magnetic resonance imaging abnormalities in congenital cytomegalovirus infection. *Neuropediatrics.* 2004;35(2):113–119.

15. Malinger G, Lev D, Lerman-Sagie T. Imaging of fetal cytomegalovirus infection. *Fetal Diagn Ther.* 2011;29(2):117–126.

16. Noyola DE, et al. Early predictors of neurodevelopmental outcome in symptomatic congenital cytomegalovirus infection. *J Pediatr.* 2001;138(3):325–331.

17. Guerra B, et al. Ultrasound prediction of symptomatic congenital cytomegalovirus infection. *Am J Obstet Gynecol.* 2008;198(4):380.e1–380.e7.

18. Gonce A, et al. Maternal IgM antibody status in confirmed fetal cytomegalovirus infection detected by sonographic signs. *Prenat Diagn.* 2012;32(9):817–821.

19. Nigro G, et al. Passive immunization during pregnancy for congenital cytomegalovirus infection. *N Engl J Med.* 2005;353(13):1350–1362.

20. Jacquemard F, et al. Maternal administration of valaciclovir in symptomatic intrauterine cytomegalovirus infection. *BJOG.* 2007;114(9):1113–1121.

21. Puliyanda DP, et al. Successful use of oral ganciclovir for the treatment of intrauterine cytomegalovirus infection in a renal allograft recipient. *Transpl Infect Dis.* 2005;7(2):71–74.

22. Negishi H, et al. Intraperitoneal administration of cytomegalovirus hyperimmunoglobulin to the cytomegalovirus-infected fetus. *J Perinatol.* 1998;18(6, pt 1):466–469.

23. Sato A, et al. Intrauterine therapy with cytomegalovirus hyperimmunoglobulin for a fetus congenitally infected with cytomegalovirus. *J Obstet Gynaecol Res.* 2007;33(5):718–721.

24. Japanese Congenital Cytomegalovirus Infection Immunoglobulin Fetal Therapy Study Group. A trial of immunoglobulin fetal therapy for symptomatic congenital cytomegalovirus infection. *J Reprod Immunol.* 2012;95(1–2):73–79.

25. Matsuda H, Kawakami Y, Furuya K, et al. Intrauterine therapy for a cytomegalovirus-infected symptomatic fetus. *BJOG.* 2004;111(7):756–757.

26. Buxmann H, et al. Use of cytomegalovirus hyperimmunoglobulin for prevention of congenital cytomegalovirus disease: a retrospective analysis. *J Perinat Med.* 2012;40(4):439–446.

27. Brown T, et al. Intrauterine parvovirus infection associated with hydrops fetalis. *Lancet.* 1984;2(8410):1033–1034.

28. Heegaard ED, Brown KE. Human parvovirus B19. *Clin Microbiol Rev.* 2002;15(3):485–505.

29. Dembinski J, et al. Long term follow up of serostatus after maternofetal parvovirus B19 infection. *Arch Dis Child.* 2003;88(3):219–221.

30. Chisaka H, et al. Parvovirus B19 and the pathogenesis of anaemia. *Rev Med Virol.* 2003;13(6):347–359.

31. Nyman M, et al. Detection of human parvovirus B19 infection in first-trimester fetal loss. *Obstet Gynecol.* 2002;99(5, pt 1):795–798.

32. Wattre P, et al. A clinical and epidemiological study of human parvovirus B19 infection in fetal hydrops using PCR Southern blot hybridization and chemiluminescence detection. *J Med Virol.* 1998;54(2):140–144.

33. Yaegashi N, et al. The frequency of human parvovirus B19 infection in nonimmune hydrops fetalis. *J Perinat Med.* 1994;22(2):159–163.

34. Rodis JF. Parvovirus infection. *Clin Obstet Gynecol.* 1999;42(1):107–120.

35. Enders M, et al. Fetal morbidity and mortality after acute human parvovirus B19 infection in pregnancy: prospective evaluation of 1018 cases. *Prenat Diagn.* 2004;24(7):513–518.

36. Miller E, et al. Immediate and long term outcome of human parvovirus B19 infection in pregnancy. *BJOG.* 1998;105(2):174–178.

37. DeHann T, Oepkes D, Beersma MFC. Aetiology, diagnosis and treatment of hydrops foetalis. *Curr Pediatr Rev.* 2005;1:63–72.

38. Jordan J, et al. Human parvovirus B19: prevalence of viral DNA in volunteer blood donors and clinical outcomes of transfusion recipients. *Vox Sang.* 1998;75(2):97–102.

39. Torok T. Human Parvovirus B19. In: Remington JS, Klein JO, eds. *Infectious Disease of the Fetus and Newborn Infant.* 4th ed. Philadelphia, PA: Saunders; 1995:668–702.

40. Rouger P, Gane P, Salmon C. Tissue distribution of H, Lewis and P antigens as shown by a panel of 18 monoclonal antibodies. *Rev Fr Transfus Immunohematol.* 1987;30(5):699–708.

41. Jordan JA, Butchko AR. Apoptotic activity in villous trophoblast cells during B19 infection correlates with clinical outcome: assessment by the caspase-related M30 Cytodeath antibody. *Placenta.* 2002;23(7):547–553.

42. Prospective study of human parvovirus (B19) infection in pregnancy. Public Health Laboratory Service Working Party on Fifth Disease. *BMJ.* 1990;300(6733):1166–1170.

43. Koch WC, et al. Serologic and virologic evidence for frequent intrauterine transmission of human parvovirus B19 with a primary maternal infection during pregnancy. *Pediatr Infect Dis J.* 1998;17(6):489–494.

44. de Jong EP, et al. Parvovirus B19 infection in pregnancy. *J Clin Virol.* 2006;36(1):1–7.

45. Anderson MJ, et al. Experimental parvoviral infection in humans. *J Infect Dis.* 1985;152(2):257–265.

46. Beersma MF, et al. Parvovirus B19 viral loads in relation to VP1 and VP2 antibody responses in diagnostic blood samples. *J Clin Virol.* 2005;34(1): 71–75.

47. Cosmi E, et al. Noninvasive diagnosis by Doppler ultrasonography of fetal anemia resulting from parvovirus infection. *Am J Obstet Gynecol.* 2002;187(5):1290–1293.

48. Ergaz Z, Ornoy A. Parvovirus B19 in pregnancy. *Reprod Toxicol.* 2006;21(4):421–435.

49. Markenson G, et al. Parvoviral infection associated with increased nuchal translucency: a case report. *J Perinatol.* 2000;20(2):129–131.

50. Simchen MJ, et al. Fetal hepatic calcifications: prenatal diagnosis and outcome. *Am J Obstet Gynecol.* 2002;187(6):1617–1622.

51. Yaron Y, et al. Evaluation of fetal echogenic bowel in the second trimester. *Fetal Diagn Ther.* 1999;14(3):176–180.

52. Zerbini M, et al. Intra-uterine parvovirus B19 infection and meconium peritonitis. *Prenat Diagn.* 1998;18(6):599–606.

53. Mari G, et al; for the Collaborative Group for Doppler Assessment of the Blood Velocity in Anemic Fetuses. Noninvasive diagnosis by Doppler ultrasonography of fetal anemia due to maternal red-cell alloimmunization. *N Engl J Med.* 2000;342(1):9–14.

54. Fairley CK, et al. Observational study of effect of intrauterine transfusions on outcome of fetal hydrops after parvovirus B19 infection. *Lancet.* 1995;346(8986):1335–1337.

55. Dembinski J, et al. Neurodevelopmental outcome after intrauterine red cell transfusion for parvovirus B19-induced fetal hydrops. *BJOG.* 2002;109(11): 1232–1234.

56. Isumi H, et al. Fetal brain infection with human parvovirus B19. *Pediatr Neurol.* 1999;21(3):661–663.

57. Lindenburg IT, et al. Long-term neurodevelopmental outcome after intrauterine transfusion for hemolytic disease of the fetus/newborn: the LOTUS study. *Am J Obstet Gynecol.* 2012;206(2):141.e1–141.e8.

58. Weisse ME. The fourth disease, 1900–2000. *Lancet.* 2001;357(9252):299–301.

59. Zimmerman L, Reef S. Congenital rubella syndrome. In: *VPD Surveillance Manual.* 3rd ed. Washington, DC: Centers for Disease Control and Prevention; 2002.

60. Centers for Disease Control and Prevention. Epidemiology and Prevention of Vaccine-Preventable Disease. Atkinson W, Hamborsky J, Wolfe S, et al, eds. 12th ed. Second printing. Washington DC: Public Health Foundation, 2012

61. Ciofi Degli Atti ML, et al. Pediatric sentinel surveillance of vaccine-preventable diseases in Italy. *Pediatr Infect Dis J.* 2002;21(8):763–768.

62. Gabutti G, et al. Epidemiology of measles, mumps and rubella in Italy. *Epidemiol Infect.* 2002;129(3):543–550.

63. Best JM, Bantavala J. Rubella. In: Pattison JR, ed. *Principles and Practice of Clinical Virology.* 4th ed. New York: John Wiley & Sons; 2000:387–418.

64. Horstmann DM, Liebhaber H, Kohorn EI. Post-partum vaccination of rubella-susceptible women. *Lancet.* 1970;2(7681):1003–1006.

65. Miron D, On A. Congenital rubella syndrome after maternal immunization [in Hebrew]. *Harefuah.* 1992;122(5):291–293.

66. Enders G, et al. Outcome of confirmed periconceptional maternal rubella. *Lancet.* 1988;1(8600):1445–1447.

67. Remington J. *Infectious Diseases of the Fetus and Newborn Infant.* 5th ed. Philadelphia, PA: WB Saunders; 2001.

68. Best JM, et al. Interpretation of rubella serology in pregnancy—pitfalls and problems. *BMJ.* 2002;325(7356):147–148.

69. Bosma TJ, et al. PCR for detection of rubella virus RNA in clinical samples. *J Clin Microbiol.* 1995;33(5):1075–1079.

70. Hudson P, Morgan-Capner P. Evaluation of 15 commercial enzyme immunoassays for the detection of rubella-specific IgM. *J Clin Virol.* 1996;5(1):21–26.

71. Almeida JD, Griffith AH. Viral infections and rheumatic factor. *Lancet.* 1980;2(8208–8209):1361–1362.

72. Akingbade D, Cohen BJ, Brown DW. Detection of low-avidity immunoglobulin G in oral fluid samples: new approach for rubella diagnosis and surveillance. *Clin Diagn Lab Immunol.* 2003;10(1):189–190.

73. Ben Salah A, et al. Validation of a modified commercial assay for the detection of rubella-specific IgG in oral fluid for use in population studies. *J Virol Methods.* 2003;114(2):151–158.

74. World Health Organization. *Report of a Meeting on Preventing Congenital Rubella Syndrome: Immunization Strategies, Surveillance Needs.* Geneva, Switzerland: World Health Organization; 2000:12–14.

75. Ramsay ME, et al. Salivary diagnosis of rubella: a study of notified cases in the United Kingdom, 1991–4. *Epidemiol Infect.* 1998;120(3):315–319.

76. Terry GM, et al. First trimester prenatal diagnosis of congenital rubella: a laboratory investigation. *Br Med J (Clin Res Ed).* 1986;292(6525):930–933.

77. Migliucci A, et al. Prenatal diagnosis of congenital rubella infection and ultrasonography: a preliminary study. *Minerva Ginecol.* 2011;63(6):485–489.

78. Ugurbas SH, et al. Microphthalmos: clinical and ultrasonographic findings. *Ann Ophthalmol (Skokie).* 2007;39(2):112–122.

79. Boyle MK, Pretorius DH. Fetal infections. In: Nyberg DA, McGahan JP, Pretorius DH, et al, eds. *Diagnostic Imaging of Fetal Anomalies.* Philadelphia, PA: Lippincott Williams & Wilkins; 2003:756.

80. Andrade J. Congenital Rubella syndrome and fetal exencephaly: a case report. *Ultrasound Obstet Gynecol.* 2000;16(suppl S1):72.

81. Ferreira SM, et al. Semilunar valvar stenosis associated with congenital Rubella syndrome. *Braz J Infect Dis.* 1998;2(5):256–259.

82. Moore JW, Mullins CE. Severe subaortic stenosis associated with congenital rubella syndrome: palliation by percutaneous transcatheter device occlusion of a patent ductus arteriosus. *Pediatr Cardiol.* 1986;7(4):221–223.

83. Varghese PJ, Izukawa T, Rowe RD. Supravalvular aortic stenosis as part of rubella syndrome, with discussion of pathogenesis. *Br Heart J.* 1969;31(1):59–62.

84. Wui ET, Ling LH, Yang H. Severe aortic regurgitation: an exceptional cardiac manifestation of congenital rubella syndrome. *Int J Cardiol.* 2006;113(2):e46–e47.

85. Levy-Bruhl D, Six C, Parent I. Rubella control in France. *Euro Surveill.* 2004;9(4):15–16.

86. Centers for Disease Control and Prevention. Seroprevalence of herpes simplex virus type 2 among persons aged 14–49 years: United States, 2005–2008. *MMWR Morb Mortal Wkly Rep.* 2010;59(15):456–459.

87. Whitley R, Davis EA, Suppapanya N. Incidence of neonatal herpes simplex virus infections in a managed-care population. *Sex Transm Dis.* 2007;34(9):704–708.

88. Clinical manifestations and diagnosis of genital herpes simplex virus infection. *UpToDate.* 2011. http://www.uptodate.com/contents/epidemiology-clinical-manifestations-and-diagnosis-of-genital-herpes-simplex-virus-infection.

89. Dickson N, et al. Risk of herpes simplex virus type 2 acquisition increases over early adulthood: evidence from a cohort study. *Sex Transm Infect.* 2007;83(2):87–90.

90. Lanouette JM, et al. Prenatal diagnosis of fetal herpes simplex infection. *Fetal Diagn Ther.* 1996;11(6):414–416.

91. Jayaram PM, Wake CR. A rare case of absent corpus callosum with severe ventriculomegaly due to congenital herpes simplex infection. *J Obstet Gynaecol.* 2010;30(3):316.

92. Diguet A, et al. Prenatal diagnosis of an exceptional intrauterine herpes simplex type 1 infection. *Prenat Diagn.* 2006;26(2):154–157.

93. Duin LK, et al. Major brain lesions by intrauterine herpes simplex virus infection: MRI contribution. *Prenat Diagn.* 2007;27(1):81–84.

94. World Health Organization. Global summary of the AIDS epidemic: 2009. http://data.unaids.org/pub/report/2009/jc1700_epi_update_2009_en.pdf.

95. World Health Organization. Towards universal access: scaling up priority HIV/AIDS interventions in the health sector. Progress Rep. 2010:97. http://whqlibdoc.who.int/publications/2010/9789241500395_eng.pdf.

96. Branson BM, Handsfield HH, Lampe MA, et al; Centers for Disease Control and Prevention. Revised recommendations for HIV testing of adults, adolescents, and pregnant women in health-care settings. *MMWR Recomm Rep.* 2006;55:1–17.

97. Center, N.H.A.C.C., Compendium of State HIV Testing Laws. 2011. www.hivlawandpolicy.org/.../compendium-state-hiv-testing-laws-quick-reference-guide-clinicians-national-hivaids.

98. Ray N, Doms RW. HIV-1 coreceptors and their inhibitors. *Curr Top Microbiol Immunol.* 2006;303:97–120.

99. Joao EC, et al. Maternal antiretroviral use during pregnancy and infant congenital anomalies: the NISDI perinatal study. *J Acquir Immune Defic Syndr.* 2010;53(2):176–185.

100. Cotter AM, et al. Is antiretroviral therapy during pregnancy associated with an increased risk of preterm delivery, low birth weight, or stillbirth? *J Infect Dis.* 2006;193(9):1195–1201.

101. Kourtis AP, et al. Use of antiretroviral therapy in pregnant HIV-infected women and the risk of premature delivery: a meta-analysis. *AIDS.* 2007;21(5):607–615.

102. Szyld EG, et al. Maternal antiretroviral drugs during pregnancy and infant low birth weight and preterm birth. *AIDS.* 2006;20(18):2345–2353.

103. Tuomala RE, et al. Improved obstetric outcomes and few maternal toxicities are associated with antiretroviral therapy, including highly active antiretroviral therapy during pregnancy. *J Acquir Immune Defic Syndr.* 2005;38(4):449–473.

104. Palaii N. Late intrauterine growth restriction in HIV pregnant women in developed countries. *Ultrasound Obstet Gynecol.* 2009;34(S1):151.

105. Aaron E, et al. Small-for-gestational-age births in pregnant women with HIV, due to severity of HIV disease, not antiretroviral therapy. *Infect Dis Obstet Gynecol.* 2012;2012:135030.

106. Savvidou MD, et al. First trimester maternal uterine artery Doppler examination in HIV-positive women. *HIV Med.* 2011;12(10):632–636.

107. Davies G, et al. Amniocentesis and women with hepatitis B, hepatitis C, or human immunodeficiency virus. *J Obstet Gynaecol Can.* 2003;25(2):145–148, 149–152.

108. Opinion AC, Scheduled cesarean delivery and the prevention of vertical transmission of HIV infection. *Int J Gynaecol Obstet.* 2001;73:279–281.

109. Davis JA, Yawetz S. Management of HIV in the pregnant woman. *Clin Obstet Gynecol.* 2012;55(2):531–540.

110. Department of Health and Human Services, P.o.A.G.f.A.a.A.,Guidelines for the Use of Antiretroviral Agents in Pediatric HIV Infection. 2011:1–268. http://aidsinfo.nih.gov/contentfiles/PediatricGuidelines003005.pdf.

111. Enders G, Miller E. Varicella and herpes zoster in pregnancy and the newborn. In: Arvin AM, Gershon AA, editors. *Varicella-Zoster Virus Virology and Clinical Management.* Cambridge, England: Cambridge University Press; 2000:317–347.

112. Lamont RF, et al. Varicella-zoster virus (chickenpox) infection in pregnancy. *BJOG.* 2011;118(10):1155–1162.

113. Laforet EG, Lynch CL Jr. Multiple congenital defects following maternal varicella; report of a case. *N Engl J Med.* 1947;236(15):534–537.

114. Paryani SG, Arvin AM. Intrauterine infection with varicella-zoster virus after maternal varicella. *N Engl J Med.* 1986;314(24):1542–1546.

115. Smith CK, Arvin AM. Varicella in the fetus and newborn. *Semin Fetal Neonatal Med.* 2009;14(4):209–217.

116. Gardella C, Brown ZA. Managing varicella zoster infection in pregnancy. *Cleve Clin J Med.* 2007;74(4):290–296.

117. Enders G, et al. Consequences of varicella and herpes zoster in pregnancy: prospective study of 1739 cases. *Lancet.* 1994;343(8912):1548–1551.

118. Miller E, Cradock-Watson JE, Ridehalgh MK. Outcome in newborn babies given anti-varicella-zoster immunoglobulin after perinatal maternal infection with varicella-zoster virus. *Lancet.* 1989;2(8659):371–373.

119. Sauerbrei A, Wutzler P. Neonatal varicella. *J Perinatol.* 2001;21(8):545–549.

120. Mandelbrot L. Fetal varicella: diagnosis, management, and outcome. *Prenat Diagn.* 2012;32(6):511–518.

121. Leung J, et al. Evaluation of laboratory methods for diagnosis of varicella. *Clin Infect Dis.* 2010;51(1):23–32.

122. Mendelson E, et al. Laboratory assessment and diagnosis of congenital viral infections: rubella, cytomegalovirus (CMV), varicella-zoster virus (VZV), herpes simplex virus (HSV), parvovirus B19 and human immunodeficiency virus (HIV). *Reprod Toxicol.* 2006;21(4):350–382.

123. Koren G. Congenital varicella syndrome in the third trimester. *Lancet.* 2005;366(9497):1591–1592.

124. Mouly F, et al. Prenatal diagnosis of fetal varicella-zoster virus infection with polymerase chain reaction of amniotic fluid in 107 cases. *Am J Obstet Gynecol.* 1997;177(4):894–898.

125. Tan M, Koren G. Chickenpox in pregnancy: revisited. *Reprod Toxicol.* 2006: 410–420.

126. Verstraelen H, et al. Prenatal ultrasound and magnetic resonance imaging in fetal varicella syndrome: correlation with pathology findings. *Prenat Diagn.* 2003;23:705–709.

127. Fernandez-Aguilar S, et al. Congenital pulmonary airway malformation and congenital varicella infection—a possible association. *Ultrasound Obstet Gynecol.* 2005;26(6):680–682.

128. Watson B, et al. Validity of self-reported varicella disease history in pregnant women attending prenatal clinics. *Public Health Rep.* 2007;122(4):499–506.

129. Salisbury D, Ramsay M, Noakes K. *Immunisation Against Infectious Disease: The Green Book.* 3rd ed. London, England: The Department of Health; 2006:421–442.

130. Balducci J, Rodis JF, Rosengren S, et al. Pregnancy outcome following first-trimester varicella infection. *Obstet Gynecol.* 1992;79:5–6.

131. Siegel M. Congenital malformations following chickenpox, measles, mumps and hepatitis. *JAMA.* 1973;226:1521–1524.

132. Darfour P, de Bievre P, Vinatier N, et al. Varicella and pregnancy. *Eur J Obstet Gynecol Reprod Biol.* 1996;66:119–123.

133. Michie CA, Acolet D, Charlton R, et al. Varicella-zoster contracted in the second trimester of pregnancy. *Pediatr Infect Dis J.* 1992;11:1050–1053.

134. Kotchmar GS Jr, Grose C, Brunell PA. Complete spectrum of the varicella congenital defects syndrome in 5-year-old child. *Pediatr Infect Dis.* 1984;3(2):142–145.

135. Schulze A, Dietzsch HJ. The natural history of varicella embryopathy: a 25-year follow-up. *J Pediatr.* 2000;137(6):871–874.

136. Meyers JD. Congenital varicella in term infants: risk reconsidered. *J Infect Dis.* 1974;129(2):215–217.

137. Elfving M, et al. Maternal enterovirus infection during pregnancy as a risk factor in offspring diagnosed with type 1 diabetes between 15 and 30 years of age. *Exp Diabetes Res.* 2008;2008:271958.

138. Alford CA Jr, Stagno S, Reynolds DW. Congenital toxoplasmosis: clinical, laboratory, and therapeutic considerations, with special reference to subclinical disease. *Bull N Y Acad Med.* 1974;50(2):160–181.

139. Guerina NG, et al. Neonatal serologic screening and early treatment for congenital *Toxoplasma gondii* infection. The New England Regional Toxoplasma Working Group. *N Engl J Med.* 1994;330(26):1858–1863.

140. Kimball AC, Kean BH, Fuchs F. Congenital toxoplasmosis: a prospective study of 4,048 obstetric patients. *Am J Obstet Gynecol.* 1971;111(2):211–218.

141. Dubey JP. Toxoplasmosis. *J Am Vet Med Assoc.* 1994;205(11):1593–1598.

142. Jones JL, et al. Congenital toxoplasmosis: a review. *Obstet Gynecol Surv.* 2001;56(5):296–305.

143. Vogel N, et al. Congenital toxoplasmosis transmitted from an immunologically competent mother infected before conception. *Clin Infect Dis.* 1996;23(5):1055–1060.

144. Dunn D, et al. Mother-to-child transmission of toxoplasmosis: risk estimates for clinical counselling. *Lancet.* 1999;353(9167):1829–1833.

145. Foulon W, et al. Treatment of toxoplasmosis during pregnancy: a multicenter study of impact on fetal transmission and children's sequelae at age 1 year. *Am J Obstet Gynecol.* 1999;180(2, pt 1):410–415.

146. Montoya JG. Laboratory diagnosis of *Toxoplasma gondii* infection and toxoplasmosis. *J Infect Dis.* 2002;185(suppl 1):S73–S82.

147. Wilson M, et al. Evaluation of six commercial kits for detection of human immunoglobulin M antibodies to *Toxoplasma gondii*. The FDA Toxoplasmosis Ad Hoc Working Group. *J Clin Microbiol*. 1997;35(12):3112–3115.

148. Administration, FDA public health advisory: limitations of toxoplasmosis IgM commercial test kits. 1997. http://www.fda.gov/MedicalDevices/Safety/AlertsandNotices/PublicHealthNotifications/ucm062411.htm.

149. Montoya JG, et al. VIDAS test for avidity of *Toxoplasma*-specific immunoglobulin G for confirmatory testing of pregnant women. *J Clin Microbiol*. 2002;40(7):2504–2508.

150. Hohlfeld P, et al. Prenatal diagnosis of congenital toxoplasmosis with a polymerase-chain-reaction test on amniotic fluid. *N Engl J Med*. 1994;331(11):695–699.

151. Foulon W, et al. Prenatal diagnosis of congenital toxoplasmosis: a multicenter evaluation of different diagnostic parameters. *Am J Obstet Gynecol*. 1999;181(4):843–847.

152. Hohlfeld P, et al. Fetal toxoplasmosis: ultrasonographic signs. *Ultrasound Obstet Gynecol*. 1991;1(4):241–244.

153. Malinger G, et al. Prenatal brain imaging in congenital toxoplasmosis. *Prenat Diagn*. 2011;31(9):881–886.

154. Cuillier F. Case of the week #168. TheFetus.net. 2006-02-27. http://sonoworld.com/fetus/case.aspx?id=1696.

155. Garel C. MRI ot the fetal brain. In: *Normal Development and Cerebral Pathologies*. Springer: Berlin; 2004.

156. Gay-Andrieu F, et al. Fetal toxoplasmosis and negative amniocentesis: necessity of an ultrasound follow-up. *Prenat Diagn*. 2003;23(7):558–560.

157. Becker LE. Infections of the developing brain. *AJNR Am J Neuroradiol*. 1992;13(2):537–549.

158. Baron J, et al. The incidence of cytomegalovirus, herpes simplex, rubella, and toxoplasma antibodies in microcephalic, mentally retarded, and normocephalic children. *Pediatrics*. 1969;44(6):932–939.

159. ACOG Practice Bulletin. Perinatal viral and parasitic infections. Number 20, September 2000. (Replaces educational bulletin number 177, February 1993). American College of Obstetrics and Gynecologists.

160. Newton LH, Hall SM. Survey of local policies for prevention of congenital toxoplasmosis. *Commun Dis Rep CDR Rev*. 1994;4(10):R121–R124.

161. Aspock H, Pollak A. Prevention of prenatal toxoplasmosis by serological screening of pregnant women in Austria. *Scand J Infect Dis Suppl*. 1992;84:32–37.

162. Lopez A, et al. Preventing congenital toxoplasmosis. *MMWR Recomm Rep*. 2000;49(RR-2):59–68.

163. Dorangeon PH, et al. The risks of pyrimethamine-sulfadoxine combination in the prenatal treatment of toxoplasmosis. *J Gynecol Obstet Biol Reprod (Paris)*. 1992;21(5):549–556.

164. Remington J. Toxoplasmosis. In: Remington JS, Klein J, eds. *Infectious Diseases of the Fetus and Newborn Infant*. 5th ed. Philadelphia, PA: WB Saunders; 2001:205–346.

165. Gilbert R, Gras L. Effect of timing and type of treatment on the risk of mother to child transmission of *Toxoplasma gondii*. *BJOG*. 2003;110(2):112–120.

166. Foulon W, et al. Impact of primary prevention on the incidence of toxoplasmosis during pregnancy. *Obstet Gynecol*. 1988;72(3, pt 1):363–366.

167. Wilson CB, et al. Development of adverse sequelae in children born with subclinical congenital *Toxoplasma* infection. *Pediatrics*. 1980;66(5):767–774.

168. Chigozie JU. Impact of placental *Plasmodium falciparum* malaria on pregnancy and perinatal outcome in Sub-Saharan Africa. *Yale J Biol Med*. 2007;80(3):95–103.

169. Desai M, et al. Epidemiology and burden of malaria in pregnancy. *Lancet Infect Dis*. 2007;7(2):93–104.

170. Poespoprodjo JR, et al. Vivax malaria: a major cause of morbidity in early infancy. *Clin Infect Dis*. 2009;48(12):1704–1712.

171. Bittencourt AL, et al. Placental involvement in schistosomiasis mansoni: report of four cases. *Am J Trop Med Hyg*. 1980;29(4):571–575.

172. World Health Organization. The global elimination of congenital syphilis: rationale and strategy for action. 2007. http://www.who.int/reproductivehealth/publications/rtis/9789241595858/en/.

173. Centers for Disease Control and Prevention. Sexually transmitted diseases surveillance. 2010. http://www.cdc.gov/STD/stats10/default.htm.

174. World Health Organization. Towards eliminating congenital syphilis. 2011. http://www.who.int/reproductivehealth/topics/rtis/cs_regional_updates/en/.

175. Hawkes S, et al. Effectiveness of interventions to improve screening for syphilis in pregnancy: a systematic review and meta-analysis. *Lancet Infect Dis*. 2011;11(9):684–691.

176. Centers for Disease Control and Prevention. Syphilis. CDC Fact Sheet. 2012.

177. Ingall D. Syphilis. In: Remington JS, Klein JO, eds. *Infectious Diseases of the Fetus and Newborn Infant*. 5th ed. Philadelphia, PA: WB Saunders; 2001:643–681.

178. Kent ME, Romanelli F. Reexamining syphilis: an update on epidemiology, clinical manifestations, and management. *Ann Pharmacother*. 2008;42(2):226–236.

179. Hallak M, et al. Nonimmune hydrops fetalis and fetal congenital syphilis: a case report. *J Reprod Med*. 1992;37(2):173–176.

180. Nathan L, et al. Fetal syphilis: correlation of sonographic findings and rabbit infectivity testing of amniotic fluid. *J Ultrasound Med*. 1993;12(2):97–101.

181. Satin AJ, Twickler DM, Wendel GD Jr. Congenital syphilis associated with dilation of fetal small bowel: a case report. *J Ultrasound Med*. 1992;11(1):49–52.

182. Hill LM, Maloney JB. An unusual constellation of sonographic findings associated with congenital syphilis. *Obstet Gynecol*. 1991;78(5, pt 2):895–897.

183. D'Aunoy R, Pearson B. Intestinal lesions in congenital syphilis. *Arch Pathol*. 1939;27:239–248.

184. Wendel G, Gilstrap LC. Syphilis during pregnancy. In: Gillstrap LC, Faro S, eds. *Infections in Pregnancy*. New York: Alan R. Liss; 1990:115–125.

185. Lucas MJ, Theriot SK, Wendel GD Jr. Doppler systolic-diastolic ratios in pregnancies complicated by syphilis. *Obstet Gynecol*. 1991;77(2):217–222.

186. Schulman H, Miller JN, Dolisi F. The pathophysiology of acute syphilitic funisitis. *Ultrasound Obstet Gynecol*. 1991;1:353–356.

187. Araujo Júnior E, et al. Prenatal diagnosis of congenital syphilis using two- and three-dimensional ultrasonography: case report. *Case Rep Infect Dis*. 2012;2012:478436.

188. Radcliffe M. et al. Single-dose benzathine penicillin in infants at risk of congenital syphilis—results of a randomised study. *S Afr Med J*. 1997;87(1):62–65.

189. Workowski K. Sexually transmitted diseases treatment guidelines. *MMWR Morb Mortal Wkly Rep*. 2010;59(RR-12):1–113.

190. Saloojee H. The prevention and management of congenital syphilis: an overview and recommendations. *Bull World Health Organ*. 2004;82(6):424–430.

191. Jover-Diaz F, et al. Q fever during pregnancy: an emerging cause of prematurity and abortion. *Infect Dis Obstet Gynecol*. 2001;9(1):47–49.

192. Shinar S, Skornick-Rapaport A, Rimon E. Placental abruption remote from term associated with Q fever infection. *Obstet Gynecol*. 2012;120(2, pt 2):503–505.

193. Peker E, Bozdogan E, Dogan M. A rare tuberculosis form: congenital tuberculosis. *Tuberk Toraks*. 2010;58(1):93–96.

194. Carter EJ, Mates S. Tuberculosis during pregnancy: the Rhode Island experience, 1987 to 1991. *Chest*. 1994;106(5):1466–1470.

195. Hamadeh MA, Glassroth J. Tuberculosis and pregnancy. *Chest*. 1992;101(4):1114–1120.

196. Llewelyn M, et al. Tuberculosis diagnosed during pregnancy: a prospective study from London. *Thorax*. 2000;55(2):129–132.

197. Abramowsky CR, Gutman J, Hilinski JA. *Mycobacterium tuberculosis* infection of the placenta: a study of the early (innate) inflammatory response in two cases. *Pediatr Dev Pathol*. 2012;15(2):132–136.

198. Peng W, Yang J, Liu E. Analysis of 170 cases of congenital TB reported in the literature between 1946 and 2009. *Pediatr Pulmonol*. 2011;46(12):1215–1224.

199. Rivera-Alsina ME, et al. Listeria monocytogenes: an important pathogen in premature labor and intrauterine fetal sepsis. *J Reprod Med*. 1983;28(3):212–214.

200. Cheng BR, Kuo DM, Hsieh TT. Perinatal listeriosis: a case report. *Chang Gung Med J*. 1990;13(2):152–156.

201. Valkenburg MH, Essed GG, Potters HV. Perinatal listeriosis underdiagnosed as a cause of pre-term labour? *Eur J Obstet Gynecol Reprod Biol*. 1988;27(4):283–288.

202. Nolla-Salas J, et al. Perinatal listeriosis: a population-based multicenter study in Barcelona, Spain (1990–1996). *Am J Perinatol*. 1998;15(8):461–467.

203. Cassell G. Mycoplasmal infections. In: Remington JS, Klein JO, eds. *Infectious Diseases of the Fetus and Newborn Infant*. 5th ed. Philadelphia, PA: WB Saunders; 2001:733–767.

204. Cassell GH, et al. Ureaplasma urealyticum intrauterine infection: role in prematurity and disease in newborns. *Clin Microbiol Rev*. 1993;6(1):69–87.

205. Cassell GH, et al. Isolation of *Mycoplasma hominis* and *Ureaplasma urealyticum* from amniotic fluid at 16–20 weeks of gestation: potential effect on outcome of pregnancy. *Sex Transm Dis*. 1983;10(4 suppl):294–302.

206. Benacerraf BR, Gatter MA, Ginsburgh F. Ultrasound diagnosis of meconium-stained amniotic fluid. *Am J Obstet Gynecol*. 1984;149(5):570–572.

207. DeVore GR, Platt LD. Ultrasound appearance of particulate matter in amniotic cavity: vernix or meconium? *J Clin Ultrasound*. 1986;14(3):229–230.

208. Romero R, et al. What is amniotic fluid "sludge"? *Ultrasound Obstet Gynecol*. 2007;30(5):793–798.

209. Sherer DM, et al. Sonographically homogeneous echogenic amniotic fluid in detecting meconium-stained amniotic fluid. *Obstet Gynecol*. 1991;78(5, pt 1):819–822.

# First Trimester Values

| Table 1A | Combined Data Comparing Menstrual Age with Mean Gestational Sac Diameter, Crown-Rump Length, and Human Chorionic Gonadotropin (HCG) Levels |

| Menstrual Age (d) | Menstrual Age (wk) | Gestational Sac Size (mm) | Crown-Rump Length (mm) | HCG Level (First IRP), Mean (U/L) | HCG Level (First IRP), Range (U/L) |
|---|---|---|---|---|---|
| 30 | 4.3 | — | — | — | — |
| 31 | 4.4 | — | — | — | — |
| 32 | 4.6 | 3 | — | 1,710 | (1,050–2,800) |
| 33 | 4.7 | 4 | — | 2,320 | (140–3,760) |
| 34 | 4.9 | 5 | — | 3,100 | (1,940–4,980) |
| 35 | 5 | 5.5 | — | 4,090 | (2,580–6,330) |
| 36 | 5.1 | 6 | — | 5,340 | (3,400–8,450) |
| 37 | 5.3 | 7 | — | 6,880 | (4,420–10,810) |
| 38 | 5.4 | 8 | — | 8,770 | (5,680–13,660) |
| 39 | 5.6 | 9 | — | 11,040 | (7,220–17,050) |
| 40 | 5.7 | 10 | 0.2 | 13,730 | (9,050–21,040) |
| 41 | 5.9 | 11 | 0.3 | 15,300 | (10,140–23,340) |
| 42 | 6 | 12 | 0.4 | 16,870 | (11,230–25,640) |
| 43 | 6.1 | 13 | 0.4 | 30,480 | (13,750–30,880) |
| 44 | 6.3 | 14 | 0.5 | 24,560 | (16,650–36,750) |
| 45 | 6.4 | 15 | 0.6 | 29,110 | (19,910–43,220) |
| 46 | 6.6 | 16 | 0.7 | 34,100 | (25,530–50,210) |
| 47 | 6.7 | 17 | 0.8 | 39,460 | (27,470–57,640) |
| 48 | 6.9 | 18 | 0.9 | 45,120 | (31,700–65,380) |
| 49 | 7 | 19 | 1.0 | 50,970 | (36,130–73,280) |
| 50 | 7.1 | 20 | 1.0 | 56,900 | (40,700–81,150) |
| 51 | 7.3 | 21 | 1.1 | 62,760 | (45,300–88,790) |
| 52 | 7.4 | 22 | 1.2 | 68,390 | (49,810–95,990) |
| 53 | 7.6 | 23 | 1.3 | 73,640 | (54,120–102,540) |
| 54 | 7.7 | 24 | 1.4 | 78,350 | (58,100–108,230) |
| 55 | 7.9 | 25 | 1.5 | 82,370 | (61,640–112,870) |
| 56 | 8 | 26 | 1.6 | 85,560 | (64,600–116,310) |
| 57 | 8.1 | 26.5 | 1.7 | — | — |
| 58 | 8.3 | 27 | 1.8 | — | — |
| 59 | 8.4 | 28 | 1.9 | — | — |
| 60 | 8.6 | 29 | 2.0 | — | — |
| 61 | 8.7 | 30 | 2.1 | — | — |
| 62 | 8.9 | 31 | 2.2 | — | — |
| 63 | 9 | 32 | 2.3 | — | — |
| 64 | 9.1 | 33 | 2.4 | — | — |
| 65 | 9.3 | 34 | 2.5 | — | — |
| 66 | 9.4 | 35 | 2.6 | — | — |
| 67 | 9.6 | 36 | 2.8 | — | — |
| 68 | 9.7 | 37 | 2.9 | — | — |
| 69 | 9.9 | 38 | 3.0 | — | — |
| 70 | 10 | 39 | 3.1 | — | — |
| 71 | 10.1 | 40 | 3.2 | — | — |
| 72 | 10.3 | 41 | 3.4 | — | — |
| 73 | 10.4 | 42 | 3.5 | — | — |
| 74 | 10.6 | 43 | 3.7 | — | — |
| 75 | 10.7 | 44 | 3.8 | — | — |
| 76 | 10.9 | 45 | 4.0 | — | — |
| 77 | 11 | 46 | 4.1 | — | — |
| 78 | 11.1 | 47 | 4.2 | — | — |
| 79 | 11.3 | 48 | 4.4 | — | — |
| 80 | 11.4 | 49 | 4.6 | — | — |
| 81 | 11.6 | 50 | 4.8 | — | — |
| 82 | 11.7 | 51 | 5.0 | — | — |
| 83 | 11.9 | 52 | 5.2 | — | — |
| 84 | 12 | 53 | 5.4 | — | — |

IRP, international reference preparation.

Reproduced with permission from Nyberg DA, Hill LM, Bohm-Velez M. *Transvaginal Ultrasound.* St Louis, MO: Mosby-Year Book; 1992; Hadlock FP, Shah YP, Kanon DJ, et al. Crown-rump length: reevaluation of relation to menstrual age (5–18 weeks) with high-resolution real-time US. *Radiology.* 1992;182:501; and Robinson HP. "Gestational sac" volumes as determined by sonar in the first trimester of pregnancy. *BJOG.* 1975;82:100; and data from Daya S, Woods S. Transvaginal ultrasound scanning in early pregnancy and correlation with human chorionic gonadotropin levels. *J Clin Ultrasound.* 1991;19:139.

| Table 1B | Relationship between Mean Sac Diameter and Menstrual Age | |
|---|---|---|
| **Mean Sac Diameter** | **Predicted Age in Days** | **95% CI** |
| 2 | 34.9 | 34.3–35.5 |
| 3 | 35.8 | 35.2–36.3 |
| 4 | 36.6 | 36.1–37.2 |
| 5 | 37.5 | 37.0–38.0 |
| 6 | 38.4 | 37.9–38.9 |
| 7 | 39.3 | 38.9–39.7 |
| 8 | 40.2 | 39.8–40.6 |
| 9 | 41.1 | 40.7–41.4 |
| 10 | 41.9 | 41.6–42.3 |
| 11 | 42.8 | 42.5–43.2 |
| 12 | 43.7 | 43.4–44.0 |
| 13 | 44.6 | 44.3–44.9 |
| 14 | 45.5 | 45.2–45.8 |
| 15 | 46.3 | 46.0–46.6 |
| 16 | 47.2 | 46.9–47.5 |
| 17 | 48.1 | 47.8–48.4 |
| 18 | 49 | 48.6–49.4 |
| 19 | 49.9 | 49.5–50.3 |
| 20 | 50.8 | 50.3–51.2 |
| 21 | 51.6 | 51.2–52.1 |
| 22 | 52.5 | 52.0–53.0 |
| 23 | 53.4 | 52.9–53.9 |
| 24 | 54.3 | 53.7–54.8 |

## Table 2 — Predicted Menstrual Age from Crown-Rump Length Measurements

| Crown-Rump Length (mm) | Menstrual Age (wk) | Crown-Rump Length (mm) | Menstrual Age (wk) |
|---|---|---|---|
| 0.2 | 5.7 | 4.2 | 11.1 |
| 0.3 | 5.9 | 4.4 | 11.3 |
| 0.4 | 6.0 | 4.6 | 11.4 |
| 0.4 | 6.1 | 4.8 | 11.6 |
| 0.5 | 6.3 | 5.0 | 11.7 |
| 0.6 | 6.4 | 5.2 | 11.9 |
| 0.7 | 6.6 | 5.4 | 12.0 |
| 0.8 | 6.7 | 5.5 | 12.1 |
| 0.9 | 6.9 | 5.6 | 12.2 |
| 1.0 | 7.0 | 5.7 | 12.3 |
| 1.0 | 7.1 | 5.8 | 12.3 |
| 1.1 | 7.3 | 5.9 | 12.4 |
| 1.2 | 7.4 | 6.0 | 12.5 |
| 1.3 | 7.6 | 6.1 | 12.6 |
| 1.4 | 7.7 | 6.2 | 12.6 |
| 1.5 | 7.9 | 6.3 | 12.7 |
| 1.6 | 8.0 | 6.4 | 12.8 |
| 1.7 | 8.1 | 6.5 | 12.8 |
| 1.8 | 8.3 | 6.6 | 12.9 |
| 1.9 | 8.4 | 6.7 | 13.0 |
| 2.0 | 8.6 | 6.8 | 13.1 |
| 2.1 | 8.7 | 6.9 | 13.1 |
| 2.2 | 8.9 | 7.0 | 13.2 |
| 2.3 | 9.0 | 7.1 | 13.3 |
| 2.4 | 9.1 | 7.2 | 13.4 |
| 2.5 | 9.3 | 7.3 | 13.4 |
| 2.6 | 9.4 | 7.4 | 13.5 |
| 2.8 | 9.6 | 7.5 | 13.6 |
| 2.9 | 9.7 | 7.6 | 13.7 |
| 3.0 | 9.9 | 7.7 | 13.8 |
| 3.1 | 10.0 | 7.8 | 13.8 |
| 3.2 | 10.1 | 7.9 | 13.9 |
| 3.4 | 10.3 | 8.0 | 14.0 |
| 3.5 | 10.4 | 8.1 | 14.1 |
| 3.7 | 10.6 | 8.2 | 14.2 |
| 3.8 | 10.7 | 8.3 | 14.2 |
| 4.0 | 10.9 | 8.4 | 14.3 |
| 4.1 | 11.0 | — | — |

Reproduced with permission from Hadlock FP, Shah YP, Kanon DJ, et al. Fetal crown-rump length: reevaluation of relation to menstrual age (5–18 weeks) with high-resolution real-time US. *Radiology.* 1992;182:501–505.

## Table 3 — Reference Values for Crown-Rump Length Compared with Gestational Sac Size

| Gestational Sac (mm)[a] | Crown-Rump Length (mm)[b] Percentiles 5th | 50th | 95th |
|---|---|---|---|
| 10 | 0 | 4 | 8 |
| 11 | 0 | 5 | 9 |
| 12 | 0 | 5 | 10 |
| 13 | 1 | 5 | 10 |
| 14 | 1 | 6 | 11 |
| 15 | 1 | 7 | 12 |
| 16 | 1 | 7 | 13 |
| 17 | 2 | 8 | 14 |
| 18 | 2 | 8 | 15 |
| 19 | 2 | 9 | 15 |
| 20 | 3 | 10 | 16 |
| 21 | 3 | 10 | 17 |
| 22 | 4 | 11 | 18 |
| 23 | 4 | 12 | 19 |
| 24 | 5 | 12 | 20 |
| 25 | 5 | 13 | 21 |
| 26 | 6 | 14 | 22 |
| 27 | 6 | 15 | 24 |
| 28 | 7 | 16 | 25 |
| 29 | 7 | 17 | 26 |
| 30 | 8 | 18 | 27 |
| 31 | 9 | 18 | 28 |
| 32 | 9 | 19 | 29 |
| 33 | 10 | 20 | 31 |
| 34 | 11 | 21 | 32 |
| 35 | 12 | 22 | 33 |
| 36 | 12 | 23 | 34 |
| 37 | 13 | 25 | 36 |
| 38 | 14 | 26 | 37 |
| 39 | 15 | 27 | 38 |
| 40 | 16 | 28 | 40 |
| 41 | 17 | 29 | 41 |
| 42 | 18 | 30 | 43 |
| 43 | 19 | 31 | 44 |
| 44 | 20 | 33 | 46 |
| 45 | 21 | 34 | 47 |
| 46 | 22 | 35 | 49 |
| 47 | 23 | 37 | 50 |
| 48 | 24 | 38 | 52 |
| 49 | 25 | 39 | 54 |
| 50 | 26 | 41 | 55 |

[a]Standard deviation = 0.9185 + 0.1599 × gestational sac size.
[b]Crown-rump length = 0.012 × gestational sac size$^2$ + 0.9708 + 0.192 × gestational sac size.
Adapted from Grisolia G, Milano V, Pilu G, et al. Biometry of early pregnancy with transvaginal sonography. *Ultrasound Obstet Gynecol.* 1993;3:403–411.

## Amniotic Fluid Index

| Table 4A | Amniotic Fluid Index (AFI) Values in Centimeters during Normal Pregnancy | | | | |
|---|---|---|---|---|---|
| Gestational Age (wk) | 5th Percentile | 10th Percentile | 50th Percentile | 90th Percentile | 95th Percentile |
| 18 | 4.6 | 5.1 | 6.8 | 9.7 | 11.1 |
| 19 | 5.1 | 5.6 | 7.4 | 10.4 | 12 |
| 20 | 5.5 | 6.1 | 8 | 11.3 | 12.9 |
| 21 | 5.9 | 6.6 | 8.7 | 12.2 | 13.9 |
| 22 | 6.3 | 7.1 | 9.3 | 13.2 | 14.9 |
| 23 | 6.7 | 7.5 | 10 | 14.2 | 15.9 |
| 24 | 7 | 7.9 | 10.7 | 15.2 | 16.9 |
| 25 | 7.3 | 8.2 | 11.4 | 16.1 | 17.8 |
| 26 | 7.5 | 8.4 | 12 | 17 | 18.7 |
| 27 | 7.6 | 8.6 | 12.6 | 17.8 | 19.4 |
| 28 | 7.6 | 8.6 | 13 | 18.4 | 19.9 |
| 29 | 7.6 | 8.6 | 13.4 | 18.8 | 20.4 |
| 30 | 7.5 | 8.5 | 13.6 | 18.9 | 20.6 |
| 31 | 7.3 | 8.4 | 13.6 | 18.9 | 20.6 |
| 32 | 7.1 | 8.1 | 13.6 | 18.7 | 20.4 |
| 33 | 6.8 | 7.8 | 13.3 | 18.2 | 20 |
| 34 | 6.4 | 7.4 | 12.9 | 17.7 | 19.4 |
| 35 | 6 | 7 | 12.4 | 16.9 | 18.7 |
| 36 | 5.6 | 6.5 | 11.8 | 16.2 | 17.9 |
| 37 | 5.1 | 6 | 11.1 | 15.3 | 16.9 |
| 38 | 4.7 | 5.5 | 10.3 | 14.4 | 15.9 |
| 39 | 4.2 | 5 | 9.4 | 13.7 | 14.9 |
| 40 | 3.7 | 4.5 | 8.6 | 12.9 | 13.9 |
| 41 | 3.3 | 4 | 7.8 | 12.3 | 12.9 |

Data from Magann EF, Sanderson M, Martin JN, et al. The amniotic fluid index, single deepest pocket, and two-diameter pocket in normal human pregnancy. *Am J Obstet Gynecol*. 2000;182(6):1581–1588.

| Table 4B | Maximal Vertical Pocket (SDP) Values in Centimeters during Normal Pregnancy | | | | |
|---|---|---|---|---|---|
| Gestational Age (wk) | 5th Percentile | 10th Percentile | 50th Percentile | 90th Percentile | 95th Percentile |
| 18 | 2.7 | 2.9 | 4.1 | 5.9 | 6.4 |
| 19 | 2.8 | 3.1 | 4.3 | 6.1 | 6.6 |
| 20 | 2.9 | 3.2 | 4.4 | 6.2 | 6.7 |
| 21 | 2.9 | 3.3 | 4.5 | 6.3 | 6.8 |
| 22 | 3 | 3.3 | 4.6 | 6.3 | 6.8 |
| 23 | 3 | 3.4 | 4.6 | 6.3 | 6.8 |
| 24 | 3.1 | 3.4 | 4.7 | 6.3 | 6.8 |
| 25 | 3 | 3.3 | 4.7 | 6.3 | 6.8 |
| 26 | 3 | 3.3 | 4.8 | 6.4 | 6.8 |
| 27 | 3 | 3.3 | 4.8 | 6.4 | 6.9 |
| 28 | 3 | 3.3 | 4.8 | 6.4 | 6.9 |
| 29 | 2.9 | 3.3 | 4.8 | 6.4 | 6.9 |
| 30 | 2.9 | 3.3 | 4.8 | 6.4 | 6.9 |
| 31 | 2.9 | 3.2 | 4.8 | 6.5 | 7 |
| 32 | 2.9 | 3.2 | 4.8 | 6.6 | 7.1 |
| 33 | 2.9 | 3.2 | 4.82 | 6.6 | 7.2 |
| 34 | 2.8 | 3.2 | 4.8 | 6.6 | 7.2 |
| 35 | 2.8 | 3.1 | 4.7 | 6.6 | 7.2 |
| 36 | 2.7 | 3.1 | 4.7 | 6.6 | 7.1 |
| 37 | 2.6 | 2.9 | 4.5 | 6.5 | 7 |
| 38 | 2.4 | 2.8 | 4.4 | 6.3 | 6.8 |
| 39 | 2.3 | 2.7 | 4.2 | 6.1 | 6.6 |
| 40 | 2.1 | 2.5 | 3.9 | 5.8 | 6.2 |
| 41 | 1.9 | 2.2 | 3.7 | 5.4 | 5.7 |

Data from Magann EF, Sanderson M, Martin JN, et al. The amniotic fluid index, single deepest pocket, and two-diameter pocket in normal human pregnancy. *Am J Obstet Gynecol*. 2000;182(6):1581–1588.

## Basic Ultrasound Biometry

| Table 5 | Predicted Fetal Measurements at Specific Gestational Age (GA) | | | |
|---|---|---|---|---|
| GA (wk) | Biparietal Diameter (cm)[a] | Head Circumference (cm)[b] | Femur Length (cm)[c] | Abdominal Circumference (cm)[d] |
| 12 | 1.7 | 6.8 | 0.7 | 4.6 |
| 13 | 2.1 | 8.2 | 1.1 | 6.0 |
| 14 | 2.5 | 9.7 | 1.4 | 7.3 |
| 15 | 2.9 | 11.1 | 1.7 | 8.6 |
| 16 | 3.2 | 12.4 | 2.1 | 9.9 |
| 17 | 3.6 | 13.8 | 2.4 | 11.2 |
| 18 | 3.9 | 15.1 | 2.7 | 12.5 |
| 19 | 4.3 | 16.4 | 3.0 | 13.7 |
| 20 | 4.6 | 17.7 | 3.3 | 15.0 |
| 21 | 5.0 | 18.9 | 3.6 | 16.2 |
| 22 | 5.3 | 20.1 | 3.8 | 17.4 |
| 23 | 5.6 | 21.3 | 4.1 | 18.5 |
| 24 | 5.9 | 22.4 | 4.4 | 19.7 |
| 25 | 6.2 | 23.5 | 4.6 | 20.8 |
| 26 | 6.5 | 24.6 | 4.9 | 21.9 |
| 27 | 6.8 | 25.6 | 5.1 | 23.0 |
| 28 | 7.1 | 26.6 | 5.4 | 24.0 |
| 29 | 7.3 | 27.5 | 5.6 | 25.1 |
| 30 | 7.6 | 28.4 | 5.8 | 26.1 |
| 31 | 7.8 | 29.3 | 6.1 | 27.1 |
| 32 | 8.0 | 30.1 | 6.3 | 28.1 |
| 33 | 8.3 | 30.8 | 6.5 | 29.1 |
| 34 | 8.5 | 31.5 | 6.7 | 30.0 |
| 35 | 8.7 | 32.2 | 6.9 | 30.9 |
| 36 | 8.8 | 32.8 | 7.1 | 31.8 |
| 37 | 9.0 | 33.3 | 7.2 | 32.7 |
| 38 | 9.2 | 33.8 | 7.4 | 33.6 |
| 39 | 9.3 | 34.2 | 7.6 | 34.4 |
| 40 | 9.4 | 34.6 | 7.7 | 35.3 |

[a]Biparietal diameter $= -3.08 + 0.41 \times GA - 0.000061 \times GA^2$ (standard deviation, 3 mm).

[b]Head circumference $= -11.48 + 1.56 \times GA - 0.0002548 \times GA^2$ (standard deviation, 1 cm).

[c]Femur length $= -3.91 + 0.427 \times GA - 0.0034 \times GA^2$ (standard deviation, 3 mm).

[d]Abdominal circumference $= -13.3 + 1.61 \times GA - 0.00998 \times GA^2$ (standard deviation, 1.34 cm).

Data from Hadlock FP, Deter RL, Harrist RB, et al. Estimating fetal age: computer assisted analysis of multiple fetal growth parameters. *Radiology.* 1984;152:497–501.

| Table 6 | Reference Values for Abdominal Circumference | | | | |
|---|---|---|---|---|---|
| | Abdominal Circumference (cm) | | | | |
| Menstrual Age (wk) | Percentiles | | | | |
| | 3rd | 10th | 50th | 90th | 97th |
| 14.0 | 6.4 | 6.7 | 7.3 | 7.9 | 8.3 |
| 15.0 | 7.5 | 7.9 | 8.6 | 9.3 | 9.7 |
| 16.0 | 8.6 | 9.1 | 9.9 | 10.7 | 11.2 |
| 17.0 | 9.7 | 10.3 | 11.2 | 12.1 | 12.7 |
| 18.0 | 10.9 | 11.5 | 12.5 | 13.5 | 14.1 |
| 19.0 | 11.9 | 12.6 | 13.7 | 14.8 | 15.5 |
| 20.0 | 13.1 | 13.8 | 15.0 | 16.3 | 17.0 |
| 21.0 | 14.1 | 14.9 | 16.2 | 17.6 | 18.3 |
| 22.0 | 15.1 | 16.0 | 17.4 | 18.8 | 19.7 |
| 23.0 | 16.1 | 17.0 | 18.5 | 20.0 | 20.9 |
| 24.0 | 17.1 | 18.1 | 19.7 | 21.3 | 22.3 |
| 25.0 | 18.1 | 19.1 | 20.8 | 22.5 | 23.5 |
| 26.0 | 19.1 | 20.1 | 21.9 | 23.7 | 24.8 |
| 27.0 | 20.0 | 21.1 | 23.0 | 24.9 | 26.0 |
| 28.0 | 20.9 | 22.0 | 24.0 | 26.0 | 27.1 |
| 29.0 | 21.8 | 23.0 | 25.1 | 27.2 | 28.4 |
| 30.0 | 22.7 | 23.9 | 26.1 | 28.3 | 29.5 |
| 31.0 | 23.6 | 24.9 | 27.1 | 29.4 | 30.6 |
| 32.0 | 24.5 | 25.8 | 28.1 | 30.4 | 31.8 |
| 33.0 | 25.3 | 26.7 | 29.1 | 31.5 | 32.9 |
| 34.0 | 26.1 | 27.5 | 30.0 | 32.5 | 33.9 |
| 35.0 | 26.9 | 28.3 | 30.9 | 33.5 | 34.9 |
| 36.0 | 27.7 | 29.2 | 31.8 | 34.4 | 35.9 |
| 37.0 | 28.5 | 30.0 | 32.7 | 35.4 | 37.0 |
| 38.0 | 29.2 | 30.8 | 33.6 | 36.4 | 38.0 |
| 39.0 | 29.9 | 31.6 | 34.4 | 37.3 | 38.9 |
| 40.0 | 30.7 | 32.4 | 35.3 | 38.2 | 39.9 |

Adapted from Hadlock FP, Deter RL, Harrist RB, et al. Estimating fetal age: computer-assisted analysis of multiple fetal growth parameters. *Radiology.* 1984;152:497–501.

| Table 7 | Reference Values for Head Circumference | | | | |
|---|---|---|---|---|---|

| | Head Circumference (cm) | | | | |
| | Percentiles | | | | |
| Menstrual Age (wk) | 3rd | 10th | 50th | 90th | 97th |
|---|---|---|---|---|---|
| 14.0 | 8.8 | 9.1 | 9.7 | 10.3 | 10.6 |
| 15.0 | 10.0 | 10.4 | 11.0 | 11.6 | 12.0 |
| 16.0 | 11.3 | 11.7 | 12.4 | 13.1 | 13.5 |
| 17.0 | 12.6 | 13.0 | 13.8 | 14.6 | 15.0 |
| 18.0 | 13.7 | 14.2 | 15.1 | 16.0 | 16.5 |
| 19.0 | 14.9 | 15.5 | 16.4 | 17.4 | 17.9 |
| 20.0 | 16.1 | 16.7 | 17.7 | 18.7 | 19.3 |
| 21.0 | 17.2 | 17.8 | 18.9 | 20.0 | 20.6 |
| 22.0 | 18.3 | 18.9 | 20.1 | 21.3 | 21.9 |
| 23.0 | 19.4 | 20.1 | 21.3 | 22.5 | 23.2 |
| 24.0 | 20.4 | 21.1 | 22.4 | 23.7 | 24.3 |
| 25.0 | 21.4 | 22.2 | 23.5 | 24.9 | 25.6 |
| 26.0 | 22.4 | 23.2 | 24.6 | 26.0 | 26.8 |
| 27.0 | 23.3 | 24.1 | 25.6 | 27.0 | 27.9 |
| 28.0 | 24.2 | 25.1 | 26.6 | 28.1 | 29.0 |
| 29.0 | 25.0 | 25.9 | 27.5 | 29.1 | 30.0 |
| 30.0 | 25.8 | 26.8 | 28.4 | 30.0 | 31.0 |
| 31.0 | 26.7 | 27.6 | 29.3 | 31.0 | 31.9 |
| 32.0 | 27.4 | 28.4 | 30.1 | 31.8 | 32.8 |
| 33.0 | 28.0 | 29.0 | 30.8 | 32.6 | 33.6 |
| 34.0 | 28.7 | 29.7 | 31.5 | 33.3 | 34.3 |
| 35.0 | 29.3 | 30.4 | 32.2 | 34.1 | 35.1 |
| 36.0 | 29.9 | 30.9 | 32.8 | 34.7 | 35.8 |
| 37.0 | 30.3 | 31.4 | 33.3 | 35.2 | 36.3 |
| 38.0 | 30.8 | 31.9 | 33.8 | 35.8 | 36.8 |
| 39.0 | 31.1 | 32.2 | 34.2 | 36.2 | 37.3 |
| 40.0 | 31.5 | 32.6 | 34.6 | 36.6 | 37.7 |

Adapted from Hadlock FP, Deter RL, Harrist RB, et al. Estimating fetal age: computer-assisted analysis of multiple fetal growth parameters. *Radiology*. 1984;152:497–501.

| Table 8 | Reference Values for Femur Length |
|---------|-----------------------------------|

| Menstrual Age (wk) | Femur Length (cm) | | | | |
|---|---|---|---|---|---|
| | Percentiles | | | | |
| | 3rd | 10th | 50th | 90th | 97th |
| 14.0 | 1.2 | 1.3 | 1.4 | 1.5 | 1.6 |
| 15.0 | 1.5 | 1.6 | 1.7 | 1.9 | 1.9 |
| 16.0 | 1.7 | 1.8 | 2.0 | 2.2 | 2.3 |
| 17.0 | 2.1 | 2.2 | 2.4 | 2.6 | 2.7 |
| 18.0 | 2.3 | 2.5 | 2.7 | 2.9 | 3.1 |
| 19.0 | 2.6 | 2.7 | 3.0 | 3.3 | 3.4 |
| 20.0 | 2.8 | 3.0 | 3.3 | 3.6 | 3.8 |
| 21.0 | 3.0 | 3.2 | 3.5 | 3.8 | 4.0 |
| 22.0 | 3.3 | 3.5 | 3.8 | 4.1 | 4.3 |
| 23.0 | 3.5 | 3.7 | 4.1 | 4.5 | 4.7 |
| 24.0 | 3.8 | 4.0 | 4.4 | 4.8 | 5.0 |
| 25.0 | 4.0 | 4.2 | 4.6 | 5.0 | 5.2 |
| 26.0 | 4.2 | 4.5 | 4.9 | 5.3 | 5.6 |
| 27.0 | 4.4 | 4.6 | 5.1 | 5.6 | 5.8 |
| 28.0 | 4.6 | 4.9 | 5.4 | 5.9 | 6.2 |
| 29.0 | 4.8 | 5.1 | 5.6 | 6.1 | 6.4 |
| 30.0 | 5.0 | 5.3 | 5.8 | 6.3 | 6.6 |
| 31.0 | 5.2 | 5.5 | 6.0 | 6.5 | 6.8 |
| 32.0 | 5.3 | 5.6 | 6.2 | 6.8 | 7.1 |
| 33.0 | 5.5 | 5.8 | 6.4 | 7.0 | 7.3 |
| 34.0 | 5.7 | 6.0 | 6.6 | 7.2 | 7.5 |
| 35.0 | 5.9 | 6.2 | 6.8 | 7.4 | 7.8 |
| 36.0 | 6.0 | 6.4 | 7.0 | 7.6 | 8.0 |
| 37.0 | 6.2 | 6.6 | 7.2 | 7.9 | 8.2 |
| 38.0 | 6.4 | 6.7 | 7.4 | 8.1 | 8.4 |
| 39.0 | 6.5 | 6.8 | 7.5 | 8.2 | 8.6 |
| 40.0 | 6.6 | 7.0 | 7.7 | 8.4 | 8.8 |

Adapted from Hadlock FP, Deter RL, Harrist RB, et al. Estimating fetal age: computer-assisted analysis of multiple fetal growth parameters. *Radiology*. 1984;152:497–501.

| Table 9 | Reference Values for Abdominal Circumference (AC), Head Circumference (HC), Biparietal Diameter (BPD), and Femur Length (FL) | | | | | | | | | | | |
|---|---|---|---|---|---|---|---|---|---|---|---|---|

| | AC (mm) | | | HC (mm) | | | BPD (mm) | | | FL (mm) | | |
| | Percentiles | | | Percentiles | | | Percentiles | | | Percentiles | | |
| GA (wk) | 5th | 50th | 95th | 5th | 50th | 95th | 5th | 50th | 95th | 5th | 50th | 95th |
|---|---|---|---|---|---|---|---|---|---|---|---|---|
| 14 | 76 | 86 | 97 | 97 | 105 | 113 | 27 | 30 | 32 | 13 | 16 | 18 |
| 15 | 84 | 95 | 107 | 106 | 115 | 123 | 30 | 32 | 35 | 16 | 18 | 21 |
| 16 | 92 | 104 | 117 | 116 | 125 | 134 | 32 | 35 | 38 | 18 | 21 | 23 |
| 17 | 100 | 113 | 127 | 126 | 135 | 146 | 35 | 38 | 41 | 20 | 23 | 26 |
| 18 | 109 | 123 | 138 | 136 | 146 | 157 | 38 | 41 | 45 | 23 | 26 | 29 |
| 19 | 118 | 133 | 150 | 146 | 157 | 170 | 41 | 44 | 48 | 25 | 28 | 32 |
| 20 | 127 | 144 | 162 | 157 | 169 | 182 | 44 | 48 | 52 | 28 | 31 | 35 |
| 21 | 137 | 155 | 174 | 168 | 181 | 195 | 47 | 51 | 55 | 30 | 34 | 37 |
| 22 | 147 | 166 | 187 | 179 | 192 | 207 | 50 | 54 | 59 | 33 | 36 | 40 |
| 23 | 157 | 178 | 200 | 190 | 204 | 220 | 53 | 57 | 62 | 35 | 39 | 43 |
| 24 | 168 | 189 | 213 | 201 | 216 | 233 | 56 | 61 | 66 | 38 | 42 | 46 |
| 25 | 178 | 201 | 226 | 212 | 228 | 246 | 59 | 64 | 69 | 41 | 44 | 49 |
| 26 | 189 | 213 | 239 | 222 | 240 | 258 | 62 | 67 | 73 | 43 | 47 | 51 |
| 27 | 199 | 225 | 253 | 233 | 251 | 270 | 65 | 70 | 76 | 45 | 50 | 54 |
| 28 | 210 | 237 | 266 | 243 | 262 | 282 | 67 | 73 | 80 | 48 | 52 | 57 |
| 29 | 220 | 248 | 279 | 253 | 272 | 293 | 70 | 76 | 83 | 50 | 55 | 59 |
| 30 | 230 | 260 | 292 | 262 | 282 | 304 | 73 | 79 | 86 | 52 | 57 | 61 |
| 31 | 240 | 271 | 305 | 270 | 291 | 314 | 75 | 82 | 89 | 54 | 59 | 64 |
| 32 | 250 | 282 | 317 | 278 | 300 | 323 | 78 | 84 | 92 | 56 | 61 | 66 |
| 33 | 259 | 292 | 329 | 285 | 308 | 331 | 80 | 87 | 94 | 58 | 63 | 68 |
| 34 | 268 | 302 | 340 | 292 | 314 | 339 | 82 | 89 | 97 | 60 | 65 | 70 |
| 35 | 276 | 312 | 350 | 297 | 320 | 345 | 84 | 91 | 99 | 62 | 67 | 72 |
| 36 | 284 | 320 | 360 | 302 | 325 | 350 | 85 | 93 | 101 | 64 | 68 | 74 |
| 37 | 291 | 328 | 369 | 305 | 329 | 354 | 86 | 94 | 102 | 65 | 70 | 75 |
| 38 | 297 | 336 | 377 | 307 | 331 | 357 | 88 | 95 | 103 | 66 | 71 | 77 |
| 39 | 303 | 342 | 384 | 309 | 333 | 358 | 88 | 96 | 105 | 67 | 73 | 78 |
| 40 | 307 | 347 | 390 | 309 | 333 | 359 | 89 | 97 | 105 | 69 | 74 | 79 |

*Note:* $\text{Log}_{10}(AC + 9) = 1.3257977 + 0.0552337 \times GA - 0.0006146 \times GA^2$ (SD = 0.02947); $\text{Log}_{10}(HC + 1) = 1.3369692 + 0.0596493 \times GA - 0.0007494 \times GA^2$ (SD = 0.01887); $\text{Log}_{10}(BPD + 5) = 0.9445108 + 0.0509883 \times MA - 0.0006097 \times GA^2$ (SD = 0.02056); and $FL^5 = -1.1132444 + 0.4263429 \times A33 - 0.0045992 \times GA^2$ (SD = 0.1852).

GA, gestational age; MA, menstrual age.

Reproduced with permission from Snijders RJM, Nicolaides KH. Fetal biometry at 14–40 weeks' gestation. *Ultrasound Obstet Gynecol.* 1994;4:34–38.

| Table 10 | Normal Biometric Ratios of Head Circumference (HC)/Abdominal Circumference (AC), AC/Femur Length (FL), and Biparietal Diameter (BPD)/FL |
|---|---|

| GA (wk) | HC/AC[a] | | | AC/FL[b] | | | BPD/FL[c] | | |
|---|---|---|---|---|---|---|---|---|---|
| | 5th | 50th | 95th | 5th | 50th | 95th | 5th | 50th | 95th |
| 14 | 1.13 | 1.23 | 1.34 | 4.93 | 5.51 | 6.16 | 1.75 | 1.92 | 2.11 |
| 15 | 1.12 | 1.22 | 1.33 | 4.73 | 5.29 | 5.92 | 1.66 | 1.82 | 2.00 |
| 16 | 1.11 | 1.21 | 1.32 | 4.57 | 5.11 | 5.71 | 1.58 | 1.74 | 1.91 |
| 17 | 1.10 | 1.20 | 1.31 | 4.43 | 4.95 | 5.54 | 1.52 | 1.67 | 1.83 |
| 18 | 1.09 | 1.19 | 1.30 | 4.32 | 4.83 | 5.40 | 1.47 | 1.61 | 1.77 |
| 19 | 1.08 | 1.18 | 1.29 | 4.23 | 4.73 | 5.29 | 1.42 | 1.56 | 1.71 |
| 20 | 1.07 | 1.17 | 1.28 | 4.16 | 4.65 | 5.20 | 1.39 | 1.52 | 1.67 |
| 21 | 1.06 | 1.17 | 1.27 | 4.11 | 4.59 | 5.13 | 1.36 | 1.49 | 1.64 |
| 22 | 1.05 | 1.16 | 1.26 | 4.07 | 4.55 | 5.08 | 1.34 | 1.47 | 1.61 |
| 23 | 1.04 | 1.15 | 1.25 | 4.04 | 4.52 | 5.05 | 1.32 | 1.45 | 1.59 |
| 24 | 1.03 | 1.14 | 1.24 | 4.03 | 4.50 | 5.03 | 1.30 | 1.43 | 1.57 |
| 25 | 1.02 | 1.13 | 1.23 | 4.02 | 4.50 | 5.03 | 1.29 | 1.42 | 1.56 |
| 26 | 1.01 | 1.12 | 1.22 | 4.03 | 4.50 | 5.03 | 1.29 | 1.41 | 1.55 |
| 27 | 1.00 | 1.11 | 1.21 | 4.04 | 4.51 | 5.04 | 1.28 | 1.41 | 1.54 |
| 28 | 0.99 | 1.10 | 1.20 | 4.05 | 4.53 | 5.06 | 1.28 | 1.40 | 1.54 |
| 29 | 0.98 | 1.09 | 1.19 | 4.07 | 4.55 | 5.09 | 1.28 | 1.40 | 1.54 |
| 30 | 0.97 | 1.08 | 1.18 | 4.10 | 4.58 | 5.12 | 1.27 | 1.40 | 1.53 |
| 31 | 0.96 | 1.07 | 1.17 | 4.12 | 4.61 | 5.15 | 1.27 | 1.40 | 1.53 |
| 32 | 0.95 | 1.06 | 1.16 | 4.15 | 4.64 | 5.18 | 1.27 | 1.39 | 1.53 |
| 33 | 0.94 | 1.05 | 1.16 | 4.17 | 4.67 | 5.22 | 1.27 | 1.39 | 1.52 |
| 34 | 0.94 | 1.04 | 1.15 | 4.20 | 4.69 | 5.24 | 1.26 | 1.38 | 1.52 |
| 35 | 0.93 | 1.03 | 1.14 | 4.21 | 4.71 | 5.27 | 1.25 | 1.37 | 1.51 |
| 36 | 0.92 | 1.02 | 1.13 | 4.23 | 4.73 | 5.28 | 1.24 | 1.36 | 1.50 |
| 37 | 0.91 | 1.01 | 1.12 | 4.23 | 4.73 | 5.29 | 1.23 | 1.35 | 1.48 |
| 38 | 0.90 | 1.00 | 1.11 | 4.23 | 4.73 | 5.29 | 1.21 | 1.33 | 1.46 |
| 39 | 0.89 | 0.99 | 1.10 | 4.22 | 4.71 | 5.27 | 1.19 | 1.30 | 1.43 |
| 40 | 0.88 | 0.98 | 1.09 | 4.19 | 4.69 | 5.24 | 1.16 | 1.28 | 1.40 |

[a]HC/AC = $0.3668952 - 0.0096 \times GA$ (SD = 0.064) (modified formula to fit published tabular data).
[b]Log (AC/FL) = $1.3260806 - 0.0693157 \times GA + 0.0023154 \times GA^2 - 0.0000248 \times GA^3$ (SD = 0.02942).
[c]Log (BPD/FL) = $1.0205449 - 0.0865895 \times GA + 0.0028771 \times GA^2 - 0.0000321 \times GA^3$ (SD = 0.02458).
GA, gestational age.
Reproduced with permission from Snijders RJM, Nicolaides KH. Fetal biometry at 14–40 weeks' gestation. *Ultrasound Obstet Gynecol*. 1994;4:34–38.

| Table 11 | Estimated Fetal Weight (in Grams) Based on Femur Length (FL) and Abdominal Circumference (AC) |

| | AC (cm) | | | | | | | | | | | | | |
| FL (cm) | 15 | 15.5 | 16 | 16.5 | 17 | 17.5 | 18 | 18.5 | 19 | 19.5 | 20 | 20.5 | 21 | 21.5 |
|---|---|---|---|---|---|---|---|---|---|---|---|---|---|---|
| 3 | 325 | 340 | 356 | 373 | 390 | 409 | 428 | 448 | 469 | 491 | 514 | 538 | 563 | 590 |
| 3.1 | 334 | 350 | 366 | 383 | 401 | 420 | 440 | 460 | 481 | 504 | 527 | 552 | 578 | 604 |
| 3.2 | 345 | 360 | 377 | 394 | 413 | 432 | 452 | 472 | 494 | 517 | 541 | 566 | 592 | 619 |
| 3.3 | 355 | 371 | 388 | 406 | 424 | 444 | 464 | 485 | 507 | 531 | 555 | 580 | 607 | 634 |
| 3.4 | 366 | 382 | 399 | 418 | 436 | 456 | 477 | 498 | 521 | 544 | 569 | 595 | 622 | 650 |
| 3.5 | 377 | 394 | 411 | 430 | 449 | 469 | 490 | 512 | 535 | 559 | 584 | 610 | 637 | 666 |
| 3.6 | 388 | 405 | 423 | 442 | 462 | 482 | 503 | 526 | 549 | 573 | 599 | 625 | 653 | 682 |
| 3.7 | 400 | 417 | 436 | 455 | 475 | 495 | 517 | 540 | 564 | 588 | 614 | 641 | 669 | 699 |
| 3.8 | 412 | 430 | 448 | 468 | 488 | 509 | 531 | 555 | 579 | 604 | 630 | 657 | 686 | 716 |
| 3.9 | 424 | 442 | 461 | 481 | 502 | 524 | 546 | 570 | 594 | 620 | 646 | 674 | 703 | 733 |
| 4 | 437 | 456 | 475 | 495 | 516 | 538 | 561 | 585 | 610 | 636 | 663 | 691 | 720 | 751 |
| 4.1 | 450 | 469 | 489 | 509 | 531 | 553 | 576 | 601 | 626 | 652 | 680 | 709 | 738 | 769 |
| 4.2 | 464 | 483 | 503 | 524 | 546 | 569 | 592 | 617 | 643 | 504 | 697 | 726 | 757 | 788 |
| 4.3 | 478 | 497 | 518 | 539 | 561 | 585 | 609 | 634 | 660 | 504 | 715 | 745 | 776 | 808 |
| 4.4 | 492 | 512 | 533 | 555 | 577 | 601 | 625 | 651 | 677 | 504 | 734 | 764 | 795 | 827 |
| 4.5 | 507 | 527 | 549 | 571 | 594 | 618 | 643 | 668 | 695 | 504 | 753 | 783 | 815 | 847 |
| 4.6 | 522 | 543 | 565 | 587 | 611 | 635 | 660 | 687 | 714 | 504 | 772 | 803 | 835 | 868 |
| 4.7 | 538 | 559 | 581 | 604 | 628 | 653 | 678 | 705 | 733 | 504 | 792 | 823 | 856 | 889 |
| 4.8 | 554 | 576 | 598 | 621 | 646 | 671 | 697 | 724 | 752 | 504 | 812 | 844 | 877 | 911 |
| 4.9 | 571 | 593 | 616 | 639 | 664 | 690 | 716 | 744 | 772 | 504 | 833 | 865 | 899 | 933 |
| 5 | 588 | 610 | 634 | 658 | 683 | 709 | 736 | 764 | 793 | 504 | 855 | 887 | 921 | 956 |
| 5.1 | 606 | 628 | 652 | 677 | 702 | 729 | 756 | 785 | 814 | 504 | 877 | 910 | 944 | 980 |
| 5.2 | 624 | 647 | 671 | 696 | 722 | 749 | 777 | 806 | 836 | 504 | 899 | 933 | 967 | 1,003 |
| 5.3 | 643 | 666 | 691 | 716 | 743 | 770 | 798 | 828 | 858 | 504 | 922 | 956 | 992 | 1,028 |
| 5.4 | 662 | 686 | 711 | 737 | 764 | 791 | 820 | 850 | 881 | 504 | 946 | 981 | 1,016 | 1,053 |
| 5.5 | 682 | 706 | 732 | 758 | 785 | 814 | 843 | 873 | 904 | 504 | 970 | 1,005 | 1,041 | 1,079 |
| 5.6 | 702 | 727 | 753 | 780 | 808 | 836 | 866 | 897 | 928 | 504 | 995 | 1,031 | 1,067 | 1,105 |
| 5.7 | 724 | 749 | 775 | 802 | 831 | 860 | 890 | 921 | 953 | 504 | 1,021 | 1,057 | 1,094 | 1,132 |
| 5.8 | 745 | 771 | 798 | 826 | 854 | 884 | 914 | 946 | 979 | 504 | 1,047 | 1,084 | 1,121 | 1,160 |
| 5.9 | 768 | 794 | 821 | 849 | 878 | 908 | 939 | 971 | 1,005 | 504 | 1,074 | 1,111 | 1,149 | 1,188 |
| 6 | 791 | 818 | 845 | 874 | 903 | 934 | 965 | 998 | 1,031 | 504 | 1,102 | 1,139 | 1,178 | 1,217 |
| 6.1 | 815 | 842 | 870 | 899 | 929 | 960 | 992 | 1,025 | 1,059 | 504 | 1,130 | 1,168 | 1,207 | 1,247 |
| 6.2 | 839 | 867 | 895 | 925 | 955 | 987 | 1,019 | 1,052 | 1,087 | 504 | 1,160 | 1,198 | 1,237 | 1,278 |
| 6.3 | 865 | 893 | 922 | 951 | 982 | 1,014 | 1,047 | 1,081 | 1,116 | 504 | 1,189 | 1,228 | 1,268 | 1,309 |
| 6.4 | 891 | 919 | 949 | 979 | 1,010 | 1,042 | 1,076 | 1,110 | 1,146 | 504 | 1,220 | 1,259 | 1,299 | 1,341 |
| 6.5 | 918 | 946 | 976 | 1,007 | 1,039 | 1,072 | 1,105 | 1,140 | 1,176 | 504 | 1,251 | 1,291 | 1,332 | 1,373 |
| 6.6 | 945 | 975 | 1,005 | 1,036 | 1,068 | 1,101 | 1,136 | 1,171 | 1,207 | 504 | 1,284 | 1,323 | 1,365 | 1,407 |
| 6.7 | 974 | 1,004 | 1,034 | 1,066 | 1,099 | 1,132 | 1,167 | 1,203 | 1,240 | 504 | 1,317 | 1,357 | 1,399 | 1,441 |
| 6.8 | 1,003 | 1,033 | 1,065 | 1,097 | 1,130 | 1,164 | 1,199 | 1,235 | 1,273 | 504 | 1,351 | 1,391 | 1,433 | 1,477 |
| 6.9 | 1,033 | 1,064 | 1,096 | 1,128 | 1,162 | 1,196 | 1,232 | 1,269 | 1,306 | 504 | 1,385 | 1,427 | 1,469 | 1,513 |
| 7 | 1,064 | 1,096 | 1,128 | 1,161 | 1,195 | 1,230 | 1,266 | 1,303 | 1,341 | 504 | 1,421 | 1,463 | 1,506 | 1,550 |
| 7.1 | 1,096 | 1,128 | 1,161 | 1,194 | 1,229 | 1,264 | 1,301 | 1,338 | 1,377 | 504 | 1,458 | 1,500 | 1,543 | 1,588 |
| 7.2 | 1,129 | 1,162 | 1,195 | 1,229 | 1,264 | 1,299 | 1,336 | 1,374 | 1,414 | 504 | 1,495 | 1,538 | 1,581 | 1,626 |
| 7.3 | 1,163 | 1,196 | 1,230 | 1,264 | 1,299 | 1,336 | 1,373 | 1,412 | 1,451 | 504 | 1,534 | 1,577 | 1,621 | 1,666 |
| 7.4 | 1,199 | 1,232 | 1,266 | 1,300 | 1,336 | 1,373 | 1,411 | 1,450 | 1,490 | 504 | 1,573 | 1,616 | 1,661 | 1,707 |
| 7.5 | 1,235 | 1,268 | 1,303 | 1,338 | 1,374 | 1,411 | 1,450 | 1,489 | 1,529 | 504 | 1,614 | 1,657 | 1,702 | 1,749 |
| 7.6 | 1,272 | 1,306 | 1,341 | 1,376 | 1,413 | 1,451 | 1,490 | 1,529 | 1,570 | 504 | 1,655 | 1,699 | 1,745 | 1,791 |
| 7.7 | 1,310 | 1,345 | 1,380 | 1,416 | 1,453 | 1,491 | 1,531 | 1,571 | 1,612 | 504 | 1,698 | 1,742 | 1,788 | 1,835 |
| 7.8 | 1,350 | 1,384 | 1,420 | 1,457 | 1,494 | 1,533 | 1,573 | 1,613 | 1,655 | 504 | 1,741 | 1,786 | 1,833 | 1,880 |
| 7.9 | 1,390 | 1,426 | 1,462 | 1,499 | 1,537 | 1,576 | 1,616 | 1,657 | 1,699 | 504 | 1,786 | 1,832 | 1,878 | 1,926 |
| 8 | 1,432 | 1,468 | 1,505 | 1,542 | 1,580 | 1,620 | 1,660 | 1,702 | 1,744 | 504 | 1,832 | 1,878 | 1,925 | 1,973 |
| 8.1 | 1,475 | 1,511 | 1,549 | 1,586 | 1,625 | 1,665 | 1,706 | 1,748 | 1,791 | 504 | 1,879 | 1,926 | 1,973 | 2,021 |
| 8.2 | 1,520 | 1,556 | 1,594 | 1,632 | 1,671 | 1,712 | 1,753 | 1,795 | 1,838 | 504 | 1,928 | 1,974 | 2,022 | 2,070 |
| 8.3 | 1,566 | 1,603 | 1,640 | 1,679 | 1,719 | 1,759 | 1,801 | 1,844 | 1,887 | 504 | 1,977 | 2,024 | 2,072 | 2,121 |

*(continued)*

| Table 11 | Estimated Fetal Weight (in Grams) Based on Femur Length (FL) and Abdominal Circumference (AC) *(continued)* |
|---|---|

| FL (cm) | 22 | 22.5 | 23 | 23.5 | 24 | 24.5 | 25 | 25.5 | 26 | 26.5 | 27 | 27.5 | 28 | 28.5 |
|---|---|---|---|---|---|---|---|---|---|---|---|---|---|---|
| 3 | 618 | 647 | 677 | 709 | 742 | 777 | 814 | 852 | 892 | 934 | 978 | 1,024 | 1,072 | 1,122 |
| 3.1 | 633 | 662 | 693 | 725 | 759 | 794 | 831 | 870 | 910 | 953 | 997 | 1,044 | 1,092 | 1,143 |
| 3.2 | 648 | 678 | 709 | 742 | 776 | 812 | 849 | 888 | 929 | 972 | 1,017 | 1,064 | 1,113 | 1,164 |
| 3.3 | 663 | 694 | 725 | 758 | 793 | 829 | 867 | 907 | 948 | 991 | 1,037 | 1,084 | 1,134 | 1,185 |
| 3.4 | 679 | 710 | 742 | 776 | 811 | 847 | 886 | 926 | 968 | 1,011 | 1,057 | 1,105 | 1,155 | 1,207 |
| 3.5 | 695 | 727 | 759 | 793 | 829 | 866 | 905 | 945 | 987 | 1,032 | 1,078 | 1,126 | 1,177 | 1,229 |
| 3.6 | 712 | 744 | 777 | 811 | 847 | 885 | 924 | 965 | 1,008 | 1,052 | 1,099 | 1,148 | 1,199 | 1,252 |
| 3.7 | 729 | 761 | 795 | 830 | 866 | 904 | 944 | 985 | 1,028 | 1,073 | 1,121 | 1,170 | 1,221 | 1,275 |
| 3.8 | 747 | 779 | 813 | 848 | 885 | 924 | 964 | 1,006 | 1,049 | 1,095 | 1,143 | 1,192 | 1,244 | 1,298 |
| 3.9 | 765 | 798 | 832 | 868 | 905 | 944 | 984 | 1,027 | 1,071 | 1,117 | 1,165 | 1,215 | 1,267 | 1,322 |
| 4 | 783 | 816 | 851 | 887 | 925 | 964 | 1,006 | 1,048 | 1,093 | 1,139 | 1,188 | 1,238 | 1,291 | 1,346 |
| 4.1 | 802 | 836 | 871 | 907 | 946 | 986 | 1,027 | 1,070 | 1,115 | 1,162 | 1,211 | 1,262 | 1,315 | 1,371 |
| 4.2 | 821 | 855 | 891 | 928 | 967 | 1,007 | 1,049 | 1,093 | 1,138 | 1,186 | 1,235 | 1,287 | 1,340 | 1,396 |
| 4.3 | 841 | 875 | 912 | 949 | 988 | 1,029 | 1,071 | 1,116 | 1,162 | 1,209 | 1,259 | 1,311 | 1,365 | 1,422 |
| 4.4 | 861 | 896 | 933 | 971 | 1,010 | 1,051 | 1,094 | 1,139 | 1,185 | 1,234 | 1,284 | 1,336 | 1,391 | 1,448 |
| 4.5 | 882 | 917 | 954 | 993 | 1,033 | 1,074 | 1,118 | 1,163 | 1,210 | 1,259 | 1,309 | 1,362 | 1,417 | 1,474 |
| 4.6 | 903 | 939 | 976 | 1,015 | 1,056 | 1,098 | 1,142 | 1,187 | 1,235 | 1,284 | 1,335 | 1,388 | 1,444 | 1,501 |
| 4.7 | 924 | 961 | 999 | 1,038 | 1,079 | 1,122 | 1,166 | 1,212 | 1,260 | 1,310 | 1,361 | 1,415 | 1,471 | 1,529 |
| 4.8 | 947 | 984 | 1,022 | 1,062 | 1,103 | 1,146 | 1,191 | 1,237 | 1,286 | 1,336 | 1,388 | 1,442 | 1,498 | 1,557 |
| 4.9 | 969 | 1,007 | 1,046 | 1,086 | 1,128 | 1,171 | 1,216 | 1,263 | 1,312 | 1,363 | 1,415 | 1,470 | 1,527 | 1,585 |
| 5 | 993 | 1,030 | 1,070 | 1,111 | 1,153 | 1,197 | 1,242 | 1,290 | 1,339 | 1,390 | 1,443 | 1,498 | 1,555 | 1,615 |
| 5.1 | 1,016 | 1,055 | 1,095 | 1,136 | 1,179 | 1,223 | 1,269 | 1,317 | 1,367 | 1,418 | 1,471 | 1,527 | 1,584 | 1,644 |
| 5.2 | 1,041 | 1,080 | 1,120 | 1,162 | 1,205 | 1,250 | 1,296 | 1,344 | 1,395 | 1,446 | 1,500 | 1,556 | 1,614 | 1,674 |
| 5.3 | 1,066 | 1,105 | 1,146 | 1,188 | 1,232 | 1,277 | 1,324 | 1,373 | 1,423 | 1,476 | 1,530 | 1,586 | 1,644 | 1,705 |
| 5.4 | 1,091 | 1,131 | 1,172 | 1,215 | 1,259 | 1,305 | 1,352 | 1,401 | 1,452 | 1,505 | 1,560 | 1,617 | 1,675 | 1,736 |
| 5.5 | 1,118 | 1,158 | 1,199 | 1,242 | 1,287 | 1,333 | 1,381 | 1,431 | 1,482 | 1,535 | 1,591 | 1,648 | 1,707 | 1,768 |
| 5.6 | 1,144 | 1,185 | 1,227 | 1,271 | 1,316 | 1,362 | 1,411 | 1,461 | 1,513 | 1,566 | 1,622 | 1,679 | 1,739 | 1,801 |
| 5.7 | 1,172 | 1,213 | 1,255 | 1,299 | 1,345 | 1,392 | 1,441 | 1,491 | 1,544 | 1,598 | 1,654 | 1,712 | 1,772 | 1,834 |
| 5.8 | 1,200 | 1,242 | 1,284 | 1,329 | 1,375 | 1,422 | 1,472 | 1,523 | 1,575 | 1,630 | 1,686 | 1,744 | 1,805 | 1,867 |
| 5.9 | 1,229 | 1,271 | 1,314 | 1,359 | 1,406 | 1,454 | 1,503 | 1,554 | 1,608 | 1,662 | 1,719 | 1,778 | 1,839 | 1,902 |
| 6 | 1,258 | 1,301 | 1,345 | 1,390 | 1,437 | 1,485 | 1,535 | 1,587 | 1,641 | 1,696 | 1,753 | 1,812 | 1,873 | 1,936 |
| 6.1 | 1,289 | 1,331 | 1,376 | 1,421 | 1,469 | 1,518 | 1,568 | 1,620 | 1,674 | 1,730 | 1,787 | 1,847 | 1,908 | 1,972 |
| 6.2 | 1,319 | 1,363 | 1,408 | 1,454 | 1,501 | 1,551 | 1,602 | 1,654 | 1,709 | 1,765 | 1,823 | 1,882 | 1,944 | 2,008 |
| 6.3 | 1,351 | 1,395 | 1,440 | 1,487 | 1,535 | 1,585 | 1,636 | 1,689 | 1,744 | 1,800 | 1,858 | 1,919 | 1,981 | 2,045 |
| 6.4 | 1,384 | 1,428 | 1,473 | 1,520 | 1,569 | 1,619 | 1,671 | 1,724 | 1,779 | 1,836 | 1,895 | 1,955 | 2,018 | 2,082 |
| 6.5 | 1,417 | 1,461 | 1,507 | 1,555 | 1,604 | 1,655 | 1,707 | 1,760 | 1,816 | 1,873 | 1,932 | 1,993 | 2,056 | 2,121 |
| 6.6 | 1,451 | 1,496 | 1,542 | 1,590 | 1,640 | 1,691 | 1,743 | 1,797 | 1,853 | 1,911 | 1,970 | 2,031 | 2,094 | 2,160 |
| 6.7 | 1,486 | 1,531 | 1,578 | 1,626 | 1,676 | 1,727 | 1,780 | 1,835 | 1,891 | 1,949 | 2,009 | 2,070 | 2,134 | 2,199 |
| 6.8 | 1,521 | 1,567 | 1,614 | 1,663 | 1,713 | 1,765 | 1,818 | 1,873 | 1,930 | 1,988 | 2,048 | 2,110 | 2,174 | 2,240 |
| 6.9 | 1,558 | 1,604 | 1,652 | 1,701 | 1,752 | 1,804 | 1,857 | 1,913 | 1,970 | 2,028 | 2,089 | 2,151 | 2,215 | 2,281 |
| 7 | 1,595 | 1,642 | 1,690 | 1,740 | 1,791 | 1,843 | 1,897 | 1,953 | 2,010 | 2,069 | 2,130 | 2,192 | 2,256 | 2,322 |
| 7.1 | 1,633 | 1,681 | 1,729 | 1,779 | 1,830 | 1,883 | 1,938 | 1,994 | 2,051 | 2,110 | 2,171 | 2,234 | 2,299 | 2,365 |
| 7.2 | 1,673 | 1,720 | 1,769 | 1,819 | 1,871 | 1,924 | 1,979 | 2,035 | 2,093 | 2,153 | 2,214 | 2,277 | 2,342 | 2,408 |
| 7.3 | 1,713 | 1,761 | 1,810 | 1,861 | 1,913 | 1,966 | 2,021 | 2,078 | 2,136 | 2,196 | 2,258 | 2,321 | 2,386 | 2,453 |
| 7.4 | 1,754 | 1,802 | 1,852 | 1,903 | 1,955 | 2,009 | 2,065 | 2,122 | 2,180 | 2,240 | 2,302 | 2,365 | 2,431 | 2,498 |
| 7.5 | 1,796 | 1,845 | 1,895 | 1,946 | 1,999 | 2,053 | 2,109 | 2,166 | 2,225 | 2,285 | 2,347 | 2,411 | 2,476 | 2,543 |
| 7.6 | 1,839 | 1,888 | 1,939 | 1,990 | 2,043 | 2,098 | 2,154 | 2,211 | 2,270 | 2,331 | 2,393 | 2,457 | 2,523 | 2,590 |
| 7.7 | 1,883 | 1,933 | 1,983 | 2,035 | 2,089 | 2,144 | 2,200 | 2,258 | 2,317 | 2,378 | 2,440 | 2,504 | 2,570 | 2,638 |
| 7.8 | 1,928 | 1,978 | 2,029 | 2,082 | 2,135 | 2,190 | 2,247 | 2,305 | 2,365 | 2,426 | 2,488 | 2,552 | 2,618 | 2,686 |
| 7.9 | 1,975 | 2,025 | 2,076 | 2,129 | 2,183 | 2,238 | 2,295 | 2,353 | 2,413 | 2,474 | 2,537 | 2,602 | 2,668 | 2,735 |
| 8 | 2,022 | 2,072 | 2,124 | 2,177 | 2,231 | 2,287 | 2,344 | 2,403 | 2,463 | 2,524 | 2,587 | 2,652 | 2,718 | 2,785 |
| 8.1 | 2,071 | 2,121 | 2,173 | 2,227 | 2,281 | 2,337 | 2,394 | 2,453 | 2,513 | 2,575 | 2,638 | 2,702 | 2,769 | 2,837 |
| 8.2 | 2,120 | 2,171 | 2,224 | 2,277 | 2,332 | 2,388 | 2,446 | 2,504 | 2,565 | 2,626 | 2,690 | 2,754 | 2,821 | 2,889 |
| 8.3 | 2,171 | 2,222 | 2,275 | 2,329 | 2,384 | 2,440 | 2,498 | 2,557 | 2,617 | 2,679 | 2,742 | 2,807 | 2,874 | 2,942 |

| Table 11 | Estimated Fetal Weight (in Grams) Based on Femur Length (FL) and Abdominal Circumference (AC) *(continued)* |

| FL (cm) | AC (cm) | | | | | | | | | | | | | |
|---|---|---|---|---|---|---|---|---|---|---|---|---|---|---|
| | 29 | 29.5 | 30 | 30.5 | 31 | 31.5 | 32 | 32.5 | 33 | 33.5 | 34 | 34.5 | 35 | 35.5 |
| 3 | 1,175 | 1,230 | 1,288 | 1,349 | 1,412 | 1,479 | 1,548 | 1,621 | 1,697 | 1,777 | 1,860 | 1,948 | 2,039 | 2,135 |
| 3.1 | 1,196 | 1,252 | 1,310 | 1,371 | 1,435 | 1,502 | 1,572 | 1,645 | 1,722 | 1,802 | 1,886 | 1,973 | 2,065 | 2,161 |
| 3.2 | 1,218 | 1,274 | 1,333 | 1,394 | 1,458 | 1,526 | 1,596 | 1,669 | 1,746 | 1,827 | 1,911 | 1,999 | 2,092 | 2,188 |
| 3.3 | 1,239 | 1,296 | 1,355 | 1,417 | 1,482 | 1,550 | 1,620 | 1,694 | 1,772 | 1,853 | 1,937 | 2,026 | 2,118 | 2,215 |
| 3.4 | 1,262 | 1,319 | 1,378 | 1,441 | 1,506 | 1,574 | 1,645 | 1,720 | 1,797 | 1,879 | 1,964 | 2,052 | 2,145 | 2,242 |
| 3.5 | 1,284 | 1,342 | 1,402 | 1,465 | 1,530 | 1,599 | 1,670 | 1,745 | 1,823 | 1,905 | 1,990 | 2,079 | 2,172 | 2,270 |
| 3.6 | 1,307 | 1,365 | 1,426 | 1,489 | 1,555 | 1,624 | 1,696 | 1,771 | 1,850 | 1,932 | 2,017 | 2,107 | 2,200 | 2,298 |
| 3.7 | 1,331 | 1,389 | 1,450 | 1,514 | 1,580 | 1,649 | 1,722 | 1,797 | 1,876 | 1,959 | 2,045 | 2,134 | 2,228 | 2,326 |
| 3.8 | 1,354 | 1,413 | 1,475 | 1,539 | 1,606 | 1,675 | 1,748 | 1,824 | 1,903 | 1,986 | 2,072 | 2,162 | 2,256 | 2,354 |
| 3.9 | 1,379 | 1,438 | 1,500 | 1,564 | 1,632 | 1,702 | 1,775 | 1,851 | 1,931 | 2,014 | 2,101 | 2,191 | 2,285 | 2,383 |
| 4 | 1,403 | 1,463 | 1,525 | 1,590 | 1,658 | 1,729 | 1,802 | 1,879 | 1,959 | 2,042 | 2,129 | 2,220 | 2,314 | 2,413 |
| 4.1 | 1,429 | 1,489 | 1,551 | 1,617 | 1,685 | 1,756 | 1,830 | 1,907 | 1,987 | 2,071 | 2,158 | 2,249 | 2,344 | 2,442 |
| 4.2 | 1,454 | 1,515 | 1,578 | 1,644 | 1,712 | 1,783 | 1,858 | 1,935 | 2,016 | 2,100 | 2,187 | 2,278 | 2,373 | 2,472 |
| 4.3 | 1,480 | 1,541 | 1,605 | 1,671 | 1,740 | 1,812 | 1,886 | 1,964 | 2,045 | 2,129 | 2,217 | 2,308 | 2,404 | 2,503 |
| 4.4 | 1,507 | 1,568 | 1,632 | 1,699 | 1,768 | 1,840 | 1,915 | 1,993 | 2,074 | 2,159 | 2,247 | 2,339 | 2,434 | 2,533 |
| 4.5 | 1,534 | 1,596 | 1,660 | 1,727 | 1,797 | 1,869 | 1,944 | 2,023 | 2,104 | 2,189 | 2,278 | 2,370 | 2,465 | 2,565 |
| 4.6 | 1,561 | 1,623 | 1,688 | 1,756 | 1,826 | 1,898 | 1,974 | 2,053 | 2,135 | 2,220 | 2,309 | 2,401 | 2,497 | 2,596 |
| 4.7 | 1,589 | 1,652 | 1,717 | 1,785 | 1,855 | 1,928 | 2,004 | 2,084 | 2,166 | 2,251 | 2,340 | 2,432 | 2,528 | 2,628 |
| 4.8 | 1,618 | 1,681 | 1,746 | 1,814 | 1,885 | 1,959 | 2,035 | 2,115 | 2,197 | 2,283 | 2,372 | 2,464 | 2,560 | 2,660 |
| 4.9 | 1,647 | 1,710 | 1,776 | 1,845 | 1,916 | 1,990 | 2,066 | 2,146 | 2,229 | 2,315 | 2,404 | 2,497 | 2,593 | 2,693 |
| 5 | 1,676 | 1,740 | 1,806 | 1,875 | 1,947 | 2,021 | 2,098 | 2,178 | 2,261 | 2,347 | 2,437 | 2,530 | 2,626 | 2,726 |
| 5.1 | 1,706 | 1,770 | 1,837 | 1,906 | 1,978 | 2,053 | 2,130 | 2,210 | 2,294 | 2,380 | 2,470 | 2,563 | 2,659 | 2,760 |
| 5.2 | 1,737 | 1,801 | 1,868 | 1,938 | 2,010 | 2,085 | 2,163 | 2,243 | 2,327 | 2,413 | 2,503 | 2,597 | 2,693 | 2,794 |
| 5.3 | 1,768 | 1,833 | 1,900 | 1,970 | 2,043 | 2,118 | 2,196 | 2,277 | 2,360 | 2,447 | 2,537 | 2,631 | 2,727 | 2,828 |
| 5.4 | 1,799 | 1,865 | 1,933 | 2,003 | 2,076 | 2,151 | 2,229 | 2,310 | 2,394 | 2,482 | 2,572 | 2,665 | 2,762 | 2,863 |
| 5.5 | 1,832 | 1,897 | 1,966 | 2,036 | 2,109 | 2,185 | 2,264 | 2,345 | 2,429 | 2,516 | 2,607 | 2,700 | 2,797 | 2,898 |
| 5.6 | 1,864 | 1,931 | 1,999 | 2,070 | 2,143 | 2,219 | 2,298 | 2,380 | 2,464 | 2,552 | 2,642 | 2,736 | 2,833 | 2,933 |
| 5.7 | 1,898 | 1,964 | 2,033 | 2,104 | 2,178 | 2,254 | 2,333 | 2,415 | 2,500 | 2,587 | 2,678 | 2,772 | 2,869 | 2,969 |
| 5.8 | 1,932 | 1,999 | 2,068 | 2,139 | 2,213 | 2,290 | 2,369 | 2,451 | 2,536 | 2,624 | 2,714 | 2,808 | 2,905 | 3,006 |
| 5.9 | 1,966 | 2,034 | 2,103 | 2,175 | 2,249 | 2,326 | 2,405 | 2,488 | 2,573 | 2,660 | 2,751 | 2,845 | 2,942 | 3,043 |
| 6 | 2,002 | 2,069 | 2,139 | 2,211 | 2,286 | 2,363 | 2,442 | 2,525 | 2,610 | 2,698 | 2,789 | 2,883 | 2,980 | 3,080 |
| 6.1 | 2,038 | 2,105 | 2,175 | 2,248 | 2,323 | 2,400 | 2,480 | 2,562 | 2,647 | 2,736 | 2,827 | 2,921 | 3,018 | 3,118 |
| 6.2 | 2,074 | 2,142 | 2,212 | 2,285 | 2,360 | 2,438 | 2,518 | 2,600 | 2,686 | 2,774 | 2,865 | 2,959 | 3,056 | 3,156 |
| 6.3 | 2,111 | 2,180 | 2,250 | 2,323 | 2,398 | 2,476 | 2,556 | 2,639 | 2,724 | 2,813 | 2,904 | 2,998 | 3,095 | 3,195 |
| 6.4 | 2,149 | 2,218 | 2,289 | 2,362 | 2,437 | 2,515 | 2,595 | 2,678 | 2,764 | 2,852 | 2,943 | 3,037 | 3,134 | 3,235 |
| 6.5 | 2,187 | 2,256 | 2,328 | 2,401 | 2,477 | 2,555 | 2,635 | 2,718 | 2,804 | 2,892 | 2,983 | 3,077 | 3,174 | 3,274 |
| 6.6 | 2,227 | 2,296 | 2,367 | 2,441 | 2,517 | 2,595 | 2,675 | 2,759 | 2,844 | 2,933 | 3,024 | 3,118 | 3,215 | 3,315 |
| 6.7 | 2,267 | 2,336 | 2,408 | 2,481 | 2,557 | 2,636 | 2,716 | 2,800 | 2,885 | 2,974 | 3,065 | 3,159 | 3,256 | 3,355 |
| 6.8 | 2,307 | 2,377 | 2,449 | 2,523 | 2,599 | 2,677 | 2,758 | 2,841 | 2,927 | 3,015 | 3,107 | 3,200 | 3,297 | 3,397 |
| 6.9 | 2,348 | 2,418 | 2,490 | 2,564 | 2,641 | 2,719 | 2,800 | 2,884 | 2,969 | 3,058 | 3,149 | 3,242 | 3,339 | 3,438 |
| 7 | 2,391 | 2,461 | 2,533 | 2,607 | 2,683 | 2,762 | 2,843 | 2,926 | 3,012 | 3,101 | 3,191 | 3,285 | 3,381 | 3,481 |
| 7.1 | 2,433 | 2,504 | 2,576 | 2,650 | 2,727 | 2,806 | 2,887 | 2,970 | 3,056 | 3,144 | 3,235 | 3,328 | 3,424 | 3,523 |
| 7.2 | 2,477 | 2,547 | 2,620 | 2,694 | 2,771 | 2,850 | 2,931 | 3,014 | 3,100 | 3,188 | 3,279 | 3,372 | 3,468 | 3,567 |
| 7.3 | 2,521 | 2,592 | 2,664 | 2,739 | 2,816 | 2,895 | 2,976 | 3,059 | 3,145 | 3,233 | 3,323 | 3,416 | 3,512 | 3,610 |
| 7.4 | 2,566 | 2,637 | 2,710 | 2,785 | 2,861 | 2,940 | 3,021 | 3,105 | 3,190 | 3,278 | 3,368 | 3,461 | 3,557 | 3,655 |
| 7.5 | 2,612 | 2,683 | 2,756 | 2,831 | 2,908 | 2,987 | 3,068 | 3,151 | 3,236 | 3,324 | 3,414 | 3,507 | 3,602 | 3,700 |
| 7.6 | 2,659 | 2,730 | 2,803 | 2,878 | 2,955 | 3,034 | 3,115 | 3,198 | 3,283 | 3,371 | 3,461 | 3,553 | 3,648 | 3,745 |
| 7.7 | 2,707 | 2,778 | 2,851 | 2,926 | 3,002 | 3,081 | 3,162 | 3,245 | 3,330 | 3,418 | 3,508 | 3,600 | 3,694 | 3,791 |
| 7.8 | 2,755 | 2,826 | 2,899 | 2,974 | 3,051 | 3,130 | 3,211 | 3,294 | 3,379 | 3,466 | 3,555 | 3,647 | 3,741 | 3,838 |
| 7.9 | 2,805 | 2,876 | 2,949 | 3,024 | 3,100 | 3,179 | 3,260 | 3,343 | 3,427 | 3,514 | 3,604 | 3,695 | 3,789 | 3,885 |
| 8 | 2,855 | 2,926 | 2,999 | 3,074 | 3,151 | 3,229 | 3,310 | 3,392 | 3,477 | 3,564 | 3,653 | 3,744 | 3,837 | 3,933 |
| 8.1 | 2,906 | 2,977 | 3,050 | 3,125 | 3,202 | 3,280 | 3,360 | 3,443 | 3,527 | 3,614 | 3,702 | 3,793 | 3,886 | 3,981 |
| 8.2 | 2,958 | 3,029 | 3,102 | 3,177 | 3,253 | 3,332 | 3,412 | 3,494 | 3,578 | 3,664 | 3,752 | 3,843 | 3,935 | 4,030 |
| 8.3 | 3,011 | 3,082 | 3,155 | 3,230 | 3,306 | 3,384 | 3,464 | 3,546 | 3,630 | 3,716 | 3,803 | 3,893 | 3,985 | 4,080 |

*(continued)*

| Table 11 | **Estimated Fetal Weight (in Grams) Based on Femur Length (FL) and Abdominal Circumference (AC)** *(continued)* |
|---|---|

| | AC (cm) | | | | | | | | | | | | | | |
|---|---|---|---|---|---|---|---|---|---|---|---|---|---|---|---|
| FL (cm) | 36 | 36.5 | 37 | 37.5 | 38 | 38.5 | 39 | 39.5 | 40 | 40.5 | 41 | 41.5 | 42 | 42.5 | 43 |
| 3 | 2,236 | 2,341 | 2,451 | 2,566 | 2,687 | 2,813 | 2,945 | 3,083 | 3,228 | 3,380 | 3,539 | 3,705 | 3,880 | 4,062 | 4,253 |
| 3.1 | 2,262 | 2,367 | 2,478 | 2,593 | 2,714 | 2,840 | 2,972 | 3,111 | 3,256 | 3,407 | 3,566 | 3,732 | 3,906 | 4,087 | 4,278 |
| 3.2 | 2,289 | 2,394 | 2,505 | 2,620 | 2,741 | 2,868 | 3,000 | 3,138 | 3,283 | 3,434 | 3,593 | 3,758 | 3,932 | 4,113 | 4,303 |
| 3.3 | 2,316 | 2,422 | 2,532 | 2,648 | 2,769 | 2,896 | 3,028 | 3,166 | 3,311 | 3,462 | 3,620 | 3,785 | 3,958 | 4,139 | 4,328 |
| 3.4 | 2,344 | 2,450 | 2,560 | 2,676 | 2,797 | 2,924 | 3,056 | 3,194 | 3,339 | 3,489 | 3,647 | 3,812 | 3,985 | 4,165 | 4,353 |
| 3.5 | 2,371 | 2,478 | 2,588 | 2,704 | 2,825 | 2,952 | 3,084 | 3,222 | 3,367 | 3,517 | 3,675 | 3,839 | 4,011 | 4,191 | 4,379 |
| 3.6 | 2,399 | 2,506 | 2,617 | 2,733 | 2,854 | 2,981 | 3,113 | 3,251 | 3,395 | 3,545 | 3,703 | 3,867 | 4,038 | 4,217 | 4,404 |
| 3.7 | 2,428 | 2,534 | 2,646 | 2,762 | 2,883 | 3,010 | 3,142 | 3,280 | 3,424 | 3,574 | 3,731 | 3,894 | 4,065 | 4,244 | 4,430 |
| 3.8 | 2,457 | 2,563 | 2,675 | 2,791 | 2,912 | 3,039 | 3,171 | 3,309 | 3,452 | 3,602 | 3,759 | 3,922 | 4,093 | 4,270 | 4,456 |
| 3.9 | 2,486 | 2,593 | 2,704 | 2,821 | 2,942 | 3,068 | 3,200 | 3,338 | 3,481 | 3,631 | 3,787 | 3,950 | 4,120 | 4,297 | 4,482 |
| 4 | 2,515 | 2,622 | 2,734 | 2,850 | 2,972 | 3,098 | 3,230 | 3,367 | 3,511 | 3,660 | 3,816 | 3,978 | 4,148 | 4,324 | 4,508 |
| 4.1 | 2,545 | 2,652 | 2,764 | 2,880 | 3,002 | 3,128 | 3,260 | 3,397 | 3,540 | 3,689 | 3,845 | 4,007 | 4,175 | 4,351 | 4,534 |
| 4.2 | 2,575 | 2,683 | 2,794 | 2,911 | 3,032 | 3,159 | 3,290 | 3,427 | 3,570 | 3,719 | 3,874 | 4,035 | 4,203 | 4,378 | 4,561 |
| 4.3 | 2,606 | 2,713 | 2,825 | 2,942 | 3,063 | 3,189 | 3,321 | 3,458 | 3,600 | 3,748 | 3,903 | 4,064 | 4,231 | 4,406 | 4,588 |
| 4.4 | 2,637 | 2,744 | 2,856 | 2,973 | 3,094 | 3,220 | 3,351 | 3,488 | 3,630 | 3,778 | 3,933 | 4,093 | 4,260 | 4,434 | 4,614 |
| 4.5 | 2,668 | 2,776 | 2,888 | 3,004 | 3,125 | 3,251 | 3,383 | 3,519 | 3,661 | 3,809 | 3,962 | 4,122 | 4,288 | 4,461 | 4,641 |
| 4.6 | 2,700 | 2,807 | 2,919 | 3,036 | 3,157 | 3,283 | 3,414 | 3,550 | 3,692 | 3,839 | 3,992 | 4,151 | 4,317 | 4,489 | 4,668 |
| 4.7 | 2,732 | 2,839 | 2,951 | 3,068 | 3,189 | 3,315 | 3,446 | 3,582 | 3,723 | 3,870 | 4,022 | 4,181 | 4,346 | 4,517 | 4,696 |
| 4.8 | 2,764 | 2,872 | 2,984 | 3,100 | 3,221 | 3,347 | 3,478 | 3,613 | 3,754 | 3,901 | 4,053 | 4,211 | 4,375 | 4,546 | 4,723 |
| 4.9 | 2,797 | 2,905 | 3,017 | 3,133 | 3,254 | 3,379 | 3,510 | 3,645 | 3,786 | 3,932 | 4,083 | 4,241 | 4,404 | 4,574 | 4,751 |
| 5 | 2,830 | 2,938 | 3,050 | 3,166 | 3,287 | 3,412 | 3,542 | 3,677 | 3,818 | 3,963 | 4,114 | 4,271 | 4,434 | 4,603 | 4,779 |
| 5.1 | 2,864 | 2,972 | 3,083 | 3,200 | 3,320 | 3,445 | 3,575 | 3,710 | 3,850 | 3,995 | 4,145 | 4,302 | 4,464 | 4,632 | 4,806 |
| 5.2 | 2,898 | 3,005 | 3,117 | 3,233 | 3,354 | 3,479 | 3,608 | 3,743 | 3,882 | 4,027 | 4,177 | 4,332 | 4,494 | 4,661 | 4,835 |
| 5.3 | 2,932 | 3,040 | 3,152 | 3,268 | 3,388 | 3,513 | 3,642 | 3,776 | 3,915 | 4,059 | 4,208 | 4,363 | 4,524 | 4,690 | 4,863 |
| 5.4 | 2,967 | 3,075 | 3,186 | 3,302 | 3,422 | 3,547 | 3,676 | 3,809 | 3,948 | 4,091 | 4,240 | 4,394 | 4,554 | 4,720 | 4,891 |
| 5.5 | 3,002 | 3,110 | 3,221 | 3,337 | 3,457 | 3,581 | 3,710 | 3,843 | 3,981 | 4,124 | 4,272 | 4,426 | 4,584 | 4,749 | 4,920 |
| 5.6 | 3,037 | 3,145 | 3,257 | 3,372 | 3,492 | 3,616 | 3,744 | 3,877 | 4,015 | 4,157 | 4,304 | 4,457 | 4,615 | 4,779 | 4,948 |
| 5.7 | 3,073 | 3,181 | 3,293 | 3,408 | 3,527 | 3,651 | 3,779 | 3,911 | 4,048 | 4,190 | 4,337 | 4,489 | 4,646 | 4,809 | 4,977 |
| 5.8 | 3,110 | 3,218 | 3,329 | 3,444 | 3,563 | 3,686 | 3,814 | 3,946 | 4,082 | 4,224 | 4,370 | 4,521 | 4,677 | 4,839 | 5,006 |
| 5.9 | 3,147 | 3,254 | 3,365 | 3,480 | 3,599 | 3,722 | 3,849 | 3,981 | 4,117 | 4,257 | 4,403 | 4,553 | 4,709 | 4,869 | 5,036 |
| 6 | 3,184 | 3,291 | 3,402 | 3,517 | 3,636 | 3,758 | 3,885 | 4,016 | 4,151 | 4,291 | 4,436 | 4,586 | 4,740 | 4,900 | 5,065 |
| 6.1 | 3,222 | 3,329 | 3,440 | 3,554 | 3,673 | 3,795 | 3,921 | 4,052 | 4,186 | 4,326 | 4,470 | 4,618 | 4,772 | 4,931 | 5,095 |
| 6.2 | 3,260 | 3,367 | 3,478 | 3,592 | 3,710 | 3,832 | 3,957 | 4,087 | 4,222 | 4,360 | 4,503 | 4,651 | 4,804 | 4,962 | 5,125 |
| 6.3 | 3,299 | 3,406 | 3,516 | 3,630 | 3,747 | 3,869 | 3,994 | 4,124 | 4,257 | 4,395 | 4,537 | 4,684 | 4,836 | 4,993 | 5,154 |
| 6.4 | 3,338 | 3,445 | 3,555 | 3,668 | 3,785 | 3,906 | 4,031 | 4,160 | 4,293 | 4,430 | 4,572 | 4,718 | 4,868 | 5,024 | 5,185 |
| 6.5 | 3,377 | 3,484 | 3,594 | 3,707 | 3,824 | 3,944 | 4,069 | 4,197 | 4,329 | 4,465 | 4,606 | 4,751 | 4,901 | 5,056 | 5,215 |
| 6.6 | 3,418 | 3,524 | 3,633 | 3,746 | 3,863 | 3,983 | 4,106 | 4,234 | 4,365 | 4,501 | 4,641 | 4,785 | 4,934 | 5,087 | 5,245 |
| 6.7 | 3,458 | 3,564 | 3,673 | 3,786 | 3,902 | 4,021 | 4,144 | 4,271 | 4,402 | 4,537 | 4,676 | 4,819 | 4,967 | 5,119 | 5,276 |
| 6.8 | 3,499 | 3,605 | 3,714 | 3,826 | 3,941 | 4,060 | 4,183 | 4,309 | 4,439 | 4,573 | 4,711 | 4,854 | 5,000 | 5,151 | 5,307 |
| 6.9 | 3,541 | 3,646 | 3,754 | 3,866 | 3,981 | 4,100 | 4,222 | 4,347 | 4,477 | 4,610 | 4,747 | 4,888 | 5,034 | 5,184 | 5,338 |
| 7 | 3,583 | 3,688 | 3,796 | 3,907 | 4,022 | 4,139 | 4,261 | 4,386 | 4,514 | 4,647 | 4,783 | 4,923 | 5,067 | 5,216 | 5,369 |
| 7.1 | 3,625 | 3,730 | 3,837 | 3,948 | 4,062 | 4,180 | 4,300 | 4,425 | 4,552 | 4,684 | 4,819 | 4,958 | 5,101 | 5,249 | 5,400 |
| 7.2 | 3,668 | 3,772 | 3,880 | 3,990 | 4,103 | 4,220 | 4,340 | 4,464 | 4,591 | 4,721 | 4,855 | 4,994 | 5,136 | 5,282 | 5,432 |
| 7.3 | 3,712 | 3,815 | 3,922 | 4,032 | 4,145 | 4,261 | 4,380 | 4,503 | 4,629 | 4,759 | 4,892 | 5,029 | 5,170 | 5,315 | 5,464 |
| 7.4 | 3,756 | 3,859 | 3,965 | 4,075 | 4,187 | 4,303 | 4,421 | 4,543 | 4,668 | 4,797 | 4,929 | 5,065 | 5,205 | 5,348 | 5,496 |
| 7.5 | 3,800 | 3,903 | 4,009 | 4,118 | 4,230 | 4,344 | 4,462 | 4,583 | 4,708 | 4,835 | 4,966 | 5,101 | 5,240 | 5,382 | 5,528 |
| 7.6 | 3,845 | 3,948 | 4,053 | 4,161 | 4,272 | 4,386 | 4,504 | 4,624 | 4,747 | 4,874 | 5,004 | 5,137 | 5,275 | 5,415 | 5,560 |
| 7.7 | 3,891 | 3,993 | 4,098 | 4,205 | 4,316 | 4,429 | 4,545 | 4,665 | 4,787 | 4,913 | 5,042 | 5,174 | 5,310 | 5,449 | 5,592 |
| 7.8 | 3,937 | 4,039 | 4,143 | 4,250 | 4,359 | 4,472 | 4,587 | 4,706 | 4,827 | 4,952 | 5,080 | 5,211 | 5,346 | 5,484 | 5,625 |
| 7.9 | 3,984 | 4,085 | 4,188 | 4,295 | 4,404 | 4,515 | 4,630 | 4,748 | 4,868 | 4,992 | 5,118 | 5,248 | 5,381 | 5,518 | 5,658 |
| 8 | 4,031 | 4,131 | 4,234 | 4,340 | 4,448 | 4,559 | 4,673 | 4,790 | 4,909 | 5,031 | 5,157 | 5,286 | 5,417 | 5,553 | 5,691 |
| 8.1 | 4,079 | 4,179 | 4,281 | 4,386 | 4,493 | 4,603 | 4,716 | 4,832 | 4,950 | 5,072 | 5,196 | 5,323 | 5,454 | 5,587 | 5,724 |
| 8.2 | 4,127 | 4,226 | 4,328 | 4,432 | 4,539 | 4,648 | 4,760 | 4,875 | 4,992 | 5,112 | 5,235 | 5,361 | 5,490 | 5,622 | 5,758 |
| 8.3 | 4,176 | 4,275 | 4,376 | 4,479 | 4,585 | 4,693 | 4,804 | 4,918 | 5,034 | 5,153 | 5,275 | 5,399 | 5,527 | 5,658 | 5,791 |

*Note:* $\text{Log}_{10} = 1.3598 + (0.051 \times AC) + (0.1844 \times FL) - (0.0037 \times AC \times FL)$.

Reproduced with permission from Hadlock FP, Harrist RB, Carpenter RJ, et al. Sonographic estimation of fetal weight. *Radiology*. 1984;150:535–540.

| Table 12 | Neonatal Birth Weights and Percentiles Based on Gestational Age (GA) Derived by First-Trimester Ultrasound (Males and Females Combined) |
|---|---|

| | Neonatal Weight Percentiles (g) | | | | | | |
|---|---|---|---|---|---|---|---|
| GA (wk) | 5th | 10th | 25th | 50th | 75th | 90th | 95th |
| 25 | 450 | 489 | 564 | 660 | 772 | 890 | 968 |
| 26 | 523 | 568 | 652 | 760 | 885 | 1,016 | 1,103 |
| 27 | 609 | 659 | 754 | 875 | 1,015 | 1,160 | 1,257 |
| 28 | 707 | 764 | 870 | 1,005 | 1,161 | 1,323 | 1,430 |
| 29 | 820 | 884 | 1,003 | 1,153 | 1,327 | 1,505 | 1,623 |
| 30 | 947 | 1,019 | 1,152 | 1,319 | 1,511 | 1,707 | 1,836 |
| 31 | 1,090 | 1,170 | 1,317 | 1,502 | 1,713 | 1,928 | 2,070 |
| 32 | 1,249 | 1,337 | 1,499 | 1,702 | 1,933 | 2,167 | 2,321 |
| 33 | 1,422 | 1,519 | 1,696 | 1,918 | 2,168 | 2,422 | 2,588 |
| 34 | 1,607 | 1,713 | 1,906 | 2,146 | 2,416 | 2,688 | 2,865 |
| 35 | 1,804 | 1,918 | 2,126 | 2,383 | 2,671 | 2,960 | 3,148 |
| 36 | 2,006 | 2,128 | 2,350 | 2,622 | 2,927 | 3,231 | 3,428 |
| 37 | 2,210 | 2,339 | 2,572 | 2,859 | 3,177 | 3,493 | 3,698 |
| 38 | 2,409 | 2,544 | 2,786 | 3,083 | 3,412 | 3,737 | 3,947 |
| 39 | 2,595 | 2,734 | 2,984 | 3,288 | 3,622 | 3,952 | 4,164 |
| 40 | 2,762 | 2,903 | 3,156 | 3,462 | 3,798 | 4,128 | 4,340 |
| 41 | 2,900 | 3,041 | 3,293 | 3,597 | 3,929 | 4,255 | 4,462 |
| 42 | 3,002 | 3,141 | 3,388 | 3,685 | 4,008 | 4,323 | 4,523 |
| 43 | 3,060 | 3,195 | 3,433 | 3,717 | 4,026 | 4,325 | 4,515 |

*Note:* $Ln\,(Wt) = 5.5952 - 0.16626 \times GA + 0.011973 \times GA^2 - 0.0001555 \times GA^3$; and SD of $Ln\,(Wt) = 0.39269 - 0.0063838 \times GA$.
Ln, natural log; Wt, weight.
Data from Doubilet PM, Benson CB, Nadel AS, et al. Improved birth weight table for neonates developed from gestations dated by early ultrasonography. *J Ultrasound Med.* 1997;16:241–249.

| Table 13 | Gender-Specific Reference Values for Neonatal Birth Weights Based on Gestational Age (GA) Derived by First-Trimester Ultrasound |
|---|---|

| | Birth Weights (g) | | | | | | | | | | | | | |
|---|---|---|---|---|---|---|---|---|---|---|---|---|---|---|
| | Males[a] | | | | | | | Females[b] | | | | | | |
| | Percentiles | | | | | | | Percentiles | | | | | | |
| GA (wk) | 5th | 10th | 25th | 50th | 75th | 90th | 95th | 5th | 10th | 25th | 50th | 75th | 90th | 95th |
| 25 | 460 | 501 | 577 | 676 | 791 | 911 | 992 | 450 | 487 | 557 | 646 | 749 | 856 | 927 |
| 26 | 533 | 578 | 664 | 773 | 901 | 1,034 | 1,123 | 526 | 568 | 647 | 748 | 864 | 984 | 1,064 |
| 27 | 617 | 668 | 764 | 886 | 1,028 | 1,175 | 1,273 | 613 | 662 | 751 | 865 | 995 | 1,130 | 1,219 |
| 28 | 715 | 772 | 879 | 1,015 | 1,173 | 1,335 | 1,443 | 713 | 768 | 869 | 997 | 1,144 | 1,294 | 1,393 |
| 29 | 827 | 891 | 1,011 | 1,162 | 1,336 | 1,515 | 1,634 | 827 | 889 | 1,002 | 1,146 | 1,309 | 1,477 | 1,587 |
| 30 | 955 | 1,027 | 1,160 | 1,327 | 1,519 | 1,716 | 1,846 | 955 | 1,024 | 1,151 | 1,311 | 1,493 | 1,678 | 1,800 |
| 31 | 1,099 | 1,179 | 1,326 | 1,511 | 1,722 | 1,937 | 2,078 | 1,097 | 1,174 | 1,316 | 1,493 | 1,694 | 1,898 | 2,032 |
| 32 | 1,259 | 1,348 | 1,510 | 1,713 | 1,943 | 2,177 | 2,331 | 1,253 | 1,339 | 1,496 | 1,691 | 1,911 | 2,135 | 2,281 |
| 33 | 1,435 | 1,532 | 1,710 | 1,931 | 2,181 | 2,434 | 2,599 | 1,423 | 1,517 | 1,689 | 1,902 | 2,143 | 2,385 | 2,543 |
| 34 | 1,625 | 1,731 | 1,924 | 2,164 | 2,433 | 2,704 | 2,881 | 1,603 | 1,706 | 1,893 | 2,125 | 2,384 | 2,646 | 2,815 |
| 35 | 1,827 | 1,941 | 2,149 | 2,406 | 2,693 | 2,982 | 3,169 | 1,792 | 1,904 | 2,105 | 2,354 | 2,632 | 2,911 | 3,092 |
| 36 | 2,036 | 2,159 | 2,380 | 2,653 | 2,957 | 3,260 | 3,456 | 1,986 | 2,105 | 2,321 | 2,586 | 2,881 | 3,176 | 3,366 |
| 37 | 2,248 | 2,377 | 2,611 | 2,897 | 3,215 | 3,530 | 3,734 | 2,180 | 2,306 | 2,534 | 2,813 | 3,123 | 3,431 | 3,630 |
| 38 | 2,455 | 2,591 | 2,834 | 3,130 | 3,458 | 3,783 | 3,991 | 2,368 | 2,500 | 2,738 | 3,029 | 3,350 | 3,669 | 3,874 |
| 39 | 2,651 | 2,790 | 3,040 | 3,343 | 3,677 | 4,006 | 4,217 | 2,544 | 2,681 | 2,926 | 3,225 | 3,554 | 3,880 | 4,088 |
| 40 | 2,826 | 2,967 | 3,220 | 3,525 | 3,860 | 4,189 | 4,398 | 2,701 | 2,841 | 3,091 | 3,394 | 3,727 | 4,054 | 4,264 |
| 41 | 2,971 | 3,112 | 3,364 | 3,667 | 3,997 | 4,320 | 4,525 | 2,831 | 2,972 | 3,223 | 3,526 | 3,858 | 4,184 | 4,391 |
| 42 | 3,078 | 3,216 | 3,462 | 3,757 | 4,078 | 4,389 | 4,587 | 2,928 | 3,068 | 3,316 | 3,615 | 3,941 | 4,259 | 4,462 |
| 43 | 3,138 | 3,271 | 3,507 | 3,790 | 4,094 | 4,390 | 4,577 | 2,986 | 3,122 | 3,364 | 3,654 | 3,968 | 4,275 | 4,470 |

[a]Males: $Ln\,(Wt) = 6.5464 - 0.24681 \times GA + 0.014222 \times GA^2 - 0.00017596 \times GA^3$; SD of $Ln\,(Wt) = 0.39791 - 0.0065856 \times GA$.
[b]Females: $Ln\,(Wt) = 4.4807 - 0.0689 \times GA + 0.0091683 \times GA^2 - 0.00012913 \times GA^3$; SD of $Ln\,(Wt) = 0.35439 - 0.0053902 \times GA$.
Ln, natural log; Wt, weight.
Data from Doubilet PM, Benson CB, Nadel AS, et al. Improved birth weight table for neonates developed from gestations dated by early ultrasonography. *J Ultrasound Med.* 1997;16:241–249.

| Table 14 | Fetal Weight Percentiles by Gestational Age |
| --- | --- |

| | Fetal Weight Percentiles (g) | | | | |
| --- | --- | --- | --- | --- | --- |
| GA (wk) | 3rd | 10th | 50th | 90th | 97th |
| 10 | 26 | 29 | 35 | 41 | 44 |
| 11 | 34 | 37 | 45 | 53 | 56 |
| 12 | 43 | 48 | 58 | 68 | 73 |
| 13 | 54 | 61 | 73 | 85 | 92 |
| 14 | 69 | 77 | 93 | 109 | 117 |
| 15 | 87 | 97 | 117 | 137 | 147 |
| 16 | 109 | 121 | 146 | 171 | 183 |
| 17 | 135 | 150 | 181 | 212 | 227 |
| 18 | 166 | 185 | 223 | 261 | 280 |
| 19 | 204 | 227 | 273 | 319 | 342 |
| 20 | 247 | 275 | 331 | 387 | 415 |
| 21 | 298 | 331 | 399 | 467 | 500 |
| 22 | 357 | 397 | 478 | 559 | 599 |
| 23 | 424 | 472 | 568 | 664 | 712 |
| 24 | 500 | 556 | 670 | 784 | 840 |
| 25 | 586 | 652 | 785 | 918 | 984 |
| 26 | 681 | 758 | 913 | 1,068 | 1,145 |
| 27 | 787 | 876 | 1,055 | 1,234 | 1,323 |
| 28 | 903 | 1,005 | 1,210 | 1,415 | 1,517 |
| 29 | 1,029 | 1,145 | 1,379 | 1,613 | 1,729 |
| 30 | 1,163 | 1,294 | 1,559 | 1,824 | 1,955 |
| 31 | 1,306 | 1,454 | 1,751 | 2,048 | 2,196 |
| 32 | 1,457 | 1,621 | 1,953 | 2,285 | 2,449 |
| 33 | 1,613 | 1,795 | 2,162 | 2,529 | 2,711 |
| 34 | 1,773 | 1,973 | 2,377 | 2,781 | 2,981 |
| 35 | 1,936 | 2,154 | 2,595 | 3,036 | 3,254 |
| 36 | 2,098 | 2,335 | 2,813 | 3,291 | 3,528 |
| 37 | 2,259 | 2,514 | 3,028 | 3,542 | 3,797 |
| 38 | 2,414 | 2,687 | 3,236 | 3,785 | 4,058 |
| 39 | 2,563 | 2,852 | 3,435 | 4,018 | 4,307 |
| 40 | 2,700 | 3,004 | 3,619 | 4,234 | 4,538 |
| 41 | 2,825 | 3,144 | 3,787 | 4,430 | 4,749 |
| 42 | 2,935 | 3,266 | 3,934 | 4,602 | 4,933 |

*Note:* Ln (Wt) $= 0.578 + 0.332$ MA $- 0.00354 \times$ MA$^2$; standard deviation $= 12.7\%$ of predicted weight.
Ln, natural log; MA, menstrual age; Wt, weight.
Reproduced with permission from Hadlock FP, Harrist RB, Marinez-Poyer J. In utero analysis of fetal growth: a sonographic weight standard. *Radiology*. 1991;181:129–133, extrapolated to 42 weeks from 40 weeks.

| Table 15 | Fitted Percentiles for Fractional Arm Volume |

| Menstrual Age (wk) | Fractional Arm Volume (m) | | | | | | | |
|---|---|---|---|---|---|---|---|---|
| | *n* | 5th | 10th | 25th | 50th | 75th | 90th | 95th | 1 SD |
| 18–18.9 | 16 | 1.3 | 1.4 | 1.6 | 1.9 | 2.2 | 2.6 | 2.8 | 1.27 |
| 19–19.9 | 12 | 1.5 | 1.7 | 1.9 | 2.3 | 2.7 | 3.1 | 3.4 | 1.27 |
| 20–20.9 | 11 | 1.9 | 2.1 | 2.4 | 2.9 | 3.3 | 3.8 | 4.2 | 1.26 |
| 21–21.9 | 17 | 2.3 | 2.5 | 2.9 | 3.4 | 4.0 | 4.6 | 5.0 | 1.26 |
| 22–22.9 | 15 | 2.7 | 2.9 | 3.4 | 3.9 | 4.6 | 5.3 | 5.8 | 1.26 |
| 23–23.9 | 12 | 3.4 | 3.7 | 4.3 | 5.0 | 5.8 | 6.7 | 7.3 | 1.26 |
| 24–24.9 | 10 | 3.8 | 4.1 | 4.8 | 5.5 | 6.4 | 7.4 | 8.0 | 1.25 |
| 25–25.9 | 14 | 4.6 | 5.0 | 5.7 | 6.7 | 7.8 | 8.9 | 9.6 | 1.25 |
| 26–26.9 | 13 | 5.4 | 5.9 | 6.7 | 7.8 | 9.1 | 10.4 | 11.3 | 1.25 |
| 27–27.9 | 12 | 6.3 | 6.8 | 7.8 | 9.0 | 10.5 | 12.0 | 13.0 | 1.25 |
| 28–28.9 | 14 | 7.2 | 7.8 | 8.9 | 10.3 | 11.9 | 13.6 | 14.7 | 1.24 |
| 29–29.9 | 11 | 8.2 | 8.9 | 10.1 | 11.7 | 13.6 | 15.5 | 16.8 | 1.24 |
| 30–30.9 | 14 | 9.5 | 10.3 | 11.7 | 13.6 | 15.7 | 17.9 | 19.3 | 1.24 |
| 31–31.9 | 13 | 10.8 | 11.7 | 13.4 | 15.4 | 17.8 | 20.3 | 22.0 | 1.24 |
| 32–32.9 | 15 | 12.5 | 13.5 | 15.4 | 17.8 | 20.5 | 23.3 | 25.2 | 1.24 |
| 33–33.9 | 14 | 14.3 | 15.4 | 17.5 | 20.2 | 23.3 | 26.5 | 28.6 | 1.24 |
| 34–34.9 | 9 | 15.3 | 16.5 | 18.8 | 21.6 | 24.9 | 28.3 | 30.6 | 1.23 |
| 35–35.9 | 13 | 17.3 | 18.7 | 21.2 | 24.4 | 28.1 | 32.0 | 34.5 | 1.23 |
| 36–36.9 | 13 | 19.7 | 21.3 | 24.1 | 27.7 | 31.9 | 36.2 | 39.1 | 1.23 |
| 37–37.9 | 15 | 22.0 | 23.7 | 26.9 | 30.9 | 35.6 | 40.3 | 43.5 | 1.23 |
| 38–38.9 | 45 | 25.0 | 27.0 | 30.6 | 35.1 | 40.3 | 45.7 | 49.2 | 1.23 |
| 39–39.9 | 49 | 26.9 | 28.9 | 32.8 | 37.6 | 43.2 | 48.9 | 52.7 | 1.23 |
| 40–40.9 | 9 | 29.4 | 31.6 | 35.8 | 41.1 | 47.1 | 53.3 | 57.4 | 1.23 |
| 41–41.9 | 13 | 33.6 | 36.1 | 40.8 | 46.8 | 53.7 | 60.7 | 65.3 | 1.22 |
| 42–42.9 | 8 | 35.0 | 37.7 | 42.6 | 48.8 | 55.9 | 63.2 | 68.0 | 1.22 |

Reproduced with permission from Lee W, Balasubramaniam M, Deter RL, et al. Fractional limb volume—a soft tissue parameter of fetal body composition: validation, technical considerations and normal ranges during pregnancy. *Ultrasound Obstet Gynecol.* 2009;33:427–440.

| Table 16 | Fitted Percentiles for Fractional Thigh Volume |
| --- | --- |

| Menstrual Age (wk) | n | Fractional Thigh Volume (m) | | | | | | | |
| --- | --- | --- | --- | --- | --- | --- | --- | --- | --- |
| | | 5th | 10th | 25th | 50th | 75th | 90th | 95th | 1 SD |
| 18–18.9 | 16 | 2.4 | 2.6 | 2.9 | 3.4 | 3.9 | 4.4 | 4.7 | 1.23 |
| 19–19.9 | 12 | 2.9 | 3.2 | 3.6 | 4.1 | 4.7 | 5.4 | 5.8 | 1.23 |
| 20–20.9 | 11 | 3.7 | 4.0 | 4.6 | 5.3 | 6.1 | 6.9 | 7.4 | 1.23 |
| 21–21.9 | 17 | 4.5 | 4.9 | 5.6 | 6.4 | 7.4 | 8.4 | 9.1 | 1.23 |
| 22–22.9 | 15 | 5.3 | 5.7 | 6.5 | 7.5 | 8.6 | 9.8 | 10.6 | 1.24 |
| 23–23.9 | 12 | 6.9 | 7.4 | 8.4 | 9.7 | 11.2 | 12.8 | 13.8 | 1.24 |
| 24–24.9 | 10 | 7.6 | 8.2 | 9.4 | 10.8 | 12.5 | 14.2 | 15.4 | 1.24 |
| 25–25.9 | 14 | 9.3 | 10.1 | 11.5 | 13.3 | 15.3 | 17.5 | 18.9 | 1.24 |
| 26–26.9 | 13 | 11.1 | 12.0 | 13.7 | 15.8 | 18.3 | 20.8 | 22.5 | 1.24 |
| 27–27.9 | 12 | 13.0 | 14.0 | 16.0 | 18.5 | 21.3 | 24.3 | 26.3 | 1.24 |
| 28–28.9 | 14 | 14.9 | 16.1 | 18.3 | 21.2 | 24.5 | 27.9 | 30.2 | 1.24 |
| 29–29.9 | 11 | 17.2 | 18.6 | 21.2 | 24.5 | 28.4 | 32.3 | 35.0 | 1.24 |
| 30–30.9 | 14 | 20.1 | 21.8 | 24.8 | 28.7 | 33.2 | 37.9 | 41.0 | 1.24 |
| 31–31.9 | 13 | 23.1 | 25.0 | 28.6 | 33.1 | 38.3 | 43.7 | 47.2 | 1.24 |
| 32–32.9 | 15 | 26.9 | 29.2 | 33.3 | 38.5 | 44.6 | 50.9 | 55.1 | 1.24 |
| 33–33.9 | 14 | 31.0 | 33.5 | 38.3 | 44.3 | 51.4 | 58.7 | 63.5 | 1.24 |
| 34–34.9 | 9 | 33.3 | 36.1 | 41.2 | 47.8 | 55.4 | 63.2 | 68.4 | 1.24 |
| 35–35.9 | 13 | 38.0 | 41.2 | 47.0 | 54.5 | 63.2 | 72.2 | 78.2 | 1.25 |
| 36–36.9 | 13 | 43.6 | 47.2 | 54.0 | 62.6 | 72.6 | 83.0 | 89.9 | 1.25 |
| 37–37.9 | 15 | 49.1 | 53.1 | 60.8 | 70.5 | 81.8 | 93.5 | 101.3 | 1.25 |
| 38–38.9 | 45 | 56.2 | 61.0 | 69.7 | 80.9 | 93.9 | 107.4 | 116.4 | 1.25 |
| 39–39.9 | 49 | 60.6 | 65.7 | 75.1 | 87.2 | 101.3 | 115.9 | 125.6 | 1.25 |
| 40–40.9 | 9 | 66.6 | 72.2 | 82.6 | 95.9 | 111.4 | 127.5 | 138.2 | 1.25 |
| 41–41.9 | 13 | 76.7 | 83.2 | 95.2 | 110.7 | 128.6 | 147.2 | 159.6 | 1.25 |
| 42–42.9 | 8 | 80.2 | 87.0 | 99.6 | 115.8 | 134.5 | 154.0 | 167.0 | 1.25 |

Reproduced with permission from Lee W, Balasubramaniam M, Deter RL, et al. Fractional limb volume—a soft tissue parameter of fetal body composition: validation, technical considerations and normal ranges during pregnancy. *Ultrasound Obstet Gynecol*. 2009;33:427–440.

## Ultrasound Extremity Measurements

| Table 17 | Ultrasound Reference Values of Major Long Bones |
|---|---|

| GA (wk) | Femur (mm)[a] | | | | Tibia (mm)[b] | | | | Fibula (mm)[c] | | | |
|---|---|---|---|---|---|---|---|---|---|---|---|---|
| | Percentiles | | | | Percentiles | | | | Percentiles | | | |
| | 5th | 50th | 95th | SD | 5th | 50th | 95th | SD | 5th | 50th | 95th | SD |
| 12 | 3.9 | 8.1 | 12.3 | 2.5 | 3.3 | 7.2 | 11.2 | 2.4 | 1.7 | 5.7 | 9.6 | 2.4 |
| 13 | 6.8 | 11.0 | 15.2 | 2.5 | 5.6 | 9.6 | 13.6 | 2.4 | 4.7 | 8.7 | 12.7 | 2.4 |
| 14 | 9.7 | 13.9 | 18.1 | 2.6 | 8.1 | 12.0 | 16.0 | 2.4 | 7.7 | 11.7 | 15.6 | 2.4 |
| 15 | 12.6 | 16.8 | 21.0 | 2.6 | 10.6 | 14.6 | 18.6 | 2.4 | 10.6 | 14.6 | 18.6 | 2.4 |
| 16 | 15.4 | 19.7 | 23.9 | 2.6 | 13.1 | 17.1 | 21.2 | 2.5 | 13.3 | 17.4 | 21.4 | 2.5 |
| 17 | 18.3 | 22.5 | 26.8 | 2.6 | 15.6 | 19.7 | 23.8 | 2.5 | 16.1 | 20.1 | 24.2 | 2.5 |
| 18 | 21.1 | 25.4 | 29.7 | 2.6 | 18.2 | 22.3 | 26.4 | 2.5 | 18.7 | 22.8 | 26.9 | 2.5 |
| 19 | 23.9 | 28.2 | 32.6 | 2.6 | 20.8 | 24.9 | 29.0 | 2.5 | 21.3 | 25.4 | 29.5 | 2.5 |
| 20 | 26.7 | 31.0 | 35.4 | 2.7 | 23.3 | 27.5 | 31.6 | 2.5 | 23.8 | 27.9 | 32.0 | 2.5 |
| 21 | 29.4 | 33.8 | 38.2 | 2.7 | 25.8 | 30.0 | 34.2 | 2.5 | 26.2 | 30.3 | 34.5 | 2.5 |
| 22 | 32.1 | 36.5 | 40.9 | 2.7 | 28.3 | 32.5 | 36.7 | 2.5 | 28.5 | 32.7 | 36.9 | 2.5 |
| 23 | 34.7 | 39.2 | 43.6 | 2.7 | 30.7 | 34.9 | 39.1 | 2.6 | 30.8 | 35.0 | 39.2 | 2.6 |
| 24 | 37.4 | 41.8 | 46.3 | 2.7 | 33.1 | 37.3 | 41.6 | 2.6 | 33.0 | 37.2 | 41.5 | 2.6 |
| 25 | 39.9 | 44.4 | 48.9 | 2.7 | 35.4 | 39.7 | 43.9 | 2.6 | 35.1 | 39.4 | 43.6 | 2.6 |
| 26 | 42.4 | 46.9 | 51.4 | 2.7 | 37.6 | 41.9 | 46.2 | 2.6 | 37.2 | 41.5 | 45.7 | 2.6 |
| 27 | 44.9 | 49.4 | 53.9 | 2.8 | 39.8 | 44.1 | 48.4 | 2.6 | 39.2 | 43.5 | 47.8 | 2.6 |
| 28 | 47.3 | 51.8 | 56.4 | 2.8 | 41.9 | 46.2 | 50.5 | 2.6 | 41.1 | 45.4 | 49.7 | 2.6 |
| 29 | 49.6 | 54.2 | 58.7 | 2.8 | 43.9 | 48.2 | 52.6 | 2.6 | 42.9 | 47.2 | 51.6 | 2.6 |
| 30 | 51.8 | 56.4 | 61.0 | 2.8 | 45.8 | 50.1 | 54.5 | 2.7 | 44.7 | 49.0 | 53.4 | 2.7 |
| 31 | 54.0 | 58.6 | 63.2 | 2.8 | 47.6 | 52.0 | 56.4 | 2.7 | 46.3 | 50.7 | 55.1 | 2.7 |
| 32 | 56.1 | 60.7 | 65.4 | 2.8 | 49.4 | 53.8 | 58.2 | 2.7 | 47.9 | 52.4 | 56.8 | 2.7 |
| 33 | 58.1 | 62.7 | 67.4 | 2.8 | 51.1 | 55.5 | 60.0 | 2.7 | 49.5 | 53.9 | 58.4 | 2.7 |
| 34 | 60.0 | 64.7 | 69.4 | 2.9 | 52.7 | 57.2 | 61.6 | 2.7 | 50.9 | 55.4 | 59.9 | 2.7 |
| 35 | 61.8 | 66.5 | 71.2 | 2.9 | 54.2 | 58.7 | 63.2 | 2.7 | 52.3 | 56.8 | 61.3 | 2.7 |
| 36 | 63.5 | 68.3 | 73.0 | 2.9 | 55.8 | 60.3 | 64.8 | 2.8 | 53.6 | 58.2 | 62.7 | 2.8 |
| 37 | 65.1 | 69.9 | 74.7 | 2.9 | 57.2 | 61.8 | 66.3 | 2.8 | 54.9 | 59.4 | 64.0 | 2.8 |
| 38 | 66.6 | 71.4 | 76.2 | 2.9 | 58.7 | 63.2 | 67.8 | 2.8 | 56.0 | 60.6 | 65.2 | 2.8 |
| 39 | 68.0 | 72.8 | 77.7 | 2.9 | 60.1 | 64.7 | 69.3 | 2.8 | 57.1 | 61.7 | 66.3 | 2.8 |
| 40 | 69.3 | 74.2 | 79.0 | 3.0 | 61.5 | 66.1 | 70.7 | 2.8 | 58.1 | 62.8 | 67.4 | 2.8 |

| GA (wk) | Humerus (mm)[d] | | | | Radius (mm)[e] | | | | Ulna (mm)[f] | | | |
|---|---|---|---|---|---|---|---|---|---|---|---|---|
| | Percentiles | | | | Percentiles | | | | Percentiles | | | |
| | 5th | 50th | 95th | SD | 5th | 50th | 95th | SD | 5th | 50th | 95th | SD |
| 12 | 4.8 | 8.6 | 12.3 | 2.3 | 3.0 | 6.9 | 10.8 | 2.4 | 2.9 | 6.8 | 10.7 | 2.4 |
| 13 | 7.6 | 11.4 | 15.1 | 2.3 | 5.6 | 9.5 | 13.4 | 2.4 | 5.8 | 9.7 | 13.7 | 2.4 |
| 14 | 10.3 | 14.1 | 17.9 | 2.3 | 8.1 | 12.0 | 16.0 | 2.4 | 8.6 | 12.6 | 16.6 | 2.4 |
| 15 | 13.1 | 16.9 | 20.7 | 2.3 | 10.5 | 14.5 | 18.5 | 2.4 | 11.4 | 15.4 | 19.4 | 2.4 |
| 16 | 15.8 | 19.7 | 23.5 | 2.3 | 12.9 | 16.9 | 20.9 | 2.4 | 14.1 | 18.1 | 22.1 | 2.4 |
| 17 | 18.5 | 22.4 | 26.3 | 2.4 | 15.2 | 19.3 | 23.3 | 2.5 | 16.7 | 20.8 | 24.8 | 2.5 |
| 18 | 21.2 | 25.1 | 29.0 | 2.4 | 17.5 | 21.5 | 25.6 | 2.5 | 19.3 | 23.3 | 27.4 | 2.5 |
| 19 | 23.8 | 27.7 | 31.6 | 2.4 | 19.7 | 23.8 | 27.9 | 2.5 | 21.8 | 25.8 | 29.9 | 2.5 |
| 20 | 26.3 | 30.3 | 34.2 | 2.4 | 21.8 | 25.9 | 30.0 | 2.5 | 24.2 | 28.3 | 32.4 | 2.5 |
| 21 | 28.8 | 32.8 | 36.7 | 2.4 | 23.9 | 28.0 | 32.2 | 2.5 | 26.5 | 30.6 | 34.8 | 2.5 |
| 22 | 31.2 | 35.2 | 39.2 | 2.4 | 25.9 | 30.1 | 34.2 | 2.5 | 28.7 | 32.9 | 37.1 | 2.5 |
| 23 | 33.5 | 37.5 | 41.6 | 2.4 | 27.9 | 32.0 | 36.2 | 2.5 | 30.9 | 35.1 | 39.3 | 2.5 |
| 24 | 35.7 | 39.8 | 43.8 | 2.5 | 29.7 | 34.0 | 38.2 | 2.6 | 33.0 | 37.2 | 41.5 | 2.6 |
| 25 | 37.9 | 41.9 | 46.0 | 2.5 | 31.6 | 35.8 | 40.0 | 2.6 | 35.1 | 39.3 | 43.5 | 2.6 |
| 26 | 39.9 | 44.0 | 48.1 | 2.5 | 33.3 | 37.6 | 41.9 | 2.6 | 37.0 | 41.3 | 45.6 | 2.6 |
| 27 | 41.9 | 46.0 | 50.1 | 2.5 | 35.0 | 39.3 | 43.6 | 2.6 | 38.9 | 43.2 | 47.5 | 2.6 |
| 28 | 43.7 | 47.9 | 52.0 | 2.5 | 36.7 | 41.0 | 45.3 | 2.6 | 40.7 | 45.0 | 49.3 | 2.6 |
| 29 | 45.5 | 49.7 | 53.9 | 2.5 | 38.3 | 42.6 | 46.9 | 2.6 | 42.5 | 46.8 | 51.1 | 2.6 |
| 30 | 47.2 | 51.4 | 55.6 | 2.6 | 39.8 | 44.1 | 48.5 | 2.7 | 44.1 | 48.5 | 52.8 | 2.7 |

*(continued)*

| GA (wk) | Humerus (mm)[d] | | | | Radius (mm)[e] | | | | Ulna (mm)[f] | | | |
|---|---|---|---|---|---|---|---|---|---|---|---|---|
| | Percentiles | | | | Percentiles | | | | Percentiles | | | |
| | 5th | 50th | 95th | SD | 5th | 50th | 95th | SD | 5th | 50th | 95th | SD |
| 31 | 48.9 | 53.1 | 57.3 | 2.6 | 41.2 | 45.6 | 50.0 | 2.7 | 45.7 | 50.1 | 54.5 | 2.7 |
| 32 | 50.4 | 54.7 | 58.9 | 2.6 | 42.6 | 47.0 | 51.4 | 2.7 | 47.2 | 51.6 | 56.1 | 2.7 |
| 33 | 52.0 | 56.2 | 60.5 | 2.6 | 44.0 | 48.4 | 52.8 | 2.7 | 48.7 | 53.1 | 57.5 | 2.7 |
| 34 | 53.4 | 57.7 | 62.0 | 2.6 | 45.2 | 49.7 | 54.1 | 2.7 | 50.0 | 54.5 | 59.0 | 2.7 |
| 35 | 54.8 | 59.2 | 63.5 | 2.6 | 46.4 | 50.9 | 55.4 | 2.7 | 51.3 | 55.8 | 60.3 | 2.7 |
| 36 | 56.2 | 60.6 | 64.9 | 2.6 | 47.6 | 52.1 | 56.6 | 2.7 | 52.6 | 57.1 | 61.6 | 2.7 |
| 37 | 57.6 | 62.0 | 66.4 | 2.7 | 48.7 | 53.2 | 57.7 | 2.8 | 53.7 | 58.2 | 62.8 | 2.8 |
| 38 | 59.0 | 63.4 | 67.8 | 2.7 | 49.7 | 54.2 | 58.8 | 2.8 | 54.8 | 59.3 | 63.9 | 2.8 |
| 39 | 60.4 | 64.8 | 69.3 | 2.7 | 50.6 | 55.2 | 59.8 | 2.8 | 55.8 | 60.4 | 64.9 | 2.8 |
| 40 | 61.9 | 66.3 | 70.8 | 2.7 | 51.5 | 56.2 | 60.8 | 2.8 | 56.7 | 61.3 | 65.9 | 2.8 |

[a]Femur (mean) = $-25.252 + 2.555 \times GA + 0.027566 \times GA^2 - 0.00073286 \times GA^3$ (Jeanty et al., 1984).
[b]Tibia (mean) = $5.555 - 0.915554 \times GA + 0.23359 \times GA^2 - 0.00638 \times GA^3 + 0.000055801 \times GA^4$ (Jeanty et al., 1984).
[c]Fibula (mean) = $-36.563 + 3.963 \times GA - 0.037 \times GA^2$ (Exacoustos et al., 1991).
[d]Humerus (mean) = $-16.24 + 0.76315 \times GA + 0.1683 \times GA^2 - 0.0056212 \times GA^3 + 0.000055666 \times GA^4$.
[e]Radius (mean) = $-29.09 + 3.371 \times GA - 0.031 \times GA^2$ (Exacoustos et al., 1991).
[f]Ulna (mean) = $-34.313 + 3.8685 \times GA - 0.036949 \times GA^2$ (Jeanty et al., 1984).
GA, gestational age.
Derived from compilation of data: Jeanty P, Cousaert E, Cantraine F, et al. A longitudinal study of fetal limb growth. *Am J Perinatol*. 1984;1:136–144; Merz E, Grubner A, Kern F. Mathematical modeling of fetal limb growth. *J Clin Ultrasound*. 1989;17:179–185; and Exacoustos C, Rosati P, Rizzo G, et al. Ultrasound measurements of fetal limb bones. *Ultrasound Obstet Gynecol*. 1991;1:325–330.

**Table 18**    **Ultrasound Reference Values for Foot Length**

| GA (wk) | Foot Length (mm) | | |
|---|---|---|---|
| | −2 SD | Mean | +2 SD |
| 12 | 7 | 8 | 9 |
| 13 | 10 | 11 | 12 |
| 14 | 13 | 15 | 16 |
| 15 | 16 | 18 | 20 |
| 16 | 19 | 21 | 23 |
| 17 | 21 | 24 | 27 |
| 18 | 24 | 27 | 30 |
| 19 | 27 | 30 | 33 |
| 20 | 30 | 33 | 37 |
| 21 | 32 | 36 | 40 |
| 22 | 35 | 39 | 43 |
| 23 | 37 | 42 | 46 |
| 24 | 40 | 45 | 49 |
| 25 | 42 | 47 | 52 |
| 26 | 44 | 50 | 55 |
| 27 | 47 | 53 | 58 |
| 28 | 49 | 55 | 61 |
| 29 | 51 | 58 | 64 |
| 30 | 53 | 60 | 66 |
| 31 | 56 | 62 | 69 |
| 32 | 58 | 65 | 72 |
| 33 | 60 | 67 | 74 |
| 34 | 62 | 69 | 77 |
| 35 | 63 | 71 | 79 |
| 36 | 65 | 74 | 81 |
| 37 | 67 | 76 | 84 |
| 38 | 69 | 78 | 86 |
| 39 | 71 | 80 | 88 |
| 40 | 72 | 81 | 90 |

*Note:* Modified formula to fit tabular data: foot length = $-0.02728 \times GA^2 + 4.045 \times GA - 36.74$ (range ± 11%).
GA, gestational age.
Reproduced with permission from Mercer BM, Sklar S, Shariatmadar A, et al. Fetal foot length as a predictor of gestational age. *Am J Obstet Gynecol*. 1987;156:350–355.

**Table 19**    **Ultrasound Scapular Length (±2 SD) Compared with Gestational Age**

| Gestational Age (wk) | Scapular Length (mm) | | |
|---|---|---|---|
| | −2 SD | Mean | +2 SD |
| 14 | 10 | 10 | 10 |
| 15 | 11 | 11 | 11 |
| 16 | 12 | 12 | 12 |
| 17 | 13 | 13 | 13 |
| 18 | 14 | 14 | 14 |
| 19 | 14 | 15 | 15 |
| 20 | 15 | 16 | 16 |
| 21 | 16 | 17 | 17 |
| 22 | 17 | 18 | 18 |
| 23 | 18 | 19 | 19 |
| 24 | 19 | 20 | 20 |
| 25 | 20 | 21 | 21 |
| 26 | 21 | 22 | 22 |
| 27 | 22 | 23 | 23 |
| 28 | 23 | 23 | 24 |
| 29 | 24 | 24 | 25 |
| 30 | 25 | 25 | 26 |
| 31 | 26 | 26 | 27 |
| 32 | 27 | 27 | 28 |
| 33 | 28 | 28 | 29 |
| 34 | 29 | 29 | 30 |
| 35 | 30 | 30 | 31 |
| 36 | 31 | 31 | 32 |
| 37 | 32 | 32 | 32 |
| 38 | 33 | 33 | 33 |
| 39 | 34 | 34 | 34 |
| 40 | 35 | 35 | 35 |
| 41 | 35 | 36 | 36 |
| 42 | 36 | 37 | 37 |

Data from Sherer DM, Plessinger MA, Allen TA. Fetal scapular length in the ultrasonographic assessment of gestational age. *J Ultrasound Med*. 1994;13:523–528.

| Table 20 | Ultrasound Reference Values of Clavicle Length |

| GA (wk) | Jeanty[a] Percentiles | | | Yarkoni[b] Percentiles | | |
|---|---|---|---|---|---|---|
| | 5th | 50th | 95th | 5th | 50th | 95th |
| 12 | 8 | 13 | 18 | — | — | — |
| 13 | 10 | 15 | 20 | — | — | — |
| 14 | 11 | 16 | 21 | — | — | — |
| 15 | 12 | 17 | 22 | 11 | 16 | 21 |
| 16 | 13 | 18 | 23 | 12 | 17 | 22 |
| 17 | 14 | 19 | 24 | 13 | 18 | 23 |
| 18 | 15 | 20 | 25 | 14 | 19 | 24 |
| 19 | 16 | 21 | 26 | 15 | 20 | 25 |
| 20 | 17 | 22 | 27 | 16 | 21 | 26 |
| 21 | 18 | 23 | 28 | 17 | 22 | 27 |
| 22 | 20 | 25 | 30 | 18 | 23 | 28 |
| 23 | 21 | 26 | 31 | 19 | 24 | 29 |
| 24 | 22 | 27 | 32 | 20 | 25 | 30 |
| 25 | 23 | 28 | 33 | 21 | 26 | 31 |
| 26 | 24 | 29 | 34 | 22 | 27 | 32 |
| 27 | 25 | 30 | 35 | 23 | 28 | 33 |
| 28 | 26 | 31 | 36 | 24 | 29 | 34 |
| 29 | 27 | 32 | 37 | 25 | 30 | 35 |
| 30 | 29 | 34 | 39 | 26 | 31 | 36 |
| 31 | 30 | 35 | 40 | 27 | 32 | 37 |
| 32 | 31 | 36 | 41 | 28 | 33 | 38 |
| 33 | 32 | 37 | 42 | 29 | 34 | 39 |
| 34 | 33 | 38 | 43 | 30 | 35 | 40 |
| 35 | 34 | 39 | 44 | 31 | 36 | 41 |
| 36 | 35 | 40 | 45 | 32 | 37 | 42 |
| 37 | 36 | 41 | 46 | 33 | 38 | 43 |
| 38 | 37 | 42 | 47 | 34 | 39 | 44 |
| 39 | 39 | 44 | 49 | 35 | 40 | 45 |
| 40 | 40 | 45 | 50 | 36 | 41 | 46 |

*Note:* Used modified formula to fit tabular data. Clavicle = 1.118303 + 0.988639 × GA (SD = 2.920)
[a]From Jeanty et al.
[b]Reproduced with permission from Yarkoni S, Schmidt W, Jeanty P, et al. Clavicular measurement: a new biometric parameter for fetal evaluation. *J Ultrasound Med.* 1985;4:467–470.
GA, gestational age.

| Table 21 | Ultrasound Reference Values for Rib Length |

| GA (wk) | Rib Length (mm) Percentiles | | |
|---|---|---|---|
| | 5th | 50th | 95th |
| 14 | 1.4 | 2.3 | 3.1 |
| 15 | 1.6 | 2.5 | 3.3 |
| 16 | 1.8 | 2.7 | 3.5 |
| 17 | 2.0 | 2.9 | 3.7 |
| 18 | 2.2 | 3.1 | 3.9 |
| 19 | 2.5 | 3.3 | 4.1 |
| 20 | 2.7 | 3.5 | 4.3 |
| 21 | 2.9 | 3.7 | 4.5 |
| 22 | 3.1 | 3.9 | 4.7 |
| 23 | 3.3 | 4.1 | 4.9 |
| 24 | 3.5 | 4.3 | 5.1 |
| 25 | 3.7 | 4.5 | 5.3 |
| 26 | 3.9 | 4.7 | 5.5 |
| 27 | 4.1 | 4.9 | 5.7 |
| 28 | 4.3 | 5.1 | 5.9 |
| 29 | 4.5 | 5.3 | 6.1 |
| 30 | 4.7 | 5.5 | 6.3 |
| 31 | 4.9 | 5.7 | 6.5 |
| 32 | 5.1 | 5.9 | 6.7 |
| 33 | 5.3 | 6.1 | 6.9 |
| 34 | 5.5 | 6.3 | 7.1 |
| 35 | 5.7 | 6.5 | 7.3 |
| 36 | 5.9 | 6.7 | 7.5 |
| 37 | 6.1 | 6.9 | 7.8 |
| 38 | 6.3 | 7.1 | 8.0 |
| 39 | 6.5 | 7.3 | 8.2 |
| 40 | 6.7 | 7.5 | 8.4 |

*Note:* Rib length = −0.5834 + 0.203 × GA (SD = 0.5).
GA, gestational age.
Adapted from Abuhamad AZ, Sedule-Murphy SJ, Kolm P, et al. Prenatal ultrasonographic fetal rib length measurement: correlation with gestational age. *Ultrasound Obstet Gynecol.* 1996;7:193–196.

## Brain and Face Measurements

| Table 22 | Ultrasound Transcerebellar Diameter Measurements | |
|---|---|---|
| **GA** | **Mean (cm)** | **SD (cm)** |
| 15 | 1.46 | 0.14 |
| 16 | 1.61 | 0.1 |
| 17 | 1.71 | 0.1 |
| 18 | 1.83 | 0.12 |
| 19 | 1.94 | 0.11 |
| 20 | 2.03 | 0.12 |
| 21 | 2.14 | 0.13 |
| 22 | 2.28 | 0.18 |
| 23 | 2.43 | 0.16 |
| 24 | 2.59 | 0.17 |
| 25 | 2.76 | 0.16 |
| 26 | 2.91 | 0.18 |
| 27 | 3.08 | 0.17 |
| 28 | 3.25 | 0.18 |
| 29 | 3.41 | 0.21 |
| 30 | 3.6 | 0.22 |
| 31 | 3.78 | 0.24 |
| 32 | 3.92 | 0.24 |
| 33 | 4.14 | 0.26 |
| 34 | 4.29 | 0.27 |
| 35 | 4.47 | 0.3 |
| 36 | 4.66 | 0.34 |
| 37 | 4.8 | 0.32 |
| 38 | 4.98 | 0.33 |

GA, gestational age; SD, standard deviation.
Adapted from Chaves MR, Ananth CV, Smulian JC, et al. Fetal transcerebellar diameter nomogram in singleton gestations with special emphasis in the third trimester: a comparison with previously published nomograms. *Am J Obstet Gynecol.* 2003;189:1021.

| Table 23 | **Ultrasound Reference Intervals for the Cerebellar Vermis, Basilar Pons, and the Brain Stem** |
|---|---|

| | **Vermis** | | | | | | | | |
|---|---|---|---|---|---|---|---|---|---|
| **GA** | **Sagittal CC (mm)** | | | **Sagittal AP (mm)** | | | **Sagittal Surface Area (cm²)** | | |
| **(wk)** | **5%** | **50%** | **95%** | **5%** | **50%** | **95%** | **5%** | **50%** | **95%** |
| 18–19 | 8.4 | 9.2 | 11.3 | 7.8 | 8.8 | 10.6 | 0.61 | 0.65 | 0.80 |
| 20–21 | 10.0 | 12.2 | 14.0 | 8.3 | 10.0 | 13.2 | 0.80 | 1.06 | 1.34 |
| 22–23 | 11.3 | 13.4 | 15.1 | 11.2 | 12.6 | 15.5 | 1.07 | 1.25 | 1.56 |
| 24–25 | 14.6 | 15.7 | 17.3 | 13.3 | 14.7 | 16.9 | 1.32 | 1.63 | 1.87 |
| 26–27 | 15.6 | 17.3 | 18.6 | 13.7 | 16.2 | 18.7 | 1.9 | 2.20 | 2.50 |
| 28–29 | 16.4 | 18.5 | 22.2 | 16.1 | 18.6 | 20.6 | 1.73 | 2.48 | 2.97 |
| 30–31 | 19.1 | 20.3 | 22.8 | 16.5 | 19.1 | 22.8 | 2.59 | 3.12 | 3.52 |
| 32–33 | 19.6 | 22.3 | 23.5 | 18.3 | 20.2 | 22.4 | 2.84 | 3.27 | 3.90 |
| 34–35 | 20.6 | 22.1 | 25.4 | 18.6 | 22.0 | 23.6 | 3.12 | 3.81 | 4.38 |
| 36–37 | 22.0 | 24.7 | 27.1 | 20.5 | 24.7 | 26.0 | 3.71 | 4.00 | 4.78 |
| 38–39 | 24.3 | 26.5 | 28.2 | 18.8 | 22.7 | 25.8 | 4.30 | 4.64 | 5.02 |

| | **Pons** | | | | | | | | |
|---|---|---|---|---|---|---|---|---|---|
| **GA** | **Sagittal CC (mm)** | | | **Sagittal AP (mm)** | | | **Sagittal Surface Area (cm²)** | | |
| **(wk)** | **5%** | **50%** | **95%** | **5%** | **50%** | **95%** | **5%** | **50%** | **95%** |
| 18–19 | 4.5 | 5.5 | 6.8 | 3.4 | 4.2 | 4.7 | 0.13 | 0.22 | 0.28 |
| 20–21 | 4.8 | 6.7 | 8.4 | 4.3 | 5.2 | 6.7 | 0.22 | 0.30 | 0.39 |
| 22–23 | 5.8 | 7.1 | 9.3 | 3.6 | 5.2 | 6.5 | 0.30 | 0.40 | 0.56 |
| 24–25 | 7.4 | 8.6 | 10.9 | 5.4 | 6.3 | 8.0 | 0.41 | 0.48 | 0.54 |
| 26–27 | 6.4 | 9.1 | 10.9 | 4.7 | 5.9 | 7.7 | 0.40 | 0.69 | 0.86 |
| 28–29 | 9.3 | 10.1 | 14.1 | 5.8 | 7.6 | 9.5 | 0.50 | 0.69 | 0.78 |
| 30–31 | 10.0 | 12.3 | 13.9 | 6.7 | 7.9 | 9.9 | 0.62 | 0.83 | 0.98 |
| 32–33 | 11.2 | 13.1 | 15.7 | 7.9 | 8.9 | 10.5 | 0.75 | 0.99 | 1.23 |
| 34–35 | 11.5 | 13.5 | 15.1 | 7.6 | 8.6 | 10.3 | 0.92 | 1.11 | 1.37 |
| 36–37 | 12.1 | 13.7 | 14.4 | 6.8 | 8.9 | 10.1 | 1.00 | 1.28 | 1.35 |
| 38–39 | 12.5 | 13.4 | 14.0 | 9.3 | 9.4 | 10.1 | 1.20 | 1.51 | 1.67 |

| | **Brainstem** | | |
|---|---|---|---|
| **GA** | **Sagittal Surface Area (cm²)** | | |
| **(wk)** | **5%** | **50%** | **95%** |
| 18–19 | 1.08 | 1.26 | 1.66 |
| 20–21 | 1.51 | 1.75 | 1.98 |
| 22–23 | 1.66 | 2.14 | 2.57 |
| 24–25 | 1.89 | 2.34 | 2.92 |
| 26–27 | 2.62 | 3.09 | 3.61 |
| 28–29 | 2.85 | 3.74 | 4.40 |
| 30–31 | 3.15 | 4.00 | 4.58 |
| 32–33 | 3.59 | 4.36 | 5.08 |
| 34–35 | 3.59 | 4.72 | 5.56 |
| 36–37 | 5.04 | 5.26 | 5.59 |
| 38–39 | 4.76 | 5.02 | 5.57 |

Reproduced from Ginath S, Lerman-Sagie T, Haratz Krajden K, et al. The fetal vermis, pons and brainstem: normal longitudinal development as shown by dedicated neurosonography. *J Matern Fetal Neonatal Med.* 2013;26:757–762, with permission.

**Table 24** **MRI Measurements of the Fetal Brain**

## FRONTO-OCCIPITAL DIAMETER (FOD)

Between extreme points of frontal and occipital lobes (sagittal).

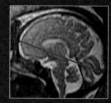

| GA | 16 | 17 | 18 | 19 | 20 | 21 | 22 | 23 | 24 | 25 | 26 | 27 | 28 | 29 | 30 | 31 | 32 | 33 | 34 | 35 | 36 | >37 |
|---|---|---|---|---|---|---|---|---|---|---|---|---|---|---|---|---|---|---|---|---|---|---|
| # | 15 | 12 | 18 | 19 | 25 | 19 | 13 | 13 | 16 | 13 | 14 | 13 | 15 | 14 | 13 | 12 | 11 | 13 | 14 | 16 | 13 | 14 |
| Ave | 35.38 | 38.39 | 44.02 | 47.75 | 51.57 | 57.41 | 59.59 | 64.92 | 66.90 | 69.98 | 74.99 | 77.56 | 79.36 | 84.94 | 87.35 | 91.10 | 92.22 | 92.73 | 99.18 | 101.60 | 102.56 | 104.96 |
| SD | 1.72 | 2.00 | 2.28 | 2.74 | 2.62 | 2.53 | 3.00 | 1.93 | 1.60 | 3.44 | 2.92 | 3.45 | 3.50 | 2.21 | 3.58 | 4.37 | 1.57 | 4.13 | 3.74 | 5.21 | 4.15 | 4.22 |

## CEREBAL BIPARIETAL DIAMETER (C-BPD)

Greatest transverse diameter of brain at level of temporal lobes (coronal).

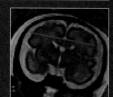

| GA | 16 | 17 | 18 | 19 | 20 | 21 | 22 | 23 | 24 | 25 | 26 | 27 | 28 | 29 | 30 | 31 | 32 | 33 | 34 | 35 | 36 | >37 |
|---|---|---|---|---|---|---|---|---|---|---|---|---|---|---|---|---|---|---|---|---|---|---|
| # | 15 | 12 | 18 | 18 | 24 | 18 | 14 | 13 | 16 | 13 | 14 | 14 | 15 | 15 | 13 | 12 | 11 | 13 | 14 | 18 | 13 | 14 |
| Ave | 29.06 | 31.29 | 34.42 | 36.23 | 38.85 | 42.04 | 44.61 | 47.80 | 49.23 | 51.07 | 55.41 | 59.05 | 60.43 | 65.23 | 67.16 | 69.72 | 74.09 | 74.91 | 79.33 | 79.45 | 82.50 | 83.90 |
| SD | 0.94 | 1.12 | 1.98 | 1.77 | 2.33 | 2.85 | 1.89 | 1.07 | 1.79 | 4.87 | 2.66 | 3.81 | 2.20 | 2.03 | 2.25 | 3.01 | 3.42 | 2.27 | 3.90 | 4.60 | 4.57 | 5.86 |

## BONE BIPARIETAL DIAMETER (B-BPD)

Greatest transverse diameter of skull at level of temporal lobes (coronal)

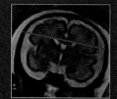

| GA | 16 | 17 | 18 | 19 | 20 | 21 | 22 | 23 | 24 | 25 | 26 | 27 | 28 | 29 | 30 | 31 | 32 | 33 | 34 | 35 | 36 | >37 |
|---|---|---|---|---|---|---|---|---|---|---|---|---|---|---|---|---|---|---|---|---|---|---|
| # | 15 | 12 | 18 | 18 | 24 | 19 | 14 | 13 | 15 | 13 | 14 | 13 | 14 | 15 | 13 | 12 | 11 | 13 | 13 | 18 | 13 | 14 |
| Ave | 32.93 | 35.25 | 39.20 | 42.50 | 45.64 | 50.45 | 51.39 | 56.88 | 57.18 | 60.86 | 64.31 | 67.26 | 68.22 | 73.25 | 75.04 | 78.16 | 81.56 | 83.29 | 85.64 | 86.60 | 90.75 | 90.88 |
| SD | 1.46 | 1.39 | 2.43 | 1.92 | 2.44 | 3.00 | 4.19 | 2.59 | 2.44 | 4.91 | 4.01 | 3.55 | 2.46 | 2.48 | 3.66 | 4.07 | 4.04 | 2.31 | 3.46 | 5.45 | 7.23 | 7.07 |

## CRANIOCEREBRAL INDEX  Bone BPD – cerebral BPD/ bone BPD.

| GA | 16 | 17 | 18 | 19 | 20 | 21 | 22 | 23 | 24 | 25 | 26 | 27 | 28 | 29 | 30 | 31 | 32 | 33 | 34 | 35 | 36 | >37 |
|---|---|---|---|---|---|---|---|---|---|---|---|---|---|---|---|---|---|---|---|---|---|---|
| Index | 11.75 | 11.23 | 12.20 | 14.76 | 14.87 | 16.68 | 13.19 | 15.96 | 13.91 | 16.09 | 13.85 | 12.21 | 11.43 | 10.94 | 10.49 | 10.79 | 9.16 | 10.06 | 7.37 | 8.26 | 9.09 | 7.68 |

## LENGTH OF CORPUS CALLOSUM (LCC)

Between genu and splenium of CC (sagittal)

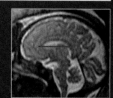

| GA | 16 | 17 | 18 | 19 | 20 | 21 | 22 | 23 | 24 | 25 | 26 | 27 | 28 | 29 | 30 | 31 | 32 | 33 | 34 | 35 | 36 | >37 |
|---|---|---|---|---|---|---|---|---|---|---|---|---|---|---|---|---|---|---|---|---|---|---|
| # | 15 | 12 | 16 | 16 | 20 | 16 | 13 | 12 | 15 | 11 | 12 | 14 | 13 | 14 | 13 | 12 | 11 | 12 | 13 | 16 | 13 | 14 |
| Ave | 7.53 | 9.73 | 13.64 | 16.44 | 20.01 | 22.93 | 23.99 | 27.83 | 28.05 | 31.25 | 32.52 | 32.68 | 34.44 | 36.14 | 36.60 | 37.29 | 37.79 | 39.40 | 40.05 | 41.37 | 42.18 | 45.02 |
| SD | 0.61 | 1.03 | 2.53 | 2.02 | 1.16 | 1.42 | 1.76 | 1.96 | 1.16 | 2.44 | 2.02 | 1.87 | 1.95 | 2.06 | 1.63 | 2.44 | 2.92 | 1.63 | 1.54 | 2.66 | 3.32 | 2.28 |

**Table 24** | **MRI Measurements of the Fetal Brain** *(continued)*

## LCC/FOD RATIO

| GA | 16 | 17 | 18 | 19 | 20 | 21 | 22 | 23 | 24 | 25 | 26 | 27 | 28 | 29 | 30 | 31 | 32 | 33 | 34 | 35 | 36 | >37 |
|---|---|---|---|---|---|---|---|---|---|---|---|---|---|---|---|---|---|---|---|---|---|---|
| Ratio | 21.29 | 25.34 | 30.98 | 34.44 | 38.80 | 39.94 | 40.26 | 42.86 | 41.93 | 44.65 | 43.36 | 42.14 | 43.40 | 42.54 | 41.90 | 40.93 | 40.98 | 42.48 | 40.38 | 40.72 | 41.13 | 42.89 |

## AP VERMIS

Greatest AP diameter measured from median part of 4<sup>th</sup> ventricle's roof (fastigial point) posteriorly (sagittal)

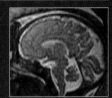

| GA | 16 | 17 | 18 | 19 | 20 | 21 | 22 | 23 | 24 | 25 | 26 | 27 | 28 | 29 | 30 | 31 | 32 | 33 | 34 | 35 | 36 | >37 |
|---|---|---|---|---|---|---|---|---|---|---|---|---|---|---|---|---|---|---|---|---|---|---|
| # | 15 | 12 | 17 | 17 | 24 | 16 | 12 | 10 | 15 | 13 | 14 | 14 | 15 | 14 | 13 | 12 | 12 | 13 | 12 | 14 | 13 | 14 |
| Ave | 3.51 | 4.15 | 4.87 | 5.45 | 6.17 | 6.49 | 7.41 | 8.21 | 8.57 | 9.65 | 9.71 | 10.45 | 11.09 | 11.82 | 12.00 | 12.83 | 12.93 | 13.89 | 14.90 | 14.90 | 16.48 | 16.96 |
| SD | 0.31 | 0.32 | 0.43 | 0.54 | 0.65 | 0.76 | 0.44 | 1.12 | 0.58 | 1.24 | 0.96 | 1.15 | 1.08 | 1.03 | 0.68 | 0.96 | 1.50 | 1.12 | 0.60 | 0.88 | 0.91 | 2.18 |

## HEIGHT OF VERMIS

Greatest height of vermis, parallel to axis of brainstem (sagittal)

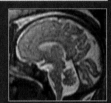

| GA | 16 | 17 | 18 | 19 | 20 | 21 | 22 | 23 | 24 | 25 | 26 | 27 | 28 | 29 | 30 | 31 | 32 | 33 | 34 | 35 | 36 | >37 |
|---|---|---|---|---|---|---|---|---|---|---|---|---|---|---|---|---|---|---|---|---|---|---|
| # | 15 | 12 | 17 | 17 | 24 | 17 | 13 | 12 | 15 | 13 | 14 | 14 | 15 | 14 | 13 | 12 | 12 | 13 | 13 | 15 | 13 | 14 |
| Ave | 4.73 | 5.65 | 6.70 | 7.19 | 8.11 | 8.96 | 9.97 | 11.23 | 11.84 | 12.05 | 13.54 | 14.87 | 15.38 | 15.87 | 16.64 | 17.51 | 18.31 | 19.12 | 19.79 | 20.09 | 22.32 | 22.33 |
| SD | 0.43 | 0.39 | 0.63 | 0.80 | 1.07 | 1.45 | 1.00 | 1.32 | 0.83 | 0.84 | 1.19 | 0.88 | 1.46 | 0.98 | 1.55 | 0.82 | 1.58 | 0.97 | 1.30 | 1.29 | 3.10 | 1.97 |

## TRANSCEREBELLAR DIAMETER

Greatest transverse diameter of cerebellum (axial)

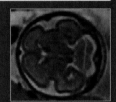

| GA | 16 | 17 | 18 | 19 | 20 | 21 | 22 | 23 | 24 | 25 | 26 | 27 | 28 | 29 | 30 | 31 | 32 | 33 | 34 | 35 | 36 | >37 |
|---|---|---|---|---|---|---|---|---|---|---|---|---|---|---|---|---|---|---|---|---|---|---|
| # | 15 | 12 | 18 | 18 | 24 | 17 | 14 | 13 | 15 | 13 | 13 | 13 | 15 | 15 | 13 | 12 | 11 | 12 | 14 | 17 | 13 | 14 |
| Ave | 14.73 | 15.94 | 17.16 | 17.92 | 19.32 | 20.39 | 21.91 | 24.32 | 25.33 | 27.42 | 28.12 | 30.25 | 32.68 | 34.92 | 35.94 | 38.06 | 40.33 | 40.98 | 44.34 | 45.78 | 48.12 | 49.83 |
| SD | 0.70 | 0.60 | 1.35 | 1.30 | 1.45 | 1.38 | 1.81 | 1.40 | 1.83 | 2.75 | 1.31 | 1.95 | 1.21 | 1.40 | 2.23 | 1.77 | 2.57 | 1.85 | 3.31 | 2.19 | 3.82 | 3.44 |

## AP PONS

Maximal AP diameter of pons (midline sagittal)

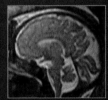

| GA | 16 | 17 | 18 | 19 | 20 | 21 | 22 | 23 | 24 | 25 | 26 | 27 | 28 | 29 | 30 | 31 | 32 | 33 | 34 | 35 | 36 | >37 |
|---|---|---|---|---|---|---|---|---|---|---|---|---|---|---|---|---|---|---|---|---|---|---|
| # | 15 | 12 | 15 | 15 | 23 | 12 | 12 | 12 | 15 | 13 | 13 | 15 | 14 | 12 | 12 | 12 | 13 | 13 | 15 | 13 | 14 |
| Ave | 5.02 | 5.44 | 6.14 | 6.18 | 6.29 | 6.39 | 6.48 | 7.77 | 7.78 | 8.11 | 8.99 | 9.19 | 10.08 | 10.85 | 11.22 | 11.57 | 11.97 | 12.28 | 12.75 | 13.25 | 13.54 | 13.86 |
| SD | 0.34 | 0.26 | 0.43 | 0.61 | 0.64 | 0.58 | 0.72 | 0.39 | 0.46 | 0.83 | 0.65 | 1.14 | 1.05 | 0.84 | 0.53 | 0.73 | 1.47 | 1.31 | 0.81 | 0.83 | 1.74 | 1.39 |

*(continued)*

**Table 24**    **MRI Measurements of the Fetal Brain** *(continued)*

## DIAMETER THIRD VENTRICLE (DV3)
Maximal transverse diameter (coronal)

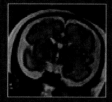

| GA | 16 | 17 | 18 | 19 | 20 | 21 | 22 | 23 | 24 | 25 | 26 | 27 | 28 | 29 | 30 | 31 | 32 | 33 | 34 | 35 | 36 | >37 |
|---|---|---|---|---|---|---|---|---|---|---|---|---|---|---|---|---|---|---|---|---|---|---|
| # | 15 | 12 | 18 | 16 | 24 | 18 | 13 | 12 | 16 | 13 | 14 | 14 | 15 | 14 | 13 | 12 | 12 | 13 | 14 | 17 | 13 | 14 |
| Ave | 2.04 | 2.07 | 2.13 | 1.91 | 1.75 | 2.13 | 1.84 | 2.09 | 2.03 | 2.01 | 1.99 | 2.16 | 2.06 | 2.09 | 2.04 | 2.22 | 2.03 | 2.81 | 2.50 | 2.37 | 2.42 | 2.35 |
| SD | 0.31 | 0.26 | 0.49 | 0.48 | 0.38 | 0.40 | 0.32 | 0.36 | 0.56 | 0.43 | 0.45 | 0.50 | 0.50 | 0.49 | 0.73 | 0.84 | 0.68 | 0.48 | 0.62 | 0.68 | 0.70 | 0.87 |

## DIAMETER FOURTH VENTRICLE (DV4)
Maximal AP diameter (midline sagittal)

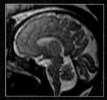

| GA | 16 | 17 | 18 | 19 | 20 | 21 | 22 | 23 | 24 | 25 | 26 | 27 | 28 | 29 | 30 | 31 | 32 | 33 | 34 | 35 | 36 | >37 |
|---|---|---|---|---|---|---|---|---|---|---|---|---|---|---|---|---|---|---|---|---|---|---|
| # | 15 | 12 | 17 | 18 | 25 | 17 | 13 | 12 | 15 | 13 | 13 | 14 | 15 | 14 | 13 | 12 | 12 | 13 | 13 | 15 | 13 | 14 |
| Ave | 2.51 | 2.63 | 2.87 | 2.52 | 2.33 | 2.44 | 2.43 | 2.52 | 2.88 | 2.68 | 2.76 | 2.89 | 3.54 | 3.33 | 3.21 | 3.20 | 3.50 | 4.00 | 3.60 | 3.79 | 4.05 | 4.35 |
| SD | 0.46 | 0.32 | 0.75 | 0.58 | 0.69 | 0.52 | 0.43 | 0.51 | 0.60 | 0.79 | 0.54 | 0.82 | 0.60 | 0.79 | 0.47 | 0.55 | 0.69 | 0.50 | 0.80 | 0.86 | 0.53 | 0.95 |

## INTERHEMISPHERIC DISTANCE (IHD)
Between internal edges of lateral hemispheres (coronal)

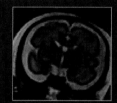

| GA | 16 | 17 | 18 | 19 | 20 | 21 | 22 | 23 | 24 | 25 | 26 | 27 | 28 | 29 | 30 | 31 | 32 | 33 | 34 | 35 | 36 | >37 |
|---|---|---|---|---|---|---|---|---|---|---|---|---|---|---|---|---|---|---|---|---|---|---|
| # | 15 | 12 | 18 | 19 | 25 | 19 | 13 | 13 | 15 | 13 | 14 | 14 | 15 | 15 | 13 | 12 | 12 | 13 | 14 | 17 | 13 | 14 |
| Ave | 2.61 | 2.80 | 2.57 | 2.72 | 2.66 | 3.09 | 2.77 | 2.94 | 2.49 | 2.42 | 2.89 | 2.70 | 2.69 | 2.45 | 2.42 | 2.28 | 2.62 | 2.51 | 2.81 | 2.76 | 2.26 | 2.45 |
| SD | 0.55 | 0.53 | 0.61 | 0.57 | 0.92 | 0.63 | 0.83 | 0.59 | 0.52 | 0.71 | 0.87 | 0.75 | 0.61 | 0.65 | 0.60 | 0.72 | 0.90 | 0.47 | 0.73 | 0.60 | 0.80 | 0.77 |

## IHD/C-BPD INDEX

| GA | 16 | 17 | 18 | 19 | 20 | 21 | 22 | 23 | 24 | 25 | 26 | 27 | 28 | 29 | 30 | 31 | 32 | 33 | 34 | 35 | 36 | 37-39 |
|---|---|---|---|---|---|---|---|---|---|---|---|---|---|---|---|---|---|---|---|---|---|---|
| Index | 8.98 | 8.95 | 7.46 | 7.51 | 6.86 | 7.34 | 6.21 | 6.15 | 5.05 | 4.74 | 5.21 | 4.58 | 4.45 | 3.76 | 3.61 | 3.27 | 3.53 | 3.35 | 3.54 | 3.47 | 2.74 | 2.92 |

## AP INTEROPERCULAR DISTANCE
Distance between anterior and posterior edge of sylvian fissure
at most external point, at level of third ventricle (axial)

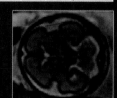

| GA | 16 | 17 | 18 | 19 | 20 | 21 | 22 | 23 | 24 | 25 | 26 | 27 | 28 | 29 | 30 | 31 | 32 | 33 | 34 | 35 | 36 | >37 |
|---|---|---|---|---|---|---|---|---|---|---|---|---|---|---|---|---|---|---|---|---|---|---|
| # | 15 | 11 | 18 | 18 | 19 | 18 | 14 | 12 | 16 | 12 | 14 | 13 | 16 | 11 | 12 | 10 | 12 | 12 | 14 | 16 | 12 | 13 |
| Ave | 9.54 | 10.31 | 10.52 | 10.40 | 10.76 | 11.31 | 11.10 | 11.56 | 13.38 | 11.96 | 13.17 | 12.65 | 13.86 | 12.38 | 11.22 | 9.46 | 9.63 | 9.94 | 9.78 | 10.02 | 6.95 | 7.65 |
| SD | 1.04 | 0.77 | 1.34 | 2.50 | 2.05 | 2.59 | 1.83 | 2.11 | 2.56 | 2.57 | 3.00 | 2.25 | 2.10 | 2.97 | 1.10 | 2.36 | 1.63 | 2.30 | 2.42 | 4.09 | 1.90 | 2.42 |

| Table 24 | MRI Measurements of the Fetal Brain *(continued)* |
|---|---|

## CRANIOCAUDAL INTEROPERCULAR DISTANCE
Distance between superior and inferior edge of sylvian
fissure at most external point, at level of third ventricle (axial)

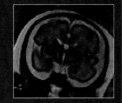

| GA | 16 | 17 | 18 | 19 | 20 | 21 | 22 | 23 | 24 | 25 | 26 | 27 | 28 | 29 | 30 | 31 | 32 | 33 | 34 | 35 | 36 | >37 |
|---|---|---|---|---|---|---|---|---|---|---|---|---|---|---|---|---|---|---|---|---|---|---|
| # | 15 | 12 | 14 | 15 | 21 | 18 | 14 | 13 | 15 | 13 | 14 | 13 | 15 | 13 | 13 | 11 | 12 | 12 | 14 | 17 | 12 | 14 |
| Ave | 6.46 | 7.59 | 7.98 | 8.49 | 7.72 | 7.56 | 8.04 | 7.02 | 8.76 | 6.25 | 6.11 | 5.23 | 5.41 | 3.95 | 3.43 | 3.50 | 2.62 | 2.85 | 2.77 | 2.64 | 1.97 | 2.25 |
| SD | 0.53 | 0.83 | 1.48 | 1.85 | 1.99 | 1.39 | 1.84 | 1.99 | 1.72 | 1.07 | 1.36 | 1.81 | 1.49 | 0.91 | 1.70 | 1.06 | 0.82 | 0.95 | 0.83 | 0.62 | 0.77 | 1.09 |

## CISTERNA MAGNA (CM)
From posterior aspect cerebellum to inner table skull (axial)

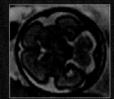

| GA | 16 | 17 | 18 | 19 | 20 | 21 | 22 | 23 | 24 | 25 | 26 | 27 | 28 | 29 | 30 | 31 | 32 | 33 | 34 | 35 | 36 | >37 |
|---|---|---|---|---|---|---|---|---|---|---|---|---|---|---|---|---|---|---|---|---|---|---|
| # | 15 | 12 | 17 | 18 | 24 | 18 | 13 | 13 | 15 | 13 | 14 | 14 | 15 | 14 | 12 | 10 | 12 | 13 | 13 | 16 | 12 | 14 |
| Ave | 4.47 | 6.11 | 6.02 | 6.39 | 5.20 | 5.08 | 5.65 | 4.52 | 5.27 | 4.92 | 4.61 | 6.04 | 6.84 | 6.25 | 5.43 | 5.74 | 4.84 | 6.20 | 6.11 | 5.89 | 4.77 | 5.59 |
| SD | 1.31 | 1.43 | 1.61 | 2.15 | 1.49 | 1.39 | 1.28 | 0.92 | 1.59 | 1.41 | 1.63 | 1.51 | 2.32 | 2.09 | 1.98 | 1.55 | 1.89 | 2.23 | 1.44 | 2.19 | 1.94 | 1.59 |

## HEIGHT PONS
Maximal height of pons (midline sagittal)

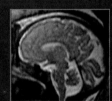

| GA | 16 | 17 | 18 | 19 | 20 | 21 | 22 | 23 | 24 | 25 | 26 | 27 | 28 | 29 | 30 | 31 | 32 | 33 | 34 | 35 | 36 | >37 |
|---|---|---|---|---|---|---|---|---|---|---|---|---|---|---|---|---|---|---|---|---|---|---|
| # | 15 | 12 | 15 | 13 | 19 | 13 | 13 | 12 | 12 | 12 | 13 | 13 | 15 | 14 | 12 | 11 | 12 | 13 | 13 | 15 | 13 | 14 |
| Ave | 5.01 | 5.56 | 5.89 | 5.93 | 6.34 | 6.60 | 6.76 | 7.87 | 8.48 | 8.58 | 8.96 | 10.07 | 10.32 | 11.15 | 11.74 | 12.17 | 12.29 | 12.52 | 13.01 | 13.11 | 13.64 | 14.56 |
| SD | 0.57 | 0.68 | 0.63 | 0.62 | 0.92 | 1.37 | 1.20 | 1.03 | 0.87 | 2.11 | 2.70 | 1.54 | 0.66 | 0.68 | 1.36 | 1.12 | 0.85 | 1.23 | 1.14 | 1.17 | 2.15 | 1.26 |

Revised from Egloff A, Hoshim H, Bulas D, Vezina G M MRI Measurements of the Fetal Brain abstract European Society of Pediatric Radiology June 2009, Istanbul, Turkey.
Additional biometry provided by Beth M. Kline-Fath and Constance Bitters

| Table 25A | **Ultrasound Reference Values for Binocular Diameter, Interocular Diameter, and Ocular Diameter by Gestational Age** |
|-----------|-------------------------------------------------------------------------------------------|

| | Binocular Diameter (mm) | | | Interocular Diameter (mm) | | | Ocular Diameter (mm) | | |
|---|---|---|---|---|---|---|---|---|---|
| | Percentiles | | | Percentiles | | | Percentiles | | |
| GA (wk) | 5th | 50th | 95th | 5th | 50th | 95th | 5th | 50th | 95th |
| 11 | 5 | 13 | 20 | — | — | — | — | — | — |
| 12 | 8 | 15 | 23 | 4 | 9 | 13 | 1 | 3 | 6 |
| 13 | 10 | 18 | 25 | 5 | 9 | 14 | 2 | 4 | 7 |
| 14 | 13 | 20 | 28 | 5 | 10 | 14 | 3 | 5 | 8 |
| 15 | 15 | 22 | 30 | 6 | 10 | 14 | 4 | 6 | 9 |
| 16 | 17 | 25 | 32 | 6 | 10 | 15 | 5 | 7 | 9 |
| 17 | 19 | 27 | 34 | 6 | 11 | 15 | 5 | 8 | 10 |
| 18 | 22 | 29 | 37 | 7 | 11 | 16 | 6 | 9 | 11 |
| 19 | 24 | 31 | 39 | 7 | 12 | 16 | 7 | 9 | 12 |
| 20 | 26 | 33 | 41 | 8 | 12 | 17 | 8 | 10 | 13 |
| 21 | 28 | 35 | 43 | 8 | 13 | 17 | 8 | 11 | 13 |
| 22 | 30 | 37 | 44 | 9 | 13 | 18 | 9 | 12 | 14 |
| 23 | 31 | 39 | 46 | 9 | 14 | 18 | 10 | 12 | 15 |
| 24 | 33 | 41 | 48 | 10 | 14 | 19 | 10 | 13 | 15 |
| 25 | 35 | 42 | 50 | 10 | 15 | 19 | 11 | 13 | 16 |
| 26 | 36 | 44 | 51 | 11 | 15 | 20 | 12 | 14 | 16 |
| 27 | 38 | 45 | 53 | 11 | 16 | 20 | 12 | 14 | 17 |
| 28 | 39 | 47 | 54 | 12 | 16 | 21 | 13 | 15 | 17 |
| 29 | 41 | 48 | 56 | 12 | 17 | 21 | 13 | 15 | 18 |
| 30 | 42 | 50 | 57 | 13 | 17 | 22 | 14 | 16 | 18 |
| 31 | 43 | 51 | 58 | 13 | 18 | 22 | 14 | 16 | 19 |
| 32 | 45 | 52 | 60 | 14 | 18 | 23 | 14 | 17 | 19 |
| 33 | 46 | 53 | 61 | 14 | 19 | 23 | 15 | 17 | 19 |
| 34 | 47 | 54 | 62 | 15 | 19 | 24 | 15 | 17 | 20 |
| 35 | 48 | 55 | 63 | 15 | 20 | 24 | 15 | 18 | 20 |
| 36 | 49 | 56 | 64 | 16 | 20 | 25 | 16 | 18 | 20 |
| 37 | 50 | 57 | 65 | 16 | 21 | 25 | 16 | 18 | 21 |
| 38 | 50 | 58 | 65 | 17 | 21 | 26 | 16 | 18 | 21 |

Reproduced with permission from Romero R, Pilu G, Jeanty F, et al. *Prenatal Diagnosis of Congenital Anomalies.* Norwalk, CT: Appleton & Lange; 1988:83.

| Table 25B | **Reference Ranges for Fetal Optic Tract Diameter (in mm)** |
|-----------|-------------------------------------------------------------|

| | Centile | | | | |
|---|---|---|---|---|---|
| GA (wk) | 3rd | 5th | 50th | 95th | 97th |
| 21 | 1.6 | 1.7 | 2.0 | 2.3 | 2.3 |
| 22 | 1.7 | 1.8 | 2.1 | 2.4 | 2.4 |
| 23 | 1.8 | 1.9 | 2.2 | 2.5 | 2.5 |
| 24 | 1.9 | 2.0 | 2.3 | 2.6 | 2.6 |
| 25 | 2.0 | 2.1 | 2.4 | 2.6 | 2.7 |
| 26 | 2.1 | 2.2 | 2.5 | 2.7 | 2.8 |
| 27 | 2.2 | 2.3 | 2.5 | 2.8 | 2.9 |
| 28 | 2.3 | 2.4 | 2.6 | 2.9 | 3.0 |
| 29 | 2.4 | 2.4 | 2.7 | 3.0 | 3.1 |
| 30 | 2.5 | 2.5 | 2.8 | 3.1 | 3.2 |
| 31 | 2.6 | 2.6 | 2.9 | 3.2 | 3.3 |
| 32 | 2.7 | 2.7 | 3.0 | 3.3 | 3.3 |
| 33 | 2.8 | 2.8 | 3.1 | 3.4 | 3.4 |
| 34 | 2.9 | 2.9 | 3.2 | 3.5 | 3.5 |
| 35 | 2.9 | 3.0 | 3.3 | 3.6 | 3.6 |
| 36 | 3.0 | 3.1 | 3.4 | 3.7 | 3.7 |

Reproduced from Bault JP, Salomon LJ, Guibaud L, et al. Role of three-dimensional ultrasound measurement of the optic tract in fetuses with agenesis of the septum pellucidum. *Ultrasound Obstet Gynecol.* 2011;37(5):570–575. Copyright © International Society of Ultrasound in Obstetrics and Gynecology. With permission of John Wiley & Sons Ltd.

| Table 26 | MRI Reference Values for Binocular Diameter, Interocular Diameter, and Ocular Diameter by Gestational Age |

| Gestational Age (wk) | No. of Fetuses | No. of Observations | BOD | | | IOD | | | OD | | |
|---|---|---|---|---|---|---|---|---|---|---|---|
| | | | 5% | 50% | 95% | 5% | 50% | 95% | 5% | 50% | 95% |
| 15 | | | 16.6 | 20.8 | 21.4 | 7.4 | 9.8 | 12.3 | 3.4 | 5.5 | 6.4 |
| 16 | 2 | 2 | 19.0 | 22.8 | 24.0 | 8.2 | 10.6 | 13.3 | 4.2 | 6.1 | 7.1 |
| 17 | 1 | 3 | 21.3 | 24.8 | 26.5 | 9.0 | 11.4 | 14.3 | 5.0 | 6.7 | 7.9 |
| 18 | | | 23.4 | 26.8 | 28.9 | 9.7 | 12.1 | 15.2 | 5.7 | 7.3 | 8.5 |
| 19 | 3 | 9 | 25.4 | 28.7 | 31.1 | 10.4 | 12.9 | 16.1 | 6.4 | 7.9 | 9.2 |
| 20 | 6 | 11 | 27.3 | 30.5 | 33.2 | 11.1 | 13.6 | 16.9 | 7.0 | 8.5 | 9.8 |
| 21 | 14 | 40 | 29.1 | 32.3 | 35.2 | 11.7 | 14.3 | 17.6 | 7.6 | 9.0 | 10.4 |
| 22 | 9 | 28 | 30.8 | 34.1 | 37.1 | 12.3 | 14.9 | 18.4 | 8.2 | 9.6 | 10.9 |
| 23 | 8 | 29 | 32.4 | 35.8 | 38.9 | 12.8 | 15.6 | 19.1 | 8.8 | 10.1 | 11.4 |
| 24 | 8 | 46 | 34.0 | 37.4 | 40.7 | 13.4 | 16.2 | 19.8 | 9.3 | 10.6 | 11.9 |
| 25 | 4 | 14 | 35.5 | 39.0 | 42.4 | 13.9 | 16.8 | 20.4 | 9.8 | 11.1 | 12.4 |
| 26 | 10 | 36 | 37.0 | 40.6 | 44.0 | 14.4 | 17.4 | 21.0 | 10.3 | 11.6 | 12.9 |
| 27 | 5 | 23 | 38.4 | 42.1 | 45.5 | 14.9 | 17.9 | 21.6 | 10.8 | 12.0 | 13.3 |
| 28 | 7 | 27 | 39.7 | 43.5 | 47.0 | 15.3 | 18.5 | 22.2 | 11.3 | 12.5 | 13.8 |
| 29 | 9 | 22 | 41.0 | 44.9 | 48.5 | 15.8 | 19.0 | 22.8 | 11.7 | 12.9 | 14.2 |
| 30 | 1 | 4 | 42.3 | 46.3 | 49.9 | 16.2 | 19.5 | 23.3 | 12.1 | 13.4 | 14.6 |
| 31 | 4 | 6 | 43.5 | 47.6 | 51.2 | 16.6 | 19.9 | 23.8 | 12.5 | 13.8 | 15.0 |
| 32 | 3 | 5 | 44.6 | 48.8 | 52.5 | 17.0 | 20.4 | 24.3 | 12.9 | 14.2 | 15.4 |
| 33 | 6 | 19 | 45.8 | 50.0 | 53.8 | 17.4 | 20.8 | 24.8 | 13.3 | 14.6 | 15.7 |
| 34 | 5 | 17 | 46.9 | 51.2 | 55.0 | 17.8 | 21.2 | 25.3 | 13.7 | 15.0 | 16.1 |
| 35 | 5 | 9 | 48.0 | 52.3 | 56.2 | 18.2 | 21.5 | 25.7 | 14.1 | 15.3 | 16.4 |
| 36 | | | 49.0 | 53.3 | 57.3 | 18.5 | 21.9 | 26.2 | 14.4 | 15.7 | 16.7 |
| 37 | 1 | 3 | 50.0 | 54.4 | 58.5 | 18.9 | 22.2 | 26.6 | 14.8 | 16.0 | 17.1 |
| 38 | | | 51.0 | 55.3 | 59.6 | 19.2 | 22.5 | 27.0 | 15.1 | 16.3 | 17.4 |
| 39 | | | 52.0 | 56.2 | 60.6 | 19.5 | 22.7 | 27.4 | 15.4 | 16.6 | 17.7 |
| 40 | | | 52.9 | 57.1 | 61.7 | 19.9 | 23.0 | 27.8 | 15.8 | 16.9 | 18.0 |
| Total | 111 | 353 | | | | | | | | | |

Reproduced with permission from Robinson AJ, Blaser S, Toi A, et al. MRI of the fetal eyes: morphologic and biometric assessment for abnormal development with ultrasonographic and clinicopathologic correlation. *Pediatr Radiol.* 2008;38:971–981.

| Table 27 | Ultrasound Percentile Reference Values for Ear Length |

| Gestational Age (wk) | Ear Length (mm) | | |
| | Percentiles | | |
| | 5th | 50th | 95th |
|---|---|---|---|
| 15 | 7 | 9 | 11 |
| 16 | 8 | 10 | 12 |
| 17 | 9 | 11 | 13 |
| 18 | 10 | 12 | 14 |
| 19 | 11 | 13 | 16 |
| 20 | 11 | 15 | 17 |
| 21 | 12 | 16 | 18 |
| 22 | 13 | 17 | 19 |
| 23 | 14 | 18 | 21 |
| 24 | 15 | 19 | 22 |
| 25 | 16 | 20 | 24 |
| 26 | 17 | 22 | 26 |
| 27 | 18 | 23 | 27 |
| 28 | 18 | 24 | 28 |
| 29 | 19 | 25 | 29 |
| 30 | 20 | 26 | 30 |
| 31 | 21 | 27 | 31 |
| 32 | 22 | 28 | 32 |
| 33 | 22 | 28 | 33 |
| 34 | 23 | 29 | 34 |
| 35 | 24 | 30 | 35 |
| 36 | 25 | 30 | 36 |
| 37 | 25 | 31 | 37 |
| 38 | 26 | 31 | 37 |
| 39 | 27 | 32 | 38 |
| 40 | 27 | 32 | 38 |

*Note:* Ratio biparietal diameter/ear length is 3.03 (SD, 0.29), independent of gestational age.
Modified data, smoothed and rounded to nearest millimeter, from Chitkara U, Lee L, El-Sayed YY, et al. Ultrasonographic ear length measurement in normal second- and third-trimester fetuses. *Am J Obstet Gynecol.* 2000;183:230–234. Reproduced with permission from Shimizu T, Salvador L, Allanson J, et al. Ultrasonographic measurements of fetal ear. *Obstet Gynecol.* 1992;80:381–384.

| Table 28 | Ultrasound Reference Values for Mandible Length |

| MA (wk) | Mandible Length (mm) | | |
| | Percentiles | | |
| | 5th | 50th | 95th |
|---|---|---|---|
| 15 | 11 | 14 | 18 |
| 16 | 13 | 17 | 20 |
| 17 | 15 | 19 | 22 |
| 18 | 17 | 21 | 24 |
| 19 | 19 | 23 | 26 |
| 20 | 21 | 25 | 28 |
| 21 | 23 | 26 | 30 |
| 22 | 25 | 28 | 32 |
| 23 | 27 | 30 | 33 |
| 24 | 28 | 32 | 35 |
| 25 | 30 | 33 | 37 |
| 26 | 31 | 35 | 38 |
| 27 | 33 | 36 | 40 |
| 28 | 34 | 38 | 41 |
| 29 | 36 | 39 | 43 |
| 30 | 37 | 41 | 44 |
| 31 | 39 | 42 | 45 |
| 32 | 40 | 43 | 47 |
| 33 | 41 | 45 | 48 |
| 34 | 42 | 46 | 49 |
| 35 | 43 | 47 | 50 |
| 36 | 44 | 48 | 51 |
| 37 | 45 | 49 | 52 |
| 38 | 46 | 50 | 53 |
| 39 | 47 | 51 | 54 |

*Note:* Mandible length (mm) = $-20.41 + 2.97 \times GA - 0.027 \times GA^2$ (SD = 2.077). GA, gestational age; MA, menstrual age.
Reproduced with permission from Otto C, Platt LD. The fetal mandible measurement: an objective determination of fetal jaw size. *Ultrasound Obstet Gynecol.* 1991;1:12–17.

| Table 29 | Ultrasound Reference Values for Length of Nasal Bone |

| Gestational Age (wk) | Length of Nasal Bone (mm) | | |
| | −2 SD | Mean | +2 SD |
|---|---|---|---|
| 14 | 3.3 | 4.2 | 5.0 |
| 16 | 3.1 | 5.2 | 7.3 |
| 18 | 5.0 | 6.3 | 7.6 |
| 20 | 5.7 | 7.6 | 9.5 |
| 22 | 6.0 | 8.2 | 10.4 |
| 24 | 6.8 | 9.4 | 12.0 |
| 26 | 7.2 | 9.7 | 12.3 |
| 28 | 7.8 | 10.7 | 13.6 |
| 30 | 8.3 | 11.3 | 14.4 |
| 32 | 8.0 | 11.6 | 15.2 |
| 34 | 7.5 | 12.3 | 17.0 |

Reproduced with permission from Guis F, Ville Y, Vincent Y, et al. Ultrasound evaluation of the length of the fetal nasal bones throughout gestation. *Ultrasound Obstet Gynecol.* 1995;5:304–307.

## Neck and Chest Measurements

| Table 30 | Ultrasound Thyroid Circumference Based on Biparietal Diameter (BPD) | | | | |
|---|---|---|---|---|---|
| **BPD (cm)** | **Thyroid Circumference by Percentile (cm)** | | | | |
| | **5th** | **10th** | **50th** | **90th** | **95th** |
| 3.50 | 1.5 | 1.7 | 2.3 | 2.8 | 3.0 |
| 3.75 | 1.6 | 1.8 | 2.3 | 2.9 | 3.1 |
| 4.00 | 1.6 | 1.8 | 2.4 | 3.0 | 3.2 |
| 4.25 | 1.7 | 1.8 | 2.5 | 3.1 | 3.3 |
| 4.50 | 1.7 | 1.9 | 2.5 | 3.2 | 3.4 |
| 4.75 | 1.8 | 2.0 | 2.6 | 3.3 | 3.5 |
| 5.00 | 1.9 | 2.1 | 2.8 | 3.4 | 3.6 |
| 5.25 | 2.0 | 2.2 | 2.9 | 3.6 | 3.8 |
| 5.50 | 2.1 | 2.3 | 3.0 | 3.7 | 3.9 |
| 5.75 | 2.2 | 2.4 | 3.1 | 3.9 | 4.1 |
| 6.00 | 2.3 | 2.5 | 3.3 | 4.0 | 4.3 |
| 6.25 | 2.4 | 2.7 | 3.4 | 4.2 | 4.4 |
| 6.50 | 2.6 | 2.8 | 3.6 | 4.4 | 4.6 |
| 6.75 | 2.7 | 3.0 | 3.8 | 4.6 | 4.8 |
| 7.00 | 2.9 | 3.1 | 4.0 | 4.8 | 5.0 |
| 7.25 | 3.1 | 3.3 | 4.2 | 5.0 | 5.2 |
| 7.50 | 3.2 | 3.5 | 4.4 | 5.2 | 5.5 |
| 7.75 | 3.4 | 3.7 | 4.6 | 5.5 | 5.7 |
| 8.00 | 3.6 | 3.9 | 4.8 | 5.7 | 6.0 |
| 8.25 | 3.8 | 4.1 | 5.0 | 6.0 | 6.2 |
| 8.50 | 4.1 | 4.3 | 5.3 | 6.2 | 6.5 |
| 8.75 | 4.3 | 4.6 | 5.5 | 6.5 | 6.8 |
| 9.00 | 4.5 | 4.8 | 5.8 | 6.8 | 7.0 |

Reproduced from Ranzini AC, Anath CV, Smulian JC, et al. Ultrasonography of the fetal thyroid: monograms based on biparietal diameter and gestational age. *J Ultrasound Med.* 2001;20(6):613–617, with permission from the American Institute for Ultrasound in Medicine.

| Table 31 | Ultrasound Thyroid Circumference Based on Gestational Age | | | | | |
|---|---|---|---|---|---|---|
| **Gestational Age (wk)** | **No. of Patients** | **Thyroid Circumference by Percentile (cm)** | | | | |
| | | **5th** | **10th** | **50th** | **90th** | **95th** |
| 16 | 5 | 1.3 | 1.7 | 2.3 | 2.8 | 3.0 |
| 17 | 5 | 1.4 | 1.8 | 2.3 | 2.9 | 3.1 |
| 18 | 14 | 1.5 | 1.8 | 2.4 | 3.0 | 3.2 |
| 19 | 10 | 1.7 | 1.8 | 2.5 | 3.1 | 3.3 |
| 20 | 25 | 1.8 | 1.9 | 2.5 | 3.2 | 3.4 |
| 21 | 13 | 1.9 | 2.0 | 2.6 | 3.3 | 3.5 |
| 22 | 11 | 2.1 | 2.1 | 2.8 | 3.4 | 3.6 |
| 23 | 4 | 2.2 | 2.2 | 2.9 | 3.6 | 3.8 |
| 24 | 11 | 2.3 | 2.3 | 3.0 | 3.7 | 3.9 |
| 25 | 11 | 2.5 | 2.4 | 3.1 | 3.9 | 4.1 |
| 26 | 15 | 2.6 | 2.5 | 3.3 | 4.0 | 4.3 |
| 27 | 7 | 2.7 | 2.7 | 3.4 | 4.2 | 4.4 |
| 28 | 10 | 2.9 | 2.8 | 3.6 | 4.4 | 4.6 |
| 29 | 9 | 3.0 | 3.0 | 3.8 | 4.6 | 4.8 |
| 30 | 6 | 3.1 | 3.1 | 4.0 | 4.8 | 5.0 |
| 31 | 5 | 3.3 | 3.3 | 4.2 | 5.0 | 5.2 |
| 32 | 9 | 3.4 | 3.5 | 4.4 | 5.2 | 5.5 |
| 33 | 11 | 3.5 | 3.7 | 4.6 | 5.5 | 5.7 |
| 34 | 1 | 3.7 | 3.9 | 4.8 | 5.7 | 6.0 |
| 35 | 7 | 3.8 | 4.1 | 5.0 | 6.0 | 6.2 |
| 36 | 7 | 3.9 | 4.3 | 5.3 | 6.2 | 6.5 |
| 37 | 4 | 4.1 | 4.6 | 5.5 | 6.5 | 6.8 |

Reproduced from Ranzini AC, Anath CV, Smulian JC, et al. Ultrasonography of the fetal thyroid: monograms based on biparietal diameter and gestational age. *J Ultrasound Med.* 2001;20(6):613–617, with permission from the American Institute for Ultrasound in Medicine.

| Table 32 | Ultrasound Reference Values for Thyroid Volume | |
|---|---|---|
| **GA (wk)** | **Thyroid Volume (cm³)** | |
| | **Mean** | **Range** |
| 20–23 | 0.08 | ±0.05 |
| 24–27 | 0.15 | ±0.09 |
| 28–31 | 0.24 | ±0.10 |
| 32–35 | 0.42 | ±0.21 |
| >35 | 0.63 | ±0.22 |

*Note:* Volume $= 0.38 - 0.02 \times GA + 0.3 \times EFW$.
EFW, estimated fetal weight; GA, gestational age.
Reproduced with permission from Ho SSY, Metreweli C. Normal thyroid volume. *Ultrasound Obstet Gynecol.* 1998;11:118–122.

| Table 33 | Ultrasound Percentile Reference Values for Thoracic Circumference |
|---|---|

| Gestational Age (wk) | n | Predictive Percentiles | | | | | | | | |
|---|---|---|---|---|---|---|---|---|---|---|
| | | 2.5th | 5th | 10th | 25th | 50th | 75th | 90th | 95th | 97.5th |
| 16 | 6 | 5.9 | 6.4 | 7.0 | 8.0 | 9.1 | 10.3 | 11.3 | 11.9 | 12.4 |
| 17 | 22 | 6.8 | 7.3 | 7.9 | 8.9 | 10.0 | 11.2 | 12.2 | 12.8 | 13.3 |
| 18 | 31 | 7.7 | 8.2 | 8.8 | 9.8 | 11.0 | 12.1 | 13.1 | 13.7 | 14.2 |
| 19 | 21 | 8.6 | 9.1 | 9.7 | 10.7 | 11.9 | 13.0 | 14.0 | 14.6 | 15.1 |
| 20 | 20 | 9.5 | 10.0 | 10.6 | 11.7 | 12.8 | 13.9 | 15.0 | 15.5 | 16.0 |
| 21 | 30 | 10.4 | 11.0 | 11.6 | 12.6 | 13.7 | 14.8 | 15.8 | 16.4 | 16.9 |
| 22 | 18 | 11.3 | 11.9 | 12.5 | 13.5 | 14.6 | 15.7 | 16.7 | 17.3 | 17.8 |
| 23 | 21 | 12.2 | 12.8 | 13.4 | 14.4 | 15.5 | 16.6 | 17.6 | 18.2 | 18.8 |
| 24 | 27 | 13.2 | 13.7 | 14.3 | 15.3 | 16.4 | 17.5 | 18.5 | 19.1 | 19.7 |
| 25 | 20 | 14.1 | 14.6 | 15.2 | 16.2 | 17.3 | 18.4 | 19.4 | 20.0 | 20.6 |
| 26 | 25 | 15.0 | 15.5 | 16.1 | 17.1 | 18.2 | 19.3 | 20.3 | 21.0 | 21.5 |
| 27 | 24 | 15.9 | 16.4 | 17.0 | 18.0 | 19.1 | 20.2 | 21.3 | 21.9 | 22.4 |
| 28 | 24 | 16.8 | 17.3 | 17.9 | 18.9 | 20.0 | 21.2 | 22.2 | 22.8 | 23.3 |
| 29 | 24 | 17.7 | 18.2 | 18.8 | 19.8 | 21.0 | 22.1 | 23.1 | 23.7 | 24.2 |
| 30 | 27 | 18.6 | 19.1 | 19.7 | 20.7 | 21.9 | 23.0 | 24.0 | 24.6 | 25.1 |
| 31 | 24 | 19.5 | 20.0 | 20.6 | 21.6 | 22.8 | 23.9 | 24.9 | 25.5 | 26.0 |
| 32 | 28 | 20.4 | 20.9 | 21.5 | 22.6 | 23.7 | 24.8 | 25.8 | 26.4 | 26.9 |
| 33 | 27 | 21.3 | 21.8 | 22.5 | 23.5 | 24.6 | 25.7 | 26.7 | 27.3 | 27.8 |
| 34 | 25 | 22.2 | 22.8 | 23.4 | 24.4 | 25.5 | 26.6 | 27.6 | 28.2 | 28.7 |
| 35 | 20 | 23.1 | 23.7 | 24.3 | 25.3 | 26.4 | 27.5 | 28.5 | 29.1 | 29.6 |
| 36 | 23 | 24.0 | 24.6 | 25.2 | 26.2 | 27.3 | 28.4 | 29.4 | 30.0 | 30.6 |
| 37 | 22 | 24.9 | 25.5 | 26.1 | 27.1 | 28.2 | 29.3 | 30.3 | 30.9 | 31.5 |
| 38 | 21 | 25.9 | 26.4 | 27.0 | 28.0 | 29.1 | 30.2 | 31.2 | 31.9 | 32.4 |
| 39 | 7 | 26.8 | 27.3 | 27.9 | 28.9 | 30.0 | 31.1 | 32.2 | 32.8 | 33.3 |
| 40 | 6 | 27.7 | 28.2 | 28.8 | 29.8 | 30.9 | 32.1 | 33.1 | 33.7 | 34.2 |

*Note:* Measurements in centimeters.

Reproduced with permission from Chitkara U, Rosenberg J, Chervenak FA, et al. Prenatal sonographic assessment of the fetal thorax: normal values. *Am J Obstet Gynecol.* 1987;156:1069–1074.

| Table 34 | Reference Values for Lung Volumes Calculated by 3D Ultrasound |
|---|---|

| | Lung Volume (cm³) | | |
| | Percentiles | | |
| GA (wk) | 5th | 50th | 95th |
|---|---|---|---|
| 14 | 0.3 | 3.9 | 11.6 |
| 15 | 0.7 | 5.3 | 14.1 |
| 16 | 1.2 | 6.8 | 16.9 |
| 17 | 2.0 | 8.6 | 20.0 |
| 18 | 2.9 | 10.6 | 23.3 |
| 19 | 3.9 | 12.8 | 26.8 |
| 20 | 5.1 | 15.2 | 30.7 |
| 21 | 6.5 | 17.8 | 34.7 |
| 22 | 8.1 | 20.7 | 39.0 |
| 23 | 9.8 | 23.7 | 43.6 |
| 24 | 11.7 | 26.9 | 48.4 |
| 25 | 13.7 | 30.4 | 53.5 |
| 26 | 16.0 | 34.0 | 58.9 |
| 27 | 18.3 | 37.9 | 64.5 |
| 28 | 20.9 | 42.0 | 70.3 |
| 29 | 23.6 | 46.2 | 76.4 |
| 30 | 26.5 | 50.7 | 82.7 |
| 31 | 29.5 | 55.4 | 89.3 |
| 32 | 32.8 | 60.3 | 96.2 |
| 33 | 36.1 | 65.4 | 103.3 |
| 34 | 39.7 | 70.7 | 110.7 |
| 35 | 43.4 | 76.2 | 118.3 |
| 36 | 47.3 | 82.0 | 126.2 |
| 37 | 51.3 | 87.9 | 134.3 |
| 38 | 55.5 | 94.0 | 142.7 |
| 39 | 59.9 | 100.4 | 151.3 |
| 40 | 64.4 | 107.0 | 160.2 |

*Note:* Mean volume$^{0.5}$ = $-2.538094 + 0.322 \times$ GA.

GA, gestational age.

Reproduced with permission from Lee A, Kratochwil A, Stumpflen I, et al. Fetal lung volume determination by three-dimensional ultrasonography. *Am J Obstet Gynecol*. 1996;175(3, pt 1):588–592.

## Table 35 — Reference Values for the Right Lung Volume Calculated by 3D Ultrasound

| EFW (g) | n | Lung Volume (cm³) | | | | | | | |
| | | Percentiles | | | | | | | |
| | | 2.5th | 5th | 10th | 50th | 90th | 95th | 97.5th | SD |
|---|---|---|---|---|---|---|---|---|---|
| 200 | 23 | 0.48 | 0.92 | 1.42 | 3.99 | 6.56 | 7.07 | 7.50 | 1.566 |
| 300 | 27 | 1.42 | 1.97 | 2.60 | 5.85 | 9.10 | 9.74 | 10.28 | 1.980 |
| 400 | 28 | 2.35 | 3.02 | 3.78 | 7.71 | 11.63 | 12.41 | 13.07 | 2.393 |
| 500 | 17 | 3.28 | 4.07 | 4.97 | 9.57 | 14.17 | 15.08 | 15.86 | 2.806 |
| 600 | 20 | 4.22 | 5.12 | 6.15 | 11.43 | 16.71 | 17.74 | 18.64 | 3.219 |
| 700 | 16 | 5.15 | 6.17 | 7.33 | 13.29 | 19.25 | 20.41 | 21.43 | 3.633 |
| 800 | 13 | 6.09 | 7.22 | 8.51 | 15.15 | 21.78 | 23.08 | 24.21 | 4.046 |
| 900 | 15 | 7.02 | 8.27 | 9.70 | 17.01 | 24.32 | 25.75 | 27.00 | 4.459 |
| 1,000 | 16 | 7.96 | 9.32 | 10.88 | 18.87 | 26.86 | 28.42 | 29.78 | 4.872 |
| 1,100 | 11 | 8.89 | 10.37 | 12.06 | 20.73 | 29.40 | 31.09 | 32.57 | 5.286 |
| 1,200 | 10 | 9.82 | 11.42 | 13.24 | 22.59 | 31.94 | 33.76 | 35.36 | 5.699 |
| 1,300 | 9 | 10.76 | 12.47 | 14.42 | 24.45 | 34.47 | 36.43 | 38.14 | 6.112 |
| 1,400 | 12 | 11.69 | 13.52 | 15.61 | 26.31 | 37.01 | 39.10 | 40.93 | 6.525 |
| 1,500 | 13 | 12.63 | 14.57 | 16.79 | 28.17 | 39.55 | 41.77 | 43.71 | 6.939 |
| 1,600 | 8 | 13.56 | 15.62 | 17.97 | 30.03 | 42.09 | 44.44 | 46.50 | 7.352 |
| 1,700 | 8 | 14.50 | 16.67 | 19.15 | 31.89 | 44.62 | 47.11 | 49.28 | 7.765 |
| 1,800 | 14 | 15.43 | 17.72 | 20.34 | 33.75 | 47.16 | 49.78 | 52.07 | 8.179 |
| 1,900 | 6 | 16.36 | 18.77 | 21.52 | 35.61 | 49.70 | 52.45 | 54.86 | 8.592 |
| 2,000 | 7 | 17.30 | 19.82 | 22.70 | 37.47 | 52.24 | 55.12 | 57.64 | 9.005 |
| 2,100 | 5 | 18.23 | 20.87 | 23.88 | 39.33 | 54.78 | 57.79 | 60.43 | 9.418 |
| 2,200 | 6 | 19.17 | 21.92 | 25.07 | 41.19 | 57.31 | 60.46 | 63.21 | 9.832 |
| 2,300 | 4 | 20.10 | 22.97 | 26.25 | 43.05 | 59.85 | 63.13 | 66.00 | 10.249 |
| 2,400 | 5 | 21.04 | 24.02 | 27.43 | 44.91 | 62.39 | 65.80 | 68.78 | 10.658 |

EFW, estimated fetal weight.
Reproduced with permission from Gerards FA, Engels MAJ, Twisk JWR, et al. Normal fetal lung volume measured with three-dimensional ultrasound. *Ultrasound Obstet Gynecol.* 2006;27:134–144.

## Table 36 — Reference Values for the Left Lung Volume Calculated by 3D Ultrasound

| EFW (g) | n | Lung Volume (cm³) | | | | | | | |
| | | Percentiles | | | | | | | |
| | | 2.5th | 5th | 10th | 50th | 90th | 95th | 97.5th | SD |
|---|---|---|---|---|---|---|---|---|---|
| 200 | 23 | 0.41 | 0.77 | 1.18 | 3.30 | 5.42 | 5.84 | 6.19 | 1.291 |
| 300 | 27 | 1.19 | 1.63 | 2.14 | 4.73 | 7.32 | 7.82 | 8.27 | 1.582 |
| 400 | 28 | 1.98 | 2.50 | 3.10 | 6.15 | 9.20 | 9.80 | 10.32 | 1.862 |
| 500 | 17 | 2.77 | 3.37 | 4.06 | 7.57 | 11.08 | 11.78 | 12.37 | 2.143 |
| 600 | 20 | 3.55 | 4.23 | 5.00 | 9.00 | 12.99 | 13.76 | 14.45 | 2.434 |
| 700 | 16 | 4.34 | 5.10 | 5.97 | 10.42 | 14.87 | 15.74 | 16.50 | 2.714 |
| 800 | 13 | 5.12 | 5.96 | 6.92 | 11.84 | 16.76 | 17.72 | 18.56 | 3.000 |
| 900 | 15 | 5.91 | 6.83 | 7.88 | 13.27 | 18.66 | 19.70 | 20.63 | 3.286 |
| 1,000 | 16 | 6.70 | 7.70 | 8.84 | 14.69 | 20.54 | 21.68 | 22.68 | 3.566 |
| 1,100 | 11 | 7.48 | 8.56 | 9.79 | 16.11 | 22.43 | 23.66 | 24.74 | 3.852 |
| 1,200 | 10 | 8.27 | 9.43 | 10.75 | 17.54 | 24.33 | 25.64 | 26.81 | 4.138 |
| 1,300 | 9 | 9.05 | 10.29 | 11.71 | 18.96 | 26.21 | 27.63 | 28.87 | 4.423 |
| 1,400 | 12 | 9.84 | 11.16 | 12.67 | 20.38 | 28.09 | 29.61 | 30.92 | 4.704 |
| 1,500 | 13 | 10.63 | 12.03 | 13.63 | 21.81 | 29.99 | 31.59 | 32.99 | 4.990 |
| 1,600 | 8 | 11.41 | 12.89 | 14.58 | 23.23 | 31.88 | 33.57 | 35.05 | 5.275 |
| 1,700 | 8 | 12.20 | 13.76 | 15.54 | 24.65 | 33.76 | 35.55 | 37.10 | 5.556 |
| 1,800 | 14 | 12.98 | 14.62 | 16.49 | 26.08 | 35.67 | 37.53 | 39.18 | 5.847 |
| 1,900 | 6 | 13.77 | 15.49 | 17.45 | 27.50 | 37.55 | 39.51 | 41.23 | 6.128 |
| 2,000 | 7 | 14.57 | 16.36 | 18.41 | 28.92 | 39.43 | 41.49 | 43.27 | 6.408 |
| 2,100 | 5 | 15.34 | 17.22 | 19.36 | 30.35 | 41.34 | 43.47 | 45.36 | 6.699 |
| 2,200 | 6 | 16.14 | 18.09 | 20.32 | 31.77 | 43.22 | 45.45 | 47.40 | 6.980 |
| 2,300 | 4 | 16.93 | 18.96 | 21.28 | 33.19 | 45.10 | 47.43 | 49.45 | 7.260 |
| 2,400 | 5 | 17.70 | 19.81 | 22.23 | 34.61 | 46.99 | 49.41 | 51.52 | 7.551 |

EFW, Estimated Fetal Weight
Reproduced with permission from Gerards FA, Engels MAJ, Twisk JWR, et al. Normal fetal lung volume measured with three-dimensional ultrasound. *Ultrasound Obstet Gynecol.* 2006;27:134–144.

| Table 37 | MRI Reference Values for Lung Volumes |
|---|---|

| GA (wk) | n | FLV Range (mL) | Mean FLV (mL) | Median FLV (mL) | SD | Skewness | 95% CI |
|---|---|---|---|---|---|---|---|
| 21.0–25.0 | 13 | 16–48 | 26.15 | 24 | 9.15 | 1.18 | 13.00–47.55 |
| 26.0–27.5 | 29 | 23–66 | 38.83 | 37 | 10.12 | 0.57 | 22.33–63.27 |
| 28.0–30.0 | 34 | 29–89 | 52.97 | 53 | 14.20 | 0.59 | 29.73–88.00 |
| 31.0–31.5 | 26 | 35–101 | 65.04 | 64 | 15.91 | 0.18 | 37.71–105.53 |
| 32.0 | 32 | 38–109 | 70.22 | 67.5 | 18.16 | 0.41 | 40.30–114.62 |
| 32.5–33.0 | 34 | 47–110 | 72.29 | 69 | 17.18 | 0.69 | 44.38–111.73 |
| 33.5–35.0 | 30 | 52–129 | 80.73 | 77.50 | 24.32 | 0.73 | 43.34–138.38 |
| 35.5–38.0 | 16 | 38–150 | 88.63 | 77.50 | 31.77 | 0.42 | 39.45–175.58 |

FLV, fetal lung volume; SD, standard deviation; CI, confidence interval.
Reproduced with permission from Rypens F, Metens T, Rocourt N, et al. Fetal lung volume: estimation at MR Imaging—initial results. *Radiology*. 2001;219:236–241.

## Abdominal Measurements

| Table 38 | Ultrasound Reference Values for Renal Length |
|---|---|

| GA (wk) | N | Fitted Centiles | | | | | |
|---|---|---|---|---|---|---|---|
| | | 3rd | 10th | 50th | 90th | 97th | SD[a] |
| 14 | 3 | 7.5 | 8.0 | 9.3 | 10.8 | 11.6 | 0.12 |
| 15 | 3 | 8.8 | 9.5 | 11.0 | 12.8 | 13.7 | 0.12 |
| 16 | 2 | 10.2 | 11.0 | 12.7 | 14.8 | 15.8 | 0.12 |
| 17 | 12 | 11.6 | 12.5 | 14.5 | 16.8 | 18.1 | 0.12 |
| 18 | 10 | 13.1 | 14.1 | 16.3 | 18.9 | 20.3 | 0.12 |
| 19 | 15 | 14.6 | 15.6 | 18.2 | 21.1 | 22.6 | 0.12 |
| 20 | 15 | 16.1 | 17.2 | 20.0 | 23.2 | 24.9 | 0.12 |
| 21 | 15 | 17.5 | 18.8 | 21.8 | 25.4 | 27.2 | 0.12 |
| 22 | 14 | 19.0 | 20.4 | 23.6 | 27.4 | 29.4 | 0.12 |
| 23 | 16 | 20.4 | 21.9 | 25.4 | 29.5 | 31.6 | 0.12 |
| 24 | 17 | 21.8 | 23.4 | 27.1 | 31.5 | 33.8 | 0.12 |
| 25 | 18 | 23.1 | 24.8 | 28.8 | 33.4 | 35.8 | 0.12 |
| 26 | 20 | 24.4 | 26.2 | 30.4 | 35.3 | 37.8 | 0.12 |
| 27 | 24 | 25.6 | 27.5 | 31.9 | 37.1 | 39.7 | 0.12 |
| 28 | 18 | 26.8 | 28.7 | 33.4 | 38.7 | 41.5 | 0.12 |
| 29 | 19 | 27.9 | 29.9 | 34.7 | 40.3 | 43.2 | 0.12 |
| 30 | 19 | 28.9 | 31.0 | 36.0 | 41.8 | 44.8 | 0.12 |
| 31 | 23 | 29.9 | 32.1 | 37.2 | 43.2 | 46.3 | 0.12 |
| 32 | 23 | 30.8 | 33.0 | 38.3 | 44.5 | 47.7 | 0.12 |
| 33 | 22 | 31.6 | 33.9 | 39.4 | 45.7 | 49.0 | 0.12 |
| 34 | 19 | 32.4 | 34.7 | 40.3 | 46.8 | 50.2 | 0.12 |
| 35 | 20 | 33.1 | 35.4 | 41.1 | 47.8 | 51.2 | 0.12 |
| 36 | 23 | 33.7 | 36.1 | 41.9 | 48.7 | 52.2 | 0.12 |
| 37 | 14 | 34.2 | 36.7 | 42.6 | 49.4 | 53.0 | 0.12 |
| 38 | 17 | 34.7 | 37.2 | 43.2 | 50.1 | 53.8 | 0.12 |
| 39 | 13 | 35.1 | 37.6 | 43.7 | 50.7 | 54.4 | 0.12 |
| 40 | 14 | 35.4 | 38.0 | 44.1 | 51.2 | 54.9 | 0.12 |
| 41 | 26 | 35.7 | 38.3 | 44.5 | 51.6 | 55.4 | 0.12 |
| 42 | 17 | 36.0 | 38.6 | 44.8 | 52.0 | 55.7 | 0.12 |

[a]SD, standard deviation of log of measurement (constant).
Reproduced with permission from Chitty LS, Altman DG. Charts of fetal size: kidney and renal pelvis measurements. *Prenat Diagn*. 2003;23:891–897.

| Table 39 | Reference Values for Renal Volumes Based on 3D Ultrasound |
| --- | --- |

| | Renal Volumes (cm$^3$) | | | | | | | | | |
| --- | --- | --- | --- | --- | --- | --- | --- | --- | --- | --- |
| | Right Kidney | | | | | | Left Kidney | | | |
| | Percentiles | | | | | | Percentiles | | | |
| GA (wk) | 5th | 10th | 50th | 90th | 95th | | 5th | 10th | 50th | 90th | 95th |
| 20 | 0.3 | 0.6 | 1.5 | 2.4 | 2.7 | | 0.6 | 0.9 | 1.8 | 2.7 | 3.0 |
| 21 | 0.8 | 1.1 | 2.2 | 3.3 | 3.6 | | 1.2 | 1.5 | 2.6 | 3.6 | 4.0 |
| 22 | 1.4 | 1.7 | 3.0 | 4.2 | 4.6 | | 1.7 | 2.1 | 3.3 | 4.6 | 4.9 |
| 23 | 1.9 | 2.3 | 3.7 | 5.1 | 5.5 | | 2.3 | 2.7 | 4.1 | 5.5 | 5.9 |
| 24 | 2.4 | 2.9 | 4.5 | 6.0 | 6.5 | | 2.8 | 3.3 | 4.8 | 6.4 | 6.9 |
| 25 | 3.0 | 3.5 | 5.2 | 6.9 | 7.4 | | 3.4 | 3.9 | 5.6 | 7.3 | 7.8 |
| 26 | 3.5 | 4.0 | 5.9 | 7.8 | 8.4 | | 4.0 | 4.6 | 6.5 | 8.4 | 9.0 |
| 27 | 4.0 | 4.6 | 6.7 | 8.7 | 9.3 | | 4.5 | 5.1 | 7.1 | 9.2 | 9.8 |
| 28 | 4.5 | 5.2 | 7.4 | 9.7 | 10.3 | | 5.0 | 5.6 | 7.9 | 10.1 | 10.8 |
| 29 | 5.1 | 5.8 | 8.2 | 10.6 | 11.2 | | 5.6 | 6.3 | 8.7 | 11.0 | 11.7 |
| 30 | 5.6 | 6.3 | 8.9 | 11.5 | 12.2 | | 6.1 | 6.9 | 9.4 | 12.0 | 12.7 |
| 31 | 6.1 | 6.9 | 9.6 | 12.4 | 13.1 | | 6.7 | 7.4 | 10.2 | 12.9 | 13.7 |
| 32 | 6.7 | 7.5 | 10.4 | 13.3 | 14.1 | | 7.2 | 8.0 | 10.9 | 13.8 | 14.6 |
| 33 | 7.2 | 8.1 | 11.1 | 14.2 | 15.0 | | 7.8 | 8.6 | 11.7 | 14.7 | 15.6 |
| 34 | 7.7 | 8.6 | 11.9 | 15.1 | 16.0 | | 8.3 | 9.2 | 12.5 | 15.7 | 16.6 |
| 35 | 8.3 | 9.2 | 12.6 | 16.0 | 16.9 | | 8.9 | 9.8 | 13.2 | 16.6 | 17.6 |
| 36 | 8.8 | 9.8 | 13.3 | 16.9 | 17.9 | | 9.4 | 10.4 | 14.0 | 17.5 | 18.5 |
| 37 | 9.3 | 10.4 | 14.1 | 17.8 | 18.9 | | 10.0 | 11.0 | 14.7 | 18.4 | 19.5 |
| 38 | 9.8 | 11.0 | 14.8 | 18.7 | 19.8 | | 10.5 | 11.6 | 15.5 | 19.4 | 20.5 |
| 39 | 10.4 | 11.5 | 15.6 | 19.6 | 20.7 | | 11.1 | 12.2 | 16.3 | 20.3 | 21.4 |
| 40 | 10.9 | 12.1 | 16.3 | 20.5 | 21.7 | | 11.8 | 13.0 | 17.2 | 21.4 | 21.7 |

*Note:* Volume can be estimated by length × height × width × 0.52.

Data adapted from Yu C, Chang F, Ko H, et al. Fetal renal volume in normal gestation: a three-dimensional ultrasound study. *Ultrasound Med Biol.* 2000;26:1253–1256.

| Table 40 | Reference Values of Fetal Liver Volume Determined by 3D Ultrasound Compared with Estimated Fetal Weight |

| Estimated Fetal Weight (g) | Liver Volume (cm³) | | |
|---|---|---|---|
| | Percentiles | | |
| | 5th | 50th | 95th |
| 400 | 5 | 17 | 29 |
| 500 | 9 | 21 | 33 |
| 600 | 12 | 24 | 37 |
| 700 | 16 | 28 | 40 |
| 800 | 19 | 32 | 44 |
| 900 | 23 | 35 | 47 |
| 1,000 | 27 | 39 | 51 |
| 1,100 | 30 | 42 | 55 |
| 1,200 | 34 | 46 | 58 |
| 1,300 | 37 | 50 | 62 |
| 1,400 | 41 | 53 | 65 |
| 1,500 | 45 | 57 | 69 |
| 1,600 | 48 | 60 | 73 |
| 1,700 | 52 | 64 | 76 |
| 1,800 | 55 | 68 | 80 |
| 1,900 | 59 | 71 | 83 |
| 2,000 | 63 | 75 | 87 |
| 2,100 | 66 | 78 | 91 |
| 2,200 | 70 | 82 | 94 |
| 2,300 | 73 | 86 | 98 |
| 2,400 | 77 | 89 | 101 |
| 2,500 | 81 | 93 | 105 |
| 2,600 | 84 | 96 | 109 |
| 2,700 | 88 | 100 | 112 |
| 2,800 | 91 | 104 | 116 |
| 2,900 | 95 | 107 | 119 |
| 3,000 | 99 | 111 | 123 |

*Note:* Liver volume $= 2.79 + 0.036 \times GA$ (SD $= 7.44$).
Data from Laudy JAM, Janssen MMM, Struykk PC, et al. Fetal liver volume measurement by three-dimensional ultrasonography: a preliminary study. *Ultrasound Obstet Gynecol.* 1009;12:93–96.

| Table 41 | Fetal Ultrasound Liver Length[a] Compared with Gestational Age | | |
|---|---|---|---|

| | Liver Length (mm) | | |
| | Percentiles | | |
| GA (wk) | 5th | 50th | 95th |
|---|---|---|---|
| 13 | 10 | 13 | 16 |
| 14 | 11 | 14 | 18 |
| 15 | 13 | 16 | 19 |
| 16 | 13 | 17 | 21 |
| 17 | 14 | 19 | 23 |
| 18 | 16 | 20 | 25 |
| 19 | 18 | 22 | 28 |
| 20 | 18 | 24 | 30 |
| 21 | 20 | 26 | 32 |
| 22 | 22 | 28 | 34 |
| 23 | 23 | 29 | 36 |
| 24 | 25 | 31 | 38 |
| 25 | 26 | 33 | 41 |
| 26 | 28 | 35 | 43 |
| 27 | 29 | 37 | 45 |
| 28 | 30 | 39 | 47 |
| 29 | 32 | 40 | 50 |
| 30 | 33 | 42 | 52 |
| 31 | 34 | 43 | 53 |
| 32 | 35 | 45 | 55 |
| 33 | 36 | 46 | 56 |
| 34 | 37 | 47 | 58 |
| 35 | 38 | 48 | 60 |
| 36 | 38 | 49 | 62 |
| 37 | 39 | 50 | 63 |
| 38 | 39 | 50 | 63 |
| 39 | 40 | 51 | 64 |
| 40 | 40 | 51 | 64 |

[a]Values are approximate, based on graphic data only.
Reproduced with permission from Roberts AB, Mitchell JM, Pattison NS. Fetal liver length in normal and isoimmunized pregnancies. *Am J Obstet Gynecol.* 1989;161:42–46.

| Table 42 | Ultrasound Reference Values for Splenic Length | | |
|---|---|---|---|

| | Splenic Length (mm) | | |
| | Percentiles | | |
| Gestational Age (wk) | 5th | 50th | 95th |
|---|---|---|---|
| 18 | 7 | 14 | 21 |
| 20 | 11 | 18 | 26 |
| 22 | 15 | 22 | 29 |
| 24 | 19 | 25 | 32 |
| 26 | 20 | 27 | 34 |
| 28 | 24 | 31 | 38 |
| 30 | 27 | 34 | 41 |
| 32 | 31 | 28 | 45 |
| 34 | 35 | 43 | 50 |
| 36 | 41 | 48 | 55 |
| 38 | 47 | 54 | 62 |
| 40 | 55 | 62 | 70 |

Reproduced with permission from Schmidt W, Yarkoni S, Jeanty P, et al. Sonographic measurement of the fetal spleen: clinical implications. *J Ultrasound Med.* 1985;4:667.

| Table 43 | Ultrasound Reference Values for Splenic Circumference between 18 and 37 Weeks | |
|---|---|---|

| | Splenic Circumference | |
| | Percentiles | |
| GA (wk) | 50th | 95th |
|---|---|---|
| 18 | 30.7 | 39.7 |
| 19 | 33.9 | 43.8 |
| 20 | 37.2 | 48.0 |
| 21 | 40.4 | 52.2 |
| 22 | 43.6 | 56.3 |
| 23 | 46.9 | 60.5 |
| 24 | 50.1 | 64.7 |
| 25 | 53.3 | 68.9 |
| 26 | 56.6 | 73.0 |
| 27 | 59.8 | 77.1 |
| 28 | 63.1 | 81.3 |
| 29 | 66.3 | 85.5 |
| 30 | 69.5 | 89.6 |
| 31 | 72.8 | 93.8 |
| 32 | 76.0 | 97.9 |
| 33 | 79.7 | 102.1 |
| 34 | 82.5 | 106.3 |
| 35 | 85.7 | 110.4 |
| 36 | 88.9 | 114.6 |
| 37 | 92.2 | 118.7 |

*Note:* Splenic circumference = $-27.569 + 3.23654 \times GA$.
GA, gestational age.
Reproduced with permission from Bahado-Singh R, Oz U, Mari G, et al. Fetal splenic size in anemia due to Rhalloimmunization. *Obstet Gynecol.* 1998;92:828–832.

| Table 44 | Normal Ultrasound Colon Diameters | | |
|---|---|---|---|

| Gestational Age (wk) | Colon Diameters (mm) | | |
| | −2 SD | Mean | +2 SD |
|---|---|---|---|
| 22 | 2 | 4 | 6 |
| 24 | 3 | 5 | 7 |
| 26 | 4 | 6 | 9 |
| 28 | 4 | 7 | 10 |
| 30 | 5 | 8 | 11 |
| 32 | 6 | 9 | 12 |
| 34 | 7 | 10 | 13 |
| 36 | 8 | 12 | 16 |
| 38 | 9 | 14 | 18 |
| 40 | 10 | 16 | 20 |

Data adapted from Harris RD, Nyberg DA, Mack LA, et al. Anorectal atresia: prenatal sonographic diagnosis. *AJR Am J Roentgenol.* 1987;149:395–400.

## Cardiac Measurements

| Table 45 | Reference Values for Aortic Root Internal Diameter, Pulmonary Artery, Left Ventricle, Right Ventricle, Left Atrium, and Right Atrium (Values Are Shown for 5th, 50th, and 95th Percentiles) |
|---|---|

| GA (wk) | Aortic Root (mm)[a] | | | Pulmonary Artery (mm)[b] | | | Left Ventricle (mm)[c] | | |
|---|---|---|---|---|---|---|---|---|---|
| | 5th | 50th | 95th | 5th | 50th | 95th | 5th | 50th | 95th |
| 14.0 | 1.2 | 1.8 | 2.4 | 1.3 | 1.9 | 2.5 | 1.2 | 2.3 | 3.5 |
| 15.0 | 1.4 | 2.0 | 2.7 | 1.6 | 2.2 | 2.8 | 1.8 | 3.0 | 4.3 |
| 16.0 | 1.6 | 2.3 | 2.9 | 1.8 | 2.5 | 3.1 | 2.4 | 3.7 | 5.0 |
| 17.0 | 1.9 | 2.5 | 3.2 | 2.1 | 2.8 | 3.4 | 2.9 | 4.3 | 5.8 |
| 18.0 | 2.1 | 2.8 | 3.5 | 2.3 | 3.0 | 3.8 | 3.4 | 5.0 | 6.5 |
| 19.0 | 2.3 | 3.0 | 3.7 | 2.6 | 3.3 | 4.1 | 3.9 | 5.6 | 7.2 |
| 20.0 | 2.5 | 3.3 | 4.0 | 2.8 | 3.6 | 4.4 | 4.4 | 6.1 | 7.9 |
| 21.0 | 2.8 | 3.5 | 4.3 | 3.1 | 3.9 | 4.7 | 4.8 | 6.7 | 8.5 |
| 22.0 | 3.0 | 3.8 | 4.6 | 3.3 | 4.2 | 5.0 | 5.2 | 7.2 | 9.2 |
| 23.0 | 3.2 | 4.0 | 4.8 | 3.6 | 4.5 | 5.3 | 5.6 | 7.7 | 9.8 |
| 24.0 | 3.4 | 4.3 | 5.1 | 3.8 | 4.7 | 5.6 | 6.0 | 8.2 | 10.4 |
| 25.0 | 3.6 | 4.5 | 5.4 | 4.1 | 5.0 | 5.9 | 6.4 | 8.7 | 11.0 |
| 26.0 | 3.9 | 4.8 | 5.6 | 4.4 | 5.3 | 6.3 | 6.7 | 9.1 | 11.5 |
| 27.0 | 4.1 | 5.0 | 5.9 | 4.6 | 5.6 | 6.6 | 7.0 | 9.5 | 12.0 |
| 28.0 | 4.3 | 5.3 | 6.2 | 4.9 | 5.9 | 6.9 | 7.3 | 9.9 | 12.5 |
| 29.0 | 4.5 | 5.5 | 6.5 | 5.1 | 6.2 | 7.2 | 7.6 | 10.3 | 13.0 |
| 30.0 | 4.8 | 5.7 | 6.7 | 5.4 | 6.4 | 7.5 | 7.8 | 10.6 | 13.4 |
| 31.0 | 5.0 | 6.0 | 7.0 | 5.6 | 6.7 | 7.8 | 8.0 | 10.9 | 13.9 |
| 32.0 | 5.2 | 6.2 | 7.3 | 5.9 | 7.0 | 8.1 | 8.2 | 11.2 | 14.3 |
| 33.0 | 5.4 | 6.5 | 7.5 | 6.1 | 7.3 | 8.4 | 8.4 | 11.5 | 14.7 |
| 34.0 | 5.7 | 6.7 | 7.8 | 6.4 | 7.6 | 8.8 | 8.5 | 11.8 | 15.0 |
| 35.0 | 5.9 | 7.0 | 8.1 | 6.6 | 7.9 | 9.1 | 8.6 | 12.0 | 15.4 |
| 36.0 | 6.1 | 7.2 | 8.4 | 6.9 | 8.1 | 9.4 | 8.7 | 12.2 | 15.7 |
| 37.0 | 6.3 | 7.5 | 8.6 | 7.1 | 8.4 | 9.7 | 8.8 | 12.4 | 16.0 |
| 38.0 | 6.5 | 7.7 | 8.9 | 7.4 | 8.7 | 10.0 | 8.9 | 12.5 | 16.2 |
| 39.0 | 6.8 | 8.0 | 9.2 | 7.6 | 9.0 | 10.3 | 8.9 | 12.7 | 16.5 |
| 40.0 | 7.0 | 8.2 | 9.4 | 7.9 | 9.3 | 10.6 | 8.9 | 12.8 | 16.7 |

| GA (wk) | Right Ventricle (mm)[d] | | | Left Atrium (mm)[e] | | | Right Atrium (mm)[f] | | |
|---|---|---|---|---|---|---|---|---|---|
| | 5th | 50th | 95th | 5th | 50th | 95th | 5th | 50th | 95th |
| 14.0 | 1.4 | 2.5 | 3.5 | 2.2 | 3.2 | 4.2 | 2.4 | 3.5 | 4.7 |
| 15.0 | 2.0 | 3.1 | 4.3 | 2.8 | 3.9 | 5.0 | 3.0 | 4.2 | 5.4 |
| 16.0 | 2.5 | 3.8 | 5.1 | 3.3 | 4.5 | 5.7 | 3.5 | 4.8 | 6.2 |
| 17.0 | 3.0 | 4.4 | 5.8 | 3.8 | 5.1 | 6.4 | 4.0 | 5.5 | 6.9 |
| 18.0 | 3.6 | 5.1 | 6.6 | 4.3 | 5.7 | 7.1 | 4.6 | 6.1 | 7.6 |
| 19.0 | 4.0 | 5.7 | 7.3 | 4.8 | 6.3 | 7.8 | 5.1 | 6.7 | 8.3 |
| 20.0 | 4.5 | 6.3 | 8.0 | 5.3 | 6.9 | 8.4 | 5.6 | 7.3 | 9.0 |
| 21.0 | 5.0 | 6.9 | 8.7 | 5.7 | 7.4 | 9.1 | 6.0 | 7.9 | 9.7 |
| 22.0 | 5.5 | 7.4 | 9.4 | 6.2 | 8.0 | 9.7 | 6.5 | 8.5 | 10.4 |
| 23.0 | 5.9 | 8.0 | 10.1 | 6.6 | 8.5 | 10.3 | 7.0 | 9.0 | 11.1 |
| 24.0 | 6.3 | 8.5 | 10.7 | 7.0 | 9.0 | 10.9 | 7.4 | 9.6 | 11.7 |
| 25.0 | 6.7 | 9.1 | 11.4 | 7.5 | 9.5 | 11.5 | 7.8 | 10.1 | 12.4 |
| 26.0 | 7.1 | 9.6 | 12.0 | 7.8 | 10.0 | 12.1 | 8.3 | 10.6 | 13.0 |
| 27.0 | 7.5 | 10.1 | 12.6 | 8.2 | 10.5 | 12.7 | 8.7 | 11.1 | 13.6 |
| 28.0 | 7.9 | 10.6 | 13.3 | 8.6 | 10.9 | 13.2 | 9.1 | 11.6 | 14.2 |
| 29.0 | 8.3 | 11.0 | 13.8 | 8.9 | 11.4 | 13.8 | 9.5 | 12.1 | 14.8 |
| 30.0 | 8.6 | 11.5 | 14.4 | 9.3 | 11.8 | 14.3 | 9.8 | 12.6 | 15.4 |
| 31.0 | 8.9 | 12.0 | 15.0 | 9.6 | 12.2 | 14.8 | 10.2 | 13.1 | 16.0 |
| 32.0 | 9.2 | 12.4 | 15.5 | 9.9 | 12.6 | 15.3 | 10.5 | 13.5 | 16.5 |
| 33.0 | 9.6 | 12.8 | 16.1 | 10.2 | 13.0 | 15.8 | 10.9 | 14.0 | 17.1 |
| 34.0 | 9.8 | 13.2 | 16.6 | 10.5 | 13.4 | 16.2 | 11.2 | 14.4 | 17.6 |
| 35.0 | 10.1 | 13.6 | 17.1 | 10.8 | 13.7 | 16.7 | 11.5 | 14.8 | 18.1 |

| Table 45 | Reference Values for Aortic Root Internal Diameter, Pulmonary Artery, Left Ventricle, Right Ventricle, Left Atrium, and Right Atrium (Values Are Shown for 5th, 50th, and 95th Percentiles) *(continued)* |
|---|---|

| GA (wk) | Right Ventricle (mm)[d] | | | Left Atrium (mm)[e] | | | Right Atrium (mm)[f] | | |
|---|---|---|---|---|---|---|---|---|---|
| | 5th | 50th | 95th | 5th | 50th | 95th | 5th | 50th | 95th |
| 36.0 | 10.4 | 14.0 | 17.6 | 11.0 | 14.1 | 17.1 | 11.8 | 15.2 | 18.6 |
| 37.0 | 10.6 | 14.4 | 18.1 | 11.2 | 14.4 | 17.6 | 12.1 | 15.6 | 19.1 |
| 38.0 | 10.9 | 14.7 | 18.6 | 11.5 | 14.7 | 18.0 | 12.4 | 16.0 | 19.6 |
| 39.0 | 11.1 | 15.1 | 19.0 | 11.7 | 15.0 | 18.4 | 12.7 | 16.4 | 20.1 |
| 40.0 | 11.3 | 15.4 | 19.5 | 11.9 | 15.3 | 18.8 | 12.9 | 16.7 | 20.6 |

[a]Aorta $= 0.247 \times GA - 1.6638$ (SD $= 0.0146 \times GA + 0.16$).
[b]Pulmonary artery $= 0.283 \times GA - 2.055$ (SD $= 0.018 \times GA + 0.11$).
[c]Left ventricle (end diastole) $= -0.01152 \times GA^2 + 1.024 \times GA - 9.735$ (SD $= 0.065 \times GA - 0.234$).
[d]Right ventricle (end diastole) $= -0.006848 \times GA^2 + 0.866 \times GA - 8.306$ (SD $= 0.071 \times GA - 0.359$).
[e]Left atrium $= -0.00698 \times GA^2 + 0.8422 \times GA - 7.2$ (SD $= 0.05677 \times GA - 0.18$).
[f]Right atrium $= -0.00587 \times GA^2 + 0.8246 \times GA - 6.846$ (SD $= 0.0634 \times GA - 0.21$).
GA, gestational age.
Data adapted from Shapiro I, Degani S, Leibovitz Z, et al. Fetal cardiac measurements derived by transvaginal and transabdominal cross-sectional echocardiography from 14 weeks of gestation to term. *Ultrasound Obstet Gynecol.* 1998;12:404–418.

| Table 46 | Reference Values for E/A Ratio of Mitral Valve and Tricuspid Valve |
|---|---|

| GA (wk) | Mitral Valve[a] | | | Tricuspid Valve[b] | | |
|---|---|---|---|---|---|---|
| | Percentiles | | | Percentiles | | |
| | 5th | 50th | 95th | 5th | 50th | 95th |
| 20 | 0.47 | 0.59 | 0.71 | 0.51 | 0.62 | 0.74 |
| 21 | 0.48 | 0.60 | 0.72 | 0.52 | 0.63 | 0.75 |
| 22 | 0.48 | 0.61 | 0.73 | 0.53 | 0.64 | 0.76 |
| 23 | 0.49 | 0.62 | 0.74 | 0.54 | 0.65 | 0.77 |
| 24 | 0.50 | 0.63 | 0.76 | 0.55 | 0.66 | 0.78 |
| 25 | 0.51 | 0.64 | 0.77 | 0.56 | 0.67 | 0.79 |
| 26 | 0.52 | 0.65 | 0.78 | 0.57 | 0.68 | 0.80 |
| 27 | 0.53 | 0.66 | 0.79 | 0.58 | 0.69 | 0.81 |
| 28 | 0.53 | 0.67 | 0.81 | 0.59 | 0.70 | 0.82 |
| 29 | 0.54 | 0.68 | 0.82 | 0.60 | 0.71 | 0.83 |
| 30 | 0.55 | 0.69 | 0.83 | 0.61 | 0.72 | 0.84 |
| 31 | 0.56 | 0.70 | 0.85 | 0.62 | 0.73 | 0.84 |
| 32 | 0.57 | 0.71 | 0.86 | 0.63 | 0.74 | 0.85 |
| 33 | 0.58 | 0.73 | 0.87 | 0.64 | 0.75 | 0.86 |
| 34 | 0.59 | 0.74 | 0.89 | 0.65 | 0.76 | 0.87 |
| 35 | 0.60 | 0.75 | 0.90 | 0.66 | 0.77 | 0.88 |
| 36 | 0.61 | 0.76 | 0.92 | 0.67 | 0.78 | 0.89 |
| 37 | 0.62 | 0.77 | 0.93 | 0.68 | 0.79 | 0.90 |
| 38 | 0.63 | 0.79 | 0.95 | 0.69 | 0.80 | 0.91 |
| 39 | 0.64 | 0.80 | 0.96 | 0.70 | 0.81 | 0.92 |
| 40 | 0.65 | 0.81 | 0.98 | 0.71 | 0.82 | 0.93 |

*Note:* E/A ratio is equal to the peak velocity of E wave during early diastole/peak velocity with a wave during atrial contraction.
[a]Mitral valve $\log_{10}$ (E/A ratio) $= -0.3699 + 0.007 \times GA$ (SD $= 0.0687$ transformed).
[b]Tricuspid valve E/A ratio $= 0.428 + 0.0098 \times A14$ (SD $= 0.0687$).
GA, gestational age.
Data from Hecher K, Campbell S, Snijders R, et al. Reference ranges for fetal venous and atrio-ventricular blood flow parameters. *Ultrasound Obstet Gynecol.* 1994;4:381–390.

| Table 47 | Normal Doppler Echocardiography in the Fetus |
|---|---|

| Valve | Tricuspid | Mitral | Pulmonary | Aorta |
|---|---|---|---|---|
| Maximal velocity (cm/s) | 51 ± 4 | 47 ± 4 | 60 ± 4 | 70 ± 3 |
| Mean velocity (cm/s) | 12 ± 1 | 11 ± 1 | 16 ± 2 | 18 ± 2 |
| Valve diameter (mm)[a] | 8 ± 0.5 | 6.6 ± 0.4 | 7.6 ± 0.3 | 6.7 ± 0.2 |
| Cardiac output (mL/kg/min)[a] | 307 ± 30 | 232 ± 25 | 312 ± 11 | 250 ± 9 |
| A/E ratio[a] | 1.29 ± 0.04 | 1.35 ± 0.01 | — | — |
| Deceleration time (ms)[a] | 97 ± 29 | 110 ± 31 | — | — |
| Acceleration time (ms)[a] | — | — | 50.6 ± 12.0 | 46.7 ± 9.1 |

A/E, atrial contraction/early diastole.
[a]Varies with gestational age.
Reproduced with permission from Reed KL. Fetal Doppler echocardiography. *Clin Obstet Gynecol.* 1989;32:728–737.

**Doppler**

| Table 48 | Reference Intervals for Mean Uterine Artery Pulsatility Index | | |
|---|---|---|---|
| | **Percentiles** | | |
| **GA (wk)** | **5th** | **50th** | **95th** |
| 11 | 1.18 | 1.79 | 2.7 |
| 12 | 1.11 | 1.68 | 2.53 |
| 13 | 1.05 | 1.58 | 2.38 |
| 14 | 0.99 | 1.49 | 2.24 |
| 15 | 0.94 | 1.41 | 2.11 |
| 16 | 0.89 | 1.33 | 1.99 |
| 17 | 0.85 | 1.27 | 1.88 |
| 18 | 0.81 | 1.2 | 1.79 |
| 19 | 0.78 | 1.15 | 1.7 |
| 20 | 0.74 | 1.1 | 1.61 |
| 21 | 0.71 | 1.05 | 1.54 |
| 22 | 0.69 | 1 | 1.47 |
| 23 | 0.66 | 0.96 | 1.41 |
| 24 | 0.64 | 0.93 | 1.35 |
| 25 | 0.62 | 0.89 | 1.3 |
| 26 | 0.6 | 0.86 | 1.25 |
| 27 | 0.58 | 0.84 | 1.21 |
| 28 | 0.56 | 0.81 | 1.17 |
| 29 | 0.55 | 0.79 | 1.13 |
| 30 | 0.54 | 0.77 | 1.1 |
| 31 | 0.52 | 0.75 | 1.06 |
| 32 | 0.51 | 0.73 | 1.04 |
| 33 | 0.5 | 0.71 | 1.01 |
| 34 | 0.5 | 0.7 | 0.99 |
| 35 | 0.49 | 0.69 | 0.97 |
| 36 | 0.48 | 0.68 | 0.95 |
| 37 | 0.48 | 0.67 | 0.94 |
| 38 | 0.47 | 0.66 | 0.92 |
| 39 | 0.47 | 0.65 | 0.91 |
| 40 | 0.47 | 0.65 | 0.9 |
| 41 | 0.47 | 0.65 | 0.89 |

Reproduced with permission from Gómez O, Figueras F, Fernández S, et al. Reference ranges for uterine artery mean pulsatility index at 11–41 weeks of gestation. *Ultrasound Obstet Gynecol.* 2008;32(2):128–132.

| Table 49 | **Uterine Artery Doppler Resistance Index and Pulsatility Index by Placental and Nonplacental Location** |
|---|---|

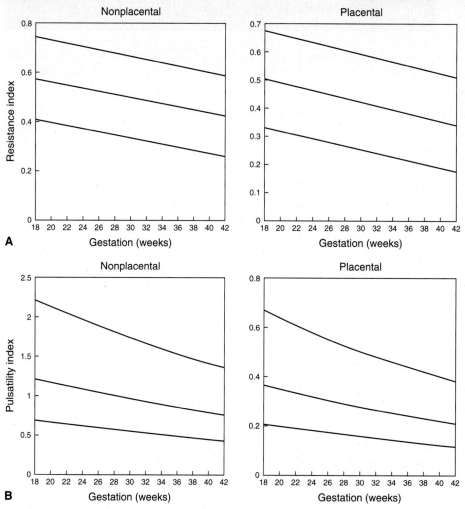

Following placental site determination, if the placenta was deviated to one side, then the uterine artery on that side was referred to as "Placental".

Reproduced with permission from Bower S, Vyas S, Campbell S, et al. Color Doppler imaging of the uterine artery in pregnancy: normal ranges of impedance to blood flow, mean velocity and volume of flow. *Ultrasound Obstet Gynecol.* 1992;2:261–265.

## Table 50    Reference Values for Umbilical Artery S/D Ratio

| GA (wk) | Percentile | | | | | | | | |
|---|---|---|---|---|---|---|---|---|---|
| | 2.5th | 5th | 10th | 25th | 50th | 75th | 90th | 95th | 97.5th |
| 19 | 2.73 | 2.93 | 3.19 | 3.67 | 4.28 | 5 | 5.75 | 6.26 | 6.73 |
| 20 | 2.63 | 2.83 | 3.07 | 3.53 | 4.11 | 4.8 | 5.51 | 5.99 | 6.43 |
| 21 | 2.51 | 2.7 | 2.93 | 3.36 | 3.91 | 4.55 | 5.22 | 5.67 | 6.09 |
| 22 | 2.43 | 2.6 | 2.83 | 3.24 | 3.77 | 4.38 | 5.03 | 5.45 | 5.85 |
| 23 | 2.34 | 2.51 | 2.72 | 3.11 | 3.62 | 4.21 | 4.82 | 5.22 | 5.61 |
| 24 | 2.25 | 2.41 | 2.62 | 2.99 | 3.48 | 4.04 | 4.63 | 5.02 | 5.38 |
| 25 | 2.17 | 2.33 | 2.52 | 2.88 | 3.35 | 3.89 | 4.45 | 4.83 | 5.18 |
| 26 | 2.09 | 2.24 | 2.43 | 2.78 | 3.23 | 3.75 | 4.3 | 4.66 | 5 |
| 27 | 2.02 | 2.17 | 2.35 | 2.69 | 3.12 | 3.63 | 4.15 | 4.5 | 4.83 |
| 28 | 1.95 | 2.09 | 2.27 | 2.6 | 3.02 | 3.51 | 4.02 | 4.36 | 4.67 |
| 29 | 1.89 | 2.03 | 2.2 | 2.52 | 2.92 | 3.4 | 3.89 | 4.22 | 4.53 |
| 30 | 1.83 | 1.96 | 2.13 | 2.44 | 2.75 | 3.2 | 3.67 | 3.98 | 4.27 |
| 31 | 1.77 | 1.9 | 2.06 | 2.36 | 2.75 | 3.2 | 3.67 | 3.98 | 4.27 |
| 32 | 1.71 | 1.84 | 2 | 2.29 | 2.67 | 3.11 | 3.57 | 3.87 | 4.16 |
| 33 | 1.66 | 1.79 | 1.94 | 2.23 | 2.6 | 3.03 | 3.48 | 3.77 | 4.06 |
| 34 | 1.61 | 1.73 | 1.88 | 2.16 | 2.53 | 2.95 | 3.39 | 3.68 | 3.96 |
| 35 | 1.57 | 1.68 | 1.83 | 2.11 | 2.46 | 2.87 | 3.3 | 3.59 | 3.86 |
| 36 | 1.52 | 1.64 | 1.78 | 2.05 | 2.4 | 2.8 | 3.23 | 3.51 | 3.78 |
| 37 | 1.48 | 1.59 | 1.73 | 2 | 2.34 | 2.74 | 3.15 | 3.43 | 3.69 |
| 38 | 1.44 | 1.55 | 1.69 | 1.95 | 2.28 | 2.67 | 3.08 | 3.36 | 3.62 |
| 39 | 1.4 | 1.51 | 1.64 | 1.9 | 2.23 | 2.61 | 3.02 | 3.29 | 3.54 |
| 40 | 1.36 | 1.47 | 1.6 | 1.85 | 2.18 | 2.56 | 2.96 | 3.22 | 3.48 |
| 41 | 1.33 | 1.43 | 1.56 | 1.81 | 2.13 | 2.5 | 2.9 | 3.16 | 3.41 |

Reproduced from Acharya G, Wilsgaard T, Berntsen GK, et al. Reference ranges for serial measurements of umbilical artery Doppler indices in the second half of pregnancy. *Am J Obstet Gynecol.* 2005;192(3):937–944.

## Table 51    Reference Values for Umbilical Artery Pulsatility Index

| GA (wk) | Percentile | | | | | | | | |
|---|---|---|---|---|---|---|---|---|---|
| | 2.5th | 5th | 10th | 25th | 50th | 75th | 90th | 95th | 97.5th |
| 19 | 0.97 | 1.02 | 1.08 | 1.18 | 1.3 | 1.44 | 1.57 | 1.66 | 1.74 |
| 20 | 0.94 | 0.99 | 1.04 | 1.14 | 1.27 | 1.4 | 1.54 | 1.62 | 1.7 |
| 21 | 0.9 | 0.95 | 1 | 1.1 | 1.22 | 1.36 | 1.49 | 1.58 | 1.65 |
| 22 | 0.87 | 0.92 | 0.97 | 1.07 | 1.19 | 1.32 | 1.46 | 1.54 | 1.62 |
| 23 | 0.84 | 0.89 | 0.94 | 1.04 | 1.15 | 1.29 | 1.42 | 1.5 | 1.58 |
| 24 | 0.81 | 0.86 | 0.91 | 1 | 1.12 | 1.25 | 1.38 | 1.47 | 1.55 |
| 25 | 0.78 | 0.83 | 0.88 | 0.97 | 1.09 | 1.22 | 1.35 | 1.44 | 1.51 |
| 26 | 0.76 | 0.8 | 0.85 | 0.94 | 1.06 | 1.19 | 1.32 | 1.41 | 1.48 |
| 27 | 0.73 | 0.77 | 0.82 | 0.92 | 1.03 | 1.16 | 1.29 | 1.38 | 1.45 |
| 28 | 0.71 | 0.75 | 0.8 | 0.89 | 1 | 1.13 | 1.26 | 1.35 | 1.43 |
| 29 | 0.68 | 0.72 | 0.77 | 0.86 | 0.98 | 1.1 | 1.23 | 1.32 | 1.4 |
| 30 | 0.66 | 0.7 | 0.75 | 0.84 | 0.95 | 1.08 | 1.21 | 1.29 | 1.37 |
| 31 | 0.64 | 0.68 | 0.73 | 0.82 | 0.93 | 1.05 | 1.18 | 1.27 | 1.35 |
| 32 | 0.62 | 0.66 | 0.7 | 0.79 | 0.9 | 1.03 | 1.16 | 1.25 | 1.32 |
| 33 | 0.6 | 0.64 | 0.68 | 0.77 | 0.88 | 1.01 | 1.14 | 1.22 | 1.3 |
| 34 | 0.58 | 0.62 | 0.66 | 0.75 | 0.86 | 0.99 | 1.12 | 1.2 | 1.28 |
| 35 | 0.56 | 0.6 | 0.64 | 0.73 | 0.84 | 0.97 | 1.09 | 1.18 | 1.26 |
| 36 | 0.54 | 0.58 | 0.63 | 0.71 | 0.82 | 0.95 | 1.07 | 1.16 | 1.24 |
| 37 | 0.53 | 0.56 | 0.61 | 0.69 | 0.8 | 0.93 | 1.05 | 1.14 | 1.22 |
| 38 | 0.51 | 0.55 | 0.59 | 0.68 | 0.78 | 0.91 | 1.04 | 1.12 | 1.2 |
| 39 | 0.49 | 0.53 | 0.57 | 0.66 | 0.76 | 0.89 | 1.02 | 1.1 | 1.18 |
| 40 | 0.48 | 0.51 | 0.56 | 0.64 | 0.75 | 0.87 | 1 | 1.09 | 1.17 |
| 41 | 0.47 | 0.5 | 0.54 | 0.63 | 0.73 | 0.85 | 0.98 | 1.07 | 1.15 |

Reproduced from Acharya G, Wilsgaard T, Berntsen GK, et al. Reference ranges for serial measurements of umbilical artery Doppler indices in the second half of pregnancy. *Am J Obstet Gynecol.* 2005;192:937–944.

| Table 52 | Reference Values for Umbilical Artery Resistance Index |
|---|---|

| GA (wk) | Percentile | | | | | | | | |
|---|---|---|---|---|---|---|---|---|---|
| | 2.5th | 5th | 10th | 25th | 50th | 75th | 90th | 95th | 97.5th |
| 19 | 0.64 | 0.66 | 0.68 | 0.72 | 0.77 | 0.81 | 0.85 | 0.88 | 0.9 |
| 20 | 0.63 | 0.65 | 0.67 | 0.71 | 0.75 | 0.8 | 0.84 | 0.87 | 0.89 |
| 21 | 0.62 | 0.64 | 0.66 | 0.7 | 0.74 | 0.79 | 0.83 | 0.85 | 0.88 |
| 22 | 0.6 | 0.62 | 0.65 | 0.68 | 0.73 | 0.78 | 0.82 | 0.84 | 0.87 |
| 23 | 0.59 | 0.61 | 0.63 | 0.67 | 0.72 | 0.76 | 0.81 | 0.83 | 0.86 |
| 24 | 0.58 | 0.6 | 0.62 | 0.66 | 0.71 | 0.75 | 0.8 | 0.82 | 0.85 |
| 25 | 0.56 | 0.58 | 0.61 | 0.65 | 0.69 | 0.74 | 0.79 | 0.81 | 0.84 |
| 26 | 0.55 | 0.57 | 0.59 | 0.64 | 0.68 | 0.73 | 0.78 | 0.8 | 0.83 |
| 27 | 0.54 | 0.56 | 0.58 | 0.62 | 0.67 | 0.72 | 0.77 | 0.79 | 0.82 |
| 28 | 0.53 | 0.55 | 0.57 | 0.61 | 0.66 | 0.71 | 0.76 | 0.78 | 0.81 |
| 29 | 0.51 | 0.53 | 0.56 | 0.6 | 0.65 | 0.7 | 0.75 | 0.77 | 0.8 |
| 30 | 0.5 | 0.52 | 0.54 | 0.59 | 0.64 | 0.69 | 0.74 | 0.76 | 0.79 |
| 31 | 0.49 | 0.51 | 0.53 | 0.58 | 0.63 | 0.68 | 0.73 | 0.76 | 0.78 |
| 32 | 0.47 | 0.5 | 0.52 | 0.56 | 0.61 | 0.67 | 0.72 | 0.75 | 0.77 |
| 33 | 0.46 | 0.48 | 0.51 | 0.55 | 0.6 | 0.66 | 0.71 | 0.74 | 0.77 |
| 34 | 0.45 | 0.47 | 0.5 | 0.54 | 0.59 | 0.65 | 0.7 | 0.73 | 0.76 |
| 35 | 0.44 | 0.46 | 0.48 | 0.53 | 0.58 | 0.64 | 0.69 | 0.72 | 0.75 |
| 36 | 0.42 | 0.45 | 0.47 | 0.52 | 0.57 | 0.63 | 0.68 | 0.71 | 0.74 |
| 37 | 0.41 | 0.43 | 0.46 | 0.51 | 0.56 | 0.62 | 0.67 | 0.7 | 0.73 |
| 38 | 0.4 | 0.42 | 0.45 | 0.5 | 0.55 | 0.61 | 0.66 | 0.7 | 0.73 |
| 39 | 0.39 | 0.41 | 0.44 | 0.48 | 0.54 | 0.6 | 0.65 | 0.69 | 0.72 |
| 40 | 0.38 | 0.4 | 0.43 | 0.47 | 0.53 | 0.59 | 0.65 | 0.68 | 0.71 |
| 41 | 0.36 | 0.39 | 0.41 | 0.46 | 0.52 | 0.58 | 0.64 | 0.67 | 0.7 |

Reproduced with permission from Acharya G, Wilsgaard T, Berntsen GK, et al. Reference ranges for serial measurements of umbilical artery Doppler indices in the second half of pregnancy. *Am J Obstet Gynecol.* 2005;192:937–944.

| Table 53 | Reference Values for Peak Systolic Velocity of the Middle Cerebral Artery |

| | Peak Systolic Velocity (cm/s) | | | | |
|---|---|---|---|---|---|
| | Multiples of the Median | | | | |
| GA (wk) | 1 | 1.3 | 1.5 | 1.7 | 2 |
| 15 | 20 | 26 | 30 | 34 | 40 |
| 16 | 21 | 27 | 32 | 36 | 42 |
| 17 | 22 | 29 | 33 | 37 | 44 |
| 18 | 23 | 30 | 35 | 39 | 46 |
| 19 | 24 | 31 | 36 | 41 | 48 |
| 20 | 25 | 33 | 38 | 43 | 50 |
| 21 | 26 | 34 | 39 | 44 | 52 |
| 22 | 28 | 36 | 42 | 48 | 56 |
| 23 | 29 | 38 | 44 | 49 | 58 |
| 24 | 30 | 39 | 45 | 51 | 60 |
| 25 | 32 | 42 | 48 | 54 | 64 |
| 26 | 33 | 43 | 50 | 56 | 66 |
| 27 | 35 | 46 | 53 | 60 | 70 |
| 28 | 37 | 48 | 56 | 63 | 74 |
| 29 | 38 | 49 | 57 | 65 | 76 |
| 30 | 40 | 52 | 60 | 68 | 80 |
| 31 | 42 | 55 | 63 | 71 | 84 |
| 32 | 44 | 57 | 66 | 75 | 88 |
| 33 | 46 | 60 | 69 | 78 | 92 |
| 34 | 48 | 62 | 72 | 82 | 96 |
| 35 | 50 | 65 | 75 | 85 | 100 |
| 36 | 53 | 69 | 80 | 90 | 106 |
| 37 | 55 | 72 | 83 | 94 | 110 |
| 38 | 58 | 75 | 87 | 99 | 116 |
| 39 | 61 | 79 | 92 | 104 | 122 |
| 40 | 63 | 82 | 95 | 107 | 126 |

*Note:* Peak systolic velocity (cm/s) $= e^{(2.31 + 0.046 \times GA)}$.
GA, gestational age.
Reproduced with permission from Mari G, Deter RL, Carpenter RL, et al. Noninvasive diagnosis by Doppler ultrasonography of fetal anemia due to maternal red-cell alloimmunization. Collaborative Group for Doppler Assessment of the Blood Velocity in Anemic Fetuses. *N Engl J Med.* 2000;342:9–14.

| Table 54 | Middle Cerebral Artery Pulsatility Index |

| | Middle Cerebral Artery Pulsatility Index | | | | |
|---|---|---|---|---|---|
| | Percentile | | | | |
| GA (wk) | 5th | 10th | 50th | 90th | 95th |
| 21 | 1.18 | 1.26 | 1.6 | 2.04 | 2.19 |
| 22 | 1.25 | 1.33 | 1.69 | 0.15 | 2.30 |
| 23 | 1.32 | 1.41 | 1.78 | 2.25 | 2.41 |
| 24 | 1.38 | 1.47 | 1.86 | 2.36 | 2.52 |
| 25 | 1.44 | 1.54 | 1.94 | 2.45 | 2.62 |
| 26 | 1.50 | 1.6 | 2.01 | 2.53 | 2.71 |
| 27 | 1.55 | 1.65 | 2.06 | 2.60 | 2.78 |
| 28 | 1.58 | 1.69 | 2.11 | 2.66 | 2.84 |
| 29 | 1.61 | 1.71 | 2.15 | 2.70 | 2.88 |
| 30 | 1.62 | 1.73 | 2.16 | 2.72 | 2.90 |
| 31 | 1.62 | 1.73 | 2.16 | 2.71 | 2.90 |
| 32 | 1.61 | 1.71 | 2.14 | 2.69 | 2.87 |
| 33 | 1.58 | 1.68 | 2.10 | 2.64 | 2.82 |
| 34 | 1.53 | 1.63 | 2.04 | 2.57 | 2.74 |
| 35 | 1.47 | 1.56 | 1.96 | 2.47 | 2.64 |
| 36 | 1.39 | 1.48 | 1.86 | 2.36 | 2.52 |
| 37 | 1.30 | 1.39 | 1.75 | 2.22 | 2.38 |
| 38 | 1.20 | 1.29 | 1.63 | 2.07 | 2.22 |
| 39 | 1.1 | 1.18 | 1.49 | 1.91 | 2.05 |

Reproduced with permission from Ebbing C, Rasmussen S, Kiserud T. Middle cerebral artery blood flow velocities and pulsatility index and the cerebroplacental pulsatility ratio: longitudinal reference ranges and terms for serial measurements. *Ultrasound Obstet Gynecol.* 2007;30:287–296.

## Table 55 — Pulsatility Index in the Umbilical and Middle Cerebral Arteries and Cerebroplacental Doppler Ratio

| GA (wk) | N | Umbilical Artery Mean | Umbilical Artery SD | Middle Cerebral Artery Mean | Middle Cerebral Artery SD | CPR Mean | CPR SD |
|---------|---|------|------|------|------|------|------|
| 20 | 25 | 1.31 | 0.26 | 1.76 | 0.24 | 1.37 | 0.40 |
| 21 | 15 | 1.27 | 0.18 | 1.79 | 0.20 | 1.44 | 0.25 |
| 22 | 9 | 1.28 | 0.17 | 1.87 | 0.33 | 1.48 | 0.29 |
| 23 | 11 | 1.12 | 0.12 | 1.65 | 0.16 | 1.49 | 0.23 |
| 24 | 21 | 1.21 | 0.14 | 1.85 | 0.21 | 1.53 | 0.22 |
| 25 | 13 | 1.13 | 0.16 | 2.03 | 0.41 | 1.83 | 0.48 |
| 26 | 14 | 1.11 | 0.13 | 2.09 | 0.43 | 1.92 | 0.55 |
| 27 | 17 | 1.07 | 0.17 | 2.18 | 0.68 | 2.12 | 0.61 |
| 28 | 17 | 1.05 | 0.13 | 2.21 | 0.41 | 2.13 | 0.52 |
| 29 | 17 | 1.11 | 0.19 | 2.02 | 0.31 | 1.86 | 0.43 |
| 30 | 12 | 1.04 | 0.23 | 2.34 | 0.33 | 2.34 | 0.55 |
| 31 | 19 | 0.99 | 0.13 | 2.21 | 0.31 | 2.29 | 0.34 |
| 32 | 10 | 0.93 | 0.19 | 1.81 | 0.19 | 2.03 | 0.48 |
| 33 | 17 | 0.92 | 0.17 | 1.90 | 0.38 | 2.10 | 0.40 |
| 34 | 21 | 0.89 | 0.13 | 1.79 | 0.27 | 2.10 | 0.45 |
| 35 | 13 | 0.91 | 0.11 | 1.81 | 0.31 | 2.01 | 0.34 |
| 36 | 19 | 0.93 | 0.18 | 1.80 | 0.27 | 2.01 | 0.46 |
| 37 | 6 | 0.95 | 0.24 | 2.06 | 0.68 | 2.25 | 0.66 |
| 38 | 11 | 0.89 | 0.16 | 1.66 | 0.30 | 1.90 | 0.41 |
| 39 | 8 | 1.01 | 0.17 | 1.64 | 0.26 | 1.64 | 0.29 |
| 40 | 11 | 0.75 | 0.16 | 1.29 | 0.21 | 1.80 | 0.44 |

CPR, cerebroplacental Doppler ratio; SD, standard deviation.
Reproduced with permission from Baschat AA, Gembruch U. The cerebroplacental Doppler ratio revisited. *Ultrasound Obstet Gynecol.* 2003;21:124–127.

## Table 56 — Reference Ranges for the Systolic-to-Atrial Ratio of the Ductus Venosus

| GA (wk) | Percentile 5th | Percentile Mean | Percentile 95th |
|---------|------|------|------|
| 14 | 3.583 | 4.497 | 5.78 |
| 15 | 3.153 | 4.047 | 5.304 |
| 16 | 2.767 | 3.641 | 4.871 |
| 17 | 2.44 | 3.295 | 4.497 |
| 18 | 2.171 | 3.007 | 4.182 |
| 19 | 1.955 | 2.771 | 3.919 |
| 20 | 1.785 | 2.582 | 3.703 |
| 21 | 1.654 | 2.432 | 3.526 |
| 22 | 1.557 | 2.315 | 3.381 |
| 23 | 1.486 | 2.225 | 3.264 |
| 24 | 1.437 | 2.157 | 3.169 |
| 25 | 1.406 | 2.107 | 3.092 |
| 26 | 1.389 | 2.07 | 3.028 |
| 27 | 1.382 | 2.044 | 2.974 |
| 28 | 1.383 | 2.025 | 2.929 |
| 29 | 1.39 | 2.013 | 2.889 |
| 30 | 1.401 | 2.005 | 2.854 |
| 31 | 1.415 | 1.999 | 2.821 |
| 32 | 1.431 | 1.996 | 2.791 |
| 33 | 1.449 | 1.994 | 2.762 |
| 34 | 1.467 | 1.993 | 2.734 |
| 35 | 1.486 | 1.993 | 2.706 |
| 36 | 1.505 | 1.993 | 2.678 |
| 37 | 1.524 | 1.992 | 2.651 |
| 38 | 1.543 | 1.992 | 2.624 |
| 39 | 1.563 | 1.992 | 2.597 |
| 40 | 1.582 | 1.992 | 2.57 |
| 41 | 1.601 | 1.992 | 2.542 |

Modified from Bahlmann F, Wellek S, Reinhardt I, et al. Reference values of ductus venosus flow velocities and calculated waveform indices. *Prenat Diagn.* 2000;20:623–634.

| Table 57 | Reference Ranges for the Pulsatility Index for Veins (PIV) of the Ductus Venosus |
| --- | --- |

| | Percentile | | | | | | | | |
| --- | --- | --- | --- | --- | --- | --- | --- | --- | --- |
| GA (wk) | 2.5th | 5th | 10th | 25th | 50th | 75th | 90th | 95th | 97.5th |
| 21 | 0.27 | 0.32 | 0.38 | 0.47 | 0.57 | 0.68 | 0.77 | 0.83 | 0.88 |
| 22 | 0.28 | 0.32 | 0.38 | 0.47 | 0.57 | 0.68 | 0.77 | 0.83 | 0.88 |
| 23 | 0.28 | 0.32 | 0.38 | 0.47 | 0.57 | 0.68 | 0.77 | 0.83 | 0.88 |
| 24 | 0.27 | 0.32 | 0.38 | 0.47 | 0.57 | 0.68 | 0.77 | 0.83 | 0.88 |
| 25 | 0.27 | 0.32 | 0.37 | 0.47 | 0.57 | 0.67 | 0.77 | 0.83 | 0.88 |
| 26 | 0.27 | 0.31 | 0.37 | 0.46 | 0.57 | 0.67 | 0.77 | 0.82 | 0.87 |
| 27 | 0.26 | 0.31 | 0.36 | 0.46 | 0.56 | 0.67 | 0.76 | 0.82 | 0.87 |
| 28 | 0.26 | 0.31 | 0.36 | 0.45 | 0.56 | 0.66 | 0.76 | 0.81 | 0.86 |
| 29 | 0.25 | 0.30 | 0.35 | 0.45 | 0.55 | 0.65 | 0.75 | 0.81 | 0.86 |
| 30 | 0.25 | 0.29 | 0.35 | 0.44 | 0.54 | 0.65 | 0.74 | 0.80 | 0.85 |
| 31 | 0.24 | 0.28 | 0.34 | 0.43 | 0.53 | 0.64 | 0.73 | 0.79 | 0.84 |
| 32 | 0.23 | 0.28 | 0.33 | 0.42 | 0.53 | 0.63 | 0.73 | 0.78 | 0.83 |
| 33 | 0.22 | 0.27 | 0.32 | 0.41 | 0.52 | 0.62 | 0.72 | 0.77 | 0.82 |
| 34 | 0.21 | 0.26 | 0.31 | 0.40 | 0.51 | 0.61 | 0.71 | 0.76 | 0.81 |
| 35 | 0.20 | 0.25 | 0.30 | 0.39 | 0.50 | 0.60 | 0.70 | 0.75 | 0.80 |
| 36 | 0.19 | 0.24 | 0.29 | 0.38 | 0.49 | 0.59 | 0.69 | 0.74 | 0.79 |
| 37 | 0.18 | 0.23 | 0.28 | 0.37 | 0.48 | 0.58 | 0.67 | 0.73 | 0.78 |
| 38 | 0.17 | 0.22 | 0.27 | 0.36 | 0.46 | 0.57 | 0.66 | 0.72 | 0.77 |
| 39 | 0.16 | 0.21 | 0.26 | 0.35 | 0.45 | 0.56 | 0.65 | 0.71 | 0.76 |

Modified from Kessler J, Rasmussen S, Hanson M, et al. Longitudinal reference ranges for ductus venosus flow velocities and waveform indices. *Ultrasound Obstet Gynecol.* 2006;28:890–898.

## Aneuploidy Tables

| Table 58 | Comparison of Likelihood Ratios Reported for Sonographic Markers of Fetal Aneuploidy from Two Studies and from a Meta-analysis Study |
| --- | --- |

| Sonographic Marker | Nyberg et al.[a] Likelihood Ratios (95% CI) | Bromley et al.[b] Likelihood Ratios | Smith-Bindman et al.[c] Likelihood Ratios (95% CI) |
| --- | --- | --- | --- |
| Nuchal thickening | 11.0 (5.5–22.0) | 12 | 17 (8–38) |
| Hyperechoic bowel | 6.7 (2.7–16.8) | — | 6.1 (3–12.6) |
| Short humerus | 5.1 (1.6–16.5) | 6 | 7.5 (4.7–12) |
| Short femur | 1.5 (0.8–2.8) | 1 | 2.7 (1.2–6) |
| Echogenic intracardiac focus | 1.8 (1.0–3.0) | 1.2 | 2.8 (1.5–5.5) |
| Pyelectasis | 1.5 (0.6–3.6) | 1.3 | 1.9 (0.7–5.1) |
| Normal ultrasound | 0.36 | 0.2 | — |

CI, confidence interval.
[a]Reproduced with permission from Nyberg DA, Souter VL, El-Bastawissi A, et al. Isolated sonographic markers for detection of fetal Down syndrome in the second trimester of pregnancy. *J Ultrasound Med.* 2001;20:1053–1063.
[b]Reproduced with permission from Bromley B, Lieberman E, Shipp T, et al. The genetic sonogram: a method of risk assessment for Down syndrome in the mid-trimester. *J Ultrasound Med.* 2002;21:1087–1096.
[c]Reproduced with permission from Smith-Bindman R, Hosmer W, Feldstein VA, et al. Second-trimester ultrasound to detect fetuses with Down syndrome: a meta-analysis. *JAMA.* 2001;285:1044–1055.

| Table 59 | Maternal Age–Specific Odds (1:___) of Fetal Down Syndrome during the Second Trimester Based on Sonographic Markers of Fetal Aneuploidy |
|---|---|

| Maternal Age (wk) | Preultrasound Odds (1:___) | Normal Ultrasound (1:___) LR 0.36 | Nuchal Thickness (1:___) LR 11.0 | Hyperechoic Bowel (1:___) LR 6.7 | Short Femur Length (1:___) LR 1.5 | Short Humerus Length (1:___) LR 5.1 | Echogenic Intracardiac Focus (1:___) LR 1.8 | Renal Pelvis (1:___) LR 1.5 |
|---|---|---|---|---|---|---|---|---|
| 20 | 1,176 | 3,265 | 108 | 176 | 784 | 231 | 654 | 784 |
| 21 | 1,160 | 3,220 | 106 | 174 | 774 | 228 | 645 | 774 |
| 22 | 1,136 | 3,154 | 104 | 170 | 758 | 224 | 632 | 758 |
| 23 | 1,114 | 3,093 | 102 | 167 | 743 | 219 | 619 | 743 |
| 24 | 1,087 | 3,018 | 100 | 163 | 725 | 214 | 604 | 725 |
| 25 | 1,040 | 2,887 | 95 | 156 | 694 | 205 | 578 | 694 |
| 26 | 990 | 2,748 | 91 | 149 | 660 | 195 | 550 | 660 |
| 27 | 928 | 2,576 | 85 | 139 | 619 | 183 | 516 | 619 |
| 28 | 855 | 2,373 | 79 | 128 | 570 | 168 | 475 | 570 |
| 29 | 760 | 2,109 | 70 | 114 | 507 | 150 | 423 | 507 |
| 30 | 690 | 1,915 | 64 | 104 | 460 | 136 | 384 | 460 |
| 31 | 597 | 1,657 | 55 | 90 | 398 | 118 | 332 | 398 |
| 32 | 508 | 1,409 | 47 | 77 | 339 | 100 | 283 | 339 |
| 33 | 421 | 1,168 | 39 | 64 | 281 | 83 | 234 | 281 |
| 34 | 342 | 948 | 32 | 52 | 228 | 68 | 190 | 228 |
| 35 | 274 | 759 | 26 | 42 | 183 | 55 | 153 | 183 |
| 36 | 216 | 598 | 21 | 33 | 144 | 43 | 120 | 144 |
| 37 | 168 | 465 | 16 | 26 | 112 | 34 | 94 | 112 |
| 38 | 129 | 357 | 13 | 20 | 86 | 26 | 72 | 86 |
| 39 | 98 | 270 | 10 | 15 | 66 | 20 | 55 | 66 |
| 40 | 74 | 204 | 8 | 12 | 50 | 15 | 42 | 50 |
| 41 | 56 | 154 | 6 | 9 | 38 | 12 | 32 | 38 |
| 42 | 42 | 115 | 5 | 7 | 28 | 9 | 24 | 28 |
| 43 | 31 | 84 | 4 | 5 | 21 | 7 | 18 | 21 |
| 44 | 23 | 62 | 3 | 4 | 16 | 5 | 13 | 16 |

*Note:* Assuming LRs of Nyberg et al. in Table 58.
Odds ratio (O) based on formula O (Down syndrome) = O (maternal age)/LR + 1 − 1/LR.
LR, likelihood ratio.
Reproduced with permission from Nyberg DA, Souter VL, El-Bastawissi A, et al. Isolated sonographic markers for detection of fetal Down syndrome in the second trimester of pregnancy. *J Ultrasound Med.* 2001;20:1053–1063.

## First Trimester Values

1A. Combined data comparing menstrual age with mean gestational sac diameter, crown-rump length, and human chorionic gonadotropin (HCG) levels
1B. Relationship between mean sac diameter and menstrual age
 2. Predicted menstrual age from crown-rump length measurements
 3. Reference values for crown-rump length compared with gestational sac size

## Amniotic Fluid Index

4A. Amniotic fluid index (AFI) values in centimeters during normal pregnancy
4B. Maximal vertical pocket (SDP) values in centimeters during normal pregnancy

## Basic Ultrasound Biometry

 5. Predicted fetal measurements at specific gestational age (GA)
 6. Reference values for abdominal circumference
 7. Reference values for head circumference
 8. Reference values for femur length
 9. Reference values for abdominal circumference (AC), head circumference (HC), biparietal diameter (BPD), and femur length (FL)
10. Normal biometric ratios of head circumference (HC)/abdominal circumference (AC), AC/femur length (FL), and biparietal diameter (BPD)/FL
11. Estimated fetal weight (in Grams) based on femur length (FL) and abdominal circumference (AC)
12. Neonatal birth weights and percentiles based on gestational age (GA) derived by first-trimester ultrasound (males and females combined)
13. Gender-specific reference values for neonatal birth weights based on gestational age (GA) derived by first-trimester ultrasound
14. Fetal weight percentiles by gestational age
15. Fitted percentiles for fractional arm volume
16. Fitted percentiles for fractional thigh volume

## Ultrasound Extremity Measurements

17. Ultrasound reference values of major long bones
18. Ultrasound reference values for foot length
19. Ultrasound scapular length ($\pm 2$ SD) compared with gestational age
20. Ultrasound reference values of clavicle length
21. Ultrasound reference values for rib length

## Brain and Face Measurements

22. Ultrasound transcerebellar diameter measurements
23. Ultrasound reference intervals for the cerebellar vermis, basilar pons, and the brain stem
24. MRI measurements of the fetal brain

25A. Ultrasound reference values for binocular diameter, interocular diameter, and ocular diameter by gestational age
25B. Reference ranges for fetal optic tract diameter (in mm)
 26. MRI reference values for binocular diameter, interocular diameter, and ocular diameter by gestational age
 27. Ultrasound percentile reference values for ear length
 28. Ultrasound reference values for mandible length
 29. Ultrasound reference values for length of nasal bone

## Neck and Chest Measurements

30. Ultrasound thyroid circumference based on biparietal diameter (BPD)
31. Ultrasound thyroid circumference based on gestational age
32. Ultrasound reference values for thyroid volume
33. Ultrasound percentile reference values for thoracic circumference
34. Reference values for lung volumes calculated by 3D ultrasound
35. Reference values for the right lung volume calculated by 3D ultrasound
36. Reference values for the left lung volume calculated by 3D ultrasound
37. MRI reference values for lung volumes

## Abdominal Measurements

38. Ultrasound reference values for renal length
39. Reference values for renal volumes based on 3D ultrasound
40. Reference values of fetal liver volume determined by 3D ultrasound compared with estimated fetal weight
41. Fetal ultrasound liver length[a] compared with gestational age
42. Ultrasound reference values for splenic length
43. Ultrasound reference values for splenic circumference between 18 and 37 weeks
44. Normal ultrasound colon diameters

## Cardiac Measurements

45. Reference values for aortic root internal diameter, pulmonary artery, left ventricle, right ventricle, left atrium, and right atrium (values are shown for 5th, 50th, and 95th percentiles)
46. Reference values for E/A ratio of mitral valve and tricuspid valve
47. Normal doppler echocardiography in the fetus

## Doppler

48. Reference intervals for mean uterine artery pulsatility index
49. Uterine artery doppler resistance index and pulsatility index by placental and nonplacental location
50. Reference values for umbilical artery S/D ratio
51. Reference values for umbilical artery pulsatility index
52. Reference values for umbilical artery resistance index
53. Reference values for peak systolic velocity of the middle cerebral artery

## Aneuploidy Tables

Note: Page numbers followed by f denote figures; those followed by t denote tables.